Neuromuscular Function and Disease

Neuromuscular Function and Disease

Basic, Clinical, and Electrodiagnostic Aspects

Volume 2

William F. Brown, M.D., F.R.C.P.(C.)

Professor of Neurology

Tufts University School of Medicine

Head of Neurology

New England Medical Center

Boston, Massachusetts

Charles F. Bolton, M.D., C.M., M.S., F.R.C.P.(C.)

Professor of Neurology

Mayo Medical School

Rochester, Minnesota

Formerly Chief of Clinical Neurological Sciences and Director of the Electromyography Laboratory

Victoria Hospital

London, Ontario, Canada

Michael J. Aminoff, M.D., D.Sc., F.R.C.P.

Professor of Neurology

University of California, San Francisco, School of Medicine

Attending Physician and Director of the Clinical Neurophysiology Laboratories

UCSF Medical Center

San Francisco, California

W.B. Saunders Company

An Imprint of Elsevier Science

Philadelphia   London   New York   St. Louis   Sydney   Toronto

W.B. SAUNDERS COMPANY
An Imprint of Elsevier Science

The Curtis Center
Independence Square West
Philadelphia, Pennsylvania 19106

Library of Congress Cataloging-in-Publication Data

Neuromuscular function and disease: basic, clinical, and electrodiagnostic aspects/
[edited by] William F. Brown, Charles F. Bolton, Michael J. Aminoff.—1st ed.

p. ; cm.

ISBN 0–7216–8922-1

1. Neuromuscular diseases. 2. Efferent pathways. 3. Neuromuscular transmission. 4.
Nerves, Peripheral. I. Brown, William F. (William Frederick) II. Bolton, Charles
Francis III. Aminoff, Michael J. (Michael Jeffrey)
[DNLM: 1. Neuromuscular Diseases. 2. Motor Neurons—physiology. 3.
Muscles—physiology. 4. Peripheral Nervous System—physiology. WE 550 N4945 2002]

RC925 .N446 2002 616.74′4—dc21

2001032284

Acquisitions Editor: Susan Pioli
Developmental Editor: Joanne Husovski
Project Manager: Lee Ann Draud
Production Manager: Natalie Ware
Illustration Coordinator: Walt Verbitski

Neuromuscular Function and Disease: Basic, Clinical, and
Electrodiagnostic Aspects

Volume 1: Part no. 9997627814
Volume 2: Part no. 9997627822
Two Volume Set: ISBN 0–7216–8922–1

Printed in the United States of America.

Last digit is the print number: 9   8   7   6   5   4   3   2   1

To our students, teachers, and colleagues
in the neurological sciences
who have been our inspiration over the years
and to our families
who have endured our preoccupation
with this book

Section Editors

Robert H. Brown, Jr., M.D., Ph.D.
Professor of Neurology, Harvard Medical School;
Director, Cecil B. Day Neuromuscular Research
Laboratory, Massachusetts General Hospital, Boston,
Massachusetts
*Section XI: Genetic and Molecular Basis for Neuromuscular
Diseases*

William W. Campbell, M.D., M.S.H.A.
Professor, Department of Neurology, Uniformed
Services University of the Health Sciences F. Edward
Hébert School of Medicine, Bethesda, Maryland;
Chief, Clinical Neurophysiology, Walter Reed Army
Medical Center, Washington, District of Columbia
Section XVII: Polyneuropathies

Jasper R. Daube, M.D.
Professor, Department of Neurology, Mayo Medical
School; Consultant, Department of Neurology, Mayo
Clinic and Mayo Foundation, Rochester, Minnesota
*Section XXV: Electrophysiological Studies in the
Operating Room*

Timothy J. Doherty, M.D., Ph.D., F.R.C.P.(C.)
Assistant Professor Department of Physical Medicine
and Rehabilitation, University of Western Ontario
Faculty of Medicine & Dentistry; Consultant
Physiatrist, London Health Sciences Centre and St.
Joseph's Health Care, London, Ontario, Canada
Section IV: Peripheral Motor System

Andrew A. Eisen, M.D., F.R.C.P.(C.)
Professor and Head, Department of Neurology,
University of British Columbia Faculty of Medicine;
Head, Neuromuscular Diseases Unit, Vancouver
General Hospital, Vancouver, British Columbia,
Canada
Section XV: Radiculopathies and Plexopathies

Aaron G. Filler, M.D., Ph.D., F.R.C.S.(S.N.)
Director, Institute for Nerve Medicine, Santa Monica,
California
*Section XII: Imaging Techniques Applied to Investigation
of Neuromuscular Diseases*

Mark Hallett, M.D.
Chief, Medical Neurology Branch, National Institute
of Neurological Disorders and Strokes, National
Institutes of Health, Bethesda, Maryland
Section III: Central Motor System
Section XXIV: Central Motor Disorders

C. Michel Harper, M.D.
Associate Professor, Department of Neurology, Mayo
Medical School; Consultant, Department of
Neurology, Mayo Clinic, Rochester, Minnesota
Section XXI: Myopathies

H. Royden Jones, Jr., M.D.
Clinical Professor, Department of Neurology, Harvard
Medical School, Boston; Jamie Ortiz-Patiño Chair in
Neurology, Lahey Clinic, Burlington, Massachusetts
Section XXIII: Pediatric Neuromuscular Disorders

Jan Lexell, M.D., Ph.D.
Adjunct Professor of Clinical Neuroscience,
Department of Health Sciences, Luleå University of
Technology, Boden; Associate Professor of
Rehabilitation Medicine, Lund University Medical
Faculty; Medical Director and Chief of Staff, Brain
Injury Unit, and Director, Neuromuscular Research
Laboratory, Department of Rehabilitation, Lund
University Hospital, Lund, Sweden
*Section X: Age-Related Changes in the Neuromuscular
System*

Hiroshi Mitsumoto, M.D.
Professor, Department of Neurology, Columbia
University College of Physicians and Surgeons;
Director, Neuromuscular Division, and Director,
Eleanor and Lou Gehrig MDA/ALS Center,
Columbia-Presbyterian Medical Center, New York,
New York
Section XVIII: Motor Neuron Diseases

Sanjeev D. Nandedkar, Ph.D.
Clinical Applications Manager, Oxford Instruments,
Hawthorne, New York
Section XIII: Basic Instrumentation

Richard K. Olney, M.D.
Professor, Department of Neurology, University of
California, San Francisco, School of Medicine;
Director, EMG Laboratory, and Director ALS Center
at UCSF, UCSF Medical Center, San Francisco,
California
*Section XXVI: Clinical Trials and Clinical
Electrophysiological Studies*

Bram W. Ongerboer de Visser, M.D., Ph.D.
Professor, Department of Clinical Neurophysiology,
University of Amsterdam School of Medicine;
Neurologist, Academic Medical Center, Amsterdam,
The Netherlands
Section VI: Cranial Nerves
Section VII: Late Responses
Section XIV: Disorders of the Cranial Nerves

Donald B. Sanders, M.D.
Professor, Department of Medicine, Division of
Neurology, Duke University School of Medicine,
Durham, North Carolina
Section V: Neuromuscular Transmission
Section XX: Neuromuscular Transmission Disorders

David M. Simpson, M.D.
Associate Professor, Department of Neurology, Mount Sinai School of Medicine of New York University; Director, Clinical Neurophysiology Laboratories, Mount Sinai Hospital, New York, New York
Section XIX: Neuromuscular Disorders Associated with Human Immunodeficiency Virus

Erik V. Stålberg, M.D., Ph.D.
Professor Emeritus, Department of Clinical Neurophysiology, University Hospital, Uppsala, Sweden
Section V: Neuromuscular Transmission
Section XX: Neuromuscular Transmission Disorders

Daniel W. Stashuk, Ph.D.
Associate Professor, Department of Systems Design Engineering, University of Waterloo, Waterloo, Ontario, Canada
Section IV: Peripheral Motor System

John D. Stewart, M.B., B.S., F.R.C.P.(C.)
Professor, Department of Neurology and Neurosurgery, McGill University Faculty of Medicine; Neurologist, Montreal Neurological Hospital and Institute, Montreal, Quebec, Canada
Section XVI: Mononeuropathies

Jože V. Trontelj, M.D., D.Sc.
Professor, Department of Neurology, University of Ljubljana Medical Faculty; Neurologist and Senior Consultant, Institute of Clinical Neurophysiology, Department of Neurology, University Medical Center, Ljubljana, Slovenia
Section V: Neuromuscular Transmission
Section XX: Neuromuscular Transmission Disorders

Anthony A. Vandervoort, Ph.D.
Professor, Schools of Physical Therapy and Kinesiology, and Kinesiology Graduate Program Chair, University of Western Ontario Faculty of Medicine & Dentistry, London, Ontario, Canada
Section X: Age-Related Changes in the Neuromuscular System

Douglas W. Zochodne, M.D., F.R.C.P.(C.)
Professor, Department of Neurology, University of Calgary Faculty of Medicine; Neurologist, Foothills Hospital, Calgary, Alberta, Canada
Section VIII: Autonomic Nervous System

Contributors

Michael A. Adams, Ph.D.
Professor, Department of Pharmacology and
Toxicology, Queen's University Faculty of Health
Sciences, Kingston, Ontario, Canada
Physiological Aspects of Sexual Function and Dysfunction

James W. Albers, M.D., Ph.D.
Professor, Department of Neurology, Co-Director of
Neurobehavioral Toxicology, University of Michigan
Medical School; Director, EMG Laboratory, University
of Michigan Health System, Ann Arbor, Michigan
Industrial and Environmental Toxic Neuropathies

Anthony A. Amato, M.D.
Associate Professor, Department of Neurology,
Harvard Medical School; Vice-Chairman, Department
of Neurology; Chief, Neuromuscular Division;
Director, and Clinical Neurophysiology Laboratory,
Brigham and Women's Hospital, Boston, Massachusetts
*Inherited Peripheral Neuropathies: Classification, Clinical
Features, and Review of Molecular Pathophysiology;
Peripheral Nervous System Diseases Associated with
Malignancy; Endocrine Myopathies and Toxic Myopathies*

Michael J. Aminoff, M.D., D.Sc., F.R.C.P.
Professor of Neurology, University of California, San
Francisco, School of Medicine; Attending Physician
and Director of the Clinical Neurophysiology
Laboratories, UCSF Medical Center, San Francisco,
California
Clinical Applications of Somatosensory Evoked Potentials

Majid Aramideh, M.D., Ph.D.
Neurologist and Clinical Neurophysiologist,
Department of Neurology, Alkmaar Medical Center,
The Netherlands
*Cranial Nerves and Brainstem Reflexes: Electrodiagnostic
Techniques, Physiology, and Normative Data; Assessment of
Disorders of the Cranial Nerves*

Reiner Benecke, Prof. Dr.
Director, Clinic of Neurology, University of Rostock
Medical Faculty, Rostock, Germany
Tone and Its Disorders

Timothy J. Benstead, M.D., F.R.C.P.(C.)
Professor, Department of Medicine, Division of
Neurology, Dalhousie University Faculty of Medicine,
Halifax, Nova Scotia, Canada
Radial Nerve

Alfredo Berardelli, M.D.
Professor, Department of Neurology, University of
Rome "La Sapienza," Rome; I.N.M. Neuromed
I.R.C.C.S., Pozzilli, Italy
Voluntary Movement Disorders

Shawn J. Bird, M.D.
Associate Professor, Department of Neurology,
University of Pennsylvania School of Medicine;
Director, Electromyography Laboratory, Hospital of
the University of Pennsylvania, Philadelphia,
Pennsylvania
Myopathies and Disorders of Neuromuscular Transmission

Charles F. Bolton, M.D., C.M., M.S., F.R.C.P.(C.)
Professor of Neurology, Mayo Medical School,
Rochester, Minnesota; formerly Chief of Clinical
Neurological Sciences and Director of the
Electromyography Laboratory, Victoria Hospital,
London, Ontario, Canada
*Peripheral Neuropathy in Systemic Disease; Assessment of
Patients in the Intensive Care Unit; Role of Electromyography
for the Acutely Paralyzed Child and the Intensive Care Unit;
Appendix: Normal Values*

Pierre Bourque, M.D.
Associate Professor of Medicine, Department of
Neurology, University of Ottawa Faculty of Medicine;
Neurologist, Ottawa Hospital, Ottawa, Ontario,
Canada
Other Mononeuropathies of the Upper Limbs

Deborah Young Bradshaw, M.D.
Clinical Associate Professor, Department of Neurology,
State University of New York Upstate Medical
University, Syracuse, New York
Peripheral Sensory Receptors and Sensation

Mark B. Bromberg, M.D., Ph.D.
Professor, Department of Neurology, University of
Utah School of Medicine, Salt Lake City, Utah
*Acute and Chronic Dysimmune Polyneuropathies; Amyotrophic
Lateral Sclerosis; Quantitative Motor Function Testing in
Clinical Trials*

Robert H. Brown, Jr., M.D., Ph.D.
Professor of Neurology, Harvard Medical School;
Director, Cecil B. Day Laboratory for Neuromuscular
Research, Massachusetts General Hospital, Boston,
Massachusetts
*Inherited Peripheral Neuropathies: Classification, Clinical
Features, and Review of Molecular Pathophysiology; Inherited
Disorders of Muscle: Classification, Clinical Features, and
Review of Molecular Pathophysiology*

William F. Brown, M.D., F.R.C.P.(C.)
Professor of Neurology, Tufts University School of
Medicine; Head of Neurology, New England Medical
Center, Boston, Massachusetts
*Transmembrane Potential and Action Potential; Recording of
Electrical Activity in Nerve Trunks and Conduction in
Human Sensory and Motor Nerve Fibers; Pathophysiology of
Conduction in Peripheral Neuropathies; Volume Conduction;
Motor Neurons, Motor Units, and Motor Unit Recruitment;
Motor Unit Number Estimation: Methods and Applications;
Quantitative Electromyography; Normal and Abnormal
Spontaneous Activity in Muscle; Negative Signs and
Symptoms of Peripheral Nerve and Muscle Disease*

William W. Campbell, M.D., M.S.H.A.
Professor, Department of Neurology, Uniformed
Services University of the Health Sciences F. Edward
Hébert School of Medicine, Bethesda, Maryland;
Chief, Clinical Neurophysiology, Walter Reed Army
Medical Center, Washington, District of Columbia
Ulnar Nerve

K. Ming Chan, M.D., F.R.C.P.(C.)
Assistant Professor, Division of Physical Medicine and
Rehabilitation/University Centre for Neuroscience,
University of Alberta Faculty of Medicine and
Dentistry, Edmonton, Alberta, Canada
*Motor Neurons, Motor Units, and Motor Unit Recruitment;
Needle EMG Abnormalities in Neurogenic and Muscle
Diseases; Underlying Mechanisms of Muscle Contraction and
Force Production and Peripheral and Central Mechanisms of
Muscle Fatigue*

Jeffrey M. Chavin, M.D.
Assistant Professor, Department of Neurology, Tufts
University School of Medicine; Assistant Professor,
Department of Neurology, New England Medical
Center, Boston, Massachusetts
*Normal and Abnormal Spontaneous Activity in Muscle;
Negative Signs and Symptoms of Peripheral Nerve and
Muscle Disease*

Robert Chen, M.A., M.B., B.Chir., M.Sc., F.R.C.P.(C.)
Assistant Professor, University of Toronto Faculty of
Medicine; Attending Neurologist, Toronto Western
Hospital, University Health Network, Toronto,
Ontario, Canada
Anatomy and Physiology of Respiration

Sudhansu Chokroverty, M.D.
Professor, Department of Neurology, New York
Medical College, Valhalla, New York; Clinical
Professor, Department of Neurology, University of
Medicine and Dentistry of New Jersey Robert Wood
Johnson Medical School, New Brunswick, New Jersey;
Program Director and Associate Chairman,
Department of Neurology; Chairman, Division of
Neurophysiology; and Director, Center of Sleep
Medicine, Saint Vincents Catholic Medical Centers,
New York, New York
Lumbosacral Radiculopathies

Joseph Classen, M.D.
Lecturer in Neurology, Clinic of Neurology, University
of Rostock Medical Faculty, Rostock, Germany
Tone and Its Disorders

Michael P. Collins, M.D.
Assistant Professor, Department of Neurology, Division
of Neuromuscular Diseases, Ohio State University
School of Medicine and Public Health; Attending
Physician, Department of Neurology, Ohio State
University Medical Center, Columbus, Ohio
*Peripheral Nervous System Diseases Associated with
Malignancy*

Robin A. Conwit, M.D.
Assistant Professor, Department of Neurology, Johns
Hopkins University School of Medicine; Director,
EMG Laboratory, Johns Hopkins Bayview Medical
Center, Baltimore, Maryland
Age-Related Changes in Peripheral and Central Conduction

Thomas O. Crawford, M.D.
Associate Professor, Department of Neurology and
Pediatrics, Johns Hopkins University School of
Medicine, Baltimore, Maryland
*Spinal Muscular Atrophies and Other Disorders of the Motor
Neuron*

Giorgio Cruccu, M.D., Ph.D.
Professor and Neurologist, Department of
Neurological Science, University of Rome "La
Sapienza," Rome, Italy
*Cranial Nerves and Brainstem Reflexes: Electrodiagnostic
Techniques, Physiology, and Normative Data; Assessment of
Disorders of the Cranial Nerves*

Brian A. Crum, M.D.
Instructor, Department of Neurology, Mayo Graduate
School of Medicine; Associate Consultant, Mayo
Clinic, Rochester, Minnesota
Peripheral Neuropathy in Systemic Disease

Antonio Currà, M.D.
Assistant Professor, University of Rome "La Sapienza,"
Rome; I.N.M. Neuromed I.R.C.C.S., Pozzilli, Italy
Voluntary Movement Disorders

Basil T. Darras, M.D.
Associate Professor in Neurology (Pediatrics), Harvard
Medical School; Director, Neuromuscular Program,
Children's Hospital, Boston, Massachusetts
*Pediatric Electromyography: Clinical Indications and
Methodology; Myopathies and Arthrogryposis Multiplex
Congenita; Role of Electromyography for the Acutely
Paralyzed Child and the Intensive Care Unit*

Jasper R. Daube, M.D.
Professor, Department of Neurology, Mayo Medical
School; Consultant, Department of Neurology, Mayo
Clinic and Mayo Foundation, Rochester, Minnesota
*Cranial Nerve Monitoring; Monitoring Spinal Function
During Surgery; Monitoring Peripheral Nerves During
Surgery*

Marie-An C. J. de Letter, M.D., Ph.D.
St. Antonius Hospital, Nieuwegein, The Netherlands
Acute Polyneuropathies Encountered in the Intensive Care Unit

Günther Deuschl, M.D.
Chairman, Department of Neurology, Christian-
Albrechts-Universität Kiel, Kiel, Germany
Tremor

Alessandro Di Rocco, M.D.
Associate Professor, Department of Neurology, Albert
Einstein College of Medicine of Yeshiva University,
Bronx; Associate Attending, Beth Israel Medical
Center, New York, New York
AIDS-Associated Myelopathies

Timothy J. Doherty, M.D., Ph.D., F.R.C.P.(C.)
Assistant Professor, Department of Physical Medicine
and Rehabilitation, University of Western Ontario
Faculty of Medicine & Dentistry; Consultant
Physiatrist, London Health Sciences Centre and St.
Joseph's Health Care, London, Ontario, Canada
*Motor Neurons, Motor Units, and Motor Unit Recruitment;
Motor Unit Number Estimation: Methods and Applications;
Normal Motor Unit Action Potential*

Peter D. Donofrio, M.D.
Professor, Department of Neurology, Wake Forest
University School of Medicine; Associate Chief of
Professional Services, North Carolina Baptist Hospital,
Winston-Salem, North Carolina
Drug-Related Neuropathies

John W. Downie, Ph.D.
Professor, Department of Pharmacology, and Assistant
Professor, Department of Urology, Dalhousie
University Faculty of Medicine, Halifax, Nova Scotia,
Canada
Physiology and Pharmacology of the Bladder

Dirk Dressler, M.D.
Senior Lecturer, Rostock University Medical Faculty;
Consultant Neurologist, Department of Neurology,
Rostock University Hospital, Rostock, Germany
Tone and Its Disorders

Richard M. Dubinsky, M.D.
Associate Professor, Department of Neurology,
University of Kansas School of Medicine, Kansas City,
Kansas
Botulinum Toxin Treatment

Andrew A. Eisen, M.D., F.R.C.P.(C.)
Professor and Head, Department of Neurology,
University of British Columbia Faculty of Medicine;
Head, Neuromuscular Diseases Unit, Vancouver
General Hospital, Vancouver, British Columbia,
Canada
Cervical Radiculopathies; Thoracic Radiculopathies

Rodger J. Elble, M.D., Ph.D.
Professor and Chair, Department of Neurology, and
Director, Center for Alzheimer Disease and Related
Disorders, Southern Illinois University School of
Medicine, Springfield, Illinois
Tremor

Ronald G. Emerson, M.D.
Professor, Department of Clinical Neurology,
Columbia University College of Physicians and
Surgeons, New York, New York
Physiological Basis of Somatosensory Evoked Potentials

Diana M. Escolar, M.D.
Associate Professor of Neurology and Assistant
Professor of Pediatrics, George Washington University
School of Medicine and Health Sciences; Director,
Pediatric Neuromuscular Service and EMG
Laboratory, and Co-Director, Muscular Dystrophy
Clinic, Children's National Medical Center,
Washington, District of Columbia
Pediatric Mononeuropathies of the Lower Extremity

Kevin J. Felice, D.O.
Associate Professor, Department of Neurology,
University of Connecticut School of Medicine;
Director, Neuromuscular Program, University of
Connecticut Health Center, Farmington, Connecticut
Upper Extremity Mononeuropathies in Infants and Children

Aaron G. Filler, M.D., Ph.D., F.R.C.S.(S.N.)
Medical Director, Institute for Nerve Medicine, Santa
Monica, California
*Magnetic Resonance Neurography: Principles of Nerve
Imaging; Clinical Applications of MRI Neurography and
MRI of Denervated Muscle*

Morris A. Fisher, M.D.
Professor, Department of Neurology, Loyola
University Stritch School of Medicine, Maywood;
Attending Neurologist, Loyola University Medical
Center and Hines Veterans Administration Hospital,
Hines, Illinois
F Waves

Mary Kay Floeter, M.D., Ph.D.
Chief, Electromyography Section and Human Spinal
Cord Physiology Unit, National Institute of
Neurological Disorders and Stroke, National Institutes
of Health, Bethesda, Maryland
Physiology and Assessment of the Spinal Cord

Roy Freeman, M.D.
Associate Professor, Department of Neurology, Harvard Medical School; Autonomic and Peripheral Nerve Laboratory, Department of Neurology, Beth Israel Deaconess Medical Center, Boston, Massachusetts
Quantitative Sensory Testing; Autonomic Testing

Clifton L. Gooch, M.D.
Associate Clinical Professor, Department of Neurology, Columbia University College of Physicians and Surgeons; Director, Electromyography Laboratory, Columbia-Presbyterian Medical Center, New York, New York
Hereditary Motor Neuron Diseases; Infectious, Syndromic, and Systemic Disorders

Douglas S. Goodin, M.D.
Associate Professor, Department of Neurology, University of California, San Francisco, School of Medicine; Attending Physician, UCSF Medical Center, San Francisco, California
Clinical Applications of Somatosensory Evoked Potentials

Ian A. Grant, M.D., F.R.C.P.(C.)
Assistant Professor, Division of Neurology, Dalhousie University Faculty of Medicine, Halifax, Nova Scotia, Canada
Radial Nerve

Mark Hallett, M.D.
Chief, Medical Neurology Branch, National Institute of Neurological Disorders and Stroke, National Institutes of Health, Bethesda, Maryland
Myoclonus and Other Involuntary Movements

C. Michel Harper, M.D.
Associate Professor, Department of Neurology, Mayo Medical School; Consultant, Department of Neurology, Mayo Clinic, Rochester, Minnesota
Congenital Myopathies and Muscular Dystrophies; Congenital Myasthenic Syndromes; Monitoring Peripheral Nerves During Surgery

Jeremy P. W. Heaton, M.D.
Professor, Department of Urology and Department of Pharmacology and Toxicology, Queen's University Faculty of Health Sciences; Staff Urologist, Kingston General Hospital, Kingston, Ontario, Canada
Physiological Aspects of Sexual Function and Dysfunction

Robert C. Hermann, Jr., M.D.
Assistant Professor, Department of Neurology, Mayo Medical School; Mayo Clinic, Rochester, Minnesota
Inflammatory and Infiltrative Myopathies

Anton A. J. Hilgevoord, M.D., Ph.D.
Clinical Neurophysiologist, Department of Clinical Neurophysiology/Neurology, Academic Medical Center, Amsterdam, The Netherlands
H Reflex, Muscle Stretch Reflex, and Axon Reflex

Max J. Hilz, M.D., Ph.D.
University Professor of Neurology and Director of Clinical Neurophysiology, Department of Neurology, University of Erlangen-Nuremberg, Erlangen, Germany; Associate Professor of Neurology, New York University School of Medicine; Attending Neurologist, Tisch Hospital, New York, New York
Quantitative Autonomic Functional Testing in Clinical Trials

James F. Howard, Jr., M.D.
Professor, Department of Neurology, University of North Carolina at Chapel Hill School of Medicine; Chief, Neuromuscular Disorders Section, University of North Carolina Hospitals, Chapel Hill, North Carolina
Neuromuscular Transmission

Charles Jablecki, M.D.
Clinical Professor, Department of Neurosciences, University of California, San Diego, School of Medicine, San Diego, California
Median Nerve

H. Royden Jones, Jr., M.D.
Clinical Professor, Department of Neurology, Harvard Medical School, Boston; Jamie Ortiz-Patiño Chair in Neurology, Lahey Clinic, Burlington, Massachusetts
Pediatric Electromyography: Clinical Indications and Methodology; The Floppy Infant; Spinal Muscular Atrophies and Other Disorders of the Motor Neuron; Disorders of Plexus and Nerve Root; Upper Extremity Mononeuropathies in Infants and Children; Pediatric Mononeuropathies of the Lower Extremity; Polyneuropathies in Children; Infantile Botulism and Other Acquired Neuromuscular Junction Disorders of Infancy and Childhood; Myopathies and Arthrogryposis Multiplex Congenita; Role of Electromyography for the Acutely Paralyzed Child and the Intensive Care Unit

Bashar Katirji, M.D., F.A.C.P.
Professor, Department of Neurology, Case Western Reserve University School of Medicine; Chief, Division of Neuromuscular Diseases, and Director, EMG Laboratory, University Hospitals of Cleveland, Cleveland, Ohio
Peroneal Nerve

John J. Kelly, M.D.
Professor and Chairman, Department of Neurology, George Washington University School of Medicine and Health Sciences, Washington, District of Columbia
Peripheral Neuropathies Associated with Paraproteinemias and Amyloidosis

John C. Kincaid, M.D.
Kenneth L. and Selma G. Earnest Professor of Neurology, Indiana University School of Medicine, Indianapolis, Indiana
Ulnar Nerve

David A. Krendel, M.D.
North Georgia Neurological Clinic, Lawrenceville, Georgia
Diabetic Neuropathy

Dale J. Lange, M.D.
Associate Professor, Department of Neurology, and Director, Division of Neuromuscular Disease and EMG Laboratory, Mount Sinai Medical Center, New York, New York
Infections and Peripheral Neuropathy

Kerry H. Levin, M.D.
Department of Neurology, Cleveland Clinic Foundation, Cleveland, Ohio
Tibial Neuropathies

Richard A. Lewis, M.D.
Professor, Department of Neurology, Wayne State University School of Medicine, Detroit, Michigan
Inherited Neuropathies

Jan Lexell, M.D., Ph.D.
Adjunct Professor of Clinical Neuroscience, Department of Health Sciences, Luleå University of Technology, Boden; Associate Professor of Rehabilitation Medicine, Lund University Medical Faculty; Medical Director and Chief of Staff, Brain Injury Unit, and Director, Neuromuscular Research Laboratory, Department of Rehabilitation, Lund University Hospital, Lund, Sweden
Age-Related Changes in the Neuromuscular System

Alan E. Lomax, Ph.D.
Research Fellow, Heart and Stroke Foundation of Canada and Alberta Heritage Foundation for Medical Research, University of Calgary, Faculty of Medicine, Calgary, Alberta, Canada
Structure and Function of the Enteric Nervous System: Neurological Disease and Its Consequences for Neuromuscular Function in the Gastrointestinal Tract

Barend P. Lotz, M.D., M.Med. (Pret.), F.C.P.(S.A.)
Professor, University of Wisconsin Medical School, Madison, Wisconsin
Metabolic Myopathies

Philip G. McManis, M.D., F.R.A.C.P.
Senior Lecturer, University of Sydney Faculty of Medicine; Director, Clinical Neurophysiology, Royal North Shore Hospital, Sydney, New South Wales, Australia
Channelopathies

E. Jeffrey Metter, M.D.
Associate Professor, Johns Hopkins University School of Medicine; Medical Director, Baltimore Longitudinal Studies of Aging, National Institutes of Aging, Baltimore, Maryland
Age-Related Changes in Peripheral and Central Conduction

Michelle M. Mezei, M.D., C.M., F.R.C.P.(C.)
Clinical Instructor, Division of Neurology, University of British Columbia Faculty of Medicine; Academic Director, Neuromuscular Diseases Unit, Vancouver General Hospital, Vancouver, British Columbia, Canada
Thoracic Radiculopathies

Thomas A. Miller, M.D., F.R.C.P.(C.)
Associate Professor, Department of Physical Medicine and Rehabilitation, University of Western Ontario Faculty of Medicine and Dentistry; Consultant Physiatrist, Hand and Upper Limb Centre; Co-director, Peripheral Nerve Clinic; and Director, Electrodiagnostic Laboratory, St. Joseph's Health Care, London, Ontario, Canada
Disorders of Plexus and Nerve Root

Hiroshi Mitsumoto, M.D.
Professor, Department of Neurology, Columbia University College of Physicians and Surgeons; Director, Neuromuscular Division, and Director, Eleanor and Lou Gehrig MDA/ALS Center, Columbia-Presbyterian Medical Center, New York, New York
Infectious, Syndromic, and Systemic Disorders

Nahid K. Nainzadeh, M.D.
Clinical Associate Professor and Director of Electrodiagnostic Laboratory, Department of Rehabilitation Medicine, Mount Sinai School of Medicine of New York University; Associate Attending, Mount Sinai Hospital, New York, New York
Technical Aspects of Intraoperative Electromyography and Somatosensory Evoked Potential Monitoring

Sanjeev D. Nandedkar, Ph.D.
Clinical Applications Manager, Oxford Instruments, Hawthorne, New York
Basic Instrumentation; Computers in the Neurophysiology Laboratory

Richard K. Olney, M.D.
Professor, Department of Neurology, University of California, San Francisco, School of Medicine; Director, EMG Laboratory, and Director, ALS Center at UCSF, UCSF Medical Center, San Francisco, California
Quantitative Measurement of Sensory Function in Clinical Trials

Gilmore O'Neill, M.B., M.R.C.P.I.
Instructor in Neurology, Harvard Medical School;
Assistant Neurologist, Massachusetts General Hospital,
Boston, Massachusetts
Inherited Disorders of Muscle: Classification, Clinical Features, and Review of Molecular Pathophysiology

Bram W. Ongerboer de Visser, M.D., Ph.D.
Professor, Department of Clinical Neurophysiology,
University of Amsterdam School of Medicine;
Neurologist, Academic Medical Center, Amsterdam,
The Netherlands
Cranial Nerves and Brainstem Reflexes: Electrodiagnostic Techniques, Physiology, and Normative Data; H Reflex, Muscle Stretch Reflex, and Axon Reflex; Assessment of Disorders of the Cranial Nerves

Matthew Pitt, M.D., F.R.C.P.
Consultant Paediatric Neurophysiologist, Great
Ormond Street Hospital, London, England
Polyneuropathies in Children

Rahman Pourmand, M.D.
Professor, Department of Neurology, State University
of New York at Stony Brook, Health Sciences Center
School of Medicine, Stony Brook, New York
Paraneoplastic Peripheral Neuropathies

Francis Renault, M.D.
Associate Professor, Université Pierre et Marie Curie;
Head, Pediatric Neurophysiology Unit, Hôpital
d'Enfants Armand-Trousseau, Paris, France
Facial and Bulbar Weakness

Devon I. Rubin, M.D.
Assistant Professor, Department of Neurology, Mayo
Medical School; Mayo Clinic, Rochester, Minnesota
Inflammatory and Infiltrative Myopathies

Howard W. Sander, M.D.
Associate Professor of Clinical Neurology and
Associate Director, Peripheral Neuropathy Center,
Cornell University Joan and Sanford I. Weill Medical
College, New York; Adjunct Associate Professor,
Department of Neurology, New York University
School of Medicine, New York; Adjunct Associate
Professor, Department of Neurology, New York
Medical College, Valhalla, New York
Lumbosacral Radiculopathies

Donald B. Sanders, M.D.
Professor, Department of Medicine, Division of
Neurology, Duke University School of Medicine,
Durham, North Carolina
Electrophysiological Methods for Assessing Neuromuscular Transmission; Diseases Associated with Disorders of Neuromuscular Transmission

Marc H. Schieber, M.D., Ph.D.
Associate Professor, Departments of Neurology and of
Neurobiology and Anatomy, University of Rochester
School of Medicine and Dentistry; Attending
Physician, Brain Injury Rehabilitation Unit, St. Mary's
Hospital, Rochester, New York
Basic Physiology of the Central Motor System

Keith A. Sharkey, Ph.D.
Professor, University of Calgary Faculty of Medicine,
Calgary, Alberta, Canada
Structure and Function of the Enteric Nervous System: Neurological Disease and Its Consequences for Neuromuscular Function in the Gastrointestinal Tract

Susan J. Shefchyk, Ph.D.
Professor, Department of Physiology, University of
Manitoba Faculty of Medicine, Winnipeg, Manitoba,
Canada
Physiology and Pharmacology of the Bladder

Jeremy M. Shefner, M.D., Ph.D.
Professor, Department of Neurology, State University
of New York, Upstate Medical University, Syracuse,
New York
Peripheral Sensory Receptors and Sensation; Peripheral Sensory Conduction

Robert W. Shields, Jr., M.D.
Staff Neurologist, Cleveland Clinic Foundation,
Cleveland, Ohio
Alcoholic and Nutritional Polyneuropathies; Postpolio Syndrome

Michael E. Shy, M.D.
Professor, Department of Neurology, and Center for
Molecular Medicine and Genetics, Wayne State
University School of Medicine, Detroit, Michigan
Inherited Neuropathies

David M. Simpson, M.D.
Associate Professor, Department of Neurology, Mount
Sinai School of Medicine of New York University;
Director, Clinical Neurophysiology Laboratories,
Mount Sinai Hospital, New York, New York
HIV-Related Neuropathies and Myopathies

Yuen T. So, M.D., Ph.D.
Associate Professor, Department of Neurology and
Neuroscience, Stanford University, School of
Medicine; Director, Neurological Clinics, Stanford
University Medical Center, Stanford, California
Sciatic Nerve

Erik V. Stålberg, M.D., Ph.D.
Professor Emeritus, Department of Clinical
Neurophysiology, University Hospital, Uppsala,
Sweden
Electrophysiological Methods for Assessing Neuromuscular Transmission

Daniel W. Stashuk, Ph.D.
Associate Professor, Department of Systems Design
Engineering, University of Waterloo, Waterloo,
Ontario, Canada
*Normal Motor Unit Action Potential; Quantitative
Electromyography*

John D. Stewart, M.B., B.S., F.R.C.P.(C.)
Professor, Department of Neurology and
Neurosurgery, McGill University Faculty of Medicine;
Neurologist, Montreal Neurological Hospital and
Institute, Montreal, Quebec, Canada
*Quantitative Sensory Testing; Median Nerve; Other
Mononeuropathies of the Lower Limb*

Jeffrey A. Strommen, M.D.
Instructor in Physical Medicine and Rehabilitation,
Mayo Medical School; Consultant, Section of
Electromyography and Department of Physical
Medicine and Rehabilitation, Mayo Clinic and Mayo
Foundation, Rochester, Minnesota
Cranial Nerve Monitoring

Peter Styles, M.D.
Founder and Former Technical Director, Medelec Ltd.
(now Oxford Instruments, Medical Division), Old
Woking, Surrey, United Kingdom
Safety in the Electromyography Laboratory

Austin J. Sumner, M.D.
Richard M. Paddison Professor and Chairman,
Department of Neurology, Louisiana State University
School of Medicine in New Orleans, New Orleans,
Louisiana
Inherited Neuropathies

Kathryn J. Swoboda, M.D.
Assistant Professor, Department of Neurology, and
Adjunct Assistant Professor, Department of Pediatrics;
University of Utah School of Medicine; Primary
Children's Medical Center, Salt Lake City, Utah
The Floppy Infant

Michele Tagliati, M.D.
Assistant Professor, Department of Neurology, Albert
Einstein College of Medicine of Yeshiva University,
Bronx; Attending, Beth Israel Medical Center, New
York, New York
AIDS-Associated Myelopathies

Eugene Tolunsky, M.D.
Fellow in Neuromuscular Disease, Department of
Neurology, Mount Sinai Medical Center, New York,
New York
Infections and Peripheral Neuropathy

Jože V. Trontelj, M.D., D.Sc.
Professor, Department of Neurology, University of
Ljubljana Medical Faculty; Neurologist and Senior
Consultant, Institute of Clinical Neurophysiology,
Department of Neurology, University Medical Center,
Ljubljana, Slovenia
*Electrophysiological Methods for Assessing Neuromuscular
Transmission*

Josep Valls-Solé, M.D., Ph.D.
University Lecturer, University of Barcelona Faculty of
Medicine; Consultant Neurologist, EMG Unit,
Neurologic Service, Hospital Clinic, Barcelona, Spain
*Cranial Nerves and Brainstem Reflexes: Electrodiagnostic
Techniques, Physiology, and Normative Data; Assessment of
Disorders of the Cranial Nerves*

Anthony A. Vandervoort, Ph.D.
Professor, Schools of Physical Therapy and
Kinesiology, and Kinesiology Graduate Program Chair,
University of Western Ontario Faculty of Medicine &
Dentistry, London, Ontario, Canada
Age-Related Changes in the Neuromuscular System

Leo H. Visser, M.D., Ph.D.
St. Elizabeth's Hospital, Tilburg, The Netherlands
Acute Polyneuropathies Encountered in the Intensive Care Unit

John J. Wald, M.D.
Clinical Associate Professor, Department of Neurology,
University of Michigan Medical School; University of
Michigan Health System, Ann Arbor, Michigan
Industrial and Environmental Toxic Neuropathies

Annabel K. Wang, M.D.
Assistant Professor, Department of Neurology, Mount
Sinai School of Medicine of New York University;
Assistant Attending Physician, Department of
Neurology, Mount Sinai Hospital, New York,
New York
HIV-Related Neuropathies and Myopathies

Bradley V. Watson, B.Sc.
Laboratory Coordinator, Electromyography
Laboratory, London Health Sciences Centre, London,
Ontario, Canada
*Recording of Electrical Activity in Nerve Trunks and
Conduction in Human Sensory and Motor Nerve Fibers;
Pathophysiology of Conduction in Peripheral Neuropathies;
Volume Conduction*

Markus Weber, M.D.
Department of Neurology, Kantonsspital St. Gallen,
St. Gallen, Switzerland
Lumbosacral Plexopathies

Asa J. Wilbourn, M.D.
Clinical Professor, Department of Neurology, Case Western Reserve University School of Medicine; Director, EMG Laboratory, Neurology Department, Cleveland Clinic, Cleveland, Ohio
Brachial Plexopathies; Peripheral Neuropathies Associated with Vascular Diseases and the Vasculitides

Enrique A. Wulff, M.D., Ph.D.
Pediatric Neurology, University of Florida College of Medicine–Jacksonville; Adult and Pediatric Neurology, Baptist Hospital and Memorial Hospital, Jacksonville, Florida
HIV-Related Neuropathies and Myopathies

Ulf Ziemann, M.D.
Assistant Professor, Department of Neurology, University of Frankfurt Faculty of Medicine; University Hospital J. W. Goethe, Frankfurt am Main, Germany
Assessment of Motor Cortex and Descending Motor Pathways

Udo A. Zifko, M.D.
University Lecturer, University of Vienna Faculty of Medicine, Vienna; Attending, University Clinic, Vienna; Head, Neurological Rehabilitation Center, Pirawarth Clinic, Bad Pirawarth, Austria
Clinical and Electrophysiological Assessment; Intensive Care– and Critical Illness–Related Neuromuscular Disorders: Ventilator Disorders

Douglas W. Zochodne, M.D., F.R.C.P.(C.)
Professor, Department of Neurology, University of Calgary Faculty of Medicine; Neurologist, Foothills Hospital, Calgary, Alberta, Canada
Overview of the Autonomic Nervous System: Anatomy and Physiology

Preface

The last decade has seen truly remarkable progress in our understanding of the function of the neuromuscular system, the many ways by which such function becomes disordered, and the accurate diagnosis and treatment of many neuromuscular diseases. Such has been the pace of advances in understanding the basic molecular, metabolic, structural, and pathophysiological features of many neuromuscular diseases that clinicians, neuromuscular specialists, and scientists working in the field have become lost in the bewildering mass of accumulating literature that is widely dispersed in a variety of medical and scientific journals. A completely new text has therefore become necessary to summarize advances in the field. It is the purpose of this book to provide a convenient summary of neuromuscular function and the basic, clinical, and electrodiagnostic aspects of neuromuscular diseases. We hope that it will appeal to clinicians, clinical neurophysiologists, and others concerned with patients who have neuromuscular diseases, as well as to basic scientists who work on the fundamental aspects of disordered neuromuscular function and require a comprehensive, multifaceted text that deals with these disorders.

We have attempted to provide, in a single, encompassing, two-volume text, an account of the essential molecular, physiological, and anatomical underpinnings of the peripheral and related central components of the neuromuscular system; the pathophysiology of neuromuscular disorders; the clinical features and differential diagnoses of the various neuromuscular diseases; and, finally, the place of electrophysiological testing in the diagnosis and management of the foregoing neuromuscular diseases. Some overlap between chapters was inevitable in the effort to produce a book comprehensive in scope and of practical utility.

Volume I provides the essential underpinnings for understanding the molecular, physiological, and pathophysiological bases of neuromuscular diseases. It also includes sections on the autonomic and respiratory systems, imaging techniques, and age-related changes in the neuromuscular system as well as sections on the technical aspects of neuromuscular testing. Volume II focuses more directly on the clinical features of the neuromuscular diseases and on the practical applications of electrophysiological tests to their diagnosis and management.

Electrophysiological studies are important in the identification, localization, and characterization of the major pathophysiological features of neuromuscular diseases, but they must be interpreted in the clinical context in which they were obtained as well as in association with other laboratory tests, imaging studies, and various immunological assays and genetic studies. Clinical neurophysiology is an expanding field, and technical advances and newer clinical applications of electrophysiological studies are emphasized. Modern computers have caught up with the technical demands of analyzing electrophysiological signals in real time. This fact and the power of newly developed software have brought hitherto unavailable measures of power and portability to clinical examinations of the neuromuscular system, enhancing the ability of clinical neurophysiologists to detect and analyze neuromuscular disorders.

We are grateful to the many contributors to this book for taking time from their already crowded schedules to provide readers with an up-to-date, detailed, and critical review of the subject. The individual authors were chosen because of their experience and expertise in their particular fields. A project of this size has, of necessity, required that we enlist the assistance of section editors, and we are greatly indebted to them for their wisdom, advice, and help. We also very much appreciate the unfailing courtesy and assistance of Allan Ross, Senior Medical Editor, Joannne Husovski, Senior Developmental Editor, Dolores Meloni, Associate Acquisitions Editor, and Gina Scala, former Copy Editing Supervisor, at Elsevier Science in seeing this project through to its completion. Finally, the understanding and support of our families made the project possible, and it is not possible to express adequately our gratitude to them.

William F. Brown, M.D.
Charles F. Bolton, M.D.
Michael J. Aminoff, M.D.

Contents

POLYNEUROPATHIES

Inherited Neuropathies

Richard A. Lewis, Austin J. Sumner, and Michael E. Shy

This chapter reviews the clinical, electrodiagnostic, and genetic aspects of the inherited neuropathies. The explosion of new information regarding these disorders is remarkable. In particular, the genetic mutations leading to these disorders are being identified so quickly that the reader is referred to the medical literature for up-to-date information. Nevertheless, the framework for a modern understanding of these disorders is presented. The elec-trodiagnostic aspects of these neuropathies, particularly those in which myelin is affected, are emphasized.

HISTORY

Charcot and Marie in France (1886) and Tooth in England (1886) described the inherited neuropathies now known as *Charcot-Marie-Tooth disease* (CMT), although the syndrome may actually have been reported 13 years earlier by Friedreich, whose descriptions included pathological peripheral nerve abnormalities (Friedreich, 1873). Although early investigators recognized the weakness and atrophy of muscles innervated by the peroneal nerve, characteristic foot abnormalities, and the familial nature of the disease, it was also soon recognized that inherited disorders of peripheral nerves made up a heterogeneous group. Dejerine and Sottas (1893) described cases that were more severe, with an onset in infancy, and Roussy and Levy (1926) described cases associated with tremor, ataxia, areflexia, and pes cavus. Rather than clarifying the inherited neuropathies, however, these classifications actually increased nosological confusion concerning the disorders owing to overlapping clinical and pathological features, as well as a lack of precise diagnostic criteria for each of these entities (reviewed in Harding and Thomas, 1980; Harding, 1995).

With the advent of nerve conduction velocity (NCV) testing, this nosological confusion began to dissipate. Early studies suggested that most CMT patients could be divided into one group with slow NCV and pathological evidence of a hypertrophic demyelinating neuropathy (CMT 1) and a second group with relatively normal NCV and axonal degeneration (CMT 2) (Dyck and Lambert, 1968; Thomas and Calne, 1974; Buchthal and Behse, 1977). The clinical features of CMT 1 and CMT 2 patients were outlined in a pair of landmark publications in which Harding and Thomas reported the genetic (1980a) and clinical (1980b) characteristics of more than 200 patients with CMT 1 and CMT 2. CMT 1 patients were found to have median motor NCVs (MNCVs) of less than 38 m per second, whereas median MNCVs of more than 38 m per second characterized CMT 2 patients. NCVs in CMT 1 patients have subsequently been shown to be uniformly slowed along individual nerves and between different nerves of an individual patient, distinguishing CMT 1 patients from those with acquired demyelinating neuropathies such as Guillain-Barré syndrome or chronic inflammatory demyelinating polyneuropathy (Lewis and Sumner, 1982; Kaku et al., 1993). Most CMT 1 patients were found to have an autosomal dominant pattern of inheritance; they also developed clinical evidence of disease within the first two decades of life, associated with weakness and sensory loss occurring predominantly in the distal legs and wasting in the distribution of weakened muscles (Harding and Thomas, 1980a, 1980b). In the series of Harding and Thomas (1980b), the clinical phenotype of patients with CMT 2 was quite similar to that of patients with CMT 1 with a few minor exceptions. For example, patients with CMT 2 were more likely to have preserved tendon reflexes than were patients with CMT 1, and some patients with CMT 2 appeared to have milder phenotypes. However, it is not possible to distinguish patients with CMT 1 from those with CMT 2 with certainty based only on neurological

examination. Specific genetic testing now permits the accurate diagnosis of most CMT 1 patients, but as yet, no genetic testing is available for CMT 2.

NOMENCLATURE

In part because much of the nomenclature for inherited neuropathies was developed before specific genetic causes of the diseases had been identified, the classification of inherited neuropathies has been a source of confusion. Dawidenkow (1927a, 1927b) may have been the first to propose a classification system based on clinical and genetic features. Before 1991, most practitioners used the classification system of Dyck and Lambert (Dyck and Lambert, 1968; Dyck, 1984) (Table 57–1) to categorize different forms of inherited neuropathies. This was very useful because it separated the inherited disorders into hereditary motor and sensory neu-

Table 57–1. Dyck and Lambert Classification of Hereditary Motor and Sensory Neuropathies

Type of Hereditary Motor and Sensory Neuropathy	Features
1A and 1B dominantly inherited hypertrophic neuropathy	Slow nerve conduction velocities; Distal weakness, mild sensory loss; Palpable nerves; Decreased reflexes; Pathology demonstrating segmental demyelination, remyelination, onion bulb formation, and axonal loss; Autosomal dominant
II neuronal type of peroneal muscular atrophy	Normal nerve conduction velocities; Distal weakness, mild sensory loss; Nonpalpable nerves; Pathology demonstrating degeneration of motor and sensory nerves; Autosomal dominant
III hypertrophic neuropathy of infancy (Dejerine-Sottas)	Delayed motor development; Severe motor sensory loss; Slow nerve conduction velocities; Autosomal recessive
IV hypertrophic neuropathy (Refsum) associated with phytanic acid excess	Refsum's disease
V associated with spastic paraplegia	Spastic paraplegia present
VI with optic atrophy	Optic atrophy present
VII	Retinitis pigmentosa present

From Dyck PJ, Lambert EH: Lower motor and primary sensory neuron diseases with peroneal muscular atrophy. I: Neurologic, genetic, and electrophysiologic findings in hereditary polyneuropathies. Arch Neurol 1968; 18:603–618; and Bergoffen J, Scherer SS, Wang S, et al: Connexin mutations in X-linked Charcot-Marie-Tooth disease. Science 1993;262:3039–3042.

ropathies (HMSNs), pure hereditary motor neuropathies (HMNs), and pure hereditary sensory neuropathies (HSNs) and was able to organize each of these based on distinctive clinical patterns. However, once specific genetic causes for the neuropathies were identified, problems with this classification system began to develop. First, different mutations in the same gene, such as the peripheral myelin protein 22-kd gene *(PMP22),* can cause a milder HMSN I phenotype (Roa et al., 1993; Nelis et al., 1994), the more severe Dejerine-Sottas disease (D-S) (Hoogendijk et al., 1993; Roa et al., 1993; Ionasescu et al., 1995; Valentijn et al., 1995; Tyson et al., 1997; Marques et al., 1998), or even a phenotype that resembles hereditary neuropathy with liability to pressure palsy (HNPP) (Garcia et al., 1995). Second, CMT X does not fit easily into the Dyck and Lambert classification, both because of its X-linked inheritance pattern and because of its intermediately slowed NCVs, as is discussed later. Third, different mutations in the same gene, such as the protein 0 gene *(P0),* may cause slow nerve conductions characteristic of HMSN I (Bird et al., 1997) or velocities more typical of HMSN II (Marrosu et al., 1998). Finally, severe forms of disease clinically typical of D-S can be inherited in dominant as well as recessive patterns and in neuronal as well as demyelinating forms.

Although classification based on clinical features remains useful, particularly in differentiating among pure motor, pure sensory, and mixed disorders, newer classifications are needed as the specific genetic defects underlying the inherited neuropathies are identified. In this review, we classify families as having CMT 1 based on slow nerve conduction velocities and a dominant pattern of inheritance, as having CMT X based on an X-linked inheritance pattern, and as having CMT 2 based on a dominant pattern of inheritance (with no male-to-male transmission) and normal NCVs but reduced motor or sensory amplitudes. CMT 1 cases, as discussed earlier, are subdivided on the basis of mutations in defined myelin genes such as *PMP22* (CMT 1A) and *P0* (CMT 1B). Cases of CMT 2 are subdivided on the basis of differences in linkage studies, because specific mutations causing CMT 2 have not been identified. The designation D-S is used simply to identify severe clinical forms of disease that begin in infancy without regard to whether the inheritance is dominant or recessive or whether the neuropathy is demyelinating or axonal.

The chapter concentrates on the electrodiagnostic features of these disorders. We first review the inherited demyelinating disorders, then CMT 2, and then the other hereditary disorders.

INHERITED DEMYELINATING NEUROPATHIES

The inherited demyelinating neuropathies include those that have carried a CMT classification, such

Table 57–2. Gene Defects in Inherited Demyelinating Neuropathies

Neuropathy	Gene Defects
CMT 1A	Duplication on chromosome 17 (region containing PMP22 gene), point mutations in PMP22 gene
CMT 1B	Point mutations in P0 gene
Hereditary neuropathy with liability to pressure palsies	Deletion on chromosome 17 (same region that is duplicated in CMT 1A)
CMT X	Point mutations in connexin 32
Dejerine-Sottas	Point mutations in PMP22 gene
	Point mutations in P0 gene
	Point mutations in EGR2
	Other undetermined causes
Congenital hypomyelination	Point mutations in P0 gene
	Point mutations in EGR2
Not named at present	Point mutations in EGR2
Pelizaeus-Merzbacher disease	PLP null mutations
CMT 4A	8q13-q21.1
CMT 4B	11q23 (MTMR2)
CMT 4C	5q23-33
CMT 4D	8q24 (NDRG1)

PMP, peripheral myelin protein; CMT, Charcot-Marie-Tooth disease; *EGR2,* early growth response 2; PLP, proteolipid protein.

as CMT 1A, CMT 1B, and CMT X, each of which has a specific mutation identified with it. In addition, there are neuropathies associated with point mutations of *PMP22, P0,* and early growth response 2 gene *(EGR2)* that have not been as well characterized or clearly classified (Table 57–2). There also are disorders of both central and peripheral myelin, which are considered here.

Overview of the Electrophysiological Aspects of Inherited Demyelinating Neuropathies

The contribution of electrophysiology to our understanding of the inherited demyelinating neuropathies cannot be overemphasized. It remains one of the crowning clinical achievements of electromyography.

Slowing of conduction velocities in patients with peroneal muscular atrophy was independently described by Henrickson (1956), Lambert (1956), and Gilliatt and Thomas (1957). Dyck and Lambert (1963) described in more detail the conduction abnormalities in CMT 1, demonstrating the marked slowing of conduction in a large kinship with the disorder. These observations were extended by these authors and others to demonstrate markedly slow conduction velocities in CMT 1 and relatively normal velocities in CMT 2. A few groups recognized families with intermediate conduction changes with velocities between 35 and 45 m per second (Brust et al., 1978; Davis et al., 1978). Although these families were thought to have autosomal dominant inheritance owing to female involvement, it has become clear that most of these families had CMT X.

The slowing of conduction in CMT 1 was further defined when Lewis and Sumner (1982) compared the electrodiagnostic features of inherited demyelinating neuropathies with those of acquired demyelinating neuropathies. This study demonstrated that patients with CMT with slow conduction velocities (HMSN 1 or CMT 1) had uniformly slow conduction velocities. In contrast, patients with chronic acquired demyelinating neuropathies, particularly chronic inflammatory demyelinating polyneuropathy, typically had multifocal conduction changes with nonuniform conduction slowing. Similar observations were made by Wilbourn in 1977. At the time of these reports, the diagnostic criteria for chronic inflammatory demyelinating polyneuropathy were just being considered, and the genetic causes of CMT were unknown. The distinction between familial and acquired disorders had some practical clinical value and allowed the clinician to use electrodiagnostic testing to assist in making diagnostic and therapeutic decisions. These observations were followed by a report that extended the observation of uniform conduction slowing to include not only CMT but also other disorders of central and peripheral myelin, metachromatic leukodystrophy, Cockayne's syndrome, and Krabbe's disease (Miller et al., 1985).

Uniform Conduction Slowing

The term *uniform conduction slowing* has been used to describe disorders in which the physiological changes suggest that all myelinated nerve fibers are affected along the entire length of the nerve, from the nerve root to the distal nerve segment. In contrast to disorders that have multifocal or segmental changes, the electrodiagnostic studies in patients with uniform conduction slowing have similar velocity changes when different nerves are compared and when different segments of nerves are compared. This includes distal latencies, forelimb velocities, proximal velocities, and F-wave latencies. Some have used the terminal latency index (Kaku et al., 1994; Amato et al., 1996) to compare the distal motor latency (DML) with forearm conduction. Conduction block and excessive temporal dispersion are characteristic of multifocal disorders and are not noted in disorders with uniform conduction slowing. Temporal dispersion, in which the duration of the compound motor action potential (CMAP) becomes prolonged on proximal stimulation compared with distal stimulation, is indicative of excessive conduction slowing of intermediate nerve fibers and points to nonuniform conduction changes. Although there is some temporal dispersion on proximal stimulation in normal subjects and in patients with uniform conduction slowing, excessive temporal dispersion (usually defined as >20% increase in duration for the median, peroneal, and ulnar nerves and >30%

for the tibial nerve) (Weber, 1997) is indicative of nonuniform disorders.

At the time of these reports, there remains some question as to whether the hypertrophic form of CMT (CMT 1) was primarily axonal or demyelinating. The extensive pathological study of Dyck and colleagues (1974) suggested that axonal atrophy, which had a proximal-to-distal gradient, along with secondary demyelination, might be responsible for the conduction slowing. However, the studies of Aguayo and associates (1978), which showed that when Schwann cells from a patient with CMT were grafted into the nerves of immunosuppressed mice, the cells failed to myelinate the normal mouse axons. This strongly implicated the Schwann cell in the pathogenesis of the disease (Aguayo et al., 1978). Because all myelinating Schwann cells are presumably affected in the disease, these findings were in keeping with the uniform slowing of nerve conduction described previously.

Since the late 1980s, there has been a dramatic increase in knowledge of the specific genetic abnormalities that underlie the different forms of inherited demyelinating neuropathy. In many of these, specific mutations in myelin genes have been shown to cause the disease. However, we still do not understand the mechanisms by which these mutations cause the electrophysiological and pathological features of demyelination. In addition, new genetic disorders of peripheral myelin have been discovered in which slowing of nerve conduction velocities is nonuniform and similar to that found in the acquired demyelinating neuropathies. Thus, patterns and features of demyelination in inherited neuropathies appear to be more complex than was previously recognized. Table 57–3 outlines the inherited disorders of myelin that have uniform conduction slowing, those that appear to be multifocal, and those for which the physiological characteristics remain to be determined.

Despite clinical similarities among CMT 1 patients, it was soon discovered that the group was genetically heterogeneous, as linkage studies demonstrated loci on both chromosome 1 (Bird et al., 1982) and chromosome 17 (Raeymaekers et al., 1989; Vance et al., 1989; Middleton et al., 1990). In 1991, two groups of investigators showed that the most common form of CMT 1, CMT 1A, was associated with a 1.5-Mb duplication within chromosome 17p11.2 (Lupski et al., 1991; Raeymaekers et al., 1991). It is estimated that 60% to 90% of CMT 1 patients have this duplication (Brice et al., 1992; Hallum et al., 1992; Wise et al., 1993; Patel and Lupski, 1994). The extra copy of *PMP22* contained within the 1.5-Mb duplication on chromosome 17 is likely to cause the neuropathy for two reasons. First, missense mutations in *PMP22* have been demonstrated to cause demyelinating neuropathies in Trembler (Suter et al., 1992a) and Trembler J (Suter et al., 1992b) mice, as well as in some families with a CMT 1 phenotype (Valentijn et al., 1992; Nelis et al., 1994). Second, transgenic mice (Huxley et al., 1996; Magyar

---

Table 57–3. Inherited Disorders of Myelin

Inherited Disorders with Uniform Conduction Slowing
  CMT 1A
  CMT 1B
  Dejerine-Sottas disease
  Metachromatic leukodystrophy
  Cockayne's disease
  Krabbe's disease
Inherited Disorders with Multifocal Conduction Slowing
  Hereditary neuropathy with liability to pressure palsies
  CMT X
  Adrenomyeloneuropathy
  Pelizaeus-Merzbacher disease with PLP null mutation
  Refsum's disease
Inherited Demyelinating Disorders with a Yet to Be
    Determined Electrophysiology
  PMP22 point mutations
  P0 point mutations
  Adult-onset leukodystrophies
  Merosin deficiency
  Early growth response 2 gene mutations
  CMT 4A
  CMT 4B
  CMT 4C
  CMT 4D

CMT, Charcot-Marie-Tooth; PLP, proteolipid protein; PMP, peripheral myelin protein.

et al., 1996) and rats (Sereda et al., 1996) that overexpress PMP22 develop neuropathies that resemble CMT 1.

Reports of other genetic defects associated with hereditary neuropathies followed. CMT 1B, which was linked to chromosome 1, was found to be associated with mutations in the P0 glycoprotein (Hayasaka et al., 1993), and an X-linked neuropathy, CMT X, was found to be due to mutations in the connexin 32 (Cx32) protein on the X chromosome (Bergoffen et al., 1993). Deletion of the *PMP22* gene locus was associated with HNPP (Chance et al., 1993), and D-S, a severe infantile neuropathy, was associated with mutations in *PMP22* (Nelis et al., 1996; De Jonghe et al., 1997; Reilly, 1998) or *P0* (Warner et al., 1996). Mutations in *EGR2* were found in families with the CMT 1 phenotype or with congenital hypomyelinating neuropathy (Warner et al., 1998). Table 57–2 summarizes the CMT disorders associated with known genetic mutations.

Peripheral Nervous System Myelin Proteins

Peripheral nervous system (PNS) myelin is a multilamellar structure composed of a spiral of specialized membrane that surrounds axons. The *PNS myelin internode,* or segment of myelin generated by an individual myelinating Schwann cell, can be divided into a domain of compact myelin and a domain of noncompact myelin. Compact myelin, which constitutes the bulk of the internode, consists of successive wraps of the Schwann cell plasma membrane around the axon in which the ensheath-

ing membranes adhere to each other at both their extracellular (intraperiod line) and cytoplasmic (major dense line) surfaces. In noncompact myelin, the cytoplasmic membranes of the myelin wraps are not tightly opposed. These noncompacted regions include the inner and outer mesaxon, the paranodal loops adjacent to nodes of Ranvier, and the Schmidt-Lanterman incisures (the continuous channels of cytoplasm extending from the periaxonal surface of myelin to the cell soma) (Raine, 1984).

Although myelin is mainly composed of lipids, PNS myelin contains a unique set of proteins that are thought to play key roles in the myelin sheath. The main proteins in PNS myelin, including P0, PMP22, and myelin basic protein, are localized to compact myelin. Other proteins, including the myelin-associated glycoprotein and Cx32, are restricted to regions of noncompact myelin. Proteolipid protein (PLP), the main protein in central nervous system (CNS) compact myelin, is also expressed by myelinating Schwann cells although at much lower levels than in the CNS. However, whether PNS PLP is localized in compact myelin, noncompact myelin, or the perinuclear Schwann cell cytoplasm remains unclear (Garbern et al., 1997; Griffiths et al., 1998).

Peripheral Myelin Protein 22 Disorders

CHARCOT-MARIE-TOOTH TYPE 1A WITH PERIPHERAL MYELIN PROTEIN 22 DUPLICATION

The genetic defect causing CMT 1A has been shown to be a duplication on chromosome 17p11.2, which includes the gene for the myelin protein PMP22. PMP22 is a small integral membrane protein contained in compact myelin of PNS but not CNS myelin. Although some studies have suggested that PMP22 can function in cell proliferation, its function in PNS myelin remains unknown. Studies have demonstrated that PMP22 and P0 may form complexes together in PNS myelin, suggesting that their functions are interrelated (D'Urso et al., 1999). Although patients with point mutations in *PMP22* have also been classified as having CMT 1A (Nelis et al., 1994; Harding, 1995; Ionasescu, 1995), clinical descriptions of CMT 1A patients are usually limited to patients with the duplication. The duplication accounts for more than 60% of patients with inherited sensory and motor neuropathy and probably more than 80% of CMT 1 patients and is the most extensively studied.

The information that is available clearly demonstrates uniform conduction slowing in patients with CMT 1A. The conduction changes in CMT 1A were first reported by Kaku and colleagues (1993). In a study of 82 patients with CMT 1A and of 47 additional patients with CMT 1 without genetic identification, they showed uniform conduction slowing in ulnar, median, and peroneal nerves, including proximal and distal conduction velocities and F-wave latencies. The F-wave findings were consistent with previous reports in CMT 1 (Kimura, 1974; Mongia et al., 1978). As opposed to the reports of Oh and Chang (1987) and Hoogendijk and associates (1992), Kaku and colleagues did not find evidence of conduction block. The discrepancy between these reports is probably accounted for by different definitions of conduction block, as well as by important technical considerations. The threshold for stimulation in patients with CMT 1A can be exceptionally high, and supramaximal stimulation cannot always be determined. In addition, in nerves with low CMAP amplitude or severe chronic denervation/reinnervation, amplitude reductions may be more affected by excessive phase cancellation and temporal dispersion (Rhee et al., 1990; Cornblath et al., 1991). The available data suggest that if conduction block occurs, it is most unusual, may at times reflect superimposed entrapment, and is unlikely to be related to the underlying pathophysiology of this disorder.

The range of median and ulnar conduction velocities in the CMT 1A patients studied by Kaku and associates (1993) was between 10 and 42 m per second. Other studies (Hoogendijk et al., 1993; Killian et al., 1996; Thomas et al., 1997; Krajewski et al., 2000) have reported ranges between 10 and 38 m per second, with most patients having conduction velocities between 15 and 30 m per second. However, an occasional patient may have conduction velocities of greater than 40 m per second (Kaku et al., 1993; Krampitz et al., 1998). The lack of marked conduction slowing does not preclude the diagnosis of CMT 1A, and genetic testing should be considered in the appropriate clinical situation. Although the electrodiagnostic studies can provide valuable diagnostic clues, they are not, in and of themselves, diagnostic.

Longitudinal studies have shown that conduction velocity remains relatively stable for at least 20 years. Killian and associates (1996) showed that compared with values in 8 patients with CMT 1A who were previously studied in 1967, studies in 1989 showed only 2 to 3 m per second greater slowing. This confirmed, in patients with known duplications, what had previously been shown in the less specific group of CMT 1 patients (Davis et al., 1978; Gutmann et al., 1983; Roy et al., 1989). The conduction slowing has been shown to evolve over the first 3 to 5 years of age (Gutmann et al., 1983; Garcia et al., 1998) and does not appreciably change after the age of 5. Garcia and associates (1998) noted conduction changes with slowing of motor conduction velocity and DMLs before the age of 3 years. In two infants studied serially when less than 12 months old, prolonged DMLs were demonstrated in both and slow motor velocity was demonstrated in one. One infant had a prolonged DML at birth.

The longitudinal studies of CMT 1 are less clear as to the degree of clinical progression after childhood. Most studies (Harding and Thomas, 1980; Berciano et al., 1989; Dyck et al., 1989; Roy et al., 1989; Garcia et al., 1998) have noted mild progression over years,

whereas Killian and associates (1996) found that only one of eight patients had evidence of worsening on examination over 22 years, although half the patients complained of increased weakness. In CMT 1A, Garcia and colleagues (1998) suggested that clinical signs are seen in 42% by the age of 5 years. Although the neurological deficits increased in all age groups, the progression was greatest in the second decade of life.

In earlier studies of CMT 1, there had been relatively poor correlation of severity of weakness with conduction velocity (Dyck and Lambert, 1968; Davis et al., 1978; Harding and Thomas, 1980; Berciano et al., 1989), although some had noted that more weakness develops in patients with slower velocities (Dyck et al., 1989). However, longitudinal studies in CMT 1 have shown velocities to remain unchanged over decades but CMAP amplitudes to decrease (Roy et al., 1989). Dyck and associates (1989) noted that peroneal CMAP amplitudes declined when patients were restudied over an average of 31 years. However, ulnar CMAP amplitudes did not significantly change. They suspected that the severity of conduction slowing may be useful in predicting clinical severity but that the amplitude reduction, as a marker of axonal loss, is more closely linked with disability. In their study of patients with the 17p11.2 duplication, Hoogendijk and associates (1994) suggested that there was an inverse correlation between the strength component of the neurological disability score and median conduction slowing. Birouk and colleagues (1997) noted an inverse correlation of "high functional disability" (the more severely affected patients) with conduction velocity but not with CMAP amplitude. The correlation of velocity and disability, however, has not been found in other studies (Thomas et al., 1997; Krajewski et al., 2000). Part of the problem with attempts at the correlation of CMAP amplitude with strength and disability is that the muscles examined electrophysiologically—the extensor digitorum brevis in the foot and the abductor digiti minimi and abductor pollicis brevis in the hand—have only limited influence on strength and disability. Reductions in the CMAP amplitude of these muscles may not indicate changes in other muscles that are more directly related to function. Functional assessment scales may not be the optimal way of correlating disability with electrophysiological parameters. In addition, CMAP amplitudes may remain high despite severe axonal loss, owing to collateral sprouting and motor unit reconfiguration. Other electrophysiological correlates of axonal loss, such as motor unit number estimates, may provide a better appreciation of the true physiological aspects of the clinical condition.

There is good reason to suspect that disability in CMT 1A would correlate better with axonal degeneration than with slow nerve conduction, because weak muscles are typically atrophied, and pathological analyses of nerve biopsy samples of patients demonstrate axonal degeneration (Davis et al., 1978;

Bouche et al., 1983; Berciano et al., 1989; Combarros et al., 1989; Dyck et al., 1989). Consistent with this hypothesis, Sahenk and colleagues (1999) have shown that xenograft transplants of CMT 1A Schwann cells into sciatic nerve of nude mice reduced the caliber of regenerating axons. In a series of 42 patients with CMT 1A, we found that neurological disability correlates with reductions in CMAP and sensory nerve action potential (SNAP) amplitudes but not with slowing of NCVs (Krajewski et al., 2000). How the primary Schwann cell disorder relates to the apparent progressive axonal loss, whether axonal atrophy (Dyck et al., 1974) is important in this process, and the important axon–Schwann cell interactions that may be altered in CMT 1A are crucial issues that need to be understood.

Although affected members of a family all have conduction slowing, the slowing is variable even within families without relationship to age, gender, severity of the disease, or length of time with symptomatic disease (Kaku et al., 1993; Killian et al., 1996). A study of two sets of identical twins (Garcia et al., 1995) revealed concordance of electrodiagnostic findings within each pair of twins despite significant discordance of clinical dysfunction. There appear to be modifying factors that influence the severity of the clinical disorder.

The changes in sensory conduction have not been emphasized. Distal sensory responses are frequently absent (Kaku et al., 1993; Thomas et al., 1997; Krajewski et al., 2000). However, when obtained, sensory conduction slowing is to the same extent as motor conduction slowing. Sensory potentials may be difficult to obtain, in part owing to the phase cancellation, which has a more profound effect on sensory studies than on motor conduction. However, there also is significant clinical distal sensory involvement in CMT 1A, and the inability to obtain sensory potentials appears to correspond to the clinical disease (Krajewski et al., 2000).

HEREDITARY NEUROPATHY WITH LIABILITY TO PRESSURE PALSIES WITH PERIPHERAL MYELIN PROTEIN 22 DELETION

HNPP is defined clinically as an autosomal dominantly inherited disorder characterized by nonuniform slowing of NCVs and a predisposition to the development of pressure palsies. The electrophysiological findings in HNPP are therefore in striking contrast to the uniform conduction slowing seen in CMT 1A, with duplication of 17p11.2. Most cases of HNPP are associated with a deletion of the same 17p11.2 region that is duplicated in CMT 1A, leaving patients with only a single allele expressing *PMP22* (Chance et al., 1993; Verhalle et al., 1994). The underexpression of *PMP22* has been correlated with the severity of the clinical disease and the extent of axonal atrophy but not with the electrodiagnostic findings or degree of tomaculum formation (Schenone et al., 1997). Heterozygous *PMP22* knockout

mice, in which one of the two *PMP22* alleles has been deleted, develop a similar neuropathy (Adlkofer et al., 1995). These studies suggest it is the absence of *PMP22* that causes the neuropathy, that axonal diameter may be affected by the underexpression of *PMP22,* and that the traditional hallmarks of HNPP—tomaculum formation and conduction changes at sites of compression—may be related to other factors. Although the deletion of 17p11.2 is found in the majority of cases, there are families with HNPP who do not have this deletion (Mariman et al., 1994; Nicholson et al., 1994). Some of these cases are caused by *PMP22* point mutations resulting in truncated proteins and functional deletions of *PMP22* (Nicholson et al., 1994). At least one *PMP22* missense mutation has been reported to cause HNPP. Sahenk and associates (1998) reported an asymptomatic woman with a Val30Met missense mutation. The electrodiagnostic studies (not reported in detail) were suggestive of multiple entrapments, and the sural nerve biopsy had tomaculous changes, which the authors considered to be an HNPP phenotype. Nerve xenograft studies showed a delay in myelination and axonal neurofilament density increase (Nelis et al., 1994).

NCVs in patients with HNPP associated with the 17p deletion have been characterized by nonuniform slowing, with segmental slowing in the peroneal and ulnar nerves at sites of compression, but only mild slowing in forearm segments of median and ulnar nerves. DML prolongation is characteristic (Debruyne et al., 1980; Gouider et al., 1995; Amato et al., 1996; Schenone et al., 1997; Andersson et al., 2000), and the degree of prolongation is frequently out of proportion to forelimb conduction slowing. Terminal latency indexes are abnormal even if the median nerve is excluded from analysis (Amato et al., 1996; Andersson et al., 2000). This has raised the speculation that there may be a distally accentuated myelinopathy (Amato et al., 1996; Andersson et al., 2000). Focal slowing and distal latency prolongation can be seen in asymptomatic patients, including 5- and 6-year-olds (Uncini et al., 1995; Amato et al., 1996). Median, ulnar, and peroneal nerve conduction velocities are otherwise only mildly affected (Debruyne et al., 1980; Magistris and Roth, 1985; Sellma and Mayer, 1987; Uncini et al., 1995; Amato et al., 1996; Andersson et al., 2000). Prolonged F-wave latencies are common (Andersson et al., 2000). Thus, it appears that there are electrodiagnostic changes consistent with an underlying multifocal demyelinating neuropathy independent of superimposed compression. The conduction slowing is disproportionately distal and involves both sensory and motor fibers.

Conduction block, when defined as amplitude and/or area reduction of greater than 50%, was uncommon in most reported series of patients with HNPP (Magistris and Roth, 1985; Sellman and Mayer, 1987; Gouider et al., 1995), ranging from 6% to 22% of nerves studied. However, when smaller-amplitude decrements were used as criteria, conduction block was more common. Magistris and Roth (1985) found a much higher incidence of conduction block than that reported by others, noting 29 focal blocks in 12 patients (the total number of nerves studied is not mentioned). Eleven of these blocks (excluding 2 from a sporadic case) were with amplitude reductions of over 70%, and 10 blocks were with reductions of 40% to 70%. Six of the blocks were of the ulnar nerve at the elbow, 2 were peroneal at the knee, and 3 were determined to be of the median nerve at the wrist. Uncini and associates (1995) compared the incidence of block in HNPP and CMT 1A using two different criteria of block—one with a 20% drop in amplitude and area, and the other with a 50% drop. With use of the less stringent criteria, there was a 21% incidence of block in the CMT 1A patients and a 25% incidence in the HNPP patients. With the more stringent criteria of 50% drop, none of the CMT 1A patients had block and only 6% of the HNPP patients had block. The authors concluded that the more stringent criteria provided more specific evidence of conduction block and that lesser degrees of amplitude reduction may overestimate the incidence of block. Thus, there is no consensus regarding the incidence of conduction block. Clearly, the lack of block does not preclude the possibility of HNPP. Even in symptomatic nerves, focal conduction slowing at sites of compression may be the predominant electrodiagnostic feature rather than conduction block. Whether conduction block is the cause of the focal weakness in HNPP is unclear. In a well-documented case (1985), Magistris and Roth show persistent block for up to 10 years. Ulnar nerve transposition resulted in partial improvement of the block in 3 days and complete reversal of the block in 1 month, coinciding with symptomatic improvement. Sellman and Mayer (1987) noted appropriate neurological findings associated with the block and relatively normal function when only conduction slowing was present. However, Gouider and colleagues (1995) described a patient who was studied 3 days after partial peroneal nerve palsy; the authors documented focal slowing across the fibula head but no amplitude reduction while the patient had a foot drop. Thus, it appears that in many patients, focal weakness may correspond to conduction block, but in some, weakness may be apparent without block.

PERIPHERAL MYELIN PROTEIN GENE POINT MUTATIONS

There have been a number of point mutations of *PMP22*. Gabreels-Festen and colleagues (1995) suggested that patients with *PMP22* point mutations develop more severe neuropathies with slower nerve conduction velocities than those in patients with the 17p duplication. However, a review of the literature suggests that different *PMP22* mutations may affect NCVs to different degrees. Nicholson and colleagues (1994) reported a patient with a point mutation that caused a frame-shift mutation and a

premature termination that resulted in essentially a null mutation. As expected, the phenotype was consistent with HNPP. Other mutations have had clinical and electrophysiological changes consistent with CMT 1A (Nelis et al., 1994) or CMT III (D-S) (Hoogendijk et al., 1993; Roa et al., 1993; Ionasescu et al., 1995; Valentijn et al., 1995; Tyson et al., 1997; Marques et al., 1998), as described in other sections of this chapter. Why some mutations cause a more severe phenotype than that associated with others is not known. Interestingly, virtually all *PMP22* point mutations that cause neuropathy are located in putative transmembrane domains. Detailed electrophysiological data on most patients with *PMP22* point mutations are not available. When described, NCVs for patients with milder, or CMT 1A, phenotypes range from 10 to 25 m per second within the same family (Roa et al., 1993). For patients with D-S phenotypes, routine NCVs are either unobtainable (Tyson et al., 1997) or less than 5 m per second (Roa et al., 1993; Marques et al., 1998). However, median motor conduction velocities as high as 21 m per second have been described in some patients with D-S (Roa et al., 1993).

Protein 0 Disorders

CHARCOT-MARIE-TOOTH TYPE 1B WITH PROTEIN 0 GENE POINT MUTATIONS

CMT 1B was the first CMT disorder to have an identified gene locus when it was linked to the Duffy locus (Bird et al., 1982). However, this is a much less common disorder than CMT 1A. The CMT 1B locus has been mapped to the centromeric region of chromosome 1q21-23 and involves the gene encoding the major PNS myelin protein, P0.

P0 is a single-transmembrane protein with a highly basic 69-residue intracellular domain and a 124-residue extracellular domain that shows sequence similarity to immunoglobulins. It makes up 60% of all PNS myelin proteins. An essential function of P0 is to mediate adhesion between adjacent wraps of myelin, forming the intraperiod line. P0-mediated adhesion appears to require both the extracellular and intracellular portions of the molecule (Shapiro et al., 1996). Mutations affecting each of these portions, as well as the transmembrane domain, have been shown to cause the various clinical presentations of CMT 1B, including a classic CMT phenotype, a D-S phenotype, a congenital hypomyelination phenotype, and possibly a CMT 2 phenotype. Preliminary evaluations suggest that certain mutations may cause more severe clinical phenotypes than others (Warner et al., 1996; Pareyson et al., 1999), although this needs to be evaluated in greater detail. Similarly, preliminary results suggest that certain mutations disrupt NCVs much more profoundly than do others.

Bird and colleagues (1997) reported a 20-year study of the original CMT 1B family that was demon-

strated to have linkage to the Duffy blood group locus on chromosome 1 (Bird et al., 1982). The mutation has subsequently been mapped to Asp61Glu. Conduction velocities were uniformly very slow, from 5 to 15 m per second—significantly slower than those for patients with CMT 1A. Children were affected at an early age with slow conduction velocities noted in 4- and 6-year-olds. There was significant clinical variation, and although the clinical severity was greater than that for most patients with CMT 1A, the authors believed that the disorder overlapped with CMT 1A and was not as severe as most cases of D-S. Sindou and associates (1999) described two patients with different autosomal dominant mutations, also involving the extracellular domain of P0. The nerve conduction changes were uniformly slow (15 to 17 m per second for one patient and 21 to 30 m per second for the other) with sensory conduction slowing consistent with the motor. However, Marrosu and colleagues (1998) describe a Sardinian family with an autosomal dominant P0 mutation with electrophysiological findings suggestive of a primary axonal disorder as seen in CMT 2. Distal latencies were normal and velocities were normal or near normal despite distal denervation on electromyography. However, nerve biopsy samples were not obtained, and there was electrophysiological variability from patient to patient. Heterozygous patients with Phe35 deletion (Warner et al., 1996) and Thr95Met mutations were also characterized as having CMT 2 phenotypes based on normal or near-normal conduction velocities (Chapon et al., 1999; De Jonghe et al., 1999). Nevertheless, physiological and pathological analyses remain inconclusive, and whether any P0 mutation causes a true axonal neuropathy, independent of demyelination, remains to be convincingly demonstrated. Part of the confusion is based on the attempts to classify patients on the basis of NCVs alone. De Jonghe and colleagues (1999) classified their CMT 2 patients on the basis of at least one patient in each family having an MNCV of greater than 38 m per second. In the patients with the Thr95Met mutation, a number of patients had an MNCV of less than 35 m per second, and those with a normal NCV had normal amplitudes. The slower conduction velocities suggest a demyelinating disorder. The normal velocities may be due to minimal disease. The classification of CMT 2 or any axonal disorder should be based on normal or near-normal conduction velocities despite significant denervation and/or low CMAP amplitudes in the corresponding muscles.

Dejerine-Sottas and Congenital Hypomyelination Neuropathy

Before the identification of specific myelin gene disorders, D-S was considered to be an autosomal recessive disorder with a severe phenotype that manifested in young children with delayed motor milestones, leading to an inability to walk. Studies before identification of specific gene defects demonstrated uniform conduction slowing below 10 m per second in all nerves tested. Testing of proximal nerves, including the musculocutaneous nerve, revealed slowing that was similar to that of more distal nerves (Benstead et al., 1990). Nerves were difficult to stimulate, and supramaximal stimulation was not always possible. Marked temporal dispersion was noted, but conduction slowing was consistent between different nerves. The authors recognized that because of the severe slowing, the reduced amplitudes, and the difficulty in obtaining supramaximal stimulation, the usual criteria for temporal dispersion and conduction block were not valid for D-S. They thought that in this disorder, both the temporal dispersion and amplitude drop did not necessarily indicate multifocal demyelination, and that the disorder was most likely uniform but very severe.

Congenital hypomyelination neuropathy is a term used to describe a disorder in which children present in the neonatal period with hypotonia, weakness, and dysphagia. Some have arthrogryposis (Guzzetta et al., 1982). The children either die in infancy or are severely disabled. The pathology of the nerves is remarkable for hypomyelination and onion bulb formation. Whether congenital hypomyelination neuropathy constitutes one end of the spectrum of D-S or represents different genetic mutations is not clear.

It is now apparent that the D-S phenotype can be caused by both autosomal dominant and autosomal recessive mutations (Hayasaka et al., 1993; Roa et al., 1993; Tyson et al., 1997). Tyson and associates (1997) describe nine patients with hereditary demyelinating neuropathy of infancy with D-S phenotype. Four patients (two were mother and son) demonstrated novel missense mutations of *PMP22*, all in exon 3, whereas two patients had novel *P0* mutations and three had no demonstrable abnormality of *P0* or *PMP22*. There was consanguinity in these three cases, and they were suspected to be autosomal recessive disorders with an unidentified locus. At least three of the patients had neonatal symptoms. Two of these three had *PMP22* mutations, and one had an unidentified mutation. The electrophysiological features of the nine patients were remarkable for marked slowing of motor conduction velocities to below 10 m per second in one of four with the PMP mutation, both patients with the P0 mutations, and one of the recessive cases. The other two patients with the autosomal recessive form had velocities of 15 to 17 m per second, and the other three patients with *PMP22* mutations had unexcitable nerves.

The available data suggest that the electrodiagnostic features of D-S include severe conduction slowing, usually below 10 m per second, which is consistent in all nerves from which responses can be obtained. Nerves are difficult to stimulate, and there may be marked temporal dispersion and amplitude reduction on proximal stimulation. However, these latter findings are not due to nonuniform conduction but instead represent changes due to severe slowing and axonal loss.

Charcot-Marie-Tooth Type X with Connexin 32 Disorders

Although reports of X-linked CMT date back to 1889 (Herringham, 1889), it was considered a rare disorder until the identification of genetic defects on the proximal long arm of the X chromosome (Gal et al., 1985), with localization to Xq13.1 (Fishbeck et al., 1986). It has now been established that this is the locus of the gene encoding the Cx32 protein, which is expressed by myelinating Schwann cells (Bergoffen et al., 1993). Cx32 belongs to a family of proteins, all of which have a similar structure. When connexins meet at opposed cell membranes, channels, called *gap junctions,* can form, through which ions and small molecules can pass (Scherer, 1996). Each connexin protein has four membrane-spanning domains connected by two extracellular loops and one intracellular loop. Six connexin molecules assemble to form a connexon, with the third transmembrane domain lining the central pore. The six cysteine residues in Cx32 are necessary to maintain the structure of the extracellular loops. It has been suggested that mutations affecting only the second transmembrane domain or cytoplasmic loop, or both, may be associated with a milder clinical phenotype (Hahn et al., 1999). However, detailed, individual descriptions of genotype/phenotype correlations are not available for many of the patients with CMT X mutations. As a result, it is not possible to correlate specific mutations with severity of disease.

More than 150 different mutations of the gene for connexin 32 have been identified. It appears that CMT X is the second most common form of CMT (Nicholson and Nash, 1993) and may be the disease variant in some families formerly considered to have CMT 2 (Timmerman et al., 1996). The electrodiagnostic findings in patients with CMT X remain somewhat confusing. In part, this is because females with the mutation may manifest symptoms, but the clinical and electrophysiological features are not consistent in males. The conduction velocities in men are usually between 30 and 40 m per second, values that would be considered an intermediate range (Hahn et al., 1990; Birouk et al., 1998; Nicholson et al., 1998; Lewis and Shy, 1999) between CMT 1 and CMT 2. Before gene localization, some authors (Brust et al., 1978; Davis et al., 1978) recognized a group of CMT patients with intermediate conduction velocities, but because of frequent female involvement, this intermediate form was considered autosomal dominant, rather than X-linked. It is increasingly apparent that CMT X is the form of the disease in a majority of CMT patients with intermediate conduction slowing. Birouk and colleagues (1998) noted that 90% of the 21 males with CMT X that they studied had median MNCVs in the intermediate range, whereas only 40% of the 27 females had intermediate slowing. Of the females, 24% had mild slowing (in a range considered typical of CMT 2) and 36% were normal. This variability in females, noted by others (Rozear et al., 1987; Hahn et al., 1990; Nicholson and Corbett, 1996; Nicholson et al., 1998; Lewis and Shy, 1999), which is also apparent clinically, partially explains why some female patients classified as having CMT 2 may in fact have CMT X. It is likely that the lack of conduction slowing in some females may be related to the expression of normal Cx32 from the other normal X chromosome. Thus, females with relatively normal conduction studies may have CMT X, whereas both males and females with slow or intermediate velocities may have Cx32 mutations. The clinician should suspect CMT X in any familial neuropathy without male-to-male transmission.

The electrophysiological changes have suggested to some investigators that the disorder may be primarily axonal rather than a disorder of myelin (Hahn et al., 1990; Timmerman et al., 1996; Birouk et al., 1998). They note that CMAP amplitudes are all reduced in the nerves with intermediate slowing as well as in patients with relatively normal velocities. This was interpreted as demonstrating a primary axonal disorder. Moreover, studies in xenographs have confirmed that Cx32 mutations can cause axonal degeneration in an experimental model (Sahenk and Chen, 1998). Hahn and colleagues (1990) initially considered their patients to have electrophysiological changes of an axonal disorder based on peroneal nerve conduction studies of 57 patients from one kindred. However, when they looked at 116 patients from 13 families (including the patients from the previous report) and studied the median as well as the peroneal nerve, they recognized changes in conduction velocity, DMLs, and F-wave latencies that were consistent with demyelination (Hahn et al., 1999). Peroneal conduction studies can be difficult to interpret when comparing conduction slowing with amplitude reduction and may overemphasize the axonal pathology. There are other studies (Lewis and Shy, 1999; Tabaraud et al., 1999; Gutierrez et al., 2000) that have reported that the electrodiagnostic findings not only pointed to a primary demyelinating disorder but also suggested nonuniform conduction slowing. The patients of Lewis and Shy (1999) had distal latencies that were not always prolonged despite moderate forearm slowing. Gutierrez and colleagues (2000) reported excessive temporal dispersion, possible conduction block, and differential slowing of conduction velocities in a three-generation family with CMT X. Sural nerve biopsy showed loss of large myelinated fibers and onion bulb formation. Tabaraud and associates (1999) reported a female CMT X patient who was initially thought to have chronic inflammatory demyelinating polyneuropathy because of the multifocal conduction changes. These reports of differential slowing in different segments of nerves strongly suggest that segmental demyelination is a significant aspect of the disorder in at least some families.

Whether CMT X is primarily axonal or demyelinat-

ing remains to be determined. Although investigations that use electrophysiological criteria can be very helpful, the interpretation of the conduction changes in CMT X based on grouped data should be done with caution. Because the conduction velocities are intermediate between normal and those of CMT 1A, are possibly nonuniform and sometimes differ between males and females within the same family, an analysis of grouped data may be misleading. To best understand the relationship between the electrophysiology and the pathophysiology of CMT X, it is preferable to examine the conduction studies of individuals, with particular attention to differential slowing, rather than to look at the mean conduction velocities of a group of patients.

Some pathological studies (Hahn et al., 1990; Birouk et al., 1998) have tended to suggest an axonal neuropathy with evidence of loss of myelinated fibers; minimal, if any, onion bulbs; and no evidence on teased fiber analysis of segmental demyelination or remyelination. Other histopathological studies have revealed thinly myelinated fibers (Sander et al., 1998), onion bulb formations (Fishbeck et al., 1986; Sander et al., 1998), and marked variation of myelin thickness (Sander et al., 1998), suggesting a primary demyelinating process.

The confusion regarding the primary pathophysiology of Cx32 disorders may be caused in part by the number of different mutations that have been identified in CMT X. It is possible that some mutations affect the channel properties of Cx32 and may not affect conduction velocity as much as they influence Schwann cell–axonal interactions. Others may affect conduction to a greater extent. It is anticipated that further genotype, phenotype, electrophysiological, and pathological correlations will shed more light on the true nature of the pathophysiology of Cx32 disorders.

Cx32 is also expressed in the CNS, and some patients with CMT X have been noted to have mild hearing loss (Nicholson et al., 1996, 1998). Brainstem auditory evoked response testing demonstrated prolonged central conduction times in males with CMT X. Wave I was normal, but all central latencies were significantly slow. Females also showed statistically significant central latency prolongation but not as severe or as consistent as did the males. This is distinctly different from the findings in CMT 1A, in which wave I was prolonged but central conduction was normal (Nicholson et al., 1996, 1998).

Pelizaeus-Merzbacher Disease and Proteolipid Protein Mutations

Pelizaeus-Merzbacher disease (PMD) is an X-linked disorder of myelin caused by mutations in *PLP* (Garbern et al., 1997). PLP is an integral membrane protein constituting approximately 50% of the total protein mass of CNS myelin. PLP is thought to

compose the intraperiod line of CNS myelin (Griffiths et al., 1998). It has been proposed to act both as an adhesion molecule and as an ion channel, but its actual function in oligodendrocytes remains unknown (Knapp, 1996; Griffiths et al., 1998). PLP is also expressed by myelinating Schwann cells, although its precise location within the myelin sheath remains uncertain.

PMD had been considered a disorder confined to the CNS. Classic forms of PMD involve infants and children with spasticity, ataxia, nystagmus, optic atrophy, and delayed psychomotor development with evidence of widespread CNS demyelination (Seitelberger, 1970, 1995). Some forms of hereditary spastic paraparesis have been linked to PLP mutations (Cambi et al., 1996). With the discovery of the specific gene for PLP, it has become apparent that most disorders are due to duplications or missense mutations. A family with a unique mutation leading to the absence of PLP protein expression was described (Garbern et al., 1997) in which the affected members of the family had a CNS disorder similar to, but less severe than, other cases of PMD. In addition, they were noted to have a demyelinating peripheral neuropathy. The electrodiagnostic findings were consistent with a nonuniform conduction disorder with median and ulnar nerve conduction velocities that varied from 37 to 52 m per second in the forearm segments. A few patients had significant conduction slowing across the elbow, and distal latencies were variably slow, more frequently in the median than in the ulnar nerve. These changes were seen in both the clinically affected males and the relatively asymptomatic females. The abnormalities suggested a multifocal disorder with a possible predilection for changes at sites of compression. Teased fiber analysis of axillary and sciatic nerves obtained from an autopsy of one of the affected males revealed paranodal and segmental demyelination. Other families with null mutations have had similar phenotype with milder CNS disease but evidence of peripheral nerve involvement (Raskind et al., 1991; Sistermans et al., 1996; Garbern et al., 1997).

It is of interest that in this genetic disorder involving a myelin protein that is a relatively minor constituent of peripheral nerve myelin, missense mutations and duplications appear to have little phenotypic expression in peripheral nerve, whereas null mutations or the complete absence of protein expression adversely affects peripheral nerve myelin function. In the CNS, where PLP is the major myelin protein, duplications and missense mutations appear to cause more severe CNS disease than that associated with null mutations. If *PLP* accounts for 50% of CNS myelin protein, how does some of the myelin continue to function when no PLP is made? Are other myelin protein genes upregulated? It will require further investigation of the different mutations of *PLP* in patients and animal models to better understand the role of PLP in peripheral and central myelin in the normal and diseased state.

Early Growth Response 2 *(krox20)*

Studies have shown that mutations in *EGR2,* or *krox20,* cause a novel form of CMT. *EGR2* functions as a transcription factor as it binds to specific DNA sequences on the promoter region of genes whose expression it regulates (Topilko et al., 1994). *EGR2* is expressed in developing Schwann cells at a time when future myelinating Schwann cells have established a 1:1 ratio with axons and have made the commitment to myelinate. During this same period, the expression of *PMP22, P0,* and other myelin-specific genes is also upregulated. It is attractive to think that *EGR2* may be directly responsible for binding to the promoters of, and upregulating the expression of, myelin genes such as *PMP22* and *P0.* However, as yet no definite binding of *EGR2* to promoters of myelin-specific genes has been established.

Warner and associates (1998) identified two families with clinical signs and symptoms of CMT 1 caused by a point mutation in *EGR2.* Each of these *EGR2* mutations segregated as an autosomal dominant trait, and both were found to affect the zinc finger region of the protein, which is the region that directly binds to DNA. Median and ulnar conduction velocities were 25 to 30 m per second. A third family with a congenital hypomyelinating neuropathy caused by an *EGR2* mutation was also identified. This mutation, however, segregated as an autosomal recessive trait and was located in a region of the protein outside of the DNA-binding domain (Nicholson and Nash, 1993; Hahn et al., 1999). Limited electrophysiological studies of these patients were reported. NCVs, when obtainable, were between 3 and 7 m per second. However, both CMAP and SNAP were often absent, or amplitudes were significantly reduced (Hahn et al., 1999). At this time, there is insufficient information to further characterize the electrophysiological characteristics of these disorders.

INHERITED DEMYELINATING NEUROPATHIES CAUSED BY MUTATIONS NOT AFFECTING MYELIN-SPECIFIC PROTEINS

The following disorders are primary demyelinating disorders that affect both the CNS and the PNS. However, the genetic defects do not primarily affect the myelin proteins but cause the neuropathy by accumulating various substances in myelinated nerve fibers. As in PMD, patients with these disorders are typically more affected by the CNS disorder than by the peripheral neuropathy. However, occasional patients may manifest more striking PNS signs. The neuromuscular disease clinician and the electromyographer should be familiar with these disorders.

Adrenoleukodystrophy and Adrenomyeloneuropathy

Adrenoleukodystrophy (ALD) is an X-linked recessive paroxysmal disease characterized by the accumulation of elevated concentrations of saturated very long chain fatty acids. Different phenotypes have been described, with the most common being childhood ALD (a rapidly progressive CNS disorder in early childhood) and adrenomyeloneuropathy (AMN) (a chronic disorder of adults) (Moser et al., 1992; Chaudhry et al., 1996). Peripheral nerve involvement is a prominent feature of AMN but not of ALD. Chaudhry and colleagues (1996) studied 99 men and 38 women with symptomatic AMN. Eighty-seven percent of men and 67% of women had at least one conduction abnormality. Motor nerve conduction abnormalities were more severe than sensory abnormalities (80% versus 39%), with peroneal F-wave latency, peroneal velocity, and tibial H-reflex slowing being the most common abnormalities. Conduction slowing (80%) was more frequent than amplitude reduction (29%). With the use of research criteria for demyelination (Cornblath et al., 1991) in which conduction velocity less than 70% of normal and distal motor latency and F-wave latency of more than 125% of normal were necessary for the disorder to be considered demyelinating, only 26% of patients (31% of men and 12% of women) had any value that would meet these criteria for demyelination. These changes were not thought to be uniform, with some patients having prolonged distal latencies present without peroneal velocity slowing; 32 had velocity slowing but normal distal latency. In men, the level of very long chain fatty acids correlated with peroneal amplitude, tibial H-reflex latency, median velocity, DML, and median F-wave latency. The authors concluded that these conduction changes were consistent with multifocal demyelination as well as axonal loss. Similar conclusions were suggested by Van Geel and colleagues (1996). The prolongation of late responses, F-wave latencies, and H-reflex latencies was emphasized in the case of a 15-year-old (Case records of the Massachusetts General Hospital, 1982). The presence of demyelination as well as axonal loss was confirmed by findings on sural nerve biopsy (Tanaka et al., 1985).

Metachromatic Leukodystrophy, Krabbe's Disease, and Cockayne's Syndrome

Metachromatic leukodystrophy is caused by an inherited deficiency of arylsulfatase A. This causes an accumulation of galactosyl sulfatide in nerve tissue as well as in other organs. Peripheral nerve involvement has been noted most commonly in the childhood forms but has also been noted in some, but not all, patients with adult onset. The occasional adult patient may present with peripheral neuropathy (Fressinaud et al., 1992).

Krabbe's disease is an autosomal recessive disorder caused by a deficiency of the enzyme galactocerebroside galactosidase. Although this usually causes symptoms before the age of 1 year, there are juvenile and later-onset forms. Peripheral nerve involvement has been demonstrated in all forms of the disease but is usually overshadowed by the CNS disorder. However, the occasional patient may have prominent peripheral nerve symptoms and signs (Marks et al., 1997).

Cockayne's syndrome is an autosomal recessive multisystem disorder that causes ataxia, weakness, growth retardation, developmental delay, and dysmorphic features. The exact cause of the disorder remains unclear, but there appear to be abnormalities of DNA repair mechanisms. Peripheral nerve involvement has been recognized, and in a review of 25 cases, nerve conduction slowing was identified in more than 80% of the patients studied (Ozdirim et al., 1996).

All of these disorders have been described as showing uniform conduction slowing (Miller et al., 1985), but there have been only a few patients whose electrodiagnostic studies have been described in sufficient detail to determine whether this holds true for the majority of patients regardless of age at onset or length of time with the disease.

Refsum's Disease

Refsum's disease is an autosomal recessive disorder characterized by peripheral neuropathy, night blindness, and ataxia. Phytanic acid accumulation occurs in tissues secondary to the blockade of mitochondrial oxidation of fatty acids. Segmental demyelination has been noted on biopsy studies (Refsum et al., 1984; Kuntzer et al., 1993), although the degree of demyelination varies. Electrophysiological changes also appear to vary. Kuntzer and associates (1983) reported a 21-year study of an individual with Refsum's disease who displayed relatively nonuniform conduction changes in motor and sensory nerves. Distal latencies were mildly prolonged, and F-wave latencies were slow. Median conduction velocity was 33 to 36 m per second, whereas the ulnar velocity was 44 m per second below the elbow but 29 m per second across the elbow. Peroneal conduction was 10 to 12 m per second, but amplitudes were less than 1 mV. The authors noted that the patient had episodic weakness that remitted. CMAPs were reduced on distal stimulation, but no proximal conduction block was found. Dietary restrictions led to clinical improvement. With improvement in strength, CMAP amplitude improved, but there was a general progression of weakness (Kuntzer et al., 1993).

Autosomal Recessive Demyelinating Neuropathies (Charcot-Marie-Tooth Type 4)

Autosomal recessive sensorimotor demyelinating neuropathies (CMT 4) are proving to be a heterogeneous group of disorders, with at least four distinct genetic loci already identified. CMT 4A is linked to a 5-cM region of 8q13-q21.1. The disorder was first described in four highly inbred families in Tunisia. Clinical onset was in the first 2 years of life, with delayed achievement of developmental milestones such as sitting or walking. Weakness spread to proximal muscles by the end of the first decade of life, and many patients became wheelchair dependent (Ben Othmane, 1990; Ben Othmane et al., 1995). Sensory loss was mild, deep tendon reflexes were absent, and motor conduction velocities slowed to an average of 30 m per second in the upper limbs. Pathological studies from sural nerve biopsies showed a loss of large-diameter myelinated fibers, hypomyelination, and no abnormalities of myelin folding. "Basal lamina" onion bulbs, characterized by concentric layers of basal lamina without intervening regions of Schwann cell cytoplasm, have been described in biopsy reports (Garbern et al., 1997; Sander et al., 1998). *PMP2,* localized in this region, has been excluded as a candidate gene for CMT 4A (Ben Othmane et al., 1995).

Kalaydjieva and colleagues (1996) reported a separate disorder with linkage to chromosome 8q24 in a Gypsy population with an autosomal recessive inheritance pattern (classified as CMT 4D). The mutation has been found to alter the N-*myc*-downstream-regulated gene 1 (*NDRG1*) that is expressed in Schwann cells (Kalaydjieva et al., 2000). Patients with this neuropathy presented with distal wasting of muscle and weakness, sensory loss, foot and hand deformities, and loss of deep tendon reflexes. Disability appears to begin in the first decade of life, and patients are often significantly disabled by the fifth decade. NCVs are severely reduced in median, ulnar, tibial, and peroneal nerves of younger patients and are unobtainable after 15 years of age (Kalaydjieva et al., 1996). Neuropathological studies have demonstrated a decreased number of myelinated fibers along with abnormally thin myelin ensheathing other axons. Onion bulbs have been identified in at least one patient (Kalaydjieva et al., 1996). Deafness is invariant and usually develops by the third decade. Brainstem auditory evoked responses are markedly abnormal with prolonged interpeak latencies (Kalaydjieva et al., 1996). Ionasescu and colleagues (1996) described a black U.S. family with linkage in a similar region but with an autosomal dominant pedigree. The proband in this family presented with a D-S phenotype characterized by a clinical onset at the age of 2 years. Features of the disease included pes cavus, hammer toes, claw hands, and severe atrophy and weakness of muscles in the distal legs. Most CMAPs and SNAPs were unobtainable; DMLs innervating proximal muscles were prolonged. Hearing loss was not mentioned. Thus, as in some families with CMT 1 caused by *EGR2* mutations, there may be a gene in the region expressed in myelinating Schwann cells that causes either recessive or dominant inherited neuropathies, depending on where it is mutated.

CMT 4B has been defined as hereditary motor and sensory neuropathy with focally folded myelin sheaths (Gambardella et al., 1999). Studies from one large family with 10 patients demonstrated linkage at chromosome 11q23 (Gambardella et al., 1999). This has been identified as the gene *MTMR2*, which encodes the myotubularin-related protein 2, a dual-specificity phosphatase (Bolino et al., 2000). However, in a second family with a similar clinical and pathological presentation, the defect does not map to this region, although no other locus has been identified for the two affected individuals (Gambardella et al., 1997). The patients from both families presented in early childhood, with an average age at clinical onset of 34 months, although early milestones such as walking appear to be normal (Gambardella et al., 1997). Unlike in most forms of CMT, proximal as well as distal weakness is prominent. Several patients with CMT 4B have died before age 40, perhaps of respiratory failure (Bolino et al., 2000). Motor conduction velocities are typically 14 to 17 m per second, but unlike in most forms of demyelinating CMT, they display temporal dispersion. CMAPS have been reduced, and SNAPs have usually been absent. Brainstem auditory evoked responses frequently show prolonged interpeak latencies between waves 1 and 3 (Gambardella et al., 1997). Some patients have noted mild hearing loss. Pathologically, teased fiber studies from sural nerve biopsy samples demonstrate segmental demyelination with redundant loops of myelin. Semithin sections demonstrate a decreased number of myelinated fibers (Gambardella et al., 1997).

An additional autosomal recessive form of demyelinating CMT classified as CMT 4C has been identified at chromosome 5q23-33 by homozygosity mapping in two large Algerian families with extensive consanguinity (LeGuern et al., 1996; Guilbot et al., 1999). Patients developed a sensorimotor neuropathy with onset in childhood or adolescence. Pes cavus and scoliosis were frequent. Mild walking disability typically occurred after 15 years. Investigators have noted a discrepancy between a rapid worsening of deformities and the slow progression of the motor deficits. Cutaneous sensation is impaired initially, followed by abnormalities in vibratory and then joint position sensation. Median MNCVs are 20 to 30 m per second, and SNAPs are absent. Pathologically, in sural nerve biopsy samples, there is a loss of myelinated fibers, remaining axons have thin myelin sheaths, and typical onion bulbs may be present (Guilbot et al., 1999).

INHERITED NEUROPATHIES AFFECTING NEURONS OR AXONS

There are many inherited disorders that are not related to abnormalities of myelin proteins or are not secondary to accumulations of substances that cause demyelination. The sensorimotor disorders are discussed as CMT 2.

The electrophysiologic features of these disorders are similar. Sensory and motor conduction velocities are normal or minimally slow and can always be accounted for by loss of the largest-diameter fibers. Temporal dispersion is usually less than 10% unless severe axonal loss is present, in which case the degree of temporal dispersion is difficult to interpret. Conduction block is inconsistent with the concept of an axonal disorder, and if present, it suggests a superimposed compression or immune-mediated disorder. Distal amplitude reductions of CMAPs and SNAPs on nerve conduction studies, the physiological markers of axonal loss, are usually striking despite the relatively preserved velocities. On occasion, the CMAPs may be normal or near normal despite significant axonal loss. Collateral sprouting, particularly in these very chronic and insidious neuropathies, can produce giant motor units (similar to those seen in "old polio"), which can preserve the CMAP amplitude. Needle electromyography of these muscles can provide important information as to the extent of denervation. Motor unit number estimates may provide a more accurate sense of motor unit loss than will CMAP amplitude reduction.

Charcot-Marie-Tooth Type 2 (Hereditary Motor and Sensory Neuropathy Type II)

At present, four subtypes of CMT 2—CMT 2A, 2B, 2C, and 2D—have been identified by linkage analysis, although there is some confusion about forms CMT 2B and CMT 2D, as is discussed here.

CMT 2A has been mapped to chromosome 1p36 (Pericak-Vance et al., 1997; Saito et al., 1997). Clinically, patients develop sensorimotor neuropathies. Clinical onset has been reported as early as age 7 or 8 years (Saito et al., 1997). However, the clinical phenotype in CMT 2A may vary even more than that of CMT 1, so the onset of symptoms in older, or even younger, patients is likely (Vance, 1999).

CMT 2B has been mapped to chromosome 3q (Kwon et al., 1995). Patients present with severe sensory abnormalities leading to foot ulcerations and even amputations. Although motor abnormalities may be present, they are mild compared with sensory deficits. Affected family members have been noted to have high-arched feet, hammer toes, and decreased reflexes in addition to their sensory abnormalities. In these patients, CMAP amplitudes were reduced, and denervation was described on electromyographic studies. However, no clinical weakness was described (Kwon et al., 1995). Because of the predominance of sensory findings, it has been suggested that CMT 2B may better be classified as an example of hereditary sensory and autonomic neuropathy (HSAN) type 1 (Vance et al., 1996), an autosomal dominant sensory disorder that is discussed later here.

CMT 2C is a rare disorder in which patients have respiratory distress in addition to conduction velocities characteristic of CMT 2. As appears to be the rule with inherited neuropathies, there is clinical variability in the severity of disease within affected families. Some patients develop weakness or sensory loss in childhood, whereas in other patients, the clinical onset is during adult years (Dyck et al., 1994). Typical presenting features are an "altered voice," shortness of breath, or "asthma." Paresis of vocal cords has been detected in several patients. Abnormal inspiratory and expiratory pressures are usually detected on pulmonary function testing. On electrophysiological testing, phrenic nerve CMAP amplitudes have been reduced or absent (Dyck et al., 1994). The second most frequent symptom has been hand weakness, particularly involving functions that require fine movement, such as turning keys or buttoning. When examined, however, these patients also have had leg weakness, which, unlike in most forms of inherited neuropathy, may be proximal (Dyck et al., 1994). Loss of vibration and temperature sensations is noted in patients with severe disability. NCVs are normal, whereas both CMAP and SNAP amplitudes are likely to be reduced or absent (Dyck et al., 1994). There remains some question as to whether vocal cord paralysis identifies a distinct disorder or whether it may be present in patients with a variety of forms of CMT. Until there is identification of a specific gene mutation for CMT 2C, this classification will remain in doubt.

CMT 2D was originally reported in a large family with weakness and sensory loss whose symptoms began in the hands and in whom linkage was found on chromosome 7p (Ionasescu et al., 1996). Similar linkage was detected in other families, although weakness did not begin in the hands in these patients (reviewed in Vance, 1999). Confusion has developed about the nomenclature for this disorder, however, as families with a form of spinal muscular atrophy (SMA), or distal HMN, have demonstrated linkage to the same region (HMN type V; see later). One reported family contains affected individuals with the pure motor syndrome and others with sensory loss, suggesting that the two disorders are likely to be different phenotypes of the same disease (Sambuughin et al., 1998).

Distal Hereditary Motor Neuronopathies

HMNs are a heterogeneous group of disorders, often referred to as the SMAs. The most frequent forms of HMN have been classified as proximal HMN and include disorders such as SMA1 (Werdnig-Hoffmann disease) and SMA2 (Kugelberg-Welander disease) (reviewed in Harding, 1993). The X-linked bulbospinal neuronopathy (Kennedy's disease) is also a member of this group. These disorders are often thought of as motor neuron disorders and are discussed in Chapter 69.

The electrodiagnostic characteristics of the HMNs reveal normal or near-normal sensory amplitudes and latencies. Motor conduction velocities are also normal or minimally slow despite clinical evidence of significant weakness and atrophy and electromyographic evidence of denervation-reinnervation. The possibility of relatively preserved CMAPs despite marked denervation mentioned earlier holds true for these disorders as well. Although fasciculations may be encountered, they are not nearly as prominent as those seen in amyotrophic lateral sclerosis. Presumably, the insidious and chronic nature of these disorders makes it unlikely that one will encounter many fasciculations.

The distal HMNs, often referred to as the "spinal form of CMT," are often included with the inherited neuropathies and are discussed later. This group of disorders composes about 10% of the total HMNs (Pearn and Hudgson, 1979) and has been tentatively classified into seven subtypes on the basis of clinical phenotype, age at onset, and mode of inheritance (Harding, 1993). Four of the subtypes have autosomal dominant modes of inheritance, with the first two being juvenile-onset (type I) and adult-onset (type II) disorders with clinical onset in the lower extremities. The third autosomal dominant form, type V, is characterized by onset in the upper extremities. Type VII is an autosomal dominant form associated with vocal cord paralysis. The three autosomal recessive forms of distal HMN—types III, IV, and VI—are distinguished on the basis of age at onset and severity, and all begin with distal weakness in the lower extremities. Based on the clinical variability demonstrated in patients with inherited neuropathies whose genetic cause is known, the classification of the recessive forms may need to be revised when the gene or genes that cause the disorders are identified. The three subtypes may prove to be variable phenotypes caused by different mutations of the same gene. In general, the recessive forms of distal HMN begin earlier and are more severe than the dominant forms. Genetic loci for several subtypes of distal HMN have been identified and are discussed later. As mentioned previously, sometimes distinctions between distal HMN and more traditional forms of CMT can be confusing. Patients with traditional CMT 2 may have mild sensory loss and normal NCVs with distally reduced CMAPs. They can thus be difficult to distinguish from patients with distal HMN, as the following example illustrates. In 1995, a large Bulgarian family was identified as having distal HMN type V (Christodoulou et al., 1995). The following year, Ionasescu and colleagues described CMT 2D with linkage to the same region in patients with sensory loss in addition to weakness (Ionasescu et al., 1996). Subsequently the two "distinct" disorders were found to segregate within the same large kindred, mapping to the same 7p15 region, demonstrating that the two disorders were examples of phenotypic variability of the same disease (Sambuughin et al., 1998).

Distal HMN type II, an "adult-onset" form, is an autosomal dominantly inherited disorder. Patients usually present with weakness in the lower extremities around the age of 15 to 20 years. Weakness begins first in toe extensors and then affects the foot muscles of dorsiflexion. Progression rapidly develops in the feet so that all intrinsic foot muscles are paralyzed within 5 years. Later, weakness may involve the hands and proximal leg muscles. Wheelchair dependence in older age does occur in some patients but is not invariant. Sensory abnormalities are usually absent, although some older patients may have mild decreases in vibratory sensation. Motor and sensory NCVs are normal, whereas needle electromyography reveals evidence of chronic denervation. Linkage studies in a large Belgian family suggest a locus on chromosome 12q24.3 (Timmerman et al., 1999).

Distal HMN type V is an autosomal dominant form that affects primarily upper limbs, does not prevent ambulation, and does not shorten life expectancy (Harding, 1993). Christodoulou and colleagues (1995) evaluated a multigeneration Bulgarian family of 114 members with 30 affected patients. Linkage in the family has been localized to chromosome 7p. The mean age at onset in the family is 17, with the typical presentation being selective wasting of the thenar eminence and first dorsal interosseous region of the hands. Although 40% of patients develop foot problems within 2 years, progression is slow and patients remain ambulatory at age 60. With the exception of mild, probably age-related loss of vibratory sense, there are no clinical sensory abnormalities. One branch of the family has been noted to have mild pyramidal features on neurological examination, including, rarely, Babinski signs. Motor and sensory nerve conduction studies are normal except in wasted muscles, where CMAP amplitudes are reduced (Christodoulou et al., 1995).

A novel form of autosomal recessive distal HMN has been termed the Jerash type by L.T. Middleton and colleagues (1999), after the Jerash region in Jordan where 27 affected patients were detected (Ozdirim et al., 1996). The HMN-Jerash locus has been mapped to chromosome 9p21.1-p12 (Middleton et al., 1999). Patients present with gait instability and foot drop between the ages of 6 and 10. Of the 27 patients in the series, all had wasting and weakness of distal foot muscles, and 23 had weakness of intrinsic hand muscles. Patients over the age of 12 to 14 developed hand weakness. Three patients over the age of 50 developed mild sensory symptoms. In the early stages of disease, patients were noted to have upper motoneuron signs, including diffuse hyperreflexia, mild spasticity, and upgoing toes. Subsequently, ankle reflexes were lost, and plantar reflexes became downgoing, although patellar reflexes frequently remained hyperactive. The course of the disorder is benign, with the oldest affected patient remaining ambulatory at age 80 (Middleton et al., 1999). Neurophysiological and pathological results are said to be consistent with HMN (Middleton et al., 1999).

An additional distal motor syndrome was mapped to chromosome 9, although in this case the linkage is to 9q34 (Chance et al., 1998). The vast majority of patients have upper motoneuron as well as lower motoneuron signs, so the disorder has been characterized as an autosomal dominant form of juvenile amyotrophic lateral sclerosis by the authors. Patients develop weakness in the second decade of life that usually manifests with problems in walking, followed by wasting and weakness of muscles in the feet and hands. Proximal weakness develops in the fourth to fifth decade of life, with many patients becoming wheelchair dependent. By the sixth decade, patients have lost useful hand function (Chance et al., 1998). Eighty-six percent of patients were said to have pathologically brisk reflexes, and 17% have Babinski signs. Sensory examination has been normal except for mild decreases in vibratory sensation with increasing age. NCVs in five patients were normal, with the exception of decreased CMAP amplitudes recorded over wasted muscles. Needle electromyography demonstrated chronic partial denervation that is greatest in distal muscles. An autopsy was reported for an 80-year-old affected woman who died of a myocardial infarction. Results demonstrated atrophy of both ventral and dorsal roots, loss of anterior horn cells, chromatolysis, and axonal swellings in ventral and dorsal roots (Chance et al., 1998).

INHERITED SENSORY AND AUTONOMIC NEUROPATHIES

Rare cases of heritable sensory neuropathies, often with autonomic features, have been described with various inheritance patterns. These patterns, along with clinical features, have been used to subclassify these disorders (reviewed in Dyck, 1993). As was the case with CMT 1, this subclassification is likely to be modified in the future as specific genetic mutations causing the sensory neuropathies are identified. A discussion of Friedreich's ataxia and the other spinocerebellar ataxias is beyond the scope of this chapter and is not presented here, although in some respects, they may be considered HSANs.

HSAN type 1 is characterized by an autosomal dominant pattern of inheritance, a symmetrical predominantly small-fiber sensory loss mainly involving the lower extremities, with onset between the second and fourth decades of life. The disorder is slowly progressive. Typically, patients present with plantar ulcers, neuropathic pain, sensory loss, and, in some cases, autonomic symptoms. Symptoms usually involve small-fiber pain and temperature modalities but may involve large-fiber modalities such as vibration and position sense. On neurological examination, in addition to a length-dependent sensory loss, patients are likely to have plantar ulcers and decreased deep tendon reflexes (particularly in the lower extremities); they may have some distal muscle atrophy and pes cavus (Dyck, 1993). NCVs are normal or demonstrate reduced SNAPs. Pathological studies reveal what is described as a primary degeneration of spinal ganglion neurons with subsequent length-dependent degeneration of small-fiber axons, although all size classes of axons are affected to some degree. Disorders resembling HSAN I but associated with deafness or weakness have been described, as have cases in which patients develop primarily burning feet without other clinical features of neuropathy.

HSAN II is distinguished from type I by its early, severe onset and by its apparent autosomal recessive inheritance pattern. Fingers as well as toes are frequently involved, and patients develop paronychia, whitlows, and ulcerations of the fingers in addition to the ulcerations of the feet (Dyck, 1993). Sensory loss affects both small- and large-fiber modalities. Sweating is reduced, although patients do not develop orthostatic hypotension, sphincter dysfunction, or (in males) impotence (Dyck, 1993). Nerve conduction testing reveals absent SNAPs, and sural nerve biopsies demonstrate an absence of myelinated fibers and reductions in nonmyelinated fibers (Dyck, 1993). Although HSANs I and II may be separate disorders, it is well to keep in mind that D-S was previously thought to be a disorder distinct from HMSN I, or CMT 1, and it is now known that different mutations in the same gene can cause either phenotype. Thus, a true understanding of differences between the inherited sensory neuropathies will have to await identification of the genetic defects that cause the neuropathies. Linkage studies have identified a locus on chromosome 9 (9q22) in several Australian families with autosomal dominant sensory neuropathies (Nicholson et al., 1996).

Familial dysautonomia (HSAN III), or the Riley-Day syndrome, is a severe disorder, inherited in an autosomal recessive pattern, that appears particularly frequently in the Ashkenazi Jewish population. Some estimates have placed the frequency of carriers in Israel as high as 18 per 100,000 (Moses et al., 1967). Linkage analysis has localized the genetic defect to chromosome 9 (9q31-33) (Blumenfeld et al., 1993, 1999; Axelrod, 1998). Clinically, patients display abnormalities from birth, including an absence of fungiform papillae on the tongue, poor sucking, difficulty swallowing, frequent vomiting, alacrima (absence of overflow tears), and blotching of the skin with emotion. Many patients have kyphoscoliosis (Dyck, 1993). Autonomic abnormalities include labile blood pressure, with severe postural hypotension, and both excesses and decreases of sweating. Intradermal injections of histamine fail to produce the characteristic "histamine flare." Deep tendon reflexes are typically decreased. Most patients have loss of pain and temperature sensation. Corneal reflexes are absent, consistent with trigeminal nerve involvement. Vibration and position sense are also abnormal in some patients. Motor nerve conduction may be mildly slowed, and sensory amplitudes may be reduced. Morphological studies have shown a significant loss of neurons in cervical and thoracic sympathetic ganglia. Decreased numbers of small, unmyelinated fibers have been described in sural nerve biopsies (Dyck, 1993).

Congenital insensitivity to pain with anhidrosis (CIPA) has been classified as HSAN-IV (Ben Othmane, 1990). The entity was first described by Swanson and colleagues (1963, 1965), and a review of 31 patients with the disorder was published by Rosemberg and associates (1994). Patients present with congenital insensitivity to pain and anhidrosis, despite normal-appearing sweat glands on skin biopsy. Temperature sensation is also defective, and 20% of patients die because of hyperpyrexia, usually before the age of 3 (Rosemberg, 1994). One of the initial patients described with CIPA died after a 24-hour illness in which his temperature reached 109°C (Swanson et al., 1965). Patients appear insensitive to pain and have been noted to bite off the tip of the tongue when they develop dentition and to self-mutilate the lips and tips of the fingers (Rosemberg et al., 1994). Most children are mentally retarded with IQs between 41 and 78 (Rosemberg et al., 1994). In the studies of Yagev and associates (1999), 10 of 15 Bedouin children with CIPA developed corneal opacities. Pathologically, sural nerve biopsies reveal a reduction in the number of myelinated and nonmyelinated fibers (Langer et al., 1981). An absence of eccrine sweat gland innervation has also been reported (Ismail et al., 1998). *TrkA* knockout mice, in which the tyrosine kinase receptor for nerve growth factor has been deleted, also appear to have congenital insensitivity to pain (Smeyne et al., 1994). Investigators have begun to study the human homologue of *TrkA, NTRK1*, as a candidate gene for CIPA. In three unrelated patients, Indo and colleagues (1996) detected a missense mutation in the tyrosine kinase region of the molecule, a splice site abnormality, and a deletion of the gene. These findings suggest that mutations in *NTRK1* cause CIPA and that the nerve growth factor–tyrosine kinase system is crucial to the development of nociception in humans as well as in establishing thermal regulation through sweating.

Neuropathy, Ataxia, and Retinitis Pigmentosa (NARP Syndrome)

Peripheral neuropathies are increasingly recognized as components of mitochondrial disease. In the disorder comprising neuropathy, ataxia, and retinitis pigmentosa (NARP syndrome), described by Holt and colleagues (1990), a missense mutation at nucleotide 8993 resulted in a change from a highly conserved leucine to an arginine in subunit 6 of mitochondrial H^+-ATPase. The patient was a 47-year-old woman in whom night blindness developed as a child as a result of retinitis pigmentosa, who had seizures in her 20s, and who had unsteadiness of gait in her 30s. Electrophysiological studies demonstrated a reduction in SNAP amplitudes. A quadriceps biopsy demonstrated partial denervation and collateral regeneration. In the patient's daughter, only retinitis pigmentosa developed, but severe disease developed in the daughter's daughter, including gait and limb ataxia, by age 3.

HEREDITARY BRACHIAL PLEXUS NEUROPATHY–HEREDITARY NEURALGIC AMYOTROPHY

This is a relatively rare disorder in which patients present with episodes of pain, weakness, and sensory loss. In almost all cases, the onset of weakness is preceded by pain in the affected arm. Onset is typically in the second or third decade. Recovery usually occurs, beginning several weeks to months after the initial symptoms. Attacks may subsequently occur in the same or opposite arm. NCVs have been reported as normal (Pellegrino et al., 1996), demonstrating pressure palsies (Windebank et al., 1995) or demonstrating axonal loss in a brachial plexus distribution (Windebank, 1993). Tomacula have been found on sural nerve biopsy samples; hence, the other name for the disorder is used: tomaculous neuropathy. Because of the presence of tomacula, which is also present in HNPP, it was initially thought that hereditary brachial plexus neuropathy was simply a variant of HNPP. However, linkage analysis has demonstrated that the hereditary brachial plexus neuropathy locus does not involve *PMP22*. The locus for hereditary brachial plexus neuropathy has also been mapped to chromosome 17 (17q24-25) (Windebank et al., 1995; Pellegrino et al., 1996, 1997). Several minor dysmorphic features, including short stature, hypotelorism, epicanthal folds, and cleft palate, have been associated with hereditary brachial plexus neuropathy (Windebank et al., 1995; Pellegrino et al., 1996, 1997), but a clear association of these features with the neuropathy has not yet been proved.

GIANT AXONAL NEUROPATHY

Giant axonal neuropathy is a rare, autosomal recessive disorder that was first characterized by Asbury and colleagues in 1972. In addition to the characteristic pathology of peripheral nerves, patients often have characteristic kinky hair and are likely to have CNS abnormalities, including mental retardation. Clinically, the disease presents in childhood and is steadily progressive until death occurs by the end of the third decade (Flanigan et al., 1998). Neuropathy symptoms and signs include prominent large-fiber sensory loss and distal weakness (Tandan et al., 1987). Electrophysiological studies reveal a severe axonal neuropathy with evidence of active denervation, although there may also be evidence of mild demyelination (Tandan et al., 1987). The pathological hallmarks of the disease are found on sural nerve biopsy; these include axonal swellings that contain masses of tightly woven neurofilaments.

These swellings, greatly enlarging the axon caliber, are often found near nodes of Ranvier (Asbury et al., 1972; Tandan et al., 1987; Flanigan et al., 1998). Abnormalities in the organization of intermediate neurofilaments are also found in other organs and are probably responsible for the characteristic hair pattern. The pathogenesis of the disease is thought to involve a defect in the generalized processing of neurofilaments (Tandan et al., 1987; Flanigan et al., 1998). Linkage studies localize the genetic defect to chromosome 16 (16q24) (Flanigan et al., 1998).

FAMILIAL AMYLOIDOTIC POLYNEUROPATHY

Familial amyloidotic polyneuropathy (FAP) refers to a hereditary autosomal dominant neuropathy characterized by systemic deposition of amyloid with special involvement of peripheral nerves (reviewed in Saraiva, 1996). The disorder was first described in northern Portugal; the onset of symptoms typically began in the third to fourth decades of life and included impairment of pain and temperature sensation in the feet, along with evidence of autonomic dysfunction (Andrade, 1952). The genetic mutation causing FAP in virtually all Portuguese FAP kindreds is a point mutation in the plasma protein transthyretin (TTR) gene in which a valine is changed to a methionine (TTR Met30–associated FAP). In other parts of the world, many other mutations in TTR have been associated with FAP; in some cases, patients develop familial amyloid cardiomyopathies without neuropathic involvement (reviewed in Saraiva, 1996).

As noted previously, small-fiber sensory abnormalities beginning with paresthesias and dysesthesias are usually the earliest symptoms, with involvement of the upper extremities at about the time lower extremity sensory abnormalities have risen to the level of the knees. Within 2 to 3 years, motor abnormalities begin, characterized by length-dependent atrophy and weakness (Saraiva, 1996). Autonomic neuropathy is particularly severe in Portuguese FAP patients and may be the presenting feature. Gastrointestinal abnormalities consisting of alternating constipation and diarrhea and of gastric stasis, nausea, and vomiting are frequent. Both urinary and fecal sphincter dysfunction are frequent, as is impotence. Cardiac conduction disturbances, including branch blocks (requiring pacemakers), often occur, and orthostatic hypotension is common (Chance et al., 1998). Progression of the disease is inexorable, leading to death in 10 to 15 years. Mutations in the apolipoprotein A1 (FAP type III) and gelsolin (FAP type IV) genes can also cause FAP.

NCVs may demonstrate axonal changes in both motor and sensory nerves. Pathologically, amyloid deposits may be found in the epineurium, perineurium, and endoneurium, as well as in the basal lamina of Schwann cells. A loss of both myelinated and nonmyelinated fibers may occur, and there is degeneration of both axons and myelin. Amyloid deposition in peripheral nerves is not always detectable in genetically diagnosed patients (Saraiva, 1996). Amyloid deposits may be found in the leptomeninges, ependyma, choroid plexus, sympathetic chain, dorsal root ganglia, and intrinsic nervous system of the gastrointestinal tract (Saraiva, 1996). Treatment of FAP is largely symptomatic. The role of liver transplantation in the prevention or treatment of FAP is under investigation.

PORPHYRIAS

The porphyrias are a group of rare inherited diseases that lead to defects in heme synthesis. Three of these cause peripheral neuropathy, along with disorders of mentation: variegate porphyria, acute intermittent porphyria, and hereditary coproporphyria. Each of these three disorders is caused by enzyme deficiencies in the production of heme from succinyl coenzyme A and glycine. Variegate porphyria is caused by a deficiency of protoporphyrinogen oxidase, blocking the transition between protoporphyrinogen IX to protoporphyrin IX; acute intermittent porphyria is caused by abnormalities of porphobilinogen deaminase, which blocks the conversion of porphobilinogen to hydroxymethylbilane; and hereditary coproporphyria is caused by deficiency of coproporphyrinogen oxidase, which prevents the conversion of coproporphyrinogen III to protoporphyrinogen IX. All three of these disorders are inherited as autosomal dominant disorders.

The peripheral neuropathy is similar in all three diseases and usually begins 2 to 3 days after attacks of abdominal pain and psychiatric disturbances. The abdominal pain is typically acute and colicky; the psychiatric disturbance may range from restlessness and agitation to frank psychosis with hallucinations, and may even include seizures. The neuropathy is known to mimic Guillain-Barré syndrome because the onset is acute and may primarily involve motor nerves. Pain may present early in the legs or back. The weakness is often asymmetrical. Nerves innervating proximal muscles are often affected early. Respiratory distress may occur, and autonomic abnormalities (including tachycardia, difficulties with urination, constipation, and pupillary dilatation) are frequent. Electrophysiological studies, which can be normal in the first few days, demonstrate axonal loss rather than demyelination, which helps distinguish the disorder from Guillain-Barré syndrome. The diagnosis depends on identification of the appropriate metabolic abnormality. Recovery from the neuropathy depends on the degree of axonal damage, although at least some recovery is the rule (reviewed in Windebank and Bonkovsky, 1993).

References

Adlkofer K, Martini R, Aguzzi A, et al: Hypermyelination and demyelinating peripheral neuropathy in Pmp22-deficient mice. Nat Genet 1995;11:274–280.

Aguayo A, Perkins S, Duncan I, Bray G: Human and animal neuropathies in experimental nerve transplants. In Canal N, Pozza G (eds): Peripheral Neuropathies. Amsterdam, Elsevier North-Holland, 1978; 37–48.

Amato AA, Gronseth GS, Callerme KJ, et al: Tomaculous neuropathy: A clinical and electrophysiological study in patients with and without 1.5-Mb deletions in chromosome 17p11.2. Muscle Nerve 1996;19:16–22.

Andersson PB, Yuen E, Parko K, So YT: Electrodiagnostic features of hereditary neuropathy with liability to pressure palsies. Neurology 2000;54:40–44.

Andrade C: A peculiar form of peripheral neuropathy: Familial atypical generalized amyloidosis with special involvement of the peripheral nerves. Brain 1952;75:408–427.

Asbury AK, Gale MK, Cox SC, et al: Giant axonal neuropathy: A unique case with segmental neurofilamentous masses. Acta Neuropathy 1972;70:237–247.

Axelrod FB: Familial dysautonomia: A 47 year perspective: How technology confirms clinical acumen. J Pediatr 1998;132:S2–S5.

Ben Othmane K, Loeb D, Hayworth-Hodgte R, et al: Physical and genetic mapping of the CMT4A locus and exclusion of PMP-2 as the defect in CMT4A. Genomics 1995;28:286–290.

Ben Othmane K: Formes Pures de la Maladie de Charcot-Marie-Tooth (HMSN) en Tunesie: Etude Clinique, Genealogique, Electrophysiologique et Histologique de 82 Familles. MD thesis, Tunisia, Faculte de Medecine de Tunis, 1990.

Benstead TJ, Kuntz NL, Miller RG, Daube JR: The electrophysiologic profile of Dejerine-Sottas disease (HMSN III). Muscle Nerve 1990;13:586–592.

Berciano J, Combarros O, Calleja J, et al: The application of nerve conduction and clinical studies to genetic counseling in hereditary motor and sensory neuropathy type 1. Muscle Nerve 1989;12:302–306.

Bergoffen J, Scherer SS, Wang S, et al: Connexin mutations in X-linked Charcot-Marie-Tooth disease. Science 1993;262:3039–3042.

Bird TD, Kraft GH, Lipe HP, et al: Clinical and pathological phenotype of the original family with Charcot-Marie-Tooth type 1B: A 20-year study. Ann Neurol 1997;41:463–469.

Bird TD, Ott J, Giblett ER: Evidence for linkage of Charcot-Marie-Tooth neuropathy to the Duffy locus on chromosome 1. Am J Hum Genet 1982;34:388–394.

Birouk N, LeGuern E, Maisonobe T, Rouger H: X-linked Charcot-Marie-Tooth disease with connexin 32 mutations: Clinical and electrophysiologic study. Neurology 1998;50:1074–1082.

Birouk X, Gouider R, Le Guern E, et al: Charcot Marie Tooth disease type 1A with 17p11.2 duplication: Clinical and electrophysiological phenotype study and factors influencing disease severity in 119 cases. Brain 1997;120:813–823.

Blumenfeld A, Slaugenhaupt SA, Axelrod FB, et al: Localization of the gene for familial dysautonomia on chromosome 9 and definition of DNA markers for genetic diagnosis. Nat Genet 1993;4:160–164.

Blumenfeld A, Slaugenhaupt SA, Liebert CB, et al: Precise genetic mapping and haplotype analysis of the familial dysautonomia gene on human chromosome 9q31. Am J Hum Genet 1999;64:1110–1118.

Bolino A, Muglia M, Conforti FL, et al: Charcot-Marie-Tooth type 4B is caused by mutations in the gene encoding myotubularin-related protein-2. Nat Genet 2000;25:17–19.

Bouche P, Gherardi R, Cathala HP, et al: Peroneal muscular atrophy: Part 1. Clinical and elecrophysiological study. J Neurol Sci 1983;61:389–399.

Brice A, Ravise N, Stevanin G, et al: Duplication within chromosome 17p11.2 in 12 patients of French ancestry with Charcot Marie Tooth disease type 1a. J Med Genet 1992;29:807–812.

Brust JCM, Lovelace RE, Devi S: Clinical and electrodiagnostic features of Charcot-Marie-Tooth syndrome. Acta Neurol Scand 1978;suppl 68:1–142.

Buchthal F, Behse F: Peroneal muscular atrophy (PMA) and related disorders: I. Clinical manifestations as related with biopsy findings, nerve conduction and electromyography. Brain 1977;100:41–66.

Cambi F, Tang XM, Cordray P, et al: Refined genetic mapping and proteolipid point mutation analysis in X-linked pure hereditary spastic paraplegia. Neurology 1996;46:1112–1117.

Case records of the Massachusetts General Hospital: Weekly clinicopathological exercises: A 15-year-old boy with slowly progressive dementia. N Engl J Med 1982;306:286–293.

Chance PF, Alderson MK, Leppig KA, et al: DNA deletion associated with hereditary neuropathy with liability to pressure palsies. Cell 1993;72:143–151.

Chance PF, Rabin BA, Ryan SG, et al: Linkage of the gene for an autosomal dominant form of juvenile amyotrophic lateral sclerosis to chromosome 9q34. Am J Hum Genet 1998;62:633–640.

Chapon F, Latour P, Diraison P, et al: Axonal phenotype of Charcot-Marie-Tooth disease associated with a mutation in the myelin protein zero gene. J Neurol Neurosurg Psychiatr 1999;66:779–782.

Charcot JM, Marie P: Sur une forme particulaire d'atrophie musculaire progressive souvent familial debutant par les pieds et les jambes et atteingnant plus tard les mains. Rev Med 1886;6:97–138.

Chaudhry V, Moser HW, Cornblath DR: Nerve conduction studies in adrenomyeloneuropathy. J Neurol Neurosurg Psychiatr 1996;61:181–185.

Christodoulou K, Kyriakides T, Hristova AH, et al: Mapping of a distal form of spinal muscular atrophy with upper limb predominance to chromosome 7p. Hum Mol Genet 1995;4:1629–1632.

Combarros O, Calleja J, Polo JM: Prevalence of hereditary motor and sensory neuropathy in Cantabria. Acta Neurol Scand 1989;75:9–12.

Cornblath DR, Asbury AK, Albers JW, et al: Research criteria for diagnosis of chronic inflammatory demyelinating polyneuropathy (CIDP). Neurology 1991;41:617–618.

Cornblath DR, Sumner AJ, Daube J, et al: Conduction block in clinical practice. Muscle Nerve 1991;14:869–871.

Davis CJF, Bradley WG, Madrid R: The peroneal muscular atrophy syndrome: Clinical, genetic, electrophysiological and nerve biopsy findings and classification. J Genet Hum 1978; 26:311–349.

Dawidenkow S: Uber die neurotische Muskelatrophie Charcot-Marie: Klinisch-genetische Studien. Z Neurol 1927a;107:259.

Dawidenkow S: Uber die neurotische Muskelatrophie Charcot-Marie: Klinisch-genetische Studien. Z Neurol 1927b;108:344.

Debruyne J, Dehaene I, Martin JJ: Hereditary pressure-sensitive neuropathy. J Neurol Sci 1980;47:385–394.

Dejerine H, Sottas J: Sur la nevritte interstitielle, hypertrophique et progressive de l'enfance. C R Soc Biol (Paris) 1893;45:63–96.

DeJonghe P, Timmerman V, Ceuterick C, et al: The Thr124Met mutation in the peripheral myelin protein zero (MPZ) gene is associated with a clinically distinct Charcot-Marie-Tooth phenotype. Brain 1999;122:281–290.

DeJonghe P, Timmerman V, Fitzpatrick D, et al: Charcot Marie Tooth disease and related peripheral neuropathies. J Periph Nerv Syst 1997;2:370–387.

D'Urso D, Ehrhardt P, Muller HW: Peripheral myelin protein 22 and protein zero: A novel association in peripheral nervous system myelin. J Neurosci 1999;19:3396–3403.

Dyck PJ: Inherited neuronal degeneration and atrophy affecting peripheral motor, sensory, and autonomic neurons. In Dyck PJ, Thomas PK, Lambert EH, Bunge RE (eds): Peripheral Neuropathy. Philadelphia, WB Saunders, 1984; 1600–1642.

Dyck PJ: Neuronal atrophy and degeneration predominantly affecting peripheral sensory and autonomic neurons. In Dyck P, Thomas P, Griffin J, et al (eds): Peripheral Neuropathy. Philadelphia, WB Saunders, 1993; 1065–1093.

Dyck PJ, Karnes JL, Lambert EH: Longitudinal study of neuropathic deficit and nerve conduction abnormalities in hereditary motor and sensory neuropathy type 1. Neurology 1989;39:1302–1308.

Dyck PJ, Lais AC, Offord KP: The nature of myelinated nerve fiber degeneration in dominantly inherited hypertrophic neuropathy. Mayo Clin Proc 1974;49:34–39.

Dyck PJ, Lambert EH: Lower motor and primary sensory neuron diseases with peroneal muscular atrophy: I. Neurologic, genetic, and electrophysiologic findings in hereditary polyneuropathies. Arch Neurol 1968;18:603–618.

Dyck PJ, Lambert EH, Mulder DW: Charcot-Marie-Tooth disease: Nerve conduction and clinical studies of a large kinship. Neurology 1963;13:1.

Dyck PJ, Litchy WJ, Minnerath S, et al: Hereditary motor and sensory neuropathy with diaphragm and vocal cord paresis. Ann Neurol 1994;35:608–615.

Fishbeck KH, al-Rushdi N, Pericak-Vance M, et al: X-linked neuropathy: Gene localization with DNA probes. Ann Neurol 1986;20:527–532.

Flanigan KM, Crawford TO, Griffin JW, et al: Localization of the giant axonal neuropathy gene to chromosome 16q24. Ann Neurol 1998;43:143–148.

Fressinaud C, Vallat JM, Masson M, Jauberteau MO: Adult-onset metachromatic leukodystrophy presenting as isolated peripheral neuropathy. Neurology 1992;42:1396–1398.

Friedreich N: Uber progressive Muskelatrophie, uber wahre und falsche Muskelhypertrophie. Berlin, Hirschwald, 1873.

Gabreels-Festen AAWM, Bolhuis PA, Hoogendijk JE, et al: Charcot-Marie-Tooth disease type 1A: Morphological phenotype of the 17p duplication versus PMP22 point mutations. Acta Neuropathol 1995;90:645–649.

Gal A, Mucke J, Theile H, et al: X-linked dominant Charcot-Marie-Tooth disease: Suggestion of linkage with a cloned DNA sequence from the proximal Xq. Hum Genet 1985;70:38–42.

Gambardella A, Bolino A, Muglia M, et al: Genetic heterogeneity in autosomal recessive motor and sensory neuropathy with focally folded myelin sheaths (CMT4B). Neurology 1997;50:799–801.

Gambardella A, Bono F, Muglia M, et al: Autosomal recessive motor and sensory neuropathy with focally folded myelin sheaths (CMT4B). Ann N Y Acad Sci 1999;883:47–55.

Garbern JY, Cambi F, Tang X-E, et al: Proteolipid protein is necessary in peripheral as well as central myelin. Neuron 1997;19:205–218.

Garcia A, Combarros O, Calleja J, Berciano J: Charcot-Marie-Tooth disease type 1A with 17p duplication in infancy and early childhood: A longitudinal clinical and electrophysiologic study. Neurology 1998;50:1061–1067.

Garcia CA, Malamut RE, England JD, et al: Clinical variability in two pairs of identical twins with the Charcot-Marie-Tooth disease type 1A duplication. Neurology 1995;45:2090–2093.

Gilliatt RW, Thomas PK: Extreme slowing of nerve conduction in peroneal muscular atrophy. Ann Phys Med 1957;4:104–106.

Gouider R, LeGuern E, Gugenheim M, et al: Clinical, electrophysiologic and molecular correlations in 13 families with hereditary neuropathy with liability to pressure palsies and a chromosome 17p11.2 deletion. Neurology 1995;45:2018–2023.

Griffiths I, Klugmann M, Anderson T, et al: Current concepts of PLP and its role in the nervous system. Microsc Res Tech 1998;41:344–358.

Guilbot A, Kesali M, Ravise N, et al: The autosomal recessive form of CMT linked to chromosome 5q23-5q33. Ann N Y Acad Sci 1999;883:56–59.

Gutierrez A, England JD, Ferer SS, et al: Unusual electrophysiological findings in X-linked dominant Charcot-Marie-Tooth disease. Muscle Nerve 2000;23:182–188.

Gutmann L, Fakadej A, Riggs J: Evolution of nerve conduction abnormalities in children with dominant hypertrophic neuropathy of the Charcot-Marie-Tooth type. Muscle Nerve 1983;6:515–519.

Guzzetta F, Ferrière G, Lyon G: Congenital hypomyelination polyneuropathy—pathological findings compared with polyneuropathies starting later in life. Brain 1982;105:395–416.

Hahn AF, Bolton CF, White CM, et al: Genotype/phenotype correlations in X-linked Charcot-Marie-Tooth disease. Ann N Y Acad Sci 1999;883:366–382.

Hahn AF, Brown WF, Koopman WJ, Feasby TE: X-linked dominant hereditary motor and sensory neuropathy. Brain 1990;113:1511–1525.

Hallum PJ, Harding AE, Berciano J, et al: Duplication of part of chromosome 17 is commonly associated with hereditary motor and sensory neuropathy type I (Charcot-Marie-Tooth disease type 1). Ann Neurol 1992;31:570–572.

Harding AE: From the syndrome of Charcot, Marie and Tooth to disorders of peripheral myelin proteins. Brain 1995;118:809–818.

Harding AE: Inherited neuronal atrophy and degeneration predominantly of lower motor neurons. In Peripheral Neuropathy. Philadelphia, WB Saunders, 1993; 1051–1064.

Harding AE, Thomas PK: Genetic aspects of hereditary motor and sensory neuropathy (types I and II). J Med Genet 1980a; 176:329–336.

Harding AE, Thomas PK: The clinical features of hereditary motor and sensory neuropathy types I and II. Brain 1980b;103:259–280.

Hayasaka K, Himoro M, Sawaishi Y, et al: De novo mutation of the myelin P-0 gene in Dejerine-Sottas disease (hereditary motor and sensory neuropathy type III). Nat Genet 1993;5:266–268.

Hayasaka K, Ohnishi A, Takada G, et al: Mutation of the myelin P0 gene in Charcot-Marie-Tooth neuropathy type-1. Biochem Biophys Res Commun 1993;194:1317–1322.

Henrickson JD: Conduction velocity of motor nerves in normal subjects, and patients with neuromuscular disorders. Thesis, University of Minnesota, 1956.

Herringham WP: Muscular atrophy of the peroneal type affecting many members of a family. Brain 1889;11:230–236.

Holt IJ, Harding AE, Petty RKH, Morgan-Hughes JA: A new mitochondrial disease associated with mitochondrial DNA heteroplasmy. Am J Hum Genet 1990;46:428–433.

Hoogendijk JE, de Visser M, Bolhuis PA, et al: Hereditary motor and sensory neuropathy type I: Clinical and neurographical features of the 17P duplication subtype. Muscle Nerve 1994; 17:85–90.

Hoogendijk JE, de Visser M, Bour LJ, Ongerboer BW: Conduction block in hereditary motor and sensory neuropathy type 1. Muscle Nerve 1992;15:520–521.

Hoogendijk JE, Janssen EAM, Gabreels-Festen AAWM, et al: Allelic heterogeneity in hereditary motor and sensory neuropathy type 1A (Charcot-Marie-Tooth disease type 1A). Neurology 1993;43:1010–1015.

Huxley C, Passage E, Manson A, et al: Construction of a mouse model of Charcot Marie Tooth disease type 1A by pronuclear injection of human YAC DNA. Hum Mol Genet 1996;5:563–569.

Indo Y, Tsuruta M, Hayashida Y, et al: Mutations in the TRKA/NGF receptor gene in patients with congenital insensitivity to pain with anhidrosis. Nat Genet 1996;13:485–488.

Ionasescu VV: Charcot-Marie-Tooth neuropathies: From clinical description to molecular genetics. Muscle Nerve 1995;18:267–275.

Ionasescu VV, Ionasescu R, Searby C, Neahring R: Dejerine-Sottas disease with the de novo dominant point mutation of the PMP22 gene. Neurology 1995;45:1766–1767.

Ionasescu VV, Kimura J, Searby C, et al: A Dejerine-Sottas neuropathy family with a gene mapped on chromosome 8. Muscle Nerve 1996;19:319–323.

Ionasescu VV, Searby C, Sheffield VC, et al: Autosomal dominant Charcot Marie Tooth axonal neuropathy mapped on chromosome 7p (CMT2D). Hum Mol Genet 1996;5:1373–1375.

Ismail EAR, Al-Shammari N, Anim JT, Moosa A: Congenital insensitivity to pain with anhidrosis: Lack of eccrine sweat gland innervation confirmed. J Child Neurol 1998;13:243–246.

Kaku DA, England JD, Sumner AJ: Distal accentuation of conduction slowing in polyneuropathy with antibodies to myelin-associated glycoprotein and sulphated glucuronyl paragloboside. Brain 1994;117:941–947.

Kaku DA, Parry GS, Malamut R, et al: Nerve conduction studies in Charcot-Marie-Tooth polyneuropathy associated with a segmental duplication of chromosome 17. Neurology 1993;443: 1806–1808.

Kaku DA, Parry GJ, Malamut R, et al: Uniform slowing of conduction velocities in Charcot-Marie-Tooth disease polyneuropathy type 1. Neurology 1993;434:2664–2667.

Kalaydjieva L, Hallmayer J, Chandler D, et al: Gene mapping in Gypsies identifies a novel demyelinating neuropathy on chromosome 8q24. Nat Genet 1996;14:214–217.

Kalaydjieva L, Gresham D, Gooding R, et al: N-myc downstream-regulated gene is mutated in hereditary motor and sensory neuropathy-Lom. Am J Hum Genet 2000;67:47–58.

Killian JM, Tiwari PS, Jacobson S, et al: Longitudinal studies of the duplication form of Charcot-Marie-Tooth polyneuropathy. Muscle Nerve 1996;19:74–78.

Kimura J: F-wave velocity in the central segment of the median and ulnar nerves. Neurology 24:1974;539–546.

Knapp PE: Proteolipid protein: Is it more than just a structural protein of myelin? Dev Neurosci 1996;18:297–308.

Krajewski K, Lewis R, Fuerst DR, et al: Neurological dysfunction and axonal degeneration in Charcot-Marie-Tooth disease type 1A. Brain 2000;123:1516–1527.

Krampitz DE, Wolfe GI, Fleckenstein JL, Barohn RJ: Charcot-Marie-Tooth disease type 1A presenting as calf hypertrophy and muscle cramps. Neurology 1998;51:1508–1509.

Kuntzer T, Ochsner F, Schmid F, Regli F: Quantitative EMG analysis and longitudinal nerve conduction studies in a Refsum's disease patient. Muscle Nerve 1993;16:857–863.

Kwon JM, Elliott JL, Yee WC, et al: Assignment of a second Charcot-Marie-Tooth type II locus to chromosome 3q. Am J Hum Genet 1995;57:853–858.

Lambert EH: Electromyography and electric stimulation of peripheral nerves and muscle. In Clinical Examinations in Neurology. Philadelphia, WB Saunders, 1956; 287–317.

Langer J, Goebel HH, Veit S: Eccrine sweat glands are not innervated in hereditary sensory neuropathy type IV: An electron-microscopic study. Acta Neuropathol 1981;54:199–202.

LeGuern E, Guilbot A, Kessali M, et al: Homozygosity mapping of an autosomal recessive form of demyelinating Charcot-Marie-Tooth disease to chromosome 5q23-5q33. Hum Mol Genet 1996; 10:1685–1688.

Lewis RA, Shy ME: Electrodiagnostic findings in CMT X: a disorder of the Schwann cell and peripheral nerve myelin. Proc N Y Acad Sci 1999;883:504–508.

Lewis RA, Sumner AJ: The electrodiagnostic distinctions between chronic familial and acquired demyelinating neuropathies. Neurology 1982;32:592–596.

Lupski J, Montes de Oca-Luna R, et al: DNA duplication associated with Charcot-Marie-Tooth disease type 1A. Cell 1991;66:219–232.

Magistris M, Roth G: Long-lasting conduction block in hereditary neuropathy with liability to pressure palsies. Neurology 1985; 35:1639–1641.

Magyar AP, Martini R, Ruelicke T, et al: Impaired differentiation of Schwann cells in transgenic mice with increased PMP22 gene dosage. J Neurosci 1996;16:5351–5360.

Mariman EC, Gabreëls-Festeen, AA, van Beersum SE, et al: Prevalence of the 1.5 Mb 17p deletion in families with hereditary neuropathy with liability to pressure palsies. Ann Neurol 1994; 36:650–655.

Marks HG, Scavina MT, Kolodny EH, et al: Krabbe's disease presenting as a peripheral neuropathy. Muscle Nerve 1997;20: 1024–1028.

Marques W Jr, Thomas PK, Sweene MG, et al: Dejerine-Sottas neuropathy and PMP22 point mutations: A new base pair substitution and a possible "hot spot" on ser72. Ann Neurol 1998; 43:680–683.

Marrosu MG, Vaccargiu S, Marrosu G, Vannelli A: Charcot-Marie-Tooth disease type 2 associated with mutation of the myelin protein zero gene. Neurology 1998;50:1397–1401.

Middleton LT, Christodoulou K, Mubaidin A, et al: Distal hereditary motor neuronopathy of the Jerash type. Ann N Y Acad Sci 1999;883:65–68.

Middleton PHR, Harding AE, Monteiro C, et al: Linkage of hereditary motor and sensory neuropathy type I to the pericentromeric region of chromosome 17. Am J Hum Genet 1990;46:92–4.

Miller RG, Gutmann L, Lewis RA, Sumner AJ: Acquired versus familial demyelinative neuropathies in children. Muscle Nerve 1985;8:205–210.

Mongia SK, Ghanem Q, Preston D, et al: Dominantly inherited hypertrophic neuropathy. Can J Neurol Sci 1978;5:239–246.

Moser HW, Moser AB, Smith KD, et al: Adrenoleukodystrophy: Phenotypic variability and implications for therapy. J Inherit Metab Dis 1992;15:645–664.

Moses SW, Rotem, Jagoda N, et al: A clinical, genetic and biochemical study of familial dysautonomia in Israel. Isr J Med Sci 1967; 3:358.

Nelis E, Timmerman V, De Jonghe P, et al: Rapid screening of myelin genes in CMT1 patients by SSCP analysis: Identification of new mutations and polymorphisms in the p-0 gene. Hum Genet 1994;94:653–657.

Nelis E, Timmerman V, De Jonghe P, Van Broeckhoven C: Identification of a 5′ splice site mutation in the PMP-22 gene in autosomal dominant Charcot-Marie-Tooth disease type 1. Hum Mol Genet 1994;3:515–516.

Nelis E, Van Broeckhoven C, De Jonghe P, et al: Estimation of the mutation frequencies in Charcot-Marie-Tooth disease type 1 and hereditary neuropathy with liability to pressure palsies: A European collaborative study. Eur J Hum Genet 1996;4:25–33.

Nicholson G, Corbett A: Slowing of central conduction in X-linked Charcot-Marie-Tooth neuropathy shown by brain stem auditory evoked responses. J Neurol Neurosurg Psychiatr 1996;61:43–46.

Nicholson G, Nash J: Intermediate nerve conduction velocities define X-linked Charcot-Marie-Tooth neuropathy families. Neurology 1993;43:2558–2564.

Nicholson GA, Dawkins JL, Blair IP, et al: The gene for hereditary sensory neuropathy type I (HSN-1) maps to chromosome 9q22.1-q22.3. Nat Genet 1996;13:101–104.

Nicholson GA, Valentijn LJ, Cherryson ML, et al: A frame shift mutation in the PMP 22 gene in hereditary neuropathy with liability to pressure palsies. Nat Genet 1994;6:263–266.

Nicholson GA, Yeung L, Corbett A: Efficient neurophysiologic selection of X-linked Charcot-Marie-Tooth families: Ten novel mutations. Neurology 1998;51:1412–1416.

Oh SJ, Chang CW: Conduction block and dispersion in hereditary motor and sensory neuropathy. Muscle Nerve 1987;10:656.

Ozdirim E, Topcu M, Ozon A, Cila A: Cockayne syndrome: Review of 25 cases. Pediatr Neurol 1996;15:312–316.

Pareyson D, Menichella D, Botti S, et al: Heterozygous null mutation in the P0 gene associated with mild Charcot-Marie-Tooth disease. Ann N Y Acad Sci 1999;883:477–481.

Patel PI, Lupski JR: Charcot-Marie-Tooth disease—a new paradigm for the mechanism of inherited disease. Trends Genet 1994;10:128–133.

Pearn J, Hudgson P: Distal spinal muscular atrophy: A clinical and genetic study in 8 kindreds. J Neurol Sci 1979;43:183–191.

Pellegrino JE, George RAV, Biegel J, et al: Hereditary neuralgic amyotrophy: Evidence for genetic homogeneity and mapping to chromosome 17q25. Hum Genet 1997;101:277–283.

Pellegrino JE, Rebbeck TR, Brown MJ, et al: Mapping of hereditary neuralgic amyotrophy (familial brachial plexus neuropathy) to distal chromosome 17q. Neurology 1996;46:1128–1132.

Pericak-Vance MA, Speer MC, Lennon F, et al: Confirmation of a second locus for CMT2 and evidence for additional genetic heterogeneity. Neurogenetics 1997;1:89–93.

Raeymaekers P, De JP, Backhovens H, et al: Absence of genetic linkage of Charcot-Marie-Tooth disease (HMSN Ia) with chromosome 1 gene markers. Neurology 1989;39:844–846.

Raeymaekers P, Timmerman V, Nelis E, et al: Duplication in chromosome 17p11.2 in Charcot-Marie-Tooth neuropathy type 1a (CMT 1a): The HMSN Collaborative Research Group. Neuromuscul Disord 1991;1:93–97.

Raine CS: Morphology of myelin and myelination. In Morrell P (ed): Myelin. New York, Plenum, 1984; 1–41.

Raskind WH, Williams CA, Hudson LD, Bird TD: Complete deletion of proteolipid protein gene (PLP) in a family with X-linked Pelizaeus-Merzbacher disease. Am J Hum Genet 1991;49:1355–1360.

Refsum S, Stokke O, Eldjarn L, Fardeau M: Heredopathia atactica poyneuritiformis (Refsum's disease). In Dyck PJ, Thomas PK, Lambert EH, Bunge R (eds): Peripheral Neuropathy. Philadelphia, WB Saunders, 1984; 1680–1703.

Reilly MM: Genetically determined neuropathies. J Neurol 1998; 245:6–13.

Rhee EK, England JD, Sumner AJ: A computer simulation of conduction block: Effects produced by actual block versus interphase cancellation. Ann Neurol 1990;28:146–156.

Roa BB, Dyck PJ, Marks HG, et al: Dejerine-Sottas syndrome associated with point mutation in the peripheral myelin protein 22 (PMP22) gene. Nat Genet 1993;5:269–273.

Roa BB, Garcia CA, Suter U, et al: Charcot-Marie-Tooth disease type-1A: Association with a spontaneous point mutation in the PMP22 gene. N Engl J Med 1993;329:96–101.

Rosemberg S, Nagahashi Marie SK, Kliemann S: Congenital insensitivity to pain with anhidrosis (hereditary sensory and autonomic neuropathy type IV). Pediatr Neurol 1994;11:50–56.

Roussy G, Levy G: A sept cas d'une maladie familiale particuliare. Rev Neurol 1926;33:427–450.

Roy EP, Gutmann L, Riggs JE: Longitudinal conduction studies in hereditary motor and sensory neuropathy type 1. Muscle Nerve 1989;12:52–55.

Rozear MP, Pericak-Vance MA, Fishbeck KH, et al: Hereditary motor and sensory neuropathy, X-linked: A half century follow-up. Neurology 1987;37:1460–1465.

Sahenk Z, Chen L: Abnormalities in the axonal cytoskeleton induced by a connexin 32 mutation in nerve xenographs. J Neurosci Res 1998;51:174–184.

Sahenk Z, Chen L, Freimer M: A novel PMP22 point mutation causing HNPP phenotype. Neurology 1998;51:702–707.

Sahenk Z, Chen L, Mendell JR: Effects of PMP22 duplication and deletions on the axonal cytoskeleton. Ann Neurol 1999;45:16–24.

Saito M, Hayashi Y, Tanaka H, et al: Linkage mapping of the gene for Charcot Marie Tooth disease type 2 to chromosome 1p (CMT2A) and the clinical features of CMT2A. Neurology 1997; 49:1630–1635.

Sambuughin N, Sivakumar K, Selenge B, et al: Autosomal dominant spinal muscular atrophy type V (dSMA-V) and Charcot-Marie-Tooth disease type 2D (CMT2D) segregate within single large kindred and map to a refined region on chromosome 7p15. J Neurol Sci 1998;161:23–28.

Sander S, Nicholson GA, Ouvrier RA, McLeod JG: Charcot-Marie-Tooth disease: Histopathological features of the peripheral myelin protein (PMP22) duplication (CMT1A) and connexin32 mutations (CMTX1). Muscle Nerve 1998;21:217–225.

Saraiva MJM: Molecular genetics of familial amyloidotic polyneuropathy. J Peripher Nerv Syst 1996;1:179–188.

Schenone A, Nobbio L, Caponnetto C, et al: Correlation between PMP-22 messenger RNA expression and phenotype in hereditary neuropathy with liability to pressure palsies. Ann Neurol 1997;42:866–872.

Scherer SS: Molecular specializations at nodes and paranodes in peripheral-nerve. Microsc Res Tech 1996;34:452–461.

Seitelberger F: Neuropathology and genetics of Pelizaeus-Merzbacher disease. Brain Pathol 1995;5:267–273.

Seitelberger F: Pelizaeus-Merzbacher disease. In Vinken PJ, Bruyn GW (eds): Handbook of Clinical Neurology. Amsterdam, Elsevier North Holland, 1970; 150–220.

Sellman MS, Mayer RF: Conduction block in hereditary neuropathy with susceptibility to pressure palsies. Muscle Nerve 1987; 10:621–625.

Sereda M, Griffiths I, Puhlhofer A, et al: A transgenic rat model of Charcot-Marie-Tooth disease. Neuron 1996;16:1049–1060.

Shapiro L, Doyle JP, Hensley P, et al: Crystal structure of the extracellular domain from P0, the major structural protein of peripheral nerve myelin. Neuron 1996;17:435–448.

Sindou P, Vallat J-M, Chapon F, et al: Ultrastructural protein zero expression in Charcot-Marie-Tooth type 1B disease. Muscle Nerve 1999;22:99–104.

Sistermans EA, Dewijs IJ, Decii RF, et al: A (G-to-A) mutation in the initiation codon of the proteolipid protein gene causing a relatively mild form of Pelizaeus-Merzbacher disease in a Dutch family. Hum Genet 1996;97:337–339.

Smeyne RJ, Klein R, Schnapp A, et al: Severe sensory and sympathetic neuropathies in mice carrying a disrupted Trk/NGF receptor gene. Nature 1994;368:246–249.

Suter U, Moskow JJ, Welcher AA, et al: A leucine-to-proline mutation in the putative 1st transmembrane domain of the 22-kDa peripheral myelin protein in the Trembler-J mouse. Proc Natl Acad Sci U S A 1992a;89:4382–4386.

Suter U, Welcher AA, Ozcelik T, et al: Trembler mouse carries a point mutation in a myelin gene. Nature 1992b;356:241–244.

Svaren J, Sevetson BR, Apel ED, et al: NAB2, a corepressor of NGFI-A (Egr-1) and Krox20, is induced by proliferative and differentiative stimuli. Mol Cell Biol 1996;16:3545–3553.

Swanson AG: Congenital insensitivity to pain with anhydrosis: A unique syndrome in two male children. Arch Neurol 1963; 8:299–306.

Swanson AG, Buchan GC, Alvord ECJ: Anatomic changes in congenital insensitivity to pain: Absence of small primary sensory neurons in ganglia, roots and Lissauer's tract. Arch Neurol 1965;12:12–18.

Tabaraud F, Lagrange E, Sindou P, et al: Demyelinating X-linked Charcot-Marie-Tooth disease: Unusual electrophysiological features, Muscle Nerve 1999;22:1442–1447.

Tanaka K, Koyama A, Koike R, et al: Adrenomyeloneuropathy: A report of a family and electron microscopic findings in peripheral nerve. J Neurol 1985;232:73–78.

Tandan R, Little BW, Emery ES, et al: Childhood giant axonal neuropathy: Case report and review of the literature. J Neurol Sci 1987;82:205–228.

Thomas PK, Calne DB: Motor nerve conduction velocity in peroneal muscular atrophy: Evidence for genetic heterogeneity. J Neurol Neurosurg Psychiatr 1974;37:68–74.

Thomas PK, Marques W Jr, Davis MB, et al: The phenotypic manifestations of chromosome 17p11.2 duplication. Brain 1997; 120:465–478.

Timmerman V, Beuten J, Irobi J, et al: Distal hereditary motor neuropathy type II (distal HMN type II): Phenotype and molecular genetics. Ann N Y Acad Sci 1999;883:60–64.

Timmerman V, De Jonghe P, Spoelders P, Simokovic S: Linkage and mutation analysis of Charcot-Marie-Tooth neuropathy type 2 families with chromosomes 1p35-36 and Xq13. Neurology 1996;46:1311–1318.

Tooth HH: The Peroneal Type of Progressive Muscular Atrophy. London, Lewis, 1886.

Topilko P, Schneider-Maunoury S, Levi G, et al: Krox-20 controls myelination in the peripheral nervous system. Nature 1994; 371:396–399.

Tyson J, Ellis D, Fairbrother U, King RHM, et al: Hereditary demyelinating neuropathy of infancy: A genetically complex syndrome. Brain 1997;120:47–63.

Uncini A, Di Guglielmo, Di Muzio A, et al: Differential electrophysiological features of neuropathies associated with 17p11.2 deletion and duplication. Muscle Nerve 1995;18:628–635.

Valentijn LJ, Baas F, Wolterman RA, et al: Identical point mutations of PMP-22 in Trembler-J mouse and Charcot-Marie-Tooth disease type-1A. Nat Genet 1992;2:288–291.

Valentijn LJ, Ouvrier RA, van den Bosch NH, et al: Dejerine-Sottas neuropathy is associated with a de novo PMP22 mutation. Hum Mutat 1995;5:76–80.

Van Geel BM, Koelman JHTM, Barth PG, et al: Peripheral nerve abnormalities in adrenomyeloneuropathy: A clinical and electrodiagnostic study. Neurology 1996;46:112–118.

Vance JM: Charcot-Marie-Tooth disease type II. Ann N Y Acad Sci 1999;883:42–46.

Vance JM, Nicholson GA, Yamaoka LH, et al: Linkage of Charcot-Marie-Tooth neuropathy type 1a to chromosome 17. Exp Neurol 1989;104:186–189.

Vance JM, Speer MC, Stajich JM, et al: Misclassification and linkage of hereditary sensory and autonomic neuropathy type 1 as Charcot-Marie-Tooth disease, type 2B. Am J Hum Genet 1996; 59:258–260.

Verhalle D, Lofgren A, Nelis E, et al: Deletion in the CMT 1A locus on chromosome 17p11.2 in hereditary neuropathy with liability to pressure palsies. Ann Neurol 1994;35:704–708.

Warner LE, Hilz MJ, Appel SH, et al: Clinical phenotypes of different MPZ (P-0) mutations may include Charcot-Marie-Tooth type 1B, Dejerine-Sottas, and congenital hypomyelination. Neuron 1996;17:451–460.

Warner LE, Mancias P, Butler IJ, et al: Mutations in the early growth response 2 (EGR2) gene are associated with hereditary myelinopathies. Nat Genet 1998;18:382–384.

Weber F: Conduction block and abnormal temporal dispersion: Diagnostic criteria. Electromyogr Clin Neurophysiol 1997;37: 305–309.

Wilbourn AJ: Differentiating acquired from familial segmental demyelinating neuropathies by EMG. Electroencephalogr Clin Neurophysiol 1977;43:616.

Windebank AJ: Inherited recurrent focal neuropathies. In Dyck PJ, Thomas PK, Griffin JW, et al (eds): Peripheral Neuropathy. Philadelphia, WB Saunders, 1993; 1137–1148.

Windebank AJ, Bonkovsky HL: Porphyric neuropathy. In Dyck PJ, Thomas PK, Griffin J, et al (eds): Peripheral Neuropathy. Philadelphia, WB Saunders, 1993; 1161–1168.

Windebank AJ, Schenone A, Dewald GW: Hereditary neuropathy with liability to pressure palsies and inherited brachial plexus neuropathy: Two genetically distinct disorders. Mayo Clin Proc 1995;70:743–746.

Wise CA, Garcia CA, Davis SN, et al: Molecular analyses of unrelated Charcot-Marie-Tooth (CMT) disease patients suggest a high frequency of the CMTIA duplication. Am J Hum Genet 1993;53:853–863.

Yagev R, Levy J, Shorer Z, Lifshitz T: Congenital insensitivity to pain with anhidrosis: Ocular and systemic manifestations. Am J Ophthal 1999;127:322–326.

Acute and Chronic Dysimmune Polyneuropathies

Mark B. Bromberg

Demyelinating neuropathies, from the clinical neurophysiological perspective, represent a category of neuropathies characterized by electrophysiological evidence of slowed or blocked nerve conduction. The underlying disorder is presumed to be immune-mediated demyelination, but other processes may be involved, such as antibody-mediated channel blockade and axonal damage. Demyelinating neuropathies have various clinical presentations, including acute and chronic time courses, and motor and sensory nerve fibers can be involved, both together and separately. Autonomic nerves may be included. Clinical neurophysiology has a prominent role in diagnosing demyelinating neuropathies because nerve conduction studies are a practical means of obtaining evidence of demyelinating disorders. Nerve biopsy is less diagnostic because of sampling limitations. Obtaining evidence of primary demyelination by clinical neurophysiological testing has therapeutic implications, because demyelinating neuropathies are believed to be immune mediated and amenable to immunomodulating therapy.

Obtaining and evaluating neurophysiological evidence of demyelination can be challenging, because the degree of demyelination varies within and among different types of inflammatory neuropathies. It is important to appreciate underlying pathological changes to interpret neurophysiological data accurately. This chapter first describes the clinical features of different types of demyelinating neuropathies. Next, a review of pathological findings in the various forms of demyelinating neuropathies is presented as an aid to understanding the objectives and limitations of clinical neurophysiological testing. It is also important to have an understanding of the principles and practice of nerve conduction recording as they relate to identifying primary demyelination and diagnostic criteria for primary demyelination, and these issues are reviewed. The next section presents the clinical neurophysiological experience with the various clinical forms of demyelinating neuropathies. The final section is an algorithm to consider in evaluating neuropathies for demyelinating components.

CLINICAL FORMS OF DEMYELINATING NEUROPATHIES

Certain demyelinating neuropathies are recognized by clinical features. Although the underlying pathological mechanisms of demyelination may differ within and among the forms, clinical neurophysiological principles are similar. It will be useful to review the clinical features of the major forms of demyelinating neuropathies before discussing electrophysiological details, because all clinical neurophysiological data must be interpreted in the clinical context. The first clinical division is based on time course, with acute and chronic forms. The acute form is frequently referred to as *Guillain-Barré syndrome* (GBS). The chronic form is referred to as *chronic inflammatory demyelinating polyradiculoneuropathy* (CIDP). A rare and unique form of inflammatory neuropathy is *multifocal motor neuropathy.* CIDP and multifocal motor neuropathy may represent two ends of a spectrum of chronic inflammatory neuropathies (Chaudhry et al., 1993; Krendel and Costigan, 1993). Several variants of chronic demyelinating neuropathies are also recognized.

The term *Guillain-Barré syndrome* describes several clinical entities characterized by acute ascending paralysis (Griffin et al., 1996). Various forms are recognized based on the pattern of nerve involvement and severity of weakness (Table 58–1).

Acute Inflammatory Demyelinating Polyradiculoneuropathy

Acute inflammatory demyelinating polyradiculoneuropathy (AIDP) is the most common form in North America and Europe. Clinical diagnostic criteria have been formulated that include a set of neurophysiological criteria (Asbury and Cornblath, 1990). Acute inflammatory demyelinating polyradiculoneuropathy is characterized by progressive weakness and sensory loss, reaching a nadir within 4 weeks of symptom onset. Weakness is both distal and proximal. Tendon reflexes are absent, or at least distal reflexes are absent and proximal reflexes are reduced. Supportive laboratory findings include ele-

vated cerebrospinal fluid protein in association with a mild elevation of white blood cells, usually less but occasionally more than five cells. These spinal fluid findings occur in most but not all patients, and they may not be apparent early in the course of the disease (Ropper et al., 1991). Variants of AIDP with focal involvement, such as pure motor, pharyngeal-cervical-brachial, and pure pandysautonomia, may be challenging to recognize clinically as demyelinating polyradiculoneuropathy (Ropper et al., 1991). AIDP is a monophasic immune-mediated neuropathy preceded by an acute infectious illness in two thirds of patients. There is a high association with *Campylobacter jejuni* gastroenteritis, with strong evidence of molecular mimicry between epitopes on the bacterium and peripheral nerve to account for pathological damage to myelin (Hartung et al., 1995). The degree of myelin and axon damage varies, and it results in weakness ranging from mild (difficulties with ambulation) to severe (requiring ventilator support). The short-term outcome can be improved by treatment with plasma exchange (two to four exchanges) or intravenous immune globulin (2 g/kg) administered within 2 weeks of symptom onset (The Guillain-Barré Syndrome Study Group, 1985; van der Meché et al., 1992; Hartung et al., 1995). The long-term outcome depends on the severity, with good recovery following mild weakness and with residual weakness in patients requiring ventilatory support (Visser et al., 1999; Fletcher et al., 2000).

Acute Motor and Sensory Axonal Neuropathy

A severe variant of Guillain-Barré syndrome referred to as *axonal Guillain-Barré syndrome* (Feasby et al., 1986), and now called *acute motor and sensory axonal neuropathy* (AMSAN), has a fulminant course leading to limb paralysis and respiratory failure over several days. These patients have high morbidity rates from medical complications associated with prolonged ventilatory support and hospitalization (Ropper et al., 1991). Recovery is slow and incomplete despite treatment with plasma exchange and intravenous immune globulin.

Table 58–1. Proposed Relationship Among Forms of Guillain-Barré Syndrome

Guillain-Barré Syndrome			
Acute demyelinating pattern (AIDP)	Fisher's syndrome (variant of AIDP)	Acute axonal motor and sensory pattern	Acute axonal motor pattern
⇓			
Increasing severity of immune attack			
⇓			
Secondary axonal damage			

Modified from Griffin J, Li C, Ho T, et al.: Pathology of the motor-sensory axonal Guillain-Barré syndrome. Ann Neurol 1996;39:17–28.

Acute Motor Axonal Neuropathy

A unique form of Guillain-Barré syndrome, called *acute motor axonal neuropathy* (AMAN), has been described most frequently in northern China, but a similar neuropathy is described outside of China (McKhann et al., 1993). It is characterized by rapid onset of severe weakness suggesting axonal disease, but prognosis is better than in AMSAN, a finding indicating a different disorder. Acute motor axonal neuropathy has a higher incidence in the summer and is strongly associated with *C. jejuni* infections. Treatment is supportive, and recovery is remarkably good (McKhann et al., 1993).

Fisher's Syndrome

Fisher's syndrome classically includes the triad of ophthalmoplegia, ataxia, and areflexia, with little clinical weakness (Fisher, 1956). Prognosis is usually good, with complete recovery without treatment. However, the triad can represent an early distribution of symptoms that progresses to an acute inflammatory demyelinating polyradiculoneuropathy pattern of weakness (Ropper et al., 1991). In these patients, the degree of weakness and recovery is proportional to the degree of axonal damage. Fisher's syndrome is associated with unique antibodies to the GQ 1b ganglioside found in both nerves and the cerebellum, a feature that likely accounts for the spectrum of symptoms of neuropathy and ataxia (Kornberg et al., 1996; Kusunoki et al., 1999). Treatment of classic Fisher's syndrome or in association with limb involvement has not been formally studied, but plasma exchange and intravenous immune globulin have been effective (Ropper et al., 1991).

The acute nature of Guillain-Barré syndrome helps to exclude many other forms of peripheral neuropathy. However, the varied presentations of Guillain-Barré syndrome should open the differential diagnosis to include central nervous system, infectious, and toxic causes of acute symptoms (Ropper et al., 1991). From the neurophysiological perspective, other causes of acute motor and sensory neuropathy include electrophysiological evidence of segmental demyelination, and these conditions should be considered in the differential diagnosis (Donofrio and Albers, 1990). Among them are acute neuropathies from arsenic, amiodarone, glue sniffing, and acquired immunodeficiency.

Chronic Inflammatory Demyelinating Polyradiculoneuropathy

Acute and chronic inflammatory demyelinating polyradiculoneuropathies have similar clinical neurophysiological features, but they are different disorders (chronic inflammatory demyelinating polyra-diculoneuropathy is not chronic Guillain-Barré syndrome). By definition, symptoms of chronic inflammatory demyelinating polyradiculoneuropathy progress over at least a 2-month period. The natural time course is prolonged and includes relapses and remissions, steady progression, and stepwise disease progression (Dyck et al., 1975). However, remissions and relapses are more commonly the result of changes in immunosuppressive medication regimens. Clinical diagnostic criteria are available that include sets of neurophysiological criteria (Ad Hoc Subcommittee of the American Academy of Neurology, 1991). CIDP is characterized by weakness involving both distal and proximal muscles and symptoms of sensory loss. Tendon reflexes are reduced or absent. Supportive laboratory findings are elevated cerebrospinal fluid protein with less than 10 white blood cells. The diagnostic criteria are guidelines, and clinical variants of chronic inflammatory demyelinating polyradiculoneuropathy occur. CIDP is generally considered to be a symmetrical disorder in distribution of symptoms and signs, but it may be more focal in onset, and the demyelinating nature may be challenging to determine (Thomas et al., 1996).

The most common laboratory-based variant is chronic inflammatory demyelinating polyradiculoneuropathy with *monoclonal gammopathy of uncertain significance* (MGUS). Rarely, CIDP may be the presenting symptom of plasma cell dyscrasias (osteosclerotic myeloma, multiple myeloma, and Waldenström's macroglobulinemia) (Kelly, 1985). Because clinical signs of these disorders may not be apparent, serum immunofixation and urine electrophoresis should be performed as part of the evaluation when CIDP is diagnosed (Bromberg et al., 1992).

Chronic inflammatory demyelinating polyradiculoneuropathy and its variants respond to numerous treatment modalities. However, many patients require a combination of treatment modalities, and the selection of modalities and doses must be tailored to the individual patient. The primary therapies of plasma exchange, corticosteroids (prednisone), and intravenous immune globulin have been demonstrated to be efficacious in randomized controlled trials. Plasma exchange (two to three times per week until improvement is established, then tapered over months) induces a temporary improvement in most patients (Dyck et al., 1986; Hahn et al., 1996a). Patients who do not respond to plasma exchange or who are unstable in their response and require frequent exchanges need immunosuppressive therapy. Prednisone alone (120 mg orally q.o.d. for 1 week, followed by a taper to 0 mg over 3 months) results in clinical improvement (Dyck et al., 1982). Prednisone in lower doses (60 mg orally q.d. followed by a taper over months) is used as adjuvant therapy with plasma exchange. Intravenous immune globulin (in varying doses and regimens from 0.4 g/kg weekly for several weeks, to 2 g/kg over 2 days followed by 1 g/kg at 3 weeks, to 2 g/kg in divided doses over 5 days) is also effective (Dyck et al., 1994; Hahn et al., 1996b; Mendell et al., 2001).

Both the short-term (initial) and the long-term (years) responses to treatment are good, but CIDP and its variants remain chronic disorders, and some symptoms and signs may persist despite treatment (Simmons et al., 1993; Simmons et al., 1995). Patients with CIDP who have monoclonal gammopathy of uncertain significance experience a smaller degree of improvement, but they are generally less severely impaired (Simmons et al., 1995). Children with CIDP respond to plasma exchange, corticosteroids, and intravenous immune globulin, but with a long-term prognosis that is generally better than that in adults (Simmons et al., 1997a; Simmons et al., 1997b).

Distal Acquired Demyelinating Symmetrical Neuropathy

Distal acquired demyelinating symmetrical neuropathy is a chronic neuropathy that has been distinguished from classic CIDP based on clinical symptoms and signs and laboratory findings (Katz et al., 2000). As in CIDP, there is evidence of demyelination, but sensory symptoms in a symmetrical distribution predominate, and weakness is found in distal muscles in a length-dependent fashion. Furthermore, there is a high incidence of a monoclonal protein (most frequently the immunoglobulin M class) and antibodies reactive against myelin-associated glycoprotein (anti-MAG antibodies). Treatment responses from uncontrolled trials suggest that plasma exchange, prednisone, and immune globulin may be effective, but less so among patients with distal acquired demyelinating symmetrical neuropathy who have a monoclonal protein (Katz et al., 2000; Saperstein et al., 2001).

Multifocal Motor Neuropathy

Multifocal motor neuropathy is a rare and unique neuropathy characterized by focal motor nerve conduction block at sites away from common points of entrapment (Lewis et al., 1982; Parry and Clarke, 1988; Pestronk et al., 1988). Despite focal weakness, little or no sensory involvement occurs at sites of conduction block. Nerves and sites in which focal conduction block occurs with high frequency include the ulnar and median nerves and less so the tibial and peroneal nerves. Conduction block may occur proximally, in the brachial plexus, and occasionally in the cranial nerves (Kaji et al., 1992; Katz et al., 1997). Multifocal motor neuropathy is a chronic disease, generally with slow progression. Clinically, there is usually little muscle atrophy despite considerable weakness. Muscle cramps and fasciculations can occur in involved muscles. Multifocal motor neuropathy is sometimes confused with amyotrophic lateral sclerosis, but a distinguishing feature is reduced or tendon reflexes in affected

regions. Antibodies to GM1 gangliosides are frequently elevated in multifocal motor neuropathy (high antibody titers are uncommon in other disorders), and their presence is helpful in making the diagnosis (Pestronk et al., 1988; Pestronk, 1998). Treatment is unique in that prednisone and plasma exchange are generally not effective, and patients have shown clinical deterioration (Pestronk et al., 1988). Intravenous immune globulin (initial treatment 0.4 g/kg for 5 days) has been shown to be effective in randomized controlled trials (Federico et al., 2000). Multifocal motor neuropathy is a chronic disease, and despite the requirement for long-term therapy with immune globulin, there may be a slow deterioration of function (Taylor et al., 2000).

The issue of sensory involvement with multifocal motor nerve conduction block is controversial (Parry, 1999). A distinction has been proposed, with multifocal motor neuropathy defined as an entity without clinical or neurophysiological sensory involvement. *Multifocal acquired demyelinating sensory and motor neuropathy* (also referred to as Lewis-Sumner syndrome) is a newly determined entity defined as having both prominent motor conduction block and evidence of demyelination in sensory nerves, as well as the rare occurrence of anti–GM1 gangliosides (Saperstein et al., 1999). Therapeutic implications for this separation have been raised because multifocal acquired demyelinating sensory and motor neuropathy may be responsive to prednisone, in contradistinction to multifocal motor neuropathy, which is not responsive. However, the separation of these two entities has not been resolved (Lewis, 1999).

PATHOLOGICAL FINDINGS

General Findings

Pathological changes in demyelinating polyradiculoneuropathies are believed to be immune-mediated destruction of myelin at multiple sites along nerve roots and nerves. Specific information is sparse and largely inferential, based on autopsy cases, nerve biopsies, and experimental allergic animal models. This section presents an overview of pathological changes to provide a basis for understanding the neurophysiological changes, and vice versa, and to provide an understanding of what neurophysiological changes to look for to demonstrate demyelinating disease. This discussion focuses on the pathological changes and does not consider immunological mechanisms.

Sites of demyelination are focal in distribution, including roots and spinal nerves, peripheral nerves, and intramuscular branches (Ropper et al., 1991). Destructive processes involve loss of myelin, but Schwann cell nuclei and basement membranes remain intact, to allow for remyelination. During remyelination, Schwann cell nuclei proliferate, leading to shorter myelin internode lengths (Kimura, 1989).

The immunological processes of demyelination may result in secondary axonal damage that will slow the restoration of nerve conduction.

Acute Inflammatory Demyelinating Polyradiculoneuropathy

Most information on the pathological processes in AIDP is from autopsy studies of affected patients dying at different intervals after symptom onset and from experimental allergic neuritis (Ropper et al., 1991; Arnason and Soliven, 1993). Gross inspection of nerves is unremarkable. Perivenular cellular infiltrates are distributed randomly in cranial nerves, dorsal and ventral roots, plexuses, peripheral nerves, and intramuscular nerve branches. Sympathetic nerves and ganglia may be involved. The belief was that roots were preferentially involved, but detailed study of peripheral nerves indicates diffuse involvement.

Infiltrates on microscopic inspection are observed around endoneural vessels, primarily small veins. Infiltrates consist of lymphocytes and macrophages. These changes are observed within days of symptom onset. Macrophages are important in myelin destruction, and they increase in numbers over several weeks. Segmental demyelination is found adjacent to the area of inflammation. Data from experimental allergic neuritis indicate early retraction of myelin at the nodes of Ranvier. This process leads to a separation of myelin lamellae and the formation of myelin ovoids. Macrophages are involved in these processes, including removal of myelin debris. Denuded axons are observed in association with Schwann cell nuclei and intact basement membranes. Axonal damage can be observed at sites of intense inflammation in association with polymorphonuclear lymphocytes. This finding supports the concept that axonal damage is a secondary or bystander effect.

Nerve biopsy data, primarily from sensory nerves (sural nerve), show patchy demyelination in about half the nerves studied (Dyck et al., 1975). Nerves that have normal nerve conduction values are usually normal at biopsy.

Acute Motor and Sensory Axonal Neuropathy

Controversy surrounds the entity of *primary axonal acute motor and sensory polyradiculoneuropathies* (Dyck, 1993; Feasby, 1994; Yuki, 1994). The neurophysiological findings of inexcitable motor and sensory nerves may be accounted for by primary axonal damage or distal conduction block with or without secondary axonal damage (Brown et al., 1993). The clinical outcome of fulminant Guillain-Barré syndrome varies from poor recovery supporting early and severe axonal involvement, to intermediate recovery supporting a mixture of conduction block and secondary axonal damage, to good recovery supporting primary conduction block (Triggs et al., 1992). From the neurophysiological perspective, it is not possible to correlate electrophysiological findings with disease accurately at the time of diagnosis. It is reasonable to consider fulminant cases of Guillain-Barré syndrome as representing a spectrum of pathological involvement with demyelination and axonal damage (see Table 58–1) (Dyck, 1993; Griffin et al., 1996).

Acute Motor Axonal Neuropathy

This unique form of Guillain-Barré syndrome is characterized by a severe degree of motor weakness and widespread denervation on neurophysiological testing, yet it has a good prognosis (McKhann et al., 1993). Autopsy findings do not fully explain the clinical or neurophysiological findings. Pathological changes in cases of severe weakness with death from 5 to 12 days from symptom onset include wallerian-like degeneration of ventral roots, but essentially normal dorsal roots and sensory nerves (Griffin et al., 1995). Rare internodal demyelination and widening of the internodal space are observed. The pathological changes are modest compared with the degree of weakness. Possible explanations for this discrepancy include conduction block resulting from paranodal demyelination or antibody binding or degeneration of motor nerve terminals (Ho et al., 1997). Evidence of intramuscular changes comes from motor point muscle biopsy specimens, in which terminal degeneration has been observed (Ho et al., 1997).

Chronic Inflammatory Demyelinating Polyradiculoneuropathy

Chronic inflammatory demyelinating polyradiculoneuropathy is a chronic disease, and nerve biopsy and autopsy samples are obtained at markedly different times during the natural and treatment-modulated course of the disease. Autopsy samples show patchy groups of mononuclear cells in roots, in dorsal root ganglia and pia arachnoid matter, and occasionally in proximal nerve segments (Dyck et al., 1975; Dyck et al., 1993). Changes in the spinal cord include loss of fibers in the dorsal column and lateral columns and loss of anterior horn cells. Nerve roots and peripheral nerves show a loss of large-diameter fibers. Sural nerve biopsy specimens show perivascular mononuclear cells in the epineurium and endoneurium and edema between the endoneurium and perineurium. Onion bulb formations are also observed, but infrequently. Teased fiber preparations show segmental demyelination, linear rows of myelin ovoids, and segmental remyelination with internodes, with myelin of varying thickness and frequent evidence of wallerian degeneration and regeneration of fibers (Bouchard et al., 1999).

Multifocal Motor Neuropathy

Multifocal motor neuropathy is a challenging disorder to define pathologically, because lesions are very focal and largely confined to motor nerves. Peripheral nerve enlargement has been observed on magnetic resonance imaging studies (Kaji et al., 1993; Van den Berg-Vos et al., 2000). Biopsies of involved nerve segments show inflammation (Van den Berg-Vos et al., 2000), scattered demyelinated axons with onion bulb formations, and relatively little axonal loss (Auer et al., 1989; Kaji et al., 1993). Sensory nerve biopsies in the proposed entity of multifocal acquired demyelinating sensory and motor neuropathy include fiber loss and demyelination-remyelination in teased fiber preparations (Saperstein et al., 1999).

NEUROPHYSIOLOGICAL PRINCIPLES IN DEMYELINATION

Myelinated nerve fibers conduct by saltatory conduction, in which the nerve impulse moves rapidly along internodal segments and undergoes a slower regenerative process at nodes of Ranvier. The rate of conduction is proportional to fiber diameter and internode length, and larger-diameter axons are associated with longer internode lengths (Kimura, 1989). Whole nerves contain many nerve fibers and a range of fiber diameters, leading to a range of nerve fiber conduction velocities within a nerve. An important concept in assessing nerve conduction data is temporal dispersion of the response. During nerve conduction studies, all nerve fibers are activated by supramaximal electrical stimulation. This initiates a volley of nerve impulses moving along the nerve at different conduction velocities and arriving at the recording electrode at different times. This represents the normal temporal dispersion of the response. A measure of temporal dispersion is the duration of the negative peak of the *compound muscle action potential* (CMAP). The duration of dispersion will increase with longer conduction distances. One analogy is to consider nerve impulses as a group of runners that includes fast 6-minute milers, slow 7-minute milers, and a range of runners running at speeds in between. In a 1-mile race there will be a 1-minute temporal dispersion of the group, whereas over a 10-mile race there will be a 10-minute dispersion. In nerve conduction studies, normal temporal dispersion is tight. Motor nerve fibers have a conduction velocity range of approximately 13 m per second, and sensory nerve fibers have a range of approximately 25 m per second (Olney et al., 1987). Normal temporal dispersion of motor

nerves results in a less than 10% increase in compound muscle action potential duration over long distances with stimulation at Erb's point compared with stimulation at the wrist (Kimura, 1989).

Clinical neurophysiology assesses the state of a nerve by measures of the rate of conduction and the number of activated nerve fibers. Measures of conduction speed include distal latency, conduction velocity, F-wave latency, and negative peak duration. CMAP amplitude is a measure of the number of activated fibers. Most measures of conduction are of the largest and fastest conduction fibers. The remaining fibers contribute to the amplitude and duration of the response.

Nerve conduction tests in demyelinating neuropathies focus mainly on large myelinated motor nerves and less on sensory nerves. This results from the intrinsic properties of motor and sensory nerve recording arrangements. Motor responses are recorded as the CMAP, which represents the sum of muscle fiber action potentials in the innervated muscle. Muscle fibers serve as surrogates for recording directly from motor nerves, because the nerve innervating a muscle contains both motor efferent and motor afferent fibers that cannot be separated except by recording the efferent component from the muscle. The sensory response is recorded as the *sensory nerve action potential* (SNAP), which represents the sum of nerve fiber action potentials. The sensory component of a mixed nerve can be easily isolated from the motor component by recording electrode placement. SNAPs can be recorded from orthodromic or antidromic conduction. Both provide identical information, but antidromic responses are of higher amplitude because nerves are closer to the surface at distal locations (Kimura, 1989).

Both muscle and nerve fiber action potentials are primarily biphasic, with an initial negative phase followed by a positive phase. Muscle fiber action potentials have a duration of approximately 4 ms, whereas sensory nerve action potentials have a duration of less than 1 ms (Kimura, 1989). Temporal dispersion of arriving action potentials results in a shift of the initial negative phase of later action potentials so that they begin to arrive during the positive phase of the earlier arriving action potentials (Fig. 58–1). Because the CMAP and the SNAP represent the algebraic summation of action potentials, some degree of negative and positive cancellation will reduce the CMAP and SNAP amplitudes compared with simple summations (Kimura, 1989). This is called *phase cancellation*. The degree of phase cancellation depends on the duration of the negative and positive waveform components of the action potentials and the degree of temporal dispersion. Because of the short duration of sensory nerve action potentials and the greater range of conduction velocities of sensory nerve fibers, phase cancellation will affect sensory nerve action potential amplitude to a greater degree. The longer duration of muscle fiber action potentials and the narrow range of conduction velocities of motor nerve fibers will

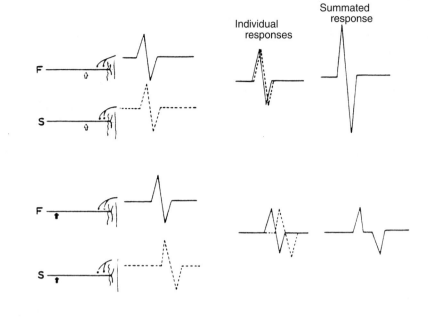

Figure 58–1. Schematic diagram showing the effect of temporal dispersion and phase cancellation with nerve conduction over longer distance. *Top,* Sensory nerve action potentials have short duration, and temporal dispersion from longer conduction distances is associated with marked phase cancellation that greatly reduces sensory nerve action potential amplitude. *Bottom,* Muscle fiber action potentials have longer duration, and temporal dispersion is associated with less marked phase cancellation with less of an effect on compound muscle action potential amplitude. (From Kimura J, Machida M, Ishida T, et al.: Relation between size of compound sensory or motor action potentials and length of nerve segment. Neurology 1986;36:647–652.)

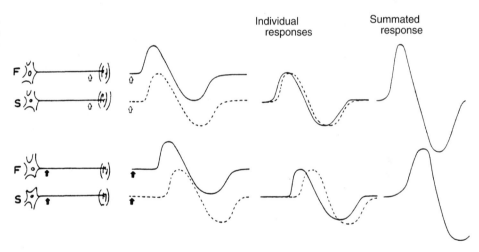

reduce CMAP amplitude to a lesser degree (Fig. 58–2 and see Fig. 58–1). The effects of temporal dispersion from conduction over long distances will therefore reduce SNAP amplitude more than compound muscle action potential amplitude, and the SNAP may be lost in bioelectric background noise when long conduction distances are involved (Kimura et al., 1986).

The neurophysiological changes following demyelination are an increase in capacitance across the internodal membrane and greater current leakage along the axon (Brown, 1984). This will change action potential propagation from saltatory conduction to slower continuous conduction along the demyelinated segments. Demyelination of paranodal regions may be more important because of the dis-

tribution of sodium and potassium ion channels. Demyelination exposes potassium channels in the paranodal axon and slows and reduces the degree of depolarization, a process leading to conduction block. Individual myelin segments may be affected in a discontinuous pattern along the nerve, with a resulting multifocal pattern of demyelination. It follows that more segments will be affected over longer lengths of the nerve. Demyelination of consecutive internodes increases the probability of blocked action potential propagation.

Nerve conduction changes expected in demyelinating neuropathies are slowed conduction and conduction block, and secondary axonal loss is common. These changes result in prolonged distal latency, slowed conduction velocity, abnormal tem-

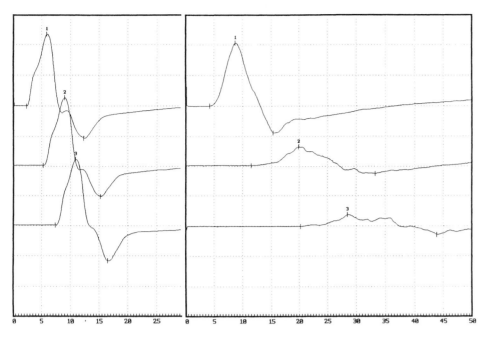

Figure 58–2. Motor nerve conduction waveforms in response to stimulation at the wrist, below the elbow, and above the elbow. *Left,* Normal change in compound muscle action potential amplitude and waveform. *Right,* Abnormal compound muscle action potential amplitude drop and change in waveform resulting from abnormal temporal dispersion in a patient with chronic inflammatory demyelinating polyradiculoneuropathy.

poral dispersion, conduction block, and prolonged F- and H-wave latencies. The degree of these changes will vary with the degree and distribution of demyelinating lesions. Specifically, the degree of conduction slowing depends on the involvement of large-diameter fibers, because measures of distal latencies and conduction velocity are based on the fastest fibers. Slowing of smaller-diameter fibers causes abnormal temporal dispersion. The effects of abnormal temporal dispersion are observed by comparing the CMAPs generated from proximal stimulation sites; there will be an increase in the negative peak duration, a greater loss of CMAP amplitude, and irregularities in the CMAP waveform (see Fig. 58–2).

Demyelinating neuropathies are to be compared with axonal neuropathies. Axonal neuropathies without demyelination will slow nerve conduction because of the loss of large-diameter fibers. The ability to distinguish between axonal and demyelinating neuropathies is based on "estimating a degree of slowing that is greater than expected for the degree of axonal loss." Clinical experience supports the principle that pure axonal neuropathies result in only mild conduction slowing. However, the limits of slowing attributable to axonal loss alone are estimates that have been derived empirically, and there are differences of opinion on the limits that distinguish primary demyelination from primary axonal loss. This has led to several sets of electrodiagnostic criteria for acute (Alam et al., 1998) and chronic inflammatory demyelinating polyradiculoneuropathy (Bromberg, 1991). The limits distinguishing primary demyelination from primary axonal neuropathies are based on laboratory limits of normal for the measures of compound muscle action potential distal latency, conduction velocity, and F-wave latency. The sets of criteria also require demonstration of abnormalities in several measures in two or more nerves. Some sets of criteria include adjustments based on the amplitude of the response to require a greater degree of slowing with more axonal loss.

There are separate criteria for neuropathies with focal conduction block (Lange et al., 1992). Conduction block is recognized by a lower CMAP amplitude and area following stimulation proximal to the block than the amplitude and area of the response following stimulation distal to the block. The obvious technical factor of submaximal stimulation at the proximal stimulation site must be considered, as well as the anatomical features of anomalous innervation. Another cause of reduced CMAP amplitude to proximal stimulation is abnormal temporal dispersion and phase cancellation (Rhee et al., 1990). The degree of abnormal temporal dispersion is proportional to the number of demyelinated segments and the length of nerve between the distal and proximal stimulation sites. The optimal distance to show focal conduction block and to minimize the effects of abnormal temporal dispersion is about 4 cm (Cornblath et al., 1991). Distinguishing between pure conduction block and abnormal temporal dispersion is aided by considering not only compound muscle action potential amplitude changes between proximal and distal stimulation sites but also negative peak CMAP area and duration changes (Olney et al., 1987; Oh et al., 1994). Relative preservation of negative peak CMAP area with prolongation of negative peak duration favors abnormal temporal dispersion, whereas reduction of negative peak area and relative preservation of negative peak duration favor conduction block. Many neuropathies include a combination of conduction block and abnormal temporal dispersion, and an accurate distinction between the two may not be clinically important. An

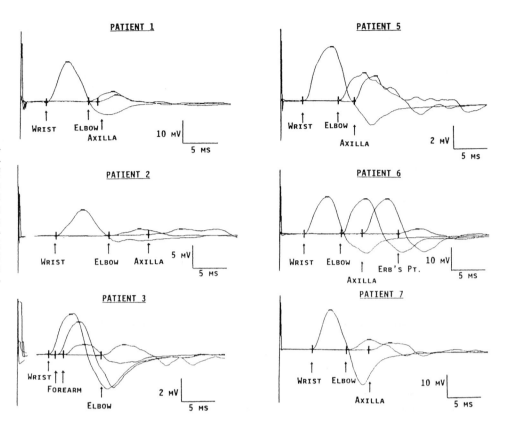

Figure 58–3. Motor nerve conduction waveforms showing focal conduction block. Sites of stimulation are marked with *arrows*. Sites of conduction block may be distal (forearm in patient 3) or proximal (between the axilla and Erb's point in patient 6). (From Chaudhry V, Corse A, Cornblath D, et al.: Multifocal motor neuropathy: Electrodiagnostic features. Muscle Nerve 1994;17:198–205.)

exception is distinguishing between CIDP and multifocal motor neuropathy. In multifocal motor neuropathy, the CMAP amplitude change occurs focally, with little evidence of abnormal temporal dispersion (Fig. 58–3). In CIDP, the length-dependent drop in proximal CMAP amplitude is progressive at more proximal stimulation sites, and there is associated evidence of abnormal temporal dispersion (see Fig. 58–2).

One clinical condition that could be mistaken for multifocal motor neuropathy or chronic inflammatory demyelinating polyradiculoneuropathy is *hereditary neuropathy with liability of pressure palsies* (HNPP). HNPP is a genetic disorder associated with deletions in the peripheral myelin protein 22 (PMP 22) gene on chromosome 17 (Chance et al., 1993), but it also occurs without a deletion (Amato et al., 1996). This disorder is characterized by prolonged distal latencies in a diffuse distribution and focal conduction block, most frequently at common sites of nerve entrapment (Gouider et al., 1995; Amato et al., 1996; Andersson et al., 2000).

NEUROPHYSIOLOGICAL FINDINGS IN DEMYELINATING POLYNEUROPATHIES

Neurophysiological identification of primary demyelination in acute and chronic inflammatory demyelinating polyradiculoneuropathies is based on empirical observations. The various forms of Guil-lain-Barré syndrome have unique electrophysiological characteristics that help one to distinguish among them. The diagnostic issue in CIDP is obtaining evidence of primary demyelination, in contradistinction to primary axonal neuropathy. This section reviews the various sets of electrophysiological criteria and their sensitivity and specificity.

Acute Inflammatory Demyelinating Polyradiculoneuropathy

Acute inflammatory demyelinating polyradiculoneuropathy is characterized by slowed motor nerve conduction values, including prolonged distal latency, slow nerve conduction velocity, and prolonged F-wave latency. At least six sets of neurophysiological criteria have been proposed to aid in the diagnosis (Albers et al., 1985; Albers and Kelly, 1989; Cornblath, 1990; Ho et al., 1995; Meulstee et al., 1995; The Italian Guillain-Barré Study Group, 1996). Two representative sets are shown in Table 58–2. The various sets are similar in that they focus on detecting certain measures of slowed conduction away from entrapment sites, and they require abnormalities in two or more nerves. They differ in the limiting values needed to distinguish primary demyelination and the number of abnormal nerves required. Limiting nerve conduction values are based on exceeding a percentage of the upper limits of normal for distal latency and F-wave latency or being less than a percentage of the lower limit of normal for

Table 58–2. Two Sets of Neurophysiological Criteria for Acute Inflammatory Demyelinating Polyradiculoneuropathy*

Criteria A from Albers et al. Demonstrate at least one of the following abnormalities in two or more nerves.		Criteria B from Cornblath. Demonstrate at least three of the following abnormalities in two or more nerves.		
Conduction velocity	*Amp >50% LLN* <95% LLN	*Amp <50% LLN* <85% LLN	*Amp >80% LLN* <80% LLN	*Amp <80% LLN* <70% LLN	Two or more nerves
Distal latency	*Amp >LLN* >110% ULN	*Amp <LLN* >120% ULN	*Amp >80% LLN* >125% ULN	*Amp <LLN* >150% ULN	Two or more nerves
Temporal dispersion	Dispersion or P:D Amp ratio <.7		Dispersion or partial conduction block		One or more nerves
F-wave latency	>120% ULN		*Amp >80% LLN* >120% ULN	*Amp <80% LLN* >150% ULN	Two or more nerves

*Exceptions include abnormalities at common sites of nerve entrapment and anomalous innervation.

Amp, amplitude; LLN, lower limits of normal; ULN, upper limits of normal.

Criteria A from Albers J, Donofrio P, McGonagle T: Sequential electrodiagnostic abnormalities in acute inflammatory demyelinating polyradiculoneuropathy. Muscle Nerve 1985;8:528–539; criteria B from Cornblath D: Electrophysiology in Guillain-Barré syndrome. Ann Neurol 1990;27(suppl):S17–S20.

conduction velocity and the proximal-to-distal CMAP amplitude ratio.

A comparison of six sets of criteria on data from 43 patients with AIDP recorded an average of 13.4 days from symptom onset indicates considerable differences in sensitivity among the six sets of criteria (Alam et al., 1998). The highest fulfillment value was 72% for set A in Table 58–2, and the lowest value was 21% for set B. A separate evaluation of patients less than 18 years old revealed a slightly higher percentage of children who fulfilled diagnostic criteria.

The evolution of neurophysiological changes has been studied by evaluating data from patients with a firm clinical diagnosis of AIDP. In a review using set A in Table 58–2, the time course of neurophysiological abnormalities in 70 patients was assessed by serial studies timed from symptom onset (Albers et al., 1985). Table 58–3 shows that during the first 2 weeks, 50% of patients fulfill criteria, whereas 38% are indeterminate. At 3 weeks, the criteria are the most sensitive, with 85% fulfilling criteria. Conduction abnormalities partially resolve between weeks 4 and 25, but 20% to 25% of patients remain sufficiently abnormal at 1 year to fulfill criteria.

On needle electromyography, reduced motor unit recruitment is the earliest neurophysiological change, occurring in both proximal and distal muscles, and it was found in all patients at the time of initial examination (Albers et al., 1985). The interpretation of reduced recruitment is fewer numbers of motor fibers conducting to the muscle because of blocked conduction. Other electromyographic abnormalities are frequently recorded in AIDP. Abnormal spontaneous activity (fibrillation potentials and positive waves) appears between weeks 2 and 4 simultaneously in distal and proximal muscles. Spontaneous activity is the most profuse between weeks 6 and 10 for proximal muscles and between weeks 11 and 15 for distal muscles. Motor unit complexity (polyphasia) is observed between weeks 9 and 15. Motor unit abnormalities resolve slowly over a time course of 1 to 3 years.

Unusual needle electromyography findings have been observed in AIDP. Myokymic discharges can be recorded as a transient phenomenon during the first 3 weeks. Electrical discharges have been recorded in muscles with and without clinical myokymia (Albers et al., 1985).

A review of motor nerve conduction abnormalities has been made to determine which is the most commonly abnormal in AIDP. Data from 210 patients tested within 30 days of symptom onset (75% within the first 15 days) indicate that an abnormal F-wave latency is the most common abnormality (46%), followed by distal motor latency (40%), proximal-to-distal CMAP ratio (30%), conduction velocity (24%), and CMAP amplitude (20%) (Cornblath et al., 1988).

Sensory nerve conduction studies are less informative for primary demyelination for several reasons. Sensory nerve responses are less homogeneously affected than motor nerve responses, and they may be normal in some nerves and absent in others (Albers et al., 1985). An absent response provides no information on whether underlying disease is demyelinating with conduction block or

Table 58–3. Percentage of Patients with Acute Inflammatory Demyelinating Polyradiculoneuropathy Fulfilling Neurodiagnostic Criteria in Set A at Various Time Periods from Symptom Onset (Data from 80 Patients)

Weeks from Symptom Onset	1 (%)	2 (%)	3 (%)	4 (%)	5 (%)	6–25 (%)	36–50 (%)
Yes	50	50	85	68	63	63	20–25
No	12	28	7.5	16	11	16–33	50–80
Indeterminate	38	28	7.5	16	26	21	0–25

Modified from Albers J, Donofrio P, McGonagle T: Sequential electrodiagnostic abnormalities in acute inflammatory demyelinating polyradiculoneuropathy. Muscle Nerve 1985;8:528–539.

axonal. However, a pattern of sensory nerve abnormalities has been observed in demyelinating neuropathies, in the form of an abnormal median and normal sural response (Murray and Wade, 1980; Albers et al., 1985). The sensitivity of this pattern for demyelination was assessed in a comparison of different neuropathies. The abnormal median and normal sural response pattern was more common in primary demyelinating neuropathies (39% in AIDP and 28% in CIDP compared with 23% in mild diabetic neuropathy and 22% in amyotrophic lateral sclerosis) (Bromberg and Albers, 1993). The opposite pattern, a normal median and abnormal sural response, was rare in demyelinating neuropathies (3% in AIDP and 7% in CIDP) and more common in mild diabetic neuropathy (18%). An explanation is a predilection in demyelinating neuropathies for involvement of distal sensory nerve segments. The typical sural nerve recording electrode arrangement picks up activity from more proximal nerve segments, whereas the typical digital ring recording electrodes for the median nerve picks up activity from more distal nerve segments. In support of this length-dependent pattern is a normal radial sensory response recorded at the snuff box and an abnormal median response recorded at the digit (Fraser, 1994).

Cranial nerves are affected in many patients with AIDP, and the seventh nerve is weak in approximately 50% at an early stage of the disease (Ropper et al., 1991). Cranial nerve involvement can be assessed by facial nerve conduction studies of the seventh nerve and blink reflex studies that measure conduction over the fifth and seventh cranial nerves and brainstem synaptic connections between them (Kimura, 1989). The direct facial nerve response latency is prolonged in up to 80% of patients (Kimura, 1971). Blink reflexes are prolonged in approximately half the patients with AIDP in association with clinical facial weakness (Kimura, 1971; Ropper et al., 1991).

Neurophysiology can also be used for prognosis. In a review of 210 patients who received standardized neurophysiological testing, multivariate analysis of motor nerve measures revealed that average CMAP amplitude is the most predictive measure of long-term clinical outcome (Cornblath et al., 1988). Average CMAP amplitude, expressed as a percentage of the lower limit of normal for a nerve, is calculated as the sum of individual CMAP values divided by the number of nerves tested. Average CMAP amplitudes less than 20% of the lower limit of normal are associated with a markedly increased probability of a poor outcome. Low CMAP amplitude is thought to reflect axonal loss. However, distal conduction block can also produce low CMAP amplitudes, and low average amplitude does not preclude a good clinical outcome.

Acute inflammatory demyelinating polyradiculoneuropathy also occurs in children, and clinical and electrophysiological evaluation can be challenging. A review of 43 children (many less than 3 years old) revealed that during the first week after symptom onset, a prolonged F-wave latency was the most common abnormality (88%), followed by prolonged distal latency (75%) and motor slowed conduction velocity (50%) (Delanoe et al., 1998). Later in the course of the disease, reduced CMAP amplitude was observed in all patients, with the lowest average values at 3 weeks. Conduction velocities continue to fall and reach the lowest values at 5 weeks. The median sensory nerve was more often abnormal than the sural nerve. From these data, specific electrophysiological criteria for children have been proposed (Table 58–4). When these criteria are applied retrospectively, 90% of children fulfill them (Delanoe et al., 1998). This criteria set includes both motor and sensory nerve conduction testing.

The typical pattern of disease progression in AIDP is symmetrical ascending paralysis. The sets of neurophysiological criteria discussed assume a generalized pathological process, with multiple nerves involved and available for testing. However, some AIDP variants begin focally and remain localized, including pharyngeal-cervical-brachial and paraparetic limb weakness (Ropper, 1986). In these rare examples, only regionally involved nerves have nerve conduction abnormalities supportive of primary demyelination.

Table 58–4. Motor and Sensory Nerve Conduction Criteria for the Diagnosis of Acute Inflammatory Demyelinating Polyradiculoneuropathy in Children*

Motor and sensory conduction velocities	*Amp >80% LLN* <80% LLN	*Amp <80% LLN* <70% LLN	Two or more nerves
Motor distal latency	*Amp >80% LLN* >125% ULN	*Amp <LLN* >150% ULN	Two or more nerves
Motor conduction block	>20% amp with <15% duration increase		Two or more nerves
Motor temporal dispersion	>15% duration increase		Two or more nerves
F-wave latency	*Amp >20% LLN* >120% ULN or absent response		Two or more nerves
Motor and sensory nerve amplitudes	Reduced amplitudes to >20%		Two or more nerves

*Demonstrate at least four abnormal variables in three nerves (at least two motor nerves and one sensory nerve).
Amp, amplitude; LLN, lower limits of normal; ULN, upper limits of normal.
Modified from Delanoe C, Sebire G, Landrieu P, et al.: Acute inflammatory demyelinating polyradiculopathy in children: Clinical and electrodiagnostic studies. Ann Neurol 1998;44:350–356.

Acute Motor and Sensory Axonal Neuropathy

The concept of an axonal form of Guillain-Barré syndrome arose from descriptions of acute weakness developing over 5 to 9 days associated with inexcitable motor nerves, reduced or absent sensory nerve responses, and profuse and widespread fibrillation potentials within 2 to 3 weeks (Feasby et al., 1986). The poor prognosis of these patients argues for severe axonal loss. Severe axonal loss may be a primary pathological process or secondary to an inflammatory-demyelinative process (Feasby et al., 1993). However, early in the course of AIDP distal conduction block occurs, as do fibrillation potentials. Accordingly, some patients with inexcitable motor nerves early in the course of the disease may follow a course of recovery more typical of AIDP than of acute motor and sensory axonal neuropathy (Triggs et al., 1992). For example, some motor nerves judged inexcitable after stimulation at routine distal stimulation sites (70 to 90 mm proximal to the motor point) may show a small response with more distal stimulation (Brown et al., 1993). Whether this small response reflects only conduction block or a combination of axonal degeneration and block cannot be determined neurophysiologically. The presence or absence of sensory responses does not enable one to distinguish between axonal degeneration and demyelination (van der Meché et al., 1991). An axonal form of Guillain-Barré syndrome, or acute motor and sensory axonal neuropathy (AMSAN), remains a controversial entity that cannot be readily resolved neurophysiologically at the initial study. It is more important to document the progressive loss of CMAP amplitude with serial studies. Severe secondary axonal loss can be best demonstrated by serial studies showing the progressive loss of CMAP amplitude (Triggs et al., 1992).

Acute Motor Axonal Neuropathy

Neurophysiological findings are reduced CMAP responses and normal sensory responses. Formal criteria to distinguish acute motor axonal neuropathy from *acute inflammatory demyelinating polyradiculoneuropathy* include finding no evidence of primary demyelination and compound muscle action potential amplitudes less than 80% of the lower limit of normal (Ho et al., 1995).

Fisher's Syndrome

Fisher's syndrome can be considered a variant of AIDP. As such, there will be a range of neurophysiological abnormalities. In pure Fisher's syndrome, neurophysiological studies show marked involvement of sensory nerves, with absent or reduced SNAP amplitude and mild slowing (Fross and Daube, 1987). Motor nerves show mild reduction in CMAP amplitude, mild prolongation of distal latency, and slowing of conduction velocity. There is evidence of axonal involvement on needle electromyography in cranial and limb muscles. Blink reflexes are absent or prolonged in half of these patients, a finding associated with reduced facial nerve responses. Patients who have both ophthalmoplegia and other signs of AIDP may have significant sensory nerve involvement, with absent sensory responses (Jacobs et al., 1997).

Chronic Inflammatory Demyelinating Polyradiculoneuropathy

Neurophysiological findings in *chronic inflammatory demyelinating polyradiculoneuropathy* are similar to those in AIDP. The chronic nature of CIDP means that patients will be evaluated at different times after symptom onset. The chronic nature also allows time for secondary axonal involvement, and many nerve responses may be absent. Absent responses do not provide information on the nature of the pathological process. As in AIDP, several sets of neurophysiological criteria have been proposed and compared for sensitivity. A comparison of three sets of criteria (Albers and Kelly, 1989; Barohn et al., 1989, Ad Hoc Subcommittee of the American Academy of Neurology AIDS Task Force, 1991) in 70 pa-

---

Table 58–5. Two Sets of Neurophysiological Criteria for Chronic Inflammatory Demyelinating Polyradiculoneuropathy*

Criteria A modified from Albers et al. Demonstrate three of the following abnormalities.			Criteria B modified from Barohn et al. Demonstrate the following abnormalities in two nerves.		
Conduction velocity	<75% LLN	Two or more nerves	Conduction velocity	<70% LLN	Two or more nerves
Distal latency	>130% ULN	Two or more nerves			
Temporal dispersion	Dispersion or P:D amp ratio <.7	One or more nerves			
F-wave latency	>130% ULN	One or more nerves			

*Exceptions include abnormalities at common sites of nerve entrapment and anomalous innervation.

Amp, amplitude; LLN, lower limits of normal; ULN, upper limits of normal.

Criteria A modified from Albers J, Kelly J: Acquired inflammatory demyelinating polyneuropathies: Clinical and electrodiagnostic features. Muscle Nerve 1989;12:435–451; criteria B modified from Barohn R, Kissel J, Warmolts J, Mendell J: Chronic inflammatory demyelinating polyradiculoneuropathy. Arch Neurol 1989;46:878–884.

tients with CIDP revealed sensitivities between 64% (set A in Table 58–5) and 43% (set B in Table 58–5) (Bromberg, 1991). One set of criteria made adjustments in the limits of conduction values based on CMAP amplitude, to account for natural slowing resulting from axonal loss (Ad Hoc Subcommittee of the American Academy of Neurology AIDS Task Force, 1991). Sensitivity was not improved by making adjustments. An exploration of the data was made to see how changes in the limiting values could affect sensitivity and specificity. Specificity was assessed by applying the sets of criteria to data from patients with mild diabetic neuropathy

(neuropathy with axonal and demyelinating features) and amyotrophic lateral sclerosis (neuropathy with primary axonal loss). Adjustments in the limiting values did not increase sensitivity for CIDP to higher than 66% without reducing specificity (Bromberg, 1991). The reason for an upper limit of 66% sensitivity is that nerve conduction values overlap among the three types of neuropathies (Fig. 58–4).

Chronic inflammatory demyelinating polyradiculoneuropathy variants are associated with several medical disorders, and differences in nerve conduction measures have been sought that would distin-

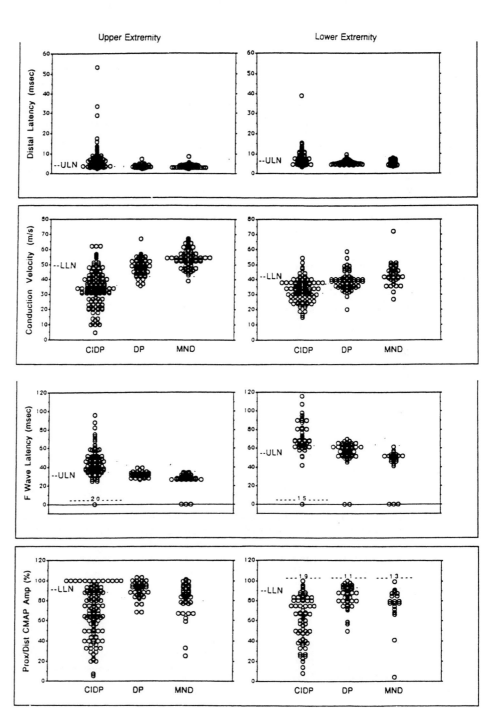

Figure 58–4. Distribution of values for motor nerve conduction measures. Values are for upper and lower extremity nerves. The *horizontal lines* at the *left* mark the upper and lower limits of normal (ULN and LLN, respectively). Values are from patients with chronic inflammatory demyelinating polyradiculoneuropathy (CIDP), diabetic polyneuropathy (DP), and motor neuron disease (MND). (From Bromberg M: Comparison of electrodiagnostic criteria for primary demyelination in chronic polyneuropathy. Muscle Nerve 1991; 14:968–976.)

guish or predict the presence of these disorders. The most common associated medical disorder is monoclonal gammopathy of uncertain significance. More patients with CIDP who do not have monoclonal gammopathy of uncertain significance than those with monoclonal gammopathy of uncertain significance fulfill neurophysiological criteria for primary demyelination, but the difference is not statistically significant (Bromberg et al., 1992). Comparisons of nerve conduction data from patients with CIDP and monoclonal gammopathy of uncertain significance reveal differences between immunoglobulin M and G gammopathies, but the differences are not clinically important (Gosselin et al., 1991). An interesting nerve conduction finding reported in some patients with immunoglobulin M monoclonal protein who also have antibodies against myelin-associated glycoprotein is a prolonged distal motor latency out of proportion to conduction velocity slowing measured along more proximal segments (Kaku et al., 1994). Focal distal slowing can be expressed as a terminal latency index, defined as distal conduction distance in millimeters/proximal conduction velocity in meters per second/distal motor latency in milliseconds (Shahani et al., 1979). This finding of prolonged distal motor latencies may be transient and can resolve when it is tested at a later time (Ponsford et al., 2000).

Nerve conduction studies in patients with CIDP who have associated plasma cell dyscrasias show various patterns, from primary demyelination to primary axonal features (Kelly, 1983). In one series, all patients with osteosclerotic myeloma fulfilled a set of neurophysiological criteria for primary demyelination, most patients with primary systemic amyloidosis fulfilled criteria for primary axonal loss, and patients with multiple myeloma had heterogeneous findings (Kelly, 1983).

Orthodromic mixed nerve responses have been studied in dysimmune neuropathies (CIDP without and with monoclonal gammopathy of uncertain significance). It is possible with orthodromic recording in the median and ulnar nerves along forearm segments to obtain information about sensory nerve conduction changes in demyelinating neuropathies, especially when distal sensory responses are reduced or absent. Findings in patients with CIDP are lower-amplitude mixed nerve responses and evidence of abnormal temporal dispersion (Luciano et al., 1995). Abnormal temporal dispersion is attributed to slowing of smaller sensory fibers, because motor nerve conduction velocities are believed to be too slow to contribute to the dispersed mixed nerve waveform.

Other variant forms of CIDP have been described. These include patients with focal involvement supported by demyelination on clinical neurophysiological studies of affected nerves and at biopsy and response to treatment (Midroni and Dyck, 1996). Thus, it is important to seek evidence of disproportionate conduction slowing, conduction block, and abnormal temporal dispersion in unusual clinical situations. Distal acquired demyelinating symmetrical polyneuropathy is characterized by prolonged distal latencies and low terminal latency index values, but the neurophysiological values are not distinguishable from those seen in CIDP (Katz et al., 2000).

Chronic Inflammatory Demyelinating Polyradiculoneuropathy Versus Hereditary Neuropathy

Hereditary neuropathies can be divided into two classes based on nerve conduction velocities (Dyck and Lambert, 1968a, 1968b). *Hereditary motor sensory neuropathy* (HMSN) or *Charcot-Marie-Tooth disease* (CMT) *type I* is considered to be a hypertrophic neuropathy associated with motor nerve conduction velocities less than 38 m per second. Hereditary motor sensory neuropathy or Charcot-Marie-Tooth disease type II is considered to be an axonal neuropathy with normal or near-normal conduction velocities (Harding and Thomas, 1980). Despite similar conduction velocity values in acquired and hereditary demyelinating neuropathies, neurophysiological features can help separate the two forms. In hereditary hypertrophic (type I) neuropathies, slowing is uniform along nerve fibers, resulting in slow conduction with normal temporal dispersion (Fig. 58–5) (Lewis and Sumner, 1982). This is in contrast

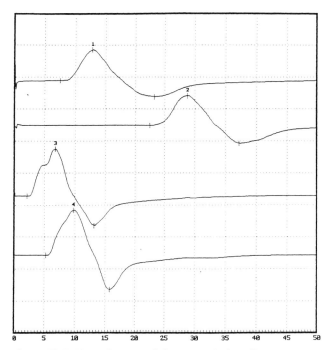

Figure 58–5. Normal temporal dispersion in hereditary neuropathy. *Top traces:* Charcot-Marie-Tooth disease type I with slow nerve conduction velocity (18 m per second) but normal amplitude change to proximal stimulation indicating normal temporal dispersion. *Bottom traces:* Normal subject showing similar amplitude change to proximal stimulation.

to CIDP, in which abnormal temporal dispersion and conduction block are observed. However, abnormal temporal dispersion can be observed in hereditary neuropathies when conduction velocities and CMAP amplitudes are extremely low (Lewis et al., 2000). Thus, it is important to review the family history and to look for clinical features of foot deformities.

Recognition of different types of hereditary neuropathy has led to genotype-neurophysiology comparisons. In X-linked Charcot-Marie-Tooth disease, motor and sensory nerve conduction velocities vary within affected males, and slow values are also recorded in many female carriers who may be asymptomatic (Nicholson and Nash, 1993). Detailed analysis of motor nerve conduction studies in both affected males and female carriers shows evidence of nonuniform demyelinating abnormalities that include abnormal temporal dispersion (Gutierrez et al., 2000). It is important to consider X-linked Charcot-Marie-Tooth disease in any patient with a slowly progressive, unexplained neuropathy (Tabaraud et al., 1999; Lewis, 2000).

In hereditary neuropathy with a predisposition to pressure palsies, neurophysiological findings include slowing at common sites of entrapment. However, reduced or absent sensory nerve responses, prolonged distal motor latencies and F-wave latencies, and nonuniform slowing are also observed (Gouider et al., 1995; Mouton et al., 1999; Lewis et al., 2000). Conduction block may also be present (Sellman and Mayer, 1987). Asymmetrical carriers as young as age 5 years usually show nerve conduction abnormalities (Gouider et al., 1995; Mouton et al., 1999). Comparisons of neurophysiological findings with CIDP reveal that hereditary neuropathy with liability of pressure palsies is associated with slow sensory nerve conduction velocity in a diffuse distribution and prolonged distal motor latencies with relatively minor slowing of conduction velocity (Andersson et al., 2000). Not all patients with hereditary neuropathy with liability of pressure palsies have deletions of the PMP-22 gene, but neurophysiological findings are indistinguishable (Amato et al., 1996).

Chronic Inflammatory Demyelinating Polyradiculoneuropathy and Diabetes Mellitus

Clinical data support an increased incidence of CIDP among patients with *diabetes mellitus* (Krendel et al., 1995). Fourteen patients with diabetes and neuropathy who fulfilled clinical and research criteria for CIDP (Albers and Kelly, 1989) were compared with 60 patients with idiopathic CIDP (Gorson et al., 2000). The 14 patients with diabetes and a CIDP-like neuropathy showed clinical improvement with treatment resembling that in patients with idiopathic CIDP, but the magnitude of the improvement

was less. Motor nerve conduction findings were similar between the two groups, but several features were noteworthy. There was a trend for average SNAP and CMAP amplitudes to be lower in the patients with diabetes. Conduction block was equally common in the patients with diabetes. Sural nerve responses were absent in all patients with diabetes compared with 41% of patients with CIDP. The degree of denervation on needle electromyography was similar. These findings indicate that patients with diabetes who have clinical features of a rapid loss of strength should be considered for an inflammatory neuropathy. An investigation with a set of nerve conduction criteria for CIDP can distinguish those who can respond to immunosuppressive therapy.

Multifocal Motor Neuropathy

Multifocal motor neuropathy is characterized by focal conduction block at multiple sites along a motor nerve, away from common entrapment sites (Pestronk et al., 1988). Identification of conduction block may be challenging, and there are technical considerations (Cornblath et al., 1991). Neurophysiological criteria to distinguish pure conduction block from apparent conduction block caused by abnormal temporal dispersion have been proposed (Table 58–6) (Lange et al., 1992). Concerns exist that patients with lesser degrees of conduction block may be misdiagnosed as not having multifocal motor neuropathy, and a dual set of neurophysiological criteria has been proposed to distinguish definite from probable conduction block (see Table 58–6) (Van den Berg-Vos et al., 2000). Many reported cases of multifocal motor neuropathy reveal features of diffuse demyelination and abnormal temporal dispersion as well as conduction block in illustrative waves (Pestronk et al., 1988; Lange et al., 1992; Chaudhry et al., 1994). Furthermore, there are patients who are considered to have clinical features of multifocal motor neuropathy but without neurophysiological evidence of focal motor conduction block (Katz et al., 1997; Pakiam and Parry, 1998). When conduction block is described, it is focal in distribution (over several centimeters), and sensory conduction across the same segment in the same nerve is normal (see Fig. 58–3). However, the proposed subtype of multifocal acquired demyelinating sensory and motor neuropathy includes sensory nerve conduction abnormalities (Saperstein et al., 1999). Certain nerves are more often involved, and they include ulnar and median more commonly than peroneal and tibial (Katz et al., 1997). Because motor neuropathy is multifocal, nerves on both sides of the body should be studied.

DIAGNOSTIC ALGORITHMS

Several sets of electrodiagnostic criteria have been proposed to aid in the diagnosis of AIDP and

Table 58–6. Neurophysiological Criteria to Distinguish Motor Nerve Conduction Block from Abnormal Temporal Dispersion from Submaximal Stimulation*

Criteria A modified from Lange et al.	Proximal CMAP amplitude	Proximal CMAP area	Proximal CMAP negative peak duration
Conduction block	<50%	<50%	≤30%
Conduction block or abnormal temporal dispersion	<50%	<50%	<30%
Temporal dispersion	<50%	>50%	<30%
Submaximal stimulation	<50%	<50%	≤30%
Criteria B from Van den Berg-Vos et al.	Distal CMAP amplitude	Proximal CMAP amplitude	
Definite conduction block	≥1 mV	≤50% over long segments ≤30% over short segments (2.5 cm)	
Probable conduction block	≥1 mV	≤30% over long segments	

*Changes in CMAP amplitude, negative peak area, and negative peak duration are from proximal stimulation sites compared with distal stimulation.
CMAP, compound muscle action potential.
Criteria A modified from Lange D, Trojaborg W, Latov N, et al.: Multifocal motor neuropathy with conduction block: Is it a distinct clinical entity? Neurology 1992;42:497–505; criteria B modified from Van den Berg-Vos R, Van den Berg L, Franssen H, et al.: Multifocal inflammatory demyelinating neuropathy: A distinct clinical entity? Neurology 2000;54:26–32.

CIDP. As discussed previously, diagnostic sensitivity varies markedly among sets for AIDP and CIDP, and it is not possible to design a set of neurophysiological criteria that will have both high sensitivity and high specificity (see Fig. 58–4). Two points to keep in mind are a clinical suspicion of a demyelinating neuropathy and an understanding of the neurophysiological features that support primary demyelination. What follows is an algorithmic approach to neurophysiological testing for the results of AIDP, AMSAN, CIDP, and multifocal motor neuropathy. The diagnostic criteria represent sets that have been tested for sensitivity for the respective neuropathies. However, these represent guidelines, and clinical interpretation is essential. It is assumed that routine recording techniques will be used, with attention to proper limb temperature, adequate stimulation intensity but without overstimulation that could activate neighboring nerves, and interpretation of results in the context of common sites of nerve entrapment and anomalous innervation patterns.

Acute Inflammatory Demyelinating Polyradiculoneuropathy

1. Sensory nerve studies:
   Record from the sural and digital median nerves.
   Assess for the pattern of involvement:
   Abnormal median and normal sural responses are supportive.
2. Motor nerve studies:
   Record from the peroneal, tibial, ulnar, and median nerves. AIDP is usually symmetrical, and sampling nerves on one side is usually sufficient. Stimulate the ulnar nerve proximally, including the axilla.
   Assess for the following abnormalities (two or more abnormalities in each of two nerves are supportive):
   Distal latency greater than 125% of the upper limits of normal

Conduction velocity less than 75% of the lower limits of normal
F-wave latency greater than 125% of the upper limits of normal
Proximal-to-distal amplitude ratio less than 50%
Proximal-to-distal negative peak duration ratio greater than 20%
Evidence of abnormal temporal dispersion in compound muscle action potential waveform shape
If the CMAP amplitude is low or absent from distal stimulation sites use inch stimulating electrode distally to determine whether the amplitude increases.
3. Blink reflex studies:
   Record blink reflexes.
   Assess R1 and R2 response latencies:
   Prolonged or absent R1 and R2 responses are supportive.
4. Needle electromyography study:
   Record from a distal and a proximal muscle in an arm and a leg.
   Assess for the following abnormalities:
   Abnormal spontaneous activity (fibrillation and positive wave potentials) indicating axonal involvement is supportive.
   Decreased motor unit recruitment with normal motor units (motor units larger in amplitude than expected) supports conduction block.

Acute Motor and Sensory Axonal Neuropathy

1. Sensory nerve studies:
   Record from the sural and digital median nerves.
   Assess for sensory nerve involvement:
   Low or absent responses are supportive.
2. Motor nerve studies:
   Record from the peroneal, tibial, ulnar, and me-

dian nerves. These disorders are usually symmetrical in distribution, and sampling nerves on one side is usually sufficient.

Assess for the following abnormalities:

Low or absent responses are supportive.

Lower values or values that remain low with repeat studies are supportive.

3. Needle electromyography study:

Record from a distal and a proximal muscle in an arm and a leg.

Assess for the following abnormalities:

Profuse, abnormal spontaneous activity (fibrillation and positive wave potentials) indicating axonal involvement is supportive.

Decreased or absent motor unit recruitment with normal motor units indicating conduction block or denervation is supportive.

Acute Motor Axonal Neuropathy

1. Sensory nerve studies:

Record from the sural and digital median nerves.

Assess for sensory nerve involvement:

Normal responses are supportive.

2. Motor nerve studies:

Record from the peroneal, tibial, ulnar, and median nerves. These disorders are usually symmetrical in distribution, and sampling nerves on one side is usually sufficient.

Assess for the following abnormalities:

Low or absent responses are supportive.

Lower values or values that remain low with repeat studies are supportive.

3. Needle electromyography study:

Record from a distal and a proximal muscle in an arm and a leg.

Assess for the following abnormalities:

Profuse, abnormal spontaneous activity (fibrillation and positive wave potentials) indicating axonal involvement is supportive.

Decreased or absent motor unit recruitment with normal motor units indicating conduction block or denervation is supportive.

Chronic Inflammatory Demyelinating Polyradiculoneuropathy

1. Sensory nerve studies:

Record from the sural and digital median nerves.

Assess for the pattern of involvement:

Abnormal median and normal sural responses are supportive.

2. Motor nerve studies:

Record from the peroneal, tibial, ulnar, and me-

dian nerves. These disorders are usually symmetrical in distribution, and sampling nerves on one side is usually sufficient.

Assess for the following abnormalities (two or more abnormalities in each of two nerves is supportive):

Distal latency greater than 130% of the upper limits of normal

Conduction velocity less than 75% of the lower limits of normal

F-wave latency greater than 130% of the upper limits of normal

Proximal-to-distal amplitude ratio less than 70%

Proximal-to-distal negative peak duration ratio greater than 20%

Evidence of abnormal temporal dispersion in CMAP waveform shape

If the CMAP amplitude is low or absent from distal stimulation sites use inch stimulating electrode distally to determine whether the amplitude increases.

3. Needle electromyography study:

Record from a distal and a proximal muscle in an arm and a leg.

Assess for the following abnormalities:

Abnormal spontaneous activity (fibrillation and positive wave potentials) indicating axonal involvement is supportive.

Decreased motor unit recruitment with normal motor units (motor units may be larger in amplitude than expected) supports conduction block.

Multifocal Motor Neuropathy

1. Sensory nerve studies:

Record from the sural and digital median nerves and across segments showing motor conduction block.

Assess for sensory nerve involvement:

Normal responses are supportive.

Normal response across the segment showing motor block is supportive.

2. Motor nerve studies:

Record from the peroneal, tibial, ulnar, and median nerves. Multifocal motor neuropathy is usually asymmetrical, and sampling nerves on both sides is necessary.

Assess for the following abnormalities:

Distal latency normal

Conduction velocity normal

F-wave latency normal

Proximal-to-distal amplitude ratio less than 50% over long distances

Proximal-to-distal negative peak duration ratio less than 30%

Inching technique to narrow the focal site of conduction block with proximal-to-distal ratio less than 30% over short distances

3. Needle electromyography study:

Record from muscles innervated by nerves showing focal conduction block.
Assess for the following abnormalities:
Abnormal spontaneous activity (fibrillation and positive wave potentials) indicating axonal involvement is supportive.
Decreased motor unit recruitment with normal motor units indicates conduction block is supportive.

References

Ad Hoc Subcommittee of the American Academy of Neurology AIDS Task Force: Research criteria for diagnosis of chronic inflammatory demyelinating polyneuropathy (CIDP). Neurology 1991;41:617–618.

Alam T, Chaudhry V, Cornblath D: Electrophysiological studies in the Guillain-Barré syndrome: Distinguishing subtypes by published criteria. Muscle Nerve 1998;21:1275–1279.

Albers J, Donofrio P, McGonagle T: Sequential electrodiagnostic abnormalities in acute inflammatory demyelinating polyradiculoneuropathy. Muscle Nerve 1985;8:528–539.

Albers J, Kelly J: Acquired inflammatory demyelinating polyneuropathies: Clinical and electrodiagnostic features. Muscle Nerve 1989;12:435–451.

Amato A, Gronseth G, Callerame K, et al: Tomaculous neuropathy: A clinical and electrophysiological study in patients with and without 1.5-Mb deletions in chromosome 17P11.2. Muscle Nerve 1996;19:16–22.

Andersson P-B, Yuen E, Parko K, So Y: Electrodiagnostic features of hereditary neuropathy with liability to pressure palsies. Neurology 2000;54:40–44.

Arnason B, Soliven B: Acute inflammatory demyelinating polyradiculoneuropathy. In Dyck P, Thomas P (eds): Peripheral Neuropathy. Philadelphia, WB Saunders, 1993; 1437–1497.

Asbury A, Cornblath D: Assessment of current diagnostic criteria for Guillain-Barré syndrome. Ann Neurol 1990;27(suppl):S21–S24.

Auer R, Bell R, Lee M: Neuropathy with onion bulb formation and pure motor manifestations. Can J Neurol Sci 1989;16:194–197.

Barohn R, Kissel J, Warmolts J, Mendell J: Chronic inflammatory demyelinating polyradiculoneuropathy. Arch Neurol 1989;46:878–884.

Bouchard C, Lacroix C, Planté V, et al: Clinicopathologic findings and prognosis of chronic inflammatory demyelinating polyneuropathy. Neurology 1999;52:498–503.

Bromberg M: Comparison of electrodiagnostic criteria for primary demyelination in chronic polyneuropathy. Muscle Nerve 1991;14:968–976.

Bromberg M, Feldman E, Albers J: Chronic inflammatory demyelinating polyradiculoneuropathy: Comparison of patients with and without an associated monoclonal gammopathy. Neurology 1992;42:1157–1163.

Bromberg M, Albers J: Patterns of sensory nerve conduction abnormalities in demyelinating and axonal peripheral nerve disorders. Muscle Nerve 1993;16:262–266.

Brown W: The Physiological and Technical Basis of Electromyography. Boston, Butterworth, 1984.

Brown W, Feasby T, Hahn A: Electrophysiological changes in the acute "axonal" form of Guillain-Barré syndrome. Muscle Nerve 1993;16:200–205.

Chance P, Alderson M, Leppig K, et al: DNA deletion associated with hereditary neuropathy with liability to pressure palsies. Cell 1993;72:143–151.

Chaudhry V, Cornblath D, Griffin J, et al: Multifocal motor neuropathy or CIDP? A reply. Ann Neurol 1993;34:750–751.

Chaudhry V, Corse A, Cornblath D, et al: Multifocal motor neuropathy: Electrodiagnostic features. Muscle Nerve 1994;17:198–205.

Cornblath D, Mellits E, Griffin J, et al: Motor conduction studies in Guillain-Barré syndrome: Description and prognostic value. Ann Neurol 1988;23:354–359.

Cornblath D: Electrophysiology in Guillain-Barré syndrome. Ann Neurol 1990;27(suppl):S17–S20.

Cornblath D, Sumner A, Daube J, et al: Conduction block in clinical practice. Muscle Nerve 1991;14:869–871.

Delanoe C, Sebire G, Landrieu P, et al: Acute inflammatory demyelinating polyradiculopathy in children: Clinical and electrodiagnostic studies. Ann Neurol 1998;44:350–356.

Donofrio P, Albers J: AAEM minimonograph 34: Polyneuropathy: Classification by nerve conduction studies and electromyography. Muscle Nerve 1990;13:889–903.

Dyck P, Lambert E: Lower motor and primary sensory neuron diseases with peroneal muscular atrophy. I. Neurologic, genetic, and electrophysiologic findings in hereditary polyneuropathies. Arch Neurol 1968a;18:603–681.

Dyck P, Lambert E: Lower motor and primary sensory neuron diseases with peroneal muscular atrophy. II. Neurologic, genetic, and electrophysiologic findings in various neuronal degenerations. Arch Neurol 1968b;18:619–621.

Dyck P, Lais A, Ohta M, et al: Chronic inflammatory polyradiculoneuropathy. Mayo Clin Proc 1975;50:621–636.

Dyck P, O'Brien P, Oviatt K, et al: Prednisone improves chronic inflammatory demyelinating polyradiculoneuropathy more than no treatment. Ann Neurol 1982;11:136–141.

Dyck P, Daube J, O'Brien P, et al: Plasma exchange in chronic inflammatory demyelinating polyradiculoneuropathy. N Engl J Med 1986;314:461–465.

Dyck P: Is there an axonal variety of GBS? Neurology 1993;43:1277–1280.

Dyck P, Prineas J, Pollard J: Chronic inflammatory demyelinating polyradiculoneuropathy. In Dyck P, Thomas P (eds): Peripheral Neuropathy. Philadelphia, WB Saunders, 1993; 1498–1517.

Dyck P, Litchy W, Kratz K, et al: A plasma exchange versus immune globulin infusion trial in chronic inflammatory demyelinating polyradiculoneuropathy. Ann Neurol 1994;36:838–845.

Feasby T, Gilbert J, Brown W, et al: An acute axonal form of Guillain-Barré polyneuropathy. Brain 1986;109:1115–1126.

Feasby T, Hahn A, Brown W, et al: Severe axonal degeneration in acute Guillain-Barré syndrome: Evidence of two different mechanisms? J Neurol Sci 1993;116:185–192.

Feasby T: Axonal Guillain-Barré syndrome. Muscle Nerve 1994;17:678–679.

Federico P, Zochodne D, Hahn A, et al: Multifocal motor neuropathy improved by IVIg: Randomized, double-blind, placebo-controlled study. Neurology 2000;55:1256–1262.

Fisher M: An unusual variant of acute idiopathic polyneuritis (syndrome of ophthalmoplegia, ataxia and areflexia). N Engl J Med 1956;255:57–65.

Fletcher D, Lawn N, Wolter T, Wijdicks F: Long-term outcome in patients with Guillain-Barré syndrome requiring mechanical ventilation. Neurology 2000;54:2311–2315.

Fraser J: Distal sensory fiber involvement in inflammatory demyelinating polyneuropathy. Muscle Nerve 1994;17:112–113.

Fross R, Daube J: Neuropathy in the Miller Fisher syndrome: Clinical and electrophysiologic findings. Neurology 1987;37:1493–1498.

Gorson K, Ropper A, Adelman L, Weinberg D: Influence of diabetes mellitus on chronic inflammatory demyelinating polyneuropathy. Muscle Nerve 2000;23:37–43.

Gosselin S, Kyle R, Dyck P: Neuropathy associated with monoclonal gammopathies of undetermined significance. Arch Neurol 1991;30:54–61.

Gouider R, LeGuern E, Gugenheim M, et al: Clinical, electrophysiologic, and molecular correlations in 13 families with hereditary neuropathy with liability to pressure palsies and a chromosome 17p11.2 deletion. Neurology 1995;45:2018–2023.

Griffin J, Li C, Ho T, et al: Guillain-Barré syndrome in northern China: The spectrum of neuropathological changes in clinically defined cases. Brain 1995;118:577–595.

Griffin J, Li C, Ho T, et al: Pathology of the motor-sensory axonal Guillain-Barré syndrome. Ann Neurol 1996;39:17–28.

The Guillain-Barré Syndrome Study Group: Plasmapheresis and acute Guillain-Barré syndrome. Neurology 1985;35:1096–1104.

The Italian Guillain-Barré Study Group: The prognosis and main prognostic indicators of Guillain-Barré syndrome: A multicentre prospective study of 297 patients. Brain 1996;119:2053–2061.

Gutierrez E, Sumner A, Ferer S, et al: Unusual electrophysiological findings in X-linked dominant Charcot-Marie-Tooth disease. Muscle Nerve 2000;23:182–188.

Hahn A, Bolton C, Pillay N, et al: Plasma-exchange therapy in chronic inflammatory demyelinating polyneuropathy: A double-blind, sham-controlled, cross-over study. Brain 1996a;119:1055–1066.

Hahn A, Bolton C, Zochodne D, Feasby T: Intravenous immunoglobulin treatment in chronic inflammatory demyelinating polyneuropathy: A double-blind, placebo-controlled, cross-over study. Brain 1996b;119:1067–1077.

Harding A, Thomas P: The clinical features of hereditary motor and sensory neuropathy types I and II. Brain 1980;103:259–280.

Hartung H-P, Pollard J, Harvey G, Toyka K: Immunopathogenesis and treatment of the Guillain-Barré syndrome. Part II. Muscle Nerve 1995;18:154–164.

Ho R, Mishu B, Li C, et al: Guillain-Barré syndrome in northern China. Relationship to *Campylobacter jejuni* infection and anti-glycolipid antibodies. Brain 1995;118:597–605.

Ho T, Li C, Cornblath D, et al: Patterns of recovery in the Guillain-Barré syndromes. Neurology 1997;48:695–700.

Jacobs B, Meulstee J, van Doorn P, van der Meché F: Electrodiagnostic findings related to anti-G$_{M1}$ and anti-GQ1b antibodies in Guillain-Barré syndrome. Muscle Nerve 1997;20:446–452.

Kaji R, Shibasaki H, Kimura J: Multifocal demyelinating motor neuropathy: Cranial nerve involvement and immunoglobulin therapy. Neurology 1992;42:506–509.

Kaji R, Oka N, Tsuji T, et al: Pathological findings at the site of conduction block in multifocal motor neuropathy. Ann Neurol 1993;33:152–158.

Kaku D, England J, Sumner A: Distal accentuation of conduction slowing in polyneuropathy associated with antibodies to myelin-associated glycoprotein and sulphated glucuronyl paragloboside. Brain 1994;117:941–947.

Katz J, Wolfe G, Bryan W, et al: Electrophysiologic findings in multifocal motor neuropathy. Neurology 1997;48:700–707.

Katz J, Saperstein D, Gronseth G, et al: Distal acquired demyelinating symmetric neuropathy. Neurology 2000;54:615–620.

Kelly J: The electrodiagnostic findings in peripheral neuropathy associated with monoclonal gammopathy. Muscle Nerve 1983;6:504–509.

Kelly J: Peripheral neuropathies associated with monoclonal proteins: A clinical review. Muscle Nerve 1985;8:138–150.

Kimura J: An evaluation of the facial and trigeminal nerves in polyneuropathy: Electrodiagnostic study in Charcot-Marie-Tooth disease, Guillain-Barré syndrome, and diabetic neuropathy. Neurology 1971;21:745–752.

Kimura J, Machida M, Ishida T, et al: Relation between size of compound sensory or motor action potentials and length of nerve segment. Neurology 1986;36:647–652.

Kimura J: Electrodiagnosis in Diseases of Nerve and Muscle: Principles and Practice. Philadelphia, FA Davis, 1989.

Kornberg A, Pestronk A, Blume G, et al: Selective staining of the cerebellar molecular layer by serum IgG in Miller-Fisher and related syndromes. Neurology 1996;47:1317–1320.

Krendel D, Costigan D: Multifocal motor neuropathy of CIDP? Ann Neurol 1993;34:750.

Krendel D, Costigan D, Hopkins L: Successful treatment of neuropathies in patients with diabetes mellitus. Arch Neurol 1995;52:1053–1061.

Kusunoki S, Chiba A, Kanazawa I: Anti-GQ1b antibody is associated with ataxia as well as ophthalmoplegia. Muscle Nerve 1999;22:1071–1074.

Lange D, Trojaborg W, Latov N, et al: Multifocal motor neuropathy with conduction block: Is it a distinct clinical entity? Neurology 1992;42:497–505.

Lewis R, Sumner A: The electrodiagnostic distinctions between chronic familial and acquired demyelinative neuropathies. Neurology 1982;32:592–596.

Lewis R, Sumner A, Brown M, Asbury A: Multifocal demyelinating neuropathy with persistent conduction block. Neurology 1982;32:958–964.

Lewis R: Multifocal motor neuropathy and Lewis Sumner syndrome. Two distinct entities. Muscle Nerve 1999;22:1738–1739.

Lewis R: The challenge of CMTX and connexin 32 mutations. Muscle Nerve 2000;23:147–149.

Lewis R, Sumner A, Shy M: Electrophysiological features of inherited demyelinating neuropathies: A reappraisal in the era of molecular diagnosis. Muscle Nerve 2000;23:1472–1487.

Luciano C, Gilliatt R, Conwit R: Mixed nerve action potentials in acquired demyelinating polyneuropathy. Muscle Nerve 1995;18:85–92.

McKhann G, Cornblath D, Griffin J, et al: Acute motor axonal neuropathy: A frequent cause of acute flaccid paralysis in China. Ann Neurol 1993;33:333–342.

Mendell J, Barohn R, Freimer M, et al: Randomized controlled trial of IVIg in untreated chronic inflammatory demyelinating polyradiculoneuropathy. Neurology 2001;56:445–449.

Meulstee J, van der Meché F: Electrodiagnostic criteria for polyneuropathy and demyelination: Application in 135 patients with Guillain-Barré syndrome. Dutch Guillain-Barré Study Group. J Neurol Neurosurg Psychiatry 1995;59:482–486.

Midroni G, Dyck P: Chronic inflammatory demyelinating polyradiculoneuropathy: Unusual clinical features and therapeutic responses. Neurology 1996;46:1206–1212.

Mouton P, Tardieu S, Gouider R, et al: Spectrum of clinical and electrophysiologic features in HNPP patients with the 17p11.2 deletion. Neurology 1999;52:1440–1446.

Murray N, Wade D: The sural sensory action potential in Guillain-Barré syndrome. Muscle Nerve 1980;3:444.

Nicholson G, Nash J: Intermediate nerve conduction velocities define X-linked Charcot-Marie-Tooth neuropathy families. Neurology 1993;43:2558–2564.

Oh S, Kim D, Kuruoglu H: What is the best diagnostic index of conduction block and temporal dispersion? Muscle Nerve 1994;17:489–493.

Olney R, Budingen H, Miller R: The effect of temporal dispersion on compound action potential area in human peripheral nerve. Muscle Nerve 1987;10:728–733.

Pakiam A, Parry G: Multifocal motor neuropathy without overt conduction block. Muscle Nerve 1998;21:243–245.

Parry G, Clarke S: Multifocal acquired demyelinating neuropathy masquerading as motor neuron disease. Muscle Nerve 1988;11:103–107.

Parry G: Are multifocal motor neuropathy and Lewis-Sumner syndrome distinct nosologic entities? Muscle Nerve 1999;22:557–559.

Pestronk A, Cornblath D, Ilyas A, et al: A treatable multifocal motor neuropathy with antibodies to G$_{M1}$ ganglioside. Neurology 1988;24:73–78.

Pestronk A: Multifocal motor neuropathy: Diagnosis and treatment. Neurology 1998;51(suppl 5):S22–S24.

Ponsford W, Willison H, Veitch J, et al: Long-term clinical and neurophysiological follow-up of patients with peripheral neuropathy associated with benign monoclonal gammopathy. Muscle Nerve 2000;23:164–174.

Rhee E, England J, Sumner A: A computer simulation of conduction block: Effects produced by actual block versus interphase cancellation. Ann Neurol 1990;28:146–156.

Ropper A: Unusual clinical variants and signs in Guillain-Barré syndrome. Arch Neurol 1986;43:1150–1152.

Ropper A, Wijdicks E, Truax B: Guillain-Barré Syndrome. Philadelphia, FA Davis, 1991.

Saperstein D, Amato A, Wolfe G, et al: Multifocal acquired demyelinating sensory and motor neuropathy: The Lewis-Sumner syndrome. Muscle Nerve 1999;22:560–566.

Saperstein D, Katz J, Amato A, Barohn R: Clinical spectrum of chronic acquired demyelinating polyneuropathies. Muscle Nerve 2001;24:311–324.

Sellman M, Mayer R: Conduction block in hereditary neuropathy with susceptibility to pressure palsies. Muscle Nerve 1987;10:621–625.

Shahani B, Young R, Potts F, Maccabee P: Terminal latency index (TLI) and late response studies in motor neuron disease (MND), peripheral neuropathies, and entrapment syndromes. Acta Neurol Scand Suppl 1979;73:118.

Simmons Z, Albers J, Bromberg M, Feldman E: Presentation and initial clinical course in patients with chronic inflammatory demyelinating polyradiculoneuropathy: Comparison of patients without and with monoclonal gammopathy. Neurology 1993;43:2202–2209.

Simmons Z, Albers J, Bromberg M, Feldman E: Long-term follow-up of patients with chronic inflammatory demyelinating polyradiculoneuropathy, without and with monoclonal gammopathy. Brain 1995;118:359–368.

Simmons Z, Wald J, Albers J: Chronic inflammatory demyelinating polyradiculoneuropathy in children. I. Presentation, electrodiagnostic studies, and initial clinical course with comparison to adults. Muscle Nerve 1997a;20:1008–1015.

Simmons Z, Wald J, Albers J: Chronic inflammatory demyelinating polyradiculoneuropathy in children. II. Long-term follow-up, with comparison to adults. Muscle Nerve 1997b;20:1569–1575.

Tabaraud F, Lagrange E, Sindou P, et al: Demyelinating X-linked Charcot-Marie-Tooth disease: Unusual electrophysiological findings. Muscle Nerve 1999;22:1442–1447.

Taylor B, Wright R, Harper C, Dyck P: Natural history of 46 patients with multifocal motor neuropathy with conduction block. Muscle Nerve 2000;23:900–908.

Thomas P, Claus D, Jaspert A, et al: Focal upper limb demyelinating neuropathy. Brain 1996;119:765–774.

Triggs W, Cros D, Gominak S, et al: Motor nerve inexcitability in Guillain-Barré syndrome. Brain 1992;115:1291–1302.

Van den Berg-Vos R, Van den Berg L, Franssen H, et al: Multifocal inflammatory demyelinating neuropathy: A distinct clinical entity? Neurology 2000;54:26–32.

van der Meché F, Meulstee J, Kleyweg R: Axonal damage in Guillain-Barré syndrome. Muscle Nerve 1991;14:997–1002.

van der Meché F, Schmitz P: A randomized trial comparing intravenous immune globulin and plasma exchange in Guillain-Barré syndrome. Dutch Guillain-Barré Study Group. N Engl J Med 1992;326:1123–1129.

Visser L, Schmitz P, Meulstee J, et al: Prognostic factors of Guillain-Barré syndrome after intravenous immunoglobulin or plasma exchange. Neurology 1999;53:598–604.

Yuki N: Pathogenesis of axonal Guillain-Barré syndrome: Hypothesis. Muscle Nerve 1994;17:680–682.

Diabetic Neuropathy

David A. Krendel

EPIDEMIOLOGY

Diabetes mellitus is the most common cause of peripheral neuropathy in North America today. Elsewhere, the prevalence of diabetic neuropathy is similar, but in some tropical countries, leprosy supersedes diabetes as the most common cause of neuropathy. The prevalence of diabetes in the United States has been estimated to be 1% to 2%, with type 2 diabetes being three to seven times more prevalent than type 1 diabetes and with the percentage of patients with type 2 increasing with age (Dyck et al., 1993; Foster, 1998). Estimates of the prevalence of peripheral neuropathy in diabetic patients have varied depending in part on the criteria used to determine the presence of neuropathy, including the sensitivity of tests that are used.

Using only clinical criteria in 4,400 patients, Pirart (1978) found evidence of neuropathy in 7.5% of diabetic patients at the time of diagnosis, but this increased to 45% after 25 years of disease. In addition to clinical signs and symptoms, Dyck and colleagues (1993) used sensitive quantitative techniques to determine the prevalence of diabetic neuropathy in the population of Rochester, Minnesota. These techniques included nerve conduction studies, quantitative sensory testing, and testing for autonomic dysfunction by beat-to-beat cardiac interval variability with deep breathing or Valsava maneuver. They found that 1.3% of the Rochester population (870 of 64,573) had diabetes and that about 44% (380) of these persons were enrolled in the study. Of those enrolled, 27% (102) had type 1 and 73% (278) had type 2. Some form of neuropathy was detectable in 66% of patients with type 1 and in 59% of those with type 2 diabetes. The types of abnormalities detected were similar in type 1 and type 2 patients, with the most common being polyneuropathy (noted in about 50% of enrolled patients); however, severe symptomatic neuropathy was uncommon and more frequent in type 1 than in type 2 (6% versus 1%). Severity of polyneuropathy increased with the duration of diabetes but was not judged to be of a degree sufficient to cause disability in any of the patients. Thus, the authors concluded that although peripheral neuropathy is very common in diabetic persons, being detectable in more than half of their study population, it is symptomatic in only about 20%, most of whom have only mild symptoms.

Dyck and colleagues (1993) also found that slowing of median nerve conduction at the wrist typical of carpal tunnel syndrome was very common, being detectable in about 32% of diabetic patients, but only 11% with type 1 and 6% of type 2 patients were symptomatic. Autonomic neuropathy was detected in 6% to 7%. Proximal diabetic neuropathy was diagnosed in 4 (1%) with type 2 and in 1 (1%) with type 1 diabetes. Both autonomic neuropathy and carpal tunnel slowing were statistically more common in patients with polyneuropathy. Diabetic nephropathy and retinopathy were also positively correlated with polyneuropathy.

The positive correlation between peripheral neuropathy and the other major complications of diabetes was confirmed by the findings of the Diabetes Control and Complications Trial (DCCT) research group (1993, 1995). They recruited 1441 patients with type 1 diabetes, roughly half of whom had no retinopathy or nephropathy (primary prevention cohort), with the others having minimal to moderate abnormalities (secondary intervention cohort). At baseline, only 3.5% of the primary prevention cohort was judged to have "confirmed clinical" neuropathy defined as clinical evidence of neuropathy confirmed by abnormal nerve conduction studies or autonomic testing. Among those with some evidence of retinal or renal involvement, however, the prevalence of "confirmed clinical" neuropathy was 9.4%.

Also in agreement with the findings of Dyck and colleagues, asymptomatic neuropathy was much more prevalent than symptomatic neuropathy among the DCCT patients. If the requirement for symptoms is dropped from their definition and neuropathy is then defined as abnormal nerve conduction in at least two nerves, the prevalence of neuropathy among diabetics with no detectable renal or retinal involvement jumps to about 20% from 3.5%. In those with some retinopathy or nephropathy, about 45% had neuropathy detectable on nerve conduction studies, but only 9.4% also had symptoms or signs.

In summary, peripheral neuropathy is a very common complication of this very common disease. A majority of diabetics will eventually have some evidence of neuropathy, but most will be asymptomatic. Symptoms are severe in only a small percentage (1% to 6%), and disabling neuropathy is relatively rare. This implies that only a small minority of patients with diabetic neuropathy are likely to be referred to neurologists or to undergo electrophysiological testing.

CLASSIFICATION

The study of diabetic neuropathy is somewhat hampered by the fact that it is not a single disease but instead consists of a group of diseases with different clinical features and pathogenetic mechanisms. Consequently, one should expect prognosis and approach to treatment to vary between specific subtypes. This has been particularly true as therapeutic options have expanded, giving classification an increasingly important role in the clinical evaluation of diabetic patients with peripheral neuropathy. Traditional classification based entirely on clinical characteristics has resulted in the naming of a large list of syndromes, many with overlapping clinical features. A classification based on pathogenesis would be preferable, but the precise cause of any form of diabetic neuropathy is unknown. Nevertheless, basic pathophysiological mechanisms can be divided into three broad categories: metabolic, vascular, and inflammatory/immune.

The most common form of neuropathy to which diabetics are predisposed, diabetic polyneuropathy, can be best classified as metabolic. Extensive evidence now points to hyperglycemia itself as the primary underlying mechanism responsible for this typically mild disorder (Low, 1987; Sima, 1996). Most convincing has been a large, prospective, controlled study showing that polyneuropathy can be prevented or that its course can be improved by maintaining serum glucose levels at normal or near-normal levels (Diabetes Control and Complications Study Group, 1993, 1995). There is some evidence suggesting that ischemia due to diabetic microvasculopathy may play an etiological role (Low, 1987; Thomas et al., 1993; Sima, 1996; Thomas, 1999), and there is some evidence for an immune/inflammatory contribution (Thomas et al., 1993; Sima, 1996; Younger et al., 1996).

Vascular neuropathies in diabetics include the relatively uncommon focal, multifocal, and proximal neuropathies to which diabetics are predisposed. Evidence showing nerve infarction due to small vessel occlusion comes from studies of autopsy and biopsy specimens from patients with syndromes in this category (Raff et al., 1968; Asbury et al., 1970; Bradley et al., 1984; Costigan et al., 1990; Krendel et al., 1995; Younger et al., 1996; Llewelyn et al., 1998; Dyck et al., 1999). Studies have shown inflammation of small vessels in nerve biopsy samples from patients with proximal diabetic neuropathy (Bradley et al., 1984; Costigan et al., 1990; Said et al., 1994; Krendel et al., 1995; Younger et al., 1996; Llewelyn et al., 1998; Dyck et al., 1999), and several uncontrolled studies have suggested that immunosuppressive treatment can be beneficial (Bradley et al., 1984; Costigan et al., 1990; Engel and Prentice, 1993; Said et al., 1994; Krendel et al., 1995; Pascoe et al., 1997). Although these syndromes occur in only a small percentage of diabetic patients, they affect a disproportionately large percentage of those referred to neurologists because they tend to be disabling. Included in this category are the largest number of named diabetic neuropathic syndromes, probably at least in part because different clinical syndromes result when different nerves are infarcted. Names applied to these syndromes include *diabetic amyotrophy* (Garland, 1961), *proximal diabetic neuropathy* (Asbury, 1977), *subacute proximal neuropathy* (Pascoe et al., 1997), *diabetic polyradiculopathy* (Bastron and Thomas, 1981), *diabetic mononeuropathy multiplex* (Raff et al., 1968), *diabetic femoral neuropathy* (Cappack and Watkins, 1991), *diabetic thoracoabdominal neuropathy* (Sun and Streib, 1981), and *diabetic cranial neuropathies* (most commonly, third nerve palsy) (Asbury et al., 1970).

In addition to the inflammatory vasculopathy associated with proximal diabetic neuropathy just noted, some diabetics appear to have immune-mediated demyelinating neuropathy that shares clinical and electrodiagnostic characteristics with chronic inflammatory demyelinating polyradiculoneuropathy (CIDP) (Costigan et al., 1990; Krendel et al., 1995; Stewart et al., 1996; Simpson, 1997; Baruah, 1998; Krendel and Skehan, 1998; Cross et al., 1999; Sharma et al., 1999). CIDP would be expected to occur in some patients with diabetes by chance association alone, but there is some evidence suggesting that diabetics, especially those with type 1 diabetes, are predisposed to CIDP (Krendel and Skehan, 1998). Diabetic polyneuropathy typically does not show electrodiagnostic evidence of demyelination, and the finding of such evidence in an individual patient should at least prompt the consideration of CIDP in a diabetic, just as it should in a patient without diabetes.

In this chapter, I divided diabetic peripheral neuropathies into three main groups: (1) diffuse metabolic neuropathies, (2) vascular neuropathies, and (3) demyelinating neuropathy. Inflammatory/immune mechanisms appear to be important in the latter two groups, and the roles of vascular or immune mechanisms in the first category remain to be determined.

DIFFUSE METABOLIC NEUROPATHIES

Diabetic Polyneuropathy

This is the most common type of peripheral neuropathy throughout most of the world today, eventually affecting more than half of all patients with diabetes mellitus (Pirart, 1978; Dyck et al., 1993; Foster, 1998; Diabetes Control and Complications Study Group, 1993, 1995). Fortunately, as noted earlier, it is usually asymptomatic or minimally symptomatic. Nevertheless, diabetic polyneuropathy tends to be progressive, particularly when blood sugar control is less than optimal, and distressing or even disabling symptoms eventually develop in a significant minority.

CLINICAL FEATURES

The clinical features of diabetic polyneuropathy are like those to be expected in any mild, chronic, distal sensory and motor peripheral neuropathy. The most common symptom is numbness or paresthesia of the toes, gradually ascending over years to involve more proximal areas of the feet and then the ankles. Mild asymmetry is not uncommon in diabetics with polyneuropathy, but asymmetry or focality should at least prompt consideration of a different or coexisting process such as an entrapment neuropathy. Loss of pain perception due to neuropathy contributes to the development of foot ulcers and infections because breaks in the skin may go unnoticed and therefore unprotected. Numbness of the fingers directly attributable to polyneuropathy occurs only in more advanced cases, but this symptom is commonly caused by carpal tunnel syndrome, to which diabetics, particularly those with polyneuropathy, are highly susceptible.

Less common in diabetic polyneuropathy but much more troublesome is pain. This involves only the feet in most cases and is usually described as burning, but sometimes as stinging, pricking, electrical, or unlike any sensation with which the patient was previously familiar. Sudden shock-like or stabbing pains may occur. Patients with foot pain due to polyneuropathy almost always find that it is most severe or bothersome when they are in bed trying to sleep. This is probably because without the distractions of daytime activity to inhibit the perception of pain, it occupies the patient's full attention. Other causes of foot pain, such as plantar fasciitis, arthritis, or plantar nerve compression, can usually be distinguished by their tendency to be worse while the patient is standing or walking.

Sensory ataxia due to loss of proprioceptive input sometimes occurs in diabetics with advanced polyneuropathy ("diabetic pseudotabes"). However, because proprioceptive information is transmitted via large, myelinated axons, disabling or disproportionate sensory ataxia should prompt consideration of a demyelinating process, particularly CIDP.

Clinically important weakness due to diabetic polyneuropathy is also unusual. Atrophy of intrinsic foot muscles is not uncommon but is rarely noticed by the patient. If significant weakness of the lower extremities occurs in a patient with diabetic polyneuropathy, it usually involves ankle dorsiflexion, ultimately resulting in a gait disturbance caused by the need to step abnormally high to avoid tripping over the toes. However, one should be disinclined to attribute this degree of disability to diabetic polyneuropathy and should instead consider other causes such as peroneal nerve compression, L5 radiculopathy, or concurrent inflammatory or hereditary neuropathy. The same is true of intrinsic hand muscle weakness in a diabetic, which more often results from focal median or ulnar nerve lesions than directly from diabetic polyneuropathy.

PATHOGENESIS

Although the pathogenesis of diabetic polyneuropathy is unknown, the importance of hyperglycemia in its causation can be inferred by the proven preventative or ameliorative effect of maintaining blood glucose levels as close to normal as possible (Reeves et al., 1984; Diabetes Control and Complications Study Group, 1993, 1995). The mechanism by which hyperglycemia might cause peripheral neuropathy has been the subject of extensive research.

One theory invokes the upregulation of the enzyme aldose reductase (Greene, 1986; Low, 1987; Dyck et al., 1988; Thomas et al., 1993; Sima, 1996; Greene et al., 1999; Thomas, 1999). This enzyme is inactive except under conditions of hyperglycemia, when it provides for metabolism of glucose through the polyol pathway. This results in the production of sorbitol and fructose and the depletion of myoinositol. Depletion of endoneurial myoinositol with resultant impairment of axonal sodium-potassium ATPase activity was advanced as an etiological factor for diabetic polyneuropathy based on experiments in animals (Greene, 1986). However, the reduction of myoinositol in animal nerves was found to abate with time, and myoinositol levels proved not to be reduced in human nerves affected by diabetic polyneuropathy (Dyck et al., 1988). Nevertheless, the polyol pathway might still play a pathogenetic role, because sorbitol and fructose do accumulate in diabetic nerve and because sorbitol content correlates well with the severity of neuropathy (Dyck et al., 1988; Greene et al., 1999).

Another theory invokes nonenzymatic glycation, in which structural proteins bind glucose or other reducing sugars, potentially interfering with function (Brownlee, 1991; Sima, 1996). Glycation of neurofilaments or neurotubules might interfere with axonal transport, which is known to be impaired in animal models of diabetic neuropathy (Yagihashi, 1995). Myelin proteins are also abnormally glycated under hyperglycemic conditions, and altered myelin proteins might become antigenic. Glycation of perineurial collagen and capillary basement membrane could contribute to increased permeability and permit large, potentially harmful molecules to enter the endoneurium. Glycation of endothelial cell components has been implicated as a possible contributing factor in the development of diabetic microvasculopathy, which also has been theorized to contribute to the development of diabetic polyneuropathy (Giannini and Dyck, 1995).

Abnormal fatty acid metabolism in diabetic rats has been shown to reduce endoneurial blood flow and conduction velocity by decreasing production of vasoactive prostaglandins (Sima, 1996; Thomas, 1999). Hyperglycemia in rats inhibits conversion of linoleic to γ-linoleic acid, thereby diminishing the production of arachidonic acid, precursor to prostaglandins. Endoneurial blood flow and conduction velocity are restored when rats are fed γ-linoleic acid or evening primrose oil (Stevens et al., 1993). However, no benefit has been shown in humans.

Microvascular disease resulting in nerve ischemia has long been suspected to play a role in the development of diabetic polyneuropathy, although this has been convincingly established for only some of the focal and multifocal neuropathies to which diabetics are predisposed. Diabetic rats are known to have diminished perfusion and oxygenation of nerves, and the animals show some improvement in conduction velocity when maintained in an oxygen-rich environment (Low et al., 1984). In humans, multifocal fiber loss typical of small vessel ischemia has been seen at autopsy and sural nerve biopsy in some patients with diabetic polyneuropathy (Sugimura and Dyck, 1982). However, multifocal fiber loss is not entirely specific for ischemia, and ischemic lesions in elderly patients with atherosclerosis might not reflect the true cause of typical diabetic polyneuropathy. Other observations favoring an ischemic mechanism are the frequently seen thickened endoneurial capillary basement membranes and occluded endoneurial capillaries, findings that some have found to correlate with severity of the neuropathy (Giannini and Dyck, 1995).

Axonal regeneration is impaired in diabetes, and this might contribute to the severity of diabetic polyneuropathy (Bradley et al., 1995). It has been theorized that deficiency of nerve growth factor, which has been noted in both experimental and human diabetes, might be important in that regard (Mitsumoto et al., 1999). Nerve growth factor is pro-duced by target tissues and taken up by the axons of small sensory and sympathetic neurons, supporting their growth and regeneration. In diabetic mice, the administration of nerve growth factor restores c-fiber function (Elias et al., 1998), but the results of a multicenter study in humans were disappointing (Apfel et al., 1998; Mitsumoto et al., 1999).

Immune-mediated mechanisms have also been suspected of contributing to the pathogenesis of peripheral neuropathy in diabetics. Although more widely accepted for proximal, multifocal, and demyelinating diabetic neuropathies, it has been suggested that the immune system might also play a role in causation of diabetic polyneuropathy (Thomas and Tomlinson, 1993; Sima, 1996; Younger et al., 1996). Type 1 diabetes is an autoimmune disease (Atkinson and Maclaren, 1994), and diabetics are predisposed to other autoimmune conditions, possibly including peripheral neuropathy. Some immune cross-reactivity might be expected between endocrine (pancreatic islet) cells and neurons because of their common embryological origin and functional similarities. In that regard, cytotoxicity of diabetic sera against neuroblastoma cells has been shown to correlate with the severity of peripheral neuropathy (Pittenger et al., 1999). Also, antibodies to sympathetic ganglia have been detected in patients with diabetes (Schnell et al., 1996), and inflammatory infiltrates have been seen at autopsy in autonomic ganglia in patients diagnosed with diabetic autonomic neuropathy (Duchen et al., 1980). Younger and colleagues (1996) found inflammatory cells in nerve biopsy specimens from individuals diagnosed with diabetic polyneuropathy, in excess of those seen in patients with other forms of chronic neuropathy. Patients who have undergone a biopsy tended to have unusually severe neuropathy, as would be expected in a cohort referred for neurological consultation, so the findings might not directly apply to mild polyneuropathy, which is much more common in diabetics. Nevertheless, the evidence suggests that autoimmunity and inflammation do play a role in exacerbation, if not in basic pathogenesis, of diabetic polyneuropathy.

ELECTROPHYSIOLOGY

Electrodiagnostic studies of diabetic polyneuropathy have yielded varying results depending on how diabetic subjects were ascertained. When subjects were referred to neurologists or to neurodiagnostic laboratories for symptoms related to peripheral neuropathy, nerve conduction studies have tended to be more abnormal. This is because most patients with diabetic neuropathy are asymptomatic or minimally symptomatic and would be unlikely to see a specialist.

The DCCT (1993, 1995) provides particularly useful information on the expected nerve conduction abnormalities in young patients with relatively uncomplicated type 1 diabetes, because symptoms or signs of neuropathy were not considered in recruitment of subjects. One thousand four hundred forty-one type 1 diabetics were studied, ranging in age from 13 to 39 years. They were divided into two groups, one of which included patients with no retinopathy and diabetes for 1 to 5 years (primary prevention cohort), and another group with minimal to moderate nonproliferative retinopathy and diabetes for 1 to 15 years (secondary intervention cohort). Sural and median sensory and peroneal and median motor nerve conduction velocity results were reported at baseline and at 1, 2, and 9 years. Results for patients receiving conventional therapy were compared with results for those receiving intensive insulin therapy. Values were reported as median and 25th and 75th percentiles. For the primary prevention cohort, these values for both motor and sensory conduction remained within the normal range regardless of therapy. In the secondary prevention cohort, the motor velocity values were also all normal except that the 25th percentile for the peroneal nerve was 2.5% below normal (39 m per second) at baseline in the intensive therapy group. Sensory conduction velocities in the secondary intervention cohort were more often abnormal, with the 25th percentile value for median sensory velocity dropping to 15% below the normal limit and the 25th percentile for sural sensory velocities being 5% below normal at 1 and 2 years for the conventional therapy group. The patients who received intensive insulin therapy on average showed smaller declines in nerve conduction velocities and more of a tendency to stabilize or improve over the course of the study. This was statistically significant, but the differences between the two treatment group means were small in absolute terms (2 to 5 m per second for motor and 2 to 6 m per second for sensory conduction), and they occurred mainly within the limits of normal.

Motor and sensory amplitudes in the DCCT were measured but not specifically reported. It was noted, however, that there were no significant differences in amplitude between treatment groups. There was statistically less prolongation of F-wave latencies in the intensive treatment group over time.

Because the nerve conduction velocities reported from the DCCT were only those between the 25th and 75th percentiles, we do not know the full range of values. Some abnormality in nerve conduction in at least two nerves was measured in about 20% of patients in the primary prevention cohort and about in 45% of the secondary intervention cohort at baseline. At 5 years, in the primary prevention cohort, only 16% of patients who received intensive insulin therapy had abnormal nerve conduction, compared with 40% of those on conventional therapy. In the secondary intervention cohort, abnormal nerve conduction was measured in 33% on intensive treatment compared with 52% of those on conventional treatment after 5 years.

Reeves and colleagues (1984) had studied 10 patients with type 1 diabetes for whom, as in the DCCT, neuropathy was not considered as a criterion for selection. These patients had minimal or no clinical evidence of peripheral neuropathy and, as in the DCCT, were subjected to intensive insulin therapy to keep blood sugar levels as normal as possible. They had had diabetes for a mean duration of 8.4 years, and their mean age was 21.4 years. In this group, the mean values for ulnar and tibial motor conduction studies and sural sensory studies were within the normal range at baseline and remained so throughout the 6-month study. As in the DCCT, there were small but significant increases in the mean velocities after 6 months of intensive therapy, and a few individual patients had initial velocities that were below the lower limit of normal, becoming normal after 6 months. Most impressive, however, were the results of medial plantar sensory conduction studies. Medial plantar potentials were unobtainable in 7 of the 10 patients initially, and all could be obtained after 6 months of intensive insulin treatment. In addition to providing evidence of the beneficial effect of good blood sugar control, these findings imply that the medial plantar sensory conduction study is a very sensitive test for the detection of early diabetic polyneuropathy.

Hendriksen and colleagues (1992) reported nerve conduction study results in 52 type 1 and 36 type 2 diabetics who had evidence of peripheral neuropathy on examination but no symptoms. They had been hospitalized for other reasons by internists. Because evidence of neuropathy on examination was a condition for inclusion, this group would be expected to show more abnormal results than in the two studies discussed earlier. The results support this supposition. About 75% had abnormal tibial nerve conduction velocity, and there was no response in about 10%. Sural nerve sensory conduction was abnormal in 60%, with no recordable response in 40%. The ulnar nerve motor study was abnormal in about 25% but never unrecordable, and the ulnar nerve sensory study was abnormal in about 35%, with 7% having no recordable potential. The mean tibial nerve motor conduction velocity was about 15% below the lower limit of normal at 33.9 m per second, with a standard deviation of 7.7 m per second, but the mean ulnar nerve motor velocity was within the normal range at 53.5 ± 5.6 m per second. There was no significant difference between type 1 and type 2 diabetics. Although abnormalities were more severe and more prevalent in this group with clinically manifest asymptomatic neuropathy than in the DCCT or the group studied by Reeves and associates (1984), conduction velocities were more than 80% of the lower limit of normal and therefore did not suggest primary demyelination (Cornblath et al., 1991). This is consistent with the prevailing concept that axonal degeneration is the predominant basic mechanism underlying diabetic polyneuropathy.

Abu-Shakra and colleagues (1991) addressed the question of whether primary demyelination is important in the pathogenesis of diabetic polyneuropathy. They studied 24 diabetic patients referred to their electromyography laboratory, a group that presumably consisted of patients with symptomatic neuropathy severe enough to warrant referral and therefore even more likely to show abnormal results. They looked for conduction block, defined as a drop of more than 20% in amplitude on proximal compared with distal motor nerve stimulation (excluding amplitude loss due to temporal dispersion) in 76 nerve segments. A single instance of conduction block was found in 6 of the 24 patients, all located in nerve segments not commonly susceptible to compression. These included the median nerve in the forearm in 1 patient, the ulnar nerve in the forearm in 3 patients, and the peroneal nerve below the fibular head in 2 patients. The authors also reported ranges of conduction velocity (38 to 63 m per second median forearm, 32 to 74 m per second ulnar forearm, and 23 to 48 m per second peroneal below fibular head) that included some that were less than 80% of the lower limit of normal and therefore possibly reflected primary demyelination. Very low amplitudes were also reported, which could account for some of the low velocities based on axon loss, but amplitudes are mentioned separately from velocities and not correlated. These workers did not find slowing in the demyelinating range across segments with conduction block. They thought that their findings weighed against an important role for demyelination in diabetic polyneuropathy, because conduction block was found in only 6 of their patients (25%). However, one might argue that a prevalence of 25% is not negligible and that there might well be a predisposition to focal demyelination, possibly immune mediated, in this group. It should be remembered that their study group was representative not of patients with typical diabetic polyneuropathy but rather of that small subset of diabetics with neuropathy severe enough to warrant referral to an electromyography laboratory. Superimposed inflammatory neuropathy is probably more prevalent in this group than in the general population of patients with diabetic polyneuropathy.

Aside from patient selection on the basis of clinical neuropathy, results of electrophysiological studies of diabetic polyneuropathy are strongly influenced by inclusion or exclusion of patients with other significant complications of diabetes, most notably renal involvement.

Navarro and colleagues (1997) studied a group with a high prevalence of end-stage nephropathy but without selection bias related to peripheral neuropathy. One hundred fifteen patients were studied before and at intervals after pancreatic transplantation for period of 10 years. They were compared with a well-matched control group of 92 patients. From 30% to 40% from each group had renal transplantation. One hundred percent of patients in the pancreatic transplantation and control group had clinical evidence of peripheral neuropathy, and all except four patients had electrophysiological evidence of neuropathy. The mean ulnar, median, peroneal, and tibial motor conduction velocities were

below normal at baseline for both groups, as were median and sural sensory velocities and amplitudes. Mean compound muscle action potential amplitudes were in the low-normal range for hand muscles and below normal for foot muscles at entry. All except 7 of the 92 patients who did not undergo pancreatic transplantation (controls) had electrophysiological evidence of neuropathy. The control subjects tended to show progressive declines in conduction velocity, so that after 10 years, the mean median conduction velocity had declined from 46.9 to 44.9 m per second, and if the standard deviation of 3.34 m per second is subtracted, a velocity of 41.6 m per second is obtained. This value is close to 80% of the lower limit, so at least some of these patients probably had slowing in the demyelinating range. Amplitudes declined proportionately less, and similar results were obtained for ulnar and peroneal conduction. The remarkable finding of this study was that instead of deteriorating, nerve conduction parameters improved in the patients who had successful pancreatic transplantation.

Trojaborg and colleagues (1994) studied 26 insulin-dependent diabetics with end-stage nephropathy. Sixty-nine percent of these patients had signs and symptoms of peripheral neuropathy, whereas signs and symptoms of peripheral neuropathy are present in only about 20% of unselected patients (Dyck et al., 1993), approximately 10% with albuminuria of less than 200 mg/24 hr and minimal-moderate nonproliferative retinopathy and 3.5% with neither retinopathy nor nephropathy (Diabetes Control and Complications Study Group, 1993, 1995). In the group with renal failure studied by Trojaborg and colleagues (1994), the authors found nerve conduction abnormalities in two or more nerves in 100%, regardless of whether neuropathy was clinically manifest. From the graphic depiction of their data (Trojaborg, 1996), it is evident that a significant proportion of conduction velocities fell within a range suggestive of demyelination. At least 37% of the peroneal and 8% of the median motor conduction velocities were below 80% of the lower limit of normal. Amplitudes corresponding to these velocities are not given, but the author suggested that much of slowing might have been due to axon loss and reinnervation.

A recent study evaluated a group of 94 diabetics who were scheduled for renal transplantation (Krendel and Skehan, 1998). The patients included all diabetics scheduled for renal transplantation during a period of several years, regardless of the presence or severity of neuropathy. Seventy-seven had type 1 diabetes, and of those, 44% met criteria for demyelination as proposed for the diagnosis of CIDP by Cornblath and associates (1991). Of the 17 patients with type 2 diabetes, 6% met criteria for demyelinating neuropathy. Therefore, when renal failure is present, nerve conduction studies in type 1 diabetics commonly show evidence of demyelination. Whether this represents a predisposition to autoimmune demyelination (CIPD) or occurs through some other mechanism remains to be determined.

In summary, nerve conduction studies in diabetics are frequently abnormal, even in the absence of clinical neuropathy. Abnormalities are almost always mild and not suggestive of demyelination in unselected diabetics with normal or mildly impaired renal function. The population of diabetics seen by neurologists represents a small subset with unusually severe neuropathy. These patients often show more severe electrophysiological abnormalities, sometimes suggestive of demyelination. Diabetics with renal failure also have a high prevalence of severely abnormal nerve conduction, commonly suggestive of demyelination.

TREATMENT

The beneficial effect of good blood sugar control on diabetic polyneuropathy is well established (Diabetes Control and Complications Study Group, 1993, 1995). This applies both to patients with early, relatively uncomplicated diabetes and to patients with long-standing diabetes complicated by renal failure (Navarro et al., 1997). The findings of DCCT show that the prevention of symptomatic polyneuropathy should be attainable for many if euglycemia is maintained by means of an implanted insulin pump or intensive injected insulin therapy. The benefits must be weighed against the risk of hypoglycemia. Unfortunately, not all patients are capable of complying with these relatively rigorous forms of treatment.

Still more rigorous but of proven efficacy in arresting progression or improving diabetic polyneuropathy is pancreatic transplantation (Navarro et al., 1997). Significant differences between 115 transplanted patients and 92 control subjects were recorded over a period of 9 years for neurological examination, nerve conduction studies, and, to a lesser extent, tests of autonomic function. Transplant recipients generally showed improvement in mean values, whereas control subjects deteriorated. Immunosuppression is required after transplantation, and its effect should be considered because there might be an autoimmune contribution to the cause of some forms of diabetic neuropathy (Krendel, 1998). However, patients immunosuppressed after renal transplantation who did not undergo pancreatic transplantation showed deterioration comparable to that of nonimmunosuppressed control subjects (Navarro and Kennedy, 1998). Therefore, the maintenance of euglycemia is more likely to be the main explanation for the beneficial effect of pancreatic transplantation on diabetic polyneuropathy.

The effects of aldose reductase inhibitors on diabetic polyneuropathy have been studied based on the theoretically detrimental effect of activation of the polyol shunt (controlled by aldose reductase) by hyperglycemia (Greene, 1986; Dyck et al., 1988; Greene et al., 1999). Results in humans had been disappointing, but a study using zenarestat, a potent inhibitor of aldose reductase, showed significant benefit (Greene et al., 1999). Two hundred eight patients with diabetes complicated by peripheral neuropathy were randomized to receive different doses of zenarestat or placebo. Motor and sensory nerve conduction velocities were followed, and sural biopsies were performed at 6 and 52 weeks. Nerve conduction velocities improved in a dose-dependent manner in the treatment groups, increasing by a mean of 1 to 1.5 m per second in the group given the highest dose (600 mg b.i.d.). Velocities declined in the placebo group. Also, there was an increased density of small myelinated fibers between the 6- and 52-week sural nerve biopsy specimens from subjects receiving the higher doses of zenarestat. This was interpreted as indicating axonal regeneration and was correlated with a reduction in nerve sorbitol content by more than 80% of control levels. The necessity of this high degree of aldose reductase inhibition might explain the less impressive results for less potent inhibitors used in prior studies. Unfortunately, in three patients in the treatment group, non-Hodgkin's lymphoma developed, although it might have been preexisting in two of the patients.

Promising results were reported for an angiotensin-converting enzyme inhibitor in the treatment of diabetic neuropathy (Malik et al., 1998). Angiotensin-converting enzyme inhibition has been shown to improve or delay nephropathy and retinopathy through its beneficial effects on diabetic microvasculopathy. Improvement in nerve blood flow in diabetic rats has also been found, so angiotensin-converting enzyme inhibitors have been tested in humans based on the theory that microvasculopathy contributes to the causation of diabetic polyneuropathy. In a placebo-controlled study of 41 diabetics with mild neuropathy, there was modest but significant improvement in nerve conduction velocities and sural sensory potential amplitude after 1 year in patients treated with trandolapril. There was no clinical improvement, but it is hoped that clinical benefit will be seen in a larger study of longer duration.

Immunosuppression has been used in diabetic patients with severe peripheral neuropathy, and improvement has been reported in uncontrolled studies (Bradley et al., 1984; Costigan et al., 1990; Engel and Prentice, 1993; Said et al., 1994; Krendel et al., 1995; Younger et al., 1996; Pascoe et al., 1997). This has been based mainly on findings of inflammation involving nerve and epineurial vessels in biopsy specimens from diabetics with severe neuropathy. Most patients have had proximal diabetic neuropathy or amyotrophy and have shown vascular inflammation. Some have had demyelinating neuropathy and likely coexisting CIDP (Costigan et al., 1990; Krendel et al., 1995; Stewart et al., 1996; Simpson, 1997; Baruah, 1998; Krendel and Skehan, 1998; Cross et al., 1999; Sharma et al., 1999). There is no convincing support for the use of immunosuppressive treatments in typical diabetic polyneuropathy.

Aside from striving for optimal blood sugar control, treatments for diabetic polyneuropathy are mainly symptomatic. The most common symptom for which treatment is sought is neuropathic pain, usually in the feet. Numerous medications have been reported to alleviate pain in diabetic neuropathy.

Topical capsaicin cream is sometimes effective (Capsaicin Study Group, 1991; Tandan et al., 1992). Capsaicin is the active substance in hot peppers, producing the sensation of burning pain when eaten but causing no tissue damage. The effect is produced through the stimulation of afferent small axons that mediate pain and is thought to involve substance P. Patients should be warned that they may experience a warm or burning sensation during the first week or two of regular use, but this usually subsides as the analgesic effect becomes apparent. Severe pain results if capsaicin comes into contact with the eyes or other sensitive areas. The cream must be applied to the painful areas three or four times daily. The main advantage of this method of treatment is its lack of systemic toxicity, but in a large multicenter study (Capsaicin Study Group, 1991), only 10% to 15% of patients experienced more benefit than from a placebo cream. It is worth trying for patients who tolerate medication poorly or who are at increased risk of toxic effects or drug-drug interactions. It can also provide additional relief when added to existing pain control regimens.

Tricyclic antidepressants have been a mainstay in the treatment of neuropathic pain for many years. These substances have analgesic effects in addition to and independent of their potential beneficial effect on mood. Amitriptyline has been studied most extensively (Max et al., 1987, 1992), and provides about 33% benefit over placebo. Other tricyclics, such as desipramine, are also effective, but newer antidepressants that selectively block serotonin reuptake (selective serotonin reuptake inhibitors) are less effective. The selective serotonin reuptake inhibitor fluoxetine had no benefit over placebo in one study (Max et al., 1992), and citalopram had modest benefit, although it was judged to be less effective but better tolerated than the tricyclic imipramine (Sindrup et al., 1992). The sedative effect of tricyclics can be used to advantage because neuropathic pain is usually most bothersome at bedtime and commonly interferes with sleep. The effective dose of amitriptyline varies but often is less than the dose that would be required for the treatment of depression. An initial dose of 25 mg at bedtime, or 10 mg in elderly patents or in patients with a history of increased sensitivity to central nervous system–active medications, is commonly used, with increases of 10 to 25 mg every 3 to 7 days. The mean effective dose was about 50 mg in one study (Morello et al., 1999) and approximately 100 mg in another study (Max et al., 1992). If unwanted daytime sedation occurs, it will usually resolve if the dose is not increased after 1 to 2 weeks of treatment. Weight gain, dry mouth, and urinary retention can be problematic.

Anticonvulsants also have been proved to reduce pain due to diabetic neuropathy (McQuay et al., 1995). Carbamazepine and phenytoin have been used for many years, but the newer anticonvulsant gabapentin is gaining favor (Backonja et al., 1998). Gabapentin is usually better tolerated than carbamazepine or phenytoin, having fewer potential toxic effects or interactions with other drugs. Gabapentin sometimes causes unwanted sedation or dizziness, but these symptoms tend to abate with continued use and are less likely to occur with gradual dose titration. In one study (Morello et al., 1999), gabapentin was as effective as amitriptyline, the drug that probably has been studied most thoroughly and shown benefit most consistently. The authors of that study found amitriptyline and gabapentin to be equally well tolerated, although gabapentin has been better tolerated in my experience. The authors point out that gabapentin is more expensive than amitriptyline, so amitriptyline should be tried first when cost is a consideration. The effective dose of gabapentin varies and can be as high as 2.7 g daily. It is taken three times daily, usually beginning with 300 or 400 mg (100 mg in elderly patients or when sedation is likely to be a problem) at each dosing and is increased as tolerated over several weeks. Other, newer anticonvulsants are also being tested (Edwards et al., 1998) in patients with chronic painful conditions, including diabetic neuropathy.

The antiarrhythmic agent mexiletine initially showed some promise (Stracke et al., 1992) in the management of neuropathic pain and is helpful in some cases, but it has not gained widespread acceptance. It is similar to lidocaine and may relieve pain when administered systemically via a mechanism like that of locally applied lidocaine, by hindering conduction along unmyelinated or thinly myelinated afferent axons through sodium channel blockade. Intravenous lidocaine (Kastrup et al., 1987; Galer et al., 1993) may be more effective, presumably because of higher tissue levels, but skilled professionals are required for administration, so it is of limited practical value in the management of chronic pain. It may be useful for patients whose pain is refractory to other modalities.

Conventional analgesics can be useful, but most patients have tried over-the-counter analgesics before consulting a specialist. Gastrointestinal and renal toxicity from nonsteroidal anti-inflammatory agents is common in patients with chronic pain. Hepatotoxicity due to acetaminophen is also a concern, particularly if an acetaminophen-containing narcotic preparation is also prescribed. The relatively nonaddictive opiate analogue tramadol has been studied in painful diabetic neuropathy and found to be effective (Harati et al., 1998). Conventional opiate analgesics can be effective in painful diabetic neuropathy, as in any painful condition. Constipation, nausea, urinary retention, and unwanted sedation or cognitive difficulty can be problematic. Tolerance and physical dependence are expected with chronic therapy, but these are usually acceptable if pain is effectively relieved. Preparations that contain acetaminophen should usually be avoided if opiate tolerance is anticipated because tolerance to the hepatotoxicity of acetaminophen does not develop.

AUTONOMIC NEUROPATHY

After pain, autonomic symptoms are probably the most common problems associated with diabetic polyneuropathy for which patients seek treatment. The degree and prevalence of autonomic nervous system involvement increase with the duration of diabetes and severity of polyneuropathy, being detectable by abnormal beat-to-beat cardiac variability with respiration or Valsalva maneuver in approximately 30% of diabetics after 10 to 15 years of disease (Low, 1996).

Among the 380 subjects in the Rochester Diabetic Study (Dyck et al., 1993), impotence, the most common autonomic symptom in men, was reported in 13% of men with type 1 and 8% with type 2 diabetes. However, this is significantly lower than the prevalence reported in other studies. The prevalence of any degree of erectile dysfunction in men with or without diabetes between the ages of 40 and 70 years was found to be 52% in the Massachusetts Male Aging Study (Feldman et al., 1994), and the prevalence of complete impotence (no erections) was 10%, increasing from 5% at age 40 to 15% at age 70. Among diabetics in that study, the overall prevalence of complete impotence was about three times higher (28%) and also increased with age. The prevalence of erectile dysfunction in diabetics has been estimated to be between 35% and 75% in other studies, with higher rates in older patients (McCullock et al., 1980). Not all erectile dysfunction in diabetics is due to diabetic autonomic neuropathy (Rubin and Babbott, 1958; Zemel, 1988), as is evident from the high prevalence of this symptom in nondiabetic men. Atherosclerosis is also a factor if there is involvement of the internal pudendal artery. Medications can impair sexual function—notably, antidepressants and narcotic analgesics that may have been prescribed for neuropathic pain. Psychological factors are always important to consider in the evaluation of sexual dysfunction.

Treatment of erectile dysfunction in diabetics with the drug sildenafil has been shown to be helpful in about 50% of patients (Rendell et al., 1999). Its mechanism of action is based on the fact that cyclic guanosine monophosphate (cGMP)–mediated relaxation of corpus cavernosal smooth muscle is necessary for the initiation and maintenance of an erection. Sexual stimulation results in the release of nitric oxide from nerve endings and arteriolar endothelial cells in the penis. Nitric oxide activates guanylate cyclase, resulting in the production of cGMP. Sildenafil increases the concentration of cGMP within the corpus cavernosum by inhibiting cGMP phospodiesterase, which catalyzes its hydrolysis.

In a placebo-controlled study of 252 diabetics with erectile dysfunction, 56% of the patients taking 25 to 100 mg of sildenafil 1 hour before intercourse reported improved erections compared with 10% of the placebo group (Rendell et al., 1999). However, sildenafil is not as effective for neurogenic erectile dysfunction as it is for other types. In a study that compared its efficacy for erectile dysfunction of various etiologies, 58% of diabetics and 56% of nondiabetics with neurogenic erectile dysfunction reported satisfaction compared with 89% of patients with psychogenic and 86% with vasculogenic erectile dysfunction (Jarow et al., 1999). The group with the worst response had dysfunction caused by nerve damage during prostate surgery (35%). This might be predicted because release of nitric oxide from nerves is important for initiation of cGMP formation, so inhibition of cGMP hydrolysis will be ineffective if the nerves are sufficiently damaged. Nevertheless, a response rate of more than 50% in diabetics significantly exceeds success rates for older pharmacological treatments such as oral yohimbine or the injection of papaverine or prostaglandin E into the corpus cavernosum (Jarow et al., 1999). Sildenafil was tolerated reasonably well by patients with diabetes, although 16% developed symptoms related to the medication, most commonly headache, nausea, and nasal congestion. Cardiovascular symptoms were not more common with sildenafil than with placebo. Chest pain occurred in four patients who took placebo and in none of the sildenafil group (Rendell et al., 1999). The drug is contraindicated in patients taking nitrates because severe, sometimes fatal hypotension can result. If pharmacological treatment is unsatisfactory or contraindicated, a surgically implanted penile prosthesis can be considered.

After impotence, the next most common complaints referable to diabetic autonomic neuropathy result from involvement of the gastrointestinal tract. The alimentary tract can be involved at any level from the esophagus to the rectum, but the most common symptom is constipation, which can result from colonic denervation (Low, 1996). However, this symptom is so common in the general population that it is difficult to attribute it to diabetes in an individual patient.

Chronic severe intermittent diarrhea, particularly when nocturnal, is a more distinctive symptom of diabetic gastroenteropathy. The prevalence of chronic diarrhea among 861 patients attending a diabetes clinic was found to be 3.7%. Diabetic diarrhea, in which autonomic neuropathy is frequently implicated, was much more common in type 1 (5%) than in type 2 (0.4%) diabetics, in whom the most common cause of diarrhea was the oral hypoglycemic agent metformin (Lysy et al., 1999). Bacterial overgrowth within the small intestine has been shown to be present in almost 50% of patients diagnosed with diabetic diarrhea (Ogbonnaya and Arem, 1990; Valdovinos et al., 1993; Virally-Monod et al., 1998). Diminished motility due to autonomic neuropathy permits excessive proliferation of intestinal flora, leading to malabsorption. Antibiotic treatment (e.g., amoxicillin–clavulinic acid at 1.5 g/24 hr for 10 days) has been reported to produce a dramatic therapeutic response in 75% of patients in whom bacterial overgrowth was proved by glucose-hydrogen breath testing (Virally-Monod, 1998). It is important to maintain a high index of suspicion for vitamin B_{12} deficiency due to malabsorption in this group, particularly because vitamin B_{12} deficiency would be likely to speed progression of neuropathy. A Schilling's test will usually distinguish between vitamin B_{12} deficiency due to bacterial overgrowth from that due to autoimmune pernicious anemia, to which diabetics are also predisposed.

Celiac disease is common in diabetics, with histological evidence of the disease reported in 6% of type 1 diabetics (Greenberger and Isselbacher, 1998). Serological evidence of celiac disease (antiendomysial, anti-reticulin, or anti-gliadin antibodies) was found in 4% of 211 diabetic children with gastrointestinal symptoms in one study (Rossi et al., 1993). It is important to consider this diagnosis in diabetic patients with malabsorptive diarrhea because institution of a gluten-free diet is almost always effective in this group. Occasionally, diabetic patients have malabsorption due to abnormal function of the exocrine pancreas, and if so, pancreatic enzyme preparations are helpful (Greenberger and Isselbacher, 1998).

Unfortunately, in almost 50% of cases, no specific treatable explanation can be found for diabetic diarrhea, and abnormal motility or secretion due to autonomic neuropathy is suspected (Valdovinos et al., 1993). Anticholinergics and opioids can provide some symptomatic relief, and clonidine or somatostatin analogues such as octreotide have proved to be effective in refractory cases (Walker and Kaplan, 1993).

Diabetic gastroparesis results from autonomic neuropathy involving the stomach. It is detectable through the measurement of delayed gastric emptying in about 50% of diabetics, but it usually is not symptomatic (Kong et al., 1999). Esophageal motility is also commonly impaired in these patients. Symptomatic patients with gastroparesis may complain of anorexia, nausea, vomiting, abdominal pain, early satiety, or bloating.

Drugs that enhance gastric motility are useful in the treatment of diabetic gastroparesis. Metoclopramide (10 mg before meals) is often effective (Brunton, 1996). Its mechanism of action is thought to involve dopamine receptor antagonism in the upper gastrointestinal tract, which is known to enhance motility. It may also stimulate the release or enhance the activity of acetylcholine. Central nervous system toxicity, consisting mainly of extrapyramidal symptoms, limits its usefulness. This is particularly true in elderly patients, in whom parkinsonism is more likely to occur. Cisapride (Brunton, 1996) lacks extrapyramidal effects, being devoid of dopamine-blocking activity. It is thought to increase motility by enhancing the release of myenteric acetylcholine. Unfortunately, its use has been curtailed because it has been associated with sudden death and life-threatening cardiac arrhythmias. It should not be used in patients with heart disease that would predispose them to arrhythmias or who are taking medication that can prolong the QT interval (including tricyclic antidepressants). Domperidone blocks D_2 dopamine receptors and has been shown to be as effective as metoclopramide in the treatment of diabetic gastroparesis but with a lower incidence of central nervous system side effects (Brunton, 1996; Patterson et al., 1999). This is because it does not penetrate the blood-brain barrier well. Unfortunately, domperidone is not approved for use in the United States despite extensive worldwide marketing since 1978 (Barone, 1999). The gastrointestinal peptide motilin promotes gastric emptying, and erythromycin has been shown to stimulate motilin receptors. Oral erythromycin has been shown to improve gastric emptying in diabetics (Janssens et al., 1990; Brunton, 1996), but it is poorly tolerated because it tends to cause nausea and diarrhea. Intravenous erythromycin has been shown to be effective in severe, refractory cases (DiBaise and Quigley, 1999), but this mode of administration obviously limits its practical usefulness. Nevertheless, because patients with very severe gastroparesis sometimes require intravenous hyperalimentation, intravenous erythromycin may be a reasonable way to avoid that drastic step in selected patients.

Involvement of the bladder was present in 14% of patients with diabetic neuropathy reported by Rundles (1945). It typically results in bladder atony. Patients progressively lose the sensation of the need to void, and the length of time between voiding increases. Stretching of the bladder wall and loss of parasympathetic innervation of the detrusor result in a weak, intermittent stream and incomplete emptying. Overflow incontinence can eventually occur, and patients are at high risk for the development of urinary tract infections (Thomas and Tomlinson, 1993; Low, 1996).

Initial treatment consists of scheduled voiding. Manual pressure applied to the lower abdomen can improve emptying and reduce postvoid residual volume. The cholinergic agent bethanechol is sometimes helpful. Intermittent self-catheterization may be necessary, but sterile technique is very important. In men, transurethral resection of the prostate can improve bladder emptying. Urinary tract infections should be treated promptly. Chronic suppression of bacterial growth by nitrofurantoin is sometimes recommended, but this medication can cause or exacerbate peripheral neuropathy, so it should be avoided in patients with diabetic neuropathy.

Symptomatic orthostatic hypotension was present in 6% of 125 patients with diabetic neuropathy reported by Rundles (1945) and in 31% of 73 patients with diabetic autonomic neuropathy reported by Ewing and colleagues (1980). An additional 14% of the patients of Ewing and colleagues had asymptomatic drops of at least 30 mm Hg in systolic pressure on standing. Patients risk injury due to falls, and ischemic stroke can occur during hypotension, particularly in the presence of significant cerebrovascular disease with impaired vascular autoregulation.

Treatment (Thomas and Tomlinson, 1993; Low, 1996) should first address potentially exacerbating factors. Antihypertensive medication can usually be discontinued. Fluid and salt intake should be encouraged. Elevation of the head of the bed can lessen the adjustment required when the erect posture is assumed, with symptoms usually being worst on first arising in the morning. This position also helps avoid supine hypertension. Support stockings can be helpful. Caffeine-containing beverages at meals can limit postprandial hypotension.

Fludrocortisone, a mineralocorticoid, is useful when nonmedical treatment is not satisfactory. The initial dose is 0.1 mg daily, which can be cautiously increased, but the dose should not exceed 0.6 mg daily. Supine hypertension, fluid retention with cardiac decompensation, and hypokalemia are potential problems. Midodrine is a short-acting α-adrenergic agonist that was introduced for the treatment of orthostatic hypotension. Because its duration of action is 3 to 4 hours, it can be taken shortly before the patient expects to be standing and avoided 3 to 4 hours before bedtime, reducing the risk of supine hypertension.

Hyperglycemic Neuropathy

Nerve conduction velocity increases acutely after the treatment of severe hyperglycemia. Gregerson (1968) studied 14 newly diagnosed diabetics, most of whom had blood sugar levels in the range of 300 to 500 mg/dL initially. Virtually all patients showed increased peroneal conduction velocities, beginning within 2 days of the start of insulin therapy, corresponding to improvements in blood sugar levels. In six patients from whom insulin was subsequently withheld, velocities promptly decreased again as blood sugar values increased. However, no clinical correlation could be made, because there was no significant change in vibration sensation threshold. No patient had severely reduced velocities at diagnosis, as initial measurements were in the minimally reduced–low-normal range. The clinical significance of this acutely reversible effect of severe hyperglycemia on nerve conduction is uncertain, but it might explain the occasional newly diagnosed diabetic who reports acral pain or dysesthesia that quickly resolves with the establishment of normoglycemia. The term *hyperglycemic neuropathy* (Thomas, 1999) has been applied to this syndrome.

Insulin Neuritis

Paradoxically, some patients develop burning, dysesthetic skin soon after beginning insulin treatment (Caravati, 1933). This is said to usually involve the feet and legs (Thomas and Tomlinson, 1993), but in my experience (three patients), it has been more generalized, prominently involving the chest and back where even the touch of clothing is very uncomfortable. Nerve conduction studies and electromyography results have been normal or mildly abnormal, and Achilles tendon reflexes can be retained consistent with involvement of small cutaneous nerve fibers.

A sural nerve biopsy taken soon after onset in one reported case (Llewelyn et al., 1986) showed only chronic neuropathy with axonal regeneration. The authors postulated that the establishment of euglycemia in a patient with chronic neuropathy may have permitted axonal regeneration and that the pain originated from newly regenerated axons.

Some authors have noted a tendency for this syndrome to resolve with continued insulin treatment (Thomas and Tomlinson, 1993; Pourmand, 1997) and have postulated that delayed adjustment to lower but normal glucose concentrations can cause transiently impaired energy metabolism in peripheral nerves. However, in my experience, burning pain and dysesthesia persisted for 3 years in one patient with type 2 diabetes, subsiding promptly when insulin (human recombinant) was discontinued and hyperglycemia was managed by diet alone. Blood glucose levels were slightly higher without insulin treatment, so the patient's cutaneous nerves might have had an idiosyncratic, persistent requirement for higher glucose concentrations. Although he used human recombinant insulin, it is also possible that this was an immune reaction to exogenous insulin, as originally proposed by Caravati (1933). The pain of Caravati's patient also promptly subsided when insulin was discontinued. Fortunately, this syndrome is rare and may not always have the same pathophysiological basis.

Hypoglycemic Neuropathy

This is a rarely reported entity, and its existence has not been firmly established. Hypoglycemia usually does not result in peripheral neuropathy because the sensitivity of the brain to low levels of circulating glucose far exceeds that of the peripheral nervous system. In the brain, neurons are essentially dependent on circulating glucose for energy metabolism, whereas spinal cord neurons and peripheral axons are able to utilize fatty acids and amino acids. Hypoglycemia in animals and in humans can cause devastating, irreversible brain damage without affecting peripheral nerves. With more protracted, severe hypoglycemia, spinal neurons are affected, with anterior horn cells being most sensitive (Winkelman and Moore, 1940).

Most reports of "hypoglycemic neuropathy" have been of patients with insulinomas (Danta, 1969; Harrison, 1976; Jaspan et al., 1982) who develop a distal, symmetrical polyneuropathy, often with distal pain and paresthesia. Onset has usually been acute or subacute, but the development of peripheral neuropathy in these patients was not always correlated with individual episodes of hypoglycemia. It is possible that peripheral neuropathy in these patients was a paraneoplastic phenomenon rather than a result of hypoglycemia. Paraneoplastic neurological diseases result from the reaction of the immune system to a tumor. They are caused by autoimmune attack against normal neuronal components that are similar to tumor antigens. Endocrine cells bear many similarities to neurons, both being of similar embryological origin, so a paraneoplastic syndrome associated with islet cell tumors would be consistent with this mechanism. The tumor most commonly associated with paraneoplastic syndromes is small cell carcinoma of the lung, also of neuroendocrine origin. The disproportionately large number of reported patients with insulinoma who develop neuropathy despite the rarity of this tumor and the common occurrence of hypoglycemia due to other causes also favors a mechanism specifically related to the tumor other than hypoglycemia.

In one patient (Harrison, 1976), also with insulinoma, distal muscle wasting occurred during prolonged hypoglycemic coma, and nerve conduction studies and electromyography were more consistent with anterior horn cell damage than with peripheral neuropathy. As mentioned, anterior horn cell bodies within the spinal cord are more sensitive to glucose deprivation than are peripheral axons.

Another group often cited as providing evidence for hypoglycemic neuropathy is the psychiatric patients who were treated with insulin-induced hypoglycemia in the 1940s and 1950s (Stern et al., 1942; Zeigler, 1954). Sensory symptoms developed in 10 of 103 patients reported by Stern and colleages (1942) at some time during the course of insulin therapy, and Zeigler (1954) found this in 13 of 24 patients. Numbness usually involved the hands and often the nose or other areas of the face. No patient had objective weakness or wasting, findings that were prominent in the insulinoma group. The sensory symptoms were commonly transient. Transient subjective numbness in the hands and face is known to commonly occur among anxious patients who have not had insulin therapy and is usually attributed to hyperventilation. Thus, the existence of a syndrome that can properly be called *hypoglycemic neuropathy* remains to be proved.

VASCULAR NEUROPATHIES

Although the role of ischemia in the pathogenesis of diabetic polyneuropathy is debated, it has been well established for certain distinctive focal, multifocal, and proximal neuropathies to which diabetics are predisposed.

Diabetic Inflammatory Vasculopathy

CLINICAL FEATURES

Garland (1955) used the term *diabetic amyotrophy* to describe a syndrome that is now known to be characterized pathologically by inflammation of small epineurial blood vessels and by nerve infarctions. The patients reported by Garland (1955, 1961) had pain and progressive weakness and atrophy of lower extremity muscles, evolving over weeks to months. The quadriceps were most commonly affected, but involvement of other proximal as well as distal muscles was also described. Deep tendon reflexes related to weak muscles were lost. In some of his patients, the weakness was bilateral, but if so, it was asymmetrical, and in some, there was involvement of shoulder girdle muscles. Subsequent reports have mentioned occasional involvement of thoracic or abdominal regions. The involvement of one lower extremity is often followed by the involvement of the contralateral limb after several weeks or months (Chokroverty et al., 1977; Said et al., 1994; Krendel et al., 1995; Dyck et al., 1999). Weight loss has also come to be recognized as a common feature, sometimes reaching cachectic proportions and arousing the suspicion of malignancy (Bastron and Thomas, 1981; Subharmony and Wilborn, 1982; Krendel et al., 1995; Dyck et al., 1999). Garland (1955) found that men were affected about twice as often as were women and that most patients were older than 50, a consistent finding in most studies that address the epidemiology of this syndrome (Bastron and Thomas, 1981; Krendel et al., 1995; Dyck et al., 1999). The prognosis was generally favorable in Garland's opinion, as all of his patients ultimately improved to some extent and some recovered completely, but he did not provide further details. For treatment, he recommended optimizing blood sugar control (good advice for diabetics under any circumstances), despite reporting several patients who "continued to deteriorate in an alarming fashion for some months after diabetes was fully controlled." Garland and, later, others recognized the syndrome occasionally in patients without diabetes (Bradley et al., 1984; Triggs et al., 1997; Verma and Bradley, 1994), and he suggested that "one of the collagen diseases" might be have been the cause in such cases. Garland (as well as Bradley et al., 1984; Triggs et al., 1997; and Verma and Bradley, 1994) recommended a therapeutic trial of immunosuppressive (steroid) treatment for nondiabetics. Since Garland's description of diabetic amyotrophy, other authors have often used alternate names for this syndrome, albeit sometimes to distinguish clinical variations; these have included *proximal diabetic neuropathy* (Asbury, 1977; Said et al., 1994), *diabetic mononeuropathy multiplex* (Raff et al., 1968), *diabetic polyradiculopathy* (Bastron and Thomas, 1981), *diabetic femoral neuropathy* (Coppack and Watkins, 1991), *diabetic neuropathic cachexia* (Ellenberg, 1974), and *diabetic lumbosacral radiculoplexus neuropathy* (Dyck et al., 1999).

This syndrome is uncommon in comparison with diabetic polyneuropathy, being found in only 2% of 380 unselected diabetics reported by Dyck and associates (1993). However, it is quite common among patients with diabetic neuropathy who are referred to a tertiary center for neurological consultation. In one series, this syndrome was identified in about 85% of 55 prospectively ascertained diabetics who were referred for neuromuscular consultation because of peripheral neuropathy severe enough to cause disabling weakness (Krendel et al., 1997). This is because it accounts for a disproportionately high percentage of patients with severe, disabling neuropathy. Also, referring physicians are less likely to easily attribute proximal or multifocal neuropathies to diabetes, in part because the severity of the neuropathy does not match the severity of the diabetes. It tends to occur in type 2 diabetics (about 80%), often soon after or before the diagnosis, and sometimes worsens despite meticulous blood sugar control (Bradley et al., 1984; Garland, 1961). Also unlike diabetic polyneuropathy, it does not tend to be associated with other diabetic complications (Chokroverty et al., 1977; Bastron and Thomas, 1981; Dyck et al., 1999). In a series of 33 patients (Dyck et al., 1999), only 4 had retinopathy (nonproliferative) and 2 had nephropathy.

PATHOGENESIS

Histopathological studies have consistently shown evidence of nerve infarction. Raff and colleagues (1968) reported a detailed postmortem histological study of lower extremity nerves from a man with this syndrome who died unexpectedly 9.5 weeks after the onset. The patient had been clinically stable for 6 weeks before his cardiac arrest. Focal zones of apparent loss or discontinuity in axons and myelin were interpreted as infarctions. An artery occluded by organized thrombus was seen in the obturator nerve, providing further evidence of ischemic pathogenesis. The cause of the thrombosis was not apparent. A lymphocytic infiltrate involving a small epineurial vessel was present, but it was relatively mild and was not considered to be significant. However, subsequent biopsy studies (Bradley et al., 1984; Costigan et al., 1990; Said et al., 1994; Krendel et al., 1995; Younger et al., 1996; Llewelyn et al., 1998; Dyck et al., 1999) have shown that inflammation of small vessels is a common and characteristic finding, possibly because biopsies are more likely to be performed at an active phase of the disease process when clinical decisions are being made.

Vascular inflammation in biopsy samples has been seen in about 50% of patients in most series. This has most commonly consisted of perivascular collections of lymphocytes, with actual vasculitis being reported in 10% to 50%. Vasculitis has usually been seen as transmural lymphocytic infiltration of small epineurial arteries or arterioles, but fibrinoid necrosis has been reported in a few specimens (Dyck et al., 1999).

Bradley and colleagues (1984) found lymphocytic infiltrates surrounding small epineurial arterioles in sural nerve biopsy samples from six patients with painful lumbosacral plexopathy. Focal involvement of nerve fascicles consistent with infarction was seen in three. Three of the six patients were diabetic but were not thought to have diabetic plexopathy because they worsened despite good diabetic control (a clinical phenomenon originally described by Garland in several patients whom he considered to have diabetic amyotrophy). Bradley and colleagues treated all three diabetics with prednisone and also treated two with cyclophosphamide. All three appeared to respond favorably.

Said and colleagues (1994) took biopsy samples of cutaneous nerves from the thighs of 10 patients with proximal diabetic neuropathy and found vasculitis in 2 and perivascular inflammation in 4.

In another series (Krendel et al., 1995), vasculitis was found in 2 of 15 patients and perivascular inflammation in 5 patients. Vascular inflammation was found in the epineurium of the sural nerve in 3, a femoral cutaneous branch in 2, and in the quadriceps muscle in 2 patients.

Llewelyn and colleagues (1998) found microvasculitis or epineurial inflammatory infiltrates in 4 of 15 patients with proximal diabetic neuropathy.

Younger and colleagues (1996) found microvasculitis in sural nerve biopsy samples from 6 of 12 patients with proximal diabetic neuropathy. The remaining 6 patients with proximal neuropathy all showed perivascular inflammation. Both of the patients with mononeuropathy multiplex and 2 of 6 patients with distal symmetrical polyneuropathy also had microvasculitis. The occasional occurrence of distal symmetrical neuropathy is not unexpected, because this pattern occurs in about 40% of nondiabetic patients with neuropathy due to vasculitis (Kissel et al., 1985; Dyck et al., 1987). Multiple random small lesions in nerve trunks might preferentially affect axons destined to reach distal muscles, because those axons traverse the longest segments of the nerves.

Dyck and colleagues (1999) published findings in distal cutaneous nerve biopsy specimens from 33 patients with this syndrome and reported perivascular inflammation in all 33, compared with 6 of 21 with diabetic polyneuropathy and 2 of 14 normal control subjects. A total of 15 of the 33 patients with proximal diabetic neuropathy had inflammation of the vessel walls, with fibrinoid necrosis of the vascular walls in 2, compared with none in biopsy samples from patients with diabetic polyneuropathy or from normal control subjects. In addition, patients with proximal diabetic neuropathy had a significantly higher prevalence of microscopic findings suggesting ischemic damage such as focal nerve fiber loss.

Thus, small vessel inflammation with associated

nerve infarction is well established to be the typical pathological finding in this syndrome, implying that it is caused by an inflammatory vasculopathy.

In addition to nerve, vessels within muscle can be involved, sometimes associated with muscle cell necrosis resembling polymyositis (Krendel, 1997). It appears that this is primarily a disease of small blood vessels rather than of nerve. The reason for its predilection to involve nerves and muscles or, more specifically, nerves and muscles in the thighs is unknown; perhaps the vascular supply to these structures is relatively tenuous.

Laboratory findings in this syndrome are not distinctive. As mentioned, renal function is not usually impaired. Bradley and associates (1984) emphasized elevation of the sedimentation rate in all three of their diabetic patients with lumbosacral plexopathy as evidence supporting an inflammatory process rather than a metabolic cause. I find an elevated sedimentation rate in about half of the patients in whom it is measured. Cerebrospinal fluid is usually normal except for elevated protein (Dyck et al., 1999; Garland, 1961; Bastron and Thomas, 1981; Subharmony and Wilborn, 1982), as originally noted by Garland (1961). Dyck and colleagues (1999) found a median cerebrospinal fluid protein level of 89 g/dL with a range of 44 to 214 g/dL.

ELECTROPHYSIOLOGY

Electrophysiological studies in diabetic patients with proximal or multifocal neuropathies typically show evidence of axon loss in the affected area, and often in areas that are not clinically involved. Although the weight of evidence favors axon loss as the basic pathological mechanism, in about 2% of patients with clinically typical proximal diabetic neuropathy, nerve conduction study results meet criteria for demyelinating neuropathy as proposed for CIDP (Cornblath et al., 1991). Electromyography usually shows evidence of denervation, with fibrillations and reduced recruitment (Chokroverty et al., 1977; Bastron and Thomas, 1981; Subharmony and Wilborn, 1982; Dyck et al., 1999; Krendel et al., 1999), but myopathic changes are occasionally seen (i.e., small, complex, easily recruited motor unit potentials) (Lamontagne and Buchthal, 1970; Krendel et al., 1995). This probably reflects the myopathic changes sometimes seen in muscle biopsy samples (Krendel, 1997) and supports the idea that inflammatory vasculopathy can damage muscle as well as nerve. Alternatively, ischemic damage to terminal branches of motor axons could produce a myopathic electromyographic pattern by reducing the size of individual motor unit potentials.

Subharmony and Wilbourn (1982) studied 27 patients with proximal diabetic neuropathy and compared 17 patients who had associated distal symmetrical polyneuropathy (presumed diabetic polyneuropathy) with 10 patients who did not. Patients with coexisting polyneuropathy tended to have a more gradual onset and to have both clinical and electrodiagnostic evidence of bilateral disease, whereas onset was abrupt and weakness was unilateral in all except 1 of 10 patients without polyneuropathy. In addition to denervation in limb muscles, paraspinal muscles showed fibrillations in 15 of 16 patients with and 3 of 10 patients without polyneuropathy. The finding of paraspinal fibrillations correlated with elevated cerebrospinal fluid protein. This might reflect nerve root involvement due to proximal diabetic neuropathy, but elevated cerebrospinal fluid protein is common in diabetics with (but not those without) polyneuropathy (Madonick and Margolis, 1952). Fibrillations in the paraspinal muscles could be produced by ischemic damage to branches of the posterior rami within the paraspinal muscles themselves. The finding of Chokroverty and associates (1977) of variable slowing among different branches of the femoral nerve lends support to the idea that lesions are located in intramuscular nerve branches.

The thoracic or abdominal region is affected in a significant proportion of patients with proximal diabetic neuropathy, being involved in 4 of 33 patients (Dyck et al., 1999) and in 9 of 47 patients (Krendel et al., 1997). When these areas are involved in isolation, the terms *diabetic thoracic radiculopathy* and *thoracoabdominal* or *truncal neuropathy* have been applied (Longstretch and Newcomber, 1977; Sun and Streib, 1981; Stewart, 1989). Because of their common association, the pathogenesis of truncal neuropathy is probably the same as that for proximal neuropathy. Abdominal or chest pain is the most prominent clinical feature, often leading to a mistaken diagnosis of visceral pain. Abdominal muscle denervation can sometimes be recognized clinically as a hernia-like bulge over the weakened area when the patient attempts to sit up. The location of the lesion, as with other manifestations of proximal neuropathy, is probably in cutaneous or intramuscular nerve branches rather than in roots. The distribution of sensory loss usually corresponds to a distal branch of an intercostal nerve (Stewart, 1989), and skin biopsy samples from affected areas have shown loss of nerve fibers, indicating lesions distal to the dorsal root ganglia (Lauria et al., 1998). Fibrillations are commonly found in thoracic paraspinal muscles, possibly reflecting damage at the root level. However, lesions involving the dorsal rami probably account for this finding in many cases, because sensory disturbances may be confined to the sensory distribution of the dorsal rami. Also, fibrillations are sometimes found in abdominal muscles but not in paraspinal muscles, consistent with intracostal nerve or nerve branch rather than thoracic root involvement (Sun and Streib, 1981).

TREATMENT

The potential for spontaneous improvement or recovery was strongly emphasized by Garland (1961) when he wrote, "It can be categorically stated that even the bed-ridden patient may make a full

Lamontagne A, Buchthal F: Electrophysiologic studies in diabetic neuropathy. J Neurol Neurosurg Psychiatry 1970;33:442–452.

Lauria G, McArthur JC, Hauser PE, et al: Neuropathological alterations in diabetic truncal neuropathy: Evaluation by skin biopsy. J Neurol Neurosurg Psychiatry 1998;65:762–766.

Llewelyn JG, Thomas PK, Fonseca V, et al: Acute painful diabetic neuropathy precipitated by strict glycaemic control. Acta Neuropathol 1986;72:157–163.

Llewelyn JG, Thomas PK, King RH: Epineurial microvasculitis in proximal diabetic neuropathy. J Neurol 1998;245:159–165.

Longstretch GF, Newcomber AD: Abdominal pain caused by diabetic radiculopathy. Ann Intern Med 1977;86:166–186.

Low PA, Tuck RR, Dyck PJ, et al: Prevention of some electrophysiologic and biochemical abnormalities with oxygen supplementation in experimental diabetic neuropathy. Proc Natl Acad Sci U S A 1984;81:6894.

Low PA: Recent advances in the pathogenesis of diabetic neuropathy. Muscle Nerve 1987;10:121–128.

Low PA: Diabetic autonomic neuropathy. Semin Neurol 1996;16:143–151.

Lysy J, Isreli E, Goldin E: The prevalence of chronic diarrhea among diabetic patients. Am J Gastroenterol 1999;94:2165–2170.

Madonick MJ, Margolis J: Protein content of spinal fluid in diabetes mellitus: report on one hundred cases. Arch Neurol Psychiatry 1952;68:641–644.

Malik RA, Williamson S, Abbott C, Carrington AL, et al: Effect of angiotensin-converting enzyme (ACE) inhibitor trandolapril on human diabetic neuropathy: Randomized double-blind controlled trial. Lancet 1998;352:1978–1981.

Max MB, Culnane M, Schager SC, et al: Amitriptyline relieves diabetic neuropathy pain in patients with normal or depressed mood. Neurology 1987;37:589–596.

Max MB, Lynch SA, Muire J, et al: Effects of desipramine, amitriptyline, and fluoxetine on pain in diabetic neuropathy. N Engl J Med 1992;326:1250–1256.

McCulloch DK, Campbell IW, Wu FC, et al: The prevalence of diabetic impotence. Diabetologia 1980;18:279–283.

McQuay H, Carroll D, Jadad AR, et al: Anticonvulsant drugs for management of pain: A systematic review. BMJ 1995;311:1047–1052.

Menkes DL, Hood DC, Balleseros RA: Root stimulation improves the detection of acquired demyelinating polyneuropathies. Muscle Nerve 1998;21:298–308.

Mitsumoto H, Tsuzaka K: Neurotrophic factors and neuromuscular disease: 1. Gereral comments, the neurotrophin family, and neuropoietic cytokines. Muscle Nerve 1999;22:983–999.

Morello CM, Leckband SG, Stoner CP, et al: Randomized double-blind study comparing the efficacy of gabapentin with amitriptyline on diabetic peripheral neuropathy pain. Arch Intern Med 1999;159:1931–1937.

Navarro X, Sutherland DER, Kennedy WR: Long-term effects of pancreatic transplantation on diabetic neuropathy. Ann Neurol 1997;42:727–736.

Navarro X, Kennedy WR: Benefit of pancreatic transplantation on diabetic neuropathy: Euglycemia or immunosuppression [reply]? Ann Neurol 1998;44:149–150.

Ogbonnaya KI, Arem R: Diabetic diarrhea: Pathophysiology, diagnosis, and management. Arch Intern Med 1990;150:262–267.

Pascoe, MK, Low PA, Windebank AJ: Subacute diabetic proximal neuropathy. Mayo Clin Proc 1997;72:1123–1132.

Patterson D, Abell T, Rothstein R, et al: A double-blind multicenter comparison of domperidone and metoclopramide in the treatment of diabetic patients with symptoms of gastroparesis. Am J Gastroenterol 1999;94:1230–1234.

Pirart J: Diabetes mellitus and its degenerative complications: A prospective study of 4400 patients observed between 1947 and 1973. Diabetes Care 1978;1:168–188, 252–263.

Pittenger GL, Malik RA, Burcus N, et al: Specific fiber deficits in sensorimotor diabetic neuropathy correspond to cytotoxicity against neuroblastoma cells of sera from patients with diabetes. Diabetes Care 1999;22:1839–1844.

Pourmand R: Diabetic neuropathy. Neurol Clin North Am 1997;15:569–576.

Raff MC, Sangalang V, Asbury AK: Ischemic mononeuropathy multiplex associated with diabetes mellitus. Arch Neurol 1968;18:487–499.

Reeves ML, Seigler DE, Ayyar DR, et al: Medial plantar sensory response: Sensitive indicator of peripheral nerve dysfunction in patients with diabetes mellitus. Am J Med 1984;76:842–846.

Rendell MS, Rajfer J, Wicker PA, et al: Sildenafil for treatment of erectile dysfunction in men with diabetes: A randomized controlled trial. JAMA 1999;281:421–426.

Rossi TM, Albini CH, Kumar V: Incidence of celiac disease identified by the presence of serum endomysial antibodies in children with chronic diarrhea, short stature, or insulin-dependent diabetes mellitus. J Pediatr 1993;123:262–264.

Rubin A, Babbott D: Impotence in diabetes mellitus. JAMA 1958;168:498–500.

Rundles RW: Diabetic neuropathy. Medicine (Balt) 1945;24:11–159.

Said G, Goulongoeau C, Lacroix C, et al: Nerve biopsy findings in different forms of proximal diabetic neuropathy. Ann Neurol 1994;35:559–569.

Said G: Painful proximal diabetic neuropathy: Inflammatory nerve lesions and spontaneous favorable outcome. Ann Neurol 1997;41:762–770.

Schnell O, Muhr D, Dresel S, et al: Autoantibodies against sympathetic ganglia and evidence of cardiac sympathetic dysinnervation in newly diagnosed and long-term IDDM patients. Diabetologia 1996;39:970–975.

Sharma KR, Cross J, Ayar DR, et al: Diabetic demyelinating neuropathy responsive to intravenous immunoglobin. Neurology 1999;52:A121.

Sima AF: Metabolic alterations of peripheral nerve in diabetes. Semin Neurol 1996;16:129–137.

Simpson DA: Diabetic autoimmune neuropathies: Response to intravenous gammaglobulin. Muscle Nerve 1997;20:1069–1070.

Sindrup SH, Bjerre U, Dejgaard A, et al: The selective serotonin reuptake inhibitor citalopram relieves the symptoms of diabetic neuropathy. Clin Pharm Ther 1992;52:547–552.

Souaya N, Krendel DA: Central nervous system demyelination in diabetes mellitus. Neurology 2000;51:441–442.

Stern K, Dancey TE, McNauton FL: Sensory disturbances following insulin treatment of psychoses. J Nerv Ment Dis 1942;95:183–191.

Stevens EJ, Carrington AL, Tomlinson DR: Prostacyclin release in experimental diabetes: Effect of evening primrose oil. Br J Pharmacol 1993;107:276P.

Stewart JD: Diabetic truncal neuropathy: Topography of the sensory deficit. Ann Neurol 1989;25:233–238.

Stewart JD, McKelvey R, Durcan L, et al: Chronic inflammatory demyelinating polyneuropathy (CIDP) in diabetics. J Neurol Sci 1996;142:59–64.

Stracke H, Meyer UE, Shumacher HE, et al: Mexiletine in the treatment of diabetic neuropathy. Diabetes Care 1992;15:1550–1555.

Subharmony SH, Wilbourn AJ: Diabetic proximal neuropathy: Clinical and electromyographic studies. J Neurol Sci 1982;53:293–304.

Sugimura K, Dyck PJ: Multifocal fiber loss in proximal sciatic nerve in symmetric distal diabetic neuropathy. J Neurol Sci 1982;53:501–509.

Sun SF, Streib EW: Diabetic thoracoabdominal neuropathy: Clinical and electrodiagnostic features. Ann Neurol 1981;9:75–79.

Tandan R, Lewis GA, Krusinski PB, et al: Topical capsaicin in painful diabetic neuropathy: Controlled study with long-term follow-up. Diabetes Care 2992;15:8–14.

Thomas PK, Tomlinson DR: Diabetic and hypoglycemic neuropathy. In Dyck PJ, Thomas PK, Low PA, Podulso JF (eds): Peripheral Neuropathy. Philadelphia, WB Saunders, 1993;1216–1250.

Thomas PK: Diabetic neuropathy: Mechanisms and future treatment options. J Neurol Neurosurg Psychiat 1999;67:277–279.

Triggs WJ, Young MS, Eskin T, et al: Treatment of idiopathic lumbosacral plexopathy. Muscle Nerve 1997;20:244–246.

Trojaborg W, Smith T, Jakobsen J, et al: Cardiorespiratory reflexes, vibratory and thermal thresholds, sensory and motor conduction in diabetic patients with end-stage nephropathy. Acta Neurol Scand 1994;90:1–4.

Trojaborg W: The electrophysiologic profile of diabetic neuropathy. Semin Neurol 1996;16:123–128.

Valdovinos MA, Camilleri M, Zimmerman BR: Chronic diarrhea in diabetes mellitus: Mechanisms and an approach to diagnosis and treatment. Mayo Clinic Proc 1993;68:691–702.

Verma A, Bradley WG: High-dose intravenous immunoglobin therapy in chronic progressive lumbosacral plexopathy. Neurology 1994;44:248–250.

Virally-Monod M, Tielmans D, Kevorkian JP, et al: Chronic diarrhea and diabetes mellitus: Prevalence of small intestinal bacterial overgrowth. Diabetes Metab 1998;24:530–536.

Walker JJ, Kaplan DS: Efficacy of the somatostatin analog octreotide in the treatment of two patients with refractory diabetic diarrhea. Am J Gastroenterol 1993;88:765–767.

Westfall SG, Felten DL, Mandelbaum JA, et al: Degenerative neuropathy in insulin treated diabetic rats. J Neurol Sci 1983; 61:93–107.

Winkelman NW, Moore MT: Neurohistopathologic changes with metrazol and insulin shock therapy. Arch Neurol Psychiat 1940; 43:1108–1137.

Yagihashi S: Pathology and pathogenic mechanisms in diabetic neuropathy. Diabetes Metab Rev 1995;11:193–227.

Younger DS, Rosoklija G, Hays AP, et al: Diabetic peripheral neuropathy: A clinicopathologic and immunohistochemical study of sural nerve biopsies. Muscle Nerve 1996;19:722–727.

Zeigler DK: Minor neurologic signs and symptoms following insulin coma. J Nerv Ment Dis 1954;120:76–78.

Zemel P: Sexual dysfunction in the diabetic patient with hypertension. Am J Cardiol 1988;61:27H–33H.

Peripheral Neuropathy in Systemic Disease

Brian A. Crum and Charles F. Bolton

Neurological complications of systemic disease are common and vital to recognize. These complications may be the first manifestation of a more systemic disease process, and the early detection of this process can then lead to prompt treatment and avoidance of further complications. In terms of peripheral neuropathy, diagnosis of a systemic disorder that is causative may offer the opportunity to reverse or halt progression of the neuropathy and, again, to potentially prevent further neurological and systemic complications. (See other chapters in this Section, and Chapters 74 and 82.)

HYPOTHYROIDISM

The thyroid gland develops embryologically from pharyngeal epithelium and lateral pharyngeal pouches and descends to its final position leaving the thyroglossal duct behind. The normal adult thyroid is a bilobed structure joined by an isthmus that lies directly anterior to the laryngeal cartilage. It responds to thyroid-stimulating hormone (thyrotropin), which is released from the anterior pituitary gland in response to thyrotropin-releasing hormone

from the hypothalamus. The thyroid gland secretes L-thyroxine and triiodothyronine.

Thyroid hormones regulate growth and development of cells and tissues in several ways. The primary mechanism of action of thyroxine and triiodothyronine is through binding to intracellular receptors. These receptor complexes then bind to regulatory sites of chromosomes to affect genomic expression. There may also be regulation of mitochondrial function and regulation of the activity of ionized calcium adenosine triphosphatase (Ca^{2+}-ATPase). Thyroid hormone is also important in mobilizing mucopolysaccharides and in preventing their deposition in skin and other tissues.

Hypothyroidism is the result of impaired secretion of the active thyroid hormones from the thyroid gland. Most often, this is the result of failure of the thyroid gland itself (*primary hypothyroidism*). Suprathyroid origins account for up to 5% of cases and are caused by failure of the anterior pituitary or hypothalamus. *Cretinism* is the term given to congenital hypothyroidism resulting in developmental abnormalities. *Myxedema* refers to severe hypothyroidism in which there is thickening of facial features and a doughy texture to the skin caused by accumulation of mucopolysaccharides in subcutaneous tissues.

The clinical manifestations of hypothyroidism depend in some degree on the age at onset of the illness. In cretinism, shortly after birth, jaundice, hoarse cry, constipation, somnolence, and feeding problems are noted. With time, developmental delay occurs, and the physical characteristics of cretinism appear: short stature, coarse facies, dry skin, and delayed dentition, as well as impaired mental development. In older children, cognitive deficiency and delayed growth are most likely to occur (Wartofsky, 1998).

Symptoms and signs develop insidiously in the adult patient with hypothyroidism. Slowness, lethargy, fatigue, constipation, cold intolerance, increased weight, loss of hair, dryness of skin, and a deeper, hoarse voice all may appear. Without detection and treatment, hypothyroidism progresses, leading to myxedema with periorbital puffiness, large tongue, dull facies, sparse hair, and typical skin changes. Psychiatric symptoms or cerebellar ataxia may also be present. The end stage of myxedema is a hypothermic, stuporous, or comatose state that may be fatal. Central nervous system manifestations include depressed mental status, seizures, headaches, and ataxia. Weakness, usually proximal, and myopathic changes on electromyography occur in these patients. Disorders of neuromuscular transmission can occur in hypothyroid patients. Complaints of paresthesias and clinical and electrophysiological evidence of mononeuropathies (predominantly carpal tunnel syndrome) and peripheral neuropathies are also seen (Rao et al., 1980).

One interesting clinical sign is that of the *myoedema reflex,* first described in 1884 (Ord, 1884). This term refers to the prolongation of muscle contraction and relaxation that occurs when the examiner elicits muscle stretch reflexes, especially at the ankle. The decreased function of the calcium adenosine triphosphatase, which clears calcium from the cytoplasm after muscle contraction, may be the explanation for the delayed relaxation. Myoedema is due to electrically silent muscle contraction, leading to a mounding up of muscle, brought on by percussion or irritation of muscle. This is seen in up to one third of patients with hypothyroidism and may be related to the same mechanism of rippling muscle disease. *Hoffman's syndrome* is a condition seen in adults with hypothyroidism in which muscles are hypertrophied and become painful and stiff with exercise. This muscle activity, as in myoedema, is electrically silent. Muscle enlargement in children with hypothyroidism, termed *Kocher-Debré-Sémélaigne syndrome,* is not associated with muscle pain (Laycock and Pascuzzi, 1991; Wartofsky, 1998).

Much of the literature on peripheral neuropathy in hypothyroidism is gleaned from those patients with more severe disease, or myxedema, which is not as common today with more sophisticated testing and screening. Paresthesias without objective peripheral or central nervous system signs are frequently present. Mononeuropathies, most often median neuropathy at the wrist (carpal tunnel syndrome), and length-dependent, sensorimotor peripheral neuropathy are the most common peripheral neuropathic complications seen in hypothyroidism.

Carpal Tunnel Syndrome

The median nerve travels through an anatomical tunnel in the volar proximal wrist; this tunnel, made up of carpal bones and ligaments, is called the carpal tunnel. Increases in pressure within the canal lead to the common *carpal tunnel syndrome.* Typical clinical symptoms include paresthesias in the distal median nerve sensory distribution, wrist pain, nocturnal exacerbation, and clumsiness of the hand and fingers. Signs on neurological examination include loss of sensation over the volar aspect of the first three digits, thenar muscle weakness and atrophy, Tinel's and Phalen's signs, and positive results on the carpal tunnel compression test. Electromyography is important in confirming the diagnosis, in grading the severity, and in eliminating other possible disorders (i.e., cervical radiculopathy, brachial plexopathy, proximal median neuropathy).

Patients with hypothyroidism frequently complain of paresthesias in the hands, typically bilaterally. In one third of patients, thenar muscle atrophy is seen (Murray and Simpson, 1958). No consistent correlation is found between the severity of myxedema and the presence of carpal tunnel syndrome (Murray and Simpson, 1958; Purnell et al., 1961). Studies have quoted a prevalence of carpal tunnel syndrome in hypothyroidism of 2% to 20% (Murray and Simpson, 1958; Scarpalezos et al., 1973; Rao et al., 1980). In the study by Rao et al., whereas only 15% of patients had symptoms of carpal tunnel syndrome, nearly half of the 20 patients had electrophysiological evidence of median neuropathy at the wrist (in six it was a subclinical median neuropathy at the wrist) (Rao et al., 1980). One prospective study of 24 patients with newly diagnosed hypothyroidism found that 29% had clinical signs of carpal tunnel syndrome (often bilateral), whereas only 25% of all the patients had electrophysiological signs of carpal tunnel syndrome (Duyff et al., 2000).

Pathological findings in patients with carpal tunnel syndrome have included edematous synovial tissue and fibrosis (Purnell et al., 1961) and soft tissue deposition of a mucinous material (Nickel et al., 1961) within the carpal tunnel itself, features suggesting an explanation for mechanical compression of the median nerve. Increase in weight, edema (anasarca), and joint effusions are other hypothesized mechanisms. There is improvement or elimination of symptoms with treatment of the underlying hypothyroidism, and therefore, carpal tunnel release surgery is usually not necessary (Purnell et al., 1961).

Other Mononeuropathies

Hypothyroidism can lead to *anosmia,* and it has been shown in mice to cause a loss of development of neural olfactory epithelium (Mackay-Sim and Beard et al., 1987). Anosmia also improves after hormone replacement. *Hearing loss* can occur in hypothyroidism and may be related to fluid accumulation in the inner ear or changes in the spiral ganglion or the organ of Corti. Hearing usually improves after hormone replacement. *Hoarseness* and *dysarthria* occur in hypothyroidism, but they are probably related to mucopolysaccharide deposition within the larynx, vocal cords, and tongue, and not to cranial nerve dysfunction (Ritter, 1967). There have been reports of isolated *cranial nerve palsies:* II, V, VII, and VIII (Nickel et al., 1961; Nickel and Frame, 1961; Abend and Tyler, 1989), as well as phrenic neuropathy (Hamley et al., 1975; Laroche et al., 1988) and megacolon related to infiltration of Auerbach's plexus (Borrie et al., 1983). In a patient with hypothyroidism and pretibial pitting edema, a deep peroneal palsy was present (Yasuoka et al., 1993). Conduction block was seen on nerve conduction studies without other mononeuropathies or peripheral neuropathy. The patient's palsy completely resolved 2 months after treatment with levothyroxine. It is unclear whether this mononeuropathy was related to direct damage to nerve (or myelin) or whether this was a consequence of local edema and nerve impingement. Distal tibial neuropathy *(tarsal tunnel syndrome)* has been associated with hypothyroidism. The basis of this diagnosis was tingling in the sole of the foot aggravated by walking, with sensory loss in the distribution of the medial plantar nerve and prolongation of the tibial motor distal latency. A diffuse peripheral neuropathy was not, however, completely excluded by neurophysiological studies (Schwartz et al., 1983).

Peripheral Neuropathy

Distal paresthesias occur commonly in hypothyroid patients, but electrodiagnostically proven sensorimotor peripheral neuropathy is less frequent. Distal sensory symptoms are much more common than the complaint of distal weakness. Crevasse and Logue (1959) reported that nearly half (31 of 65) of their patients with hypothyroidism complained of distal paresthesias or lancinating pains, some resembling radicular pain. These symptoms, which resolved after hormone replacement, actually helped lead to the diagnosis in three patients (Crevasse and Logue, 1959). All 25 patients in the study by Nickel et al. (1961) complained of distal paresthesias. Between 10% and 71% of patients have clinical evidence of peripheral neuropathy, most commonly with distal sensory loss or depressed ankle reflexes (Murray and Simpson, 1958; Nickel et al., 1961; Rao et al., 1980; Shinoda et al., 1987a; Duyff et al., 2000). Hypothyroid patients often complain of weakness, which is more often proximal and related to myopathy (Nickel et al., 1961; Nickel and Frame, 1961; Rao et al., 1980; Duyff et al., 2000).

Nerve conduction studies are abnormal in 10% to 50% of patients with hypothyroidism and show predominantly axonal features—low sensory and motor evoked amplitudes, slightly slowed sensory and motor conduction velocities, and occasionally prolonged motor and sensory distal latencies, mostly in the median nerve (Dyck and Lambert, 1970; Martin et al., 1983; Yamamoto et al., 1983; Nemni et al., 1987; Duyff et al., 2000). Proximal nerve segments may be affected, with prolonged F wave and H reflexes. On needle examination, moderate to severe neurogenic changes were noted in 61% of patients, whereas myopathic changes occurred in 39% (Shinoda et al., 1987a). Slowing of conduction has been demonstrated in vitro, as well, and it was not the result of decreased temperature of tissue (Dyck and Lambert, 1970). Electrophysiological changes of peripheral neuropathy, unrelated to any neurological complaints, occur in patients with clinical hypothyroidism (Yamamoto, 1983) and subclinical hypothyroidism (Misiunas et al., 1995).

The pathology of hypothyroid neuropathy has been studied for more than a century (Ord, 1897). Initial observations suggested a deposition of mucinous material in endoneurium and perineurium that was thought to disrupt nerves mechanically. Some damage to myelin sheath and axonal degeneration was also noted (Nickel et al., 1961). This observation of mucinous deposition has not been well corroborated, and more evidence of demyelination and remyelination as well as axonal degeneration has been seen (Pollard et al., 1982).

Dyck and Lambert (1970) reported pathological findings in two patients with peripheral neuropathy. These investigators found an accumulation of glycogen aggregates in Schwann cells, in capillaries, or in the cytoplasm of perineural cells. Glycogen was also found within both myelinated and unmyelinated axons. Accompanying these glycogen aggregates in Schwann cells were mitochondrial aggregates, lamellar bodies, or lipid droplets. Widespread segmental demyelination was seen and was thought to be most indicative of Schwann cell dysfunction, whereas some degree of primary axonal damage, which could account for some of the findings of segmental demyelination, was also found (Dyck and Lambert, 1970).

Primary segmental demyelination was described in another patient (Shirabe et al., 1975). Other pathological studies have supported primary axonal damage as the underlying pathogenic mechanism (Meier and Bischoff, 1977; Pollard et al., 1982; Nemni et al., 1987), and one additionally commented on endoneurial vessel involvement similar to that seen in diabetes mellitus (Cavaletti et al., 1987). Shinoda et al. found axonal degeneration with what they postulated was secondary demyelination (Shinoda et al., 1987b). Mucinous depositions within nerve were not a prominent feature in the more recent pathological studies, and mechanical disruption of nerve is therefore not thought to be the cause of peripheral neuropathy in hypothyroidism.

The pathophysiology underlying the peripheral neuropathy in hypothyroidism is undetermined. It is clear that mucinous deposition in or around nerve is not the primary mechanism. There is evidence that lack of thyroid hormone may cause a defect in microtubule assembly and in slow axonal transport, at least in rats (Sidenius et al., 1987). As mentioned earlier, a primary insult to the endoneurial vessels and subsequent nerve fiber involvement is also possible. Glycogen aggregates signal some form of abnormal glycogen metabolism; this is probably a result of hypothyroidism itself and may potentially also be related to the cause of peripheral neuropathy (Simpson, 1962; Shinoda et al., 1987b). Given the recovery from clinical symptoms and electrophysiological abnormalities on replacement therapy, especially early in the course of the disease, some type of functional defect as opposed to a completely persistent degenerative or structural disturbance is likely (Crevasse and Logue, 1959; Purnell et al., 1961; Dyck and Lambert, 1970; Shinoda et al., 1987a, 1987b).

In summary, hypothyroid peripheral neuropathy can occur but is rarely severe. It is usually manifested by a preponderance of mild sensory symptoms. A few patients have electrophysiological evidence of an axonal sensorimotor peripheral neuropathy; the sensory abnormalities may be more marked than the motor changes. Carpal tunnel syndrome may also be present either with or without a superimposed peripheral neuropathy. Pathological findings indicative of both axonal degeneration and demyelination (possibly secondary to axonal loss) are seen. With hormone replacement therapy, especially given early in the disease course, significant improvement or complete resolution is to be expected.

Treatment of hypothyroidism requires replacement of thyroid hormone, typically with L-thyroxine. This is usually begun at 25 μg once a day and titrated upward by 25 to 50 μg every 4 weeks until a normal metabolic state is achieved. Monitoring thyroid-stimulating hormone levels is ideal for most hypothyroid patients. For patients in myxedematous coma, intravenous infusion of 3 to 4 μg/kg of L-thyroxine is followed by daily infusions of 100 μg of L-thyroxine. Additional infusion of liothyronine (which causes more immediate rise in triiodothyronine levels) and hydrocortisone is recommended (Wartofsky, 1998).

HYPERTHYROIDISM

Hyperthyroidism refers to a state in which tissues are exposed to an excess of thyroid hormone. Common causes include excess production of thyroid hormone (thyrotoxicosis), as in Graves' disease, and leakage of thyroid hormone, as in subacute thyroiditis. Other less common causes are exogenous thyroid intake and overproduction of thyroid-stimulating hormone by pituitary tumors. The main systemic manifestations of hyperthyroidism include nervousness, insomnia, tremor, sweating, weight loss, and heat intolerance. Ocular signs include a wide palpebral fissure, lid lag, and the classic ophthalmopathy.

Complaints of weakness are frequent in hyperthyroidism, and clinical findings of proximal muscle weakness are seen in up to 62% of patients, although electrophysiological evidence of a myopathy is less common (Duyff et al., 2000). Hypokalemic periodic paralysis and myasthenia gravis can also complicate hyperthyroidism (Swanson et al., 1981). The occurrence of peripheral nerve disease, however, is less common.

Carpal Tunnel Syndrome

Carpal tunnel syndrome in conjunction with hyperthyroidism typically resolves with treatment of the underlying disorder (Beard et al., 1985; Roquer and Cano, 1993). Patients with hyperthyroidism rarely, however, manifest symptoms of carpal tunnel syndrome. No patients (of 21 total patients) in one study (Duyff et al., 2000) and only 3 of 60 in another (Roquer and Cano, 1992) had symptoms of carpal tunnel syndrome. More often, but still infrequent, is subclinical median neuropathy at the wrist.

It has been suggested that the pathogenetic mechanism of carpal tunnel syndrome in hyperthyroidism probably involves an infiltration of the tendon sheaths with mucopolysaccharides in the carpal tunnel, perhaps similar to what is seen in hypothyroidism (Beard et al., 1985). Another point is that treatment of hyperthyroidism can result in iatrogenic hypothyroidism, which as discussed earlier can predispose to carpal tunnel syndrome.

Peripheral Neuropathy

Generalized *peripheral neuropathy* is thought to be less common in hyperthyroidism than in hypothyroidism. Acute neuropathy with paraplegia or quadriplegia has been reported in patients with severe hyperthyroidism or thyroid storm. This was first commented on by Charcot (1889), who noted flaccid paraplegia with absent reflexes, occasional sensory disturbance, and preserved sphincter function. The term *Basedow's paraplegia* was used by Joffroy (1894); this disorder bears a close resemblance to Guillain-Barré syndrome (Bronsky et al., 1964). Several reports of patients with this syndrome exist (Feibel and Campa, 1976), but one case was described (Pandit et al., 1998), and, for the first time, nerve pathology was included. A 47-year-old woman developed flaccid, areflexic quadriparesis in the midst of thyroid storm; she improved markedly on endocrinological treatment. Electrophysiological studies showed an asymmetrical, mixed axonal and demyelinating, sensorimotor peripheral neuropathy. Sural nerve biopsy was most remarkable for abnormalities in mitochondria and cytoskeletal elements without significant segmental demyelination or inflammation. Similarities to hyperthyroid myopathy (Engel, 1966) and hypothyroid peripheral neuropathy (see earlier) were thus noted.

Other investigators have made the association between hyperthyroidism and peripheral neuropathy (Lundin et al., 1969; Chollet et al., 1971). In the series of Duyff et al., clinical findings suggesting peripheral neuropathy (stocking-and-glove sensory loss and decreased ankle muscle stretch reflexes) were seen in 19% of patients with hyperthyroidism, whereas electrophysiological evidence of peripheral neuropathy (slowed conduction velocities or fibrillation potentials) was present in 24%. All sensory complaints resolved on appropriate treatment. No detailed electrophysiological data or pathological observations were included in this study (Duyff et al., 2000). A reversible loss in the number of motor unit (based on estimates) has been described in patients with thyrotoxicosis (McComas et al., 1974). Other associations have been made with a disorder mimicking amyotrophic lateral sclerosis (Fisher et al., 1985), polyradiculomyopathy (Birket-Smith and Olivarius, 1957), and multiple mononeuropathies affecting peroneal and lateral femoral cutaneous nerves (Ijichi et al., 1990).

ACROMEGALY

Growth hormone (somatotropin) is secreted by the anterior pituitary gland and is necessary for linear growth. Excess growth hormone secretion before epiphyseal closure leads to gigantism. *Acromegaly* is caused by excessive growth hormone secretion after epiphyseal closure and causes bone and soft tissue overgrowth. The common phenotype is that of increased hand, foot, and head size with prognathism, coarse facial features, and wide spacing of the teeth. Complaints of arthralgias, distal paresthesias, and proximal muscle weakness are common (Biller and Daniels, 1998). Clinical and electrophysiological evidence of proximal myopathy can be found in approximately half of those patients with acromegaly (Pickett et al., 1975).

Carpal Tunnel Syndrome

The syndrome of acromegaly was first recognized and reported by Marie in 1886 (Marie, 1886). The first of these patients reported probably had *carpal tunnel syndrome* (Marie and Souza-Leite, 1891). Marie and Foix were the first to report the autopsy findings of a thickened transverse carpal ligament in median neuropathy (Marie and Foix, 1913). The incidence of carpal tunnel syndrome in acromegaly ranges from 35% to 64% (O'Duffy et al., 1973; Pickett et al., 1975; Baum et al., 1986), and, in a few cases, this was the

presenting symptom of acromegaly (Baum et al., 1986). Asymptomatic median neuropathy at the wrist, usually bilateral, was reported in 13 of 16 (81%) patients with acromegaly (Kameyama et al., 1993).

Shortly after pituitary surgery, electrophysiological parameters may improve (Baum et al., 1986), whereas some electrophysiological abnormalities may persist (Pickett et al., 1975; Kameyama et al., 1993; Jenkins et al., 2000), a finding suggesting some irreversible carpal tunnel narrowing or persistent demyelination. Following appropriate endocrinological treatment (including hypophysectomy), however, the clinical symptoms of carpal tunnel syndrome typically abate or completely resolve.

Various causes of carpal tunnel syndrome in acromegaly have been proposed. Patients with underlying peripheral neuropathy may be at increased risk of focal compression mononeuropathies. This scenario occurs in half of patients with acromegaly and carpal tunnel syndrome. The other half, therefore, have an entrapment neuropathy independent of any generalized process (Jamal et al., 1987). Alteration of components within the carpal tunnel has been suggested. This includes bone and soft tissue overgrowth, edema from sodium and water retention, and enlargement of the median nerve from hypertrophic neuropathy, all of which have been suggested (Brain, 1947; Johnston, 1960; Pickett et al., 1975). A magnetic resonance imaging study of the distal median nerve through the carpal tunnel in patients with acromegaly found increased median nerve size and signal intensity, a finding suggesting nerve edema, in symptomatic patients in comparison with asymptomatic patients. No change in the overall volume of the carpal tunnel or of its components, other than the median nerve, was observed. Following treatment, symptoms of carpal tunnel syndrome resolved, and the abnormal imaging characteristics improved (Jenkins et al., 2000). The persistence of symptoms with treatment of the underlying disorder, however, may again suggest some degree of irreversible narrowing of the carpal tunnel. A direct correlation between the decrease in the level of growth hormone and clinical and electrophysiological improvement has been seen in some patients (Baum et al., 1986), but not others (Jenkins et al., 2000). The symptoms of carpal tunnel syndrome paralleled disease activity in one study (O'Duffy et al., 1973).

Peripheral Neuropathy

Peripheral neuropathy in patients with acromegaly was first reported in 1891 (Marie and Marinesco, 1891). Studies since then have found that nearly half to two thirds of patients suffer from peripheral neuropathy (Low et al., 1974; Dinn and Dinn, 1985; Jamal et al., 1987). Clinical manifestations have varied from mild distal paresthesias to mild distal sensory and motor loss to, rarely, severely incapacitating sensorimotor neuropathy. Most commonly, patients complain of distal paresthesias and are found to have mild sensory loss and decreased reflexes on examination with or without minimal toe weakness. Another interesting clinical finding is that of enlarged peripheral nerves. This has typically been described in the ulnar and lateral popliteal nerves. Nearly half of patients with acromegaly have nerve hypertrophy (Low et al., 1974; Jamal et al., 1987), although some investigators have not observed this finding (Dinn and Dinn, 1985). The nerve hypertrophy may occur even in those patients without peripheral neuropathy.

Electrophysiological findings have included mild reduction in motor and sensory amplitudes and conduction velocities. The decrease in motor and sensory amplitudes was more significant than the slowing of conduction velocities (Low et al., 1974; Jamal et al., 1987). As discussed earlier, median neuropathy at the wrist, either symptomatic or asymptomatic, is often also found. Abnormal thermal thresholds also implicate damage to distal small fibers in addition to large, myelinated fibers (Jamal et al., 1987).

Pathological studies of sural nerve biopsies in patients with acromegaly and peripheral neuropathy have shown segmental demyelination, a reduction in density of nerve fibers, and an increase in size of nerve fascicles related to increase in subperineurial and endoneurial tissue (Low et al., 1974). Some investigators have concluded that the primary pathological abnormality was segmental demyelination without axonal damage (Dinn and Dinn, 1985). Onion bulbs were found in those patients with more chronic underlying disease lasting at least 1 year. No comment was made regarding increase in perineurial or endoneurial tissue, and no patients had clinically palpable nerves. In addition, no patients had evidence of carbohydrate intolerance, which may coexist with acromegaly and may confound conclusions regarding peripheral neuropathy and acromegaly (Dinn and Dinn, 1985). Correlation between levels of growth hormone and the presence or severity of peripheral neuropathy or median neuropathy has not been found (Low et al., 1974; Pickett et al., 1975; Jamal et al., 1987). Persistently elevated growth hormone may be related to more severe peripheral neuropathic complications (Dinn and Dinn, 1985). An association between total exchangeable body sodium and neurophysiological abnormalities was found in one study (Jamal et al., 1987).

The mechanism whereby excess growth hormone leads to generalized peripheral neuropathy is unclear, but it is clearly independent of glucose intolerance or hypothyroidism. The cause may be multifactorial because nerve hypertrophy with electrolyte and water retention may combine to render nerves susceptible to damage. Although symptoms of carpal tunnel syndrome improve on treatment of acromegaly, little has been published on the course of peripheral neuropathy and its response to treatment.

OTHER ENDOCRINOLOGICAL DISORDERS

There are rare reports, mostly single cases, of peripheral neuropathic complications of other endocrinological disorders. Few detailed electrophysiological data are provided in these reports.

Hyperparathyroidism

Carpal tunnel syndrome caused by calcific deposits within the carpal tunnel was the presenting symptom in a patient found to have secondary *hyperparathyroidism* from chronic renal failure (Firooznia et al., 1981). Carpal tunnel syndrome has occurred following parathyroid adenoma resection for hyperparathyroidism. Median motor and sensory distal latencies were prolonged, and evoked amplitudes were reduced (Valenta, 1975). A patient with pseudogout and hyperparathyroidism developed carpal tunnel syndrome (Weinstein et al., 1968). A patient with hyperparathyroidism developed peripheral neuropathy and electrophysiologically was found to have an axonal polyneuropathy and bilateral median neuropathies at the wrist. A nerve biopsy showed segmental demyelination without inflammation (Gentric et al., 1993). Other mononeuropathies in the form of ulnar neuropathy at the elbow and posterior tibial neuropathy have been seen (Turken et al., 1989).

Symptoms of paresthesias or cramps are not uncommon in patients with hyperparathyroidism. Approximately 30% of patients have clinical findings of peripheral neuropathy on examination (Turken et al., 1989). Electrophysiological studies show mild slowing of conduction velocities and relative preservation of sensory and motor amplitudes (Gerster and Gauthier, 1969/1970; Turken et al., 1989). Improvement in peripheral neuropathy occurred following treatment. Other investigators have found peripheral neuropathy in hyperparathyroidism (Patten et al., 1974), and some have hypothesized that the weakness seen in these patients has its origin in abnormal neuromuscular transmission (Kaplan et al., 1982). Guillain-Barré syndrome occurred simultaneously with hyperparathyroidism as a result of parathyroid adenoma in one patient (Vallat et al., 1982).

Addison's Disease

Guillain-Barré syndrome presented simultaneously with *Addison's disease* in one patient (Abbas et al., 1977). Adrenomyeloneuropathy is an X-linked disorder of peroxisomal long-chain fatty acid metabolism that causes adrenal failure and a demyelinating peripheral neuropathy. Adrenal insufficiency and peripheral neuropathy coexist in combination with multisystem disease (pigmentary retinopathy, hearing loss, seizures, and hepatosplenomegaly) in young children as a result of an unknown type of lipid metabolism dysfunction (Dyck et al., 1981; Federico et al., 1988). A different syndrome of adrenal insufficiency and peripheral neuropathy with multisystemic manifestations (achalasia, alacrima, and microcephaly) has been reported (Tsao et al., 1994).

POEMS Syndrome

A symmetrical, length-dependent, sensorimotor peripheral neuropathy is one component of the *POEMS syndrome* (*p*olyneuropathy, *o*rganomegaly, *e*ndocrine dysfunction, *m*onoclonal protein, and *s*kin changes) in which the endocrine dysfunction includes diabetes mellitus, hyperprolactinemia, hyperestrogenemia, hypogonadism, and hypothyroidism. Often, more than one endocrine disturbance is present. Electrophysiological studies often reveal mixed axonal and demyelinating neuropathy but, in a few patients, pure demyelinating neuropathy is seen (Soubrier et al., 1994).

HEPATIC DISEASE

Peripheral nervous system involvement in *hepatic disease* can occur as a direct result of a primary hepatic disease. It can also be part of a more systemic disease process affecting both liver and peripheral nervous system independently. Examples of this latter category include systemic vasculitis (specifically as in polyarteritis nodosa), cytomegalovirus infection, Sjögren's syndrome, chronic alcohol consumption, porphyria, and amyloidosis. In this section, emphasis is on those primary hepatic disorders that lead to peripheral nervous system diseases. In addition, certain treatments of these underlying hepatic disorders (specifically viral hepatitis) need to be considered, as they can damage the peripheral nervous system. Peripheral nervous system involvement can also occur as a distant complication of primary hepatic neoplasms in a paraneoplastic syndrome.

Chronic Hepatic Disease

SENSORIMOTOR PERIPHERAL NEUROPATHY

An association between *peripheral neuropathy* and chronic hepatic disease has been recognized for many years (Dayan and Williams, 1967; Knill-Jones et al., 1972). This peripheral neuropathy is often minimally symptomatic (sensory complaints more common than motor ones) or asymptomatic. Detection is therefore most often by electrophysiological studies or nerve biopsy.

The prevalence of peripheral neuropathy in chronic hepatic disease has varied in studies from 14% to 89% (Knill-Jones et al., 1972; Chari et al.,

1977; Perretti et al., 1995; Oliver et al., 1997; Chaudry et al., 1999). The most common complaints are those of distal paresthesias. On examination, patients demonstrate glove-and-stocking distribution sensory loss, reduced to absent distal muscle stretch reflexes, and less commonly muscle weakness or wasting.

Electrophysiological studies reveal subclinical neuropathy in up to 40% of patients (Chaudry et al., 1999). Conduction velocity slowing was noted in early studies; however, the slowing was not necessarily into the demyelinating range. Sensory and motor amplitudes were generally not mentioned (Knill-Jones et al., 1972; Chari et al., 1977). More recent studies describe decreased motor and sensory nerve amplitudes as well as mild slowing of conduction velocities, a pattern more in keeping with length-dependent, axonal, sensorimotor peripheral neuropathy (Perretti et al., 1995; Oliver et al., 1997; Chaudry et al., 1999). One third of patients are found to have median neuropathy at the wrist (Chaudry et al., 1999).

Autoimmune chronic active hepatitis was associated with sensory neuronopathy predominantly affecting the upper extremities in one patient. Large-fiber sensory dysfunction was evident in the arms and legs. Sensory nerve action potentials were absent in the arms but present and normal in the legs, with normal trigeminal blink reflexes (Merchut et al., 1993).

Past studies suggested that hepatic peripheral neuropathy is a primary demyelinating process. Nerve conduction studies revealed slowing of conduction velocities, and sural nerve biopsies show thinly myelinated fibers, short internodes, and segmental demyelination and remyelination (Knill-Jones et al., 1972; Chari et al., 1977). In contrast with these reports, Chaudry and colleagues found features on nerve conduction studies supporting a primary axonal process, in view of the minimal conduction velocity slowing seen. Their interpretation of the previous studies was that the changes seen were, in fact, most probably related to a primary axonal dying-back peripheral neuropathy. Severity of the peripheral neuropathy, in terms of the total neuropathy score, was greater the more severe the underlying hepatic disease (Perretti et al., 1995; Chaudry et al., 1999). Other investigators, however, have not found a correlation between hepatic disease severity and clinical, electrophysiological, or pathological findings of peripheral neuropathy (Knill-Jones et al., 1972; Chari et al., 1977; Chopra et al., 1980).

The underlying pathogenesis of the neuropathy in chronic hepatic disease is unclear. Chopra and colleagues studied two groups of patients, one with nonalcoholic cirrhosis and one with idiopathic portal fibrosis without deterioration of hepatic function. Clinical signs of peripheral neuropathy were rare (being seen in 14% and none of the patients, respectively), whereas pathological changes on sural nerve biopsy were common (in 100% and 91%, respectively). The most striking pathological finding was myelinated fiber loss and segmental demyelination and remyelination. The authors proposed that the existence of both portosystemic shunting and hepatocellular damage played a role in the development of neuropathy that may ultimately be caused by an alteration in nitrogen metabolism (Chopra et al., 1980). Other investigators, however, have not found an association between the presence or absence of portacaval shunting and electrophysiological findings (Chari et al., 1977). Experimental studies of portacaval anastomosis in rats suggest that hepatocellular damage, not portosystemic shunting, is the primary mechanism of peripheral neurotoxicity (Hindfelt and Holmin, 1980). Finally, an abnormal immune response triggered by hepatic cirrhosis has also been proposed (Knill-Jones et al., 1972; Golding et al., 1973).

CARPAL TUNNEL SYNDROME

Carpal tunnel syndrome can be seen in patients with cirrhosis (Chaudry et al., 1999) and inflammatory hepatic disease (Massey et al., 1979). Carpal tunnel syndrome developed in 1.5% of patients after orthotopic liver transplantation. All but one patient with carpal tunnel syndrome received a transplant for primary biliary cirrhosis, and all were taking cyclosporine (Grant et al., 1998).

AUTONOMIC DYSFUNCTION

Autonomic dysfunction, either with or without superimposed sensorimotor peripheral neuropathy, occurs in conjunction with hepatic disease. Its presence is important to recognize because it identifies those patients who probably have a poor prognosis (Johnson and Robinson, 1988; Hendrickse et al., 1992; Fleckenstein et al., 1996).

Autonomic neuropathy occurs in most patients with chronic hepatic disease and is unrelated to alcohol use (Kempler et al., 1989; Trevisani et al., 1996). Symptoms and signs are typically absent, and the abnormalities are detected by electrophysiological testing of the autonomic nervous system. Rarely are symptoms of autonomic neuropathy severe (Oliver et al., 1997). Peripheral and autonomic neuropathy coexist in most, but not all, patients. Parasympathetic dysfunction (reduced heart rate variation with deep breathing and abnormal Valsalva ratio) is much more common than sympathetic dysfunction (blood pressure drop with tilt table testing) (Thuluvath and Triger, 1989; Chaudry et al., 1999).

The underlying pathogenesis of autonomic dysfunction is unknown, and postulated mechanisms include effects of toxic metabolites and dysimmune mechanisms. The cause, although uncertain, may be similar to that of somatic peripheral neuropathy. Some patients develop autonomic neuropathy and have extrahepatic portal vein thrombosis without laboratory markers for hepatocellular damage. Hepatocellular damage therefore may not be necessary for autonomic neuropathy. In these cases, variations in intravascular volume and local hepatic or portal vein autonomic receptor alterations may lead to the autonomic neuropathy (Voigt et al., 1997).

A correlation between the severity of hepatic disease and the presence of autonomic neuropathy has been recognized by some (Hendrickse et al., 1992; Chaudry et al., 1999) but not all (Oliver et al., 1997) authors. Patients with chronic hepatic disease and autonomic dysfunction have a worse prognosis than that in patients without autonomic dysfunction (Hendrickse et al., 1992).

The significance of peripheral or autonomic neuropathy in terms of predicting morbidity, mortality, or the likelihood of reversal after hepatic transplantation is unknown. Liver transplantation in endstage liver disease can be lifesaving. In eight patients undergoing liver transplantation, two had peripheral neuropathy, and both improved after transplantation (Hockerstedt et al., 1992).

Hepatocellular Carcinoma

Hepatocellular carcinoma can be a complication of chronic cirrhosis and may be related to infection with hepatitis B or C virus. Rare neurological complications have been reported in association with hepatocellular carcinoma. The first report was of a patient with hepatocellular carcinoma and severe sensory greater than motor peripheral neuropathy. Sensory potentials were absent, and motor studies showed low-amplitude responses with slowed conduction velocities in the upper extremities (Calvey et al., 1983).

Severe axonal sensorimotor peripheral neuropathy has been described in two patients with the diagnosis of hepatocellular carcinoma. The diagnosis came several months later (Hatzis et al., 1998) or at autopsy despite a thorough search for neoplasm during life (Nishiyama et al., 1993). Chronic inflammatory demyelinating polyradiculoneuropathy has been associated with hepatocellular carcinoma (Abe and Sugai, 1998) and cholangiocarcinoma (Antoine et al., 1996). Finally, Guillain-Barré syndrome has occurred as a possible paraneoplastic manifestation in one patient with gallbladder adenocarcinoma (Phan et al., 1999).

Primary Biliary Cirrhosis

Primary biliary cirrhosis can lead to chronic hepatic failure and peripheral neuropathy. A unique feature of the neuropathy is the small-fiber involvement leading to autonomic dysfunction and predominantly sensory complaints.

The earliest description of peripheral neuropathy in primary biliary cirrhosis was by Thomas and Walker in 1965. They described two patients with painful paresthesias and a xanthomatous neuropathy. Nerve conduction studies showed minimal low-amplitude sensory nerve action potentials in the upper extremities and absent lateral popliteal responses. Motor studies were normal. Histologically, deposition of lipid in the perineurium was seen. Serum cholesterol was markedly elevated in these patients (Thomas and Walker, 1965).

Asymmetrical sensory neuropathy can occur as the presenting feature of primary biliary cirrhosis (Charron et al., 1980; Illa et al., 1989). In one patient, central and peripheral sensory evoked potentials were absent, whereas motor studies were normal. A 50% reduction in the number of myelinated fibers was seen in sural nerve biopsy. Xanthomatous infiltrations were not seen in these patients, and an immunological mechanism, perhaps similar to that of Sjögren's syndrome, was postulated. The conclusion of these two reports was that the cause of the sensory neuropathy was either distal axonopathy or sensory neuronopathy, with the latter favored by Illa and coworkers.

Patients with primary biliary cirrhosis commonly have cardiovascular autonomic, predominantly parasympathetic, abnormalities, although sympathetic abnormalities can occur (Hendrickse and Triger, 1993; Kempler et al., 1994). The existence of autonomic disturbance closely correlates with the presence of peripheral neuropathy. This peripheral neuropathy is seen in half of patients with autonomic neuropathy and is usually asymptomatic. Autonomic and peripheral nerve dysfunctions correlate with albumin and bilirubin, but not vitamin E, levels. The corrected QT interval may be prolonged when compared with that in controls, again indicating significant autonomic impairment (Kempler et al., 1994).

Patients with primary biliary cirrhosis are also at risk of developing vitamin E deficiency from malabsorption. The neurological syndrome in children with chronic cholestatic liver disease and vitamin E deficiency includes proximal weakness, areflexia, and large-fiber sensory loss. Vitamin E deficiency has also been reported in adults with primary biliary cirrhosis. Electrophysiological studies have shown low-amplitude sensory nerve action potentials and abnormal central conduction on somatosensory evoked potentials. Motor evoked amplitudes may be slightly reduced, and electromyography reveals occasional increased spontaneous activity with both small and large motor unit action potentials. In one patient, muscle biopsy revealed neurogenic changes, and sural nerve biopsy showed mild changes of axonal degeneration and segmental demyelination. No xanthomatous infiltrations were seen (Knight et al., 1986; Jeffrey et al., 1987).

Viral Hepatitis

Peripheral neuropathy, especially that in *Guillain-Barré syndrome,* has long been associated with viral hepatitis. Less frequent associations are with length-dependent peripheral neuropathies and mononeu-

ritis multiplex. Several complicating factors must be taken into consideration in a discussion of the association of viral hepatitis and peripheral neuropathy. The existence of cryoglobulinemia in hepatitis, either B or C, is associated with peripheral neuropathy. *Polyarteritis nodosa* is a systemic form of vasculitis that can be seen in those with hepatitis B and can directly cause vasculitic peripheral neuropathy, typically mononeuritis multiplex. Other viral infections, such as cytomegalovirus infection, can result in both hepatitis and peripheral neuropathic complications. Chronic viral hepatitis can also lead to hepatic cirrhosis and peripheral neuropathy (discussed previously). Finally, treatment of viral hepatitis with interferon has been associated with peripheral neuropathy.

GUILLAIN-BARRÉ SYNDROME

Acute infection with hepatitis A has been associated with *Guillain-Barré syndrome.* The onset of Guillain-Barré syndrome is typically 3 days to 2 weeks after the appearance of the hepatitis symptoms (Tabor, 1987). Several single cases have been reported since Tabor's review (Endoh et al., 1991; Ono et al., 1994; Lee et al., 1997; Mihori et al., 1998; Azuri et al., 1999). The neurological syndrome does not differ significantly from non–hepatitis A–related Guillain-Barré syndrome. Men are more frequently affected than women, and facial weakness and loss of proprioception may be more prominent. Recovery is good, regardless of the degree of hepatic impairment (Ono et al., 1994). Anti–hepatitis A immunoglobulin M antibody has been detected in the cerebrospinal fluid of one patient, the titer of which declined with neurological improvement (Endoh et al., 1991). One study, however, did not find an increased incidence of Guillain-Barré syndrome during a hepatitis A outbreak (Xie et al., 1988). Other investigators have also disputed the causal association between hepatitis A and Guillain-Barré syndrome (Murthy, 1994).

Tabor reviewed instances in which Guillain-Barré syndrome followed acute hepatitis B infection (Tabor, 1987). Neurological symptoms typically began 3 to 9 weeks after the onset of hepatitis. Neurological symptoms can develop before hepatitis (Ng et al., 1975; Berger et al., 1981). In some patients, increased levels of hepatitis B surface antigen–immune complexes in sera and cerebrospinal fluid were seen. In addition, hepatitis B surface antigen–positive immunofluorescence around endoneurial blood vessels and in endoneurium was detected (Tsukada et al., 1987). Immune complexes containing hepatitis B surface antigen were also detected in serum and cerebrospinal fluid of a patient with Guillain-Barré syndrome that followed acute hepatitis B infection. The disappearance of these immune complexes coincided with neurological improvement and was thought to represent repair of a damaged blood-brain barrier (Penner et al., 1982). An attack of Guillain-Barré syndrome has been associated with an acute exacerbation of chronic hepatitis B (Han et al., 1999), and it has been noted in acute δ hepatitis virus superinfection (Lin et al., 1989).

Guillain-Barré syndrome can present as a manifestation of acute hepatitis C infection (De Klippel et al., 1993). It has also been described in two patients with chronic hepatitis C (Lacaille et al., 1998). One of these patients, however, had previously been treated with interferon. Guillain-Barré syndrome has occurred in association with non-A, non-B hepatitis, possibly representing hepatitis C (McLeod, 1987; Tabor, 1987).

Many investigators believe that the association between Guillain-Barré syndrome and viral hepatitis probably reflects an underlying dysimmune mechanism. This may be triggered by the viral infection and can lead to damage by immune complexes in the serum or cerebrospinal fluid (Ng et al., 1975; Penner et al., 1982; Tsukada et al., 1987). Most authors recommend obtaining liver enzymes and viral hepatitis serological studies in patients presenting with Guillain-Barré syndrome.

MONONEUROPATHIES

Mononeuropathies have occurred in association with acute hepatitis A infection (lateral cutaneous nerve of the thigh and peripheral facial palsy) and acute hepatitis B infection (axillary and median neuropathy). These mononeuropathies occurred acutely and followed jaundice in the cases of hepatitis A and preceded jaundice in the cases of hepatitis B (Pelletier et al., 1985). Isolated abducens and facial nerve palsies were seen in a patient with acute hepatitis B (Kuriakose and Pawar, 1994).

MONONEURITIS MULTIPLEX

Mononeuritis multiplex is a disorder characterized by an asymmetrical, often painful, motor and sensory neuropathy beginning with multiple mononeuropathies (e.g., footdrop, wristdrop). Its association with viral hepatitis in the absence of cryoglobulinemia or systemic vasculitis is discussed.

Left ulnar and right lateral femoral cutaneous mononeuropathies occurred in a patient recovering from an acute attack of hepatitis. These did develop, however, 10 days into hospitalization and after 10 kg of weight loss, and no electrophysiological confirmation was provided (Safadi et al., 1996). In a patient with acute hepatitis B and multiple mononeuropathies (bilateral ulnar, median, and left lateral femoral cutaneous nerves), electrophysiological studies showed bilateral, nonlocalized median and ulnar neuropathies with axonal loss. A skin biopsy demonstrated vasculitis (Cohen et al., 1990). Three other patients with mononeuritis multiplex and hepatitis B infection showed histological evidence of small-vessel vasculitis without cryoglobulinemia (Tsukada et al., 1983). A patient with chronic hepatitis C infection had recurrent asymmetrical median, ulnar, and radial neuropathies without cryoglobulinemia (Kashihara et al., 1995).

CHRONIC INFLAMMATORY DEMYELINATING POLYNEUROPATHY

Chronic inflammatory demyelinating polyneuropathy occurred in a patient 6 weeks after hepatitis B infection (Colarian et al., 1989) and in another patient who had chronic hepatitis B that was responsive to plasmapheresis (Inoue et al., 1998). Immune complexes of hepatitis B surface antigen were seen around endoneurial vessels and in the endoneurium. A third patient with hepatitis B and chronic inflammatory demyelinating polyradiculoneuropathy had no abnormal immune complexes in serum, but this patient did express hepatitis B surface antigen on the peripheral nerve as detected by Western blot analysis of a sural nerve biopsy (Inoue et al., 1994). Chronic inflammatory demyelinating polyneuropathy has been described in patients with chronic hepatitis C (Cacoub et al., 1999), as well as in a patient with both chronic hepatitis B and C (Ohyama et al., 1995).

SENSORIMOTOR PERIPHERAL NEUROPATHY

Chronic *sensorimotor peripheral neuropathy* has been associated with chronic viral hepatitis (Vasilescu et al., 1978; Berkompas, 1990). Detailed electrophysiological studies reveal slowing of conduction velocities in both distal and proximal segments of nerves and marked reduction in both sensory and motor evoked potentials. Fibrillation potentials and neurogenic motor unit action potentials are frequently seen. These results are interpreted as a dying-back neuropathy affecting sensory greater than motor nerves with axonal degeneration and secondary segmental demyelination (Vasilescu et al., 1978).

Peripheral neuropathy occurs in association with chronic hepatitis B (Tsukada et al., 1983; Koh et al., 1988). Peripheral neuropathy is also associated with hepatitis C infection and can be severe with inexcitable motor and sensory nerves. Many of these patients, however, have vasculitic changes on nerve biopsy and cryoglobulinemia (Ripault et al., 1998; Heckmann et al., 1999). Peripheral neuropathy can be found in patients with acute viral hepatitis, in whom electrophysiological testing reveals abnormalities (slowing of motor conduction velocities) in up to 42% of patients (Chari et al., 1977).

PATHOGENESIS

It is clear that acute infectious viral hepatitis can be associated with attacks of Guillain-Barré syndrome and multiple mononeuropathies, likely the result of some immunological mechanism. Chronic hepatitis may cause peripheral neuropathy on the basis of hepatocellular failure or by some mechanism again based on disordered immune function, such as vasculitis, or by deposition of immune complexes in nerve (Tsukada et al., 1983, 1987).

Demyelination associated with viral infections

may result from several pathogenic mechanisms. There may be direct damage to the peripheral Schwann cell by the virus itself. There may be cross-reactivity between the Schwann cell or myelin and the viral antigen *(molecular mimicry)*. The immune system may be abnormally sensitized to damaged myelin or virus antigen-antibody immune complexes in or around nerves. Immune complex deposition may also spark vasculitis around nerve (Pelletier et al., 1985; Tsukada et al., 1983, 1987; Tabor, 1987).

Course and Treatment

The course of Guillain-Barré syndrome occurring in the setting of acute viral hepatitis is similar to that occurring without the preceding infection, and the disorder can be treated in a similar fashion, including plasmapheresis (Lee et al., 1997). Recovery occurs within several months after onset of neurological symptoms; however, most reports predate the use of the aggressive therapies used currently. Mononeuropathies typically are mild and resolve spontaneously. The treatment of mononeuritis multiplex in patients with hepatitis C infection, many of whom have cryoglobulinemia, may be successful with prednisone or interferon-α (IFN-α) (Scelsa et al., 1998; Heckmann et al., 1999). Treatment of chronic inflammatory demyelinating polyradiculoneuropathy in hepatitis B has included prednisolone (Inoue et al., 1994) and plasmapheresis (Inoue et al., 1998).

Finally, the effect of treatment of the underlying viral or nonviral hepatic disease on the peripheral nervous system is addressed. Earlier treatment of chronic hepatitis B infection involved adenine arabinoside monophosphate. In one study, nearly one fourth of the patients treated with this drug developed painful dysesthesia in the feet and predominantly sensory neuropathy on examination. This usually developed near the end of the course of treatment and persisted for up to 7 months after treatment (Lok et al., 1984).

IFN-α has been used more recently as a treatment for viral hepatitis. A patient with hepatitis C developed chronic inflammatory demyelinating polyradiculoneuropathy after 6 weeks of treatment with this drug, which subsequently responded to drug withdrawal and a course of plasmapheresis (Meriggioli and Rowin, 2000). In another patient with hepatitis C, chronic inflammatory demyelinating polyradiculoneuropathy developed 4 months after treatment with IFN-α (Marzo et al., 1998). Other conditions associated with IFN-α treatment for hepatitis C are severe acute axonal neuropathy (Negoro et al., 1994), chronic axonal peripheral neuropathy (Tambini et al., 1997), axonal sensory neuropathy (Quattrini et al., 1997), mononeuritis multiplex (Sakajiri and Takamori, 1992), and worsening of a pre-existing mononeuritis multiplex (Maeda et al., 1995). In most cases, the symptoms of neuropathy occurred within several weeks of IFN-α therapy and resolved after discontinuation. Concomitant cryoglobulinemia was absent in all the preceding cases, except one (Maeda et al., 1995).

RENAL FAILURE

Renal failure has widespread effects on both peripheral nerve and muscle. Manifestations include uremic polyneuropathy, several types of mononeuropathy, and various primary myopathies.

Peripheral Neuropathy

The toxins of renal failure induce a generalized effect on peripheral nerves. The degree of dysfunction is determined by the severity of the renal failure and the effects of various forms of treatment. Thus, neuropathy is absent or mild during the acute or the early stages of renal failure, although Brismar and Tegnèr (1984) have shown evidence of neuropathy in acute renal failure in an animal model. By the time end-stage renal disease is reached, however, 50% of patients have polyneuropathy. It tends to stabilize during treatment with chronic hemodialysis or peritoneal hemodialysis and then regularly resolves with successful renal transplantation (Bolton and Young, 1990).

Clinical Manifestations

Common and early signs and symptoms are restless legs syndrome, muscle cramping, and distal paresthesias, not always resulting from the neuropathy but at times resulting from transient metabolic disturbances. The *burning foot syndrome,* caused by a deficiency of the water-soluble B vitamins, which are washed out during the hemodialysis procedure, is now rarely seen because of proper vitamin supplementation. In more severe neuropathies, distal weakness (most marked in the legs), a stocking-and-glove loss of sensation to all modalities, and an unsteady gait occur.

The earliest signs of uremic polyneuropathy are loss of vibration sense in toes and reduction of deep tendon reflexes, beginning with ankle jerks (Jennekens et al., 1971). Severe cases of polyneuropathy causing quadriplegia are now rarely seen because of early institution of hemodialysis or peritoneal dialysis. When such cases do occur, the clinician should be suspicious that intercurrent infection may be the important factor; it is now known that sepsis itself can induce a polyneuropathy called *critical illness polyneuropathy* (Zochodne et al., 1987).

The cerebrospinal fluid protein level in uremia may be normal or elevated, and the degree of elevation bears some relation to the severity of the polyneuropathy (Jennekens et al., 1971). The cell counts are normal.

Overt clinical signs of autonomic dysfunction are probably uncommon, but more careful testing reveals abnormalities in a high percentage of patients. This appears to affect both the sympathetic and the

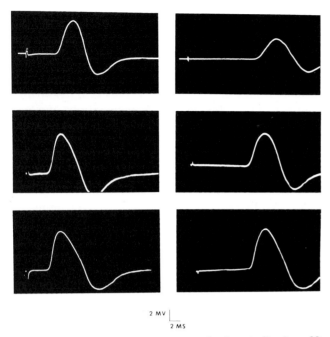

2 MV

2 MS

Figure 60–1. Median nerve motor conduction studies in a 38-year-old man with severe uremic polyneuropathy. Studies were performed at 3 months before *(upper traces),* and at 15 and 27 months after *(middle and lower traces),* successful renal transplantation. Conduction velocities were 42, 47, and 53 m per second, respectively, with reversal of the dispersed compound muscle action potential. (Case 1, from Bolton CF, Baltzan MA, Baltzan RB: Effects of renal transplantation on uremic neuropathy: A clinical and electrophysiologic study. N Engl J Med 1971;284: 1170–1175. Copyright © 1971 Massachusetts Medical Society. All rights reserved.)

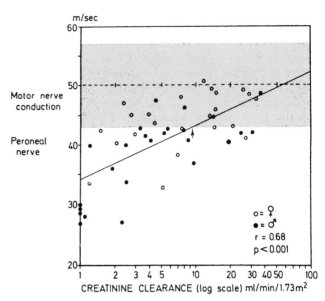

Figure 60–2. Fall in nerve conduction as kidney function declined in 56 patients before the institution of hemodialysis. The *arrow* indicates when 50% of patients showed abnormal values. The conduction velocities tended to be lower in male than in female patients ($P < 0.001$). (From Neilsen VK: The peripheral nerve function in chronic renal failure. VI. The relationship between sensory and motor nerve conduction and kidney function, azotemia, sex and clinical neuropathy. Acta Med Scand 1973;194:455–462.)

parasympathetic nervous systems (Solders et al., 1985). The normal variation in the cardiac RR interval tends to decrease; the more severe the renal failure, the more marked is the decrease. Sympathetic system abnormalities may be demonstrated by the Valsalva test, the tilt test, the forced handgrip test, the cold pressor test, the mental stress test, and the sweat test. Autonomic system neuropathy in uremia can be stabilized by chronic hemodialysis, and it regularly regresses after successful renal transplantation (Fig. 60–1).

NEUROPHYSIOLOGICAL STUDIES

Motor and sensory nerve conduction studies remain the best method of documenting the incidence and severity of polyneuropathy. Conduction velocity decreases in parallel with renal function, as measured by the creatinine clearance test (Nielsen, 1973b) (Fig. 60–2). Compound muscle and sensory nerve action potential amplitudes decrease because of dispersion from secondary demyelination or fall-out of larger myelinated axons from a primary axonal degeneration (Nielsen, 1973a; Bolton, 1976). Changes on needle electromyography may be distinctive. Fibrillation potentials and positive sharp waves may be relatively absent in human uremic muscle, possibly because of the inhibition of extrajunctional acetylcholine receptors. This may also explain failure of collateral reinnervation of muscle,

which depends on the presence of these receptors (Bolton et al., 1997b) (Fig. 60–3). Thus, there may be little spontaneous activity, and motor unit potentials may be decreased in number, small in size, but polyphasic, a finding suggesting myopathy (as discussed later).

Computer analysis (Hansen and Ballantyne, 1978) showed that the number of motor unit potentials is reduced to one third of the normal value. Single-fiber electromyographic studies (Theile and Stålberg, 1975; Konishi et al., 1982) indicated that the density of muscle fibers within a unit is normal; this finding suggests a failure of collateral reinnervation. The variation in the interval between the firing of single-muscle fiber potentials, so-called *jitter,* is probably related to peripheral demyelination. Somatosensory evoked potential studies reveal that conduction is slowed along both the peripheral and the central segments or primary sensory neurons, including transcallosal conduction (Serra et al., 1979; Vaziri et al., 1981). H-reflex and F-wave studies, which measure conduction in motor fibers both proximally and distally, have shown some prolongation of latencies in up to 85% of patients in end-stage renal failure, particularly those undergoing long-term hemodialysis (Panayiotopoulous and Laxos, 1980).

Disordered sensation is the earliest symptom in uremic polyneuropathy. Studies by Nielsen (1975) and Tegnèr and Lindholm (1985), using hand-held vibrators, have shown elevated thresholds in 83% of patients in end-stage renal failure. Quantitative sensory testing shows abnormalities in 39% of pa-

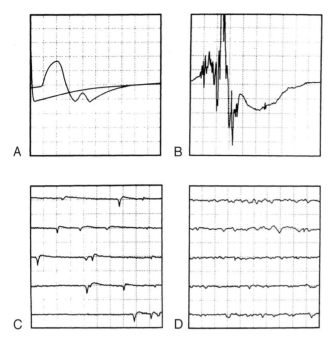

Figure 60–3. Electrophysiological studies illustrating almost total absence of denervation potentials in a 32-old man undergoing long-term hemodialysis who had severe trauma to the right femoral nerve. Studies at 2 and 5 months were similar. *A,* Supramaximal stimulation of the right femoral nerve at the inguinal ligament evoked no response from the right vastus lateralis muscle *(lower trace),* but a normal response on the left *(upper trace,* 5 mV, 5 ms per division). *B,* Monopolar needle electromyography of the right vastus lateralis muscle recorded normal insertional activity, but no positive sharp waves or fibrillation potentials (100 μV, 10 ms per division) on multiple passes of the electrode, except for *(C)* one area of positive sharp waves. *D,* No motor unit potentials were recorded on voluntary activation (low-amplitude activity is from thigh muscles not innervated by the femoral nerve). Thus, all clinical and electrophysiological features pointed to total denervation of the quadriceps muscles, but there was an unusual absence of denervation potentials. (From Bolton CF, Remtulla H, Toth B, et al: Distinctive electrophysiological features of denervated muscle in uremic patients. J Clin Neurophysiol 1997;14:539–542.)

tients with uremic neuropathy, and an unusual perception of heat in response to *low* temperature stimuli in 42% is an early sign (Yosipovitch et al., 1995).

PATHOPHYSIOLOGY

Although the cause of uremic neuropathy is still not understood, much is known of the pathology and basic physiology (Bolton and Young, 1990). Conduction velocity is slowed in motor and sensory fibers, both large and small, along proximal and distal segments. There is clearly an underlying demyelination because conduction velocity is slowed more than would be expected from pure axonal degeneration. Moreover, there is a relative preservation of compound muscle action potential amplitudes, which are often dispersed on more proximal stimulation. However, conduction block has not been seen. There is also elevation of excitation thresholds, a prolonged refractory period, abnormal responses to changes in limb temperature and ische-

mia, and evidence from voltage-clamp studies of a decrease in excitability and in the specific sodium permeability F-nodal membrane. Nielsen theorized that uremic toxin inhibits the ouabain-sensitive sodium-potassium adenosine triphosphatase (Na^+, K^+-ATPase), with resulting reduced flux, increased intracellular sodium concentration, and decrease in transmembrane potential difference (Nielsen, 1973a, 1974, 1978). Several investigations in animals tend to support this theory. As noted earlier, uremic toxins may also inhibit the occurrence of fibrillation potentials and positive sharp waves in uremic through suppression of extrajunctional acetylcholine receptors.

Morphological studies of peripheral nerve in humans (Asbury et al., 1963; Dyck et al., 1971; Thomas et al., 1971) indicated a primary axonal degeneration of motor and sensory fibers with secondary segmental demyelination. Small and unmyelinated fibers were also involved. However, there was nothing in the pathological features that appeared to be peculiar to uremic neuropathy.

Many different specific etiological factors have been considered. There appears to be no definite evidence of any of the following: deficiency of B vitamins, deficiency of biotin, accelerated breakdown of muscle protein, or accumulation of certain "toxins" such as myoinositol, urea, and creatinine (see earlier). More plausible has been the theory that proteins in the middle molecular mass range (500 to 500,000 daltons) may accumulate and may be toxic to peripheral nerve. The toxicity of the b4-2 or C7 fraction may be even more specific.

Finally, although no vascular changes have been clearly seen in nerve, microangiopathy has been demonstrated in skin that, in serial studies, did not improve during dialysis but did so after successful renal transplantation (Gilchrest et al., 1980).

PREVENTION AND TREATMENT

During the early stages of renal failure, all methods used to treat the underlying cause of the kidney disease and the various systemic effects of renal failure benefit the neuropathy, because it has been shown that conduction velocity falls in parallel with a decrease in renal function, as measured by the creatinine clearance. Such conservative measures include attention to nutrition (Rudman and Williams, 1985).

When end-stage renal disease has been reached, the patient undergoes either long-term hemodialysis or peritoneal dialysis. It has been shown that both of these methods of treatment halt the progress of uremic polyneuropathy, and a few patients demonstrate either mild improvement or mild deterioration (Bolton and Young, 1990). It is important to start such treatment early enough; if some renal function is preserved beforehand, the degree of uremic neuropathy will be less. There is no good evidence, however, that specifically manipulating the various hemodialysis schedules necessarily alters the course of uremic polyneuropathy. For example, hemodialysis techniques that clear middle molecular mass fractions do not necessarily lessen the severity of uremic polyneuropathy, although it is still an important area of research.

Patients undergoing peritoneal dialysis seem to have the same incidence and severity of uremic polyneuropathy as in those receiving hemodialysis (Bolton and Young, 1990). Because patients with diabetes achieve better control of blood sugar with peritoneal dialysis than with hemodialysis, the former method is now more frequently used for those patients. The neuropathy, however, does not regress with this treatment, although it does stabilize (Amair et al., 1982).

Kidney transplantation has been shown to produce a much better quality of life than that obtainable with dialysis, and the procedure is much more cost effective (Eggers, 1988). Renal function becomes relatively normal within 1 month of transplantation, and 1-year survival rate of the transplanted kidney is 68% (Bolton and Young, 1990). The symptoms of uremic neuropathy improve within a few days or weeks (Nielsen, 1974). The lessening of the distal numbness and tingling coincides with improvement in nerve conduction velocity, as well as in vibratory perception. This improvement is much more protracted when the uremic neuropathy is more severe, and residual clinical signs and symptoms may remain (Bolton et al., 1971). Should the transplanted kidney undergo rejection, the neuropathy regresses with a successful second renal transplantation. Mononeuropathies (of a compressive nature) of the ulnar nerve at the elbow or peroneal nerve at the fibular head also resolve after successful renal transplantation. Symptoms of autonomic insufficiency, including impotence and infertility, resolve completely (Bolton et al., 1971).

The electrophysiological studies normalize in parallel with resolution of the clinical signs and symptoms. The conduction velocities and distal latencies rise toward normal. The compound muscle (Fig. 60–4) and sensory nerve action potential amplitudes also rise but not to the same extent in more severe neuropathies. Needle electromyographic abnormalities eventually disappear. Autonomic function, as assessed by heart rate variability measurements, also improves (Yildiz et al., 1998). The only exception to this improvement in uremic neuropathy occurs in patients who also have diabetes. In these patients, neuropathy shows little improvement (Kennedy et al., 1990), a finding suggesting that the underlying cause of the neuropathy is mainly diabetes mellitus. However, with combined renal and pancreatic transplantation, mild but definite improvement has been demonstrated in prolonged follow-up (Navarro et al., 1997).

Combined Diabetic and Uremic Peripheral Neuropathy

With the increasing number of patients with diabetes receiving long-term dialysis and transplantation,

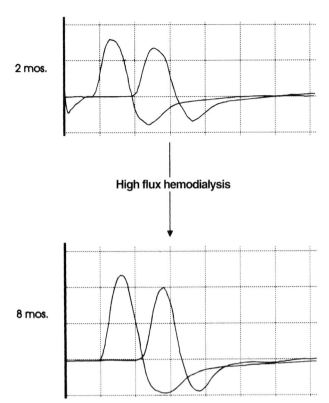

Figure 60–4. Median nerve motor conduction studies in a 68-year-old man with subacute uremic and diabetic polyneuropathy. Clinical improvement and a rise in compound muscle action potential amplitude occurred after treatment with high-flux hemodialysis (calibration, 5 mV and 5 ms per division). (From Bolton CF, McKeown MJ, Chen R, et al: Subacute uremic and diabetic neuropathy. Muscle Nerve 1997;20:59–64.)

the problem of *combined diabetic and uremic polyneuropathy* is more prevalent. Both neuropathies manifest as a symmetrical motor and sensory polyneuropathy with reduced deep tendon reflexes and varying degrees of ataxia, the distal parts of the limbs being particularly involved. However, diabetic neuropathy is more likely to induce the compressive palsies of ulnar neuropathy at the elbow, carpal tunnel syndrome, and common peroneal nerve palsy; autonomic disturbances and a tendency to multifocal involvement of peripheral nerves are more characteristic. There are also electrophysiological differences: conduction velocities tend to be lower in patients with chronic renal failure and diabetes mellitus (Hansen and Ballentyne, 1978), and in uremia, attempts at reinnervation of muscle (i.e., the re-establishment of nerve supply) are not as successful as they are in diabetic neuropathy (Mitz et al., 1984).

A distinctive variant is subacute uremic and diabetic polyneuropathy (Bolton et al., 1997a). Weakness develops over 2 to 4 months, and clinical and electrophysiological features suggest myopathy (with the unusual feature of sparse fibrillation potentials and positive sharp waves, as noted previously). Creatine kinase is only mildly elevated, and muscle biopsy indicates denervation. Accumulation of advanced glycosylated end products may be a mechanism of this neuropathy, a process reversed by high-flux hemodialysis (see Fig. 60–4) or combined renal and pancreatic transplantation (or renal transplantation alone) both of which may help to reverse the neuropathy in these patients. This neuropathy may be similar to the one described by Ropper, except that Ropper's patients had a more acute onset (Ropper, 1993).

Uremic Mononeuropathies

The dysfunction of peripheral nerves that occurs in a generalized fashion in chronic renal failure renders these nerves susceptible to local compression (Bolton and Young, 1990). Thus, with the cachexia associated with chronic renal failure, the ulnar nerves at the elbow or the common peroneal nerves at the fibular head are likely to be traumatized. At the time of transplant surgery, compression may occur by operating room equipment. The brachial plexus and radial nerves are particularly susceptible if the patient's arm is kept in an abducted position during anesthesia and surgery. These compressive palsies will not resolve during dialysis but will after successful renal transplantation.

Nerves may also be compressed as part of a compartment syndrome; for example, bleeding into the iliopsoas muscle causes acute swelling with compression of the femoral nerves. The process is demonstrated most effectively by computed tomographic scanning; electrophysiological studies are of little value in the acute stage. This is an emergency situation that requires surgical decompression.

The most common mononeuropathy is *carpal tunnel syndrome.* As in the patient with normal renal function, it may be caused by narrowing of the carpal tunnel from old age, rheumatism, or other factors. In the patient with renal failure, however, it is particularly likely to occur distal to a Cimino-Brescia forearm arteriovenous shunt used for access during hemodialysis. Here, there is a combination of venous congestion and arterial ischemia.

The signs and symptoms of carpal tunnel syndrome are remarkably similar to those in otherwise healthy persons, except that in uremic patients, the symptoms are more pronounced during each hemodialysis procedure. Electrophysiological studies aid greatly in diagnosis by showing prolonged conduction in both motor and sensory fibers through the carpal tunnel region.

Decompressive surgery, with sectioning of the flexor retinaculum, has been found to be an effective method of treatment, particularly if the carpal tunnel syndrome occurs in the arm not containing a Cimino-Brescia forearm fistula. In the case of such a fistula, carpal tunnel surgery itself may not be effective, and consideration may have to be given to either discontinuing or altering the degree of forearm shunting.

It was previously believed that these were the

only mechanisms of carpal tunnel syndrome, but it is known that patients who have received hemodialysis with a Cuprophan membrane for more than 10 years are susceptible to amyloidosis (Gejyo et al., 1986). The amyloid deposit is composed of β_2-microglobulin, which is normally present in small amounts in the serum and other body fluids in healthy persons. It is normally catabolized by the kidneys and, consequently, it rises progressively during renal failure. Such a rise may not occur if dialysis is performed with a newer AN-69-polyacrylonitrile membrane. Levels of α_2-microglobulin may be just as high in patients receiving chronic ambulatory peritoneal dialysis; as yet, carpal tunnel syndrome has not been reported in this condition, perhaps because patients have not used this form of dialysis for a sufficient period. Methods of hemodialysis are now being altered to prevent this serious complication, which may cause amyloid deposition not only in the carpal tunnel area but also in the bones and joints, particularly of the upper limbs (Bardin et al., 1986). This more widespread distribution causes severe arthropathy and intractable pain. Moreover, decompressive carpal tunnel surgery may not relieve the situation; if there is relief, it may be only transient, with a tendency for the syndrome to recur later (Fig. 60–5).

Mononeuropathies of a more diffuse nature may occur in the median and ulnar nerves as a result of Cimino-Brescia arteriovenous forearm fistulas. Although these conditions are usually mild and subclinical and are demonstrated only by careful electrophysiological techniques, some dysfunction may occur in up to three fourths of patients (Knezevic and Mastaglia, 1984). However, shunts located more proximally in the arms, between the brachial artery and antecubital vein, may sometimes produce acute, severe, and painful neuropathies involving median, ulnar, and radial nerves (Bolton et al., 1979). This is an emergency situation in which electrophysiological studies are not of much value, and the diagnosis must rely on clinical examination. Consideration should be given to taking down the shunt on an emergency basis, or severe and possible permanent neuropathy may result. The clinical and electrophysiological studies of these neuropathies are typical of acute nerve ischemia, with a resulting primary axonal degeneration of motor and sensory fibers.

Cochlear and vestibular dysfunction may occur in chronic renal failure as a result of treatment by antibiotics, notably erythromycin and aminoglycosides, and also by diuretic drugs. Uremic toxicity itself, however, is probably also a factor. Eighth cranial nerve dysfunction may improve during long-term hemodialysis and is most likely to do so after successful renal transplantation.

Myopathy

A defect in neuromuscular transmission does not occur as a direct manifestation of uremic toxicity,

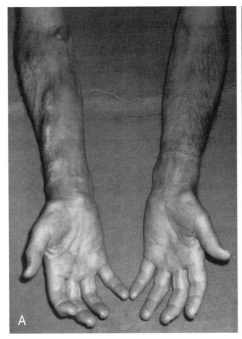
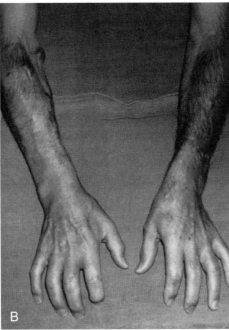

Figure 60–5. The upper limbs of a patient who had β₂-microglobulin amyloidosis. It caused bilateral carpal tunnel syndrome (note proximal thenar wasting, *A*) and right ulnar neuropathy (note the wasting of the interosseous muscles, *B*). Tissue from biopsy at the time of the carpal tunnel surgery revealed infiltration of blood vessels with amyloid. The pain may have been caused by arthropathy (note thickening and flexion contraction of interphalangeal joints) and periodic nerve ischemia. Repeated surgical procedures for carpal tunnel syndrome provided only transient relief. (The Cimino-Brescia forearm fistula caused the dilated veins in the right forearm.) (From Bolton CF, Young GB: Neurological Complications of Renal Disease. Stoneham, MA, Butterworth-Heinemann, 1990; 110.)

but it may occur as a complication of aminoglycoside antibiotics. Repetitive nerve stimulation studies show an incrementing response typical of the presynaptic defect in this complication. Discontinuance of the drug results in improvement.

Myoglobinuria (Penn, 1986) is an important cause of acute renal failure and may have various origins. The clinical picture is mainly determined by the underlying disease. The urine is red, and special tests reveal myoglobin in the urine. The muscles themselves have been traditionally described as weak, swollen, and painful, but they may be surprisingly normal on examination. The creatine kinase level is invariably elevated. The muscle disease and the kidney disease are both potentially reversible. Dialysis, or possibly plasmapheresis, may be effective.

Other relatively acute forms of myopathy associated with renal failure are those caused by water and electrolyte disturbances. If muscle weakness occurs in acute attacks, periodic paralysis associated with potassium disturbance should be considered. Hypocalcemia may occur and may be manifested as tetany, but this is rare because of the often associated acidosis in renal failure.

More chronic myopathy may be induced as a complication of steroid therapy. The chief conditions to be considered in chronic myopathies are, first, the nonspecific cachexia associated with chronic renal failure, and second, perhaps more frequently, the type of myopathy that may be associated with a remarkable proximal wasting of muscle in the limbs (Bolton and Young, 1990). It is associated with underlying bone disease that is caused by either secondary hyperparathyroidism or aluminum accumulation (Fig. 60–6). In both types of cachexia, needle electromyography reveals no clear-cut abnormalities, the creatine kinase levels are usually normal, and biopsy reveals some atrophy of type II muscle fibers.

SARCOIDOSIS

Sarcoidosis is a systemic granulomatous disease of undetermined origin that is characterized pathologically by noncaseating granulomas. Systemic involvement typically includes hilar lymphadenopathy, pulmonary infiltrates, and ocular or skin lesions.

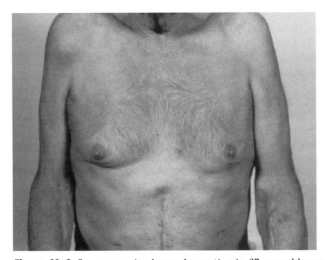

Figure 60–6. Severe proximal muscle wasting in 67-year-old man who had received long-term hemodialysis for 7 years. He had progressive bone disease and dementia; aluminum intoxication was never proved. Electromyographic findings were consistent with primary myopathy of the cachectic type. (From Bolton CF, Young GB: Neurological Complications of Renal Disease. Stoneham, MA, Butterworth-Heinemann, 1990; 158.)

Neurological manifestations of sarcoidosis (neurosarcoidosis) occur in approximately 5% of patients according to large studies (Maycock et al., 1963; Delaney, 1977; Stern et al., 1985; Chen and McLeod, 1989). Neurosarcoidosis can occur in patients who have systemic sarcoidosis or in those with no known previous diagnosis of sarcoidosis. This latter scenario occurs in 48% to 65% of patients with neurosarcoidosis, and, often there is laboratory or radiological evidence of systemic sarcoidosis. Additionally, in some patients, systemic signs of sarcoidosis may not develop (Delaney, 1977; Stern et al., 1985; Chapelon et al., 1990).

Central nervous system involvement in neurosarcoidosis can take many forms. These include aseptic meningitis secondary to leptomeningeal disease and intracranial lesions (especially hypothalamic, pituitary, and periventricular). Encephalopathy, seizures, hydrocephalus, and intraspinal lesions are less common. In general, most patients with neurosarcoidosis have a favorable prognosis, even though some experience relapsing neurological dysfunction. Treatment with prednisone in doses of approximately 40 mg per day is typically met with good success, although some patients improve spontaneously (Stern et al., 1985).

The peripheral nervous system is affected in about 4% to 15% of patients with neurosarcoidosis (Wiederholt and Siekert, 1965; Delaney, 1977; Stern et al., 1985). Cranial neuropathies predominate in all studies, whereas mononeuritis multiplex, polyradiculopathy, and symmetrical peripheral neuropathy also occur. The interval between the onset of neurological symptoms and the diagnosis of sarcoidosis is much longer when the initial manifestation is peripheral neuropathy (Chapelon et al., 1990).

Cranial Neuropathy

Cranial neuropathies are the most common neurological complications of sarcoidosis. These occur in 48% to 73% of patients with neurosarcoidosis, and in approximately half, multiple cranial neuropathies exist at presentation (Colover, 1948; Wiederholt and Siekert, 1965; Delaney, 1977; Stern et al., 1985). The facial nerve is most commonly affected. Bilateral involvement, either simultaneous or sequential, frequently occurs. Recovery usually takes place, and relapses rarely occur. The cause of facial neuropathy was initially thought to be parotid gland involvement by sarcoid. This hypothesis has proved to be incorrect, however, given the more proximal involvement causing stapedial and taste dysfunction and the lack of association with clinical parotiditis. Brainstem auditory evoked potentials have shown abnormalities in these patients, a finding suggesting lesions at the level of the brainstem (Oksanen, 1987). The optic, vestibulocochlear, glossopharyngeal, and vagus are the next most commonly involved cranial nerves. The other cranial nerves are rarely affected. In the study by Stern et al. (1985), of 16 patients whose presenting symptom of sarcoidosis was neurological, 13 had cranial neuropathies. Outlook in these patients is good, and response to steroid treatment is favorable (Stern et al., 1985).

Peripheral Neuropathy

The association of peripheral neuropathy and sarcoidosis was first made by Winkler in 1905 (Winkler, 1905). In large studies of neurosarcoidosis, peripheral neuropathy is uncommon, occurring in only 4% to 7% of patients (Wiederholt and Siekert, 1965; Delaney, 1977; Stern et al., 1985). Peripheral nerve involvement can take several forms, including symmetrical sensory, motor, or sensorimotor peripheral neuropathy. In addition, mononeuritis multiplex or polyradiculopathy occasionally mimicking Guillain-Barré syndrome can be seen. Intercostal neuritis characterized by spotty, painful patches over the thorax with loss of abdominal reflexes has been described (Colover, 1948).

SENSORIMOTOR PERIPHERAL NEUROPATHY

Sensorimotor peripheral neuropathy in sarcoidosis typically presents clinically with distal paresthesias and mild distal weakness. Neurological signs are stocking-and-glove sensory loss, decreased vibratory sensation distally, decreased or absent ankle reflexes, and variable distal weakness (Oh, 1980; Nemni et al., 1981; Galassi et al., 1984; Zuniga et al., 1991; Scott et al., 1993). Symmetrical sensorimotor peripheral neuropathy can occur as the initial manifestation of sarcoidosis (Oh, 1980; Nemni et al., 1981), shortly after diagnosis, or many years later. Simultaneous central nervous system involvement is rare. The peripheral neuropathy may follow a relapsing course (Silverstein et al., 1965; Sharma and Anders, 1985;).

Electrophysiological examination has revealed reduction of motor and sensory amplitudes and variable, usually mild slowing of conduction velocities. Sural sensory responses are typically absent. Changes suggestive of active denervation by needle examination are usually found in distal muscles. The interpretation is that of length-dependent, axonal, sensorimotor peripheral neuropathy (Oh, 1980; Nemni et al., 1981; Galassi et al., 1984; Zuniga et al., 1991; Scott et al., 1993). The importance of performing needle examination has been stressed because it may give clues to the asymmetry or multifocality of the process (Scott et al., 1993).

Sarcoidosis is also associated with pure sensory neuropathy (Payne et al., 1980; Vital et al., 1982; Chapelon et al., 1990; Zuniga et al., 1991). One patient had experienced numbness and paresthesias in the upper extremities for 18 years before the diagnosis of sarcoidosis. Examination disclosed distal sensory loss with normal strength and reflexes. Nerve conduction studies showed absent or low-amplitude sensory nerve action potentials and normal motor studies and needle electromyography. Rapid improvement followed on steroid treatment (Payne et al., 1980). Pure motor neuropathy can occur in sarcoidosis (Silverstein et al., 1965; Chapelon et al., 1990).

MONONEURITIS MULTIPLEX

Mononeuritis multiplex can occur as a complication of sarcoidosis, commonly affecting cranial and peripheral nerves. Colover (1948) summarized many early cases of "polyneuritis" in sarcoidosis and found patients with asymmetrical, predominantly motor or sensory, multifocal neuropathies. Muscle stretch reflexes were lost in asymptomatic areas, and sensory complaints did not always correspond to peripheral nerve territories or dermatomes (Colover, 1948). Multiple mononeuropathies often involve both cranial and peripheral nerves, although there have been patients reported with bilateral median neuropathies or thoracic radiculopathy with peroneal neuropathy (Kompf et al., 1986). The ulnar and peroneal nerves are more commonly affected along with the cranial nerves (Sharma and Anders, 1985; Chapelon et al., 1990; Zuniga et al., 1991). Lumbosacral plexopathy superimposed on chronic, sensorimotor, peripheral neuropathy has also been associated with sarcoidosis (Zuniga et al., 1991).

Twenty-nine patients with sarcoidosis who had no symptoms or signs of peripheral nerve disease were studied electrophysiologically. Nerve conduction studies showed at least one abnormal sensory nerve amplitude in 66% of patients. In addition, the mean sensory nerve action potential amplitudes for the median, ulnar, and sural nerves were all lower than those in a control population. Motor studies and needle electromyography were normal in all patients. Although some patients had abnormal sural responses, suggesting a length-dependent peripheral neuropathy, many had isolated abnormalities in the median or ulnar nerves. The authors suggested this may be related to subclinical multiple sensory mononeuropathies, possibly caused by compression of nerves by sarcoid granulomas (Challenor et al., 1984).

POLYRADICULOPATHY

Subacute or chronic *polyradiculopathy,* not infrequently manifesting as a cauda equina syndrome, occurs in sarcoidosis and may even be the initial presentation of the disease (Wiederholt and Siekert, 1965; Campbell et al., 1977; Chamaillard et al., 1990; Zajicek, 1990; Abrey et al., 1998). Systemic signs of sarcoidosis may be lacking, and the diagnosis of neurosarcoidosis may be made only by nerve root or meningeal biopsy (Campbell et al., 1977; Zajicek, 1990). In a review of patients with sarcoidosis and polyradiculopathy, most presented with lower extremity weakness (71%) and low back or leg pain (47%). Weakness was often more prominent in proximal muscles. Sphincter dysfunction was reported in

35%, and muscle reflexes were absent in the legs in 59%. Cerebrospinal fluid analysis typically showed elevated protein (mean, 326 mg/dL) and white blood cells (mean, 156 cells/mm³). Hypoglycorrhachia (cerebrospinal fluid glucose concentration lower than 40 mg/dL) was seen in 73%. Magnetic resonance imaging of the lumbosacral spine demonstrates enhancement of the cauda equina and, occasionally, the conus medullaris (Koffman et al., 1999). Myelography shows contour irregularities of the cauda equina with fusiform thickening or nodularity (Marra, 1982). The radiographic appearance can resemble that in leptomeningeal malignant disease in some cases (Abrey et al., 1998). The cervical spine was affected in only 1 of 17 patients reviewed by Koffman et al. This finding, coupled with the finding that the basal meninges are the most affected part of the intracranial meninges, suggests that gravity may play a role in determining the site of active granulomatous disease.

Nerve conduction abnormalities in polyradiculopathy caused by sarcoidosis are rarely mentioned, and studies are often normal when reported (Marra, 1982; Koffman et al., 1999). There can be prolongation of peroneal or median F waves or absent H reflexes (Zajicek, 1990; Scott et al., 1993). Needle examination may be more helpful because thoracic and upper to middle lumbar myotomes are most severely affected, with detection of fibrillation potentials and neurogenic motor units. Abnormalities on needle examination can also been seen in asymptomatic regions (upper thoracic paraspinals, upper extremities) and may add valuable information in categorizing the type of neuropathy present (Marra, 1982; Scott et al., 1993; Koffman et al., 1999).

Patients presenting with Guillain-Barré syndrome have been described in sarcoidosis. This has occurred simultaneously with the diagnosis of sarcoidosis (LeLuyer et al., 1983; Sharma and Anders, 1985; Miller et al., 1989; Zuniga et al., 1991) or has followed it by 2 months (Schott et al., 1968) or 2 years (Strickland and Moser, 1967). Some investigators have questioned whether the association of Guillain-Barré syndrome and sarcoidosis may be only a chance occurrence (Miller et al., 1989).

PATHOLOGY

Early pathological studies in sarcoid peripheral neuropathy described spindle-shaped swellings of the median, ulnar, and radial nerves, with endothelioid cells, lymphocytes, mononuclear cells, plasma cells, and giant cells between nerve fibers (Mazza, 1908). The hallmark finding in nerve biopsy is the noncaseating granuloma (Fig. 60–7). More recent descriptions of peripheral nerve pathology have shown predominant damage to large, myelinated fibers as well as some other conflicting findings. A patient with relatively severe sarcoid peripheral neuropathy was found to have granulomas in perineurium and, in less frequently, epineurium. Periangiitis, panangiitis, and axonal degeneration were also

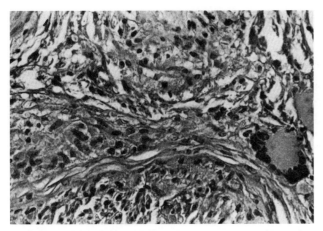

Figure 60–7. Sural nerve biopsy in a patient with sarcoidosis demonstrating noncaseating granuloma within the nerve. (Courtesy of Peter James Dyck.)

seen. The cause of the axonal neuropathy was postulated to be the angiitis as well as compression by sarcoid granulomas (Oh, 1980). Another patient had numerous granulomas in the endoneurium with evidence of both primary demyelination and axonal degeneration. No angiopathic signs were detected. The investigators in this case believed that the neuropathy was probably a direct consequence of the sarcoid granulomas (Nemni et al., 1981). Two additional patients with sarcoid peripheral neuropathy were studied with sural nerve biopsies. One had epineurial granulomas surrounding and invading arterioles with occasional fibrinoid necrosis and severe ultrastructural damage to myelinated and unmyelinated fibers. The second patient showed minimal ultrastructural alterations and some epineurial granulomas encroaching on the walls of arterioles. The conclusion was that the degree of damage to nerve fibers depended on the amount of arteriolar involvement (Vital et al., 1982). Epineurial and perineurial granulomas with angiitis were found in two patients with moderately severe sensorimotor peripheral neuropathy. It was thought, however, that neither compression from granulomas nor the angiitis was the sole cause of the neuropathy. The heterogeneous effects of sarcoidosis on myelinated fibers, blood vessels, and the interstitium of nerve were thought to combine to cause peripheral neuropathy (Galassi et al., 1984).

EVALUATION AND TREATMENT

In a patient with peripheral neuropathy of unknown origin, in whom the diagnosis of sarcoidosis is considered, appropriate screening studies should include chest radiography and ophthalmological examination. Serum angiotensin-converting enzyme can be measured, but typically is elevated only in active pulmonary sarcoidosis and is not indicative of neurological involvement (Oksanen, 1987). Computed tomography of the chest and gallium scanning can also be considered. Analysis of cerebrospinal

fluid can be done, especially in cases of polyradiculopathy. Supportive evidence from cerebrospinal fluid includes elevated protein and white blood cells, low glucose, and negative cytology. Fungal and mycobacterial cultures are negative. Cerebrospinal fluid abnormalities may even be seen in patients with peripheral neuropathy, about half of whom have elevated protein and, occasionally, mild lymphocytic pleocytosis (Scott, 1993). An elevation of cerebrospinal angiotensin-converting enzyme can be seen in neurosarcoidosis affecting the central nervous system, and it may be a useful index of disease activity in neurosarcoidosis, as serum angiotensin-converting enzyme level is for pulmonary sarcoidosis. Its utility in evaluation of polyradiculopathy and peripheral neuropathy, however, is unclear (Oksanen, 1987). If a patient has pathologically proven sarcoidosis from other sources (e.g., lung, conjunctiva, skin, lymph node) and other common causes of peripheral neuropathy can be excluded, a diagnosis of sarcoid peripheral neuropathy can be made without nerve biopsy. If, however, pathological confirmation is not found, nerve biopsy is then indicated. Laminectomy may be performed in cases of polyradiculopathy, first to obtain tissue for biopsy, and second to decompress the spinal canal in cases of mass effect. In a patient with polyradiculopathy who has known, biopsy-proven systemic sarcoidosis and appropriate cerebrospinal fluid findings, additional tissue confirmation with nerve root or meningeal biopsy is not necessary.

Although no clinical trials on treatment of peripheral neuropathy (including Guillain-Barré syndrome) in sarcoidosis with corticosteroids exist, this approach is generally recommended (Stern et al., 1985). Most patients respond to prednisone with initial doses ranging from 30 to 100 mg a day (Oh, 1980; Nemni et al., 1981), although some show no response (Zuniga et al., 1991). Some patients may experience a relapse of symptoms (Scott et al., 1993).

The outcome in patients with sarcoidosis and peripheral neuropathy is good. In one study, 42% recovered, and another 42% improved. Most were treated with steroids. Occasionally, patients with peripheral neuropathy required higher doses of oral or intravenous steroids (Chapelon et al., 1990). The addition of azathioprine was beneficial in one patient with polyradiculopathy (Koffman et al., 1999).

CELIAC DISEASE

Celiac disease is a disorder characterized by symptoms and signs of diarrhea, malabsorption, and weight loss that typically resolve on a gluten-free diet. Villous atrophy, crypt hyperplasia, and intraepithelial lymphocytes are seen on small bowel mucosal biopsy. The disease is thought to result from a heightened immunological responsiveness to ingested gluten. Patients often have antigliadin, antiendomysial, and antireticulum antibodies. There also is an association with certain HLA class II types (DQ2 and less commonly DQ8) (Hadjivassiliou et al., 1998). Neurological dysfunction related to celiac disease includes a wide variety of disorders such as brain atrophy, dementia, ataxia, myopathy, myelopathy, epilepsy with or without occipital calcifications, progressive multifocal leukoencephalopathy, and central nervous system vasculitis (Cooke and Smith, 1966; Hall, 1968; Kepes et al., 1975; Chapman et al., 1978; Rush et al., 1986; Collin et al., 1991; Gobbi et al., 1992).

Various peripheral neuropathic complications have been described, including large-fiber sensorimotor or motor peripheral neuropathy (Cooke and Smith, 1966; Polizzi et al., 2000), painful small-fiber neuropathy (Murphy et al., 1998; Luostarinen et al., 1999), and mononeuritis multiplex (Kelkar et al., 1996). Patients with known celiac disease may develop peripheral neuropathic complications, or patients may present with peripheral neuropathy and may be found subsequently to have celiac disease by biopsy. In one study, 7% of patients newly diagnosed with celiac disease initially presented with neurological complaints, and 1.5% of patients with peripheral neuropathy of unknown origin were subsequently found to have celiac disease (Luostarinen et al., 1999).

There is also a group of patients presenting with neurological complaints who have antigliadin antibodies but no gastrointestinal symptoms. Small bowel biopsy may or may not show typical pathological changes of celiac disease. The diagnosis of *gluten sensitivity* has been given to this group of patients. This diagnosis can occasionally be made in patients with neurological dysfunction of unknown cause, especially cerebellar ataxia and peripheral neuropathy (Hadjivassiliou et al., 1996).

Peripheral Neuropathy

Paresthesias occur in up to one third of patients with celiac disease, although often the neurological examination fails to disclose evidence of peripheral neuropathy (Benson et al., 1964; Morris et al., 1970). No patients in two studies reported by Benson (1964) and Morris (1970) and their respective colleagues showed electrophysiological abnormalities of peripheral neuropathy on nerve conduction studies. Other studies have described patients with celiac disease who complain of distal paresthesias and numbness. On examination, these patients have distal sensory loss, hyporeflexia, sensory ataxia, and varying degrees of weakness. Electrophysiological studies are consistent with a length-dependent axonal peripheral neuropathy mainly affecting sensory fibers (Binder et al., 1967; Banerji and Hurwitz, 1971; Kaplan et al., 1988; Luostarinen et al., 1999). As mentioned, gastrointestinal symptoms may be absent. The gluten sensitivity in these patients is underscored by the finding that neuropathic symptoms may begin when a gluten-free diet is stopped

and that most patients show a favorable response to gluten restriction.

The heightened sensitivity to gluten in celiac disease is further exemplified by a case of a girl with celiac disease since the age of 6 months who experienced two bouts of an acute sensorimotor peripheral neuropathy after accidental reintroduction of gluten into her diet. The electrophysiological characteristics were those of a predominantly motor demyelinating neuropathy with marked slowing of motor conduction velocities in the legs with prolonged distal latencies and F waves. The neuropathy completely resolved after elimination of gluten from the diet (Polizzi et al., 2000).

Patients with primary neurological complaints can be found to harbor antigliadin antibodies, and subsequently asymptomatic celiac disease is confirmed by small bowel biopsy. This was the case in a study of nine patients with neuromuscular disorders of unknown cause. These patients were found to have antigliadin antibodies, prompting small bowel biopsy, which was diagnostic of celiac disease. Six patients had generalized peripheral neuropathy, four with sensorimotor and two with motor neuropathies. Nerve conduction studies in these patients revealed low motor and sensory evoked potential amplitudes with minimal or no slowing of conduction velocities. Myopathy was also seen in two patients with peripheral neuropathy; one had polymyositis, and the other had inclusion body myositis. Finally, there was one case each of mononeuritis multiplex, neuromyotonia, and Guillain-Barré syndrome (Hadjivassiliou et al., 1997).

Patients may additionally present with neurological complaints and gluten sensitivity as evidenced by the presence of antigliadin antibodies but without histological evidence of celiac disease. In a study of patients with a variety of neurological disorders of unknown cause, Hadjivassiliou found that 30 of 53 patients (57%) had positive antigliadin immunoglobulin A or G antibodies. Ataxia and peripheral neuropathy were the most common manifestations (in 25 and 20 patients, respectively). Mononeuritis multiplex (in five patients) and pure motor neuropathy (in three patients) also occurred. Only 1 of these 30 patients was found to have a vitamin deficiency (B_{12}), and only three patients had gastrointestinal symptoms. Duodenal biopsy was performed in 26 of these patients, and, in 7, the results were normal (Hadjivassiliou et al., 1996).

Nerve biopsy findings in patients with peripheral neuropathy often show axonal degeneration (Kaplan et al., 1988; Simonati et al., 1998), although distal nerve terminal axonal degeneration (Cooke et al., 1966) and segmental demyelination (Binder et al., 1967) have also been described.

The origin of the peripheral neuropathy is unclear. Cooke and Smith (1966) hypothesized that a pyridoxine deficiency existed, because some of their patients treated with supplements of this vitamin made complete recoveries. No relationship was found between neuropathy and the levels of folate or vitamin B_{12}. Gluten restriction did not affect the neuropathy (Cooke and Smith, 1966). Peripheral neuropathy may precede a state of malabsorption, however, and many patients have no demonstrable deficiency of vitamin B or E (Kaplan et al., 1988; Hadjivassiliou et al., 1997; Luostarinen et al., 1999). Dietary elimination of gluten has been shown to improve recovery from peripheral neuropathy (Kaplan et al., 1988; Polizzi et al., 2000). The neuropathy may also be present in cases with no histological changes of celiac disease, a finding essentially eliminating the possibility of a malabsorptive state. In addition, peripheral neuropathy can develop in patients with stable celiac disease who follow gluten-free diets. Immunological mechanisms have therefore been proposed to include direct or indirect neurotoxicity of antigliadin antibodies. T cells activated in the small bowel by gliadin may circulate, initiating an immune response in peripheral nerve tissue (Hadjivassiliou et al., 1997). Clinical improvement following steroid administration also supports an immune-mediated cause (Kelkar et al., 1996).

CHRONIC OBSTRUCTIVE PULMONARY DISEASE

Chronic obstructive pulmonary disease has long been associated with clinical and electrophysiological evidence of peripheral nerve dysfunction. Although detailed electrophysiological analysis of groups of patients with chronic obstructive pulmonary disease have been reported in the literature, comparison of the groups is difficult because of the differences in disease severity and electrophysiological parameters measured. In addition, when nerve conduction abnormalities are limited to one nerve (e.g., median, ulnar, or peroneal nerve), other factors need to be considered. These include the age of the patients studied, and the possibility of other confounding variables such as alcohol consumption, radiculopathies, or the presence of focal compression neuropathies in these chronically ill patients, some of whom are thin or have experienced significant weight loss.

Several studies of patients with chronic obstructive pulmonary disease have been performed to assess the prevalence and type of peripheral neuropathy (Appenzeller et al., 1968; Narayan and Ferranti, 1978; Faden et al., 1981; Valli et al., 1984; Paramelle et al., 1986; Jarrat et al., 1992). Overall, it is rare for patients to volunteer symptoms of neuropathy. In one study, 11% of patients mentioned distal paresthesias or muscle cramps (Pfeiffer et al., 1990). Objective clinical findings of peripheral neuropathy are more common and occur in 10% to 80% of patients.

Electrophysiological findings are more common in sensory than in motor nerves and in lower than in upper extremities. Conduction velocities may be slowed, on average by 20% (Narayan and Ferranti, 1978), and sensory amplitudes may be reduced. Abnormal findings in two or more nerves may be seen in up to three fourths of patients (Paramelle et al., 1986). Needle electromyographic examination typically reveals neurogenic changes in distal lower extremity muscles. Quantitative electromyography was performed in one study, with 95% of patients demonstrating neurogenic changes, most often an increase in the percentage of polyphasic motor units. This, coupled with the findings on nerve conduction studies of predominantly motor abnormalities, led the authors to suggest that there was selective damage to motor neurons in patients with chronic obstructive pulmonary disease (Valli et al., 1984). Median neuropathy at the wrist and peroneal neuropathy at the knee have each been found in about 10% of patients (Jarratt et al., 1992).

In summary, although symptoms of peripheral neuropathy in patients with chronic obstructive pulmonary disease are rare, signs of neuropathy may be present on examination. Electrophysiological testing reveals many patients with subclinical axonal, length-dependent sensorimotor neuropathy.

Most studies have found a significant association between the degree and duration of hypoxemia in chronic obstructive pulmonary disease and peripheral neuropathy (Narayan and Ferranti, 1978; Valli et al., 1984; Paramelle et al., 1986; Pfeiffer et al., 1990; Jarratt et al., 1992). Age (Paramelle et al., 1986; Jarratt et al., 1992), malnutrition (Appenzeller et al., 1968), hypercapnia (Stoebner et al., 1989), and cigarette smoking (Faden et al., 1981) have also been implicated as causative factors in development of peripheral neuropathy.

Pathological studies of endoneurial vessels have shown basement membrane thickening, narrowing of vessel lumina, and mural pericytic debris deposits (Stoebner et al., 1989). Endothelial proliferation of the vasa nervorum has also been reported (Church et al., 1988). Studies of experimental diabetic neuropathy have implicated endoneurial hypoxia as a likely cause of this disorder (Tuck et al., 1984). Experiments in rats subjected to chronic hypoxia have noted neuropathic changes (Low et al., 1986). These findings all suggest that the peripheral neuropathy seen in patients with chronic obstructive pulmonary disease, like that in patients with diabetes, may be caused by chronic hypoxia.

PORPHYRIA

Porphyria is a hereditary disorder of heme biosynthesis. *Heme* is synthesized via certain cytosolic and mitochondrial reactions involving modifications of molecules called *porphyrins*. Excess porphyrins created via normal metabolism are excreted in urine (aminolevulinic acid, porphobilinogen, and coproporphyrinogen), feces (protoporphyrin), or both (coproporphyrin). Interruptions in heme biosynthesis lead to abnormal accumulation of excess porphyrins, which exert their toxicity on skin, liver, and central and peripheral nervous systems.

Porphyrias are separated into erythropoietic and

hepatic types, depending on the locus of the enzymatic deficiency. *Erythropoietic porphyrias* cause photosensitivity but typically do not lead to neurological dysfunction. Patients with erythropoietic protoporphyria associated with proximal, motor-predominant, neuropathy have been described in the setting of hepatic failure (Muley et al., 1998). *Hepatic porphyrias* include acute intermittent porphyria, coproporphyria, variegate porphyria, porphyria cutanea tarda, and aminolevulinic acid dehydratase deficiency. *Porphyria cutanea tarda* is a chronic porphyria that may be either genetic or acquired and is usually associated with photosensitivity and hepatic dysfunction. Acute attacks do not occur, and although reports of axonal peripheral neuropathy (Enriquez de Salamanca et al., 1985) and carpal tunnel syndrome (Massey, 1980) exist, neuropathy is generally thought not to be directly associated with the disease. The other hepatic porphyrias are considered further.

The genetic porphyrias are each caused by specific enzyme defects and are typically inherited in an autosomal dominant pattern. Most affected carriers, between 60% and 90%, do not manifest attacks of the disease (Moore et al., 1990; Goren and Chen, 1991). *Acute intermittent porphyria* results from a deficiency of porphobilinogen deaminase (also known as uroporphyrinogen I synthetase). *Coproporphyria* is caused by deficiency of coproporphyrinogen oxidase. *Variegate porphyria* is caused by a defect in protoporphyrinogen oxidase. The only autosomal recessive disorder is *aminolevulinic acid dehydratase deficiency.* Clinically, these disorders are difficult to distinguish, although the presence of photosensitivity is helpful because it occurs only in variegate porphyria and coproporphyria, not acute intermittent porphyria. Biochemical analysis of urine and fecal samples is required to make a definitive diagnosis based on the known patterns of increased porphyrins present. Assays of specific enzymatic activity also help to confirm the diagnosis.

Drugs, alcohol, starvation, or hormonal changes often precipitate clinical attacks. The initial symptoms of an attack are acute abdominal pain and psychiatric disturbance. Acute neuropathy may develop within 2 to 3 days. The neurological manifestations of these different types of porphyria are identical in most cases (Windebank and Bonovsky, 1993).

Peripheral neuropathy is present in two thirds of attacks, but severe, progressive neuropathy develops in only approximately 5% (McEneaney et al., 1993). The severe neuropathy in porphyria is heralded by proximal weakness, often in the shoulder girdles. Weakness of cranial nerve–innervated muscles and respiratory muscles can occur. Sensory loss may also be present and, again, can be more prominent proximally. Some have used the term *bathing-trunk sensory loss* to describe this pattern (Ridley, 1969). Distal sensory loss in a *stocking-and-glove distribution* also occurs. A predominantly sensory neuropathy manifesting with patchy numbness of the genitals, buttocks, posterior thigh, and ankle

has been reported to occur (Goren and Chen, 1991). Clinical signs of mild sensorimotor peripheral neuropathy (Wikberg et al., 2000) and mild slowing of motor and sensory nerve conduction velocities (Mustajoki and Seppalainen, 1975) can be detected in patients with latent or quiescent acute intermittent porphyria.

The acute neuropathy seen in porphyria can resemble Guillain-Barré syndrome. In porphyritic neuropathy, however, there is typically preservation of reflexes in clinically unaffected or minimally affected muscles, although not always (McEneaney et al., 1993), and cerebrospinal fluid is normal. As in Guillain-Barré syndrome, cardiovascular lability with tachycardia can be present and is thought to represent autonomic overactivity (Ridley et al., 1968). It is present before neurological deterioration, and its resolution often signals recovery from the attack. This autonomic overactivity may also explain abdominal pain in these patients and may cause hypertension, constipation, nausea, and vomiting (McDougall and McLeod, 1996).

Electrophysiological studies may be normal, especially early in the attack. Nerve conduction studies of distal nerves and muscles may not be contributory if weakness is in proximal muscles; therefore, needle examination may be more helpful in the diagnosis. Albers and colleagues showed a common pattern with needle electromyography in patients with acute intermittent porphyria and quadriparesis. The early findings were reduced recruitment in weak muscles with mild fibrillation potentials in paraspinal muscles. With time, an increase in fibrillation potentials in proximal muscles and an appearance of fibrillation potentials in distal muscles occurred. By 6 months, there was evidence of reinnervation with a decrease in the amount of fibrillation potentials and the presence of large, polyphasic motor unit action potentials. Nerve conduction studies revealed some low-amplitude motor and sensory responses but no evidence of segmental or proximal slowing of conduction. All findings suggested a primary axonal process localized to the root or cord level (Albers et al., 1978). Other investigators have described this pattern of prominent fibrillation potentials and neurogenic changes on needle electromyography in proximal greater than distal muscles, with little or no change in nerve conduction studies (Nagler, 1971; Defanti et al., 1985).

Another series of electrophysiological studies on patients with acute intermittent porphyria showed mainly low-amplitude or absent motor responses with slowing of conduction velocity commensurate with the degree of amplitude reduction, a finding suggesting an axonal neuropathy (Flugel and Druschky, 1977). A patient with coproporphyria demonstrated some electrophysiological suggestion of demyelination with prolonged F-wave latencies, distal latencies, and temporal dispersion in one nerve. Other changes of low motor and sensory amplitudes and needle electromyographic findings of fibrillation potentials at rest and decreased number of voluntary motor units with long duration motor units suggested some axonal contribution to the neuropathy (Barohn et al., 1994).

Pathological studies in acute intermittent porphyria have revealed isolated axonal degeneration (Pellissier et al., 1987; Barohn et al., 1994) or a combination of both axonal and demyelinating changes (Anzil and Dozic, 1978).

The pathogenesis of the neuropathy in porphyria is not clearly known. Some investigators have proposed that aminolevulinic acid is a neurotoxin, given its highly elevated levels in patients with neuropathy and its in vitro effect on neurophysiological parameters. This toxin could be taken up in the periphery by axons or nerve terminals and then be transported proximally and exert its effect on the neuron cell body. The shorter distance to these neuron cell bodies may be a possible explanation for the proximal preponderance in this neuropathy. A mouse model of acute porphyria has been developed to investigate the pathogenesis of porphyric neuropathy. Electrophysiological and pathological studies in these porphobilinogen-deficient mice reveal a motor neuropathy with axonal features. High levels of aminolevulinic acid in serum, urine, or peripheral tissue were not seen, thus casting doubt on the role of aminolevulinic acid in the pathogenesis of porphyric complications. These authors hypothesized that heme deficiency and dysfunction of hemoproteins, such as mitochondrial cytochromes, caused porphyric neuropathy (Lindberg et al., 1999).

Avoidance of offending drugs is the most important way to prevent an attack. Once an attack occurs, treatment includes both supportive and specific therapies. Pain, nausea, and vomiting are treated symptomatically. Narcotics and phenothiazines are considered safe to administer to patients with porphyria. Treatment with intravenous hematin infusions can reverse an attack. Screening of at-risk family members with erythrocyte porphobilinogen deaminase should be performed. In this way, carriers can be warned against taking potentially offending medications and can be encouraged to avoid (Windebank and Bonovsky, 1993; Barohn et al., 1994).

References

Abbas DH, Schlagenhauff RE, Strong HE: Polyradiculoneuropathy in Addison's disease. Neurology 1977;27:494–495.

Abe K, Sugai F: Chronic inflammatory demyelinating polyneuropathy accompanied by carcinoma [Letter]. J Neurol Neurosurg Psychiatry 1998;65:403–404.

Abend WK, Tyler HR: Thyroid disease and the nervous system. In Aminoff MJ (ed): Neurology in General Medicine. New York, Churchill Livingstone, 1989; 257–271.

Abrey LE, Rosenblum MK, DeAngelis LM: Sarcoidosis of the cauda equina mimicking leptomeningeal malignancy. J Neurooncol 1998;39:261–265.

Albers JW, Robertson WC, Daube JR: Electrodiagnostic findings in acute porphyric neuropathy. Muscle Nerve 1978;1:292–296.

Amair P, Khanna R, Leibel B, et al: Continuous ambulatory peritoneal dialysis in diabetics with end-stage renal disease. N Engl J Med 1982;306:625–630.

Antoine JC, Mosnier JF, Lapras J, et al: Chronic inflammatory demyelinating polyneuropathy associated with carcinoma. J Neurol Neurosurg Psychiatry 1996;60:188–190.

Anzil AP, Dozic S: Peripheral nerve changes in porphyric neuropathy: Findings in a sural nerve biopsy. Acta Neuropathol (Berl) 1978;42:121–126.

Appenzeller O, Parks RD, MacGee J: Peripheral neuropathy in chronic disease of the respiratory tract. Am J Med 1968;44:873–880.

Asbury AK, Victor M, Adams RD: Uremic polyneuropathy after successful renal transplantation. Arch Neurol 1963;8:413–428.

Azuri J, Lerman-Sagie T, Mizrahi A, et al: Guillain-Barré syndrome following serological evidence of hepatitis A in a child [Letter]. Eur J Pediatr 1999;158:341–342.

Banjeri NK, Hurwitz LJ: Neurological manifestations in adult steatorrhea. J Neurol Sci 1971;14:125–141.

Bardin T, Zingraff J, Kuntz D, et al: Dialysis-related amyloidosis. Nephrol Dial Transplant 1986;1:151–154.

Barohn RJ, Sanchez JA, Anderson KE: Acute peripheral neuropathy due to hereditary coproporphyria. Muscle Nerve 1994; 17:793–799.

Baum H, Ludecke DK, Herrmann HD: Carpal tunnel syndrome and acromegaly. Acta Neurochir (Wien) 1986;83:54–55.

Beard L, Kumar A, Estep HL: Bilateral carpal tunnel syndrome caused by Graves' disease. Arch Intern Med 1985;145:345–346.

Benson GD, Kowlessar OD, Sleisenger MH: Adult celiac disease with emphasis upon response to the gluten-free diet. Medicine (Baltimore) 1964;43:1–40.

Berger JR, Ayyar DR, Sheremata WA: Guillain-Barré syndrome complicating acute hepatitis B: A case with detailed electrophysiological and immunological studies. Arch Neurol 1981; 38:366–368.

Berkompas R: A case of peripheral neuropathy and hepatitis. J Tenn Med Assoc 1990;83:191.

Biller BMK, Daniels GH, Bolton CF: In Fauci A, Braunwald E, Esselbucher KJ, et al (eds): Harrison's Principles of Internal Medicine, 14th ed. New York, McGraw-Hill, 1997; 1978–1983.

Binder HJ, Solitaire GB, Spiro HM: Neuromuscular disease in patients with steatorrhea. Gut 1967;8:605–611.

Birket-Smith E, Olivarius BDF: Polyradiculo-myopathia in transient thyrotoxicosis. Dan Med Bull 1957;4:217–219.

Bolton CF, Baltzan MA, Baltzan RB: Effects of renal transplantation on uremic neuropathy: A clinical and electrophysiologic study. N Engl J Med 1971;284:1170–1175.

Bolton CF: Electrophysiological changes in uremic neuropathy following successful renal transplantation. Neurology 1976;26: 152–161.

Bolton CF, Driedger AA, Lindsay RM: Ischemic neuropathy in uremic patients due to arteriovenous fistulas. J Neurol Neurosurg Psychiatry 1979;42:810–814.

Bolton CF, Young GB: Neurological Complications of Renal Disease. Stoneham, MA, Butterworth-Heinemann, 1990.

Bolton CF, McKeown MJ, Chen R, et al: Subacute uremic and diabetic neuropathy. Muscle Nerve 1997a;20:59–64.

Bolton CF, Remtulla H, Toth B, et al: Distinctive electrophysiological features of denervated muscle in uremic patients. J Clin Neurophysiol 1997b;14:539–542.

Borrie MJ, Cape RDT, Troster MM, et al: Myxedema megacolon after external neck irradiation. J Am Geriatr Soc 1983;31:228–230.

Brain WR, Wright AD, Wilkinson M: Spontaneous compression of both median nerves in the carpal tunnel. Lancet 1947;1:277–282.

Brismar T, Tegnèr R: Experimental uremic neuropathy. Part II. Sodium permeability decrease and inactivation in potential clamped nerve fibers. J Neurol Sci 1984;65:37–45.

Bronsky D, Kaganiee GI, Waldstein SS: An association between the Guillain-Barré syndrome and hyperthyroidism. Am J Med Sci 1964;247:196.

Cacoub P, Sbai A, Wechsler B, et al: Chronic inflammatory polyradiculoneuropathy and hepatitis C virus. Rev Med Interne 1999; 20:1146–1147.

Calvey HD, Melia WM, Williams R: Polyneuropathy: An unreported non-metastatic complication of primary hepatocellular carcinoma. Clin Oncol 1983;9:199–202.

Campbell JN, Black P, Ostrow PT: Sarcoid of the cauda equina. J Neurosurgery 1977;47:109–112.

Cavaletti G, Guazzi M, Marcucci A, et al: Endoneural vessel involvement in hypothyroidism. Ital J Neurol Sci 1987;8:259–264.

Challenor YB, Felton CP, Brust JCM: Peripheral nerve involvement in sarcoidosis: An electrodiagnostic study. J Neurol Neurosurg Psychiatry 1984;47:1219–1222.

Chamaillard S, Dubas F, Penisson-Besnier I: Cauda equina syndrome in sarcoidosis: Report of a case. Rev Rhum 1990;57:901–903.

Chapelon C, Ziza JM, Piette JC, et al: Neurosarcoidosis: Signs, course and treatment in 35 confirmed cases. Medicine (Baltimore) 1990;69:261–276.

Chapman RWG, Laidlow JM, Colin-Jones D, et al: Increased prevalence of epilepsy in coeliac disease. BMJ 1978;2:250–251.

Charcot J: Nouveaux signes de la maladie de Basedow. Bull Med 1889;3:147–149.

Chari VR, Katiyar BC, Rastogi BL, et al: Neuropathy in hepatic disorders. J Neurol Sci 1977;31:93–111.

Charron L, Peyronnard JM, Marchand L: Sensory neuropathy associated with primary biliary cirrhosis. Arch Neurol 1980;37:84–87.

Chaudhry V, Corse AM, O'Brian R, et al: Autonomic and peripheral (sensorimotor) neuropathy in chronic liver disease: A clinical and electrophysiologic study. Hepatology 1999;29:1698–1703.

Chen RCY, McLeod JG: Neurological complications of sarcoidosis. Clin Exp Neurol 1989;26:99–112.

Chollet P, Rigal JP, Pignide L: Une complication méconnue de l'hyperthyroidie: La neuropathie périphérique. Presse Med 1971;79:145.

Chopra JS, Samanta AK, Murthy JMK, et al: Role of portasystemic shunt and hepatocellular damage in the genesis of hepatic neuropathy. Clin Neurol Neurosurg 1980;82:37–44.

Church S, Manson EA, Boulton AJM, et al: Functional and morphological characteristics of peripheral neuropathy in chronic lung disease. Thorax 1988;43:858.

Cohen JA, Wilborn SL, Rector WG, et al: Mononeuropathy multiplex associated with acute hepatitis B infection. Muscle Nerve 1990;13:195–198.

Colarian J, Eisenstadt J, LaFave L: Hepatitis B–associated chronic inflammatory polyradiculoneuropathy [Letter]. Am J Gastroenterol 1989;84:1586–1587.

Collin P, Pirttila T, Nurmikko T, et al: Celiac disease, brain atrophy, and dementia. Neurology 1991;41:372–375.

Colover J: Sarcoidosis with involvement of the nervous system. Brain 1948;71:451–475.

Cooke WT, Johnson AG, Woolf AL: Vital staining and electron microscopy of the intramuscular nerve endings in the neuropathy of adult coeliac disease. Brain 1966;89:663–682.

Cooke WT, Smith WT: Neurological disorders associated with adult celiac disease. Brain 1966;89:683–722.

Crevasse LE, Logue BR: Peripheral neuropathy in myxedema. Ann Intern Med 1959;50:1433–1437.

Dayan AD, Williams R: Demyelinating peripheral neuropathy and liver disease. Lancet 1967;2:133–134.

Defanti CA, Sghirlanzoni A, Bottacchi E, et al: Porphyric neuropathy: A clinical, neurophysical and morphological study. Ital J Neurol Sci 1985;6:521–526.

De Klippel N, Hautekeete ML, De Keyser J, et al: Guillain-Barré syndrome as the presenting manifestation of hepatitis C infection. Neurology 1993;43:2143.

Delaney P: Neurologic manifestations in sarcoidosis. Ann Intern Med 1977;87:336–345.

Dinn JJ, Dinn EI: Natural history of acromegalic peripheral neuropathy. Q J Med 1985;57:833–842.

Duyff RF, Van den Bosch J, Laman DM, et al: Neuromuscular findings in thyroid dysfunction: A prospective clinical and electrodiagnostic study. J Neurol Neurosurg Psychiatry 2000;68:750–755.

Dyck PJ, Johnson WJ, Lambert EH, O'Brien PC: Segmental demyelination secondary to axonal degeneration in uremic neuropathy. Mayo Clin Proc 1971;46:400–531.

Dyck PJ, Lambert EH: Polyneuropathy associated with hypothyroidism. J Neuropathol Exp Neurol 1970;29:631–658.

Dyck PJ, Yao JK, Knickerbocker DE, et al: Multisystem neuronal degeneration, hepatosplenomegaly, and adrenocortical deficiency associated with reduced tissue arachidonic acid. Neurology 1981;31:925–934.

Eggers PW: Effect of transplantation on the Medicare end-stage renal disease program. N Engl J Med 1988;318:223–229.

Endoh J, Ogasawara N, Mushimoto M: Guillain-Barré syndrome following acute hepatitis A. Rinsho Shinkeigaku 1991;31:210–212.

Engel AG: Electron microscopic observation in thyrotoxic and corticosteroid-induced myopathies. Mayo Clin Proc 1966;41:785.

Enriquez de Salamanca R, Cocero E, Jimenez LC, et al: Electroneurophysiological abnormalities in porphyria cutanea tarda. Clin Exp Dermatol 1985;10:438–443.

Faden A, Mendoza E, Flynn F: Subclinical neuropathy associated with chronic obstructive pulmonary disease. Arch Neurol 1981;38:639–642.

Federico A, Baracchini G, Dotti MT, et al: Infanto-juvenile encephaloneuropathy and pigmentary retinopathy in a girl associated with congenital adrenal insufficiency and altered plasma medium-chain fatty acid levels. J Inherit Metab Dis 1988;11:178–182.

Feibel JH, Campa JF: Thyrotoxic neuropathy (Basedow's paraplegia). J Neurol Neurosurg Psychiatry 1976;39:491–497.

Firooznia H, Golimbu C, Rafii M: Carpal tunnel syndrome as a manifestation of secondary hyperparathyroidism [Letter]. Arch Intern Med 1981;141:959.

Fisher M, Mateer JE, Ullrich I, et al: Pyramidal tract deficits and polyneuropathy in hyperthyroidism: Combination clinically mimicking amyotrophic lateral sclerosis. Am J Med 1985;78:1041–1044.

Fleckenstein JF, Frank SM, Thuluvath PJ: Presence of autonomic neuropathy is a poor prognostic indicator in patients with advanced liver disease. Hepatology 1996;23:471–475.

Flugel KA, Druschky K-F: Electromyogram and nerve conduction in patients with acute intermittent porphyria. J Neurol 1977;214:267–279.

Galassi G, Gibertoni M, Mancini A, et al: Sarcoidosis of the peripheral nerve: Clinical, electrophysiological and histological study of two cases. Eur Neurol 1984;23:459–465.

Gejyo F, Jonna N, Suxuki Y, et al: Serum levels of beta₂ microglobin as a new form of amyloid protein in patients undergoing long-term hemodialysis [Letter]. N Engl J Med 1986;314:585–586.

Gentric A, Jezequel J, Pennec YL: Severe neuropathy related to primary hyperparathyroidism cured by parathyroidectomy. J Am Geriatr Soc 1993;41:759.

Gerster JC, Gauthier G: Polyneuropathy in a case of primary hyperparathyroidism: Disappearance of the neurological picture after surgical correction of the hyperparathyroidism. Helv Med Acta 1969/70;35:296–303.

Gilchrest BA, Rowe JW, Mihm MC Jr: Clinical and histological skin changes in CRF: Evidence for a dialysis-resistant, transplant-responsive microangiopathy. Lancet 1980;2:1271–1275.

Gobbi G, Bouquet F, Greco L, et al: Coeliac disease, epilepsy, and cerebral calcifications. Lancet 1992;340:439–443.

Golding PL, Smith M, Williams R: Mutisystem involvement in chronic liver disease. Am J Med 1973;55:772–782.

Goren MD, Chen C: Acute intermittent porphyria with atypical neuropathy. South Med J 1991;84:668–669.

Grant AJ, Buckels JA, Neuberger J: Symptomatic carpal tunnel syndrome after orthotropic liver transplantation: A retrospective analysis. Transplantation 1998;65:442–444.

Hadjivassiliou M, Chattopadhyay AK, Davies-Jones GAB, et al: Neuromuscular disorder as a presenting feature of coeliac disease. J Neurol Neurosurg Psychiatry 1997;63:770–775.

Hadjivassiliou M, Gibson A, Davies-Jones GAB, et al: Does cryptic gluten sensitivity play a part in neurological illness? Lancet 1996;347:369–371.

Hadjivassiliou M, Grunewald RA, Chattopadhyay AD, et al: Clinical, radiological, neurophysiological, and neuropathological characteristics of gluten ataxia. Lancet 1998;352:1582–1585.

Hall WH: Proximal muscle atrophy in adult celiac disease. Am J Dig Dis 1968;13:697–704.

Hamley FH, Timms RT, Mign VD, et al: Bilateral phrenic nerve paralysis in myxedema [Abstract]. Am Rev Respir Dis 1975; 111:A911.

Han H-F, Wu J-C, Huo T-I, et al: Chronic hepatitis B exacerbated by Guillain-Barré syndrome: A report of two cases. Chin Med J (Taipei) 1999;62:652–656.

Hansen S, Ballantyne JP: A quantitative electrophysiological study of uremic neuropathy: Diabetic and renal neuropathies compared. J Neurol Neurosurg Psychiatry 1978;41:128–134.

Hatzis GS, Delladetsima I, Koufos C: Hepatocellular carcinoma presenting with paraneoplastic neurologic syndrome in a hepatitis B surface antigen–positive patient. J Clin Gastroenterol 1998;26:144–147.

Heckmann JG, Kayser C, Heuss D, et al: Neurological manifestations of chronic hepatitis C. J Neurol 1999;246:486–491.

Hendrickse MT, Thuluvath PJ, Triger DR: Natural history of autonomic neuropathy in chronic liver disease. Lancet 1992;339: 1462–1464.

Hendrickse MT, Triger DR: Autonomic and peripheral neuropathy in primary biliary cirrhosis. J Hepatol 1993;19:401–407.

Hindfelt B, Holmin T: Experimental porta-caval anastomosis and motor nerve conduction velocity in the rat. J Neurol 1980; 223:171–175.

Hockerstedt K, Kajaste S, Muuronen A, et al: Encephalopathy and neuropathy in end-stage liver disease before and after liver transplantation. J Hepatol 1992;16:31–37.

Ijichi S, Niina K, Tara M, et al: Mononeuropathy associated with hyperthyroidism. J Neurol Neurosurg Psychiatry 1990;53:1109–1110.

Illa I, Graus F, Ferrer I, et al: Sensory neuropathy as the initial manifestation of primary biliary cirrhosis [Letter]. J Neurol Neurosurg Psychiatry 1989;52:1307.

Inoue A, Koh CS, Yahikozawa H, et al: A pathogenic study of chronic inflammatory demyelinating polyradiculoneuropathy in a patient with hepatitis B infection. Jpn J Allergol 1994; 43:585–589.

Inoue A, Oguchi K, Iwahashi T, et al: Prominent effect of immunoadsorption plasmapheresis therapy in a patient with chronic inflammatory demyelinating polyneuropathy associated with hepatitis B infection. Ther Apheresis 1998;2:305–307.

Jamal GA, Kerr DJ, McLellan AR, et al: Generalised peripheral nerve dysfunction in acromegaly: A study by conventional and neurophysiological techniques. J Neurol Neurosurg Psychiatry 1987;50:886–894.

Jarratt JA, Morgan CN, Twomey JA, et al: Neuropathy in chronic obstructive pulmonary disease: A multicentre electrophysiological and clinical study. Eur Respir J 1992;5:517–524.

Jeffrey GP, Muller DPR, Burroughs AK, et al: Vitamin E deficiency and its clinical significance in adults with primary biliary cirrhosis and other forms of chronic liver disease. J Hepatol 1987; 4:307–317.

Jenkins PJ, Sohaib SA, Akker S, et al: The pathology of median neuropathy in acromegaly. Ann Intern Med 2000;133:197–201.

Jennekens FGI, Mees EJ, van der Most van Spijk D: Clinical aspects of uraemic polyneuropathy. Nephron 1971;8:414–426.

Joffroy MA: Hospice de la Salpetrière, Clinique nerveuse: Leçons faites en décembre. Prog Med 1894;22:61–62.

Johnson RH, Robinson BJ: Mortality in alcoholics with autonomic neuropathy. J Neurol Neurosurg Psychiatry 1988;51:476–480.

Johnston AW: Acroparesthesias and acromegaly. BMJ 1960;1: 1616–1618.

Kameyama S, Tanaka R, Hasegawa A, et al: Subclinical carpal tunnel syndrome in acromegaly. Neurol Med Chir (Tokyo) 1993; 33:547–551.

Kaplan JG, Pack, D, Horoupian, D, et al: Distal axonopathy associated with chronic gluten enteropathy: A treatable disorder. Neurology 1988;38:642–645.

Kaplan PE, Hines JR, Leestma JE, et al: Neuromuscular junction transmission dysfunction in primary hyperparathyroidism: A new hypothesis. Electromyogr Clin Neurophysiol 1982;22:239–242.

Kashihara K, Terai T, Shomori T: Relapsing neuropathy associated with hepatitis C virus infection. Intern Med 1995;34:265–266.

Kelkar P, Ross MA, Murray J: Mononeuropathy multiplex associated with celiac sprue. Muscle Nerve 1996;19:234–236.

Kempler P, Varadi A, Kadar E, et al: Autonomic and peripheral

neuropathy in primary biliary cirrhosis: Evidence of small sensory fibre damage and prolongation of the QT interval [Letter]. J Hepatol 1994;21:1150–1151.

Kempler P, Varadi A, Szalay F: Autonomic neuropathy in liver disease [Letter]. Lancet 1989;2:1332.

Kennedy WR, Navarro X, Goetz FC, et al: Effects of pancreatic transplantation on diabetic neuropathy. N Engl J Med 1990;12: 1031–1037.

Kepes JJ, Chou SM, Price LW: Progressive multifocal leukoencephalopathy with 10-year survival in a patient with non-tropical sprue. Neurology 1975;25:1006–1012.

Knezevic W, Mastaglia FL: Neuropathy associated with Brescia-Cimino arteriovenous fistulas. Arch Neurol 1984;41:1184–1186.

Knight RE, Bourne AJ, Newton M, et al: Neurologic syndrome associated with low levels of vitamin E in primary biliary cirrhosis. Gastroenterology 1986;91:209–211.

Knill-Jones RP, Goodwill CJ, Dayan AD, et al: Peripheral neuropathy in chronic liver disease: Clinical, electrophysiologic, and nerve biopsy findings. J Neurol Neurosurg Psychiatry 1972; 35:22–30.

Koffman B, Junck L, Elias SB, et al: Polyradiculopathy in sarcoidosis. Muscle Nerve 1999;22:608–613.

Koh C, Tsukada N, Tanaka Y, et al: A case of chronic polyneuropathy associated with chronic type B hepatitis. No To Shinkei 1988;40:721–725.

Kompf D, Neudorfer B, Kayser-Gatchalian C, et al: Mononeuritis multiplex bei Boeckscher Sarkoidose. Nervenarzt 1986;47:687–689.

Konishi T, Nishitani H, Motomura S: Single fiber electromyography in CRF. Muscle Nerve 1982;5:458–461.

Kuriakose P, Pawar GP: Cranial nerve palsy associated with acute hepatitis B. Ind J Gastroenterol 1994;13:101.

Lacaille F, Zylberberg J, Hagege H, et al: Hepatitis C associated with Guillain-Barré syndrome. Liver 1998;18:49–51.

Laroche CM, Cairns T, Moxham J, et al: Hypothyroidism presenting with respiratory muscle weakness. Am Rev Respir Dis 1988;138:472–474.

Laycock MA, Pascuzzi RM: The neuromuscular effects of hypothyroidism. Semin Neurol 1991;11:288–294.

Lee DK, Do JK, Kim YJ: Guillain-Barré like syndrome associated with acute renal failure and thrombocytopenia following acute viral hepatitis A. J Korean Med Sci 1997;12:151–156.

LeLuyer B, Devaux AM, Dailly R, et al: Polyradiculonevrite revelatrice d'une sarcoidose de l'enfant. Arch Fr Pediatr 1983;40:175–178.

Lin S, Ryu S, Liaw Y: Guillain-Barré syndrome associated with acute delta hepatitis virus superinfection. J Med Virol 1989; 28:144–145.

Lindberg RLP, Martini R, Baumgartner M, et al: Motor neuropathy in porphobilinogen deaminase-deficient mice imitates the peripheral neuropathy of human acute porphyria. J Clin Invest 1999;103:1127–1134.

Lok ASF, Wilson LA, Thomas HC: Neurotoxicity associated with adenine arabinoside monophosphate in the treatment of chronic hepatitis B virus infection. J Antimicrob Chemother 1984;14:93–99.

Low PA, McLeod JG, Turtle JR, et al: Peripheral neuropathy in acromegaly. Brain 1974;97:139–152.

Low PA, Schmelzer JD, Ward KK, et al: Experimental chronic hypoxic neuropathy: Relevance to diabetic neuropathy. Am J Physiol 1986;250:E94–E99.

Lundin HP, Spiess H, Koenig MP: Neuromuscular dysfunction associated with thyrotoxicosis. Eur Neurol 1969;2:269–278.

Luostarinen L, Pirttila T, Collin P: Coeliac disease presenting with neurological disorders. Eur Neurol 1999;42:132–135.

Mackay-Sim A, Beard MD: Hypothyroidism disrupts neural development in the olfactory epithelium of adult mice. Brain Research 1987;433:190–198.

Maeda M, Ohkoshi N, Hisahara S, et al: Mononeuropathy multiplex in a patient receiving interferon alpha therapy for chronic hepatitis C. Clin Neurol 1995;35:1048–1050.

Marie P: Sur deux cas d'acromegalie: Hypertrophie singuliere, non congenitale, des extremities superieures, inferieures et cephalique. Rev Med (Paris) 1886;6:297–333.

Marie P, Foix C: Atrophie isolee de l'eminence thenar d'origine nevritique: Role du ligament annulaire anterieur du carpe dans la pathogenie de la lesion. Rev Neurol 1913;26:647–649.

Marie P, Marinesco G: Sur l'anatomie pathologique de l'acromegalie. Arch Med Exp Anat Pathol 1891;3:539–565.

Marie P, Souza-Leite JD: Essays on Acromegaly: With Bibliography and Appendix of Cases by Other Authors. London, New Sydenham Society, 1891;137.

Marra TR: Sarcoid polyradiculoneuropathy with myelographic confirmation. Wisc Med J 1982;81:21–24.

Martin J, Tomkin GH, Hutchinson M: Peripheral neuropathy in hypothyroidism: An association with spurious polycythaemia (Gaisbock's syndrome). J R Soc Med 1983;76:187–189.

Marzo ME, Tintore M, Fabregues O, et al: Chronic inflammatory demyelinating polyneuropathy during treatment with interferon-alpha [Letter]. J Neurol Neurosurg Psychiatry 1998;65:604–615.

Massey EW: Carpal tunnel syndrome in porphyria [Letter]. Lancet 1980;2:808.

Massey EW, Folger WN, Holohan T, et al: Carpal tunnel syndrome in hepatic disease [Letter]. South Med J 1979;72:1030.

Maycock RL, Bertrand P, Morrison CE, et al: Manifestations of sarcoidosis. Am J Med 1963;35:67–89.

Mazza G: Über das multiple benigne Sarkoid der Haut. Arch Dermatol Syphilol Wien 1908;91:57–78.

McComas AJ, Sca REP, McNabb AR, et al: Evidence for reversible motoneurone dysfunction in thyrotoxicosis. J Neurol Neurosurg Psychiatry 1974;37:548–558.

McDougall AJ, McLeod JG: Autonomic neuropathy. II. Specific peripheral neuropathies. J Neurol Sci 1996;138:1–13.

McEneaney D, Hawkins S, Trimble E, et al: Porphyric neuropathy: A rare and often neglected differential diagnosis of Guillain-Barré syndrome. J Neurol Sci 1993;114:231–232.

McLeod WN: Sporadic non-A, non-B hepatitis and Epstein-Barr hepatitis associated with the Guillain-Barré syndrome. Arch Neurol 1987;44:438–442.

Meier C, Bischoff A: Polyneuropathy in hypothyroidism. J Neurol 1977;215:103–114.

Merchut MP, Adams EM, Morrissey M: Sensory neuronopathy in autoimmune chronic active hepatitis. Neurology 1993;43:2410–2411.

Meriggioli MN, Rowin J: Chronic inflammatory demyelinating polyneuropathy after treatment with interferon-alpha. Muscle Nerve 2000;23:433–435.

Mihori A, Nakayama M, Ono S, et al: Ataxic form of Guillain-Barré syndrome associated with acute hepatitis A: A case report. Rinsho Shinkeigaku 1998;38:242–245.

Miller R, Sheron N, Semple S: Sarcoidosis presenting with an acute Guillain-Barré syndrome. Postgrad Med 1989;65:765–767.

Misiunas A, Niepomniszcze H, Ravera B, et al: Peripheral neuropathy in subclinical hypothyroidism. Thyroid 1995;5:283–286.

Mitz M, Benedetto MD, Kleinbeil GE, et al: Neuropathy in end-stage renal disease secondary to primary renal disease and diabetes. Arch Phys Med Rehabil 1984;65:235–238.

Moore KE, McColl KEL, Fitzsimmons EJ, et al: The porphyrias. Blood Rev 1990;4:88–96.

Morris JS, Ajdukiewicz AB, Read AE: Neurological disorders and adult coeliac disease. Gut 1970;11:549–554.

Muley SA, Midani HA, Rank JM, et al: Neuropathy in erythropoietic protoporphyrias. Neurology 1998;51:262–265.

Murphy D, Laffy J, O'Keeffe D: Electrical spinal cord stimulation for painful peripheral neuropathy secondary to coeliac disease. Gut 1998;42:448–449.

Murray IPC, Simpson JH: Acroparesthesiae in myxoedema: A clinical and electromyographic study. Lancet 1958;1:1360–1363.

Murthy JM: Guillain-Barré syndrome following specific viral infections: An appraisal. J Assoc Physicians India 1994;42:27–29.

Mustajoki P, Seppalainen AM: Neuropathy in latent hereditary hepatic porphyria. BMJ 1975;2:310–312.

Nagler W: Peripheral neuropathy in acute intermittent porphyrias. Arch Phys Med Rehabil 1971;52:426–431.

Narayan M, Ferranti R: Nerve conduction impairment in patients with respiratory insufficiency and severe chronic hypoxemia. Arch Phys Med Rehabil 1978;59:188–192.

Navarro X, Sutherland DER, Kennedy WR: Long-term effects of pancreatic transplantation on diabetic neuropathy. Ann Neurol 1997;42:727–736.

Negoro K, Fukusako T, Morimatsu M, et al: Acute axonal polyneuropathy during interferon alpha-2A therapy for chronic hepatitis type C. Muscle Nerve 1994;17:1351–1352.

Nemni R, Bottacchi E, Fazio R, et al: Polyneuropathy in hypothyroidism: Clinical, electrophysiological and morphological findings in four cases. J Neurol Neurosurg Psychiatry 1987;50:1454–1460.

Nemni R, Galassi G, Cohen M, et al: Symmetric sarcoid polyneuropathy: Analysis of a sural nerve biopsy. Neurology 1981;31:1217–1223.

Ng PL, Powell LW, Cambell CB: Guillain Barré syndrome during the pre-icteric phase of acute type B viral hepatitis. Aust N Z J Med 1975;5:367–369.

Nickel SN, Frame B: Nervous and muscular systems in myxedema. J Chronic Dis 1961;14:570–581.

Nickel SN, Frame B, Bebin J, et al: Myxedema neuropathy and myopathy. Neurology 1961;11:125–137.

Nielsen VK: The peripheral nerve function in CRF. V. Sensory and motor conduction velocity. Acta Med Scand 1973a;194:455–462.

Nielsen VK: The peripheral nerve function in CRF. VI. The relationship between sensory and motor nerve conduction and kidney function, azotemic, age, sex and clinical neuropathy. Acta Med Scand 1973b;194:455–462.

Nielsen VK: The peripheral nerve function in CRF. VIII. Recovery after renal transplantation: Clinical aspects. Acta Med Scand 1974;195:163–170.

Nielsen VK: The vibration stimulus: Effects of viscous-elastic resistance of skin on the amplitude of vibrations. Electroencephalogr Clin Neurophysiol 1975;38:647–652.

Nielsen VK: Pathophysiological aspects of uremic neuropathy. In Canal N, Pozza G (eds): Peripheral Neuropathies. New York, Elsevier North Holland Biomedical Press, 1978; 197–210.

Nishiyama K, Kurisaki H, Masuda N, et al: Carcinomatous neuropathy associated with hepatic cell carcinoma: An autopsy case report. Neuromusc Disord 1993;3:227–229.

O'Duffy JD, Randall RY, MacCarty CS: Median neuropathy (carpal tunnel syndrome) in acromegaly. Ann Intern Med 1973;78:379–383.

Oh SJ: Sarcoid polyneuropathy: A histologically proved case. Ann Neurol 1980;7:178–181.

Ohyama T, Okiyama R, Yamada M, et al: Chronic inflammatory demyelinating polyneuropathy associated with chronic liver disease due to type B and type C hepatitis virus. No To Shinkei 1995;47:161–165.

Oksanen V: New cerebrospinal fluid, neurophysiological and neuroradiological examinations in the diagnosis and follow-up of neurosarcoidosis. Sarcoidosis 1987;4:105–110.

Oliver MI, Miralles R, Rubies-Prat J, et al: Autonomic dysfunction in patients with non-alcoholic chronic liver disease. J Hepatol 1997;26:1242–1248.

Ono S, Chida K, Takasu T: Guillain-Barré syndrome following fulminant viral hepatitis A. Intern Med 1994;33:799–801.

Ord WM: On some disorders of nutrition related with affections of nervous system. BMJ 1884;2:205–211.

Panayiotopoulous CP, Laxos G: Tibial nerve H-reflex and F-wave studies in patients with uremic neuropathy. Muscle Nerve 1980;3:423–426.

Pandit L, Shankar SK, Gayathri N, et al: Acute thyrotoxic neuropathy: Basedow's paraplegia revisited. J Neurol Sci 1998;155:211–214.

Paramelle B, Vila A, Pollack P, et al: Frequence des polyneuropathies dan les bronchopneumopathies chroniques obstructives. Presse Med 1986;15:563–567.

Patten BM, Bilezikian JP, Mallette LE, et al: Neuromuscular disease in primary hyperparathyroidism. Ann Intern Med 1974;80:182–193.

Payne CR, Tait D, Batten JC: Sarcoidosis and chronic sensory neuropathy. Postgrad Med J 1980;56:781–782.

Pelletier G, Elghozi D, Trepo C, et al: Mononeuritis in acute viral hepatitis. Digestion 1985;32:53–56.

Pellissier JF, Serratrice G, Toga M: Pathologie de la neuropathie porphyrique. Arch Anat Cytol Pathol 1987;35:173–177.

Penn AS: Myoglobinuria. In Engle AG, Banker BQ (eds): Myology. New York, McGraw-Hill, 1986.

Penner E, Maida E, Mamoli B, et al: Serum and cerebrospinal fluid immune complexes containing hepatitis B surface antigen in Guillain-Barré syndrome. Gastroenterology 1982;82:576–580.

Perretti A, Gentile S, Balbi P, et al: Peripheral neuropathy in liver cirrhosis: A clinical and electrophysiological study. Ital J Gastroenterol 1995;27:349–354.

Pfeiffer G, Kunze K, Bruch M, et al: Polyneuropathy associated with chronic hypoxaemia: Prevalence in patients with chronic obstructive pulmonary disease. J Neurol 1990;237:230–233.

Phan TG, Hersch M, Zagami AS: Guillain-Barré syndrome and adenocarcinoma of the gallbladder: A paraneoplastic phenomenon? [Letter] Muscle Nerve 1999;22:141–142.

Pickett JBE III, Layzer RB, Levin SR, et al: Neuromuscular complications of acromegaly. Neurology 1975;25:638–645.

Polizzi A, Finocchiaro M, Parano E, et al: Recurrent peripheral neuropathy in a girl with celiac disease. J Neurol Neurosurg Psychiatry 2000;68:104–105.

Pollard JD, McLeod JG, Angel Honnibal TG, et al: Hypothyroid polyneuropathy: Clinical, electrophysiological and nerve biopsy findings in two cases. J Neurol Sci 1982;53:461–471.

Purnell DC, Daly DD, Lipscomb PR: Carpal-tunnel syndrome associated with myxedema. Arch Intern Med 1961;108:151–156.

Quattrini A, Comi G, Nemni R, et al: Axonal neuropathy associated with interferon-alpha treatment for hepatitis C: HLA-DR immunoreactivity in Schwann cells. Acta Neuropathol (Berl) 1997;94:504–508.

Rao SN, Katiyar BC, Nair KRP, et al: Neuromuscular status in hypothyroidism. Acta Neurol Scand 1980;61:167–177.

Ridley A: The neuropathy of acute intermittent porphyria. Q J Med 1969;38:307–333.

Ridley A, Hierons R, Cavanagh JB: Tachycardia and the neuropathy of porphyria. Lancet 1968;2:708–710.

Ripault MP, Borderie C, Dumas P, et al: Peripheral neuropathies and chronic hepatitis C: A frequent association? Gastroenterol Clin Biol 1998;22:891–896.

Ritter FN: The effects of hypothyroidism upon the ear, nose, and throat: A clinical and experimental study. Laryngoscope 1967;77:1427–1479.

Ropper AH: Accelerated neuropathy of renal failure. Arch Neurol 1993;50:536–539.

Roquer J, Cano JF: Carpal tunnel syndrome and hyperthyroidism: A prospective study. Acta Neurol Scand 1993;88:149–152.

Rudman D, Williams PJ: Pathophysiologic principles in nutrition. In Smith LH (ed): Pathophysiology: The Biologic Principles of Disease, 2nd ed. Philadelphia, WB Saunders, 1985.

Rush PJ, Inman R, Bernstein M, et al: Isolated vasculitis of the central nervous system in a patient with coeliac disease. Am J Med 1986;81:1092–1094.

Safadi R, Ben-Hur T, Shouval D: Mononeuritis multiplex: A rare complication of acute hepatitis A. Liver 1996;16:288–289.

Said G: Acquired neuropathies (2): Kidney failure, hypothyroidism and hypoglycemia. Rev Neurol (Paris) 1987;143:785–790.

Sakajiri K, Takamori M: Multiple mononeuropathy during recombinant interferon-alpha 2a therapy for chronic hepatitis C. Clin Neurol 1992;32:1041–1043.

Scarpalezos SC, Lygidakis C, Papageorgou C, et al: Neural and muscular manifestation of hypothyroidism. Arch Neurol 1973;29:140–143.

Schott PMM, Michel D, Lejeune E, et al: Polyradiculoneurites au cours de la maladie de Besnier-Boeck-Schaumann. J Med Lyon 1968;49:931–937.

Schwartz MS, Mackworkth-Young CG, McKeran RO: The tarsal tunnel syndrome in hypothyroidism. J Neurol Neurosurg Psychiatry 1983;46:440–442.

Sclesa SN, Herskovitz S, Reichler B: Treatment of mononeuropathy multiplex in hepatitis C virus and cryoglobulinemia. Muscle Nerve 1998;21:1526–1529.

Scott TF: Neurosarcoidosis: Progress and clinical aspects. Neurology 1993;43:8–12.

Scott TF, Brillman J, Gross JA: Sarcoidosis of the peripheral nervous system. Neurol Res 1993;15:389–390.

Serra C, D'Angelillo A, Facciolla D, et al: Somatosensory cerebral evoked potentials in uremic polyneuropathy. Acta Neurol (Napoli) 1979;34:1–14.

Sharma OP, Anders A: Neurosarcoidosis: A report of ten patients illustrating some usual and unusual manifestations. Sarcoidosis 1985;2:96–106.

Shinoda K, Takamatsu J, Mozai T: Peripheral neuropathy in hypothyroidism. I. Clinical and electrophysiologic study. Bull Osaka Med School 1987a;33–2:137–148.

Shinoda K, Hosokawa S, Mozai T: Peripheral neuropathy in hypothyroidism. II. Morphometric and electron microscopical studies on sural nerve in hypothyroidism and axonal atrophy in hypothyroid polyneuropathy. Bull Osaka Med School 1987b;33–2:149–163.

Shirabe T, Tawara S, Terao A, et al: Myxoedematous polyneuropathy: A light and electron microscopic study of the peripheral nerve and muscle. J Neurol Neurosurg Psychiatry 1975;38:241–247.

Sidenius P, Nagel P, Larsen JR, et al: Axonal transport of slow component a in sciatic nerves of hypo- and hyperthyroid rats. J Neurochem 1987;49:1790–1795.

Silverstein A, Feuer MM, Siltzbach LE: Neurologic sarcoidosis. Arch Neurol 1965;12:1–11.

Simonati A, Battistella PA, Guariso G, et al: Coeliac disease associated with peripheral neuropathy in a child: A case report. Neuropediatrics 1998;29:155–158.

Simpson JA: Conduction velocity of peripheral nerve in human metabolic disorders. Electroencephalogr Clin Neurophysiol 1962;22:6–42.

Solders G, Persson A, Gutierrez A: Autonomic dysfunction in nondiabetic terminal uremia. Acta Neurol Scand 1985;71:321–327.

Soubrier MJ, Dubost J, Sauvezie BJM, et al: POEMS syndrome: A study of 25 cases and a review of the literature. Am J Med 1994;97:543–553.

Stern BJ, Krumholz A, Johns C, et al: Sarcoidosis and its neurological manifestations. Arch Neurol 1985;42:909–917.

Stoebner P, Mezin P, Vila A, et al: Microangiopathy of endoneurial vessels in hypoxemic chronic obstructive pulmonary disease (COPD): A quantitative ultrastructural study. Acta Neuropathol (Berl) 1989;78:388–395.

Strickland GT, Moser KM: Sarcoidosis with a Landry-Guillain-Barré syndrome and clinical response to corticosteroids. Am J Med 1967;43:131–135.

Swanson JW, Kelly JJ, McConahey WM: Neurologic aspects of thyroid dysfunction. Mayo Clin Proc 1981;56:504–512.

Tabor E: Guillain-Barré syndrome and other neurologic syndromes in hepatitis A, B, and non-A, non-B. J Med Virol 1987;21:207–216.

Tambini R, Quattrini A, Fracassetti O, et al: Axonal neuropathy in a patient receiving interferon-alpha therapy for chronic hepatitis C [Letter]. J Rheumatol 1997;24:1656–1657.

Tegnèr R, Lindholm B: Vibratory perception threshold compared with nerve conduction velocity in the evaluation of uraemic neuropathy. Acta Neurol Scand 1985;71:284–289.

Thiele B, Stålberg E: Single fibre EMG findings in polyneuropathies of different aetiology. J Neurol Neurosurg Psychiatry 1975;38:881–887.

Thomas PK, Hollinrake K, Lascelles RG, et al: The polyneuropathy of CRF. Brain 1971;94:761–780.

Thomas PK, Walker JG: Xanthomatous neuropathy in primary biliary cirrhosis. Brain 1965;88:1079–1088.

Thuluvath PJ, Triger DR: Autonomic neuropathy in chronic liver disease. Q J Med 1989;72:737–747.

Trevisani F, Sica G, Bernardi M: Autonomic neuropathy in advanced liver disease [Letter]. Hepatology 1996;24:1549.

Tsao CY, Romshe CA, Lo WD, et al: Familial adrenal insufficiency, achalasia, alacrima, peripheral neuropathy, microcephaly, normal plasma very long chain fatty acids, and normal muscle mitochondrial respiratory chain enzymes. J Child Neurol 1994;9:135–138.

Tsukada N, Koh C, Inoue A, et al: Demyelinating neuropathy associated with hepatitis B virus infection. J Neurol Sci 1987;77:203–216.

Tsukada N, Koh C, Owa A, et al: Chronic neuropathy associated with immune complexes of hepatitis B virus. J Neurol Sci 1983;61:193–211.

Tuck RR, Schmelzer JD, Low PA: Endoneurial blood flow and oxygen tension in the sciatic nerves of rats with experimental diabetic neuropathy. Brain 1984;107:935–950.

Turken SA, Cafferty M, Silverberg SJ, et al: Neuromuscular involvement in mild asymptomatic primary hyperparathyroidism. Am J Med 1989;87:553–557.

Valenta LJ: Hyperparathyroidism due to parathyroid adenoma and carpal tunnel syndrome [Letter]. Ann Intern Med 1975; 82:541–542.

Vallat JM, Poumier C, Dumas M, et al: Guillain-Barré syndrome and parathyroid adenoma [Letter]. Arch Neurol 1982;39:322.

Valli G, Barbieri S, Sergi P, et al: Evidence of motor neuron involvement in chronic respiratory insufficiency. J Neurol Neurosurg Psychiatry 1984;47:1117–1121.

Vasilescu C, Florescu A, Balta N: Electroneurographic evidence of polyneuropathy in chronic liver disease. Arch Psychiatry Neurol Sci 1978;225:87–96.

Vaziri D, Pratt H, Saiki JD, et al: Evaluation of somatosensory pathway by short latency evoked potentials in patients with end-stage renal disease maintained on hemodialysis. Int J Artif Organs 1981;4:17–21.

Vital C, Aubertin J, Ragnault JM, et al: Sarcoidosis of the peripheral nerve: A histological and ultrastructural study of two cases. Acta Neuropathol (Berl) 1982;58:111–114.

Voigt MD, Trey G, Levitt NS, et al: Autonomic neuropathy in extra-hepatic portal vein thrombosis: Evidence for impaired autonomic reflex arc. J Hepatol 1997;26:634–641.

Wartofsky L: Diseases of the thyroid. In Fauci A, Braunwald E, Esselbacher KJ, et al (eds): Harrison's Principles of Internal Medicine, 14th ed. New York, McGraw-Hill, 1997; 2012–2023.

Weinstein JD, Dick HM, Grantham SA: Pseudogout, hyperparathyroidism, and carpal tunnel syndrome: A case report. J Bone Joint Surg Am 1968;50:1669–1674.

Wiederholt WC, Siekert RG: Neurological manifestations of sarcoidosis. Neurology 1965;15:1147–1154.

Wikberg A, Andersson C, Lithner F: Signs of neuropathy in the lower legs and feet of patients with acute intermittent porphyria. J Intern Med 2000;248:27–32.

Windebank AJ, Bonkovsky HL: Porphyric neuropathy. In Dyck PJ, Thomas PK, et al (eds): Peripheral Neuropathy, 3rd ed. Philadelphia, WB Saunders, 1993; 1161–1168.

Winkler M: Beitrag zur Frage der "Sarkoide" (Boeck), resp. der subkutanen nodulären Tuberkulide. Arch Dermatol Syphilol Wien 1905;77:3–24.

Xie J, Cai Y, Davis L: Guillain-Barré syndrome and hepatitis A: Lack of association during a major epidemic. Ann Neurol 1988; 24:697–698.

Yamamoto K, Saito K, Takai T, et al: Unusual manifestations in primary hypothyroidism. Prog Clin Biol Res 1983;116:169–187.

Yasuoka T, Yokota T, Tsukagoshi H: Deep peroneal nerve palsy associated with hypothyroidism. No To Shinkei 1993;45:563–566.

Yildiz A, Sever MS, Demirel S, et al: Improvement in autonomic function after renal transplantation: A heart rate variability study. Nephron 1998;80:57–60.

Yosipovitch G, Yarnitisky D, Mermelstein V, et al: Paradoxical heat sensation in uremic polyneuropathy. Muscle Nerve 1995; 18:768–771.

Zajicek J: Sarcoidosis of the cauda equina: A report of three cases. J Neurol 1990;237:424–426.

Zochodne DW, Bolton CF, Wells GA, et al: Polyneuropathy associated with critical illness: A complication of sepsis and multiple organ failure. Brain 1987;110:819–842.

Zuniga G, Ropper A, Frank J: Sarcoid peripheral neuropathy. Neurology 1991;41:1558–1561.

CHAPTER 61

Alcoholic and Nutritional Polyneuropathies

Robert W. Shields, Jr.

Polyneuropathies resulting from dietary nutritional deficiency are relatively rare in developed countries but may still occur in developing countries, particularly in the setting of famines (Roman, 1994). However, polyneuropathy resulting from dietary nutritional deficiency that occurs in the setting of chronic alcoholism remains a relatively common nutritional disorder (Victor and Adams, 1953, 1961; Victor et al., 1971). Most nutritional deficiency–associated polyneuropathies that are not related to alcoholism are caused not by dietary deficiency but by malabsorption of single or multiple vitamins resulting from specific disorders, such as pernicious anemia, sprue, and malabsorption that may follow gastrectomy. It has been pointed out that polyneuropathies resulting from nutritional deficiency are more likely to occur in the setting of imbalance of nutrition rather than in a state of complete deficiency that could occur in starvation (Victor, 1983). Furthermore, there is compelling evidence that nutritional deficiency–associated polyneuropathies are more likely to be caused by multiple vitamin deficiencies rather than by deficiency of an isolated single vitamin (Victor, 1983). This chapter reviews the major polyneuropathies resulting from nutritional deficiency, including alcoholic polyneuropathy.

NEUROPATHIC BERIBERI

Historical Review

Beriberi may represent the first disorder attributed to a nutritional deficiency. As far back as the 1600s, *dry beriberi* or *neuropathic beriberi* was recog-

nized as a condition resulting in generalized weakness (Victor, 1983). *Wet beriberi* was identified as a cardiac disease causing a clinical picture of tachycardia, dyspnea, and peripheral edema. Detailed clinical descriptions of both wet and dry forms of beriberi appeared in the medical literature by the middle to late 1800s (Carter, 1977; Victor, 1983), and it was widely recognized that both forms of beriberi did, in fact, represent different manifestations of the same underlying disease (Victor, 1983). However, beriberi remained a relatively uncommon disorder until the latter part of the nineteenth century, when it reached epidemic proportions in many areas of the world in which rice was the mainstay of the diet. The beriberi epidemic was the product of the industrialization of the processing of rice. The introduction of steam-powered rice mills to "polish" rice to impart a more desirable texture inadvertently resulted in the separation of the pericarp and germ from the rice shaft. This process rendered the rice deficient in thiamine and other nutrients (Carpenter and Sutherland, 1995). Unfortunately, the nutritional origin of beriberi was not discovered until many years later. Initially, beriberi was believed to be the result of an infection or possibly an intoxication (Carter, 1977). Nevertheless, clues to the nutritional origin of beriberi were emerging by the late 1800s. A Dutch naval physician, VanLeent, reported in 1879 that the mortality rate from beriberi appeared higher among the native Indian crews of the Dutch navy operating in the East Indies compared with the European crews (Victor, 1983). He observed that the diets of the two crews were different and recommended changing the diet of the Indian crews to a more varied diet similar to that of the European crews. When this dietary adjustment was made, the incidence of beriberi was clearly reduced (Carter, 1977; Victor, 1983). Apparently, VanLeent's observations were not widely recognized.

Nearly a decade later, Admiral Kanehiro Takaki of the Japanese navy reported his observations regarding the potential role of nutrition in the beriberi epidemic that was ravaging the Japanese navy (Carter, 1977; Victor, 1983; Jukes, 1989). Takaki noted that deaths from beriberi occurred more often among sailors and cadets than in officers. A detailed analysis of the potential differences in diet and environment that could occur during a long cruise led Takaki to conclude that the difference in diet between the two groups was the most likely cause of the widely different incidences of beriberi. By altering the diet of the sailors and cadets to the diet consumed by the officers, Admiral Takaki essentially eradicated beriberi from the Japanese navy (Itokowa, 1976; Carter, 1977; Victor, 1983; Jukes, 1989). The precise dietary deficiency causing beriberi was not identified, and Takaki incorrectly presumed that a protein deficiency was responsible.

The discovery that beriberi was indeed a nutritional deficiency has been credited to Christiaan Eijkman, a Dutch military surgeon, who traveled to the Dutch East Indies to study beriberi. While attempting to develop an animal model of beriberi, Eijkman discovered that a disease similar to beriberi occurred in birds that were fed a diet of steam-cooked polished rice, as opposed to crude rice (Carter, 1977; Victor, 1983; Jukes, 1989; Carpenter and Sutherland, 1995). Although Eijkman initially speculated that the rice husks that were removed in the polishing process contained a substance that countered a toxin in polished rice, he subsequently concluded with others that certain foods may contain protective substances that are essential for health (Carter, 1977; Carpenter and Sutherland, 1995).

The next major advancement in the understanding of beriberi came from Casimir Funk, a physician working in the Lister Institute in London. Funk was successful in isolating a water-soluble substance from rice polishings that appeared to represent an essential neurotrophic factor (Funk, 1911; Griminger, 1972; Carter, 1977; Jukes, 1989). Funk subsequently demonstrated that a disorder similar to beriberi could be produced in pigeons fed a diet deficient in this water-soluble substance (Griminger, 1972; Carter, 1977). He named this substance *vitamine* and suggested that other diseases including pellagra, rickets, and scurvy could also result from a deficiency of this particular vitamin or other vitamins that were yet to be discovered (Funk, 1912; Griminger, 1972; Carter, 1977; Victor, 1983). Funk coined the term *vitamine* to describe "vital amines," which he believed were the essential nutrients in the diet. Subsequently, it was discovered that these nutrients were not invariably amines, and the term was later changed to *vitamin.* In 1926, Jansen and Donath isolated the *antineuritic vitamin,* (Jansen and Donath, 1926), and in 1936 it was synthesized and named

thiamine by Williams (Williams, 1936). In 1929, Christiaan Eijkman and Frederick Hopkins were awarded the Nobel prize in physiology and medicine for their work on vitamins.

The discovery of thiamine revolutionized the management of wet beriberi because thiamine quickly reversed the cardiac manifestations of the disease (Joliffe, 1939). However, it was more difficult to demonstrate the beneficial effects of thiamine on the peripheral neuropathy of neuropathic beriberi (Victor, 1983). This observation led some investigators to speculate that thiamine deficiency was not the cause of neuropathic or dry beriberi (Victor, 1983). This speculation was further supported by the difficulty noted by early investigators who attempted to develop an animal model of neuropathic beriberi by inducing isolated thiamine deficiency (Victor, 1983). Nevertheless, animal models were eventually developed that clearly demonstrated that isolated thiamine deficiency could result in polyneuropathy (North and Sinclair, 1956; Kunze and Muskat, 1969; Prineas, 1970; Victor, 1983).

Etiology and Pathogenesis

As noted in the preceding section, convincing evidence indicates that the polyneuropathy associated with *neuropathic beriberi* is caused by thiamine deficiency. *Thiamine,* or *vitamin B_1,* is a pyrimidyl-substituted thiazole (McCormick and Greene, 1999). The principal coenzyme form of thiamine is the pyrophosphate ester, thiamine pyrophosphate. Thiamine is found in small concentrations in most plant and animal tissues, but it is found abundantly in unrefined cereal grains, soybean flour, wheat germ, yeast, and pork. The recommended daily allowance for thiamine ranges from 1.0 mg for older women to 1.5 mg for young men (McCormick and Greene, 1999). Thiamine is absorbed in the small intestine by an active transport process as well as by passive diffusion (McCormick and Greene, 1999). Phosphorylation takes place in the jejunal mucosa, and this produces thiamine pyrophosphate. Thiamine and thiamine pyrophosphate are primarily involved in carbohydrate metabolism. The two main chemical reactions in humans in which thiamine pyrophosphate functions in active aldehyde transfers are the oxidative decarboxylation of α-keto acids and the formation of α-ketols catalyzed by transketolase (McCormick and Greene, 1999). Thus, as dietary carbohydrate increases, the nutritional requirement for thiamine also increases. The precise mechanism by which thiamine deficiency causes peripheral nerve injury is unknown, but it is likely that it is mediated via altered carbohydrate metabolism in peripheral nerves (Windebank, 1993).

Neuropathic beriberi from dietary deficiency is rarely observed in developed countries, except in the context of the nutritional deficiency state that may occur in severe chronic alcoholism (Victor, 1983). In fact, it has been observed that the clinical features of neuropathic beriberi are essentially identical to those of alcoholic polyneuropathy (Shattuck, 1928), and, furthermore, the polyneuropathy associated with chronic alcoholism may be a manifestation of thiamine deficiency (Strauss, 1935). These issues are discussed later. Outside the setting of chronic alcoholism, neuropathic beriberi may represent an iatrogenic disorder that may be observed in the setting of total parenteral nutrition (Zak et al., 1991; Kitamura et al., 1996; Hahn et al., 1998).

Clinical Features

The most detailed and methodical clinical descriptions of beriberi may be found in the writings of Pekelharing and Winkler (Pekelharing and Winkler, 1887; Victor, 1983). These authors traveled to the Dutch East Indies during the beriberi epidemic to study this disease and to determine its origin (Victor, 1983; Carter, 1997). The cardinal features of neuropathic beriberi include a nonspecific clinical syndrome characterized by painful paresthesias, muscular aches and pains, and limb weakness (Victor, 1983). These symptoms most often conform to a relatively symmetrical pattern with a distal to proximal gradient of involvement. The symptoms typically evolve slowly over many weeks or months, but, on occasion, they have been noted to evolve rapidly over several days (Victor, 1983). Sometimes, pain may dominate the clinical picture. In these situations, the clinical features resemble those of a typical painful small-fiber neuropathy, including a remarkable hypersensitivity of the involved areas, which has been termed *painful anesthesia*. Numerous symptoms and signs referable to cranial nerve involvement have been reported as relatively rare manifestations of beriberi. These symptoms have included deafness, facial numbness, and facial weakness. Retrobulbar optic neuropathy, typically manifested by a central or a centrocecal scotoma, has been encountered as a rare manifestation of beriberi. It has been suggested that the occurrence of optic neuropathy in beriberi is evidence of a separate deficiency syndrome, most likely Strachan's syndrome, especially when it occurs in the setting of orogenital dermatitis and a predominantly sensory polyneuropathy (Denny-Brown, 1947). In some reports, the occurrence of ocular motor involvement, nystagmus, and confusional states appears to represent Wernicke's disease as opposed to a thiamine deficiency state causing peripheral and cranial nerve involvement. However, the occurrence of hoarseness has been regarded as a relatively common manifestation of neuropathic beriberi, particularly in children and infants. This manifestation is secondary to involvement of the recurrent laryngeal nerve (Novak and Victor, 1974). The clinical features of beriberi neuropathy may be associated with cardiac manifestations including peripheral edema, palpitations that are particularly excessive on mild physical activity, and shortness of breath.

Electrodiagnostic Features

There are relatively few modern descriptions of the electrodiagnostic findings in neuropathic beriberi (Ohnishi et al., 1980; Hong, 1986; Djoenaidi and Notermans, 1990; Djoenaidi et al., 1995). The typical pattern of abnormality conforms to a generalized and symmetrical axonal degeneration. Signs of active motor fiber loss manifested by fibrillation potentials are often noted in the intrinsic foot muscles and other distal lower extremity muscles. In addition, the sural sensory response is frequently reduced or absent, and abnormalities of motor conduction studies of the peroneal and tibial nerves are also noted. Motor conduction studies typically disclose mild slowing of conduction velocity and reduction in the motor response, depending on the severity of the polyneuropathy. F-wave latencies and H-reflex latencies are typically prolonged to a modest degree. An electrodiagnostic study of ex-prisoners of war who had been diagnosed with beriberi neuritis 47 years earlier disclosed persistent electrodiagnostic abnormalities indicating mild axonal degeneration polyneuropathy (Hong, 1986).

Diagnosis

The diagnosis of neuropathic beriberi is usually considered in the context of significant malnutrition, often in the setting of chronic alcoholism, in patients who are nutritionally at risk by receiving total parenteral nutrition without vitamin supplementation, or in patients who are malnourished by a diet principally of polished rice. Because the clinical features of neuropathic beriberi are nonspecific, many other generalized sensorimotor polyneuropathies must be considered in the differential diagnosis (Table 61–1). Electrodiagnostic studies, as noted earlier, are nonspecific and tend to disclose features of a general-

Table 61–1. Generalized Sensorimotor Polyneuropathies

Acute Polyneuropathies
Guillain-Barré syndrome
Porphyric neuropathy
Metal neuropathy
Chronic Polyneuropathies
Diabetic polyneuropathies
Alcoholic-nutritional polyneuropathy
Uremic polyneuropathy
Chronic inflammatory demyelinating polyradiculoneuropathy
Paraneoplastic neuropathies
Myeloma and dysproteinemic polyneuropathies
Drug- and toxin-induced neuropathies
Amyloid neuropathy
Endocrine polyneuropathies
Infectious polyneuropathies
Polyneuropathies associated with human immunodeficiency virus infection
Sarcoid neuropathy
Vasculitic polyneuropathies
Familial polyneuropathies

ized axonal degeneration polyneuropathy. Cerebrospinal fluid examinations are usually unremarkable (Ohnishi et al., 1980). The pathological features of neuropathic beriberi are also relatively nonspecific and tend to conform to axonal degeneration (Takahashi and Nakamura, 1976; Ohnishi et al., 1980; Victor, 1983). Because of the relatively nonspecific clinical, pathological, and electrodiagnostic features of neuropathic beriberi, emphasis has been placed on documenting thiamine deficiency to help confirm this diagnosis. Unfortunately, attempts to measure thiamine in the blood have not provided consistent and reliable results (Burch et al., 1950; Victor, 1983; Windebank, 1993; McCormick and Greene, 1999). An indirect measure of thiamine involves the determination of the activity of transketolase, a thiamine-dependent enzyme, in blood and red blood cells (Brin et al., 1960; Brin, 1962; Jeyasingham et al., 1987a, 1987b; McCormick and Greene, 1999). In the setting of chronic thiamine deficiency, transketolase activity is reduced (Brin, 1962). Although reduced blood or red blood cell transketolase activity has provided a method for the assessment of thiamine deficiency, it has not been studied extensively enough to precisely establish its sensitivity and specificity (Windebank, 1993). In addition, transketolase activity may normalize rapidly following dietary supplementation, thus making the test a less practical and reliable indicator of chronic thiamine deficiency (McLaren et al., 1981; Jeyasingham et al., 1987a, 1987b). Because thiamine deficiency prevents pyruvate from entering the Krebs cycle, it may result in elevations of both pyruvate and lactate in the blood. Unfortunately, these findings have proved to be too nonspecific for diagnostic purposes (Williams et al., 1943; Victor et al., 1957; Windebank, 1993).

Therapy

Management of neuropathic beriberi involves replenishing the thiamine stores as quickly as possible. Often, thiamine therapy is initiated with intramuscular or intravenous thiamine at a dosage of 100 mg daily. It is essential that parenteral thiamine therapy be continued until adequate general nutrition is restored. In most patients, improvement in the polyneuropathy is anticipated following thiamine replacement therapy. However, patients with severe axonal degeneration polyneuropathies may have a limited potential for a full recovery. Furthermore, persistent axonal degeneration polyneuropathy can be observed for many years following the nutritional deficiency (Hong, 1986).

ALCOHOLIC POLYNEUROPATHY

Historical Review

The first descriptions of polyneuropathy occurring in the setting of *chronic alcoholism* have been credited to Lettsom in 1787 (Lettsom, 1787) and later to Jackson in 1822 (Jackson, 1822). These early reports were followed by numerous accounts of similar cases, so that by the late nineteenth century, the clinical entity of alcoholic polyneuropathy was clearly defined and widely known (Victor, 1983). During this era, there was a general consensus that polyneuropathy occurring in the setting of chronic alcoholism was the result of a toxic effect of alcohol on peripheral nerves. It was not until 1928 that Shattuck first introduced the concept that polyneuropathy seen in the context of chronic alcoholism was the product of nutritional deficiency of vitamin B and thus should be regarded as a manifestation of beriberi (Shattuck, 1928). Considerable evidence has been gathered over the years to support Shattuck's proposal that chronic alcoholism accompanied by nutritional deficiency is the primary pathogenic mechanism of alcoholic polyneuropathy (Minot et al., 1933; Wechsler, 1933; Strauss, 1935; Williams et al., 1943; Victor and Adams, 1953, 1961; Denny-Brown, 1958; Victor et al., 1971; McLeod, 1982; Victor, 1983; Hallett et al., 1987). Nevertheless, controversy has persisted up to the present time regarding the issue of whether alcohol may also act as a toxin to peripheral nerves, and in some patients with alcoholism may represent the principal pathogenic mechanism of their polyneuropathy (Behse and Buchthal, 1977; Bosch et al., 1979; Juntunen et al., 1983; Claus et al., 1985; Monforte et al., 1995). This controversy is discussed in greater detail later in the chapter.

Alcoholic polyneuropathy represents a relatively common disorder. Although the precise incidence is unknown, it has been reported in approximately 9% of patients with alcoholism who were admitted to hospital for alcoholism-related disorders (Victor and Laureno; Victor and Adams, 1953;). The true incidence of alcoholic polyneuropathy may be better appreciated by its frequent occurrence in otherwise asymptomatic patients with alcoholism, in whom it may be manifested by physical signs of polyneuropathy (Victor and Laureno, 1978; Victor, 1983), abnormalities on nerve conduction studies (Jurko et al., 1964; Wanamaker and Skillman, 1964; Blackstock et al., 1972; Willer and Dehen, 1977; Lefebvre D'Amour et al., 1979), or alterations on autonomic nervous system testing indicating autonomic neuropathy (Duncan et al., 1980; Monforte et al., 1995; Agelink et al., 1998).

Etiology and Pathogenesis

The concept that alcoholic polyneuropathy is in fact a nutritional disorder as opposed to a disorder related to the toxic effect of alcohol on peripheral nerves was supported by the observation that the clinical syndrome in alcoholic polyneuropathy is identical to that of neuropathic beriberi (Shattuck, 1928; Victor, 1983). It is evident that patients with alcoholism, because of their nutritional deficiency caused by alcohol displacing essential nutrients from the diet, may develop both wet and dry forms of beriberi (Minot et al., 1933; Blakenhorn, 1945; Lahey et al., 1953; Victor, 1983). However, the most compelling clinical evidence in support of the nutritional deficiency origin of alcoholic polyneuropathy may be found in the writings of Victor and Adams, who methodically studied hundreds of patients with alcoholism with various neurological complications including polyneuropathy (Victor and Adams, 1953, 1961; Victor et al., 1971). These authors documented a history of poor nutrition in every patient with alcoholic polyneuropathy in whom an accurate nutritional history could be obtained (Victor, 1983).

Direct clinical evidence supporting a nutritional origin of alcoholic polyneuropathy is provided by an experiment performed by Strauss in 1935 (Strauss, 1935). This experiment encompassed 10 patients with alcoholic polyneuropathy who were hospitalized and who were allowed to continue consuming alcohol, provided that they ate a nutritious and balanced diet. These patients continued consuming alcohol according to their preadmission habit, which ranged between 1 pint to 1 quart of whiskey per day. These patients were carefully examined during their hospital stay, which ranged between 14 and 129 days, with a mean duration of 64 days. Despite their continued heavy alcohol consumption, all 10 patients showed clear, clinical improvement in their polyneuropathy during the hospitalization. Further clinical evidence comes from a study by Victor and Adams, that encompassed 10 patients with alcoholism and alcoholic polyneuropathy who were hospitalized (Victor and Adams, 1961). These patients were provided nutritious diets that were deficient in thiamine for 5 consecutive days following admission. None of the 10 patients showed any signs of remission of their polyneuropathy until thiamine was subsequently added to their diet (Victor and Adams, 1961).

The clinical evidence that alcoholic polyneuropathy is related to a toxic effect of alcohol comes from the observations that polyneuropathy may occur in patients with alcoholism who do not appear malnourished (Behse and Buchthal, 1977; Claus et al., 1985; Monforte et al., 1995). However, a persistent criticism of these observations is that the criteria used to assess and define nutritional deficiency may not have been sufficient to exclude completely the possibility of a nutritional deficiency as a pathogenic factor in the genesis of the polyneuropathy.

One of the most widely cited studies supporting the toxic origin of alcoholic polyneuropathy was reported by Behse and Buchthal in 1977 (Behse and Buchthal, 1977). These authors performed careful clinical and electrodiagnostic examinations as well as pathological studies of sural nerve biopsies on 37 patients with alcoholism and polyneuropathy. Twenty-three of the patients had no clinical evidence of nutritional deficiency as defined by a history of adequate dietary intake and normal weight, whereas 14 patients had overt evidence of nutritional deficiency as manifested by a marked weight loss. Because the clinical, electrodiagnostic, and pathological features of polyneuropathy in both groups of alcoholic patients were identical, Behse and Buchthal concluded that malnutrition was not a requirement for alcoholic polyneuropathy. Furthermore, these investigators concluded that alcohol must act as a toxin on peripheral nerves in those patients with adequate nutrition (Behse and Buchthal, 1977). However, the methods used in this study to assess nutritional status were dependent on the patients' own history as well as on their weight. Because most of the patients in this study were beer drinkers, weight was not a reliable indicator of adequate nutrition.

A more recent study by Monforte et al. concluded that alcoholic polyneuropathy is related to the cumulative toxic effect of the total lifetime dose of alcohol (Monforte et al., 1995). These authors performed careful clinical surveys and examinations, electrodiagnostic studies, and autonomic nervous system testing to assess both somatic and autonomic nerve function in 107 patients with alcoholism and in 61 control subjects. The history of alcohol consumption, dietary habit, and nutritional status was assessed with standard questionnaires confirmed with family members. Although the assessment of alcohol intake was estimated over a lifetime, the details of the nutritional history extended only 2 months before hospital admission. Despite the findings that patients with alcoholism had a thinner tricipital skin fold, a smaller arm circumference, and a significantly lower mean percentage of ideal body weight, findings suggesting nutritional deficiency, a multivariate analysis showed that the only significant independent variable related to polyneuropathy was the total lifetime dose of alcohol. However, this study failed to take into account that the nutritional deficiency that may occur in alcoholic polyneuropathy may be the product of a cumulative effect that may span many months or years. The assessment of a lifetime dose of alcohol without a similar measure of nutritional status does not permit a comparable analysis of these two variables in the genesis of the alcoholic polyneuropathy. Clearly, these issues require further study.

The pathogenesis of alcoholic polyneuropathy has also been studied using animal models. Several studies employing different animal models of alcoholism reported evidence that alcohol may indeed act as a toxin on peripheral nerves (Juntunen et al., 1978, 1983; Bosch et al., 1979; Claus et al., 1985). However, in nearly all these studies, the animals lost substantial weight, a finding indicating a coexistent nutritional insult that could have contributed to the peripheral nerve damage. Windebank and colleagues performed a careful study using a rat model of alcoholism (Windebank, 1993). In their study, which involved eight control rats and eight rats given 16.8 g/kg body weight of alcohol per day, weight remained stable in both groups. However, when peripheral nerves were analyzed at 3 and 9 months into the study, there was no evidence of polyneuropathy on 1-μm-thin sections or on teased nerve fiber analysis (Windebank, 1993). Hallett and collaborators performed two studies of alcoholic polyneuropathy in primate models (Hallett et al., 1987). In one study, five male monkeys were given a diet in which 50% of their calories were derived from alcohol. Four control monkeys ate a balanced diet. At the conclusion of the study, 5 years later, there was no histological or electrophysiological evidence of polyneuropathy in either group. In a similar study of 19 female monkeys in which 9 monkeys derived 30% of their calories from alcohol, there was no histological or electrophysiological evidence of polyneuropathy after 3 years (Hallett et al., 1987). Thus, in experimental models of alcoholic polyneuropathy, there is no clear or convincing evidence that alcohol acts as a toxin on peripheral nerves.

The clinical and experimental evidence noted earlier provides compelling evidence that alcoholic polyneuropathy occurs in the setting of nutritional deficiency. Although the potential of alcohol to cause a toxic effect on peripheral nerve cannot be totally excluded, the weight of clinical and experimental evidence at this time continues to favor a nutritional origin for alcoholic polyneuropathy.

Clinical Features

The most comprehensive description of the clinical features of alcoholic polyneuropathy may be found in the writings of Victor and colleagues (Victor and Adams, 1953, 1961; Victor et al., 1971; Victor, 1983). These authors carefully and methodically analyzed the clinical features of patients with alcoholism and polyneuropathy and other alcohol-nutrition–related disorders. These investigators found that alcoholic polyneuropathy is associated with serious, chronic alcoholism, which is invariably associated with nutritional deficiency resulting from alcohol displacing essential nutrients in the diet (Victor and Adams, 1953; Victor et al., 1971; Victor, 1983). In most patients with alcoholism, weight loss provides an accurate assessment of the severity of nutritional deficiency. Weight loss is often profound, typically in the range of 30 to 40 pounds, or at least 10% of body weight. Nevertheless, weight loss cannot be used as the sole index of nutritional deficiency in patients with alcoholism, particularly in patients who consume large quantities of beer, who may, in fact, be obese (Victor, 1983). Nutritional deficiency can usually be documented in nearly all patients with alcoholism and polyneuropathy if a careful nutritional history can be obtained (Victor, 1983). Alcoholic polyneuropathy is not observed in the spree or periodic drinker who is able to maintain proper nutrition between episodes of alcohol consumption. Even though the non-nutritional complications of alcoholism are noted to occur predominantly in men, alcoholic polyneuropathy is observed in men and women equally (Victor and Adams,

1953). The precise reason for the increased incidence of alcoholic polyneuropathy in women is unclear.

The symptoms of alcoholic polyneuropathy conform to a relatively nonspecific pattern of a generalized sensorimotor polyneuropathy. Both sensory and motor symptoms tend to develop in a relatively symmetrical pattern. However, in nearly one of four patients, a syndrome consistent with painful, small-fiber neuropathy may be observed in which severe, dysesthetic burning pain dominates the clinical picture (Victor and Adams, 1953; Victor, 1983). The severity of the polyneuropathy spans a considerable range from subclinical polyneuropathy that can be detected only on careful neurological examination, or possibly electrodiagnosis, to severe polyneuropathy resulting in profound physical disability. Although overt symptoms and signs of autonomic involvement are not frequently noted, subclinical autonomic dysfunction is frequently observed on quantitative autonomic nervous system testing (Low et al., 1975; Duncan et al., 1980; Monforte et al., 1995; McDougall and McLeod, 1996; Agelink et al., 1998). In most patients, the polyneuropathy tends to evolve in a slow fashion, typically over weeks, months, or even years. However, an acute or subacute syndrome may develop on the background of chronic polyneuropathy (Victor, 1983) that may mimic Guillain-Barré syndrome (Wöhrle et al., 1998).

The neurological findings are consistent with a generalized and symmetrical sensorimotor polyneuropathy (Victor, 1983). Typically, sensory loss is noted in the lower extremities in a distal to proximal gradient, with all modalities affected to a relatively equal degree. Hyperpathia or allodynia are observed in those patients with a small-fiber neuropathy presentation. In many patients, tenderness of muscles to palpation, especially in the feet and legs, is regarded as a classic finding (Shattuck, 1928; Denny-Brown, 1958; Victor, 1983). Weakness is usually symmetrical and is distributed in a distal to proximal gradient with reduced or absent tendon reflexes. Occasionally, proximal lower extremity weakness may be relatively prominent, thus giving the false impression of chronic alcoholic myopathy (Faris and Reyes, 1971; Laureno, 1979; Victor, 1983). Many patients with alcoholic polyneuropathy manifest other clinical features of alcoholism-related nutritional disorders including Wernicke-Korsakoff syndrome and cerebellar degeneration (Victor and Adams, 1953; Victor et al., 1971; Victor, 1983). In addition, the clinical stigmata of chronic alcoholism and liver disease may also be evident (Kemppainen et al., 1982; Victor, 1983).

Electrodiagnostic Features

The electrodiagnostic findings in alcoholic polyneuropathy usually conform to a generalized and symmetrical axon loss sensorimotor polyneuropathy (Mawdsley and Mayer, 1965, 1966; Casey and

LeQuesne, 1972; Behse and Buchthal, 1977; Lefebvre D'Amour et al., 1979; Shields, 1985). Typically, nerve conduction studies disclose low or absent sensory responses in the lower extremities (Behse and Buchthal, 1977; Willer and Dehen, 1977; Lefebvre D'Amour et al., 1979), mild slowing of motor conduction velocities (Mawdsley and Mayer, 1965; Behse and Buchthal, 1977; Willer and Dehen, 1977), prolongation of distal sensory and motor latencies (Mawdsley and Mayer, 1965; Behse and Buchthal, 1977; Willer and Dehen, 1977), and, in more advanced disease, a reduction in or absence of motor responses. As in most generalized sensorimotor polyneuropathies, these findings are first observed in the lower extremities, and with increasing severity of disease may be observed in the upper extremities as well. Late responses are also frequently abnormal. The latencies of F waves and H reflexes are typically increased, or these responses may be absent (Mawdsley and Mayer, 1965; Willer and Dehen, 1977; Lefebvre D'Amour et al., 1979). The needle electrode examination often reveals findings consistent with a distal to proximal gradient of motor axon loss. These findings include fibrillation potentials, chronic neurogenic motor unit potential alterations, and reduced interference patterns (Shields, 1985). Single-fiber electromyography discloses increased fiber density and jitter, consistent with axonal degeneration and reinnervation (Thiele and Stalberg, 1975).

Diagnosis

The diagnosis of alcoholic polyneuropathy is usually made in the context of a characteristic clinical syndrome of sensorimotor polyneuropathy occurring in a patient with chronic sustained alcoholism and malnutrition. However, the clinical and laboratory features of alcoholic polyneuropathy are relatively nonspecific, and thus many other chronic axon loss sensorimotor polyneuropathies need to be considered in the differential diagnosis (see Table 61–1). General laboratory studies may disclose features consistent with chronic malnutrition and liver disease, including macrocytic anemia and altered liver function tests (Kemppainen et al., 1982; Victor, 1983; Windebank, 1993). Because alcoholic polyneuropathy has been regarded as a manifestation of beriberi, efforts have been directed at assessing thiamine status. However, because of the difficulties in developing methods for the direct assay of thiamine in the blood and urine (Burch et al., 1950; Victor, 1983; Windebank, 1993; McCormick and Greene, 1999), thiamine deficiency has been assessed indirectly via measurement of transketolase activity in the blood or red blood cells (Brin, 1962; Blass and Gibson, 1977; Baines and Davies, 1988; McCormick and Greene, 1999). Transketolase activity is reduced in thiamine deficiency (Brin, 1962), and this finding has been observed in patients with alcoholism and polyneuropathy (Jeyasingham et al., 1987a, 1987b). However, transketolase activity may quickly improve following dietary supplementation (McLaren et al., 1981; Jeyasingham et al., 1987a, 1987b; Windebank, 1993). This and other factors have made the transketolase assessment a less reliable and practical diagnostic aid to document thiamine deficiency in patients with alcoholism (Windebank, 1993). Although elevated pyruvate levels have been observed in thiamine deficiency (Victor et al., 1957), particularly following glucose loading (Williams et al., 1943), the value of this test in the diagnosis of thiamine deficiency is limited by its lack of specificity (Victor, 1983).

The pathological findings in peripheral nerve are nonspecific and conform to an axonal degeneration polyneuropathy (Walsh and McLeod, 1970; Victor, 1983). Electron microscopic findings include reduced numbers of myelinated and unmyelinated fibers, degenerative changes in myelinated and unmyelinated fibers, and some regenerative changes, all typical of an axonal degeneration polyneuropathy (Tredici and Minazzi, 1975).

Therapy

The principal goal of managing the patient with alcoholic polyneuropathy is to reinstitute proper nutrition and to provide a suitable environment for the alcoholic patient to abstain from continued alcohol abuse. Often, it is valuable to initiate nutritional therapy with parenteral multivitamins until the patient can maintain an adequate nutritional intake. Typically, patients with mild or modest polyneuropathy demonstrate significant improvement in their symptoms and signs over the weeks and months that follow the restoration of proper balanced nutrition. Patients with more severe and chronic polyneuropathies have a less favorable prognosis and are likely to have chronic or residual symptoms and signs of their polyneuropathy. Ultimately, the rehabilitation of the patient with chronic alcoholism is the key goal of therapy, because persistent, continued abstinence from alcohol is essential to reestablish balanced nutrition.

VITAMIN B$_{12}$ DEFICIENCY

The neurological disorder associated with *vitamin B$_{12}$ (cobalamin) deficiency* was first described by Lichtheim in 1887 (Lichtheim, 1887; Kass, 1976). Over the ensuing years, numerous similar cases were reported of progressive myelopathy occurring in the setting of pernicious anemia (Victor and Lear, 1956; Pant et al., 1968). Neuropathological examinations documented that the principal pathological alterations conformed to a vacuolar myelopathy primarily involving the posterior columns and cortical spinal tracts in the cervical and upper thoracic spinal cord (Russell, 1900; Kass, 1976). This unique pathological pattern was termed *subacute combined degeneration of the cord* (Russell, 1900). The clinical features of this disorder, particularly the sensory symptoms and signs, are similar to the symptoms of polyneuropathy; thus, it is difficult on clinical grounds to clearly delineate a superimposed peripheral nerve disorder. Nevertheless, there is compelling evidence that peripheral nerves may be involved in vitamin B_{12} deficiency (Mayer, 1965; Cox-Klazinga and Endtz, 1980; Fine and Hallett, 1980; Victor, 1983; McCombe and McLeod, 1984; Fine et al., 1990). However, the clinical features of polyneuropathy probably constitute only a minor component of the sensory and motor features caused by the spinal cord disease (Woltman, 1919; Victor, 1983).

Etiology and Pathogenesis

Vitamin B_{12}, or cobalamin, is a complex corrinoid compound with a central cobalt atom surrounded by a planar corrin ring composed of four pyrrole rings (Tefferi and Pruthi, 1994; Markle, 1996). Cobalamin is required for two enzymatic reactions in humans. Adenosylcobalamin is a cofactor for methylmalonyl coenzyme A mutase, an enzyme that converts methylmalonic coenzyme A to succinyl coenzyme A, which ultimately enters the Krebs cycle (Tefferi and Pruthi, 1994; Green, 1995). Methylcobalamin is essential for methionine synthase, the enzyme that catalyzes the reaction between homocysteine and methyltetrahydrofolate, which results in the formation of methionine and tetrahydrofolate. Thus, cobalamin deficiency may result in accumulation of both methylmalonic acid and homocysteine in the blood. Assays for these metabolites in the plasma and urine provide additional sensitive measures of cobalamin deficiency (Green, 1995). Cobalamin is formed only in cobalamin-producing microorganisms, and thus animal products are the sole dietary source for mammals (Pruthi and Tefferi, 1994). It has been estimated that the average Western diet provides 5 to 15 µg of vitamin B_{12} per day. The recommended daily requirement of vitamin B_{12} is approximately 1 µg (Herbert, 1987).

An acidic environment in the stomach is necessary for cobalamin to be released from its dietary protein-bound state, a process required for proper absorption of cobalamin from the diet (Pruthi and Tefferi, 1994). Cobalamin, which is initially bound to R proteins in the salvia and gastric juice, is liberated from the R proteins by pancreatic proteases in the duodenum. At this point, cobalamin is then bound by an intrinsic factor, a glycoprotein secreted by gastric parietal cells. The cobalamin–intrinsic factor complex then passes into the terminal ileum, where it is absorbed via active transport across the enterocyte. In the blood, cobalamin is bound to transcobalamin II, a transport protein. It then may be absorbed via endocytosis into various tissues and converted intracellularly into its two coenzyme forms, adenosylcobalamin and methylcobalamin.

The most common cause of vitamin B_{12} deficiency is *pernicious anemia,* an autoimmune disorder associated with intrinsic factor antibodies. Pernicious anemia results in a selective defect in vitamin B_{12} absorption from failure of the gastric parietal cells to secrete intrinsic factor (Pruthi and Tefferi, 1994; Savage and Lindenbaum, 1995). Other less common causes of vitamin B_{12} deficiency include ileal or gastric resection (Best, 1959; Knox and Delamore, 1960), infection with the fish tapeworm, *Diphyllobothrium latum* (Bjorkenheim, 1966), strict vegetarian diets, and severe steatorrhea (Britt et al., 1971). Subacute combined degeneration of the cord may also result from rare genetic disorders involving the binding protein required in vitamin B_{12} transport (Sigal et al., 1987) and methionine synthase (Carmel et al., 1988). In addition, this syndrome may follow exposure to nitrous oxide (Layzer, 1978; Heyer et al., 1986; Holloway and Alberico, 1990; Nestor and Stark, 1996). Nitrous oxide oxidizes cobalamin from an active monovalent state to an inactive trivalent state, and this results in permanent inactivation of the enzyme vitamin complex. Recovery requires synthesis of new methionine synthase (Holloway and Alberico, 1990).

The precise mechanism by which vitamin B_{12} deficiency causes polyneuropathy and subacute combined degeneration of the cord is unknown. However, investigators have proposed that the inhibition of methionine synthase may play a pathogenic role (Metz, 1992; Weir and Scott, 1995; Green, 1996). The pathological features of the spinal cord disease are composed of axon loss and demyelination in the posterior columns, primarily involving the lower cervical and thoracic segments. These pathological changes may extend up and down the spinal cord as well as into the lateral and anterior columns (Pant et al., 1968). Peripheral nerves have not been studied as comprehensively as the spinal cord (Victor, 1983; Windebank, 1993). Pathological changes in peripheral nerves consist of axonal degeneration and modest demyelination (Pant et al., 1968; McCombe and McLeod, 1984).

Clinical Features

The neurological symptoms associated with vitamin B_{12} deficiency are predominantly sensory and are usually paresthesias, which begin in the feet and legs that may extend into the upper extremities (Victor and Lear, 1956; Healton et al., 1991). Other sensory symptoms include numbness, stiffness, tightness, feelings of heat or cold, formication, and shooting pains (Victor and Lear, 1956). At times, the sensory symptoms can be distressing and uncomfortable. As the disorder progresses, generalized weakness may develop, initially in the lower extremities and later in the upper extremities. Weakness is often accompanied by stiffness resulting from spasticity. Neurological findings early in the course of the disease, especially when paresthesias are the only symptom, may be modest, or the examination findings may be entirely normal. More often, however, sensory findings reflect posterior column involvement manifested by loss of vibratory sense and joint position sense (Victor and Lear, 1956; Healton et al., 1991). Motor signs are those referable to involvement of the cortical spinal tract and consist of spasticity, hyperreflexia, and extensor plantar responses. On occasion, the Achilles tendon reflexes may be depressed or absent. This finding, coupled with the prominent sensory complaints that are often noted in a distal to proximal gradient, has provided clinical evidence that a coexisting peripheral nerve disorder may be present (Windebank, 1993).

Electrodiagnostic Features

One of the earliest electrodiagnostic observations in vitamin B_{12} deficiency was reported by Gilliatt et al. (1961). These authors documented abnormal lateral popliteal nerve action potentials in three of four patients with B_{12} deficiency and clinical features of myelopathy (Gilliatt et al., 1961). Another early electrodiagnostic study was reported by Mayer, who examined 32 patients with symptoms and signs of vitamin B_{12} deficiency and noted slowing of sensory conduction velocities of median and ulnar nerves, as well as an increase in H-reflex latencies (Mayer, 1965). Subsequently, there have been numerous observations using more modern electrodiagnostic techniques documenting typical findings of a sensorimotor axon loss polyneuropathy (Kayser-Gatchalian and Neundorfer, 1977; Cox-Klazinga and Endtz, 1980; Fine and Hallett, 1980; McCombe and McLeod, 1984; Heyer et al., 1986; Steiner et al., 1988; Fine et al., 1990; Healton et al., 1991). Electrodiagnostic features include reduced sensory and motor amplitudes (Fine and Hallett, 1980; Fine et al., 1990; Healton et al., 1991), mild reductions in sensory and motor conduction velocities (Kayser-Gatchalian and Neundorfer, 1977; Cox-Klazinga and Endtz, 1980; Fine and Hallett, 1980; McCombe and McLeod, 1984; Heyer et al., 1986; Steiner et al., 1988; Fine et al., 1990; Healton et al., 1991), modest prolongations of F-wave latencies (Fine and Hallett, 1980; Heyer et al., 1986; Fine et al., 1990), modest prolongations of H-wave latencies (Steiner et al., 1988; Fine et al., 1990), and active and chronic motor fiber loss manifested by fibrillation potentials and neurogenic motor unit potential remodeling in distal muscles (Kayser-Gatchalian and Neundorfer, 1977; Fine et al., 1990; Healton et al., 1991). Somatosensory evoked potentials, particularly of the lower extremity nerves, are often abnormal (Dick et al., 1988; Fine et al., 1990). Visual evoked potentials may also be abnormal (Fine et al., 1990), but auditory evoked potentials are typically normal (Fine et al., 1990).

Diagnosis

The diagnosis of the neurological disorders associated with B_{12} deficiency is usually considered in the differential diagnosis of generalized predominately sensory polyneuropathy or in the setting of myelopathy with predominant involvement of the cortical spinal tracts and posterior columns. Because of the ease of diagnosing vitamin B_{12} deficiency and the potential for an excellent prognosis with early detection and treatment, it is prudent to screen all patients presenting with polyneuropathy and myelopathy for vitamin B_{12} deficiency. Although megaloblastic anemia often occurs in vitamin B_{12} deficiency, it is not invariably present even in those patients with prominent neurological manifestations (Victor and Lear, 1956; Mayer, 1965; Lindebaum et al., 1988). Vitamin B_{12} deficiency can be diagnosed accurately by a direct assay of vitamin B_{12} in the blood (Green, 1996; Green and Kinsella, 1996). However, adding additional serum assays for homocysteine and, in particular, methylmalonic acid, metabolites that are often increased in the serum of patients with vitamin B_{12} deficiency states, will increase sensitivity for detecting a vitamin B_{12} deficiency state (Green, 1995, 1996; Green and Kinsella, 1996). The presence of biochemical evidence of vitamin B_{12} deficiency, coupled with the typical clinical profile and electrodiagnostic findings, makes the diagnosis of these disorders straightforward. The etiology of the vitamin B_{12} deficiency should be pursued with anti–intrinsic factor antibody assay and Schilling test or other studies to determine the mechanism of vitamin B_{12} malabsorption.

Therapy

Numerous treatment guidelines have been proposed for the management of vitamin B_{12} deficiency states (Beck, 1991; Pruthi and Tefferi, 1994; Savage and Lindenbaum, 1995; Swain, 1995). Most plans begin with intramuscular injections of cobalamin, usually at doses of 100 µg to 1,000 µg given daily for 2 weeks and then twice weekly until neurological symptoms and signs have abated or stabilized and the hematological abnormalities, if present, have been corrected (Shields and Harris, 1987). Cobalamin injections are then continued at a dosage of 100 µg to 1,000 µg monthly for the remainder of the patient's life, depending on the specific etiology of the vitamin B_{12} deficiency state. However, there is evidence that high doses of oral cobalamin of 1,000 µg per day may be effective in treating patients with pernicious anemia (Berlin et al., 1968; Kuzminski et al., 1998). Effective oral treatment occurs because approximately 1% of ingested cobalamin may be absorbed by passive diffusion. The prognosis for the neurological disorder associated with vitamin B_{12} deficiency is excellent if treatment is initiated early in the course of the deficiency (Healton et al., 1991). However, it has been observed that patients who have significant symptoms and signs lasting 6 months or longer may have incomplete recovery despite replenishment of the vitamin B_{12} stores (Healton et al., 1991).

VITAMIN E DEFICIENCY

The first report linking vitamin E deficiency to neurological deficits was published in 1928 by Evans and Burr, who documented paralysis in the suckling offspring of mother rats deficient in vitamin E (Evans and Burr, 1928). Subsequently, other reports were published that documented various neurological disorders in animal models of vitamin E deficiency (Sokol, 1990). Despite these early observations in animal models, it was not until 1965 that vitamin E deficiency was proposed as a pathogenic mechanism for the neurological disorder associated with abetalipoproteinemia (Kayden et al., 1965). Since that time, numerous reports have established that vitamin E deficiency is a key pathogenic mechanism resulting in a variety of neurological disorders associated with chronic lipid malabsorption (Binder et al., 1967; Harries and Muller, 1971; Muller et al., 1974; Cavalier and Gambetti, 1981; Rosenblum et al., 1981; Sokol, 1988).

Etiology and Pathogenesis

Vitamin E is found in four major forms: α-, γ-, β-, and δ-tocopherol (Sokol, 1990). Of these four major forms, α-tocopherol has the most biological activity. Vitamin E is biosynthesized in plants and is particularly abundant in wheat germ and vegetable oils (McCormick and Greene, 1999). The recommended daily allowances for vitamin E are 10 mg of α-tocopherol for boys 11 years and older and men and 8 mg for girls 11 years and older and women. Additional allowances of 4 mg per day are recommended for pregnant and lactating women. The recommended daily allowance for children less than 11 years of age is 6 to 7 mg per day (McCormick and Greene, 1999). It has been estimated that 7 to 13 mg of α-tocopherol can be expected in balanced diets supplying 1,800 to 3,000 calories per day (McCormick and Greene, 1999). Approximately 20% to 40% of dietary vitamin E in the form of α- and γ-tocopherol is absorbed (Sokol, 1990). Because vitamin E is a lipid-soluble molecule, it must be solubilized into mixed micelles by bile acids secreted by the liver. Vitamin E is absorbed into the intestinal mucosa by a non–carrier-mediated passive diffusion process (Sokol, 1990). Vitamin E is then incorporated within the enterocyte into chylomicrons with other products of lipid digestion and is transported via enteric lymphatics into the systemic circulation (Sokol, 1990). Although vitamin E may be transferred to target tissues in this state, the residual vitamin E in chylomicrons is transported to the liver, where the α-tocopherol is secreted again as a component of very low-density lipoproteins and high-density lipoproteins, and the γ-tocopherol is metabolized or excreted (Sokol, 1990). Vitamin E appears to function as an antioxidant, but it may also have an important role in maintaining the structure of cell membranes (Tappel, 1962).

Table 61–2. Causes of Vitamin E Deficiency

Hereditary
Abetalipoproteinemia
Cystic fibrosis
Isolated vitamin E malabsorption (α-tocopherol transfer protein mutation)
Homozygous hypobetaliproteinemia
Alagille's syndrome
Acquired
Cholestatic liver disease
Short bowel syndrome
Postgastrectomy states
Crohn's disease
Celiac disease
Chronic pancreatitis
Tropical sprue
Neonatal hepatitis
Congenital extrahepatic biliary atresia
Total parenteral nutrition

Because vitamin E is widely distributed in vegetable oils, grains, and animal fat, dietary deficiency of vitamin E is rarely seen in developed countries (Sokol, 1990). More commonly, disorders of lipid malabsorption are responsible for chronic vitamin E deficiency (Binder et al., 1967; Harries and Muller, 1971; Muller et al., 1974; Geller et al., 1977; Guggenheim et al., 1982; Harding et al., 1982; Howard et al., 1982; Sokol, 1988, 1990). In addition, there are rare disorders in which a selective vitamin E deficiency syndrome may occur (Harding et al., 1985; Krendel et al., 1987; Yokota et al., 1987; Sokol, 1988; Jackson et al., 1996). Both acquired and inherited or familial disorders may result in vitamin E deficiency states (Table 61–2). Inherited or familial disorders include *abetalipoproteinemia,* a relatively rare autosomal recessive disorder characterized by progressive ataxia, steatorrhea, pigmentary retinopathy, and acanthocytosis (Muller et al., 1974; Kayden et al., 1983). *Cystic fibrosis* represents another autosomal recessive disorder associated with steatorrhea and vitamin E malabsorption (Geller et al., 1977; Elias et al., 1981). In addition, there are rare familial disorders in which there is selective malabsorption of vitamin E without evidence of more widespread lipid malabsorption (Harding et al., 1985; Yokota et al., 1987). These disorders, which may be autosomal recessive, X-linked, or autosomal dominant, may be associated with a mutation on the α-tocopherol transfer protein gene on chromosome 8q13 (Gotoda et al., 1995; Ouahchi et al., 1995). In addition to these rare inherited disorders, vitamin E deficiency may occur as a result of numerous, more common *chronic cholestatic hepatobiliary disorders* including idiopathic neonatal hepatitis, Alagille's syndrome, paucity of interlobular bile ducts, and extrahepatic biliary atresia (Binder et al., 1967; Harries and Muller, 1971; Rosenblum et al., 1981; Guggenheim et al., 1982; Harding et al., 1982; Sokol et al., 1983; Jeffrey et al., 1987, 1988). In addition, vitamin E deficiency may result from the *short bowel syndrome* that may occur following small bowel resections for treatment of various intestinal disorders (Harding et al., 1982; Howard et al., 1982; Satya-Murti et al., 1986).

The typical pathological features of vitamin E deficiency are found in the spinal cord. Features of axonal dystrophy are noted in the posterior columns, Clarke's column, and the dorsal and ventral spinocerebellar tracts (Sung and Stadlan, 1966; Geller et al., 1977; Rosenblum et al., 1981; Sokol et al., 1983; Weder et al., 1984; Landrieu et al., 1985). In addition, axonal spheroids are noted in the cuneate and gracile nuclei of the brain stem. Pathological findings in peripheral nerves include loss of large-caliber myelinated sensory axons (Geller et al., 1977; Burck et al., 1981; Rosenblum et al., 1981; Landrieu et al., 1985; Wichman et al., 1985; Sokol et al., 1988). These findings correlate with the observation that the dorsal root ganglion cell may be the primary target in vitamin E deficiency (Windebank, 1993).

Clinical Features

The principal clinical features of vitamin E deficiency are referable to progressive cerebellar ataxia, clinical deficits resulting from posterior column dysfunction, and hyporeflexia (Rosenblum et al., 1981; Guggenheim et al., 1982; Harding et al., 1982; Howard et al., 1982; Muller et al., 1983; Weder et al., 1984; Alvarez et al., 1985; Jeffrey et al., 1987; Yokota et al., 1987; Sokol, 1988, 1990; Jackson et al., 1996). Rarely, vitamin E deficiency may present as an isolated sensorimotor axonal degeneration polyneuropathy (Binder et al., 1967; Palmucci et al., 1988). Typically, the spinocerebellar features are coupled with other neurological manifestations that may include dysarthria (Muller et al., 1983; Krendel et al., 1987; Yokota et al., 1987; Jackson et al., 1996), dystonia and bradykinesia (Krendel et al., 1987), ptosis (Muller et al., 1983), ophthalmoplegia (Rosenblum et al., 1981; Guggenheim et al., 1982; Muller et al., 1983; Weder et al., 1984; Alvarez et al., 1985; Sokol, 1990), visual loss from pigmented retinopathy (Howard et al., 1982; Muller et al., 1983; Satya-Murti et al., 1986; Sokol, 1990), and generalized or proximal weakness secondary to myopathy (Burck et al., 1981; Neville et al., 1983).

Electrodiagnostic Studies

The electrodiagnostic features seen in the neurological syndromes associated with vitamin E deficiency are indicative of a predominantly sensory axonal polyneuropathy. Most often, the electrodiagnostic features include reduced or absent sensory responses with intact responses on motor nerve conduction studies and normal findings on needle electromyography (Guggenheim et al., 1982; Wiehman et al., 1985; Brin et al., 1986; Satya-Murti et al., 1986; Krendel et al., 1987). F responses are usually preserved, but H reflexes may be absent or prolonged (Brin et al., 1986). This constellation of electrodiagnostic findings is consistent with pure sensory neuropathy or sensory neuronopathy implying involvement of the dorsal root ganglion cells (Windebank, 1993). In some cases, motor fiber involvement is also noted by virtue of mild alterations in motor nerve conduction studies as well as signs of active and chronic motor fiber loss noted on needle electromyography (Brin et al., 1986; Jeffrey et al., 1987). In some circumstances, particularly in adult-onset vitamin E deficiency, findings on electrodiagnostic studies may be normal, disclosing no features of sensory or motor fiber involvement (Harding et al., 1985; Yokota et al., 1987). The electrodiagnostic abnormalities referable to spinal cord involvement consist of abnormal somatosensory evoked potentials manifested by a delay in conduction or failure to conduct beyond cervical segments (Harding et al., 1982, 1985; Howard et al., 1982; Weder et al., 1984; Brin et al., 1986; Satya-Murti et al., 1986; Krendel et al., 1987; Yokota et al., 1987). Patients with significant pigmented retinopathy may have abnormal electroretinograms, and in some of these patients the visual evoked potentials may also be abnormal (Brin et al., 1986). However, auditory evoked potentials are typically preserved (Brin et al., 1986).

Diagnosis

The diagnosis of the spinocerebellar degeneration and the peripheral neuropathy associated with vitamin E deficiency is usually straightforward when these clinical syndromes occur in the setting of chronic fat malabsorption. Nevertheless, other disorders with similar clinical features must be considered in the differential diagnosis (Subramony and Nance, 1998). This is particularly important when evidence of malabsorption may be less prominent or not apparent. Documenting a deficiency of vitamin E can be accomplished by direct measurement of α-tocopherol in the serum. This measurement is usually obtained by high-performance liquid chromatography (Sokol, 1990). The clinical features of vitamin E deficiency may not be prominent until several years after the onset of the deficiency, and progression and evolution of the neurological disease tend to be slow. For example, it may take 5 to 10 years of vitamin E depletion before symptoms develop in adults. Children, however, tend to develop symptoms after shorter intervals of time. The normal vitamin E blood level for adults and children 12 years of age and older is 5 μg/mL (Farrell et al., 1978). The normal vitamin E blood level for children 6 months to 12 years old is 3 to 4 μg/mL or higher (Farrell et al., 1978). Vitamin E concentrations in the blood may appear normal in hyperlipidemic states despite a true deficiency (Sokol et al., 1984). The reason for this false-negative result is that vitamin E may be present in serum lipoproteins. To address this issue, it has been recommended that the ratio of the total serum vitamin E to the total serum lipid concentration be used as a more accurate assessment of vitamin E status (Sokol et al., 1984). Using this method, normal values for children 1 to 12 years of age are less than 0.6 mg of total tocopherol per gram of total lipid (Farrell et al., 1978). For older children and adults, the normal limit of the ratio is less than 0.8 mg/g (Farrell et al., 1978). Often, the α-tocopherol level in patients with chronic vitamin E deficiency is undetectable (Sokol, 1988).

Therapy and Prognosis

Treatment of vitamin E deficiency consists of high doses of oral vitamin E supplementation. The principal goal of treatment is to replenish vitamin E stores and to prevent further progression of the neurological disorder. Specific treatment guidelines have been created depending on the underlying disorder that is responsible for the vitamin E deficiency. In disorders associated with isolated vitamin E deficiency, treatment usually begins with 1 to 4 g of oral vitamin E per day in divided doses (Sokol, 1990). However, in the setting of chronic cholestasis, treatment consists of 50 IU/kg per day of oral vitamin E. Once initiated, this dose may be increased by 50 IU/kg increments up to a total dose of 200 IU/kg per day depending on normalization of the tocopherol-to-lipid ratio in the blood (Sokol, 1990). For patients with cystic fibrosis who are receiving oral pancreatic enzymes, vitamin E is administered at doses of 5 to 10 IU/kg per day (Sokol, 1990). However, in patients with cystic fibrosis who have prominent cholestasis, treatment guidelines are identical to those for patients with chronic cholestasis and vitamin E deficiency. Vitamin E is administered in doses of 200 to 3,600 mg per day to patients with short bowel syndrome (Harding et al., 1982; Weder et al., 1984; Brin et al., 1985; Satya-Murti et al., 1986; Sokol, 1990).

In abetalipoproteinemia, treatment typically is initiated with 100 to 200 mg/kg per day of oral vitamin E in divided doses. Because vitamin E levels do not typically improve following successful therapy of this condition, alternative methods are used to assess adequate vitamin E replacement. These methods include erythrocyte hydrogen peroxide hemolysis testing (Muller et al., 1983), serial needle aspirate biopsies of adipose tissue for analysis of vitamin E stores (Kayden et al., 1983), and serial electrophysiological studies. In addition to vitamin E therapy, these patients are also treated with vitamin A using doses of 15 to 20,000 IU per day with monitoring of the vitamin A concentrations (Bishara et al., 1982). With this combination therapy, patients with abetalipoproteinemia may have their neurological syndrome stabilized, and when the diagnosis is made early, before the onset of neurological features, this regimen may entirely avert neurological disease.

VITAMIN B$_6$ DEFICIENCY AND TOXICITY

Vitamin B$_6$, pyridoxine, has the unusual distinction of causing polyneuropathy as a result of a deficiency state (Vilter et al., 1953) and of having a direct toxic effect on peripheral nerve (Schaumberg et al., 1983; Albin et al., 1987; Dalton and Dalton, 1987). Although dietary deficiency as a cause of vitamin B$_6$ deficiency is relatively uncommon in developed countries, it may occur in the context of the general malnutrition observed in patients with alcoholism (Bonjour, 1980). However, pyridoxine deficiency–induced polyneuropathy is more often associated with antituberculosis drug therapy with isoniazid or with therapy with the chemically related antihypertensive drug hydralazine (Selikoff et al., 1952; Gammon et al., 1953; Lubing, 1953). Isoniazid results in a marked increase in the excretion of pyridoxine (Biehl and Vilter, 1954), and it inhibits the phosphorylation of pyridoxine, with a resulting reduction in pyridoxine stores (Dreyfus and Geel, 1972). However, it was observed that cotreatment with pyridoxine could prevent isoniazid-induced polyneuropathy (Biehl and Vilter, 1954).

The clinical features of vitamin B$_6$ deficiency are nonspecific and conform to a generalized symmetrical sensorimotor polyneuropathy (Gammon et al., 1953; Lubing, 1953). Confirmation of vitamin B$_6$ deficiency can be obtained with direct measurement of vitamin B$_6$ in the blood by a variety of different microbiological and chemical assay methods (McCormick and Greene, 1999). The typical replacement therapy for vitamin B$_6$ deficiency is oral supplementation at a dosage of 50 to 100 mg of vitamin B$_6$ per day. This dosage is also recommended for patients treated with isoniazid and hydralazine (Windebank, 1993).

The neuropathy that follows excessive dietary intake of vitamin B$_6$ conforms to a pure sensory neuronopathy manifested electrodiagnostically by reduced or absent sensory responses with relatively well-preserved motor responses and no significant abnormalities on needle electromyography. Selective sensory fiber involvement has been confirmed in an animal model (Windebank et al., 1985). However, some elements of motor fiber involvement may be observed (Albin et al., 1987). The dosage required for a toxic effect on peripheral nerve may be as low as 200 mg per day (Parry and Bredesen, 1985). The prognosis for the toxic sensory neuronopathy is relatively poor. However, reversal of modest motor fiber involvement on electrodiagnostic studies has been reported (Albin and Albers, 1990).

PELLAGRA

Pellagra, the nutritional disorder caused by *niacin deficiency,* may produce a wide array of neurological manifestations. It was first described by Casal, a physician at the royal court of Spain in 1735 (Etheridge, 1993). Although pellagra has essentially been eradicated in many Western countries by the practice of enriching bread with niacin, it still occurs in malnourished patients, particularly in the setting of chronic alcoholism (Serdaru et al., 1988). In addition, pellagra may be observed in developing parts of the world where corn remains the principal source of carbohydrates in the diet. More recently, pellagra has been observed in India and Egypt, where it has been associated with diets based on jowar, a type of millet or sorghum (Etheridge, 1993).

Pellagra is classically described as a disorder consisting of dermatitis, diarrhea, and dementia (Victor, 1983). The characteristic skin manifestations consist of hyperkeratotic and reddish-brown lesions distributed in a classic distribution over the face, neck, and dorsal surfaces of the limbs (Isaac, 1998), often resembling a sunburn. Diarrhea and other gastrointestinal manifestations are typically associated with weight loss and general fatigue. The neurological disorders associated with pellagra are diverse and appear to result from involvement of the brain, spinal cord, and peripheral nerves. When peripheral nerve involvement occurs as a more isolated clinical picture, it usually indicates a relatively mild form of the disease (Lewy et al., 1940). The peripheral neuropathy of pellagra shares many clinical features with beriberi (Lewy et al., 1940; Victor, 1983). The pathological changes in peripheral nerves are those of nonspecific axonal degeneration. Although it has been clearly established that treatment with niacin reverses most of the clinical manifestations of pellagra, treatment with niacin alone does not always reverse the peripheral nerve symptoms (Jolliffe, 1939; Ruffin and Smith, 1939; Sebrell and Butler, 1939; Lewy et al., 1940). This finding has led to speculation that some of the apparent neurological manifestations of pellagra result from coexisting deficiencies of thiamine and pyridoxine (Victor, 1983). Niacin supplementation typically consists of daily doses of 40 to 250 mg.

STRACHAN'S SYNDROME

Strachan's syndrome refers to a constellation of neurological symptoms and signs encompassing painful polyneuropathy, orogenital dermatitis, and amblyopia. This syndrome was described by Strachan, first in 1888 and later in 1897 (Strachan, 1888, 1897). Because Strachan initially described this clinical syndrome in Jamaican sugarcane workers, it later became known as peripheral neuritis of Jamaica. A similar clinical syndrome was described by Scott in 1918 (Scott, 1918). Although Strachan speculated that this disorder was caused by malaria, it was subsequently regarded as a nutritional deficiency disorder. In the years that followed, numerous reports appeared in the literature describing similar clinical syndromes with the cardinal features of polyneuropathy and optic neuropathy (Pallister, 1940; Victor, 1983). The polyneuropathy of Strachan's syndrome is typically a painful, predominantly sensory neuropathy (Strachan, 1888, 1897). The optic neuropathy results in a central or centrocecal scotoma (Victor, 1983). The orogenital dermatitis may be manifested by excoriation at the

corners of the mouth, prepuce, anus, and vulva. In addition, stomatoglossitis and corneal degeneration may also occur.

The pathological features of Strachan's syndrome were studied in Canadians held prisoners of war during World War II (Fisher, 1955). The most prominent findings were demyelination and axon loss in the posterior columns of the spinal cord and the columns of Goll. In addition, there was degeneration of fibers in the optic nerves referable to the papillomacular bundle (Fisher, 1955). No apparent peripheral nerve involvement was noted in this study, but clearly a comprehensive analysis of peripheral nerve pathology was not pursued. In fact, there are no comprehensive or definitive pathological studies on peripheral nerves in Strachan's syndrome (Victor, 1983; Windebank, 1993).

A clinical syndrome resembling Strachan's syndrome occurred in an epidemic in Cuba in 1992 and 1993 (Roman, 1994). This syndrome consisted of painful sensory polyneuropathy, sensorineural hearing loss, optic neuropathy, and dorsal lateral myeloneuropathy (Roman, 1994). The features of the myeloneuropathy consisted of posterior column abnormalities, including sensory ataxia as well as mild cortical spinal tract signs (Roman, 1994). Tinnitus and sensorineural hearing loss were often noted. Optic neuropathy as an isolated feature or in combination with myeloneuropathy and other variations was also observed (Roman, 1994). Sural nerve biopsies disclosed an axonal neuropathy predominantly affecting large-diameter myelinated axons (Borrajero et al., 1994). The precise origin of this epidemic is unclear, but it is believed to represent a deficiency of micronutrients including thiamine, cobalamin, folate, and sulfur amino acids (Roman, 1994). Most patients in this epidemic responded to treatment with B group vitamins and folate. These observations prompted the belief that Strachan's syndrome and the myeloneuropathic syndrome in the Cuban epidemic are probably related to multiple deficiencies of thiamine, niacin, riboflavin, pyridoxine, and cobalamin. In Strachan's syndrome, treatment with riboflavin (vitamin B_2) may rapidly reverse the orogenital dermatitis, but it does not appear to have a beneficial effect on the optic neuropathy or myeloneuropathy (Windebank, 1993).

References

Agelink MW, Malessa R, Weisser U, et al: Alcoholism, peripheral neuropathy (PNP) and cardiovascular autonomic neuropathy (CAN). J Neurol Sci 1998;161:135–142.

Albin RL, Albers JW: Long-term follow-up of pryidoxine-induced acute sensory neuropathy-neuronopathy. Neurology 1990;40:1319.

Albin RL, Albers JW, Greenberg HS, et al: Acute sensory neuropathy-neuronopathy from pyridoxine overdose. Neurology 1987;37:1729–1732.

Alvarez F, Landrieu P, Feo C, et al: Vitamin E deficiency is responsible for neurologic abnormalities in cholestatic children. J Pediatr 1985;107:422–425.

Baines M, Davies G: The evaluation of erythrocyte thiamin diphosphate as an indicator of thiamin status in man, and its comparison with erythrocyte transketolase activity measurements. Ann Clin Biochem 1988;25:698–705.

Beck WS: Neuropsychiatric consequences of cobalamin deficiency. Adv Intern Med 1991;36:33–56.

Behse F, Buchthal F: Alcoholic neuropathy: Clinical, electrophysical and biopsy findings. Ann Neurol 1977;2:95–110.

Berlin H, Berlin R, Brante G: Oral treatment of pernicious anemia with high doses of vitamin B$_{12}$ without intrinsic factor. Acta Med Scand 1968;184:247–258.

Best CN: Subacute combined degeneration of the spinal cord after extensive resection of ileum in Crohn's disease. BMJ 1959; 2:862–864.

Biehl JP, Vilter RW: The effect of isoniazid on vitamin B$_6$ metabolism, and its possible significance in producing isoniazid neuritis. Proc Soc Exp Biol Med 1954;85:389–392.

Binder HJ, Solitare GB, Spiro HM: Neuromuscular disease in patients with steatorrhea. Gut 1967;8:605–611.

Bishara S, Merin S, Cooper M, et al: Combined vitamin A and E therapy prevents retinal electrophysiological deterioration in abetalipoproteinemia. Br J Ophthalmol 1982;66:767–770.

Bjorkenheim B: Optic neuropathy caused by vitamin B$_{12}$ deficiency in carriers of the fish tapeworm, *Diphyllobothrium latum.* Lancet 1966;1:688–690.

Blackstock E, Rushworth G, Gath D: Electrophysiological studies in alcoholism. J Neurol Neurosurg Psychiatry 1972;35:326–334.

Blankenhorn MA: The diagnosis of beriberi heart disease. Ann Intern Med 1945;23:398–404.

Blass JP, Gibson GE: Abnormality of a thiamine-requiring enzyme in patients with Wernicke-Korsakoff syndrome. N Engl J Med 1977;297:1367–1170.

Bonjour JP: Vitamins and alcoholism. III. Vitamin B$_6$. Int J Vitam Nutr Res 1980;50:215–230.

Borrajero I, Perez JL, Dominguez C, et al: Epidemic neuropathy in Cuba: Morphological characterization of peripheral nerve lesions in sural nerve biopsies. J Neurol Sci 1994;127:68–76.

Bosch EP, Pelham RW, Rasool CG, et al: Animal models of alcoholic neuropathy: Morphologic, electrophysiologic, and biochemical findings. Muscle Nerve 1979;2:133–144.

Brin M: Erythrocyte transketolase in early thiamine deficiency. Ann NY Acad Sci 1962;98:528–541.

Brin M, Tai M, Ostashever AS, et al: The effect of thiamine deficiency on the activity of erythrocyte hemolysate transketolase. J Nutr 1960;712:273–281.

Brin MF, Fetell MR, Green PH, et al: Blind loop syndrome, vitamin E malabsorption, and spinocerebellar degeneration. Neurology 1985;35:338–342.

Brin MF, Pedley TA, Lovelace RE, et al: Electrophysiologic features of abetalipoproteinemia: Functional consequences of vitamin E deficiency. Neurology 1986;36:669–673.

Britt RP, Harper C, Spray GH: Megaloblastic anemia among Indians in Britain. Q J Med 1971;40:499–520.

Burch HB, Salcedo J, Carrasco EO, et al: Nutrition survey and tests in Bataan, Philippines. J Nutr 1950;42:9–29.

Burck U, Goebel HH, Kuhlendahl HD, et al: Neuromyopathy and vitamin E deficiency in man. Neuropediatrics 1981;12:267–278.

Carmel R, Watkins D, Goodman SI, et al: Hereditary defect of cobalamin metabolism (cblG mutation) presenting as a neurologic disorder in adulthood. N Engl J Med 1988;318:1738–1741.

Carpenter KJ, Sutherland B: Eijkman's contribution to the discovery of vitamins. J Nutr 1995;125:155–163.

Carter KC: The germ theory, beriberi and the deficiency theory of disease. Med Hist 1977;21:119–136.

Casey EB, LeQuesne PM: Electrophysiological evidence for a distal lesion in alcoholic neuropathy. J Neurol Neurosurg Psychiatry 1972;35:624–630.

Cavalier SJ, Gambetti P: Dystrophic axons and spinal cord demyelination in cystic fibrosis. Neurology 1981;31:714–718.

Claus D, Eggers R, Engelhardt A, et al: Ethanol and polyneuropathy. Acta Neurol Scand 1985;72:312–316.

Cox-Klazinga M, Endtz LJ: Peripheral nerve involvement in pernicious anemia. J Neurol Sci 1980;45:367–371.

Dalton K, Dalton MJ: Characteristics of pyridoxine overdose neuropathy syndrome. Acta Neurol Scand 1987;76:8–11.

Denny-Brown DE: Neurological conditions resulting from prolonged and severe dietary restriction. Medicine (Baltimore) 1947;26:41–113.

Denny-Brown DE: The neurological aspects of thiamine deficiency. Fed Proc 1958;17:35–39.

Dick JPR, Smaje JC, Crawford P, et al: Delayed somatosensory evoked potentials in pernicious anemia with intact peripheral nerves. J Neurol Neurosurg Psychiatry 1988;51:1105–1106.

Djoenaidi W, Notermans SLH: Electrophysiologic evaluation of beri-beri polyneuropathy. Electromyogr Clin Neurophysiol 1990;30:97–103.

Djoenaidi W, Notermans SLH, Lilisantoso AH: Electrophysiologic examination of subclinical beriberi polyneuropathy. Electromyogr Clin Neurophysiol 1995;35:439–442.

Dreyfus PM, Geel SE: Vitamin and nutritional deficiencies. In Albers RW, Siegel GJ, Katzman R, Agranoff BW (eds): Basic Neurochemistry. Boston, Little, Brown, 1972; 517–535.

Duncan G, Johnson RH, Lambie DG, et al: Evidence of vagal neuropathy in chronic alcoholics. Lancet 1980;2:1053–1057.

Elias E, Muller DPR, Scott J: Association of spinocerebellar disorders with cystic fibrosis or chronic childhood cholestasis and very low serum vitamin E. Lancet 1981;2:1319–1321.

Etheridge E: Pellagra. In Kiple KF (ed): The Cambridge World History of Human Disease. Cambridge, Cambridge University Press, 1993; 918–924.

Evans HM, Burr GO: Development of paralysis in the suckling young of mothers deprived of vitamin E. J Biol Chem 1928; 76:273–297.

Faris AA, Reyes MG: Reappraisal of alcoholic myopathy. J Neurol Neurosurg Psychiatry 1971;34:86–92.

Farrell PM, Levine SL, Murphy MD, et al: Plasma tocopherol levels and tocopherol-lipid relationships in a normal population of children as compared to healthy adults. Am J Clin Nutr 1978; 31:1720–1726.

Fine EJ, Hallett M: Neurophysiological study of subacute combined degeneration. J Neurol Sci 1980;45:331–336.

Fine EJ, Soria E, Paroski MW, et al: The neurophysiological profile of vitamin B$_{12}$ deficiency. Muscle Nerve 1990;13:158-164.

Fisher CM: Residual neuropathological changes in Canadians held prisoners of war by the Japanese. Can Serv Med J 1955;11:157–199.

Funk C: On the chemical nature of the substance which cures polyneuritis in birds induced by a diet of polished rice. J Physiol (Lond) 1911;43:395–400.

Funk C: The etiology of the deficiency diseases: Beri-beri, polyneuritis in birds, epidemic dropsy, scurvy, experimental scurvy in animals, infantile scurvy, ship beri-beri, pellagra. J State Med 1912;20:341–368.

Gammon GD, Burge FW, King G: Neural toxicity in tuberculous patients treated with isoniazid (isonicotinic acid hydrazide). Arch Neurol Psychiatry 1953;70:64–69.

Geller A, Gilles F, Shwachman H: Degeneration of fasciculus gracilis in cystic fibrosis. Neurology 1977;27:185–187.

Gilliatt RW, Goodman HV, Willison RG: The recording of lateral popliteal nerve action potentials in man. J Neurol Neurosurg Psychiatry 1961;24:305–318.

Gotoda T, Arita M, Arai H, et al: Adult-onset spinocerebellar dysfunction caused by a mutation in the gene for the alpha-tocopherol-transfer protein. N Engl J Med 1995;333:1313–1318.

Green R: Metabolite assays in cobalamin and folate deficiency. Baillieres Clin Haematol 1995;8:533–566.

Green R: Screening for vitamin B$_{12}$ deficiency: Caveat emptor. Ann Intern Med 1996;124:509–511.

Green R, Kinsella LJ: Current concepts in the diagnosis of cobalamin deficiency. Neurology 1995;45:1435–1440.

Griminger P: Casimir Funk: A biographical sketch (1884–1967). J Nutr 1972;102:1105–1113.

Guggenheim MA, Ringel SP, Silverman A, et al: Progressive neuromuscular disease in children with chronic cholestasis and vitamin E deficiency: Diagnosis and treatment with alpha tocopherol. J Pediatr 1982;100:51–58.

Hahn JS, Berquist W, Alcorn DM, et al: Wernicke encephalopathy and beriberi during total parenteral nutrition attributable to multivitamin infusion shortage. Pediatrics 1998;101:E10.

Hallett M, Fox JG, Rogers AE, et al: Controlled studies on the effects of alcohol ingestion on peripheral nerves of macaque monkeys. J Neurol Sci 1987;80:65–71.

Harding AE, Matthews S, Jones S, et al: Spinocerebellar degeneration associated with a selective defect of vitamin E absorption. N Engl J Med 1985;313:32–35.

Harding AE, Muller DPR, Thomas PK, et al: Spinocerebellar degeneration secondary to chronic intestinal malabsorption: A vitamin E deficiency syndrome. Ann Neurol 1982;12:419–424.

Harries JT, Muller DPR: Absorption of vitamin E in children with biliary obstruction. Gut 1971;12:579–584.

Healton EB, Savage DG, Brust JCM, et al: Neurologic aspects of cobalamin deficiency. Medicine (Baltimore) 1991;70:229–245.

Herbert V: Recommended dietary intakes (RDI) of vitamin B-12 in humans. Am J Clin Nutr 1987;45:671–678.

Heyer EJ, Simpson DM, Bodis-Wollner I, et al: Nitrous oxide: Clinical and electrophysiologic investigation of neurologic complications. Neurology 1986;36:1618–1622.

Holloway KL, Alberico AM: Postoperative myeloneuropathy: A preventable complication in patients with B₁₂ deficiency. J Neurosurg 1990;72:732–736.

Hong C-Z: Electrodiagnostic findings of persisting polyneuropathies due to previous nutritional deficiency in former prisoners of war. Electromyogr Clin Neurophysiol 1986;26:351–363.

Howard L, Ovensen L, Satya-Murti S, et al: Reversible neurological symptoms caused by vitamin E deficiency in a patient with short bowel syndrome. Am J Clin Nutr 1982;36:1243–1249.

Isaac S: The "gauntlet" of pellagra. Int J Dermatol 1998;37:599.

Itokawa Y: Kanehiro Takaki (1849–1920): A biographical sketch. J Nutr 1976;106:581–588.

Jackson CE, Amato AA, Barohn RJ: Isolated vitamin E deficiency. Muscle Nerve 1996;19:1161–1165.

Jackson J: On a peculiar disease resulting from the use of ardent spirits. N Engl J Med Surg 1822;11:351–353.

Jansen BCP, Donath WF: On the isolation of anti-beriberi vitamin. Proc K Ned Akad Wet 1926;29:1390.

Jeffrey GP, Muller DPR, Burroughs AK, et al: Vitamin E deficiency and its clinical significance in adults with primary biliary cirrhosis and other forms of chronic liver disease. J Hepatol 1987; 4:307–317.

Jeyasingham MD, Pratt OE, Burns A, et al: The activation of red blood cell transketolase in groups of patients especially at risk from thiamin deficiency. Psychol Med 1987a;17:311–318.

Jeyasingham MD, Pratt OE, Shaw GK, et al: Changes in the activation of red blood cell transketolase of alcoholic patients during treatment. Alcohol Alcohol 1987b;22:359–365.

Jolliffe N: The diagnosis, treatment and prevention of vitamin B₁ deficiency. Bull NY Acad Med 1939;15:469–478.

Jukes TH: The prevention and conquest of scurvy, beri-beri, and pellagra. Prev Med 1989;18:877–883.

Juntunen J, Matikainen E, Nickels J, et al: Alcoholic neuropathy and hepatopathy in mice, an experimental study. Acta Pathol Microbiol Immunol Scand 1983;91:137–144.

Juntunen J, Teräväinen H, Eriksson K, et al: Experimental alcoholic neuropathy in the rat: Histological and electrophysiological study on the myoneural junctions and the peripheral nerves. Acta Neuropathol (Berl) 1978;41:131–137.

Jurko MF, Currier RD, Foshee DP: Peripheral nerve changes in chronic alcoholics: A study of conduction velocity in motor nerves. J Nerv Ment Dis 1964;139:488–490.

Kass L: Pernicious anemia. In Smith LH (ed): Major Problems in Internal Medicine, vol 7. Philadelphia, WB Saunders, 1976; l–62.

Kayden HJ, Hatam LJ, Traber MG: The measurement of nanograms of tocopherol from needle aspiration biopsies of adipose tissue: Normal and abetalipoproteinemic subjects. J Lipid Res 1983;24:652–656.

Kayden HJ, Silber R, Kossmann CE: The role of vitamin E deficiency in the abnormal autohemolysis of acanthocytosis. Trans Assoc Am Physicians 1965;78:334–342.

Kayser-Gatchalian MC, Neundorfer B: Peripheral neuropathy with vitamin B₁₂ deficiency. J Neurol 1977;214:183–193.

Kemppainen R, Juntunen J, Hillbom M: Drinking habits and peripheral alcoholic neuropathy. Acta Neurol Scand 1982;65:11–18.

Kitamura K, Yamaguchi T, Tanaka H, et al: TPN-induced fulminant beriberi: A report on our experience and a review of the literature. Surg Today 1996;26:769–776.

Knox JDE, Delamore IW: Subacute combined degeneration of the cord after partial gastrectomy. BMJ 1960;2:1494–1496.

Krendel DA, Gilchrist JM, Johnson AO, et al: Isolated deficiency of vitamin E with progressive neurologic deterioration. Neurology 1987;37:538–540.

Kunze K, Muskat E: Thiamine deficiency neuropathy in rats. Electroencephalogr Clin Neurophysiol 1969;27:721.

Kuzminski AM, Del Giacco EJ, Allen RH, et al: Effective treatment of cobalamin deficiency with oral cobalamin. Blood 1998;92: 1191–1198.

Lahey WJ, Arst DB, Silver M, et al: Physiologic observations on a case of beriberi heart disease, with a note on the acute effects of thiamine. Am J Med 1953;14:248–255.

Landrieu P, Selva J, Alvarez F, et al: Peripheral nerve involvement in children with chronic cholestasis and vitamin E deficiency: A clinical, electrophysiological and morphological study. Neuropediatrics 1985;16:194–201.

Laureno R: Alcoholic myopathy. N Engl J Med 1979;301:1239.

Layzer RB: Myeloneuropathy after prolonged exposure to nitrous oxide. Lancet 1978;2:1227–1230.

Lefebvre D'Amour M, Shahani BT, Young RR, et al: The importance of studying sural nerve conduction and late responses in the evaluation of alcoholic subjects. Neurology 1979;29:1600–1604.

Lettsom JC: Some remarks on the effects of lignum quassiae amarae. Mem Med Soc Lond 1787;1:128.

Lewy FH, Spies TD, Aring CD: The incidence of neuropathy in pellagra: The effect of cocarboxylase upon its neurologic signs. Am J Med Sci 1940;199:840–849.

Lichtheim L: Zur Kermtoriss der perniciösen Anäemie. Munch Med Wochenschr 1887;34:300–306.

Lindenbaum J, Healton EB, Savage DG, et al: Neuropsychiatric disorders caused by cobalamin deficiency in the absence of anemia or macrocytosis. N Engl J Med 1988;318:1720–1728.

Low PA, Walsh JC, Huang CY, et al: The sympathetic nervous system in alcoholic neuropathy: A clinical and pathological study. Brain 1975;98:357–364.

Lubing HN: Peripheral neuropathy in tuberculosis patients with isoniazid. Am Rev Tuberc 1953;68:458–461.

Markle HV: Cobalamin. Crit Rev Clin Lab Sci 1996;33:247–356.

Mawdsley C, Mayer RF: Nerve conduction in alcoholic polyneuropathy. Brain 1965;88:335–356.

Mayer RF: Peripheral nerve function in vitamin B₁₂ deficiency. Arch Neurol 1965;13:355–362.

Mayer RF: Peripheral nerve conduction in alcoholics. Psychosom Med 1966;28:475–483.

McCombe PA, McLeod JG: The peripheral neuropathy of vitamin B₁₂ deficiency. J Neurol Sci 1984;66:117–126.

McCormick DB, Greene HL: Vitamins. In Burtis CA, Ashwood ER (eds): Tietz Textbook of Clinical Chemistry, Philadelphia, WB Saunders, 1999; 999–1028.

McDougall AJ, McLeod JG: Autonomic neuropathy. II. Specific peripheral neuropathies. J Neurol Sci 1996;138:1–13.

McLaren DS, Docherty MA, Boyd DH: Plasma thiamin pyrophosphate and erythrocyte transketolase in chronic alcoholism. Am J Clin Nutr 1981;34:1031–1033.

McLeod JG: Alcohol, nutrition, and the nervous system: Alcoholic neuropathy. Med J Aust 1982;2:274–275.

Metz J: Cobalamin deficiency and the pathogenesis of nervous system disease. Annu Rev Nutr 1992;12:59–79.

Minot GR, Strauss MB, Cobb S: "Alcoholic" polyneuritis: Dietary deficiency as a factor in its production. N Engl J Med 1933;208: 1244–1249.

Monforte R, Estruch R, Valls-Solé J, et al: Autonomic and peripheral neuropathies in patients with chronic alcoholism. A dose-related toxic effect of alcohol. Arch Neurol 1995;52:45–51.

Muller DPR, Harries JT, Lloyd JK: The relative importance of the factors involved in the absorption of vitamin E in children. Gut 1974;15:966–971.

Muller DPR, Lloyd JK, Wolff OH: Vitamin E and neurological function. Lancet 1983;1:225–228.

Nestor PJ, Stark RJ: Vitamin B₁₂ myeloneuropathy precipitated by nitrous oxide anesthesia. Med J Aust 1996;165:174.

Neville HE, Ringel SP, Guggenheim MA, et al: Ultrastructural and histochemical abnormalities of skeletal muscle in patients with chronic vitamin E deficiency. Neurology 1983;33:483–488.

North JDK, Sinclair HM: Nutritional neuropathy: Chronic thiamine deficiency in the rat. AMA Arch Pathol 1956;62:341–353.

Novak DJ, Victor M: The vagus and sympathetic nerves in alcoholic polyneuropathy. Arch Neurol 1974;30:273–284.

Ohnishi A, Tsuji S, Igisu H, et al: Beriberi neuropathy. Morphometric study of sural nerve. J Neurol Sci 1980;45:177–190.

Ouahchi K, Arita M, Kayden H, et al: Ataxia with isolated vitamin E deficiency is caused by mutations in the alpha-tocopherol transfer protein. Nat Genet 1995;9:141–145.

Pallister RA: Ataxia paraplegia occurring amongst Chinese in Malaya. Trans R Soc Trop Med Hyg 1940;34:203–211.

Palmucci L, Doriguzzi C, Orsi L, et al: Neuropathy secondary to vitamin E deficiency in acquired intestinal malabsorption. Ital J Neurol Sci 1988;9:599–602.

Pant SS, Asbury AK, Richardson EP Jr: The myelopathy of pernicious anemia: A neuropathological reappraisal. Acta Neurol Scand 1968;44[Suppl 5]:1–36.

Parry GJ, Bredesen DE: Sensory neuropathy with low-dose pyridoxine. Neurology 1985;35:1466–1468.

Pekelharing CA, Winkler C: Mittheilung uber die Beriberi. Dtsch Med Wochenschr 1887;13:845. Beriberi: Researches concerning its nature and cause, and the means of its arrest. Translation by J Cantlie. London, John Bale Sons and Daniellson, 1893.

Prineas J: Peripheral nerve changes in thiamine-deficient rats: An electron microscopic study. Arch Neurol 1970;23:541–548.

Pruthi RK, Tefferi A: Pernicious anemia revisited. Mayo Clin Proc 1994;69:144–150.

Roman GC: An epidemic in Cuba of optic neuropathy, sensorineural deafness, peripheral sensory neuropathy and dorsolateral myeloneuropathy. J Neurol Sci 1994;127:11–28.

Rosenblum JL, Keating JP, Prensky AL, et al: A progressive neurologic syndrome in children with chronic liver disease. N Engl J Med 1981;304:503–508.

Ruffin JM, Smith DT: Treatment of pellagra with special reference to the use of nicotinic acid. South Med J 1939;32:40–47.

Russell JSR, Batten FE, Collier J: Subacute combined degeneration of the spinal cord. Brain 1900;23:39–110.

Satya-Murti S, Howard L, Krohel G, et al: The spectrum of neurologic disorder from vitamin E deficiency. Neurology 1986;36:917–921.

Savage DG, Lindenbaum J: Neurological complications of acquired cobalamin deficiency: Clinical aspects. Baillieres Clin Haematol 1995;8:657–677.

Schaumburg H, Kaplan J, Windebank A, et al: Sensory neuropathy from pyridoxine abuse: A new megavitamin syndrome. N Engl J Med 1983;309:445–448.

Scott HH: An investigation into an acute outbreak of "central neuritis." Ann Trop Med Parasitol 1918;12:109–196.

Sebrell WH, Butler RE: Riboflavin deficiency in man (ariboflavinosis). Public Health Rep 1939;54:2121–2131.

Selikoff IJ, Robitzek EH, Ornstein GG: Treatment of pulmonary tuberculosis with hydrazide derivatives of isonicotinic acid. JAMA 1952;150:973–980.

Serdaru M, Hausser-Hauw C, Laplane D, et al: The clinical spectrum of alcoholic pellagra encephalopathy: A retrospective analysis of 22 cases studied pathologically. Brain 1988;111:829–842.

Shattuck GC: The relation of beri-beri to polyneuritis from other causes. Am J Trop Med 1928;8:539–543.

Shields RW: Alcoholic polyneuropathy. Muscle Nerve 1985;8:183–187.

Shields RW, Harris JW: Subacute combined degeneration of the spinal cord and brain. In Johnson RT (ed): Current Therapy in Neurologic Disease. Toronto, BC Decker, 1987; 310–313.

Sigal SH, Hall CA, Antel JP: Plasma R binder deficiency and neurologic disease. N Engl Med 1987;317:1330–1332.

Sokol RJ: Vitamin E deficiency and neurologic disease. Annu Rev Nutr 1988;8:351–373.

Sokol RJ: Vitamin E and neurologic deficits. Adv Pediatr 1990;37:119–148.

Sokol RJ, Heubi JE, Iannaccone ST, et al: Mechanism causing vitamin E deficiency during chronic childhood cholestasis. Gastroenterology 1983;85:1172–1182.

Sokol RJ, Heubi JE, Iannaccone ST, et al: Vitamin E deficiency with normal serum vitamin E concentrations in children with chronic cholestasis. N Engl J Med 1984;310:1209–1212.

Sokol RJ, Kayden HJ, Bettis DB, et al: Isolated vitamin E deficiency in the absence of fat malabsorption, familial and sporadic cases: Characterization and investigation of causes. J Lab Clin Med 1988;111:548–559.

Steiner I, Kidron D, Soffer D, et al: Sensory peripheral neuropathy of vitamin B_{12} deficiency: A primary demyelinating disease? J Neurol 1988;235:163–164.

Strachan H: Malarial multiple peripheral neuritis. Annu Univ Med Sci 1888;1:139–142.

Strachan H: On a form of multiple neuritis prevalent in the West Indies. Practitioner 1897;59:477–484.

Strauss MB: The etiology of alcoholic polyneuritis. Am J Med Sci 1935;189:378–382.

Subramony SH, Nance M: Diagnosis and management of the inherited ataxias. Neurologist 1998;4:327–338.

Sung JH, Stadlan EM: Neuraxonal dystrophy in congenital biliary atresia. J Neuropathol Exp Neurol 1966;25:341–361.

Swain R: An update on vitamin B_{12} metabolism and deficiency states. J Fam Pract 1995;41:595–600.

Takahashi K, Nakamura H: Axonal degeneration in beriberi neuropathy. Arch Neurol 1976;33:836–841.

Tappel AL: Vitamin E as the biological lipid oxidant. Vitam Horm 1962;20:493–510.

Tefferi A, Pruthi RK: The biochemical basis of cobalamin deficiency. Mayo Clin Proc 1994;69:181–186.

Thiele B, Stalberg E: Single fibre EMG findings in polyneuropathies of different aetiology. J Neurol Neurosurg Psychiatry 1975;38:881–887.

Tredici G, Minazzi M: Alcoholic neuropathy: An electron-microscopic study. J Neurol Sci 1975;25:333–346.

Victor M: Polyneuropathy due to nutritional deficiency and alcoholism. In Dyck PJ, Lambert EH, Thomas PK, Bunge R (eds): Peripheral Neuropathy, 2nd ed, vol 2. Philadelphia, WB Saunders, 1983; 1899–1940.

Victor M, Adams RD: The effect of alcohol on the nervous system. Res Publ Assoc Res Nerv Ment Dis 1953;32:526–573.

Victor M, Adams RD: On the etiology of the alcoholic neurologic diseases. With special references to the role of nutrition. Am J Clin Nutr 1961;9:379–397.

Victor M, Adams RD, Collins GH: The Wernicke-Korsakoff Syndrome: A Clinical and Pathological Study of 245 patients, 82 With Post-mortem Examinations. Philadelphia, FA Davis, 1971.

Victor M, Altschule MD, Holliday PD, et al: Carbohydrate metabolism in brain disease. VIII. Carbohydrate metabolism in Wernicke's encephalopathy associated with alcoholism. Arch Intern Med 1957;99:28–39.

Victor M, Laureno R: Neurologic complications of alcohol abuse: Epidemiologic aspects. Adv Neurol 1978;19:603–617.

Victor M, Lear AA: Subacute combined degeneration of the spinal cord: Current concepts of the disease process. Value of serum B_{12} determinations in clarifying some of the common clinical problems. Am J Med 1956;20:896–911.

Vilter RW, Mueller JF, Glazer HS, et al: The effect of vitamin B_6 deficiency induced by desoxypyridoxine in human beings. J Lab Clin Med 1953;42:335–953.

Walsh JC, McLeod JG: Alcoholic neuropathy: An electrophysiological and histological study. J Neurol Sci 1970;10:457–469.

Wanamaker WM, Skillman TG: Motor nerve conduction in alcoholics. Q J Stud Alcohol 1966;27:16–22.

Wechsler IS: Etiology of polyneuritis. Arch Neurol Psychiatry 1933;29:813–827.

Weder B, Meienberg O, Wildi E, et al: Neurologic disorder of vitamin E deficiency in acquired intestinal malabsorption. Neurology 1984;34:1561–1565.

Weir DG, Scott JM: The biochemical basis of the neuropathy in cobalamin deficiency. Baillieres Clin Haematol 1995;8:479–497.

Wichman A, Buchthal F, Pezeshkpour GH, et al: Peripheral neuropathy in abetalipoproteinemia. Neurology 1985;35:1279–1289.

Willer JC, Dehen H: Respective importance of different electrophysiological parameters in alcoholic neuropathy. J Neurol Sci 1977;33:387–396.

Williams RD, Mason HL, Power MH, et al: Induced thiamine (vitamin B_1) deficiency in man: Relation of depletion of thiamine to development of biochemical defect and of polyneuropathy. Arch Intern Med 1943;71:38–53.

Williams RR: Structure of vitamin B_1. J Am Chem Soc 1936;58:1063–1064.

Windebank AJ: Polyneuropathy due to nutritional deficiency and alcoholism. In Dyck PJ, Thomas PK, Griffin JW, et al (eds): Peripheral Neuropathy, 3rd ed, vol 2. Philadelphia, WB Saunders, 1993; 1310–1321.

Windebank AJ, Low PA, Blexrud MD, et al: Pyridoxine neuropathy in rats: Specific degeneration of sensory axons. Neurology 1985; 35:1617–1622.

Wöhrle JC, Spengos K, Steinke W, et al: Alcohol-related acute axonal polyneuropathy: A differential diagnosis of Guillain-Barré syndrome. Arch Neurol 1998;55:1329–1334.

Woltmann HW: The nervous symptoms in pernicious anemia: An analysis of one hundred and fifty cases. Am J Med Sci 1919; 172:400–409.

Yokota T, Wada Y, Furukawa T, et al: Adult-onset spinocerebellar syndrome with idiopathic vitamin E deficiency. Ann Neurol 1987;22:84–87.

Zak J, Burns D, Lingenfelser T, et al: Dry beriberi: Unusual complication of prolonged parenteral nutrition. JPEN J Parenter Enteral Nutr 1991;15:200–201.

Drug-Related Neuropathies

Peter D. Donofrio

ALLOPURINOL
ALMITRINE
AMIODARONE
AMITRIPTYLINE
CHLORAMPHENICOL
CLIOQUINOL
COLCHICINE
CYANATE
DAPSONE
DISULFIRAM
ETHAMBUTOL

ETHIONAMIDE
GOLD
GLUTETHIMIDE
HYDRALAZINE
INDOMETHACIN
ISONIAZID
LITHIUM
METHAQUALONE
METRONIDAZOLE
MISONIDAZOLE
NITROFURANTOIN
NITROUS OXIDE

PERHEXILINE
PHENYTOIN
PYRIDOXINE
STATINS
SURAMIN
THALIDOMIDE
ZIMELDINE
MISCELLANEOUS DRUGS
INADVERTENT POISONING FROM
    MEDICATIONS

The presentation of patients with symptoms and signs of a drug-related or -induced polyneuropathy does not differ from that of patients with most chronic length-dependent neuropathies, with a few exceptions. The peripheral nervous system reacts to toxins in a limited manner. Schaumburg and Spencer hypothesized that most toxins, including medications, produce damage in one of four regions of the peripheral nerve: (1) the distal sensory and motor axon (axonopathy); (2) the Schwann cell, leading to demyelinating neuropathy; (3) the dorsal root ganglion (ganglionopathy or neuronopathy); and (4) the anterior horn cell or motor neuron. In keeping with this classification, most medication-induced neuropathies can be grouped into one of four categories, depending on the region of the peripheral nervous system where the primary pathological process occurs (Table 62–1). As in most attempts to categorize biological systems, the classification is not perfect and can be imprecise when applied, particularly when the toxic process occurs at more than one site or in both the peripheral nervous system and the central nervous system. Table 62–1 groups medication-induced neuropathies by the major anatomical site of disease. Amiodarone is included in both the axonopathy and Schwann cell lists because the medication can cause neuropathy by either mechanism. When no nerve conduction study or nerve pathology information is known, the neuropathy is listed under axonopathy because of the strong likelihood that axon damage is the primary pathogenesis.

In this chapter, each medication and its associated neuropathy are discussed separately. It is not the intent in this chapter to review mononeuropathies that are caused by medications, injections, implantations, local reactions, or vaccinations.

ALLOPURINOL

Allopurinol was first described as a potential cause of polyneuropathy in 1966 (Glyn and Crofts, 1966). Since that description, researchers have published several other reports that associate allopurinol with the development of polyneuropathy (Azulay and colleagues, 1993). Azulay and colleagues described a man who noted dysesthesias 8 years after beginning therapy with allopurinol (Azulay et al., 1993). The physical examination abnormalities included stocking hypesthesia, a tremor, absent ankle reflexes, and mild proximal muscle weakness. Cerebrospinal fluid analysis showed no cells and a protein level of 480 mg/dL. Nerve conduction studies documented markedly prolonged motor nerve distal latencies, and slowed conduction velocities, findings suggestive of a demyelinating polyneuropathy. All electrophysiological results improved within 8 months after discontinuation of allopurinol, a finding paralleling the patient's clinical improvement. The authors also demonstrated that the autonomical nervous system was affected by showing abnormalities in sinus arrhythmia and Valsalva ratio testing.

ALMITRINE

Almitrine bismesylate was introduced in Europe in the 1980s as an agent for improving arterial blood gas concentrations and for increasing tissue oxygen-

Table 62–1. Drug-Induced Neuropathies: Anatomical Site of Disease

Axonopathy	Anterior Horn Cell
Almitrine	Dapsone
Amiodarone	**Dorsal Root Ganglion**
Amitriptyline	Pyridoxine
Carbamide	**Schwann Cell**
Chloramphenicol	Allopurinol
Chloroquine	Amiodarone
Clioquinol	Indomethacin
Colchicine	Perhexiline
Cyanate	Suramin
Disopyramide	Zimeldine
Disulfiram	Gentamicin
Ethambutol	Streptokinase
Ethionamide	Eosinophilia-myalgia syndrome
Hydralazine	
Gold	
Glutethimide	
Isoniazid	
Lithium	
Methaqualone	
Metronidazole	
Misonidazole	
Nitrofurantoin	
Nitrous oxide	
Phenytoin	
Sulfapyridine	
Sulfasalazine	
Statins	
Thalidomide	
Vancomycin	

ation in patients with chronic respiratory insufficiency. Soon thereafter, there were reports that related almitrine to symptoms and signs of polyneuropathy (Chedru et al., 1985; Gherardi et al., 1985). Chedru and colleagues reported four patients with chronic obstructive pulmonary disease who developed symptoms of paresthesia and pain in the distal legs after taking 100 to 150 mg of almitrine for 4 to 7 months. The neuropathy tends to affect sensory fibers more than motor fibers, and it typically begins between 2 and 25 months after the drug is taken (Bouche et al., 1989). The most common symptoms are distal paresthesia, pain, burning, diminished sensation, and unexplained weight loss (4 to 15 kg). Weakness is rare. Nerve conduction studies typically show reduced sensory nerve action potentials and compound muscle action potential amplitudes and relatively preserved or slightly slowed conduction velocities. Nerve biopsy shows reductions in the density of the myelinated nerve fiber, axon degeneration, and clusters of regenerating myelinated fibers, features consistent with a distal axonopathy (Chedru et al., 1985). Most patients have a modest elevation of cerebrospinal fluid protein (48 to 60 mg/dL). The condition of all patients improved when almitrine was discontinued, most within 6 months and almost all within 12 months.

AMIODARONE

Amiodarone is a diiodated benzofuran derivative that was first introduced as a cardiac antiarrhythmic

agent in 1964. The most noted neurological adverse effects are tremor, optic neuropathy, and peripheral neuropathy (Meier et al., 1979; Feiner et al., 1987). The neuropathy typically begins between 5 and 12 months after amiodarone is first taken. Unlike most toxic neuropathies, polyneuropathy related to amiodarone may differ among patients in its electrophysiological and pathological features. The neuropathy may be primarily axon loss or demyelination, or a combination (Jacobs and Costa-Jussa, 1985; Zea et al., 1985). Nerve biopsy shows severe loss of large and small myelinated fibers as well as unmyelinated fibers (Meier et al., 1979). Electron microscopy has shown many empty stacks of Schwann cell processes (Meier et al., 1979), electron-dense bodies within the Schwann cells, endothelial and pericyte cells, perineurial cells, and fibroblasts (Jacobs and Costa-Jussa, 1985).

AMITRIPTYLINE

Amitriptyline is a tricyclic antidepressant that over time has become a well-accepted treatment for neuropathic pain. Its attractiveness stems from its low cost, one-time dosing, effectiveness, and capability to induce sleep in patients with nocturnal pain. Ironically, amitriptyline has been associated with the development of peripheral neuropathy in several case reports (Meadows et al., 1982; Zampollo et al., 1988). Zampollo and associates reported a man who developed lower limb paresthesias, distal hypesthesia, and reduced ankle reflexes after taking a daily dose of 150 mg of amitriptyline uninterrupted for 2 years. Motor and sensory amplitudes were reduced, latencies were normal or prolonged, and conduction velocities were slowed, findings consistent with diffuse axon loss. When amitriptyline was discontinued, symptoms, signs, and electrophysiological abnormalities normalized within 3 years. Meadows and colleagues reported a woman who developed amitriptyline-induced neuropathy and whose symptoms remitted when she was treated with pyridoxine, 500 mg per day. The authors hypothesized that amitriptyline produces polyneuropathy in the same way as does isoniazid, by depleting the availability of pyridoxal phosphate (Meadows et al. 1982). In a separate article, Leys and colleagues described a patient who experienced features of a polyradiculoneuropathy after an overdose of amitriptyline (Leys et al., 1987).

CHLORAMPHENICOL

Chloramphenicol is an antibiotic first extracted from *Streptomyces venezuelae* in 1947. Although chloramphenicol is rarely used at present, it was a prominent antibiotic for many decades because of its effectiveness against gram-negative organisms. Its most feared adverse effects are bone marrow suppression and aplastic anemia. A few cases of sensory peripheral neuropathy and optic neuritis beginning 3 to 10 months after the prescription of chloramphenicol therapy were described (Wallenstein and Snyder, 1952; Joy et al., 1960; Wilson, 1962). The clinical features were optic neuritis, paresthesias in the lower extremities, and loss of deep tendon reflexes. No pathological features or nerve conduction studies were reported. Good recovery occurred in all patients. In one instance, the patient improved when vitamin B therapy was advised despite this patient's continuing to take chloramphenicol. The amelioration suggests either that the neuropathy was not caused by chloramphenicol or that chloramphenicol produces neurotoxicity by interfering with vitamin B metabolism.

CLIOQUINOL

Clioquinol is a halogenated hydroxyquinoline used primarily as an intestinal antiseptic. In the late 1940s, it was first reported that clioquinol caused a syndrome of myelopathy, peripheral neuropathy, optic neuropathy, and abdominal symptoms. This presentation was most commonly observed in children who were prescribed clioquinol for acrodermatitis enteropathica. Children were found to have a constellation of neurological complications that covered the spectrum from isolated optic atrophy to myelo-optic neuropathy, myelopathy and neuropathy, isolated myelopathy, isolated neuropathy, and neuropathy and optic atrophy (Baumgartner et al., 1979). Combined myelopathy and neuropathy constituted the rarest complications. In the most severe forms, patients had impaired vision, sensory deficits over the legs and lower trunk, painful dysesthesias, spastic paraparesis, pathologically brisk knee reflexes, absent ankle reflexes, and Babinski signs. Some authors referred to this condition as *subacute myelo-opticoneuropathy*. Despite the presence of clinical signs that suggested involvement of the distal sensory nerve, pathological and electrophysiological evidence verifying a neuropathy remains meager (Baumgartner et al., 1979). A report by Tsubaki and colleagues described axonal damage and demyelination of the optic nerve, lateral and posterior columns of the spinal cord, and peripheral nerves in patients with subacute myelo-opticoneuropathy, but these investigators did not describe the pathological features in greater detail, nor were prints of the pathological findings published (Tsubaki et al., 1971). In 1970, the Ministry of Health and Welfare of Japan prohibited further production and selling of clioquinol in Japan, a change that led to a marked drop in the number of patients who developed subacute myelo-opticoneuropathy. This ban on clioquinol during a period when nerve conduction studies were not commonly performed probably explains the absence of peripheral electrophysiological data in this disease.

COLCHICINE

In 1986, Riggs and colleagues first described a relationship between *colchicine* and neuropathy and myopathy (Riggs et al., 1986). Their patient had taken large doses of colchicine for 5 years. Her neurological examination was consistent with a severe sensory and motor neuropathy and mild proximal myopathy. Nerve conduction studies demonstrated small compound muscle action potential amplitudes, absent to small sensory nerve action potentials, mildly or moderately prolonged distal latencies, and mildly slowed conduction velocities. The muscle biopsy showed an increase in the variability of myofiber size, rounded and atrophic myofibers, muscle fibers that contained small vacuoles and subsarcolemmic deposits, and uneven staining of central muscle fibers. Electron microscopy revealed myofibrillar derangement and deposits of osmiophilic granular material. After discontinuing colchicine, the patient recovered well, except for persistent gait ataxia and distal hand weakness. In a larger study of 12 patients with colchicine myopathy and neuropathy, Kuncl and associates found similar abnormalities of nerve conduction (Kuncl et al., 1987). Sural nerve biopsy in one patient identified mild loss of large myelinated axons, degenerating axons, and regenerating axon clusters. Biopsies of proximal muscles showed a distinctive vacuolar myopathy, in which the vacuoles were distributed either centrally or in the region of the subsarcolemma. After discontinuation of colchicine, the patients' neurological function returned to normal within 4 weeks, except for symptoms and signs of mild neuropathy (Kuncl et al., 1987). The authors related the colchicine neuropathy and myopathy to renal dysfunction, because the adverse effect occurred only in patients with elevated serum creatinine who were taking therapeutic doses of colchicine.

CYANATE

Sodium cyanate has been used experimentally to treat sickle cell anemia because of its ability to inhibit sickling of erythrocytes. Initial studies of oral and intravenous cyanate in humans showed little toxicity except for weight loss. When large doses were prescribed over 1 to 2 years, a severe motor and sensory polyneuropathy developed in two patients (Peterson et al., 1974). Nerve biopsy showed a decrease in the density of large and small myelinated fibers (Ohnishi et al., 1975). Teased-fiber preparation demonstrated segmental demyelination and remyelination in one patient and linear rows of myelin ovoids in the other (Ohnishi et al., 1975). In a separate study of 27 patients who had been taking sodium cyanate for 47 to 749 days, nerve conduction abnormalities were detected in 16 patients (Peterson et al., 1974). The abnormalities consisted of slight prolongation of motor and sensory distal latency and slight slowing of conduction velocity, abnormalities most easily explained by a process of axon loss. Amplitudes were not reported. A correlation was found between the number of patients with nerve conduction abnormalities and longer duration of therapy and higher dosing of cyanate. Recovery was almost complete 3 months after discontinuation of the cyanate.

DAPSONE

Dapsone is commonly used to treat several dermatological disorders, such as dermatitis herpetiformis, pyoderma gangrenosum, acne conglobata, alopecia mucinosa, and leprosy. The first report of peripheral neuropathy as a complication of dapsone treatment appeared in 1969. In subsequent years, several other patients were described who developed a polyneuropathy that was more motor than sensory and distal more than proximal after taking dapsone (Rapoport and Guss, 1972; Waldinger et al., 1984). The neuropathy has been found in patients taking doses ranging from 100 to 600 mg per day for periods of several weeks up to 16 years. Neuropathic involvement is typically greatest in the hands. Nerve conduction studies typically show normal to low-normal conduction velocities, normal to prolonged distal latencies, and reduced compound muscle action potential amplitudes (Gutmann et al., 1976). Needle examination demonstrates findings consistent with acute and chronic denervation, greater distally than proximally (Gutmann et al., 1976). Gutmann and colleagues followed a single patient with a polyneuropathy for 5 years after dapsone was discontinued. Initially, distal latencies were either normal or slightly prolonged, and conduction velocities were normal or slightly slowed. Over time, all conduction rates returned to normal or high-normal values, and all distal latencies normalized. Compound muscle action potential amplitudes rose from profoundly depressed to normal values. The authors proposed that dapsone has its primary effect on the motor soma and axons of the motor neuron.

Marked improvement has occurred in the conditions of all patients after discontinuation of dapsone. Similar to isoniazid, dapsone is metabolized by acetylation. Slow acetylation of the drug and accumulation of toxic blood and tissue levels have been implicated as the initiating steps in the development of the neuropathy (Koller et al., 1977; Waldinger et al., 1984). Other investigators have shown that the rate of acetylation of dapsone is parallel to that of isoniazid and sulfamethazine, and the acetylation rate of dapsone metabolism varies among individual patients (Gelber et al., 1971).

DISULFIRAM

Disulfiram has been used since the 1940s as an agent to aid in the detoxification of patients with chronic alcoholism. In 1966, Bradley and Hewer re-ported a patient who developed, over 48 hours, a severe peripheral neuropathy manifested as foot-drop, weak hands, and numbness and paresthesia in the elbows and the knees (Bradley and Hewer, 1966). The patient had been taking disulfiram for 9 months. Nerve conduction studies showed moderately prolonged distal motor latencies and H-reflex latencies in the lower extremities. The abnormalities were interpreted as too prolonged for toxic neuropathy from chronic alcohol abuse. Within 2 months after stopping the disulfiram, marked improvement was noted in the patient's strength and sensation.

Mokri and colleagues reported four patients with a disulfiram-induced polyneuropathy (Mokri et al., 1981). The initial symptoms of the neuropathy developed between several weeks and 4 months after beginning the disulfiram. All patients were found to have symmetrical motor and sensory polyneuropathy, varying from mild to severe. Nerve conduction studies showed absent sensory nerve action potentials, reduced compound muscle action potentials, and slightly diminished nerve conduction velocities. The needle examination demonstrated findings consistent with active and chronic denervation. In one patient, repeat nerve conduction studies at 1 year showed partial recovery of the sensory nerve action potential in the median nerve and normalization of the conduction velocity in the motor fibers of the median and ulnar nerves. In two of their patients, the investigators observed a decrease in both large and small myelinated fibers and axon degeneration in the sural nerve biopsy.

ETHAMBUTOL

Ethambutol is a medication commonly used with isoniazid and tobramycin as triple therapy for tuberculosis. Optic neuritis is a well-known adverse effect of ethambutol therapy. Tugwell and James described three patients who developed polyneuropathy 5 to 9 months after initiation of ethambutol therapy (Tugwell and James, 1972). The timing of the evolution of the polyneuropathy was similar to the interval delay for optic neuritis. All patients had features consistent with a sensory neuropathy more so than a motor neuropathy. Nerve conduction studies showed reduced sensory nerve action potential amplitudes and slightly prolonged distal sensory latencies. Motor amplitudes were normal, and motor conduction velocities were either normal or slightly reduced. In two patients who were taking isoniazid in combination therapy with ethambutol, the neuropathy did not resolve when isoniazid was stopped in one patient, and the dose was considered too low in the other patient to implicate isoniazid. The conditions of all three patients improved when the ethambutol was discontinued. An unpublished series of more than 1,000 patients taking ethambutol reported 15 patients who complained of numbness in the extremities at some time while they took the medication.

ETHIONAMIDE

Ethionamide is a derivative of isonicotinic acid and shares chemical similarities with isoniazid. Ethionamide was commonly prescribed in the past for the treatment of tuberculosis. Poole and Schneeweiss report a patient who developed myeloneuropathy 5 months after taking ethionamide (Poole and Schneeweiss, 1961). The physical examination disclosed tender lower extremity muscles, impaired vibration sense from the toes to the pelvis, abnormal joint position sense in the feet, exaggerated upper extremity and knee tendon reflexes, and absent ankle reflexes. Spinal fluid analysis showed a protein level of 80 mg/dL. Substantial improvement was observed when ethionamide was discontinued. Leggat described a patient who developed generalized weakness, burning in the feet, and tingling in the hands and feet 7 months after daily therapy with ethionamide (Leggat, 1962). The physical examination was normal. Five days after stopping ethionamide, the patient experienced full resolution of symptoms. There are no reports on the nerve pathological features or electrophysiological results of patients with ethionamide-induced neuropathy.

GOLD

In 1941, Sundelin commented on the development of paresthesias in the fingers and toes of three patients who were undergoing *gold therapy* for the treatment of rheumatoid arthritis (Sundelin, 1941). In 1950, Doyle and Cannon reported the first extensive description of polyneuritis as an adverse reaction to gold therapy (Doyle and Cannon, 1950). They described a man who developed features of a severe motor and sensory polyneuropathy after receiving a cumulative dose of 900 mg of Myochrysine (450 mg of gold). At the peak of the neuropathy, the patient could not feed himself and complained of paresthesias from the feet to the rib cage. The physical examination revealed findings consistent with severe motor and sensory polyneuropathy as well as marked incoordination, dysmetria, writhing movements of the hands, and gait ataxia. The patient improved rapidly once the gold injections were discontinued. Nerve conduction studies and biopsy were not performed. Walsh was the first to describe nerve conduction data in gold neuropathy. He reported his results in a woman who developed a polyneuropathy after receiving a total of 85 mg of gold (Walsh, 1970). All sensory responses were absent. Motor latencies and conduction velocities were normal, except for an ulnar nerve conduction velocity of 40 m per second. A sural nerve biopsy showed loss of large- and small-diameter myelinated fibers. Teased-fiber preparations demonstrated that most fibers were undergoing active axon degeneration. Only rare fibers showed segmental demyelination (Walsh, 1970).

Katrak and colleagues reported electrophysiological and nerve biopsy results in three patients with gold-induced peripheral neuropathy (Katrak et al., 1980). In two of the cases, myokymia was observed in leg muscles. In one patient, nerve conduction studies were normal, whereas the needle examination showed spontaneous motor unit potentials in the form of doublets, triplets, and quadruplets in two muscles. In the other two patients, abnormalities were recorded in almost all nerves tested. Many of the conduction rates (prolonged latencies and slowed conduction velocities) were sufficiently severe to suggest a demyelinating process. Nerve biopsy in two patients showed findings confirming axon degeneration. In the third patient, nerve pathological study revealed a striking increase in internodes and a 50% or greater reduction in myelin thickness. In all three patients, improvement occurred when the gold therapy was discontinued. Two of the patients had residual leg weakness, and one patient had bilateral footdrop.

GLUTETHIMIDE

Glutethimide is a sedative that is chemically similar to thalidomide, an agent well known for its propensity to cause peripheral neuropathy. As is the case with thalidomide toxicity, patients may show palmar erythema and nail splitting (Spencer and Schaumberg, 1980). Haas and Marasigan reported three patients who developed polyneuropathy and prominent cerebellar dysfunction after long-term treatment with glutethimide (Haas and Marasigan, 1968). The physical examination showed severe cerebellar dystaxia, hyporeflexia, areflexia or dysarthric speech, dilated pupils, nystagmus, and distal sensory loss in all extremities. Nerve conduction studies showed absent sensory potentials and slightly reduced motor conduction velocities. Recovery was incomplete in two patients with severe gait ataxia manifesting as the major residual deficit.

HYDRALAZINE

Hydralazine is a chelating agent and a carbonyl reagent that has been shown to form complexes with sulfhydryl groups. It inhibits enzymes involved in pyridoxine metabolism and blocks the conversion of pyridoxine to its metabolite, 4-pyridoxic acid (Kirdendall and Page, 1962). Similar to isoniazid, its capability to inhibit pyridoxine probably accounts for the development of peripheral neuropathy in some patients who take hydralazine. Although hydralazine is infrequently used for the treatment of hypertension at present, it was a mainstay of therapy several decades ago. Its most feared adverse effect is the development of a drug-induced, lupus-like reaction.

In 1962, Kirkendall and Page reported two patients who developed symptoms and signs of polyneuropathy after taking hydralazine for 3 to 8 months. In one patient, the neuropathy appeared to be primarily sensory. In the other, the neurological deficits were left footdrop and pronounced sensory symptoms and signs from the toes to the upper third of the legs. In both patients, hydralazine discontinuation and the addition of pyridoxine therapy led to improvement in symptoms and strength within 2 to 4 weeks (Kirkendall and Page, 1962). Raskin and Fishman reported two additional patients with pyridoxine deficiency polyneuropathy resulting from hydralazine, one who developed symptoms after 7 days and the other who noted symptoms after 10 years (Raskin and Fishman, 1965). There are no reports of nerve conduction or nerve pathological findings in hydralazine neuropathy.

INDOMETHACIN

In 1975, Eade and colleagues described the complication of polyneuropathy in four patients who were treated with *indomethacin* for one of the following conditions: myalgias, osteoarthritis, or seronegative rheumatoid arthritis (Eade et al., 1975). The onset of the neuropathic symptoms in the four patients began 2 days to 6 months after indomethacin was prescribed. All patients had sensory symptoms, and one patient was weak to the point where he lost the ability to climb stairs and required support to walk. Nerve conduction studies in this last patient showed severe slowing of conduction velocity in the peroneal nerve (27 m per second) and in the median (32 m per second) and ulnar (33 m per second) nerves, values suggestive of a demyelinating process. The patient was clinically normal 4 months after the indomethacin was stopped. Comparative electrophysiological studies at that time showed a return to normal of the ulnar nerve conduction velocity and marked improvement in the other two nerve conduction velocities.

ISONIAZID

Isoniazid is a hydrazide of isonicotinic acid. Its major route of metabolism is through acetylation to acetyl isoniazid (Blakemore, 1980). This process is mediated by *N*-acetyltransferase, an enzyme located in hepatic cells and the same enzyme that acetylates dapsone and sulfamethazine. Isoniazid has been one of the mainstays of tuberculosis treatment since the 1950s.

Isoniazid is another medication that causes peripheral neuropathy through its effect on pyridoxine metabolism. Isoniazid inhibits pyridoxal phosphokinase, the enzyme that phosphorylates pyridoxal to produce the active coenzyme. In addition, isoniazid chelates with pyridoxal phosphokinase, and the resulting aggregate is more active against pyridoxal phosphokinase than is isoniazid alone (Blakemore, 1980). Studies have shown that a large variation exists among humans in the metabolism of isoniazid,

and the distribution is bimodal. With the use of metabolic testing, patients can be categorized into rapid or slow inactivators of isoniazid (Evans, 1963), and this bimodality is genetically determined. Hughes and colleagues investigated whether the development of isoniazid polyneuropathy could be related to the metabolism of the drug (Hughes et al., 1954). They identified polyneuropathy in 6 of 17 patients taking isoniazid, 4 of whom were slow inactivators of isoniazid. Although the number of patients was small, there was a suggestion that slow inactivators are more predisposed than rapid inactivators to the development of polyneuropathy after treatment with isoniazid. Other investigators have shown that the metabolism of isoniazid is inherited as an autosomal trait (Blakemore, 1980). Slow acetylators have the recessive trait, and their inability to metabolize isoniazid quickly leads to high blood levels and a greater propensity to develop toxic neuropathy.

One of the first comprehensive studies of isoniazid-induced neuropathy was published by Money (Money, 1959). He reported 84 patients with pulmonary tuberculosis who were receiving antituberculous therapy with isoniazid and *para*-aminosalicylic acid. Sixteen patients developed neurologically adverse effects that spanned the spectrum from neurasthenia, painful feet syndrome, and polyneuropathy to myelopathy, retrobulbar neuritis, and encephalopathy. Polyneuropathy was the most common of the neurological adverse effects. In almost all cases, the neurological adverse effect did not develop until 6 months after the beginning of isoniazid therapy. In the case of polyneuropathy, sensory symptoms and signs were more common than weakness, and the lower extremities were affected more frequently than the upper ones. Nerve conduction studies and nerve pathological findings were not reported. The conditions of most patients improved when they were prescribed vitamin B supplementation despite the maintenance of isoniazid therapy. Three other patients were found to have myelopathy, heralded by difficulty in walking and painful feet. This condition improved once isoniazid was withdrawn and vitamin B was prescribed as a supplement to the diet.

Ochoa described the neuropathological findings in nine patients with isoniazid-induced neuropathy (Ochoa, 1970). Using light and electron microscopy, he observed a marked reduction in the number of myelinated fibers, the presence of denervated Schwann cell bands, and regenerated myelinated fibers. He noted less impressive changes in unmyelinated fibers. Mild slowing of nerve conduction velocities in the ulnar and peroneal nerves was reported in six of the nine patients.

Thiazina is a combination medication containing isoniazid 100 mg and thocetazone. It was the standard treatment for tuberculosis in Kenyan adults in the early 1980s. In most patients, it was given without pyridoxine prophylaxis. Bahemuka and colleagues reported the electrophysiological findings in

27 asymptomatic patients who had taken thiazina for at least 10 months (Bahemuka et al., 1982). These investigators showed that the mean ulnar and peroneal conduction velocities were slower in the patients receiving thiazina than in a control population without tuberculosis.

LITHIUM

Lithium in toxic doses can lead to severe polyneuropathy. Vanhooren and colleagues reported two patients who developed acute motor and sensory polyneuropathy as the result of lithium intoxication (Vanhooren et al., 1990). Both patients initially presented with central nervous system manifestations including coma, hypertonia, conjugate eye deviation, Babinski signs, hemiparesis, and extrapyramidal signs. When consciousness was regained, one patient was found to have proximal weakness, and the other had flaccid paralysis in the legs and areflexia. Motor nerve conduction studies showed reduced compound muscle action potential amplitudes and either normal or diminished conduction velocities. In one patient, the sural response was absent. The needle examination revealed abnormal resting activity and polyphasic motor units. Several months after clearance of the intoxication, improvement was documented in sensory and motor amplitudes. Sural nerve biopsy in one patient identified a moderate loss of myelinated fibers, mild endoneural fibrosis, and scattered vacuolated macrophages in which myelin debris was observed (Vanhooren et al., 1990). Both patients rebounded from lithium intoxication, but only incompletely. One regained strength and sensation yet continued to be ataxic. The other patient had, as a result, an intention tremor, truncal ataxia, and dysarthria.

METHAQUALONE

Methaqualone is a hypnotic and tranquilizing agent that is sometimes packaged in combination with an antihistamine. In 1975, Hoaken reported a patient who developed paresthesias of the feet and lower legs after taking Mandrax, a combination product containing methaqualone and diphenhydramine hydrochloride, for several months (Hoaken, 1975). This report followed a more detailed description of seven patients by Finke and Spiegelberg in the German literature (Finke and Spiegelberg, 1973). The physical examination showed reduced or absent knee and ankle reflexes and a gradient loss of large- and small-fiber modalities in the distal legs. The patient experienced abatement of her symptoms several days after discontinuing the medication. The results of nerve conduction studies were not published. Several years before, Kunze and colleagues had disputed whether methaqualone caused polyneuropathy (Kunze et al., 1967). In 44 of their patients, nerve conduction studies and electromyo-

graphic findings were normal, and in the one patient who showed abnormalities of nerve conduction, the causal relationship of the polyneuropathy to methaqualone was unclear. Marks and Sloggem reported three additional patients who complained of either paresthesias or weakness several days after beginning methaqualone treatment (Marks and Sloggem, 1976). In each case, the symptoms resolved 24 to 48 hours after discontinuation of the hypnotic agent. Nerve conduction study results have not been reported in methaqualone neuropathy, because of the brevity of the symptoms.

METRONIDAZOLE

Metronidazole is a 5-nitromidazole and is an antimicrobial used in the treatment of protozoan infections (trichomoniasis, giardiasis, and amebiasis) and as a bactericidal agent in anaerobic infection. It is sometimes prescribed in high doses for treating Crohn's disease (Bradley et al., 1977). Several authors have reported a primarily sensory neuropathy or neuronopathy in patients receiving metronidazole for the treatment of Crohn's disease (Coxon and Pallis, 1976; Bradley et al., 1977). Patients typically complain of paresthesias in the feet and hands. Sensory examination shows a distal gradient loss of small-fiber perception more than large-fiber perception in the setting of preserved strength. Ankle reflexes may be present or absent. Nerve conduction studies show absent to reduced sensory nerve action potential amplitudes, normal sensory conduction velocities, and normal motor conduction studies (Coxon and Pallis, 1976; Bradley et al., 1977). Sural nerve biopsy in the patient reported by Bradley and colleagues identified a loss of many myelinated fibers and axon degeneration in all the remaining sensory fiber sizes, findings interpreted as consistent with chronic, active axonal polyneuropathy (Bradley et al., 1977). When metronidazole was discontinued in the three patients reported by Coxon and Pallis, the sensory neuropathy improved completely in one, it improved partially in another, and it remained static in the third.

Coxon and Pallis advised that the dose of metronidazole used for treating trichomonal or giardial infections, 12 g over 5 days, is probably safe and is unlikely to cause polyneuropathy. Their two patients with polyneuropathy had been prescribed a cumulative dose of 30.6 and 114 g of metronidazole, respectively, for the management of Crohn's disease (Coxon and Pallis, 1976).

MISONIDAZOLE

Misonidazole is a 2-nitromidazole that is used as a red blood cell sensitizer before radiation therapy, particularly for patients with carcinoma of the pharynx, larynx, and lung. Melgaard and associates reported eight patients who developed severe subacute sensory polyneuropathy after treatment with misonidazole for 3 to 5 weeks (Melgaard et al., 1982). The total dose of misonidazole varied between 17.0 and 22.0 g. All patients except one complained of severe pain and paresthesias in the feet and hands. Strength was rarely affected, and deep tendon reflexes were preserved. On sensory testing, touch, pain sensation, vibration, and joint position sense were affected more in the feet than in the hands. Three to five months after discontinuation of the misonidazole, three patients had died of the underlying carcinoma, the condition of one patient was unchanged, and four experienced improvement.

Nerve conduction studies were consistent with a severe, primarily sensory neuropathy. Sensory nerve action potentials were affected more in the feet than in the hands and were moderately to markedly reduced. Motor amplitudes and distal latencies were normal, and motor conduction velocities were normal or slightly slowed. Nerve biopsies in three patients showed a diminution of myelinated fibers, myelin debris, and clumps of disorganized myelin.

NITROFURANTOIN

Nitrofurantoin is a synthetic bacteriostatic antimicrobial agent created by the attachment of a nitro group to furan and a side chain of hydantoin (Morris, 1966). In years past, it was used to treat a wide range of gram-positive and gram-negative organisms, and it was frequently prescribed for urinary tract infections.

In 1956, several authors described toxic neuropathy temporally related to the use of nitrofurantoin. The neuropathy can present as early as 1 to 2 weeks after initiation of nitrofurantoin therapy. The major manifestations are distal paresthesias, loss of sensory perception in the hands and feet, mild to moderate distal weakness, and areflexia (Loughridge, 1962). The neuropathy may resolve over time, or it may be irreversible (Ellis, 1962). Nerve biopsy shows features of wallerian degeneration (Loughridge, 1962). Ellis reported six patients who developed an acute form of nitrofurantoin-induced polyneuropathy. Three of the patients died of complications of the polyneuropathy because the relation to nitrofurantoin was not recognized, and nitrofurantoin therapy was continued until death. The other three patients made partial recoveries. Ellis remarked that all six patients had renal insufficiency, an observation also noted by Loughridge and other authors. This observation led to the recommendation that nitrofurantoin be used with caution in patients with renal insufficiency, and the potential development of a peripheral neuropathy should be considered in patients receiving prophylactic nitrofurantoin (Ellis, 1962; Loughridge, 1962). Craven reported five patients who developed polyneuropathy after they received treatment with nitrofurantoin (Craven, 1971). All five patients had normal blood urea nitrogen levels when the drug was first prescribed and were determined to have only mild renal insufficiency at the time the neuropathy developed clinically. A similar experience was reported in two other patients (Jacknowitz et al., 1977).

In 1973, Toole and Parrish reviewed the world literature on nitrofurantoin neuropathy (Toole and Parrish, 1973). Most patients experienced the onset of neuropathic symptoms within the first 6 weeks of treatment. The daily dose prescribed was 100 to 800 mg. Of the patients for whom follow-up information was available, approximately one third experienced complete resolution of symptoms and signs, one half had residual disease, and one sixth remained unchanged.

There are no reports of the nerve conduction study findings in nitrofurantoin-induced polyneuropathy. Morris stated that electromyography in his first patient showed extensive fibrillation and a poor volitional pattern. Nerve biopsy tissue showed atrophy of the peripheral nerves; the muscle biopsy was interpreted as normal (Morris, 1966).

In 1954, nitrofurantoin was shown to inhibit carbohydrate metabolism. Paul and colleagues demonstrated in vitro that nitrofurantoin reversibly inhibits the formation of citrate at the stage of generation of acetyl coenzyme A from pyruvate and coenzyme A (Paul et al., 1954). Inhibition should be greater when the blood level of nitrofurantoin is higher, a condition that exists in renal insufficiency.

NITROUS OXIDE

In 1978, Layzer and colleagues reported three patients, two dentists and a hospital technician, who presented with symptoms of numbness and the sensation of an electric shock passing from the toes to the neck after flexion of the neck (reverse Lhermitte's sign) (Layzer et al., 1978). Neurological examination revealed incoordination in the hands, hypoactive reflexes, and a stocking-and-glove loss of sensation to vibration and position sense in the hands and feet. All three patients gave a common history of excessive recreational use of *nitrous oxide.* Layzer and colleagues proposed that the combination of distal numbness, hypoactive reflexes, and the reverse Lhermitte sign forms an unusual neurological constellation characteristic of nitrous oxide abuse.

Motor nerve conduction studies in nitrous oxide toxicity show mildly slowed to normal velocities and distal latencies at the upper end of normal. Sensory nerve action potentials are reduced.

In the same year, Layzer described 15 patients with the same condition. He characterized the clinical presentation as that of myeloneuropathy because of the combination of peripheral and central nervous system findings (Layzer, 1978). All his patients were dentists except for one. All had abused nitrous oxide recreationally, except for two, who were exposed to the inhalant professionally. In each case, the patients improved after cessation of nitrous oxide use. A total of 5 of the 15 patients continued to have moderate disability 6 weeks to 3 years after discontinuation of nitrous oxide. The similarity of this condition to subacute combined degeneration prompted Layzer to speculate that nitrous oxide could interfere with vitamin B_{12} metabolism. This hypothesis was furthered when Amess and colleagues showed, in patients undergoing cardiac bypass surgery, that nitrous oxide inhalation produced a deoxyuridine suppression test result identical to that found in patients with vitamin B_{12} deficiency (Amess et al., 1978). Given that all their patients had normal vitamin B_{12} concentrations, the data imply that nitrous oxide interferes with vitamin B_{12} function. Dinn and colleagues were able to produce the biochemical changes, the neurological signs, and the spinal cord features of subacute combined degeneration after they exposed a monkey to 50% nitrous oxide and 50% oxygen for 2 months (Dinn et al., 1978). Thus, nitrous oxide appears to produce neurological dysfunction by interfering with vitamin B_{12} metabolism, a process leading to an illness mimicking subacute combined degeneration.

Sahenk and associates described one patient who developed a toxic polyneuropathy after inhaling nitrous oxide cartridges through a whipped-cream dispenser (Sahenk et al., 1978). Toxicological analysis showed that 23 additional compounds were present in the inhalant, including three well-known neurotoxins: phenol, trichloroethylene, and toluene. In this patient, nerve conduction studies showed normal results in motor nerves and mild slowing of conduction velocities in sensory nerves. Sural nerve biopsy showed a normal number of nerve fibers, varying degrees of myelin ovoid formation, and rare fibers exhibiting focal areas of axon swelling and denuded myelin.

PERHEXILINE

Perhexiline maleate is a 2-(2,2-dicyclohexylethyl) piperidine that was introduced in the 1970s to treat coronary artery disease. Its use produces direct coronary artery vasodilatation and slowing of the heart rate via its effect on the sinoatrial node. Soon after it began to be used, several reports appeared describing severe motor and sensory polyneuropathy beginning 4 months to 3 years after prescription of perhexiline (Lhermitte et al., 1976; Said, 1978; Fardeau et al., 1979). Patients commonly complained of calf pain, paresthesias, weakness, and difficulty in walking. The findings on neurological examination were consistent with severe sensory and motor polyneuropathy. In a series of five patients reported by Said, one patient presented with facial diplegia and hypesthesia of the forehead, another had bilateral papilledema, and a third was noted to have discoloration of the right optic disc. The cerebrospinal fluid protein level was elevated (55 to 85 mg/dL) in four of the five patients. Nerve conduction velocities were moderately to markedly slow. Pero-

neal motor nerve conduction velocities were recorded as low as 17 m per second, and distal latencies were as long as 15 ms. A sensory conduction velocity was found to be 25 m per second in one patient. In Said's manuscript, no comment was made about motor and sensory amplitudes and whether conduction block or temporal dispersion was observed. Sural nerve biopsies showed severe loss of myelinated axons in all five patients, segmental demyelination in 16% to 90% of the fibers, and wallerian degeneration in 3% to 20%. Improvement occurred in all patients between several weeks and 6 months after discontinuation of perhexiline. In one patient, the conduction velocity of the peroneal nerve improved from 33 to 37 m per second 4 months after cessation of perhexiline. Lhermitte and colleagues reported similar electrophysiological and nerve pathological findings in their patient with perhexiline-induced neuropathy (Lhermitte et al., 1976).

Fardeau and associates described equally profound slowing of conduction velocities in four patients with perhexiline-induced polyneuropathy (Fardeau et al., 1979). As was the case in the journal article by Said, no comment was made about the presence of conduction block or temporal dispersion. Nerve biopsies disclosed a loss of myelinated fibers, particularly large fibers; an increase of collagen in the endoneurium and the perineurium; and numerous calcium-containing dark, round granules in the cytoplasm of Schwann cells. Teased–nerve fiber preparations showed abnormalities predicted by the electrophysiological findings. There were numerous thinly myelinated or demyelinated segments, sometimes extending along several consecutive internodes. The authors were able to identify similar dark, round inclusions in the Schwann cells of mice given perhexiline for 13 to 18 weeks. No reductions were counted in the number of nerve fibers, nor were abnormalities observed in the teased–nerve fiber preparations in the mice model of perhexiline.

When they analyzed the major lipid classes in human peripheral nerve biopsies, Pollet and colleagues determined that the concentration of neuraminic acid level was considerably increased in the nerves of patients with perhexiline-induced polyneuropathy (Pollet et al., 1979). This finding is of uncertain biochemical and clinical significance.

PHENYTOIN

Phenytoin has been the drug of choice for the treatment of several types of epilepsy since its introduction in 1938 (Lovelace and Horwitz, 1968). Lovelace and Horwitz published the first extensive study of the association between peripheral neuropathy and phenytoin. They identified 26 of 50 patients taking phenytoin who had peripheral neuropathy by clinical examination and electrophysiological study. All patients had absent deep tendon reflexes in the lower extremities. No other cause was apparent for the peripheral neuropathy. Conduction velocities in the lower extremities ranged from 30 to 40 m per second in most affected patients, and the sensory and motor amplitudes were often low in amplitude, long in duration, and complex. The authors determined that the neuropathy was more likely to occur in patients who had taken phenytoin for more than 10 years. There was no correlation between the dosage of phenytoin and the development of polyneuropathy.

Other authors have reported results contradicting those of Lovelace and Horwitz. Swift and colleagues noted a 16.7% prevalence of peripheral neuropathy in 186 patients with epilepsy who were taking various anticonvulsants (Swift et al., 1981). Peripheral neuropathy was not more common in patients taking phenytoin than in patients taking a combination of multiple anticonvulsants.

Shorvon and Reynolds followed 51 patients with epilepsy prospectively for 5 years who were prescribed either phenytoin or carbamazepine monotherapy (Shorvon and Reynolds, 1982). None of the patients receiving carbamazepine developed either clinical or electrophysiological features suggestive of diffuse polyneuropathy. In the phenytoin-treated group, none who were taking therapeutic doses developed clinical evidence of neuropathy. Eighteen percent showed mild electrophysiological abnormalities. The authors further demonstrated that slowing of sensory conduction occurred during phenytoin and long-term barbiturate intoxication in patients with chronic epilepsy, and sural sensory conduction velocities improved by 22% and median sensory conduction velocity by 11% when therapeutic levels were achieved. Motor nerve conduction studies were not reported. In the group of patients taking phenytoin who developed polyneuropathy, review of the medical records uncovered recurrent toxic drug levels and low folic acid levels. The authors concluded that previously reported cases of polyneuropathy in patients taking multiple agents could as easily be attributed to phenobarbital or primidone toxicity as to the implied association with phenytoin.

PYRIDOXINE

Pyridoxine is an essential vitamin that has been taken in large doses by persons to aid in bodybuilding, and it has been prescribed as a treatment for premenstrual syndrome, carpal tunnel syndrome, schizophrenia, autism, and hyperkinesis. One of its medicinal uses is to treat intoxication with the false morel mushroom *Gyromitra esculenta* (Albin et al., 1987). In 1980, Krinke and associates showed that large doses of pyridoxine produced sensory neuronopathy in dogs (Krinke et al., 1980). Spinal cord pathological examination showed widespread neuronal degeneration in the dorsal root ganglia, as well as in the sensory nerve fibers in the peripheral nerves, the dorsal columns of the spinal cord, and

the descending spinal tract of the trigeminal nerves. Schaumburg and colleagues reported two patients who began to experience an ascending numbness 3 and 11 months after they consumed large doses of pyridoxine (2 and 3 g) daily (Schaumburg et al., 1982). Neurological examination demonstrated normal strength, loss of ankle reflexes, and a distal gradient loss of vibration, pinprick, temperature, and touch sense. Neither patient improved when the pyridoxine was discontinued and after 1 year of follow-up. In their patients, motor nerve conduction studies were normal. Sural responses were absent, and median sensory responses were markedly reduced. Schaumburg and colleagues reported a larger cohort of patients who developed severe sensory neuropathy after taking 2 to 6 g of pyridoxine daily for 2 to 40 months (Schaumburg et al., 1983). One patient manifested Lhermitte's sign and pseudoathetosis of outstretched arms. He could walk only with the aid of a cane and could not walk with his eyes closed. Two other patients had Lhermitte's signs. All patients showed profound loss of most sensory modalities and were areflexic. The nerve conduction abnormalities were characteristic of a severe sensory neuropathy or neuronopathy. Sensory responses were absent, whereas motor amplitudes and conduction rates were normal. Somatosensory evoked potentials in the arms and legs were either absent or markedly reduced in amplitude. The conditions of all patients improved when pyridoxine use was stopped. Two patients experienced almost complete recovery after 2 to 3 years of follow-up. The authors concluded that vitamin B_6 in toxic doses was probably toxic to the dorsal root ganglia.

Albin and associates reported two patients (husband and wife) who were given large doses of pyridoxine for treating the symptoms of nausea, vomiting, and diarrhea arising from intoxication from the false morel *Gyromitra esculenta* (Albin et al., 1987). On examination, the patients manifested blurred vision, slurred speech, dysphagia, nystagmus, facial diplegia, proximal muscle weakness, appendicular ataxia, autonomic dysfunction, diminished sensation in a stocking-and-glove distribution, and a profound loss of vibration and joint position sense. Unique to their patients was the presence of autonomic dysfunction, mild proximal weakness, and nystagmus. Serial nerve conduction studies measured at seven intervals over 1 year showed complete loss of all sensory responses in the setting of relatively preserved compound muscle action potential amplitudes and mild to moderate slowing of motor conduction rates. One year after the intoxication with pyridoxine, neither patient could walk or had regained joint position sense.

STATINS

The statins are inhibitors of 3-hydroxy-3-methylglutaryl-coenzyme A reductase, an enzyme that regulates the synthesis of cholesterol. Although these agents are usually well tolerated, adverse effects include nausea, vomiting, rash, headaches, myalgias, myopathy, and elevated liver function tests. In 1994, Jacobs reported the development of sensory polyneuropathy in a patient who was treated with lovastatin for 2 years (Jacobs, 1994). The patient's symptoms abated when lovastatin was discontinued, but they returned within 2 weeks when pravastatin was substituted for lovastatin. The following year, Ahmad reported two patients with lovastatin-induced neuropathy. Although nerve conduction data were not described in the article, the results in one patient were described as consistent with mild sensory and motor axonal neuropathy (Ahmad, 1995).

Nerve conduction study results were published in four patients with polyneuropathy caused by simvastatin (Phan et al., 1995). Compound muscle action potential amplitudes were reduced in three of the four patients, and all patients had absent or reduced sensory nerve action potential amplitudes. Sensory latencies were normal, and motor and sensory conduction velocities were either normal or slightly slowed. The authors proposed that the simvastatin could produce toxicity through an adverse reaction on mitochondrial function. Inhibitors of 3-hydroxy-3-methyl-glutaryl-coenzyme A reductase, in addition to blocking cholesterol synthesis, also block synthesis of dolichol and ubiquinone. A deficiency of ubiquinone, a key enzyme in the mitochondrial respiratory chain, could interfere with the energy use of the neuron and, in turn, could produce reversible polyneuropathy.

Jeppesen and colleagues reported electrophysiological results similar to those of Phan and associates in seven patients who developed polyneuropathy after taking one of the following statin medications: lovastatin, fluvastatin, pravastatin, or simvastatin (Jeppesen et al., 1999). Four of their patients had irreversible neuropathy, a finding that the authors attributed to a longer exposure to the statins (4 to 7 years compared with 1 to 2 years).

Substitution of one statin that causes polyneuropathy for another may not prevent the recurrence of drug-induced neuropathy. Ziajka and Wehmeier reported a patient who developed neuropathy after taking lovastatin and whose symptoms returned when this patient was treated individually with simvastatin, pravastatin, and atorvastatin (Ziajka and Wehmeier, 1998).

SURAMIN

Suramin is a polysulfonated naphthylurea that has been used to treat African trypanosomiasis since the 1920s. In addition, suramin has therapeutic benefit for the treatment of prostate cancer, nodular lymphoma, and adrenocortical carcinoma. In 1990, four patients were described who developed severe flaccid motor and sensory polyneuropathy after they received parenteral suramin (La Rocca et al.,

1990). Two of the patients experienced bulbar and respiratory dysfunction to the point that intubation was necessary. Serial nerve conduction studies showed a progressive loss of compound muscle action potential amplitudes and slowing of conduction velocity that attained levels as low as 25 m per second in the ulnar nerve by 7 to 12 weeks. Conduction blocks of more than 50% were recorded in the ulnar and peroneal nerves in two patients. F-wave responses were lost in nerves in which the responses had been recorded earlier. All four patients had an elevation of cerebrospinal fluid protein during the acute phase of the illness, and in all cases the protein returned to normal as the disease activity abated. The onset of the neuropathy correlated with the maximal plasma level of suramin. Improvement varied between complete recovery and severe residual dysfunction.

THALIDOMIDE

Thalidomide was initially manufactured as a sedative and hypnotic. In 1961, it was withdrawn from use because of its teratogenesis and propensity to cause phocomelia in neonates. Thalidomide is now undergoing a resurgence as an effective treatment for numerous dermatological conditions, such as complex aphthous ulcers, Behçet's disease, prurigo nodularis, discoid lupus erythematosus, and erythema nodosum leprosum.

Thalidomide was first described as causing sensory and motor polyneuropathy in the early 1960s. The neuropathy is often associated with erythema of the hands and brittle fingernails. Ochonisky and colleagues reported a 21% incidence of neuropathy (based on both clinical and electrophysiological abnormalities) in their patients who were prescribed thalidomide (Ochonisky et al., 1994). Another 29% had either clinical symptoms or electrophysiological abnormalities. The occurrence of neuropathy was not related to the daily dose of the drug or the duration of treatment. Women and elderly patients were the most prone to developing the neuropathy. Most of the patients complained of paresthesias, hypesthesias, and leg cramps. Patients with electrophysiological evidence of neuropathy were found to have reductions in sural and median sensory nerve action potentials in the setting of normal or only slightly abnormal motor nerve conduction study results (Lagueny et al., 1986; Ochonisky et al., 1994). In the study of 13 patients reported by Lagueny and colleagues, amplitude reduction was recorded in the sural and median sensory fibers, but not in the superficial radial sensory fibers. Hess and colleagues documented the development of a polyneuropathy in five of the nine patients who were studied serially before and after treatment with thalidomide (Hess et al., 1986). Only slight nerve conduction velocity deterioration was recorded, a finding that did not reach statistical significance. The authors emphasized that without pretreatment nerve conduction data, one of the five patients may not have been discovered to have neuropathy, and another would have been predetermined to have neuropathy before treatment. Partial recovery is the rule when thalidomide is withdrawn, yet in some patients, the nerve conduction abnormalities worsen even when no further deterioration is detected on clinical examination (Lagueny et al., 1986).

Sural nerve biopsies have demonstrated a reduction of large-diameter fibers and an increase in the number of small fibers (Fullerton and O'Sullivan, 1968). No segmental demyelination has been observed. Fullerton and O'Sullivan attributed the absence of recovery in their patients with thalidomide-induced neuropathy to irreversible degeneration of the dorsal root ganglion and fiber tracts in the peripheral and central nervous systems.

In experimentally induced thalidomide neuropathy in female New Zealand white rabbits, Schroder and Matthiesen showed that the predominant pathological finding in sural nerve fibers was a reduction of the mean myelin thickness (Schroder and Matthiesen, 1985). Axon diameters were not significantly altered.

ZIMELDINE

Zimeldine was a selective serotonin reuptake inhibitor introduced in Sweden in 1982 (Fagius et al., 1985). Within 18 months after prescribing zimeldine, 13 cases of Guillain-Barré syndrome were reported in patients who had taken the drug, a finding prompting the manufacturer to withdraw zimeldine from the market. The clinical presentation was stereotyped as patients developing influenza-type symptoms 6 to 17 days after beginning treatment with zimeldine. Approximately 1 to 20 days later, all 13 patients showed signs of widespread symmetrical polyneuropathy. Ten patients displayed classic findings of Guillain-Barré syndrome, one had bifacial weakness and symmetrical sensory loss, and the remaining two had a protracted course that lasted for 4.5 months before recovery occurred. Nerve conduction velocities were reported as reduced in the six patients in whom the studies were performed. No data were reported describing motor and sensory amplitudes, distal latencies, specific values for the conduction velocities, and characteristics such as conduction block and temporal dispersion. Cerebrospinal fluid showed cytoalbumin dissociation and protein values varying from 60 to 180 mg/dL. The authors estimated that the risk of developing Guillain-Barré syndrome was increased 25-fold in patients who were prescribed zimeldine. The authors hypothesized that zimeldine probably triggered an immunological reaction that culminated in multifocal demyelinating polyradiculoneuropathy.

MISCELLANEOUS DRUGS

The neurological literature is replete with single case reports of patients who developed polyneurop-

athy temporally related to the use of a specific medicinal agent and resolution of the neuropathy when the agent was withdrawn. In some cases, the patient had risk factors for neuropathy, such as chronic diabetes or long-term alcohol abuse. It is unclear whether these medicinal agents cause neuropathy because of the infrequency of reports and complicating factors.

In 1976, Reilly described a middle-aged man who developed sensory symptoms and weakness in the hands after taking *citrated calcium carbamide* for approximately 9 months (Reilly, 1976). The patient denied any problems in the lower extremities. All features of the neuropathy resolved 3 days after the citrated calcium carbamide was stopped. Nerve conduction studies were not performed. Citrated calcium carbamide had been prescribed as an alcohol-sensitizing agent, and it is known that the biochemical action of citrated calcium carbamide resembles that of disulfiram.

Chloroquine is a known cause of myopathy. Marks reported the rapid onset and progression of motor neuropathy in a woman with seropositive rheumatoid arthritis (Marks, 1979). Over 10 days, she became weak in the arms and flaccid in the lower extremities. Other features of her clinical presentation were nystagmus and an elevated cerebrospinal fluid protein level of 130 mg/dL. Nerve conduction studies of the popliteal nerve showed slight slowing (no specific values reported). Denervation was recorded on the needle examination. Other electrodiagnostic parameters were not described. The patient recovered substantially within 1 month of stopping chloroquine.

Disopyramide is a medication used to treat intractable cardiac arrhythmias. Most of its adverse effects are related to its anticholinergic properties. Dawkins and Gibson reported a patient who began to experience burning in the feet 3 weeks after the prescription of disopyramide for atrial fibrillation (Dawkins and Gibson, 1978). Her symptoms worsened for 3 weeks until disopyramide was discontinued. Examination showed proximal and distal weakness in the lower extremities, profoundly reduced vibratory perception from the toes to the iliac crest, and loss of joint position sense in the toes and feet. The authors described the nerve conduction study results as compatible with sensory and motor neuropathy primarily affecting the large fibers. The patient made a complete recovery 4 months after withdrawal of the disopyramide.

Hormigo and Alves reported a patient who complained of paresthesias of the hands and feet beginning 18 months after taking *enalapril* for the treatment of hypertension (Hormigo and Alves, 1992). The physical examination documented the loss of large- and small-fiber function in a stocking-and-glove distribution in the setting of preserved strength and reflexes. Nerve conduction studies demonstrated diminished sural amplitudes and slowing of peroneal motor and sural conduction velocities. Six months after stopping enalapril, the patient was asymptomatic for neuropathy, and all nerve conduction studies had normalized.

Gentamicin is an aminoglycoside antibiotic that is highly effective against gram-negative bacteria. A well-known adverse effect is interference with neuromuscular junction transmission. Martens and Ansink described a patient who developed symptoms and signs suggestive of myasthenia gravis 2 months after undergoing treatment for tibia osteomyelitis. The infection had been managed by placing 120 polymethylmethacrylate beads, each impregnated with 7.5 mg of gentamicin, into the area of the osteomyelitis (Martens and Ansink, 1979). Motor nerve conduction studies revealed a conduction velocity of 27 m per second in the peroneal nerve and 43 m per second in the median nerve. Sensory nerve conduction studies were normal. Surprisingly, repetitive nerve stimulation of the facial and ulnar nerves did not show a significant decrement. The patient's only clinical findings suggestive of polyneuropathy were hypoactive reflexes in the arms and absent reflexes in the right knee and left ankle. Nerve conduction studies normalized 15 months after removal of all but one of the gentamicin beads.

Barnes and Hughes reported a patient who experienced classic symptoms and signs of Guillain-Barré syndrome 3 weeks after receiving an intravenous injection of *streptokinase* for the treatment of a myocardial infarction (Barnes and Hughes, 1992). The authors commented on four similar cases previously reported in the neurological literature. In the patient reported by Barnes and Hughes, motor nerve conduction velocity was slowed to 41 m per second in the median nerve and 29 m per second in the peroneal nerve. All F waves were unobtainable, and the compound muscle action potential amplitudes were small and dispersed. The patient recovered to independent ambulation 3 months after the streptokinase infusion. The authors hypothesized that Guillain-Barré syndrome may have arisen from an immunological reaction provoked by a foreign protein in the streptokinase.

Several reports can be found that relate the onset of peripheral neuropathy to the use of *sulfa-containing medications*. Volden described one patient who developed paresthesias of the hands after taking sulfapyridine and an occasional sulfoxone dose over 22 years for the treatment of dermatitis herpetiformis (Volden, 1977). The physical examination was normal except for hypesthesia of the hands. Electromyography was reported as normal. The paresthesias disappeared when the sulfa preparations were discontinued. Price reported a woman who experienced severe sensory and motor polyneuropathy 3 weeks after taking sulfasalazine for ulcerative colitis (Price, 1985). At the height of the illness, sensation was reduced below the knees and elbows, and the patient was flaccidly weak in the legs. She partially recovered 3 months after stopping the sulfasalazine. Nerve conduction studies were not described.

Vancomycin, the drug of choice for methicillin-resistant staphylococcal infections, is considered relatively free from neurological toxicity. In a brief report, Leibowitz and colleagues described a woman who began to experience tinnitus and right leg weakness after taking vancomycin for 1 month (Leibowitz et al., 1990). Nerve conduction studies showed right peroneal mononeuropathy and bilateral tibial mononeuropathies.

INADVERTENT POISONING FROM MEDICATIONS

On rare occasions, peripheral neuropathy that appears to be temporally related to the prescription of a medication can be traced to toxins within the preparation. Two prominent examples are *mercury toxicity* and the contamination associated with L-*tryptophan* manufacturing.

Matheson and colleagues reported a patient with a rash, flushed cheeks, photophobia, irritability, a tremor, and abnormal sensation (Matheson et al., 1980). The patient was eventually determined to have a polyneuropathy from merthiolate, a mercury-containing compound used as a bacteriostatic agent in the gammaglobulin product that he had been receiving for 15 years to treat congenital agammaglobulinemia. Nerve conduction velocity was reported as slowed. Analysis of blood and urine identified that both organic and inorganic mercury levels were elevated for weeks after an infusion of the gammaglobulin.

Topical mercurial salts are popular in many parts of the world as an ingredient in traditional remedies and in over-the-counter dermatological products. Deleu and associates reported sensory polyneuropathy in a patient with oxyuriasis who had been applying, for 2 years to the rectal area, an ointment containing 5% ammoniated inorganic mercury (Deleu et al., 1998). The patient had been complaining of burning, lack of sensation, and paresthesias in the hands, feet, and face for the preceding 2 months. Blood and urine samples showed a marked elevation in mercury levels. Nerve conduction studies revealed absent tibial sensory responses, a prolonged sural distal latency and slowed conduction velocity, a reduced sensory median nerve action potential, a diminished peroneal compound muscle action potential amplitude, and prolonged distal latency. The sural nerve biopsy demonstrated abnormalities consistent with a demyelinating and axon loss polyneuropathy. Two years after discontinuation of the topical agent and after treatment with D-penicillamine, the patient was markedly improved, but he was left with residual numbness, anhidrosis, and impotence. Repeat nerve conduction studies showed improvement in most conduction parameters, yet the tibial sensory responses remained absent, the peroneal compound muscle action potential amplitude was again reduced, and the conduction velocity was slowed. Chu and colleagues reported a much more severe case of polyneuropathy in a man who had been prescribed a mixed herbal drug for 6 months to treat visual hallucinations (Chu et al., 1998). The concoction contained a droplet of mercury from 10 broken thermometers. The patient was quadriplegic at the time of presentation. Two years later, he was areflexic and had experienced little improvement in strength and sensation.

L-Tryptophan is an over-the-counter medication that has been self-prescribed by patients to treat depression, premenstrual symptoms, insomnia, anxiety, tremor, pain, and obesity. In the late 1980s, a group of patients presented with a constellation of symptoms including myalgias, arthralgias, paresthesias, weakness, shortness of breath, cough, weight loss, fever, edema, rash, ecchymoses, and alopecia (Kaufman et al., 1990). The laboratory finding of profound eosinophilia, sometimes exceeding 10,000/mm^3, accompanied these symptoms and signs. For this reason, the condition became known as the *eosinophilia-myalgia syndrome.* Approximately one fourth to two thirds of the patients with eosinophilia-myalgia syndrome progressed to severe myopathy and chronic inflammatory neuropathy. Nerve conduction studies were typical of those recorded in multifocal demyelinating polyneuropathy and were similar to those reported in patients with acute arsenic poisoning and diphtheritic polyneuropathy (Donofrio et al., 1992). Although eosinophilia-myalgia syndrome was initially thought to result from a toxic reaction to L-tryptophan, the disease was eventually traced to a contaminant, a di-L-tryptophan aminal of acetaldehyde, a byproduct that had been accidentally introduced into the manufacturing process of L-tryptophan.

References

Ahmad S: Lovastatin and peripheral neuropathy. Am Heart J 1995; 130:1321.

Albin RL, Albers JW, Greenberg HS, et al: Acute sensory neuropathy-neuronopathy from pyridoxine overdose. Neurology 1987; 37:1729–1732.

Amess JAL, Burman JF, Rees GM, et al: Megaloblastic haemopoiesis in patients receiving nitrous oxide. Lancet 1978;1:339–342.

Azulay JP, Blin O, Valentin P, et al: Regression of allopurinol-induced peripheral neuropathy after drug withdrawal. Eur Neurol 1993;33:193–194.

Bahemuka M, Kioy PM, Wanjama M, et al: Electrophysiological evidence of peripheral nerve damage in patients treated with thiazina. East Afr Med J 1982;59:798–802.

Barnes D, Hughes RAC: Guillain-Barré syndrome after treatment with streptokinase. BMJ 1992;304:1225.

Baumgartner G, Gawel MJ, Kaeser HE, et al: Neurotoxicity of halogenated hydroxyquinolines: Clinical analysis of cases reported outside Japan. J Neurol Neurosurg Psychiatry 1979;42:1073–1083.

Blakemore WF: Isoniazid: Experimental and Clinical Neurotoxicology. Baltimore, Williams & Wilkins, 1980; 476–489.

Bouche P, Lacomblez L, Leger JM, et al: Peripheral neuropathies during treatment with almitrine: Report of 46 cases. J Neurol 1989;236:29–33.

Bradley WG, Hewer RL: Peripheral neuropathy due to disulfiram. BMJ 1966;2:449–450.

Bradley WG, Karlsson IJ, Rassol CG: Metronidazole neuropathy. BMJ 1977;2:610–611.

Chedru F, Nodzenski R, Dunand JF, et al: Peripheral neuropathy during treatment with almitrine. BMJ 1985;290:896.

Chu CC, Huang CC, Ryu SJ, et al: Chronic inorganic mercury induced peripheral neuropathy. Acta Neurol Scand 1998;98:461–465.

Coxon A, Pallis CA: Metronidazole neuropathy. J Neurol Neurosurg Psychiatry 1976;39:403–405.

Craven RS: Furadantin neuropathy. Aust NZ J Med 1971;3:246–249.

Dawkins KD, Gibson J: Peripheral neuropathy with disopyramide. Lancet 1978;1:329.

Deleu D, Hanssens Y, Al-Salmy HS, et al: Peripheral polyneuropathy due to chronic use of topical ammoniated mercury. Clin Toxicol 1998;36:233–237.

Dinn JJ, McCann S, Wilson P, et al: Animal model for subacute combined degeneration. Lancet 1978;11:1154.

Donofrio PD, Stanton C, Miller VS, et al: Demyelinating polyneuropathy in eosinophilia-myalgia syndrome. Muscle Nerve 1992; 15:796.

Doyle JB, Cannon EF: Severe polyneuritis following gold therapy for rheumatoid arthritis. Ann Intern Med 1950;33:1468–1472.

Eade OE, Acheson ED, Cuthbert MF, et al: Peripheral neuropathy and indomethacin. BMJ 1975;2:66–67.

Ellis FG: Acute polyneuritis after nitrofurantoin therapy. Lancet 1962;2:1136–1138.

Evans DAP: Pharmacogenetics. Am J Med 1963;34:639–662.

Fagius J, Osterman PO, Siden A, et al: Guillain-Barré syndrome following zimeldine treatment. J Neurol Neurosurg Psychiatry 1985;48:65–69.

Fardeau M, Tome FMS, Simon P: Muscle and nerve changes induced by perhexiline maleate in man and mice. Muscle Nerve 1979;2:24–36.

Feiner LA, Younge BR, Kazmier FJ, et al: Optic neuropathy and amiodarone therapy. Mayo Clin Proc 1987;62:702–717.

Finke J, Spiegelberg U: Polyneuropathy nach Methaqualone. Nervenarzt 1973;44:104.

Fullerton PM, O'Sullivan DJ: Thalidomide neuropathy: A clinical, electrophysiological, and histological follow-up study. J Neurol Neurosurg Psychiatry 1968;31:543.

Gelber R, Peters JH, Gordon R, et al: The polymorphic acetylation of dapsone in man. Clin Pharmacol Ther 1971;12:225–238.

Gherardi R, Benvenuti C, Lejonc, JL, et al: Peripheral neuropathy in patients treated with almitrine dimesylate. Lancet 1985;1:1247–1249.

Glyn JH, Crofts PA: Peripheral neuropathy due to allopurinol. BMJ 1966;2:1531.

Gutmann L, Martin JD, Welton W: Dapsone motor neuropathy: An axonal disease. Neurology 1976;26:514–516.

Haas DC, Marasigan A: Neurological effects of glutethimide. J Neurol Neurosurg Psychiatry 1968;31:561.

Hess CW, Hunziker T, Kupfer A, et al: Thalidomide-induced peripheral neuropathy. J Neurol 1986;233:83.

Hoaken PCS: Adverse effect of methaqualone. Can Med Assoc J 1975;112:685.

Hormigo A, Alves M: Peripheral neuropathy in a patient receiving enalapril. BMJ 1992;305:1332.

Hughes HB, Biehl JP, Jones AP, et al: Metabolism of isoniazid in man as related to the occurrence of peripheral neuritis. Am Rev Tuberc 1954;70:266.

Jacknowitz AI, Le Frock JL, Prince RA: Nitrofurantoin polyneuropathy: Report of two cases. Am J Hosp Pharm 1977;34:759–762.

Jacobs JM, Costa-Jussa FR: The pathology of amiodarone neurotoxicity. Brain 1985;108:753–769.

Jacobs MB: HMG-CoA reductase inhibitor therapy and peripheral neuropathy. Ann Intern Med 1994;120:970.

Jeppesen U, Gaist D, Smith T, et al: Statins and peripheral neuropathy. J Clin Pharmacol 1999;54:835–838.

Joy RJT, Scalettar R, Sodee DB: Optic and peripheral neuritis: Probable effect of prolonged chloramphenicol therapy. JAMA 1960;173:1731–1734.

Katrak SM, Pollock M, O'Brien CP, et al: Clinical and morphological features of gold neuropathy. Brain 1980;103:671–693.

Kaufman LD, Seidman RJ, Gruber BL: L-Tryptophan–associated eosinophilic perimyositis, neuritis, and fasciitis: A clinicopathologic and laboratory study of 25 patients. Medicine (Baltimore) 1990;69:187–199.

Kirkendall WM, Page EB: Polyneuritis occurring during hydralazine therapy. JAMA 1962;167:427–432.

Koller WC, Gehlmann LK, Malkinson FD, et al: Dapsone-induced peripheral neuropathy. Arch Neurol 1977;34:644–646.

Krinke G, Schaumburg HH, Spencer PS, et al: Pyridoxine megavitaminosis produces degeneration of peripheral sensory neurons (sensory neuronopathy) in the dog. Neurotoxicology 1980;2:13–24.

Kuncl RW, Duncan G, Watson D, et al: Colchicine myopathy and neuropathy. N Engl J Med 1987;316:1562–1568.

Kunze K, Noelle H, Prull G: Untersuchungen uber die Wirkung und Vertraglichkeit von Methaqualone bei neurologischen Krankheiten. Arneimittelforschung 1967;17:1052.

Lagueny A, Rommel A, Vignolly B, et al: Thalidomide neuropathy: An electrophysiologic study. Muscle Nerve 1986;9:837.

La Rocca RV, Meer J, Gilliatt RW, et al: Suramin-induced polyneuropathy. Neurology 1990;40:954–960.

Layzer RB: Myeloneuropathy after prolonged exposure to nitrous oxide. Lancet 1978;11:1227–1230.

Layzer RB, Fishman RA, Schafer JA: Neuropathy following abuse of nitrous oxide. Neurology 1978;28:504–506.

Leggat PO: Ethionamide neuropathy. Tubercle 1962;43:95–96.

Leibowitz G, Golan D, Jeshurun D, et al: Mononeuritis multiplex associated with prolonged vancomycin treatment. BMJ 1990;300:1344.

Leys D, Pasquier F, Lamblin MD, et al: Acute polyradiculoneuropathy after amitriptyline overdose. BMJ 1987;294:608.

Lhermitte F, Fardeau M, Chedru F, et al: Polyneuropathy after perhexiline maleate therapy. BMJ 1976;1:1256.

Loughridge LW: Peripheral neuropathy due to nitrofurantoin. Lancet 1962;2:1133–1135.

Lovelace RE, Horwitz SJ: Peripheral neuropathy in long-term diphenylhydantoin therapy. Arch Neurol 1968;18:69–77.

Marks JS: Motor polyneuropathy and nystagmus associated with chloroquine phosphate. Postgrad Med J 1979;55:569.

Marks P, Sloggem J: Peripheral neuropathy caused by methaqualone. Am J Med Sci 1976;272:323–326.

Martens EIF, Ansink BJJ: A myasthenia-like syndrome and polyneuropathy: Complications of gentamicin therapy. Clin Neurol Neurosurg 1979;81:241–246.

Matheson DS, Clarkson TW, Gelfand EW: Mercury toxicity (acrodynia) induced by long-term injection of gammaglobulin. J Pediatr 1980;97:153–155.

Meadows GG, Huff MR, Fredericks S: Amitriptyline-related peripheral neuropathy relieved during pyridoxine hydrochloride administration. Drug Intell Clin Pharm 1982;16:876–877.

Meier C, Kauer B, Muller U, et al: Neuromyopathy during chronic amiodarone treatment: A case report. J Neurol 1979;220:231–239.

Melgaard B, Hansen HS, Zamieniecka Z, et al: Misonidazole neuropathy: A clinical, electrophysiological, and histological study. Ann Neurol 1982;12:10–17.

Mokri B, Ohnishi A, Dyck PJ: Disulfiram neuropathy. Neurology 1981;31:730–735.

Money GL: Isoniazid neuropathies in malnourished tuberculous patients. J Trop Med 1959;62:198–202.

Morris JS: Nitrofurantoin and peripheral neuropathy with megaloblastic anaemia. J Neurol Neurosurg Psychiatry 1966;29:224–228.

Ochoa J: Isoniazid neuropathy in man: Quantitative electron microscopic study. Brain 1970;93:831–850.

Ochonisky S, Verroust J, Bastuji-Garin S, et al: Thalidomide neuropathy incidence and clinicoelectrophysiologic findings in 42 patients. Arch Dermatol 1994;130:66.

Ohnishi A, Peterson CM, Dyck PJ: Axonal degeneration in sodium cyanate-induced neuropathy. Arch Neurol 1975;32:530–534.

Paul MF, Paul HE, Kopko F, et al: Inhibition by Furacin of citrate formation in testis preparations. J Biol Chem 1954;206:491–497.

Peterson CM, Tsairis P, Ohnishi A, et al: Sodium cyanate induced polyneuropathy in patients with sickle-cell disease. Ann Intern Med 1974;81:152–158.

Phan T, McLeod JG, Pollard JD, et al: Peripheral neuropathy associated with simvastatin. J Neurol Neurosurg Psychiatry 1995;58:625–628.

Pollet S, Hauw JJ, Turpin JC, et al: Analysis of the major lipid classes in human peripheral nerve biopsies. J Neurol Sci 1979;41:199–206.

Poole GW, Schneeweiss J: Peripheral neuropathy due to ethionamide. Annu Rev Respir Dis 1961;84:890–892.

Price TR: Sensorimotor neuropathy with sulphasalazine. Postgrad Med J 1985;61:147–148.

Rapoport AM, Guss SB: Dapsone-induced peripheral neuropathy. Arch Neurol 1972;27:184–185.

Raskin NH, Fishman RA: Pyridoxine-deficiency neuropathy due to hydralazine. N Engl J Med 1965;273:1182–1185.

Reilly TM: Peripheral neuropathy associated with citrated calcium carbamide. Lancet 1976;1:911–912.

Riggs JE, Schochet SS, Gutmann L, et al: Chronic human colchicine neuropathy and myopathy. Arch Neurol 1986;43:521–523.

Sahenk Z, Mendell JR, Couri D, et al: Polyneuropathy from inhalation of N₂O cartridges through a whipped-cream dispenser. Neurology 1978;28:485–487.

Said G: Perhexiline neuropathy: A clinicopathological study. Ann Neurol 1978;3:259–266.

Schaumburg H, Kaplan J, Rasmus S, et al: Pyridoxine megavitaminosis produces sensory neuropathy (?neuronopathy) in humans. Ann Neurol 1982;12:107–108.

Schaumburg H, Kaplan J, Windebank A, et al: Sensory neuropathy from pyridoxine abuse. N Engl J Med 1983;309:445–448.

Schroder JM, Matthiesen T: Experimental thalidomide neuropathy: The morphological correlate of reduced conduction velocity. Acta Neuropathol (Berl) 1985;65:285–292.

Shorvon SD, Reynolds EH: Anticonvulsant peripheral neuropathy: A clinical and electrophysiological study of patients on single drug treatment with phenytoin, carbamazepine or barbiturates. J Neurol Neurosurg Psychiatry 1982;45:620–626.

Spencer PS, Schaumburg HH: Experimental and Clinical Neurotoxicology. Baltimore, Williams & Wilkins, 1980; 599.

Sundelin F: Die Boldbehandlung der chronischen Arthritis unter besonderer Berucksichtigung der Komplikationen. Acta Med Scand Suppl 1941;117:1–291.

Swift TR, Gross JA, Ward C, et al: Peripheral neuropathy in epileptic patients. Neurology 1981;31:826–831.

Toole JF, Parrish ML: Nitrofurantoin polyneuropathy. Neurology 1973;23:554.

Tsubaki T, Honma Y, Hoshi M: Neurological syndrome associated with clioquinol. Lancet 1971;1:696–697.

Tugwell P, James SL: Peripheral neuropathy with ethambutol. Postgrad Med J 1972;48:667–670.

Vanhooren G, Dehaene I, Van Zandycke M, et al: Polyneuropathy in lithium intoxication. Muscle Nerve 1990;13:204.

Volden G: Peripheral neuropathy: A side effect of sulphones. BMJ 1977;1:1193.

Waldinger TP, Siegle RJ, Weber W, et al: Dapsone-induced peripheral neuropathy. Arch Dermatol 1984;120:356–359.

Wallenstein L, Snyder J: Neurotoxic reaction to chloromycetin. Ann Intern Med 1952;36:1526–1528.

Walsh JC: Gold neuropathy. Neurology 1970;20:455–458.

Wilson W: Toxic amblyopia due to chloramphenicol. Scot Med J 1962;7:90–95.

Zampollo A, Sozzi G, Basso F: Amitriptyline-related peripheral neuropathy: Case report. Ital J Neurol Sci 1988;9:89–91.

Zea BL, Leonard JA, Donofrio PD: Amiodarone producing an acquired demyelinating and axonal polyneuropathy. Muscle Nerve 1985;8:612.

Ziajka PE, Wehmeier T: Peripheral neuropathy and lipid-lowering therapy. South Med J 1998;91:667–668.

Industrial and Environmental Toxic Neuropathies

James W. Albers and John J. Wald

This chapter reviews the application of conventional clinical electrophysiology, as described in Volume I of this text, to the evaluation of patients with suspected neuropathy, particularly forms associated with industrial or environmental exposures. Many chemicals have known peripheral neurotoxicity, whereas others have been implicated as potential neurotoxins only on the basis of isolated case reports or cross-sectional epidemiological studies showing minor but statistically significant differences of uncertain importance between exposed and nonexposed persons. Clinically significant toxic neuropathies occur infrequently compared with those related to hereditary, metabolic, or inflammatory causes. In general, clinical, electrodiagnostic, and laboratory results are not unique for a toxic origin in general, let alone suggestive of a particular toxin. The electrodiagnostic evaluation of a suspected chemically induced toxic neuropathy is identical to the evaluation performed for any neuropathy, regardless of its suspected or actual cause. In other words, the cause of the neuropathy does not have to be known for the practitioner to perform the appropriate clinical and electrodiagnostic evaluations.

The diagnostic expression *toxic-metabolic neuropathy* is frequently and perhaps excessively used by electrodiagnosticians, in particular, and clinicians, in general. The expression usually is used in the context of nonspecific sensorimotor neuropathy of the axonal type when no apparent cause of the neuropathy has been identified. Frequently, a "toxic" explanation is attributed to long-term or excessive alcohol ingestion, although even this seemingly straightforward explanation is controversial. The controversy reflects uncertainty about whether alcohol alone explains the neuropathy or whether additional components, such as genetic susceptibility or nutritional impairment, are required. Most neurologists do have considerable experience with peripheral neurotoxins. However, this experience relates to adverse effects of medication, not to industrial or environmental toxins, because medications represent a common cause of toxic neuropathy. In fact, the major dose-limiting effect of several medications, particularly the chemotherapy agents cisplatin and vincristine, is peripheral neurotoxicity.

Neuropathies associated with industrial exposures exist, but they are uncommon and appear to occur infrequently compared with the numbers expressed in reports from the early twentieth century. This apparent decline in frequency undoubtedly represents increased awareness of the neurotoxic potential of numerous chemicals used in the manufacturing process of products important in our society, and it probably reflects increased emphasis on appropriate industrial hygiene and worker protection. For example, numerous reports of industrial lead-induced neuropathy exist. Yet few patients with lead neuropathy have ever been reported in the literature using modern evaluation techniques, and most neurologists never identify a patient with lead neuropathy.

Toxic neuropathies related to environmental exposures are of potential concern but are probably less common than industrial neuropathies. Yet evaluations searching for occult environmental exposures, including 24-hour urine samples for heavy metals and arsenic, are among the most common laboratory studies performed in the evaluation of cryptogenic neuropathy. These evaluations are often requested routinely, even when no associated systemic abnormalities suggest a toxic cause or even an elevated clinical suspicion of such an exposure. Excluding homicidal intoxications, the most common "positive" results for toxic exposures reflect slight elevations of substances, such as organic mercury associated with high levels of seafood ingestion (Buchet et al., 1996). These findings are infrequently a likely cause of the patient's neuropathy.

Why is there this discrepancy between the large amount of information about industrial and environmental toxic neuropathies and the infrequent identification of patients with industrial or environmental exposures producing neuropathy? The obvious explanation is that such neuropathies are exceedingly rare. Although they are rare, the search for them is appropriately fueled by the fear of overlooking such easily treated disorders. In almost all but the most severe intoxications, treatment of the resulting neuropathy consists of removal of the patient from additional exposure. Of potentially greater importance, identification of a patient with an industrial or environmental neuropathy increases the likelihood that others can avoid similar exposure. Furthermore, information about the pathogenesis of any toxic neuropathy may lead to understanding other forms of neuropathy, including those far more commonly seen. An additional reason for the large number of descriptions of toxic neuropathy is the increased likelihood that a patient identified with a toxic neuropathy will be reported in the literature, not only because of the importance of the observation but also because of the rarity of the disorder.

Most clinicians will never see all the disorders discussed in this chapter. Yet it is probable that all neurologists experience a sense of concern that they are simply not identifying such patients. Familiarity with the examples provided should reinforce the importance of using standard clinical and electrodiagnostic methods in the evaluation of neuropathy. Occasionally, the practitioner substantiates the correct diagnosis only after identifying a source of exposure and demonstrating improvement after removal of the patient from additional exposure. However, even this additional information does not establish a definite toxic origin. Alternatively, progression of the disorder in the absence of further or ongoing patient exposure renders the initial diagnosis of a toxic neuropathy incorrect.

METHODOLOGY

In the context of the evaluation of a patient with suspected polyneuropathy of any cause, the most important responsibility of the physician is to use the results of the history, neurological examination, and electrodiagnostic evaluation to confirm localization to the peripheral nervous system, to identify the peripheral components involved (anterior horn cells, nerve roots, sensory or motor axons, muscle fibers, or neuromuscular junctions), and to provide a reasonable differential diagnosis of the resulting findings. The differential diagnosis may or may not include a toxic origin. The electrodiagnostic results rarely establish the cause of neuropathy, but they are not interpreted in isolation. Instead, the combined information derived from the clinical and electrodiagnostic examinations is used to direct the subsequent evaluation, usually to include additional laboratory studies. The additional information is used to refine the differential diagnosis. This iterative technique ideally terminates with a final diagnosis that explains the patient's neurological problem. Frequently, the final diagnosis identifies a disorder not considered in the initial differential diagnosis. It is the method of iterative clinical problem solving and diagnostic reasoning that is important in deriving a final diagnostic impression.

The inability to identify the cause of a given neuropathy should not suggest that the electrodiagnostic examination has a limited role in the evaluation of toxic neuropathy. On the contrary, the electrodiagnostic examination plays a major role in the diagnosis of toxic neuropathy, and it is recognized as the "gold standard" in the preliminary evaluation of suspected neuropathy. The electrodiagnostic data are of established sensitivity, specificity, and reproducibility, and they are used to localize lesions within the nervous system to an extent not clinically possible. When the electrodiagnostic examination is properly performed, its major limitation is the inability to distinguish among competing causes of neuropathy. The findings are exceptionally helpful in reducing the list of possible causes of a given neuropathy. For example, documentation of substantial motor conduction slowing in the presence of severe sensorimotor neuropathy greatly limits the number of diagnostic possibilities and excludes many toxic disorders from consideration.

The technique of performing the electrodiagnostic evaluation is reviewed elsewhere in this volume. Suffice it to say that the electrodiagnostic information is useful only when it is collected appropriately. The method includes using proper stimulation and recording techniques, carefully measuring distances, monitoring limb temperatures and warming cool

Table 63–1. Basic Questions That Should Be Addressed by the Electrodiagnostic Study in the Evaluation of Peripheral Dysfunction

Is there evidence of the following:
  Polyneuropathy, mononeuropathy multiplex, or polyradiculopathy?
  Sensory, motor, or combined involvement?
  Substantial conduction slowing (myelin or membrane) or amplitude loss (axon)?
  Impaired neuromuscular transmission?
  Isolated muscle fiber involvement?

Modified from Aminoff MJ, Albers JW: Electrophysiologic techniques in the evaluation of patients with suspected neurotoxic disorders. In Aminoff MJ (ed): Electrodiagnosis in Clinical Neurology. New York, Churchill Livingstone, 1999; 721.

limbs as necessary to attain temperatures of at least 31° to 32°C, performing sufficient evaluation to document the problem and exclude alternative explanations (errors of omission), and ensuring that electrodiagnostic results are consistent with the clinical findings. In addition to documenting the distribution and magnitude of abnormality, the electrodiagnostic information helps to identify the prominent pathophysiology, another important step in focusing the differential diagnosis. Basic questions involving the evaluation of neuropathy that should be addressed by the electrodiagnostic study are listed in Table 63–1, and expectations of the electromyographic evaluation of suspected neuropathy are listed in Table 63–2.

In the evaluation of suspected neuropathy, the results of nerve conduction studies are especially important with regard to identifying the presence or absence of involvement of the dorsal root ganglia or distal sensory axons. The needle electromyographic examination plays a relatively minor role in the eval-

Table 63–2. Expectations for the Electromyographic Evaluation of Neuropathy

Document evidence of a peripheral abnormality:
  Detection of presence
  Documentation of location (diffuse, focal, multifocal)
Identify the peripheral modalities involved:
  Sensory fibers
  Motor fibers
  Autonomic fibers
Identify the predominant pathophysiology:
  Axonal loss lesions
  Uniform demyelination
  Multifocal demyelination with partial or complete conduction block
  Conduction slowing suggestive of membranopathy
  Combination of above
Establish a temporal profile when possible (acute, chronic, old, ongoing).
Exclude accompanying or alternative disorders.
Determine the prognosis.

Modified from Albers JW: Numbness, tingling, and weakness: Making sense of the neuropathies. In Denys EH (ed): Numbness, Tingling, Pain and Weakness: 1994 AAEM Course for Primary Care Physicians. Rochester, MN, American Association of Electrodiagnostic Medicine, 1994; 27.

uation of neuropathy compared with nerve conduction studies, although it is a sensitive indicator of ongoing or prior axonal degeneration. The needle examination also can identify findings representative of polyradiculopathy to a greater extent than is possible clinically by identifying paraspinal muscle involvement. The major limitation of the needle examination is the inability to distinguish denervation resulting from abnormality of anterior horn cells within the spinal cord, the intradural or extradural ventral nerve roots, or more peripheral disorders of the motor nerve axon. Characterizing the distribution of abnormality does help in this determination, but the interpretation is not absolute for identifying neuropathy. The needle examination also provides information important in establishing the duration of abnormality. This is occasionally helpful in the evaluation of suspected toxic neuropathy when the time of onset relative to neurotoxic exposure is at issue. For example, following acute motor axon degeneration, fibrillation potentials appear in approximately 3 weeks. Over time, the amplitude of fibrillation potentials decreases in concert with muscle fiber atrophy. Reinnervation of muscle fibers by collateral sprouting may result in reduction or disappearance of fibrillation potentials, but after extensive denervation and clinically complete reinnervation, evidence of minute fibrillation potentials frequently remains decades after the initial event. A representative electrodiagnostic protocol for evaluating suspected peripheral neuropathy is shown in Table 63–3.

ESTABLISHING CAUSATION

The clinical, electrodiagnostic, and laboratory evaluations frequently, but not always, establish the cause of a polyneuropathy. Establishing the immediate, if not the ultimate, cause of toxic neuropathy is particularly problematic, because the diagnosis itself suggests that the cause is known (e.g., arsenical neuropathy). Unfortunately, few toxic neuropathies have characteristic features sufficient to be considered pathognomonic. Furthermore, for many common, readily diagnosed neuropathies, the actual cause of the neuropathy is unknown. An example of this seeming paradox is hereditary neuropathy. Although much is known about many of these neuropathies, the ultimate biochemical or metabolic defect is rarely known, and it is only through identification of similarly involved family members (a finding that could be explained on occasion by a common environmental exposure) or genetic testing that the diagnosis is established.

Physicians evaluating patients with neuropathy must be alert for potential industrial, recreational, and environmental exposures, as well as for new epidemics with new or old chemicals. However, simply identifying a potential neurotoxic exposure does not ensure that the toxin produced the neuropathy. Most examiners are familiar with the method used

Table 63–3. Representative Electrodiagnostic Protocol for Evaluating Suspected Peripheral Neuropathy

Nerve conduction studies*
1. Test the most involved site if clinically mild or moderate and the least involved site if severe.
2. Evaluate the peroneal motor nerve (extensor digitorum brevis); stimulate the ankle and below the fibular head. Measure the F-wave latency.†
3. If the peroneal study is abnormal, evaluate the tibial motor nerve (abductor hallucis); stimulate the ankle and knee. Measure the F-wave latency.
4. If motor response amplitudes are low or absent for peroneal or tibial nerve studies, evaluate the following:
   a. The peroneal motor nerve (anterior tibialis); stimulate below the fibular head and above the knee.
   b. The ulnar motor nerve (hypothenar); stimulate the wrist and below the elbow. Measure the F-wave latency.
   c. The median motor nerve (thenar); stimulate the wrist and elbow. Measure the F-wave latency.
5. Evaluate the sural nerve (ankle); stimulate the calf.
6. Evaluate the median sensory nerve (index finger); stimulate the wrist and elbow. If a response is absent or focal entrapment is suspected, record from the wrist and stimulate the midpalm; evaluate the ulnar sensory nerve (fifth digit); stimulate the wrist.
7. Additional nerves can be evaluated if findings are equivocal. Definite abnormalities should result in the following:
   a. Evaluation of the contralateral extremity
   b. Evaluation of a specific suspected abnormality

Needle examination
1. Examine the anterior tibialis, medial gastrocnemius, vastus lateralis, biceps brachii, first dorsal interosseous (hand), and lumbar paraspinal muscles.
2. Any abnormality should be confirmed by examination of at least one contralateral muscle to look for symmetry.

*Muscles in parentheses indicate recording sites for conduction studies.
†All F-wave latency measurements are for distal stimulation sites. Record as absent if no response after 10 to 15 stimulations.

Modified from Albers JW, Donofrio PD, McGonagle TK: Sequential electrodiagnostic abnormalities in acute inflammatory demyelinating polyradiculopathy. Muscle Nerve 1985;8:528, with permission of John Wiley & Sons, Inc. Copyright © 1985.

to establish the cause of a patient's problem, because this method is applied routinely in clinical practice. Clinical neurology is based on the scientific method of hypothesis generation and testing, and most clinicians apply general scientific principles in the formulation of a differential diagnosis without giving thought to the process. Yet the problem of establishing causation in suspected toxic neuropathy is seldom straightforward. Even after neuropathy has been identified, the neurologist's ability to establish a neurotoxic cause is limited by several factors, including the frequent absence of a definite measure of exposure (Taubes, 1995). Most diagnostic impressions rely heavily on the temporal association between exposure to a potential neurotoxin and the subsequent development of neuropathy. A temporal association is obviously important, but it is only one of several considerations used to establish causation. The problem of establishing causation is further complicated by the problem that many forms of neuropathy are idiopathic and of unknown origin.

Although it is difficult to establish the cause of

Table 63–4. Questions Useful in Establishing a Toxic Origin (Bradford Hill Criteria)

Appropriate timing of exposure and signs?
High relative risk based on epidemiological studies or case reports?
Biologically plausible?
Dose-response relationship?
Removal from exposure modifies effect?
Existence of an animal model?
Consistency among studies conducted at different times and in different settings?
Relative specificity of cause and effect?
Evidence of analogous problems caused by similar agents?
Other causes eliminated?

Modified from Hill AB: The environment and disease: Association or causation? Proc R Soc Med 1965;58:295.

some toxic neuropathies, some criteria are useful. One such method is based on a series of questions referred to as the *Bradford Hill criteria* (Hill, 1965). A similar method has direct application to the evaluation of infectious diseases, and the method represents a didactic exercise similar to the process clinicians use daily in identifying the cause of any clinical problem. Table 63–4 lists questions important in establishing a toxic origin for a given syndrome (e.g., is a certain toxin capable of causing the patient's neuropathy?), modified from those outlined by Hill. These questions have their greatest utility in distinguishing causation from association. The Hill criteria essentially use temporal association, the presence of an appropriate exposure, biological plausibility, and the elimination of competing causes to establish a neurotoxic origin. Of these, the most difficult diagnostic step, and the one that requires the greatest clinical experience, is the requirement to address competing causes. The term *consistent with* is frequently used in clinical electrodiagnostic reports to link a particular finding to a toxic exposure, without recognizing or acknowledging that the clinical or electrodiagnostic findings are "consistent with" other causes. The patient who develops subacute pure sensory neuropathy in the setting of excessive alcohol exposure may have alcohol-associated sensory neuropathy. However, a clinically indistinguishable neuropathy occurs in association with Sjögren's syndrome, neoplasm, human immunodeficiency virus (HIV), idiopathic sensory ganglionitis, vitamin E deficiency, the Fisher variant of Guillain-Barré syndrome, and several peripheral neurotoxins, including Vacor, cisplatin, metronidazole, pyridoxine, styrene, thalidomide, and thallium (Donofrio and Albers, 1990; Albers, 1993). In this context, the application of the differential diagnosis process, eliminating competing causes, is the most important and most difficult of the questions implied by the Bradford Hill criteria.

CLUES SUGGESTING A TOXIC ORIGIN

Before examining specific examples of toxic neuropathy, one should consider the clinical or electrodiagnostic features suggesting the possibility of a toxic origin. Proposing a toxic origin when no other cause is immediately apparent (as in probable toxic-metabolic neuropathy) rarely results in identification of the correct diagnosis. Unfortunately, there is no guarantee that the only cause considered (e.g., possible toxin exposure) is the explanation for the patient's problem. The initial clue suggesting a toxic origin may be recognition of some cardinal systemic feature suggesting exposure to a specific toxin, such as identifying a characteristic rash or Mees' lines in the fingernails. Such recognition usually stems from a high level of suspicion. Unfortunately, only rarely are clinical findings characteristic enough to suggest a specific disorder. Occasionally, the results of a laboratory test, such as basophilic stippling of red blood cells, suggest toxic exposure. In the appropriate clinical setting, specific laboratory tests may be useful in establishing an increased body burden of a potential neurotoxin or in identifying other pathological features of toxic exposure.

In the context of industrial or environmental neuropathy, identification of an "outbreak" or a cluster of persons in the workplace or residential area who develop neuropathy should raise clinical suspicion of a common cause. Following a common environmental exposure, development of neuropathy would be expected to occur within a brief interval. The same may be true of industrial exposure, although a particular job could have unusually high exposure to some neurotoxin that produces neuropathy in a single worker. It would not be until a similarly exposed individual, perhaps a replacement worker, developed neuropathy that a toxic cause would be suspected.

The diagnosis of chemically induced neuropathy depends on thorough clinical, electrodiagnostic, and laboratory evaluations. The remainder of this chapter emphasizes the method used to evaluate patients with suspected peripheral neurotoxic disorders and reviews selected examples of chemicals used in industry or present in the environment and thought to produce neuropathy, including several whose neurotoxicity remains controversial.

SELECTED EXAMPLES

The examples that follow serve several purposes. First, individual examples demonstrate the application of the electrodiagnostic evaluation in refining the differential diagnosis. For each example, alternative diagnoses are possible. Second, several of the examples demonstrate the process of establishing causation, with the recognition that opportunity for exposure or even evidence of an increased body burden of a given neurotoxin does not guarantee that exposure to the toxin causes the patient's problem. Third, the accompanying discussion summarizes available information about the selected neurotoxins, usually, but not always, based on epidemiological evaluations. In this context, the

chapter answers the types of question faced by the clinical neurologist, rather than concentrating on large group evaluations. We have tried to highlight examples of toxic neuropathy produced by acute exposure as well as provide examples of neuropathy produced by chronic, low-level exposure to the same chemicals. Several chemicals found in the workplace and environment known to cause neuropathy are reviewed, as are several chemicals whose neurotoxicity is controversial.

Arsenic

Arsenic is a metalloid with a long history of medicinal and homicidal applications (Poklis and Saady, 1990; Barton et al., 1992). Industrial exposure occurs in copper and lead smelting processes and in the pesticide-manufacturing process. Environmental exposure results from contact with numerous arsenic-containing compounds, such as some pesticides, paints, wood preservatives, and mordants (Feldman et al., 1979; Manzo et al., 1985; Windebank, 1993). After absorption, arsenic is excreted in the urine, with a half-life of about 3 weeks (Cavanagh, 1984). Blood levels are not helpful because of rapid clearance. Small amounts of arsenic bind to keratin in growing tissues, and exposure can be documented by accumulation in hair or nails (Politis et al., 1980).

ACUTE EXPOSURE

Arsenic ingestion is a common means of attempted homicide, but exposures occur in other situations, such as inhalation of arsenic fumes from burning wood treated with an arsenic preservative. Acute exposure produces a combination of systemic and neurological symptoms, some of which are suggestive of Guillain-Barré syndrome. For example, the initial gastrointestinal symptoms resemble gastroenteritis, a common antecedent illness preceding development of Guillain-Barré syndrome. The symmetrical sensorimotor neuropathy develops 5 to 10 days after a single exposure, progresses over days to weeks, and frequently requires assisted ventilation (Heyman et al., 1956; Jenkins, 1966; Chhuttani and Chopra, 1979; Windebank, 1993). Laboratory studies demonstrate elevated cerebrospinal fluid protein, and electrodiagnostic studies performed early in the course of illness, when the diagnosis is in question, demonstrated findings typical of acquired demyelination, with conduction slowing and partial conduction block or abnormal temporal dispersion. Because these neurological and laboratory findings are indistinguishable from those associated with Guillain-Barré syndrome (Greenberg, 1996), the possibility of arsenic intoxication is not always suspected unless additional systemic features not explained by Guillain-Barré syndrome are recognized. A typical patient with acute arsenic intoxication is summarized in Case 1.

Case 1

A 31-year-old man awoke with severe nausea, vomiting, and diarrhea (Donofrio et al., 1987). These symptoms persisted for 1 week, and his physician attributed them to gastroenteritis. As the patient began to feel better, he developed numbness and tingling of his feet, with progression over days to involve the legs and hands. He also developed unsteady gait and limb weakness that progressed over days. His medical history was otherwise unremarkable. He was taking no medications. No other family members were ill. Examination demonstrated mild respiratory difficulty and a weak cough. He had distal greater than proximal limb weakness and bifacial weakness. Reflexes were hypoactive in the arms and absent in the legs. Pinprick sensation was normal, but he had markedly impaired vibration and joint position sensations distally. Admission laboratory evaluation identified pancytopenia (white blood cell count of 1,250) and mildly abnormal liver function, both of which were attributed to a presumed viral infection. The amylase level was elevated, and the Westergren erythrocyte sedimentation rate (WESR) was 70 mm per hour. The cerebrospinal fluid protein was elevated (270 mg/dL), with a normal cell count and glucose level.

Electrodiagnosis

Initial nerve conduction studies 11 days after onset of sensory symptoms were interpreted as consistent with acquired sensorimotor neuropathy of the demyelinating type, although rigid criteria for acquired demyelination were not fulfilled. Abnormalities included absent sural and low-amplitude median sensory responses. Motor responses demonstrated reduced amplitudes with borderline-abnormal conduction velocities and distal latencies. F waves were unobtainable. Partial conduction block was demonstrated in two motor nerves, a finding supporting the diagnosis of acquired demyelination. Subsequent nerve conduction studies demonstrated absent motor and sensory responses 6 weeks after onset, and needle electromyographic examination demonstrated profuse fibrillation potentials in all muscles examined, with decreased motor unit recruitment. In distal-extremity muscles, no voluntary motor units were present.

Clinical Course

The diagnosis was presumed to be Guillain-Barré syndrome, and treatment was with plasma exchange. During the first week of hospitalization, progressive respiratory difficulty resulted in intubation and ventilator support. Sequential chest radiographs demonstrated progressive cardiomegaly with bilateral pleural effusions. Bone marrow examination, performed because of persistent pancytopenia, showed hypocellular marrow with megaloblastic changes and basophilic stippling of red blood cells. Almost coincident with identification of basophilic

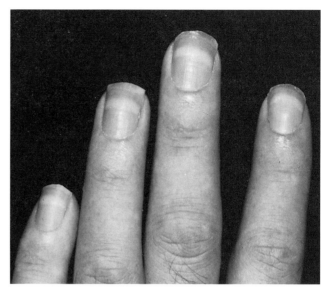

Figure 63–1. Mees' lines in the nails of a patient following arsenic intoxication resulting in severe sensorimotor neuropathy. (From Albers JW, Bromberg MB: Neuromuscular emergencies. In Schwartz GR [ed]: Principles and Practice of Emergency Medicine, 3rd ed. Philadelphia, Lea & Febiger, 1992; 1544.)

stippling, a 24-hour urine evaluation identified an arsenic level of 1,500 μg/dL (normal is less than 10 μg/dL and up to 50 μg/dL in an occupational setting). Over the next several weeks, a brownish desquamated palm and sole rash appeared, as did fingernail and toenail Mees' lines (Fig. 63–1). Slow recovery took place over several years. The source of arsenic was never identified.

Neuropathy constitutes only one component of an acute systemic illness following arsenic exposure. Other features of arsenic intoxication include nausea, vomiting, abdominal pain, diarrhea, dermatitis, cardiomyopathy, pancytopenia, basophilic stippling of red blood cells, and abnormal liver function tests. Mees' lines appear at the nail base about 1 month after isolated ingestion, too late to be helpful during the initial presentation but potentially helpful in the diagnosis of patients who have had multiple exposures. Features of neuropathy develop in 5 to 10 days after a single exposure and progress for several weeks. Neurological symptoms include paresthesias, unsteady gait, myalgia, muscle cramping, and weakness. Signs include ascending length-dependent limb weakness, prominent loss of vibration and joint position sensations, and hypoactive or absent reflexes. The severity of the neuropathy depends on the magnitude of arsenic exposure, varying from mild sensory loss with distal paresthesias to severe sensory loss, dysautonomia, quadriplegia, and respiratory failure.

Electromyographic studies performed within days of onset of neurological symptoms may show only decreased motor unit recruitment. Within the first weeks, however, electrodiagnostic abnormalities include low-amplitude or absent sensory and motor responses, slowed motor nerve conduction velocity, prolonged or absent F-wave latencies, and increased temporal dispersion and partial conduction block along motor nerves (Gherardi et al., 1990). Motor nerve abnormalities may fulfill criteria suggestive of acquired demyelination (Donofrio et al., 1987; Oh, 1991). Serial electrodiagnostic evaluations become more typical of a severe dying-back axonal neuropathy. Studies performed late in the clinical course often show only absent sensory and motor responses and profuse fibrillation potentials with markedly decreased motor unit recruitment, as in Case 1. It is likely that the initial findings suggestive of demyelination are secondary, appearing just before generalized axonal failure. Similar findings have been reported in association with acute nerve infarction, as seen in vasculitis. Nerve pathological examination shows axonal degeneration involving larger diameter fibers to a greater degree than the small fibers (Windebank, 1993). The diagnostic confusion with Guillain-Barré syndrome is substantial, and it is based on similar clinical, electrodiagnostic, and laboratory abnormalities. Unfortunately, this confusion has at times resulted in litigation based on failures to diagnose arsenic intoxication and to prevent subsequent exposure of the patient.

CHRONIC EXPOSURE

There are numerous industrial and environmental opportunities for chronic, low-level arsenic exposure, including herbal health food preparations (Tay and Seah, 1975). Such exposure produces systemic symptoms such as mucosal irritation, hyperpigmentation, hyperkeratosis, hepatic injury, and peripheral vascular disease ("black foot disease"), as well as neuropathy that can affect cranial nerves (Landrigan, 1981). Mees' lines are usually not seen with chronic exposure. The best documented industrial exposures occur in the smelting industry. The presence of subclinical sensory neuropathy was suggested on the basis of findings from discriminate analysis of electrodiagnostic measures and arsenic load in a blinded evaluation of arsenic smelter workers, although in these groups the individual nerve conduction data may be normal (Feldman et al., 1979; Blom et al., 1985). A 5-year follow-up study of one group of smelter workers who initially had slight subclinical neuropathy found significant negative correlations between cumulative exposure and nerve conduction velocities and sensory amplitudes, a finding supporting the concept that chronic low-dose exposure can produce neuropathy (Blom et al., 1985; Lagerkvist and Zetterlund, 1994). A patient with isolated macrocytosis and neuropathy but without anemia was found to have chronic arsenic intoxication related to chronic pesticide exposure (Heaven et al., 1994). The similarities between the symptoms of chronic arsenic toxicity and thiamine and riboflavin deficiency suggest that the mechanism of neurotoxicity may relate to arsenic's disruption of the Krebs cycle (Sexton and Gowdey, 1963). Neuropathies associated with arsenic intoxication are characterized by symmetrical sensory symptoms, usually numbness and paresthesias of the distal extremities. Neurophysiological and histological studies show variable results, a finding reflecting a significant dose-response relationship between arsenic load and evidence of neuropathy.

Mercury

Mercury is another neurotoxic metal that, like arsenic, was once a widely prescribed medication. It exists in three oxidation states (elemental, mercurous, and mercuric mercury), with toxicity in part dependent on the state. Organic mercury, bound to alkyl or aryl groups, is also toxic, again with toxicity dependent on the organic ligand (Atchison and Hare, 1994). Elemental mercury is found in thermometers; inorganic mercury is found in many devices (batteries), procedures (plating processes, tanning, and felt manufacturing), and dental amalgam (Albers and Bromberg, 1995). Occupational mercury exposure most commonly occurs in the chloralkali industry, where exposure is associated with a higher prevalence of reduced distal sensation, postural tremor, a positive Romberg sign, and impaired coordination among exposed persons compared with the referents many years after exposure has ceased (Albers et al., 1988; Andersen et al., 1993). Although these mercury-associated signs may persist, the abnormalities are typically mild and in most cases cannot be classified as disease (Andersen et al., 1993). Organic mercury exposure occurs with contamination, such as fish from the Minimata Bay of Japan in the 1950s. The long-term pathological changes of this exposure have been reviewed (Eto, 1997). The mechanism of mercury intoxication is not known, but it is thought to combine and interfere with sulfhydryl groups in enzymes or structural proteins (Windebank, 1993). The symptoms of acute inorganic mercury exposure include encephalopathy and neuropathy. Chronic inorganic mercury intoxication may also cause neuropathy (Chu et al., 1998). In addition, nonspecific sensorimotor neuropathy has been associated with chronic occupational mercury exposure (Albers et al., 1982, 1988; Andersen et al., 1993; Windebank, 1993; Chu et al., 1998). Long-term mercury toxicity affecting motor nerves has been considered a potential origin of motor neuron disease (Pamphlett and Waley, 1996); however, mercury has been found in control groups at a rate similar to that in patients with motor neuron disease (Pamphlett and Waley, 1998). The potential toxicity of low-dose mercury exposure has been reviewed (Cranmer et al., 1996).

n-Hexane and Related Hexacarbons

n-Hexane is a six-member carbon chain hexacarbon used in industrial and household glues. Methyl-*n*-butylketone is another common substituted hexacarbon. Both compounds are absorbed across respiratory membranes and skin, and both produce neuropathy following intoxication. Oxidative metabolism to 2,5-hexanedione takes place in the liver. Neurotoxicity of these and other neurotoxic carbon compounds, such as 2,5-heptanedione and 3,6-octanedione, is probably related to their metabolism to 2,5-hexanedione, the probable neurotoxic agent (DiVincenzo et al., 1980; O'Donoghue and Krasavage, 1980). A similar substituted hexacarbon, methylethylketone, is not neurotoxic, but it may promote neuropathy resulting from other hexacarbons (Altenkirch et al., 1977).

Subacute High-Level Exposure

Several organic solvents, including *n*-hexane and methyl-*n*-butylketone, produce neuropathy following recreational (huffing) use (Kuwabara et al., 1993, 1999) or occupational exposures (Herskowitz et al., 1971; Spencer et al., 1975; Paulson and Waylonis, 1976; Scelsi et al., 1981; Iida, 1982 Chang et al., 1993). The dying-back, length-dependent neuropathy is characterized by distal weakness, stocking-and-glove sensory loss, and absent ankle reflexes. The type and magnitude of clinical impairment are related to the potency, dose, and duration of exposure (Spencer and Schaumburg, 1985). A patient with a representative *n*-hexane neuropathy is described in the following case presentation (Case 2).

Case 2

A 25-year-old man experienced progressive weakness, sensory loss, and limb pain over several months (Smith and Albers, 1997). These neurological symptoms developed in association with a 25-pound weight loss over the previous 3 months despite reportedly good nutrition. He had a past history of schizophrenia and auditory hallucinations, successfully treated with chlorpromazine (Thorazine) and fluoxetine (Prozac). He also acknowledged polysubstance abuse, including crack cocaine, amphetamines, and occasional glue sniffing, but he denied use of recreational drugs within the preceding 12 months. The only abnormalities on examination involved his peripheral nervous system. He had distal weakness (graded 2+ and 3+ on the Medical Research Council scale) and decreased touch, vibration, joint position, pinprick, and temperature sensations to the midlimb level. He was hyporeflexic in the arms and areflexic in the legs. Initial laboratory testing was unremarkable, including liver function, human immunodeficiency virus antibodies, and phosphate and glucose levels. He had normal serum protein electrophoresis and no evidence suggesting vasculitis. Twenty-four–hour urine measurements for arsenic, mercury, and lead were normal, and he had a negative "toxicology screen." The cerebrospinal fluid protein was slightly elevated (60 mg/dL), with normal glucose level and a normal cell count.

Electrodiagnosis

Electrodiagnostic testing performed about 1 month after the onset of weakness demonstrated slightly reduced sensory amplitudes, including the sural response. Motor responses, however, were moderately reduced in amplitude, and there was further loss of amplitude with proximal stimulation consistent with abnormal temporal dispersion or partial conduction block. Nerve conduction velocities were reduced (e.g., median 44 m per second and ulnar 28 m per second). Motor distal latencies were prolonged to an extent greater than what could be explained by axonal loss alone. F waves were unobtainable. The needle electromyographic examination showed profuse fibrillation potentials in distal muscles, decreased motor unit recruitment, and slightly increased motor unit amplitude and duration.

Clinical Course

Weakness progressed during the first 3 weeks of hospitalization to less than antigravity function in his legs and hands, and this markedly interfered with activities of daily living. He also complained of severe burning and electric shock–like pain in his extremities. Approximately 4 weeks after admission, the pain decreased, with stabilization of sensory and motor function. Sural nerve biopsy demonstrated decreased density of large myelinated fibers without evidence of vasculitis. Several axons demonstrated focal swellings suggestive of *n*-hexane exposure (Fig. 63–2). He acknowledged a recent dramatic increase in glue sniffing, in which he huffed into a plastic bag more than 40 4-oz bottles of rubber cement during the month before his admission. The rubber cement contained *n*-hexane. He continued huffing after onset of his weakness, but not after admission to the hospital. Approximately 1 year after discharge, he had minimal distal weakness and sensory loss with normal reflexes. Sequential electrodiagnostic evalua-

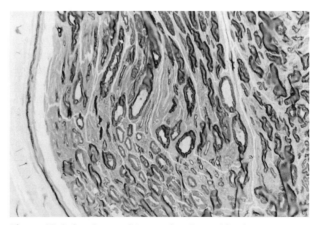

Figure 63–2. Sural nerve biopsy of patient with *n*-hexane neuropathy demonstrating a loss of large myelinated fibers and axonal swellings. (From Albers JW: Toxic Neuropathies. In Mancall EL [ed]: Neurotoxicology: Continuum 1999. Baltimore, Lippincott–Williams & Wilkins, 1999; 27.)

tions demonstrated progressive improvement in nerve conduction studies, with increased sensory and motor amplitudes.

This patient is representative of most reported patients who develop neuropathy after voluntary inhalation of glue or thinner containing *n*-hexane. Although some reports emphasize the prominent motor nerve findings, others document distal sensory abnormalities (Oh and Kim, 1976; Lalloo et al., 1981; Tenenbein et al., 1984; Kuwabara et al., 1993). Pure motor neuropathy would be inconsistent with the abnormalities reported on sural nerve biopsy. The symptoms of neuropathy may develop over weeks to months, often escalating or intensifying over time, as in this case. Continued progression for several weeks after cessation of exposure ("coasting") is typical of this and many other toxic neuropathies (Schaumburg and Spencer, 1984).

Nerve conduction abnormalities associated with *n*-hexane intoxication include reduced sensory and motor amplitudes and reduced conduction velocities, up to 40% of the lower limit of normal. This degree of conduction slowing is sufficient to suggest demyelination (Yokoyama et al., 1990; Smith and Albers, 1997). Other abnormalities, such as partial conduction block or abnormal temporal dispersion, commonly exist (Kuwabara et al., 1993; Chang et al., 1998), a finding supporting demyelination with superimposed axonal degeneration. Whereas demyelinating neuropathy is not commonly thought of as toxically induced, features of acquired demyelination were observed in the first two toxic neuropathies described in this chapter. *n*-Hexane neuropathy, like arsenic neuropathy, is another exception to the rule that toxic neuropathies are purely axonal (Sumner, 1980). In Case 2, the differential diagnosis included peripheral vasculitis, paraneoplastic disorder, chronic inflammatory demyelinating polyneuropathy, and *n*-hexane neuropathy. *n*-Hexane neuropathy was initially thought to be unlikely because of the patient's convincing denial of exposure. Support for a diagnosis of acquired demyelinating neuropathy included the electrodiagnostic findings and a slightly elevated cerebrospinal fluid protein level early in the course of the illness.

Sural nerve biopsy in *n*-hexane neuropathy demonstrates multifocal axonal distention with paranodal swelling and neurofilamentous masses that are sufficiently characteristic to suggest the diagnosis (Yokoyama et al., 1990; Chang et al., 1993; Kuwabara et al., 1993). The axonal swellings consist of neurofilament aggregates, which may accumulate because of abnormalities of axonal transport (Korobkin et al., 1975; Spencer et al., 1975; Griffin, 1981). Covalent interaction with lysyl residues causes cross-linking of axonal neurofilaments and disruption of axonal flow (Couri and Milks, 1985). Unlike arsenical neuropathy, in which the conduction abnormalities are thought to represent generalized axonal failure, the conduction abnormalities in *n*-hexane neuropathy are thought to represent secondary myelin sheath damage from focal axonal swellings. The electromyo-

graphic needle examination demonstrates evidence of superimposed axonal degeneration. Improvement follows removal from exposure, although conduction slowing and unobtainable responses may persist in patients with the most severe involvement. Abnormal spontaneous activity completely or partially resolves, and reinnervation is demonstrated by the presence of large-amplitude motor unit action potentials (Iida, 1982).

CHRONIC LOW-LEVEL EXPOSURE

Occupational exposure to *n*-hexane has been associated with a dying-back sensorimotor neuropathy, characterized by stocking-and-glove sensory loss, distal weakness, and absent ankle reflexes (Paulson and Waylonis, 1976; Ruff et al., 1981). Examples of pure motor or motor-predominant neuropathy associated with occupational hexacarbon exposure are unusual (Spencer et al., 1980; Lalloo et al., 1981). Herskowitz and associates reported three cabinet finishers who had prolonged occupational exposure to *n*-hexane (Herskowitz et al., 1971). These workers developed distal weakness, sensory loss, and areflexia, in association with moderate slowing of motor conduction velocities. This differs slightly from the motor greater than sensory neuropathy associated with acute, high-level *n*-hexane exposure, and it reflects a spectrum of findings based on the severity of neuropathy. For example, nerve conduction studies recorded from asymptomatic, hexacarbon-exposed workers may be normal or may suggest the existence of subclinical neuropathy in the form of mildly slowed motor conduction velocities (Buiatti et al., 1978), whereas symptomatic exposed workers demonstrate reduced motor and sensory amplitudes in addition to slowed conduction velocities (Oh and Kim, 1976; Scelsi et al., 1981). Evaluation of *n*-hexane–exposed printers who had symptoms and signs of sensorimotor neuropathy demonstrated a spectrum of electrodiagnostic abnormalities, ranging from reduced sensory amplitudes in workers with mild neuropathy to reduced motor amplitudes, decreased conduction velocities, and evidence of axonal degeneration in workers more severely involved (Chang et al., 1993).

The neuropathy associated with chronic methyl-*n*-butylketone exposure initially results in slowly progressive sensory impairment characterized by acral and pedal numbness with mild loss of touch, pin, and vibration sensations (Allen et al., 1975). Reflexes may be preserved, but ankle reflexes are usually reduced or absent. With disease progression, weakness and atrophy of intrinsic hand and foot muscles occur.

Trichloroethylene and Related Solvent Mixtures

Trichloroethylene is a chlorinated hydrocarbon with extensive use as a cleaner, solvent, and degreasing agent. It has been used in industry, in the home, and as a surgical anesthetic, including use as self-administered anesthesia (Waters et al., 1977). As many as 60,000 patients a year were estimated to have received trichloroethylene as an anesthetic agent, and the National Institute for Occupational Safety and Health reported that the total number of persons exposed to trichloroethylene may have exceeded 3.6 million in 1974 (National Institute for Occupational Safety and Health, 1974). Trichloroethylene also was used as a treatment for trigeminal neuralgia after it was found to produce relatively selective trigeminal mononeuropathy (described later). Trichloroethylene is primarily absorbed by inhalation, but it is also absorbed orally and through the skin. It is metabolized in the liver to chlorohydrate and, subsequently, to trichloroethanol and trichloroacetic acid, more water-soluble products that are excreted in the urine (Wells, 1982). Occupational exposure can be monitored by urinary excretion of these trichloroethylene metabolites (Jacobson et al., 1990).

Acute High-Level Exposure

Trichloroethylene has anesthetic properties, and acute, high-level exposure produces narcosis, altered consciousness, and respiratory depression. If the exposure is sufficient, respiratory depression produces hypoxia, hypoxic encephalopathy, and even death. When it is administered as an anesthetic, respiratory function is monitored and hypoxia is avoided. Trichloroethylene has been associated with multiple cranial nerve abnormalities, as reported by Feldman and associates and highlighted in Case 3.

Case 3

A 26-year-old man attempted to repair a degreasing machine that was used in a carburetor reconditioning shop (Feldman, 1999). He was unaware of necessary precautions, and he wore no protective equipment. Within minutes, he became lightheaded and dizzy, and he obtained an ill-fitting mask containing a potassium superoxide canister but no fresh air supply. He returned to his work, but after 90 minutes he became lightheaded, confused, and stuporous. He was hospitalized for somnolence, apathy, and difficulty in following commands. Over days, he developed numbness of the face and oral cavity, with difficulty in articulating and chewing. Examination at that time showed asymmetrical pupillary responses, impaired eye movements, asymmetrical ptosis, absent corneal reflexes, anesthesia to pinprick in a trigeminal nerve distribution, and weakness of facial and jaw muscles. Reflexes and extremity strength and sensation were normal. Difficulty in concentrating cleared over weeks.

Electrodiagnosis

Needle electrode nerve conduction studies showed abnormal facial nerve conduction. Blink reflex studies showed prolonged R1 latencies, well above the upper limit of normal.

Facial anesthesia improved over about 18 months, as did other symptoms and signs. Additional electrodiagnostic studies performed several years after exposure, however, showed evidence of sensorimotor neuropathy. Even 18 years after exposure, some abnormalities persisted, including malar hypalgesia, facial myokymia, and an asymmetrical pupillary light response with a tonic pupil.

This syndrome of multiple cranial mononeuropathies was reported by other investigators (Bauer and Rabins, 1977). Two of four trichloroethylene-exposed workers reported by Buxton and Hayward had ptosis, reduced eye movements, facial and bulbar muscle weakness, and findings of trigeminal nerve dysfunction (Buxton and Hayward, 1967). One of the four developed severe multiple cranial mononeuropathies and reduced reflexes. The syndrome of multiple cranial mononeuropathy also occurred when trichloroethylene was used for general anesthesia, a problem attributed by some investigators to a breakdown product (dichloroacetylene) that results from a reaction between trichloroethylene and soda lime (Selby, 1984). When contact with soda lime was avoided, trichloroethylene was regarded as a safe anesthetic agent (Mitchell and Parsons-Smith, 1969). Nevertheless, the effects of impure trichloroethylene on the trigeminal nerve were sufficiently predictable that it was used in the treatment of trigeminal neuralgia (Schaumburg et al., 1983).

The term *neuropathy* is used to describe the findings associated with acute trichloroethylene exposure. However, evidence of sensory or sensorimotor neuropathy is sparse, and *multiple cranial mononeuropathy* is a more appropriate description. The association of trichloroethylene and bilateral trigeminal mononeuropathy is unusual, and the trigeminal nerve is not a common neurotoxic target (Selby, 1984).

The pathological process underlying trichloroethylene-associated cranial nerve dysfunction is unclear. Necropsy examination of one of the patients with trigeminal dysfunction reported by Buxton and Hayward showed abnormalities involving the brainstem nuclei and tracts, the trigeminal nerve, and sensory roots (Buxton and Hayward, 1967). It has been suggested that the trigeminal mononeuropathy associated with trichloroethylene exposure is not a direct neurotoxic effect, but rather it reflects a chemically induced reactivation of latent orofacial herpes simplex virus (Cavanagh and Buxton, 1989).

Chronic Low-Level Exposure

Unlike the case with *n*-hexane, in which evidence of a dose-related neuropathy is well documented, the association of a clinically significant peripheral neuropathy after chronic, low-level exposure to solvents such as trichloroethylene or related solvents such as trichloroethane, perchloroethylene, mineral spirits, or similar solvents, alone or in combination, is controversial (Herskowitz et al., 1971; Spencer et al., 1975; Paulson and Waylonis, 1976; Scelsi et al., 1981; Iida, 1982; Maizlish et al., 1987; Bleecker et al., 1991; Chang et al., 1993). Existing descriptions are often uncontrolled, with some studies describing neuropathy and others showing no evidence of neuropathy. A distinction between clinical and subclinical neuropathy is not always clear, and this makes interpretation and comparisons difficult (Baker and Fine, 1986). To date, neuropathological and experimental animal studies are inconclusive or lacking (Spencer and Schaumburg, 1985; Seppalainen, 1986; Baker, 1994). The controversy over trichloroethylene-associated neuropathy reflects questions about trichloroethylene neurotoxicity in general, particularly in relation to the question of chronic solvent-induced encephalopathy. A common problem in any review of occupational solvent exposure relates to exposure documentation (type and amount). In most industrial settings, various solvents are available. In the review that follows, trichloroethylene is frequently identified, but it is by no means the only solvent in the studies.

Some studies identified mild neuropathies in 60% of 87 workers diagnosed with chronic occupational solvent intoxication (Seppalainen and Antti-Poika, 1983). Electrodiagnostic evaluations included conduction velocity measures, but no mention of amplitude, a sensitive indicator of axonal loss lesions. Limb temperatures were not described. Evidence of mild neuropathy was based on reduced conduction velocities, but there was no evidence of a dose-response effect, and termination of exposure did not influence the findings. In a comparison of 32 solvent-exposed persons with solvent-induced toxic encephalopathy with 50 unexposed control subjects, reduced sensory amplitudes were found for exposed persons, but quantitative vibration thresholds and motor nerve conduction study results did not differ between the groups (Orbaek et al., 1988). Sensory nerve conduction group differences were described as small, but they were thought to reflect mild axonal sensory neuropathy. However, only two persons had absent lower extremity reflexes, a finding making clinically significant neuropathy unlikely. Limb temperature and anthropometric features were not reported.

Other investigators reported significant correlations between increasing occupational exposure to mixed solvents and increased vibration thresholds (Bleecker et al., 1991). All findings were subclinical, and typical neuropathy symptoms were absent. The mild abnormalities consistent with neuropathy detected by Fine and associates in 16% of workers with occupational exposure to mixed solvents disappeared when multiple linear regression models controlled for the effects of age, sex, alcohol intake, and examiner (Maizlish et al., 1987). This study used conventional clinical criteria and quantitative sensory testing for detection of neuropathy, and it raised doubt about the presence of clinically significant polyneuropathy in association with occupational exposure to a mixed solvent.

The diagnosis of neuropathy is relatively objective and is not influenced by the numerous factors such as education, anxiety, and motivation that make examination of the central nervous system difficult. It therefore seems surprising that controversy exists over the presence or absence of neuropathy in association with chronic, low-level occupational exposure to solvents such as trichloroethylene. We therefore evaluated whether objective evidence of neuropathy existed among workers who had been diagnosed with solvent-induced toxic encephalopathy by either a neurologist or an occupational medicine physician, because these workers would be the ones most likely to have a solvent-induced neuropathy (Albers et al., 1999). Several of the workers, in fact, had been diagnosed with toxic neuropathy by the same physicians. All these workers were evaluated in the context of litigation related to solvent neurotoxicity. All these workers described long-term occupational solvent exposure, averaging 20 years (range, 10 to 29 years), and they all described solvent exposures that produced acute intoxication on a regular basis.

Among the 32 workers, only three fulfilled conventional clinical criteria for neuropathy. The single worker fulfilling nerve conduction criteria for neuropathy had diabetes mellitus, a common cause of neuropathy. Mean nerve conduction values for most measures were similar to control values. The few existing group differences among sensory amplitudes, similar in magnitude to those described in some previous reports, disappeared when compared with an unexposed worker control group matched by gender, age, and body mass index. Furthermore, nerve conduction measures were not influenced significantly by duration of employment or job title, two surrogates of exposure magnitude. After separation into groups based on the presence or absence of symptoms, previous diagnosis of neuropathy, disability status, and severity or type of encephalopathy, there still were no significant nerve conduction differences. Overall, there were neither clinical signs nor nerve conduction study findings of clinical or subclinical neuropathy that could be related to occupational solvent exposure. It was concluded that the complaints of these workers claiming neurotoxic injury from occupational solvent exposure were not explained by peripheral neuropathy.

Blink reflex latencies have been used to assess potential trichloroethylene neurotoxicity following occupational or environmental exposures. For example, Feldman and associates reported that average blink reflex latencies for a group of persons exposed to trichloroethylene through public drinking water were significantly longer than control latencies (Feldman et al., 1989). Not all similar evaluations have found comparable results. For example, examination of 31 printing workers with long-term solvent exposure at about the threshold limit value did demonstrate an equivocal reduction in mean sural conduction velocity compared with age-matched control subjects, but no abnormality of blink reflexes (Ruijten et al., 1991). We reviewed blink reflexes recorded from 51 workers with long-term occupational exposure to solvents including trichloroethylene who were diagnosed by others with solvent-induced toxic encephalopathy (an extension of the group of solvent-exposed workers described earlier) (Albers et al., 2000). No worker had evidence or a history of trigeminal mononeuropathy. All had normal R1 and R2 blink reflex latencies, and R1 latencies correlated significantly with several nerve conduction measures, findings suggesting that some of the intersubject variability reflected intrinsic conduction properties. Although all individual values were normal, the workers' mean R1 latencies were prolonged compared with historical controls, including gender-matched control subjects of similar mean age (11.2 ms versus 9.9 ms; $P < .0001$). This observation is similar to that reported previously by Feldman (1994). In our study, stepwise multiple regression models demonstrated significant associations of R1 latency with age and with the use of central nervous system–active prescription medications ($P = .003$). However, the duration (years) of solvent exposure did not enter into the regression models. Unexpectedly and somewhat paradoxically, workers using central nervous system–active medications had significantly shorter R1 latencies than those of workers who did not use such medications (10.9 versus 11.7 ms; $P = .01$). Job title, a potential surrogate of exposure, was not significantly related to reflex latencies. The overall results were inconclusive with regard to the use of blink reflex latencies to document suspected solvent exposure. They did not entirely exclude a possible relationship between subclinical blink reflex abnormalities and occupational solvent exposure. However, the small group differences in R1 latency between exposed and unexposed workers were of no diagnostic importance for individual subjects. It was concluded that the small differences likely reflected some confounders and technical factors that remained unrecognized in the study.

Organophosphorus Compounds

Organophosphorus compounds are used in a variety of industrial and commercial applications, including pesticides, hydraulic fluids, lubricants, fuel additives, plasticizers, and flame retardants. Organophosphorus pesticides exert their effects by inactivation (slowly reversible) of acetylcholine esterase, producing accumulation of acetylcholine at cholinergic synapses and inhibition of plasma butyrylcholinesterase (pseudocholinesterase) and red blood cell cholinesterase. Other nonpesticide organophosphorus compounds do not inhibit acetylcholine esterase. Organophosphorous pesticides are widely used to control a broad spectrum of insects in ag-

ricultural and urban settings (Koller and Klawans, 1979; Davis et al., 1985; Gutmann and Besser, 1990). They are absorbed across respiratory, gastrointestinal, and dermal membranes. Gastrointestinal absorption is rapid, with peak metabolite levels reached in hours; dermal absorption is slower, reaching peak levels about 24 hours after application. Butyrylcholinesterase inhibition is the most sensitive indication of organophosphorus pesticide exposure, and exposures that do not inhibit butyryl and red blood cell cholinesterase levels to less than 30% of baseline values are probably not associated with symptoms. Most organophosphorus pesticides require bioactivation in the liver to the active moiety. The bioactive oxon is inactivated by hydrolysis to products that no longer inhibit cholinesterase. These metabolites are excreted in the urine.

Accidental exposure to organophosphorus compounds occurs during manufacture and application, although organophosphorus poisoning as a result of accidental exposure is uncommon and serious examples are rarely seen (Gutmann and Besser, 1990). Because organophosphorus pesticides are readily available, intentional ingestion is a common means of attempted suicide, particularly in India (Wadia et al., 1987). Although exposures of the type described in this discussion are rare, the resulting neuropathy is one of the classic and best-studied neurotoxic disorders.

ORGANOPHOSPHORUS INSECTICIDE

Case 4

A 42-year-old man ingested an unknown amount of an organophosphorus insecticide (Lotti et al., 1986). On admission to the hospital, he was unconscious and required intubation for ventilatory support. He was treated with atropine to control muscarinic cholinergic signs, and he received pralidoxime (2-PAM), a cholinesterase reactivator. Plasma butyrylcholinesterase and red blood cell cholinesterase levels were markedly reduced when these levels were measured soon after the poisoning. Following a period of intensive care and respiratory support, he slowly recovered. Three weeks after admission, he was asymptomatic.

Electrodiagnosis

Nerve conduction studies before discharge were normal, including repetitive motor nerve stimulation studies. Shortly after discharge, however, he developed leg weakness and paresthesias. These symptoms were accompanied by weakness with impaired gait, diminished vibration sensation in the legs, and loss of reflexes. Repeat nerve conduction studies showed low-amplitude sensory and motor responses, with reduced motor conduction velocities, compared with the initial evaluation. The needle electromyographic examination showed fibrillation potentials in distal lower limb muscles.

Organophosphorus Pesticides

Acute effects of organophosphorus intoxication producing substantial cholinesterase inhibition include muscarinic overactivity characterized by miosis, increased secretions, sweating, gastric hyperactivity, and bradycardia, as well as central effects of anxiety, headaches, confusion, and sometimes convulsions during acute intoxication. Nicotinic overactivity produces fasciculations, muscle twitching, and weakness. Respiratory failure may result from weakness of respiratory muscles and airway obstruction, but there also is depression of medullary respiratory centers (Grob, 1963; Stewart and Anderson, 1968). Additional reports exist of unsuccessful suicide attempts using organophosphorus pesticides (Osterloh et al., 1983; Lotti et al., 1986). In patients with severe organophosphorus intoxication, butyrylcholinesterase cholinesterase activity is often undetectable or markedly reduced, and red blood cell cholinesterase inhibition may persist beyond 1 month after poisoning.

If the organophosphorus exposure is not fatal, the acute cholinergic effects of organophosphorus intoxication resolve, usually within several days, but occasionally longer (Lotti et al., 1986). As the acute cholinergic phase resolves, there may be evidence of prominent proximal weakness involving predominantly the head, neck, and proximal limb muscles. This reversible weakness represents an "intermediate" syndrome (Senanayake and Karalliedde, 1987). It develops 24 to 96 hours after acute organophosphorus intoxication during the initial recovery from the acute cholinergic phase. This syndrome likely represents a depolarizing blockade of neuromuscular transmission, similar to that seen in patients with myasthenia gravis who receive too much pyridostigmine, a rapidly reversible cholinesterase inhibitor. The weakness associated with the intermediate syndrome also resolves, usually within days.

Exposure to some organophosphorus compounds may be followed by rapidly progressive neuropathy that develops a few weeks after the acute exposure, as in Case 4. This neuropathy is referred to as *organophosphorus-induced delayed neurotoxicity*. Although it has been widely studied in laboratory animals (Capodicasa et al., 1991; Lotti, 1991; Richardson, 1995), organophosphorus-induced delayed neurotoxicity has only rarely been observed in humans. When it occurs, it is most common after massive organophosphorus exposure, sufficient to require intensive medical treatment and respiratory support and produce substantial inhibition of plasma butyrylcholinesterase and red blood cell cholinesterase levels (Moretto and Lotti, 1998). Such exposures typically occur in association with suicidal ingestion, as in Case 4. Organophosphorus-induced delayed neurotoxicity is thought by some investigators to occur more often with subacute or chronic organophosphorus exposure than after a single large dose (Senanayake and Johnson, 1982; Gutmann and Besser, 1990). Recovery, at times in-

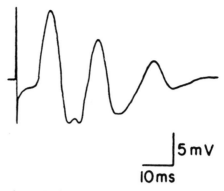

Figure 63–3. Repetitive discharges following the initial compound muscle action potential in response to a single supramaximal stimulation from a patient with acute organophosphorus intoxication. (From Gutmann L, Besser R: Organophosphate intoxication: Pharmacologic, neurophysiologic, clinical, and therapeutic considerations. Semin Neurol 1990;10:48, with permission of Thieme Medical Publishers, Inc., copyright © 1990.)

complete, occurs followed by spasticity, a prominent late feature resulting from corticospinal fiber involvement (Aring, 1942).

Electrodiagnostic abnormalities associated with organophosphorus intoxication depend on the amount of exposure and when the study is performed relative to the acute intoxication. Immediate abnormalities are similar to those associated with cholinesterase intoxication occasionally seen in patients with myasthenia gravis. When they are severe, one sees complete depolarizing blockade of neuromuscular transmission and absent motor responses. With less severe involvement, repetitive discharges are seen, again similar to those observed in patients with myasthenia gravis who are intoxicated by anticholinesterase medications (Grob, 1963). These repetitive discharges occur in response to a single depolarizing stimulus of the motor nerve (Fig. 63–3), presumably in association with recurrent depolarization of the postsynaptic end-plate by excessive acetylcholine, which produces a prolonged end-plate potential (Blaber and Bowman, 1963). In addition, persistent acetylcholine may interact with receptors on the terminal axon just distal to the last myelinated node (Gutmann and Besser, 1990). Activation of these receptors probably accounts for antidromic backfiring of the motor axon, thus producing spontaneous fasciculations; repetitive, spontaneous discharges to a single action potential; and perhaps repetitive discharges to a single supramaximal stimulus. The repetitive discharges are recorded with surface electrodes in response to a single stimulus. Each sequential discharge is of smaller amplitude than the preceding discharge.

With excess acetylcholine insufficient to produce a complete depolarizing blockade, there may be incomplete impairment of neuromuscular transmission. Partially impaired neuromuscular transmission results in a decremental response to repetitive motor nerve stimulation, analogous to the decrement seen in myasthenia gravis. The decrement is maximal between the first and second stimuli, and it is followed by stabilization or even a slight increase in the response amplitude toward the baseline response. The response in organophosphorus intoxication differs from that in myasthenia, however, because the decrement is most pronounced at high stimulation rates (Selevan et al., 1985). This decremental motor response is consistent with a partial postsynaptic neuromuscular blockade seen during the *intermediate syndrome* (Senanayake and Karalliedde, 1987; Wadia et al., 1987; Van den Neucker et al., 1991).

Electrodiagnostic studies of patients with severe organophosphorus intoxication demonstrate an initially severe block, a subsequent decremental response with repetitive discharges (during the intermediate syndrome), and later improvement of neuromuscular transmission. Figure 63–4 shows an example of this, with sequential repetitive stimulation studies (20-Hz median nerve stimulation) for a patient with organophosphorus intoxication (Selevan et al., 1985). The first recordings demonstrate an initial depolarizing block (day 3), followed by a decremental response and repetitive discharges to a single stimulus (day 4), and subsequent improvement (day 12).

In organophosphorus-induced delayed neurotoxicity, electrodiagnostic results are consistent with sensorimotor polyneuropathy characterized by axonal degeneration. Conduction velocity remains essentially normal, but motor and sensory response amplitudes are reduced. The electromyographic needle examination demonstrates evidence of severe dener-

vation characterized by fibrillation potentials and decreased recruitment (LeQuesne, 1978; Senanayake and Johnson, 1982; Van den Neucker et al., 1991). Neuropathological features of organophosphorus-induced delayed neurotoxicity include evidence of central and peripheral distal axonopathy; in peripheral nerves there is axonal degeneration of motor and sensory fibers, and in the central nervous system there is loss of corticospinal tract fibers and sensory fibers in the dorsal column nuclei (Cavanagh, 1954; Bischoff, 1967).

Much of what is known about organophosphorus-induced delayed neurotoxicity derives from experimental animal studies. Organophosphorus compounds producing organophosphorus-induced delayed neurotoxicity inhibit neuropathic esterase (neurotoxic esterase), the presumed target for organophosphorus-induced delayed neurotoxicity (Davis and Richardson, 1980; Lotti et al., 1984). Neurotoxic esterase is distributed in the central and peripheral nervous systems and binds to neurotoxic organophosphorus compounds, although the steps leading to axonal degeneration are not established (Johnson, 1974). The relative potency of an organophosphorus compound to cause organophosphorus-induced delayed neurotoxicity is a function of its ability to inhibit neurotoxic esterase by phosphorylation and then cause it to undergo "aging." This is the permanent alteration of neurotoxic esterase through loss of an alkyl group producing a negatively charged phosphorylated neurotoxic esterase (Van den Neucker et al., 1991). Organophosphorus compounds that inhibit neurotoxic esterase but do not age may cause organophosphorus-induced delayed neurotoxicity at high levels of neurotoxic esterase inhibition. Organophosphorus agents that inhibit neurotoxic esterase but do not age may protect against development of organophosphorus-induced delayed neurotoxicity if they are administered at low doses before the neuropathic organophosphorus compound. Nevertheless, this same compound, which provides protection by blocking the active site of neurotoxic esterase, is capable of initiating or promoting organophosphorus-induced delayed neurotoxicity if it is administered after the neuropathic compound.

Motor nerve recordings from asymptomatic workers who had subclinical organophosphorus exposures were reported to show low amplitudes and a decremental response even after single exposures (Jager et al., 1970). However, interpretation of these subclinical findings is unclear, given the absence of clinically evident weakness. Other studies of neuromuscular transmission under similar conditions of organophosphorus exposure, including single-fiber electromyographic studies, identified no abnormalities (Stalberg et al., 1978; Clarke et al., 1997).

A few reports of primary sensory neuropathy appearing in association with possible organophosphorus exposures exist (Kaplan et al., 1993), but none of the patients had acute cholinergic symptoms, organophosphorus exposures were not con-

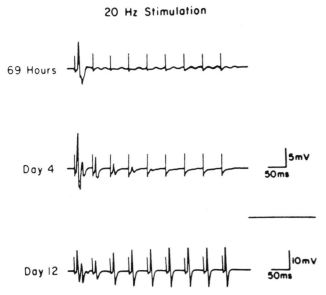

20 Hz Stimulation

69 Hours

Day 4 5mV 50ms

Day 12 10mV 50ms

Figure 63–4. Decrement-increment response to 20-Hz supramaximal median stimulation (recording thenar muscles) and repetitive compound muscle action potential discharges recorded from a patient with organophosphorus intoxication 3, 4, and 12 days after intoxication. (From Gutmann L, Besser R: Organophosphate intoxication: Pharmacologic, neurophysiologic, clinical, and therapeutic considerations. Semin Neurol 1990;10:49, with permission of Thieme Medical Publishers, Inc., copyright © 1990.)

firmed, and electrodiagnostic findings were equivocal. Furthermore, alternative explanations for the patients' symptoms were not well addressed. There are reports of impaired vibration sensation in exposed persons with documented cholinesterase inhibition compared with control subjects in cross-sectional studies (Steenland et al., 1994). Stokes and associates similarly attributed decreased vibration sensation to long-term organophosphorus exposure, as assessed by questionnaire (Stokes et al., 1995). These findings could represent mild sensory neuropathy, but in isolation they are of limited clinical importance. Although organophosphorus-induced sensory neuropathy has not been verified in subsequent reports, the question of potential sensory neuropathy was addressed by Morretto and Lotti (Moretto and Lotti, 1998). They confirmed that sensorimotor neuropathy can develop after severe organophosphorus poisoning. However, neuropathy developed only in patients with severe cholinergic toxicity occurring weeks before onset of neuropathy. In all identified patients, the sensory signs were less apparent than the motor signs, and sensory neuropathy was not identified in isolation. These investigators concluded that primary sensory neuropathy in the absence of cholinergic toxicity and motor involvement is inconsistent with the syndrome of organophosphorus-induced delayed neurotoxicity.

How do we reconcile the paucity of reports associating neuropathy with organophosphorus pesticide exposure given the widespread availability of this compounds? First, it is established that all organophosphorus compounds do not have equal neurotoxicity. It also is known that for available organophosphorus pesticides, organophosphorus-induced delayed neurotoxicity occurs only in the setting of severe intoxication, usually in relation to suicidal ingestion. In this context, the acute muscarinic symptoms are severe, and these patients require intensive medical care to support life. These are not casual exposures. Even in this setting, the world literature includes only a few documented patients with organophosphorus-induced delayed neurotoxicity related to pesticide exposure, most of them from Europe, where ingestion of pesticides is a common means of attempted suicide.

Triorthocresyl Phosphate

"Outbreaks" of organophosphorus-induced delayed neurotoxicity have been attributed to massive ingestion of *triorthocresyl phosphate,* a neuropathic organophosphorus compound. These outbreaks followed ingestion of adulterated Jamaican ginger extract in the United States (Jamaican ginger palsy, or "jake paralysis") or cooking oil contaminated by triorthocresyl phosphate in Morocco (Aring, 1942; Smith and Spalding, 1959). The neuropathy associated with adulterated Jamaican ginger was heralded by dysesthesias, followed by progressive weakness most prominent in distal muscles. In spite of subjec-

tive pain, other sensory symptoms and signs were minor unless the neuropathy was severe. Sensory loss did not occur in isolation. Reflexes were reduced at the ankles but were normal or brisk elsewhere. Recovery was often incomplete, and spasticity was a prominent feature, occurring long after the onset (Aring, 1942; Morgan and Penovich, 1978). The combined findings are suggestive of central and peripheral nervous system involvement. Organophosphorus-induced delayed neurotoxicity is uncommon in spite of the widespread use of organophosphorus pesticides.

Thallium

Thallium is a toxic heavy metal that was accidentally discovered by William Crookes in 1861 by burning the dust from a sulfuric acid industrial plant (Galvan-Arzate and Santamaria, 1998). It has industrial applications, including the manufacture of glass and optical lenses, semiconductors, scintillation counters, switching devices, and some fireworks; as a chemical catalyst and an insecticide; and in rodent control (Bank, 1980; Moore et al., 1993). It was banned as a rodent poison in the United States in 1972 (Desenclos et al., 1992). Like many neurotoxic substances, thallium has had medicinal applications, including past treatment of sexually transmitted diseases, tuberculosis, and ringworm (Bank, 1980; Windebank, 1993). At present, thallium isotopes are used in cardiac scanning (Moore et al., 1993). Thallium salts are water soluble and are readily absorbed across respiratory, gastrointestinal, and dermal membranes (Cavanagh, 1984). Following absorption, thallium is distributed uniformly throughout the body and is eliminated in the stool and in the urine (Bank, 1980). The pathways of absorption and excretion follow those of potassium, and it enters cells through potassium channels (Cavanagh, 1984). The toxic effects of thallium may be cumulative, because the elimination half-life of thallium is long, varying between 2 and 30 days, depending on the chronicity of ingestion (Moore et al., 1993).

Thallium poisoning most commonly involves intentional (suicidal or homicidal) or accidental ingestion of rat poison (Rangel-Guerra et al., 1990; Villanueva et al., 1990; Desenclos et al., 1992; Meggs et al., 1994; Kubis et al., 1997). Thallium poisoning has resulted from nasal insufflation of cocaine that had been adulterated with thallium (Insley et al., 1986). Industrial or environmental intoxication is uncommon, but intoxication has been reported after inhalation of contaminated dust from pyrite burners, in zinc and lead smelting, and in the manufacture of cadmium, as well as after dermal absorption through protective rubber gloves (Moore et al., 1993). An example of industrial intoxication was reported by Hirata and associates and involved a manufacturing company (Hirata et al., 1998). One worker who handled thallium-containing raw materials over a period of 4 years developed alopecia, abdominal pain, diarrhea, and paresthesias with signs of a stocking-and-glove neuropathy. A diagnosis of neuropathy from chronic thallium intoxication was considered probable, based on elevated thallium levels in hair. Nevertheless, the neuropathy was not characteristic of most descriptions related to acute or subacute thallium intoxication, as in Case 5.

Case 5

Over a period of 3 weeks, a 20-year-old man developed painful sensory neuropathy associated with diffuse alopecia (Kubis et al., 1997). On examination 6 weeks after the first symptoms, he had hypoesthesia of the distal limbs and distal weakness, but reflexes were normal. Electrodiagnostic testing showed mainly axonal motor neuropathy. Based on the combined findings, thallium poisoning was suspected, and this was confirmed by elevated thallium concentrations in plasma, urine, hair, and nails. The source of thallium was identified as rat poison.

In many ways, the early symptoms of thallium intoxication resemble those of arsenic poisoning. The neurotoxic effects of thallium are well documented (Bank, 1980; Windebank, 1993). The main neurological manifestation of thallium intoxication is mixed neuropathy, presenting in association with abdominal pain, nausea, vomiting, diarrhea, and alopecia (Herrero et al., 1995). Pain and paresthesias develop in the distal extremities within hours to days, followed by distal limb weakness or even quadriparesis and respiratory failure if the neuropathy is severe (Andersen, 1984; Cavanagh, 1984). The neuropathy presents as a painful stocking-and-glove sensory loss, with subsequent dysautonomia manifested as abdominal pain, constipation, urinary retention, and anhidrosis (Kalantri and Kurtz, 1988). Occasionally, distal weakness is present, but motor symptoms or signs are minor compared with the painful dysesthesias. In some patients, symptoms and signs of small-fiber neuropathy are apparent (Herrero et al., 1995). In these patients, pin-pain sensation is markedly impaired, and reflexes remain normal. Associated signs of cardiovascular autonomic neuropathy also are reported (Nordentoft et al., 1998).

Additional systemic manifestations include nephropathy, anemia, and hepatotoxicity, but the hallmark of thallium intoxication is alopecia developing several weeks after acute intoxication (Bank, 1980; Windebank, 1993). Some investigators believe that the combination of rapid, diffuse alopecia and neurological and gastrointestinal involvement is pathognomonic for thallium toxicity (Feldman and Levisohn, 1993). All patients with confirmed thallium poisoning (23 accidents, 21 suicide attempts, 5 homicides) reported by Rangel-Guerra and colleagues demonstrated alopecia (Rangel-Guerra et al., 1990). Mees' lines may also develop, but they are not apparent until alopecia is present (Passarge and Weink, 1965). Although they are important features, alopecia and Mees' lines are not diagnostically helpful in the immediate stages of toxicity, when the diagnosis is in question. In fact, early in the clinical course, the combined symptoms and signs are suggestive of Guillain-Barré syndrome. Preserved reflexes, at least initially, may be useful in differentiating thallium-induced neuropathy from acute sensory greater than motor Guillain-Barré syndrome. The differential diagnosis also should include one of the hepatic porphyrias, because the combination of abdominal pain, autonomic dysfunction, and progressive neuropathy is similar to abnormalities caused by acute porphyric neuropathy. Urinary excretion of porphobilinogen and δ-aminolevulinic acid is normal in thallium neuropathy (Bank, 1980). The basic neurotoxic mechanism of thallium intoxication is unknown, although thallium is believed to interfere with oxidative phosphorylation (Cavanagh, 1984). It also may interfere with the sodium/potassium–adenosine triphosphatase system, in relation to binding of sulfhydryl groups (Windebank, 1993). The prognosis for complete recovery is good, even in patients requiring prolonged therapeutic support, including mechanical ventilation (Vergauwe et al., 1990).

There are few electrodiagnostic descriptions of thallium-induced neuropathy and few electrophysiological studies of groups of workers with occupational exposure. Electrophysiological information in thallium intoxication is frequently untimely, limited in extent, and uninformative. Sequential evaluations of a victim of an apparent attempted homicidal poisoning exist (Kalantri and Kurtz, 1988; Dumitru and Kalantri, 1990). Ten days after the onset of symptoms, the plantar nerves in the foot showed profound axonal loss while the sural and peroneal nerves were essentially normal. The latter two nerves subsequently underwent a decline in response amplitude. All findings were consistent with axonal sensorimotor neuropathy (axonopathy), significantly worse in the lower extremities. Recovery required more than 2 years. Neuropathology in thallium neuropathy also demonstrates distal axonal degeneration with evidence of chromatolysis in dorsal root ganglion and anterior horn cells (Cavanagh, 1984). These combined findings are consistent with dying-back axonopathy involving sensory and motor nerves.

Lead

Lead is a widely used, nonferrous toxic metal that is ubiquitous in our environment (Fischbein, 1983). Lead is absorbed across respiratory and gastrointestinal membranes, and it is excreted in the urine. It has a long biological half-life, and about 90% of the total body burden is stored in bone (Conradi et al., 1982). The history of lead toxicity *(plumbism)* begins in ancient times, and it is intertwined with the development of industry in general and metallurgy in particular. Bone lead levels have increased since the beginning of the industrial revolution, and present-day bone samples contain about two orders of magnitude more lead than prehistoric human skeletons (Grandjean, 1978). Lead levels can be measured in blood and urine. Body stores can be measured indirectly in urine after chelation by Calcium Disodium Versenate (Whitaker et al., 1962). There are several measures of lead's effect on heme synthesis, and an elevation of free erythroporphyrin is thought to reflect altered iron incorporation to heme at the mitochondrial level. This produces microcytic, hypochromic anemia, with basophilic stippling of red cells (Baloh, 1974). Like porphyria, lead toxicity causes abnormal excretion of heme precursors (Moore et al., 1987).

Diet is a major source of lead, especially among children who ingest lead pigment–based paint (pica) (Anonymous, 1998). Leaded fuel was a major source of environmental pollution that decreased in the United States following the ban on leaded gasoline. Consumption of illicit whiskey made in lead-lined stills is a declining but continuing source of lead exposure (Ellis and Lacy, 1998). Occasional exposure derives from the use of glaze pigments in ceramic dishes or lead shot (Tavolato et al., 1980; Wu et al., 1995; Phan et al., 1998). Occupational exposures occur in association with smelting, reprocessing of lead-containing products such as batteries, demolition of lead-painted structures, manufacturing of paint pigments, and repair of automobile radiators (Conradi et al., 1982).

In addition to its neurotoxic potential, lead is a systemic poison with hematological, renal, hepatic, endocrine, cardiovascular, and reproductive effects. Acute intoxication causes abdominal cramps, constipation, and anorexia; chronic exposure results in a gingival lead line, weight loss, constipation, and anemia (Feldman et al., 1977). Lead intoxication in children may cause encephalopathy (Needleman et al., 1979). Anemia is a prominent finding, but anemia in a person with lead levels of up to 80 µg/dL should not be attributed to lead toxicity until other causes have been excluded (Froom et al., 1999).

Lead neuropathy is a complicated and controversial disorder, and most physicians never see a patient with lead neurotoxicity. Our current experience with lead neuropathy is anecdotal, much of it related to consumption of illicit whiskey made in lead-lined stills or reprocessing of lead-containing products. The classic picture of asymmetrical weakness with wrist or footdrop dates to the nineteenth century, when lead neuropathy was a conspicuous and frequent expression of plumbism (Beritic, 1984). This motor neuropathy typically is asymmetrical, involves upper extremities before lower, and shows preferential involvement of extensor muscles, a description atypical of other forms of neuropathy (Aub et al., 1925; Seto and Freeman, 1964). This weakness is not length dependent (Ehle, 1986). It is unclear whether the findings are explained by predisposition to local trauma or pressure, but some animal models have suggested a differential susceptibility of different nerve fiber populations, perhaps related to pref-erential entry of lead into different nerves (Bouldin et al., 1985). In humans, lead produces axonal degeneration, not demyelination (Ehle, 1986). Although examples of overt lead neuropathy are hard to find, consider the following case presentation, taken from the literature and purporting to represent neuropathy attributable to lead.

Case 6

A 25-year-old man worked for 2 years at a vinyl chloride resin factory where he was exposed to lead stearate, a stabilizer of resin (Kajiyama et al., 1993). Neurological examination revealed atrophy of small hand muscles, especially in the left dorsal interossei (his dominant hand). Sensation was intact, and there was no evidence of a generalized neuropathy.

Electrodiagnosis

Nerve conduction studies showed evidence of partial conduction block at the elbow, a finding indicating possible compressive mononeuropathy related to cubital tunnel syndrome. Within months following chelation therapy, the patient had progressive recovery of ulnar motor evoked amplitude, conduction velocity, and diminution of the conduction block at the elbow.

In this case, the differential diagnosis includes compressive ulnar neuropathy at the elbow or, given the normal sensory responses, a form of multifocal motor neuropathy. The coexistence of elevated lead levels was taken to indicate a potential relationship between lead intoxication and the mononeuropathy. Furthermore, it was suggested that lead intoxication made nerves vulnerable to mechanical trauma at sites of entrapment (Kajiyama et al., 1993). Yet in group comparisons of lead-exposed workers and controls, no differences were found among ulnar nerve conduction studies (Paulev et al., 1979). This example highlights the problems involved in determining the "cause" of the patient's problem. At present, overt lead neuropathy is considered a rarity (Beritic, 1984). There have been few studies of lead neuropathy using modern electrodiagnostic techniques, and between 1949 and 1989, fewer than 10 cases of lead neuropathy were identified among 3,500,000 new patient evaluations at the Mayo Clinic (Windebank, 1993). Based on evaluation of exposed workers, it seems certain that clinically overt neuropathy attributable to lead is essentially nonexistent in populations having blood lead concentrations below 60 µg/dL (Ehle, 1986). However, the advent of electrophysiology, instead of clarifying the issue, has provided conflicting and inconsistent findings with regard to overt and latent lead neuropathies, as described later (Beritic, 1984).

Subclinical Lead Neuropathy. The question related to the existence of a subclinical lead neuropathy has been difficult to assess, and the results have been controversial (He et al., 1988). Most studies have relied on electrodiagnostic evaluations of asymptomatic subjects who have industrial or environmental lead exposures. These predominantly cross-sectional studies have evaluated dose-response relationships between estimates of lead exposure or body burden and nerve conduction study results (Seppalainen, 1982; Beritic, 1984; Ehle, 1986). The reported findings show disparate results and include evidence of abnormal temporal dispersion or partial conduction block (Catton et al., 1970), slowing of motor or sensory conduction velocities (Feldman et al., 1977; Aashby, 1980), and preferential conduction slowing along the small motor nerve fibers (Bordo et al., 1982). Needle electromyographic studies are not frequently performed, but in severe cases, results have provided evidence of axonal degeneration, with abnormal spontaneous activity and mild abnormalities of motor unit action potentials (Seppalainen and Hernberg, 1972; Seppalainen et al., 1975). These changes may be present in some persons with systemic evidence of lead toxicity and blood lead concentrations higher than 80 μg/dL (Ehle, 1986). Selected studies are summarized in the following paragraphs.

In a comparison of 40 lead smelter workers and 50 nonexposed control subjects, few significant correlations were identified between blood lead levels and nerve conduction measures, and the few identified did not demonstrate a relationship with exposure duration (He et al., 1988). Conversely, comprehensive health surveys of 41 lead-exposed automobile workers and 31 control subjects showed that exposed workers had reduced sensory and motor conduction velocities, but the median motor conduction velocity was inversely associated with duration of exposure (Singer et al., 1983). Similar findings were reported after study of 202 5- to 9-year-old children living near a primary lead smelter (Landrigan et al., 1976). Among these children, 22% with blood lead levels higher than 80 μg/dL, a significant negative correlation was found between blood lead levels and motor nerve conduction velocity ($R = 0.38$; $P < .02$). None of the children had symptomatic neuropathy. In further analyses of these same data, the investigators confirmed that increased lead absorption caused slowing of nerve conduction in the absence of symptoms, but they also indicated that conduction velocity measures are an insensitive screen for low-level lead toxicity (Schwartz et al., 1988). Division of asymptomatic lead workers into groups with blood lead levels less and more than 30 μg/dL showed relative slowing of several nerve conduction velocities in the arms but not the legs, with the clearest difference noted in median nerve conduction velocities (Seppalainen and Hernberg, 1980). However, in all these cross-sectional studies, it is difficult to determine whether the effects are related to unidentified confounders or to lead exposure.

In general, it has been difficult to demonstrate evidence of subclinical neuropathy in subjects with serum lead levels lower than 60 μg/dL. Studies of subjects with this level of exposure have shown no significant changes in conduction velocity compared with unexposed control populations (Triebig et al., 1984), compared with the normal population conduction velocity range (He et al., 1988), or over time (Seppalainen et al., 1979). Evaluation of lead-exposed foundry employees with previous blood lead levels less than or equal to 90 μg/dL and unexposed workers found no characteristic weakness such as wrist extensor weakness, no gastrointestinal symptoms, and no sural nerve conduction abnormalities (Baker et al., 1984). Evaluation of workers with exposure for more than 9 years, whose blood lead concentrations were less than or slightly more than 70 μg/dL (the hygienic border value) failed to identify clinical evidence of neuropathy (Nielsen et al., 1982). Furthermore, quantitative sensory and electrodiagnostic evaluations were normal when compared with age-matched control subjects, findings suggesting that peripheral lead neuropathy is unusual when blood lead levels are kept to less than 70 μg/dL. It is not clear whether there is a threshold lead level, lower than which evidence of subclinical neuropathy does not exist. Studies have shown evidence of slowed conduction velocities among subjects with mean serum lead levels of 80 μg/dL (Aashby, 1980), 70 μg/dL (Seppalainen et al., 1975), and 50 μg/dL (Seppalainen et al., 1979). One study of lead-battery manufacturing workers that was designed to determine a "no effect" cumulative dose with nerve conduction measures concluded that a blood lead level of less than 40 μg/dL maintained for 1 year resulted in no significant effects on median or ulnar nerves (Chia et al., 1996). It is questionable whether small changes in conduction velocity, which are within the normal range, can be used to suggest subclinical lead neuropathy in an asymptomatic person (Catton et al., 1970). Furthermore, sural nerve biopsies, obtained from lead-exposed workers who showed slowed sural nerve conduction velocity, demonstrated no histological abnormalities, findings making it questionable whether the slight slowing of conduction in lead-exposed persons should be classified as subclinical neuropathy (Buchthal and Behse, 1979).

Similarities between the primarily motor neuropathy caused by lead and motor neuron disease (amyotrophic lateral sclerosis) have been noted, and a relationship between heavy metal exposure or occult plumbism and motor neuron disease has been questioned (Campbell et al., 1970; Roelofs-Iverson et al., 1984). Lead has been identified in some case studies as being weakly associated with some neurodegenerative diseases, including amyotrophic lateral sclerosis (Armon et al., 1991). This association is controversial and remains an unproven hypothesis, with many studies failing to confirm an association. Even if there is an association, this does not mean that lead caused the disorder. At present, the cause of most neurodegenerative disorders, such as amyotrophic lateral sclerosis, is unknown, although existing evidence suggests a multifactorial origin, as opposed to a single cause.

Acrylamide

Acrylamide is a vinyl monomer that polymerizes into polyacrylamide at high temperatures. It is used in soil grouting for stabilization, in waterproofing, and as a flocculator. Whereas polyacrylamide is nontoxic, it can be contaminated with acrylamide, particularly when it is used as a flocculator (Mulloy, 1996). The neurotoxicity of acrylamide is well described; it has been used in models of distal axonal neurotoxic injury. Acrylamide is taken up through oral, dermal, and respiratory absorption. It is water soluble and accumulates distally in nerves, where the initial disease is seen (Ko et al., 1999). Metabolism is via the cytochrome P-450 system to glycidamide, which is also neurotoxic; both substances are detoxified by conjugation with glutathione (Smith and Oehme, 1991). Because of these methods of metabolism and elimination, concomitant exposure to substances detoxified by glutathione or that induce the cytochrome P-450 system can increase acrylamide toxicity.

Acute acrylamide exposure produces dermal irritation and central nervous system disturbances, and chronic exposure causes signs and symptoms typical of axonal neuropathy. Peripheral signs include weakness, distal sensory loss, and areflexia, as well as autonomic dysfunction with excessive sweating (LeQuesne, 1985). Vibration sensation loss may be an early marker of neuropathy that correlates with the early involvement of fibers to pacinian corpuscles. As with other toxic neuropathies, subclinical abnormalities can be detected using quantitative electrodiagnostic and sensory measures (He et al., 1989; Myers and Macun, 1991, Deng et al., 1993).

The pathophysiology of acrylamide- and glycidamide-induced axonal injury is related to disruption of anterograde and retrograde axonal transport, with altered neurofilament transport and decreased delivery of neurotrophic substances to Schwann cells (Harris et al., 1994). Acrylamide and glycidamide also increase calmodulin-dependent protein phosphorylation, which also potentially interferes with axonal transport (Reagan et al., 1995).

Ethylene Oxide

Ethylene oxide is a reactive epoxide and potent biocide used in sterilization for heat-sensitive materials that is produced as a precursor to industrial chemicals (Gross et al., 1979; Windebank and Blexrud, 1989). It is readily absorbed across respiratory membranes. Ethylene oxide is water soluble and reacts in water to form ethylene glycol.

Ethylene oxide is neurotoxic to the central and peripheral nervous systems (Hollingsworth et al., 1956; Windebank and Blexrud, 1989), and there are reports of human toxicity following subacute (weeks) and chronic (months) occupational exposure (Gross et al., 1979; Finelli et al., 1983). In humans, the most common adverse neurotoxic effect of ethylene oxide exposure is neuropathy, occurring at exposure levels that do not affect other tissues (Windebank and Blexrud, 1989). Several cases of ethylene oxide–associated neuropathy have been reported. A representative example follows.

Case 7

A 27-year-old man who worked as a sterilizer operator for 2 years developed headaches, extremity numbness, and limb weakness (Gross et al., 1979). Examination showed distal sensory impairments, with slightly reduced pin-pain sensation and absent vibration at the toes and ankles, mild weakness of intrinsic hand and foot muscles, a wide-based gait, and absent ankle reflexes. The cerebrospinal fluid was normal.

Electrodiagnosis

Nerve conduction studies showed an absent sural response and low-amplitude peroneal response with mildly prolonged distal latency and moderately reduced conduction velocity. The needle electromyographic examination showed fibrillation potentials in intrinsic foot muscles. The findings were attributed to a generalized sensorimotor neuropathy of the axonal type.

It was discovered that this patient had been exposed for 3 weeks to a sterilizer that was leaking ethylene oxide. Following the patient's removal from exposure, subjective improvement was noted in weeks, corroborated by clinical and electrodiagnostic improvement. Repeat nerve conduction studies 10 months after the initial examination showed essentially normal results.

Chronic exposure of rats to ethylene oxide causes a primarily sensory neuropathy or neuronopathy of the axonal type (Nagata et al., 1992). Gross and associates reported three workers, in addition to the foregoing case, who also were exposed to ethylene oxide (Gross et al., 1979). In total, three of four developed peripheral neuropathy (symptomatic in two). The neuropathy was characterized by distal extremity numbness, weakness, and areflexia. Similar patients were reported by others (Finelli et al., 1983). In both reports, removal from exposure resulted in progressive improvement, and even patients with the most severe involvement demonstrated normal examinations, except for absent ankle reflexes (one patient) and difficulty in heel walking (one patient). Based on in vitro evidence of ethylene oxide neurotoxicity, Windebank and Blexrud suggested that residual ethylene oxide in dialyzers after sterilization may contribute to progressive neuropathy in patients receiving long-term hemodialysis (Windebank and Blexrud, 1989).

Electrodiagnostic studies of ethylene oxide–associated neuropathy are most consistent with distal axonopathy and secondary demyelination (Finelli et al., 1983). Abnormalities include low-amplitude responses, mild motor conduction velocity slowing (none slower than 80% of the lower limit of normal), and needle electromyographic evidence of positive waves and fibrillation potentials with polyphasic motor units. Abnormalities are most prominent in the lower extremities. Patients re-evaluated after removal from exposure demonstrate resolution or improvement in the amount of denervation potentials and increased motor unit amplitude, consistent with ongoing reinnervation (Finelli et al., 1983). As in Case 7, clinical signs and electrodiagnostic abnormalities vary among reported patients, findings likely reflecting differential exposures as opposed to differences in vulnerability.

Sural nerve biopsies from two workers who developed sensorimotor neuropathy in association with repeated exposures over 2 months showed axonal degeneration with mild changes of the myelin sheath (Kuzuhara et al., 1983). Unmyelinated fibers were also involved. Muscle biopsies showed typical denervation atrophy. The mechanisms of neurotoxicity are unknown, although some substance or substances produced in the cell body and transported down the nerve axon may be involved (Windebank and Blexrud, 1989).

Carbon Disulfide

Carbon disulfide has had widespread industrial application for over a century. It was initially used as a phosphorus solvent in match making, but it is now used in the production of viscose rayon fiber, cellophane, plywood, vulcanized rubber, and pesticides (Allen, 1979; Seppalainen and Haltia, 1980). Carbon disulfide can be absorbed by inhalation or skin contact (Allen, 1979). The mechanism of neurotoxicity is unknown, but it is associated with giant axonal swellings, similar to findings in several other toxic neuropathies (e.g., *n*-hexane neuropathy described earlier) (Schaumburg and Spencer, 1984). Absorbed carbon disulfide is biotransformed and excreted in the urine, where metabolites can be measured to document exposure (Seppalainen and Haltia, 1980).

Reports in the late nineteenth century described signs of encephalopathy, extrapyramidal dysfunction, and peripheral neuropathy after high-level occupational exposure to carbon disulfide (Lewey, 1941; Allen, 1979). Disulfiram (Antabuse) is metabolized to carbon disulfide and is associated with similar neuropathy (Olney and Miller, 1980).

Case 8

A 32-year-old man experienced insidious, progressive numbness and tingling in his legs; clumsiness and numbness of his hands; and weakness of his feet. When evaluated several weeks after the onset of symptoms, he demonstrated orthostatic hypotension, stocking-and-glove sensory loss, distal weakness with inability to walk on his toes or heels, and absent ankle reflexes. His only medication was disulfiram, which he had taken for many years to help to control alcohol abuse. He denied recent alcohol ingestion. Disulfiram was discontinued, but his symptoms progressed.

Examination 6 weeks later showed progression of neuropathy characterized by a wide-based, unsteady gait; bilateral footdrop; distal hand weakness; and absent ankle reflexes.

Electrodiagnosis

Electrodiagnostic examination showed absent sensory responses and absent or markedly reduced-amplitude motor responses in the legs. Motor conduction velocity was reduced, and distal latency was prolonged to about 90% of the lower and upper limits of normal, respectively. Although strict criteria for acquired demyelination were not fulfilled, this diagnosis was considered because some motor responses demonstrated abnormal temporal dispersion. Needle electromyographic examination showed profuse fibrillation potentials and positive waves and reduced motor unit recruitment in distal leg muscles.

Clinical improvement was first noted several months later, first in his hands. The sensation in his legs slowly improved, as did his strength. Examination several years later was normal, except for mild weakness and atrophy of the intrinsic foot muscles. Repeat electrodiagnostic evaluation at that time showed evidence of mild motor greater than sensory axonal neuropathy.

Development of fulminant neuropathy, such as that described earlier in association with industrial carbon disulfide exposure, is uncommon, with reports of carbon disulfide neurotoxicity attributed to chronic low-level occupational exposures (Allen, 1979). With such exposures, symptoms and signs of neuropathy often occur together with extrapyramidal symptoms and nonspecific neurasthenia (Vigliani, 1954; Seppalainen and Haltia, 1980; Peters et al., 1982, 1988). Symptoms suggestive of neuropathy include numbness and weakness of the lower more than upper extremities; signs include distal weakness, absent lower extremity reflexes, and impaired pinprick, touch, and vibration sensations (Schaumburg and Spencer, 1984).

Several studies support the association of neuropathy with occupational carbon disulfide exposure, with reports of workers whose findings were similar to those described in Case 8. For example, 10 of 16 viscose rayon plant workers, all of whom had at least 10 years of exposure to carbon disulfide, showed clinical and electrodiagnostic evidence of neuropathy (Aaserud et al., 1990). For seven of these affected patients, no cause other than carbon disulfide exposure could be identified. An outbreak of neuropathy involving nine workers in a viscose rayon factory was attributed to carbon disulfide exposure (Chu et al., 1995). These workers had overt neuropathy, with significantly reduced conduction velocities compared with asymptomatic coworkers and other controls. The neuropathies were related to higher concentrations of carbon disulfide in fiber-cutting areas, with peak exposures of 150 to 300 ppm and 8-hour time-weighted averages of 40 to 67 ppm. One worker with mixed axonal and demyelinating neuropathy had a sural nerve biopsy. His biopsy showed loss of large myelinated fibers, ongoing axonal degeneration, demyelination, and remyelination (Chu et al., 1996). After removal from exposure, he showed partial clinical recovery of strength over several years and improvement in serial nerve conduction studies.

In another report, only marginal abnormalities were found among workers with low levels of exposure to carbon disulfide, generally less than 20 ppm (Putz-Anderson et al., 1983). Furthermore, symptom prevalence was not consistently related to exposure levels. At higher exposure levels (up to 40 ppm), other investigators demonstrated slowing of lower extremity conduction velocity, a finding suggesting subclinical neuropathy (Seppalainen and Tolonen, 1974). Similar evidence of conduction slowing has been shown for carbon disulfide–exposed workers compared with unexposed control workers (Johnson et al., 1983). These small differences among asymptomatic workers are of questionable clinical significance. They are supported by a dose-response relationship between conduction velocity and cumulative carbon disulfide exposure, but such findings are potentially confounded by age effects.

Similar cross-sectional findings have been reported by other investigators (Corsi et al., 1983). However, in one study, re-examination of 12 subjects with neuropathy removed from exposure for 4 years showed no improvement in conduction velocity. This finding was interpreted as evidence of permanent axonal damage. This interpretation is suspect because conduction velocity measures are a poor reflection of the magnitude of axonal degeneration or regeneration, and the findings could have reflected pre-existing group differences unrelated to carbon disulfide exposure.

The overall clinical and electrodiagnostic findings associated with carbon disulfide exposure are consistent with mild, distal axonal sensorimotor neuropathy, characteristic of many toxic neuropathies. In laboratory animals, carbon disulfide exposure induces neuropathy characterized by ongoing axonal degeneration with paranodal and internodal swellings (Gottfried et al., 1985). The swellings appear to represent neurofilament accumulations, similar to those associated with *n*-hexane and acrylamide neuropathies. Recovery from carbon disulfide neuropathy may be slow and sometimes incomplete (Schaumburg and Spencer, 1984).

Unrecognized Toxic Neuropathies?

For as many as 20% of patients with clinical neuropathy, a specific cause is never established. Is it possible that some of these patients have a form of toxic neuropathy related to environmental exposures? Could these patients represent a subset of the population sensitive to some common environmental, industrial, or biological toxin? The answers to these questions are unknown. Certainly, most patients with undiagnosed neuropathy are elderly. Only recently has it been recognized that there is a difference between peripheral nervous system effects of "normal" and "successful" aging. The expected distal sensory loss and reflex loss associated with advanced age, though common, are not universal. Most investigators consider these changes a component of apoptosis or programmed cell death, perhaps influenced by a multitude of potential cumulative neurotoxic exposures. Most clinicians would likely agree with the observation that elderly persons who do not develop evidence of neuropathy are typified by overall good health. Conversely, elderly persons who are chronically ill, possibly with nutritional compromise, are more likely to demonstrate peripheral neuropathy. This statement represents an untested hypothesis, but, if correct, it would seemingly argue against some heretofore unidentified environmental toxin. Similarly, the absence of any credible evidence of regional or geographic associations makes it unlikely that some agricultural or urban pollutant is contributing to clinically significant neuropathy.

SUMMARY

Identification of toxic neuropathy associated with industrial or environmental exposure is an important but sometimes difficult task. The task is simplified by establishing reliable standards for identifying the presence and severity of neuropathy and establishing the underlying pathophysiology. Most chemically induced neuropathies are symmetrical, with a stocking or stocking-and-glove pattern of sensory and motor involvement. Large axons are commonly involved, and distal vibration sensory loss and diminished or absent reflexes are reliable early signs of neuropathy. Preserved ankle reflexes are incompatible with the diagnosis of clinically significant neuropathy, the only exceptions being isolated small-fiber neuropathies and some motor neuronopathies early in their course. Toxins are not common causes of either of these neuropathies.

The underlying pathophysiology of any neuropathy is investigated most frequently and most reliably using electrodiagnostic measures. Because most toxic neuropathies are characterized by axonal loss, evidence of reduced sensory or motor response amplitudes on nerve conduction studies and evidence of distal fibrillation potentials on needle electromyographic examination are among the most sensitive and reliable indicators of neuropathy. The most specific finding consistent with sensorimotor neuropathy is abnormal sensory evoked amplitudes; this localizes the lesion to the peripheral nervous system at or distal to the dorsal root ganglia. Findings suggestive of primary demyelination are considered rare in toxic neuropathy, although several toxic neuropathies, such as those associated with arsenic or n-hexane, produce nerve conduction findings suggestive of acquired demyelination and are particularly difficult to diagnose. The distribution and pattern of electrodiagnostic abnormality are also important. Toxic neuropathies are characterized by distal predominant and symmetrical abnormalities. Nevertheless, there is no electrodiagnostic finding specifically diagnostic of a toxic origin.

Clinical and electrodiagnostic findings of neuropathy should result in additional medical and laboratory investigations to identify systemic disorders associated with neuropathy or systemic findings associated with specific toxins. Individual responses to neurotoxic exposure occasionally differ, although these differences usually reflect the magnitude of exposure necessary to produce involvement rather than a difference in the type of symptoms or neurological findings. There may be substantially different neurological responses in the same person to increasing dosage. For example, low-level exposure may produce symptoms and signs of neuropathy, whereas higher exposures produce superimposed evidence of encephalopathy, coma, and even death.

The method described in this chapter is applicable to the evaluation of any patient with suspected neuropathy. The most important consideration is to use the results of the clinical and electrodiagnostic evaluations to develop an appropriate differential diagnosis. At times, a toxic explanation should be part of that differential diagnosis. Failure to consider the possibility of a toxic exposure makes it unlikely that such a cause will be identified unless it is accidentally "discovered" on the basis of an abnormal laboratory test or identification of another exposed person with a similar neuropathy. Realizing that the toxicity of an individual chemical cannot be predicted by chemical structure and recognizing that several forms of toxic neuropathy, particularly those related to medication use, may escape identification by conventional toxicology studies, the clinician must be alert to new agents that produce neuropathy. It would be unreasonable to presume that future medicinal, industrial, or environmental chemicals that produce neuropathy will not be introduced into society. Rapid identification of potential new syndromes will undoubtedly require recognition by some astute clinician.

ACKNOWLEDGMENTS

This work was funded in part by CSX Transportation, Inc. and a SPHERE (Supporting Public Health and Environmental Research Efforts) Award from Dow Chemical Company Foundation.

DISCLOSURE

We have at times been retained as consultants by firms or companies concerned with the manufacture or use of chemicals discussed in this chapter.

References

Aaserud O, Hommeren OJ, Tvedt B, et al: Carbon disulfide exposure and neurotoxic sequelae among viscose rayon workers. Am J Ind Med 1990;18:25.

Aashby JS: A neurological and biochemical study of early lead poisoning. Br J Ind Med 1980;37:133.

Albers JW: Clinical neurophysiology of generalized polyneuropathy. J Clin Neurophysiol 1993;10:149.

Albers JW, Bromberg MB: Chemically induced toxic neuropathy. In Rosenberg NL (ed): Occupational and Environmental Neurology. Boston, Butterworth-Heinemann, 1995; 175.

Albers JW, Cavender GF, Levine SP, Langolf GD: Asymptomatic sensorimotor polyneuropathy in workers exposed to elemental mercury. Neurology 1982;32:1168.

Albers JW, Kallenbach LR, Fine LJ, et al: Neurological abnormalities associated with remote occupational elemental mercury exposure. Ann Neurol 1988;24:651.

Albers JW, Wald JJ, Werner RA, et al: Absence of polyneuropathy among workers previously diagnosed with solvent-induced toxic encephalopathy. J Occup Environ Med 1999;41:500.

Albers JW, Wald JJ, Garabrant DH, et al: Neurologic evaluation of workers previously diagnosed with solvent-induced toxic encephalopathy. J Occup Environ Med 2000;42:410–423.

Allen N, Mendell JR, Billmaier DJ, et al: Toxic polyneuropathy due to methyl N-butyl ketone: An industrial outbreak. Arch Neurol 1975;32:209.

Allen N: Solvents and other industrial organic compounds. In Vinken PJ, Bruyn GW (eds): Handbook of Clinical Neurology. Amsterdam, Elsevier/North-Holland Biomedical Press, 1979; 361.

Altenkirch R, Mager J, Stoltenburg G, Helmbrecht J: Toxic neuropathies after sniffing a glue thinner. J Neurol 1977;214:137.

Andersen A, Ellingsen DG, Morland T, Kjuus H: A neurological and neurophysiological study of chloralkali workers previously exposed to mercury vapour. Acta Neurol Scand 1993;88:427.

Andersen O: Clinical evidence and therapeutic indications in neurotoxicology, exemplified by thallotoxicosis. Acta Neurol Scand Suppl 1984;70:185.

Anonymous: Lead poisoning associated with imported candy and powdered food coloring: California and Michigan. MMWR Morb Mortal Wkly Rep 1998;47:1041.

Aring CD: The systemic nervous affinity of triorthocresyl phosphate (Jamaica ginger palsy). Brain 1942;65:34.

Armon C, Kurland LT, Daube JR, O'Brien PC: Epidemiologic correlates of sporadic amyotrophic lateral sclerosis. Neurology 1991;41:1077.

Atchison WD, Hare MF: Mechanisms of methylmercury-induced neurotoxicity. FASEB J 1994;8:622.

Aub JC, Fairhall LT, Minot AS, Reznikoff P: Lead poisoning. Medicine (Baltimore) 1925;4:1.

Baker EL, Feldman RG, White RA, et al: Occupational lead neurotoxicity: A behavioural and electrophysiological evaluation. Study design and year one results. Br J Ind Med 1984;41:352.

Baker EL, Fine LJ: Solvent neurotoxicity: The current evidence. J Occup Med 1986;28:126.

Baker EL: A review of recent research on health effects of human occupational exposure to organic solvents: A critical review. J Occup Med 1994;36:1079.

Baloh RW: Laboratory diagnosis of increased lead absorption. Arch Environ Health 1974;28:198.

Bank WJ: Thallium. In Spencer PS, Schaumburg HH (eds): Experimental and Clinical Neurotoxicology. Baltimore, Williams & Wilkins, 1980; 570.

Barton EN, Gilbert DT, Raju K, Morgan OS: Arsenic: The forgotten poison? West Indian Med J 1992;41:36.

Bauer M, Rabins SF: Trichlorethylene toxicity: Review. Int J Dermatol 1977;16:113.

Beritic T: Lead neuropathy. CRC Crit Rev Toxicol 1984;12:149.

Bischoff A: The ultrastructure of tri-ortho-cresyl phosphate-poisoning. Acta Neuropathol (Berl) 1967;9:159.

Blaber LC, Bowman WC: Studies on the repetitive discharges evoked in motor nerve and skeletal muscles after injection of anticholinesterase drugs. Br J Pharmacol 1963;20:326.

Bleecker ML, Bolla KI, Agnew J, Schwartz BS: Dose-related subclinical neurobehavioral effects of chronic exposure to low levels of organic solvents. Am J Ind Med 1991;19:715.

Blom S, Lagerkvist B, Linderholm H: Arsenic exposure to smelter workers: Clinical and neurophysiological studies. Scand J Work Environ Health 1985;11:265.

Bordo BM, Filippini G, Massetto N, et al: Electrophysiological study of subjects occupationally exposed to lead and with low levels of lead poisoning. Scand J Work Environ Health 1982; 8(suppl 1):142.

Bouldin TW, Meighan ME, Gaynor JJ, et al: Differential vulnerability of mixed and cutaneous nerves in lead neuropathy. J Neuropathol Exp Neurol 1985;44:384.

Buchet JP, Lison D, Ruggeri M, et al: Assessment of exposure to inorganic arsenic, a human carcinogen, due to the consumption of seafood. Arch Toxicol 1996;70:773.

Buchthal F, Behse F: Electrophysiology and nerve biopsy in men exposed to lead. Br J Ind Med 1979;36:135.

Buiatti E, Cecchini S, Ronchi O, et al: Relationship between clinical and electromyographic findings and exposure to solvents, in shoe and leather workers. Br J Ind Med 1978;35:168.

Buxton PH, Hayward M: Polyneuritis cranialis associated with industrial trichloroethylene poisoning. J Neurol Neurosurg Psychiatry 1967;30:511.

Campbell AMG, Williams ER, Barltrop D: Motor neurone disease and exposure to lead. J Neurol Neurosurg Psychiatry 1970; 33:877.

Capodicasa E, Scapellato ML, Moretto A, et al: Chlorpyrifos-induced delayed polyneuropathy. Arch Toxicol 1991;65:150.

Catton MJ, Harrison MJG, Fullerton PM, Kazantzis G: Subclinical neuropathy in lead workers. BMJ 1970;2:80.

Cavanagh JB: The toxic effects of tri-ortho-cresyl phosphate on the nervous system. J Neurol Neurosurg Psychiatry 1954;17: 163.

Cavanagh JB: Neurotoxic effects of metal and their interaction. In Galli CL, Manzo L, Spencer PS (eds): Recent Advances in Nervous System Toxicology: NATO ASI Series. New York, Plenum Press, 1984; 177.

Cavanagh JB, Buxton PH: Trichloroethylene cranial neuropathy: Is it really a toxic neuropathy or does it activate latent herpes virus? J Neurol Neurosurg Psychiatry 1989;52:297.

Chang AP, England JD, Garcia CA, Sumner AJ: Focal conduction block in *n*-hexane polyneuropathy. Muscle Nerve 1998;21:964.

Chang CM, Yu CW, Fong KY, et al: *n*-Hexane neuropathy in offset printers. J Neurol Neurosurg Psychiatry 1993;56:538.

Chia SE, Chia HP, Ong CN, Jeyaratnam J: Cumulative blood lead levels and nerve conduction parameters. Occup Med 1996; 46:59.

Chu CC, Huang CC, Chen RS, Shih TS: Polyneuropathy induced by carbon disulphide in viscose rayon workers. Occup Environ Med 1995;52:404.

Chu CC, Huang CC, Chu NS, Wu TN: Carbon disulfide induced polyneuropathy: Sural nerve pathology, electrophysiology, and clinical correlation. Acta Neurol Scand 1996;94:258.

Chu CC, Huang CC, Ryu SJ, Wu TN: Chronic inorganic mercury induced peripheral neuropathy. Acta Neurol Scand 1998;98:461.

Chuttani PN, Chopra JS: Arsenic poisoning. In Vinkin PJ, Bruyn GW (eds): Handbook of Clinical Neurology, vol 36. Amsterdam, Elsevier/North-Holland Biomedical Press, 1979; 199.

Clarke EE, Levy LS, Spurgeon A, Calvert IA: The problems associated with pesticide use by irrigation workers in Ghana. Occup Med 1997;47:301.

Conradi S, Ronnevi LO, Norris FH: Motor neuron disease and toxic metals. Adv Neurol 1982;36:201.

Corsi G, Maestrelli GC, Picotti G, et al: Chronic peripheral neuropathy in workers with previous exposure to carbon disulfide. Br J Ind Med 1983;40:209.

Couri D, Milks MM: Hexacarbon neuropathy: Tracking a toxin. Neurotoxicology 1985;6:65.

Cranmer M, Gilbert S, Cranmer J: Neurotoxicity of mercury: Indicators and effects of low-level exposure: Overview. Neurotoxicology 1996;17:9.

Davis CS, Richardson RJ: Organophosphorus compounds. In Spencer PS, Schaumburg HH (eds): Experimental and Clinical Toxicology. Baltimore, Willians & Wilkins, 1980; 527.

Davis CS, Johnson MK, Richardson DJ: Organophosphorus com-

pounds. In O'Donoghue JL (ed): Neurotoxicity of Industrial and Commercial Chemicals, vol 2. Boca Raton, FL, CRC, 1985; 1.

Deng H, He F, Zhang S, et al: Quantitative measurements of vibration threshold in healthy adults and acrylamide workers. Int Arch Occup Environ Health 1993;65:53.

Desenclos JC, Wilder MH, Coppenger GW, et al: Thallium poisoning: An outbreak in Florida, 1988. South Med J 1992;85:1203.

DiVincenzo GD, Hamilton ML, Kapalan CJ, Dedinas J: Characterization of the metabolites of methyl *N*-butyl ketone. In Spencer PS, Schaumburg HH (eds): Experimental and Clinical Neurotoxicology. Baltimore, Williams & Wilkins, 1980; 846.

Donofrio PD, Wilbourn AJ, Albers JW, et al: Acute arsenic intoxication presenting as Guillain-Barré–like syndrome. Muscle Nerve 1987;10:114.

Donofrio PD, Albers JW: Polyneuropathy: Classification by nerve conduction studies and electromyography. Muscle Nerve 1990; 13:889.

Dumitru D, Kalantri A: Electrophysiologic investigation of thallium poisoning. Muscle Nerve 1990;13:433.

Ehle AL: Lead neuropathy and electrophysiological studies in low level lead exposure: A critical review. Neurotoxicology 1986; 7:203.

Ellis T, Lacy R: Illicit alcohol (moonshine) consumption in west Alabama revisited. S Med J 1998;91:858.

Eto K: Pathology of Minamata disease. Toxicol Pathol 1997;25:614.

Feldman J, Levisohn DR: Acute alopecia: Clue to thallium toxicity. Pediatr Dermatol 1993;10:29.

Feldman RG, Hayes MK, Younes R, Aldrich FD: Lead neuropathy in adults and children. Arch Neurol 1977;34:481.

Feldman RG, Niles CA, Kelly Hayes M, et al: Peripheral neuropathy in arsenic smelter workers. Neurology 1979;29:939.

Feldman RG, Chirico-Post J, Niles C, Proctor SP: Blink reflex as a measure of trichloroethylene exposure in individual and population studies Neurology 1989;39(suppl 1):181.

Feldman RG: Occupational exposure to trichloroethylene: Controversies concerning neurotoxicity. In Mehlman MA, Upton A (eds): The Identification and Control of Environmental and Occupational Disease. Princeton, NJ, Princeton Scientific, 1994.

Feldman RG: Trichloroethylene. In Occupational and Environmental Neurotoxicology. Philadelphia, Lippincott-Raven, 1999; 189.

Finelli PF, Morgan TF, Yaar I, Granger CV: Ethylene oxide–induced polyneuropathy: A clinical and electrophysiologic study. Arch Neurol 1983;40:419.

Fischbein A: Environmental and occupational lead exposure. Environ Occup Med 1983;57:433.

Froom P, Kristal-Boneh E, Benbassat J, et al: Lead exposure in battery-factory workers is not associated with anemia. J Occup Environ Med 1999;41:120.

Galvan-Arzate S, Santamaria A: Thallium toxicity. Toxicol Lett 1998;99:1.

Gherardi RK, Chariot P, Vanderstigel M, et al: Organic arsenic-induced Guillain-Barré syndrome due to melarsoprol: A clinical, electrophysiological, and pathological study. Muscle Nerve 1990;13:637.

Gottfried MR, Graham DG, Morgan M, et al: The morphology of carbon disulfide neurotoxicity. Neurotoxicology 1985;6:89.

Grandjean P: Widening perspectives of lead toxicity: A review of health effects of lead exposure in adults. Environ Res 1978; 17:303.

Greenberg SA: Acute demyelinating polyneuropathy with arsenic ingestion. Muscle Nerve 1996;19:1611.

Griffin JW: Hexacarbon neurotoxicity. Neurobehav Toxicol Teratol 1981;3:437.

Grob D: Anticholinesterase intoxication in man and its treatment. In Koelle GB (ed): Cholinesterase and Anticholinesterase Agents: Handbuch der Experimentellen Pharmakologie, vol 15. Berlin, Springer-Verlag, 1963; 989.

Gross JA, Haas ML, Swift TR: Ethylene oxide neurotoxicity: Report of four cases and review of the literature. Neurology 1979; 29:978.

Gutmann L, Besser R: Organophosphate intoxication: Pharmacologic, neurophysiologic, clinical, and therapeutic considerations. Semin Neurol 1990;10:46.

Harris CH, Gulati AK, Friedman MA, Sickles DW: Toxic neurofilamentous axonopathies and fast axonal transport. V. Reduced bidirectional vesicle transport in cultured neurons by acrylamide and glycidamide. J Toxicol Environ Health 1994;42:343.

He FS, Zhang SL, Li G, et al: An electroneurographic assessment of subclinical lead neurotoxicity. Int Arch Occup Environ Health 1988;61:141.

He FS, Zhang SL, Wang HL, et al: Neurological and electroneuromyographic assessment of the adverse effects of acrylamide on occupationally exposed workers. Scand J Work Environ Health 1989;15:125.

Heaven R, Duncan M, Vukelja SJ: Arsenic intoxication presenting with macrocytosis and peripheral neuropathy, without anemia. Acta Haematol 1994;92:142.

Herrero F, Fernandez E, Gomez J, et al: Thallium poisoning presenting with abdominal colic, paresthesia, and irritability. J Toxicol Clin Toxicol 1995;33:261.

Herskowitz A, Ishii N, Schaumburg HH: n-Hexane neuropathy: A syndrome occurring as a result of industrial exposure. N Engl J Med 1971;285:82.

Heyman A, Pfeiffer JB, Willett RW, Taylor HM: Peripheral neuropathy caused by arsenic intoxication. N Engl J Med 1956;254:401.

Hill AB: The environment and disease: Association or causation? Proc R Soc Med 1965;58:295.

Hirata M, Taoda K, Ono-Ogasawara M, et al: A probable case of chronic occupational thallium poisoning in a glass factory. Ind Health 1998;36:300.

Hollingsworth RL, Rowe UK, Oyen F: Toxicity of ethylene oxide determined on experimental animals. Arch Ind Health 1956;13:217.

Iida M: Neurophysiological studies in n-hexane polyneuropathy in the sandal factory. Electroencephalogr Clin Neurophysiol 1982;36(suppl):671.

Insley BM, Grufferman S, Ayliffe HE: Thallium poisoning in cocaine abusers. Am J Emerg Med 1986;4:545.

Jacobson JL, Jacobson SW, Humphrey HEB: Effects of in utero exposure to polychlorinated biphenyls and related contaminants on cognitive functioning in young children. J Pediatr 1990;116:38.

Jager KW, Roberts DV, Wilson A: Neuromuscular function in pesticide workers. Br J Ind Med 1970;27:273.

Jenkins RB: Inorganic arsenic and the nervous system. Brain 1966;89:479.

Johnson BL, Boyd J, Burg JR, et al: Effects on the peripheral nervous system of workers' exposure to carbon disulfide. Neurotoxicology 1983;4:53.

Johnson MK: The primary biochemical lesion leading to the delayed neurotoxic effects of some organophosphorus esters. J Neurochem 1974;23:785.

Kajiyama K, Doi R, Sawada J, et al: Significance of subclinical entrapment of nerves in lead neuropathy. Environ Res 1993;60:248.

Kalantri A, Kurtz E: Electrodiagnosis in thallium toxicity: A case report [Abstract]. Muscle Nerve 1988;11:968A.

Kaplan JG, Rosenberg NL, Pack D, Schaumburg HH: Sensory neuropathy associated with Dursban (chlorpyrifos) exposure. Neurology 1993;43:2193.

Ko MH, Chen WP, Lin-Shiau SY, Hsieh ST: Age-dependent acrylamide neurotoxicity in mice: Morphology, physiology, and function. Exp Neurol 1999;158:37.

Koller WC, Klawans HL: Organophosphorus intoxication. In Vinken PJ, Bruyn GW (eds): Handbook of Clinical Neurology, vol 37. Amsterdam, North Holland, 1979; 541.

Korobkin R, Asbury AK, Sumner AJ, Nielsen SL: Glue-sniffing neuropathy. Arch Neurol 1975;32:158.

Kubis N, Talamon C, Smadja D, Said G: Peripheral neuropathy caused by thallium poisoning. Rev Neurol (Paris) 1997;153:599.

Kuwabara S, Nakajima M, Tsuboi Y, Hirayama K: Multifocal conduction block in n-hexane neuropathy. Muscle Nerve 1993;16:1416.

Kuwabara S, Kai MR, Nagase H, Hattori T: n-Hexane neuropathy caused by addictive inhalation: clinical and electrophysiological features. Eur Neurol 1999;41:163.

Kuzuhara S, Kanazawa I, Nakanishi T, Egashira T: Ethylene oxide polyneuropathy. Neurology 1983;33:377.

Lagerkvist BJ, Zetterlund B: Assessment of exposure to arsenic among smelter workers: A five-year follow-up. Am J Ind Med 1994;25:477.

Lalloo M, Cosnett JE, Moosa A: Benzine-sniffing neuropathy. S Afr Med J 1981;59:522.

Landrigan PJ, Baker EL Jr, Feldman RG, et al: Increased lead absorption with anemia and slowed nerve conduction in children near a lead smelter. J Pediatr 1976;89:904.

Landrigan PJ: Arsenic: State of the art. Am J Ind Med 1981;2:5.

LeQuesne PM: Neuropsychological investigations of subclinical and minimal toxic neuropathies. Muscle Nerve 1978;1:392.

LeQuesne PM: Clinical and morphological findings in acrylamide toxicity. Neurotoxicology 1985;6:17.

Lewey FH: Neurological, medical, and biochemical signs and symptoms indicating chronic industrial carbon disulfide absorption. Ann Intern Med 1941;15:869.

Lotti M, Becker CE, Aminoff MJ: Organophosphate polyneuropathy: Pathogenesis and prevention. Neurology 1984;34:658.

Lotti M, Moretto A, Zoppellari R, et al: Inhibition of lymphocytic neuropathy target esterase predicts the development of organophosphate-induced delayed polyneuropathy. Arch Toxicol 1986;59:176.

Lotti M: The pathogenesis of organophosphate polyneuropathy. Crit Rev Toxicol 1991;21:465.

Maizlish NA, Fine LJ, Albers JW, et al: A neurological evaluation of workers exposed to mixtures of organic solvents. Br J Ind Med 1987;44:14.

Manzo L, Blum K, Sabbioni E: Neurotoxicity of selected metals. In Blum K, Manzo L (eds): Neurotoxicology. New York, Marcel Dekker, 1985; 385.

Meggs WJ, Hoffman RS, Shih RD, et al: Thallium poisoning from maliciously contaminated food. J Toxicol Clin Toxicol 1994;32:723.

Mitchell ABS, Parsons-Smith BG: Trichloroethylene neuropathy. BMJ 1969;1:422.

Moore D, House I, Dixon A: Thallium poisoning: Diagnosis may be elusive but alopecia is the clue. BMJ 1993;306:1527.

Moore MR, McColl KEL, Rimington C, Goldberg SA: Disorders of Porphyrin Metabolism. New York, Plenum Medical, 1987; 18.

Moretto A, Lotti M: Poisoning by organophosphorus insecticides and sensory neuropathy. J Neurol Neurosurg Psychiatry 1998;64:463.

Morgan JP, Penovich P: Jamaica ginger paralysis. Arch Neurol 1978;35:530.

Mulloy KB: Two case reports of neurological disease in coal mine preparation plant workers. Am J Ind Med 1996;30:56.

Myers JE, Macun I: Acrylamide neuropathy in a South African factory: An epidemiologic investigation. Am J Ind Med 1991;19:487.

Nagata H, Ohkoshi N, Kanazawa I, et al: Rapid axonal transport velocity is reduced in experimental ethylene oxide neuropathy. Mol Chem Neuropathol 1992;17:209.

National Institute for Occupational Safety and Health: National Occupational Hazards Survey, vol 1. Washington, DC, US Department of Health, Education and Welfare, 1974; 74.

Needleman HL, Gunnoe C, Leviton A: Deficits in psychologic and classroom performance of children with elevated dentine lead levels. N Engl J Med 1979;300:689.

Nielsen CJ, Nielsen VK, Kirkby H, Gyntelberg F: Absence of peripheral neuropathy in long-term lead-exposed subjects. Acta Neurol Scand 1982;65:241.

Nordentoft T, Andersen EB, Mogensen PH: Initial sensorimotor and delayed autonomic neuropathy in acute thallium poisoning. Neurotoxicology 1998;19:421.

O'Donoghue JL, Krasavage WJ: Identification and characterization of methyl N-butyl ketone neurotoxicity in laboratory animals. In Spencer PS, Schaumburg HH (eds): Experimental and Clinical Neurotoxicology. Baltimore, Williams & Wilkins, 1980; 856.

Oh SJ, Kim JM: Giant axonal swelling in "huffer's" neuropathy. Arch Neurol 1976;33:583.

Oh SJ: Electrophysiological profile in arsenic neuropathy. J Neurol Neurosurg Psychiatry 1991;54:1103.

Olney RK, Miller RG: Peripheral neuropathy associated with disulfiram administration. Muscle Nerve 1980;3:172.

Orbaek P, Rosen I, Svensson K: Electroneurographic findings in patients with solvent induced central nervous system dysfunction. Br J Ind Med 1988;45:409.

Osterloh J, Lotti M, Pond SM: Toxicologic studies in a fatal overdose of 2,4-D, MCPP, and chlorpyrifos. J Anal Toxicol 1983;7:125.

Pamphlett R, Waley P: Motor neuron uptake of low dose inorganic mercury. J Neurol Sci 1996;135:63.

Pamphlett R, Waley P: Mercury in human spinal motor neurons. Acta Neuropathol (Berl) 1998;96:515.

Passarge C, Weick HH: [Polyneuritis due to thallium.] Fortschr Neurol Psychiatr Grenzgeb 1965;33:477.

Paulev PE, Gry C, Dossing M: Motor nerve conduction velocity in asymptomatic lead workers. Int Arch Occup Environ Health 1979;43:37.

Paulson GW, Waylonis GW: Polyneuropathy due to n-hexane. Arch Intern Med 1976;136:880.

Peters HA, Levine RL, Matthews CG, et al: Carbon disulfide–induced neuropsychiatric changes in grain storage workers. Am J Ind Med 1982;3:373.

Peters HA, Levine RL, Matthews CG, Chapman LJ: Extrapyramidal and other neurologic manifestations associated with carbon disulfide fumigant exposure. Arch Neurol 1988;45:537.

Phan TG, Estell J, Duggin G, et al: Lead poisoning from drinking Kombucha tea brewed in a ceramic pot. Med J Aust 1998;169:644.

Poklis A, Saady JJ: Arsenic poisoning: Acute or chronic? Suicide or murder? Am J Forensic Med Pathol 1990;11:226.

Politis MJ, Schaumburg HH, Spencer PS: Neurotoxicity of selected chemicals. In Spencer PS, Schaumburg HH (eds): Experimental and Clinical Neurotoxicology. Baltimore, Williams & Wilkins, 1980; 613.

Putz-Anderson V, Albright BE, Lee ST, et al: A behavioral examination of workers exposed to carbon disulfide. Neurotoxicology 1983;4:67.

Rangel-Guerra R, Martinez HR, Villarreal HJ: Thallium poisoning: Experience with 50 patients. Gac Med Mex 1990;126:487.

Reagan KE, Wilmarth KR, Friedman MA, Abou-Donia MB: In vitro calcium and calmodulin-dependent kinase-mediated phosphorylation of rat brain and spinal cord neurofilament proteins is increased by glycidamide administration. Brain Res 1995;671:12.

Richardson RJ: Assessment of the neurotoxic potential of chlorpyrifos relative to other organophosphorus compounds: A critical review of the literature. J Toxicol Environ Health 1995;44:135.

Roelofs-Iverson RA, Mulder DW, Elveback LR: ALS and heavy metals: A pilot case-control study. Neurology 1984;34:393.

Ruff RL, Petito CK, Acheson LS: Neuropathy associated with chronic low level exposure to n-hexane. Clin Toxicol 1981;18:515.

Ruijten MW, Verberk MM, Salle HJ: Nerve function in workers with long term exposure to trichloroethene. Br J Ind Med 1991;48:87.

Scelsi R, Poggi P, Fera L, Gonella G: Industrial neuropathy due to n-hexane: Clinical and morphological findings in three cases. Clin Toxicol 1981;18:1387.

Schaumburg HH, Spencer PS, Thomas PK: Toxic neuropathy: Occupational, biological and environmental agents. In Schaumburg HH, Spencer PS, Thomas PK (eds): Disorders of Peripheral Nerves. Philadelphia, FA Davis, 1983; 131.

Schaumburg HH, Spencer PS: Human toxic neuropathy due to industrial agents. In Dyck PJ, Thomas PK, Lambert EH, Bunge R (eds): Peripheral Neuropathy, 2nd ed. Philadelphia, WB Saunders, 1984; 2115.

Schwartz J, Landrigan PJ, Feldman RG, et al: Threshold effect in lead-induced peripheral neuropathy. J Pediatr 1988;112:12.

Selby G: Diseases of the fifth cranial nerve. In Dyck PJ, Thomas PK, Lambert EH, Bunge R (eds): Peripheral Neuropathy, 2nd ed. Philadelphia, WB Saunders, 1984; 1224.

Selevan SG, Lindbohm M-L, Hornung RW, Hemminki K: A study of occupational exposure to antineoplastic drugs and fetal loss in nurses. N Engl J Med 1985;313:1173.

Senanayake N, Johnson MK: Acute polyneuropathy after poisoning by a new organophosphate insecticide. N Engl J Med 1982;306:155.

Senanayake N, Karalliedde L: Neurotoxic effects of organophosphorus insecticides. N Engl J Med 1987;316:761.

Seppalainen AM, Hernberg S: Sensitive technique for detecting subclinical lead neuropathy. Br J Ind Med 1972;29:443.

Seppalainen AM, Tolonen M: Neurotoxicity of long term exposure to carbon disulfide in the viscose rayon industry: A neurophysiological study. Work Environ Health 1974;11:145.

Seppalainen AM, Tola S, Hernberg S, Kock B: Subclinical neuropathy at "safe" levels of lead exposure. Arch Environ Health 1975;30:180.

Seppalainen AM, Hernberg S, Kock B: Relationship between lead levels and nerve conduction velocities. Neurotoxicology 1979;1:313.

Seppalainen AM, Haltia M: Carbon disulfide. In Spencer PS, Schaumburg HH (eds): Experimental and Clinical Neurotoxicology. Baltimore, Williams & Wilkins, 1980; 356.

Seppalainen AM, Hernberg S: Subclinical lead neuropathy. Am J Ind Med 1980;1:413.

Seppalainen AM: Lead poisoning: Neurophysiological aspects. Occup Neurol 1982;66:177.

Seppalainen AM, Antti-Poika M: Time course of electrophysiological findings for patients with solvent poisoning: A descriptive study. Scand J Work Environ Health 1983;9:15.

Seppalainen AM: Neurotoxicity of organic solvents in occupational exposure. Scand J Work Environ Health 1986;11(Suppl):61.

Seto DSY, Freeman JM: Lead neuropathy in childhood. Am J Dis Child 1964;107:337.

Sexton GB, Gowdey CW: Relation between thiamine and arsenical toxicity. Arch Dermatol Syphilol 1963;56:634.

Singer R, Valciukas JA, Lilis R: Lead exposure and nerve conduction velocity: The differential time course of sensory and motor nerve effects. Neurotoxicology 1983;4:193.

Smith AG, Albers JW: n-Hexane neuropathy due to rubber cement sniffing. Muscle Nerve 1997;20:1445.

Smith EA, Oehme FW: Acrylamide and polyacrylamide: A review of production, use, environmental fate and neurotoxicity. Rev Environ Health 1991;9:215.

Smith HV, Spalding JMK: Outbreak of paralysis in Morocco due to ortho-cresyl phosphate poisoning. Lancet 1959;2:1019.

Spencer PS, Schaumburg HH, Raleigh RL, Terhaar CJ: Nervous system degeneration produced by the industrial solvent methyl N-butyl ketone. Arch Neurol 1975;32:219.

Spencer PS, Schaumburg HH, Sabri MI, Veronesi B: The enlarging view of hexacarbon neurotoxicity. In DiVincenzo GD (ed): CRC Critical Reviews in Toxicology. Boca Raton, FL, CRC, 1980; 279.

Spencer PS, Schaumburg HH: Organic solvent neurotoxicity: Facts and research needs. Scand J Work Environ Health 1985;11(suppl 1):53.

Stalberg E, Hilton-Brown P, Kolmodin-Hedman B, et al: Effect of occupational exposure to organophosphorus insecticides on neuromuscular function. Scand J Work Environ Health 1978;4:255.

Steenland K, Jenkins B, Ames RG, et al: Chronic neurological sequelae to organophosphate pesticide poisoning. Am J Public Health 1994;84:731.

Stewart WG, Anderson EA: Effect of a cholinesterase inhibitor when injected into the medulla of the rabbit. J Pharmacol Exp Ther 1968;162:309.

Stokes L, Stark A, Marshall E, Narang A: Neurotoxicity among pesticide applicators exposed to organophosphates. Occup Environ Med 1995;52:648.

Sumner AJ: Physiological consequences of distal axonopathy. In Spencer PS, Schaumburg HH (eds): Experimental and Clinical Neurotoxicology. Baltimore, Williams & Wilkins, 1980; 220.

Taubes G: Epidemiology faces its limits. Science 1995;269:164.

Tavolato B, Licandro AC, Argentiero V: Lead polyneuropathy of nonindustrial origin. Eur Neurol 1980;19:273.

Tay CH, Seah CS: Arsenic poisoning from anti-asthmatic herbal preparations. Med J Aust 1975;2:424.

Tenenbein M, deGroot W, Rajani KR: Peripheral neuropathy following intentional inhalation of naphtha fumes. Can Med Assoc J 1984;131:1077.

Triebig G, Weltle D, Valentin H: Investigations on neurotoxicity of chemical substances at the workplace. V. Determination of the motor and sensory nerve conduction velocity in persons occupationally exposed to lead. Int Arch Occup Environ Health 1984;53:189.

Van den Neucker K, Vanderstraeten G, De Muynck M, De Wilde V: The neurophysiologic examination in organophosphate ester poisoning: Case report and review of the literature. Electromyogr Clin Neurophysiol 1991;31:507.

Vergauwe PL, Knockaert DC, Van Tittelboom TJ: Near fatal subacute thallium poisoning necessitating prolonged mechanical ventilation. Am J Emerg Med 1990;8:548.

Vigliani EC: Carbon disulfide poisoning in viscose rayon factories. Br J Ind Med 1954;11:235.

Villanueva E, Hernandez-Cueto C, Lachica E, et al: Poisoning by thallium: A study of five cases. Drug Saf 1990;5:384.

Wadia RS, Chitra S, Amin RB, et al: Electrophysiological studies in acute organophosphate poisoning. J Neurol Neurosurg Psychiatry 1987;50:1442.

Waters EM, Gerstner HB, Huff JE: Trichloroethylene. I. An overview. J Toxicol Environ Health 1977;2:671.

Wells JCD: Abuse of trichloroethylene by oral self-administration. Anesthesia 1982;37:440.

Whitaker JA, Austin W, Nelson JD: Edathamil calcium disodium (versenate) diagnostic test for lead poisoning. Pediatrics 1962; 29:384.

Windebank AJ, Blexrud MD: Residual ethylene oxide in hollow fiber hemodialysis units is neurotoxic in vitro. Ann Neurol 1989; 26:63.

Windebank AJ: Metal neuropathy. In Dyck PJ, Thomas PK, Griffin JW, Low PA, Poduslo JF (eds): Peripheral Neuropathy, 3rd ed. Philadelphia, WB Saunders, 1993; 1549.

Wu PB, Kingery WS, Date ES: An EMG case report of lead neuropathy 19 years after a shotgun injury. Muscle Nerve 1995;18:326.

Yokoyama K, Feldman RG, Sax DS, Salzsider BT, Kucera J: Relation of distribution of conduction velocities to nerve biopsy findings in *n*-hexane poisoning. Muscle Nerve 1990;13:314.

CHAPTER 64

Peripheral Neuropathies Associated with Paraproteinemias and Amyloidosis

John J. Kelly

Polyneuropathies have always been a source of frustration to clinicians. Almost three decades ago, when I started my training, if the cause of a polyneuropathy was not immediately obvious, a definitive diagnosis was unlikely with additional testing. As a result, fewer than half of all neuropathies were diagnosed. However, since then, owing to the work of many investigators, this picture has changed dramatically. Now, a patient who undergoes a thorough evaluation, including referral to a regional academic peripheral neuropathy center if necessary, has an 80% to 90% chance of a definitive diagnosis. Patients whose neuropathy still resists diagnosis are most likely to be elderly patients with mild sensory-dominant neuropathies.

Most of the advances have been made with better understanding of the mechanisms and treatment of previously recognized neuropathies and the description of newly recognized syndromes. The former group includes inherited neuropathies and autoimmune inflammatory, diabetic, and vasculitic neuropathies. Newer varieties include autoimmune neuropathies, atypical forms of Guillain-Barré syndrome (GBS), neuropathies that complicate medical illnesses such as human immunodeficiency virus (HIV) infection, and neuropathies associated with paraproteinemias. This chapter outlines the current state of knowledge regarding the paraprotein group and gives a practical clinical approach to these patients.

BACKGROUND

Evidence suggesting a relationship between paraproteinemias and neuropathies appeared in case reports in the earlier part of the 20th century. Several

Table 64–1. Hematological Diagnosis of 28 Patients with Plasma Cell Dyscrasias and Polyneuropathy

Diagnosis	Number
Monoclonal gammopathy of undetermined significance	16
Primary systemic amyloidosis	7
Multiple myeloma (includes osteosclerotic myeloma)	3
Other	2

Data from Kelly JJ Jr, Kyle RA, O'Brien PC, et al: Prevalence of monoclonal protein in peripheral neuropathy. Neurology 1981;31:1480–1483.

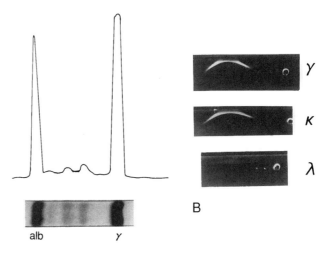

Figure 64–1. *A,* Serum protein electrophoresis showing a large "church spire" monoclonal peak for a patient with multiple myeloma. *B,* Serum immunoelectrophoresis showing a monoclonal protein that reacts with the gamma heavy chain row and the kappa light chain row, thus identifying it as IgG kappa. alb, albumin. (From Kelly JJ Jr, Kyle RA, Latov N: Polyneuropathies Associated with Plasma Cell Dyscrasias. Boston, Martinus Nijhoff, 1987, with permission.)

authors (Davison and Balser, 1937; Scheinker, 1938; Victor et al., 1958) described patients with plasma cell dyscrasias (PCDs) that appeared to be temporally related to the development of polyneuropathy. DeNavasquez and Treble (1938) described a patient with amyloidosis and polyneuropathy. Logothetis et al. (1968) described the first patient with a malignant PCD and neuropathy. Such observations continued, but there was no clear evidence of a connection between the two conditions. A relatively large series (Khan et al., 1980) was published in 1980 showing that 16 of 56 patients with monoclonal gammopathy (MG) had neuropathy. Similarly, in another group (Osby and Noring, 1982), 15 of 27 consecutive patients with MG had neuropathy. A larger, controlled study (Kelly et al., 1981b) investigated the frequency of neuropathy associated with PCD in a large referral center (Table 64–1). The frequency of MG in a group of patients with apparent idiopathic neuropathy was approximately 10%, statistically greater than the frequency of gammopathy in patients with neuropathy due to other causes or in matched historical control subjects. This study confirmed the findings in case reports and uncontrolled series and suggested that PCD probably had an important relationship to peripheral neuropathy.

Subsequent studies have confirmed the association of PCDs with neuropathy, described the manifestations of the neuropathies in each category of PCD, determined the pathophysiology of these neuropathies in some cases, and described effective treatment in a small number (Kelly et al., 1981b, 1987; Latov et al., 1997). Now, PCDs are firmly established as an infrequent but important cause of polyneuropathy.

The term *PCD* is synonymous with paraproteinemia and MG (Kyle, 1981). In this disorder, an expanding clone of plasma cells escapes control and produces a monoclonal immunoglobulin. This monoclonal protein (M protein) can be detected in serum or urine, or both, and consists of a single heavy chain (G, A, or M) and a single light chain (kappa or lambda). Gammopathies in which the paraproteins comprise multiple heavy and light chains are referred to as *polyclonal gammopathies* and are due to the expansion of multiple clones of plasma cells, typically associated with systemic inflammation or nonreticulolymphatic malignancy. They usually are not associated with polyneuropathies but can serve as markers for underlying autoimmune-inflammatory diseases, such as vasculitis, which can cause neuropathy.

Monoclonal proteins (M proteins) usually are detected by routine cellulose acetate serum protein electrophoresis (SPEP) (Kyle, 1981; Kelly et al., 1987) (Fig. 64–1A). Their presence is confirmed by a narrow "church spire" peak in the gamma or beta region. Sometimes, especially with malignant dyscrasias, the gamma fraction is otherwise depressed. The monoclonal nature of the peak is defined by immunoelectrophoresis (IEP) (see Fig. 64–1B) or immunofixation electrophoresis (IFE), which demonstrates that the immunoglobulin consists of a single heavy chain and a single light chain and is therefore monoclonal in origin. IEP and IFE also are more sensitive than SPEP and can occasionally detect an M protein in serum or urine when SPEP yields negative results. Therefore, in patients in whom a PCD is strongly suspected, the clinician should insist on IEP or IFE of serum or urine despite a normal SPEP result. It often is necessary to talk directly to the pathologist because the usual practice in most centers is to cancel the IEP or IFE if the SPEP is negative.

Although a M protein typically is present in serum, occasionally it occurs only in urine. In these cases, urinary protein electrophoresis or IFE of a concentrated 24-hour urine specimen may detect a monoclonal light chain in urine even when serum studies are negative. The presence of a monoclonal light chain suggests either a malignant PCD or amyloidosis. Occasionally, only the light chain or heavy chain is detected in serum (light chain or heavy chain disease). Also, there are rare cases of "nonsecretory" myeloma, with nondetectable serum com-

Table 64–2. Classification of Common Plasma Cell Dyscrasias

Disorder	Diagnostic Criteria
Monoclonal gammopathy of undetermined significance	MP in serum <3 g/dL and no malignancy or amyloid
Osteosclerotic myeloma	Solitary or multiple plasmacytomas with osteosclerotic features
Multiple myeloma	>10% abnormal plasma cells in bone marrow or plasmacytoma and MP in serum or urine or osteolytic lesions
Waldenström's macroglobulinemia	IgM-MP >3 g/dL; >10% lymphocytes or plasma cells in bone marrow
Primary systemic amyloidosis	Light chain amyloid by histological study
Gamma-heavy chain disease	Monoclonal heavy chain in serum or urine

MP, monoclonal protein.
Adapted, with permission, from Kelly JJ Jr, Kyle RA, Latov N: Polyneuropathies Associated with Plasma Cell Dyscrasias. Boston, Martinus-Nijhoff, 1987.

ponents, detectable only by immunostaining the bone marrow cells for surface immunoglobulin markers.

The size of the M-protein spike and accompanying features can help to determine subsequent evaluation (Kelly et al., 1987). If the spike is quite high (>3 g/dL) or if there are accompanying features of systemic disease, such as anemia, renal failure, cardiac involvement, bruising, high sedimentation rate, and others, the patient probably has a malignant gammopathy or amyloidosis. All patients with MG and polyneuropathy require a thorough evaluation by a hematologist. Working with a hematologist who is familiar with the neurological complications of gammopathies is most helpful because a thorough evaluation of these patients can be difficult to obtain.

When the evaluation is complete, the gammopathy should be classified into a hematological diagnostic category (Table 64–2). This is important not only for hematological and oncological reasons but also because the neurological syndromes tend to segregate with the medical disorders. The most common medical syndrome is MG of undetermined significance (MGUS), formerly known as *benign MG*.

This cumbersome name is now preferred because prolonged follow-up of these patients has shown that a significant percentage of cases eventually progress to amyloidosis or a malignancy (Kyle, 1984). Thus, when the patient is first seen, it is impossible to predict the outcome—hence the name. The other gammopathies, which are much more serious, include amyloidosis, myeloma, Waldenström's macroglobulinemia, and other lymphomas, leukemias, and malignancies marked by the secretion of M proteins. Ongoing follow-up by a neurologist and a hematologist is ideal for these patients but is often hard to achieve. It is worthwhile for neurologists interested in these disorders to cultivate an association with a hematologist and educate him or her in the neurological manifestations of PCDs.

CLINICAL SYNDROMES

The clinical syndromes are best approached in reference to the underlying hematological or oncological diagnosis. Although there is some overlap, these syndromes segregate with the medical disorders. Thus, the establishment of a clear medical diagnosis often greatly clarifies and restricts the differential diagnosis. In the next section, I discuss the neurological approach to these patients on presentation. In this section, I present an organized account of the peripheral nerve syndromes that occur in association with each PCD (Tables 64–3 and 64–4).

Monoclonal Gammopathy of Undetermined Significance

Monoclonal gammopathy of undetermined significance is the most frequent of these disorders by far, accounting for 50% or more of the cases in most series. This syndrome is not uniform and is best approached by dividing it into immunoglobulin M (IgM)-MGUS and non–IgM-MGUS (IgG or IgA).

IMMUNOGLOBULIN M MONOCLONAL GAMMOPATHY OF UNDETERMINED SIGNIFICANCE

Roughly 50% of MGUS neuropathies occur in patients with an IgM gammopathy (Kelly et al., 1988;

Table 64–3. Features of Dysproteinemic Polyneuropathy Syndromes

Class	Weakness	Sensory	Autonomic	CSF	MNCV
MGUS-IgM	+	+++	−	++	D
MGUS-IgG, -IgA	++	++	−	+	D
Amyloidosis	+/++	+++	+++	+	A or D
Osteosclerotic myeloma	+++	++	−	+++	D
Waldenström's macroglobulinemia	++	++	−	++	D or A

CSF, cerebrospinal fluid protein concentration; MNCV, motor nerve conduction velocity; MGUS, monoclonal gammopathy of undetermined significance; D, segmental demyelination pattern; A, axonal degeneration pattern.
Adapted, with permssion, from Kelly JJ Jr, Kyle RA, Latov N: Polyneuropathies Associated with Plasma Cell Dyscrasias. Boston, Martinus-Nijhoff, 1987.

Table 64–4. Major Electrodiagnostic Features of Polyneuropathy Associated with Plasma Cell Dyscrasia

Type of Polyneuropathy	Demyel	Axonal	CTS	Pure Sensory	Other
MGUS-IgM	+ + +	+	–	+ +	–
MGUS-IgG, -IgA	+ +	+ +	–	+	–
Osteosclerotic myeloma	+ + +	+	–	–	–
Primary systemic amyloidosis	–	+ + +	+ +	+	+ + +*
Multiple myeloma	+	+ +	+	+	+ +†

*Autonomic involvement.
†Root involvement and polyradiculopathies superimposed on polyneuropathy.
CTS, carpal tunnel syndrome superimposed on polyneuropathy; MGUS, monoclonal gammopathy of undetermined significance.
Data from Kelly JJ Jr: Peripheral neuropathies associated with monoclonal proteins: A clinical review. Muscle Nerve 1983;6:504–509.

Table 64–5. Antibody Activities of Monoclonal Immunoglobulin M in Peripheral Nerve Disorders

Antibody Activity	Clinical Syndrome	Pathology
Myelin-associated glycoprotein	Sensory>motor polyneuropathy	SD
Acidic glycolipids	Polyneuropathy	?
Gangliosides G_{M1} and G_{D1b}	Motor neuron disease	SD, ?AD
Chondroitin sulfate C	Sensory polyneuropathy	AD
Intermediate filaments	Polyneuropathy	SD
Neurofilament	Polyneuropathy	AD
Sulfatide	Sensory polyneuropathy	AD

SD, segmental demyelination; AD; axonal degeneration.
Data from Steck AJ, Murray N, Dellagi K, et al: Peripheral neuropathy associated with monoclonal IgM autoantibody. Ann Neurol 1987;22:764–767.

Latov et al., 1988). Because the percentage of IgM gammopathies in the general population is very low, early investigators suspected an etiological link between neuropathies and gammopathies. Subsequent studies have borne this out, and we now know that the IgM-MGUS neuropathies, in particular, often display antinerve antibody activity in their gammopathy fraction. Although not all these antinerve antibodies have been shown to be of pathological significance, some have been clearly linked to the pathophysiological process of these disorders. Anti–myelin-associated glycoprotein (MAG) polyneuropathies are the most important and the prototype for this group.

Anti–Myelin-Associated Glycoprotein Neuropathy (Latov's Syndrome)

This disorder has been the most fruitful area for research in the field of PCD neuropathies and was first described by Latov and colleagues in 1980 (Latov et al., 1980). The original description did not identify the offending immunoglobulin, but later studies by this group (Latov et al., 1981) showed that the M protein was an IgM antibody directed at MAG and other glycosphingolipids (Yu and Ariga, 1998) in the myelin sheath. This led to later discoveries of other antinerve antibodies (Steck et al., 1988) (Table 64–5), most of which were less likely to be of etiological significance.

Clinical Manifestations

Anti-MAG neuropathy has a fairly homogeneous clinical presentation (Melmed et al., 1983; Kelly et al., 1988; Latov et al., 1988; Ellie et al., 1996; Chassande et al., 1998). Typically, the patients are older (sixth through ninth decades) and present with a slowly progressive sensory neuropathy. Unlike many of the mild and painful benign neuropathies of late life, these are relatively painless. Patients instead complain of numbness and paresthesias of the feet and distal legs and gradually increasing unsteadiness due to sensory ataxia. Weakness is less prominent, although, as the disease progresses, it becomes more evident. Rare patients may present with mainly weakness, resembling chronic inflammatory demyelinating polyradiculoneuropathy (CIDP), although I have not seen such a case. An action tremor of the hands also is prominent in some patients.

Examination reveals that these patients have striking discriminative sensory loss, including loss of vibration sense in feet and impaired position sense, accounting for their sensory ataxia. This is accompanied by a classic Romberg sign. Cutaneous sensory modalities are less severely affected and autonomic dysfunction rarely occurs, helping to separate this disorder from amyloidosis. Motor strength often is impaired distally to a much lesser extent. Reflexes tend to be absent in legs and depressed in arms. Nerves often are thickened and firm to palpation, but this is difficult to appreciate unless the examiner regularly palpates nerves. The symptoms are very chronic, often present for months or years, and slowly progressive. Some patients are relatively stable for several years, but most progress slowly. When the disease is at its worst, patients are unable to walk, mostly because of sensory ataxia with varying degrees of weakness.

Laboratory Studies

The most helpful neurological test is electromyography (EMG) (Kelly, 1990; Kaku et al., 1994), which shows in all but the earliest cases the classic findings of a demyelinating polyneuropathy with marked slowing of conduction velocities, very prolonged distal latencies, and areas of conduction block and dispersion on proximal stimulation with secondary axonal degenerative changes. Sensory potentials typically are absent in the legs and absent or small in the hands. These findings, suggestive of a demyelinative process, greatly restrict the differential diagnosis. Cerebrospinal fluid (CSF) shows a high pro-

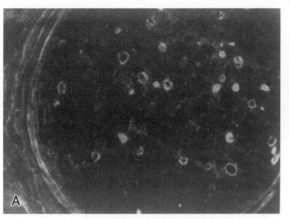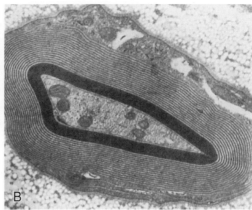

Figure 64–2. *A,* Immunohistochemistry of peripheral nerve (cross section) showing positive immunostaining of myelin sheath by IgM kappa monoclonal protein in a patient with anti–myelin-associated protein (MAG) neuropathy. *B,* Electron microscopy of peripheral nerve showing separation of the myelin lamellae characteristic of anti-MAG neuropathy. (From Latov N, Wokke JHJ, Kelly JJ Jr: Immunological and Infectious Diseases of the Peripheral Nerves. Cambridge, United Kingdom, Cambridge University Press, 1997, with permission.)

tein concentration with nonspecific features and a normal sugar and cell count. Nerve biopsy is almost pathognomonic, showing IgM deposition on the myelin sheath using immunofluorescent techniques (Fig. 64–2*A*) and splitting and separation of the outer layers of compacted myelin by electron microscopy (Nemni et al., 1983; Latov et al., 1988; Ellie et al., 1996; Jacobs, 1996) (see Fig. 64–2*B*). Results of general laboratory and hematological tests are negative in these patients, which helps to exclude the more serious gammopathies. The SPEP usually shows a small monoclonal spike in the gamma region; however, negative SPEP results may occur and should not obviate further testing in the appropriate setting. IEP or IFE confirms the presence of an IgM gammopathy, usually with kappa light chains. Further testing using enzyme-linked immunosorbent assay and Western blot assay shows that the IgM antibody reacts with MAG and other sphingoglycoli-

pid epitopes (Latov et al., 1988; Yu and Ariga, 1998), thus establishing the diagnosis.

Treatment

Treatment is problematic in these patients because the M protein is difficult to eliminate. Plasmapheresis should in theory work, but the marked chronicity of this disorder necessitates frequent and lifelong pheresis, which is not practical. However, it can be used to lower the concentration of IgM rapidly at the onset of treatment (Fig. 64–3). Likewise, intravenous gamma globulin and steroids usually are not helpful (Dalakas et al., 1996; Mariette et al., 1997). Cytotoxic drugs such as cyclophosphamide and fludarabine have been shown to be helpful in some patients (Kelly et al., 1988; Notermans et al., 1996; Wilson et al., 1999), presumably owing to the lowering of the M-protein level in serum (see Fig.

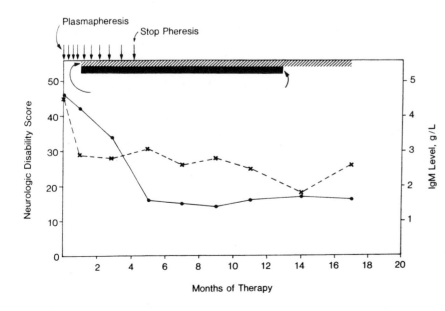

Figure 64–3. A 74-year-old woman with IgM anti-MAG neuropathy and the inability to walk was treated with plasmapheresis and oral cyclophosphamide (100 mg/day—*dark line at top*). The *y*-axis on the *left* plots the neurological disability score, and the *y*-axis on the *right* the IgM serum concentration; the *x*-axis plots the months of therapy. The serum IgM level drops rapidly with the onset of pheresis and then stays low because of the cyclophosphamide. The neurological disability score slowly improved, and she was able to walk with a cane 12 months after the beginning of treatment.

64–3). However, patients also sometimes respond without lowering of the M-protein level (Ernerudh et al., 1992; Notermans et al., 1996), perhaps because of variable antibody binding (Weiss et al., 1999), but the mechanism of action of these drugs is unclear. Toxicity clearly is the limiting factor, especially in elderly patients. In general, toxicity with monthly intravenous therapy is thought to be less than with daily oral therapy. Careful consideration in each case must be given to whether to treat and, if so, how aggressively to treat. Many patients with mild disease should not be treated aggressively unless their disease accelerates (Nobile-Orazio et al., 2000). Although some neurologists who specialize in autoimmune peripheral nerve disorders treat these patients themselves, most refer them to a hematologist/oncologist, while monitoring the patient's neurological status. There is no definitive proof of efficacy of these toxic drugs because there have been no controlled trials. However, it would be difficult to mount a controlled trial because these patients are uncommon even at academic medical centers, and such a trial would probably require a multicenter study. Clearly, better and less toxic treatments need to be developed and undoubtedly will be when we understand better the molecular pathological process of these disorders. A preliminary study found that interferon alfa seemed to help in some patients (Mariette et al., 1997).

Pathophysiology

There is now overwhelming evidence that the M protein causes the neuropathy. There is a close relationship between the clinical and the laboratory manifestations of this syndrome and the presence in serum of IgM anti-MAG antibodies. However, small studies comparing patients with IgM M protein with and without anti-MAG antibody activity could not demonstrate a difference in attributes of neuropathy between the two groups (Gosselin et al., 1991; Suarez and Kelly, 1993; Simovic et al., 1998). Laboratory data are much more convincing. The anti-MAG antibodies are deposited in the layers of the myelin (see Fig. 64–2*A*), where there is complement-mediated damage to the myelin sheath (Latov et al., 1988). Separation of the outer lamellae of myelin occurs (Latov et al., 1988; Ellie et al., 1996; Jacobs, 1996), which is presumably due to the specificity of these antibodies for the adhesion molecules of the myelin sheath (see Fig. 64–2*B*). In addition, although intraneural injections of serum in rats have not resulted in pathological changes comparable with those in humans, systemic injections into higher animals have produced identical changes (Tatum, 1993). Also, although there are exceptions, clinical improvement usually is associated with a reduction of the M-protein level in serum (Kelly et al., 1988; Notermans et al., 1996). Thus, most investigators now accept anti-MAG neuropathy as an autoimmune disease, although further work needs to be done to elucidate the specific epitopes affected and the ex-

act mechanism of the myelin damage. In addition, the presence of anti-MAG antibodies predicts future development of neuropathy in IgM M protein patients (Meucci et al. 1999).

NON–ANTI-MAG IMMUNOGLOBULIN M MONOCLONAL GAMMOPATHY OF UNDETERMINED SIGNIFICANCE

These represent the other 50% of the IgM neuropathies associated with MGUS, or approximately 25% of the total cases in the MGUS group (Kelly et al., 1987). These neuropathies tend to be more heterogeneous in type (Kelly et al., 1988), including those cases resembling the MAG group but without anti-MAG activity, and some with mostly axonal features (DiTroia et al., 1999). In addition, rare cases are associated with vasculitis, some with type 1 or 2 cryoglobulinemia (Logothetis et al., 1968).

Demyelinating Type

This neuropathy resembles the anti-MAG group and cannot be separated from the anti-MAG cases clinically without serological tests (Gosselin et al., 1991; Suarez and Kelly, 1993; Simovic et al., 1998).

Clinical Manifestations

This neuropathy is slowly progressive, sensory dominant, and distal (Kelly et al., 1987, 1988). Weakness, pain, and autonomic symptoms are less prominent than large-fiber sensory symptoms. Gait ataxia is the main symptom, as in anti-MAG neuropathy. Studies of large groups of patients with MGUS neuropathies have shown that the IgM group (MAG and non-MAG) is separable from the non-IgM group on the basis of a dominant sensory presentation with less weakness, slower nerve conduction velocities in the "demyelinating range," and a poor response to immunosuppression. However, the IgM-MAG and non-MAG groups cannot be separated by clinical, electrophysiological, and treatment response criteria (Suarez and Kelly, 1983).

Laboratory Studies

Results of laboratory tests in this group are similar to those in the MAG group unless there is an underlying disorder like amyloidosis, Waldenström's macroglobulinemia, or cryoglobulinemia. The main difference is the lack of anti-MAG activity in serum and the typical nerve histopathological changes in anti-MAG neuropathy (myelin lamellar splitting), which usually are absent in non-MAG neuropathy. Occasionally, these patients have IgM antibody activity directed at other antigens, such as sulfatides (see Table 64–5) (Steck et al., 1988). The significance of this antibody activity is uncertain because patients with non-MAG disease are less likely to respond to immunosuppressive or cytotoxic treatments and the pathological data are less compelling.

Treatment

Treatment consists of immunosuppression or cytotoxic drugs. In general, these patients respond less well to these treatments than do the patients with anti-MAG disease (Kelly et al., 1988), but there have been no controlled studies of this group. However, most patients with severe and progressive neuropathies deserve a trial of therapy.

Pathophysiology

The pathophysiological process is unknown in these patients. There is no convincing evidence that the antibody activity in the IgM fraction is the cause of the nerve damage. IgM antibody deposition in nerve is variable, and no pathognomonic pathological changes have been described. Response to lowering the antibody level in serum also is variable. More work needs to be done on this group, with careful separation of cases, to determine if there are homogeneous groups with specific pathophysiological processes and if target antigens on myelin or axons can be identified.

IMMUNOGLOBULIN A AND G MONOCLONAL GAMMOPATHY OF UNDETERMINED SIGNIFICANCE

This group accounts for approximately 50% of MGUS neuropathies (Kelly, 1985; Kelly et al., 1987). In general, these patients are quite heterogeneous and antinerve antibody activity, if found, is of unclear significance.

Chronic Inflammatory Demyelinating Polyradiculoneuropathy–Like Syndrome

Clinical Manifestations

These patients closely resemble those with idiopathic CIDP (Simmons et al., 1993a). They have a subacute, chronic progressive, or relapsing and remitting motor-dominant polyradiculoneuropathy. Sensory loss is less prominent. Weakness affects proximal and distal muscles and is symmetrical as a rule. Reflexes are reduced or absent and pain and autonomic symptoms are uncommon, except late when there has been considerable axonal damage.

Laboratory Studies

Electromyography also mirrors CIDP, with changes of a demyelinating neuropathy in most. The CSF also shows the typical albuminocytological dissociation. Nerve biopsy is nonspecific, with mixed axonal and demyelinating changes with or without inflammatory cell infiltration. However, a patient has been described (Vallat et al., 2000) with an IgA gammopathy and with IgA and complement deposition on the myelin sheath with lamellar splitting of the myelin sheath, similar to anti-MAG neuropathy but without anti-MAG or other glycolipid reactivity. Serological tests may demonstrate evidence of antinerve

antibody activity in serum in this and similar patients. However, patients with demyelinating polyneuropathy, antinerve activity on immunohistochemical staining, and myelin lamellar splitting are rare in this group.

Treatment

Therapy is similar to that for CIDP, requiring long-term immunosuppressants. These patients usually respond well and have a good prognosis if treated early before considerable axonal damage occurs.

Pathophysiology

As with CIDP, the cause is unknown.

Sensory Neuropathy

This also is a common syndrome (Gosselin et al., 1991; Suarez and Kelly, 1993; Gorson and Ropper, 1997).

Clinical Manifestations

This neuropathy usually is fairly mild in terms of deficit but disturbing in terms of symptoms (Kelly, 1985; Gorson and Ropper, 1997). These patients usually are older and complain of painful dysesthesias with or without autonomic disturbances. Motor manifestations usually are mild. This neuropathy causes considerable discomfort and often keeps the patient awake at night. It progresses very slowly and usually is more of a nuisance than a real impairment. As such, it closely resembles the many cases of idiopathic sensory neuropathy that occur in elderly patients.

Laboratory Studies

In general, results of laboratory tests, with the exception of the protein studies and EMG, are negative. The presence of anemia, an elevated erythrocyte sedimentation rate, proteinuria, or other findings should raise the question of amyloidosis or malignant PCD (Kelly et al., 1987). The SPEP typically shows a small spike and IFE confirms an IgA or IgG MG with a low concentration and no suppression of the gamma globulin fraction. EMG shows a mild axonal neuropathy with predominant sensory involvement. Nerve biopsy and CSF examination are not helpful and usually not indicated.

Treatment

Pain control is the main concern. These patients require analgesics and other pain control medications, especially at night, when the discomfort tends to keep them awake. If mild, non-narcotic analgesics such as nonsteroidal anti-inflammatory drugs are not helpful, then the tricyclic antidepressants such as amitriptyline in a dose of 25 to 75 mg at bedtime should be tried. For patients in whom this is not helpful or the side effects are limiting, gabapentin, in doses of 300 to 1200 mg three times a day, often can help and does not produce unpleasant side effects in most. Other treatments such as capsaicin occasionally are helpful, and sometimes a low dose of a long-acting narcotic at bedtime, in a medically stable and reliable patient, can help a great deal. This syndrome usually is very slowly progressive. Immunosuppression usually does not help and is not indicated in these patients.

Pathophysiology

The cause of this syndrome is unknown. Some patients have antisulfatide antibodies (Steck et al., 1988; Ilyas et al., 1992) or antibodies against other nerve antigens. However, the relevance of these antibodies to the nerve damage is not established. This may represent the chance co-occurrence of PCD and idiopathic sensory neuropathy of the elderly.

Other Disorders

This group consists of a number of other disorders that occur rarely in association with IgA or IgG M proteins. A number of these are discussed in the following sections. They include primary systemic amyloidosis (PSA), which needs to be separated from sensory neuropathy in early stages. Rapid progression, marked pain and autonomic involvement, other organ dysfunction, and abnormal laboratory study results are clues to the diagnosis. Other rare patients have myeloma, lymphoma, or cryoglobulinemia. Occasional reports cite the occurrence of a GBS-like syndrome in these patients, which may well be coincidental.

Primary Systemic Amyloidosis (Light Chain Amyloidosis)

Amyloid neuropathy is perhaps the best characterized of the polyneuropathies associated with M proteins and accounts for up to one fourth of cases in some series (Kelly et al., 1981b).

CLINICAL PRESENTATION

This neuropathy characteristically occurs in older men and is very rare before the sixth decade of life (Trotter et al., 1977; Kelly et al., 1979). Most cases are not associated with an underlying illness, but a few are associated with hematological malignancies such as myeloma and Waldenström's macroglobulinemia. PSA usually presents as a multisystem disease due to the deposition of fragments of the variable portion of a monoclonal light chain, most often lambda, in tissue.

Patients present with a medical disease with associated (sometimes incidental) polyneuropathy (60%) or severe polyneuropathy with minimal organ involvement (40%). A similar illness can occur in a

Table 64–6. Medical Syndromes in Amyloid Polyneuropathy

Syndrome	Frequency (%)
Orthostatic hypotension	42
Nephrotic syndrome	23
Cardiac failure	23
Malabsorption	16

Data from Kelly JJ Jr, Kyle RA, O'Brien PC, et al: The natural history of peripheral neuropathy in primary systemic amyloidosis. Ann Neurol 1979; 6:1–7.

variety of inherited amyloid polyneuropathies, not discussed in this chapter, caused by an abnormal circulating prealbumin (transthyretin) protein with a single amino acid substitution. Polyneuropathy does not occur in amyloidosis secondary to chronic inflammatory disease or familial central nervous system amyloidosis.

Medical syndromes (Table 64–6) include the nephrotic syndrome due to amyloid infiltration of the kidneys, cardiac failure due to amyloid cardiomyopathy, chronic diarrhea with wasting due to amyloid infiltration of the gut wall, and autonomic neuropathy with prominent orthostatic hypotension. Results of general laboratory studies reflect the medical syndromes, with proteinuria occurring in a high percentage, elevated erythrocyte sedimentation rate in approximately half, and a mild increase in benign-appearing plasma cells in bone marrow in many. As many as 90% of the patients have an M protein in serum or a monoclonal light chain in urine when thoroughly screened with serum and urine IFE (Kelly et al., 1979). Amyloid neuropathies in which an M protein is lacking, if the neuropathy is not inherited, are called *nonsecretory*, although immunocytological studies disclose that the amyloid derives from single (monoclonal) light chains (Kyle, 1999). Presumably, the serum concentration is too low for detection of light chains in these patients. The light chains are deposited in tissue, where they are digested by macrophages with the production of amyloid fibrils, which are insoluble. The resulting polyneuropathy has been well characterized (Trotter et al., 1977; Kelly et al., 1979).

Sensory symptoms typically are most prominent and the earliest to appear. Almost all patients present with numbness of the hands and legs with complaints such as burning, aching, stabbing, and shooting pains. In more than half of the patients, cutaneous sensations (light touch, pain, temperature) are more frequently and severely affected than is discriminative sensation (vibration and position sense). Some patients (approximately 20%) present with the typical symptoms of carpal tunnel syndrome, due to amyloid infiltration of the flexor retinaculum of the wrist, before distal neuropathy symptoms appear. Rare patients present with symptoms of autonomic dysfunction without symptoms of somatic sensory dysfunction. Symptoms and signs of weakness usually follow. These usually are less prominent than the sensory findings, although rare patients may present with predominantly motor findings (Quattrini et al., 1998). Patients with amyloid infiltrative myopathy occasionally present with proximal muscle weakness. Patients with malignant PCDs, such as myeloma, may present with additional compressive radiculopathies, which can mimic mononeuropathies or plexopathies. Otherwise, the findings tend to be symmetrical and predominantly distal, with gradual proximal spread. Most patients soon complain of autonomic dysfunction, with orthostatic lightheadedness and syncope, bowel and bladder disturbances, impotence, and sweating disturbances. Hypoactive pupils and an orthostatic drop in blood pressure with a fixed heart rate are the most easily detected autonomic signs at the bedside.

LABORATORY STUDIES

Electrophysiological studies (see Table 64–4) confirm the presence of a distal axonopathy, which is maximal in the legs (Kelly et al., 1979; Kelly, 1985). Motor conduction velocities in the "demyelinating" range (<60% of the mean normal for that nerve) occur rarely, and then only in severely affected nerves where the evoked compound muscle action potential is very low in amplitude. Sensory nerve action potentials usually are absent. Often, there is evidence of carpal tunnel syndrome, which can suggest the diagnosis. Needle EMG shows the changes expected of a distal axonopathy, with abundant signs of distal denervation and reinnervation. CSF usually is acellular and there usually are mild elevations of protein levels, in the range of 50 to 70 mg/dL. Diagnosis depends on the discovery of amyloid in tissue. Sural nerve biopsy is very useful for detection of amyloid in virtually all cases (Kelly et al., 1979), although occasionally it must be sought through multiple sections. One study, however, reported that 6 of 10 patients with PSA neuropathy had negative nerve biopsies (Simmons et al., 1993b), so it often is advisable to sample more than one tissue. Amorphous deposits of amyloid on Congo red or cresyl violet staining typically appear in the perivascular regions of the epineurium or occasionally in the endoneurium (Fig. 64–4). Amyloid is classically defined on Congo red staining, where it appears apple-green under polarized light. Electron microscopy also can be used to identify the characteristic β-pleated fibrils. Immunofluorescent staining for monoclonal light chain fragments is helpful but technically somewhat difficult and requires experience. Other useful tissues to sample for biopsy (Table 64–7) include rectum and other affected tissues or organs; fat pad aspiration has been reported to be 82% sensitive (Masouye, 1997). Teased fiber studies show predominant axonal degeneration. The reason for nerve fiber damage, however, is not always readily apparent in all cases. In some instances, marked axonal degeneration appears with minimal amyloid infiltration, possibly due to more proximal

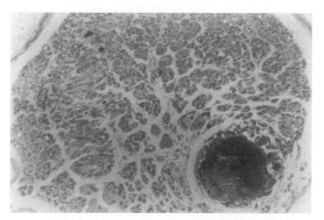

Figure 64–4. Black and white micrograph of hematoxylin and eosin–stained section of nerve showing the intense perivascular deposition of amyloid in the epineurium. With Congo red staining, this deposit would stain intensely red; under polarized light, it would appear apple-green. (From Kelly JJ Jr, Kyle RA, Latov N: Polyneuropathies Associated with Plasma Cell Dyscrasias. Boston, Martinus Nijhoff, 1987, with permission.)

amyloid infiltration, perhaps at the level of the dorsal root ganglion.

PATHOGENESIS

These findings have led to many theories of the pathogenesis of the neuropathy, including vascular and pressure changes caused by the amyloid deposits. However, direct toxic effects of the amyloid fibrils on nerve fibers and dorsal root ganglion cells seem more likely.

TREATMENT

Treatment is problematic. The amyloid fibrils are insoluble once deposited in tissue. Thus, it is unlikely that much improvement would appear even by halting amyloid deposition. Thus far, the neuropathy has resisted all attempts to halt its progression with combinations of anti-inflammatory medications, including steroids; alkylating agents, such as melphalan and cyclophosphamide, designed to slow production of the light chains; and even prolonged

Table 64–7. Results of Biopsy in Primary Amyloidosis with Neuropathy

Site	No. of Patients	Percent Positive
Rectum	25	88
Kidney	4	75
Liver	2	100
Small intestine	2	100
Bone marrow	21	33
Sural nerve	10	100
Other (skin, gingiva)	2	100

Data from Kelly JJ Jr, Kyle RA, O'Brien PC, et al: The natural history of peripheral neuropathy in primary systemic amyloidosis. Ann Neurol 1979; 6:1–7.

plasmapheresis aimed at lowering the light chain concentration in serum. However, the nephropathy due to light chain deposition has been shown to be at least partially reversible with chemotherapy (Gertz et al., 1991; Gertz and Kyle, 1994). These neuropathies usually progress inexorably, with increasing numbness and pain, autonomic failure, and weakness, with added multiorgan failure in many cases. Death typically occurs in 2 to 4 years from time of diagnosis and usually is due to major organ failure, most commonly cardiac. Overall, 85% of these patients are dead within 25 months of diagnosis (Kelly et al., 1979). Diagnosis can be delayed most in patients with relatively pure neuropathies who lack significant organ failure (median 26 months) (Rajkumar et al., 1998). One study reported some short-term reversal of neuropathy in eight patients with familial amyloid neuropathy using high-dose melphalan and autologous stem cell rescue (Gertz et al., 1999).

Multiple Myeloma Neuropathy

Multiple myeloma (MM) is a malignant PCD with high serum and urinary concentrations of M protein, infiltration of bone marrow by malignant plasma cells, and multiple bony plasmacytomas (Kyle, 1981, 1999). Most neurological complications are due to secondary effects of the tumor (hypercalcemia, infections), or to malignant infiltration of nerve roots or secondary compression of spinal cord or nerve roots because of vertebral fractures.

CLINICAL FEATURES

Polyneuropathies are uncommon. They occur in only a small percentage of patients with MM and are diverse in presentation, similar to the polyneuropathies associated with other malignancies. The exception is osteosclerotic myeloma (OSM), discussed separately in the following section. Neuropathies associated with typical lytic MM include distal sensorimotor axonopathy, a CIDP-like syndrome, and a sensory neuropathy resembling carcinomatous sensory neuropathy. In addition, these patients also may have PSA polyneuropathy due to deposition of light chain–derived amyloid in tissue. In one series, 20% of neuropathies associated with MM were due to PSA (Kelly et al., 1981a). Superimposed root involvement may confuse the clinician by suggesting a picture of mononeuritis multiplex. The root and cord compressive syndromes should be managed by conventional means but, like nonmalignant PSA, the amyloid neuropathy does not respond to chemotherapy.

Osteosclerotic Myeloma and Polyneuropathy (and Related Syndromes)

Osteosclerotic myeloma is a rare and relatively benign variant of MM (Victor et al., 1958; Kelly et al., 1981a, 1983). Less than 3% of patients with untreated myeloma have sclerotic bony lesions. In addition, although polyneuropathy is rare with typical MM, it occurs in 50% or more of reported cases with OSM. In addition, in contrast to typical MM, patients with OSM usually are not systemically ill. They present because of the neuropathy or other remote effects of the malignancy rather than as a direct effect of the malignancy. Anemia, hypercalcemia, and renal insufficiency are uncommon in OSM, the bone marrow rarely is infiltrated with malignant plasma cells, and the serum M-protein concentration is low. Finally, the course of OSM is indolent, and these patients have prolonged survival even without treatment. Thus, there is something singular about the syndrome of OSM and its paraneoplastic accompaniments. For these reasons, the syndrome can be difficult to diagnose even by experienced clinicians.

CLINICAL FEATURES

Unlike MM, the polyneuropathy accompanying OSM is distinctive and homogeneous. Deficits are mainly motor and slowly progressive without sudden changes in severity or tempo of progression. Patients present with the onset of weakness, mostly in distal limbs initially, with gradual proximal spread accompanied by reflex loss. An action tremor may appear (Bain et al., 1996). Sensory loss typically is less striking and tends to affect the larger sensory fibers disproportionately, with greater loss of discriminative than cutaneous sensation. Pain and autonomic dysfunction, with the exception of impotence (actually due to endocrine insufficiency), are very uncommon. Nerves often are palpably thickened. The deficit usually is very symmetrical and the speed of progression very slow, often over months to years. In keeping with the nature of the underlying disorder, general laboratory studies usually are relatively uninformative. The best clue to the diagnosis is the presence of a serum M protein, which is present in approximately 75% to 80% of patients. However, the M protein may be very small and obscured by the normal serum protein components isolated in the electrophoresis, emphasizing the importance of IEP or IFE in all patients with idiopathic polyneuropathy. The M protein characteristically is IgG or IgA lambda light chain (rarely kappa) and rarely present in the urine, as opposed to that in MM and amyloidosis.

LABORATORY STUDIES

Neurodiagnostic studies are helpful but nonspecific. Nerve biopsy studies disclose a reduced concentration of myelinated fibers with changes of mixed demyelination and axonal degeneration (Kelly et al., 1983). There may be mild foci of mononuclear cells in the epineurium surrounding blood vessels. These changes are nonspecific and characteristic of a number of neuropathies, including CIDP and diabetic polyneuropathy. The EMG (see Table 64–4) reveals a mixed axonal and demyelinating picture that also is nonspecific but helpful in categorizing the neuropathy into the group with clear-cut demyelinating features, so that it is more likely to be diagnosed. CSF typically discloses a normal cell count but a very high protein concentration, usually greater than 100 mg/dL and sometimes as high as several hundred milligrams per deciliter. Because all these findings are nonspecific, the diagnosis often hinges on the discovery of the characteristic bony lesions and subsequent bone biopsy (Kelly et al., 1983). The osteosclerotic lesions may be solitary or multiple. They tend to affect the axial skeleton and very proximal long bones, but spare the distal long bones and skull. They may be purely sclerotic or mixed sclerotic and lytic. Radioactive bone scans, although more sensitive than plain radiographs as a rule in detecting myeloma and other bony metastases, are not as sensitive as radiographs in detecting OSM lesions, probably because of the indolent nature of these plasmacytomas. Thus, all patients with unexplained polyneuropathies that fit the clinical profile as described previously should be screened with a radiographic skeletal survey. Occasionally, these lesions are misinterpreted by radiologists who are unfamiliar with their appearance and significance. Three of our patients (Kelly et al., 1983) were believed to have benign osteosclerotic lesions (fibrous dysplasia in a rib in two and a vertebral hemangioma in one) with negative radionuclide bone scans. We insisted on biopsy because of the clinical picture and the presence of a serum M protein, and plasmacytomas were discovered, leading to effective treatment. Thus, if there is any question of the significance of a bony lesion in a patient with a suggestive clinical picture, the neurologist should review the radiographs with the radiologist, and the lesion should be sampled if doubt remains. Open biopsy has been preferable to needle biopsy in our experience.

PATHOGENESIS

The cause of the polyneuropathy is not known, but most theories of pathogenesis have focused on some secretory product of the tumor, most likely the M protein itself. However, other secretory or autoimmune products are possible, including cytokines. One study suggested that the cytokines interleukin (IL)-1 β, tumor necrosis factor-α, and IL-6 may play a role in the pathogenesis of these neuropathies (Gherardi et al., 1996). Studies of antinerve antibody activity in the serum of these patients and immunocytochemical studies of nerves have been negative to date, although one study showed some deposition of antibody in the endoneurium in three of four cases (Adams and Said, 1998). The pathogenesis of nerve damage in this disorder and whether it is an axonopathy or a primary demyelinating disorder remain unresolved.

TREATMENT

The diagnosis of this disorder is of more than academic interest because these patients may be helped by tumoricidal treatment. Patients with solitary lesions do best. Radiation therapy in tumoricidal doses to the lesion or surgical excision results in elimination of the M protein from the serum and gradual recovery from the neuropathy and other symptoms over the ensuing months in most patients (Kelly et al., 1983). However, these patients should continue to be followed because they have a tendency to relapse with the development of new lesions months to years later. The return of the neuropathy and other symptoms and the reappearance of the serum M protein usually herald this. Patients with multiple lesions are more difficult to treat. Radiation therapy usually is not an option because of the risk of toxicity. In some cases, aggressive chemotherapy, with or without local radiation therapy to large lesions, can help these patients (Kelly et al., 1983; Donofrio et al., 1984; Kuwabara et al., 1997), but in general the outcome is less favorable than for solitary lesions. Treatment usually requires large doses of steroids and alkylating agents. Treatments that usually are effective in autoimmune inflammatory neuropathies, such as steroids, azathioprine, plasmapheresis, and intravenous immune globulin, typically are ineffective in these patients.

SYSTEMIC FEATURES

This disorder also is of considerable interest because in many of these patients, a multisystem syndrome develops that goes by a variety of names, including the *POEMS syndrome* (polyneuropathy, organomegaly, endocrinopathy, M protein, skin changes) (Bardwick et al., 1980) or the *Crow-Fukase syndrome* (Nakanishi et al., 1984). These patients have, in addition to polyneuropathy, other features (Table 64–8) suggesting the presence of an underly-

Table 64–8. Non-neurologic Abnormalities in 16 Patients with Osteosclerotic Myeloma and Polyneuropathy

Abnormality	No. of patients
Hepatomegaly	5
Hyperpigmentation	5
Edema	3
Papilledema	4
Digit clubbing	3
Hypertrichosis	3
Atrophic testes	3
Impotence	4
Polycythemia	5
Leukocytosis	3
Thrombocythemia	12
Hypotestosteronemia	5
Hyperestrogenemia	3
Other	11

Data from Kelly JJ Jr, Kyle RA, Miles JM, et al: Osteosclerotic myeloma and peripheral neuropathy. Neurology 1983;33:202–210.

ing endocrinopathy or malignancy. The reason for the endocrinopathy is unclear. Limited data suggest a disturbance of the hypothalamic–pituitary axis rather than primary end-organ failure, possibly due to antibody activity against pituitary tissue. The organomegaly usually is nonspecific pathologically. Biopsy of affected lymph nodes usually discloses hyperplastic changes, sometimes resembling the pathological findings in the syndrome of angiofollicular lymph node hyperplasia (Castleman's disease), which is a benign localized or generalized hyperplastic lymph node syndrome of unknown etiology. Patients with generalized angiofollicular lymph node hyperplasia without bony lesions also may have the manifestations of Crow-Fukase syndrome associated with serum M proteins or polyclonal gammopathies (Fig. 64–5). Thus, it is likely that the main pathogenetic determinant of these syndromes is the presence of a serum product, probably the IgG or IgA lambda M protein or polyclonal antibodies with similar specificity, directed against neural and other tissue (Adams and Said, 1998). The term *POEMS syndrome* for these patients is not entirely accurate, however, and focuses attention on a small number of these patients to the exclusion of others (Kelly et al., 1983; Miralles et al., 1992). For example, of the patients with OSM polyneuropathy, most have features other than neuropathy that are fragments of a multisystem disorder, but only a few would qualify for the term *POEMS* (see Table 64–8). Also, patients without myeloma may acquire all the features of the POEMS syndrome. Thus, I prefer the term *Crow-Fukase syndrome* for referring to patients with polyneuropathy and multisystem disorder, as suggested by Nakanishi and colleagues (1984).

Miscellaneous Syndromes

There are several uncommon syndromes with monoclonal gammopathies and peripheral neuropathy, (Kyle, 1981; Kelly et al., 1987).

WALDENSTRÖM'S MACROGLOBULINEMIA

It sometimes is difficult to separate Waldenström's macroglobulinemia from IgM-MGUS, and the latter may evolve into Waldenström's macroglobulinemia over time (Rudnicki et al., 1998). Thus, similar polyneuropathy syndromes occur. The most frequent polyneuropathy encountered is probably that associated with anti-MAG antibodies. This syndrome has the same features and clinical course as those of IgM-MGUS. One patient with anti-MAG neuropathy and Waldenström's macroglobulinemia was reported to respond to bone marrow transplantation (Rudnicki et al., 1998). Other patients may have a CIDP-like picture, a distal axonal neuropathy, typical amyloid polyneuropathy, or even the sensory neuronopathy syndrome usually seen with small cell cancer of the lung.

CRYOGLOBULINEMIA

This disorder usually is divided into three types (Logothetis et al., 1968). In type 1, the M protein itself is a cryoglobulin, present in the setting of a plasma cell disorder. In type 2, the cryoglobulin is a mixture of an M protein of IgM type with rheumatoid factor activity against polyclonal immunoglobulins, usually occurring in the setting of a lymphoproliferative disorder. Type 3 occurs in the setting of a colla-

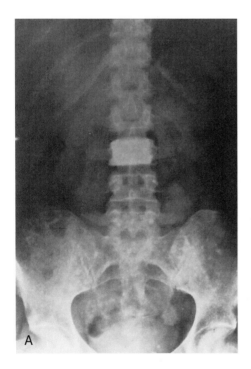

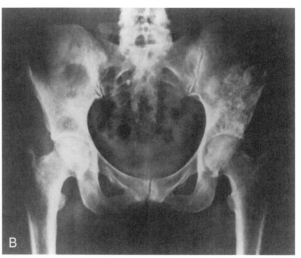

Figure 64–5. Composite showing two patients with osteosclerotic myeloma and Crow-Fukase syndrome. *A,* A dense sclerotic plasmacytoma of the L3 vertebral body ("ivory" vertebra). *B,* A mixed lytic and sclerotic plasmacytoma of the left iliac wing. (From Kelly JJ Jr, Kyle RA, Latov N: Polyneuropathies Associated with Plasma Cell Dyscrasias. Boston, Martinus Nijhoff, 1987, with permission.)

gen-vascular or other chronic inflammatory disease, and the cryoglobulin consists of polyclonal immunoglobulins. The polyneuropathy in all these syndromes is painful, symmetrical or asymmetrical, sensorimotor, and axonal. Purpura occurs in distal limbs in a high percentage of patients, and the neuropathy usually is considered to be due to a vasculopathy or vasculitis of skin and vasa nervorum.

LYMPHOMA, LEUKEMIA, AND CANCER

Malignancies (or cancers) can be associated with M protein and polyneuropathy (Kelly, 1985). In lymphoma associated with IgM M protein, the IgM may have anti-MAG activity, with the usual clinical and pathological features. Other syndromes without clear antinerve activity in the M-protein fraction may respond to ablation of the malignancy. Still others have an unclear relation to the malignancy and show little response to tumoricidal treatment or lowering of the M-protein concentration in serum.

CLINICAL APPROACH

These patients can be approached through the hematological diagnosis or through the recognition of a distinct neuropathy syndrome. Either approach works well because these disorders tend to segregate along hematological lines. Therefore, when the patient presents with a neuropathy in which the hematological disorder is well characterized, a thorough knowledge of the associated neuropathy syndromes aids diagnosis (see Tables 64–3 and 64–4).

Of course, patients often present initially without a known hematological disorder. In these situations, the neuromuscular syndrome should be classified into one of the classic neuropathy syndromes. Then, the appropriate laboratory studies should be performed as indicated by the probable choices in the differential diagnosis for each disorder. These studies should include hematological evaluation, including protein studies, as discussed previously. The discovery of an M protein or other abnormal findings on these studies should prompt further evaluation for a precise hematological diagnosis. Here, the cooperation of a hematologist-oncologist who has interest in these disorders is essential. I have seen a number of diagnoses missed despite suggestive laboratory and clinical findings because of a lack of follow-through by the physicians involved. Once the hematological diagnosis is made, the clinician can then revert to the known syndromes (see Tables 64–3 and 64–4) for the "best fit." It is likely that as further knowledge of these interesting disorders evolves, we will find other important associations between PCDs and neuropathies, and these classifications will change.

Patients also often are referred because of abnormal antinerve antibody titers, many of which are polyclonal. Deciding what to do with some of these antinerve antibody results can be a problem in some cases. This is true because many of the positive associations are not specific for individual neuropathies, are of questionable etiological importance, or simply are not helpful in the diagnosis and management of these disorders. The most helpful antinerve antibody titers are, in my opinion, the anti-MAG and antiganglioside antibody titers. Others, such as the antisulfatide antibody titers, are of unclear significance and do not add to effective therapy. The anti-*Campylobacter* and antiganglioside antibody titers in variants of GBS are of great research interest but usually are not helpful because by the time they arrive from the laboratory, the patient is improving or critical therapeutic decisions have already been made. My own approach, for clinical purposes, involves limited and directed testing only in situations where I think it will be helpful.

CONCLUSION

The topic of PCDs and neuromuscular diseases has been a fruitful area of active research since the middle 1980s. It is important to recognize these disorders because treatment may lead to remission. Also, careful study of the patients may lead to a better understanding of the pathogenesis of polyneuropathies and possibly motor neuron disease. This, in turn, may lead to effective treatment for conditions for which currently there are no effective treatments. Therefore, despite their relative infrequency, increased recognition of these disorders will continue to be a high priority both for peripheral nerve specialists and for general neurologists.

References

Adams D, Said G: Ultrastructural characterization of the M protein in nerve biopsy of patients with POEMS syndrome. J Neurol Neurosurg Psychiatry 1998;64:809–812.

Bain PG, Britton TC, Jenkins IH, et al: Tremor associated with benign IgM paraproteinemia. Brain 1996;119:789–799.

Bardwick PZ, Zvaifler NJ, Gill GN, et al: Plasma cell dyscrasia with polyneuropathy, organomegaly, endocrinopathy, M-protein and skin changes: The POEMS syndrome. Medicine (Baltimore) 1980;59:311–322.

Chassande B, Leger JM, Younes-Chennoufi AB, et al: Peripheral neuropathy associated with IgM monoclonal gammopathy: Correlations between M-protein antibody activity and clinical/electrophysiological features in 40 cases. Muscle Nerve 1998;21:55–62.

Dalakas MC, Quarles RH, Farrer RG, et al: A controlled study of intravenous immunoglobulin in demyelinating neuropathy with IgM gammopathy. Ann Neurol 1996;40:792–795.

Davison C, Balser BH: Myeloma neuropathy: Successful treatment of two patients and review of cases. Arch Surg 1937;35:913–936.

DeNavasquez S, Treble HA: A case of primary generalized amyloid disease with involvement of the nerves. Brain 1938;61:116–128.

DiTroia A, Carpo M, Meucci N, et al: Clinical features and antineural reactivity in neuropathy associated with IgG monoclonal gammopathy of undetermined significance. J Neurol Sci 1999;15:64–71.

Donofrio PD, Albers JW, Greenberg HS, et al: Peripheral neuropathy in osteosclerotic myeloma: Clinical and electrodiagnostic improvement with chemotherapy. Muscle Nerve 1984;7:137–141.

Ellie E, Vital A, Steck A, et al: Neuropathy associated with "benign" anti-myelin-associated glycoprotein IgM gammopathy: Clinical, immunological, neurophysiological and pathological findings and response to treatment in 33 cases. J Neurol 1996; 243:34–43.

Ernerudh JH, Vrethem M, Andersen O, et al: Immunochemical and clinical effects of immunosuppressive treatment in monoclonal IgM neuropathy. J Neurol Neurosurg Psychiatry 1992;55:930–934.

Gertz MA, Kyle RA, Greipp PR: Response rates and survival in primary systemic amyloidosis. Blood 1991;77:257–262.

Gertz MA, Kyle RA. Amyloidosis: Prognosis and treatment. Semin Arthritis Rheum 1994;24:124–138.

Gertz MA, Lacy MQ, Dispenzieri A: Amyloidosis: Recognition, confirmation, prognosis and therapy. Mayo Clin Proc 1999;74:490–494.

Gherardi RK, Authier FJ, Belec L: Les cytokines pro-inflammatoires: Une cle pathogenique du syndrome POEMS. Rev Neurol (Paris) 1996;64:809–812.

Gorson KC, Ropper AH: Axonal neuropathy associated with monoclonal gammopathy of undetermined significance. J Neurol Neurosurg Psychiatry 1997;63:163–168.

Gosselin S, Kyle R, Dyck P: Neuropathy associated with monoclonal gammopathies of undetermined significance. Ann Neurol 1991;30:54–61.

Ilyas AA, Cook SD, Dalakas MC, Mithen FA: Anti-MAG IgM paraproteins from some patients with polyneuropathy associated with IgM paraproteinemia also react with sulfatide. J Neuroimmunol 1992;37:85–92.

Jacobs JM: Morphological changes at paranodes in IgM paraproteinaemic neuropathy. Microsc Res Tech 1996;34:544–553.

Kaku DA, England JD, Sumner AJ: Distal accentuation of conduction slowing in polyneuropathy associated with antibodies to myelin-associated glycoprotein and sulphated glucuronyl paragloboside. Brain 1994;117:941–947.

Kelly JJ Jr, Kyle RA, O'Brien PC, et al: The natural history of peripheral neuropathy in primary systemic amyloidosis. Ann Neurol 1979;6:1–7.

Kelly JJ Jr, Kyle RA, Miles JM, et al: The spectrum of peripheral neuropathy in myeloma. Neurology 1981a;31:24–31.

Kelly JJ Jr, Kyle RA, O'Brien PC, et al: Prevalence of monoclonal protein in peripheral neuropathy. Neurology 1981b;31:1480–1483.

Kelly JJ Jr, Kyle RA, Miles JM, et al: Osteosclerotic myeloma and peripheral neuropathy. Neurology 1983;33:202–210.

Kelly JJ Jr: Peripheral neuropathies associated with monoclonal proteins: A clinical review. Muscle Nerve 1985;8:138–150.

Kelly JJ Jr, Kyle RA, Latov N: Polyneuropathies Associated with Plasma Cell Dyscrasias. Boston, Martinus Nijhoff, 1987.

Kelly JJ Jr, Adelman LS, Berkman E, et al: Polyneuropathies associated with IgM monoclonal gammopathies. Arch Neurol 1988;45:1355–1359.

Kelly JJ Jr: The electrodiagnostic findings in polyneuropathies associated with IgM monoclonal gammopathies. Muscle Nerve 1990;13:1113–1117.

Khan SN, Riches PG, Kohn J: Paraproteinemia in neurological disease: Incidence, association and classification of monoclonal immunoglobulins. J Clin Pathol 1980;33:617–21.

Kyle RA: Plasma cell dyscrasias. In Spitell JA Jr (ed): Clinical Medicine. Philadelphia, Harper & Row, 1981; 1–35

Kyle RA: "Benign" monoclonal gammopathy: A misnomer? JAMA 1984;251:1849–1854.

Kyle RA: Clinical aspects of multiple myeloma and related disorders including amyloidosis. Pathol Biol 1999;47:148–157.

Kuwabara S, Hattori T, Shimoe Y, Kamitsukasa I: Long term melphalan-prednisolone chemotherapy for POEMS syndrome. J Neurol Neurosurg Psychiatry 1997;63:385–387.

Latov N, Sherman WH, Nemni R, et al: Plasma cell dyscrasia and peripheral neuropathy with a monoclonal antibody to peripheral nerve myelin. N Engl J Med 1980;303:618–621.

Latov N, Braun PE, Gross RA, et al: Plasma cell dyscrasia and peripheral neuropathy: Identification of the myelin antigens that react with human paraproteins. Proc Natl Acad Sci U S A 1981;78:7139–7142.

Latov NR, Hays AP, Sherman WH: Peripheral neuropathy and anti-MAG antibodies. CRC Crit Rev Neurobiol 1988;3:301–332.

Latov N, Wokke JHJ, Kelly JJ Jr: Immunological and Infectious Diseases of the Peripheral Nerves. Cambridge, United Kingdom, Cambridge University Press, 1997.

Logothetis J, Kennedy WR, Ellington A, et al: Cryoglobulinemic neuropathy. Arch Neurol 1968;19:389–397.

Mariette X, Chastang C, Clavelou P, et al: A randomized clinical trial comparing interferon-alpha and intravenous immunoglobulin in polyneuropathy associated with monoclonal IgM: The IgM-associated Polyneuropathy Study Group. J Neurol Neurosurg Psychiatry 1997;63:28–34.

Masouye I: Diagnostic screening of systemic amyloidosis by abdominal fat aspiration: An analysis of 100 cases. Am J Dermatopathol 1997;19:41–45.

Melmed C, Frail DE, Duncan I, et al: Peripheral neuropathy with IgM kappa monoclonal immunoglobulin directed against myelin-associated glycoprotein. Neurology 1983;33:1397–1405.

Meucci N, Baldini L, Cappellari A, et al: Anti-myelin-associated antibodies predict the development of neuropathy in asymptomatic patients with IgM monoclonal gammopathy. Ann Neurol 1999;46:119–222.

Miralles GD, O'Fallon J, Talley NJ: Plasma cell dyscrasia with polyneuropathy: The spectrum of POEMS syndrome. N Engl J Med 1992;327:1919–1923.

Nakanishi T, Sobue I, Toyokura Y, et al: The Crow-Fukase syndrome: A study of 102 cases in Japan. Neurology 1984;34:712–720.

Nemni R, Galassi G, Latov N, et al: Polyneuropathy in non-malignant IgM plasma cell dyscrasia: A morphological study. Ann Neurol 1983;14:43–54.

Nobile-Orazio E, Meucci N, Baldini L, et al: Long-term prognosis of neuropathy associated with anti-MAG IgM M-proteins and its relationship to immune therapies. Brain 2000;123:710–717.

Notermans NC, Lokhorst HM, Franssen H, et al: Intermittent cyclophosphamide and prednisone treatment of polyneuropathy associated with monoclonal gammopathy of undetermined significance. Neurology 1996;47:1227–1233.

Osby LE, Noring L, Hast R, et al: Benign monoclonal gammopathy and peripheral neuropathy. Br J Haematol 1982;51:531–539.

Quattrini A, Nemni R, Sferrazza B, et al: Amyloid neuropathy simulating lower motor neuron disease. Neurology 1998;51:600–602.

Rajkumar SV, Gertz MA, Kyle RZ: Prognosis of patients with primary systemic amyloidosis who present with dominant neuropathy. Am J Med 1998;104:232–237.

Rudnicki SA, Harik SI, Dhodapkar M, et al: Nervous system dysfunction in Waldenström's macroglobulinemia: Response to treatment. Neurology 1998;51:1210–1213.

Scheinker I: Myelom und Nervensystem. Dtsch Z Nervenheilk 1938;147:247–273.

Simmons Z, Albers JW, Bromberg MB, et al: Presentation and initial clinical course in patients with chronic inflammatory demyelinating polyradiculoneuropathy: Comparison of patients without and with monoclonal gammopathy. Neurology 1993a; 43:2202–2209.

Simmons Z, Blaivas M, Aguilera AJ, et al: Low diagnostic yield of sural nerve biopsy in patients with peripheral neuropathy and primary amyloidosis. J Neurol Sci 1993b;120:60–63.

Simovic D, Gorson KC, Ropper AH: Comparison of IgM-MGUS and IgG-MGUS polyneuropathy. Acta Neurol Scand 1998;97:194–200.

Steck AJ, Murray N, Dellagi K, et al: Peripheral neuropathy associated with monoclonal IgM autoantibody. Ann Neurol 1987;22:764–767.

Suarez GA, Kelly JJ Jr: Polyneuropathy associated with monoclonal gammopathy of undetermined significance: Further evidence that IgM-MGUS neuropathies are different than IgG-MGUS. Neurology 1993;43:1304–1308.

Tatum AH: Experimental paraprotein neuropathy, demyelination by passive transfer of human IgM anti-myelin-associated glycoprotein. Ann Neurol 1993;33:502–506.

Trotter JL, Engel WE, Ignaczak TF: Amyloidosis with plasma cell dyscrasia: An overlooked cause of adult onset sensorimotor polyneuropathy. Arch Neurol 1947;34:209–214.

Vallat J-M, Tabaraud F, Sindou P, et al: Myelin widenings and MGUS-IgA: An immunoelectron microscopic study. Ann Neurol 2000;47:808–811.

Victor M, Banker B, Adams RD: The neuropathy of multiple my-eloma. J Neurol Neurosurg Psychiatry 1958;21:73–78.

Weiss MD, Dalakas MC, Lauter CJ, et al: Variability in the binding of anti-MAG and anti-SGPG antibodies to target antigens in demyelinating neuropathy and IgM paraproteinemias. J Neuroimmunol 1999;95:174–184.

Wilson HC, Lunn MP, Schey S, Hughes RA: Successful treatment of IgM paraproteinemia with fludarabine. J Neurol Neurosurg Psychiatry 1999;66:575–580.

Yu RK, Ariga T: The role of glycosphingolipids in neurological disorders: Mechanisms of immune action. Ann NY Acad Sci 1998;19:285–306.

CHAPTER 65

Peripheral Nervous System Diseases Associated with Malignancy

Michael P. Collins and Anthony A. Amato

Peripheral neuropathies can develop in patients with systemic malignancy as (1) a direct effect of the cancer from invasion or compression of neural structures, (2) an indirect effect of the cancer from organ failure or malnutrition, (3) an iatrogenic effect of treatment (chemotherapy, immunosuppression, radiation, or bone marrow transplantation), or (4) an immune-mediated paraneoplastic effect (Table 65–1) (Ampil, 1985). The incidence of peripheral neuropathy in patients with cancer depends on the type of malignancy, stage and location of the cancer, duration of disease, nutritional and metabolic status of the patient, neurotoxic potential of various therapies, and degree of investigatory rigor. Clinical signs and symptoms of neuropathy develop in 1% to 5% of patients (Croft and Wilkinson, 1963, 1965; Trojaborg et al., 1969; Currie et al., 1970; McLeod, 1993).

A higher frequency is obtained in studies utilizing electrophysiological techniques, with incidences in the range of 30% to 40% commonly observed (Moody, 1965; Trojaborg et al., 1969; Paul et al., 1978).

Peripheral neuropathy occurs most frequently in patients with carcinoma of the lung but is also identified in individuals suffering from hematological malignancies and carcinomas of the breast, ovaries, stomach, colon, rectum, and many other organs (Croft and Wilkinson, 1963, 1965; Currie et al., 1970; McLeod, 1993a; McLeod, 1993b). Although a paraneoplastic cause should be considered in any patient with a systemic malignancy who develops a neuropathy (Dropcho, 1999; Grisold and Drlicek, 1999), most neuropathies associated with cancer are not demonstrably paraneoplastic in origin. Many

---
Table 65–1. Etiology of Neuropathy in Patients with Malignancy

---

Direct Effect of Malignancy
  Diffuse/restricted invasion or compression of nerve roots, brachial or lumbosacral plexuses, or peripheral and cranial nerves
Iatrogenic Effect of Treatment
  Neurotoxicity of chemotherapeutic and immunosuppressive agents
  Neurotoxicity of radiation
  Surgery
  Infection
  Alteration of immune system after bone marrow transplantation
Paraneoplastic Effect
Indirect Effect of Malignancy
  Organ failure
  Malnutrition
  Malabsorption
  Critical illness
Cryptogenic Origin

---

paraneoplastic disorders involving the peripheral nervous system (PNS) have been described (all with suspected immunological mechanisms), including sensory (Horwich et al., 1977) and autonomic (Vernino et al., 1998) neuronopathies, microvasculitis-associated multifocal neuropathies, (Oh, 1997), neuromyotonia (Caress et al., 1997), motor neuron syndromes in patients with lymphoproliferative disorders (Gordon et al., 1997), chronic demyelinating polyradiculoneuropathies associated with osteosclerotic myeloma (Kelly et al., 1983) and Castleman's disease (Donaghy et al., 1989), and acute or chronic demyelinating polyradiculoneuropathies in patients with lymphomas and leukemias (Lisak et al., 1977; McLeod 1993b; Mitsui et al., 1999). Paraneoplastic, immunologically determined neuropathies are covered in another chapter of this book, as are the neuropathies associated with monoclonal gammopathies. The current discussion is limited to PNS disorders arising directly from systemic cancers or as adverse effects of cancer treatments. The material is organized by neuroanatomical principles into (1) cranial neuropathies and radiculopathies, (2) brachial plexopathies, (3) lumbosacral plexopathies, and (4) diffuse peripheral neuropathies (polyneuropathies and multifocal neuropathies).

CRANIAL NEUROPATHIES AND RADICULOPATHIES

In patients with cancer, radiculopathies and cranial neuropathies result from direct tumor involvement, late effects of radiation, opportunistic infections, and incidental processes (e.g., disk protrusions and degenerative spinal stenosis) (Stubgen and Elliot, 1997). Direct tumor effects, radiation sequelae, and one opportunistic infection—varicella-zoster virus—are discussed in this section.

Neoplastic Radiculopathies and Cranial Neuropathies

Metastatic tumor can affect spinal nerves by direct invasion or compression, most commonly as a result of local spread from neoplastic deposits in the epidural or paravertebral spaces (Posner, 1995; Stubgen and Elliot, 1997). Epidural deposits, in turn, are usually derived from metastases to vertebral bodies. Less frequently, nerve roots and dorsal root ganglia are involved by infiltration from neoplastic meningitis or by hematogenous seeding. In an analogous fashion, cranial nerves can be involved by cancers metastatic to the base of the skull, by leptomeningeal metastases, by neurotropic head and neck cancers, and (rarely) by hematogenous spread.

Radiculopathies in patients with cancer are most commonly caused by epidural spinal metastases (Rodichok et al., 1981). Of patients with systemic cancer, 1% to 5% develop spinal epidural metastases (Barron et al., 1959; Byrne, 1992; Posner, 1995). Almost any cancer can metastasize to vertebrae and the paravertebral space, but the most common to do so are breast, lung, and prostate carcinomas, multiple myeloma, and other lymphoproliferative disorders (Gilbert et al., 1978; Costans et al., 1983; Grant et al., 1991; Posner, 1995). Back pain is usually the first symptom. In cancer patients suffering from back pain, about one third have epidural tumor and another one third have vertebral metastases without epidural/neural involvement (Clouston et al., 1992). In addition to back pain and the more ominous signs of spinal cord compression, root pain and weakness develop in up to 90% of patients with epidural lesions (Gilbert et al., 1978). The thoracic spine is the most common site of epidural cord/root compression, followed by the lumbosacral spine and, finally, the cervical spine (Grant et al., 1991; Posner, 1995).

Analogous to the relationship between epidural metastases and radiculopathies at spinal levels, metastases to the base of the skull are the usual source of cranial neuropathies in patients with cancer. Skull metastases most frequently originate from breast carcinomas, but also are common with lymphoma and lung, prostate, and head and neck cancers (Vikram and Chu, 1979; Greenberg et al., 1981; Gupta et al., 1990). The cranial nerve most commonly affected is the sixth, followed by the third, fifth, and twelfth (Gupta et al., 1990). Malignant tumors of the parotid gland affect the seventh nerve preferentially.

Several neurological syndromes with localizing value have been identified in patients with base of the skull metastases (Nisce and Chu, 1968; Greenberg et al., 1981; Posner, 1995). The *middle cranial fossa syndrome* is most common (Greenberg et al., 1981; Posner, 1995; Mastronardi et al., 1997). In this syndrome, symptoms derive from tumoral involvement of the gasserian ganglion in Meckel's cave or one of the proximal divisional branches of the trigeminal nerve. The motor root of this nerve and cranial nerves VI and VII may also be affected.

Middle fossa metastases are one source of the so-called numb-chin syndrome, which is often a common harbinger of malignancy (Burt et al., 1992; Lossos and Siegal, 1992). The *jugular foramen (Vernet's) syndrome* reflects dysfunction of the ninth, tenth, and eleventh cranial nerves (Svien et al., 1963; Greenberg et al., 1981; Posner, 1996). Presenting complaints include hoarseness, dysphagia, retroauricular pain, glossopharyngeal neuralgia, and, occasionally, syncope. The *occipital condyle syndrome* is recognized by the emergence of continuous occipital and neck pains combined with unilateral tongue weakness from cranial nerve XII paralysis (arising from malignant invasion of the hypoglossal canal) (Greenberg et al., 1981; Posner, 1995; Moris et al., 1998). The *parasellar syndrome* occurs with metastases to the cavernous sinus region (sella turcica, petrous bone apex) (Roessmann et al., 1970; Thomas and Yoss, 1970; Keane, 1996). The *orbital syndrome* is rarest (Greenberg et al., 1981; Bairey et al., 1994). Metastases to the orbit produce periorbital pain, proptosis, diplopia, and, possibly, hypesthesia in the distribution of the ophthalmic division of the fifth nerve.

PERINEURAL INVASION

Some head and neck cancers have a propensity to disseminate in a perineural pattern along superficial cranial nerve branches. This includes squamous cell carcinomas of the oral cavity, pharynx, larynx, and skin; adenoid cystic carcinomas; neurotropic melanomas; and even basal cell skin carcinomas (Ballantyne et al., 1963; Carter et al., 1982; Carter et al., 1983; Morris and Joffe, 1983; Goepfert et al., 1984; Mack and Gomez, 1992; Boerman et al., 1999). Tumor cells within the nerve typically proliferate in the perineurium and adjacent epineurium, with limited endoneurial extension. Longitudinal spread along the nerve for more than 1 to 2 cm is unusual, although distances up to 14 cm are reported (Ballantyne et al., 1963; Carter et al., 1982; Carter et al., 1983). The maxillary and mandibular divisions of the trigeminal nerve, facial nerve, and glossopharyngeal nerve are most commonly involved, yielding painful dysesthesias, facial weakness, and dysphagia (Carter et al., 1982; Morris and Joffe, 1983; Goepfert et al., 1984). Perineural spread signals an aggressive tumor and is an adverse prognostic factor (Goa and Faulds, 1994; Sonobe et al., 1998).

LEPTOMENINGEAL METASTASES

Leptomeningeal metastases are another cause for cancer-related radiculopathies and cranial neuropathies (Posner, 1995; Lesser, 1996; Chamberlain, 1997; DeAngelis, 1998). Almost any cancer has the potential to spread to the leptomeninges, compressing or invading cranial nerves and nerve roots in the process. The incidence of meningeal spread at postmortem examination in patients with all types of cancer is 8% (Posner, 1978). The most common tu-

mors to seed the meninges are breast, lung (especially small cell), melanoma, leukemia, and non-Hodgkin's lymphoma (NHL), especially immunoblastic, diffuse large cell, and AIDS-related lymphomas (Little et al., 1974; Olsen et al., 1974; Posner and Chernik, 1978; Wasserstrom et al., 1982; Kaplan et al., 1990; Lesser, 1996; Chamberlain, 1997; Van Oostenbrugge and Twijnstra, 1999). Leptomeningeal metastases are frequently accompanied by metastases to other sites in the central nervous system (CNS). Particularly with solid tumors, neoplastic meningitis occurs as a late manifestation of the illness in association with progressive systemic disease (Wasserstrom et al., 1982; Lesser, 1996; Van Oostenbrugge and Twijnstra, 1999). Neoplastic cells gain access to the meninges by direct extension from CNS parenchymal or bone metastases, hematogenous dissemination, or perineural spread along craniospinal nerves (Lesser, 1996; Chamberlain, 1997).

The entire neuraxis can be affected by neoplastic meningitis, so that signs and symptoms are variable. Involvement is typically multifocal and multilevel. The most common region of involvement is the spinal roots, occurring in nearly 75% of patients (Posner, 1995). Meningeal signs, such as nuchal rigidity, are uncommon (15%) and late manifestations. The cauda equina syndrome is most characteristic, with an incidence of 30% to 40%. Symptoms usually evolve gradually, over several weeks to several months, but in rare cases acute polyradiculopathies occur, mimicking the Guillain-Barré syndrome (GBS) (Guarino et al., 1995).

Cranial neuropathies develop in 40% to 60% of patients with leptomeningeal neoplasms (Little et al., 1974; Olsen et al., 1974; Wasserstrom et al., 1982; Kaplan et al., 1990; Posner, 1995; Balm and Hammack, 1996). Diplopia is the most common symptom (20% to 30%), followed by decreased vision, impaired hearing, and facial numbness (approximately 10% each). Oculomotor weakness is the commonest examination finding (30% to 40%), with cranial nerve VI dysfunction observed most frequently. Facial palsies are seen in 25%, optic neuropathies and eighth cranial nerve abnormalities in 10% to 20%, and trigeminal neuropathies in about 10%. Multiple cranial neuropathies are the norm. Cerebral signs and symptoms commonly accompany the cranial nerve manifestations.

ELECTROPHYSIOLOGY IN NEOPLASTIC CRANIAL NEUROPATHIES AND RADICULOPATHIES

Electrophysiological studies can assist with evaluation of the extent of PNS involvement in patients with neoplastic compression or invasion of spinal nerve roots and cranial nerves (Ekholm et al., 1997), but they have a limited role in clinical management. Very little electrodiagnostic information concerning neoplastic radiculopathies and cranial neuropathies is available in the literature. For patients with facial nerve palsies resulting from cancer, the direct facial nerve conduction study may demonstrate a decreased amplitude of the compound muscle action potential (CMAP) and needle electromyography (EMG) examination of facial muscles may reveal fibrillation potentials and decreased recruitment. Similar EMG findings may appear in the masseter with trigeminal neuropathies, the tongue with hypoglossal neuropathies, and the trapezius or sternocleidomastoid with spinal accessory palsies. Because most neoplastic cranial neuropathies are rapidly evolving, significant motor unit action potential (MUAP) remodeling is not expected. Blink reflex studies may show absent or prolonged R_1 and R_2 responses if cranial nerve V or VII is involved.

In patients with neoplastic radiculopathies, routine motor and sensory nerve conduction studies are normal in the extremities, unless they are associated with severe axon loss, in which case CMAP amplitudes may be decreased and motor conduction velocities mildly reduced (Argov and Siegel, 1985). According to some investigators, prolonged or absent F waves are a sensitive early indicator of nerve root involvement in leptomeningeal cancer, occurring in approximately 75% of affected patients (Argov and Siegel, 1985). Needle EMG examination of paraspinal and limb muscles is the most sensitive indicator of nerve root dysfunction (Kaplan et al., 1990). In the only study dedicated to the assessment of EMG findings in patients with leptomeningeal metastases, all patients had fibrillation potential and positive sharp waves in multiple lumbosacral myotomes, most commonly involving the L4-S2 nerve roots (both paraspinal and limb muscles). Two thirds of patients had fibrillation potentials in cervical myotomes (Kaplan et al., 1990). For patients with spinal epidural metastases, active denervation in the paraspinal muscles may be an early sign, preceding denervation in the corresponding primary anterior ramus distribution by several weeks. In one study, paraspinal EMG was abnormal in many patients whose metastatic spine disease was occult to neurological, radiological, and scintigraphic examinations (LaBan and Grant, 1971).

Radiation-Induced Cranial Neuropathies and Radiculopathies

Late effects of ionizing radiation on the human nervous system can be divided into syndromes resulting from damage to the CNS and the PNS. Animal studies have suggested that peripheral nerves are relatively more radioresistant than CNS tissues (Caincross, 1991; Giese and Kinsella, 1991; Thomas and Holdorff, 1993). Nevertheless, many radiation-related PNS syndromes have been reported, including plexopathies, radiculopathies, and cranial neuropathies. Most common and best described are brachial plexopathies following radiation to the thorax.

Cranial Neuropathies from Radiation

The radiation tolerance threshold of PNS structures depends on several factors, including total radiation dose, fractional dose, number of fractions, and duration of treatment (Giese and Kinsella, 1991; Thomas and Holdorff, 1993). These factors are combined into the so-called nominal standard dose—expressed in units of *ret* (rad equivalent therapy)—using a formula devised by Ellis (1971). Compared with the brachial and lumbosacral plexuses, cranial nerves have a relatively high nominal standard dose of 1,800 to 2,000 ret (Berger and Bataini, 1977; Thomas and Holdorff, 1993). They are most commonly affected following radiation treatment of oropharyngeal, nasopharyngeal, and laryngeal tumors (Berger and Bataini, 1977). After megavoltage irradiation for nasopharyngeal cancer, radiation-induced cranial neuropathies occur in 10% to 20% of long-term survivors (more than 5 years) (Hoppe et al., 1976; Mesic et al., 1981; Lee et al., 1992; Chew et al., 2001). The lower five cranial nerves are most often affected (Hoppe et al., 1976; Mesic et al., 1981; Lee et al., 1992; Chew et al., 2001). Patients who develop a hypoglossal nerve palsy following radiotherapy for nasopharyngeal carcinoma usually have a postirradiation syndrome, not a tumor recurrence (King et al., 1999).

Lower cranial nerve dysfunction resulting from radiation has an onset latency ranging from 0.5 to 28 years (median 5 years) (Lee et al., 1992; Poncelet et al., 1996). There is an inverse relationship between the latency and the nominal standard dose of the radiation (Berger and Bataini, 1977). The pathogenesis of radiation-induced lower cranial nerve palsies is usually attributed to radiation fibrosis in the anterior cervical soft tissues, but vascular damage and direct neural injury are other possibilities (Cheng and Schultz, 1975; Giese and Kinsella, 1991; Posner, 1995; King et al., 1999). Delayed, progressive, radiation-induced damage to the motor branches of cranial nerves V, VII, IX, XI, and XII can produce a syndrome resembling motor neuron disease (Wang et al., 1993; Poncelet et al., 1996; Shapiro et al., 1996; Tsang et al., 1999; Glenn and Ross, 2000). Radiation-induced cases are distinguished from motor neuron disease by the presence of myokymic and neuromyotonic discharges in involved muscles.

Myokymic discharges are grouped, rhythmic potentials composed of multiple individual MUAPs within each burst (Albers et al., 1981; Gutman, 1991; Shapiro et al., 1996). Interburst frequency is 0.25 to 5 seconds. Intraburst firing rates vary from 2 to 60 Hz. Neuromyotonic discharges are single MUAPs firing repetitively at an exquisitely fast rate of 150 to 300 Hz, with a characteristic decrement in both amplitude and frequency within bursts (Lance et al., 1979; Auger, 1994; Shapiro et al., 1996). Abortive runs are manifested as doublets, triplets, and multiplets (Tsang et al., 1999). It is believed that myokymia and neuromyotonia are both generated along hyperexcitable segments of the peripheral motor axon having altered membrane channel function. Neuromyotonic discharges derive from repetitive, spontaneous depolarizations of the motor axon, with voltage-gated potassium channel dysfunction an established mechanism (Hart et al., 1997). Myokymia is attributed to spontaneously generated discharges that are ephaptically transmitted along demyelinated segments of nerve to adjacent motor units, resulting in a reverberating circuit rhythm. Myokymic and neuromyotonic discharges occur in many clinical settings (Albers et al., 1981; Gutman, 1991; Auger, 1994). Their occurrence following radiotherapy is suggestive of radiation-induced damage to PNS structures.

RADICULOPATHIES FROM RADIATION

A rare postirradiation lumbosacral polyradiculopathy or cauda equina syndrome, primarily affecting ventral roots, is well characterized (Maier et al., 1969; Sadowsky et al., 1976; Kristensen et al., 1977; Schiodt and Kristensen, 1978; Horowitz and Stewart, 1983; Lagueny et al., 1985; De Carolis et al., 1986; Gallego et al., 1986; Berlit and Schwechheimer, 1987; Feistner et al., 1989; Lamy et al., 1991; Bowen et al., 1997; Wohlgemuth et al., 1998; van der Sluis et al., 2000). For many years, the presumed locus of injury was the anterior horn cell and the entity was referred to as a postirradiation motor neuron syndrome (Sadowsky et al., 1976; Bradley et al., 1991). More recent reports have convincingly demonstrated that the disorder is due to predominant cauda equina damage (Feistner et al., 1989; Bowen et al., 1997; Wohlgemuth et al., 1998). The syndrome usually occurs after para-aortic radiation for malignant testicular tumors, although patients with Hodgkin's disease and other cancers have also been described (Gallego et al., 1986; Berlit and Schwechheimer, 1987; Lamy et al., 1991). Almost all reported patients have received a total dose of more than 4,000 cGy. The incidence increases with higher cumulative doses and dose intensities, but individual susceptibility varies. Two large series reveal a 3% to 4% overall incidence (Maier et al., 1969; Schiodt and Kristensen, 1978).

The classic presentation is subacutely or chronically progressive pure motor, flaccid paraparesis. The latency between irradiation and onset of symptoms varies widely, from 3 months to 25 years (Maier et al., 1969; Krieger et al., 1982; Bowen et al., 1997). Recent series have determined mean latencies of 5 to 6 years and a median latency of about 11 years (Bowen et al., 1997; Wohlgemuth et al., 1998). The gluteal, peroneal, and hamstring muscles (L4-S1 myotomes) are maximally involved, with distal worse than proximal weakness and atrophy. Mild motor asymmetries are routinely observed, and completely monomelic presentations can occur (Lamy et al., 1991). Muscle fasciculations are characteristically identified. Although motor predominance is a distinguishing feature, recent series have emphasized coexisting mild but often delayed sensory findings and sphincter symptoms in many patients (Bowen et al., 1997; Wohlgemuth et al., 1998). Urodynamic studies may reveal a hypotonic bladder (Maier et al., 1969). Pain is not expected. Lower limb stretch reflexes are generally absent, but cremasteric, bulbocavernosal, and anal reflexes are preserved.

Nerve conduction studies generally show normal CMAP amplitudes and normal or mildly reduced motor conduction velocities. Sensory nerve action potentials (SNAPs) are normal. F waves and H reflexes in the legs may be absent or disclose prolonged latencies (Feistner et al., 1989). Lumbar dermatomal and posterior tibial somatosensory evoked potentials sometimes show prolonged latencies of the scalp-recorded potential, confirming involvement of the sensory pathways in some patients (Feistner et al., 1989; Bowen et al., 1997; Wohlgemuth et al., 1998). Needle EMG examination reveals signs of active and chronic partial denervation in lower extremity muscles innervated by L4 to S1 nerve roots and the lower lumbosacral paraspinal muscles, with higher lumbar levels infrequently involved. Fasciculation potentials and low-frequency complex repetitive discharges may be seen. Myokymic discharges—characteristic of radiation-induced injury (see preceding)—were observed in 60% of patients in one series (Bowen et al., 1997), but not in other individual case reports (Horowitz and Stewart, 1983; Gallego et al., 1986; Feistner et al., 1989; Lamy et al., 1991).

Infectious Radiculopathies and Cranial Neuropathies

Varicella-zoster virus infection occurs more commonly in cancer and transplantation patients than in the general population and represents another potential source of radiculopathies and cranial neuropathies in patients with systemic malignancy (Straus et al., 1988; Posner, 1995; Gilden et al., 1999; Liesegang, 1999). Patients with compromised cell-mediated immunity are predisposed; those suffering from Hodgkin's disease are at highest risk (Schimpff et al., 1972; Reboul et al., 1978).

Cutaneous zoster typically presents with sensory symptoms (pain, pruritus, paresthesias) in a dermatomal distribution. Sensory symptoms are associated with clinical evidence of motor dysfunction—so-called segmental zoster paresis—in 10% of varicella-zoster virus cases (Grant and Rowe, 1961; Gupta et al., 1969; Thomas and Howard, 1972; Wiernik et al., 1987; Mondelli et al., 1996; Haanpaa et al., 1997). The presumed mechanism is spread of the virus from the dorsal root ganglion to the anterior root or anterior horn. Findings include weakness, wasting, and segmental reflex loss, usually involving muscles supplied by the nerve root(s) implicated in the cutaneous eruption. However, motor dysfunction can be more widespread than dermal involvement and, in 5% to 10% of patients with noncephalic zoster, occurs at a noncontiguous, topographically dissociated site (Thomas and Howard, 1972).

The onset of weakness is usually acute, evolving over hours or, at most, several days (Thomas and

Howard, 1972). The latency between the appearance of the rash and the development of clinical weakness ranges from hours to 5 months (Grant and Rowe, 1961), with a mean of about 20 days (Merchut and Gruener, 1996). Approximately 11% of cranial zoster patients develop motor neuropathies (Thomas and Howard, 1972; Mondelli et al., 1996a; Haanpaa et al., 1997). Fifty percent of these abnormalities are manifested as Ramsay Hunt syndrome, characterized by skin lesions in the external auditory canal, ipsilateral facial palsy, and inconstantly associated (in 50% of patients) hearing loss and vertigo (Thomas and Howard, 1972; Murakami et al., 1996).

Electrodiagnostic studies in typical patients with varicella-zoster virus infection reveal changes consistent with a sensory axonal neuropathy or neuronopathy in the involved dermatomes, often accompanied by evidence of a motor axonal neuropathy or neuronopathy (Thomas and Howard, 1972; Gardner-Thorpe et al., 1976; Greenberg et al., 1992; Cioni et al., 1994; Merchut and Gruener, 1996; Mondelli et al., 1996a; Mondelli et al., 1996b; Haanpaa et al., 1997). Low-amplitude or absent SNAPs occur in approximately 50% of patients with limb involvement (Merchut and Gruener, 1996; Mondelli et al., 1996b). Sensory conduction velocities are normal or mildly reduced. CMAP amplitudes are reduced in 5% to 10% of patients (Merchut and Gruener, 1996; Mondelli et al., 1996b; Haanpaa et al., 1997). Slow, demyelinating range motor conduction velocities are rarely reported (Gardner-Thorpe et al., 1976; Merchut and Gruener, 1996). Fifteen percent of patients have delayed or unevocable tibial H reflexes (Mondelli et al., 1996a; Mondelli et al., 1996b). Needle EMG changes are usually more prevalent and widely distributed than the clinical signs. Fibrillation potentials are identified in 40% to 50% of patients with cervical, thoracic, and lumbosacral zoster. Involved muscles are those corresponding to the segmental skin changes, with extension to contiguous myotomes in more than 50% of patients (Cioni et al., 1994; Mondelli et al., 1996a). In clinically weak muscles, fibrillation potentials, positive sharp waves, and decreased recruitment are almost always observed. Active denervation is also seen in the corresponding paraspinal muscles. Abnormal spontaneous activity usually resolves in the latter muscles by 6 months but can persist in limb muscles for several years (Cioni et al., 1994; Merchut and Gruener, 1996). Complex repetitive discharges and long-duration MUAPs occur in at least 50% of patients (Gardner-Thorpe et al., 1976; Haanpaa et al., 1997). Myokymic discharges are not reported.

In cranial zoster, 36% of patients exhibit abnormal R_1 or R_2 areas and 22% abnormal R_1 or R_2 latencies during blink reflex testing (Mondelli et al., 1996b). Neurogenic needle EMG abnormalities occur in facial nerve–supplied muscles in just 15% of patients (Mondelli et al., 1996b; Haanpaa et al., 1997). Patients with ophthalmic zoster may show signs of active denervation in the ipsilateral masseter muscle (Negrin and Peserico, 1975).

BRACHIAL PLEXOPATHIES

In patients with systemic malignancies, brachial plexopathies are usually caused by direct neoplastic plexus involvement or by radiation-induced injury (Wilbourn, 1993; Posner, 1995; Stubgen and Elliot, 1997) The true incidence of cancer-related brachial plexopathy is unknown. In one large surgical series of 1,007 brachial plexopathy cases, 4.5% of patients had metastatic or postirradiation plexopathies (Narakas, 1984). Of cancer patients with neurological symptoms seen at tertiary referral centers, 3.5% to 5.8% are diagnosed with direct neoplastic plexopathies (Clouston et al., 1992; Lassouw et al., 1992). As neoplastic lumbosacral plexopathies are nearly twice as common as neoplastic brachial plexopathies, the latter must occur in about 2% to 3% of neurologically affected cancer patients (Kori et al., 1981; Jaeckle et al., 1985; Clouston et al., 1992). Malignant brachial plexopathies are, in turn, twice as common as radiation-induced brachial plexopathies (Kori et al., 1981; Lederman and Wilbourn, 1984; Thyagarajan et al., 1995).

Malignant Brachial Plexopathies

Malignant lesions of the brachial plexus result from metastases to the lateral group of axillary lymph nodes or regional spread of a tumor located at the apex of the lung (Pancoast's syndrome) (Pancoast, 1932; Kori et al., 1981; Wilbourn, 1993; Stubgen and Elliot, 1997). Metastatic tumor plexopathies are more common than the Pancoast type. Pancoast's, or superior pulmonary sulcus, tumors produce neurological symptoms by spreading to the posterior chest wall and paravertebral space, then invading the C8 and T1 spinal nerves and primary anterior rami, sympathetic chain, and stellate ganglion (Hepper et al., 1966; Arcasoy and Jett, 1997). Breast cancers and, to a lesser extent, lung cancers are responsible for at least two thirds of neoplastic brachial plexopathy cases (Thomas and Colby, 1972; Bagley et al., 1978; Kori et al., 1981; Lederman and Wilbourn, 1984; Harper et al., 1989; Thyagarajan et al., 1995). Hodgkin's disease and non-Hodgkin's lymphomas are the next most commonly implicated tumors. Melanomas, sarcomas, myelomas, and many other types of carcinoma have also been reported. Most Pancoast tumors are non–small cell lung cancers, especially low-grade squamous cell carcinomas (Hepper et al., 1966; Arcasoy and Jett, 1997).

With the exception of Pancoast's syndrome, brachial plexopathy is seldom the first manifestation of a systemic malignancy and typically develops years after apparent successful treatment of the primary tumor (Thomas and Colby, 1972; Bagley et al., 1978; Kori et al., 1981; Lederman and Wilbourn, 1984; Harper et al., 1989). Reported latencies range from

0 months to 34 years (Harper et al., 1989), with median latencies of 1.5 to 5.5 years (Bagley et al., 1978; Kori et al., 1981; Lederman and Wilbourn, 1984; Harper et al., 1989) and mean latencies of 3 to 6.5 years (Nisce and Chu, 1968; Thomas and Colby, 1972; Kori et al., 1981; Lederman and Wilbourn, 1984). In 85% of cases, metastases occur simultaneously in other parts of the body (Kori et al., 1981).

Anatomical considerations dictate that lower trunk involvement is most common. The lateral group of axillary lymph nodes abuts the lower trunk of the plexus, and apical lung tumors have direct access to the C8 and T1 nerve roots, as noted previously (Kori et al., 1981; van den Bent et al., 1998). By combining examination data from four large series, predominant lower trunk involvement occurs in about 60% of patients, upper/middle trunk in about 10%, and all trunks in about 30% (Thomas and Colby, 1972; Kori et al., 1981; Lederman and Wilbourn, 1984; Harper et al., 1989).

Pain is the prototypical symptom of neoplastic invasion of the brachial plexus, occurring in at least 85% of patients and serving to distinguish malignant from radiation-induced etiologies (Hepper et al., 1966; Thomas and Colby, 1972; Bagley et al., 1978; Kori et al., 1981; Lederman and Wilbourn, 1984; Harper et al., 1989; Thyagarajan et al., 1995). With disease progression, plexal pain tends to become severe and debilitating. About 50% of patients complain of numbness and tingling, typically involving the medial hand and forearm, and approximately 45% report upper limb and hand weakness.

Neurological signs depend on the region of the plexus involved by tumor. Most patients exhibit combined weakness, hypesthesia, and reflex loss in a distribution corresponding to the affected trunks and/or cords. As lower trunk involvement is most common, typical findings include weakness of the intrinsic hand muscles; sensory loss in the medial hand, medial forearm, posteromedial arm, and axilla; and impairment of the finger flexor stretch reflex (Posner, 1995). Horner's syndrome, due to neoplastic invasion of the cervical sympathetic chain or upper thoracic ventral roots, occurs in about 50% of patients with tumor-related brachial plexopathies (Kori et al., 1981; Lederman and Wilbourn, 1984; Harper et al., 1989) and about 80% of patients with Pancoast's syndrome (Hepper et al., 1966), but only rarely in radiation-induced plexopathies (Harper et al., 1989). Neoplastic brachial plexopathies are generally progressive over several weeks to months. Pain often becomes intractable. Neurological deficits spread from the initial area of involvement to the entire plexus.

Magnetic resonance imaging (MRI) and computed tomography (CT) are the radiographic procedures of choice for diagnosing malignant brachial plexopathies. They have not yet been compared in a head-to-head prospective study. MRI is superior to CT for differentiating brachial plexus nerve elements from adjacent tissues because of its multiplanar capability and improved soft tissue contrast (Blair et al., 1987; Qayyum et al., 2000). Retrospective analyses suggest that MRI may be more sensitive and specific in the diagnosis of neoplastic plexopathies (Rapoport et al., 1988; Thyagarajan et al., 1995).

Radiation-Induced Brachial Plexopathies

Delayed brachial plexopathy, the most common PNS complication of radiation therapy, was not reported until the 1960s when high-voltage therapy replaced orthovoltage therapy (Stoll and Andrews, 1966; Wilbourn, 1993). Brachial plexopathies can occur after radiation treatment to the upper thorax, chest wall, axilla, or supraclavicular area. Most cases involve patients with breast cancer, but other tumors are also frequently encountered, including bronchogenic carcinoma, lymphoma, and renal cell carcinoma (Thomas and Colby, 1972; Kori et al., 1981; Lederman and Wilbourn, 1984; Harper et al., 1989; Thyagarajan et al., 1995). The risk of neural damage is influenced by such factors as cumulative radiation dose, number of fractions, fractional size, total time of therapy, field techniques, geometry, nerve length, and concomitant chemotherapy (Giese and Kinsella, 1991; Pierce et al., 1992; Olsen et al., 1993; Thomas and Holdorff, 1993; Wilbourn, 1993). Risk increases with cumulative doses greater than 5,000 cGy (Pierce et al., 1992) and fractional doses greater than 200 cGy (Olsen et al., 1993). Relatively safe doses are 5,000 cGy over 30 to 35 days at 3 to 5 fractions per week or 5,600 cGy in 28 fractions of 200 cGy over 38 days (Thomas and Holdorff, 1993). In some series, postirradiation brachial plexopathy occurs in as many as 35% to 73% of patients (Stoll and Andrews, 1966; Mondrup et al., 1990), but the reported incidence in most studies clusters in the 2% to 7% range, with a weighted average of 3.5% (Basso-Ricci et al., 1980; Barr and Kissin, 1987; Pierce et al., 1992; Olsen et al., 1993).

Radiation-induced brachial plexopathy occurs with a highly variable posttreatment latency, ranging from 0 to 570 months (Thyagarajan et al., 1995). Reported median latencies are unexpectedly diverse but show a central tendency of about 4 to 5 years (Bagley et al., 1978; Kori et al., 1981; Lederman and Wilbourn, 1984; Harper et al., 1989; Mondrup et al., 1990; Pierce et al., 1992). Mean latencies vary from 4 to 7 years (Thomas and Colby, 1972; Kori et al., 1981; Lederman and Wilbourn, 1984; Killer and Hess, 1990). Some studies have found an inverse relationship between latency and total dose (Stoll and Andrews, 1966; Kori et al., 1981; Pierce et al., 1992).

Kori et al. reported that 78% of their 22 radiation plexopathy patients had involvement of the upper plexus, the rest exhibiting diffuse involvement (Kori et al., 1981). They speculated that the lower trunk was relatively protected from radiation damage by its shorter length in the radiation port and the overlying clavicle. However, other studies have not confirmed this predilection. In fact, most report that a pan-plexopathy pattern is most common (combined incidence of about 50%, compared with about 30%

for the upper/middle trunks and about 20% for the lower trunk) (Thomas and Colby, 1972; Kori et al., 1981; Lederman and Wilbourn, 1984; Harper et al., 1989; Fardin et al., 1990; Mondrup et al., 1990; Olsen et al., 1993; Boyaciyan et al., 1996).

Pain is less common and less severe in radiation plexopathy than in metastatic plexopathy, occurring in approximately 45% of patients (Thomas and Colby, 1972; Basso-Ricci et al., 1980; Kori et al., 1981; Lederman and Wilbourn, 1984; Harper et al., 1989; Fardin et al., 1990; Killer and Hess, 1990; Mondrup et al., 1990; Esteban and Traba, 1993; Olsen et al., 1993; Thyagarajan et al., 1995). Nevertheless, some patients develop severe debilitating pain (Bagley et al., 1978; Mumenthaler, 1984). The most common symptoms of radiation-induced brachial plexopathy—noted in about 80% of patients—are progressive numbness and paresthesias of the arm. Approximately 60% complain of arm weakness. On examination, weakness, sensory loss, and reduced reflexes are all identified in 80% to 90% of patients (Thomas and Colby, 1972; Lederman and Wilbourn, 1984; Killer and Hess, 1990; Mondrup et al., 1990; Olsen et al., 1993). Unlike neoplastic plexopathies, Horner's syndrome is uncommon. Lymphedema occurs in about 35% of patients (Kori et al., 1981; Harper et al., 1989; Mondrup et al., 1990; Esteban and Traba, 1993; Thyagarajan et al., 1995). Although most investigators agree that lymphedema does not distinguish radiation from neoplastic etiologies, its appearance more than 3 years after treatment is more characteristic of tumor (Kori et al., 1981). Radiogenic skin changes are commonly present but do not distinguish radiation from metastatic plexopathies (Kori et al., 1981; Esteban and Traba, 1993).

CT or MRI of the plexus typically reveals diffuse soft tissue infiltration with loss of tissue planes, but this is also seen in metastatic plexopathies (Glazer et al., 1985; Thyagarajan et al., 1995; Qayyum et al., 2000). Areas of increased T2 signal adjacent to the plexus are usually present. In the plexus itself, T1 and T2 signal intensities are decreased. Incidental masses are sometimes seen, either primary nerve sheath tumors or radiation-induced malignancies (Thyagarajan et al., 1995).

Whereas most reports stress relentless progression over many years, culminating in a severely paretic, useless arm, several series indicate that one third to two thirds of patients eventually stabilize after 1 to 9 years of progression (Thomas and Colby, 1972; Harper et al., 1989; Killer and Hess, 1990). A less well-documented, reversible, radiation-induced brachial plexopathy can also occur, with an incidence of 1% to 2% (Stoll and Andrews, 1966; Salner et al., 1981; Pierce et al., 1992). There is no proven therapy for radiation-induced plexopathy.

Electrophysiological Testing in Cancer-Related Brachial Plexopathies

In patients with malignancy-related brachial plexopathies, electrodiagnostic testing is useful in as-

sessing the extent of involvement and differentiating neoplastic from postirradiation etiologies. Changes indicative of axon loss are usually present with both malignancy and radiation-induced processes (Albers et al., 1981; Streib et al., 1982; Lederman and Wilbourn, 1984; Levin et al., 1987; Harper et al., 1989; Fardin et al., 1990; Mondrup et al., 1990; Esteban and Traba, 1993; Boyaciyan et al., 1996). SNAP amplitude reduction, with relatively preserved conduction velocities, is the most sensitive nerve conduction parameter in detecting axon loss. Absent or low-amplitude SNAPs occur in more than 90% of patients with postirradiation plexopathies, including approximately 90% of median studies and 80% of ulnar studies (Lederman and Wilbourn, 1984; Harper et al., 1989; Esteban and Traba, 1993). Some investigators report that a low-amplitude median SNAP is the earliest alteration (Levin et al., 1987). The lateral antebrachial cutaneous SNAP was abnormal in all 10 patients tested in one report (Lederman and Wilbourn, 1984). SNAPs are less commonly affected in neoplastic plexopathies (median and ulnar responses each abnormal in about 65% of patients) (Lederman and Wilbourn, 1984; Harper et al., 1989). Median and ulnar CMAP amplitude reductions occur less frequently than do SNAP reductions in radiation-induced plexopathies (Albers et al., 1981; Lederman and Wilbourn, 1984; Harper et al., 1989; Esteban and Traba, 1993; Boyaciyan et al., 1996), but are at least as prevalent as SNAP abnormalities in malignant plexopathies due to axon loss in the lower trunk (Lederman and Wilbourn, 1984; Harper et al., 1989; Boyaciyan et al., 1996). Distal motor latencies and motor conduction velocities are usually normal. Ulnar or median F wave latencies were prolonged in about 50% of patients with both neoplastic and radiation plexopathies in one large series (Harper et al., 1989); two other groups reported a nearly 100% incidence of F-wave abnormalities (Esteban and Traba, 1993; Boyaciyan et al., 1996). Many workers feel that chronic demyelinative conduction block is also characteristic of radiation-induced brachial plexopathies (Harper et al., 1989; Esteban and Traba, 1993; Wilbourn, 1993; Boyaciyan et al., 1996). Erb's point or cervical root stimulation reveals partial or complete motor conduction block to various proximal and distal arm muscles in up to 90% to 100% of radiation plexopathy patients (Streib et al., 1982; Harper et al., 1989; Esteban and Traba, 1993). Conduction block across the plexus is less common in patients with neoplastic plexopathy (54%) (Harper et al., 1989).

Fibrillation potentials and positive sharp waves on needle EMG examination are the most sensitive early indicator of motor denervation, but do not typically appear until 3 weeks after axon disruption. Decreased recruitment of MUAPs can be seen immediately but is more difficult to identify. Fibrillation potentials are detected in at least one muscle in 80% to 85% of patients with both radiation-induced and neoplastic brachial plexopathies (Lederman and Wilbourn, 1984; Levin et al., 1987; Harper et al., 1989;

Esteban and Traba, 1993). Paraspinal muscles are more commonly involved in radiation cases than in neoplastic cases (23% versus 2%) (Harper et al., 1989). Indicative of the chronicity of the lesions at the time of diagnosis, signs of chronic reinnervation (long-duration, large-amplitude, polyphasic MUAPs) are present in an even higher proportion of patients with either plexopathy type, typically 90% to 100% of those examined (Lederman and Wilbourn, 1984; Levin et al., 1987; Harper et al., 1989; Mondrup et al., 1990; Esteban and Traba, 1993).

The one distinguishing EMG feature of radiation-induced neural injury is myokymic discharges. Unfortunately, myokymic discharges do not occur in all postirradiation brachial plexopathies. Their combined incidence, drawn from several reported series, is about 50% (Levin et al., 1987; Harper et al., 1989; Mondrup et al., 1990; Esteban and Traba, 1993; Thyagarajan, 1995; Boyaciyan et al., 1996). In contrast, myokymic discharges do not generally occur in neoplastic plexopathies. In the study by Harper et al., 2 of 50 neoplastic plexopathy patients had myokymic discharges, but the discharges were restricted to a single muscle in each patient and both patients had received radiation to the brachial plexus (Harper et al., 1989). Fasciculation potentials are also more common in radiation-induced neoplastic plexopathies than in neoplastic ones (45% versus 15%), but with less discriminative value than for myokymic discharges (Lederman and Wilbourn, 1984; Harper et al., 1989; Mondrup et al., 1990; Esteban and Traba, 1993; Boyaciyan et al., 1996). Stohr (1982) reported additional types of abnormal electrical activity in radiogenic nerve injuries (brachial and lumbosacral plexopathies), including low-frequency (<10 Hz) complex repetitive discharges in 10% of patients and myoclonus in 6% (Stohr, 1982). The complex repetitive charges had greater complexity (up to 84 phases), longer mean durations (39 msec), and greater persistence (up to 30 minutes) than those observed with complex repetitive charges in other conditions.

In upper trunk plexopathies, affected SNAPs are the lateral antebrachial cutaneous and median (thumb recorded or stimulated) (Ferrante and Wilbourn, 1995; Wilbourn, 1997). Superficial radial SNAPs are less consistently involved (60% of cases). The musculocutaneous (biceps) and axillary (deltoid) responses are the most useful motor nerve conduction studies. In middle trunk plexopathies, the most sensitive SNAPs are the median responses from the index and middle fingers. Radial SNAPs are affected 40% of the time. CMAP amplitude abnormalities may be observed in the radial motor study recorded from the extensor digitorum communis. With lower trunk plexopathies, the ulnar and medial antebrachial cutaneous SNAPs are nearly always absent or decreased in amplitude; corresponding CMAP/F-wave abnormalities may be seen in the median, ulnar, and radial (extensor indicis proprius) motor nerve conduction studies. For assessment of the three cords, the following motor and sensory studies are most useful: lateral cord (lateral antebrachial cutaneous SNAP, median [index finger/thumb/middle finger] SNAP, and musculocutaneous CMAP); posterior cord (radial SNAP, radial CMAP, and axillary CMAP); and medial cord (ulnar SNAP, medial antebrachial cutaneous SNAP, ulnar CMAP, and median CMAP).

LUMBOSACRAL PLEXOPATHIES

Malignant Lumbosacral Plexopathies

As with brachial plexopathies, lumbosacral plexopathies in patients with systemic malignancies can result from tumor invasion or radiation-induced damage (Lesser, 1996; van den Bent et al., 1998). Direct malignant involvement of the plexus is the more common cause (Pettigrew et al., 1984; Jaeckle et al., 1985; Thomas et al., 1985; Saphner et al., 1989; Taylor et al., 1997). Tumor plexopathies are caused by local spread of intrapelvic neoplasms or metastatic disease to the retroperitoneal lymph nodes, sacrum, lumbar vertebrae, and iliopsoas muscles. Direct spread or local metastasis from intrapelvic cancers is more common (73%) than metastasis from extrapelvic tumors (27%) (Jaeckle et al., 1985). The single most common tumor to produce a malignant lumbosacral plexopathy is a colorectal adenocarcinoma. Rectal tumors tend to spread lymphatically to the lumbar vertebrae or the adjacent paravertebral space, later compressing the lumbar plexus by a tumor mass, with direct nerve infiltration occurring less frequently. Other pelvic neoplasms with a propensity to the damage the lumbosacral plexus are sarcomas and carcinomas of the prostate, cervix, uterus, bladder, and ovary. Breast cancers and lymphomas are the most common metastatic tumors to produce a malignant lumbosacral plexopathy. Similar to the brachial plexus, lumbosacral plexus involvement by tumor usually occurs in patients with known cancers, but in 10% to 15% of cases, lumbosacral plexopathies are the initial manifestation of the cancer (Jaeckle et al., 1985; Taylor et al., 1997). Latency from cancer diagnosis to onset of plexopathy symptoms varies from 0 to 216 months (Saphner et al., 1989), with a median of 20 months (Saphner et al., 1989) and reported means of 23 to 56 months (Pettigrew et al., 1984; Taylor et al., 1997). The true incidence of this condition is unknown, but in patients with cervical cancer, 2% to 3% of patients are eventually affected (De Alvarez, 1953; Saphner et al., 1989). The prognosis for patients with malignant lumbosacral plexopathies is poor, consistent with their usually advanced cancer stage. Median survival is about 5 months (Saphner et al., 1989; Taylor et al., 1997; Jacobson et al., 1998), and 85% of patients are dead in 1 year (Thomas et al., 1985). Treatment of the plexopathy is palliative and typically restricted to external-beam radiation.

In tumor-induced plexopathies, the lower lumbosacral plexus (L4-S2) is involved in approximately 50% of patients, the upper plexus (L1-L4) in about 30%, and the entire plexus in about 20% (Jaeckle et al., 1985; Thomas et al., 1985; Saphner et al., 1989). Isolated mononeuropathies of nerves derived from the lumbosacral plexus can also be produced by pelvic neoplasms, including obturator (Saphner et al., 1989; Rogers et al., 1993), femoral (Geiger et al., 1998), genitofemoral (Saphner et al., 1989), and inferior gluteal/posterior femoral cutaneous (LaBan et al., 1982) neuropathies. Malignant plexopathies are usually unilateral, but about 20% have bilateral signs and symptoms with a unilateral predominance.

Patients with malignant invasion of the lumbosacral plexus present with progressive, persistent, commonly severe, lateralized pain over several weeks to several months. Pain is the first plexopathy symptom in 90% of patients and eventually develops in nearly all (Pettigrew et al., 1984; Jaeckle et al., 1985; Thomas et al., 1985; Saphner et al., 1989; Taylor et al., 1997). Lumbosacral plexal pain is apt to worsen at night and when the patient is lying supine or sitting, decreasing with standing, walking, and lying prone or semiprone. Weakness, numbness, and paresthesias are unusual presenting symptoms (10% to 15% of patients) but become more common with plexopathy progression (Jaeckle et al., 1985; Thomas et al., 1985; Saphner et al., 1989; Taylor et al., 1997). About two thirds of patients eventually complain of weakness, and just under half report numbness. Urinary incontinence and erectile dysfunction each occur in about 10% of patients, indicative of sacral plexus involvement (Jaeckle et al., 1985; Thomas et al., 1985; Saphner et al., 1989; Taylor et al., 1997). Sympathetic dysfunction, evidenced by a warm, anhidrotic foot, has been reported in a few cases (Gilchrist and Moore, 1985; Dalmau et al., 1989).

The most common neurological finding is leg weakness, identified in 85% of patients (Pettigrew et al., 1984; Jaeckle et al., 1985; Thomas et al., 1985; Saphner et al., 1989; Taylor et al., 1997). Upper plexopathies are associated with weakness of the hip flexors, hip adductors, and quadriceps muscles, and lower plexopathies with weakness of hamstring, gluteal, and ankle muscles. Sensory loss appropriate to the region of involved plexus occurs in 70% of patients. A similar percentage of patients have signs of asymmetrical reflex loss. Plain radiographs show vertebral or sacral osseous erosions in 50% to 60% of patients, and bone scans reveal abnormal uptake in these areas in 60% of patients (Jaeckle et al., 1985; Thomas et al., 1985; Saphner et al., 1989). Retrospective data suggest that MRI is the preferred neuroimaging technique for lumbosacral plexus tumors (Taylor et al., 1997).

Published experience with electrodiagnostic testing is limited (Pettigrew et al., 1984; Jaeckle et al., 1985; Thomas et al., 1985; Taylor et al., 1997). In almost all patients, needle EMG examination reveals fibrillation potentials and signs of chronic reinnervation (long-duration MUAPs). Approximately 30% of patients had denervation bilaterally in two combined series (Jaeckle et al., 1985; Taylor et al., 1997). Fibrillation potentials in paraspinal muscles occurred in approximately 25% of patients in one study (Taylor et al., 1997). Myokymic discharges are rarely reported, and then only in patients who received radiation therapy (Taylor et al., 1997). Nerve conduction studies should demonstrate asymmetrical reduction of CMAP and SNAP amplitudes in the affected nerves.

Radiation-Induced Lumbosacral Plexopathies

Radiation-induced nerve injury is less common in the lumbosacral plexus than in the brachial plexus (Contamin et al., 1978; Albers et al., 1981; Giese and Kinsella, 1991), but may develop after treatment of lymphomas, sarcomas, and cervical, uterine, bladder, colorectal, ovarian, and testicular carcinomas (Ashenhurst et al., 1977; Contamin et al., 1978; Schiodt and Kristensen, 1978; Albers et al., 1981; Aho and Sainio, 1983; Pettigrew et al., 1984; Glass et al., 1985; Thomas et al., 1985; Enevoldson et al., 1992). Plexus injury is more likely to occur with higher doses of radiation, but a safe threshold dosage has not been established (Thomas and Holdorff, 1993). The delay between treatment and first appearance of symptoms ranges from 1 month (Klaua, 1974) to 31 years (Thomas et al., 1985), with a median of 5 years (Thomas et al., 1985). Postirradiation lumbosacral plexopathies may be difficult to distinguish from the postirradiation, motor-predominant cauda equina syndrome described earlier.

As with radiation-induced brachial plexopathies, pain is an uncommon presenting feature in postirradiation lumbosacral plexopathies (10% of patients) (Thomas et al., 1985). At more advanced stages of the illness, 50% of patients report pain in the legs, but even then, pain is infrequently a major complaint (Pettigrew et al., 1984; Glass et al., 1985; Thomas et al., 1985; Georgiou et al., 1993). Leg weakness is the most common presenting symptom. Essentially all patients develop weakness with disease progression. Numbness and paresthesias are initially present in approximately one third of patients and become more common as the plexopathy evolves (Ashenhurst et al., 1977; Aho and Sainio, 1983; Thomas et al., 1985; Georgiou et al., 1993). Bowel and bladder incontinence is not expected.

On examination, all patients exhibit leg weakness, which is bilateral but asymmetrical in about 75% (Ashenhurst et al., 1977; Aho and Sainio, 1983; Pettigrew et al., 1984; Glass et al., 1985; Thomas et al., 1985; Saphner et al., 1989; Georgiou et al., 1993). Unlike neoplastic plexopathies, where pan-plexus involvement is uncommon, 80% of patients with radiation lumbosacral plexopathies show diffuse motor dysfunction, albeit with a lower plexus and distal lower limb predominance (Ashenhurst et al., 1977; Pettigrew et al., 1984; Glass et al., 1985; Thomas et al., 1985). Only 10% of patients showed isolated upper lumbar or femoral nerve involvement in the largest series (Thomas et al., 1985), although smaller series dedicated to patients with femoral palsies can be found (Laurent, 1975). Two thirds of patients have demonstrable sensory loss. Nearly all have reduced or absent stretch reflexes in the legs, usually bilaterally (ankle reflexes decreased more commonly than knee reflexes).

Electrodiagnostic findings in radiation-related lumbosacral plexopathies have been reported in a few cases (Albers et al., 1981; Aho and Sainio, 1983; Thomas et al., 1985; Enevoldson et al., 1992). Motor nerve conduction studies show normal or slightly reduced conduction velocities and inconsistently decreased CMAP amplitudes. The sural SNAP is reduced in amplitude or absent in 50% of patients, presumably those with lower plexus involvement. Needle EMG examination shows widespread fibrillation potentials and long-duration, large-amplitude MUAPs in the lower limb muscles of nearly all patients. Fibrillation potentials were observed in the lumbosacral paraspinal muscles in 50% of patients by Thomas et al. (1985), indicative of a radiculoplexopathy. Recruitment is decreased in clinically weak muscles. Myokymic discharges are noted in 60% to 65% of patients, involving both paraspinal and limb muscles (Aho and Sainio, 1983; Thomas et al., 1985). As elaborated in the section on radiation-induced brachial plexopathies, low-frequency complex repetitive discharges of abnormal complexity, duration, and persistence are also characteristic of this disorder, but occur uncommonly (Stohr 1982).

Whereas most lumbosacral radiation plexopathies evolve in a slowly progressive fashion over many years, 20% of patients progress to moderate or severe weakness in several months (Thomas et al., 1985). Some patients stabilize after 1 to 5 years (Aho and Sainio, 1983; Thomas et al., 1985; Georgiou et al., 1993), and rare patients spontaneously recover (Schiodt and Kristensen, 1978; Thomas et al., 1985; Enevoldson et al., 1992). As with brachial plexopathies, there is no established treatment for radiation injury to the lumbosacral plexus.

In summary, radiation lumbosacral plexopathies can be distinguished from their malignant counterparts by (1) lack of significant pain at onset, (2) tendency for more diffuse plexus involvement, (3) presence of bilateral signs and symptoms, (4) absence of rectal mass and leg edema, (5) tendency for slower progression over many years, (6) lack of mass lesion on pelvic imaging, (7) normal lumbar myelogram and magnetic resonance images, and (8) myokymic discharges or low-frequency, abnormally persistent complex repetitive discharges on needle EMG examination.

DIFFUSE PERIPHERAL NEUROPATHIES

Peripheral neuropathies in patients with systemic cancer can present in diverse neuroanatomical patterns and result from multiple etiologic factors. Two well-recognized categories of malignancy-related neuropathy—paraneoplastic and monoclonal gammopathy associated—are dealt with in other chapters of this book. We will concentrate instead on two other well-established mechanisms specific to cancer patients—neoplastic infiltration and peripheral neurotoxicity from chemotherapeutic agents. Post–bone marrow transplantation neuropathies and the commonly encountered cryptogenic, sensorimotor, length-dependent polyneuropathy will also be addressed. Patients with advanced malignancy are also susceptible to widespread PNS damage from many other nonspecific influences, including renal failure, hepatic insufficiency, critical illness, hypoxemia, other drug-related toxicities, malnutrition, and vitamin deficiencies; however, these topics are covered in other chapters.

Infiltrative Neoplastic Polyneuropathies

Diffuse infiltration by neoplastic cells into peripheral nerves is an uncommon cause of neuropathy in patients with systemic malignancy (Henson and Urich, 1982; van den Bent et al., 1998). However, the incidence of this phenomenon may be underestimated because (1) its clinicopathological features overlap with those of paraneoplastic/immunological neuropathies; (2) nerve biopsies are infrequently performed in advanced-stage, debilitated cancer patients; (3) sampling error may occur in those patients who are biopsied; and (4) sophisticated genetic and immunohistochemical methodologies for identifying monoclonal populations of cells are lacking in all but the most recent reports. Widespread PNS infiltration, when it occurs, is largely restricted to hematological malignancies, particularly NHL and leukemias (Henson and Urich, 1982). There are rare reports of patients with multiple myeloma (Barron et al., 1960) and Waldenström's macroglobulinemia (Abad et al., 1999) developing diffuse infiltrative neuropathies. In one reported case, malignant melanoma produced multiple mononeuropathies by invading peripheral nerves (Ogose et al., 1998). Carcinomas and sarcomas, on the other hand, do not invade nerves diffusely, instead producing focal nerve disturbances such as radiculopathies, cranial neuropathies, and limb plexus neuropathies by external compression or more restricted, short-range infiltration (Henson and Urich, 1982; van den Bent et al., 1998).

LYMPHOMA

As defined by large retrospective series, the incidence of clinically identified polyneuropathy in lymphoma patients ranges from 0.1% to 2% (Williams et al., 1959; Curriet et al., 1970; McLeod, 1993b); however, these figures undoubtedly underestimate the true incidence. In one prospective study, 8% of patients with lymphoma had signs and symptoms of a polyneuropathy and 35% had electrophysiological evidence of a generalized neuropathy (Walsh, 1971). Some of these neuropathies are produced when lymphoma cells directly infiltrate and thereby damage peripheral nerves. This is called a lymphomatous neuropathy, or neurolymphomatosis (Lhermitte and Trelles, 1934; Henson and Urich, 1982; van den Bent et al., 1998). The diagnosis of lymphomatous neuropathy rests on the demonstration of tumor cells in peripheral nerves. Judging from the number of available reports, this is a very uncommon occurrence, but the condition is probably under-recognized for the reasons outlined above. Careful autopsy studies have demonstrated neoplastic infiltrates in spinal and peripheral nerves of 35% to 40% of patients with malignant lymphoma (Dickenman and Chason, 1958; Jellinger and Radaszkiewicz, 1976).

Remote effects of lymphoma on the PNS are largely immune mediated and can be classified as (1) classic GBS in patients with Hodgkin's disease (Lisak et al., 1977; Vital et al., 1990); (2) chronic, sometimes relapsing, inflammatory, demyelinating polyradiculoneuropathy (CIDP) in both Hodgkin's disease (Croft et al., 1967) and NHL (Sumi et al., 1983; Vallat et al., 1995); (3) paraproteinemic neuropathies (especially IgM monoclonal gammopathy–associated, chronic demyelinating neuropathies) (Vallat et al., 1995); (4) paraneoplastic motor neuron syndromes associated with lymphoproliferative disorders (Gordon et al., 1997); (5) paraneoplastic vasculitic neuropathies (Oh, 1997); (6) paraneoplastic sensory neuronopathies (Plante-Bordeneuve et al., 1994); or (7) chronic demyelinating neuropathies in POEMS syndrome (characterized by polyneuropathy, organomegaly, endocrinopathy, monoclonal gammopathy, and skin changes) and Castleman's disease (Kelly et al., 1983; Donaghy et al., 1989). Paraneoplastic neuropathies are discussed in other chapters. But as a practical matter, it can occasionally be difficult to distinguish lymphomatous neuropathies from these paraneoplastic variants by clinical, electrodiagnostic, and even pathological criteria. For instance, small clonal populations of neoplastic cells can sometimes be found in peripheral nerve specimens from patients who otherwise meet criteria for an immune-mediated, inflammatory neuropathy (Vital et al., 1990; Vallat et al., 1995; Creange et al., 1996).

NEUROLYMPHOMATOSIS

Neurolymphomatosis is largely confined to NHL, as only rare reports of Hodgkin's disease infiltrating peripheral nerves are found (Barron et al., 1960; Jellinger and Radaszkiewicz, 1976). The majority of cases—at least 75%—arise from B-cell lymphomas (Diaz-Arrastia et al., 1992). Neurolymphomatosis may be the presenting feature of the cancer or the first sign of a relapse (Pietrangeli et al., 2000). The PNS may represent a site of sanctuary for tumor cells, with the blood–nerve barrier protecting them

from exposure to the systemic chemotherapy (van den Bent et al., 1995). Diaz-Arrastia et al. reviewed the literature on neurolymphomatosis in 1992 and found only 48% of patients to have known systemic lymphoma at the time of the neurological presentation; at autopsy, one third still had lymphoma restricted to the nervous system (Diaz-Arrastia et al., 1992). Seventy percent had postmortem evidence of simultaneous meningeal lymphoma.

Most patients with neurolymphomatosis present with a subacute-chronic, slowly progressive, painful, axonal, sensorimotor neuropathy or polyradiculoneuropathy (Lhermitte and Trelles, 1934; Barron et al., 1960; Guberman et al., 1978; Ince et al., 1987; Gold et al., 1988; Thomas et al., 1990; Vital et al., 1990; Atiq et al., 1992; Diaz-Arrastia et al., 1992; Vallat et al., 1995; Sonobe et al., 1998; Walk et al., 1998; van den Bent et al., 1999). In typical patients, the neuropathy is at least somewhat asymmetrical, as would be expected for an infiltrative process. Discrete multiple mononeuropathies (Krendel et al., 1991) occur less frequently than overlapping, asymmetrical profiles. Isolated mononeuropathies have been reported in a few patients (van den Bent, 1995; Quinones-Hinojosa et al., 2000). As discussed previously, lymphomas can also focally infiltrate the brachial and lumbosacral plexuses. Coexisting cranial neuropathies are present in 50% of patients (Diaz-Arrastia et al., 1992).

At presentation, the duration of symptoms is usually less than a year. Although most cases evolve over many weeks to several months, more acute, GBS-like presentations can occur. A chronic, relapsing course is also possible (Gherardi et al., 1986; Case Records MGH, 1995), but patients with a relapsing illness lasting for many years probably suffer from CIDP, not neurolymphomatosis (Borit and Altrocchi, 1971).

Analysis of cerebrospinal fluid (CSF) shows increased protein and lymphocytic pleocytosis in 60% to 70% of patients. CSF cytology demonstrates neoplastic cells in about 50% of patients (Diaz-Arrastia et al., 1992). MRI may be diagnostically useful, revealing swollen, enhancing nerves with increased T2 signal intensity (van den Bent et al., 1995; Quinones-Hinojosa et al., 2000).

Electrodiagnostic findings are usually reflective of an axonal or mixed axonal/demyelinating, asymmetrical, sensorimotor neuropathy (Guberman et al., 1978; Gherardi et al., 1986; Krendel et al., 1991; Atiq et al., 1992; Diaz-Arrastia et al., 1992; Case Records MGH, 1995; Vallat et al., 1995; van den Bent et al., 1995; Phan et al., 1998; Walk et al., 1998; van den Bent et al., 1999; Zaretsky et al., 2000). SNAP and CMAP amplitudes are diminished, with normal or mildly slowed conduction velocities and distal latencies. Needle EMG reveals fibrillation potentials and positive sharp waves in involved muscles. One patient had an axonal electrophysiological picture with preserved SNAPs, indicative of motor neuron disease, motor axonal neuropathy, or polyradiculopathy (Diaz-Arrastia et al., 1992). There are rare re-

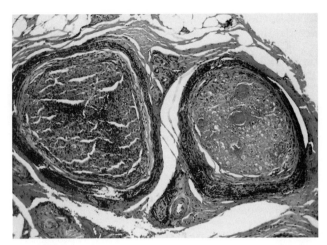

Figure 65–1. Sural nerve biopsy of a patient with non-Hodgkin's lymphoma demonstrates lymphomatous infiltration of the perineurium and endoneurium.

ports of pathologically confirmed neurolymphomatosis, with nerve conduction studies showing predominantly demyelinating characteristics, including slowed conduction velocities, prolonged F-wave latencies, abnormal temporal dispersion, and partial motor conduction block, mirroring the findings in GBS and CIDP (Ince et al., 1987; Thomas et al., 1990; Stack, 1991). Nevertheless, the presence of a demyelinating neuropathy in a patient with lymphoma is more suggestive of a paraneoplastic than a neoplastic etiology (Sumi et al., 1983).

In pathology studies, the pattern of PNS infiltration is diffuse but nonuniform (Figure 65–1) (Henson and Urich, 1982; Midroni and Bilbao, 1995). Peripheral nerves, spinal nerves, and dorsal root ganglia are commonly involved together. The distribution of involvement is patchy, with some nerves affected but not others, and differential intensity of infiltration along the course of a single nerve. Interfascicular variability is also characteristically seen, with some fascicles being destroyed by tumor and others escaping tumor altogether (van den Bent et al., 1999). The infiltration involves all three nerve compartments, with a typical perineurial predominance (Barron et al., 1960; Henson and Urich, 1982).

The nerves themselves usually exhibit a mixture of axonal and segmental demyelinating/remyelinating alterations. In adequately studied preparations, the axonal changes predominate, including wallerian-like degeneration, myelinated nerve fiber loss, and thinly myelinated regenerating axonal clusters (Guberman et al., 1978; Henson and Urich, 1982; Gherardi et al., 1986; Midroni and Bilbao, 1995). Ince et al. reported on a patient with B-cell neurolymphomatosis presenting as a primary myelinopathy (Ince et al., 1987). However, this patient also had an IgMκ monoclonal gammopathy, suggesting that the segmental demyelination resulted from local, intranerve secretion of IgM paraproteins (although no binding of IgM to peripheral nerve myelin could be demonstrated).

The mechanism of neural damage in neurolymphomatosis is unclear (Henson and Urich, 1982; Diaz-Arrastia et al., 1992; Stubgen and Elliot, 1997). Speculated pathogenetic mechanisms include external compression, local ischemia from vascular involvement, secretion of neurotoxic cytokines, secretion of antinerve antibodies, and coinfection of hematological cells and nerve fibers by an oncogenic/neurotropic virus.

The diagnosis of lymphomatous neuropathy depends on the detection of monoclonal lymphoma cells in a cutaneous nerve biopsy. Because of the segmental, nonuniform pattern of PNS infiltration, nerve biopsies are sometimes falsely negative (van den Bent et al., 1999). The sensitivity of sural and other nerve biopsies in this condition has not been analyzed. MRI may be useful in identifying affected nerves prior to biopsy (van den Bent et al., 1999). In the large literature review by Diaz-Arrastia et al., only 15 of 40 patients were diagnosed during life (Diaz-Arrastia et al., 1992).

INTRAVASCULAR LYMPHOMATOSIS (ANGIOTROPIC LARGE CELL LYMPHOMA)

Intravascular lymphomatosis (IVL) is a rare form of NHL characterized by the proliferation of large, noncohesive, malignant lymphoid cells within vascular spaces (Domizio et al., 1989; Glass et al., 1993; Demirer et al., 1994; Calamia et al., 1999). It was previously known as malignant angioendotheliomatosis and regarded as an endothelial neoplasm (Petito et al., 1978). However, with the advent of reliable immunophenotyping methods, the lymphocytic nature of the condition was confirmed (Domizio et al., 1989). Most studies have demonstrated a B-cell lineage of the neoplastic cells, but rare cases express a T-cell phenotype (Au et al., 1997). The lymphoma cells typically fill capillaries, arterioles, venules, small-to-medium sized arteries, and small veins in many different tissues. They rarely circulate in the peripheral blood and uncommonly spread to vessel walls or perivascular spaces. Vessel wall destruction does not occur. Fibrin thrombi are often associated, leading to small-vessel occlusions and ischemic infarcts in involved organs.

Most patients present with fevers and multiorgan failure, mimicking systemic vasculitis (Al-Chalabi et al., 1994). Although virtually any organ in the body can be affected, neurological and dermatological features usually predominate (Domizio et al., 1989; Glass et al., 1993). Involvement of the PNS is reported in only 5% to 10% of patients, but most studies have not addressed this complication, so that the true incidence may be higher (Glass et al., 1993). Peripheral nerve disease in IVL most characteristically takes the form of a multifocal, asymmetrical, sensorimotor neuropathy (Petito et al., 1978; Daniel et al., 1987; Glass et al., 1993; Roux et al., 1995; Levin and Lutz, 1996) or a lumbosacral polyradiculoneuropathy (cauda equina syndrome)

(Krieger et al., 1982; Sunohara et al., 1984; Lacomis et al., 1992; Al-Chalabi et al., 1994; Harris et al., 1994; Nakahara et al., 1999), but mononeuropathies (Vital et al., 1989), symmetrical sensorimotor polyneuropathies (including GBS-like presentations) (Dolman et al., 1979; Devlin et al., 1998), and motor neuron disorders (Rubio et al., 1996) have also been reported.

Only limited electrodiagnostic information is available (Petito et al., 1978; Sunohara et al., 1984; Daniel et al., 1987; Lacomis et al., 1992; Keane, 1996; Levin and Lutz, 1996; Roux et al., 1995; Rubio et al., 1996; Devlin et al., 1998). Data taken from individual case reports indicate that electrophysiological studies show changes consistent with an asymmetrical, axonal, sensorimotor neuropathy or lumbosacral polyradiculoneuropathy. Needle EMG examination reveals fibrillation potentials, long-duration large-amplitude MUAPs, and MUAP dropout in involved muscles.

Most patients (about 70%) with CNS presentations are diagnosed at autopsy (Glass et al., 1993). A diagnosis during life is more common when systemic, dermatological, and/or PNS manifestations dominate. Elevated serum lactate dehydrogenase occurs in 90% of patients and is a clue to the diagnosis, discriminating this condition from vasculitis (Calamia et al., 1999). Diagnostic biopsies have been obtained from brain, leptomeninges, skin, lung, muscle, nerve, prostate, kidney, and liver (Domizio et al., 1989; Glass et al., 1993; Liszka et al., 1994). Reported brain biopsies are nearly always positive (Smadja et al., 1991; DiGiuseppe et al., 1994; Liszka et al., 1994; Calamia et al., 1999). Muscle biopsies have been diagnostic in approximately 70% of cases (Nakahara et al., 1999). Two of three reported nerve biopsies were positive (Vital et al., 1989; Lacomis et al., 1992; Levin and Lutz, 1996).

Examination of postmortem or biopsy-obtained peripheral nerve specimens has shown intravascular collections of large lymphoid cells, primarily in the epineurial blood vessels but sometimes in the endoneurial and perineurial vasculature as well (Krieger et al., 1982; Vital et al., 1989; Lacomis et al., 1992; Harris et al., 1994; Roux et al., 1995; Levin and Lutz, 1996; Devlin et al., 1998). Epineurial vessels may be thrombosed or occluded by neoplastic cells. Axon loss and wallerian-like degeneration are typically observed, with mild segmental demyelinating/remyelinating changes. One patient with progressive lower motor neuron weakness during life was found at autopsy to have necrotic anterior horn cells and hemorrhage in the anterior horn (Al-Chalabi et al., 1994). Another such patient had degenerating motor neurons, analogous to ALS (Rubio et al., 1996).

LYMPHOMATOID GRANULOMATOSIS

Lymphomatoid granulomatosis (LYG) is a rare angiocentric and angiodestructive lymphoproliferative disorder with a propensity for pulmonary involvement (Liebow et al., 1972; Katzenstein et al., 1979; Jaffe and Wilson, 1997). Recent immunohistochemical and genotypic data have convincingly demonstrated that most cases represent Epstein-Barr virus–infected clonal B-cell proliferations, associated with an exuberant T-cell reaction and angiitis (Guinee et al., 1994; Myers et al., 1995; Wilson et al., 1996). Diffuse B-cell lymphomas emerge in 13% to 47% of patients (Katzenstein et al., 1979; Fauci et al., 1982; Pisani and DeRemee, 1990).

The PNS is affected in about 10% of patients with LYG (Israel et al., 1977; Katzenstein et al., 1979; Calatayud, et al., 1980; Fauci et al., 1982; Pisani and DeRemee, 1990; Guinee et al., 1994; Myers et al., 1995), and the same proportion of patients have cranial neuropathies (Katzenstein et al., 1979). Most series provide few clinical details on the neuropathies. On the basis of individual case reports, PNS involvement most commonly manifests as a discrete or overlapping, multifocal, sensorimotor neuropathy (Liebow et al., 1972; Gibbs, 1977; Garcia et al., 1978; Calatayud, et al., 1980; Henson and Urich, 1982; Cortes and Pazdur, 1995; Midroni and Bilbao, 1995), although patchy sensory deficits (Hogan et al., 1981) and distal, symmetrical polyneuropathies (Liebow et al., 1972; Bone et al., 1978; Richter et al., 1997) are also described. The clinical course can be acute (Calatayud, et al., 1980) or chronic (Case Records MGH, 1996).

There is no specific laboratory feature in LYG. Lumbar puncture commonly shows increased CSF protein (Jaffe and Wilson, 1997), but malignant cells are only rarely encountered (Liebow et al., 1972; Calatayud, et al., 1980). The diagnosis may be achieved by endobronchial, ear/nose/throat, skin, or brain biopsies, but open-lung biopsy is most reliable, with nearly 100% sensitivity (Pisani and DeRemee, 1990). There are scant data on peripheral nerve pathology (Liebow et al., 1972; Garcia et al., 1978; Calatayud, et al., 1980; Henson and Urich, 1982; Midroni and Bilbao, 1995). Some nerve specimens have revealed intense, angiocentric, lymphoid infiltrates—primarily T cells (Midroni and Bilbao, 1995)—interspersed with a few large atypical cells, involving all nerve compartments. More restricted endoneurial and perineurial invasion has also been observed. Perineurial thickening, marked fiber loss, wallerian-like degeneration, and focal demyelination are featured in some specimens. Epineurial vessels may be stenosed, occluded, necrotic, thrombosed, or recanalized.

Information on the electrophysiological profile of LYG is equally sparse (Calatayud, et al., 1980; Midroni and Bilbao, 1995; Wilson et al., 1996; Richter et al., 1997). Limited available data suggest that findings are typical of an active, multifocal, sensorimotor, axonal neuropathy, including low-amplitude CMAPs, mildly reduced conduction velocities, and abundant fibrillation potentials.

Leukemia

The incidence of clinically significant peripheral neuropathies in patients with leukemia is very low.

Several large series of leukemia patients reported no polyneuropathies whatsoever (Wells and Silver, 1957; Williams et al., 1959). In other retrospective studies, neuropathies have been identified in approximately 1% of patients (Schwab and Weiss, 1935; Currie et al., 1970). If attention is restricted to chronic lymphocytic leukemia (CLL), the incidence increases to about 3% (Currie et al., 1970; Walsh, 1971). However, in Walsh's prospective electrodiagnostic study, 45% of patients with CLL had nerve conduction evidence of a generalized but subclinical peripheral neuropathy (Walsh, 1971). This finding is more in keeping with two autopsy studies of leukemia patients in which 15 of 32 patients (47%) had leukemic infiltration in spinal nerve roots, dorsal root ganglia, and peripheral nerves (Dickenman and Chason, 1958; Jellinger and Radaszkiewicz, 1976).

ACUTE LEUKEMIA

For the acute leukemias, case reports of peripheral neuropathy are uncommon. Most document diffuse leukemic infiltration into the PNS as the primary pathogenetic mechanism (Henson and Urich, 1982; McLeod, 1993b; Midroni and Bilbao, 1995). In rare patients, leukemic invasion is not identified and alternate mechanisms are proposed, including (1) multifocal, subperineurial intranerve hemorrhages (Brun et al., 1964; McLeod, 1993a), (2) widespread leukostasis in the endoneurial and epineurial microvasculature, producing nerve ischemia (Sugita et al., 1973), and (3) immune-mediated, inflammatory demyelination, either acute (GBS) or chronic (CIDP) (Phanthumchinda et al., 1988; McLeod, 1993b).

The typical presentation is that of an acute or subacute, discretely multifocal or asymmetrical, sensorimotor polyneuropathy (Krendal et al., 1987; Vital et al., 1993; Kishimoto et al., 1994; Lekos et al., 1994). As with neurolymphomatosis, most leukemic neuropathies are painful. Rapidly progressive generalized yet asymmetrical weakness is commonly encountered, provoking diagnostic consideration of GBS (Aaljouanine et al., 1949; Nishi et al., 1991; Boiron et al., 1993). Acute symmetrical polyneuropathies have also been described (Buge et al., 1977). Subacute mononeuropathies occur more rarely (Muss and Moloney, 1973; Stillman et al., 1988).

Electrodiagnostic studies in acute leukemic neuropathies demonstrate findings supportive of an asymmetrical, axonal, sensorimotor neuropathy or radiculoneuropathy (Buge et al., 1977; Krendel et al., 1987; Vital et al., 1993; Kishimoto et al., 1994; Lekos et al., 1994), sometimes accompanied by superimposed demyelinating features (Krendel et al., 1987). Needle EMG examination typically shows abundant fibrillation potentials and decreased recruitment in involved muscles. MRI is not well studied in this condition; however, in one patient it revealed focal enlargement of the affected median nerve, perineural edema, and heterogeneously increased T2 signal (Lekos et al., 1994).

CHRONIC LEUKEMIA

Peripheral neuropathies are more commonly encountered in patients with CLL than in patients with acute leukemias, and the clinicopathological spectrum is more diverse (Walsh, 1971; McLeod, 1993b; Midroni and Bilbao, 1995). Unfortunately, the distinction between (1) neoplastic infiltrative and (2) paraneoplastic inflammatory neuropathies is frequently blurred in CLL (Creange et al., 1996). This is particularly true for older reports, in which modern immunophenotyping and genetic methods are not utilized.

One pattern of PNS involvement in CLL is an acute, paralytic polyradiculoneuropathy. In cases showing spontaneous recovery and demyelinating electrophysiological/neuropathological characteristics, typical immune-mediated GBS is the likely pathogenetic mechanism (Powles and Malpas, 1967; Creange et al., 1996) irrespective of the presence of small collections of clonal B cells in nerve biopsies (Creange et al., 1996). Other cases are more clearly examples of primary leukemic infiltration (Haberland et al., 1987; Thomas et al., 1990). Chronic demyelinating neuropathies that respond to immunomodulatory interventions (e.g., steroids and intravenous immunoglobulin) are also encountered in patients with CLL, probably immune-mediated and analogous to CIDP (Sumi et al., 1983; Mitsui et al., 1999). In one such patient with a chronic demyelinating neuropathy, perineurial and endoneurial lymphocytic accumulations were detected in a sural nerve biopsy, along with macrophage-mediated vesicular myelin degeneration. The lymphocytes were assumed but not proved to be of leukemic origin (Sumi et al., 1983). Acute-to-subacute, multifocal, painful, sensorimotor neuropathies also occur in patients with CLL (Ulrich and Miller, 1968; Masson et al., 1977; Creange et al., 1996). Electrophysiological studies in two such patients showed (1) an acute, axonal mononeuropathy and (2) multiple, active, axonal mononeuropathies superimposed on a chronic, sensorimotor, axonal polyneuropathy (Creange et al., 1996). Nerve/muscle biopsies have demonstrated (1) necrotizing vasculitis (Creange et al., 1996), epineurial lymphoid (?leukemic) infiltrates (Mason et al., 1977), and (3) endoneurial and perineurial leukemic infiltration with axonal degeneration (Ulrich and Miller, 1968). In the vasculitis patients, clonal B cells were identified in the biopsies using polymerase chain reaction techniques (Creange et al., 1996). Therefore, the multifocal neuropathies in these patients may have had a neoplastic, paraneoplastic, or mixed neoplastic/paraneoplastic etiology.

Other patients with CLL develop chronic, nondemyelinating, symmetrical polyneuropathies associated with leukemic infiltrates in peripheral nerves (Rowland and Schneck, 1963; Grisold et al., 1990). These neuropathies may be sensorimotor or sensory ataxic in character, with durations up to 3 years. The only reported electrodiagnostic study was essentially normal (Grisold et al., 1990). Postmortem or biopsy-derived nerve specimens showed endoneurial-predominant leukemic cells associated with mixed axonal and demyelinating nerve alterations of variable severity. Chronic, symmetrical, sensorimotor polyneuropathies with axonal or mixed axonal/demyelinating electrophysiology and neuropathology are also reported in patients with CLL with no identified etiology (Currie et al., 1970; Walsh, 1971; Case Records MGH, 1972).

Diffuse infiltrative neuropathies have also been reported with several other types of chronic leukemia, including chronic myelogenous leukemia (Barron et al., 1960), adult T-cell leukemia associated with human T-lymphocyte virus type 1 (HTLV-1) infection (Kuroda et al., 1989; Vital et al., 1993), natural killer cell leukemia (Bobker and Deloughery, 1993), and erythroleukemia (Barron et al., 1960). In contrast to the acute leukemias, infiltrative neuropathies in chronic, non-CLL leukemias generally evolve over several months and follow a distal, symmetrical, sensorimotor profile. Pain is routinely reported. Limited experience with nerve conduction studies has revealed axonal or mixed axonal/demyelinating, sensorimotor findings, with occasional asymmetries (Kuroda et al., 1989; Bobker and Deloughery, 1993). Needle EMG shows fibrillation potentials in affected muscles (Kuroda et al., 1989). In the case of chronic myelogenous leukemia reported by Barron et al., short-duration, polyphasic MUAPs were observed in a proximal muscle, but this was explained by massive infiltration of skeletal muscles detected at autopsy (Barron et al., 1960). Pathological specimens demonstrate leukemic infiltrates, accentuated in the endoneurium/subperineurial space (Kuroda et al., 1989; Bobker and Deloughery, 1993) or the epineurium/perineurium (Barron et al., 1960). Nerve fibers adjacent to these infiltrates may be normal (Bobker and Deloughery, 1993) or exhibit primary demyelinating (Barron et al., 1960), primary axonal (Kuroda et al., 1989), or mixed demyelinating/axonal changes (Barron et al., 1960).

Cryptogenic Sensorimotor Polyneuropathy

Chronic, noninfiltrative, sensorimotor polyneuropathies in patients with systemic malignancy are 2 to 4 times more common than paraneoplastic subacute sensory neuronopathies (Croft and Wilkinson, 1965; Morton et al., 1966; Croft et al., 1967). By clinical, electrophysiological, and pathological standards, these neuropathies resemble cryptogenic sensory or sensorimotor peripheral neuropathies occurring in individuals without underlying malignancies (McLeod, 1993a, 1993b; Wolfe et al., 1999). Initial symptoms are symmetrical numbness and paresthesias in the feet, which gradually progress into the distal legs and then involve the hands. Both small- and large-fiber sensory modalities are affected, but the prominent sensory ataxia observed in sensory

neuronopathies is not evident. Mild weakness in the toes and ankles eventually develops in most patients. Cranial nerves are not involved. Muscle stretch reflexes are reduced or absent in the lower limbs, particularly at the ankles.

Nerve conduction studies demonstrate features of a chronic, length-dependent, symmetrical, axonal, sensorimotor polyneuropathy (Moody, 1965; Trojaborg et al., 1969; Campbell and Paty, 1974; Paul et al., 1978; Hawley et al., 1980; Dumitru, 1995). The lower extremity SNAPs are decreased in amplitude or absent, while sensory conduction velocities are normal or slightly reduced. Lower limb CMAPs are commonly normal, but may be mildly reduced in amplitude if the neuropathy is advanced. Likewise, distal motor latencies are normal or mildly prolonged and conduction velocities normal or mildly reduced. The needle EMG examination is more sensitive than motor nerve conduction studies are, generally revealing mild active denervation and chronic reinnervation in distal lower extremity muscles. Significant asymmetries are not expected and, if found, should prompt consideration of an alternate condition or a superposed focal process such as an entrapment neuropathy or radiculopathy.

Nerve biopsies and postmortem tissue study typically reveal uniform loss of myelinated nerve fibers, signs of axonal degeneration and regeneration, and secondary demyelination with remyelination (Fisher et al., 1961; Croft et al., 1967; Case Records MGH, 1972; Henson and Urich, 1982; McLeod, 1993a). Mild, perivascular, lymphocytic infiltrates are infrequently seen in peripheral nerve specimens (Croft et al., 1967), but neoplastic cell infiltration excludes the diagnosis.

The etiology of most distal sensory and sensorimotor polyneuropathies in patients with malignancy is unknown (Henson and Urich, 1982; Dalmau et al., 1989; McLeod, 1993a; Grisold and Drlicek, 1999). Many chemotherapeutic agents are toxic to peripheral nerves (see following), but polyneuropathies also occur in untreated individuals with cancer. Metabolic factors may contribute to the peripheral nerve damage. For example, neoplasms alter normal protein and lipid metabolism in cancer patients (Costa and Holland, 1965) and may compete for metabolites and nutrients essential for normal functioning of the PNS. While deserving of further investigation, metabolic theories lack experimental support at this time. Hildebrand and Coers found an association between histological evidence of neuropathy and malignant cachexia (Hildebrand and Coers, 1967); however, their findings were not confirmed by other investigators (Croft and Wilkinson, 1963; Croft and Wilkinson, 1965; Trojaborg et al., 1969). Although weight loss frequently accompanies cancer, maintenance of a normal nutritional state neither prevents this syndrome nor alters the clinical course (Henson and Urich, 1982). Furthermore, vitamin supplementation is of no proven benefit (McLeod, 1993a). Therefore, nutritional factors are unlikely to be relevant to the development of most cancer-associated polyneuropathies. An exception occurs in patients who have received pelvic irradiation for cervical and bladder carcinomas, in whom delayed vitamin B_{12} deficiency can develop as a result of radiation-induced damage to the ileum (Anderson et al., 1981; Kinn and Lantz, 1984). Another possibility is that tumors release biological substances injurious to nervous system tissues, be they cytokines, inflammatory mediators, or trophic factors; however, experimental support is lacking. Immunological mechanisms may also be operative, but pathological changes are usually noninflammatory and specific humoral markers have not been identified.

Neuropathies Complicating Bone Marrow Transplantation

Bone marrow transplantations (BMTs) are performed for the treatment of patients with leukemia, refractory lymphoma, or various solid-organ malignancies. Peripheral and cranial neuropathies develop in approximately 25% of BMT recipients (Wiznitzer et al., 1984). Potential mechanisms include toxic effects from chemotherapeutic or immunosuppressive agents, radiation-induced damage, infections, and autoimmunity. Of these, the most common causes are varicella-zoster virus infection (see preceding section in this chapter) and chemotherapy-associated neurotoxicity (see following) (Wiznitzer et al., 1984; Davius and Patchell, 1988). Infrequently, peripheral neuropathies occur as an apparent complication of chronic graft-versus-host disease (GVHD) (Amato et al., 1993; Amato and Barohn, 1997). Chronic GVHD, which resembles many autoimmune disorders, may mediate an immunological attack directed against the PNS in selected patients (Amato and Barohn, 1997).

A wide variety of PNS disorders have been described in post-BMT patients, including cranial neuropathies (Mattsson et al., 1992), painful axonal sensory neuropathies (Greenspan et al., 1990), multifocal axonal neuropathies (Wiznitzer et al., 1984), and generalized sensorimotor polyradiculoneuropathies (Granena et al., 1983). The polyradiculoneuropathies may be acute (resembling GBS) (Johnson et al., 1987; Hagensee et al., 1994; Perry et al., 1994; Openshaw et al., 1996, 1997), subacute (Granena et al., 1983), or chronic (resembling CIDP) (Adams et al., 1995; Openshaw, 1997). Patients receiving both allogeneic and autologous BMTs are susceptible. Some of the GBS-like cases have been attributed to chemotherapy with high-dose cytosine arabinoside (ara-C; see following) (Johnson et al., 1987; Openshaw et al., 1996), CMV infection (Perry et al., 1994), or *Campylobacter jejuni* infection (Hagensee et al., 1994). Most patients with chronic polyradiculoneuropathy have concurrent chronic GVHD, supporting an immune-mediated pathogenesis.

Electrodiagnostic findings in patients with the GBS-like neuropathy reflect those observed in idiopathic GBS, indicative of an acquired demyelinating neuropathy (Hadden et al., 1998). The results of electrophysiological testing in patients with chronic polyradiculoneuropathies associated with chronic GVHD generally fail to meet research criteria for a primary chronic demyelinating neuropathy (Cornblath et al., 1911). Instead, they reveal mixed axonal and demyelinating features (Amato et al., 1993). Mixed axonal and demyelinating/remyelinating changes are also typically observed in sural nerve biopsy specimens from these patients (Amato et al., 1993). The biopsies show collections of T cells (CD8$^+$ predominance) in the endoneurium.

Toxic Polyneuropathies Secondary to Chemotherapy

Commonly used anticancer drugs that may produce a toxic neuropathy are platinum agents (e.g., cisplatin, carboplatin), vinca alkaloids (e.g., vincristine, vinorelbine), taxanes (e.g., paclitaxel, docetaxel), suramin, ara-C, etoposide (VP-16), and ifosfamide (Table 65–2) (Amato and Collins, 1998). These agents typically cause a distal axonopathy or ganglionopathy, almost always in a dose-dependent fashion. Pain and other sensory symptoms usually herald the neuropathy. With additional doses, symptoms worsen and electrodiagnostic abnormalities appear. In general, patients with pre-existing neuropathy (e.g., Charcot-Marie-Tooth disease) are at increased risk of developing a severe neuropathy from chemotherapy, as are patients treated with two neurotoxic agents simultaneously.

The medical oncologist faces a difficult decision when cancer patients develop symptoms of neuropathy while under treatment with a neurotoxic chemotherapeutic agent. Drug withdrawal or dose reduction at an early stage of the neuropathy prevents progression to a more severe grade and usually suffices to enable complete functional recovery. However, if therapy is continued and high cumulative doses are achieved, residual neuropathic deficits are inevitable, especially distal sensory loss and painful paresthesias.

Much effort has been devoted in recent years to the development of neuroprotective strategies. Amifostine is the first approved drug with demonstrated efficacy in a randomized, controlled trial to reduce the incidence and severity of cisplatin neurotoxicity, without loss of antitumor effect (Kemp et al., 1996). However, amifostine was not neuroprotective for paclitaxel in another controlled study (Gelmon et al., 1999). This agent's cytoprotective potential is specific to normal cells. Mechanisms include antioxidant effects and prevention of cisplatin-DNA adduct formation (Capizzi, 1999). Nerve growth factor, insulin-like growth factor I, other neurotrophic agents, and other antioxidants are under investigation (Windebank, 1999).

Table 65–2. Toxic Neuropathies Caused by Chemotherapy

Drug	Mechanism of Neurotoxicity	Clinical Features	Nerve Histopathology	EMG/NCS
Vinca alkaloids (vincristine, vinblastine, vindesine, vinorelbine)	Interferes with axonal microtubule assembly; impairs axonal transport	Symmetrical, sensorimotor, large/small-fiber PN; autonomic symptoms common; infrequent cranial neuropathies	Axonal degeneration of large and small myelinated and unmyelinated fibers; regenerating clusters; minimal segmental demyelination	Axonal, sensorimotor PN; H reflex preserved until late; distal denervation on EMG; abnormal QST, particularly vibratory perception
Platinum agents (cisplatin, carboplatin, oxaliplatin)	Preferential damage to DRG: ?Binds to and cross-links DNA, inducing neuronal apoptosis ?Inhibits protein synthesis ?Impairs axonal transport	Predominant large-fiber sensory neuronopathy; sensory ataxia	Loss of large > small myelinated and unmyelinated fibers; axonal degeneration; ± clusters of regenerating fibers; secondary segmental demyelination	Low-amplitude or absent SNAPs with normal CMAPs and EMG; early loss of H reflex; abnormal QST, particularly vibratory perception
Taxanes (paclitaxel, docetaxel)	Promotes axonal microtubule assembly; interferes with axonal transport	Symmetrical, sensory-predominant PN; large-fiber modalities affected more than small-fiber; ± proximal weakness (myopathic)	Loss of large > small myelinated and unmyelinated fibers; axonal degeneration; ± clusters of regenerating fibers; secondary segmental demyelination	Axonal, sensorimotor PN; distal denervation on EMG; ± proximal myopathic EMG changes; abnormal QST, particularly vibratory perception
Suramin Axonal PN	?Inhibition of neurotrophic growth factor binding ?Neuronal/Schwann cell lysosomal storage disease, with ceramide-mediated apoptosis	Symmetrical, length-dependent, sensory-predominant PN	None described	Abnormalities consistent with an axonal, sensorimotor PN
Demyelinating PN	?Immunomodulating effects ?As for axonal PN	Subacute, sensorimotor PN with diffuse proximal and distal weakness; areflexia; increased CSF protein	Loss of large and small myelinated fibers with primary demyelination and secondary axonal degeneration; ± epi- and endoneurial inflammatory cell infiltrates	Features suggestive of an acquired demyelinating sensorimotor PN (e.g., slow conduction velocities, prolonged distal latencies and F-wave latencies, conduction block, temporal dispersion)
Cytosine arabinoside (ara-C)	Unknown ?Selective Schwann cell toxicity ?Immunomodulating effects	GBS-like syndrome; pure sensory neuropathy; brachial plexopathy	Varied: loss of myelinated nerve fibers with axonal degeneration; primary segmental demyelination; or mixed demyelination and axonal degeneration; no inflammation	Varied: primary axonal, primary demyelinating, or mixed axonal/demyelinating sensorimotor PN; denervation on EMG
Etoposide (VP-16)	Unknown Inhibits topoisomerase II ?Selective DRG toxicity	Length-dependent, sensory-predominant PN; autonomic neuropathy	None described	Abnormalities consistent with an axonal sensorimotor PN

CMAP, compound muscle action potential; CSF, cerebrospinal fluid; DRG, dorsal root ganglion; EMG, electromyography; GBS, Guillain-Barré syndrome; NCS, nerve conduction studies; PN, polyneuropathy; QST, quantitative sensory testing; SNAP, sensory nerve action potential; ±, inconsistently observed.
Modified with permission from Amato AA, Collins MP. Neuropathies associated with malignancy. Semin Neurol 1998;18:125–144.

PLATINUM COMPOUNDS

Cisplatin

Cisplatin is a chemotherapeutic agent used for a wide variety of tumors, most notably ovarian, testicular, lung, bladder, head and neck, and germ cell cancers (Reed et al., 1996). Peripheral neuropathy is an important side effect and can be dose limiting. Cisplatin is believed to kill malignant cells through its ability to covalently bind DNA, creating intrastrand cross-links, which disrupt DNA function and produce DNA damage. The exact mechanism of cis-

functional recovery." Coppack and Watkins (1991) reexamined 18 patients an average of 4 years after onset and emphasized the good prognosis—none of these patients remained disabled, and residual signs and symptoms were mild. Five patients had relapses in the contralateral thigh, and two were judged to have severe relapses. Recovery did not begin until more than 3 months after onset, and sometimes recovery took more than 1.5 years.

The usually good long-term prognosis for this syndrome has encouraged physicians to use symptomatic treatment, good diabetic control, and reassurance as the mainstays of therapy. However, recognition of the inflammatory nature of this disease has lead to efforts at treatment with immunosuppression.

Garland (1961) recommended the use of corticosteroids only in nondiabetics with this syndrome, presumably because he believed that the pathological process was metabolic rather than inflammatory in diabetics.

Bradley and colleagues (1984) used prednisone and cyclophosphamide in three diabetics who had lumbosacral plexopathy and nerve biopsy samples that showed vascular inflammation. All three improved with treatment, but the authors thought that their patients did not have the diabetic syndrome because they had worsened despite good diabetic control.

Engel and Prentice (1993) reported good results in the treatment of 10 diabetics with severe progressive neuropathy, some of whom had proximal neuropathy or mononeuropathy multiplex, with immunosuppressive techniques that included plasmapheresis, prednisone, and intravenous immunoglobulin.

Costigan and colleagues (1990) treated four diabetic patients with immunosuppressive medication that included intravenous immunoglobulin, cyclophosphamide, and prednisone. Nerve biopsy samples showed vasculitis or chronic demyelination, and all patients improved with treatment. The authors suggested that an autoimmune/inflammatory process might be responsible for proximal diabetic neuropathy or mononeuropathy multiplex, because their patients had clinical features consistent with these syndromes.

Said and colleagues (1994) treated two patients who had progressive proximal neuropathy and vascular inflammation on nerve biopsy samples with prednisone. Pain quickly subsided in both, and weakness resolved over 2 to 3 months. In a subsequent report, however, Said (1997) questioned the benefit of corticosteroids because four patients in whom he had been considering the use of prednisone became free of pain without treatment soon after their biopsy samples showed vasculitis. It should be noted, however, that these patients had pain in the distributions of the nerves that underwent biopsy, so resolution of pain after removal of the nerves would not be unexpected.

Pascoe and colleagues (1997) retrospectively studied 44 patients with subacute diabetic proximal neuropathy. They found that improvement occurred in 75% of 12 patients treated with intravenous immunoglobulin, plasma exchange, or prednisone. Of 29 untreated patients, 59% also improved but more slowly.

Successful treatment of 15 patients with this syndrome has been reported with the use of various immunosuppressive medications, including prednisone, cyclophosphamide, azathioprine, and intravenous immunoglobulin (Krendel et al., 1995). All of the patients had been progressively worsening before treatment, and on treatment, all began to improve, sometimes rapidly (over 1 to 3 weeks). Two patients had a relapse 2 to 3 months after treatment, but they responded again when treatment was reinstituted. Complications of prednisone use included insomnia, depression, heart failure (fluid retention), gastrointestinal hemorrhage, and increased requirement for insulin. Intravenous immunoglobulin was better tolerated, although one patient developed a rash and one patient became septic.

In a continuation of this study, 39 of 40 patients with this syndrome began to improve within 1 month of treatment with intravenous immunoglobulin (Krendel et al., 1997). Eight patients relapsed in 1 to 8 months, of whom two recovered when treated with prednisone. For one patient, prednisone failed, but treatment with intravenous immunoglobulin resulted in improvement, and three patients improved with a second course of intravenous immunoglobulin and concurrent prednisone. Eight patients were not treated initially, and three of them improved over 1 to 3 months, one improved after 8 months, and four worsened over 1 to 7 months (of whom one was subsequently treated with intravenous immunoglobulin, and improved quickly).

Intravenous immunoglobulin can impair renal function, and although this is almost always transient, the serum creatinine level should be monitored and the treatment stopped if the level increases significantly. There have been reports of venous and arterial occlusive events in patients receiving intravenous immunoglobulin, presumably due to a hypercoagulable state resulting from hyperviscosity. The risk is low, however, and should be reduced by spreading the infusion of 2 g/kg over at least 5 days.

In summary, there is convincing histopathological evidence of an inflammatory process that involves small vessels in proximal diabetic neuropathy/amyotrophy/mononeuropathy multiplex. This, together with reports from several authors of apparently successful treatment, suggests that there is a place for immunosuppressive treatment in these patients. Because spontaneous recovery commonly occurs, treatment probably should be considered only for patients who are progressively worsening and becoming significantly impaired. In the future, controlled studies may further clarify the role of immunosuppressive therapy in this disease.

DEMYELINATING NEUROPATHY

Because diabetic polyneuropathy is typically characterized by axon loss rather than by demyelination, electrophysiological or pathological evidence of primary demyelination should have a different explanation. CIDP and Guillain-Barré syndrome are by far the most common acquired demyelinating neuropathies in nondiabetics, so these diseases might also be the most common causes of demyelinating neuropathy in persons who have diabetes. Because both diabetic polyneuropathy and CIDP are chronic and may be difficult or impossible to distinguish on clinical grounds, making a diagnosis of CIDP in a person with diabetes can be difficult. Therefore, it is likely that CIDP is underdiagnosed in diabetics. The reports in the literature of small series of diabetic patients with CIDP serve to underscore the practical need to resist automatically attributing peripheral neuropathy in a diabetic to metabolic factors (Krendel et al., 1995; Stewart et al., 1996; Cornblath et al., 1997; Simpson, 1997; Baruah, 1998; Cross et al., 1999; Sharma et al., 1999). The fact that the occurrence of CIDP in a few patients with diabetes is deemed "reportable" is, in itself, an illustration of the difficulty this diagnosis can pose and is further evidence that CIDP is probably underdiagnosed in diabetics. It is unlikely that a series of patients with CIDP associated with hypertension or migraine would be published.

Most diabetics reported to have CIDP have had type 2 diabetes (Cornblath et al., 1987; Stewart et al., 1996; Cross et al., 1999). This is probably in part because type 2 diabetes is more common than type 1. Another factor may relate to the discordance between the severity of the neuropathy and the severity of the diabetes in these patients, with type 2 diabetes generally being milder than type 1. For example, if a patient with relatively mild type 2 diabetes develops severe peripheral neuropathy, one would expect a clinician to be disinclined to attribute the neuropathy to diabetes. Conversely, severe peripheral neuropathy in a patient with severe, complicated type 1 diabetes would be more easily attributed to diabetes. Patients in this latter category are less likely to be referred to a neurologist. CIDP therefore is probably most often overlooked in this group, yet this is the group that may be most predisposed to CIDP (Krendel and Skehan, 1998).

Although few would argue that CIDP could not occasionally occur in a diabetic patient by coincidence, whether diabetics are predisposed to CIDP is more controversial. Type 1 diabetes is known to be an autoimmune disease, and it is associated with an increased risk of acquiring other autoimmune diseases, possibly including CIDP. The prevalence of CIDP in diabetes cannot be determined by studying diabetics who are referred to neurologists for symptoms related to neuropathy because this is a subset of diabetics who are likely to have unusually severe neuropathy. This group would be expected to have a relatively high prevalence of CIDP.

As recently reported, nerve conduction studies were reviewed for 94 diabetic patients referred as part of a protocol before renal transplantation rather than because of clinical questions related to neuropathy (Krendel and Skehan, 1998). Of the 94 patients, 77 had type 1 diabetes, and of these, 44% met nerve conduction criteria for demyelination as proposed by a subcommittee of the American Academy of Neurology for the diagnosis of CIDP (Cornblath et al., 1991). Of those with type 2 diabetes, 6% met those criteria. Trojaborg and colleagues also found a relatively high prevalence of conduction velocities in the demyelinating range in unselected diabetics with end-stage renal disease (Trojaborg et al., 1994; Trojaborg, 1996). Thus, although rare in uncomplicated diabetes, demyelinating neuropathy, possibly CIDP, is common in type 1 diabetics with renal failure.

Also studied were a group of diabetics referred because of disabling peripheral neuropathy and found that 13 of the 60 patients met electrophysiological criteria for CIDP. Eleven of the 13 had type 1 diabetes. In many, the neuropathy was chronic and indolent. The average duration of symptoms before presentation was 33 months, with a range of 1 to 180 months. The distribution of involvement is interesting and may differ from that of typical CIDP in nondiabetics. Intrinsic hand and forearm muscles were predominantly involved in 6 of the 13 patients. Three of the 13 had asymmetrical limb involvement with thoracic bands of pain and focal abdominal muscle denervation. One had asymmetrical thigh involvement typical of proximal diabetic neuropathy. All except two patients were treated. Seven received intravenous immunoglobulin, two received prednisone alone, one received plasma exchange and cyclophosphamide, and one received prednisone, azathioprine, and cyclophosphamide. All treated patients improved over 1 to 2 months. One untreated patient was worse after 7 months, and one patient improved spontaneously.

Stewart and colleagues (1996) reported successful treatment of seven diabetics in whom they diagnosed CIDP. They selected patients with more rapid worsening than they would have expected in typical diabetic polyneuropathy, and they used lack of retinopathy or nephropathy as evidence favoring CIDP over diabetic polyneuropathy. However, I find that a response to treatment can occur even in very chronic cases, and I suspect from the findings in renal transplant patients that diabetic complications actually make CIDP more rather than less likely.

Cornblath and colleagues (1987) reported on four patients with type 2 diabetes and Simpson (1997) reported on seven insulin-dependent diabetic patients with severe subacute motor neuropathies, all of whom improved with treatment for presumed CIDP. Sharma and associates (1999) reported improvement after treatment with intravenous immunoglobulin in 14 of 17 type 2 diabetics who met electrophysiological criteria for CIDP.

Baruah (1998) reported on 11 type 1 diabetics with demyelinating neuropathy who were treated with both high-dose intravenous methylprednisolone and intravenous immunoglobulin. All patients improved, and improvement was maintained without further treatment for 10 to 15 months. His patients all had elevated cerebrospinal fluid protein, although I find that, as in CIDP in nondiabetics, cerebrospinal fluid protein levels need not be elevated to predict treatment response. Interestingly, the cerebrospinal fluid of Baruah's patients contained oligoclonal bands, adding further support for an autoimmune pathogenesis. Jaradeh and colleagues (1999) also found oligoclonal bands in cerebrospinal fluid from 5 of 15 diabetics with progressive polyradiculoneuropathy, all of whom responded to treatment with immunosuppressive therapy that included plasma exchange, intravenous immunoglobulin, and prednisone.

The potential basis for autoimmune attack on peripheral nerve myelin in diabetics is unknown, as it is in nondiabetics. Glycosylation of proteins or lipids within myelin might cause them to become antigenic and to incite an inflammatory response, as has been theorized for components of blood vessels (Brownlee, 1991). It is even possible that central nervous system myelin is involved. White matter hyperintensities are frequently seen on magnetic resonance images from patients with diabetes, and this might not always be due to small vessel disease. The reports by Baruah (1998) and Jaradeh (1999) of oligoclonal bands in the cerebrospinal fluid of diabetics with treatment-responsive neuropathies might reflect central nervous system involvement, although it might also be explained by involvement of nerve roots.

A recent study reviewed magnetic resonance imaging findings in a group of diabetics and compared them with those in patients without diabetes but with hypertension (Souaya and Krendel, 2000). The prevalence and location of the lesions did not usually differ between the two groups, but one type 1 diabetes patient with end-stage renal disease had transiently enhancing white matter lesions more consistent with inflammatory demyelination than with small vessel ischemia. Another type 1 diabetes patient with demyelinating peripheral neuropathy had lesions in the corpus callosum oriented along the fiber tracts, also typical of inflammatory demyelination. None of the patients without diabetes had similar corpus callosal lesions or enhancing lesions. Interestingly, multiple sclerosis had not been considered as a diagnostic possibility in either patient. It is possible that, as for CIDP, multiple sclerosis is underdiagnosed in patients with diabetes, with central nervous system lesions and symptoms being more readily attributed to small vessel disease.

The detection of CIDP in a diabetic person remains a diagnostic challenge. In addition to clinical features, findings on cerebrospinal fluid examination and nerve biopsy can be helpful in individual cases, but these are commonly nonspecific. Although evidence of demyelination on nerve conduction studies is expected in CIDP, its absence does not exclude the diagnosis. Unconventional techniques have been used to detect demyelination when standard nerve conduction studies and electromyography show evidence of only axonal involvement. Menkes and colleagues (1998) were able to find evidence of proximal demyelination by nerve root stimulation in patients who had been diagnosed with "untreatable axonal diabetic neuropathy." These patients subsequently improved dramatically when treated with intravenous immunoglobulin.

In nerve biopsy samples, the most helpful marker of chronic demyelination is probably the "onion bulb" (Krendel et al., 1989). The "bulbs" are thinly myelinated or demyelinated axons surrounded by concentric layers of Schwann cell processes resulting from repeated attempts at remyelination. This finding might distinguish CIDP from diabetic neuropathy. We found onion bulbs in the sural nerve biopsy samples of all four diabetic patients who underwent biopsy and had electrophysiological evidence of demyelination. These patients improved with treatment. In one report that attributed onion bulbs to diabetic neuropathy, the diagnosis was later changed to CIDP (Thomas and Tomlinson, 1993).

Because of the limited usefulness of diagnostic tests in the detection of CIDP in diabetic patients, the diagnosis is often uncertain. Moreover, it is virtually impossible to rule out an autoimmune contribution to any clinically significant neuropathy in these patients. Therefore, I sometimes consider a trial of treatment, mainly basing the decision on the severity of the neuropathy and the potential risks and expense of treatment.

References

Abu-Shakra SR, Cornblath DR, Avila OL, et al: Conduction block in diabetic neuropathy. Muscle Nerve 1991;14:858–862.
Apfel SC, Kessler JA, Adornato BT, et al: Recombinant nerve growth factor in the treatment of diabetic polyneuropathy. Neurology 1998;51:695–702.
Asbury AK, Aldredge H, Hershberg R, et al: Oculomotor palsy in diabetes mellitus: A clinicopathological study. Brain 1970;93:555–566.
Asbury AK: Proximal diabetic neuropathy. Ann Neurol 1977;2:170–180.
Atkinson MA, Maclaren NK: The pathogenesis of insulin-dependent diabetes mellitus. N Engl J Med 1994;331:1428–1436.
Backonja M, Beydoun A, Edwards KR, et al: Gabapentin for the symptomatic treatment of painful neuropathy in patients with diabetes mellitus: A randomized controlled trial. JAMA 1998;280:1831–1836.
Barone JA: Domperidone: A peripherally acting dopamine$_2$-receptor antagonist. Ann Pharmacol 1999;33:429–440.
Baruah JK: Diabetic demyelinating polyneuropathy and response to high doses of methylprednisolone and immunoglobin therapies. Muscle Nerve 1998;21:1607.
Bastron JA, Thomas JE: Diabetic polyradiculopathy: Clinical and electromyographic findings. Mayo Clin Proc 1981;56:725–732.
Bradley JL, Thomas PK, King RHM, et al: Myelinated fiber regener-

ation: Correlation with type of diabetes. Acta Neuropathol 1995; 90:403–410.

Bradley WG, Chad D, Verghese JP, et al: Painful lumbosacral plexopathy with elevated sedimentation rate: A treatable inflammatory syndrome. Ann Neurol 1884;15:457–464.

Brownlee M: Glycosylation products as toxic mediators of diabetic complications. Annu Rev Med 1991;42:159–166.

Brunton LL: Agents affecting gastrointestinal water flux and motility. In Hardman JG, Limbird LE, Molinoff PB, et al (eds): The Pharmacological Basis of Therapeutics, 9th ed. New York, McGraw-Hill, 1996;932–934.

Capsaicin Study Group: Treatment of painful diabetic neuropathy with topical capsicin: A multicenter, double-blind, vehicle-controlled study. Arch Intern Med 1991;151:2225–2229.

Caravati CM: Insulin neuritis: A case report. Va Med Mon 1933; 60:745–746.

Chokroverty S, Reyes MG, Rubino FA: The syndrome of diabetic amyotrophy. Ann Neurol 1977;2:181–194.

Coppack SW, Watkins PJ: The natural history of diabetic femoral neuropathy. Q J Med 1991;288:307–313.

Cornblath DR, Drachman DB, Griffin JW: Demyelinating motor neuropathy in patients with diabetic polyneuropathy. Ann Neurol 1987;22:126.

Cornblath DR, Asbury AK, Albers JW, et al: Research criteria for the diagnosis of chronic inflammatory demyelinating polyneuropathy (CIDP): Report from an ad hoc subcommittee of the American Academy of Neurology AIDS Task Force. Neurology 1991;41:617–618.

Costigan DC, Krendel DA, Hopkins LC, et al: Inflammatory neuropathy in diabetes. Ann Neurol 1990;28:272.

Cross J, Sharma KR, Ayar DR: Demyelinating neuropathy in patients with type 2 diabetes mellitus. Neurology 1999;52:A85.

Danta G: Hypoglycemic peripheral neuropathy. Arch Neurol 1969; 21:121–132.

DiBaise JK, Quigley EM: Efficacy of prolonged administration of intravenous erythromycin in an ambulatory setting as treatment of severe gastroparesis: One center's experience. J Clin Gastroenterol 1999;28:131–134.

Diabetes Control and Complications Trial Research Group: The effect of intensive treatment of diabetes on the development and progression of long-term complications in insulin-dependent diabetes mellitus. N Engl J Med 1993;329:977–986.

Diabetes Control and Complications Trial Research Group: The effect of Intensive diabetes therapy on the development and progression of neuropathy. Ann Intern Med 1995;122:561–568.

Duchen LW, Anjorin A, Watkins PJ, et al: Pathology of autonomic neuropathy in diabetes. Ann Intern Med 1980;92:301–303.

Dyck PJ, Benstead TJ, Conn DL, et al: Nonsystemic vasculitic neuropathy. Brain 1987;110:843–854.

Dyck PJ, Zimmerman BR, Vilen TH, et al: Nerve glucose, fructose, sorbitol, myo-inositol, and fiber degeneration and regeneration in diabetic neuropathy. N Engl J Med 1988;319:542–548.

Dyck PJ, Kratz KM, Karnes MS, et al: The prevalence by staged severity of various types of diabetic neuropathy, retinopathy, and nephropathy in a population-based cohort: The Rochester Diabetic Neuropathy Study. Neurology 1993;43:817–824.

Dyck PJB, Norell JE, Dyck PJ: Microvasculitis and ischemia in diabetic lumbosacral radiculoplexus neuropathy. Neurology 1999;53:2113–2121.

Edwards KR, Glantz MJ, Levin P: Evaluation of Topiramate in the Management of Painful Diabetic Neuropathy. Glenville, IL, American Pain Society Program Book, 1998;120.

Elias KA, Cronin MJ, Stewart TA, Carlsen RC: Peripheral neuropathy in transgenic diabetic mice: Restoration of c-fiber function with human recombinant nerve growth factor. Diabetes 1998; 47:1637–1642.

Ellenberg M: Diabetic neuropathic cachexia. Diabetes 1974;23: 418–423.

Engel WK, Prentice AF: Some polyneuropathies in insulin-requiring adult-onset diabetes can benefit remarkably from anti-dysimmune treatment. Neurology 1993;43:A255.

Ewing DJ, Campbell IW, Clarke BF: The natural history of diabetic autonomic neuropathy. Q J Med 1980;49:95–102.

Feldman HA, Goldstein I, Hatzichristou DG, et al: Impotence and its medical and psychosocial correlates: Results of the Massachusetts Male Aging Study. J Urol 1994;151:54–61.

Foster DW: Diabetes mellitus. In Fauci AS, Braunwald E, Isselbacher KJ, et al (eds): Principles of Internal Medicine, 14th ed. New York, McGraw-Hill, 1998;2060–2080.

Galer BS, Miller KV, Rowbotham MC: Response to intravenous lidocaine differs based on clinical diagnosis and site of nervous system injury. Neurology 1993;43:1233–1235.

Garland H: Diabetic amyotrophy. Br J Clin Pract 1955;2:1287–1290.

Garland H: Diabetic amyotrophy. Br J Clin Pract 1961;15:9–14.

Giannini C, Dyck PJ: Basement membrane reduplication and pericyte degeneration precede development of diabetic polyneuropathy and are associated with its severity. Ann Neurol 1995; 37:498–504.

Greenberger NJ, Isselbacher KJ: Disorders of absorption. In Fauci AS, Braunwald E, Isselbacher KJ, et al (eds): Principles of Internal Medicine, 14th ed. New York, McGraw-Hill, 1998;1631.

Greene DA, Winegrad AI: Effects of acute experimental diabetes on composite energy metabolism in peripheral nerve axons and schwann cells. Diabetes 1981;30:967–974.

Greene DA: Sorbitol, myo-inositol and sodium-potassium ATPase in diabetic peripheral nerve. Drugs 1986;32(Suppl 2):6–14.

Greene DA, Arezzo JC, Brown MB, et al: Effect of aldose reductase inhibition on nerve conduction and morphometry in diabetic neuropathy. Neurology 1999;53:580–591.

Gregerson G: Variations in motor conduction velocity produced by acute changes in the metabolic state in diabetic patients. Diabetologica 1968;4:273–277.

Harati Y, Gooch C, Swenson M, et al: Double-blind randomized trial of tramadol for the treatment of pain of diabetic neuropathy. Neurology 1998;50:1842–1846.

Harrison MJ: Muscle wasting after prolonged hypoglycemic coma: Case report with electrophysiologic data. J Neurol Neuro Surg Psychiatry 1976;39:465–470.

Hendriksen PH, Oey PL, Wieneke GH, et al: Subclinical diabetic neuropathy: Similarities between electrophysiologic results of patients with type 1 (insulin-dependent) and type 2 (non-insulin-dependent) diabetes mellitus. Diabetologica 1992;35:690–695.

Janssens J, Peeters TL, Vantrappen G, et al: Improvement of gastric emptying in diabetic gastroparesis by erythromycin: Preliminary studies. N Engl J Med 1990;322:1028–1031.

Jaradeh SS, Thomas EP, Lobeck LJ: Progressive polyradiculoneuropathy in diabetes: Correlation of variables and clinical outcome after immunotherapy. J Neurol Neurosurg Psychiatry 1999;67:607–612.

Jarow JP, Burnett AL, Geringer AM: Clinical efficacy of sildenafil citrate based on etiology and response to prior treatment. J Urol 1999;162:722–725.

Jaspan JB, Wollman RL, Bernstein L, Rubenstein AH: Hypoglycemic peripheral neuropathy in association with insulinoma: Implication of glucopenia rather than hyperinsulinism: Case report and literature review. Medicine 1982;61:33–44.

Kastrup J, Petersen P, Dejgard A, et al: Intravenous lidocaine infusion: A new treatment for chronic painful diabetic neuropathy? Pain 1987;28:69–75.

Kissel JT, Slivka AP, Warmolts JR: The clinical spectrum of necrotizing angiopathy of the peripheral nervous system. Ann Neurol 1985;18:2521–257.

Kong MF, Horowitz M, Jones KL: Natural history of diabetic gastroparesis. Diabetes Care 1999;22:503–507.

Krendel DA, Parks HP, Anthony DC, et al: Sural nerve biopsy in chronic inflammatory demyelinating polyradiculoneuropathy. Muscle Nerve 1989;12:265–272.

Krendel DA, Costigan DA, Hopkins LC: Successful treatment of neuropathies in patients with diabetes mellitus. Arch Neurol 1995;52:1053–1061.

Krendel DA: Polymyositis-like findings in proximal diabetic neuropathy. Neurology 1997;48:A307.

Krendel DA, Zacharias A, Skehan ME: Treatment of neuropathy associated with diabetes: An analysis of 55 patients. J Neurol 1997;244:S40–S41.

Krendel DA: Benefit of pancreatic transplantation on diabetic neuropathy: Euglycemia or immunosuppression? Ann Neurol 1998;44:149.

Krendel DA, Skehan ME: Patients with type 1 diabetes are predisposed to chronic demyelinating polyneuropathy. Neurology 1998;50:A333.

platin-induced neurotoxicity is uncertain. Morphological and electrophysiological studies in humans and animals suggest that the dorsal root ganglion neuronal cell body is the primary target (Gregg et al., 1992; Krarup-Hansen et al., 1993; Krarup-Hansen et al., 1999; Cece et al., 1995). Drug-induced apoptosis of dorsal root ganglion neurons triggered by neuronal DNA binding, impaired axonal transport, and reduced protein synthesis are proposed mechanisms (Cece et al., 1995; Russel et al., 1995; Gill and Windebank, 1998).

The clinical syndrome is a symmetrical sensory neuropathy or neuronopathy, the severity of which is related to total cumulative dose (Roelofs et al., 1984; Thompson et al., 1984; Gastaut and Pellissier, 1985; Ongerboer de Visser and Tiessens, 1985; Mollman et al., 1988; Cersosimo, 1989; Gregg et al., 1992; LoMonaco et al., 1992; Pirovano et al., 1992). Neuropathies are common at doses exceeding 300 mg/m^2 of body surface (85% incidence) and nearly universal above 600 mg/m^2 (Cersosimo, 1989; Gerritsen et al., 1990; Gregg et al., 1992). Large-fiber sensory modalities are preferentially involved. Early clinical features include paresthesias in the feet, reduced vibration perception in the feet, and loss of ankle reflexes. Pain is not a prominent symptom. At higher cumulative doses, proprioceptive defects appear, occasionally of sufficient severity to produce sensory ataxia and pseudoathetoid hand movements. All stretch reflexes are eventually lost. Light touch, temperature, and pinprick sensations are only mildly affected. Weakness is very uncommon, occurring in approximately 2% of patients (Cersosimo, 1989). Autonomic symptoms are uncommon (Cersosimo, 1989). Cranial nerves are usually spared. A transient Lhermitte's sign is reported in 30% to 40% of patients (Ongerboer de Visser and Tiessens, 1985; Siegal and Haim, 1990), probably caused by demyelination in the posterior columns of the cervical cord.

An important characteristic of cisplatin neuropathies is their tendency for off-therapy deterioration. The appearance of neuropathic symptoms may be delayed for up to 8 weeks after the drug is stopped (Mollman et al., 1988). Moreover, in 30% of patients, the neuropathy continues to progress for as long as 6 months after withdrawal of cisplatin (Mollman et al., 1988; Siegal and Haim, 1990; LoMonaco et al., 1992). This is termed *coasting*. The neuropathy eventually subsides with time, albeit slowly and incompletely, as might be predicted of a dorsal root ganglionopathy. Long-term follow-up studies reveal that 40% of patients complain of residual sensory symptoms (Roth et al., 1988), two thirds have neuropathic findings on examination (Gerritsen van der Hoop et al., 1990; Krarup-Hansen et al., 1993), and 50% have abnormal sural SNAPs and vibration perception thresholds (Krarup-Hansen et al., 1993).

Sural nerve biopsies show a reduced number of large myelinated nerve fibers (Roelofs et al., 1984; Thompson et al., 1984; Ongerboer de Visser and Tiessens, 1985; Mollman et al., 1988; Krarup-Hansen et al., 1993; Krarup-Hansen et al., 1999). Small-diame-

ter nerve fibers are preserved. Wallerian-like degeneration and secondary segmental demyelination may be present. Regenerating axonal sprouts are also sometimes seen, suggesting that nerve damage is not restricted to the neuronal cell body but also involves the axons.

The predominant electrophysiological feature of cisplatin-induced neuropathy is a progressive, dose-related decrease in all SNAP amplitudes, affecting both the upper and lower extremities (Roelofs et al., 1984; Thompson et al., 1984; Gastaut and Pellissier, 1985; Ongerboer de Visser and Tiessens, 1985; Daugaard et al., 1987; Mollman et al., 1988; Riggs et al., 1988; LoMonaco et al., 1992; Pirovano et al., 1992; Fu et al., 1995). With increasing cumulative dose, sensory responses eventually disappear altogether. Distal sensory conduction velocities are also moderately reduced. Most investigators report normal motor nerve conduction studies, but a few have found mildly reduced conduction velocities in a minority of patients (Ongerboer de Visser and Tiessens, 1985; Pirovano et al., 1992; Krarup-Hansen et al., 1993). F-wave latencies are unaffected. The tibial H reflex is lost in concert with the ankle stretch reflex (Ongerboer de Visser and Tiessens, 1985; Krarup-Hansen et al., 1993). Needle EMG is usually normal, but fibrillation potentials and long-duration MUAPs are observed in distal muscles in a few patients (Roelofs et al., 1984; Ongerboer de Visser and Tiessens, 1985).

Carboplatin

Carboplatin is another platinum compound with the same spectrum of antitumor activity as that of cisplatin (Canetta et al., 1985; Reed et al., 1996). It is more myelosuppressive than cisplatin but less neurotoxic, ototoxic, and nephrotoxic. At conventional doses, neuropathies occur in only 6% of patients and are always mild (Canetta et al., 1985). However, at high doses (above 1,000 mg/m^2)—as might be employed for patients with drug-refractory cancer prior to autologous hematopoietic stem cell or bone marrow transplantation—severe neuropathies can occur, similar to cisplatin neuropathies, except for a higher incidence of motor involvement (Cavaletti et al., 1998; Heinzlef et al., 1998).

VINCA ALKALOIDS

Vincristine

The vinca alkaloids are extracts from the periwinkle plant that have been employed as anticancer agents since 1961 (Rowinsky and Donehower, 1997). Two naturally occurring alkaloids, vincristine and vinblastine, and two semisynthetic derivatives, vinorelbine and vindesine, are used clinically as chemotherapeutic agents. All but vindesine are approved for use in the United States. Vincristine is the most neurotoxic of the vinca compounds and vinorelbine the least. Whereas peripheral neurotoxicity is vincristine's dose-limiting side effect, vinblastine and vinorelbine are limited by myelotoxicity (Weiss et al., 1974; Goa and Faulds, 1994). Vincristine is most commonly utilized in the treatment of leukemia, Hodgkin's disease, and NHL, but has activity against many other tumors, including lung cancers, breast carcinoma, and several childhood tumors (Rowinsky and Donehower, 1997). Vincristine's neurotoxicity probably results from its ability to bind dimeric tubulin and, thereby, prevent its polymerization into microtubules and accelerate its depolymerization from existing microtubules (Sahenk et al., 1987; Rowinsky and Donehower, 1997). In the rat model of vincristine-induced neuropathy, the axoskeleton is disorganized, axonal microtubules are decreased in length and number, and fast axonal transport is secondarily impaired (Green et al., 1977; Sahenk et al., 1987; Tanner et al., 1998).

Vincristine produces a symmetrical, sensorimotor and autonomic, dose-related polyneuropathy in nearly all exposed patients (McLeod and Penny, 1969; Sandler et al., 1969; Bradley et al., 1970; Casey et al., 1973; Holland et al., 1973; Weiss et al., 1974; Legha, 1986; DeAngelis et al., 1991; Pal, 1999). The standard dose is 1.4 mg/m^2 (up to 2 mg) every 1 to 4 weeks (McCune and Lindley, 1997). With a weekly schedule, the maximum tolerated cumulative dose ranges from 15 to 20 mg. With less frequent administration, doses of 30 to 50 mg may be tolerated. The earliest sign of neuropathy is reduced ankle jerks, usually noted after a cumulative dose of 4 mg/m^2. At higher doses, generalized hypo- or areflexia often ensues (DeAngelis et al., 1991; Pal, 1999). The earliest symptoms, generally occurring 1 to 2 weeks after the loss of ankle jerks, are paresthesias in the hands and feet, developing in 50% to 60% of patients (Holland et al., 1973; Pal, 1999). Sensory loss on examination is usually mild, involves the hands and feet, and affects vibration (Pal, 1999) and small-fiber modalities (Casey et al., 1973), sparing joint position sensation (DeAngelis et al., 1991). Distal weakness follows the sensory loss, affecting almost all patients but becoming significant in only 25% to 35% (Sandler et al., 1969; Holland et al., 1973; DeAngelis et al., 1991). Wrist/finger extensors, hand intrinsic muscles, and toe/ankle dorsiflexors are usually the weakest muscles. Gastrointestinal autonomic toxicity occurs in 30% to 50% of patients, producing constipation, abdominal pain, and sometimes ileus (Sandler et al., 1969; Holland et al., 1973; Pal, 1999). Less common autonomic side effects are orthostatic hypotension, urinary retention, and erectile dysfunction. Cranial nerves are affected in 10% of patients, including optic neuropathies, oculomotor palsies, paroxysmal jaw pain, facial weakness, hearing loss, and laryngeal nerve palsies (Sandler et al., 1969; Holland et al., 1973; Legha, 1986). Identified risk factors for the occurrence of a severe neuropathy are hepatic failure (Sandler et al., 1969), Charcot-Marie-Tooth neuropathy (Mercuri et al., 1999), and the coadministration of hematopoietic colony-stimulating factors (Weintraub et al., 1996).

Vincristine-induced neuropathies are largely reversible after the chemotherapy is stopped (Legha, 1986), although signs and symptoms may initially continue to progress for at least 1 month (DeAngelis et al., 1991). All motor, sensory, autonomic, and cranial nerve symptoms eventually diminish over several months, but mild symptoms may persist (Sandler et al., 1969). Complete symptomatic recovery occurs in 75% to 80% (Haim et al., 1994). Some examination findings are usually permanent (e.g., loss of ankle jerks and toe extensor weakness).

Sural nerve biopsies in vincristine-treated patients demonstrate loss of both large and small myelinated fibers, prominent wallerian-like degeneration of myelinated and unmyelinated axons, occasional regenerating fibers, and little or no segmental demyelination (Gottschalk et al., 1968; McLeod and Penny, 1969; Bradley et al., 1970).

Electrophysiological studies show evidence of a distal-predominant, axonal, sensorimotor neuropathy (McLeod and Penny, 1969; Sandler et al., 1969; Bradley et al., 1970; Casey et al., 1973; Guiheneuc et al., 1980; DeAngelis et al., 1991; Pal, 1999). During successive treatment cycles, CMAP amplitudes progressively decrease, distal motor latencies become prolonged, motor conduction velocities are unchanged, and F waves remain normal. Prolongation of the distal motor latencies in the face of normal proximal motor conductions and decreasing CMAP amplitudes suggests a distal axonopathy. Sensory nerve conduction studies reveal decreased amplitudes in both upper and lower limb nerves and relatively unchanged conduction velocities. A characteristic feature of vincristine neuropathies is early preservation of the tibial H reflex in patients with absent ankle jerks (McLeod and Penny, 1969; Sandler et al., 1969; Casey et al., 1973; Pal, 1999). Guiheneuc et al. showed that the H/M amplitude ratio was increased for up to 7 days after vincristine injection, indicative of transient hyperexcitability of the monosynaptic stretch reflex arc (Guiheneuc et al., 1980). The pathophysiological basis for this H-reflex effect is unknown. The H reflex often disappears later in the course of treatment (Casey et al., 1973; Pal, 1999). Upon discontinuation of vincristine, SNAP and CMAP amplitudes partially recover but do not return to baseline (Casey et al., 1973). On EMG examination, fibrillation potentials are identified in at least 50% of patients, primarily in distal muscles, and recruitment is decreased in distal more than proximal muscles (Bradley et al., 1970; Casey et al., 1973; Pal, 1999). Eventually, motor unit remodeling occurs and leads to long-duration, large-amplitude MUAPs in distal muscles.

Vinorelbine

Vinorelbine is approved in the United States for the treatment of advanced non–small cell lung cancer. It also has established activity against metastatic breast cancer, ovarian cancer, lymphomas, cervical carcinomas, and other tumors (Goa and

Faulds, 1994; O'Reilly et al., 1994). In vitro, this agent is less effective in depolymerizing axonal microtubules and interfering with axonal transport than its parent compound, vincristine (Binet et al., 1990). As predicted from the experimental model, vinorelbine has been less PNS toxic than vincristine in clinical trials (Perol et al., 1996). Its dose-limiting toxicity is myelosuppression, which permits maximal doses of about 25 to 30 mg/m² every week.

Vinorelbine-induced neuropathies are similar in character to those produced by vincristine, having the features of a dose-related, distal, symmetrical, sensorimotor, axonal polyneuropathy (Goa and Faulds, 1994; O'Reilly et al., 1994). On the basis of data accumulated in clinical oncology trials, 20% to 30% of patients treated with this agent develop a neuropathy, which is severe in only 1% (Goa and Faulds, 1994). Early symptoms are distal sensory loss, paresthesias, and dysesthesias. On examination, both small- and large-fiber sensory modalities are affected. While sensory symptoms remain dominant, some patients develop mild distal weakness after 3 to 6 months of therapy. Constipation occurs in approximately one third of patients. Other autonomic and cranial nerve findings have not been reported.

One prospective study used neurophysiological techniques and careful charting of neurological signs and symptoms to analyze vinorelbine-induced neuropathy (Pace et al., 1997). The findings revealed a much higher incidence of neuropathy than that obtained in the clinical oncology trials. After four cycles of 25 mg/week, 87% of patients had signs and symptoms of a mild neuropathy, although only 13% had distal paresthesias. Ankle jerks were reduced or absent in about 50% of patients. After 12 cycles, 100% of patients had a clinically defined neuropathy (mild to moderate severity), approximately 50% had dysesthesias in the feet and hands, and approximately 75% exhibited diffuse tendon hypo-/areflexia. Neuropathic signs and symptoms were almost completely reversible within 6 months of stopping vinorelbine.

The only available electrodiagnostic information comes from this prospective trial (Pace et al., 1997). Serial nerve conduction studies revealed a dose-dependent decrease in peroneal CMAP, median SNAP, and sural SNAP amplitudes, with normal distal latencies and conduction velocities. Sympathetic skin responses were preserved. No EMG examinations were performed. The SNAP and CMAP amplitudes improved following withdrawal of vinorelbine. Nerve pathology has not been described.

TAXANES

Paclitaxel

Paclitaxel is derived from the bark and needles of the Pacific yew tree. It is clinically effective in the treatment of ovarian, breast, small cell and non-small cell lung, bladder, cervical, bladder, and head and neck cancers and NHL (Rowinsky, 1997). Myelosuppression is its leading toxicity, but when treatment is combined with the use of granulocyte colony-stimulating factor, peripheral neurotoxicity becomes the dose-limiting factor (Lipton et al., 1989; Rowinsky, 1997). In contrast to the vinca alkaloids, which disassemble microtubules, paclitaxel binds to dimeric tubulin and promotes microtubule assembly by enhancing tubulin polymerization. As a result, disordered microtubular bundles accumulate (Schiff et al., 1979; Rowinsky, 1997). In organotypic tissue cultures exposed to paclitaxel, abnormal microtubular bundles aggregate in axons, dorsal root ganglion neurons, satellite cells, and Schwann cells (Masurovsky et al., 1983). The axonal microtubular abnormalities may disrupt fast axoplasmic transport. Paclitaxel also inhibits regenerative responses in axons and Schwann cells after crush injuries (Vuorinen et al., 1988). Most clinical and morphological evidence points to the axon, the dorsal root ganglion neuronal cell body, or both as the primary site of paclitaxel toxicity (Lipton et al., 1989; Rowinsky et al., 1993; Chaudhry et al., 1994; Sahenk et al., 1994). Single high doses (>300 mg/m²) may have a neuronopathic effect, whereas lower doses produce a cumulative distal axonopathy (Chaudhry et al., 1994).

Paclitaxel is associated with a largely length-dependent, axonal, sensorimotor neuropathy with predominant sensory symptoms (Wiernik et al., 1987; Lipton et al., 1989; Chaudhry et al., 1994; Sahenk et al., 1994; Cavaletti et al., 1995; Postma et al., 1995; Forsyth et al., 1997; Pace et al., 1997; Iniguez et al., 1998). The severity of the neuropathy depends on cumulative dose and dose intensity per cycle (Wiernik et al., 1987; Chaudhry et al., 1994; Postma et al., 1995; Kunitoh et al., 1998). When lower doses of 135 to 200 mg/m² every 3 weeks are employed, as many as 85% of patients develop neuropathies, usually after the third to seventh cycle, but the neuropathy is generally mild or subclinical (Wiernik et al., 1987; Chaudhry et al., 1994; Postma et al., 1995; Kunitoh et al., 1998). Significant neurotoxicity occurs with single doses above 200 mg/m². For doses of 250 to 350 mg/m² every 3 weeks, neuropathies invariably develop after the first or second cycle and 70% of the neuropathies are severe, marked by intense paresthesias or sensory ataxia (Wiernik et al., 1987; Chaudhry et al., 1994; Postma et al., 1995). Paclitaxel is now conventionally dosed at 135 to 250 mg/m², infused over 3 to 24 hours, in 3-week cycles, but higher doses are under investigation. Additional risk factors for a severe neuropathy include cumulative doses above 1500 mg/m², prior exposure to other neurotoxic agents, and pre-existing diabetic or alcoholic polyneuropathy (Rowinsky et al., 1993; Chaudhry et al., 1994; Cavaletti et al., 1995; Iniguez et al., 1998).

Initial symptoms are numbness, paresthesias, and occasionally pain in the feet, sometimes also involving the hands and face. The symptoms appear within 1 to 8 days of the infusion (Iniguez et al., 1998). They may begin asymmetrically but later become symmetrical (Lipton et al., 1989). Troublesome dysesthesias occur in 22% of patients (Forsyth et al., 1997). Some patients experience severe pruritus (Glantz et al., 1996). Distal sensory symptoms may be transitory initially, but worsen with each cycle and become persistent. On examination, vibration sensation is more affected than small-fiber modalities. Joint position sensation is relatively preserved, except for severe, ataxia-producing neuropathies. Ankle jerks are typically reduced or absent early in the course, with more generalized reflex loss emerging after high single or cumulative doses. Significant weakness is uncommon, even with large doses. Mild toe extensor weakness is identified in 25% to 85% of patients (Chaudhry et al., 1994; Forsyth et al., 1997). Autonomic and cranial nerve involvement is rare at standard doses. Focal entrapment neuropathies, including carpal tunnel syndrome (Forsyth et al., 1997) and peroneal palsy at the fibular head (Chaudhry et al., 1994), are uncommonly reported. We have seen several patients with symptomatic ulnar nerve entrapments at the elbow.

Occasionally, mild proximal weakness is recognized in patients treated with high doses of paclitaxel (250 to 350 mg/m²), including approximately 20% of those in the study by Chaudhry et al. (1994). This weakness is probably due to a superimposed toxic myopathy, as the patients in the latter report all exhibited short-duration, small-amplitude MUAPs with early recruitment in proximal muscles on needle EMG examination. There was no abnormal spontaneous activity or serum creatine kinase elevation. Muscle biopsy in one patient showed dense staining with acid phosphatase (Rowinsky et al., 1993), indicative of lysosomal activation, reminiscent of the toxic vacuolar myoneuropathies caused by chloroquine (Estes et al., 1987) and colchicine (Kuncl et al., 1987). Proximal weakness resolves within several weeks of stopping therapy.

Following withdrawal of paclitaxel, the neuropathy may continue to progress for up to 4 weeks because of a coasting effect (Glantz et al., 1996; van den Bent et al., 1997). Paclitaxel-related neuropathy is at least partially reversible after discontinuation of therapy. Most patients with mild sensory symptoms recover within several months, but up to 40% have residual numbness and tingling in the toes. Vibration perception abnormalities also tend to persist (Postma et al., 1995; Glantz et al., 1996; Kunitoh et al., 1998). Severe neuropathies often leave patients with persistent sensory ataxia and weakness in the feet (Wiernik et al., 1987; Kaplan et al., 1993; Postma et al., 1995).

A few sural nerve biopsies have been reported (Sahenk et al., 1994; van den Bent et al., 1997). Findings include the loss of large more than small myelinated and unmyelinated fibers, prominent axonal atrophy, mild secondary segmental demyelination/remyelination, and occasional wallerian-like degeneration. No regenerating axonal sprouts are observed, suggesting a dorsal root ganglion cell body disorder or failure of regenerative mechanisms in the axon.

Electrophysiological studies demonstrate abnormalities indicative of a length-dependent, primarily axonal, sensorimotor neuropathy (Lipton et al., 1989; Kaplan et al., 1993; Chaudhry et al., 1994; Sahenk et al., 1994; Cavaletti et al., 1995; Pace et al., 1997; van den Bent et al., 1997; Iniguez et al., 1998). Dose-dependent reductions of SNAP amplitudes occur, involving the sural nerve more often than the upper limb nerves. Peroneal CMAP amplitudes also decrease in a dose-related fashion. Sensorimotor distal latencies and conduction velocities are usually normal or slightly slowed, but more significant slowing is infrequently observed (Lipton et al., 1989; Sahenk et al., 1994; van den Bent et al., 1997). Ulnar F waves were normal in one study (Cavaletti et al., 1995); in another, peroneal F waves were absent in most patients (Iniguez et al., 1998). Needle EMG examination shows fibrillation potentials and decreased recruitment in distal leg muscles, with long-duration MUAPs observed in patients with long-standing symptoms (Lipton et al., 1989; Kaplan et al., 1993). Cardiovascular autonomic tests and sympathetic skin responses are normal (Cavaletti et al., 1995; Ekholm et al., 1997). Patients retested 1 year after treatment commonly show normalized CMAPs and SNAPs (Pace et al., 1997).

Docetaxel

Docetaxel is a semisynthetic analogue of paclitaxel (Cortes and Pazdur, 1995; Rowinsky, 1997). Like paclitaxel, it promotes the assembly of stable microtubules while simultaneously preventing microtubular depolymerization. Docetaxel's mechanism of neurotoxicity is presumably similar to that of paclitaxel. Both drugs produce abnormal accumulations of microtubular bundles in neurons when tested in experimental models. Docetaxel has been used most extensively in metastatic breast, ovarian, and non–small cell and small cell lung cancers, but is active against a wide spectrum of tumors. The drug is usually administered in a 100 mg/m² dose over 1 hour every 21 days.

Docetaxel produces a dose-dependent, sensory-predominant polyneuropathy, which shares many characteristics with paclitaxel-induced neuropathies (Balmaceda et al., 1993; Cortes and Pazdur, 1995; Freilich et al., 1995; Hilkens et al., 1996; New et al., 1996; Fazio et al., 1999). When typical doses are employed, clinically significant neurotoxicity is less common with docetaxel than with paclitaxel (Apfel, 1996). Using data from the drug manufacturer on more than 1,300 patients treated with docetaxel in phase II trials, Cortes and Pazdur reported a 48% incidence of all grades of neuropathy and a 3.6% incidence of severe neuropathies (Cortes and Pazdur, 1995). Severe neuropathies are characterized by severe pain or paresthesias, proximal or distal weakness, gait ataxia, or loss of hand dexterity. Most, but not all, of the severe neuropathies occur with a cumulative dose above 600 mg/m² (Cortes and Pazdur, 1995; Freilich et al., 1995; Hilkens et al., 1997; Fazio et al., 1999).

Most neuropathies due to docetaxel are mild, presenting with numbness and paresthesias of the hands and feet after the third to fifth cycle of treatment. Foot and hand pains occur in about 40% of affected patients (Hilkens et al., 1996). The severity of the sensory symptoms increases with higher cumulative doses. Almost 50% of symptomatic patients develop an unsteady gait (Hilkens et al., 1996). Lhermitte's sign occurs transiently in 6% of patients (van den Bent et al., 1998). As with paclitaxel, vibration sensation is impaired most significantly, with milder impairment of pinprick and temperature perception (Balmaceda et al., 1993; New et al., 1996). Proprioception is altered only in severe cases. Ankle and knee reflexes are usually lost (Hilkens et al., 1996; New et al., 1996).

The literature on motor involvement is confusing. In studies devoted to neurological complications, weakness occurred in 6% of patients, all of whom received cumulative doses under 600 mg/m² (Hilkens et al., 1996; New et al., 1996). In one study, all 10 patients with weakness had generalized proximal and distal involvement (New et al., 1996). EMG examinations in eight of these patients showed no abnormalities in the proximally weak muscles, whereas distal muscles exhibited neurogenic changes. Serum creatine kinase levels were normal. A muscle biopsy in one patient revealed neurogenic atrophy. The authors felt that the proximal weakness was probably due to the toxic neuropathy. In a second study, all seven clinically weak patients had proximal weakness alone. Three patients had electrodiagnostic studies; two revealed findings incidental to the proximal weakness and the third showed myopathic changes in proximal muscles with fibrillation potentials in both proximal and distal muscles. Serum creatine kinase levels were normal. No muscle biopsy was performed. The authors termed the process a *motor neuropathy*. Considering that (1) docetaxel is an analogue of paclitaxel, (2) paclitaxel has been demonstrated to cause a proximal myopathy (see preceding), (3) no proximally weak muscle exhibited neurogenic changes on EMG testing, (4) one proximally weak muscle had myopathic EMG alterations, and (5) proximal weakness is more commonly myopathic than neuropathic (even in patients with superimposed distal axonopathies), docetaxel-induced proximal weakness more probably results from a toxic myopathy than from a non–length-dependent neuropathy. Proximal weakness resolves in several months after withdrawal of docetaxel. Rare patients develop moderately severe, neuropathic weakness restricted to distal lower limb muscles (Hilkens et al., 1997; Fazio et al., 1999).

After chemotherapy has been stopped, most patients begin to slowly improve, but the neuropathy may continue to progress for several months, as occasionally happens with the other neurotoxic agents (Hilkens et al., 1996; New et al., 1996). Although the majority of patients recover, some are left with residual numbness and paresthesias in the feet and hands (New et al., 1996).

Sensory nerve biopsy results have been reported for two patients. The first revealed a decreased concentration of large myelinated nerve fibers and wallerian-like degeneration (New et al., 1996). The second also demonstrated a preferential loss of large myelinated fibers, but wallerian-like degeneration was not present (Fazio et al., 1999). Abundant regenerating axonal clusters, axonal atrophy, and decreased unmyelinated nerve fibers were additional findings. The morphologic evidence of regeneration—not seen to date with paclitaxel neuropathies—suggested a distal axonopathy.

Very few reports contain electrodiagnostic information (New et al., 1996; Hilkens et al., 1997; Fazio et al., 1999). In most patients, changes consistent with an axonal sensorimotor polyneuropathy have been obtained. Sensory responses are usually low in amplitude or absent, with the sural responses affected more than the median or ulnar responses. CMAP amplitudes are also decreased, especially in the legs. Motor conduction velocities and distal latencies are normal or mildly slowed. In one report, several patients had moderately reduced motor or sensory conduction velocities, but the corresponding amplitudes were not specified (Hilkens et al., 1997). In 75% of patients, needle EMG examination shows fibrillation potentials, decreased recruitment, and long-duration, large-amplitude MUAPs in distal leg muscles (New et al., 1996).

SURAMIN

Suramin is a hexasulfonated naphthylurea introduced in the 1920s as an antiparasitic agent. Since 1987, the drug has been investigated for its antitumor properties, with phase I/II trials focusing on the treatment of hormone-refractory prostate cancer. Suramin is also active against adrenocortical, ovarian, and renal cell carcinomas, malignant thymoma, and NHL (Stein, 1993).

Peripheral neuropathy is the dose-limiting side effect of suramin (La Rocca et al., 1990). The drug produces two distinct neuropathy profiles: (1) a mild, length-dependent, axonal, sensorimotor neuropathy and (2) a subacute, demyelinating, motor-predominant polyradiculoneuropathy (Chaudhry et al., 1996; Soliven et al., 1997). The incidence of all types and severities of neuropathy in suramin-treated patients across many series ranges from 25% to 90%, with a mean of approximately 50% (Myers et al., 1992; Bitton et al., 1995; Chaudhry et al., 1996; Mirza et al., 1997; Soliven et al., 1997). Early clinical trials suggested that neurotoxicity depended on peak suramin concentration, not cumulative dose (La Rocca et al., 1990; Stein, 1993). In particular, severe demyelinating neuropathies occurred only when peak levels greater than 350 μg/mL were maintained (La Rocca et al., 1990; Stein, 1993; Chaudhry et al., 1996). However, subsequent studies have reported many exceptions to this rule, suggesting that peak plasma concentration is not the primary determinant (Bitton et al., 1995; Soliven et al., 1997; Tu et al., 1998). In one recent analysis, the following factors were identified as better predictors of serious neurotoxicity: (1) cumulative dose greater than 157 mg/kg over 8 weeks; (2) exposure to concentrations above 200 µg/mL on more than 25 days per month; and (3) area under the curve above 200 µg/mL greater than 48,000 mg·hr/L (Bitton et al., 1995).

A distal axonopathy is the most commonly encountered form of PNS neurotoxicity (Myers et al., 1992; Chaudhry et al., 1996; Soliven et al., 1997). Patients present with mild, distal numbness and paresthesias. Examination reveals decreased ankle jerks, impaired pinprick and vibration sensation in the feet, and weak toe extensors. The neuropathy is slowly reversible in most patients once suramin is withdrawn. No nerve biopsies have been reported for this type of neuropathy. Electrodiagnostic studies demonstrate length-dependent reductions of SNAP and CMAP amplitudes, predominantly involving the lower limb responses. Distal latencies and conduction velocities are relatively preserved. The little information available on needle EMG testing in this syndrome indicates that fibrillation potentials, chronic neurogenic MUAPs, and decreased recruitment may occur in distal muscles (Soliven et al., 1997).

About 10% of patients develop a more severe, subacute, motor-predominant polyradiculoneuropathy, generally emerging after 1 to 5 months of treatment (La Rocca et al., 1990; Bitton et al., 1995; Chaudhry et al., 1996; Soliven et al., 1997; Tu et al., 1998). The initial symptoms are numbness and paresthesias of the distal extremities or face, succeeded by subacutely evolving generalized, symmetrical, proximal more than distal weakness. Reflexes are globally decreased or absent. Sensory examination reveals a stocking-distribution loss involving all modalities. Twenty-five percent of patients become bedridden and require ventilatory assistance. The clinical nadir is reached 2 to 9 weeks after the onset of symptoms. CSF protein is elevated in almost all patients. Several patients have been treated with plasma exchange, with variable results (La Rocca et al., 1990; Chaudhry et al., 1996). Most patients recover over 3 to 6 months, with mild residual weakness and sensory loss. However, some patients do not recover and are left with severe weakness and incapacity (La Rocca et al., 1990; Bitton et al., 1995; Soliven et al., 1997). Sural nerve biopsies have demonstrated a mixture of axonal and demyelinating/remyelinating changes, including decreased number of large and small myelinated fibers, occasional wallerian-like degeneration, occasional thinly myelinated fibers, and mild Schwann cell proliferation (La Rocca et al., 1990; Chaudhry et al., 1996). One biopsy was normal except for segmental demyelination on teased-fiber examination (La Rocca et al., 1990). In two of four specimens, mild mononuclear inflammatory infiltrates were seen in the epineurium and endoneurium (Chaudhry et al., 1996).

Electrodiagnostic studies in patients with this subacute, motor-predominant syndrome have generally supported a primary demyelinating process, indistinguishable from classic GBS (La Rocca et al., 1990; Chaudhry et al., 1996; Soliven et al., 1997). Typical findings are prolonged distal motor latencies, prolonged or absent F waves, significantly reduced motor conduction velocities (especially tibial) (Soliven et al., 1997), low-amplitude upper and lower extremity SNAPs, reduced median sensory conduction velocity (Soliven et al., 1997), and occasional abnormal temporal dispersion and partial motor conduction block. CMAP amplitudes are also commonly decreased. In some patients, multiple nerves become inexcitable, associated with a poor outcome (La Rocca et al., 1990). Needle EMG examination demonstrates decreased recruitment in both proximal and distal muscles; in severely affected patients, abundant fibrillation potentials occur in weak distal muscles (Soliven et al., 1997).

The mechanism of neurotoxicity is unknown in both forms of suramin neuropathy. Suramin competitively inhibits growth factor interactions with their receptors, including nerve growth factor and insulin-like growth factor II (Russell et al., 1994; Sullivan et al., 1997). A recent in vitro study suggested that suramin modulation of nerve growth factor receptors, at least, is not involved in its neurotoxicity (Gill and Windebank, 1998). The drug also disrupts glycolipid metabolism in dorsal root ganglion cultures, leading to the formation of lamellar inclusion bodies in Schwann cells and neuron cell bodies, which contain G_{M1} ganglioside and ceramide, (Gill et al., 1995). In effect, a form of lysosomal storage disease is created. Suramin-induced ceramide accumulation within neurons may provoke apoptotic cell death, as ceramide is an intracellular mediator of apoptosis (Gill and Windebank, 1998). The demyelinating neuropathy may be immune mediated, triggered by suramin's known immunomodulatory effects (Czernin et al., 1993).

CYTOSINE ARABINOSIDE (ARA-C)

Ara-C is an antimetabolite used in the treatment of leukemia and NHL (Baker et al., 1991). Peripheral neuropathy is a rare complication that has occurred following cumulative doses ranging from 600 mg to 36 g/m². Pure sensory polyneuropathies (Russell and Powles, 1974), severe and acute sensorimotor polyneuropathies resembling GBS (Borgeat et al., 1986; Johnson et al., 1987; Paul et al., 1991; Openshaw et al., 1996), and bilateral brachial plexopathies are described (Scherokman et al., 1989). Symptoms begin within hours to 3 weeks after the ara-C treatment. The GBS-like neuropathies occur in approximately 1% of patients treated with high-dose ara-C (Openshaw et al., 1996). One patient with an acute polyradiculoneuropathy transiently improved after a course of plasma exchange (Openshaw et al., 1996).

SECTION XIX

NEUROMUSCULAR DISORDERS ASSOCIATED WITH HUMAN IMMUNODEFICIENCY VIRUS

CHAPTER 73

AIDS-Associated Myelopathies

Alessandro Di Rocco and Michele Tagliati

The spinal cord is commonly affected during human immunodeficiency virus (HIV) infection, and vacuolar myelopathy associated with acquired immunodeficiency syndrome (AIDS) is the most common spinal cord disease in HIV-infected individuals (Petito et al., 1985; Simpson and Tagliati, 1994). In addition to vacuolar myelopathy, HIV may also cause a rare acute myelitis. Other viral, bacterial, fungal, and parasitic infections, and vascular and neoplastic diseases, may also be infrequently encountered during the course of HIV infection.

AIDS-ASSOCIATED VACUOLAR MYELOPATHY

Although the clinical manifestations of myelopathy are not encountered as frequently as those of

neuropathy and dementia, autopsy studies have documented that white matter changes in the thoracic cord consistent with vacuolar myelopathy are present in a third or more of patients with HIV infection. In autopsy series, evidence of spinal cord disease consistent with vacuolar myelopathy is present in 20% to 55% of patients with AIDS (Petito et al., 1985; Artigas et al., 1990; Dal Pan et al., 1994). The number of HIV-infected individuals who develop the clinical manifestations of myelopathy is, however, much smaller, although there are no data on the true incidence of the disease or the impact of antiretroviral agents on the incidence of the disease (Dal Pan et al., 1994). Although vacuolar myelopathy has typical clinical features and well-defined pathological findings, it remains one of the least studied and least understood of the neurological manifestations of AIDS.

Pathology

The first large, autopsy-based series of AIDS myelopathy that described vacuolization of the spinal cord in 20 of 89 consecutive AIDS patients autopsied was reported by Petito and colleagues in 1985. These patients had various degrees of weakness, sensory abnormalities, urinary symptoms, and other clinical signs of myelopathy. The high prevalence of spinal cord vacuolization in AIDS was later reported in other large pathological series (Artigas et al., 1990; Dal Pan et al., 1994).

Vacuolar myelopathy usually affects the middle portion of the thoracic cord, but the vacuolization can be present in other portions of the thoracic cord and the cervical cord, while the lumbar cord is rarely involved (Fig. 73–1). The disease is characterized by the presence of intramyelinic and periaxonal vacuoles, often filled with foamy macrophages, in the lateral and posterior columns of the spinal cord (Petito et al., 1985; Tan et al., 1995). The axons are usually intact in areas of mild or moderate vacuolization, but in cases with more severe vacuolization the axons are disrupted (Petito et al., 1985).

The clinicopathological correlation of spinal cord vacuolization with neurological symptoms and signs of myelopathy has been difficult because of the retrospective nature of most reported series (Table 73–1) (Petito et al., 1985; Dal Pan et al., 1994; Tan et al., 1995). Myelopathic signs are infrequent in patients with mild (grade I) vacuolar myelopathy (Petito et al., 1985), in which only a few vacuoles per transverse section are present. Patients with mild vacuolar myelopathy rarely have motor signs and may present with fatigue, mild weakness, increased reflexes, and sphincter abnormalities (Petito et al., 1985; Dal Pan et al., 1994; Tan et al., 1995). In this stage of the disease, somatosensory evoked potential examination may detect subclinical forms of spinal cord structural damage (Dal Pan et al., 1994). Symptomatic myelopathy generally correlates with pathological evidence of moderate and severe vacuolar myelopathy. Approximately 20% to 60% of patients with grade II (moderate) and almost all patients with grade III (severe) vacuolar myelopathy show symptoms and signs of myelopathy, with spasticity, weakness, ataxia, and incontinence (Petito et al., 1985; Dal Pan et al., 1994; Tan et al., 1995). This may explain the relatively small number of patients who develop clinical evidence of myelopathy. In most cases, vacuolar myelopathy is a subclinical disease, manifesting only when the white matter vacuolization has become severe.

Vacuolization is less common in children with AIDS, although other pathological changes, such as diffuse loss of myelin, axonal loss, presence of multinucleated giant cells, and prominent inflammatory infiltrates, are commonly observed (Dickson et al., 1989; Sharer et al., 1990).

Pathogenesis

The pathogenesis of vacuolar myelopathy is probably related to immunological and biochemical mechanisms, rather than direct viral infection. Although there have been attempts to correlate HIV infection with the presence and severity of vacuolar myelopathy (Budka, 1990), most studies have not found evidence of a direct effect of HIV infection on the spinal cord in subjects with vacuolar myelopathy. HIV is found within macrophages, but not in neuronal cells or microglia, and there is no relationship between the presence of HIV and the development of myelopathy (Eilbott et al., 1989; Rosenblum et al., 1989; Kure et al., 1991; Petito et al., 1994; Tan et al., 1995).

Vacuolar myelopathy has striking pathological similarities to the subacute combined degeneration associated with vitamin B_{12} deficiency (Petito et al., 1985). This has led to speculation on the role of cobalamin deficiency in the pathogenesis of vacuolar myelopathy, but most investigators have found that subjects with myelopathy have a normal serum

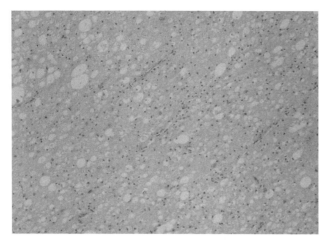

Figure 73–1. Vacuolization in the posterior columns of the spinal cord of subjects infected with human immunodeficiency virus who have myelopathy (hematoxylin & eosin).

Table 73–1. Clinicopathological Correlation in HIV-Associated Vacuolar Myelopathy

Grade	Pathological Findings	Clinical Findings
I	<15 vacuoles per transverse section	Asymptomatic
II	Numerous, nonconfluent vacuoles	Rare myelopathy (20%)
III	Areas on confluent vacuolization	Frequent myelopathy (80%)

Adapted from Dal Pan GJ, Glass JD, McArthur JC: Clinicopathologic correlation of HIV-1–associated vacuolar myelopathy: An autopsy-based case-control study. Neurology 1994;44:2159–2164.

vitamin B$_{12}$ level (Petito et al., 1985; Harriman et al., 1989; Keibutz et al., 1991), and treatment with vitamin B$_{12}$ supplementation does not affect the course of the disease (Keibutz et al., 1991). Cobalamin in the nervous system acts as a coenzyme of methionine synthetase for the production of methionine, which is then converted into S-adenosyl-L-methionine (SAM), the major methyl group donor in the nervous system (Scott et al., 1994). Methylation is essential in myelin formation, stabilization, and repair, and in the metabolism of nucleic acids and neurotransmitters. Evidence linking impaired methylation in the nervous system and neurological complications of AIDS has been documented in adults and children (Surtees et al., 1990; Castagna et al., 1995). The pathogenesis of vacuolar myelopathy may therefore be related to a complex chain of events that is initiated by the viral infection, with consequent macrophage activation and cytokine release that may ultimately lead to transmethylation impairment and myelin vacuolization and destruction.

Clinical Manifestations

Vacuolar myelopathy manifests clinically late in the course of HIV infection (Petito et al., 1985; Simpson and Tagliati, 1994; Dal Pan and Berger, 1997; Di Rocco, 1999), although there are reported cases of the early appearance of vacuolar myelopathy and cases in which myelopathy was the first clinical manifestation of AIDS (Dal Pan et al., 1994; Epstein et al., 1986; Tan and Guiloff, 1998). The disease usually develops slowly over months, and its initial symptoms are often subtle and not easily recognized. It frequently begins with constipation and urinary urgency and frequency, or erectile dysfunction in men (Yarchoan et al., 1987; Di Rocco et al., 1998). The myelopathy slowly progresses, with weakness in the lower extremities and gait abnormalities that can progress to severe paresis (Simpson and Tagliati, 1994; Di Rocco, 1999). Spasticity can be mild, with brisk reflexes at the knees and ankles, or can become a severe source of disability, with clonus and painful spasms. Often a coexisting neuropathy leads to the typical neurological findings of brisk reflexes at the knees and reduced or absent ankle reflexes. Sensory symptoms manifest with numbness and tingling in the lower extremities, but they are rarely severe. A loss of vibration and joint position sense is common, and when severe it may cause ataxia of the lower limbs and further impair gait (Petito et al., 1985; Dal Pan et al., 1994). Pain and temperature sensations are usually preserved, and their absence often indicates the presence of neuropathy. As a rule, a discrete sensory level is usually absent in vacuolar myelopathy, and its presence strongly suggests an alternative diagnosis.

Diagnosis

The diagnosis of vacuolar myelopathy is based largely on the typical symptoms and findings on neurological examination and the exclusion of other causes of spinal cord disease. Magnetic resonance imaging (MRI) studies are usually normal, except for mild atrophy of the thoracic cord or, less frequently, nonspecific areas of increased signal on T2-weighted images (Barakos et al., 1990; Santosh et al., 1995; Sartoretti-Schefer et al., 1997; Chong et al., 1999). Cerebrospinal fluid studies are usually normal or reveal mild pleocytosis (<20 cells/mm^3) and a nonspecific increase in protein content. A rapid progression of the myelopathy over days or weeks, the presence of a discrete sensory level, cerebrospinal fluid pleocytosis, and back pain are all strong evidence against a diagnosis of vacuolar myelopathy and should lead to aggressive diagnostic investigations to disclose the cause of spinal cord disease.

The differential diagnosis of vacuolar myelopathy is extensive and includes other infections, such as human T-lymphotropic virus type I or II, cytomegalovirus, herpes simplex virus type 2, *Toxoplasma*, tuberculosis, syphilis, and metabolic (vitamin B$_{12}$ deficiency) and neoplastic diseases, particularly lymphomas. Although the clinical presentation and the evolution of vacuolar myelopathy are fairly typical, the diagnosis may be difficult in patients with advanced AIDS and severe systemic disease or coexisting peripheral neuropathy and dementia (Petito et al., 1985; Simpson and Tagliati, 1994).

ELECTROPHYSIOLOGICAL STUDIES

The clinical evaluation of spinal cord diseases has been classically based on the neurological examination, combined with a neuroimaging study, including spinal MRI, computed tomography (CT), or myelography. These clinical tools provide detailed anatomic data about the spinal cord and adjacent structures; however, they fail to inform the clinician about the functional properties of the spinal cord, which can be affected in the absence of gross structural abnormalities. Electrophysiological tests are therefore a fundamental addition to the clinical and imaging assessment, as they are able to reliably measure abnormal function of central sensory and motor function. Somatosensory and motor evoked potentials have been successfully employed in the evaluation of several diseases involving the spinal cord, including multiple sclerosis, cervical myelopathy, motor neuron disease, and hereditary, traumatic, and metabolic myelopathy (Kiers and Chiappa, 1997).

Somatosensory Evoked Potentials

The clinical diagnosis of AIDS-associated myelopathy is complicated by the concurrent presence of peripheral neuropathy in more than 50% of patients (Dal Pan et al., 1994). As somatosensory evoked potentials (SSEPs) provide measurement of both peripheral and central nervous system function, this test can be particularly useful in the assessment of

HIV patients with neurological involvement of the lower limbs.

Several studies have investigated SSEP results in HIV-infected subjects, showing that posterior tibial SSEPs have the highest rate of abnormality of all evoked potential modalities in HIV-positive subjects (Hall et al., 1997). These studies were mostly performed on neurologically asymptomatic patients and, therefore, assessed the presence of subclinical disease of sensory pathways, with controversial results. While some authors reported abnormalities of peripheral (Smith et al., 1988; Jakobsen et al., 1989; Koralnik et al., 1990; Jabarri et al., 1993; Hall et al., 1997) or central SSEP components in asymptomatic HIV-infected subjects (Jabarri et al., 1993; Iragui et al., 1994), other studies have failed to demonstrate SSEP abnormalities (McAllister et al., 1992; Boccellari et al., 1993). These differences may be due, in part, to variability in patient selection.

Fewer studies have assessed SSEP in HIV-infected subjects who had symptoms of neurological dysfunction of the lower extremities. Helweg-Larsen and colleagues (1988) reported prolonged latency of tibial nerve SSEPs in 16 patients with AIDS and clinical symptoms and signs of myelopathy. Peripheral slowing of conduction could account for the conduction delay at the cortical level in five cases, while conduction slowing through the spinal cord was detected in all other cases. Median nerve central conduction time (CCT) was abnormal in only two patients, confirming the localization of the conduction defect in the spinal cord. The delay in tibial nerve SSEPs was more pronounced in patients with lower limb ataxia and/or paresis (Fig. 73–2).

The authors reviewed their SSEP data in HIV-infected patients to assess the diagnostic yield of SSEPs in AIDS-associated myelopathy (Tagliati et al., 2000). The authors recorded tibial and median nerve SSEPs in 69 HIV-infected subjects referred for evaluation of neurological abnormalities of the lower extremities. Of this group, 57 patients had peripheral neuropathy and 35 had myelopathy. In addition, 23 patients showed clinical symptoms and signs of both neuropathy and myelopathy. Patients with no response to ankle stimulation were further evaluated with stimulation of the peroneal nerve at the popliteal fossa.

Results indicated that HIV-infected subjects had significantly delayed latencies of both peripheral and central potentials, suggesting a combination of peripheral and central nervous system abnormalities. The analysis of peripheral and central latencies allowed the authors to discriminate between neuropathy and myelopathy in individual patients. There was no significant difference in median CCT between patients and control subjects.

By subtracting the median nerve CCT from the posterior tibial or peroneal nerve CCT, the authors calculated a derived spinal conduction time (SCT). They hypothesized that the subtraction of median CCT from tibial CCT would provide a better assessment of spinal cord conduction. Indeed, in the evalu-

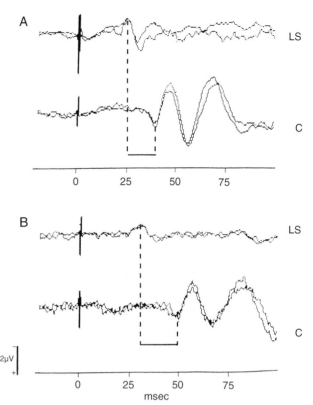

Figure 73–2. Lumbosacral (LS) and cortical (C) somatosensory evoked potential (SSEP) following tibial nerve stimulation at the ankle. *A,* Normal control subject of comparable age and height. *B,* HIV-infected patient with symptoms and signs of myelopathy and neuropathy. Peak latencies are linked to visually represent the central conduction time (CCT). The lower record shows delayed N20 and P37, with a prolonged CCT. These findings are consistent with a conduction defect of the large-fiber sensory system involving both the peripheral and the central nervous system. (From Tagliati M, Di Rocco A, Danisi F, Simpson D: The role of somatosensory evoked potentials in the diagnosis of AIDS-associated myelopathy. Neurology 2000;54:1477–1482, with permission.)

ation of individual patients, the derived SCT seemed to be a more sensitive marker of spinal cord dysfunction than tibial CCT. Abnormalities of SCT identified nine patients with abnormal conduction through the spinal cord but with "normal" tibial CCT. In the authors' opinion, SCT is a sensitive marker of spinal conduction abnormalities and improves the diagnostic yield of SSEPs in AIDS-associated myelopathy. By focusing the evaluation on the thoracolumbar segments of the spinal cord, SCT represents a more precise measure of spinal cord function in AIDS-associated myelopathy, consistent with the typical midthoracic localization of pathological lesions in vacuolar myelopathy (Petito et al., 1985).

The abnormalities of tibial CCT and SCT correlated with the clinical diagnosis of myelopathy. Patients with objective signs of myelopathy had significantly longer tibial CCT and SCT than those with only subjective neurological symptoms in the lower limbs. Abnormalities of SCT were twice as frequent as tibial CCT abnormalities in HIV-infected patients without objective signs of myelopathy, indicating a possible preclinical stage of spinal cord disease. Although longitudinal studies with systematic neuroradiological and pathological controls are needed to confirm this hypothesis, these data suggest a spectrum of spinal cord conduction abnormalities in HIV-infected patients. Clinicopathological studies of vacuolar myelopathy have demonstrated a range of abnormalities extending from mild disease with few vacuoles and mostly subjective symptoms to diffuse vacuolization of the posterior and lateral columns that leads to severe clinical myelopathy (Dal Pan et al., 1994).

In conclusion, the combination of median, posterior tibial, and peroneal SSEPs is a valuable tool in the diagnosis of AIDS-associated myelopathy, particularly when myelopathy and peripheral neuropathy coexist. The use of the derived SCT improves the diagnostic yield of SSEPs in AIDS-associated myelopathy.

Motor Evoked Potentials

The motor evoked potential (MEP) is generated by magnetic stimulation of the upper motor neurons in the motor cortex or lower motor neurons in the spinal cord enlargements. This technique provides the clinician with a reliable method of studying the function of central motor pathways in diseases affecting the pyramidal system. A central motor conduction time (CMCT) can be calculated by subtracting the peripheral motor latency from the latency of the MEP elicited by transcranial stimulation. Abnormalities of CMCT have been described in many neurological conditions affecting the spinal cord, including multiple sclerosis, cervical myelopathy, motor neuron disease, and spinocerebellar degeneration (Jakobsen et al., 1989).

Motor evoked potentials could also increase the yield for electrophysiological diagnosis. As the vacuolization can be more severe in the lateral than in the posterior columns, SSEPs may fail to detect the abnormality. Although there are no published clinical data on HIV-infected patients with myelopathy, MEPs were used to evaluate the damage to motor pathways in a simian model of neuro-AIDS. Recordings were obtained in nine monkeys that underwent transcranial electrical stimulation of the motor cortex and spinal cord before and after experimental infection with neurovirulent SIVmac R17/17E (Raymond et al., 1999). Six of the seven monkeys that developed rapidly progressive disease showed postinoculation increases in the latencies of cortical MEPs. Increases in cortical MEP latencies ranged from 21% to 97% in different monkeys. All seven of the rapidly progressing animals showed postinoculation increases in spinal cord MEP latencies, ranging from 22% to 147%. Increases in CCT ranged up to 204% and exceeded two standard deviations (SDs) of control in four monkeys. The affected monkeys showed classic AIDS-related neuropathology, although there was no consistent relationship between the severity of neuropathology and the extent of MEP abnormalities.

Treatment

There is currently no specific treatment for vacuolar myelopathy. Zidovudine (AZT) appears ineffective (Yarchoan et al., 1987), and there is no evidence that other antiretroviral drugs currently used can improve the symptoms or slow the progression of vacuolar myelopathy. Treatment with vitamin B_{12} has proved ineffective in improving the symptoms or delaying the progression of the disease (Keibutz et al., 1991). Corticosteroids and intravenous gamma globulin have also been ineffective (Dal Pan and Berger, 1997).

Based on the hypothesis that vacuolar myelopathy may be related to abnormal transmethylation metabolism, a pilot study that used high doses of oral l-methionine led to improvement in clinical and electrophysiological features of the disease in most of the patients treated (Di Rocco et al., 1998). A placebo-controlled clinical trial is currently being conducted to further assess the potential of l-methionine in the treatment of vacuolar myelopathy.

The effects of protease inhibitors and the current highly active antiretroviral therapies (HAART) on vacuolar myelopathy is unknown. To date, there has been no study describing the effect of HAART on the clinical manifestations or electrophysiological measures of vacuolar myelopathy. It is also not known whether these drugs are capable of stopping or delaying the progression of the disease, or whether the introduction of HAART has decreased the overall incidence of vacuolar myelopathy. A report described clinical improvement of myelopathy after the introduction of HAART in one patient (Staudinger and Henry, 2000). Although HAART reduced the plasma viral load, there was no cerebrospinal fluid viral load measurement, electrophysiological confirmation of the diagnosis, or improvement after therapy. The authors have encountered a similar patient who regained some strength after starting HAART. However, repeated SSEPs demonstrated worsening of CCT, thus suggesting that symptomatic improvement was related to general improvement of health, without a specific effect on the spinal cord (Di Rocco and Geraci, 2000). These cases further illustrate the role of electrophysiological studies in monitoring progression of the disease and the therapeutic effect of treatment.

OTHER MYELOPATHIES IN HIV INFECTION

A rare, acute or subacute transverse myelitis can develop as an early or late complication of AIDS and, in rare cases, can be the presenting manifestation of HIV infection. The disease is considered a direct consequence of HIV infection and is accompanied by cerebrospinal fluid pleocytosis (Denning et al., 1987; Jerez et al., 1998).

In addition to HIV, other viruses can cause spinal cord disease AIDS. Human T-lymphotropic virus type 1 or 2 (HTLV-1 or -2) is a common cause of myelopathy, and co-infection with HIV and HTLV-1 viruses has been reported in patients with myelopathy, particularly in regions with endemic HTLV-1 infection and in the drug user population (Harrison et al., 1997). The diagnosis is based on the isolation of HTLV-1 or the measurement of anti–HTLV-1 antibodies in serum and cerebrospinal fluid. Pathologically, HTLV myelopathy is characterized by inflammatory infiltrates and spongiform changes in the thoracic cord. The pathological characteristics of the myelopathy in patients co-infected with the two viruses remain undefined (Berger et al., 1991). Although it is difficult to clinically differentiate HTLV myelopathy from vacuolar myelopathy, a mild to moderate pleocytosis in the cerebrospinal fluid and demonstration of HTLV infection suggest that the myelopathy may be related to HTLV infection, rather than vacuolar myelopathy. This may have important therapeutic implications, as HTLV myelopathy may respond to steroids or high doses of interferon-α (McArthur et al., 1990; Yamasaki et al., 1997).

Cytomegalovirus (CMV) is another rare cause of myelopathy in HIV infection, and its incidence has declined significantly with the introduction of HAART (Whitley et al., 1998). Cytomegalovirus infection causes a typical radiculomyelitis, usually involving the cauda equina, with the acute or subacute development of flaccid paraplegia and incontinence. Rarely, the acute myeloradiculitis can be the initial manifestation of AIDS (Mahieux et al., 1989; Vinters et al., 1989; Chimelli et al., 1990). Cytomegalovirus myelitis and myeloradiculitis may respond to ganciclovir and cidofovir, alone or in combination (Danner, 1995; Cline and Garrett, 1997).

Herpes simplex virus type 2 (HSV-2) can cause an acute transverse myelitis (Tucker et al., 1985; Dal Pan et al., 1994; Folpe et al., 1994), and herpes zoster has been implicated in the development of meningo-myeloradiculitis. These myelopathies can be diagnosed through the HSV culture of cerebrospinal fluid and can be treated with acyclovir (Britton et al., 1985).

Other infectious causes of myelopathy include the rare toxoplasmosis of the spinal cord, tuberculosis with spinal cord tuberculomas, cryptococcosis of the spinal cord, and spinal cord aspergillosis. All these are diagnosed by appropriate serological and spinal fluid studies and are treated with the appropriate antimicrobial agents, although symptomatic treatment of spasticity and urinary symptoms may be necessary (Di Rocco, 1999). Syphilis can cause spinal cord disease, but a syphilitic myelopathy is rare in patients with HIV infection and can respond to treatment with penicillin (Di Rocco, 1999).

As discussed, electrophysiological studies do not play a major role in differentiating vacuolar myelop-

athy from these rarer causes of spinal cord disease in AIDS.

Acknowledgment

Supported in part by NIH-NS 35745.

References

Artigas J, Grosse G, Niedobitek F: Vacuolar myelopathy in AIDS: A morphological analysis. Pathol Res Pract 1990;186:228–237.

Barakos JA, Mark AS, Dillon WP, Norman D: MR imaging in acute transverse myelitis and AIDS myelopathy. J Comput Assist Tomogr 1990;14:45–50.

Berger JR, Raffanti S, Svenningison A, et al: The role of HTLV in HIV-associated neurologic disease. Neurology 1991;41:197–202.

Boccellari AA, Diley JW, Yingling CD, et al: Relationship of CD4 counts to neurophysiological function in HIV-1 homosexual men. Arch Neurol 1993;50:517–521.

Britton CB, Mesa-Tejada R, Fenoglio CM, et al: A new complication of AIDS: Thoracic myelitis caused by herpes simplex virus. Neurology 1985;35:1071–1074.

Budka H: Human immunodeficiency virus (HIV) envelope and core proteins in CNS tissues of patients with the acquired immune deficiency syndrome (AIDS). Acta Neuropathol (Berl) 1990;79:611–619.

Castagna A, Le Grazie C, Accordini A, et al: Cerebrospinal fluid S-adenosylmethionine (SAMe) and glutathione concentrations in HIV infections: Effect of parenteral treatment with SAMe. Neurology 1995;45:1678–1683.

Chimelli L, de Freitas MR, Bazin AR, et al: Cytomegalovirus encephalo-myelo-radiculitis in acquired immunodeficiency syndrome. Rev Neurol (Paris) 1990;146:354–360.

Chong J, Di Rocco A, Danisi F, et al: Atlas: MR abnormalities in AIDS-associated vacuolar myelopathy. AJNR Am J Neuroradiol 1999;20:1412–1416.

Cline JJ, Garrett AD: Combination antiviral therapy for cytomegalovirus disease in patients with AIDS. Ann Pharmacother 1997;31:1080–1082.

Dal Pan GJ, Berger JR: Spinal cord disease in human immunodeficiency virus infection. In Berger JR, Levy RM (eds): AIDS and the Nervous System, 2nd ed. Philadelphia, Lippincott-Raven, 1997; 173–187.

Dal Pan GJ, Glass JD, McArthur JC: Clinicopathologic correlation of HIV-1–associated vacuolar myelopathy: An autopsy-based case-control study. Neurology 1994;44:2159–2164.

Danner SA: Management of cytomegalovirus disease. AIDS 1995; 9(suppl 2):S3–S8.

Denning DW, Anderson J, Rudge P, Smith H: Acute myelopathy associated with primary infection with human immunodeficiency virus. BMJ 1987;294:143–144.

Di Rocco A: Diseases of the spinal cord in human immunodeficiency virus infection. Semin Neurol 1999;19:151–155.

Di Rocco A, Geraci A: Remission of HIV myelopathy after highly active antiretroviral therapy. Neurology 2000;55:456–461.

Di Rocco A, Tagliati M, Danisi F, et al: L-Methionine for AIDS-associated vacuolar myelopathy. Neurology 1998;51:266–268.

Dickson DW, Belman AL, Kim TS, et al: Spinal cord pathology in pediatric acquired immunodeficiency syndrome. Neurology 1989;39:227–235.

Eilbott DJ, Peress N, Burger H, et al: Human immunodeficiency virus type 1 in spinal cords of acquired immunodeficiency syndrome patients with myelopathy: Expression and replication in macrophages. Proc Natl Acad Sci U S A 1989;86:3337–3341.

Epstein LG, Sharer LR, Oleske JM, et al: Neurologic manifestation of human immunodeficiency virus infection in children. Pediatrics 1986;78:678–687.

Folpe A, Lapham LW, Smith HC: Herpes simplex myelitis as a cause of acute necrotizing myelitis syndrome. Neurology 1994; 44:1955–1957.

Hall CD, Messenheimer JA, Vaughn BV: Clinical neurophysiological testing in human immunodeficiency virus infection. In Berger JR, Levy RM (eds): AIDS and the Nervous System, 2nd ed. Philadelphia, Lippincott-Raven, 1997; 279–296.

Harriman GR, Smith PD, Horne MK, et al: Vitamin B_{12} malabsorption in patients with acquired immunodeficiency syndrome. Arch Intern Med 1989;149:2039–2041.

Harrison LH, Vaz B, Taveira DM, et al: Myelopathy among Brazilians coinfected with human T-cell lymphotropic virus type I and HIV. Neurology 1997;48:13–18.

Helweg-Larsen S, Jakobsen J, Boesen F, et al: Myelopathy in AIDS: A clinical and electrophysiological study of 23 Danish patients. Acta Neurol Scand 1988;77:64–73.

Iragui VJ, Kalmijn J, Thal L, Grant I, HNRC Group: Neurological dysfunction in asymptomatic HIV-1–infected men: Evidence from evoked potentials. Electroencephalogr Clin Neurophysiol 1994;92:1–10.

Jabarri B, Coats M, Salazar A, et al: Longitudinal study of EEG and evoked potentials in neurologically asymptomatic HIV-infected subjects. Electroencephalogr Clin Neurophysiol 1993;86:145–151.

Jakobsen J, Smith T, Gaub J, et al: Progressive neurological dysfunction during latent HIV infection. BMJ 1989;299:225–228.

Jerez P, Palao A, Leiva C: HIV myelopathy as the presenting symptom of acquired immunodeficiency syndrome. Rev Neurol 1998;26:1008–1010.

Keibutz KD, Giang DW, Schiffer RB, Vakil N: Abnormal vitamin B_{12} metabolism in human immunodeficiency virus infection. Arch Neurol 1991;48:312–314.

Kiers L, Chiappa KH: Motor and somatosensory evoked potentials in spinal cord disorders. In Chiappa KH (ed): Evoked Potentials in Clinical Medicine, 3rd ed. Philadelphia, Lippincott-Raven, 1997; 509–528.

Koralnik IJ, Beaumanoir A, Hausler R, et al: A controlled study of early neurological abnormalities in men with asymptomatic human immunodeficiency virus infection. N Engl J Med 1990; 323:864–870.

Kure K, Llena JF, Lyman WD, et al: Human immunodeficiency virus-1 infection of the nervous system: An autopsy study of 268 adult, pediatric and fetal brains. Hum Pathol 1991;22:700–710.

Mahieux F, Gray F, Fenelon G, et al: Acute myeloradiculitis due to cytomegalovirus as the initial manifestation of AIDS. J Neurol Neurosurg Psychiatry 1989;52:270–274.

McAllister RH, Herns MV, Harrison MJG, et al: Neurological and neuropsychological performance in HIV-seropositive men without symptoms. J Neurol Neurosurg Psychiatry 1992;55:143–148.

McArthur JC, Griffin JW, Cornblath DR, et al: Steroid-responsive myeloneuropathy in a man dually infected with HIV-1 and HTLV-I. Neurology 1990;40:938–944.

Petito CK, Navia BA, Cho ES, et al: Vacuolar myelopathy pathologically resembling subacute combined degeneration in patients with the acquired immunodeficiency syndrome. N Engl J Med 1985;312:874–879.

Petito CK, Vecchio D, Chen YT: HIV antigen and DNA in AIDS spinal cords correlate with macrophage infiltration but not with vacuolar myelopathy. J Neuropathol Exp Neurol 1994;53:86–94.

Raymond LA, Wallace D, Marcario JK, et al: Motor evoked potentials in a rhesus macaque model of neuro-AIDS. J Neurovirol 1999;5:217–231.

Rosenblum M, Scheck AC, Cronin K, et al: Dissociation of AIDS-related vacuolar myelopathy and productive HIV-1 infection of the spinal cord. Neurology 1989;39:892–896.

Santosh CG, Bell JE, Best JJ: Spinal tract pathology in AIDS: Postmortem MRI correlation with neuropathology. Neuroradiology 1995;37:134–138.

Sartoretti-Schefer S, Blattler T, Wichmann W: Spinal MRI in vacuolar myelopathy, and correlation with histopathological findings. Neuroradiology 1997;39:865–869.

Scott JM, Molloy AM, Kennedy DG, et al: Effects of destruction of transmethylation in the central nervous system: An animal model. Acta Neurol Scand Suppl 1994;154:27–31.

Sharer LR, Dowling PC, Michaels J, et al: Spinal cord disease in children with HIV-1 infection: A combined molecular biology and neuropathological study. Neuropathol Appl Neurobiol 1990; 16:317–331.

Simpson DM, Tagliati M: Neurologic manifestations of HIV infection. Ann Intern Med 1994;121:769–785.

Smith T, Jakobsen J, Gaub J, et al: Clinical and electrophysiological studies of human immunodeficiency seropositive men without AIDS. Ann Neurol 1988;23:295–297.

Staudinger R, Henry K: Remission of HIV myelopathy after highly active antiretroviral therapy. Neurology 2000;54:267–268.

Surtees R, Hyland K, Smith I: Central nervous system methyl group metabolism in children with neurological complications of HIV infection. Lancet 1990;335:619–621.

Tagliati M, Di Rocco A, Danisi F, Simpson D: The role of somatosensory evoked potentials in the diagnosis of AIDS-associated myelopathy. Neurology 2000;54:1477–1482.

Tan SV, Guiloff RJ: Hypothesis on the pathogenesis of vacuolar myelopathy, dementia, and peripheral neuropathy in AIDS. J Neurol Neurosurg Psychiatry 1998;65:23–28.

Tan SV, Guiloff RJ, Scaravilli F: AIDS-associated vacuolar myelopathy: A morphometric study. Brain 1995;118:1247–1261.

Tucker T, Dix RD, Katzen C, et al: Cytomegalovirus and herpes simplex virus ascending myelitis in a patient with acquired immune deficiency syndrome. Ann Neurol 1985;18:74–79.

Vinters HV, Kwok MK, Ho HW, et al: Cytomegalovirus in the nervous system of patients with the acquired immune deficiency syndrome. Brain 1989;112(Pt 1):245–268.

Whitley RJ, Jacobson MA, Friedberg DN, et al: Guidelines for the treatment of cytomegalovirus diseases in patients with AIDS in the era of potent antiretroviral therapy: Recommendations of an international panel. International AIDS Society–USA. Arch Intern Med 1998;158:957–969.

Yamasaki K, Kira J, Koyanagi Y, et al: Long-term, high-dose interferon-alpha treatment in HTLV-I–associated myelopathy/tropical spastic paraparesis: A combined clinical, virological and immunological study. J Neurol Sci 1997;147:135–144.

Yarchoan R, Berg G, Brouwers P, et al: Response of immunodeficiency virus–associated neurological disease to 3′-azido-3′-deoxythymidine. Lancet 1987;1:132–135.

CHAPTER 74

HIV-Related Neuropathies and Myopathies

Annabel K. Wang, Enrique A. Wulff, and David M. Simpson

NEUROPATHIES
  Distal Symmetrical Polyneuropathy
  Inflammatory Demyelinating
   Polyradiculoneuropathy
  Progressive Polyradiculopathy
  Mononeuropathy Multiplex
  Autonomic Neuropathy
  Diffuse Infiltrative Lymphocytosis Syndrome
  Ataxic Neuropathy

MYOPATHIES
  HIV-Associated Myopathy
  Zidovudine-Associated Myopathy
  HIV Wasting Syndrome
MOTOR NEURON DISEASE
CONCLUSION

Neuromuscular complications can occur at any stage of human immunodeficiency virus (HIV) infection and acquired immunodeficiency syndrome (AIDS) (Table 74–1). In one of the earliest epidemiological studies, Snider and associates identified 50 patients from a cohort of 160 AIDS patients, with central and peripheral neurologic complications (Snider et al., 1983). Eight patients had neuropathy, and one patient had polymyositis. Levy and colleagues (1985) found that 51 of 352 individuals with AIDS developed cranial nerve or neuromuscular complications, which included the following: chronic inflammatory polyneuropathy, lymphoma, Bell's palsy, distal symmetrical neuropathy, herpes zoster radiculitis, persistent myalgias, and polymyositis. Lipkin and coworkers (1985) reported 12 cases of peripheral neuropathy in patients with fever, night sweats, malaise, and general lymphadenopathy, preceding the appearance of AIDS. Nine patients with multifocal mononeuropathy and three patients with distal symmetrical polyneuropathy were identified.

Hall and colleagues identified evidence of neuropathy in 32 of 94 patients with HIV infection (Hall et al., 1991). Eighteen patients had clinical signs of neuropathy on examination, whereas 21 had electrophysiological evidence of neuropathy. Thirty-five percent of patients with nerve conduction abnormalities had clinical evidence of peripheral neuropathy. Forty-five percent of patients with neuropathy on clinical examination had nerve conduction abnormalities.

A wide spectrum of neuromuscular disorders is associated with HIV and AIDS. The forms of neuropathy include distal symmetrical polyneuropathy, acute and chronic idiopathic demyelinating polyra-

diculoneuropathy, progressive polyradiculopathy, mononeuritis multiplex, cranial neuropathy, autonomic neuropathy, diffuse infiltrative lymphocytosis syndrome, and ataxic neuropathy. The forms of myopathy include HIV-associated myopathy, zidovudine (AZT)–associated myopathy, and HIV wasting syndrome. Myasthenia gravis and motor neuron disease have also been reported in patients with HIV infection, although they likely represent chance association rather than a causal connection.

NEUROPATHIES

Distal Symmetrical Polyneuropathy

Distal symmetrical polyneuropathy (DSP), the most common form of neuropathy associated with HIV infection, most commonly occurs in late stages of HIV infection or AIDS (Lange et al., 1988; Lange, 1994). DSP is present in 10% to 49% of patients with AIDS (Cornblath and McArthur, 1988; Dalakas and Pezeshkpour, 1988; Fuller et al., 1993; Simpson et al., 1997). DSP may occur secondarily to the use of neurotoxic antiretroviral medications. DSP occurs less commonly in children, and is more common in those over the age of 14 years (Floeter et al., 1997).

The most common symptoms of DSP include pain in the feet, heightened by contact with sheets or socks, and painful paresthesias (Cornblath and McArthur, 1988; Lange et al., 1988; Miller et al., 1988; So et al., 1988; Lange, 1994; Tagliati et al., 1999). Vibration and pain thresholds are increased in the feet. Ankle reflexes are absent or reduced, whereas knee reflexes are usually normal. Symptoms are usually absent or mild in the hands. In some patients,

Neuropathological findings in sural nerve biopsies and postmortem-derived nerve specimens have been contradictory, revealing primary segmental demyelination (Openshaw et al., 1996), primary axonal degeneration (Paul et al., 1991), or mixed demyelination and wallerian-like degeneration (Borgeat et al., 1986). Electrodiagnostic studies have demonstrated equally variable results, with nerve conduction studies showing either primary axonal (Paul et al., 1991) or primary demyelinating features (Johnson et al., 1987; Openshaw et al., 1996). Partial motor conduction block may be observed in patients with the GBS-like neuropathy. Needle EMG examination shows active denervation in clinically weak muscles (Borgeat et al., 1986; Johnson et al., 1987; Openshaw et al., 1996).

The pathogenic basis for the sensory neuropathy is not known. Ara-C may inhibit the transcription of proteins important for myelin production or axonal transport (Baker et al., 1991). In the acute GBS-like neuropathies and acute brachial plexopathies, an autoimmune pathogenesis is possible. The immunomodulating effects of ara-C may lead to the disinhibition of autoreactive lymphocytes, provoking an autoimmune attack against peripheral nerve antigens. Alternately, ara-C–induced peripheral nerve damage may create or expose a novel antigen (Openshaw et al., 1996). A direct neurotoxic effect is supported by evidence from an animal model that ara-C is toxic to Schwann cells (Aguaya et al., 1975).

ETOPOSIDE (VP-16)

Etoposide is a semisynthetic derivative of podophyllotoxin used to treat patients with lymphoma, leukemia, small cell lung cancer, and testicular carcinoma. Its anticancer effect is mediated by inhibition of the DNA-unwinding enzyme topoisomerase II (Hande, 1998). A distal, axonal, predominantly sensory polyneuropathy develops in 4% to 10% of patients receiving this drug (Falkson et al., 1975; Imrie et al., 1994). The neuropathy may be severe and associated with autonomic dysfunction (e.g., postural hypotension and gastrointestinal dysmotility). The neuropathy slowly resolves over several months following discontinuation of etoposide (Imrie et al., 1994).

In mice, etoposide preferentially damages dorsal root ganglion neurons by an unknown mechanism (Bregman et al., 1994). Neuropathological studies in humans are not available. There are few descriptions of the associated electrodiagnostic abnormalities. In one study, needle EMG examination and nerve conduction studies were consistent with an axonal sensorimotor polyneuropathy (Imrie et al., 1994).

IFOSFAMIDE

Ifosfamide is an alkylating agent used for the management of testicular and cervical carcinomas, sarcomas, lymphomas, and lung cancers, with a well-established potential for causing acute CNS toxicity (Miller and Eaton, 1992). A sensory neuropathy characterized by severe pain, numbness, and paresthesias in the hands and feet occurs less commonly (Patel et al., 1994). It has been reported in 3% of patients receiving high-dose therapy (14 g/m^2 every 3 weeks) (Patel et al., 1997). Neuropathies—some of them severe—can also occur in 3% to 4% of patients treated with lower doses (Costanzi et al., 1982; Loehrer et al., 1986). Symptoms develop acutely 10 to 14 days after treatment and then gradually abate over a few days to a few weeks. They may recur if patients are rechallenged with ifosfamide (Miller and Eaton, 1992). Patients with pre-existing neuropathies are at increased risk for this side effect. Electrophysiological and pathological information is not available.

Neuropathies Secondary to Immunosuppressive Agents

Immunosuppressive agents are employed for the prevention and management of GVHD following BMT. The most common PNS complication arising from these therapies is varicella-zoster virus infection–associated radiculopathies and cranial neuropathies (see preceding). A peripheral neuropathy can also develop as a direct side effect of the immunosuppressive agents, occurring uncommonly with the immunophilin ligands tacrolimus and cyclosporine and commonly with thalidomide.

TACROLIMUS AND CYCLOSPORINE

Tacrolimus and cyclosporine are structurally dissimilar but functionally related immunosuppressive agents that modulate T-cell function. Both act by binding to intracellular proteins known as immunophilins. They are used primarily to prevent rejection after solid-organ transplants but are also effective against GVHD and various autoimmune diseases (Chaudhuri et al., 1997; Jacobson et al., 1998; Letko et al., 1999). CNS toxicity is well recognized with both agents (Gijtenbeek et al., 1999; Letko et al., 1999). Peripheral neuropathies are much more rarely reported. Many patients (10% to 20%) receiving cyclosporine and tacrolimus complain of acral paresthesias, which may reflect a mild sensory neuropathy, but this has not been investigated (McDiarmid et al., 1995; Pirsch et al., 1997).

The best characterized PNS disorder is a chronic demyelinating neuropathy associated with tacrolimus. This neuropathy can be either symmetrical (Bronster et al., 1995), resembling CIDP, or asymmetrical (Wilson et al., 1994), simulating chronic multifocal demyelinating polyradiculoneuropathy (Lewis-Sumner syndrome) (Saperstein et al., 1999). Symptom onset occurs 2 to 10 weeks after starting tacrolimus. In the symmetrical variant, initial symptoms are burning dysesthesias in the lower extremities, followed by progressive numbness of the hands and feet and distal more than proximal weakness of all four limbs. In the asymmetrical form, patients present with asymmetrical or multifocal weakness, numbness, and paresthesias in the distal lower limbs. Symptoms then spread proximally and to the upper extremities, remaining asymmetrical and distally accentuated. Irrespective of symmetry, large-fiber sensory loss exceeds pinprick impairment. Reflexes are decreased or absent, with sporadic asymmetries. Cranial nerves have been spared in the cases reported to date. Analysis of CSF reveals normal cells and increased protein. Sural nerve biopsy in one patient showed severe demyelination and axon loss (Wilson et al., 1994). Electrodiagnostic studies demonstrate features indicative of a demyelinating neuropathy. Distal motor latencies and F-wave latencies are prolonged. Some motor conduction velocities are reduced to the demyelinating range. CMAP amplitudes are commonly decreased, especially in the lower limbs. Abnormal temporal dispersion is observed. EMG examination shows active denervation in distal muscles and more widespread chronic reinnervation. Patients have slowly improved with plasma exchange, IVIg, and replacement of tacrolimus with cyclosporine.

A second PNS syndrome ascribed to tacrolimus toxicity is an acute, severe, motor-predominant, axonal polyneuropathy (Ayres et al., 1994; Wilson et al., 1994). Symptoms commence 1 to 2 weeks into the therapeutic regimen. Onset is abrupt, with full expression within one to several days. Patients experience flaccid quadriparesis, sometimes accompanied by ptosis, bilateral facial muscle weakness, lethargy, and pains in the feet. Sensory symptoms are a minor feature. CSF protein was increased in the one report with CSF data. No neuropathological information is reported. Electrophysiological studies reveal a motor-predominant, axonal neuropathy, with decreased CMAP amplitudes, normal distal motor latencies and motor conduction velocities, and relatively preserved SNAPs. On needle EMG examination, distal leg and hand muscles exhibit fibrillation potentials, decreased recruitment, and increased polyphasic MUAPs. Symptoms in two patients resolved with discontinuation or dose reduction of tacrolimus (Ayres et al., 1994). A third patient stabilized after receiving IVIg and then began to slowly improve (Wilson et al., 1994). The neuropathy may relapse if tacrolimus is reintroduced (Ayres et al., 1994).

The pathogenesis of tacrolimus-induced peripheral neuropathy is not understood. The demyelinating neuropathy is probably mediated by a dysimmune process, supported by the therapeutic responses to plasma exchange and IVIg. Tacrolimus may enhance or disinhibit a clone of autoreactive T cells directed against peripheral nerve myelin.

There are also sporadic case reports of cyclosporine-induced neuropathies. Acute, motor-predominant, generalized polyneuropathies—reminiscent of the acute axonal neuropathy associated with tacrolimus—have been described in several reports (Palmer and Toto, 1991; Guarino et al., 1996; Terro-

vitis et al., 1998). The neuropathy begins 1 to 8 weeks after treatment initiation, inconsistently associated with high levels of cyclosporine. CSF protein is normal. Electrodiagnostic studies and sural nerve biopsies yield findings supportive of an axonal or mixed axonal/demyelinating process. All patients have recovered 1 to 2 months after cyclosporine was withdrawn. There is one report of a cyclosporine-triggered bilateral brachial plexopathy (Papa et al., 1985).

THALIDOMIDE

Thalidomide was first marketed in 1957 as a sedative-hypnotic agent but was withdrawn in 1961–1962 because of teratogenicity. The drug was reintroduced in the United States in 1998 for the treatment of erythema nodosum leprosum (Calabrese and Fleischer, 2000). It is also effective for chronic GVHD (Gaziev et al., 2000), many other skin disorders, aphthous stomatitis, several HIV-associated conditions, and Behçet's disease (Tseng et al., 1996; Calabrese and Fleischer, 2000). A wide variety of immunomodulatory and anti-inflammatory properties have been identified. Down-regulation of tumor necrosis factor-α production is one important effect (Calabrese and Fleischer, 2000).

Peripheral neuropathy was recognized as a potential side effect of thalidomide as early as 1959 (Florence, 1960). The incidence of neuropathy has varied from 0.5% (Fullerton and O'Sullivan, 1968) to 100% (Wulff et al., 1985) in published series, but in most studies, symptomatic neuropathies developed in approximately 25% of patients (Knop et al., 1983; Gardner-Medwin et al., 1994; Ochonisky et al., 1994). Electrodiagnostic criteria for neuropathy are typically met in one third of patients (Gardner-Medwin et al., 1994; Ochonisky et al., 1994), although there is a tendency for sensory amplitudes to decrease in all (Gardner-Medwin et al., 1994). Data on the relationship between neuropathy risk and daily dose, cumulative dose, and duration of treatment are conflicting. Individual idiosyncratic factors are important. Slow drug acetylation may be one of these (Hess et al., 1986). Females and older patients have been shown to be at increased neuropathy risk in some studies (Fullerton and O'Sullivan, 1968; Ochonisky et al., 1994).

The neuropathy produced by thalidomide is a distal, symmetrical, axonal, sensory-predominant disorder (Gibbels, 1967; Hafstrom, 1967; Fullerton and O'Sullivan, 1968; Knop et al., 1983; Wulff et al., 1985; Lagueny et al., 1986; Gardner-Medwin et al., 1994; Ochonisky et al., 1994). Patients present with numbness and paresthesias in the feet or, less frequently, the hands. With continued treatment, sensory symptoms spread to the legs and then to the distal upper extremities, often (60% of patients) accompanied by painful dysesthesias and hyperpathia in the feet (Gibbels, 1967). Weakness in the toes and ankles occurs infrequently (in about 15% of patients) and later in the course of therapy (Gibbels, 1967; Hafstrom, 1967). Proximal limb weakness has also been reported (Lagueny et al., 1986) and was present in 25% of patients in the series of Fullerton and O'Sullivan (1968). The basis for this proximal weakness has not been established. Seventy percent of patients complain of leg cramps (Gibbels, 1967; Fullerton and O'Sullivan, 1968; Wulff et al., 1985). Examination shows distal sensory loss in a symmetrical, stocking-glove distribution. Some investigators have observed greater involvement of small-fiber modalities (Gibbels, 1967; Fullerton and O'Sullivan, 1968; Wulff et al., 1985). Position sensation is least affected. Ankle jerks are reduced or absent in 40% of patients, whereas other reflexes are typically normal or even increased (Gibbels 1967; Hafstrom, 1967; Fullerton and O'Sullivan, 1968; Wulff et al., 1985; Ochonisky et al., 1994). Extensor plantar responses may occur in severely affected patients (Fullerton and O'Sullivan, 1968).

The symptoms are usually reversible if thalidomide is withdrawn at their first appearance (Gardner-Medwin et al., 1994). However, if the drug is continued, recovery will be very slow and chronic residua can be expected. Cramps, proximal weakness, and pyramidal signs tend to remit faster and more completely than distal sensory and motor deficits. As with the chemotherapeutic agents, symptoms and electrodiagnostic findings sometimes continue to progress for several months after thalidomide is stopped (Hafstrom, 1967; Lagueny et al., 1986; Ochonisky et al., 1994). In one series with long-term follow-up, 25% of patients recovered completely, 30% improved but had residual deficits, and 45% had no recovery (Fullerton and O'Sullivan, 1968). In another report, 75% of patients showed no long-term improvement (Hafstrom, 1967).

Examination of CSF yields normal results (Hafstrom, 1967). Sural nerve biopsies and postmortem peripheral nerve examinations demonstrate a selective loss of large myelinated fibers and variable wallerian-like degeneration and regeneration, without significant segmental demyelination (Fullerton and O'Sullivan, 1968; Seitelberger, 1968; Krucke et al., 1971). Degenerative changes in the dorsal columns and dorsal root ganglia have been observed at autopsy, typical of a ganglionopathy (Fullerton and O'Sullivan, 1968). The pathogenesis of the nerve damage is poorly understood.

Electrodiagnostic studies reveal a dose-related decrease (Wulff et al., 1985) in SNAP amplitudes, with normal or mildly decreased sensory conduction velocities (Fullerton and O'Sullivan, 1968; Clemmensen et al., 1984; Hess et al., 1986; Lagueny et al., 1986; Gardner-Medwin et al., 1994; Ochonisky et al., 1994). The sural SNAP is more commonly affected than the median SNAP, which, in turn, is more commonly reduced than the ulnar or superficial radial SNAP (Wulff et al., 1985; Lagueny et al., 1986; Gardner-Medwin et al., 1994; Ochonisky et al., 1994). The disproportionate involvement of the median may result from superimposed carpal tunnel syndrome (40% of patients in two series) (Clemmensen et al.,

1984; Wulff et al., 1985). Reductions of SNAP amplitudes commonly precede the onset of sensory symptoms (Gardner-Medwin et al., 1994). Some investigators recommend serial monitoring of the sural SNAP in patients taking thalidomide, with a dose reduction mandated for amplitude decrements of 30% to 50% and drug withdrawal if the amplitude drops by more than 50% (Gardner-Medwin et al., 1994). Motor nerve conduction studies are usually normal, but decreased median and peroneal CMAP amplitudes can occur (Hess et al., 1986). F-wave latencies are normal, but F-wave chronodispersion is increased (Sadoh et al., 1999). Needle EMG examination shows decreased recruitment and long-duration, polyphasic MUAPs in distal leg muscles in one third of patients, sometimes associated with fibrillation potentials (Clemmensen et al., 1984; Wulff et al., 1985; Hess et al., 1986; Lagueny et al., 1986). SNAP amplitudes and other electrophysiological findings may improve after the drug is discontinued (Gardner-Medwin et al., 1994); however, in some patients, the abnormalities persist indefinitely (Lagueny et al., 1986).

References

Abad S, Zagdanski A-M, Brechignac S, et al: Neurolymphomatosis in Waldenström's macroglobulinemia. Br J Haematol 1999;106: 100–103.

Adams C, August CS, Maguire H, Sladky JT: Neuromuscular complications of bone marrow transplantation. Pediatr Neurol 1995; 12:58–61.

Aguaya AJ, Romine JS, Bray GM: Experimental necrosis and arrest of proliferation of Schwann cells by cytosine arabinoside. J Neurocytol 1975;4:663–674.

Aho I, Sainio K. Late irradiation-induced lesions of the lumbosacral plexus. Neurology 1983;33:953–955.

Alajouanine T, Thurel R, Castaigne P, Lhermitte F: Leucemie aigue avec syndrome polynevritique avec infiltration leucosique des nerfs. Rev Neurol 1949;81:249–261.

Albers JW, Allen AA, Bastron JA, Daube JR: Limb myokymia. Muscle Nerve 1981;4:494–504.

Al-Chalabi A, Sivakumaran M, Holton J, et al: A case of intravascular lymphomatosis (angiotropic lymphoma) with raised perinuclear antineutrophil cytoplasmic antibody titres—a hitherto unreported association. Clin Lab Haematol 1994;16:363–369.

Amato AA, Barohn RJ, Sahenk Z, et al: Polyneuropathy complicating bone marrow and solid organ transplantation. Neurology 1993;43:1513–1518.

Amato AA, Barohn RJ: Neurological complications of transplantation. In Harati Y, Rolack LA (eds): Neuroimmunology for the Clinician. Boston, Butterworth-Heinemann, 1997; 341–375.

Amato AA, Collins MP: Neuropathies associated with malignancy. Semin Neurol 1998;18:125–144.

Anderson CG, Walton KR, Chanarin I: Megaloblastic anaemia after pelvic radiotherapy for carcinoma of the cervix. J Clin Pathol 1981;34:151–152.

Apfel SC: Docetaxel. Neurology 1996;46:2–3. Editorial.

Arcasoy SM, Jett JR: Superior pulmonary sulcus tumors and Pancoast's syndrome. N Engl J Med 1997;337:1370–1376.

Argov Z, Siegel T: Leptomeningeal metastases: Peripheral nerve and root involvement: Clinical and electrophysiological study. Ann Neurol 1985;17:593–597.

Ashenhurst EM, Quartey GR, Starreveld A: Lumbo-sacral radiculopathy induced by radiation. Can J Neurol Sci 1977;4:259–263.

Atiq OT, DeAngelis LM, Rosenblum M, Portlock CS: Cutaneous T-cell lymphoma presenting with diffuse lymphomatous infiltration of the peripheral nerves: Response to combination chemotherapy. Am J Clin Oncol 1992;15:212–215.

Au WY, Shek WH, Nicholls J, et al: T-cell intravascular lymphomatosis (angiotropic lymphoma): Association with Epstein-Barr viral infection. Histopathology 1997;31:563–567.

Auger RG: AAEM minimonograph no. 44: Diseases associated with excess motor unit activity. Muscle Nerve 1994;17:1250–1263.

Ayres RC, Dousset B, Wixon S, et al: Peripheral neurotoxicity with tacrolimus. Lancet 1994;343:862–863.

Bagley FH, Walsh JW, Cady B, et al: Carcinomatous versus radiation-induced brachial plexus neuropathy in breast cancer. Cancer 1978;41:2154–2157.

Bairey O, Kremer I, Rakowsky E, et al: Orbital and adnexal involvement in systemic non-Hodgkin's lymphoma. Cancer 1994;73:2395–2399.

Baker WJ, Royer GL, Weiss RB: Cytarabine and neurologic toxicity. J Clin Oncol 1991;9:679–693.

Ballantyne AJ, McCarten AB, Ibanez ML: The extension of cancer of the head and neck through peripheral nerves. Am J Surg 1963;106:651–667.

Balm M, Hammack J: Leptomeningeal carcinomatosis: Presenting features and prognostic factors. Arch Neurol 1996;53:626–632.

Balmaceda C, Forsyth P, Seidman AD, et al: Peripheral neuropathy in patients receiving Taxotere chemotherapy. Ann Neurol 1993;34:313.

Barr LC, Kissin MW: Radiation-induced brachial plexus neuropathy following breast conservation and radical radiotherapy. Br J Surg 1987;74:855–856.

Barron KD, Hirano A, Araski S, et al: Experiences with metastatic neoplasms involving the spinal cord. Neurology 1959;9:91–106.

Barron KD, Rowland LP, Zimmerman HM: Neuropathy with malignant tumor metastases. J Nerve Ment Dis 1960;131:10–31.

Basso-Ricci S, della Costa C, Viganotti G, et al: Report on 42 cases of postirradiation lesions of the brachial plexus and their treatment. Tumori 1980;66:117–122.

Berger PS, Bataini JP: Radiation-induced cranial nerve palsy. Cancer 1977;40:152–155.

Berlit P, Schwechheimer K: Neuropathologic findings in radiation myelopathy of the lumbosacral cord. Eur Neurol 1987;27:29–34.

Binet S, Chaineau E, Fellous A, et al: Immunofluorescence study of the action of navelbine, vincristine and vinblastine on mitotic and axonal microtubules. Int J Cancer 1990;46:262–266.

Bitton RJ, Figg WD, Venzon DJ, et al: Pharmacologic variables associated with the development of neurologic toxicity in patients treated with suramin. J Clin Oncol 1995;13:2223–2229.

Blair DN, Rapoport S, Sostman HD, Blair OC: Normal brachial plexus: MR imaging. Radiology 1987;165:763–767.

Bobker DH, Deloughery TG: Natural killer cell leukemia presenting with a peripheral neuropathy. Neurology 1993;43:1853–1854.

Boerman RH, Maassen EM, Joosten J, et al: Trigeminal neuropathy secondary to perineural invasion of head and neck carcinomas. Neurology 1999;53:213–216.

Boiron JM, Ellie E, Vital A, et al: Isolated peripheral nerve relapse masquerading as Guillain-Barré syndrome in a patient with acute lymphoblastic leukemia. Leuk Lymphoma 1993;10:489–491.

Bone RC, Vernon M, Sobonya RE, Rendon H: Lymphomatoid granulomatosis. Report of a case and review of the literature. Am J Med 1978;65:709–716.

Borgeat A, de Muralt B, Stalder M: Peripheral neuropathy associated with high-dose ARA-C therapy. Cancer 1986;58:852–854.

Borit A, Altrocchi PH: Recurrent polyneuropathy and neurolymphomatosis. Arch Neurol 1971; 24:40–49.

Bowen J, Gregory R, Squier M, Donaghy M: The post-irradiation lower motor neuron syndrome: Neuronopathy or radiculopathy? Brain 1997;119:1429–1439.

Boyaciyan A, Oge AE, Yazici J, et al: Electrophysiological findings in patients who received therapy over the brachial plexus: A magnetic stimulation study. Electroencephalogr Clin Neurophysiol 1996;101:483–490.

Bradley WG, Lassman LP, Pearce GW, Walton JN: The neuromyopathy of vincristine in man: Clinical, electrophysiological and pathological studies. J Neurol Sci 1970;10:107–131.

Bradley WG, Robison SH, Tandan R, Besser D. Post-radiation motor neuron syndrome. In Rowland LP (ed): Advances in Neurology, Vol. 56. Amyotrophic Lateral Sclerosis and Other Motor Neuron Diseases. New York, Raven Press, 1991; 341–353.

Bregman CL, Buroker RA, Hirth RS, et al: Etoposide- and BMY-40481-induced sensory neuropathy in mice. Toxicol Pathol 1994;22:528–535.

Bronster DJ, Yonover P, Stein F, et al: Demyelinating sensorimotor peripheral neuropathy after administration of FK506. Transplantation 1995;59:1066–1068.

Brun A, Caviness V, Rudnick RP, Tyler HR: Hemorrhages in peripheral nerves in association with leukemia. J Neuropathol Exp Neurol 1964;23:719–725.

Buerger LF, Monteleone PN: Leukemic-lymphomatous infiltration of skeletal muscle. Systemic study of 82 autopsy cases. Cancer 1966;19:1416–1422.

Buge A, Escourolle R, Poisson M, et al: Neuropathie peripherique avec infiltration leucoblastique sur les biopsies nerveuse et musculaire. Ann Med Intern (Paris) 1977;128:137–141.

Burt RK, Sharfman WH, Karp BI, Wilson WH: Mental neuropathy (numb chin syndrome). A harbinger of tumor progression or relapse. Cancer 1992;70:877–881.

Byrne TN: Spinal cord compression from epidural metastases. N Engl J Med 1992;327:614–619.

Cairncross JG: Radiation-induced cranial neuropathy. In Rottenberg DA (ed): Neurological Complications of Cancer Treatment. Boston, Butterworth-Heinemann, 1991;63–68.

Calabrese L, Fleischer AB: Thalidomide: Current and potential clinical applications. Am J Med 2000;108:487–495.

Calamia KT, Miller A, Shuster EA, et al: Intravascular lymphomatosis: A report of ten patients with central nervous system involvement and a review of the disease process. Adv Exp Med Biol 1999;45:249–265.

Calatayud T, Vallejo AR, Dominguez L, et al: Lymphomatoid granulomatosis manifesting as a subacute polyradiculoneuropathy: A case report and review of the neurological manifestations. Eur Neurol 1980;19:213–223.

Campbell MJ, Paty DW: Carcinomatous neuromyopathy: 1. Electrophysiological studies: An electrophysiological and immunological study of patients with carcinoma of the lung. J Neurol Neurosurg Psychiatry 1974;37:131–141.

Canetta R, Rozencweig M, Carter SK: Carboplatin: The clinical spectrum to date. Cancer Treat Rep 1985;12(suppl A):125–136.

Capizzi RL: Clinical status and optimal use of amifostine. Oncology 1999;13:47–59.

Caress JB, Abend WK, Preston DC, Logigian EL: A case of Hodgkin's lymphoma producing neuromyotonia. Neurology 1997;49:258–259.

Carter RL, Pittam MR, Tanner NSB: Pain and dysphagia in patients with squamous carcinomas of the head and neck: The role of perineural spread. J R Soc Med 1982;75:598–606.

Carter RL, Foster CS, Dinsdale EA, Pittam MR: Perineural spread by squamous carcinomas of the head and neck: A morphological study using antiaxonal and antimyelin monoclonal antibodies. J Clin Pathol 1983;36:269–275.

Case Records of the Massachusetts General Hospital: Weekly clinicopathological exercises. Case 6–1972. N Engl J Med 1972;286:308–315.

Case Records of the Massachusetts General Hospital: Case 8–1995. N Engl J Med 1995;332:730–737.

Case Records of the Massachusetts General Hospital: Case 35–1996. N Engl J Med 1996;35:1514–1521.

Casey EB, Jellife AM, Le Quesne M, Millett YL: Vincristine neuropathy: Clinical and electrophysiological observations. Brain 1973;96:69–86.

Cavaletti G, Bogliun G, Marzorati L, et al: Peripheral neurotoxicity of taxol in patients previously treated with cisplatin. Cancer 1995;75:1141–1150.

Cavaletti G, Bogliun G, Zincone A, et al: Neuro- and ototoxicity of high-dose carboplatin treatment in poor prognosis ovarian cancer patients. Anticancer Res 1998;18:3797–3802.

Cece R, Petruccioli MG, Cavaletti G, et al: An ultrastructural study of neuronal changes in dorsal root ganglia (DRG) of rats after chronic cisplatin administrations. Histol Histopathol 1995;10:837–845.

Cersosimo RJ: Cisplatin neurotoxicity. Cancer Treat Rev 1989;16:195–211.

Chamberlain MC: Leptomeningeal metastases. In Vecht CJ (ed): Handbook of Clinical Neurology, Vol. 25(69): Neuro-oncology, Part III. New York, Elsevier Science, 1997; 151–165.

Chaudhry V, Rowinsky EK, Sartorius SE, et al: Peripheral neuropathy from taxol and cisplatin combination chemotherapy: Clinical and electrophysiological studies. Ann Neurol 1994;35:304–311.

Chaudhry V, Eisenberger MA, Sinibaldi VJ, et al: A prospective study of suramin-induced peripheral neuropathy. Brain 1996; 119:2039–2052.

Chaudhuri K, Torley H, Madhok R: Disease-modifying anti-rheumatic drugs: Cyclosporin. Br J Rheumatol 1997;36:1016–1021.

Cheng VS, Schultz MD: Unilateral hypoglossal nerve atrophy as a late complication of radiation therapy of head and neck carcinoma: A report of four cases and a review of the literature on peripheral and cranial nerve damages after radiation therapy. Cancer 1975;35:1537–1544.

Chew NK, Sim BF, Tan CT, et al: Delayed post-irradiation bulbar palsy in nasopharyngeal carcinoma. Neurology 2001;57:529–531.

Cioni R, Giannini F, Passero S, et al: An electromyographic evaluation of motor complications in thoracic herpes zoster. Electromyogr Clin Electrophysiol 1994;34:125–128.

Clemmensen OJ, Olsen PZ, Andersen KE: Thalidomide neurotoxicity. Arch Dermatol 1984;120:338–341.

Clouston PD, Sharpe DM, Corbett AJ, et al: Perineural spread of cutaneous head and neck cancer: Its orbital and central neurologic complications. Arch Neurol 1990;47:73–77.

Clouston PD, DeAngelis LM, Posner JB: The spectrum of neurological disease in patients with systemic cancer. Ann Neurol 1992: 31:268–273.

Contamin F, Mignot B, Ecoffet M, et al: Les atteintes plexiques post-radiothérapiques. A propos de dix-neuf cas. Sem Hop 1978; 54:1225–1229.

Cornblath DR, Asbury AK, Albers JW, et al: Research criteria for diagnosis of chronic inflammatory demyelinating polyneuropathy. Neurology 1991;41:617–618.

Cortes JE, Pazdur R: Docetaxel. J Clin Oncol 1995;13:2643–2655.

Costa G, Holland JF: Systemic effects of tumours with special reference to the nervous system. In Brain L, Norris FH (eds): The Remote Effects of Cancer on the Nervous System. New York, Grune and Stratton, 1965; 125–133.

Costans JP, de Divitiis E, Donzelli R, et al: Spinal metastases with neurological manifestations. Review of 600 cases. J Neurosurg 1983;59:111–118.

Costanzi JJ, Stephens R, O'Bryan R, Franks J: Ifosfamide in the management of malignant melanoma: A Southwest Oncology Group phase II trial. Semin Oncol 1982:9(suppl 1):93–95.

Creange A, Theodorou I, Sabourin J-C, et al: Inflammatory neuromuscular disorders associated with chronic lymphoid leukemia: Evidence for clonal B cells within muscle and nerve. J Neurol Sci 1996;137:35–41.

Croft PB, Wilkinson M: Carcinomatous neuromyopathy. Its incidence in patients with carcinoma of the lung and carcinoma of the breast. Lancet 1963; 1:184–188.

Croft PB, Wilkinson M: The incidence of carcinomatous neuromyopathy in patients with various types of carcinoma. Brain 1965; 88:427–434.

Croft PB, Urich H, Wilkinson M: Peripheral neuropathy of sensorimotor type associated with malignant disease. Brain 1967; 90: 31–66.

Currie S, Henson RA, Morgan HG, Poole AJ: The incidence of non-metastatic neurological syndromes of obscure origin in the reticuloses. Brain 1970; 93:629–640.

Czernin S, Gessl A, Wilfing A, et al: Suramin affects human peripheral blood mononuclear cells in vitro: Inhibition of T cell growth and modulation of cytokine secretion. Int Arch Allergy Immunol 1993;101:240–246.

Dalmau J, Graus F, Marco M: "Hot and dry foot" as initial manifestation of neoplastic lumbosacral plexopathy. Neurology 1989; 39:871–872.

Daniel SE, Rudge P, Scaravilli F: Malignant angioendotheliosis involving the nervous system: Support for a lymphoid origin of neoplastic cells. J Neurol Neurosurg Psychiatry 1987;50:1173–1177.

Daugaard GK, Petrera J, Trojaborg W: Electrophysiological study of the peripheral and central neurotoxic effect of cisplatin. Acta Neurol Scand 1987;76:86–93.

Davis DG, Patchell RA: Neurologic complications of bone marrow transplantation. Neurol Clin 1988;6:377–387.

De Alvarez R: The sites of metastasis in carcinoma of the cervix. West J Surg Obstet Gynecol 1953;61:623–627.

DeAngelis LM, Gnecco C, Taylor L, Warrell RP: Evolution of neuropathy and myopathy during intensive vincristine/corticosteroid chemotherapy for non-Hodgkin's lymphoma. Cancer 1991; 67:2241–2246.

DeAngelis LM: Current diagnosis and treatment of leptomeningeal metastases. J Neuro-Oncol 1998;38:245–252.

De Carolis P, Montagna P, Cipulli M, et al: Isolated motor neuron involvement following radiotherapy. J Neurol Neurosurg Psychiatry 1986;49:718–719.

Demirer TD, Dail DH, Aboulafia DM: Four varied cases of intravascular lymphomatosis and a literature review. Cancer 1994;73: 1738–1745.

Devlin T, Moll S, Hulette C, Morgenlander JC: Intravascular malignant lymphomatosis with neurologic presentation: Factors facilitating antemortem diagnosis. South Med J 1998;91:672–676.

Diaz-Arrastia R, Younger DS, Hair L, et al: Neurolymphomatosis: A clinicopathologic syndrome re-emerges. Neurology 1992;42: 1136–1142.

Dickenman RC, Chason JL: Alterations in the dorsal root ganglia and adjacent nerves in the leukemias, the lymphomas, and multiple myeloma. Am J Pathol 1958;34:349–361.

DiGiuseppe JA, Nelson WG, Seifter EJ, et al: Intravascular lymphomatosis: A clinicopathologic study of 10 cases and assessment of response to chemotherapy. J Clin Oncol 1994;12:2573–2579.

Dolman CL, Sweeny VP, Magil A: Neoplastic angioendotheliomatosis: The case of the missed primary? Arch Neurol 1979; 36:5–7.

Domizio P, Hall PA, Cotter F, et al: Angiotropic large cell lymphoma (ALCL): Morphological, immunohistochemical and genotypic studies with analysis of previous reports. Hematol Oncol 1989; 7:195–206.

Donaghy M, Hall P, Gawler J, et al: Peripheral neuropathy associated with Castleman's disease. J Neurol Sci 1989;89:253–267.

Dropcho E: Paraneoplastic neuromuscular disorders. Part 2. J Clin Neuromusc Dis 1999;1:99–108.

Dumitru D: Generalized Peripheral Neuropathies. In (ed): Electrodiagnostic Medicine. Philadelphia, Hanley and Belfus, 1995; 741–850.

Ekholm E, Rantanen V, Antila K, Salminen E: Paclitaxel changes sympathetic control of blood pressure. Eur J Cancer 1997;33: 1419–1424.

Ellis F: Nominal standard dose and the ret. Br J Radiol 1971; 44:101–108.

Enevoldson TP, Scadding JW, Rustin GJ, Senanayake LF: Spontaneous resolution of a postirradiation lumbosacral plexopathy. Neurology 1992;42:2224–2225.

Esteban A, Traba A: Fasciculation-myokymic activity and prolonged nerve conduction block. A physiopathological relationship in radiation-induced brachial plexopathy. Electroencephalogr Clin Neurophysiol 1993;89:382–391.

Estes ML, Ewing-Wilson D, Chu SM, et al: Chloroquine neuromyotoxicity. Clinical and pathologic perspective. Am J Med 1987; 82:447–455.

Falkson G, van Dyk JJ, van Eden EB, et al: A clinical trial of the oral form of 4'-demethyl-epipodophyllotoxin-β-D-ethylidene glucoside (NSC 141540) VP 16-213. Cancer 1975;35:1141–1144.

Fardin P, Lelli S, Negrin P, Maluta S: Radiation-induced brachial plexopathy: Clinical and electromyographical (EMG) considerations in 13 cases. Electromyogr Clin Neurophysiol 1990;30: 277–282.

Fauci AS, Haynes BF, Costa J, et al: Lymphomatoid granulomatosis. Prospective clinical and therapeutic experience over 10 years. N Engl J Med 1982;306:68–74.

Fazio R, Quattrini A, Bolognesi A, et al: Docetaxel neuropathy: A distal axonopathy. Acta Neuropathol 1999;98:651–653.

Feistner H, Weissenborn K, Munte TF, et al: Post-irradiation lesions of the caudal roots. Acta Neurol Scand 1989;80:277–281.

Ferrante MA, Wilbourn AJ: The utility of various sensory nerve conduction responses in assessing brachial plexopathies. Muscle Nerve 1995;18:879–889.

Fisher CM, Williams HW, Wing ES: Combined encephalopathy and neuropathy with carcinoma. J Neuropathol Exp Neurol 1961;20:535–547.

Florence AL: Is thalidomide to blame? Br Med J 1960;2:1954.

Forsyth PA, Balmaceda C, Peterson K, et al: Prospective study of paclitaxel-induced peripheral neuropathy with quantitative sensory testing. J Neuro-Oncol 1997;35:47–53.

Freilich RJ, Balmaceda C, Seidman AD, et al: Motor neuropathy due to docetaxel and paclitaxel. Neurology 1996;47:115–118.

Fu KK, Kai EF, Leung CK: Cisplatin neuropathy: A prospective clinical and electrophysiological study in Chinese patients with ovarian carcinoma. J Clin Pharm Ther 1995;20:167–172.

Fullerton PM, O'Sullivan DJ: Thalidomide neuropathy: A clinical, electrophysiological, and histological follow-up study. J Neurol Neurosurg Psychiatry 1968;31:543–551.

Gallego J, Delgado G, Tunon T, Villanueva JA: Delayed postirradiation lower motor neuron syndrome. Ann Neurol 1986;19:308–309.

Garcia CA, Hackett ER, Kirkpatrick LL: Multiple mononeuropathy in lymphomatoid granulomatosis: Similarity to leprosy. Neurology 1978;28:731–733.

Gardner-Medwin JM, Smith NJ, Powell RJ: Clinical experience with thalidomide in the management of severe oral and genital ulceration in conditions such as Behçet's disease: Use of neurophysiological studies to detect thalidomide neuropathy. Ann Rheum Dis 1994;53:828–832.

Gardner-Thorpe C, Foster JB, Barwick DD: Unusual manifestations of herpes zoster. A clinical and electrophysiological study. J Neurol Sci 1976;28:427–447.

Gastaut JL, Pellissier JF: Neuropathie au cisplatine étude clinique, electrophysiologique et morphologique. Rev Neurol 1985;141:614–626.

Gaziev D, Galimberti M, Lucarelli G, Polchi P: Chronic graft-versus-host disease: Is there an alternative to the conventional treatment? Bone Marrow Transplant 2000;25:689–696.

Geiger D, Mpinga E, Steves MA, Sugarbaker PH: Femoral neuropathy. Unusual presentation for recurrent large-bowel cancer. Dis Colon Rectum 1998;41:910–913.

Gelmon K, Eisenhauer E, Bryce C, et al: Randomized phase II study of high-dose paclitaxel with or without amifostine in patients with metastatic breast cancer. J Clin Oncol 1999;17:3038–3047.

Georgiou A, Grigsby PW, Perez CA: Radiation induced lumbosacral plexopathy in gynecologic tumors: Clinical findings and dosimetric analysis. Int J Radiat Oncol Biol Phys 1993;26:479–482.

Gerritsen van der Hoop R, van der Burg MEL, ten Bokkel Huinink WW, et al: Incidence of neuropathy in 395 patients with ovarian cancer treated with or without cisplatin. Cancer 1990;66:1697–1702.

Gherardi R, Gaulard P, Prost C, et al: T-cell lymphoma revealed by a peripheral neuropathy. A report of two cases with an immunohistologic study on lymph nodes and nerve biopsies. Cancer 1986;58:2710–2716.

Gibbels E: Toxische Schaden bei der Thalidomid-Medikation. Fortschr Neurol Psychiatr Grenzgeb 1967;35:393–411.

Gibbs AR: Lymphomatoid granulomatosis—a condition with affinities to Wegener's granulomatosis and lymphoma. Thorax 1977;32:71–79.

Giese WL, Kinsella TJ: Radiation injury to peripheral and cranial nerves. In Gutin PH, Leibel SA, Sheline GE (eds): Radiation Injury to the Nervous System. New York, Raven Press, 1991;383–403.

Gijtenbeek JM, van den Bent MJ, Vecht CJ: Cyclosporine neurotoxicity: A review. J Neurol 1999;246:339–346.

Gilbert RW, Kim J-H, Posner JB: Epidural spinal cord compression from metastatic tumor: Diagnosis and treatment. Ann Neurol 1978;3:40–51.

Gilchrist JM, Moore M: Lumbosacral plexopathy in cancer patients. Neurology 1985;35:1392. Letter.

Gilden DH, Kleinschmidt-DeMasters BK, LaGuardia JJ, et al: Neurologic complications of the reactivation of varicella-zoster virus. N Engl J Med 1999;342:635–645.

Gill JS, Hobday KL, Windebank AJ: Mechanism of suramin toxicity in stable myelinating dorsal root ganglion cultures. Exp Neurol 1995;133:113–124.

Gill JS, Windebank AJ: Activation of the high affinity nerve growth factor receptor by two polyanionic chemotherapeutic agents: Role in drug induced neurotoxicity. J Neuro-Oncol 1998;40:19–27.

Gill JS, Windebank AJ: Cisplatin-induced apoptosis in rat dorsal root ganglion neurons is associated with attempted entry into the cell cycle. J Clin Invest 1998;101:2842–2850.

Gill JS, Windebank AJ: Suramin induced ceramide accumulation leads to apoptotic cell death in dorsal root ganglion neurons. Cell Death Differ 1998;5:876–883.

Glantz MJ, Choy H, Kearns CM, et al: Phase I study of weekly outpatient paclitaxel and concurrent cranial irradiation in adults with astrocytomas. J Clin Oncol 1996;14:600–609.

Glass J, Hochberg F, Miller D. Intravascular lymphomatosis: A systemic disease with neurologic manifestations. Cancer 1993;71:3156–3164.

Glass JP, Pettigrew LC, Maor M: Plexopathy induced by radiation therapy. Neurology 1985;35:1261.

Glazer HS, Lee JK, Levitt RG, et al: Radiation fibrosis: Differentiation from recurrent tumor by MR imaging. Radiology 1985;156:721–726.

Glenn SA, Ross MA: Delayed radiation-induced bulbar palsy mimicking ALS: Muscle Nerve 2000:23:814–817.

Goa KL, Faulds D. Vinorelbine: A review of its pharmacological properties and clinical use in cancer chemotherapy. Drugs Aging 1994;5:200–234.

Goepfert H, Dichtel WJ, Median JE, et al: Perineural invasion in squamous cell skin carcinoma of the head and neck. Am J Surg 1984;148:542–54.

Gold JE, Jimenez E, Zalusky R: Human immunodeficiency virus–related lymphoreticular malignancies and peripheral neurological disease. A report of four cases. Cancer 1988;61:2318–2324.

Gordon PH, Rowland LP, Younger DS, et al: Lymphoproliferative disorders and motor neuron disease: An update. Neurology 1997;48:1671–1678.

Gottschalk PG, Dyck PJ, Kiely JM: Vinca alkaloid neuropathy: Nerve biopsy studies in rats and in man. Neurology 1968;18:875–882.

Granena A, Grau JM, Carreras E, et al: Subacute sensorimotor polyneuropathy in a recipient of an allogeneic bone marrow graft. Exp Hematol 1983;11(suppl 13):10–12.

Grant D, Rowe CR: Motor paralysis of the extremities in herpes zoster. J Bone Joint Surg Br 1961;43:885–896.

Grant R, Papadopoulos SM, Greenberg HS: Metastatic spinal cord compression. Neurol Clin 1991;9:825–841.

Green LS, Donoso JA, Heller-Bettinger IE, Samson FE: Axonal transport disturbances in vincristine-induced peripheral neuropathy. Ann Neurol 1977;1:255–262.

Greenberg HS, Deck MD, Vikram B, et al: Metastasis to the base of the skull: Clinical findings in 43 patients. Neurology 1981;31:530–537.

Greenberg MK, McVey AL, Hayes T: Segmental motor involvement in herpes zoster: An EMG study. Neurology 1992;42:1122–1123.

Greenfield MM, Stark FM: Post-irradiation neuropathy. Am J Roentgenol 1948;60:617–622.

Greenspan A, Deeg HG, Cottler-Fox M, et al: Incapacitating peripheral neuropathy as a manifestation of chronic graft-versus-host disease. Bone Marrow Transplant 1990;5:349–352.

Gregg RW, Molepo JM, Monpetit VJA, et al: Cisplatin neurotoxicity: The relationship between dosage, time, and platinum concentration in neurologic tissues, and morphologic evidence of toxicity. J Clin Oncol 1992;10:795–803.

Grisold W, Jellinger K, Lutz D. Human neurolymphomatosis in a patient with chronic lymphatic leukemia. Clin Neuropathol 1990;9:224–230.

Grisold W, Drlicek M: Paraneoplastic neuropathy. Curr Opin Neurol 1999;12:617–625.

Guarino M, Stracciari A, Cirignotta F, et al: Neoplastic meningitis presenting with ophthalmoplegia, ataxia, and areflexia (Miller-Fisher syndrome). Arch Neurol 1995;52:443–444.

Guarino M, Stracciari A, Pazzaglia P, et al: Neurological complications of liver transplantation. J Neurol 1996;243:137–142.

Guberman A, Rosenbaum H, Braciale T, Schlaepfer WW: Human neurolymphomatosis. J Neurol Sci 1978;36:1–12.

Guiheneuc P, Ginet J, Groleau JY, Rojouan J: Early phase of vincristine neuropathy in man. Electrophysiological evidence for a dying-back phenomenon, with transitory enhancement of spinal transmission of the monosynaptic reflex. J Neurol Sci 1980; 45:355–366.

Guinee D, Jaffe E, Kingma D, et al: Pulmonary lymphomatoid granulomatosis. Evidence for a proliferation of Epstein-Barr virus infected B-lymphocytes with a prominent T-cell component and vasculitis. Am J Surg Pathol 1994;18:753–764.

Gupta SK, Helal BH, Kiely P: The prognosis in zoster paralysis. J Bone Joint Surg Br 1969;51:593–603.

Gupta SR, Zdonczyk DE, Rubino FA: Cranial neuropathy in systemic malignacy in a VA population. Neurology 1990;40:997–999.

Gutman L: AAEM minimonograph no. 37: Facial and limb myokymia. Muscle Nerve 1991;14:1043–1049.

Haanpaa M, Hakkinen V, Nurmikko T: Motor involvement in acute herpes zoster. Muscle Nerve 1997;20:1433–1438.

Haberland C, Cipriani M, Kucuk O, et al: Fulminant leukemic polyradiculoneuropathy in a case of B-cell prolymphocytic leukemia. A clinicopathologic report. Cancer 1987;60:1454–1458.

Hadden RD, Cornblath DR, Hughes RA, et al: Electrophysiological classification of Guillain-Barré syndrome: Clinical associations and outcome. Plasma exchange/Sandoglobulin Guillain-Barré syndrome trial group. Ann Neurol 1998;44:780–788.

Hafstrom T: Polyneuropathy after Neurosedyn (thalidomide) and its prognosis. Acta Neurol Scand 1967;43(suppl 32):1–41.

Hagensee ME, Benyunes M, Miller JA, Spach DH. *Campylobacter jejuni* bacteremia and Guillain-Barré syndrome in a patient with GVHD after allogeneic BMT. Bone Marrow Transplant 1994;13:349–351.

Haim N, Epelbaum R, Ben-Sharar M, et al: Full dose vincristine (without 2-mg dose limit) in the treatment of lymphomas. Cancer 1994;73:2515–2519.

Hande KR: Etoposide: Four decades of development of a topoisomerase II inhibitor. Eur J Cancer 1998;34:1514–1521.

Harper CM, Thomas JE, Cascino TL, Litchy WJ: Distinction between neoplastic and radiation-induced brachial plexopathy, with emphasis on the role of EMG. Neurology 1989;39:502–506.

Harris CP, Sigman JD, Jaeckle KA: Intravascular malignant lymphomatosis: Amelioration of neurological symptoms with plasmapheresis. Ann Neurol 1994;35:357–359.

Hart IK, Waters C, Vincent A, et al: Autoantibodies detected to expressed K$^+$ channels are implicated in neuromyotonia. Ann Neurol 1997;41:238–246.

Hawley RJ, Cohen MH, Saini N, Armbrustmacher VW: The carcinomatous neuromyopathy of oat cell lung cancer. Ann Neurol 1980; 7:65–72.

Heinzlef O, Lotz J-P, Roullet E: Severe neuropathy after high dose carboplatin in three patients receiving multidrug chemotherapy. J Neurol Neurosurg Psychiatry 1998;64:667–669.

Henson RA, Urich H: Cancer and the Nervous System. The Neurological Manifestations of Malignant Disease. Oxford: Blackwell Scientific Publications, 1982.

Hepper NG, Herskovic T, Witten DM, et al: Thoracic inlet tumors. Ann Intern Med 1966;64:979–989.

Hess CW, Hunziker T, Kupfer A, Ludin HP: Thalidomide-induced peripheral neuropathy. A prospective clinical, neurophysiological and pharmacogenetic evaluation. J Neurol 1986;233:83–89.

Hildebrand J, Coers C: The neuromuscular function in patients with malignant tumors: Electromyographic and histological study. Brain 1967;90:67–82.

Hilkens PH, Verweij J, Stoter G, et al: Peripheral neurotoxicity induced by docetaxel. Neurology 1996;46:104–108.

Hilkens PH, Verweij J, Vecht CJ, et al: Clinical characteristics of severe peripheral neuropathy induced by docetaxel (Taxotere). Ann Oncol 1997;8:187–190.

Hogan PJ, Greenberg MK, McCarty GE: Neurologic complications of lymphomatoid granulomatosis. Neurology 1981;31:619–620.

Holland JF, Scharlau C, Gailani S, et al: Vincristine treatment of advanced cancer: A cooperative study of 392 cases. Cancer Res 1973;33:1258–1264.

Hopewell JW: Radiation injury to the central nervous system. Med Pediatr Oncol 1998;30(suppl 1):1–9.

Hoppe RT, Goffinet DR, Bagshaw MA: Carcinoma of the nasophar-

ynx: Eighteen years' experience with megavoltage radiation therapy. Cancer 1976;37:2605–2612.

Horowitz SL, Stewart JD. Lower motor neuron syndrome following radiotherapy. Can J Neurol Sci 1983;10:56–58.

Horwich MS, Cho L, Porro RS, Posner JB: Subacute sensory neuropathy: A remote effect of carcinoma. Ann Neurol 1977; 2:7–19.

Imrie KR, Couture F, Turner CC, et al: Peripheral neuropathy following high-dose etoposide and autologous bone marrow transplantation. Bone Marrow Transplant 1994;13:77–79.

Ince PG, Shaw PJ, Fawcett PR, Bates D. Demyelinating neuropathy due to primary IgM kappa B cell lymphoma of peripheral nerve. Neurology 1987;37:1231–1235.

Iniguez C, Larrode P, Mayordomo JI, et al: Reversible peripheral neuropathy induced by a single administration of high-dose paclitaxel. Neurology 1998;51:868–870.

Israel HL, Patchefsky AS, Saldana MJ: Wegener's granulomatosis, lymphomatoid granulomatosis, and benign lymphocytic angiitis and granulomatosis of lung. Recognition and treatment. Ann Intern Med 1977;87:691–699.

Jacobson P, Uberti J, Davis W, Ratanatharathorn V: Tacrolimus: A new agent for the prevention of graft-versus-host disease in hematopoietic stem cell transplantation. Bone Marrow Transplant 1998;22:217–225.

Jaeckle KA, Young DF, Foley KM: The natural history of lumbosacral plexopathy in cancer. Neurology 1985; 35:8–15.

Jaffe ES, Wilson WH: Lymphomatoid granulomatosis: Pathogenesis, pathology, and clinical implications. Cancer Surv 1997; 30:233–248.

Jellinger K, Radaszkiewicz T: Involvement of the central nervous system in malignant lymphomas. Virchows Arch A Pathol Anat Histol 1976;370:345–362.

Johnson NT, Crawford SW, Sargar M: Acute acquired demyelinating polyneuropathy with respiratory failure following high-dose systemic cytosine arabinoside and marrow transplantation. Bone Marrow Transplant 1987;2:203–207.

Joyce DA, Stewart-Wynne EG. Brachial plexopathy complicating central venous catheter insertion. Med J Aust 1983;1:82–83.

Kaplan JG, DeSouza TG, Farkash A, et al: Leptomeningeal metastases: Comparison of clinical features and laboratory data of solid tumors, lymphomas and leukemias. J Neuro-Oncol 1990; 9:225–229.

Kaplan JG, Portenoy RK, Pack DR, DeSouza T: Polyradiculopathy in leptomeningeal metastasis: The role of EMG and late response studies. J Neuro-Oncol 1990;9:219–224.

Kaplan JG, Einzig AI, Schaumberg HH: Taxol causes permanent large fiber peripheral nerve dysfunction: A lesson for preventative strategies. J Neuro-Oncol 1993;16:105–107.

Katzenstein A-L, Carrington CB, Liebow AA: Lymphomatoid granulomatosis: A clinicopathologic study of 152 cases. Cancer 1979;43:360–373.

Keane JR: Cavernous sinus syndrome. Analysis of 151 cases. Arch Neurol 1996;53:967–971

Kelly JJ, Kyle RA, Miles JM, Dyck PJ: Osteosclerotic myeloma and peripheral neuropathy. Neurology 1983; 33:202–210.

Kemp G, Rose P, Lurain J, et al: Amifostine pretreatment for protection against cyclophosphamide- and cisplatin-induced toxicities: Results of a randomized controlled trial in patients with advanced ovarian cancer. J Clin Oncol 1996;14:2101–2112.

Killer HE, Hess K: Natural history of radiation-induced brachial plexopathy compared with surgically treated patients. J Neurol 1990;237:247–250.

King AD, Leung SF, Teo P, et al: Hypoglossal nerve palsy in nasopharyngeal carconoma. Head Neck 1999;21:614–619.

Kinn A-C, Lantz B: Vitamin B$_{12}$ deficiency after irradiation for bladder carcinoma. J Urol 1984:131:888–890.

Kishimoto N, Shimada H, Adachi M, et al: Infiltrative peripheral neuropathy of acute monoblastic leukemia during hematologic remission (in Japanese). Rinsho Ketsueki 1994;35:876–880.

Klaua M: Uber radiogene periphere Neuropathien nach Telekobaltbestrahlung im Abdominalraum. Radiobiol Radiother (Berl) 1974;15:459–464.

Knop J, Bonsmann G, Happle R, et al: Thalidomide in the treatment of sixty cases of chronic discoid lupus erythematosus. Br J Dermatol 1983;108:461–466.

Kori SH, Foley KM, Posner JB: Brachial plexus lesions in patients with cancer: 100 cases. Neurology 1981;31:45–50.

Krarup-Hansen A, Fugleholm K, Helweg-Larsen S, et al: Examination of distal involvement in cisplatin-induced neuropathy in man. Brain 1993;116:1017–1041.

Krarup-Hansen A, Rietz B, Krarup C, et al: Histology and platinum content of sensory ganglia and sural nerves in patients treated with cisplatin and carboplatin: An autopsy study. Neuropathol Appl Neurobiol 1999;25:29–40.

Krendel D, Albright R, Graham D: Infiltrative polyneuropathy due to acute monoblastic leukemia in hematologic remission. Neurology 1987;37:474–477.

Krendel DA, Stahl RL, Chan WC: Lymphomatous polyneuropathy. Biopsy of clinically involved nerve and successful treatment. Arch Neurol 1991;48:330–332.

Krieger C, Robitaille Y, Jothy S, Elleker G: Intravascular malignant histiocytosis mimicking central nervous system vasculitis: An immunopathological diagnostic approach. Ann Neurol 1982; 12:489–492.

Kristensen O, Melgard B, Schiodt AV: Radiation myelopathy of the lumbo-sacral spinal cord. Acta Neurol Scand 1977;56:217–222.

Krucke W, von Hartrott HH, Schroder JM, et al: Licht- und elektronenmicroskopische Untersuchungen zum Spatstadium der Thalidomid-Polyneuropathie. Fortschr Neurol Psychiatr Grenzgeb 1971;39:15–50.

Kuncl RW, Duncan G, Watson D, et al: Colchicine myopathy and neuropathy. N Engl J Med 1987;316:1562–1568.

Kunitoh H, Saijo N, Noda K, Ogawa M: Neuromuscular toxicities of paclitaxel 210 mg/m^{-2} by 3-hour infusion. Br J Cancer 1998; 77:1686–1688.

Kuroda Y, Nakata H, Kakigi R, et al: Human neurolymphomatosis by adult T-cell leukemia. Neurology 1989;39:144–146.

LaBan MM, Grant AE: Occult spinal metastases: Early electromyographic manifestation. Arch Phys Med Rehabil 1971;52:223–226.

LaBan MM, Meerschaert JR, Taylor RS: Electromyographic evidence of inferior gluteal nerve compromise: An early representation of recurrent colorectal carcinoma. Arch Phys Med Rehabil 1982;63:33–35.

Lacomis D, Smith TW, Long RR: Angiotropic lymphoma (intravascular large cell lyphoma) presenting with cauda equina syndrome. Clin Neurol Neurosurg 1992;94:311–315.

Lagueny A, Aupy M, Aupy P, et al: Syndrome de la corne anterieure post-radiotherapique. Rev Neurol 1985;141:222–227.

Lagueny A, Rommel A, Vignolly B, et al: Thalidomide neuropathy: An electrophysiologic study. Muscle Nerve 1986;9:837–844.

Lamy C, Mas JL, Varet B, et al: Postradiation lower motor neuron syndrome presenting as monomelic amyotrophy. J Neurol Neurosurg Psychiatry 1991;54:648–649.

Lance JW, Burke D, Pollard J: Hyperexcitability of motor and sensory neurons in neuromyotonia. Ann Neurol 1979;5:523–532.

La Rocca RV, Meer J, Gilliatt RW, et al: Suramin-induced polyneuropathy. Neurology 1990;40:954–960.

Lassouw GMJ, Twijnstra A, Schouten LJ, van de Pol M: The neuro-oncology register. Neuroepidemiology 1992;11:261–266.

Laurent LE: Femoral neuropathy compression syndrome with paresis of the quadriceps muscle caused by radiotherapy of malignant tumors. A report of four cases. Acta Orthop Scand 1975;46:804–808.

Lederman RJ, Wilbourn AJ: Brachial plexopathy: Recurrent cancer or irradiation? Neurology 1984;34:1331–1335.

Lee AW, Law SC, Ng SH, et al: Retrospective analysis of nasopharyngeal carcinoma treated during 1976–1985: Late complications following megavoltage irradiation. Br J Radiol 1992;65:918–928.

Legha SS: Vincristine neurotoxicity: Pathophysiology and management. Med Toxicol 1986;1:421–427.

Lekos A, Katirji B, Cohen ML, et al: Mononeuritis multiplex. A harbinger of acute leukemia in relapse. Arch Neurol 1994; 51:618–622.

Lesser GJ: Neoplastic meningitis. The Neurologist 1996;2:11–24.

Letko E, Bhol K, Pinar V, et al: Tacrolimus (FK506). Ann Allergy Asthma Immunol 1999;83:179–189.

Levin KH, Lederman RJ, Wilbourn AJ: Spectrum of EMG changes in radiation brachial plexopathy. Muscle Nerve 1987;10:656.

Levin KH, Lutz G. Angiotropic large-cell lymphoma with peripheral nerve and skeletal muscle involvement: Early diagnosis and treatment. Neurology 1996;47:1009–1011.

Lhermitte J, Trelles J-O: Neurolymphomatose peripherique humaine. Presse Med 1934;42:289–292.

Liebow AA, Carrington CRB, Friedman PJ: Lymphomatoid granulomatosis. Hum Pathol 1972;3:457–558.

Liesegang TJ: Varicella-zoster viral disease. Mayo Clin Proc 1999; 74:983–998.

Lipton RB, Apfel SC, Dutcher JP, et al: Taxol produces a predominantly sensory neuropathy. Neurology 1989;39:368–373.

Lisak RP, Mitchell M, Zweiman B, et al: Guillain-Barré syndrome and Hodgkin's disease: Three cases with immunological studies. Ann Neurol 1977; 1:72–78.

Liszka U, Drlicek M, Hitzenberger P, et al: Intravascular lymphomatosis: A clinicopathological study of three cases. J Cancer Res Clin Oncol 1994;120:164–168.

Little JR, Dale AJD, Okazaki H: Meningeal carcinomatosis: Clinical manifestations. Arch Neurol 1974;30:138–143.

Loehrer PJ, Birch R, Kramer BS, et al: Ifosfamide plus *N*-acetylcysteine in the treatment of small cell and non-small cell carcinoma of the lung: A Southeastern Cancer Study Group trial. Cancer Treat Rep 1986;70:919–920.

LoMonaco M, Milone M, Batocchi AP, et al: Cisplatin neuropathy: Clinical course and neurophysiological findings. J Neurol 1992; 239:199–204.

Lossos A, Siegal T: Numb chin syndrome in cancer patients: Etiology, response to treatment, and prognostic significance. Neurology 1992;42:1181–1184.

Mack EE, Gomez EC: Neurotropic melanoma: A case report and review of the literature. J Neuro-Oncol 1992;13:165–171.

Maier JG, Perry RH, Saylor W, Sulak MH: Radiation myelitis of the dorsolumbar spinal cord. Radiology 1969;93:153–160.

Masson R, Carrier H, Barbaret C, et al: Interet de la cobaltotherapie locale dans les neuropathies peripheriques des lymphopathies chroniques (lymphoses). Deux observations avec documents histo-immunologiques et ultrastructuraux. Rev Neurol 1977;133:475–484.

Mastronardi L, Lunardi P, Farah JO, Puzzilli F: Metastatic involvement of the Meckel's cave and trigeminal nerve. A case report. J Neuro-Oncol 1997;32:87–90.

Masurovsky EB, Peterson ER, Crain SM, Horwitz SB: Morphological alterations in dorsal root ganglion neurons and supporting cells of organotypic mouse spinal cord–ganglion cultures exposed to Taxol. Neuroscience 1983;10:491–509.

Mattsson T, Arvidson K, Heimdahl A, et al: Alterations in taste acuity associated with allogeneic bone marrow transplantation. J Oral Pathol Med 1992;21:33–33.

McCune JS, Lindley C: Appropriateness of maximum-dose guidelines for vincristine. Am J Health-Syst Pharm 1997;54:1755–1758.

McDiarmid SV, Busuttil RW, Ascher NL, et al: FK506 (tacrolimus) compared with cyclosporine for primary immunosuppression after pediatric liver transplantation. Transplantation 1995;59: 530–536.

McLeod JG, Penny R: Vincristine neuropathy: An electrophysiological and histological study. J Neurol Neurosurg Psychiatry 1969;32:297–304.

McLeod JG: Paraneoplastic neuropathies. In Dyck PJ, Thomas PK, Griffin JW, et al (eds): Peripheral Neuropathy, 3rd ed. Philadelphia, WB Saunders, 1993a; 1583–1590.

McLeod JG: Peripheral neuropathy associated with lymphomas, leukemias and polycythemia vera. In Dyck PJ, Thomas PK, Griffin JW, et al. (eds): Peripheral Neuropathy, 3rd ed. Philadelphia, WB Saunders, 1993b; 1591–1598.

Merchut MP, Gruener G. Segmental zoster paresis of limbs. Electromyogr Clin Electrophysiol 1996;36:369–375.

Mercuri E, Poulton J, Buck J, et al: Vincristine treatment revealing asymptomatic hereditary motor sensory neuropathy type 1A. Arch Dis Child 1999;81:442–443.

Mesic JB, Fletcher GH, Goepfert H: Megavoltage irradiation of epithelial tumors of the nasopharynx. Int J Radiat Oncol Biol Phys 1981;7:447–453.

Midroni G, Bilbao JM: Biopsy Diagnosis of Peripheral Neuropathy. Boston, Butterworth-Heinemann, 1995.

Miller LJ, Eaton VE: Ifosfamide-induced neurotoxicity: A case report and review of the literature. Ann Pharmcother 1992; 26:183–187.

Mirza MR, Jakobsen E, Pfeiffer P, et al: Suramin in non-small cell lung cancer and advanced breast cancer: Two parallel phase II studies. Acta Oncol 1997;36:171–174.

Mitsui Y, Kusunoki S, Hiruma S, et al: Sensorimotor polyneuropathy associated with chronic lymphocytic leukemia, IgM anti-gangliosides antibody and human T-cell leukemia virus I infection. Muscle Nerve 1999;22:1461–1465.

Mollman JE, Glover DJ, Hogan M, Furman RE: Cisplatin neuropathy: Risk factors, prognosis, and protection by WR-2721. Cancer 1988;61:2192–2195.

Mondelli M, Romano C, Della Porta P, Rossi A: Electrophysiological findings in peripheral fibres of subjects with and without post-herpetic neuralgia. Electromyogr Clin Electrophysiol 1996a;101:185–191.

Mondelli M, Romano C, Passero S, et al: Effects of acyclovir on sensory axonal neuropathy, segmental motor paresis and postherpetic neuralgia in herpes zoster patients. Eur Neurol 1996b;36:288–292.

Mondrup K, Olsen NK, Pfeiffer P, Rose C: Clinical and electrodiagnostic findings in breast cancer patients with radiation-induced brachial plexus neuropathy. Acta Neurol Scand 1990; 81:153–158.

Moody JF: Electrophysiologic investigations into the neurological complications of carcinoma. Brain 1965;88:1023–1036.

Moris G, Roig C, Misiego M, et al: The distinctive headache of the occipital condyle syndrome: A report of four cases. Headache 1998;38:308–311.

Morris JG, Joffe R: Perineural spread of cutaneous basal and squamous cell carcinomas: The clinical appearance of spread into the trigeminal and facial nerves. Arch Neurol 1983;40:424–429.

Morton DL, Itabashi HH, Grimes OF: Nonmetastatic neurological complications of bronchogenic carcinoma: The carcinomatous neuromyopathies. J Thorac Cardiovasc Surg 1966;51:14–29.

Mumenthaler M: Brachial plexus neuropathies. In Dyck PJ, Thomas PK, Lambert EH, Bunge R (eds): Peripheral Neuropathy, 2nd ed. Philadelphia, WB Saunders, 1984;1383–1394.

Muss HB, Moloney WC: Chloroma and other myeloblastic tumors. Blood 1973;42:721–728.

Myers C, Cooper M, Stein C, et al: Suramin: A novel growth factor antagonist with activity in hormone-refractory metastatic prostate cancer. J Clin Oncol 1992;10:881–889.

Myers JL, Kurtin PJ, Katzenstein A-L, et al: Lymphomatoid granulomatosis. Evidence of immunophenotypic variability and relationship to Epstein-Barr virus infection. Am J Surg Pathol 1995; 19:1300–1312.

Nakahara T, Saito T, Muroi A, et al: Intravascular lymphomatosis presenting as an ascending cauda equina: Conus medullaris syndrome—remission after biweekly CHOP therapy. J Neurol Neurosurg Psychiatry 1999;67:403–406.

Negrin P, Peserico A: Complicazioni motorie in corso di Herpes zoster oftalmico studio elettromiografico di 7 casi. Riv Patol Nerv Ment 1975;96:82–86.

New PZ, Jackson CE, Rinaldi D, et al: Peripheral neuropathy secondary to docetaxel (Taxotere). Neurology 1996;46:108–111.

Nisce LZ, Chu FC: Radiation therapy of brachial plexus syndrome from breast cancer. Radiology 1968;91:1022–1025.

Nishi Y, Yufu Y, Shinomiya S, et al: Polyneuropathy in acute megakaryoblastic leukemia. Cancer 1991;68:2033–2036.

Ochonisky S, Verroust J, Bastuji-Gaarin S, et al: Thalidomide neuropathy incidence and clinicoelectrophysiologic findings in 42 patients. Arch Dermatol 1994;130:66–69.

Ogose A, Emura L, Iwabuchi Y, et al: Malignant melanoma extending along the ulnar, median, and musculocutaneous nerves: A case report. J Hand Surg [Am] 1998;23:875–878.

Oh SJ: Paraneoplastic vasculitis of the peripheral nervous system. Neuol Clin 1997;15:849–863.

Olsen ME, Chernik NL, Posner JB: Infiltration of the leptomeninges by systemic cancer: A clinical and pathological study. Arch Neurol 1974;30:122–137.

Olsen NK, Pfeiffer P, Johannsen L, et al: Radiation-induced brachial plexopathy: Neurological follow-up in 161 recurrence-free breast cancer patients. Int J Radiat Oncol Biol Phys 1993; 26:43–49.

Ongerboer de Visser BW, Tiessens G: Polyneuropathy induced by cisplatin. Prog Exp Tumor Res 1985;29:190–196.

Openshaw H, Slatkin NE, Stein AS, et al: Acute polyneuropathy after high dose cytosine arabinoside in patients with leukemia. Cancer 1996;78:1899–1905.

Openshaw H: Peripheral neuropathy after bone marrow transplantation. Biol Blood Marrow Transplant 1997;3:202–209.

O'Reilly S, Kennedy MJ, Rowinsky EK, Donehower RC: Vinorelbine and the topoisomerase 1 inhibitors: Current and potential roles in breast cancer chemotherapy. Breast Cancer Res Treat 1994;33:1–17.

Pace A, Bove L, Nistico M, et al: Vinorelbine neurotoxicity: Clinical and neurophysiological findings in 23 patients. J Neurol Neurosurg Psychiatry 1996;61:409–411.

Pace A, Bove L, Aloe A, et al: Paclitaxel neurotoxicity: Clinical and neurophysiological study of 23 patients. Ital J Neurol Sci 1997;18:73–79.

Pal PK: Clinical and electrophysiological studies in vincristine induced neuropathy. Electromyogr Clin Neurophysiol 1999; 39:323–330.

Palmer BF, Toto RD: Severe neurologic toxicity induced by cyclosporine A in three renal transplant patients. Am J Kidney Dis 1991;18:116–121.

Pancoast HK: Superior sulcus tumor. JAMA 1932;99:1391–1396.

Papa G, Biandri A, Mauro FR, et al: Cyclosporine-associated bilateral deltoid paralysis after bone marrow transplantation for chronic myelogenous leukemia. Haematologica 1985;70:273–274.

Patel SR, Forman AD, Benjamin RS: High dose ifosfamide-induced exacerbation of peripheral neuropathy. J Natl Cancer Inst 1994;86:305–306.

Patel SR, Vadhan-Raj S, Papadopoulos N, et al: High-dose ifosfamide in bone and soft tissue sarcomas: Results of a phase II and pilot studies: Dose-response and schedule dependence. J Clin Oncol 1997;15:2378–2384.

Paul M, Joshua D, Rehme N, et al: Fatal peripheral neuropathy associated with high-dose cytosine arabinoside in acute leukemia. Br J Haematol 1991;79:521–523.

Paul T, Katiyar BC, Misra S, Pant GC: Carcinomatous neuromuscular syndromes. A clinical and quantitative electrophysiological study. Brain 1978;101:53–63.

Perol M, Guerin JC, Thomas P, et al: Multicenter randomized trial comparing cisplatin-mitomycin-vinorelbine versus cisplatin-mitomycin-vindesine in advanced non–small cell lung cancer. Lung Cancer 1996;14:119–134.

Perry A, Mehta J, Iveson T, et al: Guillain-Barré syndrome after bone marrow transplantation. Bone Marrow Transplant 1994; 14:165–167.

Petito CK, Gottlieb GJ, Dougherty JH, Petito FA: Neoplastic angioendotheliomatosis: Ultrastructural study and review of the literature. Ann Neurol 1978;3:393–399.

Pettigrew LC, Glass JP, Maor M, Zornoza J: Diagnosis and treatment of lumbosacral plexopathies in patients with cancer. Arch Neurol 1984;41:1282–1285.

Phan TG, Manoharan A, Pryor D: Relapse of central nervous system Burkitt's lymphoma presenting as Guillain-Barré syndrome and syndrome of inappropriate ADH secretion. Aust N Z J Med 1998;28:223–224.

Phanthumchinda K, Intragumtornchai T, Kasantikul V: Guillain-Barré syndrome and optic atrophy in acute leukemia. Neurology 1988;38:1324–1326.

Pierce SM, Recht A, Lingos TI, et al: Long-term radiation complications following conservative surgery (CS) and radiation therapy (RT) in patients with early stage breast cancer. Int J Radiat Oncol Biol Phys 1992;23:915–923.

Pietrangeli A, Milella M, De Marco S, et al: Brachial plexus neuropathy as unusual onset of diffuse neurolymphomatosis. Neurol Sci 2000;21:241–245.

Pirovano C, Balzarini A, Bohm S, et al: Peripheral neurotoxicity following high-dose cisplatin with glutathione: Clinical and neurophysiological assessment. Tumori 1992;78:253–257.

Pirsch JD, Miller J, Deierhoi MH, et al: A comparison of tacrolimus

(FK506) and cyclosporine for immunusuppression after cadaveric renal transplantation. Transplantation 1997;63:977–983.

Pisani RJ, DeRemee RA: Clinical implications of the histopathologic diagnosis of pulmonary lymphomatoid granulomatosis. Mayo Clin Proc 1990;65:151–163.

Plante-Bordeneuve V, Baudrimont M, Gorin NC, Gherardi RK: Subacute sensory neuropathy associated with Hodgkin's disease. J Neurol Sci 1994;121:155–158.

Poncelet AN, Auger RG, Silber MH: Myokymic discharges of the tongue after radiation to the head and neck. Neurology 1996; 46:259–260.

Posner JB, Chernik NL: Intracranial metastases from systemic cancer. Adv Neurol 1978;19:579–592.

Posner JB: Neurologic Complications of Cancer. Philadelphia, FA Davis, 1995.

Postma TJ, Vermorken JB, Liefting AJ, et al: Paclitaxel-induced neuropathy. Ann Oncol 1995;6:489–494.

Powles RL, Malpas JS: Guillain-Barré syndrome associated with chronic lymphatic leukemia. Brit Med J 1967; 3:286–287.

Qayyum A, MacVicar AD, Padhani AR, et al: Symptomatic brachial plexopathy following treatment for breast cancer: Utility of MR imging with surface-coil techniques. Radiology 2000;214: 837–842.

Quinones-Hinojosa A, Friedlander RM, Boyer PJ, et al: Solitary sciatic nerve lymphoma as an initial manifestation of diffuse neurolymphomatosis. Case report and review of the literature. J Neurosurg 2000;92:165–169.

Ransom DT, Dinapoli RP, Richardson RL: Cranial nerve lesions due to base of the skull metastases in prostate carcinoma. Cancer 1990;65:586–589.

Rapoport S, Blair DN, McCarthy SM, et al: Brachial plexus: Correlation of MR imaging with CT and pathologic findings. Radiology 1988;167:161–165.

Reboul F, Donaldson SS, Kaplan HS: Herpes zoster and varicella infection in children with Hodgkin's disease: An analysis of contributing factors. Cancer 1978;41:95–99.

Reed E, Dabholkar M, Chabner BA: Platinum analogues. In Chabner BA, Longo DL (eds): Cancer Chemotherapy and Biotherapy: Principles and Practice, 2nd ed. Philadelphia, Lippincott-Raven Publishers, 1996; 357–378.

Richter C, Schnabel A, Muller KM, et al: Lymphomatoide Granulomatose-Remissionsinduktion mit Interferon-alpha 2b. Dtsch Med Wochenschr 1997;122:1106–1110.

Riggs JE, Ashraf M, Snyder RD, et al: Prospective nerve conduction studies in cisplatin therapy. Ann Neurol 1988;23:92–94.

Rodichok LD, Ruckdeschel JC, Harper GR, et al: Early diagnosis of spinal epidural metastases. Am J Med 1981:70:1181–1188.

Roelofs RI, Hrushesky W, Rogin J, Rosenberg L: Peripheral sensory neuropathy and cisplatin chemotherapy. Neurology 1984; 34:934–938.

Roessmann U, Kaufman B, Friede RL: Metastatic lesions in the sella turcica and pituitary gland. Cancer 1970;25:478–480.

Rogers LR, Borkowski GP, Albers JW, et al: Obturator mononeuropathy caused by pelvic cancer: Six cases. Neurology 1993; 43:1489–1492.

Roth BJ, Greist A, Kubilis PS, et al: Cisplatin-based combination chemotherapy for disseminated germ cell tumors: Long-term follow-up. J Clin Oncol 1988;6:1239–1247.

Roux S, Grossin M, DeBandt M, et al: Angiotropic large cell lymphoma with mononeuritis multiplex mimicking systemic vasculitis. J Neurol Neurosurg Psychiatry 1995;58:363–366.

Rowinsky EK, Chaudhry V, Cornblath DR, Donehower RC: Neurotoxicity of Taxol. Monogr Natl Cancer Inst 1993;15:107–115.

Rowinsky EK, Donehower RC: Antimicrotubule agents. In DeVita VT, Hellman S, Rosenberg SA (eds): Cancer: Principles and Practice of Oncology, 5th ed. Philadelphia, Lippincott-Raven Publishers, 1997; 467–483.

Rowinsky EK: The development and clinical utility of the taxane class of microtubule chemotherapy agents. Annu Rev Med 1997;48:353–374.

Rowland LP, Schneck SA: Neuromuscular disorders associated with malignant neoplastic disease. J Chronic Dis 1963;16:777–795.

Rubio A, Poole RM, Brara HS, et al: Motor neuron disease and angiotropic lymphoma. Arch Neurol 1996;54:92–95.

Russell JA, Powles RL: Neuropathy due to cytosine arabinoside. Br Med J 1974;4:652–653.

Russell JW, Windebank AJ, Podratz JL: Role of nerve growth factor in suramin neurotoxicity studied in vitro. Ann Neurol 1994; 36:221–228.

Russell JW, Windebank AJ, McNiven MA, et al: Effect of cisplatin and ACTH$_{4-9}$ on neural transport in cisplatin induced neurotoxicity. Brain Res 1995;676:258–267.

Sadoh DR, Hawk JL, Panayiotopoulos CP: F-chronodispersion in patients on thalidomide. Clin Neurophysiol 1999;110:735–339.

Sadowsky CH, Sachs E, Ochoa J: Postradiation motor neuron syndrome. Arch Neurol 1976;33:786–787.

Sahenk Z, Brady ST, Mendell JR: Studies on the pathogenesis of vincristine-induced neuropathy. Muscle Nerve 1987;10:80–84.

Sahenk Z, Barohn RJ, New P, Mendell JR: Taxol neuropathy: Electrodiagnostic and sural nerve biopsy findings. Arch Neurol 1994;51:726–729.

Salner AL, Botnick LE, Herzog AG, et al: Reversible brachial plexopathy following primary radiation therapy for breast cancer. Cancer Treat Rep 1981;65:797–802.

Sandler SG, Tobin W, Henderson ES: Vincristine-induced neuropathy. A clinical study of fifty leukemic patients. Neurology 1969; 19:367–374.

Saperstein DS, Amato AA, Wolfe GI, et al: Multifocal acquired demyelinating sensory and motor neuropathy: The Lewis-Sumner syndrome. Muscle Nerve 1999;22:560–566.

Saphner T, Gallion HH, van Nagell JR, et al: Neurologic complications of cervical cancer. A review of 2261 cases. Cancer 1989; 64:1147–1151.

Scherokman B, Filling-Katz MR, Tell D. Brachial plexus neuropathy following high dose cytarabine in acute monoblastic leukemia. Am J Hematol 1989;32:314–315.

Schiff PB, Fant J, Horwitz SB: Promotion of microtubule assembly in vitro by Taxol. Nature 1979;277:665–667.

Schimpff S, Serpick A, Stoler B, et al: Varicella-zoster infection in patients with cancer. Ann Intern Med 1972;76:241–254.

Schiodt AV, Kristensen O: Neurologic complications after irradiation of malignant tumors of the testis. Acta Radiol Oncol 1978; 17:369–378.

Schwab RS, Weiss S: The neurologic aspect of leukemia. Am J Med Sci 1935;189:766–778.

Seitelberger F: Thalidomid-Polyneuropathie. Klinisch-bioptische Beobachtung. Wien Klin Wochenschr 1968;80:41–43.

Shapiro BE, Rordorf G, Schwamm L, Preston DC: Delayed radiation-induced bulbar palsy. Neurology 1996;46:1604–1606.

Siegal T, Haim N: Cisplatin-induced peripheral neuropathy. Frequent off-therapy deterioration, demyelinating syndromes, and muscle cramps. Cancer 1990;66:1117–1123.

Smadja D, Mas J-L, Fallet-Bianco C, et al: Intravascular lymphomatosis (neoplastic angioendotheliosis) of the central nervous system: Case report and literature review. J Neuro-Oncol 1991; 11:171–180.

Soliven B, Dhand UK, Kobayashi K, et al: Evaluation of neuropathy in patients on suramin treatment. Muscle Nerve 1997;20:83–91.

Sonobe M, Yasuda H, Okabe H, et al: Neuropathy associated with angioimmunoblastic lymphadenopathy-like T-cell lymphoma. Intern Med 1998;37:631–634.

Stack PS: Lymphomatous involvement of peripheral nerves: Clinical and pathological features. South Med J 1991;84:512–514.

Stein CA: Suramin: A novel antineoplastic agent with multiple potential mechanisms of action. Cancer Res 1993;53:2239–2248.

Stillman MJ, Christensen W, Payne R, Foley KM: Leukemic relapse presenting as sciatic nerve involvement by chloroma (granulocytic sarcoma). Cancer 1988;62:2047–2050.

Stohr M: Special types of spontaneous electrical activity in radiogenic nerve injuries. Muscle Nerve 1982;5:S78–S83.

Stoll BA, Andrews JT: Radiation-induced peripheral neuropathy. Br Med J 1966;1:834–837.

Straus SE, Ostrove JM, Inchauspe G, et al: Varicella-zoster virus infections: Biology, natural history, treatment, and prevention. Ann Intern Med 1988;108:221–237.

Streib EW, Sun SF, Leibrock L: Brachial plexopathy in patients with breast cancer: Unusual electromyographic findings in two patients. Eur Neurol 1982;21:256–263.

Stubgen JP, Elliot JJ: Malignant radiculopathy and plexopathy. In Vecht CJ (ed): Handbook of Clinical Neurology, Vol. 25 (69), Part III. New York, Elsevier Science, 1997; 71–103.

Sugita K, Watanabe T, Niitani H, et al: Autopsy case of monocytic leukemia with severe periperal nerve disturbance (in Japanese). Rinsho Shinkeigaku 1973;13:735–744.

Sullivan KA, Kim B, Buzdon M, Feldman EL: Suramin disrupts insulin-like growth factor-II (IGF-II) mediated autocrine growth in human SH-SY5Y neuroblastoma cells. Brain Res 1997;744:199–206.

Sumi SM, Farrell DF, Knauss TA: Lymphoma and leukemia manifested by steroid-responsive polyneuropathy. Arch Neurol 1983;40:577–582.

Sunohara N, Mukoyama M, Satoyoshi E: Neoplastic angioendotheliosis of the central nervous system. J Neurol 1984;231:14–19.

Svien HJ, Baker HL, Rivers MH: Jugular foramen syndrome and allied syndromes. Neurology 1963;13:797–809.

Tanner KD, Levine JD, Topps KS: Microtubule disorientation and axonal swelling in unmyelinated sensory neurons during vincristine-induced painful neuropathy in rat. J Comp Neurol 1998;395:481–492.

Taylor BV, Kimmel DW, Krecke KN, Cascino TL: Magnetic resonance imaging in cancer-related lumbosacral plexopathy. Mayo Clin Proc 1997;72:823–829.

Terrovitis IV, Nanas SN, Rombos AK, et al: Reversible symmetric polyneuropathy with paraplegia after heart transplantation. Transplantation 1998;65:1394–1395.

Thomas FP, Vallejos U, Foitl DR, et al: B cell small lymphocytic lymphoma and chronic lymphocytic leukemia with peripheral neuropathy: Two cases with neuropathological findings and lymphocyte marker analysis. Act Neuropathol 1990;80:198–203.

Thomas JE, Yoss RE: The parasellar syndrome: Problems in determining etiology. Mayo Clin Proc 1970:45:617–723.

Thomas JE, Colby MY: Radiation-induced or metastatic brachial plexopathy? A diagnostic dilemma. JAMA 1972;222:1392–1395.

Thomas JE, Howard FM Jr: Segmental zoster paresis: A disease profile. Neurology 1972; 22:459–466.

Thomas JE, Cascino TL, Earle JD: Differential diagnosis between radiation and tumor plexopathy of the pelvis. Neurology 1985;35:1–7.

Thomas PK, Holdorff B: Neuropathy due to physical agents. In Dyck PJ, Thomas PK, Griffin JW (eds): Peripheral Neuropathy, 3rd ed. Philadelphia, WB Saunders, 1993; 990–1013.

Thompson SW, Davis LE, Kornfeld M, et al: Cisplatin neuropathy: Clinical, electrophysiologic, morphologic, and toxicologic studies. Cancer 1984;54:1269–1275.

Thyagarajan D, Cascino T, Harms G: Magnetic resonance imaging in brachial plexopathy of cancer. Neurology 1995;45:421–427.

Trojaborg W, Frantzen E, Andersen I: Peripheral neuropathy and myopathy associated with carcinoma of the lung. Brain 1969; 92:71–82.

Tsang KL, Fong KY, Ho SL: Localized neuromyotonia of neck muscles after radiotherapy for nasopharyngeal carcinoma. Mov Disord 1999;14:1047–1049.

Tseng S, Pak G, Washenik K, et al: Rediscovering thalidomide: A review of its mechanism of action, side effects, and potential uses. J Am Acad Dermatol 1996;35:969–979.

Tu SM, Pagliaro LC, Banks ME, et al: Phase I study of suramin combined with doxorubicin in the treatment of androgen-independent prostate cancer. Clin Cancer Res 1998;4:1193–1201.

Ulrich J, Miller P: Neurologische Komplikationen der Leukamien. Befall des peripheren Nervensystems und der Meningen bei einem Fall von chronischer lymphatischer Leukose. Schweiz Med Wochenschr 1968;98:580–584.

Vallat JM, de Mascarel HA, Bordessoule D, et al: Non-Hodgkin malignant lymphomas and peripheral neuropathies: 13 cases. Brain 1995;118:1233–1245.

van den Bent MJ, van Raaij-van den Aarssen VJ, Verweij J, et al: Progression of paclitaxel-induced neuropathy following discontinuation of treatment. Muscle Nerve 1997;20:750–752.

van den Bent MJ, Hilkens PH, Sillevis Smitt PA, et al: Lhermitte's sign following chemotherapy with docetaxel. Neurology 1998; 50:563–564.

van den Bent MJ, de Bruin HG, Beun GD, Vecht CJ: Neurolymphomatosis of the median nerve. Neurology 1995;45:1403–1405.

van den Bent MJ, de Bruin HG, Bos GM, et al: Negative sural nerve biopsy in neurolymphomatosis. J Neurol 1999;246:1159–1163.

van der Sluis RW, Wolfe GI, Nations SP, et al: Post-radiation lower motor neuron syndrome. J Clin Neuromusc Dis 2000;2:10–17.

Van Oostenbrugge RJ, Twijnstra A: Presenting features and value of diagnostic procedures in leptomeningeal metastases. Neurology 1999;53:382–385.

Vernino S, Adamski J, Kryzer TJ, et al: Neuronal nicotinic ACh receptor antibody in subacute autonomic neuropathy and cancer-related syndromes. Neurology 1998;50:1806–1813.

Vikram B, Chu FC: Radiation therapy for metastases to the base of the skull. Radiology 1979;130:465–468.

Vital A, Vital C, Ellie E, et al: Malignant infiltration of peripheral nerves in the course of acute myelomonoblastic leukaemia: Neuropathological study of two cases. Neuropathol Appl Neurobiol 1993;19:159–163.

Vital C, Bonnaud E, Arne L, Barrat M, Leblanc M: Polyradiculonevrite au cours d'une leucemie lymphoide chronique. Etude ultrastructurale d'une biopsie de nerf periperique. Acta Neuropathol 1975;32:169–172.

Vital C, Heraud A, Coquet M, et al: Acute mononeuropathy with angiotropic lymphoma. Acta Neuropathol 1989;78;105–107.

Vital C, Vital A, Julien J, et al: Peripheral neuropathies and lymphoma without monoclonal gammapathy: A new classification. J Neurol 1990;237:177–185.

Vital C, Vital A, Moynet D, et al: The presence of particles resembling human T-cell leukemia virus type I at ultrastructural examination of lymphomatous cells in a case of T-cell leukemia/lymphoma. Cancer 1993;71:2227–2232.

Vuorinen V, Roytta M, Raine CS: The acute effects of Taxol upon regenerating axons after nerve crush. Acta Neuropathol 1988; 76:26–34.

Walk D, Handelsman A, Beckmann E, et al: Mononeuropathy multiplex due to infiltration of lymphoma in hematologic remission. Muscle Nerve 1998;21:823–826.

Walsh JC: Neuropathy associated with lymphoma. J Neurol Neurosurg Psychiatry 1971; 34:42–50.

Wang V, Liao KK, Ju TH, et al: Myokymia and neuromyotonia of the tongue: A case report of complication of irradiation. Chung Hua I Hsueh Tsa Chih (Taipei) 1993;52:413–415.

Wasserstrom WR, Glass P, Posner JB: Diagnosis and treatment of leptomeningeal metastases from solid tumors: Experience with 90 patients. Cancer 1982;49:759–772.

Weintraub M, Adde MA, Venzon DJ, et al: Severe atypical neuropathy associated with administration of hematopoietic colony-stimulating factors and vincristine. J Clin Oncol 1996;14:935–940.

Weiss HD, Walker MD, Wiernik PH: Neurotoxicity of commonly used antineoplastic agents (second of two parts). N Engl J Med 1974;291:127–133.

Weiss S, Streifler M, Weiser HJ: Motor lesions in herpes zoster. Eur Neurol 1975;13:332–338.

Wells CE, Silver RT: The neurologic manifestations of the acute leukemias: A clinical study. Ann Intern Med 1957;46:439–449.

Wiernik PH, Schwartz EL, Strauman JJ, et al: Phase I clinical and pharmacokinetic study of Taxol. Cancer Res 1987;47:2486–2493.

Wilbourn AJ: Brachial plexus disorders. In Dyck PJ, Thomas PK, Griffin JW, et al. (eds): Peripheral Neuropathy, 3rd ed. Philadelphia, WB Saunders, 1993;911–950.

Wilbourn AJ: Assessment of the brachial plexus and the phrenic nerve. In Johson EW, Pease WS (eds): Practical Electromyography, 3rd ed. Baltimore, Williams & Wilkins, 1997; 273–310.

Williams HM, Diamond HD, Craver LF, Parsons H: Neurological Complications of Lymphomas and Leukemias. Springfield, Charles C Thomas, 1959.

Wilson JR, Conwit RA, Eidelman BH, et al: Sensorimotor neuropathy resembling CIDP in patients receiving FK506. Muscle Nerve 1994;17:528–532.

Wilson WH, Kingma DW, Raffeld M, et al: Association of lymphomatoid granulomatosis with Epstein-Barr viral infection of B lymphocytes and response to interferon-α2b. Blood 1996;87:4531–4537.

Windebank AJ: Chemotherapeutic neuropathy. Curr Opin Neurol 1999;12:565–571.

Wiznitzer M, Packer RJ, August CS, et al: Neurologic complications of bone marrow transplantation in childhood. Ann Neurol 1984;16:569–576.

Wohlgemuth WA, Rottach K, Jaenke G, Stohr M: Radiogene Amyotrophie. Cauda-equina-Lasion als Strahlenspatfolge. Nervenarzt 1998;69:1061–1065.

Wolfe GI, Baker NS, Amato AA, et al: Chronic cryptogenic sensory polyneuropathy: Clinical and laboratory characteristics. Arch Neurol 1999;56:540–547.

Wulff CH, Hoyer H, Asboe-Hansen G, Brodthagen H: Development of polyneuropathy during thalidomide therapy. Br J Dermatol 1985;112:475–480.

Zaretsky M, Pulipaka U, Schiff D, et al: Rapidly progressive, acute polyradiculopathies and cranial neuropathies resulting from leptomeningeal nasal-type NK cell lymphoma. J Clin Neuromusc Dis 2000;1:137–140.

Paraneoplastic Peripheral Neuropathies

Rahman Pourmand

Most patients with systemic cancer develop peripheral neuropathy at some point during the course of their illness. The occurrence of peripheral neuropathy in patients with known malignancy is generally related to the side effects of treatment (chemotherapy, radiation therapy, immunosuppression, bone marrow transplantation) and may be due to the direct invasion of peripheral nerves or roots by tumor cells or to systemic metabolic or nutritional deficiencies (Posner, 1995) (Table 66–1).

The term *paraneoplastic*, or *remote, effect* of carcinoma is applied when none of the aforementioned factors can explain the cause of neuropathy. Paraneoplastic neuropathies generally appear months to years before the onset of cancer. Paraneoplastic neurological syndromes are considered rare but are clinically important conditions because a careful search may lead to the early detection of a treatable tumor. The term *paraneoplastic syndrome* probably should be credited to Denny-Brown (1948). He described two patients who presented with sensory neuropathy and, at autopsy, were found to have carcinoma of the lung, with degeneration and neuronal loss in the dorsal root ganglia.

EPIDEMIOLOGY

There are several reasons why the true frequency of peripheral neuropathy in patients with systemic cancer is unknown. First, for the most part, the reported series do not address what percentage of peripheral neuropathy cases might be directly related to other causes, such as nutritional deficiencies or the side effects of treatment. Second, the series vary with regard to selection of the patient's stage and duration of cancer. Third, the percentage of cases of peripheral neuropathy would differ depending on the criteria used to define *neuropathy* (e.g., whether by clinical presentation or on the basis of results of electrophysiological testing, or a combination of the two).

According to McLeod (1993), about 5% of patients with cancer have the clinical features of peripheral neuropathy. This incidence rises to about 12% when quantitative sensory testing is used (Lipton et al., 1987, 1991) and to 40% when electrophysiological studies are added to the clinical examination (Moody, 1965; Trojaborg et al., 1969; Herishanu et al., 1970).

It has been estimated that about 10% to 15% of patients with carcinoma develop neuropathy on long-term follow-up (Prineas, 1970; Chalk et al., 1992; McLeod, 1993; Rosenfeld et al., 1997). The incidence of paraneoplastic neuropathy is probably around 2% (Elrington et al., 1991; Lim et al., 1993; von Oosterhout et al., 1996). Small cell lung cancer (SCLC) is the cancer most frequently associated with paraneoplastic sensory neuropathy, followed by gastro-

Table 66–1. Causes of Peripheral Neuropathy in Cancer Patients

Cause	Example and Mechanism
Direct invasion of peripheral nerve or compression	Infiltration of cancer cells into the nerve sheaths or compression of plexus or roots
Chemotherapy agents	Vinca alkaloids, platinum compounds, paclitaxel (Taxol), suramin, etoposide
Immunosuppressive drugs	Tacrolimus, cyclosporine, thalidomide
Radiation therapy	Radiation plexopathy
Nutritional	Vitamin deficiencies, weight loss, pressure palsy
Metabolic abnormalities	Hypothyroidism, uremia, critical illness
Paraneoplastic	Autoimmune

intestinal tract cancer and then cancers of other organs (McLeod, 1993; Hughes et al., 1996; Amato and Collins, 1998).

CLINICAL PRESENTATIONS

Motor Neuropathies

SUBACUTE MOTOR NEUROPATHY

In 1963, Rowland and Schneck described two young women with Hodgkin's lymphoma who presented with slowly progressive lower motor neuron symptoms and signs. Subsequent work established the association of this neuropathy with Hodgkin's and non-Hodgkin's lymphomas (Schold, 1979; Younger et al., 1991; Forsyth, 1997). Clinical features are usually those of lower motor neuron symptoms and signs. The symptoms may present at any stage of the tumor, but they most typically appear when the tumor is in remission. The course is often benign, and spontaneous remission can occur. Patients typically present with subacute, progressive, painless, asymptomatic weakness of the legs with diminished reflexes and minimal sensory symptoms. Involvement of bulbar muscles is rare, and fasciculations are infrequent. Although initial reports indicate this syndrome is purely a motor neuron disease, subsequent reports disclosed upper motor neuron signs in as many as 45% of patients in one series (Gordon et al., 1997). Laboratory studies in these patients often show elevation of sedimentation rates and increased cerebrospinal fluid protein concentrations with oligoclonal bands. Electrophysiological studies demonstrate relatively normal nerve conduction velocities, with decreased amplitude of motor and sensory nerve action potentials. Needle electrode examination shows denervation features, such as fibrillation potentials and positive sharp waves, but fasciculation potentials are rare. Motor unit potentials can be large and complex.

Antineuronal antibodies are rarely reported with motor neuron disease. In a series reported by Dalmau and associates (1992), 20% of 71 patients had positive anti-Hu antibodies. Other reports also show this rare association (Verma et al., 1996; Ferracci et al., 1999). The majority of these patients, however, had symptoms and signs of other types of nervous system involvement and were considered to have variants of paraneoplastic encephalomyelitis (PEM)–sensory neuronopathy, which are highly associated with SCLC and positive antibodies (Dalmau et al., 1992; Voltz et al., 1997).

Reported postmortem studies have demonstrated loss of anterior horn cells, minimal inflammation and demyelination of ventral roots and dorsal columns, and neurogenic muscle atrophy.

In the setting of carcinoma, these cases should be differentiated from postirradiation polyradiculoneuropathy (Brown et al., 1997).

MOTOR NEURON DISEASE AND AMYOTROPHIC LATERAL SCLEROSIS

The evidence for paraneoplastic motor neuron disease has been inconclusive and has long been debated; epidemiological studies show no increase in the incidence of motor neuron disease or amyotrophic lateral sclerosis in patients with cancer (Chio et al., 1988; Norris et al., 1989). An amyotrophic lateral sclerosis–like syndrome has been reported in some patients with cancer (Rosenfeld et al., 1991); the association seems to be more than just coincidence (Forsyth et al., 1977; Gordon et al., 1977). Again, most of these cases were thought to be part of PEM–paraneoplastic subacute sensory neuronopathy (PSSN), as claimed by Verma and colleagues (1996).

In a review of 442 patients with motor neuron disease, Younger and colleagues (1990) identified eight patients with lymphoma. In another series of 37 consecutive patients with motor neuron disease who underwent bone marrow biopsy because of paraproteinemia, two patients were found to have lymphoma. These studies and an editorial (Younger, 2000) suggest that a paraneoplastic work-up is probably not warranted if the patient presents with typical features of amyotrophic lateral sclerosis. On the other hand, if clinical features are somewhat atypical (e.g., pure lower motor signs or sensory symptoms), the serum paraprotein level should be checked, and if it is found to be elevated, a bone marrow biopsy should be considered.

Subacute Sensory Neuronopathy

PSSN was first described by Denny-Brown in 1948. Symptoms of PSSN may occur in the pure sensory form or as a part of PEM. The symptoms may begin several months to years before the discovery of the tumor (Chalk et al., 1992; Dalmau et al., 1992). On average, symptoms appear 4 to 5 months before tumor discovery. The onset is subacute, with pain, paresthesia, and sensory loss. The symptoms are often asymmetrical and predominantly of a distal limb distribution, with marked involvement of the arms. Sensory loss rapidly progresses to all modalities, including pain, temperature, and proprioception. The distribution of sensory loss may progress to the trunk, face, and cranial nerves (manifesting as hearing loss, facial numbness, and loss of taste). Severe proprioception sensory loss leads to sensory limb ataxia and pseudoathetoid movements of the hands and feet, which are characteristic signs of this disorder.

The majority of patients also have symptoms and signs of multifocal encephalomyelitis, presenting with an altered mental state, confusion, personality changes, dysarthria, cerebellar dysfunction, corticospinal tract dysfunction, and autonomic nervous system disturbances (Graus et al., 2001). The mean age at onset is about 59 years (Croft and Wilkinson,

1969). PSSN affects predominantly women. More than 90% of patients have SCLC (Horowich et al., 1977; Chalk et al., 1992; Dalmau et al., 1992); the next most frequent cancers in PSSN patients are ovarian cancer and breast or prostate carcinoma.

On general physical examination, many patients who are heavy smokers may have clubbed fingers. True muscle weakness and atrophy are rare. Muscle stretch reflexes are generally decreased or absent. About three fourths of patients have associated features of PEM. Associations with mononeuritis multiplex (Liang et al., 1994; Younger et al., 1994) and Lambert-Eaton myasthenic syndrome (Lennon et al., 1995) have been reported.

DIFFERENTIAL DIAGNOSIS

Any neuropathy that selectively affects sensory nerve fibers or dorsal root ganglia and manifests as pure sensory neuropathy should be considered in the differential diagnosis of PSSN. The list includes neuropathies related to pyridoxine overdose, Sjögren's syndrome, human immunodeficiency virus–related sensory neuropathy, and the sensory variant of Guillain-Barré syndrome. Idiopathic sensory neuronopathy may present acutely, subacutely, or chronically (Dalakas, 1986; Windebank et al., 1990). Patients present with numbness and paresthesias that often involve the face, trunk, and extremities. Proprioceptive loss is prominent, manifesting as sensory ataxia. The sensory complaints are generally symmetrical. Reflexes are decreased or absent. Autonomic dysfunction is uncommon.

Among patients with known cancer, sensory neuropathy due to chemotherapeutic agents should be considered in the differential diagnosis (Cavaletti et al., 1995; Hilkens et al., 1996).

Neuropathy caused by chemotherapy generally begins distally and symmetrically. Cerebrospinal fluid examination in such cases, in contrast with PSSN–PEM, shows no pleocytosis or oligoclonal banding.

DIAGNOSTIC EVALUATION

The diagnostic value of the anti-Hu antibody has been well established (Graus et al., 1986; Dalmau et al., 1992). Its specificity is about 99%, with a sensitivity of 82% in patients with PSSN–PEM (Molinuevo et al., 1998). Depending on the methodology used, a low titer of anti-Hu can be detected in as many as 40% of patients who have SCLC but no obvious clinical paraneoplastic syndrome (Dalmau et al., 1990; Dropcho and King, 1996; Verschuuren et al., 1999). A high titer with no overt paraneoplastic syndrome may occur in about 20% of patients with SCLC. The high titer is used not only as a diagnostic marker for PSSN–PEM but also to direct a search for lung cancer. The predictive value for the detection of cancer, however, differs by laboratory and meth-

odology used. The preferred methods are immunocytochemical techniques and immunoblotting (Moll et al., 1995). In patients who are strongly suspected to have PSSN and have a negative result on serum antibody testing, measurement of the cerebrospinal fluid antibody level may be considered (Vega et al., 1994).

Lung cancer is the most frequent cause of paraneoplastic neuropathy; therefore, a search for cancer cells should be continued regardless of antibody status. Chest radiographs, chest computed tomography scan, and abdomen-pelvic computed tomography scan—and a mammogram in women—should be obtained. Whole-body positron emission tomography scan can be helpful in the detection of cancer; positron emission tomography scans had a sensitivity up to 87% and a positive predictive value of 94% in one series (Hoh et al., 1993). "Blind" bronchoscopy is not warranted in the search for cancer in a patient with a negative chest computed tomography scan. There are reports that no cancer has been detected even at autopsy in patients with PSSN–progressive encephalomyelitis and positive results on anti-Hu antibody testing (Horoupian et al., 1982; Daniel et al., 1985).

Electrophysiological studies in PSSN demonstrate a decrease in amplitude or the absence of sensory potentials, with normal motor nerve conduction velocities and F-wave latencies (Horowich et al., 1977; Chalk et al., 1992; Pourmand and Maybury, 1996). Needle electrode examinations are generally normal but may show denervation potentials, such as fibrillations and positive sharp waves and neurogenic motor unit potentials, particularly when PSSN is associated with PEM. Spinal fluid examination commonly shows protein concentration elevation, with an oligoclonal band and mild pleocytosis (Dalmau et al., 1992).

PATHOLOGY

The pathological hallmarks of PSSN–PEM are degeneration and loss of primary sensory neurons of the dorsal root ganglia, with proliferation of satellite cells and secondary inflammatory response. The majority of inflammatory cells are CD8[+] lymphocytes. As the disease progresses, degeneration and demyelination of the dorsal roots and dorsal columns and sensory nerve fibers may occur (Horowich et al., 1977). Anterior roots and the anterior and lateral columns are usually spared. Patients with PEM may show variable inflammatory responses or neuronal degeneration in the cerebellum, brain stem, and autonomic ganglia. Sural nerve biopsy may demonstrate nonspecific axonal degeneration and marked loss of myelinated fibers with minor inflammation.

PATHOGENESIS

Autoimmune-mediated mechanisms have been proposed as causes of PSSN–PEM; this hypothesis is based on several observations.

- Presence of "anti-Hu" autoantibody in the serum and cerebrospinal fluid; these antibodies are usually IgG and are generally not detected in neurologically normal cancer patients (Brashear et al., 1989); Hu antigen has been shown in SCLC cells and neurons (Voltz et al., 1997; Liblau et al., 1998)
- Inflammatory cell response in dorsal root ganglia and sural nerve (Jean et al., 1994)
- Response to immunotherapy (discussed later)

THERAPY AND COURSE

PSSN–PEM has a unique, monophasic course for the most part. Patients deteriorate rather rapidly over weeks to months and generally stabilize with substantial neurological disability, even when the tumor has been treated adequately or is in remission. Sudden death can occur during the course of the illness, possibly related to acute dysautonomia (Dalmau et al., 1992; Dropcho and King, 1996). A gradual or stepwise course is less common. Some patients may show major neurological improvement with treatment of the underlying cancer. Rarely, spontaneous improvement occurs without cancer treatment (Byrne et al., 1994).

Patients who have PSSN associated with PEM and positive antibody tests generally survive longer than do patients who have SCLC and no paraneoplastic syndrome. This is because early detection of tumors in the first set of patients results in early and effective treatment (Dropcho et al., 1994).

Tumors associated with paraneoplastic syndrome are believed to be smaller than other tumors, and to have a more indolent course (Graus, 1994). The underlying cancer, when and if it is detected, should be treated promptly with the best available options. Most patients, however, remain neurologically disabled.

Immunosuppressive drug therapy, plasma exchange, and intravenous immunoglobulin are other therapeutic options that can be considered in conjunction with cancer therapy (Horowich et al., 1977; Chalk et al., 1992; Dropcho, 1999). Immunotherapy, however, is generally ineffective, because by the time patients are diagnosed, irreversible neuronal loss has occurred (Dalmau et al., 1992; Graus et al., 1994; Uchuya et al., 1996). Patients with PSSN–PEM without a confirmed tissue diagnosis of underlying cancer should not receive antitumor drugs. The neurological prognosis of patients with or without known underlying cancer is about the same (Keime-Guibert, 1999).

SENSORIMOTOR POLYNEUROPATHIES

Paraneoplastic sensorimotor polyneuropathies are not clinically different from nonparaneoplastic peripheral neuropathies. The most common form is the chronic axonal form. The onset can be acute, as in Guillain-Barré syndrome, or the condition may be chronic, such as chronic inflammatory demyelinating polyneuropathy. The acute and chronic demyelinating forms are generally associated with Hodgkin's disease and non-Hodgkin's lymphoma. Nerve conduction studies are consistent with demyelinating neuropathy, and cerebrospinal fluid examination shows elevated protein concentrations but minimal pleocytosis (Lisak et al., 1977; Vallat et al., 1995).

The patient may respond to plasma exchange, intravenous immunoglobulin, or immunosuppressive drugs. There have been reports of improvement of chronic inflammatory demyelinating polyneuropathy after tumor resection and immunotherapy (Antoine et al., 1996). In Guillain-Barré syndrome, spontaneous remission, independent of tumor treatment, can occur.

Chronic axonal sensorimotor polyneuropathies, generally associated with solid tumors, occur most frequently with SCLC and manifest clinically as symmetrical distal pain and paresthesia and decreased muscle stretch reflexes; cranial nerves are usually spared. The course is slowly progressive. This neuropathy is more common in practice than is PSSN (Croft and Wilkinson, 1969).

Chronic sensorimotor neuropathy in cancer patients is generally related to weight loss, nutritional deficiencies, and the effect of antitumor drugs. The incidence of underlying cancer in all peripheral neuropathies is about 10% to 15%, depending on the methods of investigation (Hawley et al., 1980). Sensorimotor polyneuropathy is more common in men. The symptoms of neuropathy may precede the symptoms of neoplasm by a period of 2 to 6 years. Electrophysiological studies are consistent with axonal neuropathy. Sural nerve biopsy, however, may show axonal degeneration and loss of myelinated nerve fibers (Croft and Wilkinson, 1969; Chalk et al., 1992).

VASCULITIC NEUROPATHY

Mononeuropathy multiplex due to vasculitic neuropathy has been reported to be associated with hematological and solid tumors (Johnson et al., 1979; Vincent et al., 1986; Kurzrock et al., 1994; Matsumuro et al., 1994; Younger et al., 1994). Clinical presentations are similar to those of non-neoplastic vasculitic neuropathy; painful mononeuropathies or superimposed asymmetrical generalized sensorimotor polyneuropathy. Electrophysiological tests are consistent with axonopathy. Nerve biopsy reveals vasculitis, with or without fibrinoid necrosis. Larger vessels are generally spared. Association of vasculitic neuropathy with PSSN–PEM with positive anti-Hu antibody has been reported (Johnson et al., 1979; Younger et al., 1994). Responses to immunotherapy or antitumor treatment are variable (Johnson et al., 1979; Matsumuro et al., 1994).

AUTONOMIC NEUROPATHY

Paraneoplastic autonomic neuropathy is generally associated with PSSN–PEM (Sodhi et al., 1989; Veilleux et al., 1990; Gerl et al., 1992; Riva et al., 1997). Clinical manifestations include orthostatic hypotension, urinary retention, constipation, dry mouth, pupillary abnormalities, impotence, and cardiac arrhythmias. One unique manifestation is intestinal pseudo-obstruction, which manifests as abdominal distention, nausea, and constipation. The most common associated cancer is, again, SCLC (Siemsen et al., 1963; Dalmau et al., 1992). In a few pathological reports, there were inflammatory infiltrates, neuronal loss, and glial proliferation involving dorsal root ganglia and the myenteric plexus (Chin and Schuffler, 1988; Cuirllerier et al., 1998; Vernio et al., 1998).

SUMMARY

In the setting of cancer, the development of peripheral neuropathy is commonly related to weight loss, nutritional deficiencies, and the side effects of cancer treatment. Paraneoplastic neuropathies are suspected when all other possible causes of an idiopathic polyneuropathy have been excluded. Paraneoplastic syndromes are disorders that occur at sites "remote" from the primary tumor and are not caused by metastasis or local invasion (Dalmau and Posner, 1999). Discovery of a tumor during the course of a neuropathy, however, does not necessarily indicate that the neuropathy is of paraneoplastic origin. Except for PSSN (with or without associated PEM), which has a unique etiology and clinical features, the clinical manifestations of other forms of paraneoplastic neuropathies are no different from those of neuropathies due to other causes.

Paraneoplastic neuropathies or syndromes are rare conditions, but they are clinically significant because of their frequent association with underlying carcinomas that are often curable when detected early (Liblau et al., 1998; Darnell, 1999). Most paraneoplastic neurological syndromes precede the diagnosis of cancer by months to years. Therefore, the search should be continued to detect cancer in highly suspect cases.

Paraneoplastic syndromes are now believed to be autoimmune disorders (Dalmau and Posner, 1994; Lucchinetti et al., 1998). PSSN–PEM is highly associated with anti-Hu antibody and SCLC. Only a small percentage of patients with high titers of anti-Hu have no detectable cancer even at autopsy. About 25% of patients with anti-Hu syndrome present with peripheral neuropathy as the sole manifestation of cancer (Dalmau and Posner, 1994). Low titers can be seen in cancer patients with no obvious clinical neuropathy.

The treatment of paraneoplastic neuropathy consists of treatment of the underlying cancer as soon as it is detected, with the best available methods.

Immunotherapy is of particular value for patients with a progressive course and no treatable tumor. Despite adequate cancer treatment, however, PSSN causes significant chronic neurological disability.

References

Amato AA, Collins MP: Neuropathies associated with malignancy. Semin Neurol 1998;18:125–144.

Antoine JC, Mosnier JE, Lapras J, et al: Chronic inflammatory demyelinating polyneuropathy associated with carcinoma. J Neurol Neurosurg Psychiatr 1996;46:822–824.

Brashear HR, Greenlee JE, Jaeckle KA, et al: Anti-cerebellar autoantibodies in neurologically normal patients with ovarian neoplasms. Neurology 1989;39:1650–1659.

Brown J, Gregory R, Squier M, Donaghy M: The post-irradiation lower motor neuron syndrome: Neuronopathy or radiculopathy? Brain 1997;119:1429–1439.

Byrne T, Mason WP, Posner JB, Dalmau J: Spontaneous neurological improvement in anti-Hu associated encephalomyelitis. J Neurol Neurosurg Psychiatr 1994;121:155–158.

Cavaletti G, Boglium G, Marzorati L, et al: Peripheral neuropathy of Taxol in patients previously treated with cisplatin. Cancer 1995;75:1141–1150.

Chalk CH, Windebank AJ, Kimmel DW, McManis PG: The distinctive clinical features of paraneoplastic sensory neuronopathy. Can J Neurol Sci 1992;92:346–351.

Chin JS, Schuffler MD: Paraneoplastic visceral neuropathy as a cause of severe gastrointestinal motor dysfunction. Gastroenterology 1988;95:1279–1286.

Chio A, Brignolio F, Meineri P, et al: Motor neuron disease and malignancy: Results of a population-based study. J Neurol 1988;235:374–375.

Croft PB, Wilkinson JM: The course and prognosis in some types of carcinomatous neuromyopathy. Brain 1969;92:1–8.

Cuirllerier E, Coffin B, Potet F, et al: Paraneoplastic pseudo-obstruction revealing small cell lung cancer: "The anti-Hu syndrome." Gastroenterol Clin Biol 1998;22:346–348.

Dalakas MC: Chronic idiopathic ataxic neuropathy. Ann Neurol 1986;19:545–554.

Dalmau J, Furneaux HM, Gralla RJ, et al: Detection of the anti-Hu antibody in the serum of patients with small cell lung cancer: A quantitative Western blot analysis. Ann Neurol 1990;27:544–552.

Dalmau J, Graus F, Rosenblum MK, Posner JB: Anti-Hu associated paraneoplastic encephalomyelitis, sensory neuronopathy: A clinical study of 71 patients. Medicine 1992;71:59–72.

Dalmau J, Posner JB: Neurologic paraneoplastic antibodies (anti-Yo; anti-Hu, anti-Ri): The case for a new nomenclature based on antibody and antigen specificity. Neurology 1994;44:2241–2246.

Dalmau J, Posner JB: Paraneoplastic syndromes. Arch Neurol 1999;56:405–408.

Daniel SE, Love S, Scaravilli F, Harding AE: Encephalomyeloneuropathy in the absence of a detectable neoplasm. Acta Neuropathol 1985;66:311–317.

Darnell RB: The importance of defining the paraneoplastic neurologic disorders. N Engl J Med 1999;340:1831–1833.

Denny-Brown D: Primary sensory neuropathy with muscular changes associated with carcinoma. J Neurol Neurosurg Psychiatr 1948;11:73–81.

Dropcho EJ, King PH: Autoantibodies against the Hu-N1 RNA-binding protein among patients with lung carcinoma: An association with type 1 anti-neuronal nuclear antibodies. Ann Neurol 1996;39:659–667.

Dropcho EJ: Paraneoplastic neuromuscular disorders. J Clin Neuromuscular Dis 1999;1:99–108.

Elrington GM, Murray NM, Spiro SG, Newsom-Davis J: Neurological paraneoplastic syndromes in patients with small cell lung cancer: A prospective survey of 150 patients. J Neurol Neurosurg Psychiatr 1991;54:764–767.

Ferracci F, Fassetta G, Butler MH, et al: A novel anti-neuronal antibody in motor neuron syndrome associated with breast cancer. Neurology 1999;53:852–855.

Forsyth PA, Dalmau J, Graus F, et al: Motor neuron syndromes in cancer patients. Ann Neurol 1997;41:722–730.

Gerl A, Stork M, Schalhorn A, et al: Paraneoplastic intestinal pseudo-obstruction as a rare complication of bronchial carcinoma. Gut 1992;33:1000–1003.

Gordon PH, Rowland LP, Younger DS, et al: Lymphoproliferative disorders and motor neuron disease: An update. Neurology 1997;48:1671–1678.

Graus F, Ekon KB, Gordon-Cardo C, Posner JB: Sensory neuromyopathy and small cell cancer: Anti-neuronal antibody that also reacts with the tumor. Am J Med 1986;80:45–52.

Graus F, Réné R: Paraneoplastic neuropathies. Eur Neurol 1993; 33:279–286.

Graus F, Bonivea Ventura I, Ichaya M, et al: Indolent anti-Hu associated paraneoplastic sensory neuropathy. Neurology 1994;44:2258–2261.

Graus F, Keime-Guibert F, Rene R, et al: Anti-Hu-associated paraneoplastic encephalomyetitis: Analysis of 200 patients. Brain 2001;124(Pt 6):1138–1148.

Hawley RJ, Cohen MH, Saini N, et al: The carcinomatous neuromyopathy of oat-cell lung cancer. Ann Neurol 1980;7:65.

Herishanu Y, Wolf E, Tansteim I, et al: The carcinomatous neuropathy: A clinical and electrophysiological comparative study with special reference to the effects of treatment on the nervous system. Eur Neurol 1970;4:370–374.

Hilkens PTT, Verweiji J, Stoter G, et al: Peripheral neurotoxicity induced by docetaxel. Neurology 1996;46:104–108.

Hoh CK, Hawkins RA, Glaspy JA, Dahlbom M, et al: Cancer detection with whole-body PET using 2-[18F]fluoro-2-deoxy-D-glucose. J Comput Assist Tomogr 1993;17:582–589.

Horoupian DS, Kim Y: Encephalomyeloneuropathy with ganglionitis of the myenteric plexuses in the absence of the cancer. Ann Neurol 1982;11:628–631.

Horowich MS, Cho L, Porro RS, Posner JB: Subacute sensory neuronopathy: A remote effect of carcinoma. Ann Neurol 1977; 2:7–19.

Hughes R, Sharrack B, Rubens R: Carcinoma and the peripheral nervous system. J Neurol 1996;243:371–376.

Jean WC, Dalmau J, Ho A, et al: Analysis of the IgG subclass distribution and inflammatory infiltrate in patients with anti-Hu associated paraneoplastic encephalomyelitis. Neurology 1994; 44:140–147.

Johnson PC, Rolak LA, Hamilton RH, Laguna JF: Paraneoplastic vasculitis of nerve: A remote effect of cancer. Ann Neurol 1979; 5:437–444.

Keime-Guibert F, Graus F, Broet P, et al: Clinical outcome of patients with anti-Hu associated encephalomyelitis after treatment of the tumor. Neurology 1999;53:1719–1723.

Kurzrock R, Cohen PR, Markowitz A: Clinical manifestations of vasculitis in patients with solid tumor: A case report and review of the literature. Arch Neurol 1994;54:334–340.

Lennon VA, Kryzer TJ, Greismann GE, et al: Calcium-channel antibodies in the Lambert-Eaton syndrome and other paraneoplastic neuronopathy. N Engl J Med 1995;332:1467–1474.

Liang BC, Albers JW, Sima AAF, Nostrant TT: Paraneoplastic pseudo-obstruction, mononeuropathy multiplex and sensory neuronopathy. Muscle Nerve 1994;17:91–96.

Liblau R, Benyahia B, Delattre JY: The pathophysiology of paraneoplastic neurological syndromes. Ann Intern Med 1998;149: 512–520.

Lim KP, Kwan SY, Chen SY, et al: Generalized neuropathy in Taiwan: An etiologic survey. Neuroepidemiology 1993;12:357–261.

Lipton RB, Galer BS, Datcher JP, et al: Quantitative sensory testing demonstrates that subclinical sensory neuropathy is prevalent in patients with cancer. Arch Neurol 1987;44:944–946.

Lipton RB, Galer BS, Datcher JP, et al: Large and small fiber type sensory dysfunction in patients with cancer. J Neurol Neurosurg Psychiatr 1991;54:706–709.

Lisak RP, Mitchell M, Zweiman B, et al: Guillain-Barré syndrome and Hodgkin's disease: Three causes with immunological studies. Ann Neurol 1977;1:72–78.

Lucchinetti CF, Kimmel DW, Lennon VA: Paraneoplastic and oncologic profiles of patients sero-positive for type 1 anti-neuronal nuclear autoantibodies. Neurology 1998;50:652–657.

Matsumuro K, Izuro S, Umehara F, et al: Paraneoplastic vasculitic neuropathy: Immunohistochemical studies on a biopsied nerve and postmortem explanation. J Intern Med 1994;236:225–230.

McLeod JG: Paraneoplastic neuropathies. In Dyck PJ, Thomas PK, Griffen JW, et al (eds): Peripheral Neuropathy, 3rd ed. Philadelphia, WB Saunders, 1993; 1958–1590.

Molinuevo JL, Graus F, Réné R, et al: Utility of anti-Hu antibodies in the diagnosis of paraneoplastic sensory neuronopathy. Ann Neurol 1998;44:976–980.

Moll JW, Antoine JC, Brashear HR, et al: Guidelines on the detection of paraneoplastic anti-neuronal specific antibodies. Neurology 1995;45:1937–1941.

Moody JF: Electrophysiological investigations into the neurological complications of carcinoma. Brain 1965;88:1023–1036.

Norris FH, Denys EH, Sang K, Mukai E: A population study of amyotrophic lateral sclerosis. Ann Neurol 1989;26:139–140.

Oh SJ: Paraneoplastic vasculitis of the peripheral nervous system. Neurol Clin 1997;15:849–863.

Posner JB: Neurologic Complications of Cancer. Philadelphia, FA Davis, 1995.

Pourmand R, Maybury BG: Paraneoplastic sensory neuronopathy. Muscle Nerve 1996;l19:1517–1522.

Prineas J: Polyneuropathies of undetermined cause. Acta Neurol Scand Suppl 1970;44:1–72.

Riva M, Brioshi AM, Marazzi R, et al: Immunological and endocrinological abnormalities in paraneoplastic disorders with involvement of the autonomic nervous system. Ital J Neurol Sci 1997;18:157–161.

Rosenfeld MR, Posner JB: Paraneoplastic motor neuron disease. Adv Neurol 1991;56:445–459.

Rosenfeld MR, Verschuuren J, Dalmau J: Paraneoplastic syndromes of the peripheral nervous system. Handbook Clin Neurol 1997;25:373–393.

Rowland LP, Schneck S: Neuromuscular disorders associated with malignant neoplastic disease. J Chron Dis 1963;16:777–795.

Rowland LP, Sherman WH, Latov N, et al: Amyotrophic lateral sclerosis and lymphoma: Bone marrow examination and other diagnostic tests. Neurology 1992;42:1101–1102.

Schold SC, Cho E, Somasundaram M, Posner JB: Subacute motor neuronopathy: A remote effect of lymphoma. Ann Neurol 1979; 5:271–287.

Siemsen JK, Meister L: Bronchogenic carcinoma associated with severe orthostatic hypotension. Ann Intern Med 1963;58:669–676.

Sodhi N, Camiller M, Camopiano JK, et al: Autonomic dysfunction and motility in intestinal pseudo-obstruction caused by paraneoplastic syndrome. Dig Dis Sci 1989;34:1937–1942.

Trojaborg W, Franzen E, Anderson I: Neuropathy and myopathy associated with carcinoma of the lung. Brain 1969;92:71–82.

Uchuya MF, Graus F, Vega R, et al: Intravenous immunoglobulin in paraneoplastic neurological syndrome with anti-neuronal autoantibodies. J Neurol Neurosurg Psychiatr 1996;61:388–392.

Vallat JM, De Mascared HA, Bordessoule D, et al: Non-Hodgkin's malignant lymphomas and peripheral neuropathies—13 cases. Brain 1995;118:1233–1245.

von Oosterhout AG, Van de Pol M, ten Velde GP, Twijnstra A: Neurologic disorders in 203 patients with small cell lung cancer: Results of a longitudinal study. Cancer 1996;77:1434–1441.

Vega F, Graus F, Chen QM, et al: Intrathecal synthesis of the anti-Hu antibody in patients with paraneoplastic encephalomyelitis or sensory neuronopathy: Clinical-immunologic correlations. Neurology 1994;44:21–45.

Veilleux M, Bernier JP, Lamarche JB: Paraneoplastic encephalomyelitis and subacute dysautonomia due to an occult atypical carcinoid tumour of the lung. Can J Neurol Sci 1990;17:324–328.

Verma A, Berger JR, Snodgrass S, Petito C: Motor neuron disease: A paraneoplastic process associated with anti-Hu antibody and small cell lung carcinoma. Ann Neurol 1996;40:112–116.

Vernio S, Adamski J, Kryzer TJ, et al: Neuronal nicotinic ACh receptor antibody in subacute autonomic neuropathy and cancer related syndromes. Neurology 1998;50:1806–1813.

Verschuuren JJ, Penquin M, Ten Velde G, et al: Anti-Hu antibody titer and brain metastasis before and after treatment for small cell lung cancer. J Neurol Neurosurg Psychiatr 199;67:353–357.

Vincent D, Dubas F, Hauw JJ, et al: Nerve and muscle microvasculitis in peripheral neuropathy: A remote effect of cancer. J Neurol Neurosurg Psychiatr 1986;49:1007–1010.

Voltz RD, Graus F, Posner JB, Delmau J: Paraneoplastic encephalomyelitis: An update on the effects of the anti-Hu immune response. J Neurol Neurosurg Psychiatr 1997;63:133–136.

Windebank AJ, Blexrud MD, Dyck PJ, et al: The symptoms of acute sensory neuropathy. Neurology 1990;40:584–594.

Younger DS, Rowland LP, Latov N, et al: Motor neuron disease and amyotrophic lateral sclerosis: Relation with high protein contents to paraproteinemia and clinical syndromes. Neurology 1990;40:595–599.

Younger DS, Rowland LP, Latov N, et al: Lymphoma motor neuron disease and amyotrophic lateral sclerosis. Ann Neurol 1991; 29:78–86.

Younger DS, Dalmau J, Inghirami G, et al: Anti-Hu associated peripheral nerve and microvasculitis. Neurology 1994;44:181–182.

Younger DS: Motor neuron disease and malignancy. Muscle Nerve 2000;23:658–660.

Peripheral Neuropathies Associated with Vascular Diseases and the Vasculitides

Asa J. Wilbourn

The components of the peripheral nervous system (PNS) must continually receive adequate blood flow for their integrity to be preserved. Whenever the blood supply to a portion of a nerve is insufficient in this regard, that segment is rendered ischemic. First the function and then the structure of the nerve fibers are compromised, depending principally on the severity and duration of the ischemic insult.

In general, an ischemic event of short duration produces only physiological changes; these are limited to the affected portion of the axon and manifest as an impairment (slowing or block) in its conduction properties. Once an adequate blood supply to the briefly ischemic segment is restored, normal conduction along it soon returns, and characteristically there are no apparent residuals. This type of short-lived PNS ischemia occurs as a byproduct every time tourniquets are applied to limbs to provide bloodless surgical fields.

Whenever an ischemic bout is more prolonged, however, the nerve fibers and their supporting elements begin to sustain injury to varying degrees. Unlike the situation with transient ischemia, these may cause changes that not only persist indefinitely after the local ischemia has been corrected but also may have structural effects far removed from the local site of injury, via the process of nerve fiber death, with resulting wallerian degeneration.

The fact that the first symptoms of what will soon become an established acute ischemic neuropathy are due to nonstructural injury, and are thus readily reversible, imparts an urgency to the treatment of some of these disorders that is not shared by any other type of PNS lesion (Sunderland, 1991; Wilbourn et al., 1983; Wilbourn and Levin, 1993).

ANATOMY AND PHYSIOLOGY

Peripheral nerve trunks are vascularized by superficial and deep longitudinal arterial chains, linked by an elaborate, extensive network of anastomoses in the epineurium, perineurium, and endoneurium. These are fed by a succession of nutrient arteries of varying number and size that enter at irregular intervals. Most of these are direct branches that arise from major arteries that supply the limb. However, some are subsidiary branches, derived from passing arteries that primarily supply muscles. There is considerable overlap in the distribution of the nutrient arteries that provide blood to a given nerve trunk; consequently, no single artery is responsible for the entire vascular supply of a nerve. However, the redundancy of blood supply is not complete along the entire length of many nerve trunks. As a result, some segments—which are fairly constant from one limb to another—receive essentially their entire blood flow from a single artery. These segments of the nerve trunks may be more susceptible to ischemic injury than are other segments (Richards, 1951; Sunderland, 1991).

Peripheral nerves lack autoregulation of blood flow; nevertheless, their requirements with regard to the latter are relatively low. Muscle fibers also have a well-developed collateral vascular network similar to that of nerve fibers. In addition, their resting oxygen consumption is even lower than that of peripheral nerves, and they have the capacity for autoregulation (Ritchie, 1967; Wilbourn et al., 1983; Low and Tuck, 1984). For these reasons, both nerve fibers and muscle fibers are relatively resistant to ischemic compromise. Nevertheless, both fail to function when subjected to sufficient ischemia, initially for physiological reasons and then for structural ones. Almost all the research has shown that in an ischemic environment, peripheral nerve fibers cease to conduct impulses before muscle fibers become inexcitable. Thus, there is general agreement that the threshold for ischemic dysfunction of peripheral nerve is lower than that for muscle (Chervu et al., 1989; Wilbourn and Levin, 1993). However, this consensus regarding the relative ischemic thresholds for nerve and muscle does not extend to their relative infarction thresholds. Instead, there is considerable disagreement on this point. Most animal research suggests that muscle has a lower ischemic infarction threshold than does nerve (i.e., muscle fibers degenerate before nerve fibers do so when exposed to a severe degree of ischemia) (Korthals et al., 1985). However, it is an incontrovertible fact that in humans there is at least one type of ischemic nerve disorder—ischemic monomelic neuropathy—in which the reverse is characteristic; that is, nerve fibers degenerate, whereas muscle fibers are unaffected (Wilbourn et al., 1983).

PATHOLOGY AND PATHOPHYSIOLOGY

Ischemia of a limb can simultaneously damage both nerve fibers and muscle fibers. Fortunately, these two kinds of injury can usually be distinguished from one another in the electrodiagnostic laboratory due to their differing presentations. These electrodiagnostic characteristics are discussed, beginning with the effects of ischemia on peripheral nerves.

With very few exceptions, all the electrodiagnostic abnormalities seen in patients with peripheral nerve disorders are the result of, in a broad sense, one of two types (or both) of underlying pathology: focal demyelination and axon degeneration. With focal demyelination, although the nerve fiber insult is substantial enough to damage the myelin at the site of the lesion, it does not kill the axon, and it has no effect on any portion of the segment of nerve beyond that point. In contrast, with axon degeneration, the insult is of such severity that it kills the axon at the lesion site, resulting in the entire segment of nerve distal to that point undergoing wallerian degeneration. When single axons are affected, these two fundamental types of pathology have three different pathophysiological presentations on nerve conduction studies (NCSs), as follows.

Conduction Slowing

This process results in the speed of nerve transmission being reduced as the impulse traverses the injured segment of nerve; once beyond that point, however, the speed reverts to normal. It is seen with focal demyelination.

Conduction Block

With this process, the nerve impulse is stopped at the lesion site; however, conduction remains normal along the nerve segment distal to that point. This process is seen with both demyelination (where it is referred to as a *demyelinating conduction block*) and early axon-loss lesions. With the latter, it is found only within the first week or so after axon loss has occurred, at a time when the distal stump of the fiber can still conduct impulses, even though it is actively undergoing wallerian degeneration. This type of conduction block is referred to as an *axon discontinuity conduction block*.

Conduction Failure

With this process, impulse conduction is lost along the entire segment of nerve distal to the lesion site because the axon and the myelin that envelops it have degenerated. It is seen with axon-loss lesions of more than 7 to 10 days' duration.

In the electrodiagnostic laboratory, conduction abnormalities are being detected not along single axons but rather along peripheral nerves that are composed in part of hundreds of large myelinated nerve fibers. Consequently, the number of possible pathophysiologies that may be present is expanded. With regard to conduction slowing, either conduction along all the fibers may be affected to the same degree, resulting in focal (synchronized) slowing, or conduction along the very largest fibers may be unaffected while that along the slower conducting ones is compromised to varying degrees, resulting in differential (desynchronized) slowing. Obviously, combined focal and differential slowing can readily occur. Because any number of individual axons composing a peripheral nerve can be affected by conduction block or conduction failure, at least two modifiers, at a minimum, are required to describe such lesions: *partial* and *complete*. These indicate whether all, or only some, of the axons at the injury site are affected. The electrophysiological and clinical attributes of each of the differing types of focal pathophysiology are described in Table 67–1 (Wilbourn and Ferrante, 2000).

Special circumstances apply whenever focal nerve injuries result from ischemia. The situation is complicated by the fact that although ischemia serves as one of the many causes of the two basic types of pathology described previously, it also can function, in its own right, as a focal pathological process, thereby altering physiology. It has been known since the studies of Lewis and associates (1931) that focal ischemia induced by compression can produce fleeting motor and sensory deficits. Gilliatt (1975)

Table 67–1. Electrophysiological and Clinical Manifestations of the Five Types of Pathophysiology Resulting from Focal Nerve Lesions, Recording Distal to a Significant Lesion

Type of Pathophysiology	Nerve Conduction Study Changes	Needle Electrode Examination Changes	Clinical Findings
Axon loss			
Axon discontinuity conduction block	Substantially lower-amplitude, nondispersed response on stimulating proximal, compared with distal, to lesion	Marked dropout of motor unit potentials	Weakness; sensory loss (all modalities)
Conduction failure	Equally low-amplitude responses, regardless of stimulation sites	Marked dropout of motor unit potentials; fibrillation potentials (after 3 wks)	Weakness; sensory loss (all modalities)
Demyelination			
Synchronized slowing	Response slowed (i.e., latency increased) while traversing lesion site, without configurational change	None	None
Desynchronized slowing	Response dispersed but latency unchanged while traversing lesion site; amplitude low if dispersal substantial	None	Deep tendon reflexes decreased; vibratory sense impaired
Conduction block	Substantially lower-amplitude, nondispersed response on stimulating proximal, compared with distal, to lesion	Marked dropout of motor unit potentials (often fibrillation potentials after 3 wks)	Weakness; sensory loss (position, vibration, light touch only)

© CCF, 2001.

later referred to this phenomenon as a *rapidly reversible physiological block.* This type of ischemic conduction block is presumed to be responsible for the short-lived motor and sensory deficits produced by acute trauma (e.g., compression or traction); in these instances, the episodes are simply too brief in duration to be attributed to demyelination with subsequent remyelination. Transient ischemia in certain situations is therefore the reputed pathological process underlying the clinical presentation referred to as *neurapraxia,* although focal demyelination far more often is the culprit (Seddon, 1943). Brief episodes of ischemic conduction block affecting axons that are already damaged (i.e., that have some focal demyelination along them) also are thought to cause the bouts of temporary loss of power and sensation that often are reported by patients with carpal tunnel syndrome (Gilliatt, 1975).

Even though it is well accepted that ischemia alone can produce short-lived conduction block, whether it also can cause more prolonged conduction block (i.e., one persisting for several days to several weeks) is controversial. A number of investigators have reported detecting such block along one or more nerves. In most instances, however, these were simply mentioned, without any accompanying details provided, in articles concerned with a series of patients with vasculitic neuropathy (Kissel et al., 1985; Hawke et al., 1991; Davies et al., 1996). Other investigators have disputed these findings, principally noting the following.

• The amplitudes of the motor NCS responses, on stimulation both distal and proximal to the lesion, were so small (Ropert and Metral, 1990) that the presumed conduction block was spurious, resulting from phase shift with cancellation.

• The motor NCSs were performed within a few days after an axon-loss lesion occurred, and a conduction block resulting from axon discontinuity was mistakenly attributed to focal ischemia (Cornblath and Sumner, 1990; McCluskey et al., 1999).

However, there are at least five credible reports in which neither of these objections appears to apply. In all of these reports, on NCSs performed several days after the presumed onset of nerve damage, one or more motor nerves showed very prominent conduction block, and the compound muscle action potentials (CMAPs) on distal stimulation were several millivolts in amplitude. Moreover, in most instances, the NCSs were repeated at later times, to confirm that the initial findings had not been due to an axon discontinuity conduction block (Jamieson et al., 1991; Shields et al., 1991; Gledhill and Inshasi, 1992; Homberg et al., 1992; Mohamed et al., 1998) (Table 67–2).

Given that a relatively prolonged conduction block can be caused by focal ischemia—and the evidence on this point appears rather compelling—a pertinent question arises: What is the pathogenetic mechanism underlying it? There are two separate hypotheses on this point, based in part on experimental research (the circumstances of which are very different in several respects from the clinical situations described earlier). In the first theory, it is contended that the conduction block in these instances is metabolic in origin, caused by the reduced blood flow at the lesion site. Thus, although the ischemia is not severe enough to actually kill axons, or even myelin, it is sufficient to compromise their ability to conduct nerve impulses. The majority of the authors of the five reports described earlier apparently subscribe to this hypothesis. The

Table 67–2. Reports of Prolonged Conduction Block Caused by Ischemia

Study	Patient	Underlying Disorder	Timing of Initial NCS In Relationship to Onset of Weakness	Motor Nerve Affected	NCS Amplitudes (mV) (Distal/Proximal)	Repeat NCS Amplitudes (mV) (Elapsed Time Since First NCS) (Distal/Proximal)
Shields et al., 1991	26-yr-old woman	Sickle cell anemia	± 24 d	Right median	12/4	— (21 d)
Jamieson et al., 1991	59-yr-old woman	Necrotizing angiopathy	?	Left ulnar	6/0.5	4.2/3.6 (42 d)
Gledhill and Inshasi, 1992	42-yr-old man	Presumed vasculitic process (nerve biopsy supportive)	?	Left median Left tibial	10/4.5 7.5/4.5	7.5/6.8 8/3.5 (7 d)
Homberg et al., 1992	35-yr-old woman	Ergotamine tartrate abuse	5 d	Right tibial Right peroneal	15/3.2 2.7/1.1	11.7/5.8 3.4/2.8 (+ 30 d)
Mohamed et al., 1998	67-yr-old man	Presumed vasculitic process (no nerve biopsy)	?	Right median Right ulnar	11/0.7 8.9/5.7	11.9/2.3 9.3/3.7

NCS, nerve conduction study; d = days.

experimental work they cite was performed by Parry and Linn (1988), who caused incomplete infarction of tibial nerves in 37 rats by injecting arachidonic acid into their femoral arteries. In more than 50% of the animals, there was evidence not only of substantial axon loss but also of conduction block along some of the surviving fibers. These conduction blocks were short-lived, resolving in the majority of animals by 3 days and in all except one animal by 7 days after infarction. Although the authors considered that these changes could have been due to segmental demyelination, they rejected this supposition, based on the time course of recovery and the examination of single teased fibers taken from the level of the lesion.

In the second theory, it is proposed that the conduction block is due to focal demyelination induced by ischemia. One of the principal sources of reference for this is an article by Fowler and Gilliatt (1981). They caused ischemia along the tibial branch of the sciatic nerve in 40 rabbits by ligating the major artery that supplies the limb. In nearly 25% of animals, axon loss was extensive but incomplete, and varying degrees of conduction block were present along the surviving fibers at the presumed lesion site, situated between the middle calf and upper thigh. In four animals, the conduction blocks were substantial, with distal amplitudes ranging from 2.5 to 6.8 mV and proximal amplitudes decreasing anywhere from 92% to 61%. Repeat studies revealed that these conduction blocks persisted for approximately 15 days in two animals and for approximately 24 days in two others. On histological examination, the authors found selective myelin damage at the lesion site, which they considered a more likely explanation of the conduction block than continuing ischemia. They based their reasoning on (1) the fact that the time course of changes was similar to those seen after brief periods of nerve compression that caused demyelinating conduction block and (2) the fact that the conduction block was constant and reproducible, rather than fluctuating in severity, as it should if caused by ischemia.

Most of the reported ischemia-induced conduction blocks in humans have been located along nerve segments at points where they could be detected by motor NCSs, although occasionally, with upper extremity lesions, the nerves have had to be stimulated proximal to the standard elbow stimulation sites. Even if a conduction block is situated so proximally that the nerve fibers cannot be stimulated percutaneously proximal to it (e.g., in the upper extremity at or proximal to the upper midportions of the trunks of the brachial plexus and in the lower extremity proximal to the popliteal fossa), it can still be suspected if the CMAP amplitude recorded from a weak muscle appears disproportionately high compared with both the degree of weakness manifested by that muscle on clinical examination and the marked dropout of motor unit potentials (MUPs) seen on needle electrode examination (NEE) of the muscle.

An interesting postscript is that in two of the three patients with ischemic conduction block caused by vasculitis, the lesions subsequently progressed to axon loss with resulting conduction failure, as demonstrated by motor NCSs performed later in the course of their illness (Jamieson et al., 1991; Mohamed et al., 1998).

Although nerve ischemia on rare occasions produces conduction block that persists up to several weeks, far more often it manifests as axon loss. These lesions have the same characteristics as axon damage caused by any other process. How they present on electrodiagnostic examination depends on several factors, such as their location, severity, and duration. Nevertheless, similar to any other axon-loss lesion, they affect either the NEE alone or both the NEE and the NCS, and they do so in a predictable manner. Whenever very mild axon loss involves mixed nerves, the only detectable abnormalities seen on the electrodiagnostic examination are found on the NEE, at 3 weeks or later after the onset: a minimal-to-modest number of fibrillation potentials in at least some of the muscles innervated by the damaged nerve. With more severe axon loss along mixed nerves, the NCSs, while stimulating and recording distal to the lesion, show abnormalities as well. Initially, the sensory nerve action potentials (SNAPs) are reduced in amplitude. These begin to fall 5 days after lesion onset and reach their maximal amplitude reduction at 10 to 11 days after onset. Whenever axon loss is even more substantial, the amplitudes of the CMAPs also are affected. These start to drop 2 to 3 days after onset and reach their nadir at day 7. Typically, at the point when motor NCS amplitude changes appear, additional abnormalities are noted on NEE: the MUPs are observed to fire in decreased numbers, at faster than their basal firing rate—an MUP firing pattern referred to as reduced *MUP recruitment*. After a few months, if the denervated muscle fibers are reinnervated, the number of fibrillation potentials that are present gradually decreases and highly polyphasic MUPs appear. Ultimately, after a focal nerve injury, either reinnervation can result in complete restitution of the MUPs, or if it is accomplished by substantial collateral sprouting it can end with permanently decreased MUP recruitment, with most or all of the MUPs showing chronic neurogenic changes (e.g., being of increased duration and polyphasic). Conversely, with extremely severe lesions in which no reinnervation occurs, after 1 1/2 to 2 years the denervated muscle fibers die and subsequently degenerate. At this point, no CMAP can be elicited on motor NCSs from the completely degenerated muscle, and NEE of the muscle reveals little more than electrical silence: the insertional activity is markedly decreased or absent; few, if any, fibrillation potentials are observed (and when present, they typically are minute in size); and no MUPs can be activated. After a varying interval, the denervated muscle becomes fibrotic and manifests all the NEE changes seen with end-stage ischemic muscle degeneration (discussed later). In contrast to the NCS amplitude changes and NEE findings that it produces, focal ischemia—similar to all the other axon-loss lesions—has little to no effect on those components of the NCS that are altered primarily by demyelinating conduction slowing: the latencies, the conduction velocities, and the durations of the CMAPs and SNAPs (Wilbourn and Levin, 1993; Wilbourn and Ferrante, 2000).

Direct ischemic damage of muscle, when mild, probably produces little more than a modest number of fibrillation potentials. When it is more severe, usually a mixture of fibrillating and electrically silent muscle fibers is found on NEE, at least in certain areas of the muscle. In these instances, some of the muscle fibers undergo degeneration from the ischemia, whereas others, although they survive, are denervated as a result of degeneration of the intramuscular nerve fibers that supply them (Allbrook and Aitken, 1951; Sanderson et al., 1975). Whenever some of the muscle fibers of an ischemic muscle remain viable and under voluntary control, highly polyphasic MUPs can be seen on NEE immediately after onset. This is because the muscle fiber loss has occurred in a random manner, thereby reducing the number of muscle fibers contributing to the individual MUPs; this "disintegration of the motor unit" is responsible for the "myopathic" MUP presentation that is seen. With severe ischemia, however, all the individual muscle fibers of a muscle may degenerate. In these instances, the muscle is electrically silent on NEE from onset, and no CMAP can be recorded from it on motor NCSs. If a muscle is rendered totally ischemic and its blood supply is not reestablished, it soon becomes necrotic. However, if circulation is restored at some point after permanent injury has occurred but before the development of gangrene, the degenerated muscle fibers typically undergo fibrosis; the result is end-stage ischemic muscle degeneration, which has a characteristic appearance on NEE. The muscle essentially is electrically silent or contains, at most, a minimal number of scattered, very small fibrillation potentials. The most striking finding, however, is the marked increase in mechanical resistance offered to needle electrode advancement. Frequently, because the fibrosis is not uniform throughout the muscle, abrupt changes in mechanical resistance are noted on progressive needle advancement. This is known as the "gritty feel of fibrotic muscle" and is a highly reliable sign of irreversible muscle damage (Wilbourn and Levin, 1993).

There are two situations, related principally to the duration and severity of the lesion, in which ischemic lesions of nerve and those of muscle may be difficult to distinguish from one another. The first occurs within a few weeks after a bout of ischemia, when NEE reveals highly polyphasic MUPs in a muscle near the lesion site. These may equally represent either early reinnervating MUPs resulting from nerve fiber injury or "myopathic" MUPs caused by muscle fiber injury with subsequent disintegration of the motor units. Conversely, whenever a completely atrophic muscle is encountered 1 year or longer after a severe ischemic insult, it is impossible to determine, by either NCS or NEE, whether such end-stage muscle changes were secondary to severe denervation with absence of reinnervation or were due to primary muscle degeneration caused by direct muscle fiber damage (Wilbourn and Levin, 1993).

The major vascular causes of nerve fiber injuries are discussed under four major headings: (1) vasculitic neuropathies, (2) compartment syndromes (CSs), (3) acute limb ischemia (ischemic monomelic neuropathies and acute ischemic mononeuropathies and plexopathies), and (4) chronic ischemic neuropathies.

VASCULITIC NEUROPATHIES

Vasculitis is encountered in a heterogeneous group of disorders, the majority of which are relatively uncommon. All of them, however, manifest abnormalities resulting from the same basic disease process, characterized by inflammation and structural damage that often end in necrosis of the walls of arterial vessels. With some of the disorders in this group, vasculitis is the predominant or sole process; with others, it is considered to be secondary to another process (Collins et al., 1997; Chad et al., 2001). The "pathogenesis of vasculitis is multifactorial, complex, and incompletely understood" (Chad et al., 2001). Although it is presumed to be immunologically mediated, at least five different pathogenic mechanisms have been proposed (Hawke et al., 1991; Chad et al., 2001). All of the classifications used for vasculitis are less than optimum; most are hybrids, based in part on clinical presentation and in part on pathological findings (Table 67–3). The classifications of the vasculitides are likely to remain unsettled until more is known about the responsible immunopathogenetic mechanisms (Davies, 1994; Kissel, 1994). When the pathology characteristic of vasculitis—segmental fibrinoid necrosis of blood vessel walls associated with transmural inflammatory cell infiltrate—affects the vasa nervorum, blood flow to the nerve fibers is compromised, and the resulting ischemia produces nerve infarcts (Davies, 1994; Chad et al., 2001). The blood vessels most at risk are small arteries and arterioles with diameters of 30 to 300 μm, and which are located principally in the epineurium (Davies,

1994). The two most common disorders in which vasculitis occurs are *polyarteritis nodosa* and *rheumatoid arthritis (rheumatoid vasculitis)*. The frequency with which vasculitic neuropathy is seen in patients with vasculitis varies from one disorder to another, and precise incidence figures are not available. Nevertheless, vasculitic neuropathy occurs in up to 75% of patients with primary vasculitis (Kissel, 1994). Moreover, as Kissel (1994) observed, although vasculitic neuropathy is uncommon compared with other types of neuropathy, it is important for clinicians to recognize it, because it is a potentially treatable disorder.

Ischemia, as noted in a previous section, can produce a variety of pathological and pathophysiological reactions in peripheral nerves. Depending on the severity of the damage it causes, this ranges from transient ischemic conduction block, through focal demyelinating conduction block, to conduction failure caused by axon loss. Nevertheless, in practical terms, the underlying process with vasculitic neuropathy is axon degeneration in nearly all cases. Even in the rare instance when ischemia produces prolonged conduction block, most likely on the basis of focal demyelination, often the deleterious effects progress and axon loss ultimately supervenes (Jamieson et al., 1991; Mohamed et al., 1998).

Clinically, vasculitic neuropathy typically presents with pain, paresthesias, sensory deficits, and weakness in varying combinations, depending on the particular nerve affected, the site of involvement, and the severity of the damage (Kissel et al., 2001).

For many years, vasculitic neuropathy was thought to have essentially one clinical and electrodiagnostic presentation: mononeuropathy multiplex, caused by ischemic infarction of two or more peripheral nerve trunks (Olney, 1998). It is now appreciated, however, that the pattern of involvement with vasculitic neuropathy can vary substantially, depending on the distribution, extent, and temporal progression of the ischemic process (Kissel, 1994). Three distinct presentations, which differ significantly in their appearance, generally are considered to be those most commonly seen (Fig. 67–1).

The first pattern is that of *mononeuropathy multiplex,* in which simultaneous or sequential involvement of individual major peripheral nerves occurs, typically in different limbs; most often, the symptom onset is abrupt, but more gradual evolutions have been reported (Chad et al., 2001). Although any named peripheral nerve can be damaged by vasculitis, certain ones are affected more often than are others. Several investigators have noted more frequent involvement of nerves in the lower extremity than in the upper extremity. Of the lower extremity nerves, the common peroneal is by far the most frequently affected, followed by the tibial and sural; in contrast, the femoral and sciatic nerves are seldom involved. Among the upper extremity nerves, the ulnar is most often affected, with the median less often involved and the radial nerve even less so (Davies et al., 1996; Olney, 1998; Chad et al., 2001; Kissel et al., 2001). Characteristically, ischemic

---

Table 67–3. Some Diseases in Which Vasculitic Neuropathy Occurs

Disease	Incidence (%)	Type of Neuropathy
Primary vasculitis		
Polyarteritis nodosa	50–75	MM, OMM, SSMPN
Churg-Strauss syndrome	60–75	MM
Wegener's granulomatosis	10–20	MM, SSPN
Nonsystemic (isolated) vasculitic neuropathy	100	MM, SSMPN, OMM
Connective tissue disorders		
Rheumatoid arthritis	5–10	SSMPN, MM
Systemic lupus erythematosis	10–20	SSMPN, SSPN, MM
Sjögren's syndrome	10–20	SSPN, SSMPN
Miscellaneous disorders		
Cryoglobulinemia	50	MM
Infections		
Lyme disease (bacterial)	25	SSPN, SSMPN, R
Human immunodeficiency (viral)	2	MM, SSMPN, OMM

For each disease, the incidence of vasculitic neuropathy and the most common types that occur with it (in decreasing order of frequency) are shown.

MM, mononeuropathy multiplex; OMM, overlapping (asymmetrical) multiple mononeuropathy; R, radiculopathy; SSPN, symmetrical sensory polyneuropathy; SSMPN, symmetrical sensorimotor polyneuropathy.

Compiled from Kissel et al., 2001; Fathers and Fuller, 1996; Davies, 1994; and Kissel, 1994.

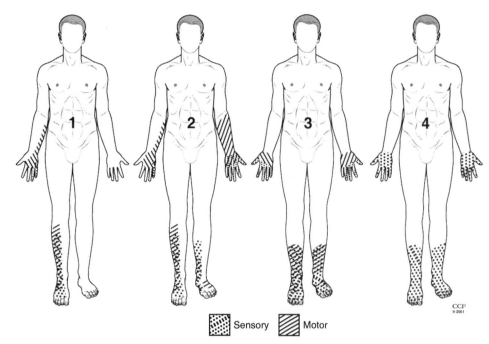

Figure 67–1. Four different patterns of peripheral nerve fiber involvement seen in patients with vasculitic neuropathy. The first three are the most common: (1) mononeuropathy multiplex, (2) overlapping multiple mononeuropathy (asymmetrical polyneuropathy), (3) symmetrical sensorimotor polyneuropathy, and (4) symmetrical sensory polyneuropathy. (Compiled from Fathers et al., 1996; Chad et al., 2001; Kissel et al., 2001; Copyright CCF, 2001.)

Sensory   Motor

damage occurs along the peripheral nerves at their "watershed zones": those regions along the nerves where they lack overlapping blood supply and are therefore at greater risk for inadequate perfusion if the blood vessel that supplies them at that point is damaged by vasculitis. In the lower extremity, these areas are situated in the middle to upper thigh, whereas in the upper extremity, they are located in the middle to upper arm region (Davies, 1994; Olney, 1998; Chad et al., 2001). Although all the axons that compose the nerve may be injured at the ischemic site, often only some of them are damaged. Thus, partial axon-loss lesions caused by ischemia are seen (Wilbourn and Levin, 1993).

The second pattern is *overlapping* or *confluent multiple mononeuropathy,* also known as *asymmetrical multifocal neuropathy* or *asymmetrical polyneuropathy.* With this presentation, so many peripheral nerves are affected, both named and unnamed, that the involvement of individual ones is obscured; the abnormalities no longer correspond to the distribution of named peripheral nerves (Kissel, 1994; Fathers and Fuller, 1996; Chad et al., 2001).

The third pattern is that of a distal, rather symmetrical, *sensorimotor polyneuropathy.* This presentation results from the peripheral nerves that supply the distal portions of the limbs being affected at multiple, more proximal levels, which produces overlapping deficits in the distal portion of the limbs (Kissel, 1994; Chad et al., 2001).

The relative frequencies of occurrence of the three main patterns of vasculitic neuropathy vary significantly among the different reported series. Nevertheless, it appears that the mononeuropathy multiplex pattern, which for many years was considered the single presentation of vasculitic neuropathy, actually serves in that capacity between 40% to

60% of the time (Wees et al., 1981; Davies, 1994; Fathers and Fuller, 1996; Chad et al., 2001). The relative incidences of all these patterns also appear to vary, depending on the particular type of vasculitic neuropathy that is present (see Table 67–3).

In addition to the three most commonly recognized presentations, at least two others have been reported: (1) a predominantly sensory polyneuropathy, which may begin asymmetrically, and (2) sensory loss in the distribution of small cutaneous nerves, especially the digital nerves in the upper extremity and the medial or lateral plantar nerves in the lower extremity that supply the sole of the foot (Moore and Fauci, 1981; Dyck et al., 1987; Kissel et al., 2001).

The particular clinical presentation of vasculitic neuropathy in the individual patient is of more than academic interest, because it is one of the factors that determine how soon the correct diagnosis is made after symptom onset. Davies (1994) noted that the mean duration of symptoms was 9.2 weeks in patients who presented with mononeuropathy multiplex, whereas it was 31.6 weeks in those presenting with asymmetrical multifocal neuropathy. Of the three major presentations, probably the most difficult to diagnose is the symmetrical sensorimotor polyneuropathy pattern, particularly when it is symmetrical from onset and has a steady progression (Kissel et al., 2001). In these instances, ischemic neuropathy shares very nonspecific clinical and electrodiagnostic manifestations with a great number of known and unknown causes for a nondescript axon-loss polyneuropathy.

Electrodiagnostic Examination

The electrodiagnostic examination is quite helpful in the evaluation of patients with suspected vasculitic neuropathy, because it can demonstrate the type, distribution (pattern), and severity of the electrophysiological abnormalities that are present (Kissel, 1994). Because the lesions characteristically are axon loss in type, both the NEE and the NCS (specifically, the amplitudes of the responses) are important. The particular abnormalities sought are (1) on the NCS, low-amplitude or unelicitable SNAPs and CMAPs, with normal or near-normal latencies and motor conduction velocities, and (2) on the NEE, fibrillation potentials, reduced MUP recruitment, and, if the process is chronic (>4 to 6 months' duration), chronic neurogenic MUP changes.

The electrodiagnostic examination has proved to be a useful diagnostic procedure with vasculitic neuropathies in three separate respects. First, it identifies the pattern of involvement of the various peripheral nerve fibers. This is especially helpful in ascertaining whether the process is symmetrical or asymmetrical and, if the latter, whether it is involving solely named peripheral nerves or has become more confluent in distribution in a given limb. To accomplish this, the electrodiagnostic studies usually must be quite extensive, focused not only on the symptomatic limb or limbs and portions of limbs but also on the asymptomatic limbs. In general, this entails, at a minimum, performing both NCSs and NEE in homologous limbs and then making side-to-side comparisons. With regard to the patterns of involvement, certain electrodiagnostic features speak against a symmetrical sensorimotor polyneuropathy: (1) asymmetry of NCS and NEE findings at the same limb level in homologous limbs, (2) more severe abnormalities in the upper extremity than in the lower extremity, and (3) substantial differences in degree of involvement of the same type of nerve (e.g., motor, sensory) at the same limb level in a single extremity (Olney, 1998).

Second, the NCS portion of the electrodiagnostic examination can help identify suitable nerves for biopsy, such as the sural or superficial radial sensory. Generally, the SNAP amplitude will be reduced when recording from a nerve affected by the vasculitic process, even if clinical sensory deficits are not present in the distribution of the nerve. Thus, the diagnostic yield of a particular sensory nerve biopsy is increased considerably if an NCS performed earlier on that nerve has demonstrated an abnormal SNAP (Wees et al., 1981; Bouche et al., 1986; Chad et al., 2001).

Third, the results of the electrodiagnostic examination can serve as a baseline concerning the severity and pattern of involvement of the ischemic neuropathy. Future electrodiagnostic examinations can then disclose whether the process is progressing, recovering, or remaining static; this information can be useful in determining the efficacy of treatment (Collins et al., 1997).

Finding abnormalities in the distribution of clinically unaffected nerves can be very helpful for diagnosis, because often this suggests that the disorder is more widespread than clinically suspected

(Bouche et al., 1986; Parry, 1986; Olney, 1998; Chad et al., 2001). Conversely, both persistent conduction block and substantial conduction slowing, when found on the NCS, speak against vasculitis as the etiology (Collins et al., 1997).

As important as the electrodiagnostic examination is in the assessment of vasculitic neuropathy—and in this regard it has been described with such adjectives as "crucial" and "imperative"—the ultimate definitive diagnosis of this disorder depends on nerve biopsy (Wees et al., 1981; Kissel, 1994). It is also pertinent to note that although the PNS manifestations of vasculitic neuropathy often respond quite well to treatment, the latter apparently does little to change the overall life expectancy of patients who have systemic vasculitis (Davies, 1994).

Unfortunately, in certain situations, the value of the NCS in the diagnosis of vasculitic neuropathy is compromised. The results of the sensory NCS are difficult to interpret in (1) elderly patients in whom the lower extremity SNAPs are bilaterally unelicitable, even when the clinical symptomatology is strictly unilateral; such NCS changes are encountered rather frequently and are considered a normal variant of the aging process, and (2) patients administered chemotherapy to treat the primary medical condition responsible for their vasculitis, in whom all the SNAPs are low in amplitude or unelicitable. Moreover, the electrodiagnostic examination, again primarily the NCS component, occasionally yields misleading information. An example of this, already mentioned, is encountered whenever motor NCSs are performed on a damaged nerve within a few days after onset of symptoms. In these instances, a prominent axon discontinuity conduction block may be demonstrated, leading to the erroneous conclusion that the underlying pathophysiology is demyelinating in nature (Collins et al., 1997; McCluskey et al., 1999). Also, in some patients in whom the distal lower extremities are affected, the sural nerves escape involvement (Hawke et al., 1991). The resulting combination of electrodiagnostic findings—normal sural SNAPs bilaterally; low-amplitude peroneal and posterior tibial motor CMAPs bilaterally, recording intrinsic foot muscles; absent H responses bilaterally; and NEE evidence of axon loss in the muscles distal to the knees—is very suggestive of a lumbar intraspinal canal lesion involving the L5 and S1 segments or roots bilaterally, with the NEE abnormalities restricted to the middle and distal muscles of the limbs (a rather common presentation). As a result of these spurious localizations, clinicians may unsuccessfully seek structural lesions in the lumbosacral regions (Battaglia et al., 1990).

COMPARTMENT SYNDROMES

The term *compartment syndrome* (CS) describes a basic pathophysiological process that is common to a number of what appear clinically to be diverse entities. These can be defined as disorders of very varied cause in which an increase in the tissue pressure within a restricted body space compromises the microcirculation, and consequently the function, of neuromuscular structures within that space. Full-blown CSs have four requisite components.

1. *A limiting envelope:* This acts as the inelastic boundary of the space. Serving in this function may be various combinations of bone, muscle, and fascia; fascia alone; epimysium; skin; or a variety of external constricting structures, such as circumferential casts, bandages, and splints.
2. *Elevated tissue pressure:* Most often, this is due to an increase in the contents of the compartment, caused by fluid accumulation. Less often, it results from boundary restriction, whereby compartment size is reduced, thus decreasing the amount of swelling necessary to elevate intracompartmental pressure.
3. *Reduced perfusion of neuromuscular structures within the compartment, because of reduced tissue circulation:* the latter most often is attributed to either microvascular occlusion (e.g., capillary closure) or a decrease in the arteriovenous gradient. Thus, in contrast to vasculitic neuropathy, the blood vessels affected by CSs are capillaries and venules rather than arterioles (Wilbourn and Levin, 1993).
4. *Neuromuscular abnormalities, resulting from the progressive ischemia*

The tissue damage caused by CSs is thought to be due to ischemia-reperfusion (incidentally, the same pathophysiological mechanism that is responsible for much of the tissue destruction that occurs during the thawing phase of frostbite injury [Wilbourn, 2001]). This theory contends that ischemia depletes intracellular energy stores. After reperfusion and the formation of toxic oxygen radicals, this depletion results in a cascade of adverse consequences, including (1) activation and adhesion of leukocytes and platelets, which narrow or occlude small blood vessels; (2) calcium influx into cells; (3) failure of cellular membrane ion pumps; and (4) transudation of fluid. Collectively, these produce both excess fluid within cells and excess interstitial fluid (i.e., edema formation), which in turn increases venous pressure within the compartment. Thus, a vicious circle is set in motion, in which increasing venous pressure produces increasing capillary pressure, which exacerbates fluid transudation and cellular swelling. Eventually, when intracompartmental pressure equals or exceeds capillary pressure, blood flow essentially stops in the small vessels. Unless it is promptly rectified, this initiates tissue infarction (Johansen and Watson, 2000). The major structures at risk with a CS are the muscles within the compartment. On occasion, major peripheral nerves also are within the compartment and therefore also are subject to injury. These nerves include the deep peroneal nerve in the anterior compartment of the leg, the lumbar plexus in the psoas compartment in the pelvis, the median nerve in the volar compart-

ment of the forearm, and various components of the infraclavicular plexus within the medial brachial fascia compartment in the axilla (which, unlike most other compartments, contains no muscle). Rarely, peripheral nerves are injured by compartment swelling, even though they are only near the affected compartment and not actually within it; this is how the sciatic nerve can be compromised by a gluteal CS (Wilbourn, 2001).

A coherent discussion of CSs must be preceded by a definition of terms. The two general types of CS are *acute* and *chronic.* Acute CS has by far the most serious adverse consequences. Evolving or developing acute CSs are labeled *incipient;* once they are full-blown, they are called *established.* Chronic CSs are referred to, variously, as *exercise-induced, exertional, intermittent,* and *recurrent* (Mubarak, 1981a; Barnes, 1997; Botte et al., 1998; Hargens and Mubarak, 1998; von Schroeder and Botte, 1998; Swain and Ross, 1999). Two major complications of acute CSs, both of which are due to irreversible ischemic damage to the muscles within the affected compartment, have special designations. The first is *Volkmann's ischemic contracture,* which is the end-stage manifestation of an acute CS in which marked necrosis of muscles and soft tissues has evolved into fibrosis and contracture. The term has been used for decades, most commonly to describe the limb deformities caused by an acute volar forearm CS. The second is *crush syndrome (Bywaters' syndrome),* which is a constellation of abnormalities that result from massive rhabdomyolysis caused by multiple simultaneous acute CSs or by a single acute CS in which a large muscle mass (e.g., gluteal muscles) is affected. These abnormalities include myoglobinemia, acidosis, hyperkalemia, and third-space fluid loss, which can produce cardiac arrhythmias, renal failure, and death (Mubarak and Owen, 1975; Garfin, 1981; Owen, 1981b; Trice and Colwell, 1998).

Because the acute CSs and the chronic CSs vary substantially in many of their features, they are discussed separately.

Acute Compartment Syndromes

Acute CSs may involve one or more of approximately 50 different compartments that have been described in the human body, but the majority affect various compartments in the leg and forearm, particularly the anterior compartment of the leg and the volar compartment in the forearm (Wilbourn, 2001).

Acute CSs can be caused by a number of traumatic and nontraumatic conditions.

- Postischemic edema, resulting from several triggering events, including arterial embolism, thrombosis, or injury; vascular surgical procedures; prolonged tourniquet use; and immobilization of the limb by compression for long periods
- Accumulation of blood or other fluids, resulting

from infiltrated transfusions, bleeding disorders, or anticoagulation
• A combination of edema and blood accumulation, produced by fractures and soft tissue injury

Overall, the most common causes of acute CSs are soft tissue damage, arterial injuries, fractures, prolonged limb compression, and burns. Noteworthy is that muscle exertion alone seldom produces acute CSs (Mubarak, 1981a; Owen, 1981a; Rorabeck, 1992; Hargens and Mubarak, 1998).

Regardless of the specific cause, ultimately one process—elevated intracompartmental pressure—decreases the arteriovenous pressure, compromises tissue perfusion, and produces ischemia (Matsen, 1975; Moore and Friedman, 1989; Hargens and Mubarak, 1998).

The first symptom of acute CS is pain—deep, persistent, and increasingly severe—localized to the affected compartment. As the process progresses, paresthesias, hyperesthesias, and finally anesthesia appear in the distribution of the nerves that traverse the involved compartment. Soon the muscles within the compartment, and those innervated by nerves that traverse it, become first paretic and then, ultimately, paralyzed. Early recognition of an evolving acute CS is vital because prompt treatment can prevent irreversible damage to muscles and nerves, and sometimes even entire limbs or portions of limbs. Acute CSs consequently are one of the very few neuromuscular disorders that can justifiably be labeled a surgical emergency. For this reason, they are cared for mainly by emergency department physicians and orthopedic surgeons. Most often, acute CSs require open decompression of the involved compartment, which usually means that a fasciotomy must be performed. At times, however, they can be treated by nonsurgical means, such as by reducing limb elevation and removing constricting structures (e.g., circumferential casts and dressings), which serve as external inelastic envelopes. In general, treatment must be quite prompt—within 4 to 6 hours after weakness of the muscles within the compartment develops—to be successful. If the elevated pressure within the compartment is reduced before the muscles and nerves within it sustain irreversible damage, all neuromuscular symptoms usually promptly resolve. In contrast, with delayed or no treatment, the results usually are permanent and severe; possible adverse results include muscle fibrosis with resulting contracture, permanent peripheral nerve deficits, limb deformities and, whenever muscle necrosis is extensive, sepsis, shock, hyperkalemia, renal failure, and death (Wilbourn, 2001).

Acute CSs are diagnosed on the basis of their clinical presentation, often supplemented by measurements of the intracompartmental pressure; the most common techniques are those that use either a slit catheter or a miniature transducer-tipped catheter (Rorabeck, 1992; Hargens and Mubarak, 1998). It has been recognized that significant pressure gradients may be present at different regions within a compartment, presumably because of local hematomas. This means that pressure measurements obtained at one site may be very misleading. As a result, two of the leading investigators in the field recommended that clinical signs be given greater weight than intracompartmental pressure measurements in the diagnosis of acute CSs (Hargens and Mubarak, 1998).

Chronic Compartment Syndromes

In contrast to acute CSs, chronic CSs are caused almost entirely by exercise and overuse, and they affect almost solely a few compartments in the leg, particularly the anterior and deep posterior. Unless they convert to acute CSs, which seldom occurs, chronic CSs do not require urgent surgical treatment, because they generally respond to rest. Consequently, most chronic CSs are managed by sports medicine physicians. Also, in contrast to acute CSs, many aspects of the pathogenesis of chronic CSs are not well understood. Most often, the only symptom of chronic CSs is pain, which usually is localized to the affected compartment, provoked by exercise, relieved by rest, and gradually worsens with exercise over time. Muscle tenderness or tenseness also may be present over the affected compartment, and occasionally there is weakness of muscles within the compartment or paresthesias in the distribution of nerves that traverse the compartment, especially noted immediately after exercise.

Most chronic CSs are diagnosed exclusively on the basis of history, because typically there are no clinical findings. Attempts usually are made to confirm the clinical diagnosis by direct measurement of intracompartmental pressure. Unfortunately, although various techniques are available for continuous pressure monitoring—not only during exercise but also before and after it—there is no consensus regarding which results are considered diagnostic (Wilbourn, 2001). A variety of treatments exist for chronic CSs. Frequently, because the condition is self-limited, patients treat themselves by stopping or reducing the activity that causes them to be symptomatic. A number of corrective factors have been attempted with chronic CSs, with limited success, including complete rest of the muscles within the compartment for prolonged periods of time. In general, the only method for the successful treatment of chronic CSs is elective fasciotomy, followed by very early limb immobilization. Occasionally, a chronic CS, when maximally symptomatic (i.e., during exercise), converts to an acute CS, with all the potential risks the latter entails. In most instances, however, the most severe adverse consequence attributable to a chronic CS is curtailment of an athletic activity, which, at worst, may prematurely terminate an athletic career (Wilbourn, 2001).

Electrodiagnostic Examination

The electrodiagnostic examination is of very limited value in the diagnosis of an evolving or a very recently established acute CS. On rare occasions, the question may arise as to whether a muscle is weak because it is being rendered ischemic by a developing acute CS or because the nerve that innervates it has been injured. In these instances, a single motor NCS may be informative, because it has been demonstrated that the initial weakness resulting from an incipient acute CS is due to conduction block developing along the large myelinated motor nerve fibers within the compartment. Thus, if the tibialis anterior muscle, for example, were quite weak, stimulation of the common peroneal nerve that innervates it, both above and below the fibular head, should resolve the question. If a conduction block pattern were demonstrated at the fibular head by this means, then the lesion would have to involve the common peroneal nerve at that point. In contrast, if stimulation at both sites yielded identical results, consisting of either no CMAPs or only very low amplitude CMAPs, the responsible lesion very likely would be an acute CS, because such findings indicate that either the common peroneal nerve has its conduction blocked distal to the fibular head or the tibialis anterior muscle has been inactivated by ischemia. In either case, the electrodiagnostic examination would help in determining the severity and location of the lesion. In practice, however, electrodiagnostic examinations usually are not conducted when incipient, acute CSs are suspected, because the examinations consume valuable time, of which there is precious little to spare if a catastrophe is to be averted. Consequently, most often they are performed on patients who have static deficits caused by a remote acute CS, to document the extent and severity of the permanent residuals. Characteristically, the involved compartment contains muscles that are completely degenerated. Consequently, CMAPs cannot be recorded from them during motor NCSs, and they demonstrate electrical silence on NEE. If electrodiagnostic examinations are performed many months after the development of acute CSs, the NEE findings usually are those of end-stage ischemic muscle degeneration, as already described.

Any peripheral nerves traversing a compartment that is the site of an acute CS are killed; most often, this means virtually all the axons that compose the nerve, as well as their supporting structures (endoneurium, perineurium, and epineurium) within the compartment. For this reason, these nerves cannot be surgically repaired. Because the nerves within the affected compartment are destroyed, any muscles innervated by them distal to the compartment are denervated. Thus, whenever an acute CS involves the anterior compartment of the leg, both the tibialis anterior and extensor digitorum brevis muscles are paralyzed, but for different reasons, as a NEE of them demonstrates. Although neither contains any MUPs, the tibialis anterior lacks fibrillation potentials as well (because its muscle fibers have degenerated), whereas the extensor digitorum

brevis fibrillates profusely (because it has been denervated) (Wilbourn and Levin, 1993).

Overall, electrodiagnostic examinations in these instances can be quite helpful in the prognosis. Obviously, whenever entire muscle groups have degenerated, the chances of any useful recovery occurring are nil.

With chronic CSs, similar to acute CSs, the electrodiagnostic examination plays a relatively minor role in the diagnosis. Occasionally, the same question arises as with acute CSs: Is the weakness present due to a primary nerve lesion or to progressive ischemia of muscle and nerve caused by a chronic CS? Very infrequently, the electromyographer can answer this question based on the electrodiagnostic findings. Also, NEE occasionally demonstrates areas of remote muscle fiber degeneration within the affected muscle. In most instances, however, electrodiagnostic examinations are unrevealing when performed on limb muscles at rest that manifest chronic CS symptoms on exercise (Wilbourn, 2001).

ACUTE LIMB ISCHEMIA

An abrupt reduction in the arterial blood supply to a limb has markedly variable consequences, depending on such factors as the exact site of the lesion, the anatomical extent of the compromise, the ability of collateral channels to compensate for the reduced blood flow, and the rapidity of treatment, which often is surgical (Richards, 1951; Sunderland, 1991; Ouriel, 2000). There are a number of causes for this type of ischemic event. Most involve the proximal arterial tree—that is, the aorta or the major limb arteries that arise from it. In some instances, the vessel is compressed by an external source, such as a hematoma, neoplasm, or bony anomaly. With the more common situation, however, arterial blood flow is reduced by some type of intrinsic obstruction, most often an embolus or thrombus, especially the latter. In contrast, two quite uncommon causes are blood diversion secondary to shunt placement and blood flow impediment due to the insertion of various devices into the vessel lumen (e.g., cannula, intra-aortic balloon pump) (Perry, 1989; Ouriel, 2000). Nevertheless, the latter two causes are important, because they have been the subject of the most extensive electrodiagnostic examinations reported on patients in this category (Richards, 1954; Wilbourn et al., 1983; Levin, 1989).

With regard to the limb itself, there are three possible outcomes after the acute cessation of arterial blood flow: (1) rapid improvement, if the circulation is promptly restored, either by effective collateral circulation or by a surgical procedure; (2) gangrene, if the ischemia persists for more than several hours; and (3) an intermediary stage between the other two stages, in which the limb remains viable but manifests various disturbances in structure and function because of prior or ongoing compromise of its blood supply (Haimovici, 1950; Richards, 1951; Sunderland, 1991).

This third outcome in turn can take several forms.

1. A limb survives as a whole, but all the structures (muscles, nerves, skin, subcutaneous tissues) in their more distal portions manifest severe effects of ischemia, producing the syndrome of ischemic paralysis. In its second, and final, stage, this consists of the skin being cool, smooth, and shiny, with a tendency to ulcerate; the soft tissues being fibrotic; muscles being fibrotic and permitting neither active nor passive movements; and the distal limb being totally anesthetic (Richards, 1954; Wilbourn and Levin, 1993). One of the first detailed descriptions of this syndrome was provided by Tinel (1917), who dealt with such injuries sustained by soldiers during World War I. A pertinent point is that peripheral nerve fibers and muscle fibers are far more vulnerable to ischemia than are skin and subcutaneous tissues. Consequently, after a prolonged bout of ischemia, occasionally a limb demonstrates surface viability in the presence of total functional loss (Ouriel, 2000).

2. A limb shows postischemic residuals and ongoing vascular insufficiency but with changes not as severe as those described above. In these extremities, there often is evidence of intermittent claudication with use, moderate-to-severe burning pain, residuals of an acute CS involving one or more limb compartments, persistent color changes and coldness of the skin, and occasional small patches of superficial gangrene. This particular combination of limb abnormalities was referred to by Haimovici (1950) as *chronic postembolic ischemia.*

3. A limb has ischemic damage to the nerve fibers but apparently none to other structures, at least not to any appreciable extent. On the basis of the literature, this is a relatively rare type of outcome. When it does occur, however, two distinct types of nerve fiber injury can be recognized. With the first, the abnormalities are strikingly length dependent, with the most severe changes being present in the most distal portion of the limb. The findings become progressively less severe proximally, so that by the midportion of the limb, essentially no abnormalities are detected. At any given level, the axon damage is present to the same degree, even though fibers from different peripheral nerve trunks are involved. This type of presentation, which has been termed *ischemic monomelic neuropathy,* has been superimposed on a backdrop of peripheral arterial disease in nearly all of the reported cases (Wilbourn et al., 1983). The second type of injury consists of nerve infarcts. Nearly all the investigators who have reported these lesions have placed them in various proximal PNS structures that supply the pelvis or lower extremity (the lumbar plexus, the sacral plexus, and the femoral, sciatic, and common peroneal nerves). With this type of injury, all the abnormalities are situated distal to a particular level and, at least initially, are present to the same degree from that point distally. The portion of the nerve immediately distal to the injury site is just as involved as the portion far distal to it; that is, there is no suggestion of distal-to-proximal shading of abnormalities. This presentation also is typically superimposed on a backdrop of peripheral arterial disease; in the majority of instances, it is triggered by arterial thrombosis.

Of the many types of lesions that compromise the circulation in major vessels, arterial embolism produces ischemia in its purest form. The obstruction is intravascular and sudden in onset and usually not accompanied by confounding factors, such as vascular compression or pre-existing vascular disease (Richards, 1951; Ouriel, 2000). More than 90% of emboli originate in the heart, and nearly that same percentage (i.e., 84%) affect lower extremity blood vessels, particularly the common femoral artery. In contrast, only 16% involve upper extremity arteries (Haimovici, 1950). Usually, emboli lodge at arterial bifurcations, obstructing flow in two parallel vascular channels and thereby producing profound ischemia (Ouriel, 2000). Unfortunately, the extent of vascular occlusion that results from an embolus does not remain limited to the size of that embolus; thus, the situation is not similar to a simple arterial ligation. Rather, a series of pathophysiological events is initiated, which aggravates the already disturbed hemodynamics.

1. The embolus, as noted, usually is situated at a site where collateral channels that arise from the artery also are blocked.
2. Marked vasospasm develops soon after the embolic event, which involves both the distal segment of the artery and the collateral branches, up to and including the arterioles.
3. After a short period, blood begins to clot proximal, and particularly distal, to the embolus, forming secondary thrombosis. As a result, a much larger segment of blood vessel than that affected by the initial mechanical obstruction is involved.
4. Structural changes soon develop in the arterial wall at the site of the embolus, consisting of an inflammatory reaction that Haimovici termed *embolic periarteritis.* The changes produced by this process rapidly become irreversible (Haimovici, 1950).
5. The tissues distal to the embolus site that are rendered ischemic begin to swell.

Ultimately, acute CSs develop, either while the ischemia persists, or soon after reperfusion occurs, or both. The end result can be a crush syndrome that has major metabolic effects (Haimovici, 1950;

Ouriel, 2000). Apparently, arterial emboli have been responsible for a relatively small minority of the PNS lesions in this category.

Arterial thrombosis may be both traumatic and nontraumatic in origin, and the former may be due to either extrinsic or intrinsic causes. One of the latter causes includes the intra-arterial injection of various medications. Nontraumatic thrombosis usually develops in an underlying atheromatous lesion located within a blood vessel or a bypass graft. Thus, it typically is the final stage in progressive peripheral arterial disease (PAD). These atheromatous plaques develop at predictable sites, with few exceptions restricted to vessels in the lower extremity and pelvic region (i.e., the distal aorta, the iliac arteries, the popliteal bifurcation, and especially the femoral artery at the adductor canal) (Ouriel, 2000). Given the arterial vessels for which PAD has a marked affinity and the fact that PAD is responsible for the majority of PNS lesions that result from compromise of large arteries, it is obvious why nearly all the reports dealing with nerve infarcts caused directly or indirectly by atherosclerosis have localized the lesions to the caudal spinal cord, spinal roots, lumbar or sacral plexus, and a few lower extremity nerves.

The two distinct types of peripheral nerve fiber damage that are caused by abrupt ischemia are discussed below.

Ischemic Monomelic Neuropathy

Ischemic monomelic neuropathy (IMN) is a relatively uncommon entity that has a highly stereotyped clinical and electrodiagnostic presentation. With all IMNs, abrupt, severe compromise of blood flow along the proximal to the midportion of the major artery of a limb causes ischemic damage to axons in the more distal portion of the limb. The degree of ischemia is such that although nerve fibers are injured, other tissues (e.g., muscle, skin) are not. The arterial compromise can be caused by diversion of the blood flow (i.e., arteriovenous shunt placement), iatrogenic intrinsic obstruction of blood flow (e.g., insertion of cannulas or intra-aortic balloon pumps), atherosclerotic thrombosis, and embolism. The specific ischemic events vary in their duration but sometimes are relatively brief (e.g., a few hours at most). The PNS lesions consist of multiple, simultaneously developing axon-loss mononeuropathies, with the nerve fiber degeneration being the most severe in the most distal portion of the limb and then gradually fading proximally. At any particular limb level, the degree of involvement of the nerve fibers invariably is uniform and unrelated to the regional distribution of any individual peripheral nerve. This striking distal-to-proximal gradient of abnormalities is the most characteristic finding with IMN, on both clinical and electrodiagnostic examination, regardless of the specific cause of the disorder or the particular limb affected. Thus, the more distal aspects of the median, ulnar, and radial nerves in the upper extremity and the peroneal, tibial, and saphenous nerves in the lower extremity are all involved, and in a very similar manner at any given limb level (see later).

Although upper extremity IMN and lower extremity IMN share the same distinctive presentation, they differ in many other respects. Upper extremity IMN is the less common of the two and nearly always is both unilateral in appearance and iatrogenic in nature (Wilbourn et al., 1983; Levin, 1989; Riggs et al., 1989). Thus, almost all of the reported cases have affected the same type of patient and have had the same proximate cause. The patients all have had end-stage diabetic nephropathy, and the initiating event has consisted of the construction of an arteriovenous shunt in the proximal arm or the antecubital fossa for dialysis purposes. Presumably, IMN occurs only in diabetics who undergo this procedure because of their extensive underlying small vessel disease (Bolton et al., 1979; Wilbourn et al., 1983; Wytrzes et al., 1987; Riggs et al., 1989; Hye and Wolf, 1994; Redfern and Zimmerman, 1995; Valji et al., 1995). A few other causes have been reported, including external compression of the subclavian artery, laceration of the brachial artery, and hypercoagulable states (Lachance and Daube, 1991). In contrast to upper extremity IMN, lower extremity IMN is somewhat more common, on occasion is bilateral, and has both iatrogenic and noniatrogenic causes, with the latter more common. Causes include insertion of an intra-aortic balloon pump or a cannula into the superficial femoral artery for cardiopulmonary bypass, thrombosis of the iliofemoral artery, and partial embolic occlusion of the proximal popliteal artery or the aortoiliac artery (Wilbourn et al., 1983; Levin, 1989). Moreover, at least two reports have described patients in whom lower extremity IMN (one unilateral and one bilateral) developed after the ingestion of ergotamine tartrate or a semisynthetic version of it (Antognini, 1991; Ghali et al., 1993). In neither patient, however, was the clinical, and particularly the electrodiagnostic, features consistent with IMN, especially with regard to the requisite prominent distal-to-proximal gradient of abnormalities.

Clinically, patients with IMN present with burning pain in the hand or foot, sensory deficits that are progressively more severe distally, and weakness of the more distal limb muscles that is much more apparent in the upper than the lower extremity (Wilbourn et al., 1983).

Electrodiagnostic Examination

On electrodiagnostic examination, the findings are identical to those seen with a severe axon-loss generalized sensorimotor polyneuropathy except that, with very few exceptions, only one extremity is involved. Thus, with upper extremity IMN, on sensory NCSs the median and ulnar nerve SNAPs, with recording from the various digits, are all equally low in amplitude or unelicitable. The superficial radial SNAP, being recorded several inches more proximally, is somewhat less affected, whereas the medial and lateral antebrachial cutaneous responses, recorded in the mid-forearm, usually are normal. With regard to the motor NCS, both the median CMAP, recording thenar, and the ulnar CMAPs, recording both hypothenar and first dorsal interosseous, usually are somewhat less affected than the SNAPs recorded from the digits, presumably because the degree of axon loss present is so dependent on nerve length. On NEE, fibrillation potentials and MUP loss are most pronounced in the intrinsic hand muscles, noticeably less prominent in the muscles assessed in the distal forearm (e.g., extensor indicis proprius, flexor pollicis longus, flexor carpi ulnaris), and either minimal in degree or absent in the muscles assessed in the proximal forearm (e.g., pronator teres, brachioradialis, flexor digitorum profundus) (Fig. 67–2). Concerning the sensory (and mixed) NCS in the lower extremity, the mixed plantar responses are more abnormal than the sural SNAP, which in turn is more abnormal than the superficial peroneal sensory SNAP. This pattern reflects the length-dependent nature of the axon loss. On the motor side, the amplitudes of the peroneal CMAPs, recording extensor digitorum brevis, and the tibial CMAPs, recording abductor hallucis or abductor digiti quinti pedis, usually are quite low or unelicitable, whereas

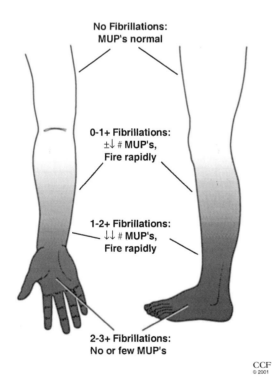

Figure 67–2. Characteristic distal-to-proximal gradient of abnormalities seen on needle electrode examination with ischemic monomelic neuropathy (IMN). (From Wilbourn AJ, Levin KH: Ischemic neuropathy. In Brown WF, Bolton CF [eds]: Clinical Electromyography, 2nd ed. Boston, Butterworth-Heinemann, 1993; 369–390, used with permission.)

the peroneal and tibial CMAPs, recording from the tibialis anterior and gastrocnemius muscles, respectively, on stimulating the same nerves in the popliteal fossa, are always much less affected. NEE of the lower extremity, similar to that of the upper extremity, vividly demonstrates the striking distal-to-proximal gradient of abnormalities. Thus, the fibrillation potentials and MUP loss are most severe in the intrinsic foot muscles, less severe in the leg muscles sampled near the ankle (extensor hallucis, flexor digitorum longus), and much less prominent in leg muscles sampled near the knee (tibialis anterior, medial gastrocnemius) (see Fig. 67–2). This pronounced distal-to-proximal shading of changes, though characteristic of IMN, is not pathognomonic of it. In the context of vascular disease that causes peripheral nerve damage, the same electrodiagnostic presentation is encountered whenever sciatic nerve infarcts located in the proximal thigh are studied many months after the event. With the latter lesion, initially it is obvious that the nerve damage is focal, because all the NEE abnormalities are located distal to a particular nerve level and because within that distal segment they are uniform in degree. With the passage of time, however, the more proximally involved muscles are reinnervated by progressive proximodistal axon regrowth or by collateral sprouting, and the sharp demarcation between normal and abnormal along the limb is lost, being replaced by a gradual shading of changes that is very similar to that seen with IMN (Wilbourn et al., 1983).

Although the underlying pathology of IMN is axon loss, it is not known with certainty exactly where this occurs along the various peripheral nerves of the limb. By far the most likely possibility is that the nerve fibers are damaged most severely in the most distal portion of the limb and progressively less in the more proximal portions, simply because the nerve fiber ischemia is more profound distally. Another possibility, however, is that the distal limb electrodiagnostic manifestations are due to proximal focal infarctions of nerve fibers, with the abnormalities accumulating along the longest axons (Wilbourn et al., 1983; Levin, 1989; Lachance and Daube, 1991).

One group of investigators has reported that the forerunner of a fully established IMN consists of conduction blocks (presumably on the basis of ischemia). They found such changes along the forearm segment of the median nerve in three patients (Kaku et al., 1993). This theory, however, is quite unlikely to be correct because it is not consistent with two basic tenets of IMN.

- The abnormalities encountered with IMN always are most severe distally and shade proximally; if the conduction block in these patients had progressed to axon loss, the abnormalities would have presented as a focal nerve infarct, rather than as IMN.
- All the nerves that supply the limb are affected, and they are affected to the same degree. However, conduction block was demonstrable only along the

median nerves, not the ulnar nerves, so if axon loss had supervened, the abnormalities would have occurred in just a median nerve distribution in the hand.

Acute Ischemic Mononeuropathies and Plexopathies

Quite infrequently, the spinal cord, roots, and plexuses, in addition to peripheral nerves, sustain acute ischemic infarcts. These can result from a variety of causes, of which one is large vessel atherosclerotic disease. Although theoretically any major neural structure could be damaged in this manner, nearly all of the reported cases have concerned pelvic and lower extremity nerve fibers. This reflects the facts that these lesions typically are caused by arterial thrombosis and that the proximal arterial system of the lower extremities, as noted previously, is quite prone to atherosclerosis (Ouriel, 2000).

The portions of the arterial system involved have included the distal aorta, the common iliac artery, the external and internal iliac arteries (especially the latter), and branches of the internal iliac artery; a pertinent point is that the last named provides the principal arterial supply to the cauda equina, the sacral plexus, and much of the lumbar plexus (Gloviczki et al., 1991; Wohlgemuth et al., 1999). The two most common precipitating causes of these acute ischemic events have been (1) atherosclerotic stenosis or occlusion of the iliac arteries or branches that arise from them, such as the femoral artery, or in grafts that have replaced portions of them, and (2) abdominal aortoiliac surgery, most often performed to treat ruptured aneurysms but sometimes performed due to graft failures or infections (in any case, operations performed to treat the complications of atherosclerosis) (Usubiaga et al., 1970; Voulters and Bolton, 1983; Boontje and Haaxma, 1987; D'Amour et al., 1987; Johnson, 1989; Gloviczki et al., 1991; Plecha et al., 1995; Robinson et al., 1997). The exact mechanism whereby these surgical procedures cause ischemic nerve fiber damage is unclear. However, it is probably multifactorial, because during these procedures, significant periods of hypotension often occur, emboli are produced, at times patients are not sufficiently heparinized, and the major vessels frequently are cross-clamped; the last may play a predominant role (Boontje and Haaxma, 1987; Plecha et al., 1995).

Most of the limited number of publications on this topic, especially those that deal with neural deficits that are first apparent in the postoperative period, have localized the responsible lesions to the caudal portion of the spinal cord. In one article, the investigators (Gloviczki et al., 1991) described nine patients who developed severe perioperative neural injuries during aortoiliac reconstruction. They localized the lesion in five patients to various regions of the caudal spinal cord; in three patients to the lumbosacral roots bilaterally plus the spinal cord,

in a "mild patchy" manner; and in the remaining patient to the lumbar plexus. On the basis of the clinical data provided in the various reports, whenever the lesions have been attributed to spinal cord involvement, such localization has appeared to be appropriate. However, it is quite a different matter when, in a relatively few articles, infarcts of the lumbar plexus, sacral plexus, femoral nerve, or sciatic nerve have been considered the cause of the neurological abnormalities. The most convincing localization in these instances has been to the femoral nerve. In a 1983 case report by Archie, the clinical description of the postoperative deficits was highly suggestive of a femoral nerve infarct. Unfortunately, localization has been much less persuasive when it has been directed toward the plexuses or sciatic nerve. At times, these structures appear to have been implicated mainly because there were no bladder abnormalities or because the symptoms involved one, rather than both, lower extremities. Unfortunately, the majority of the relatively few publications dealing with this topic contain very little or no electrodiagnostic data, presumably because electrodiagnostic examinations either were not extensive or were not performed (Ferguson and Liversedge, 1954; Archie, 1983; Boontje and Haaxma, 1987; Iliopoulos et al., 1987; Plecha et al., 1995). Moreover, in some instances, when information regarding the electrodiagnostic studies has been provided, it has been so fragmentary, or confusing, as to be inconsequential. In a 1997 article by Robinson and associates, the electrodiagnostic results are summarized in a single sentence: "Nerve conduction and electromyographic (EMG) studies demonstrated markedly reduced motor amplitudes and prolonged reflexes." In another publication, the lesion was localized to the lumbar plexus, possibly erroneously, principally because fibrillation potentials were not found in the ipsilateral lumbar paraspinal muscles (Gloviczki et al., 1991).

Localization of these lesions has faired little better when the reports have been authored by electrodiagnosticians. Thus, in a 1975 publication by Honet and colleagues, six patients were described in whom neurological deficits in one or both lower extremities developed after the use of intra-aortic balloon pumps. Although the results of the electrodiagnostic examinations were supplied for all six patients, they were not sufficient to enable the reader to localize any of the lesions. Compounding the problem, the authors provided no information regarding where they had localized the lesions or where the clinicians who cared for these patients had localized them. Consequently, although it seems probable that the neurological deficits these six patients manifested were due to infarcts of one or more PNS structures, the specific lesion locations remain unknown. Similarly, in a 1987 article by D'Amour and associates that involved six patients who had aortoiliac vascular disease, although some electrodiagnostic results were reported, they were never sufficient to permit accurate localization to be determined independently. These comments are made as observations, not as criticisms, because it can be extremely difficult at times to distinguish one proximal PNS lesion from another on the basis of clinical examination, electrodiagnostic examination, or both. This is because of the considerable amount of overlap of nerve fiber involvement between L2-4 radiculopathies, lumbar plexopathies, and femoral neuropathies on the one hand and L5-S1 radiculopathies, sacral plexopathies, and sciatic neuropathies on the other. The electrodiagnostic diagnosis of lumbar plexopathy, in particular, is always tentative at best, principally because there is no reliable sensory NCS available for assessment of fibers derived from the L3 or L4 dorsal root ganglion. If fibrillation potentials and reduced MUP recruitment are seen in the quadriceps, thigh adductors, and the ipsilateral middle and low lumbar paraspinal muscles, the responsible lesion is very likely located within the intraspinal canal, where it has affected the L2-4 roots or spinal cord segments. Conversely, if the same NEE changes are seen in various heads of the quadriceps muscles but not the ipsilateral thigh adductors or lumbar paraspinal muscles, a femoral neuropathy is very likely present. However, if the NEE changes involve the quadriceps and thigh adductors, but not the paraspinal muscles, localization is uncertain because there are always two possible diagnoses: (1) a lumbar plexopathy or (2) an L2-4 radiculopathy that lacks paraspinal fibrillation potentials. A key point is that a lumbar plexopathy can never be diagnosed by default, that is, by the absence of paraspinal fibrillation potentials. The differentiation of L5-S1 radiculopathies from sacral plexopathies and sciatic neuropathies can be a less formidable task, assuming that normal sural and superficial peroneal SNAPs are obtainable in the contralateral, asymptomatic limb. In such situations, the presence of similar SNAPs in the symptomatic limb, associated with substantial motor axon loss, would be indicative of a lumbar intraspinal canal lesion, regardless of whether ipsilateral paraspinal fibrillation potentials were present. Conversely, if in the same situation the lower extremity SNAPs were abnormal in the involved limb, the findings would be most suggestive of either a sacral plexopathy or a sciatic neuropathy. More precise localization in these instances would depend on whether NEE abnormalities were present in the glutei and tensor fascia lata. Their presence would suggest a lesion of the plexus, whereas their absence would be most consistent with a sciatic neuropathy. Unfortunately, in many patients, the sensory NCSs are unelicitable bilaterally, most often because the patients are over the age of 60 years. In these instances, localization becomes much less definite. At least one patient has been described in whom the sciatic nerve was considered the site of injury, even though an ipsilateral sural SNAP was normal and NEE revealed no abnormalities in the hamstrings (D'Amour et al., 1987). If this lack of hamstring involvement proves characteristic for sciatic nerve infarcts resulting from large vessel ischemia, it suggests that the focal damage is occurring in the more distal portion of the thigh, distal to the origin of the motor branches that supply the hamstring muscles. This would readily permit sacral plexopathies to be distinguished from sciatic neuropathies on NEE, even though all the changes on the motor and sensory NCSs, as well as on the NEE of muscles distal to the knee, would be common to both disorders. Extremely few of these reported PNS lesions have been verified at autopsy. Unfortunately, even when an autopsy is performed, confusion is not necessarily prevented. In a 1970 article by Usubiaga and colleagues, the autopsy findings on a patient who, after aortic aneurysm repair, awoke from anesthesia with total paralysis of the left lower extremity were reported to reveal "total liquefaction" of the left psoas muscle, with abnormalities of the "adjacent" left lumbosacral plexus. In the next paragraph, it was stated that the neurological symptoms could be accounted for by "infarction of the lumbosacral plexus and sciatic nerve" (Usubiaga et al., 1970). However, the lumbar plexus is not adjacent to the psoas muscle but within its substance. Moreover, the sacral plexus is a separate neural structure situated more caudally, and the sciatic nerve is much further caudally. Consequently, some questions persist regarding exactly where the responsible lesions were located that produced this patient's unilateral lower extremity nerve deficits.

Of note is that it is difficult to predict the level of vascular compromise on the basis of the particular PNS structure (e.g., lumbar plexus, femoral nerve) that is injured. Both cross-clamping of the aorta and occlusion of the common iliac artery, for example, have produced isolated ischemic femoral neuropathies (Archie, 1983; Boontje and Haaxma, 1987).

In rare instances, pelvic vascular surgery apparently can cause acute PNS abnormalities even when large vessel atherosclerosis is not present. Hefty and colleagues (1990) reported on four women, all of whom were insulin-dependent diabetics, who developed unilateral lower limb neural deficits after ipsilateral renal transplantation. In each of the four patients, the internal iliac artery had been used for revascularization of the renal allograft, and its anterior and posterior divisions had been ligated. The authors attributed their patients' symptoms to lumbosacral plexopathies caused by ischemia, which resulted from a combination of extensive small vessel disease and ligation of the internal iliac artery. Although the mechanism of injury may be accurate, the PNS localization appears speculative, based on the clinical and electrodiagnostic results provided. In one patient, the electrodiagnostic examination was reported to have documented a "sciatic nerve injury," not a lumbosacral plexopathy (Hefty et al., 1990).

Based on the above, certain facts appear evident. Whenever ischemic PNS lesions such as these are suspected, the electrodiagnostic examination must be extensive. Both lower extremity sensory NCSs—superficial peroneal sensory SNAPs and sural SNAPs—should be obtained on the symptomatic limb, because the axon loss may be incomplete, with the axons assessed by one or the other sensory NCS being relatively spared. Motor NCSs must also be performed. As with the SNAPs, both peroneal and tibial CMAPs should be obtained on the affected limb. However, the CMAPs elicited with the standard motor NCS—in which intrinsic foot muscles serve as the recorded muscles—can be misleading, because of local nerve problems (e.g., low-amplitude or unelicitable peroneal motor CMAP, recording extensor digitorum brevis, due to compression of the distal deep peroneal nerve by shoe wear; low-amplitude or unelicitable tibial CMAP, recording abductor hallucis, due to pes cavus deformity). Consequently, additional and often more reliable information can be obtained in these instances if leg, rather than foot, muscles are used for recording. Thus, peroneal CMAPs can be recorded from the tibialis anterior and peroneal muscles, and tibial CMAPs can be recorded from the gastrocnemius muscles (as the direct M component of the H response). In contrast with amplitude abnormalities seen, the latencies and conduction velocities should be normal, or nearly so. Very often, because of the patient's age, both the motor and sensory NCSs must be performed bilaterally so that side-to-side amplitude comparisons can be made. The NEE, similar to the NCS, must be extensive. It should include not only L5- and S1-innervated limb muscles but also the glutei and tensor fascia lata and the low lumbar or high sacral paraspinal muscles. At times, some muscles must be sampled in the asymptomatic contralateral limb for purposes of comparison.

Unfortunately, a confounding factor in many patients is that the lower extremity sensory NCS responses are unelicitable bilaterally, thereby seriously compromising localization, particularly for sacral plexopathies. This is because differentiation of a sacral plexopathy from L5 and S1 radiculopathies in the electrodiagnostic laboratory often rests solely on the detection of fibrillation potentials on NEE of the ipsilateral paraspinal muscles. If they are present, the lesion most likely affects the L5 and S1 roots within the intraspinal canal. However, their absence does not permit a sacral plexopathy to be diagnosed, because paraspinal fibrillation potentials are lacking in an appreciable number of proven lumbosacral radiculopathies.

As already discussed, the differentiation of long-standing (>6 to 8 months' duration) sciatic nerve infarcts from IMN can be particularly difficult. With both and for different reasons, shading of abnormalities from distal to proximal will be seen. On theoretical grounds, these two disorders should be readily separated by saphenous NCS, because the saphenous SNAP would be unelicitable with IMN but would be normal with sciatic nerve infarcts. Unfortunately, saphenous SNAPs are very difficult to obtain even in healthy, young, lean persons, and typically they are unelicitable bilaterally in most older adults, so this fact is of little more than academic interest (Wilbourn et al., 1993.)

A rare cause of acute limb ischemia has been the intra-arterial injection of various drugs, either by accident or for therapeutic purposes. The arteries involved have included the brachial, radial, ulnar, umbilical (in newborns), gluteal, and posterior tibial. These injections have caused severe thrombosis in the smaller, more distal vessels, frequently resulting in massive edema, induration, and intense pain. Among the complications reported, direct tissue injury and CSs appear to have been more prevalent than primary peripheral nerve fiber injuries. In some instances, the damage has been so severe and extensive that amputations have been necessary. Only a very few of the reports on this topic have included electrodiagnostic data; as would be expected, it was verified that the lesions were axon loss in type (Gaspar and Hare, 1972; Lachance and Daube, 1991; Chalk and Dyck, 1993; Wilbourn and Levin, 1993).

There is some confusion in the literature regarding what type of proximal vascular compromise causes the IMN pattern of nerve fiber damage (i.e., abnormalities most severe distally, shading proximally, and uniform at any given limb level) and what type causes proximal nerve infarcts (Wilbourn et al., 1983). In separate publications, Teunissen and associates (2000) and Chalk and Dyck (1993) describe the clinical and electrodiagnostic features of IMN in sections entitled "Acute Large Vessel Obstruction" and "Acute Embolism and Thrombosis," respectively. In the same publications, however, under the headings of "Ischemia after Arteriovenous Fistula" and "Iatrogenic Acute Arterial Insufficiency," the identical clinical and electrodiagnostic findings appear again, but they are not identified as being those characteristic of IMN. Thus, both reports imply, quite erroneously, that the PNS changes caused by the construction of arteriovenous shunts in the upper limbs of diabetics with renal failure are not IMN but, rather, are unique to that clinical situation (Chalk and Dyck, 1993; Teunissen et al., 2000). In fact, IMN can be produced by a variety of conditions that abruptly and severely compromise arterial blood flow in a limb, including upper extremity arteriovenous shunt construction. This point was emphasized in the 1983 article by Wilbourn and associates, in which the term *IMN* was coined: of the 14 patients reported, 4 had upper extremity IMN develop due to shunt placements, whereas 10 had lower extremity IMN develop due to cannulation, thrombosis, or embolism of various arterial structures in the pelvis or groin. Conversely, some physicians erroneously have assumed that because arterial thrombosis and embolism involving pelvic and proximal lower extremity vessels sometimes cause proximal nerve infarcts, they must always do so, even though the evidence strongly suggests that such vascular lesions can produce IMN as well as proximal nerve infarcts.

As discussed in a previous section, the peripheral nerve most frequently attacked by vasculitis is the common peroneal nerve. On rare occasions, this same nerve is injured by an embolus. The only series in the literature of such common ischemic peroneal neuropathies was reported in 1954 (Ferguson and Liversedge) and concerned nine patients. Rare instances have been reported since then (Richards, 1954). Apparently, none of the published cases have included electrodiagnostic data.

CHRONIC LIMB ISCHEMIA

Many patients, the majority of whom are elderly, experience chronic, symptomatic limb ischemia of one or both lower extremities; almost invariably, this is due to PAD (i.e., progressive, obliterative atherosclerosis). The limb structures that manifest changes resulting from the ischemia are the skin and, if the blood flow is reduced sufficiently and the limb is used, the muscles. Concerning the latter, leg pain caused by exercise and relieved by rest that results from PAD is referred to as *intermittent claudication*. Patients with these symptoms have blood flow to the limb muscles at rest that is sufficient to meet normal metabolic demands but quite inadequate to meet the increased requirements of exercise. If it is insufficient even during periods when the limb is not being exercised, rest pain ensues (TransAtlantic Inter-Society Consensus, 2000).

Beginning more than 100 years ago, various researchers have attempted to demonstrate that chronic limb ischemia affects not only skin and muscle but also peripheral nerve fibers (Chalk and Dyck, 1993). Initially with the use of clinical and pathological changes and then with electrodiagnostic findings, researchers have repeatedly tried to provide confirmation of this hypothesis, with surprisingly few unchallenged results being achieved. An apt example of the problem is the limb pain experienced with a number of peripheral vascular disorders. It has been labeled "ischemic neuritis" since 1935 because of its presumed etiology, yet almost 50 years (in 1984) after the term was first used in this manner, there still was "no direct evidence" linking it to axon damage in patients with PAD (Daube and Dyck, 1984). There are several reasons why controversy persists regarding this seemingly simple point.

- The symptoms due to nerve fiber damage (pain, sensory abnormalities, and even weakness) may be confused with those caused by ischemia of the skin and muscle (Turley and Johnson, 1991).
- Similar to the situation with acute limb ischemia, chronic limb ischemia is not stereotyped in its presentation. Rather, its severity is on a continuum ranging from being identified in an asymptomatic limb only with vascular diagnostic techniques, at the mildest extreme, to a limb that manifests impending distal gangrene as the most severe. As a result, its clinical, pathological, and electrodiagnostic manifestations also are on a continuum. Thus, Laghi Pasini and associates (1996) noted that the conduction abnormalities in affected limbs progressed as the disease was in its more advanced clinical stages.

- As Daube and Dyck (1984) observed, pathological and physiological studies concerning impaired circulation "of peripheral nerve have been meager and monotonously incomplete" compared with those that have been focused on the cerebral circulation. This most certainly accurately summarizes most of the electrodiagnostic investigations on this topic. Of 12 reports reviewed in this respect, NEEs were not performed in 8, NCSs were not performed in 1, and in the remaining 11, motor NCS amplitudes were not reported in 6 and sensory NCSs were not performed in 5. Why these electrodiagnostic investigations were so limited in their scope is unclear. Although the lack of sensory NCS can be explained by the time period in which some of them were conducted (e.g., the 1960s), there is no obvious explanation as to why CMAP amplitudes were not recorded or why NEEs were performed on only one or two muscles. In any case, the very restricted breadth of these investigations seriously compromises the value of their results as it applies to the typical patient being studied in the clinical electrodiagnostic laboratory (Miglietta and Lowenthal, 1962; Serra, 1962; Miglietta, 1966, 1967; Chopra, 1969; Chopra and Hurivitz, 1969; Kumlin et al., 1974; Hunter et al., 1988; England et al., 1992; Laghi Pasini et al., 1996; Papapetropoulou et al., 1998; Weinberg et al., 1998).
- Some of the reports have lacked adequate controls, particularly with regard to comparable ages.
- In several reports, confounding factors (e.g., diabetes, symptomatic limbs being cooler) have not been considered as possible causes for the slight changes found in the PAD limbs (Wilbourn and Levin, 1993).
- Finally, other investigators have reported contradictory results. Thus, Matsen and colleagues (1986) assessed, in the lower extremities of 176 patients with varying degrees of peripheral vascular insufficiency, the relationship of diabetes mellitus, alcoholism, and smoking to the integrity of four basic sensory modalities: joint position sense, light touch perception, sharp or dull sensation discrimination, and two-point discrimination. They found that diabetes had the most deleterious effect on sensation. In the limbs of nondiabetics, alcoholism compromised sensation the most. In the limbs of nondiabetic nonalcoholics, the severity of PAD had only a weak effect, and this was detectable only if the most strict criterion was used: the presence of an abnormality in any one of the four test procedures. The fact that the sensory acuity in limbs with severe PAD was very similar to that in limbs with moderate PAD suggests that, for sensory axons at least, chronic limb ischemia has little effect (Matsen et al., 1986).

Electrodiagnostic Examination

Despite the controversial points detailed previously, various investigators have concluded that, on electrodiagnostic studies, chronic limb ischemia alone can cause (1) mild slowing of peroneal and tibial motor conduction velocities; (2) amplitude reductions in the peroneal and tibial CMAPs, particularly the former; (3) amplitude reductions, latency prolongations, or both of the sural SNAPs; (4) absent H responses; and (5) chronic neurogenic MUP changes, fibrillation potentials, or both, in the more distal lower extremity muscles (i.e., those distal to the knee) (Miglietta and Lowenthal, 1962; Serra, 1962; Miglietta, 1966, 1967; Chopra, 1969; Chopra and Hurwitz, 1969; Kumlin et al., 1974; Hunter et al., 1988; England et al., 1992; Laghi Pasini et al., 1996; Papapetropoulou et al., 1998; Weinberg et al., 1998). Even though chronic limb ischemia may damage peripheral nerves, as asserted by these authors, unequivocal demonstration of it in a given patient assessed in the electrodiagnostic laboratory can be very difficult. Typically, confounding factors abound. In our experience, the majority of these patients are diabetic and have bilateral lower extremity symptoms. Consequently, it is almost impossible to determine the exact cause of any neurogenic abnormalities detected in the distal lower extremities. In addition, many of the patients are elderly, so the absence of H responses and lower extremity sensory NCS bilaterally is of uncertain significance. Moreover, some patients have undergone prior lumbar laminectomies, whereas others have neuroimaging evidence of lumbar canal stenosis. Thus, the chronic neurogenic MUP changes often seen in the more distal muscles in these situations have a ready explanation other than ischemia. It is pertinent to note, in this regard, that three of the five (60%) "medically normal" control patients used by 1 of the 12 groups of investigators mentioned above were shown, on routine NEE, to have evidence of L5 or S1 radiculopathies (England et al., 1992). Finally, many patients have already undergone various vascular and orthopedic surgical procedures on the affected limb at the time it is assessed, causing more uncertainty regarding the etiology of any electrodiagnostic changes that are found in it (Wilbourn and Levin, 1993). Therefore, the relevance of various electrodiagnostic abnormalities detected in limbs that manifest chronic ischemic changes is usually unclear. Probably, the conclusion of one group of investigators is most applicable in this regard: "Routine electrophysiological studies are not appropriate (sensitive enough) tests for detecting peripheral nerve . . . dysfunction associated with PAD" (Papapetropoulou et al., 1998), with the proviso that the following phrase be added: "especially when all the confounding factors encountered so frequently when assessing these patients are taken into consideration."

Lumbosacral Radiculoplexus Neuropathy

Lumbosacral radiculoplexus neuropathy is a subacute asymmetrical disorder that begins with severe pain (usually unilateral) in the thighs or legs that often progresses to a more widespread paralytic disorder involving both lower extremities. It occurs mainly in patients with diabetes mellitus (and in those patients is labeled *diabetic amyotrophy*) but may also occur in nondiabetic patients. It has been shown that both conditions are due to ischemic injury of nerve fibers as a result of microvasculitis (Dyck et al., 2001). The involved vessels are very small arterioles and venules. These conditions are usually self-limiting if left untreated, but the pain and weakness may take months to years to resolve.

CONCLUSIONS

A large number of clinical entities produce PNS abnormalities indirectly by compromising the blood supply of nerve fibers. The electrodiagnostic examination is of variable value with these disorders. With some, such as vasculitic neuropathy and IMN, it can play a principal role in diagnosis. With others, however, such as acute CSs, its major functions are to accurately catalog, after the fact, the extent and severity of the nerve (and muscle) damage and to verify its cause.

References

Allbrook DB, Aitken JT: Reinnervation of striated muscle after acute ischemia. J Anat 1951;85:376–389.
Antognini JF: Chronic pain after methysergide: A new cause for ischemic monomelic neuropathy. Reg Anesth 1991;16:337–338.
Archie JP: Femoral neuropathy due to common iliac occlusion. South Med J 1983;76:1073.
Barnes M: Diagnosis and management of chronic compartment syndromes: A review of the literature. Br J Sports Med 1997;31:21–27.
Battaglia M, Mitsumoto H, Wilbourn AJ: Utility of electromyography in the diagnosis of vasculitic neuropathy. Neurology 1990;40(suppl 1):427.
Blum L: The clinical entity of anterior crural ischemia. Arch Surg 1957;77:59–64.
Bolton CF, Driedger AA, Lindsay RM: Ischemic neuropathy in uremic patients caused by bovine arteriovenous shunt. J Neurol Neurosurg Psychiatr 1979;42:810–814.
Boontje AH, Haaxma R: Femoral neuropathy as a complication of aortic surgery. J Cardiovasc Surg 1987;28:286–289.
Botte MJ, Fronek J, Pedowitz RA, et al: Exertional compartment syndrome of the upper extremity. Hand Clin 1998;14:477–482.
Bouche P, Léger JM, Travers MA, et al: Peripheral neuropathy in systemic vasculitis: Clinical and electrophysiologic study in 22 patients. Neurology 1986;36:1598–1602.
Chad DA, Smith TW, Lacomis D: Vasculitic neuropathy: Classification, evaluation and treatment. In Cros D (ed): Peripheral Neuropathy: A Practical Approach to Diagnosis and Management. Philadelphia, Lippincott Williams & Wilkins, 2001; 160–181.
Chalk CH, Dyck PJ: Ischemic neuropathy. In Dyck PJ, Thomas PK (eds): Peripheral Neuropathy, 3rd ed. Philadelphia, WB Saunders, 1993; 980–989.
Chervu A, Moore WA, Homsher E, et al: Differential recovery of skeletal muscle and peripheral nerve function. J Surg Res 1989;47:12–19.
Chopra JS: Electromyography in diabetes mellitus and chronic occlusive peripheral vascular disease. Brain 1969;92:97–108.
Chopra JS, Hurwitz LJ: A comparative study of peripheral nerve conduction in diabetes and non-diabetic chronic occlusive peripheral vascular disease. Brain 1969;92:83–96.

Collins MP, Kissel JT, Mendell JR: Vasculitic neuropathies. In Antel JP, Birnbaum G, Harung H-P (eds): Clinical Immunology. Oxford, Blackwell Science, 1997; 316–339.

Cornblath DR, Sumner AJ: Conduction block in neuropathies with necrotizing vasculitis (letter). Muscle Nerve 1990;13:185.

D'Amour ML, Lebrun LH, Rabbat A, et al: Peripheral neurological complications of aortoiliac vascular disease. Can J Neurol Sci 1987;14:127–130.

Daube JR, Dyck PJ: Neuropathy due to peripheral vascular diseases. In Dyck PJ, Thomas PK, Lambert EH, Bunge R (eds): Peripheral Neuropathy, 2nd ed. Philadelphia, WB Saunders, 1984; 1458–1478.

Davies L: Vasculitic neuropathy. Baillieres Clin Neurol 1994;3:193–210.

Davies L, Spres JM, Pollard JD, McLeod JG: Vasculitis confined to peripheral nerve. Brain 1996;119:1441–1448.

Dyck PJ, Benstead BJ, Conn DL, et al: Nonsystemic vasculitic neuropathy. Brain 1987;110:843–854.

Dyck PJD, Norell JE, Dyck PJ: Non-diabetic lumbosacral radiculoplexus neuropathy: Natural history, outcome and comparison with the diabetic variety. Brain 2001;124:1197–1207.

England JD, Regensteiner JG, Ringel SP, et al: Muscle denervation in peripheral arterial disease. Neurology 1992;42:994–999.

Fathers E, Fuller GN: Vasculitic neuropathy. Br J Hosp Med 1996;55:643–647.

Ferguson FR, Liversedge LA: Ischaemic lateral popliteal nerve palsy. Br Med J 1954;2:333–335.

Fowler CJ, Gilliatt RW: Conduction velocity and conduction block after experimental ischaemic nerve injury. J Neurol Sci 1981;52:221–238.

Garfin SR: Historical review. In Mubarak SJ, Hargens AR (eds): Compartment Syndromes and Volkmann's Contracture. Philadelphia, WB Saunders, 1981; 6–16.

Gaspar MR, Hare RR: Gangrene due to the intra-arterial injection of drugs by drug addicts. Surgery 1972;72:573–577.

Ghali R, De Lean J, Douville Y, et al: Erythromycin-associated ergotamine intoxication: Arteriographic and electrophysiologic analysis of a rare cause of severe ischemia of the lower extremities and associated ischemic neuropathy. Ann Vasc Surg 1993;7:291–296.

Gilliatt RW: Peripheral Nerve Compression and Entrapment (The Oliver Sharpley Lecture): Eleventh Symposium on Advanced Medicine. Kent, Pitman Medical, 1975; 144–163.

Gledhill RF, Inshasi J: Conduction block in vasculitic neuropathy. Neurology 1992;42:699. Letter.

Gloviczki P, Cross SA, Stanson AW, et al: Ischemic injury to the spinal cord or lumbosacral plexus after aorto-iliac reconstruction. Am J Surg 1991;162:131–136.

Haimovici H: Peripheral arterial embolism. Angiology 1950;1:20–45.

Hargens AR, Mubarak SJ: Current concepts in the pathophysiology, evaluation, and diagnosis of compartment syndrome. Hand Clin 1998;14:371–383.

Hawke SHB, Davies L, Pamphlett R, et al: Vasculitic neuropathy: A clinical and pathologic study. Brain 1991;114:2175–2190.

Hefty TR, Nelson KA, Hatch TR, Barry JM: Acute lumbosacral plexopathy in diabetic women after renal transplant. J Urol 1990;143:107–109.

Homberg V, Reiners K, Toyka KV: Reversible conduction block in human ischemic neuropathy after ergotamine abuse. Muscle Nerve 1992;15:467–470.

Honet JC, Wajszczuk WV, Rubenfire M, et al: Neurological abnormalities in the leg(s) after use of intraaortic balloon pump: Report of six cases. Arch Phys Med Rehabil 1975;56:346–352.

Hye RJ, Wolf YG: Ischemic monomelic neuropathy: An under-recognized complication of hemodialysis access. Ann Vasc Surg 1994;8:578–582.

Hunter GC, Song GW, Nayak NN, et al: Peripheral nerve conduction abnormalities in lower extremity ischemia: The effects of revascularization. J Surg Res 1988;45:96–103.

Iliopoulos JI, Howanitz PE, Pierce GE, et al: The critical hypogastric circulation. Am J Surg 1987;154:671–675.

Jamieson PW, Giuliani MJ, Martinez AJ: Necrotizing angiopathy presenting with multifocal conduction blocks. Neurology 1991;41:442–444.

Johansen KH, Watson JC: Compartment syndrome: Pathophysiology, recognition and management. In Rutherford RB (ed): Vascular Surgery, 5th ed. Philadelphia, WB Saunders, 2000; 902–908.

Johnson KW: Nonvascular complications of vascular surgery. In Rutherford RB (ed): Vascular Surgery, 3rd ed. Philadelphia, WB Saunders, 1989; 536–540.

Kaku DA, Malamut RI, Frey DJ, Parry GJ: Conduction block as an early sign of reversible injury in ischemic monomelic neuropathy. Neurology 1993;43:1126–1130.

Kissel J: Vasculitis of the peripheral nervous system. Semin Neurol 1994;14:361–369.

Kissel JT, Collins MP, Mendell JR: Vasculitic neuropathy. In Mendell JR, Kissel JT, Cornblath DR (eds): Diagnosis and Management of Peripheral Nerve Disorders. London, Oxford University Press, 2001; 202–232.

Kissel JT, Slivka AP, Warmolts JR, Mendell JR: The clinical spectrum of necrotizing angiopathy of the peripheral nervous system. Ann Neurol 1985;18:251–257.

Korthals JK, Maki T, Gieron MA: Nerve and muscle vulnerability to ischemia. J Neurol Sci 1985;71:283–290.

Kumlin T, Seppalainen AM, Railo J: Electromyography in intermittent claudication due to obliterative arteriosclerosis. Angiology 1974;25:373–400.

Lachance DH, Daube JR: Acute peripheral artery occlusion: Electrophysiologic study of 32 cases. Muscle Nerve 1991;14:633–639.

Laghi Pasini F, Pastorelli M, Beermann U, et al: Peripheral neuropathy associated with ischemic vascular disease of the lower limbs. Angiology 1996;47:569–577.

Levin KH: AAEE case report #19: Ischemic monomelic neuropathy. Muscle Nerve 1989;12:791–795.

Lewis T, Pickering GW, Rothschild P: Centripetal paralysis arising out of arrested blood flow to the limb, including notes on a form of tingling. Heart 1931;16:1–32.

Low PA, Tuck RR: Effects of changes of blood pressure, respiratory acidosis and hypoxia on blood flow in the sciatic nerve of the rat. J Physiol 1984;347:513–524.

Matsen FA: Compartmental syndrome: A unified concept. Clin Orthop 1975;113:8–14.

Matsen FA, Wyss CR, Robertson CL, et al: Factors relating to the sensory acuity of limbs with peripheral vascular insufficiency. Surgery 1986;99:455–461.

McCluskey L, Feinberg D, Cantor C: "Pseudo-conduction block" in vasculitic neuropathy. Muscle Nerve 1999;22:1361–1366.

Miglietta O: Electrophysiological studies in chronic occlusive peripheral vascular disease. Arch Phy Med Rehabil 1967;48:89–96.

Miglietta O: Nerve motor fiber characteristics in chronic ischemia. Arch Neurol 1966;14:448–453.

Miglietta O, Lowenthal M: Nerve conduction velocity and refractory period. J Appl Physiol 1962;17:837–840.

Mohamed A, Davies L, Pollard JD: Conduction block in vasculitic neuropathy. Muscle Nerve 1998;21:1084–1088.

Moore PM, Fauci AS: Neurologic manifestations of vasculitis. Am J Med 1981;71:517–524.

Moore RE, Friedman RJ: Current concepts in pathophysiology and diagnosis of compartment syndromes. J Emerg Med 1989;7:657–662.

Mubarak S, Owen CA: Compartmental syndrome and its relation to crush syndrome: A spectrum of disease. Clin Orthop 1975;113:81–89.

Mubarak SJ: Etiologies of compartment syndromes. In Mubarak SJ, Hargans AR (eds): Compartment Syndromes and Volkmann's Contracture. Philadelphia, WB Saunders, 1981a; 71–97.

Mubarak SJ: Exertional compartment syndromes. In Mubarak SJ, Hargens AR (eds): Compartment Syndrome and Volkmann's Contracture. Philadelphia, WB Saunders, 1981b; 209–226.

Olney RK: Neuropathies associated with connective tissue disease. Semin Neurol 1998;18:63–72.

Ouriel K: Acute ischemia and its sequelae. In Rutherford RB (ed): Vascular Surgery, 5th ed. Philadelphia, WB Saunders, 2000; 813–821.

Owen CA: Clinical diagnosis of compartment syndromes. In Mubarak SJ, Hargens AR (eds): Compartment Syndromes and Volkmann's Contracture. Philadelphia, WB Saunders, 1981a: 98–105.

Owen CA: The crush syndrome. In Mubarak SJ, Hargens AR (eds): Compartment Syndromes and Volkmann's Contracture. Philadelphia, WB Saunders, 1981b; 166–182.

Papapetropoulou V, Tsolakis J, Terzis S, et al: Neurophysiologic studies in peripheral arterial disease. J Clin Neurophysiol 1998; 15:447–450.

Parry GJ, Linn DJ: Conduction block without demyelination following acute nerve infarction. J Neurol Sci 1988;84:265–273.

Parry GJG: Mononeuropathy multiplex. Muscle Nerve 1986;8:493–498.

Perry MO: Acute ischemia and its sequelae. In Rutherford RB (ed): Vascular Surgery, 3rd ed. Philadelphia, WB Saunders, 1989; 541–547.

Place EJ, Seabrook GR, Freischlag JA, Torone JB: Neurologic complications of reoperative and emergent abdominal aortic reconstruction. Ann Vasc Surg 1995;9:95–101.

Plecha EJ, Seabrook GR, Freischlag JA, Towne JB: Neurologic complications of reoperative and emergent abdominal aortic reconstruction. Ann Vasc Surg 1995;9:95–101.

Redfern AB, Zimmerman NB: Neurologic and ischemic complications of upper extremity vascular access for dialysis. J Hand Surg 1995;20A:199–204.

Richards RL: Neurovascular lesions. In Seddon HG (ed): Peripheral Nerve Injuries (Special Report 282). London, Her Majesty's Stationery Office, 1954; 186–238.

Richards RL: Ischemic lesions of peripheral nerves: A review. J Neurol Neurosurg Psychiatr 1951;14:76–87.

Riggs JE, Moss AH, Labosky DA, et al: Upper extremity ischemic monomelic neuropathy: A complication of vascular access procedures in uremic diabetic patients. Neurology 1989;39:997–998.

Ritchie JM: The oxygen consumption of mammalian non-myelinated nerve fibres at rest and during activity. J Physiol 1967; 188:309–329.

Robinson KD, Gregory RT, Gayle RG, et al: Lumbosacral plexopathy: A complication of ruptured aortic aneurysms: Three case reports. Vasc Surg 1997;31:501–507.

Ropert A, Metral S: Conduction block in neuropathies with necrotizing vasculitis. Muscle Nerve 1990;13:102–105.

Rorabeck CH: Compartment syndromes. In Browner BD, Jupiter JB, Levine AM, Trafton PG (eds): Skeletal Trauma. Philadelphia, WB Saunders, 1992; 285–309.

Sanderson RA, Foley RK, Malvor GWD, et al: Histological response of muscle to ischemia. Clin Orthop 1975;113:27–35.

Seddon HJ: Three types of nerve injury. Brain 1943;66:237–287.

Serra C: Electromyography of arterial occlusive disease. World Neurol 1962;3:664–678.

Shields RW, Harris JW, Clark M: Mononeuropathy in sickle cell anemia: Anatomical and pathophysiological basis for its rarity. Muscle Nerve 1991;14:370–374.

Sunderland S: Nerve Injuries and Their Repair. Edinburgh, Churchill Livingstone, 1991.

Swain R, Ross D: Lower extremity compartment syndrome. Postgrad Med 1999;105:159–168.

TransAtlantic Inter-Society Consensus (TASC): Management of peripheral arterial disease (PAD). Section B: Intermittent claudication. Eur J Vasc Endovasc Surg 2000;19:S47–S114.

Teunissen LL, Notermans NC, Wokke JHJ: Relationship between ischemia and neuropathy. Eur Neurol 2000;44:1–7.

Tinel J: Nerve Wounds. New York, Williams Wood and Co, 1917.

Trice M, Colwell CW: A historical review of compartment syndrome and Volkmann's ischemic contracture. Hand Clin 1998; 14:335–341.

Turley JJE, Johnson KW: Ischemic neuropathy. Semin Vasc Surg 1991;4:12–19.

Usubiaga JE, Kolodny J, Usubiaga LE: Neurological complications of prevertebral surgery under regional anesthesia. Surgery 1970;68:304–309.

Valji K, Hye RJ, Roberts AC, et al: Hand ischemia in patients with hemodialysis access grafts: Angiographic diagnosis and treatment. Radiology 1995;196:697–701.

von Schroeder HP, Botte MJ: Definitions and terminology of compartment syndrome and Volkmann's ischemic contracture of the upper extremity. Hand Clin 1998;14:331–334.

Voulters L, Bolton C: Acute lumbosacral plexopathy following vascular surgery. Can J Neurol Sci 1983;10:153.

Wees SJ, Sumvoo IN, Oh SJ: Sural nerve biopsy in systemic necrotizing vasculitis. Am J Med 1981;71:525–532.

Weinberg DH, Simovic D, Isner J: Chronic ischemic monomelic neuropathy. Neurology 1998;50:A207–A208.

Wilbourn AJ: Nonvasculitic ischemic neuropathies. In Katirji B, Kaminski HJ, Preston DC, et al (eds): Neuromuscular Disorders in Clinical Practice. Woburn, MA, Butterworth-Heinemann, 2001.

Wilbourn AJ, Ferrante MA: Clinical electromyography. In Joynt RJ, Griggs RC (eds): Baker's Clinical Neurology on CD-ROM. Philadelphia, Lippincott Williams & Wilkins, 2000, record 7592–8248.

Wilbourn AJ, Furlan AJ, Hulley W, Ruschaupt W: Ischemic monomelic neuropathy. Neurology 1983;33:447–451.

Wilbourn AJ, Levin KH: Ischemic neuropathy. In Brown WF, Bolton CF (eds): Clinical Electromyography, 2nd ed. Boston, Butterworth-Heinemann, 1993; 369–390.

Wohlgemuth WA, Rottach KG, Stoehr M: Intermittent claudication due to ischemia of the lumbosacral plexus. J Neurol Neurosurg Psychiatr 1999;67:793–795.

Wytrzes L, Markley HG, Fisher M, Alfred HJ: Brachial neuropathy after brachial artery-antecubital vein shunts for chronic dialysis. Neurology 1987;37:1398–1400.

CHAPTER 68

Infections and Peripheral Neuropathy

Dale J. Lange and Eugene Tolunsky

Invasion of the human body by infectious organisms, viral, bacterial, parasitic, or prionie, is the most common cause of human morbidity and mortality affecting the world's population. Many infections have expression in the peripheral nervous system as a result of direct infection, through an association with the direct infection, or during a postinfectious event. This chapter reviews the disorders that have direct effects on the peripheral nerve. Postinfectious polyneuropathies, neuropathies associated with infection with human immunodeficiency virus (HIV), and infections of spinal neurons are discussed elsewhere.

DIPHTHERIA

Diphtheria is a highly lethal bacterial infection that was essentially eliminated from most developed countries through effective immunization programs during childhood; however, in developing countries and those undergoing political change, such as the former Soviet Union, diphtheria continues to be a lethal childhood infection. Adults older than 30 years of age begin to lose the immune protection from childhood immunization. Therefore, older *immunized* adults are also at risk for disease during epidemics (Hann, 1999).

The infecting organism, *Corynebacterium diphtheriae,* gains access through inhalation and infection of the pharynx (particularly the tonsils) or directly through the skin. The latter infection is particularly common during warfare. The incubation period for diphtheria is short, varying between 2 and 6 days. The diagnosis is made by culturing the toxigenic bacterium from throat swabs or documenting elevated titers of diphtheria antibodies in serum (McDonald and Kocen, 1993).

Clinical Manifestations

The initial clinical manifestations consist of generalized disease (malaise, anorexia, generalized aching pain) and symptoms localized to the pharyngeal muscles, causing a sore throat. The characteristic grayish white exudates that become fixed to the mucosa develop within days. Therefore, the first manifestations include a change in voice and regurgitation of fluids from palatal paralysis. Difficulty in accommodation (reflected by difficulty in reading) may occur within 1 month of infection, but eye movements are rarely affected.

Peripheral neuropathy occurs in about 20% of infected patients. The neuropathy usually begins 6 to 8 weeks after the onset of the pharyngeal infection (Logina and Donaghy, 1999). Rarely, limb weakness and paresthesias may occur when the patient has bulbar symptoms. Limb weakness as the initial manifestation without bulbar signs has been described.

The onset of the neuropathy is usually abrupt, with progression to maximal severity over a mean of 8 days. The initial symptom is often muscle aching and tenderness. Weakness and sensory loss develop in distal portions of the arms and legs. Reflexes are absent. Limb weakness varies in severity, but one study found that 48% of patients with diphtheritic neuropathy were unable to walk when they were severely affected (Logina and Donaghy, 1999). Bulbar dysfunction, sensory symptoms, and autonomic involvement occur in 30% to 40% of affected patients.

Cerebrospinal fluid analysis shows increased levels of protein (rarely over 300 mg/dL), with little or no cellular pleocytosis (dissociation of protein and cells).

Electrodiagnostic Studies

Nerve conduction studies in patients with diphtheritic polyneuropathy show features typical of a demyelinating sensorimotor neuropathy (Creange et al., 1995). The initial abnormalities show increased distal motor latency and prolonged F-response latencies and relatively preserved sensory nerve action potentials (Kurdi and Abdul-Kader, 1979; Creange et al., 1995). As weakness progresses, conduction velocity slowing worsens and sensory nerve action potential amplitude declines. However, despite reaching maximal weakness and showing signs of improvement, the electrophysiological abnormalities may continue to worsen. The dissociation between clinical and physiological abnormalities has been confirmed in most physiological studies (Kurdi and Abdul-Kader, 1979; Creange et al., 1995; Logina and Donaghy, 1999). The dissociation has been observed early in the illness, in which conduction studies may be normal despite severe weakness.

Pathology and Pathogenesis

The neuropathy is caused by the potent toxin secreted by the *Corynebacterium diphtheriae* bacterium. The toxin, whose molecular weight is 62,000 daltons, consists of two fragments of amino acid sequences, A and B. Fragment B recognizes and attaches to specific membrane receptors. Fragment A is a potent inhibitor of protein synthesis in the infected cell. The toxin is lethal to virtually all cells to which it can attach. The toxin inhibits synthesis of myelin basic protein and myelin proteolipid protein in Schwann cells, rendering them unable to synthesize myelin. Therefore, the prominent effects of demyelination usually do not occur until the cells recycle and myelin can no longer be produced, causing delayed demyelination.

The toxin does not penetrate the blood-brain barrier but is accessible to peripheral nerves at the blood-nerve barrier (nerve roots, dorsal root ganglia, and vagus nerve ganglia). It is possible that the blood-nerve barrier is weakest in the nerve root and distal portions of peripheral nerves. This would explain why these portions of the peripheral nerve are involved earliest physiologically.

Muscle biopsy early in the disease course shows no inflammation or necrosis. Nerve biopsy shows loss of myelinated fibers and mononuclear cell infiltrates (Creange et al., 1995).

Pathological changes are most prominent in the proximal portion of the peripheral nervous system, particularly the dorsal and ventral roots. The nodal ganglion of the vagus nerve is also affected. The main pathological finding is prominent demyelination with relative axonal continuity (Fisher and Adams, 1956; Pleasure et al., 1973). However, in severe cases, axonal degeneration has been observed. There is proliferation of Schwann cells and macrophage infiltration.

The toxin's effect on myelin production is not exactly known. Injection of toxin induces demyelination. Transgenic mice that can express foreign genes in myelinating Schwann cells with a P_0 promoter show that when P_0 drives expression of diphtheria toxin A, a hypomyelinating neuropathy occurs (Messing et al., 1992). The potency of the toxin to inhibit protein synthesis has allowed the toxin to be used in other settings, including possible therapy for cancer.

Differential Diagnosis

Diphtheritic polyneuropathy is a rapidly progressive polyneuropathy that may be confused with Guillain-Barré syndrome. Both conditions may be preceded by a sore throat. However, there are prominent differences. The prevalence and severity of bulbar involvement, with limbs being relatively less affected, are more common in diphtheritic neuropathy. Also, the weakness may progress for longer than 4 weeks. There are prominent differences, however (Table 68–1).

Table 68–1. Features Differentiating Diphtheria and Guillain-Barré Syndrome

Clinical Feature	Diphtheria	GBS
Preceding infection	Sore throat	URI, sore throat
Disease course	Biphasic	Postinfectious
Accommodation	+++	+
Ocular motility disorder	++	+
Facial weakness	+++	++
Bulbar dysfunction	+++	++
Respiratory muscle weakness	++++	++
Sensory symptoms	+++	+
Autonomic involvement	+++	+++
Prolonged DML	+++	++++
Absent F	+++	++++
CSF dissociation	+++	+++

Data from Bonetti B, Scardoni M, Monaco S, et al: Hepatitis C virus infection of peripheral nerves in type II cryoglobulinemia. Virch Arch 1999;434:533–535; and Logina and Donaghy, 1999; Creange et al., 1995.

Prognosis

Polyneuropathy caused by diphtheria rarely leaves some type of residual effect in 80% of people 1 year after infection. More than 40% never return to work because of dexterity problems. Death occurs in 16% of patients with polyneuropathy. The most common cause of death is diphtheritic myocarditis. Other causes include multiple organ failure, cardiovascular disturbances, nephritis, and pneumonia.

Treatment

Treating diphtheritic polyneuropathy consists of administering antitoxin at the first sign of suspicion. Waiting for culture confirmation may cause serious delay. Duration of the effectiveness of the toxin is usually less than 48 hours, the time needed for diphtheria toxin to bind to tissue. Treatment with toxin after 48 hours seems not to prevent death or neuropathy.

LYME DISEASE

In 1975, a cluster of children with childhood arthritis were discovered in Lyme, Connecticut. Epidemiological investigation of this unusual phenomenon showed that all the children had been exposed to an *Ixodes* tick bite. The cause of their symptoms was discovered to be a spirochete bacterium called *Borrelia burgdorferi*. It is transmitted through the tick acting as a vector. *Ixodes dammini* is the primary vector in the United States. *Ixodes dammini* is also endemic to Wisconsin and Minnesota and to northern California and Oregon. The host for the tick in early development is usually a small rodent, and as the tick matures, larger animals, such as deer and bear, are preferred hosts. Therefore, the disease is most frequent in forested areas.

Borrelia infection is also present in Europe. The clinical manifestations are generically similar, with skin manifestations and neurological involvement being the most common. However, in Europe, the rash is different, being acrodermatitis chronica atrophicans and lymphocytoma cutis, whereas in the United States the characteristic rash is erythema chronicum migrans and arthritic involvement is less pronounced. The cause of the clinical difference is uncertain, but it may rest in the fact that the infecting organisms belong to different subgroups of *B. burgdorferi*. In the United States, the predominant organism is *B. burgdorferi* sensu stricto. In Europe, the most common are *B. garinii* and *B. afzelii* (Halperin et al., 1999).

Infection occurs through injection of the spirochete from the tick to the new host. The spirochete is confined to the tick's digestive system. Transmission to a new host occurs primarily during regurgitation, making rapid infection after a bite unusual.

In fact, transmission within the first 24 hours of attachment is rare.

Clinical Manifestations

The target organs during Lyme infection include the skin, heart, nervous system, and joints. The discussion in this chapter is limited to manifestations in the peripheral nervous system. Perhaps the most useful way of classifying the clinical syndrome is into early and late stages of the disease.

EARLY INFECTION

In the early stage, the characteristic skin lesion erythema migrans (EM) appears within 3 days to 3 weeks of the bite and lasts as long as 1 month. Neurological symptoms may begin while EM is still apparent or any time within the first 6 months. The neurological syndrome takes the form of multilevel polyradiculitis, cranial neuropathy, mononeuropathy multiplex, and diffuse senosorimotor peripheral neuropathy (Pachner and Steere, 1985).

Cranial neuropathy occurs in more than 50% of patients' neurological involvement within the early stages of Lyme disease. Facial palsy occurs in 3% to 10% of all patients with Lyme disease and accounts for more than 70% of all cranial neuropathies found in patients with Lyme disease (Clark et al., 1985; Halperin et al., 1988). There is no certain way of separating facial palsy caused by Lyme disease from idiopathic disease without other signs of Lyme disease, such as EM. However, as with other forms of peripheral neuropathy in Lyme disease, the clinical syndrome may occur in the absence of EM or other signs of Lyme disease (Reik et al., 1979, 1986). However, in most patients, there are other neurological signs or a lymphocytic pleocytosis (Reik, 1993). Of note, facial weakness is bilateral in about 50% of patients with facial paralysis caused by Lyme disease, occurring within 3 weeks of each other (Reik, 1993). Prognosis is good and recovery usually complete, although it may take as long as 6 months. Permanent weakness and facial hemispasm have been reported in 5% to 10% of patients. All other cranial nerves can be involved in either a mononeuritis or a mononeuritis multiplex, but these syndromes are rare. Motor neuron disease has been reported, as has increased Lyme titers, but most believe these to be coincident and not related.

Radiculitis complicates Lyme disease in more than 40% of patients (Reik, 1993). The syndrome usually begins with severe radicular pain and paresthesias within 2 months of the tick bite. The pain is usually worse at night. Asymmetrical weakness following a root or peripheral nerve distribution develops as long as 6 months after the bite; usually it is within 2 months of the tick bite. Legs are affected more than arms. The pattern of involvement is variable, including multilevel radiculopathy, lumbosacral and brachial plexitis, and mononeuropathy multiplex. Tendon reflexes are depressed.

The onset of weakness may be sudden, appearing similar to Guillain-Barré syndrome (Sternman et al., 1982). However, the main difference is the appearance of lymphocytic pleocytosis. More chronic evolution of weakness occurs in a rare manifestation of pure motor neuropathy without pain (Baumhackl et al., 1986; Scelsa et al., 1996). Symptoms of peripheral nerve dysfunction respond well to therapy, and most patients return to normal or have minimal residual weakness.

Electrodiagnostic Studies

Electrophysiological studies of the facial nerve rarely show marked prolongation of latencies to facial muscles (Wulff et al., 1983). The most common finding is low-amplitude potentials with denervation.

In the early phases of the disease, peripheral nerve conduction studies show axonal and demyelinating changes (Vallat et al., 1987). Distal motor latency is slightly prolonged, with normal or borderline normal segmental velocity. Sensory and motor amplitudes are low. F-response latencies are prolonged in 50% of patients (Halperin et al., 1987; Logigian and Steere, 1992).

LATE INFECTION

Polyneuropathy occurs in 40% to 60% of patients with Lyme disease long after the original infection. Patients complain of pain and intermittent paresthesias. Examination reveals a paucity of abnormalities, with fewer than 25% showing stocking and glove abnormalities, and these are usually mild. Significant motor weakness and sensory loss are uncommon, but central nervous system abnormalities as well as pleocytosis are seen in 25% and 40%, respectively (Reik, 1993).

Electrodiagnostic Studies

Nerve conduction studies are abnormal in as many as 70% of patients 2 to 3 years after the onset of the illness (Halperin et al., 1988). Sensory nerve conduction abnormalities were found in more than two thirds of patients, and motor system and F-response abnormalities were found in one half (Halperin et al., 1988). Focal affection of the median nerve consistent with carpal tunnel syndrome was found in about one third of patients. Treatment with antibiotics causes remission in 3 to 4 months (Reik, 1993).

Pathology and Pathogenesis

Actual spirochete infiltration of nerves has not been identified. Sural nerve biopsies show axonal degeneration, loss of large myelinated fibers, and epineurial perivasculitis (Halperin et al., 1987). Combined with the clinical pattern, a vasculitic cause of the clinical neuropathic syndrome is probable (Reik et al., 1986). Vasculitis is commonly encountered in peripheral nerve biopsy (Tezzon et al., 1991). Similar findings are seen in the experimental model of Lyme neuropathy in Rhesus monkeys (England et al., 1997). However, although inflammatory cell infiltrates were present, suggesting an immune-mediated process, no organism was identified. One patient who developed a diffuse sensorimotor polyneuropathy 4 years after the tick bite showed intense inflammatory cell infiltrates, with complement deposition strongly supporting an immune mechanism underlying the peripheral neuropathy (Maimone et al., 1997).

The laboratory diagnosis is based on the detection of a specific antibody to *B. burgdorferi* with the use of enzyme-linked immunosorbent assay (ELISA). Most patients with neuropathy have antibodies to IgG. False-positive antibodies are found in rheumatoid arthritis, tuberculous meningitis, mononucleosis, and Rocky Mountain spotted fever. Western blotting confirms the ELISA findings. The presence of antibodies in the cerebrospinal fluid is also helpful in establishing meningeal and central nervous system disease. All patients with Lyme infection do not test positive for antibodies (seronegative Lyme disease), especially in the early stages of the disease.

Treatment

Oral treatment with doxycycline or amoxicillin (500 to 1000 mg t.i.d.) for 3 weeks is the recommended therapy for early infection without evidence of cerebrospinal fluid infection (Dattwyler et al., 1990). In late infections or clinically severe disease, intravenous therapy is usually recommended, using ceftriaxone (2 g IV daily) or cefotaxime (2 g IV q8h) for 2 or 4 weeks (Wormser, 1997). They have been shown to be equally effective.

LEPROSY

Leprosy, one of the oldest diseases known to humans, still affects almost 1 million people throughout the world. It continues to be the most common cause of neuropathy in the world, being most prevalent in Southeast Asia and other tropical and subtropical areas. In the United States, leprosy is found in Hawaii, Florida, Louisiana, and Texas. Neuropathy affects 15% to 20% of infected individuals.

Leprosy is caused by the bacterium *Mycobacterium leprae*. It is one of the acid-fast organisms, morphologically indistinguishable from *M. tuberculosis*. Skin and peripheral nerves are the target tissues for *M. leprae*. *Mycobacterium leprae* reproduces best in cool temperatures (maximal reproduction frequency occurs between 27° to 30°C), accounting for its high affinity for cooler areas of the body, such as the skin, superficial nerves, nose, testes, and ears.

Leprosy is a disease primarily affecting skin and peripheral nerves. There are two main types of clinical syndrome caused by this organism, depending on the immunological status of the patient. The clinical manifestations in patients with low (host) resistance are termed *lepromatous leprosy*; in patients with high (host) resistance, the syndrome is referred to as *tuberculoid leprosy*. Patients with immune states that are in between are referred to as having *borderline leprosy*. Early in the disease, when the host immune status has yet to be determined, the illness is referred to as *indeterminate*.

Clinical Manifestations

TUBERCULOID LEPROSY

Patients with high host resistance have a form of leprosy called *tuberculoid leprosy*. Patients with turberculoid leprosy have a well-localized disease process that produces sharply demarcated skin lesions, often raised and with a central hypopigmented anesthetic area, that are few in number. The lesion is sometimes surrounded by an elevated, erythematous ring. They occur on the extensor surfaces of the arms and legs, face, and buttocks. These plaques never occur in the warmer region of the body, such as the groin or axilla. The prognosis is good, and the lesions often heal spontaneously. Pathologically, the lesion consists of an epithelioid granuloma with Langhans' giant cells. There are few acid-fast bacilli in the lesion; blood-borne spread does not occur. Accordingly, the clinical syndrome is the result primarily of the intense immune response elicited by the bacterial exposure rather than the actual infiltration of the organism itself.

LEPROMATOUS LEPROSY

Patients with low host resistance develop a form of leprosy characterized by an extensive bacterial infiltration of the skin and nerves as well as dissemination through the blood. Unlike the tuberculoid form in which the tissue damage results from the host response, in lepromatous disease the clinical signs are due to the massive infiltration of organisms in the regions of cooler temperature. The skin lesions vary in appearance, producing nodules, bullous lesions, ulcers, macules, papules, and plaques. Solitary lesions are uncommon, being present only in the early stages of the illness. Usually, the abnormalities are diffuse and often symmetrical. Sometimes there are no discrete skin abnormalities but rather a diffuse sheen to the skin due to subcutaneous tissue swelling. The involvement of the face, nose, and ears produces a generalized swelling and a characteristic facial appearance (leonine facies). The cooler testes are also involved in advanced stages of the illness, causing sterility and gynecomastia.

Biopsy of the skin shows massive infiltration of histiocytes with foamy cytoplasm, often filled with bacilli (Virchow cells). This is an advanced form of the disease, rarely encountered today because of the variety of treatments available. Rarely does it arrest spontaneously; aggressive chemotherapy is required. Left untreated, lepromatous leprosy results in the death of the patient from systemic amyloidosis and renal failure.

BORDERLINE LEPROSY

Patients with clinical disease in between the two extremes have borderline leprosy. Depending on the preponderance of types of skin lesions, patients may be borderline tuberculoid (BT) or borderline lepromatous (BL). Skin biopsy results may show similarities to both forms, with foam-filled histiotcytes as well as epithelioid cells. Clinically, this form of leprosy tends to develop into lepromatous leprosy without treatment, and it moves toward tuberculoid leprosy if treatment is administered and effective.

Clinical Manifestations

The most common symptom in patients with leprosy is sensory loss, so severe that painless injury can occur. Skin lesions are almost always present. However, rarely, leprosy may present with a pure mononeuropathy without skin lesions—the neuritic form, or pure sensory or mixed (Jacob and Mathai, 1998).

The severity of the neuropathy depends on the severity of the infection. Paralysis is rare, and sensory loss always precedes weakness. The neuropathy is due to damage inflicted in the terminal twigs of sensory nerves lying close to the skin. The most superficially located nerves in the coolest regions of the body are affected earliest. The modalities affected earliest, therefore, are nerve fibers that subserve tactile function, such as pain and temperature perception. Loss of sweating is also an early finding. As the illness progresses, nerves in deeper tissues are affected, causing a variable deficit in touch sensation. Position and vibration are entirely spared. This syndrome is called a *superficial neuropathy*, a pattern unique to leprosy. In lepromatous disease, there is little inflammation, and evolution of symptoms is slow. In tuberculoid disease, the dermal nerves are damaged by the inflammatory response, and sensory loss occurs earlier and the loss of the skin patch is more severe.

In all forms of leprosy, the trunks of peripheral nerves that are passing through the area of inflammation may be damaged, producing a mononeuropathy in the distribution of the affected nerve. Specific nerve segments are involved more frequently than others. They include the ulnar nerve at the elbow, median nerve in the forearm, peroneal nerve at the fibular head, and facial nerves. Commonly involved sensory nerves include the superficial radial at the wrist, the sural nerve, and the greater auricular nerve. Nerves are enlarged at these sites and may be palpated clinically (Brown et al., 1996).

Each form of leprosy has a common pattern of sensory loss. In the tuberculoid form, the sensory loss is patchy, affecting primarily pain and temperature sensation. Peripheral nerves passing through the affected area may be encased or destroyed by the surrounding inflammatory response, producing a characteristic pattern of localized sensory loss with remote loss of motor and sensory function in the distribution of the affected peripheral nerve trunk. Axonal loss is common in such circumstances. Pain is variably present, depending on the speed and intensity of the inflammatory response.

In some circumstances, a change in the immune responsiveness of the patient occurs, usually in reaction to effective antimicrobial therapy—a *reversal, or type I, reaction.* For example, after undergoing effective chemotherapy, a patient with tuberculoid leprosy may develop an increase in cell-mediated immunity to *M. leprae* antigen and an extremely intense inflammatory response in the affected areas. Destruction of peripheral nerve trunks passing through the involved areas causes the sudden appearance of mononeuropathy and mononeuropathy multiplex. Rapid therapy is essential to the prevention of permanent nerve damage and disability. Risk factors for the type I reaction include facial patches, enlarged ulnar nerve, lesions in two or more parts, and seropositivity to anti–phenolic glycolipid (PGL-1; Haimanot, 1990).

In patients with lepromatous leprosy, peripheral nerve affection may not be apparent early in the disease. The infiltration of the bacilli in the skin may occur with little host response and, accordingly, little neural damage. Over months to years, large areas of dysfunction occur, producing a more generalized neuropathy resembling a classic glove and stocking syndrome. Weakness occurs only when the nerves that are superficially located become affected.

In patients with lepromatous leprosy, effective therapy or stress of any kind, such as emotional disturbance or a febrile illness, may precipitate a clinical reaction called the *erythema nodosum leprosum (ENL) type 2 reaction.* This is a dangerous, potentially life-threatening complication in treated patients with lepromatous leprosy. It occurs in about 50% of patients with lepromatous leprosy. The risk of ENL increases with an increasing amount of bacterial antigen and is inversely related to patient age (Haimanot and Melaku, 2000). Areas containing large amounts of bacillary antigen develop large amounts of antibody-antigen complexes that stimulate complement and macrophage infiltration. Acute skin lesions develop, often with subcutaneous nodules. Skin and affected peripheral nerves are often very painful. Systemic signs of fever, malaise, and generalized weakness are present. Ulceration of the skin may occur. Rapid initiation of treatment (see section

on treatment that follows) is mandatory for severe reactions.

Electrodiagnostic Studies

Nerve conduction studies are a fundamental means of proving the involvement and extent of disease in peripheral nerves. Nerve conduction abnormalities have been observed in patients with both lepromatous and tuberculoid leprosy (McLeod et al., 1975). The physiological abnormalities mirror the degree of severity of clinical disease (Verghese et al., 1970). The abnormalities are more common in nerves that are most often clinically involved and hypertrophic. The ulnar nerve is the one most often found to be abnormal, usually at the elbow; the median is most affected in the distal forearm, not the wrist. In fact, most patients have normal distal motor latency in the median nerve (Hackett et al., 1968). The mechanism for slowing is primarily demyelinating because of focal slowing and excessive temporal dispersion (Antia et al., 1970). One patient was described as having presented with a pure ulnar neuropathy, but conduction studies showed maximal slowing in the distal forearm and examination showed an enlarged nerve in the ulnar groove. The radial nerve at the wrist was also thickened, raising the possibility of a more diffuse disorder. Nerve biopsy of the thickened radial nerve showed acid-fast bacilli and granuloma with epithelioid cells, compatible with tuberculoid leprosy (Jobling and Morgan-Hughes, 1965).

In lepromatous disease, the nerves most often affected are the ulnar nerve at the elbow and median nerve just proximal to the carpal tunnel on the lower third of the forearm. Medan nerve distal motor latency is usually normal. Slowing in the peroneal and tibial nerves has also been encountered. Conduction velocity correlates with weakness and nerve enlargement. Numerous studies show maximal severity of disease in specific parts of peripheral nerves that are closest to the skin. They are the distal motor latencies of the distal forearm segment of the median nerve, the ulnar nerve around the elbow, and the peroneal segment between the popliteal fossa and the tibial nerve. Specifically, the median distal motor latency was not prolonged. Facial nerve latencies are prolonged, particularly in segments that are clinically affected.

Systematic investigation of sensory abnormalities in patients with peripheral neuropathy shows an absence of potentials or reduced amplitude (Rosenberg and Lovelace, 1968). When compared with motor studies, sensory studies are more frequently nonexcitable (Ramadan et al., 2001). The sural nerve is the most frequently affected of all sensory nerves (Samant et al., 1999). Sensory studies have not been shown to correlate with clinical improvement after multiple-drug therapy (see following sections; Ramadan et al., 2001). They are also frequently affected in clinically normal lepromatous nerves, indicating that neurophysiological studies can reveal the early stages of neuropathy before it becomes evident by motor and sensory loss (Ramakrishnan and Srinivasan, 1995).

Other neurophysiological tests have also shown subclinical abnormalities. In a study of 25 patients, F-response and H-reflex latencies were the most frequently abnormal neurophysiological tests, being twice as likely to be abnormal than standard sensory and motor conduction studies (Gupta and Kochar, 1994). Somatosensory evoked responses were also more sensitive than standard studies in detecting neuropathic involvement (Kochar et al., 1997). In newly diagnosed patients with leprosy, BAER studies showed a prolongation of waves I to III (25%) and III to V (40%), and VERs showed prolonged P100 latencies in 80% (Kochar et al., 1997). The significance of these findings is uncertain. Similarly, abnormal autonomic studies were reported in asymptomatic contacts of patients with leprosy (Wilder-Smith et al., 1997).

Nerve conduction studies have been used to assess the effectiveness of therapy. At the completion of therapy, both multibacillary (MB) and paucibacillary (PB) patients showed greater sensory involvement. The sural nerve is more frequently affected than the superficial peroneal, median, ulnar, and radial nerves. In PB patients, sensory abnormalities continued to show more frequent abnormalities, but sensory nerves were affected with equal frequency. Motor nerve dysfunction was most common in the tibial nerve; the peroneal, median, and ulnar nerves were affected with equal frequency. Serial electrophysiological studies in these patients who completed multiple-drug therapy regimens show a change from 37% of tested nerves being abnormal compared with 15% 6 months after therapy. No further change was noted in the ensuing 6 months. Clinical examination also improved after therapy (Samant et al., 1999).

Pathogenesis

The occurrence of leprosy in any individual has been linked to the *NRAMP1* gene, which controls susceptibility to mycobacterial infections in mice (Abeil Sanchez et al., 1998). The target of *M. leprae* in the peripheral nervous system is the Schwann cell. The bacterium is bound to laminin-2 on the surface of the Schwann cell. Once bound, how it is actually transported within the cellular environment is not precisely known, but the organism has been identified in association with the transmembrane molecule β-dystroglycan (Rambukkana et al., 1997). The infected Schwann cells degenerate, lyse, and recruit macrophages (Griffin et al., 1996). Axonal damage is the result of the release of cytokines, causing nerve destruction and, in the case of tuberculoid leprosy, granuloma formation (Turk et al., 1991).

The different clinical manifestations in leprosy are due to the differences in the patient's immune status. Such differences may, in fact, be genetically encoded: (1) MHC class II: HLA-DR3 is more common in tuberculoid leprosy; (2) MHC class II: HLA-DQ1 is more common in lepromatous leprosy. In tuberculoid leprosy, CD4+ Th1 lymphocytes (helper-1 cells) produce interleukin-2 (IL-2) and interferon gamma (IFN-γ). These cytokines activate macrophages and promote granuloma expansion. In lepromatous leprosy, CD4+ Th2 (helper 2) cells produce interleukin-4 (IL-4), involved in humoral immunity, which inhibit macrophages, accounting for the suppressed immune response in lepromatous disease.

In reactive states, it is postulated that in tuberculoid disease, bacteria leak into the blood, causing Th1 lymphocytes to release IL-2 and IFN-γ and activated macrophages that destroy the bacilli and become new epithelioid cells. In lepromatous reactive states, new synthesis of an antibody, together with cytokines such as tumor necrosis factor–alpha (TNF-α) and IL-2, is the cause. Thalidomide is a very effective treatment for ENL, perhaps because of its ability to inhibit the mRNA of TNF-α (Abulafia and Vinale, 1999).

Diagnosis

The diagnosis of leprosy is established by identifying acid-fast organisms or granulomas in skin biopsies from affected areas. In addition to diagnosis, staining for acid-fast organisms in skin biopsies and nasal smears allows quantification of the number of bacilli that are viable. The morphological index is an indicator of the number of intact bacilli seen on microscopic evaluation. The bacterial index indicates the number of bacilli in a defined microscopic field.

An assay for antibodies to phenolic glycolipid I (PGL-I) has been shown to be a very sensitive serological test that appears to correlate with the bacterial load. It has been useful in monitoring clinical status and the response to therapy. It is most useful in MB patients, as the low bacterial load in PB patients causes a high false-negative rate.

Treatment

To assist in assessing therapeutic planning and evaluating efficacy, patients with leprosy are usually assigned to two different groups. Tuberculoid and borderline tuberculoid types, whose disease is usually caused by the immune response and therefore typically has fewer bacilli on biopsy, are referred to as paucibacillary; the subtypes in which the disease is usually caused by massive infiltration of organisms are referred to as multibacillary. The potential for nerve damage from the lepromatous process, causing sensory and motor loss, increases with age and multibacillary status (Solomon et al., 1998). In fact, multibacillary patients have nerve damage seven times more frequently than do paucibacillary patients; they also more commonly have reaction states.

Multiple-drug therapy is the most effective treatment for all forms of leprosy, having been shown to provide the best chance of controlling leprosy. Dapsone is the primary drug of choice in all forms of leprosy. It is a folate antagonist and is given in a dose of 100 mg per day. Rifampin is given in a dose of 600 mg per month and, in patients with multibacillary disease, clofazimine is recommended in a dose of 50 mg per day. The duration of treatment for PB is 6 months, and for MB it is 2 years (Nations et al., 1998). The World Health Organization (WHO) has recommended that the multiple-drug therapy for MB be shortened to 12 months, and for single-lesion PB patients a single dose of rifampin, ofloxacin, and minocycline is adequate (WHO, 1998).

Despite adequate therapy, viable organisms remain in 10% to 13% of patients who have received multiple-drug therapy 6 months to 2 years after cessation of therapy (Gupta et al., 1999). In one study following clinical and nerve conduction studies for 1 year after therapy, no patient who completed the treatment course with viable organisms present experienced recurrence (Samant et al., 1999). However, 20% showed clinical deterioration after 1 year. The mechanism of deterioration is uncertain. Reactivation of dormant infection is possible; however, one patient with neuropathy in what seemed to be inactive lepromatous leprosy was found to have a delayed vasculitis (Bowen et al., 2000).

Reversal reactions are treated with anti-inflammatory agents, analgesia, continuing antimycobacterial therapy, and physical therapy for any neurological disability encountered (Britton, 1998). Corticosteroids are given for acute nerve dysfunction. ENL is effectively treated with thalidomide; clofazimine and pentoxifylline have also been shown to be promising therapies for ENL (Welsh et al., 1999)

VIRAL HEPATITIS

Prior to serological identification of the various types of virus capable of causing hepatitis, the clinical syndrome was associated with a variety of neurological disorders, including acute inflammatory demyelinating neuropathy, chronic inflammatory demyelinating neuropathy, and mononeuropathy multiplex involving both cranial and limb peripheral nerves. Most of these conditions occurred early in the course of acute viral infection, usually in the preicteric or icteric phase of the illness. Since the incidence of neurological complications in acute viral hepatitis is low, it has been difficult to validate a true causal relationship between the neurological condition and the infectious illness.

Serologically confirmed hepatitis A has been linked in isolated case reports to peripheral neuropathy. Acute and chronic hepatitis B has been implicated as a cause of Guillain-Barré syndrome, chronic relapsing polyneuropathy, and mononeuropathy multiplex. Hepatitis C virus (HCV) has also been associated with Guillain-Barré syndrome. Overall, it is now apparent that the neurological complications of acute viral hepatitis are rare, with Guillain-Barré syndrome likely to be the least uncommon of the complications.

Perhaps the most clinically important of the viral hepatitis–induced neurological complications are those related to hepatitis C infection and mixed cryoglobulinemia. This association was initially suggested by the observation of the frequent occurrence of anti-HCV antibodies and HCV RNA in the serum of patients with mixed cryoglobulinemia (Ferri et al., 1991). Although the pathogenetic role of hepatitis B infection in cryoglobulinemia was suggested earlier by Levo and colleagues (1977), further studies revealed that hepatitis C is significantly more common in association with mixed cryoglobulinemia.

Chronic HCV infection has been associated with a high incidence of immunological abnormalities, including IgM-containing immune complexes, cold-dependent activation of complement, rheumatoid factor (70%), antitissue antibodies (40% to 50%), anticardiolipin antibodies (20%), and cryoglobulinemia (Eng et al., 2000). Overall, as many as 70% of HCV-infected patients have autoantibody formation, and 20% to 30% have clinical manifestations of autoimmunity. Although a broad spectrum of extrahepatic clinical immunological manifestations have been recognized in association with chronic HCV infection (membranoproliferative glomerulonephritis, cutaneous vasculitis, porphyria cutanea tarda, sicca syndrome, thyroiditis, rheumatoid-like polyarthritis, adult Still's disease, polyarteritis nodosa, Sjögren's syndrome, Behçet's disease, and polymyositis), the most common extrahepatic manifestation of chronic HCV infection is a mixed cryoglobulinemia. In a recent large, prospective study evaluating extrahepatic manifestations of chronic HCV infection (Cacoub et al., 2000), the incidence of mixed cryoglobulinemia was found to be 56%. Given the estimated prevalence of HCV infection of about 1% in the general population, with 50% to 80% of the infected developing persistent infection, the incidence of mixed cryoglobulinemia is expected to be significant. The prevalence of HCV infection in patients with mixed cryoglobulinemia has been estimated at 43% to 90% (Ferri et al., 1991; Disdier et al., 1991; Cacoub et al., 1994), indicating a major pathogenetic role of HCV infection in the development of mixed cryoglobulinemia.

Cryoglobulins are immunoglobulins that precipitate at low temperatures and dissolve back into solution at higher temperatures. Cryoglobulinemia has been associated with a variety of systemic illnesses, including chronic infections, malignancies, renal or hepatic dysfunction, and autoimmune disorders. The accepted classification of cryoglobulins recognizes three patterns of cryoglobulinemia: type I is a monoclonal cryoglobulinemia; type II designates a combined monoclonal and polyclonal pattern; and type III is a polyclonal pattern of cryoglobulinemia. In type II mixed cryoglobulinemia, cryoglobulins contain polyclonal IgG and monoclonal IgM; type III mixed cryoglobulinemia precipitates contain polyclonal IgM and IgG. When no underlying etiology for cryoglobulinemia is evident, the term *essential cryoglobulinemia* is used.

Clinical Manifestations

Mixed cryoglobulinemia is associated with a variety of manifestations suggestive of systemic vasculitic disease: arthralgias, arthritis, purpura, hepatosplenomegaly, glomerulonephritis, weakness, and fatigue (Gorevic et al., 1980). The association of mixed cryoglobulinemia and peripheral neuropathy is well established. Studies have cited the incidence of neuropathy in a range from 7% to 86% (Logothetis et al., 1968; Garcia-Bragado et al., 1988; Gemignani et al., 1992; Ferri et al., 1992; Ciompi et al., 1996). Peripheral neuropathy may be the presenting manifestation of mixed cryoglobulinemia. The pattern of neuropathy is variable, presenting most frequently as either mononeuropathy multiplex with acute onset or progressive distal symmetrical sensorimotor polyneuropathy occasionally combined with recognizable mononeuropathies. The latter pattern is more common. It is thought that it represents a confluence of partial vasculitis-induced mononeuropathies in multiple nerve fascicles. The neuropathy is frequently characterized by sensory loss with painful dysesthesias and paresthesias sometimes precipitated by cold. Raynaud's phenomenon can accompany the neuropathic symptoms.

Although further studies are needed, the clinical features of neuropathy in the setting of HCV infection and mixed cryoglobulinemia appear similar to the previously established clinical characteristics of essential mixed cryoglobulinemia-induced neuropathy. The patterns of chronic, mostly symmetrical sensory or sensorimotor polyneuropathy or more acute mononeuropathy multiplex sometimes superimposed over chronic sensory neuropathy are observed, with the former being more common. Sensory symptoms are often predominant, and neuropathy is sometimes manifested as a pure sensory polyneuropathy. Painful dysesthesias and paresthesias are frequently the initial symptoms and occur more prominently in the lower extremities. The serological studies, in addition to mixed cryoglobulinemia, may reveal the presence of rheumatoid factor and low levels of complements. The symptoms of arthralgia, fatigue, Raynaud's phenomenon, and cutaneous findings of purpura or erythematous exanthem may be observed.

Differential characteristics of peripheral neuropathy in the setting of HCV-related mixed cryoglobulinemia have not been well delineated. Few studies have compared the clinical features of HCV-positive and HCV-negative neuropathy in the setting of essential mixed cryoglobulinemia. One such study (Apartis et al., 1996), which reviewed 15 patients with mixed cryoglobulinemia and neuropathy and found that 10 patients were HCV-positive, suggested that HCV-infected patients had more pronounced neuropathy, mostly due to more widespread motor deficits. A total of 7 of 10 patients had polyneuropathies, and 3 had multiple mononeuropathies. Electrophysiological studies showed all neuropathies to be axonopathies. Necrotizing vasculitis was found in the biopsies of two of nine HCV-positive patients and in none of the HCV-negative patients. HCV-positive patients also revealed more frequent cryoglobulinemia-related cutaneous findings, higher serum cryoglobulin levels, lower total complement levels, and the more frequent presence of rheumatoid factor. The validity of these conclusions needs to be confirmed by larger studies.

Electrodiagnostic Studies

Electrodiagnostic studies in mixed cryoglobulinemia show an axonal neuropathy with mononeuritis multiplex (Gemignani et al., 1992; Dumitru, 1995; Cipomi et al., 1996; Steck, 1998). Demyelinating neuropathy has been reported as well, although it occurs uncommonly (Logothetis et al., 1968). Abnormal sensory conduction with absent sensory nerve action potentials and mild to moderate slowing of motor conduction and reduced compound muscle action potentials are observed. Sensory nerve conduction abnormalities are the most frequently reported electromyographic findings. Conduction blocks have been reported, although they are uncommon (Caniatti et al., 1996; Tembl et al., 1999). The nerve biopsy results reported have revealed pathological patterns similar to those seen in previously described essential cryoglobulinemia-related neuropathy. Inflammatory infiltration of the walls of the epineurial vessels without necrosis is probably the most common finding. True necrotizing vasculitis may be seen and may correlate with the clinical pattern of more acute mononeuropathy multiplex. The loss of myelinated fibers with or without axonal degeneration has been described (Tembl et al., 1999).

Nerve biopsy results reveal axonal degeneration in the setting of epineurial vasculitis and changes in the endoneurial microvessels characterized by thickening of the vessel wall and occlusion of the lumen.

Pathogenesis

The mechanism by which HCV infection induces mixed cryoglobulinemia is unclear. In the chronic phase of HCV infection, a polyclonal increase in immunoglobulins, including autoantibodies, may occur. Although the mechanism of polyclonal expansion of autoantibody production is not known, possible explanations include dysregulation of anti-idiotype networks, molecular mimicry between viral and tissue antigens, and dysregulation of T-cell suppression of B-cell antibody production due to chronic infection. Some of the produced antibodies might form cryoprecipitable immune complexes on binding to their respective antigens, leading to the development of cryoglobulinemia. Hepatitis C virus RNA and HCV antibodies have been documented in the cryoprecipitates of patients with HCV-associated mixed cryoglobulinemia in multiple studies (Pascual et al., 1990; Ferri et al., 1991; Agnello et al., 1992).

The mechanism of nerve damage in the setting of HCV-related cryoglobulinemia (and hence the development of neuropathy) is not well understood. It has been suggested that the pathogenetic role of HCV infection is probably limited to the development of an immunological response to the virus and is mediated through mixed cryoglobulinemia rather than the result of the direct cytotoxic effect of the virus itself on the nerve. The immune complexes are deposited in the vessel walls, leading to an inflammatory process partly through the activation of the complement system. This inflammatory process leads to small-vessel vasculitic changes in epineurial and endoneurial vessels, with resulting derangement of microcirculation that ultimately leads to ischemic or inflammatory nerve lesions and the development of neuropathy. Necrotizing vasculitis with acute nerve ischemia may also occur. Interestingly, there are reports of HCV-associated vasculitis with involvement of the central nervous system (Heckmann et al., 1999; Tembl et al., 1999), manifesting as encephalopathy with seizures or strokelike episodes. This mechanism of development of HCV-related neuropathy is supported by the absence of the HCV particles in the nerve biopsy of a patient reported by Khella and colleagues (1995). Frequently observed low levels of complement factors (C4, C3) in the setting of HCV cryoglobulinemic neuropathy and a case report (Murai et al., 1995) of HCV neuropathy with a good therapeutic response to cryoglobulinopheresis with improvement of hypocomplementemia highlight a role of the complement system in nerve damage.

There is, however, evidence suggesting HCV-induced neuropathy is mediated by direct HCV infection of the nerve. One study (Bonetti et al., 1999) showed by reverse transcription–polymerase chain reaction (PCR) the presence of HCV RNA in homogenates of nerve biopsies in five patients with HCV-related neuropathy. In situ reverse-transcriptase PCR was performed to exclude the possibility of tissue contamination by HCV-positive serum. Whether HCV-related neuropathy may occur without the presence of cryoglobulinemia is unclear at present. There are few reports that describe neuropathy in the setting of HCV infection without cryoglobulinemia (Kashihara et al., 1995; Caudai et al., 1997). Chronic sensory neuropathy in the setting of chronic HCV infection without cryoglobulinemia that was shown to have anti-HCV antibodies and HCV RNA in the cerebrospinal fluid has been re-

ported (Caudai et al., 1997). The exact pathogenetic roles of HCV infection and cryoglobulins in the development of neuropathy are yet to be elucidated.

Therapy

Different therapeutic regimens have been used with some success for treating HCV-related cryoglobulinemic neuropathy, including corticosteroids, cyclophosphamide, plasma exchange, and cryopheresis. The data on the therapeutic efficacy of these regimens remain anecdotal. Interferon-α has recently emerged as a therapeutic modality. It has been used successfully to treat patients with hepatitis C with or without mixed cryoglobulinemia (Durand et al., 1992; Mmisiani et al., 1994) and for essential mixed cryoglobulinemia (Casato et al., 1991). The advantage of interferon-α, if proved to be effective for HCV cryoglobulinemic neuropathy, lies in its being an established treatment for HCV hepatic disease as well as a probably efficacious treatment for mixed cryoglobulinemia. The mechanism of action of interferon-α is not well understood. Theories include various immunomodulating effects on T or B lymphocytes (inhibition of immunoglobulin synthesis by B cells, induction of helper T cells, activation of natural killer cells), enhancement of elimination of circulating cryoglobulins by stimulating macrophage function, and antiviral activity. Khella and associates (1995) reported the successful use of interferon-α specifically for HCV cryoglobulinemic neuropathy, with good symptomatic improvement. Other case series reported good results with interferon-α, some documenting an improvement in mixed cryoglobulinemia along with symptomatic improvement of neuropathy (Apartis et al., 1996; Heckman et al., 1999; Tembl et al., 1999). On the other hand, peripheral neuropathy has been shown to be a side effect of treatment of chronic viral hepatitis with interferon-α (Fattovich et al., 1996). Some reports documented worsening of existing neuropathy or a new development of neuropathy with interferon-α treatment (Zuber and Gause, 1997). Further studies are needed to establish the role of interferon-α in the treatment of HCV cryoglobulinemic neuropathy.

Patients with peripheral neuropathy and essential cryoglobulinemia should be evaluated for the presence of serum anti-HCV antibodies so that the degree of hepatic dysfunction could be evaluated and treatment for neuropathy as well as for HCV hepatitis could be rationally selected.

References

Abeil Sanchez FO, Oberti J, Thuc NV, et al: Susceptibility to leprosy is linked to the human *NRAMP1* gene. J Infect Dis 1998; 177:133–145.

Abulafia J, Vinale RA: Leprosy: Pathogenesis updated. Int J Dermatol 1999;38:321–334.

Agnello V, Chung RT, Kaplan LM: A role of hepatitis C virus

infection in type II cryoglobulinemia. N Engl J Med 1992;327: 1490–1495.

Antia NH, Pandaya SS, Dastur DK: Nerves in the arm in leprosy. I. Clinical electrodiagnostic and operative aspects. Int J Lepr 1970;38:12.

Apartis E, Leger JM, Musset L, et al: Peripheral neuropathy associated with essential mixed cryoglobulinemia: A role for hepatitis C virus infection? J Neurol Neurosurg Neuropsychiatry 1996; 60:661–666.

Bannwarth A: Chronische lymphocytare meningitis, entzudnliche polyneuritis und rheumatismus. Arch Psychiatr Nervenkr 1941; 113:284–376.

Baumhackl U, Kristoferitsch W, Sluga E, Stanek G: Neurological manifestations of *Borrelia burgdorferi* infections. Zentralbl Bakteriol Hyg [A] 1986;263:334.

Bonetti B, Scardoni M, Monaco S, et al: Hepatitis C virus infection of peripheral nerves in type II cryoglobulinemia. Virch Arch 1999;434:533–535.

Bowen JRC, McDougall AC, Morris JH, et al: Vasculitic neuropathy in a patient with inactive treated lepromatous leprosy. J Neurol Neurosurg Psychiatry 2000;68l:496–500.

Britton WJ: Management of leprosy reversal reactions. Lepr Rev 1998;69:225–234.

Brown TR, Kovinkha A, Wathanadilokkol U, et al: Lepromatous neuropathy: Correlation of clinical and electrophysiological tests. Indian J Lepr 1996;68:1–14.

Cacoub P, Lunel FF, Musset L, et al: Mixed cryoglobulinemia and hepatitis C virus. Am J Med 1994;96:124–132.

Cacoub P, Renou C, Rosenthal E, et al: Extrahepatic manifestations associated with hepatitis C virus infection. Medicine (Baltimore) 2000;79:47–56.

Camponovo F, Meier C: Neuropathy of vasculitic origin in a case of Garin-Boujadoux-Bannwarth syndrome with positive *Borrelia* antibody response. J Neurol 1986;79:271–278.

Caniatti LM, Tugnoli V, Eleopra R, et al: Cryoglobulinemic neuropathy related to hepatitis C virus infection: Clinical, laboratory and neurophysiological study. J Periph Nerv Syst 1996;1:131–138.

Casato M, Lagana B, Antonelli G, et al: Long-term results of therapy with interferon-alpha for type II essential mixed cryoglobulinemia. Blood 1991;78:3142–3147.

Caudai C, Maimone D, Almi P, et al: The potential role of hepatitis C virus in the pathogenesis of the neurological syndrome in chronic hepatitis C. Gut 1997;41:411–412.

Ciompi ML, Marini D, Siciliano G, et al: Cryoglobulinemic peripheral neuropathy: Neurophysiologic evaluation in twenty-two patients. Biomed Pharmacother 1996;50:329–336.

Clark JR, Carlson RD, Saski CT: Facial paralysis in Lyme disease. Laryngoscope 1985;95:1341–1345.

Creange A, Meyrignac D, Roualdes B, et al: Diphtheritic neuropathy. Muscle Nerve 1995;18:1460–1463.

Dattwyler RF, Volkman DJ, Conaty SM, et al: Amoxycillin plus probenecid versus doxycycline for treatment of erythema migrans borreliosis. Lancet 1990;47:586–594.

Disdier P, Harle JR, Weiller PJ: Cryoglobulinemia and hepatitis C infection. Lancet 1991;338:1151–1152.

Dumitru D: Electrodiagnostic Medicine. Philadelphia, Hanley & Belfus, 1995; 788–789.

Durand JM, Kaplanski G, Lefevre P, et al: Effect of interferon-alpha 2b on cryoglobulinemia related to hepatitis C virus infection. J Infect Dis 1992;165:778–779.

Eng MA, Kallemuchikkal U, Gorevic PD: Hepatitis C virus, autoimmunity and lymphoproliferation. Mt Sinai J Med 2000;67:120–132.

England JD, Bohm RP, Roberts ED, Philipp MT: Mononeuropathy multiplex in Rhesus monkeys with chronic Lyme disease. Ann Neurol 1997;41:375–384.

Fattovich G, Giustina G, Favarato S, Ruol A: A survey of adverse events in 11,241 patients with chronic viral hepatitis treated with alfa interferon. J Hepatol 1996;24:38–47.

Ferri C, Greco F, Longombardo G: Association between hepatitis C virus and mixed cryoglobulinemia. Clin Exp Rheumatol 1991; 9:621–624.

Ferri C, La Civita L, Cirafisi C, et al: Peripheral neuropathy in mixed cryoglobulinemia: Clinical and electrophysiologic investigations. J Rheumatol 1992;19:889–895.

Fisher CM, Adams RD: Diphtheritic polyneuritis, a pathological study. J Neuropathol Exp Neurol 1956;15:243–268.

Garcia-Bragado F, Fernandez JM, Navarro C, et al: Peripheral neuropathy in essential MC. Arch Neurol 1988;45:1210–1214.

Gemignani F, Pavesi G, Fiocchi A, et al: Peripheral neuropathy in essential mixed cryoglobulinaemia. J Neurol Neurosurg Psychiatry 1992;55(2):116–120.

Gorevic PD, Kassab HJ, Levo Y: Mixed cryoglobulinemia: Clinical aspects and long-term follow-up of 40 patients. Am J Med 1980; 69:287–308.

Griffin JW, George EB, Chaudhry V: Wallerian degeneration in peripheral nerve disease. Baillere's Clin Neurol 1996;5:65–75.

Gupta BK, Kochar DK: Int J Lepr Other Mycobact Dis 1994;62:586–593.

Gupta UD, Katoch K, Singh HB, et al: Detection of viable organisms in leprosy patients treated with multidrug therapy. Acta Lepr 1999;70:281–286.

Hackett ER, Shipley DE, Livengood R: Motor nerve conduction velocity studies in patients with leprosy. Int J Lepr 1968; 282.

Haimanot RT, Melaku Z: Leprosy. Curr Opin Neurol 2000;13:317–322.

Halperin J, Luft BJ, Volkman DJ, Dattwyler RJ: Lyme neuroborreliosis: Peripheral nervous system manifestations. Brain 1990;13: 1207–1221.

Halperin JJ, Little BW, Coyle PK, Dattwyler RJ: Lyme disease: Cause of a treatable peripheral neuropathy. Neurology 1987; 37:1700.

Halperin JJ, Pass HL, Anand AK, et al: Nervous system abnormalities in Lyme disease. Ann N Y Acad Sci 1988;539:24.

Hann AF: Resurgence of diphtheria in the newly independent states of the former Soviet Union: A reminder of risk. J Neurol Neurosurg Psychiatry 1999;67:426.

Heckmann JG, Kayser C, Heuss D, et al: Neurological manifestations of chronic hepatitis C. J Neurol 1999;246:486–491.

Jacob M, Mathai R: Diagnostic efficacy of cutaneous nerve biopsy in primary leprosy. Int J Lepr 1998;56:56–60.

Jobling WH, Morgan-Hughes JA: Pure neural tuberculoid leprosy. Br Med J 1965;2:799–800.

Kashihara K, Terai T, Shomori T: Relapsing neuropathy associated with hepatitis C virus infection. Intern Med 1995;34:265–266.

Khella SL, Frost S, Hermann GA, et al: Hepatitis C infection, cryoglobulinemia, and vasculitic neuropathy—treatment with interferon alfa: Case report and literature review. Neurology 1995;45(3 Pt 1):407–411.

Kochar DK, Gupta DV, Sandeep C, et al: Study of brain stem auditory-evoked potentials and visual evoked potentials in leprosy. Int J Lepr Other Mycobac Dis 1997;65:157–165.

Kurdi A, Abdul-Kader M: Clinical and electrophysiological studies of diphtheritic neuritis in Jordan. J Neurol Sci 1979;42:343–350.

Levo Y, Gorevic PD, Kassab HJ, et al: Association between hepatitis B virus and essential mixed cryoglobulinemia. N Engl J Med 1977;296:1501–1504.

Logigian EL, Steere AC: Clinical and electrophysiologic findings in chronic neuropathy of Lyme disease. Neurology 1992;42:303–311.

Logina I, Donaghy M: Diphtheritic polyneuropathy: A clinical study and comparison with Guillain-Barré syndrome. J Neurol Neurosurg Psychiatry 1999;67:433–438.

Logothetis J, Kennedy WR, Ellington A, Williams RC: Cryoglobulinemic neuropathy: Incidence and clinical characteristics. Arch Neurol 1968;19:389–397.

Maimone D, Villanova M, Stanta G, et al: Detection of *Borrelia burgdorferi* DNA and complement membrane attack complex deposits in the sural nerve of a patient with chronic polyneuropathy and tertiary Lyme disease. Muscle Nerve 1997;20:969–975.

McDonald WI, Kocen RS: Diphtheritic neuropathy. In Dyck PJ, Thomas PK, Griffin JW (eds): Peripheral Neuropathy, 3rd ed. Philadelphia, WB Saunders, 1993; 1412–1417.

McLeod JF, Hargrave JC, Walsh JC, et al: Nerve conduction studies in leprosy. Inst J Lepr Other Mycobact Dis 1975;43:21–31.

Messing A, Behringer RR, Hammang JP, et al: P0 promoter directs expression of reporter and toxin genes to Schwann cells of transgenic mice. Neuron 1992;8:507–520.

Mmisiani R, Bellavita P, Fenili D, et al: Interferon alfa-2a therapy in cryoglobulinemia associated with hepatitis C virus. N Engl J Med 1994;330:751–756.

Murai H, Inaba S, Kira J, et al: Hepatitis C virus–associated cryoglobulinemic neuropathy successfully treated with plasma exchange. Artific Organs 1995;19:334–338.

Nations SP, Katz JS, Lyde CB, Barohn RJ: Leprous neuropathy: An American perspective. Semin Neurol 1998;18:1997–1999.

Oey PL, Franssen H, Barnsen R, Wokke JHJ: Multifocal conduction block in a patient with *Borrelia burgdorferi* infection. Muscle Nerve 1991;14:375–377.

Pachner AR, Steere AC: The triad of neurologic manifestations of Lyme disease: Meningitis, cranial neuritis, and radiculoneuritis. Neurology 1985;35:47–53.

Pascual M, Perrin L, Giostra E, Shifferli JA: Hepatitis C virus in patients with cryoglobulinemia type II. J Infect Dis 1990; 162:569–570.

Pleasure DE, Feldmann B, Prockop DJ: Diphtheria toxin inhibits the synthesis of myelin proteolipid and basic proteins by peripheral nerve in vitro. J Neurochem 1973;20:81–90.

Ramadan W, Mourad B, Fadel W, Ghoraba E: Clinical, electrophysiological and immunopathological study of peripheral nerves in Hansen's disease. Lepr Rev 2001;72:35–49.

Ramakrishnan AG, Srinivasan TM: Electrophysiological correlates of hanseniasis. Int J Lepr Other Mycobact Dis 1995;63:395–408.

Rambukkana A, Salzer JL, Yurchenco PD, Tuomanen EL: Neural targeting of *Mycobacterium leprae* mediated by the G domain of the laminin–alpha 2 chain. Cell 1997;88:811–821.

Rambukkana A, Yamada H, Zanazzi G, et al: Role of alpha-dystroglycan as a Schwann cell receptor for *Mycobacterium leprae*. Science 1998;282:2076–2079.

Reik L, Steere AC, Bartenhagen NH: Neurologic abnormalities of Lyme disease. Medicine (Baltimore) 1979;58:281.

Reik L, Burgdorfer W, Donaldson JO: Neurologic abnormalities in Lyme disease without erythema chronicum migrans. Am J Med 1986;81:73.

Reik L: Peripheral neuropathy in Lyme disease. In Dyck PJ, Thomas PK, Griffin JW, et al (eds): Peripheral Neuropathy, 3rd ed. Philadelphia, WB Saunders, 1993; 1401–1411.

Rosenberg RN, Lovelace RE: Mononeuritis multiplex in lepromatous leprosy. Arch Neurol 1968;19:310–314.

Samant G, Shetty P, Uplekar MW, Antia NH: Clinical and electrophysiological evaluation of nerve function impairment following cessation of multidrug therapy in leprosy. Lepr Rev 1999; 70:10–20.

Scelsa SN, Herskovitz S, Befger AR: A predominantly motor polyradiculopathy of Lyme disease. Muscle Nerve 1996;19:780–783.

Solomon S, Kurian N, Ramadas P, Rao PS: Incidence of nerve damage in leprosy patients treated with MDT. Int J Lepr Other Mycobact Dis 1998;66:451–456.

Steck AJ: Neurological manifestations of malignant and non-malignant dysglobulinemias. J Neurol 1998;245:634–639.

Sternman AB, Nelson S, Barclay P: Demyelinating neuropathy accompanying Lyme disease. Neurology 1982;32:1302–1305.

Tembl JI, Ferrer JM, Sevilla MT, et al: Neurologic complications associated with hepatitis C virus infection. Neurology 1999; 53:861–864.

Tezzon F, Corrandini C, Huber R, et al: Vasculitic mononeuritis multiplex in patients with Lyme disease. Ital J Neurol Sci 1991; 12:229–232.

Turk JL, Curtis J, De Blaquiere G: Immunopathology of nerve involvement in leprosy. Indian J Lepr 1991;63:483–491.

Vallat JM, Hugon J, Lubeau M, et al: Tick-bite meningoradiculoneuritis: Clinical, electrophysiologic, and histologic findings in 10 cases. Neurology 1987;79:271–278.

Verghese M, Ithimani KV, Satyanarayan KR, et al: A study of conduction velocity of ulnar and median nerves in leprosy. Int J Lepr 1970;38:271.

Welsh O, Gomedz M, Mancias C, et al: Pharmacology and therapeutics: A new approach to type 2 leprosy reaction. Int J Dermatol 1999;38:931–933.

WHO Expert Committee on Leprosy. World Health Organ Tech Rep Ser 1998;874:1–43.

Wilder-Smith E, Wilder-Smith A, Egger M: Peripheral autonomic dysfunction in asymptomatic contacts. J Neurol Sci 1997;150: 33–38.

Wormser GP: Treatment and prevention of Lyme disease with emphasis on antimicrobial therapy for neuroborreliosis and vaccination. Semin Neurol 1997;17:45–52.

Wulff CH, Hansen K, Strange P, Trojaborg W: Multiple mononeuritis and radiculitis with erythema, pain, elevated CSF protein and pleocytosis (Bannwarth's syndrome). J Neurol Neurosurg Psychiatry 1983;46:485.

Zuber M, Gause A: Peripheral neuropathy during interferon-alpha therapy in patients with cryoglobulinemia and hepatitis virus infection. J Rheumatol 1997;24:2488–2489.

MOTOR NEURON DISEASES

chapter 69

Hereditary Motor Neuron Diseases

Clifton L. Gooch

There has been tremendous progress in unraveling the genetics of the hereditary motor neuron disorders. However, with this progress has come a significant increase in the complexity of our understanding of, and our attempts to classify, these diseases, as evidenced most dramatically by the expanding world of the spinal muscular atrophies (SMAs). In this chapter, we will review the history, clinical classification, molecular genetics, diagnosis, electrophysiology, and management of the SMAs and their variants, as well as spinal and bulbar muscular atrophy and hereditary spastic paraparesis. Familial amyotrophic lateral sclerosis, along with the sporadic form of that disease, is detailed in Chapter 72.

SPINAL MUSCULAR ATROPHY: HISTORY AND CLINICAL CLASSIFICATIONS

In late 1890, Guido Werdnig lectured at the University of Vienna "on a case of muscular dystrophy with positive spinal cord findings" (Groger and Werdnig, 1990). In 1891, a more detailed account appeared, entitled "Two early infantile hereditary cases: Progressive muscular atrophy appearing as dystrophy, but on a neuritic basis," along with another paper by Johann Hoffmann of Heidelberg University coining the term *spinal muscular atrophy.* Together, these papers described 10 affected children with initially normal development who developed proximal weakness between 5 and 9 months of age, with preservation of social and linguistic skills. In all cases weakness was progressive, with death following 1 to 4 years after symptomatic onset. Spinal cord histology revealed loss of anterior horn cells, most prominent at the cervical and lumbar levels, which correlated with concurrent atrophy in affected muscle groups (Gamstorp, 1984; Iannaccone et al., 1990). Over the next half century, further sporadic descriptions appeared, and in 1950 Brandt published a more comprehensive epidemiological study in which he reviewed 112 patients with early-onset disease in Denmark. Severe weakness at birth was present in most cases, and 87% developed symptoms before 1 year of age. Fifty-six percent survived less than 1 year and 80% survived less than 4 years (Brandt, 1950). Kugelberg and Welander described a milder form of the disease with later onset in 12 patients developing proximal weakness between 2 and 17 years; however, in contrast to the patients of Werdnig and Hoffmann, these children were able to ambulate and survived into adulthood (Kugelberg and Welander, 1956). In 1961, Byers and Banker reviewed 52 cases of infantile spinal muscular atrophy and divided them into three groups: (1) those with onset at birth or within 2 months of age with severe generalized weakness and early demise; (2) those with onset between 2 and 12 months with longer survival; and (3) those with onset in the second year of life with survival for a number of years (Byers and Banker, 1961). However, growing recognition of cases with onset in adolescence and adulthood prompted Emery to recognize four groups based on age of disease onset: infantile, intermediate, juvenile, and adult (Emery, 1971). Together with Fried, he then proposed three major clinical categories (the last of which combined juvenile and adult onset cases into one group): *type I,* beginning at birth or within the first few months, with death before age 2 years (infantile SMA or Werdnig-Hoffmann disease); *type II,* with symptomatic onset between 3 and 15 months and survival beyond 4 years (intermediate SMA); and *type III,* with symptomatic onset after 24 months and a more slowly progressive and benign course (juvenile and adult SMA, or Kugelberg-Welander disease) (Fried and Emery, 1971). During this same period, Hausmanowa-Petrusewicz et al. proposed a somewhat similar system but with four categories: *type IA,* a severe infantile variety with onset at birth and death within 2 to 4 years; *type IB,* an infantile onset form with no ambulation but survival over 10 years; *type II,* an intermediate form with onset at 2 to 6 years, loss of mobility in less than 10 years, and longer survival; and *type III,* with onset at 2 to 15 years, long survival, and a milder but progressive course (Hausmanowa-Petrusewicz et al., 1968).

Because of the lack of uniformity resulting from these competing classifications, an international workshop was called by the Muscular Dystrophy Association in December of 1990 in New York to develop a consensus classification system. At the time of the workshop, the recent mapping of the *SMA* gene to chromosome 5q reinforced the need for a clear and widely accepted system of classification to facilitate developing phenotype-to-genotype correlation. Three categories were proposed based on a combination of age at onset, highest motor milestone achieved, and age at death. *Type I* (severe SMA) begins at 0 to 6 months; these infants are never able to sit unsupported, and death ensues in less than 2 years. *Type II* (intermediate SMA) begins at less than 18 months; these children are never able to stand, and death occurs after age 2 years. *Type III* (mild SMA) begins after 18 months; these patients are ultimately able to stand unsupported and live into adulthood. These collaborative criteria have been widely used and are now employed in most studies. Unless otherwise specified, the collaborative criteria of the International SMA Consortium are used throughout this section (Munsat, 1991; Iannaccone, 1998; Strober and Tennekoon, 1999). In order to more specifically recognize the purely adult-onset disorders having an average age at onset of 37 years, some investigators have added an SMA type IV to the collaborative criteria. Others have recognized yet another separate clinical classification, with its own subdivisions, for the distal SMAs, and separate categories are sometimes applied for the scapuloperoneal spinal muscular atrophies, spinal muscular atrophy with prominent contractures, and other miscellaneous spinal muscular atrophy variants (Harding, 1993; Cole and Siddique, 1999) (Table 69–1).

PROXIMAL SPINAL MUSCULAR ATROPHIES

Epidemiology

SMA is a common disorder worldwide, with a combined incidence of 1 in 6,000 to 1 in 10,000 live births. It is the second most common disease seen in pediatric neuromuscular clinics after Duchenne's muscular dystrophy and the second most common fatal autosomal recessive disorder after cystic fibrosis, having a carrier frequency of approximately 1 in 40 (Chang et al., 1997; Talbot, 1999). Meta-analysis of the literature is challenging because of the disparate clinical definitions of the groups assessed in different studies, although several more recent studies have provided more detailed epidemiological information regarding survival in SMA using the collaborative criteria of the International SMA

Table 69–1. Spinal Muscular Atrophy

Types	Age at Onset	Inheritance	Selected Clinical Features
Type I	0–6 mo	AR (rare AD and X-linked)	Never sit, death <2 yr
Type II	0–18 mo	AR	Never stand, death >2 yr
Type III	>18 mo	AR or AD	Stand, survive to adult
Type IV	10–50 yr	AR or AD	Slow progression over decades
Distal juvenile, dominant	<10 yr	AD	Distal leg weakness, pes cavus
Distal adult	>15 yr	AD	Distal leg weakness, pes cavus
Distal mild juvenile, recessive	2–10 yr	AR	Ambulate, normal life expectancy
Distal severe juvenile, recessive	4 mo to 20 yr	AR	Ambulation lost by age 30 yr
Distal upper limb predominant	10–40 yr	AD	Ambulate into old age
Distal neonatal + diaphragmatic paralysis	1–2 mo	AR	Respiratory failure in <3 mo
Distal with vocal cord involvement	10–20 yr	Variable	Hoarseness, leg weakness at onset
Scapuloperoneal SMAs	Variable	AR or AD	Significant phenotypic variability
SMA with contractures	Infancy to childhood	Variable	Variable

AD, autosomal dominant; AR, autosomal recessive; SMA, spinal muscular atrophy.

Consortium detailed above (Munsat, 1991). The vast majority of type I patients die before the age of 2 years, most commonly as a result of respiratory failure, although a small number of patients who otherwise meet the collaborative criteria for type I disease survive beyond the 2 years stipulated as part of the definition of this category (Crawford and Pardo, 1996). In type II disease, death typically occurs between age 2 years and young adulthood, again due to respiratory failure or infection, although some patients live into the third decade. The majority of patients with type III disease reach adulthood, but longer and much more variable survival among patients in this group continues to make acquisition and analysis of long-term data difficult (Iannaccone, 1998).

Several epidemiological studies have more specifically measured survival and clinical function in patients with SMA, and some have addressed the difficulties of working within the collaborative criteria. In one large study, 445 patients were assessed (Zerres and Rudnik-Schoneborn, 1995; Strober and Tennekoon, 1999). Twenty-four percent of patients could not be categorized according to the collaborative criteria and were removed from the analysis, but survival probabilities were calculated for the remainder. For type I disease, the probability of survival to 2 years was 32%, to 4 years 18%, to 10 years 8%, and to 20 years 0%. In type II disease, survival probability to age 2 and 4 was 100%, to age 10 98%, and to age 20 77%. Again, because of greater variability and long-term survival exceeding the period of the study, detailed data for survival in type III disease were incomplete. Another study focused on the clinical features of the disease, utilizing groups that correspond roughly to those of the collaborative criteria (Hausmanowa-Petrusewicz and Fidzianska-Dolot, 1984; Wessel, 1989). Patients with acute infantile SMA (type I disease; symptomatic no later than age 6 months) accounted for approximately 23% of the total, and 95% of these cases were diagnosed in the first 3 months of life. Less than 2% were ever able to sit without support, and less than 25% were able to lift their heads off the bed. Those

with profound weakness at birth had the poorest survival, with an average life expectancy of 7 months, and the vast majority died in less than 1 year. Chronic infantile SMA (type II disease) could not be reliably distinguished from the acute, more severe form without a period of observation to enable a determination of progression rate. This variety accounted for 24% of total cases and had a much greater spectrum of variability in both severity at onset and rate of progression. Intermediate and juvenile SMA (Kugelberg-Welander syndrome) together accounted for the remaining 53% of the total (the combination of which approximates the collaborative criteria's type III disease). Twenty-one percent of total cases were defined as intermediate SMA, with onset between the ages of 2 and 6 years and immobilization after 1 to 10 years of illness, but prolonged survival. The remaining 32% of the total fell into the category of juvenile SMA, with onset between age 3 and 15 years, much milder symptoms, and a much longer survival. Ambulation in both of these groups is often preserved up to 20 to 30 years after symptomatic onset, and these patients have a nearly normal life expectancy. In a more recent study, the course of 159 patients with types II and III disease was followed, and an inverse relationship between maximum function achieved and the time course of functional loss was documented (Russman et al., 1996). Patients in this study walking independently typically had an age of onset greater than 2 years and maintained ambulation for an average of 44 years. Conversely, patients with onset before age 2 years lost ambulation at an average of age 12 years. If independent ambulation was never achieved but could be performed with assistance, it was lost at an average of 7 years, whereas when independent sitting was the maximal function achieved, it was lost at an average age of 14 years.

Clinical Features

SPINAL MUSCULAR ATROPHY TYPE I

As mentioned previously, this is the most severe variety of the disease and corresponds most closely with the original descriptions of Werdnig and Hoffmann (acute infantile SMA). Most patients present with both profound hypotonia and severe weakness at birth, and one third of mothers report decreased strength of fetal movement during the last trimester when carefully questioned. The syndrome of arthrogryposis multiplex congenita resulting from any severe intrauterine neuromuscular disorder is often caused by primary denervation, and a recent study suggests that up to 50% of such patients may carry deletions associated with SMA, reinforcing the importance of screening such patients for SMA-associated mutations (Bingham et al., 1997). The diagnosis is usually made as a consequence of poor movement, hypotonia, feeding problems, poor head control, or developmental delay. Tongue fasciculations are typically present but can easily be confused with normal tongue movement during crying, making it important that the tongue be examined at rest. Tongue atrophy, with scalloping of the labial and gingival margins, may also be observed. Weakness of the muscles of swallowing results in rapid tiring during feeding, and often weight loss ensues before inadequate nutrition becomes apparent. The extraocular and facial muscles are spared, resulting in a normal range of facial expression and a striking discrepancy between the infant's level of social interaction and paucity of motor skills. The infant also demonstrates poor head and trunk control along with a poor gag, paradoxical respirations, and a weak cry. Poor intercostal muscle strength necessitates diaphragmatic breathing, with accompanying inefficient respirations, pectus excavatum, and flailing of the lower ribs resulting in a bell-shaped deformity of the chest. Bilateral diaphragmatic paralysis may sometimes be a presenting manifestation, and both respiratory muscle weakness and malnutrition increase the risk of aspiration. Often no spontaneous movement is observed except in the hands and feet, where a fine tremor of the fingers (known as polyminimyoclonus) may be seen despite poorly developed, thin hand musculature. This movement has been attributed by some to fasciculations of the intrinsic hand musculature. Weakness is most prominent in the proximal muscle of the lower extremities, and movement in the legs is restricted to the toes and feet. The legs are often held in a flexed, abducted, and externally rotated position at the hips in what has been termed the "frog-leg" posture. Deep-tendon reflexes are absent, with intact sensation and normal sphincter tone. As symptoms may not begin until the first few months after birth, some cases may escape early detection.

SPINAL MUSCULAR ATROPHY TYPE II

This category approximately corresponds to the original descriptions of chronic infantile SMA, although occasionally cases of patients following this course are reported with onset before age 6 months. In this group most patients have normal motor milestones through 6 months, although hypotonia may be present, but symptoms begin before 18 months. The legs are more severely affected than the arms, and an inability to walk often prompts medical evaluation. Most of these patients can move their arms and legs and lift their heads, and they are usually able to achieve independent sitting and/or standing. Clubfoot deformity is noted in a few individuals, and deep-tendon reflexes are variably preserved in stronger muscle groups, although they are eventually lost. As in type I disease, polyminimyoclonus may be seen and fasciculations of the tongue may be present. Ongoing skeletal growth, in conjunction with poor muscular strength and development, produces skeletal deformities, progressive contractures, and severe kyphoscoliosis. Individual progression is very difficult to predict, with some patients manifesting relatively linear declines over several years and others entering years of apparent symptomatic plateaus followed by episodes of more sudden decline. Although most patients die in childhood, some survive well into adult life.

SPINAL MUSCULAR ATROPHY TYPE III

This category includes the former clinical categorizations of both intermediate SMA and juvenile progressive SMA (Kugelberg-Welander disease). The intermediate form included those children who developed proximal muscle weakness between the age of 2 and 6 years followed by progression and immobilization after 10 years, with long survival. These cases may be confused with limb-girdle muscular dystrophy, as they frequently have elevated serum creatine phosphokinase (CPK) levels; ambulatory patients often have a waddling gait, lumbar lordosis, and protruding abdomen and may appear unusually thin. Deep tendon reflexes are often absent, with prominent fasciculation and associated skeletal deformities (particularly scoliosis). Prognosis for independent ambulation correlates with the age at symptomatic onset, and if symptoms begin before 2 years ambulation is typically lost by age 15. If onset begins after 2 years, ambulation may persist well into the second decade (Russman et al., 1996).

In the juvenile progressive form of the disorder, patients develop symptoms between ages 3 and 15 years and usually present because of progressive difficulties with running, stair climbing, and getting up from the floor. Mild clumsiness, poor running skills, and delayed motor milestones may also prompt medical evaluation. Muscular weakness and atrophy presents in a limb-girdle distribution, and mild pseudohypertrophy of the calf muscles is also seen, which may result in confusion with Duchenne's or Becker's muscular dystrophy. Cranial nerve muscle is often spared, with weakness in only 20% of cases. Deep-tendon reflexes are often diminished or absent, but may be normal (Gross, 1966; Wessel, 1989; Iannaccone, 1998).

Adult-onset disease has sometimes also been included in this category since the adoption of the collaborative criteria, although some have proposed a separate subdivision (type IV disease) for clear adult-onset cases. Adult-onset SMAs account for less than 10% of all SMAs. They typically begin between the second and fifth decades, having an average age at onset of approximately 35 years and proximal, symmetrical, lower extremity weakness and associated atrophy. Face and tongue involvement may be seen in some cases. Progression is usually very slow over several decades, but distal weakness eventually appears as the disease advances. Considerable phenotypic variability is noted, with some cases of type I SMA also occurring in families otherwise affected by adult-onset disease (Pearn, 1978; Harding, 1993).

Molecular Genetics

SMA type I is most commonly inherited as an autosomal recessive disorder, but rare autosomal dominant and X-linked forms have been reported. SMA type II is autosomal recessive and SMA type III, as well as adult-onset SMA (type IV) and the distal SMAs, may be either autosomal dominant or autosomal recessive (Cole and Siddique, 1999). Chromosomal mapping for the SMAs (types I, II, and III) points to the same region of chromosome 5q11.2-13.3. Unfortunately, this region is quite complex, containing duplicate copies of other genes, numerous repetitive sequences, pseudogenes, and truncated genes, making further mapping quite challenging. Nevertheless, abnormalities in four genes on chromosome 5q13 have been associated with SMA. The most critical was recognized in 1995 in a region coding for the survival motor neuron (SMN) protein (Brzustowicz et al., 1990; Lefebvre et al., 1995; Burglen et al., 1996; Matthijs et al., 1996). The *SMN* gene, in the telomeric portion of the spinal muscular atrophy gene locus, encodes a 294-amino-acid polypeptide and has been designated *SMN1*. It is found in both nuclear and cytoplasmic forms and combines with a 32-kd protein known as SMN-interactive protein 1 (SIP1), which is found in association with spliceosomal small ribonuclear protein (snRNP). The resulting complex, termed SMN-SIP1, has been shown to participate in spliceosomal snRNP myogenesis (Murayama et al., 1991; Liu et al., 1997). More specifically, the SMN-SIP1 complex appears to be indirectly involved in the posttranscriptional processing of mRNA, the disturbance of which can damage the anterior horn cell. Recent studies have suggested another potential mechanism for this effect, as normal SMN also interacts with the anti-apoptotic Bcl-2, potentially providing a protective effect against in vitro apoptosis. Mutations and/or deletions in *SMN* render it incapable of this activity (Iwahashi et al., 1997). The *SMN* gene is either deleted or interrupted in virtually all patients with SMA, reducing intracellular SMN levels, and reduced SMN levels have been shown to correlate with more severe anterior horn cell injury (Lefebvre et al.,

1997, 1998; Talbot et al., 1998; Biros and Forrest, 1999; Talbot, 1999).

Several other genes in the 5q13 region may also be involved in modulating the severity of the proximal SMAs. The protein products of these candidate genes include spinal motor neuron survival protein 2 (SMN2), neuronal apoptosis inhibitory protein (NAIT) and H4F5 (Gennarelli et al., 1995; Van der Steege et al., 1995; Velasco et al., 1996; Campbell et al., 1997; Cole and Siddique, 1999; Monani et al., 1999). The telomeric copy of the gene (*SMN1*) and its centromeric copy (*SMN2*) are highly homologous, having a single-SMN-exon (exon 7) nucleotide difference between them. *SMN2* is present in at least 95% of the general population, and at least one copy is present in virtually all patients with spinal muscular atrophy. In some SMA patients, the *SMN2* gene facilitates coding of some full-length SMN at a reduced level, potentially ameliorating the effect of the loss of the *SMN1* gene (Gendron and MacKenzie, 1999). A number of lines of evidence have emerged to support the hypothesis that the number of copies of the *SMN2* gene present in a given patient correlates with disease severity, and type II and type III patients have, on average, a greater number of copies of the *SMN2* gene than type I patients (Campbell et al., 1997). At least two *SMN2* genes are necessary for survival of up to a few months in type I patients, and three *SMN2* genes correlate with still longer survival. However, a single *SMN2* gene is associated with extremely severe clinical symptomatology and an extremely poor prognosis. Those patients with SMA type II have three copies of *SMN2*, with four or more copies associated with a very mild clinical picture and a good prognosis (Vitali et al., 1999; Brahe, 2000). Consequently, induced up-regulation of *SMN2* has been proposed as a possible mechanism for gene therapy in this condition. The gene for the NAIP protein is deleted in up to 80% of SMA type I patients, as well as in some individuals with type II and type III disease. NAIP has been shown to directly inhibit caspase-3 apoptotic protease, an enzyme that normally promotes motor neuron apoptosis (Gendron and MacKenzie, 1999). Deletions of both the *SMN* and *NAIP* genes are relatively specific for SMA and do not appear to be a risk factor for the development of amyotrophic lateral sclerosis (Parboosingh et al., 1999). Although H4F5 is markedly deleted in type I SMA chromosomes and may be a potential candidate gene for this disease, the details of the possible molecular pathophysiology underlying this relationship remain to be elucidated (Scharf et al., 1998).

Diagnosis

The diagnosis of SPA remains a clinical one. However, numerous diagnostic assays, particularly genetic analysis, can be extremely helpful in confirming the initial clinical impression.

GENETIC TESTING

Patients suspected of having SPA can now be tested with a leukocyte assay for mutations in the *SMN* gene (Parano et al., 1996; Rudnik-Schoneborn et al., 1996). If this assay is positive in the appropriate clinical setting, the diagnosis is confirmed, although the absence of identified mutations by no means rules out the diagnosis. If no mutations are identified, additional workup with other diagnostic evaluations is clearly indicated. Recent data demonstrate that many asymptomatic patients in families with documented SMA and recognized mutations by genetic analysis may have subclinical disease identifiable only by detailed EMG testing (see the following), highlighting the importance of allied investigations, even in families with genetically confirmed disease.

ELECTROPHYSIOLOGY

The EMG features of SMA were reported by Buchthal and Olsen in 1970. In that study, EMG needle examination revealed changes associated with both active and chronic denervation, including increased insertional activity, abnormal spontaneous activity (fibrillations, positive sharp waves, and fasciculations), poor motor recruitment, and neurogenic-appearing motor units having increased amplitude, long duration, and increased complexity. Less prominent neurogenic features were seen in younger patients, becoming more pronounced as age increased. In addition, an unusual form of spontaneous activity consisting of an arrhythmic motor unit discharge at rest, having a frequency of 5 to 15 Hz, was also described. This activity was enhanced during slow-wave sleep and was thought to be due to the increased excitability of immature surviving motor neurons, although this proposed etiology has yet to be definitively demonstrated. The groups evaluated correspond roughly to those of the collaborative criteria. Rare fasciculations were seen in type I SMA, with more fasciculations and fibrillations in type II and type III disease. Complex repetitive discharges were never seen in patients younger than 5 to 6 years, but were seen with increasing frequency in patients older than 6 years in both type II and type III disease. In addition, as described in a number of other studies, an increased percentage of small-amplitude short-duration motor unit potentials were seen in patients with type III disease, possibly due to erroneous assessment of the late components of reenervated motor unit potentials as separate potentials, resulting in a "pseudo-myopathic" electromyogram. Linked potentials are also seen more commonly in type III patients as a consequence of chronic reinnervation (Gath et al., 1969; Mastaglia and Walton, 1971). Sensory nerve conduction studies are within normal limits and motor conduction studies may be normal, although mild slowing of motor conduction may be seen in cases of advanced disease (Gamstorp, 1967; Moosa and Dubowitz, 1976).

The EMG findings in SMA were assessed quantitatively in a larger cohort of 223 patients by Hausmanowa-Petrusewicz and Karwanska (1986). Diagnosis was based on clinical, genetic, biochemical, and electromyographic features, as well as muscle biopsy. Patients were divided into three groups, which correspond roughly with the three categories of the collaborative criteria. Quantitative electromyograms obtained over a 10-year period were reviewed and comparisons made between the proximal and distal muscles of the upper and lower extremities. Fibrillations and positive sharp waves were less common in small infants and most common in patients older than 4 years. Fasciculations were rarely observed in patients with type I disease but were seen in most patients with type III disease, most prominently in the proximal muscles, especially the quadriceps. Complex repetitive discharges were seen only in patients older than 6 years and were more pronounced in the proximal musculature. Among motor unit analysis parameters, the mean amplitude of the single-motor-unit action potential was the most useful for identifying pathology, with the most dramatic amplitude increases seen in the proximal muscles of patients older than 4 years having more chronic disease (consistent with well-established chronic reinnervation). Duration was similarly affected. The unusual spontaneous activity reported by Buchthal and Olsen (arrhythmical, 5- to 15-Hz motor unit discharges at rest) was also observed, most prominently in type I and type II patients younger than 4 years and less prominently in patients older than 4 years. In a later study that extended this initial work, 454 cases of SMA types I to III were analyzed, further confirming these findings (Hausmanowa-Petrusewicz, 1988). However, as with the initial study, a maximal-effort firing pattern was difficult to assess because of the young age of many of the subjects. Additional data were provided in the form of motor conduction velocities, which were slightly slower than in age-matched controls in type I disease. In this second study, fiber density (a quantitative electrophysiological measure of the fiber type grouping accompanying reinnervation) was also measured in selected cases and found to be increased in type III disease and normal to decreased in type I disease. These changes led to the speculation that patients with less aggressive disease have a greater capacity not only for motor neuron survival but for reinnervation, both of which may contribute to their slower rates of clinical decline.

More recently, EMG patterns in minimally symptomatic patients having the homozygous deletion of the *SMN* gene and their clinically affected siblings (with clear type II and type III disease) were compared, with interesting results (Bussaglia et al., 1997). Two patients were initially assessed: an affected 21-year-old man with type III disease with onset at age 2 who became wheelchair bound at age 17, and his 16-year-old sister, who reported nocturnal cramping but no other significant symptoms and had a normal neurological examination. Genotyping demonstrated the same deletion of exons 7 and 8 of the *SMN* gene in both patients. However, electromyographic examination of the minimally symptomatic sister demonstrated increased numbers of long-duration, large-amplitude motor unit potentials in the anterior tibialis and rectus femoris muscles, with no spontaneous activity, fasciculations, or complex repetitive discharges. In another family, two affected brothers age 54 and 52 showed the same homozygous deletion of the *SMN* gene. The older brother experienced disease onset at age 8, becoming wheelchair bound at age 12. His younger brother had symptomatic onset at age 32, with very mild weakness; his electromyogram demonstrated diffuse denervation with fibrillation potentials, long-duration motor unit action potentials (MUAPs), and decreased recruitment in all muscles examined. These studies clearly illustrate the high degree of phenotypic variability seen with the same apparent genetic mutation, as well as the utility of electrodiagnostic studies in detecting and quantitating subtle degrees of denervation in this condition. Further investigations are necessary to more fully elucidate the possible mechanisms for these observed differences. EMG examination of index SMA cases and their relatives remains important during the initial evaluation of this disorder, as it enables us to identify previously unrecognized, minimally symptomatic forms of the disease.

Central cortical motor neuron function was recently assessed in another study utilizing cortical magnetic stimulation (Gonschorek et al., 1999). The responses of a single tibialis anterior motor unit to transcranial magnetic stimulation and to a synchronized 1A volley evoked by peripheral electrical nerve stimulation were studied, both in control patients and patients with SMA. No significant differences were noted in excitatory postsynaptic potential occurrence or rise time, supporting normal spinal motor neuron function in SMA.

PATHOLOGY

Gross pathological examination demonstrates diffusely atrophic muscles with abnormally thin ventral spinal roots. Microscopic examination of the spinal cord demonstrates degeneration of the anterior horn cells, particularly in the cervical and lumbar regions, where chromatolysis and neuronal swelling are prominent (Lo et al., 1995). Neuronal loss is also noted in the brainstem, especially in the hypoglossal, ambiguous, and facial nuclei, and examination of the brain demonstrates cell loss in the posterior ventral nucleus of the thalamus (Duckett, 1995; Strober and Tennekoon, 1999). Muscle biopsy differs somewhat when the acute form of the disease is compared with the more chronic variety. Routine histological staining in acute infantile SMA (type I) typically shows large accumulations of severely atrophic fibers, juxtaposed with clumps of large, round hypertrophied fibers in the denervated fas-

ciculi. This pattern is relatively characteristic and has been referred to as "the infantile pattern of neurogenic atrophy" (Wessel, 1989; Iannaccone, 1998). Myosin ATPase reaction at pH 7.4 confirms the hypertrophied fibers to be nearly all type I. In the more chronic form of the disease (types II and III), more variable findings have been reported, although classic neurogenic changes, including those affecting angular fibers and fiber type grouping, are common. However, in at least one large series, neuropathic histological change was noted in 68% of biopsy specimens, with mixed neuropathic and myopathic features in 19% and myopathic features in 5%. The remaining 8% of biopsies demonstrated either nonspecific abnormalities or normal findings. In such cases, repeat biopsy of a different, more clinically affected muscle or biopsy at a later time following further disease progression often demonstrates clearer evidence of neurogenic atrophy (Namba et al., 1970).

Management

Unfortunately, no effective therapy currently exists for the spinal muscular atrophies; therefore, treatment remains supportive and is aimed at preventing complications and managing them as they arise (Eng et al., 1984). As there is a range of severity, treatment must be tailored to the individual patient, depending on age and clinical severity. Severe extremity and respiratory weakness has significant consequences for these patients, including respiratory insufficiency, nutritional complications, orthopedic problems, and psychosocial difficulties.

Diaphragmatic and intercostal muscle weakness results in a pattern of restrictive lung disease, which causes hypoventilation and a poor cough. Prophylaxis against respiratory infection is aided by chest percussion, assisted cough, and intermittent positive-pressure breathing. Such measures are often necessary on a chronic basis even when infection is not present (Wang et al., 1994; Iannaccone, 1998). It has been clearly demonstrated that pneumonia risk increases in a relatively linear fashion as forced vital capacity measurements decrease, even in the absence of losses in limb strength, and current recommendations include prophylaxis before the vital capacity drops to 50% of age-related normal values. As oxygen supplementation may dangerously enhance CO_2 retention due to suppression of respiratory drive in these patients, oxygen therapy is relatively contraindicated except during acute infection. In addition to routine respiratory function testing and forced vital capacity measurements, blood gas measurements are also useful to identify progressive CO_2 retention. When CO_2 retention begins, noninvasive ventilation is often required.

Adequate nutritional monitoring and supplementation is also critically important, as infants with SMA often develop failure to thrive because of difficulty with fatigability and a weak suck. Nutritionists, in consultation with occupational therapists, can determine necessary caloric intake and measures to assist with feeding, including adjustment of meal sizes, feeding frequency, food variety, and positioning during feeding. In some instances, gastrostomy tube feeding may be required due to excessive aspiration or fatigability. As osteoporosis may develop as a consequence of poor nutrition, dietary monitoring for appropriate calcium and phosphorus intake is also important. Ongoing monitoring following nutritional supplementation continues to be important in preventing excessive weight gain due to immobility.

In addition to potential osteoporosis, scoliosis develops in many patients surviving beyond early childhood, posing potentially serious problems. Abnormal curvatures appear in the thoracolumbar regions in most cases and are earlier and more severe in those patients who do not achieve ambulation. Although the use of orthotics will not slow the development of scoliosis, braces are often useful in assisting patients with sitting; however, these must also be closely monitored to ensure that pressure from the brace does not interfere with respiration. Surgical correction requires judicious monitoring so that the procedure can be performed with optimal pulmonary function, but after the patient's growth is substantial enough that the scoliosis has reached a relatively maximal level. Following spinal surgery, physical therapy is critically important to maximize recovery and prevent acceleration of weakness and loss of function (Aprin et al., 1982; Daher et al., 1985; Piasecki et al., 1986; Phillips et al., 1990). If surgery is not performed, progression of scoliosis is inevitable, with worsening respiratory function, increasing discomfort, and increasing difficulties with proper positioning and sitting. Other orthopedic complications include flexion contractures affecting the hips, knees, and ankles in particular. Range-of-motion exercises may be useful in preventing this complication, but splints and braces appear to be less effective. Clubfoot deformity is unusual, but it may appear in infantile SMA and often does not require surgical correction. Difficulties with mobility may be decreased by the use of motorized wheelchairs, tailored to the child's developmental age, as well as pneumatic lifts and other home care devices (Siegal and Silverman, 1984). As the disease progresses, additional home assistance may be required; special attention must be paid to appropriate intellectual stimulation, as many children with this disorder have reasonable levels of cognitive function. Finally, financial and familial stress in coping with the many demands of this disease are common serious problems, and families may benefit from counseling and other assistance, such as support groups, initiated soon after disease diagnosis (Iannaccone, 1998).

OTHER SPINAL MUSCULAR ATROPHIES
Distal Spinal Muscular Atrophies

In addition to the proximal SMAs detailed previously, a growing number of SMA variants continue to be described, including a variety of distal SMA syndromes. Harding proposed seven subtypes of distal SMA, organized by clinical and genetic features that provide a useful framework for categorizing the growing number of these syndromes: dominant juvenile onset, adult onset, recessive juvenile (mild), recessive juvenile (severe), upper limb predominant, neonatal with diaphragmatic paralysis, and distal SMA with vocal cord involvement (Table 69–2) (Harding, 1993). The group of distal hereditary motor neuropathies have also been referred to as the Charcot-Marie-Tooth type of progressive SMA because of the similar distribution of weakness and the slowly progressive course observed in most of these patients.

In 1969, Meadows and Marsden described a slowly progressive adult-onset distal SMA with no sensory findings and normal motor nerve conduction studies (Meadows and Marsden, 1969). Since that time, two distinct categories of predominantly distal SMA with clear autosomal dominant inheritance have been reported: type I (juvenile onset) and type II (adult onset), also known as the hereditary motor neuropathies type I and type II. Type I disease typically begins before age 10 years with gait abnormalities related to distal leg weakness and pes cavus. Most patients have a normal life span and minimal disability, although as the disease slowly progresses proximal weakness appears (Nelson and Amick, 1966; Davis et al., 1978). In 1992, type II disease was assessed by Timmerman and colleagues, who studied six generations of an affected family. Age at onset varied from 14 to 35, with a mean of 22 years. The first symptom was weakness of the toe extensor muscles, with progression over the next decade to weakness and atrophy of all distal leg muscles as well as the distal upper extremity. Vibratory sense loss was also noted in a few patients. Deep tendon reflexes were normal to decreased and were absent in some patients. As these patients aged, many required walkers for ambulation, and some became wheelchair bound. Motor and sensory nerve conduction studies were normal, and neurogenic motor units were noted in affected muscles during needle EMG. Ten clinically affected individuals were analyzed in a search for the genetic mutation responsible for this disease, and a candidate gene was identified on chromosome 12q24 at the PLA2a locus. The PLA2a gene product functions to catalyze the re-

Table 69–2. The Distal Spinal Muscular Atrophies

I	Dominant juvenile onset
II	Adult onset
III	Recessive mild juvenile
IV	Recessive severe juvenile
V	Upper limb predominant
VI	Neonatal with diaphragmatic paralysis
VII	With vocal cord involvement

Modified from Harding NE: Inherited neuronal atrophy and degeneration predominantly in lower motor neurons. In Dyck PJ, Thomas PK (eds): Peripheral Neuropathy, 3rd ed. Philadelphia, WB Saunders, 1993; 1051–1064.

lease of fatty acids from glycerol-3-phosphocholine and has also been isolated within the central nervous system, although the details of how this mutation results in this disease have not been determined (Pearn, 1978; Pearn and Hudgson, 1979; Harding and Thomas, 1980; Groen et al., 1993; Harding, 1993; Boylan et al., 1995; Timmerman et al., 1992, 1996). A rapidly progressive form of autosomal dominant adult-onset SMA was described in 1986 by Jansen et al. (1986). It begins between 30 and 60 years of age with subsequent rapid progression and death from respiratory failure within 2 years of onset. An autosomal dominant SMA with late adult onset (the Finkel variant) has also been described with a mean age of onset of 49 years, with proximal weakness and atrophy. Deep tendon reflexes are diminished, but sensory and bulbar function is within normal limits. EMG demonstrates neurogenic MU-APs with nerve conductions similar to those seen with the earlier onset proximal SMAs. There are also autosomal recessive forms of juvenile distal hereditary motor neuropathy (type III, mild, and type IV, severe). The mild variety typically begins between the ages of 2 and 10 years with prominent distal weakness with or without proximal leg weakness. Ambulation is usually preserved and life expectancy is normal. The more severe variety begins between 4 months and 20 years, but with loss of ambulation by age 30. Available data are less clear regarding survival in this form of the disease.

Several families with distal SMA syndromes having upper limb predominance have also been described (type V). These disorders typically begin between age 10 and 40, affecting primarily the hands, with disproportionate weakness in the thenar eminence compared with the dorsal interosseous muscles. They may be asymmetrical, and in 60% of patients lower extremity weakness also affects the peroneal musculature, often producing foot deformities. Proximal strength is typically normal. Mild upper motor neuron signs, including slight hypertonicity in the bilateral lower extremities and brisk deep tendon reflexes, may also be seen. Progression is very slow over several decades, and patients do not typically become significantly disabled. Unusual associated symptoms include decreased vibratory sense in the distal lower extremities and hyperhidrosis affecting the hands and feet in 40% of cases. Electrophysiological studies may demonstrate low-amplitude compound motor action potential with normal to mildly reduced motor nerve conduction velocities and mildly reduced sensory nerve conduction velocities, whereas needle EMG examination demonstrates high-amplitude MUAPs with decreased recruitment. Christodoulou and co-workers (1995) studied five generations of a large Bulgarian family having an autosomal dominant distal SMA with a mean age of onset of 17 years (Christodoulou et al., 1995). Weakness and wasting selectively involved the thenar muscles and the first dorsal interosseous muscle. Weakness of the distal legs also began in 40% of affected patients within 2 years of disease onset. A

few family members also had mild pyramidal features and Babinski signs, and a slightly reduced vibratory sense was noted in 10%. The vast majority had a very slowly progressive course with preserved ambulation into the seventh decade. Nerve conduction studies demonstrated reduced compound motor action potential amplitude with normal latencies and velocities. Genetic analysis mapped this disorder to chromosome 7p, allelic to Charcot-Marie-Tooth disease type IID (Ellsworth et al., 1999). Another family, demonstrating predominantly distal hand weakness and increased reflexes, has also been reported (Silver, 1966; Van Gent et al., 1985).

A severe infantile distal SMA with diaphragmatic paralysis (type VI) has also been described and localized to chromosome 11q13-q21 (Mellins et al., 1974; Bertini et al., 1989; Grohmann et al., 1999). Grohmann reported an autosomal recessive form of diaphragmatic distal SMA in nine patients from three families (referred to as SMARD, SMA with respiratory distress). This disorder usually begins at age 1 to 2 months with severe respiratory distress secondary to diaphragmatic paralysis and predominantly distal upper extremity weakness. Mild contractures may develop at the knees and ankles. Respiratory failure usually ensues at less than 3 months in most patients. Autopsy demonstrates neurogenic atrophy of skeletal muscle without reinnervation, as well as anterior spinal root atrophy and chromatolysis of the motor neuron. Chest radiography demonstrates diaphragmatic paralysis. Linkage to markers 11q13-q21 was noted in at least one family. An autosomal dominant upper extremity distal SMA syndrome with vocal cord involvement has also been seen. This disorder begins in adolescence with hand weakness followed by progression to lower extremity weakness and hoarseness beginning in the second decade. Respiratory failure may ensue owing to bilateral vocal cord paralysis. Young and Harper also reported a Welsh family with this syndrome and sensorineural hearing loss (Young and Harper, 1980; Serratrice et al., 1984; Boltshauser et al., 1989). Pridmore and associates reported another Welsh family with SMA and vocal cord paralysis in three successive generations (Pridmore et al., 1992).

Scapuloperoneal Spinal Muscular Atrophies

A number of scapuloperoneal syndromes have also been described, most of which are not motor neuronopathies. Scapuloperoneal muscular dystrophy types I and II, scapuloperoneal muscular dystrophy with mental retardation, scapuloperoneal muscular dystrophy with a lethal cardiomyopathy, and a scapuloperoneal peripheral neuropathy with motor and sensory involvement (Davidenkow's syndrome) have been described. However, true scapuloperoneal SMAs (SPSMAs) have also been reported. DeLong and Siddique described a family of French

Canadian descent in New England who demonstrated phenotypic heterogeneity with varying combinations of progressive scapuloperoneal atrophy, congenital absence of muscles, laryngeal palsy, and progressive distal weakness and muscle atrophy (DeLong and Siddique, 1992). It was most severe in male family members, and anticipation was suggested by increasing severity in third and fourth generations. Linkage of this syndrome to chromosome 12q24.1-q24.31 was noted in another study (Isozumi et al., 1996). Another scapuloperoneal neuronopathy is an autosomal dominant variety known as Kaeser's syndrome. Peroneal atrophy is the initial manifestation in this disorder, followed by equino-varus deformities of the foot and bilateral footdrop, progressing to shoulder girdle weakness and late bulbar involvement. In 1932, Palmer also described a family with eight affected members having scapuloperoneal SMA (Palmer, 1932), and additional cases were reported by Emery and colleagues (1968) and Schuchmann (1970). An autosomal recessive scapuloperoneal neuronopathy has also been described (Harding, 1993). Yet another autosomal dominant SMA is the fascioscapulohumeral type, described by Fenichel and coworkers in 1967. This disease typically begins in early adulthood, with weakness restricted to the face and pectoral girdle musculature. Because of this distribution and a characteristically slow progression, it can be clinically confused with fascioscapulohumeral muscular dystrophy; however, it is distinguished by electrophysiological and histological findings supportive of motor neuronopathy.

Spinal Muscular Atrophy with Prominent Contractures

An X-linked severe infantile SMA with arthrogryposis has been described and localized to Xp11.3-q11.2 (Greenberg et al., 1988; Kobayashi et al., 1995). This disorder has a pattern of weakness similar to that of Werdnig-Hoffmann disease, but with more prominent congenital contractures and fractures. Another family with arthrogryposis at birth but an autosomal dominant SMA with linkage to 12q23-q24 was reported (Fleury and Hageman, 1985; Van der Vleuten et al., 1998), and an autosomal dominant, nonprogressive congenital SMA with later contracture formation has also been described. These patients develop proximal lower extremity weakness in adolescence, with mild flexion contractures of the knees, equinovarus deformities, mild weakness of the adductor muscles, and minimal involvement of the jaw muscles and neck flexors. Sensory examination is normal, creatine kinase may be mildly elevated, EMG and nerve conduction studies reveal neurogenic changes with normal nerve conduction studies, and muscle biopsy confirms neurogenic change. It has been linked, in some families, to chromosome 12q23-q24 (Frijns et al., 1994; Van der Vleuten et al., 1998). The more global

syndrome of arthrogryposis multiplex congenita resulting from any severe intrauterine neuromuscular disorder is often caused by primary denervation, and a recent study suggests that up to 50% of such patients may carry deletions for the *SMN* gene, reinforcing the importance of screening such patients for SMA-associated mutations (Bingham et al., 1997).

Miscellaneous Spinal Muscular Atrophy Variants

A form of infantile olivopontocerebellar atrophy with SMA has also been described, inherited in an autosomal recessive fashion. These patients typically have severe hypotonia, areflexia, respiratory insufficiency, and failure to thrive, with associated hip dislocation and cardiomyopathy, typically resulting in death before age 6 months. Magnetic resonance imaging of the brain demonstrates the characteristic findings of olivopontocerebellar atrophy, and histological analysis confirms marked hypoplasia of the basis pontis and inferior olivary nuclei, as well as hypoplasia of the neocerebellum (both the cerebellar and cerebral peduncles). Anterior horn cell atrophy with associated neurogenic changes on examined proximal muscles is also seen (Chou et al., 1990).

SPINAL AND BULBAR MUSCULAR ATROPHY

In 1968, Kennedy and colleagues reported a unique form of adult-onset SMA having X-linked inheritance affecting 11 males from two families (Kennedy et al., 1968). Numerous studies since that time have confirmed and further defined this syndrome of X-linked spinal and bulbar muscular atrophy (SBMA), also known as Kennedy's disease.

Epidemiology and Clinical Features

SBMA is a relatively uncommon disorder, with a prevalence approaching 1 in 40,000 in certain areas. Many patients may present with typical clinical manifestations but no clear family history owing to the late onset of the disease and a relative lack of symptoms in heterozygous female carriers (Harding et al., 1982). It usually begins with tremor, cramps, fasciculations, or proximal weakness beginning in the third or fourth decade, with all symptoms appearing within 5 to 10 years following the initial manifestations. Fasciculations, cramps, and tremors may precede clinical weakness by a number of years in most cases, and the majority of patients present with finger tremor (postural, alternating, rapid and low amplitude) beginning in the middle of the third decade. Gynecomastia is also seen in many cases. Rarely, the disease may manifest without cramps or tremor, but fasciculations are a characteristic feature by the time limb weakness appears. Symmetrical limb weakness and atrophy typically begin between 30 and 50 years, first affecting the proximal muscles of the pelvic or shoulder girdle (although distal weakness may sometimes predominate), with slow progression thereafter. In some cases, extremity weakness may start as early as the early 20s or as late as the late 50s. Mild facial weakness is also present, but bulbar dysfunction does not typically develop until a decade or more after the onset of limb weakness. Tongue or soft palate weakness with mild wasting and/or fasciculations can be seen and is accompanied by dysarthria and dysphagia, which is usually mild but may be severe in some cases. Most patients also experience twitching of the chin produced by pursing of the lips, which is considered by many to be a pathognomonic sign. Extraocular muscle strength is normal. Vibratory sense impairment, if present, is typically a late finding, and deep tendon reflexes are usually diminished or absent, especially in the distal lower extremities. No upper motor neuron signs, central nervous system dysfunction, or autonomic abnormalities are observed. Though usually asymptomatic, female heterozygotes may sometimes be mildly clinically affected. A number of endocrinological complications have also been described, and affected males frequently have gynecomastia and other signs of androgen insensitivity, such as impotence, testicular atrophy, and decreased fertility. Diabetes mellitus also occurs in 20% to 30% of affected patients, and hyperlipidemia may also appear. Endocrinological evaluation may demonstrate increased levels of follicle-stimulating hormone, luteinizing hormone, or estradiol 17β in association with decreased levels of testosterone (Kennedy et al., 1968; Tsukagoshi et al., 1970; Stefanis et al., 1975; Ringel et al., 1978; Harding et al., 1982; Hausmanowa-Petrusewicz et al., 1983; Fleury and Hageman, 1985; Olney et al., 1991; Sobue, 1995; Fischbeck et al., 1999; Meriggioli et al., 1999).

At least two other syndromes presenting with progressive bulbar atrophy have been reported. The Vialetta-van Laere syndrome demonstrates a combination of sensorineural deafness and neurogenic muscular atrophy in a bulbospinal distribution and typically appears before age 20 years, with survival ranging from the third to the fifth decades. Only a few cases of this disorder, affecting the Portuguese and Tunisian populations and a few other ethnic groups, have been described (Summers et al., 1987). Fazio-Londe disease, or progressive bulbar paralysis of childhood, usually begins earlier with restricted bulbar weakness and does not include deafness (Fazio, 1892; Vialetta, 1936; Van Laere, 1967). It begins before age 12 years and has a more fulminant course, with most patients dying within 18 months of disease onset. Weakness usually starts before age 10 in the lower cranial nerves, particularly the face, with sparing of the extraocular muscles. The cranial nerve musculature then becomes progressively weak in a relatively selective bulbar pattern, with

very little deterioration of the anterior horn cells of the spinal cord.

Molecular Genetics

The genetic abnormality in Kennedy's syndrome has been clearly mapped to the androgen receptor gene on the X chromosome at Xq11-12 (La Spada et al., 1991). It results from a trinucleotide CAG repeat in the first exon of the androgen receptor gene near the 5' end, which is normally responsible for encoding a series of glutamine residues near the amino terminus of the androgen receptor protein, close to the domain for transcriptional activation (Fischbeck et al., 1999). Twenty CAG repeats are found in normal individuals (range, 11 to 33), but in patients affected with SBMA approximately 38 to 62 CAG repeats are seen. The mutated androgen receptor resulting from these expanded CAG repeats demonstrates reduced target gene activation, contributing to androgen insensitivity in these patients and, possibly, to motor neuron deterioration, although the precise mechanisms of this later effect are unknown (Mhatre et al., 1993). A variety of studies have demonstrated androgen binding to motor neurons, resulting in varying but predominantly trophic effects and possibly increasing survival. However, several other disorders with androgen insensitivity, such as testicular feminization syndrome, do not demonstrate motor neuron deterioration. A toxic gain of function effect has also been proposed for this aberrant repeat, and CAG repeats are associated with potentially neurotoxic protein products, such as polyglutamine tract expansions within the androgen receptor and resultant protein aggregates. Although there is a significant correlation between the number of CAG repeats and the age of onset as well as the presence of gynecomastia, other symptoms and findings, such as muscular weakness, glucose intolerance, dysphagia, and plasma creatine phosphokinase levels, do not significantly correlate with CAG repeat length (La Spada et al., 1992). Ongoing work in transgenic mouse models may shed further light on the pathophysiology of SBMA in the near future (Yu, 1989; Mendell et al., 1996; Fischbeck et al., 1999; Ikezoe et al., 1999).

Diagnosis

GENETIC TESTING

Polymerase chain reaction assays for triplicate CAG repeat expansions in the androgen receptor gene are now readily available as a commercial diagnostic test and can be performed on whole-blood samples. If expansions are present in the appropriate clinical setting, the diagnosis is confirmed. However, a recent description of an autosomal dominant form of this disorder lacking CAG repeat expansions emphasizes the continued importance of other investigations during diagnostic evaluation (Ikezoe et al., 1999).

ELECTROPHYSIOLOGY

Motor nerve conduction studies in SBMA patients are frequently within normal limits, although the sural sensory nerve action potential may be reduced in amplitude or absent. Other sensory responses may also be abnormal. Needle EMG demonstrates reduced motor unit recruitment patterns and complex motor unit potentials of long duration and increased amplitude in virtually all patients, with infrequent spontaneous activity. MUAP instability may also be seen, consistent with active reinnervation. These changes are typically widespread, affecting both the upper and the lower extremities, as well as the bulbar musculature. Heterozygous female carriers usually do not manifest substantial clinical symptomatology, but 50% may demonstrate abnormalities consistent with chronic reinnervation, including high-amplitude long-duration motor units on EMG examination and fiber type grouping on muscle biopsy (Sobue et al., 1981, 1993; Sobue, 1995). A relatively specific EMG finding may be seen in recordings from the facial and chin musculature. Grouped motor unit discharges occurring up to several times per second with mild voluntary activation of the mentalis muscle have been clearly described, having frequencies of 10 to 40 Hz within each group and group durations of 0.1 second to several seconds. Although these discharges are somewhat analogous to the syndrome of hereditary quivering of the chin, involuntary discharges are observed only with activation and not during rest (Laurance et al., 1968; Olney et al., 1991; Sobue, 1995; Meriggioli et al., 1999).

PATHOLOGY

The hypoglossal, facial, and trigeminal motor nuclei demonstrate severe neuronal depletion, with sparing of neurons in the trochlear, abducens, oculomotor, gracile, and cuneate nuclei and marked loss of large myelinated fibers and ventral horn cells throughout the spinal cord (Sobue et al., 1981, 1989). Although the dorsal spinal roots are normal on routine histological analysis, teased fiber preparations demonstrate a noticeable increase in segmental demyelination and remyelination, and sural nerve biopsy demonstrates marked reduction of myelinated fibers, particularly those of large diameter. Muscle biopsy demonstrates hypertrophic fibers with increased internal nuclei, fiber splitting, groups of atrophic fibers, and clumping of sarcolemmal nuclei. Polyglutamine tract expansions in androgen receptors result in protein aggregates within the cytoplasm. In non-neuronal tissues, nuclear inclusions of ubiquitinated androgen receptor protein have also been described (Li et al., 1998).

Treatment

Unfortunately, as with the SMAs, no effective therapy for SBMA exists. Treatment remains supportive and is directed at preventing complications and treating them as they arise. As with other progressive motor neuron diseases, the services of skilled physical, occupational, and speech therapists, as well as nutritional and other consultants, are important as bulbar and extremity weakness progress. Associated conditions, such as diabetes mellitus and hyperlipidemia, may require an internal medicine consultant.

HEREDITARY SPASTIC PARAPARESIS

Epidemiology and Clinical Classification

Strümpell initially reported two brothers who developed progressive spastic paraplegia in 1880, and numerous subsequent reports confirmed the existence of this syndrome, which was later termed *hereditary spastic paraparesis* (HSP) (Strümpell, 1880). Later epidemiological studies described not only patients with pure spastic paraparesis but also other groups with additional superimposed neurological features, prompting Harding to propose categories for both pure and complicated HSP in 1981 (Harding, 1981). Further subdivision by age at onset was also proposed, with onset before 35 years designated type I and onset after 35 years designated type II. The precise epidemiological characteristics of hereditary spastic paraparesis have proved difficult to fully define, as different studies have utilized differing diagnostic criteria. However, most studies report an incidence ranging from 2.0 to 9.6 per 100,000 (Polo et al., 1991; Filla et al., 1992; Leone et al., 1995; Silva et al., 1997).

Clinical Features

Symptomatic onset ranges from earliest childhood through the eighth decade, with significant phenotypic heterogeneity within families. The majority of patients with the pure HSP syndrome present with disturbances in ambulation, and in the form with onset in infancy walking may be delayed. Milder symptoms, such as leg stiffness and mild urinary incontinence, may occasionally be the only initial manifestations. Up to 25% of members in affected families having no clinical complaints will have symptoms and findings upon careful history and physical examination. Principal features include weakness of the bilateral legs with prominent spasticity, increased reflexes, and upper motor neuron signs. Weakness is usually most prominent in the anterior tibial and iliopsoas muscles, with occasional involvement of the knee flexors, whereas increased tone and spasticity are most prominent in the knee flexor and extensor muscles and in the ankles. Mild hyperreflexia may also be seen in the arms, but minimal spasticity or weakness is found in the upper extremities. Rarely, deep tendon reflexes at the ankles may be absent. The gait is, of course, spastic with circumduction, occasional scissoring, and toe walking. In most cases, spasticity dominates the clinical picture and is often severe enough to interfere with ambulation, even with minimal associated muscle weakness (Bickerstaff, 1950; Sutherland, 1975). Although mild muscular atrophy may be present after long disease duration (possibly secondary to disuse), prominent muscular atrophy on presentation should suggest a different etiology. Pes cavus deformity may also be seen in up to one third of patients and is usually associated with more severe or long-duration disease (Harding, 1981; Polo et al., 1993). Mild sensory abnormalities consisting of decreased vibratory and joint position sense in the distal legs may also be present in 10% to 65% of patients with the pure variety of the disease (Harding, 1981; Polo et al., 1993). Urinary frequency, hesitancy, and urgency may also appear in up to 50% of patients, with rare reports of bowel incontinence and sexual dysfunction. However, the bulbar musculature and autonomic nervous system are spared (Opjordsmoen and Nyberg-Hansen, 1980; Harding, 1981; Boustany et al., 1987; Bushman et al., 1993). There is significant inter- and intrafamily variability in disease severity, but there is a correlation between the age at onset and rate of progression, as well as extent of disability. Those patients having early-onset disease progress slowly, retaining ambulation throughout most of their lives, whereas those with much later onset disease progress rapidly, with loss of ambulation by the sixth to seventh decades (Harding, 1981; Schady and Sheard, 1990; Polo et al., 1993).

Complicated HSP is a much more diverse disorder than the pure variety and includes a number of additional features that appear in differing combinations. These additional symptoms include amyotrophy, mental retardation or dementia, deafness, seizure disorder, extrapyramidal dysfunction, cerebellar signs, sensory neuropathy, cardiac abnormalities, retinal disease (including retinal degeneration and optic atrophy), and others (McDermott et al., 2000). Varying combinations of symptoms have been reported in a wide variety of families, with specific syndromes manifesting in different pedigrees. Seizure disorders and deafness are also well-known features of several mitochondrial syndromes, raising the question of a possible contribution of mitochondrial dysfunction to some cases of complicated hereditary spastic paraparesis.

Molecular Genetics

A large and expanding number of genetic mutations are now associated with HSP and have been reported at 10 separate chromosomal loci. A number of inheritance patterns, including autosomal dominant (the most common), autosomal recessive, and X-linked, have also been described (McDermott et al., 2000). Genetic localization in autosomal dominant families includes 2p22-21, 12q13, 10q23.3-24.2, 8q24, 15q11.1, and 14q11.2-24.3, and the search for additional loci is ongoing. Most patients with the autosomal dominant form of the disease map to the 2p22-21 locus. This gene codes for the protein spastin, which mediates the cellular mechanisms involved in the assembly and function of various chaperone proteins. A number of spastin mutations have been identified in affected families, including missense, nonsense, and splice site mutations, supporting a loss of spastin function as the cause for degeneration of the cortical spinal tract in these groups (Hazan et al., 1999). Most patients with recognized autosomal dominant mutations have pure HSP, although both pure and complicated HSP may be manifested in some families. However, at least one autosomal dominant form (10q23.3-24.2) has been associated primarily with complicated HSP (Seri et al., 1999). Even in those families manifesting predominantly pure or complicated HSP, considerable phenotypic variability has been reported, the causes of which remain obscure. Although anticipation has been described in some studies, the search for a possible repeat expansion accounting for this phenomenon in affected families remains inconclusive (Nielsen et al., 1997; Benson et al., 1998).

Autosomal recessive HSP is much less common than the dominant form and has thus far been linked to chromosomes 15q13-15, 16q24.3, and 8p12-q13. The 15q and 16q loci are associated with both pure and complicated forms of HSP, whereas the 8p locus is associated only with the pure form of the disease (Hentati et al., 1994; De Michele et al., 1998; Martínez Murillo et al., 1999). The most common autosomal recessive localization is on 15q, manifesting phenotypic variability with affected family members. The 16q locus is in a region that codes for a protein known as paraplegin, a mitochondrial metalloprotease similar to proteins exhibiting both proteolytic and chaperone-like activity on the inner mitochondrial membrane. Interestingly, mitochondrial dysfunction has also been seen in muscle biopsy tissue from affected members of these families, with both negative cytochrome oxidase staining and ragged red fibers (Casari et al., 1998). However, in contrast, similar studies performed on patients having genetic abnormalities on chromosome 8q demonstrate no evidence of mitochondrial dysfunction (Hedera et al., 1999).

X-linked hereditary spastic paraparesis is rare and has been linked to two different spastic paraplegia genes, termed *SPG1* and *SPG2* (Kenwrick et al., 1986; Keppen et al., 1987). *SPG1* has been localized to chromosome Xq28 and *SPG2* has been localized to Xq22. Pure HSP has been linked only to *SPG2*, whereas complicated HSP has been linked to both *SPG1* and *SPG2*. *SPG1*-associated complicated HSP was found in one family and includes congenital abnormalities of the musculoskeletal system, with the absence of the extensor hallucis longus muscle and severe mental retardation in addition to spastic paraparesis (Kenwrick et al., 1986). A mutation in exon 6 of the L1 cell adhesion molecule gene (*L1CAM*) is responsible for this disorder. L1CAM plays an important role in axon outgrowth and as such is critical for nervous system development. It is a transmembrane glycoprotein expressed by both Schwann cells and neurons and has been associated with a variety of other neurological syndromes, such as X-linked hydrocephalus, X-linked agenesis of the corpus callosum, and the syndrome of mental retardation, aphasia, shuffling gait, and adducted thumbs (MASA). Phenotypic variability is seen among all families with diseases resulting from mutations in the *L1CAM* gene, and these different neurologic syndromes may sometimes present in the same family. Consequently, a disease category that encompasses all of these disorders, known as CRASH, has been proposed (corpus callosum hypoplasia, retardation, adducted thumbs, spastic paraplegia, and hydrocephalus) (Jouet et al., 1994; Fransen et al., 1995). Complicated HSP syndromes linked to *SPG2* include combinations of mental retardation, cerebellar dysfunction, and spastic paraparesis, with considerable phenotypic variability and occasional additional features including optic atrophy (Goldblatt et al., 1989; Bonneau et al., 1993). The *SPG2* gene codes for a protein known as the proteolipid protein (PLP), and mutations may also result in Pelizaeus-Merzbacher disease, a rapidly progressive syndrome of cerebellar and pyramidal dysfunction with death in infancy or early childhood (Kobayashi et al., 1994; Saugier-Veber et al., 1994). PLP has an important role in the maintenance of myelination as well as maturation of myelin within the central nervous system, and the absence of the PLP protein within the myelin sheath is associated with more rapid myelin turnover. PLP is also found in a different isoform (DM-20), which is reduced in both HSP and Pelizaeus-Merzbacher disease, although significantly greater reductions are noted in Pelizaeus-Merzbacher disease than in HSP. Complicated HSP linked to *SGP2* has also been described in a family without mutations in the *PLP* gene, suggesting a more complex genetic background and pathogenesis. X-linked HSP of the pure variety is rare, and only two of the five families described with this syndrome have been shown to have abnormalities in the *SPG2* locus (Keppen et al., 1987; Cambi et al., 1996).

Genome database designations are being assigned to each HPS mutation as they are described. As mentioned previously, the X-linked HSPs have been localized to Xq28 (designated *SGP1*; complicated associated HSP) and to Xq22 (*SPG2*; both pure and complicated associated HSP). The autosomal dominant defects currently include 14q11.2-24.3 (*SPG3*; pure), 2p22-21 (*SPG4*; pure), 15q11.1 (*SPG6*; pure), 8q24 (*SPG8*; pure), 10q23.3-24.2 (*SPG9*; complicated), and 12q13 (*SPG10*; pure), and the autosomal reces-

sive defects currently include 12-q13 (*SPG5*; pure), 16q24.3 (*SPG7*; both) and 15q13-15 (*SPG11*; both).

Diagnosis

GENETIC TESTING

HSP remains a diagnosis of exclusion. Genetic assays for delineation of this syndrome have been described by a number of research laboratories but are not yet widely available commercially. It is hoped that these assays will be accessible in the future.

ELECTROPHYSIOLOGY

A number of electrophysiological investigations may demonstrate central motor abnormalities, including transcortical magnetic stimulation and somatosensory evoked potential (SSEP) studies. Transcortical magnetic stimulation studies record decreased to absent central motor conduction times from the lower extremities and normal values from the upper extremities (McLeod et al., 1977; Claus et al., 1990; Pelosi et al., 1991; Schady et al., 1991; Nielsen et al., 1998), and SSEPs are reduced or absent in the lower extremities. EMG and nerve conduction study results are normal in most cases of pure HSP (McLeod et al., 1977; Schady et al., 1991).

LABORATORY FINDINGS

The results of imaging studies, including magnetic resonance imaging of the spinal cord, are typically normal, although mild spinal cord atrophy may occasionally be noted. Mild abnormalities in the white matter of the brain may also sometimes be seen, especially the corpus callosum (Ormerod et al., 1994; Nielsen et al., 1998). Although increased protein has been occasionally reported in patients with complicated HSP, usually no other significant cerebrospinal fluid abnormalities are seen.

PATHOLOGY

Few reports of the pathology of HSP are currently available, presumably due to the long duration of the disease and normal life span in most individuals. In the few reports available, the major abnormality is axonal degeneration in the terminal portions of both the corticospinal tracts and the dorsal column pathways in the spinal cord, which demonstrate both gliosis and demyelination. Most dramatically affected areas include the fasciculus gracilis fibers and the crossed and uncrossed corticospinal tracts to the lower limbs, consistent with predominant involvement of the legs in this disorder. Spinal cerebellar tract involvement may also be seen in approximately 50% of cases. Most patients have normal anterior horn cells, dorsal root ganglia, and peripheral nerves. In complicated HSP associated with dementia, a number of additional abnormalities are noted within the substance of the brain, including τ-immunoreactive neurofibrillary tangles and neuronal depletion (Behan and Maia, 1974; Sack et al., 1978; Bruyn, 1992; White et al., 2000).

Treatment

Unfortunately, no effective primary therapy for any of the HSP syndromes exists; however, ongoing research into the genetics and molecular pathogenesis of these disorders may facilitate the development of experimental therapies in the future. As patients with most of the HSPs have a very mild and slowly progressive course with a normal life span, supportive measures, such as physical therapy, and the use of such agents as baclofen and tizanidine may substantially reduce spasticity and improve the quality of life for these individuals (McDermott et al., 2000).

References

Aprin H, Bowen JR, MacEwen GD: Spine fusion in patients with spinal muscular atrophy. J Bone Joint Surg Am 1982;64:1179–1187.

Behan WM, Maia M: Strumpell's familial spastic paraplegia: Genetics and neuropathology. J Neurol Neurosurg Psychiatry 1974; 37:8–20.

Benson KF, Horwitz M, Wolff J, et al: CAG repeat expansion in autosomal dominant familial spastic paraparesis: Novel expansion in a subset of patients. Hum Mol Genet 1998;7:1779–1786.

Bertini E, Gadisseux JL, Palmieri G, et al: Distal infantile spinal muscular atrophy associated with paralysis of the diaphragm: A variant of infantile spinal muscular atrophy. Am J Med Genet 1989;33:328–335.

Bickerstaff ER: Hereditary spastic paraplegia. J Neurol Neurosurg Psychiatry 1950;13:134–135.

Bingham PM, Shen N, Rennert H, et al: Arthrogryposis due to infantile neuronal degeneration associated with deletion of the SMNT gene. Neurology 1997;49:848–851.

Biros I, Forrest S: Spinal muscular atrophy: Untangling the knot? J Med Genet 1999;36:1–8.

Boltshauser E, Lang W, Spillmann T, et al: Hereditary distal muscular atrophy with vocal cord paralysis and sensorineural hearing loss: A dominant form of spinal muscular atrophy? J Med Genet 1989;26:105–108.

Bonneau D, Rozet JM, Bulteau C, et al: X linked spastic paraplegia (SPG2): Clinical heterogeneity at a single gene locus. J Med Genet 1993;30:381–384.

Boustany RM, Fleischnick E, Alper CA, et al: The autosomal dominant form of "pure" familial spastic paraplegia: Clinical findings and linkage analysis of a large pedigree. Neurology 1987;37: 910–915.

Boylan KB, Cornblath DR, Glass JD, et al: Autosomal dominant distal spinal muscular atrophy in four generations. Neurology 1995;45:699–704.

Brahe C: Copies of the survival motor neuron gene in spinal muscular atrophy: The more, the better. Neuromusc Disord 2000;10:274–275.

Brandt S: Werdnig-Hoffmann's Infantile Progressive Muscular Atrophy: Clinical aspects, pathology, hereditary, relation to Oppenheim's amyotonia congenita and other morbid conditions with laxity of joints and muscles in infants. Copenhagen, Munksgaard, 1950.

Bruyn RP: The neuropathology of hereditary spastic paraparesis. Clin Neurol Neurosurg 1992;94(Suppl):S16–S18.

Brzustowicz LM, Lehner T, Castilla LH, et al: Genetic mapping of chronic childhood-onset spinal muscular atrophy to chromosome 5q11.2-13.3. Nature 1990;345:540–541.

Buchthal F, Olsen PZ: Electromyography and muscle biopsy in infantile spinal muscular atrophy. Brain 1970;93:15–30.

Burglen L, Lefebvre S, Clermont O, et al: Structure and organization of the human survival motor neuron (SMN) gene. Genomics 1996;32:479–482.

Bushman W, Steers WD, Meythaler JM: Voiding dysfunction in patients with spastic paraplegia: Urodynamic evaluation and response to continuous intrathecal baclofen. Neurourol Urodyn 1993;12:163–170.

Bussaglia E, Tizzano EF, Illa I, et al: Cramps and minimal EMG abnormalities as preclinical manifestations of spinal muscular atrophy patients with homozygous deletions of the SMN gene. Neurology 1997;48:1443–1445.

Byers RK, Banker BQ: Infantile muscular atrophy. Arch Neurol 1961;5:140–164.

Cambi F, Tang XM, Cordray P, et al: Refined genetic mapping and proteolipid protein mutation analysis in X-linked pure hereditary spastic paraplegia. Neurology 1996;46:1112–1117.

Campbell L, Potter A, Ignatius J, et al: Genome variation and gene conversion in spinal muscular atrophy: Implications for disease process and clinical phenotype. Am J Hum Genet 1997; 61:40–50.

Casari G, De Fusco M, Ciarmatori S, et al: Spastic paraplegia and OXPHOS impairment caused by mutations in paraplegin, a nuclear-encoded mitochondrial metalloproteinase. Cell 1998; 93:973–983.

Chang JG, Jong YJ, Lin SP, et al: Molecular analysis of survival motor neuron (SMN) and neuronal apoptosis inhibitory protein (NAIP) genes of spinal muscular atrophy patients and their parents. Hum Genet 1997;100:577–581.

Chou SM, Gilbert EF, Chun RW: Infantile olivopontocerebellar atrophy with spinal muscular atrophy (infantile OPCA + SMA). Clin Neuropathol 1990;9:21–32.

Christodoulou K, Kyriakides T, Hristova AH, et al: Mapping of a distal form of spinal muscular atrophy with upper limb predominance to chromosome 7p. Hum Mol Genet 1995;4: 1629–1632.

Claus D, Waddy HM, Harding AE, et al: Hereditary motor and sensory neuropathies and hereditary spastic paraplegia: A magnetic stimulation study. Ann Neurol 1990;28:43–49.

Cole N, Siddique T: Genetic disorders of motor neurons. Semin Neurol 1999;19:407–418.

Crawford TO, Pardo CA: The neurobiology of childhood spinal muscular atrophy. Neurobiol Dis 1996;3:97–110.

Daher YH, Lonstein JE, Winter RB, et al: Spinal surgery in spinal muscular atrophy. J Pediatr Orthop 1985;5:391–395.

Davis CJF, Bradley WG, Madrid R: The peroneal muscular atrophy syndrome: Clinical, genetic, electrophysiological and nerve biopsy studies. J Hum Genet 1978;26:311.

De Michele G, De Fusco M, Cavalcanti F, et al: A new locus for autosomal recessive hereditary spastic paraplegia maps to chromosome 16q24.3. Am J Hum Genet 1998;63:135–139.

DeLong R, Siddique T: A large New England kindred with autosomal dominant neurogenic scapuloperoneal amyotrophy with unique features. Arch Neurol 1992;49:905–908.

Duckett S: Pediatric Neuropathology. Philadelphia, Williams & Wilkins, 1995.

Ellsworth RE, Ionasescu V, Searby C, et al: The CMT2D locus: Refined genetic position and construction of a bacterial clone-based physical map. Genome Res 1999;9:568–574.

Emery AE: The nosology of the spinal muscular atrophies. J Med Genet 1971;8:481–495.

Emery ES, Fenichel GM, Eng G: A spinal muscular atrophy with scapuloperoneal distribution. Arch Neurol 1968;18:129–133.

Eng GD, Binder H, Koch B: Spinal muscular atrophy: Experience in diagnosis and rehabilitation management of 60 patients. Arch Phys Med Rehab 1984;65:549–553.

Fazio M: Ereditarieta della paralisi bulbare progressive. Riforma Med 1892;8:327.

Fenichel GM, Emery ES, Hunt P: Neurogenic atrophy simulating fascioscapulohumeral dystrophy: A dominant form. Arch Neurol 1967;17:257–260.

Filla A, De Michele G, Marconi R, et al: Prevalence of hereditary ataxias and spastic paraplegias in Molise, a region of Italy. J Neurol 1992;239:351–353.

Fischbeck KH, Lieberman A, Bailey CK, et al: Androgen receptor mutation in Kennedy's disease. Philos Trans R Soc Lond B Biol Sci 1999;354:1075–1078.

Fischbeck KH: Kennedy disease. J Inherit Metab Dis 1997;20:152–158.

Fleury P, Hageman G: A dominantly inherited lower motor neuron disorder presenting at birth with associated arthrogryposis. J Neurol Neurosurg Psychiatry 1985;48:1037–1048.

Fransen E, Lemmon V, Van Camp G, et al: CRASH syndrome: clinical spectrum of corpus callosum hypoplasia, retardation, adducted thumbs, spastic paraparesis and hydrocephalus due to mutations in one single gene, L1. Eur J Hum Genet 1995;3:273–284.

Fried K, Emery AE: Spinal muscular atrophy type II: A separate genetic and clinical entity from type I (Werdnig-Hoffmann disease) and type 3 (Kugelberg-Welander disease). Clin Genet 1971;2:203–209.

Frijns CJ, Van Deutekom J, Frants RR, et al: Dominant congenital benign spinal muscular atrophy. Muscle Nerve 1994;17:192–197.

Gamstorp I: Historical review of the progressive spinal muscular atrophies with onset in infancy or in early childhood. In Gamstorp I, Sarnath B (eds): Progressive Spinal Atrophies. New York, Raven Press, 1984; 11–18.

Gamstorp I: Progressive spinal muscular atrophy with onset in infancy or early childhood. Acta Paediatr Scand 1967;56:408–423.

Gath I, Sjaastad O, Loken AC: Myopathic electromyographic changes correlated with histopathology in Wohlfart-Kugelberg-Welander disease. Neurology 1969;19:344–352.

Gendron NH, MacKenzie AE: Spinal muscular atrophy: Molecular pathophysiology. Curr Opin Neurol 1999;12:137–142.

Gennarelli M, Lucarelli M, Capon F, et al: Survival motor neuron gene transcript analysis in muscles from spinal muscular atrophy patients. Biochem Biophys Res Commun 1995;213:342–348.

Goldblatt J, Ballo R, Sachs B, et al: X-linked spastic paraplegia: Evidence for homogeneity with a variable phenotype. Clin Genet 1989;35:116–120.

Gonschorek AS, Feistner H, Awiszus F: Spinal motoneuron function in lower motor neuron disease: Normal corticomotoneuronal and peripheral Ia EPSPs in patients with spinal muscular atrophy. Electromyogr Clin Neurophysiol 1999;39:27–32.

Greenberg F, Fenolio KR, Hejtmancik JF: X-linked infantile spinal muscular atrophy. Am J Dis Child 1988;142:217–219.

Groen RJ, Sie OG, van Weerden TW: Dominant inherited distal spinal muscular atrophy with atrophic and hypertrophic calves. J Neurol Sci 1993;114:81–84.

Groger H, Werdnig G: In Ashwold S (eds): The Founders of Child Neurology. San Francisco, Norman Publishing, 1990; 383—388.

Grohmann K, Wienker TF, Saar K, et al: Diaphragmatic spinal muscular atrophy with respiratory distress is heterogeneous, and one form is linked to chromosome 11q13-q21. Am J Hum Genet 1999;65:1459–1462.

Gross M: Proximal spinal muscular atrophy. J Neurol Neurosurg Psychiatry 1966;29:29–34.

Harding AE: Inherited neuronal atrophy and degeneration predominantly in lower motor neurons. In Dyck PJ, Thomas PK (eds): Peripheral Neuropathy, 3rd ed. Philadelphia, WB Saunders, 1993; 1051–1064.

Harding AE, Thomas PK, Baraitser M, et al: X-linked recessive bulbospinal neuronopathy: A report of ten cases. J Neurol Neurosurg Psychiatry 1982;45:1012–1019.

Harding AE, Thomas PK: Hereditary distal spinal muscular atrophy: A report on 34 cases and a review of the literature. J Neurol Sci 1980;45:337–348.

Harding AE: Hereditary "pure" spastic paraplegia: A clinical and genetic study of 22 families. J Neurol Neurosurg Psychiatry 1981;44:871–883.

Hausmanowa-Petrusewicz I, Askanas W, Badurska B, et al: Infantile and juvenile spinal muscular atrophy. J Neurol Sci 1968;6:269–287.

Hausmanowa-Petrusewicz I, Borkowska J, Janczewski Z: X-linked adult form of spinal muscular atrophy. J Neurol 1983;229:175–188.

Hausmanowa-Petrusewicz I, Fidzianska-Dolot A: Clinical features of infantile and juvenile spinal muscular atrophy. In Gamstrop I, Saranath B (eds): Progressive Spinal Muscular Atrophies. New York, Raven Press, 1984.

Hausmanowa-Petrusewicz I, Karwanska A: Electromyographic findings in different forms of infantile and juvenile proximal spinal muscular atrophy. Muscle Nerve 1986;9:37–46.

Hausmanowa-Petrusewicz I: Electrophysiological findings in childhood spinal muscular atrophies. Rev Neurol (Paris) 1988; 144:716–720.

Hazan J, Fonknechten N, Mavel D, et al: Spastin, a new AAA protein, is altered in the most frequent form of autosomal dominant spastic paraplegia. Nat Genet 1999;23:296–303.

Hedera P, DiMauro S, Bonilla E, et al: Phenotypic analysis of autosomal dominant hereditary spastic paraplegia linked to chromosome 8q. Neurology 1999;53:44–50.

Hentati A, Pericak-Vance MA, Hung WY, et al: Linkage of "pure" autosomal recessive familial spastic paraplegia to chromosome 8 markers and evidence of genetic locus heterogeneity. Hum Mol Genet 1994;3:1263–1267.

Iannaccone ST, Caneris O, Hoffmann J: In Ashwold S (eds): The Founders of Childhood Neurology. San Francisco, Norman Publishing, 1990; 278–284.

Iannaccone ST: Spinal muscular atrophy. Semin Neurol 1998;18:19–26.

Ikezoe K, Yoshimura T, Taniwaki T, et al: Autosomal dominant familial spinal and bulbar muscular atrophy with gynecomastia. Neurology 1999;53:2187–2189.

Isozumi K, DeLong R, Kaplan J, et al: Linkage of scapuloperoneal spinal muscular atrophy to chromosome 12q24.1-q24.31. Hum Mol Genet 1996;5:1377–1382.

Iwahashi H, Eguchi Y, Yasuhara N, et al: Synergistic anti-apoptotic activity between Bcl-2 and SMN implicated in spinal muscular atrophy. Nature 1997;390:413–417.

Jansen PH, Joosten EM, Jaspar HH, et al: A rapidly progressive autosomal dominant scapulohumeral form of spinal muscular atrophy. Ann Neurol 1986;20:538–540.

Jouet M, Rosenthal A, Armstrong G, et al: X-linked spastic paraplegia (SPG1), MASA syndrome and X-linked hydrocephalus result from mutations in the L1 gene. Nat Genet 1994;7:402–407.

Kennedy WR, Alter M, Sung JH: Progressive proximal spinal and bulbar muscular atrophy of late onset: A sex-linked recessive trait. Neurology 1968;18:671–680.

Kenwrick S, Ionasescu V, Ionasescu G, et al: Linkage studies of X-linked recessive spastic paraplegia using DNA probes. Hum Genet 1986;73:264–266.

Keppen LD, Leppert MF, O'Connell P, et al: Etiological heterogeneity in X-linked spastic paraplegia. Am J Hum Genet 1987;41:933–943.

Kobayashi H, Baumbach L, Matise TC, et al: A gene for a severe lethal form of X-linked arthrogryposis (X-linked infantile spinal muscular atrophy) maps to human chromosome X p11.3-q11.2. Hum Mol Genet 1995;4:1213–1216.

Kobayashi H, Hoffman EP, Marks HG: The rumpshaker mutation in spastic paraplegia. Nat Genet 1994;7:351–352.

Kugelberg E, Welander L: Heredofamilial juvenile muscular atrophy simulating muscular dystrophy. Arch Neurol 1956;75:500–509.

La Spada AR, Roling DB, Harding AE: Meiotic stability and genotype-phenotype correlation of the trinucleotide repeat in X-linked spinal and bulbar muscular atrophy. Nat Genet 1992;2:301–304.

La Spada AR, Wilson EM, Lubahn DB, et al: Androgen receptor gene mutations in X-linked spinal and bulbar muscular atrophy. Nature 1991;352:77–79.

Laurance BM, Matthews WB, Diggle JH: Hereditary quivering of the chin. Arch Dis Child 1968;43:249–251.

Lefebvre S, Burglen L, Frezal J, et al: The role of the SMN gene in proximal spinal muscular atrophy. Hum Mol Genet 1998;7:1531–1536.

Lefebvre S, Burglen L, Reboullet S, et al: Identification and characterization of the spinal muscular atrophy–determining gene. Cell 1995;80:155–165.

Lefebvre S, Burlet P, Liu Q, et al: Correlation between severity and SMN protein level in spinal muscular atrophy. Nat Genet 1997;16:265–269.

Leone M, Bottacchi E, D'Alessandro G, et al: Hereditary ataxias and paraplegias in Valle d'Aosta, Italy: A study of prevalence and disability. Acta Neurol Scand 1995;91:183–187.

Li M, Miwa S, Kobayashi Y, et al: Nuclear inclusions of the androgen receptor protein in spinal and bulbar muscular atrophy. Ann Neurol 1998;44:249–254.

Liu Q, Fischer U, Wang F, et al: The spinal muscular atrophy disease gene product, SMN, and its associated protein SIP1 are in a complex with spliceosomal snRNP proteins. Cell 1997;90: 1013–1021.

Lo AC, Houenou LJ, Oppenheim RW: Apoptosis in the nervous system: morphological features, methods, pathology, and prevention. Arch Histol Cytol 1995;58:139–149.

Mart3/4nez Murillo F, Kobayashi H, Pegoraro E, et al: Genetic localization of a new locus for recessive familial spastic paraparesis to 15q13-15. Neurology 1999;53:50–56.

Mastaglia F, Walton JN: Histological and histochemical changes in skeletal muscle from cases of chronic juvenile and early adult spinal muscular atrophy (the Kugelberg-Welander syndrome). J Neurol Sci 1971;12:15–44.

Matthijs G, Schollen E, Legius E, et al: Unusual molecular findings in autosomal recessive spinal muscular atrophy. J Med Genet 1996;33:469–474.

McDermott C, White K, Bushby K, et al: Hereditary spastic paraparesis: A review of new developments. J Neurol Neurosurg Psychiatry. 2000;69:150–160.

McLeod JG, Morgan JA, Reye C: Electrophysiological studies in familial spastic paraplegia. J Neurol Neurosurg Psychiatry 1977;40:611–615.

Meadows JC, Marsden CD: A distal form of chronic spinal muscular atrophy. Neurology 1969;19:53–58.

Mellins RB, Hays AP, Gold AP, et al: Respiratory distress as the initial manifestation of Werdnig–Hoffmann disease. Pediatrics 1974;53:33–40.

Mendell JR, Freimer M, Kissel JT: Randomized double blind crossover trial of androgen hormone deficiency and replacement in X-linked bulbar spinal muscular atrophy. Neurology 1996; 46:A469.

Meriggioli MN, Rowin J, Sanders DB: Distinguishing clinical and electrodiagnostic features of X-linked bulbospinal neuronopathy. Muscle Nerve 1999;22:1693–1697.

Mhatre AN, Trifiro MA, Kaufman M, et al: Reduced transcriptional regulatory competence of the androgen receptor in X-linked spinal and bulbar muscular atrophy. Nat Genet 1993;5:184–188.

Monani UR, Lorson CL, Parsons DW, et al: A single nucleotide difference that alters splicing patterns distinguishes the SMA gene SMN1 from the copy gene SMN2. Hum Mol Genet 1999;8: 1177–1183.

Moosa A, Dubowitz V: Motor nerve conduction velocity in spinal muscular atrophy of childhood. Arch Dis Child 1976;51:974–977.

Munsat TL: Workshop Report: International SMA collaboration. Neuromusc Disord 1991;1:81.

Murayama S, Bouldin TW, Suzuki K: Immunocytochemical and ultrastructural studies of Werdnig–Hoffmann disease. Acta Neuropathol (Berl) 1991;81:408–417.

Namba T, Aberfeld D, Grob D: Chronic proximal spinal muscular atrophy. J Neurol Sci 1970;11:401–423.

Nelson JW, Amick LD: Heterofamilial progressive spinal muscular atrophy: A clinical and electromyographic study of a kinship. J Neurology 1966:306.

Nielsen JE, Koefoed P, Abell K, et al: CAG repeat expansion in autosomal dominant pure spastic paraplegia linked to chromosome 2p21-p24. Hum Mol Genet 1997;6:1811–1816.

Nielsen JE, Krabbe K, Jennum P, et al: Autosomal dominant pure spastic paraplegia: A clinical, paraclinical, and genetic study. J Neurol Neurosurg Psychiatry 1998;64:61–66.

Olney RK, Aminoff MJ, So YT: Clinical and electrodiagnostic features of X-linked recessive bulbospinal neuronopathy. Neurology 1991;41:823–828.

Opjordsmoen S, Nyberg-Hansen R: Hereditary spastic paraplegia with neurogenic bladder disturbances and syndactylia. Acta Neurol Scand 1980;61:35–41.

Ormerod IE, Harding AE, Miller DH, et al: Magnetic resonance imaging in degenerative ataxic disorders. J Neurol Neurosurg Psychiatry 1994;57:51–57.

Palmer HD: Familial scapuloperoneal amyotrophy. Arch Neurol Psychiat 1932;28:477.

Parano E, Provone L, Falsaperla R, et al: Molecular basis of phenotypic heterogeneity in siblings with spinal muscular atrophy. Ann Neurol 1996;40:247–251.

Parboosingh JS, Meininger V, McKenna-Yasek D, et al: Deletions causing spinal muscular atrophy do not predispose to amyotrophic lateral sclerosis. Arch Neurol 1999;56:710–712.

Pearn J, Hudgson P: Distal spinal muscular atrophy: A clinical and genetic study of 8 kindreds. J Neurol Sci 1979;43:183–191.

Pearn J: Autosomal dominant spinal muscular atrophy: A clinical and genetic study. J Neurol Sci 1978;38:263–275.

Pelosi L, Lanzillo B, Perretti A, et al: Motor and somatosensory evoked potentials in hereditary spastic paraplegia. J Neurol Neurosurg Psychiatry 1991;54:1099–1102.

Phillips DT, Roye DP Jr, Farcy JP, et al: Surgical treatment of scoliosis in a spinal muscular atrophy population. Spine 1990; 15:942–945.

Piasecki JO, Mahinpour S, Levine DB: Long-term follow-up of spinal fusion in spinal muscular atrophy. Clin Orthop 1986; 207:44–54.

Polo JM, Calleja J, Combarros O, et al: Hereditary "pure" spastic paraplegia: A study of nine families. J Neurol Neurosurg Psychiatry 1993;56:175–181.

Polo JM, Calleja J, Combarros O, et al: Hereditary ataxias and paraplegias in Cantabria, Spain: An epidemiological and clinical study. Brain 1991;114(Pt 2):855–866.

Pridmore C, Baraitser M, Brett EM, et al: Distal spinal muscular atrophy with vocal cord paralysis. J Med Genet 1992;29:197–199.

Ringel SP, Lava NS, Treihaft MM, et al: Late-onset X-linked recessive spinal and bulbar muscular atrophy. Muscle Nerve 1978; 1:297–307.

Rudnik-Schoneborn S, Forkert R, Hahnen E, et al: Clinical spectrum and diagnostic criteria of infantile spinal muscular atrophy: Further delineation on the basis of SMN gene deletion findings. Neuropediatrics 1996;27:8–15.

Russman BS, Buncher CR, White M, et al: Function changes in spinal muscular atrophy II and III: The DCN/SMA Group. Neurology 1996;47:973–976.

Sack GH, Huether CA, Garg N: Familial spastic paraplegia—clinical and pathologic studies in a large kindred. Johns Hopkins Med J 1978;143:117–121.

Saugier-Veber P, Munnich A, Bonneau D, et al: X-linked spastic paraplegia and Pelizaeus-Merzbacher disease are allelic disorders at the proteolipid protein locus. Nat Genet 1994;6:257–262.

Schady W, Dick JP, Sheard A, et al: Central motor conduction studies in hereditary spastic paraplegia. J Neurol Neurosurg Psychiatry 1991;54:775–779.

Schady W, Sheard A: A quantitative study of sensory function in hereditary spastic paraplegia. Brain 1990;113(Pt 3):709–720.

Scharf JM, Endrizzi MG, Wetter A, et al: Identification of a candidate modifying gene for spinal muscular atrophy by comparative genetics. Nat Genet 1998;20:83–86.

Schuchmann L: Spinal muscular atrophy of the scapuloperoneal-type. Z Kinderheilkd 1970;109:118–123.

Seri M, Cusano R, Forabosco P, et al: Genetic mapping to 10q23.3-q24.2, in a large Italian pedigree, of a new syndrome showing bilateral cataracts, gastroesophageal reflux, and spastic paraparesis with amyotrophy. Am J Hum Genet 1999;64:586–593.

Serratrice G, Pellissier JF, Gastaut JL, et al: [Chronic spinal amyotrophy with paralysis of the vocal cords: Young-Harper syndrome]. Rev Neurol (Paris) 1984;140:657–658.

Siegal IM, Silverman M: Upright mobility system for spinal muscular atrophy patients. Arch Phys Med Rehabil 1984;65:418.

Silva MC, Coutinho P, Pinheiro CD, et al: Hereditary ataxias and spastic paraplegias: Methodological aspects of a prevalence study in Portugal. J Clin Epidemiol 1997;50:1377–1384.

Silver JR: Familial spastic paraplegia with amyotrophy of the hands. Ann Hum Genet 1966;30:69–75.

Sobue G, Doyu M, Kachi T, et al: Subclinical phenotypic expressions in heterozygous females of X-linked recessive bulbospinal neuronopathy. J Neurol Sci 1993;117:74–78.

Sobue G, Hashizume Y, Mukai E, et al: X-linked recessive bulbospinal neuronopathy. A clinicopathological study. Brain 1989; 112:209–232.

Sobue G, Matsuoka Y, Mukai E, et al: Spinal and cranial motor nerve roots in amyotrophic lateral sclerosis and X-linked recessive bulbospinal muscular atrophy: Morphometric and teased-fiber study. Acta Neuropathol (Berl) 1981;55:227–235.

Sobue G: X-linked recessive bulbospinal neuronopathy (SBMA). Nagoya J Med Sci 1995;58:95–106.

Stefanis C, Papapetropoulos Th, Scarpalezos S, et al: X-linked spinal and bulbar muscular atrophy of late onset: A separate type of motor neuron disease? J Neurol Sci 1975;24:493–503.

Strober JB, Tennekoon GI: Progressive spinal muscular atrophies. J Child Neurol 1999;14:691–695.

Strümpell A: Beitrage zur pathologie des ruckenmarkes. Arch Psychiatr Nurvenkrankenheit 1880;10:676–717.

Summers BA, Swash M, Schwartz MS, et al: Juvenile-onset bulbospinal muscular atrophy with deafness: Vialetta-van Laere syndrome or Madras-type motor neuron disease? J Neurol 1987;234:440–442.

Sutherland JM: Familial spastic paraplegia. In Vinken PJ, Bruyn JG (eds): Handbook of Clinical Neurology. Amsterdam, North Holland, 1975; 42–43.

Talbot K, Miguel-Aliaga I, Mohaghegh P, et al: Characterization of a gene encoding survival motor neuron (SMN)–related protein, a constituent of the spliceosome complex. Hum Mol Genet 1998;7:2149–2156.

Talbot K: Spinal muscular atrophy. J Inherit Metab Dis 1999;22:545–554.

Timmerman V, De Jonghe P, Simokovic S, et al: Distal hereditary motor neuropathy type II (distal HMN II): Mapping of a locus to chromosome 12q24. Hum Mol Genet 1996;5:1065–1069.

Timmerman V, Raeymaekers P, Nelis E, et al: Linkage analysis of distal hereditary motor neuropathy type II (distal HMN II) in a single pedigree. J Neurol Sci 1992;109:41–48.

Tsukagoshi H, Shoji H, Furukawa T: Proximal neurogenic muscular atrophy in adolescence and adulthood with X-linked recessive inheritance: Kugelberg-Welander disease and its variant of late onset in one pedigree. Neurology 1970;20:1188–1193.

Van der Steege G, Grootscholten PM, Van der Vlies P, et al: PCR-based DNA test to confirm clinical diagnosis of autosomal recessive spinal muscular atrophy. Lancet 1995;345:985–986.

Van der Vleuten AJ, Van Ravenswaaij-Arts CM, Frijns CJ, et al: Localisation of the gene for a dominant congenital spinal muscular atrophy predominantly affecting the lower limbs to chromosome 12q23-q24. Eur J Hum Genet 1998;6:376–382.

Van Gent EM, Hoogland RA, Jennekens FG: Distal amyotrophy of predominantly the upper limbs with pyramidal features in a large kinship. J Neurol Neurosurg Psychiatry 1985;48:266–269.

Van Laere J: [On a new case of chronic bulbopontine paralysis with deafness]. Verh K Vlaam Acad Geneeskd Belg 1967;29:288–308.

Velasco E, Valero C, Valero A, et al: Molecular analysis of the SMN and NAIP genes in Spanish spinal muscular atrophy (SMA) families and correlation between number of copies of cBCD541 and SMA phenotype. Hum Mol Genet 1996;5:257–263.

Vialetta E: Contributo alla forma ereditaria della paralisi bulbare progressiva. Riv Sper Freniatr 1936;40:1–24.

Vitali T, Sossi V, Tizziano F, et al: Detection of the survival motor neuron (SMN) genes by FISH: Further evidence for a role of SMN2 in the modulation of disease severity in SMA patients. Hum Mol Genet 1999;8:2525–2532.

Wang TG, Bach JR, Avilla C, et al: Survival of individuals with spinal muscular atrophy on ventilatory support. Am J Phys Med Rehabil 1994;73:207–211.

Wessel HB: Spinal muscular atrophy. Pediatr Ann 1989;18:421–427.

White KD, Ince PG, Lusher M, et al: Clinical and pathologic findings in hereditary spastic paraparesis with spastin mutation. Neurology 2000;55:89–94.

Young ID, Harper PS: Hereditary distal spinal muscular atrophy with vocal cord paralysis. J Neurol Neurosurg Psychiatry 1980;43:413.

Yu WH: Administration of testosterone attenuates neuronal loss following axotomy in the brain-stem motor nuclei of female rats. J Neurosci 1989;9:3908–3914.

Zerres K, Rudnik-Schoneborn S: Natural history in spinal muscular atrophy: Clinical analysis of 445 patients and suggestions for a modification of existing classifications. Arch Neurol 1995;52:518–523.

Infectious, Syndromic, and Systemic Disorders

Clifton L. Gooch and Hiroshi Mitsumoto

INFECTIOUS MOTOR NEURON DISEASES

Poliomyelitis

EPIDEMIOLOGY AND PATHOGENESIS

Over the last 50 years, tremendous progress has been made in the global eradication of poliomyelitis. Nevertheless, wild-type polio infections persist in less developed countries, and vaccine-associated polio, although rare, continues to appear. The dread of epidemic polio has largely faded from the public consciousness, but approximately 25,000 to 50,000 cases of poliomyelitis were reported annually in the United States alone prior to the advent of effective vaccination programs (Paul, 1971; Mulder, 1995; Gooch, 1996). Poliovirus is a single-stranded RNA virus belonging to the enterovirus subgroup of the picornaviruses, which primarily infects through fecal-oral contamination, often surviving in sewage or contaminated water for prolonged periods. Before the era of effective immunization, epidemics were restricted largely to northern countries with excellent sanitation systems. Populations living under less sanitary condition were more likely to be exposed to the virus during early infancy while they were still protected from more severe disease by maternal antibodies, facilitating the development of lifelong immunity. Without such inadvertent endemic immunization, populations in developed countries experienced recurrent epidemics, typically in the late summer, which appeared most commonly in infants, adolescents, and young adults. Although older patients were less likely to contract the disease after exposure, they were more likely to be severely affected (Codd et al., 1985; Nicolosi et al., 1986; Bharucha et al., 1991).

CLINICAL FEATURES

Poliovirus infection can be divided into four categories of successively greater clinical severity: *subclinical infection, abortive poliomyelitis, nonparalytic poliomyelitis with "aseptic" meningitis*, and *paralytic poliomyelitis*. Following exposure, the average incubation period is 1 to 2 weeks, but may range from as little as 4 days to as much as 5 weeks. *Subclinical infection* is marked by clinically silent disease from oral inoculation followed by infiltration of lymphatic tissue in the ileum and pharynx, subsequent dissemination throughout the lymphatic system, and, ultimately, hematogenous spread. In 90% of cases, infection is successfully eradicated by the host immune system at this level, with no further progression. *Abortive poliomyelitis* occurs when enteroviral infection becomes better established and produces fever, cough, malaise, headache, sore throat, nausea, vomiting, and diarrhea. An additional 8% of patients experience this syndrome but recover completely within 2 to 3 days. *Nonparalytic poliomyelitis with aseptic meningitis* occurs in the majority of the remaining 2%. In these cases, central nervous system infection develops, with persistence of the aforementioned systemic symptoms or recurrence in 2 to 10 days after apparent recovery, followed by worsening constant headache and meningismus. Cerebrospinal fluid studies during this stage demonstrate leukocytosis (25 to 500 cells/mm³) with early neutrophilic predominance (superseded by lymphocytic predominance within a few days), an elevated protein level (50 to 150 mg/dL), and a normal glucose content. In 90% of these cases, resolution occurs within 1 to 2 weeks without further sequelae. *Paralytic poliomyelitis* occurs in a very small minority of infected patients (approximately 0.02%). In these cases, the anterior horn cells and/or cranial motor nuclei are injured. Affected patients develop spasm, tenderness, and stiffness in the back and hamstring muscles. Weakness then appears over hours to days, concurrent with resoltion of fever. Coarse fasciculations typically accompany developing paralysis, and muscular atrophy begins within 1 to 3 weeks. Most commonly, aseptic meningitis precedes motor paralysis, although weakness may sometimes be the presenting feature of central nervous system involvement, and, in rare instances, meningitic symptoms may be delayed for as long as 2 to 3 weeks (Gooch, 1995).

In children younger than age 5 years, asymmetrical lower extremity weakness at onset of the disease is more common, whereas in older children and adolescents, arm weakness with bilateral leg weakness is more probable. In young adults, quadriplegia is more frequently observed. Early loss of deep tendon reflexes is the rule, although hyperreflexia may sometimes occur. Respiratory muscle dysfunction is the complication that causes the most concern at this stage, and respiratory capacity must be diligently followed. A total of 10% to 15% of patients with motor system involvement develop cranial nerve dysfunction, usually manifesting as pharyngeal paralysis and laryngeal weakness; facial diplegia is less common. Other symptoms may include urinary bladder dysfunction (particularly in adults); rarely, autonomic dysfunction with hypertension (due to involvement of the ventricular formation and the thalamus); myocarditis; transverse myelitis; and acute cerebellar ataxia. A total of 2% to 5% of children and 15% to 30% of adults who develop paralytic disease die, usually from complications of respiratory failure. In these cases, autopsy reveals destruction of the motor neurons supplying the intercostal and diaphragmatic muscles. Aspiration and disturbed control of vascular tone are other potentially fatal complications. In surviving patients, recovery of strength may begin 1 month after onset, with maximal improvement at 6 to 9 months, although some degree of permanent weakness persists in approximately one third of patients. Furthermore, 25% to 30% of patients with persistent weakness will develop renewed progression approximately 25 to 35 years after infection, occasionally in muscles not clinically affected at the time of their initial episode. This *postpolio syndrome* typically progresses extremely slowly, with an average decline in strength of 1% per year. Postpolio syndrome is more fully detailed in Chapter 72 (Nkowane et al., 1987).

DIAGNOSIS

The diagnosis of poliomyelitis is a clinical one, but it is supported by viral studies and electrophysiological testing. Specimens for viral culture should be taken from the stool, throat, and cerebrospinal fluid, as the virus is somewhat fastidious and may be difficult to grow from the cerebrospinal fluid alone. Tissue culture systems should enable identification of enterovirus in 3 to 4 days and more specific confirmation of poliovirus infection within 10 to 11 days. Acute and convalescent titers of serum antibody to each of the three pathogenic poliovirus strains may also be helpful, with fourfold increases supporting acute infection. As paralytic polio may occur with minimal systemic symptoms, it may be sometimes be confused with other conditions that cause acute areflexic paralysis, including Guillain-Barré syndrome, botulism intoxication, tick paralysis, heavy metal poisoning, and transverse myelitis.

ELECTROPHYSIOLOGY

Electrophysiological changes in poliovirus infection and recovery can be divided into five phases: *acute myelitis, early recovery, late recovery, functional stability,* and *late change.* Although results of sensory nerve conduction studies are usually normal, motor nerve conduction studies demonstrate loss of amplitude of compound motor action potentials (consistent with motor axon loss) and normal to slightly decreased nerve conduction velocities (Johnson and Guyton, 1960; Wiechers, 1995). During the first month following paralysis *(acute myelitis),* decreased recruitment is noted on needle electromyography examination. In some muscles, complete loss of motor unit activation is seen, which correlates with complete clinical paralysis of that muscle. In keeping with the classic evolution of electrophysiological change after acute denervation, positive sharp waves and fibrillation potentials begin to appear within 10 to 21 days following the onset of weakness. Although it is too early to see motor unit remodeling, motor unit assessment is still important at this stage, as the presence of even a few volitionally recruited motor units in a weakened or paralyzed muscle proves survival of some axons, suggesting some potential for recovery. Some early studies described an apparent preferential loss of the larger motor neurons in polio victims, which might be due to a selective vulnerability of the larger, high-threshold motor units in this condition (Hodes et al., 1947; Hodes, 1949).

The *early recovery* phase typically begins at 2 to 12 months and is characterized by the functional recovery of damaged (but not destroyed) motor neurons and the collateral reinnervation of nearby denervated muscle fibers by surviving motor neurons. These pathophysiological changes can be documented with several electrophysiological techniques. In the early months of this period, increasing numbers of voluntarily recruited motor units appear on needle examination, as formerly compromised motor axons return to full functionality. Spontaneous activity in the form of fibrillations and positive sharp waves persists, and their severity generally correlates with the number of muscle fibers denervated by the disease. Motor unit remodeling also begins at this time, with terminal axon sprouting and reinnervation starting within 3 to 5 weeks after the onset of paralysis. Fiber density studies provide an electrophysiological correlate of the process, known histologically as fiber type grouping, a hallmark of progressive reinnervation, and increased fiber density appears within 1 month after the onset of paralysis in these patients (Wiechers, 1985). Single-fiber electromyography studies demonstrate mild neuromuscular transmission abnormalities concurrent with increased fiber density, which has been attributed to the formation of new, immature neuromuscular junctions as axon sprouts make contact with formerly denervated muscle fibers (Stålberg and Trontel, 1979). Disturbances of neuromuscular junction function can also sometimes be seen on routine needle electromyography in the form of motor unit action potential (MUAP) instability (changing morphology of the MUAP with repeated firing of the motor unit during needle examination, consistent with intermittent failure of different populations of neuromuscular junctions within it from discharge to discharge), which also appears in the early recovery phase. In the later part of this phase, MUAPs begin to demonstrate increased complexity, increased amplitude, and longer duration as surviving motor axons expand their territories with ongoing reinnervation. At approximately 6 months, jitter values and MUAP instability decrease as newly formed neuromuscular junctions accompanying reinnervation reach maturity. Jitter values typically return to normal levels within 18 months, although fiber density values remain elevated (Hakelius and Stålberg, 1974; Kubo et al., 1976; Wiechers and Hubbell, 1981; Wiechers, 1990). A limited number of longitudinal studies have been performed with contemporary electromyography techniques in patients with vaccine-associated polio and have demonstrated ongoing abnormalities, including spontaneous activity with positive sharp waves and fibrillation potentials in completely denervated muscles as long as 10 years after onset. In other muscles with substantial denervation and loss of muscle fibers, the MUAPs have reportedly remained unstable and continuing abnormalities in jitter and blocking with increased fiber density have been seen (Wiechers, 1988).

In the *late recovery phase*, between 2 and 8 years after onset, patients demonstrate gains in functional strength attributed to ongoing aggressive exercise, as they learn how to substitute the function of stronger muscles for weaker ones to perform common tasks. Following this increase, strength then plateaus. Electromyography findings parallel those observed at the end of the early recovery phase, with ongoing fasciculations, positive sharp waves, fibrillations, and abundant neurogenic MUAPs in affected muscles, some of which demonstrate extremely high amplitudes of up to 30 to 40 mV (possibly due to both progressive reinnervation and the muscle hypertrophy accompanying exercise). Poor recruitment and interference patterns persist in clinically weak muscles. Although return of motor unit stability occurs in stronger muscles, those with continued weakness (especially those with MRC grades of 3/5 or less) demonstrate ongoing motor unit instability and increased jitter. The phase of *functional stability* appears approximately 8 years after onset, as maximum strength has been achieved and functional activity stabilizes, and persists for decades. Some spontaneous activity, including fasciculations, positive sharp waves, and fibrillation potentials, may continue, but at lower levels. Clear neurogenic MUAPs remain in weak muscles but can also occasionally be seen in muscles with normal strength, suggesting fully successful compensatory reinnervation. MUAPs can be divided into three categories at this phase: normal MUAPs (unaffected by the disease), stable reinnervated MUAPs (which have sprouted to supply additional muscle fibers but have not exceeded their functional capacity), and unstable reinnervated MUAPs, demonstrating increased jitter on single-fiber electromyography. This persistent MUAP instability may be due to axonal overextension during reinnervation, as axons sprout to supply a larger number of muscle fibers than they are able to properly support, resulting in ongoing motor unit injury and dysfunction. The phase of *late change* occurs more than 35 to 40 years after disease onset, and a large number of electrophysiological and other studies have been performed to further investigate this postpolio syndrome, which is fully detailed elsewhere in this volume (see Chapter 71) (Maselli et al., 1992; McComas et al., 1997). Although some older reports suggested an association between the late development of amyotrophic lateral sclerosis (ALS) and a history of polio infection, this rarely reported association has been called into question as the entity of postpolio syndrome has been more clearly defined over the last 20 years. Furthermore, meta-analysis of the available epidemiological studies suggests no consistent association (Okumura et al., 1995).

PREVENTION

As available antiviral medications have not proved effective in changing the course of poliomyelitis, appropriate vaccination remains the best means of controlling this disease. The live but attenuated *oral polio vaccine* (OPV; originally devised by Sabin) and the Formalin-*inactivated polio vaccine* (IPV; originally devised by Salk) are available, and each protects against all three antigenic types of poliovirus. OPV offers increased intestinal immunity (as well as herd immunity, owing to transfer of the virus from inoculated individuals to their close contacts) and remains the recommended regimen in the United States. Because of the extremely rare risk of paralytic disease following vaccination (1 case in 550,000 vaccinations following the first dose and 1 per 12.3 million following subsequent doses), OPV should not be given to patients whose immune systems are compromised. A new approach, adopted by several countries to reduce the risk of vaccine-associated poliomyelitis, involves the use of sequential enhanced immunogenicity—that is, enhanced inactivated polio vaccine (eIPV)—followed by OPV. One or more doses of eIPV are given prior to boosting with OPV, inducing very high levels of immunity. This combined vaccination schedule may be safer than early OPV vaccination alone, because of its potential to reduce vaccine-associated paralytic poliomyelitis, although this has not yet been definitively demonstrated (Faden, 1990; Faden et al., 1993). Current Centers for Disease Control and Prevention (CDC) vaccination recommendations include either OPV or eIPV at 2, 4, and 12 to 18 months and again at 4 to 6 years, or a combined schedule of eIPV at 2 and 4 months, followed by OPV at 12 to 18 months and 4 to 6 years. For immunocompromised individuals, only eIPV is recommended. Immunization for adults in the United States is not typically recommended unless they are planning to travel to areas endemic for wild-type poliomyelitis or are members of a community in which wild-type virus has been found. Unvaccinated adults whose children are receiving OPV and immunocompromised adults needing polio vaccination should also receive the eIPV, as well as health care workers who may be exposed to polio. As immunity may not be maintained indefinitely with eIPV, further adult inoculations may be necessary. Patients with a history of streptomycin or neomycin allergy should not receive eIPV. The oral vaccine also requires special handling prior to administration and must be stored and shipped frozen and, after thawing, must be refrigerated at temperatures less than 10°C; otherwise, it may lose its potency. It must be discarded if refrigerated for more than 30 days (CDC, 1997, 1999). Following institution of the poliomyelitis eradication program in 1988, the number of countries reporting new infections has declined from 100 to 53, while the number of infected continents has decreased from five to two. This corresponds with a 90% reduction in the incidence of polio worldwide. Eradication has proved most challenging in South Asia and Africa, where ongoing social unrest and poor health infrastructure are impeding progress. Up-to-the-minute information regarding the progress of the worldwide polio eradication program, as well as additional helpful information regarding the infection, can be found on the World Health Organization's official polio site: *www.polioeradication.org*.

Vaccine-Associated Paralytic Poliomyelitis

As mentioned previously, a rare complication of OPV is vaccine-associated paralytic poliomyelitis, which is usually associated with type II and type III strains and, less frequently, with the type I strain of attenuated virus (Friedrich, 1998). Although the last indigenous wild-type poliovirus was reported in the United States in 1979, since that time 80 vaccine-associated cases of paralytic poliomyelitis have appeared, most in immunodeficient individuals following the first or second dose of OPV (Strebel et al., 1992; Hull et al., 1994). In many instances, genomic modification, presumed to occur during multiplication after vaccination, has been confirmed by nucleotide sequencing, suggesting increased virulence due to postvaccination mutation. These changes typically consist of reverse mutations in the attenuation determinants of the more virulent strain. However, similar mutations have been seen in healthy vaccinated subjects without paralytic disease, suggesting that host factors such as immunodeficiency may play an important role in the development of infection. A number of other complications of oral poliovirus vaccination have also been reported, including headache, fever, vomiting, meningitis, encephalitis, facial paralysis, transverse myelitis, and Guillain-Barré syndrome (Friedrich, 1998).

Treatment

Therapy for poliomyelitis remains supportive. Hospitalization is recommended at the first sign of nervous system infection. Meningeal and muscle pain may respond to analgesics and hot packs. Vigilant observation for signs of early respiratory compromise (including increasing anxiety and restlessness) is crucial, and serial vital capacity measurements should be monitored and mechanical ventilation instituted when values fall below 30% to 50% of normal. Unfortunately, excessive secretions often necessitate early tracheostomy. Transient bladder paralysis (lasting days) is best treated with bethanechol (5 to 10 mg PO with titration to 10 to 50 mg PO t.i.d., or 2.5 to 5 mg SC), although catheterization may still be required in some of these patients. Enemas and stool softeners are often necessary, as abdominal muscle weakness promotes constipation. Weak and paralyzed limbs must be carefully positioned, and splints, boards, and sandbags, in conjunction with early physical therapy, are very important in minimizing contracture formation and other deformities. Despite these measures, surgical correction of developing abnormalities by an experienced orthopedist may be necessary (Gooch, 1995).

Other Infections

A variety of other viruses may cause a clinical syndrome similar to that of poliomyelitis. Infections due to the enteroviruses are clearly the most common viral infections that affect the central nervous system in this way, although the clinical and histological findings are typically much less severe with coxsackievirus and echovirus infection than with infection with poliovirus (Jubelt and Lipton, 1989; Bartfeld et al., 1995). Echovirus type 70 is most commonly associated with epidemics of acute hemorrhagic conjunctivitis, but it also causes acute paralytic disease in Asia, Africa, and Latin America. Echovirus type 71 is usually associated with aseptic meningitis or hand-foot-and-mouth disease, but it has also caused epidemic paralytic disease in Hungary and Bulgaria and, occasionally, in the United States (Schmidt et al., 1974; Wadia et al., 1981). Among the myxoviruses, influenza is a well-known cause of postencephalitic parkinsonism, but lower motor neuron disease may also appear as a late sequela as long as 18 years after the original infection in these patients. Ongoing inflammatory change in the anterior horn cells, with neuronal loss, inflammation, and perivascular lymphocyte cuffing, raises the question of possible chronic infection as a contributor to this syndrome (Greenfield and Matthews, 1954). Patients with human T-cell lymphotropic virus type I (HTLV-I)–associated tropical spastic paraparesis (TSP) may occasionally also experience wasting and fasciculations of the intrinsic hand musculature, and pathological analyses of the Japanese and Jamaican forms of this disease have demonstrated central chromatolysis of the anterior horn cells with associated mononuclear cell infiltration. HTLV-I also causes a chronic progressive myelopathy (TSP in the Caribbean; HTLV-I–associated myelopathy, or HAM, in Japan). This retrovirus is endemic in the Caribbean area, southern Japan, equatorial Africa, South Africa, and parts of Central and South America, and produces a chronic, insidiously progressive myelopathy that typically begins after age 30 years. The clinical syndrome is characterized by spastic paraparesis, paresthesias, and pain in the legs, and urinary bladder dysfunction. Sensory abnormalities may be minor. Some patients may develop optic neuropathy, cerebellar ataxia, or polyneuropathy. The definitive diagnosis of TSP, or HAM, requires HTLV-I–positive serology for the blood or cerebrospinal fluid. At present, no antiviral agents effectively treat TSP (HAM).

A number of patients with the much more prevalent retroviral human immunodeficiency virus (HIV) infection have also been reported with both upper and lower motor neuron degeneration (Huang et al., 1993; Bartfeld et al., 1995; Galassi et al., 1998). Retroviral fragments may be incorporated into the human genome following retroviral infection (endogenous retroviral elements, or ERVs) and are suspected agents in the pathogenesis of lymphomas and various degenerative and autoimmune diseases; the reported association between lymphoma and motor neuron disease suggests a possible role for ERVs in these patients (Younger et al., 1991; Rasmussen et al., 1993).

A number of cases of prion disease have also demonstrated motor neuron involvement, and some patients with Creutzfeldt-Jakob disease (CJD) will manifest progressive loss of muscle strength in an asymmetrical pattern, with associated fasciculations and atrophy (Allen et al., 1971). These syndromes typically involve both rapidly progressive dementia and early-onset lower motor neuron dysfunction, and many such cases demonstrate pathological findings similar to those described for retroviral infection (along with the more characteristic spongiform change in the cerebral hemispheres), as well as spinal neuronal loss and gliosis. At least one case of *Borrelia burgdorferi* infection was associated with the subsequent development of upper and lower motor neuron disease, although the most frequently described neurological syndromes associated with Lyme disease are meningitis, cranial neuritis, and painful radiculoneuritis. Appropriate therapy for chronic Lyme disease is the subject of ongoing debate and investigation, but treatment with 4- to 8-week courses of appropriate oral or intravenous antibiotics, including ceftriaxone and doxycycline, has been recommended (Hemmer et al., 1997).

MULTIPLE-SYSTEM DISORDERS WITH PROMINENT MOTOR SIGNS

Polyglucosan Body Disease

Adult-onset polyglucosan body disease was first described by Robitaille and colleagues in 1980 in four patients with progressive upper and lower motor neuron deficits, marked sensory loss in the legs, and neurogenic bladder; one patient also had dementia (Robitaille et al., 1980). Autopsy in two patients revealed a profusion of microscopic bodies that were termed polyglucosan bodies. Since this report, a series of cases have been reported. Patients with this syndrome are older than age 40 with slowly progressive, asymmetrical upper motor neuron and lower motor neuron signs. It is probably inherited as an autosomal recessive trait. The clinical syndrome differs from classic ALS in that patients also develop sensory loss (with peripheral neuropathy), neurogenic bladder problems, dementia, extensive leukoencephalopathy on magnetic resonance imaging, and extrapyramidal signs (Misra and Kalita, 1995; Bigio et al., 1997). Cases resembling ALS phenotypically have also been reported (Cafferty et al., 1991; McDonald et al., 1993). Spinal cord magnetic resonance imaging may reveal marked atrophy of the entire spinal cord (Negishi and Sze, 1992). The diagnostic hallmark is the presence of polyglucosan (periodic acid–Schiff [PAS]–positive) bodies in axons or Schwann cells in sural nerve biopsies, or in myoepithelial cells of the apocrine glands in axillary skin biopsies. Ultrastructural study of the central nervous system demonstrates that polyglucosan bodies are composed of aggre-

and when a patient presents with possible ALS it is imperative that the practitioner search for occult cancer. To date, Forsyth and colleagues (1997) have reported the largest number (n = 14) of cancer patients with motor neuron syndromes. They grouped these motor neuron syndromes into three categories. The first category consisted of three patients, all of whom had rapidly progressive upper motor neuron and lower motor neuron syndromes and less prominent symptoms of other neural system involvement. One of these cases was ours and occurred in a patient who developed rapidly progressive paralysis in all extremities within 3 months. Electromyography showed features of a myasthenic syndrome, in addition to generalized acute denervation. Autopsy demonstrated profound active gliosis and neuronophagia. All patients in this group had positive anti-Hu antibody, a strong indicator of a paraneoplastic syndrome. The second category consisted of five women who had breast cancer. They presented with an upper motor neuron syndrome, and a majority remained without lower motor neuron symptoms. Patients were thought to have primary lateral sclerosis, but the interval between the onset of the motor neuron syndrome and breast cancer was short. The neuropathy in this group is thought to represent a probable paraneoplastic syndrome. The last group is composed of six patients who had typical ALS and varied cancers, including lymphoma. They did not improve with treatment of the primary cancer. Anti-Hu antibody tests were negative. The relationship between the cancer and ALS in this group is considered to be coincidental. Forsyth and colleagues (1997) recommend a cancer work-up for patients who present with motor neuron symptoms of either group 1 or group 2—that is, symptoms suggesting a rapidly progressive ALS or an upper motor neuron phenotype in women. Autoantibodies are suspected to exist in patients with motor neuron disease and cancer (Dhib-Jalbut and Liwnicz, 1986). The importance of anti-Hu antibody is clear, but recently other antibodies, including anti-Yo antibody and antiaxonal antibody, have been reported in patients with paraneoplastic motor neuron disease (Khwaja et al., 1998; Ferracci et al., 1999).

In summary, paraneoplastic motor neuron disease may vary in clinical expression. An exhaustive cancer work-up is probably not necessary, but routine cancer testing should be performed in patients who are diagnosed with ALS. The work-up should include chest radiograph, breast examination and mammogram, stool guaiac test, routine complete blood counts, sedimentation rate, blood chemistry, and urinalysis.

Benign Focal Amyotrophy

BACKGROUND

Motor neuron disease often begins in a focal area in one extremity. In most cases, the disease steadily and rapidly spreads from one extremity to another. However, in the condition known as benign focal amyotrophy, muscle weakness remains focal and involves a limited number of myotomes in one extremity, particularly the upper extremities. In 1968, Hirayama and colleagues reported on 38 patients in Japan with this condition, referring to it as juvenile muscular atrophy of the distal upper extremity. This condition is often called Hiramaya's disease. More cases were reported from Asia, and later similar cases were reported from Western countries under different names (Sobue et al., 1978; Singh et al., 1980; Schlegel et al., 1987; Harding et al., 1983; Hirayama et al., 1987; Oryema et al., 1990; Neufeld et al., 1991; Serratrice, 1991). Since then, numerous terms have been proposed to describe this condition (Donofrio, 1994).

CLINICAL FEATURES

Sobue reviewed the findings in 71 patients and found that the disease had a juvenile onset at about age 20, though other studies indicate a slightly later age at onset. There is a male predominance (more than 60% of all cases). Hand and forearm atrophy is the most common initial manifestation. However, the distribution of muscle weakness varies markedly from case to case. Muscle stretch reflexes in the involved muscles are invariably hypoactive or absent. A small proportion of patients (approximately 20%) have pain and hypesthesia. The cranial nerves, pyramidal tracts, and the autonomic nervous system are spared. The condition may progress rapidly for the initial 2 to 3 years; thereafter, its course is less aggressive. Approximately three quarters of all cases involve the arms; the remaining cases involve the legs. About half of all cases remain localized, whereas the other half become multifocal and involve the contralateral extremity. In a few cases (approximately 5%), the symptoms become generalized. The original definition is now problematic because although this condition was first described in the upper extremities, clinically similar focal, segmental, and monomelic forms of benign amyotrophy involving the lower extremities are also well known (Harding et al., 1983; Gourie-Devi et al., 1984; Riggs et al., 1984; Uncini et al., 1992). The majority of cases are sporadic. However, several familial cases involving a father and his son, twin brothers, and male siblings have been reported (Sobue et al., 1978; Hirayama et al., 1987; Schlegel et al., 1987; Tandan et al., 1990; Gucuyener et al., 1991; Misra and Kalita, 1995; Robberecht et al., 1997). These reports suggest that the inheritance of this syndrome can be autosomal recessive. Another interesting family history is a report of Werdnig-Hoffmann disease found in the close relatives of a patient who had benign focal amyotrophy (Harding et al, 1983). Also, Robberecht and colleagues reported carriers of the D90A mutation (autosomal recessive ALS) who developed a clinically typical benign focal amyotrophy (Robberecht et al., 1997).

LABORATORY FEATURES

There are no specific laboratory tests for the condition. Creatine kinase levels are normal. A serum test for anti-G_{M1} antibody may exclude potentially treatable multifocal motor neuropathy. In a few cases, levels of anti-G_{M1} antibodies may be only slightly to moderately elevated. When such antibodies are elevated, careful electrodiagnostic tests should be performed to identify possible multiconduction blocks. However, in our series of more than 30 patients, none had conduction blocks (H. Mitsumoto and A. Wilbourn, 1999, unpublished observation).

ELECTRODIAGNOSTIC FEATURES

Results of motor nerve conduction studies in these patients are either normal or only slightly abnormal, with reduced compound motor action potentials. By definition, there is no conduction block in patients with this condition. In approximately one third of cases, results of sensory nerve conduction studies are slightly abnormal in the affected extremities. They may be clearly abnormal for the patient's age or reduced (although within normal limits) compared with those of the unaffected side (A. Wilbourn, M.D., unpublished observation, 1999). In the majority of cases, electromyography studies demonstrate fibrillation and fasciculation potentials in a variable number of muscles. Neurogenic motor unit changes are prominent, and changes in recruitment, with decreased numbers of rapidly firing motor units, are also noted (Donofrio, 1994). The C5 through T1 myotomes are most commonly involved when the arms are affected. The electrodiagnostic features in this circumstance are those of an anterior horn cell disorder and indistinguishable from focal-onset ALS. Clinical symptoms are unilateral in 70% of cases, but often bilateral changes are seen when the extent of the lesion is carefully evaluated with thorough electromyography studies, including paraspinal muscle examination.

NEUROIMAGING FEATURES

In benign focal amyotrophy, cervical magnetic resonance imaging may reveal a spinal cord that is normal or atrophy that is bilateral, or focal and unilateral, and corresponds to the location of amyotrophy. Postmyelogram sector scans of the cervical spinal cord also show the same changes apparent on magnetic resonance imaging scans (Biondi et al., 1989). Spondylosis and canal stenosis detected by magnetic resonance imaging should be carefully evaluated before the diagnosis of benign focal amyotrophy is established. Muscle magnetic resonance imaging of the affected extremity may reveal muscle atrophy that is more widespread than is evident clinically (Hamano et al., 1999).

DIFFERENTIAL DIAGNOSIS

Cervical radiculopathy is the most important choice in the differential diagnosis because it is treatable. Cervical or lumbosacral radiculopathy should produce symptoms other than just weakness, such as radicular pain and sensory impairment. The disease progression should be faster than that of benign focal amyotrophy, but radiculopathy can be chronic and indolent without any sensory symptoms. Neuroimaging, clinical assessment, and electromyography findings must be consistent with regard to nerve root lesion distributions. Brachial plexopathy is among the possibilities in the differential diagnosis, but the patient typically presents with pain and sensory symptoms. Detailed electromyography studies are essential in distinguishing benign focal amyotrophy from these conditions. Cervical syringomyelia or a benign tumor involving nerve roots or the spinal cord is also a possibility. Again, neuroimaging tests are important in distinguishing between these structural diseases and benign focal amyotrophy.

Multifocal motor neuropathy is characterized by slowly progressive focal weakness; thus, it may also resemble benign focal amyotrophy, and some cases previously reported as benign focal amyotrophy may actually be multifocal motor neuropathy. In addition, some patients with a diagnosis of benign focal amyotrophy have moderately elevated anti-G_{M1} ganglioside antibodies, although conduction blocks are not found. These patients have been treated with intravenous immunoglobulin, but without benefit.

Distinguishing this condition from ALS is critically important, because patients with this disorder are often misdiagnosed as having ALS and are given a dismal prognosis. Although a clear distinction might be difficult in the early stages, the possibility of benign focal amyotrophy should always be kept in mind when the clinician sees relatively young patient with this clinical presentation. The age at onset differs in ALS and benign focal amyotrophy, and the pace of progression may also differ. Focal muscle weakness and the initial progression can be confusing. However, the presence of a muscle stretch reflex in an involved extremity is a crucial finding, because it distinguishes benign focal amyotrophy from ALS. In the former, muscle stretch reflexes are always absent or diminished, whereas in classic ALS the reflexes are always abnormally brisk, despite atrophied and weak muscles. In patients with focal weakness and brisk reflexes in one extremity, even when the clinical course is stable for the first 1 or 2 years, disease almost invariably spreads to other extremities, confirming ALS. In patients with diminished or absent reflexes and a similar distribution of muscle weakness, the disease remains focal, confirming benign focal amyotrophy. The lack of diagnostic markers in these motor neuron diseases often makes confirming the diagnosis difficult. However, before one gives a diagnosis of ALS, particularly in cases with focal upper-extremity onset, the possibility of benign focal amyotrophy should be carefully considered.

PATHOLOGY AND PATHOGENESIS

Hirayama and colleagues (1987) first reported autopsy findings in this condition. Clinically, muscle weakness was unilateral, but pathologically the lesion was bilateral, although asymmetrical. The cervical spinal cord was flattened, and the anterior horn was markedly atrophied and gliotic. The numbers of both large and small motor neurons were reduced. The remaining cells showed degenerative changes, including lipofuscin accumulation, chromatolysis, and cell shrinkage. The cause of these changes could not be determined, although a circulatory insufficiency was suspected. The authors proposed a new term, *juvenile focal cervical poliopathy,* and hypothesized that local compression or circulatory failure caused by an anterior shift of the posterior dural wall during neck flexion might be responsible. Hirayama and Tokumaru (2000) studied the change in the cervical subarachnoid space on flexion using magnetic resonance neuroimaging in 73 patients with benign focal amyotrophy. They found a consistent defect of the dural sac and flattening of the corresponding spinal cord, supporting their original theory that benign focal amyotrophy is caused by cervical myelopathy. Kameyama and colleagues (1998) studied cervical magnetic resonance imaging in three patients with this condition and concluded that the pathophysiology of this syndrome may be one of multisegmental damage to the anterior horns caused by dynamic cord compression, possibly through circulatory insufficiency. In contrast, Schroder and colleagues (1999) studied cervical magnetic resonance imaging in nine patients with this syndrome and argued against a flexion-induced cervical myelopathy to support the view that Hirayama's disease is an intrinsic motor neuron disease.

The cervical myelopathy theory cannot explain a similar focal amyotrophy that involves the lower extremities. It is possible that benign focal amyotrophy may have two completely different causes that produce very similar clinical symptoms, the difference being that one condition affects the upper extremity and the other affects the lower extremities. The fact that this syndrome occurs in some families clearly suggests that some cases of benign focal amyotrophy have genetic causes. Furthermore, there is a report of three patients in whom postirradiation motor neuron syndrome manifested clinically as benign focal amyotrophy (Lamy et al., 1991). Taken together, these reports suggest that benign focal amyotrophy is a syndrome that probably has several causes.

TREATMENT

Although benign focal amyotrophy progresses slowly, it may seriously impair the involved extremi-

ties. Physical and occupational therapy can help maintain function. Appropriate splinting and bracing are essential. In selected patients with focal weakness in a group of muscles whose function is crucial for certain activities, a tendon transfer that uses spared muscle tendons can be considered.

Madras Pattern of Motor Neuron Disease

There appears to be an endemic form of MND that has been reported almost exclusively in the Madras area of India. The first case was reported by Jagannathan in 1973. It constitutes 1% to 2% of all hospital admissions in this area. The characteristic features that distinguish it from ALS or spinal muscular atrophy are (1) young age at onset, (2) absence of family history, (3) a progressive but benign course, (4) persistent asymmetrical involvement of limbs for years in more than half of the cases, and (5) lower cranial nerve involvement in more than two thirds of patients, with impairment of hearing in one third of these patients. No familial cases have been reported (Jagannathan, 1973; Jagannathan and Kumaresan, 1987; Gourie-Devi and Suresh, 1988).

Typically, the age at onset is less than 30 years, but less than 20% of patients have onset in the first decade of life. Approximately four times as many men as women are affected. Apparently, the disease evolves very slowly, because patients do not seek medical attention until an average of 5 years after onset. In addition to the lower motor cranial nerve involvement found in 30% to 45% of patients, the most characteristic feature of the Madras pattern of MND probably is neurosensory hearing loss, occurring in more than one third of patients. Such loss is the first sign of the disease in a small number of patients (8%). The motor syndrome is asymmetrical throughout the course in about half of the patients. Fasciculations are common; however, muscle stretch reflexes vary, being abnormal, normal, or absent, but in the majority of patients, plantar responses are extensor. Other central neurological systems (cerebellar, sensory, and higher cortical function) are normal. There is no evidence of neurogenic bowel or bladder dysfunction. Electromyography shows typical acute and chronic denervation, and the cerebrospinal fluid examination is normal. Other variants have been reported, including that in a patient born in India who presented with benign focal amyotrophy at age 17 years, which evolved to the Madras pattern of MND 10 years later (Massa et al., 1998).

Autopsy findings in this MND, although available for only a limited number of cases, include severe loss of anterior horn cells, diffuse but sparse microglial cell proliferation and lymphocytic infiltration, demyelination, and gliosis of the ventrolateral columns. In the brainstem, motor neuron loss is evident in the lower cranial nerve nuclei and cochlear nucleus; marked neuronal depletion and gliosis are present bilaterally, accompanied by demyelination and axonal loss in the cochlear nerve. An inflammatory cause has been proposed (Shankar et al., 2000).[104] A family study reported by Summers and colleagues suggests that the Madras pattern of MND may be hereditary, as the index patient's mother and brother each had subclinical involvement on electromyographic examination. Extensive investigations are needed to enhance our understanding of this condition, as such knowledge may have an enormous impact on our understanding of all motor neuron diseases.

References

Allen IV, Dermott E, Connolly JH, et al: A study of a patient with the amyotrophic form of Creutzfeldt-Jakob disease. Brain 1971; 94:715–724.

Ashenhurst EM, Quartey GRC, Starreveld A: Lumbo-sacral radiculopathy induced by radiation. Can J Sci Neurol 1977;4:259–263.

Banerjee P, Boyers MJ, Berry-Kravis E, et al: Preferential beta-hexosaminidase (Hex) A (alpha beta) formation in the absence of beta-Hex B (beta beta) due to heterozygous point mutations present in beta-Hex beta-chain alleles of a motor neuron disease patient. J Biol Chem 1994; 269:4819–4826.

Banerjee P, Siciliano L, Oliveri D, et al: Molecular basis of an adult form of beta-hexosaminidase B deficiency with motor neuron disease. Biochem Biophys Res Commun 1991;181:108–115.

Bartfeld H, Donnenfeld H, Kascsak R: Relevance of the post-polio syndrome to other motor neuron diseases: Relevance to viral (enteroviral) infections. Ann NY Acad Sci 1995;753:237–244.

Bharucha NF, Raven RH, Schoenberg BS: Epidemiology of infections of the nervous system. In Anderson DW, Schoenberg BS (eds): Neuroepidemiology: A Tribute to Bruce Schoenberg. Boca Raton, FL, CRC Press, 1991.

Bigio EH, Weiner MF, Bonte FJ, et al: Familial dementia due to adult polyglucosan body disease. Clin Neuropathol 1997; 16:227–234.

Biondi A, Dormont D, Weitzner I Jr, et al: MR imaging of the cervical cord in juvenile amyotrophy of distal upper extremity. Am J Neuroradiol 1989;10:263–268.

Bowen J, Gregory R, Squier M, et al: The post-irradiation lower motor neuron syndrome: Neuronopathy or radiculopathy? Brain 1996;119:1429–1439.

Bradley WG, Fewings JD, Cummings WJ, et al: Delayed myeloradiculopathy produced by spinal X-irradiation in the rat. J Neurol Sci 1977;31:63–82.

Brain L, Croft PB, Wilkinson M: Motor neurone disease as a manifestation of neoplasm: With a note on the course of classical motor neurone disease. Brain 1965;88:479–500.

Bruno C, Servidei S, Shanske S, et al: Glycogen branching enzyme deficiency in adult polyglucosan body disease. Ann Neurol 1993;33:88–93.

Cafferty MS, Lovelace RE, Hays AP, et al: Polyglucosan body disease. Muscle Nerve 1991;14:102–107.

Cavanagh JB: Corpora-amylacea and the family of polyglucosan diseases. Brain Res Rev 1999;29:265–295.

Centers for Disease Control and Prevention: Poliomyelitis prevention in the United States: Introduction of a sequential vaccination schedule with an activated poliovirus vaccine followed by oral poliovirus vaccine. Recommendations of the Advisory Committee of Immunization Practices (ACIP). MMWR Morb Mortal Wkly Rep 1997;46(RR-3):12.

Centers for Disease Control and Prevention: Recommended Childhood Immunization Schedule—United States. Recommendations of the Advisory Committee of Immunization Practices (ACIP). Morb Mortal Wkly Rep 1999;48:12.

Codd MB, Mulder DW, Kurland LT, et al: Poliomyelitis in Rochester, MN, 1935–1955: Epidemiology and long-term sequelae. In Halstead LS, Weichers (eds): Late Effects of Poliomyelitis. Miami, Symposia Foundation, 1985; 121–134.

Dhib-Jalbut S, Liwnicz BH: Immunocytochemical binding of serum IgG from a patient with oat cell tumor and paraneoplastic motoneuron disease to normal human cerebral cortex and molecular layer of the cerebellum. Acta Neuropathol 1986; 69:96–102.

Donofrio PD: AAEM case report #28: Monomelic amyotrophy. Muscle Nerve 1994;17:1129–1134.

Evans BK, Fagan C, Arnold T, et al: Paraneoplastic motor neuron disease and renal cell carcinoma: Improvement after nephrectomy. Neurology 1990;40:960–962.

Faden H: Poliovirus vaccination: A trilogy. J Infect Dis 1993;168: 25–28.

Faden H, Modlin JF, Thoms ML, et al: Comparative evaluation of immunization with live attenuated and enhanced-potency inactivated trivalent poliovirus vaccines in childhood: Systemic and local immune responses. J Infect Dis 1990;162:1291–1297.

Federico A: GM2 gangliosidosis with a motor neuron disease phenotype: Clinical heterogeneity of hexosaminidase deficiency disease. Adv Exp Med Biol 1987;209:19–23.

Federico A, Palmeri S, Malandrini A, et al: The clinical aspects of adult hexosaminidase deficiencies. Dev Neurosci 1991;13:280–287.

Ferracci F, Fassetta G, Butler MH, et al: A novel antineuronal antibody in a motor neuron syndrome associated with breast cancer. Neurology 1999;53:852–855.

Forman D, Rae-Grant AD, Matchett SC, et al: A reversible cause of hypercapnic respiratory failure: Lower motor neuronopathy associated with renal cell carcinoma. Chest 1999;115:899–901.

Forsyth PA, Dalmau J, Graus F, et al: Motor neuron syndromes in cancer patients. Ann Neurol 1997;41:722–730.

Friedrich F: Neurologic complications associated with oral poliovirus vaccine and genomic variability of the vaccine strains after multiplication in humans. Acta Virol 1998;42:187–194.

Galassi G, Gentilini M, Ferrari S, et al: Motor neuron disease and HIV-1 infection in a 30-year-old HIV-positive heroin abuser: A causal relationship? Clin Neuropathol 1998;17:131–135.

Glantz MJ, Burger PC, Friedman AH, et al: Treatment of radiation-induced nervous system injury with heparin and warfarin. Neurology 1994;44:2020–2027.

Glenn SA, Ross SA: Delayed radiation-induced bulbar palsy mimicking ALS. Muscle Nerve 2000;23:814–817.

Gooch CL: Poliomyelitis. In Samuels MA, et al (eds): Office Practice of Neurology. New York, Churchill Livingstone, 1995; 416–418.

Gordon PH, Rowland LP, Younger MD, et al: Lymphoproliferative disorders and motor neuron disease: An update. Neurology 1997;48:1671–1678.

Gourie-Devi M, Suresh TG: The Madras pattern of motor neuron disease in South India. J Neurol Neurosurg Psychiatry 1988; 51:773–777.

Gourie-Devi M, Suresh TG, Shankar SK: Monomelic amyotrophy. Arch Neurol 1984;41:388–394.

Greenfield MM, Stark FM: Post-irradiation neuropathy. Am J Roentgenol 1948;60:617–622.

Greenfield JG, Matthews WB: Post-encephalitic parkinsonism with amyotrophy. J Neurol Neurosurg Psychiatry 1954;17:1750–1756.

Gucuyener K, Aysun S, Topaloglu H, et al: Monomelic amyotrophy in siblings. Pediatr Neurol 1991;7:220–222.

Hakelius L, Stålberg E: Electromyographical studies of free autogenous muscle transplants in man. Scand J Plast Reconstr Surg 1974;8:211–219.

Hamano T, Mutoh T, Hirayama M, et al: MRI findings of benign monomelic amyotrophy of lower limb. J Neurol Sci 1999; 165:184–187.

Harding AE, Bradbury PG, Murray NMF: Chronic asymmetrical spinal muscular atrophy. J Neurol Sci 1983;59:69–83.

Hemmer B, Glocker FX, Kaiser R, et al: Generalised motor neuron disease as an unusual manifestation of *Borrelia burgdorferi* infection. J Neurol Neurosurg Psychiatry 1997;63:257–258.

Hirayama K, Tokumaru Y: Cervical dural sac and spinal cord in juvenile muscular atrophy of distal upper extremity. Neurology 2000;54:1922–1926.

Hirayama K, Tomonaga M, Kitano K, et al: Focal cervical poliopathy causing juvenile muscular atrophy of distal upper extremity: A pathological study. J Neurol Neurosurg Psychiatry 1987; 50:285–290.

Hirayama K, Tsubaki T, Toyokura Y, et al: Juvenile muscular atrophy of unilateral upper extremity. Neurology 1968;13:373–380.

Hodes R: Selective destruction of large moto-neurons by poliomyelitis virus: Conduction velocity of motor neuron fibers of chronic poliomyelitis patients. J Neurophysiol 1949;12:257–266.

Hodes R, Peacock M, Bodian D: Selected destruction of large motor neurons by polio virus. J Neurol Pathol Exp Neurol 1947; 8:400–410.

Huang PP, Chin R, Song S, et al: Lower motor neuron dysfunction associated with human immunodeficiency virus infection. Arch Neurol 1993;50:1328–1330.

Hull HF, Ward NA, Hull BP, et al: Paralytic poliomyelitis: Seasoned strategies, disappearing disease. Lancet 1994;343:1331–1337.

Hund E, Grau A, Fogel W, et al: Progressive cerebellar ataxia, proximal neurogenic weakness and ocular motor disturbances: Hexosaminidase A deficiency with late clinical onset in four siblings. J Neurol Sci 1997;145:25–31.

Jackson M: Post-radiation monomelic amyotrophy. J Neurol Neurosurg Psychiatry 1992;55:629.

Jagannathan K: Juvenile motor neurone disease. In Spillane JD (ed): Tropical Neurology. London, Oxford University Press, 1973; 127–130.

Jagannathan K, Kumaresan G: Madras pattern of motor neuron disease. In Gourie-Devi M (ed): Motor Neuron Disease. New Delhi, India, Oxford & IBH Publishing Co, 1987; 191–193.

Johnson E, Guyton J: Motor neuron conduction velocities in poliomyelitis. Arch Phys Med Rehabil 1960;41:185–190.

Johnson WG: The clinical spectrum in hexosaminidase deficiency diseases. Neurology 1981;31:1453–1456.

Johnson WG, Chutorian A, Miranda A: A new juvenile hexosaminidase deficiency disease presenting as cerebellar ataxia. Neurology 1977;27:1012–1018.

Jubelt B, Lipton HL: Enterovirus infections. In McKendall RR (ed): Handbook of Clinical Neurology, vol 56. New York, Elsevier Science Publications, 1989; 307–348.

Kameyama T, Ando T, Yanagi T, et al: Cervical spondylotic amyotrophy: Magnetic resonance imaging demonstration of intrinsic cord pathology. Spine 1998;23:448–452.

Khwaja S, Sripathi N, Ahmad BK, et al: Paraneoplastic motor neuron disease with type 1 Purkinje cell antibodies. Muscle Nerve 1998;21:943–945.

Kinoshita A, Hayashi M, Oda M, et al: Clinicopathological study of the peripheral nervous system in Machado-Joseph disease. J Neurol Sci 1995;130:48–58.

Korenke GC, Krasemann E, Meier V, et al: First missense mutation (W679R) in exon 10 of the adrenoleukodystrophy gene in siblings with adrenomyeloneuropathy. Hum Mutat 1998;1:S204–S206.

Kubo T, Ikuta Y, Tsuge K: Free muscle transplantation in dogs by microneurovascular anastomoses. Plast Reconstr Surg 1976; 57:495–501.

Lamy C, Mas JL, Varet B, et al: Service de Neurologie, Centre Raymond Garcin, CHS Sainte-Anne, Paris, France. Postradiation lower motor neuron syndrome presenting as monomelic amyotrophy. J Neurol Neurosurg Psychiatry 1991;54:648–649.

Lossos A, Meiner Z, Barash V, et al: Adult polyglucosan body disease in Ashkenazi Jewish patients carrying the Tyr329Ser mutation in the glycogen-branching enzyme gene. Ann Neurol 1998;44:867–872.

Louis ED, Hanley AE, Brannagan TH, et al: Motor neuron disease: Lymphoproliferative disease and bone marrow biopsy. Muscle Nerve 1996;19:1334–1337.

Maselli RA, Cashman NR, Wollman RL, et al: Neuromuscular transmission as a function of motor unit size in patients with prior poliomyelitis. Muscle Nerve 1992;15:648–655.

Massa R, Scalise A, Iani C, et al: Delayed focal involvement of upper motor neurons in the Madras pattern of motor neuron disease. Electroencephalogr Clin Neurophysiol 1998;109:523–526.

Matilla T, McCall A, Subramony SH, et al: Molecular and clinical correlations in spinocerebellar ataxia type 3 and Machado-Joseph disease. Ann Neurol 1995;38:68–72.

McComas AJ, Quartly C, Griggs RC: Early and late losses of motor units after poliomyelitis. Brain 1997;120(Pt 8):1415–1421.

McDonald TD, Faust PL, Bruno C, et al: Polyglucosan body disease simulating amyotrophic lateral sclerosis. Neurology 1993; 43:785–790.

Michelakakis H, Papadimitriou A, Divaris R, et al: Plasma lysosomal enzyme levels in patients with motor neuron disease. J Inherit Metab Dis 1995;18:72–74.

Misra UK, Kalita J: Central motor conduction in Hirayama disease. Electroencephalogr Clin Neurophysiol 1995;97:73–76.

Mitsumoto H, Sliman RJ, Schafer IA, et al: Motor neuron disease and adult hexosaminidase A deficiency in two families: Evidence for multisystem degeneration. Ann Neurol 1985;17:378–385.

Mulder DW: Clinical observations on acute poliomyelitis. Ann N Y Acad Sci 1995;753:1–10.

Nakano KK, Dawson DM, Spence A: Machado disease: A hereditary ataxia in Portuguese immigrants to Massachusetts. Neurology 1972;22:49–55.

Negishi C, Sze G: Spinal cord MRI in adult polyglucosan body disease. J Comput Assist Tomogr 1992;16:824–826.

Neufeld MY, Inzelberg R, Nisipeanu P, et al: Juvenile segmental muscular atrophy. Funct Neurol 1991;6:405–410.

Nicolosi A, Hauser WA, Beghi E, et al: Epidemiology of central nervous system infections in Olmsted County, Minnesota, 1950–1981. J Infect Dis 1986;154:399–408.

Nkowane BM, Wassilak SG, Orenstein WA, et al: Vaccine-associated paralytic poliomyelitis, United States: 1973 through 1984. JAMA 1987;257:1335–1340.

Norris FH, Engel WK: Carcinomatous amyotrophic lateral sclerosis. In Brain WR, Norris FH (eds): The Remote Effects of Cancer on the Nervous System. New York, Grune & Stratton, 1965; 24–34.

O'Brien JS: The gangliosidoses. In Stanbury JB, Wyngaarden JB, Fredrickson DS, et al (eds): The Metabolic Basis of Inherited Disease. New York, McGraw-Hill, 1983; 945–969.

Okumura H, Kurland LT, Waring SC: Amyotrophic lateral sclerosis and polio: Is there an association? Ann N Y Acad Sci 1995; 753:245–256.

Oryema J, Ashby P, Spiegel S: Monomelic atrophy. Can J Neurol Sci 1990;17:124–130.

Paul JR: A History of Poliomyelitis. New Haven, Yale University Press, 1971.

Perez Correa SE, Aladro Benito Y, Suarez Ortega S, et al: Sweet's syndrome and motor neuron disease associated with esophageal carcinoma. An Med Interna 1999;16:423–426.

Peters HA, Clatnoff DV: Spinal muscular atrophy secondary to macroglobulinemia: Reversal of symptoms with chlorambucil therapy. Neurology 1968;18:101–108.

Rapin I, Suzuki K, Suzuki K, et al: Atypical spinocerebeller degeneration in a sibship. Arch Neurol 1976;33:120–130.

Rasmussen HB, Perron H, Clausen J: Do endogenous retroviruses have etiological implications in inflammatory and degenerative nervous system diseases? Acta Neurol Scand 1993;88:190–198.

Riggs JE, Schochet S, Gutmann L: Benign focal amyotrophy: Variant of chronic spinal muscle atrophy. Arch Neurol 1984;41:678–679.

Robberecht W, Aguirre T, Van Den Bosch L, et al: D90A heterozygosity in the SOD1 gene is associated with familial and apparently sporadic amyotrophic lateral sclerosis. Neurology 1996; 47:1336–1339.

Robberecht W, Aguirre T, Van den Bosch L, et al: Familial juvenile focal amyotrophy of the upper extremity (Hirayama disease): Superoxide dismutase 1 genotype and activity. Arch Neurol 1997;54:46–50.

Robertson NP, Wharton S, Anderson J, et al: Adult polyglucosan body disease associated with an extrapyramidal syndrome. J Neurol Neurosurg Psychiatry 1998;65:788–790.

Robitaille Y, Carpenter S, Karpati G, et al: A distinct form of adult polyglucosan body disease with massive involvement of central and peripheral neuronal processes and astrocytes: A report of four cases and a review of the occurrence of polyglucosan bodies in other conditions such as Lafora's disease and normal ageing. Brain 1980;103:315–336.

Rosenberg RN, Nyhan WL, Bay C, et al: Autosomal dominant

striatonigral degeneration: A clinical, pathologic, and biochemical study of a new genetic disorder. Neurology 1976;26:703–714.

Rowland LP: Diagnosis of amyotrophic lateral sclerosis. J Neurol Sci 1998;160:S6–S24.

Rowland LP, Schneck SA: Neuromuscular disorders associated with malignant neoplastic disorders. J Chron Dis 1963;16:777–795.

Rowland LP, Sherman WH, Latov N, et al: Amyotrophic lateral sclerosis and lymphoma: Bone marrow examination and other diagnostic tests. Neurology 1992;42:1101–1102.

Schlegel U, Jerusalem F, Tackmann W, et al: Benign juvenile focal muscular atrophy of upper extremities: A familial case. J Neurol Sci 1987;80:351–353.

Schmidt NJ, Lennette EH, Ho HH: An apparently new enterovirus isolated from patients with disease of the central nervous system. J Infect Dis 1974;129:304–309.

Schnorf H, Gitzelmann R, Bosshard NU, et al: Early and severe sensory loss in three adult siblings with hexosaminidase A and B deficiency (Sandhoff disease). J Neurol Neurosurg Psychiatry 1995;59:520–523.

Schold SC, Cho E-S, Somasundaram M: Subacute motor neuronopathy: A remote effect of lymphoma. Ann Neurol 1979;5:271–278.

Schroder R, Keller E, Flacke S, et al: MRI findings in Hirayama's disease: Flexion-induced cervical myelopathy or instrinsic motor neuron disease? J Neurol 1999;246:1069–1074.

Serratrice G: Spinal monomelic amyotrophy. Adv Neurol 1991;56:169–173.

Shankar SK, Gourie-Devi M, Shankar L, et al: Pathology of Madras type of motor neuron disease (MMND)—histological and immunohistochemical study. Acta Neuropathol (Berl) 2000;99:428–434.

Singh N, Sachdev KK, Susheela AK: Juvenile muscular atrophy localized to arms. Arch Neurol 1980;37:297–299.

Sobue I, Saito N, Iida M, et al: Juvenile type of distal and segmental muscular atrophy of upper extremities. Ann Neurol 1978;3:429–432.

Stålberg E, Trontel J: Single Fiber EMG. Old Woking, UK, Mir Valle Press Limited, 1979.

Strebel PM, Sutter RW, Cochi SL, et al: Epidemiology of poliomyelitis in the United States one decade after the last reported case of indigenous wild virus–associated disease. Clin Infect Dis 1992;14:568–579.

Sudarsky L, Coutinho P: Machado-Joseph disease. Clin Neurosci 1995;3:17–22.

Sudarsky L, Corwin L, Dawson D: Machado-Joseph disease in New England. Movement Disord 1992;7:204–208.

Tandan R, Sharma KR, Bradley WG, et al: Chronic segmental spinal muscular atrophy of upper extremities in identical twins. Neurology 1990;40:236–239.

Uncini A, Servidei S, Delli Pizzi C, et al: Benign monomelic amyotrophy of lower limb: Report of three cases. Acta Neurol Scand 1992;85:397–400.

Wadia NH, Wadia PN, Katrak SM, et al: Neurological manifestations of acute haemorrhagic conjunctivitis. Lancet 1981;2:528–529.

Wiechers D: Single fiber EMG evaluation in denervation and reinnervation. Muscle Nerve 1990;13:829–832.

Wiechers D: Electrophysiology of acute polio revisited: Utilizing newer EMG techniques in vaccine-associated disease. Ann N Y Acad Sci 1995;753:111–119.

Wiechers DO, Hubbell SL: Late changes in the motor unit after acute poliomyelitis. Muscle Nerve 1981;4:524–528.

Wiechers DO: Acute and latent effect of poliomyelitis on the motor unit as revealed by electromyography. Orthopedics 1985;8:870–872.

Wiechers DO: New concepts of the reinnervated motor unit revealed by vaccine-associated poliomyelitis. Muscle Nerve 1988;11:356–364.

Younger DS, Rowland LP, Latov N, et al: Lymphoma, motor neuron diseases, and amyotrophic lateral sclerosis. Ann Neurol 1991;29:78–86.

Ziemssen F, Sindern E, Schroder JM, et al: Novel missense mutations in the glycogen-branching enzyme gene in adult polyglucosan body disease. Ann Neurol 2000;47:536–540.

CHAPTER 71

Postpolio Syndrome

Robert W. Shields, Jr.

HISTORICAL REVIEW
CLINICAL FEATURES
LABORATORY AND PATHOLOGICAL FEATURES
ELECTRODIAGNOSTIC FINDINGS

PATHOPHYSIOLOGY
DIAGNOSIS AND DIFFERENTIAL DIAGNOSIS
TREATMENT

Postpolio syndrome (PPS) refers to a constellation of neuromuscular and orthopedic symptoms and signs that have been noted to occur in patients with remote antecedent poliomyelitis (Halstead and Rossi, 1987; Jubelt and Cashman, 1987). Although the concept of delayed worsening of neuromuscular function after acute poliomyelitis was first described in the late 1800s (Cornil and Lepine, 1875; Raymond, 1875), it was not until nearly 100 years later that the concept of PPS was more widely recognized and defined (Mulder et al., 1972; Alter et al., 1982; Agre et al., 1991; Dalakas, 1995b; Halstead, 1998). This was due largely to the polio epidemic of the 1940s and 1950s that left between 250,000 and 640,000 polio survivors in the United States alone (Agre et al., 1991; Halstead, 1998). The virtual epidemic of PPS that occurred among these polio survivors in the 1980s and 1990s has served as a catalyst to attract medical attention to this entity and to focus research on defining its pathophysiology as well as on exploring therapeutic interventions.

HISTORICAL REVIEW

The first description of a syndrome of progressive weakness occurring in a patient with remote antecedent poliomyelitis is credited to Raymond and Charcot (1875). In this report, Charcot provided a clinical presentation and discussion of a young man who had experienced a febrile illness associated with acute weakness of the left arm and leg at the age of 6 months. At age 19, he began to experience increased weakness and atrophy of the right arm and leg, which Charcot diagnosed as an "overuse" phenomenon (Dalakas, 1995a). After that report, several additional reports of similar clinical syndromes were documented in the medical literature (Cornil and Lepine, 1875; Dalakas, 1995a). However, almost 100 years passed before more precise reports appeared in the medical literature describing the development of new neuromuscular symptoms and signs in patients with remote antecedent poliomyeli-

tis (Zilkha, 1962; Campbell et al., 1969; Anderson et al., 1972; Mulder et al., 1972; Dalakas, 1995a). By the early 1980s, a clear concept of PPS was emerging, which prompted the first international conference on PPS held at the Warm Springs Institute for Rehabilitation in 1984 (Halstead, 1998). Since that time, numerous reports and investigations have been undertaken to better define the clinical syndrome of PPS, to understand its pathophysiology, and to provide treatment guidelines (Kayser-Gatchalian, 1973; Maynard, 1985; Halstead and Rossi, 1987; Jubelt and Cashman, 1987; Frustace, 1988; Agre et al., 1991; Windebank et al., 1991; Jubelt and Drucker, 1993; Dalakas, 1995c).

Various terminologies have been proposed to describe progressive muscle weakness and the other neuromuscular symptoms believed to result from remote antecedent poliomyelitis, including *late-onset postpoliomyelitis progressive muscular atrophy* (Kurent et al., 1979), *late poliomyelitis muscular atrophy* (Dalakas et al., 1984), *late postpoliomyelitis muscular atrophy* (Dalakas et al., 1985), *progressive postpolio atrophy* (Block and Wilbourn, 1986), *progressive postpoliomyelitis muscular atrophy* (Dalakas et al., 1986), *postpoliomyelitis progressive muscular atrophy* (Jubelt and Cashman, 1987), and *postpolio syndrome* (Agre et al., 1991; Dalakas, 1995b). Over the years, *postpolio syndrome* has emerged as the preferred term for describing the various new neuromuscular and other symptoms that develop many years after acute poliomyelitis. It has been suggested that the term was coined by the patients, who were attempting to convince the medical community that this syndrome did represent a discrete clinical entity (Jubelt and Drucker, 1993; Dalakas, 1995b). *Progressive postpolio muscular atrophy* has been retained as a term for designating a syndrome of progressive weakness and atrophy that occurs as a late effect of poliomyelitis (Dalakas et al., 1986; Jubelt and Cashman, 1987; Dalakas, 1995b).

CLINICAL FEATURES

The symptoms that may occur in the setting of PPS are rather numerous and diverse (Table 71–1).

Table 71–1. Clinical Features of Postpolio Syndrome

Clinical Feature	Percent of Patients	
	Halstead and Rossi, 1987 (n = 132)	Jubelt and Agre, 2000 (n = 100)
Fatigue	89	86
Muscle pain	71	73
Joint pain	71	73
Weakness of previously affected muscle	69	88
Weakness of previously unaffected muscle	50	59
Cold intolerance	29	53
Atrophy	28	52
Respiratory insufficiency	NA	36
Dysphagia	NA	36

NA, data not available.

However, in nearly all series, fatigue appears to be the most prominent, and often the most disabling, symptom and may be recorded in as many as 89% of patients (Halstead and Rossi, 1985; Jubelt and Drucker, 1993). The fatigue may be generalized and global or relatively circumscribed to an individual muscle, a group of muscles, or a limb (Halstead et al., 1985; Agre and Rodriquez, 1991a). The global fatigue is often depicted by patients as a general exhaustion that may follow even minimal physical activity (Halstead et al., 1985; Jubelt and Cashman, 1987; Jubelt and Drucker, 1993). The term *polio wall* has been used by patients to describe the severe global disabling fatigue that may interrupt even mild physical activity, requiring that the patient stop and rest (Halstead et al., 1985). Global generalized fatigue of this severity may be observed in nearly 40% of patients and may occur on a daily basis in two thirds of these patients (Halstead et al., 1985). When fatigue is more focal and restricted, patients often report weakness and reduced function due to lack of stamina or exercise endurance (Agre, 1995). Most often, these types of symptoms occur in the lower extremities and are frequently noted in the quadriceps muscle group (Einarsson, 1991a). Typical symptoms include fatigue with prolonged standing and walking, which results in the knees becoming wobbly, with a tendency to buckle. On occasion, the degree of exercise-induced fatigue resembles that which might occur in myasthenia gravis and has been reported in amyotrophic lateral sclerosis (Mulder et al., 1959).

Another common symptom of PPS is muscle pain, typically dull and aching in character, which may be noted in as many as 73% of patients (Codd et al., 1985; Halstead and Rossi, 1985; Jubelt and Cashman, 1987). This type of pain tends to be focal and is often associated with fatigue that follows even modest physical activity (Willen and Grimby, 1998). This pain shares many features with the myalgia that occurs in the overuse syndrome (Agre, 1995). Typically, fatigue and pain associated with physical activity in PPS respond to rest, but even more so to sleep

(Jubelt and Drucker, 1993). This appears to be in contrast with the pain and fatigue encountered in chronic fatigue syndrome, which are less likely to improve after sleep (Jubelt and Drucker, 1993). In addition to myalgic pain, joint pain is a common symptom of PPS (Halstead and Rossi, 1985; Agre et al., 1989; Willen and Grimby, 1998). In fact, local joint pain represents the most common orthopedic symptom in PPS. Joint pain is often attributed to the chronic overstress of joints that may result from a host of different factors that stem from the persistent weakness that follows the remote polio (Jubelt and Cashman, 1987; Frustace, 1988). These factors include abnormal mechanics, especially involving the gait; excessive stress on tendons and ligaments; and progressive joint deformities (Perry and Fleming, 1985; Jubelt and Drucker, 1993). These musculoskeletal factors frequently lead to chronic orthopedic problems, including traumatic arthritis, joint instability, and local soft tissue inflammation, which may affect bursae, tendons, and ligaments (Jubelt and Cashman, 1987; Frustace, 1988). These types of chronic orthopedic problems may lead to reduced mobility and loss of function and have been regarded as very important pathophysiological mechanisms of PPS (Anderson et al., 1972; Jubelt and Drucker, 1993). It is important to recognize the role of these orthopedic problems in PPS, because they are often amenable to specific treatment (Kidd et al., 1997; Aurlien et al., 1999).

In addition to fatigue and pain, new weakness represents another common symptom of PPS that may be encountered in more than 80% of patients (Halstead and Rossi, 1985; Halstead et al., 1985). Although the muscles involved are more often those previously affected by the remote polio (Mulder et al., 1972; Halstead et al., 1985), more than 50% of patients will have symptoms of new weakness in apparently unaffected muscles (Halstead and Rossi, 1985; Agre et al., 1989; Jubelt and Drucker, 1993; Wekre et al., 1998). It should be noted, however, that various electromyographic studies in polio survivors have documented that muscles thought to have been unaffected by the remote polio may indeed disclose changes including chronic neurogenic motor unit potential alterations consistent with remote denervation and reinnervation (Hayward and Seaton, 1979; Wiechers, 1985; Ravits et al., 1990). Thus, it is uncertain how often a truly unaffected muscle may be involved by new muscle weakness in PPS. In approximately 50% of patients with new weakness, there may be new atrophy as well (Cashman et al., 1987; Halstead and Rossi, 1987; Agre et al., 1989). These clinical features, which are often distributed in a highly focal and circumscribed manner, have led to the special diagnostic term *progressive postpoliomyelitis muscular atrophy* (Dalakas et al., 1986; Jubelt and Cashman, 1987; Dalakas, 1995b). However, reports have suggested that progressive postpolio muscular atrophy is actually quite rare among polio survivors (Aurlien et al., 1999). Furthermore, it appears that new atrophy and weakness are often difficult to discern from the chronic symptoms of increased fatigue and myalgia that are so commonly encountered in the vast majority of patients with PPS (Dalakas, 1995b). Thus, it may be desirable to incorporate all patients, including those with possible new focal weakness and atrophy, into the more general term of PPS. Other neuromuscular symptoms frequently reported in polio survivors include muscular cramping and fasciculations (Campbell et al., 1969; Anderson et al., 1972; Mulder et al., 1972; Hayward and Seaton, 1979). These symptoms may occur in muscles that are involved by PPS as well as in muscles that appear to be stable and uninvolved by the PPS (Hayward and Seaton, 1979; Fetell et al., 1982).

Significant functional decline may appear in the course of PPS. Whether a patient with PPS experiences a substantial functional decline is related in large part to the patient's baseline function and the location and severity of the new symptoms of fatigue and weakness. When PPS involves the lower extremity muscles, it is not uncommon for patients who had ambulated independently to require the use of aids for ambulation, such as braces, canes, or walkers (Wekre et al., 1998; Ivanyi et al., 1999). On occasion, patients who may have functioned for many years with the use of braces and other aids may find that their gait deteriorates to the point that they become wheelchair bound (Wekre et al., 1998; Ivanyi et al., 1999). In patients with rather severe, chronic residual weakness, the onset of PPS may impart new disabilities with regard to transferring, turning, standing, and many of the other activities of daily living (Wekre et al., 1998). However, there is evidence that despite complaints of increasing neuromuscular symptoms and disabilities, there is no significant increase in the use of devices or in occupational disability in most patients with PPS (Ramlow et al., 1992).

When PPS involves the muscles of respiration, new symptoms of respiratory embarrassment due to progressive pulmonary insufficiency may ensue (Agre et al., 1989; Bach and Alba, 1991; Jubelt and Drucker, 1993; Dalakas, 1995b). New respiratory symptoms are typically encountered in patients who had acute polio after the age of 10 and who required respiratory support during their acute management (Dean et al., 1991). In patients with PPS with significant residual pulmonary involvement, there may be a decline of 1.9% of vital capacity per year (Bach et al., 1987). Orthopedic factors, including scoliosis, may also contribute to progressive pulmonary insufficiency in PPS (Bach and Alba, 1991; Jubelt and Drucker, 1993; Dalakas, 1995b). In addition, patients may acquire various cardiopulmonary diseases that can further compound their clinical difficulties (Jubelt and Drucker, 1993; Dalakas, 1995b). In some patients with PPS, respiratory embarrassment may be attributed to central hypoventilation due to residual damage from bulbar poliomyelitis (Plum and Swanson, 1959; Lane et al., 1974). In patients with progressive respiratory embarrassment, intervention with various devices to assist respiration may be required (Bach and Alba, 1991). In some patients, nocturnal ventilation is all that is necessary, whereas in others continuous ventilatory support is needed (Bach and Alba, 1991).

Nearly 10% to 20% of patients with remote bulbar poliomyelitis may note prominent residual dysphagia (Buchholz and Jones, 1991). Although these patients are particularly at risk for the development of progressive bulbar weakness in the setting of PPS (Agre et al., 1989; Dalakas, 1995b), this manifestation of PPS may also develop in patients without residual bulbar involvement (Dowhaniuk and Schentag, 1995; Sonies and Dalakas, 1995; Sonies, 1996). These problems typically present with a variety of symptoms related to difficulty swallowing, but frank aspiration is uncommon (Dowhaniuk and Schentag, 1995; Sonies and Dalakas, 1995; Sonies, 1996). These problems can often be managed conservatively with measures that reduce the risk of aspiration (Dalakas, 1995b; Sonies, 1996). In addition to dysphagia, other bulbar features may be noted, including alterations in speech and voice (Halstead et al., 1985; Sonies and Dalakas, 1995; Robinson et al., 1998). These symptoms include hoarseness of the voice, secondary to weakness of vocal cord opposition, and hypernasality, attributed to weakness of the posterior pharyngeal wall. Frank dysarthria, however, is a relatively uncommon symptom of PPS (Jubelt and Cashman, 1987).

Various sleep disorders, primarily sleep apnea syndromes, may occur in patients with PPS, typically in patients with previous bulbar poliomyelitis (Guilleminault and Motta, 1978; Bach and Alba, 1991; Dalakas, 1995b). Sleep apnea syndromes may be central, obstructive, or mixed (Guilleminault and Motta, 1978; Steljes et al., 1990; Jubelt and Drucker, 1993; Dean et al., 1998). Central sleep apnea has been associated with bulbar poliomyelitis and is attributed to residual dysfunction of the reticular formation, whereas obstructive sleep apnea has been associated with previous pharyngeal muscle weakness (Guilleminault and Motta, 1978; Steljes et al., 1990; Dalakas, 1995b). Obstructive sleep apnea syndrome may be compounded by other clinical features, including obesity, which is a common feature of patients with PPS who are forced to lead a more sedentary and less active life (Bach and Alba, 1991). Sleep apnea is an extremely important clinical feature of PPS, because it may be a major contributing factor to the generalized fatigue that is so common in this disorder. Identification and management of sleep apnea may provide a substantial improvement in the quality of life of the patient who is coping with PPS.

Cold intolerance is another common symptom reported by many patients with PPS (Bruno et al., 1985; Halstead and Rossi, 1987; Jubelt and Cashman, 1987; Frustace, 1988). As many as 50% of patients complain that exposure to cold worsens their symptoms of weakness and fatigue (Jubelt and Drucker, 1993), and many patients observe that their limbs may be cool and cyanotic when dependent (Jubelt and Cashman, 1987; Frustace, 1988). Involvement of the intermediolateral cell column of the spinal cord from acute poliomyelitis has been cited as the mechanism of these symptoms that have been attributed to altered thermoregulation (Smith et al., 1949; Frustace, 1988). Although signs of upper motor neuron involvement, including Babinski signs, increased tendon reflexes, and increased tone, have been reported in as many as 8% of patients with PPS, this is essentially the same prevalence as that encountered in patients with acute poliomyelitis (Jubelt and Cashman, 1987; Jubelt and Drucker, 1993). Although the precise cause of these upper motor neuron signs is unclear, they do not seem to indicate a new central nervous system component from the PPS, but rather appear to represent residual findings from the acute poliomyelitis. Although depression is not a component of PPS (Windebank, 1995; Schanke, 1997), patients with PPS are not immune to depressive reactions. Depression can result from the PPS patient having to cope with loss of function, coupled with the anxiety related to the possibility of a progressive disability. Identification and management of depression are important components to the proper management of patients with PPS, because depression may certainly compound the general fatigue that is so often cited as the principal symptom of this disorder (Windebank, 1995).

Despite the wide array of symptoms and signs that may constitute PPS, there are no clinical features on the general physical or neurological examination that can help differentiate patients who are otherwise stable and coping with the residuals of remote polio from patients with PPS. Signs, including atrophy, weakness, fasciculations, and vasomotor instability in a limb, may all be observed in stable patients with remote polio.

It has been estimated that clinical features of PPS develop in approximately 50% of polio survivors (Bruno et al., 1991; Windebank et al., 1991). Although it has been difficult to predict in which of the polio survivors PPS will develop, risk factors have been identified. The risk may be increased with advancing age (Ivanyi et al., 1999), the severity of weakness at the time of acute poliomyelitis (Halstead et al., 1985; Agre and Rodriquez, 1990; Windebank et al., 1991), the onset of acute poliomyelitis after the age of 10 (Halstead et al., 1985), and the need for ventilatory assistance during the period of acute poliomyelitis (Halstead et al., 1985). The delay between acute poliomyelitis and the onset of PPS may range from 8 to 71 years (Jubelt and Cashman, 1987), but the average interval is approximately 35 years (Halstead et al., 1985).

LABORATORY AND PATHOLOGICAL FEATURES

Routine laboratory studies, including complete blood cell count, chemistry profiles of the blood, and urinalysis, are usually normal in patients with

PPS (Campbell et al., 1969; Dalakas et al., 1984; Jubelt and Cashman, 1987). In some polio survivors, modest elevations of serum creatine kinase are noted (Nelson, 1990; Windebank et al., 1991; Willen and Grimby, 1998). This has been attributed to muscle overuse, which can occur not only in patients with PPS but also in polio survivors who are stable without progressive neuromuscular symptoms (Waring and McLaurin, 1992). Cerebrospinal fluid examinations have also been unrevealing (Campbell et al., 1969; Dalakas et al., 1984; Jubelt and Cashman, 1987) except for modest elevations of protein found in some patients (Palmucci et al., 1980). The presence of oligoclonal bands has been noted in the cerebrospinal fluid of some patients with PPS (Dalakas et al., 1986); however, the significance of this finding is unclear, because it has not been a consistent observation (Cashman et al., 1987; Salazar-Grueso et al., 1989).

Many patients with PPS have undergone muscle biopsy in an effort to rule out underlying neuromuscular disease and to attempt to explain the mechanism or pathophysiology of their condition. Biopsy findings typically disclose chronic neurogenic atrophy manifested by small, angular atrophic fibers, group atrophy, and fiber-type grouping (Jubelt and Cashman, 1987; Dalakas, 1988; Jubelt and Drucker, 1993). Immunohistochemical examination of muscle has disclosed the presence of neural cell adhesion molecules in atrophic fibers, split fibers, and nonatrophic fibers, indicating active, ongoing denervation (Cashman et al., 1987). In muscles more severely affected, connective tissue replacement and fatty infiltration are also noted. Many biopsies also reveal changes often seen in primary myopathic disorders, including variation in cross-sectional fiber diameters, muscle fiber necrosis, split fibers, and fibrosis (Dalakas, 1988). These findings have been attributed to "secondary myopathic changes" that may accompany chronic neurogenic atrophy (Drachman et al., 1967; Dalakas, 1988). Although lymphocytic infiltrates, often resembling lymphorrhages, have been reported (Dalakas, 1988), these findings are very uncommon and their precise significance remains uncertain (Jubelt and Cashman, 1987). When one contrasts the muscle biopsy findings in patients of PPS with those of stable polio survivors, there are no significant changes noted that clearly distinguish the two groups of patients (Cashman et al., 1987; Jubelt and Drucker, 1993).

In an autopsy study of polio survivors, the pathological findings noted in the spinal cord were those one might anticipate from the remote poliomyelitis (Pezeshkpour and Dalakas, 1988). These findings included a loss of motor neurons, atrophic motor neurons, gliosis, axonal spheroids, chromatolysis of motor neurons, and modest lymphocytic infiltrates in the meninges, perivascular structures, and spinal cord parenchyma (Pezeshkpour and Dalakas, 1988). The findings of axonal spheroids, neuronal atrophy, and gliosis appeared to be more prominent in patients with clinical features of progressive postpolio muscular atrophy than in polio survivors who were clinically stable at the time of their death. These authors suggested that these pathological findings in the patients with progressive postpolio muscular atrophy were consistent with dysfunction of the remaining motor neurons, as opposed to progressive neuronal death (Pezeshkpour and Dalakas, 1988). However, the precise significance of these findings is unclear.

ELECTRODIAGNOSTIC FINDINGS

The electrodiagnostic features encountered in patients with PPS are essentially identical to those in polio survivors without new weakness and fatigue (Cashman et al., 1987) (Table 71–2). The motor nerve conduction studies may disclose reduced amplitudes when recording from muscles previously affected by the acute polio. However, motor latencies and conduction velocities are usually normal unless the motor amplitude response is reduced, which can result in mild prolongation in latency and slowing of conduction velocity (Mulder et al., 1972; Cruz Martinez et al., 1983). These changes are relatively modest and are not consistent with acquired

Table 71–2. Electrodiagnostic Features in Postpolio Syndrome

Study and Features	Characteristics
Nerve conduction studies	
Sensory	Normal
Motor	Reduced compound motor action potentials
	Mild prolongation of distal latency
	Mild slowing of conduction velocity
Repetitive	Usually normal or decremental
	Incremental responses have been noted
Needle electrode examination	
Fibrillation potentials	Often present
Fasciculation potentials	Often present
Motor unit potentials	Reduced number firing rapidly
	Increased amplitude and duration
	Polyphasic
	Unstable morphology during successive discharges
Single-fiber electromyography	
Fiber density	Increased
Jitter	Increased, may be increased more in very large reinnervated motor units
Blocking	Present, but neurogenic or concomitant blocking is not seen
Macroelectromyography	
Motor Unit Potential	Increased
Amplitude	Serial studies have shown stable amplitudes, increased amplitudes, or no particular trend

segmental demyelinating changes. The results of motor nerve conduction studies over intervals of 5 years tend to be stable, with little, if any, change (Daube et al., 1995). Repetitive nerve conduction studies typically show decremental responses, but incremental responses and normal responses may be observed (Hodes, 1948; Feldman, 1985; Ravits et al., 1990). Sensory nerve conduction studies are normal (Ravits et al., 1990). The needle electrode examination, particularly in muscles that disclose persistent weakness or new fatigue, disclose findings of chronic neurogenic atrophy (Mulder et al., 1972; Hayward and Seaton, 1979; Lutschg and Ludin, 1981; Wiechers and Hubbell, 1981; Cruz Martinez et al., 1983; Maynard, 1985; Trojan et al., 1991). Typically, there is a reduction in the number of motor unit potentials recruited, and the motor unit potential parameters disclose changes typical of reinnervation (i.e., increased amplitude and duration as well as polyphasicity) (Lutschg and Ludin, 1981; Wiechers and Hubbell, 1981; Cruz Martinez et al., 1983; Maynard, 1985; Ryniewicz et al., 1990). Furthermore, many motor unit potentials will display unstable morphology during consecutive discharges, indicating altered neuromuscular transmission in these chronically reinnervated motor units (Wiechers, 1985). Modest numbers of fibrillation potentials may also be recorded despite the long interval from the onset of acute polio (Wiechers and Hubbell, 1981; Cruz Martinez et al., 1983; Cashman et al., 1987; Ravits et al., 1990). Occasionally, fasciculation potentials and cramp potentials may be recorded (Mulder et al., 1972; Hayward and Seaton, 1979; Cruz Martinez et al., 1983; Maynard, 1985) (see Table 71–2). A very important and consistent observation has been the finding of similar chronic neurogenic changes in muscles believed to have been spared or to have made a complete recovery from remote polio (Hayward and Seaton, 1979; Ravits et al., 1990). This constellation of standard electrodiagnostic findings is observed in all polio survivors and cannot be used to differentiate patients with features of PPS from those with stable residuals of remote polio (Ravits et al., 1990).

Single-fiber electromyography has been used to further characterize the nature and extent of the chronic denervation and reinnervation that follow remote polio, as well as to provide insight into potential mechanisms of fatigue and weakness seen in PPS (Wiechers and Hubbell, 1981; Cruz Martinez et al., 1984; Cashman et al., 1987; Einarsson et al., 1990; Trojan et al., 1991; Maselli et al., 1992). Single-fiber electromyography demonstrates findings consistent with remote denervation with reinnervation, including increased fiber density and increased jitter with blocking (Wiechers and Hubbell, 1981; Cruz Martinez et al., 1984; Cashman et al., 1987; Einarsson et al., 1990; Ravits et al., 1990; Ryniewicz et al., 1990). Neurogenic blocking is not seen (Wiechers and Hubbell, 1981; Ravits et al., 1990). There is some evidence that the degree of increased jitter is related to the size of the motor unit as measured by fiber density, macroelectromyographic motor unit potential amplitude, or fiber-type grouping on muscle biopsy (Cashman et al., 1987; Maselli et al., 1992). It should be emphasized, however, that these single-fiber electromyographic findings may be observed in patients with PPS as well as in those with stable residuals from remote polio (Cashman et al., 1987). None of the single-fiber electromyographic parameters are able to distinguish between these two groups of polio survivors (Cashman et al., 1987; Ravits et al., 1990).

Macroelectromyography has also been applied to quantify the extent of reinnervation that occurs after remote polio (Trojan et al., 1991; Lange, 1995; Rodriquez et al., 1995). The motor unit potentials recorded with macroelectromyography tend to be markedly increased in amplitude, with increases in the median amplitude of up to 11-fold compared with normal control subjects (Einarsson et al., 1990; Trojan et al., 1991; Rodriquez et al., 1995; Stalberg and Grimby, 1995). These findings are observed in weak muscles that may be stable after remote polio or in muscles involved with PPS (Ivanyi et al., 1994; Stalberg and Grimby, 1995). However, large macroelectromyography motor unit potentials have also been observed in apparently unaffected muscles or muscles that have made a complete recovery after the remote polio (Ivanyi et al., 1994; Lange, 1995; Luciano et al., 1996). An early report suggested that macroelectromyography motor unit potentials may be reduced in amplitude in newly weakened muscles affected by PPS and may in fact show further decrements in amplitude during serial studies (Lange et al., 1989). This observation has not been confirmed by subsequent studies that have invariably reported markedly increased amplitudes of the macroelectromyography motor unit potentials (Einarsson et al., 1990; Trojan et al., 1991; Ivanyi et al., 1994; Rodriquez et al., 1995; Stalberg and Grimby, 1995). Furthermore, in serial studies, macroelectromyography motor unit potential amplitudes have been reported to be stable (Ivanyi et al., 1994), to show no consistent trend (Maselli et al., 1992), or to increase by up to 56% after a 4-year interval (Stalberg and Grimby, 1995). Clearly, there is no convincing evidence that macroelectromyography can be used as a method of distinguishing patients with PPS from those with stable residual weakness due to remote polio (Ivanyi et al., 1994; Stalberg and Grimby, 1995; Cashman and Trojan, 1995).

PATHOPHYSIOLOGY

The precise pathophysiology of the new weakness and fatigue that occurs in PPS has not been defined, but numerous theories have been advanced to account for the various neuromuscular symptoms encountered in PPS. It has long been proposed that PPS may be the product of a persistent poliovirus infection (Jubelt and Cashman, 1987; Dalakas, 1995c). Evidence of a persistent infection or a possible immune-mediated mechanism has included peri-

vascular inflammation and active gliosis in the parenchyma of the gray matter of the spinal cord (Pezeshkpour and Dalakas, 1988), endomysial inflammation in muscle (Dalakas, 1988), the presence of anti-GM$_1$ antibodies (Illa et al., 1995), the detection of oligoclonal bands in the cerebrospinal fluid (Dalakas et al., 1984; Dalakas, 1990), and increased interleukin 2 and interleukin 2 receptors, along with poliovirus-specific immunoglobulin M bands in the cerebrospinal fluid (Sharief et al., 1991). More evidence in support of an immune-mediated mechanism includes higher levels of antineurofilament antibodies in polio survivors with PPS than those with controls, stable polio survivors, and patients with amyotrophic lateral sclerosis (Drory et al., 1998). In addition, poliovirus genomic sequences have been reported in the cerebrospinal fluid of patients with PPS but not in that of stable polio survivors (Julien et al., 1999). Although these numerous observations provide evidence in support of persistent viral infection or an immune-mediated mechanism for PPS, they are insufficient to clearly establish an immune-mediated pathophysiology (Dalakas, 1995c).

A dropout of motor neurons with aging has been proposed as an important factor in the genesis of PPS (Jubelt and Cashman, 1987). The attrition of motor neurons with aging may be due to a normal aging phenomenon (Kawamura et al., 1977; Tomlinson and Irving, 1977) or possibly a premature attrition related to persistent neuronal damage from the initial polio infection (Mulder et al., 1972; Kayser-Gatchalian, 1973). It has also been proposed that premature aging of motor neurons may occur due to increased metabolic demands on maximally reinnervated motor units that are commonly observed in PPS (Kayser-Gatchalian, 1973; McComas et al., 1973). The finding of a progressive increase in the amplitude of macroelectromyographic motor unit potentials has been interpreted as an indication of motor neuron dropout as a principal mechanism of PPS (Stalberg and Grimby, 1995). Clearly, the influence of age may be important in contributing to not only a progressive dropout of motor neurons but also other age-related factors, such as a decrease in contractile capacity and a reduction in muscle fiber size (Nordgren et al., 1997). However, it has been argued that the influence of age on motor neuron attrition is not likely to be significant before the age of 60 (McComas et al., 1973; Tomlinson and Irving, 1977). Furthermore, the onset and progression of PPS correlates more precisely with the interval of time from the acute infection than with age itself (Jubelt and Cashman, 1987). Nevertheless, it is likely that age-related changes may play some role in the genesis of PPS, but they do not appear to represent the primary pathophysiological mechanism.

The most widely held theory proposes that new weakness and fatigue encountered in PPS result from a progressive dropout of muscle fibers, particularly those in maximally reinnervated motor units (Wiechers and Hubbell, 1981; Dalakas et al., 1985, 1986). This concept has been based on the fact that maximally reinnervated motor units may incorporate as many as 10 times the number of muscle fibers normally innervated by a nonreinnervated motor unit (Stalberg and Grimby, 1995). Furthermore, these maximally reinnervated motor units may discharge at relatively high frequencies on a regular basis during routine physical activities (Borg et al., 1988). It has been suggested that the high-frequency discharges of these maximum reinnervated motor units result in excessive metabolic demands on the motor unit and muscle fibers, leading to attrition of motor units, muscle fibers, or both (Wiechers and Hubbell, 1981; Dalakas et al., 1986; Trojan et al., 1991; Cashman and Trojan, 1995; Stalberg and Grimby, 1995). There has been abundant electrophysiological evidence cited to support this mechanism. The single-fiber electromyographic findings of increased fiber density and jitter are consistent with this theory (Wiechers and Hubbell, 1981; Cashman et al., 1987; Einarsson et al., 1990). Furthermore, there is an absence of neurogenic or concomitant blocking on single-fiber electromyographic examinations that implies that the increased jitter is due to abnormalities at the very distal nerve fiber rather than a dropout of motor neurons (Wiechers and Hubbell, 1981). Of particular interest is the observation that jitter may be increased to a greater extent in the largest motor units, implying that the most maximally reinnervated motor units have the least effective neuromuscular transmission (Cashman et al., 1987; Maselli et al., 1992). Additional single-fiber electromyographic evidence in support of this theory comes from a stimulation single-fiber electromyographic study (Trojan et al., 1993a; Cashman and Trojan, 1995). This technique permits the electromyographer to control the rate of motor unit discharge and to assess the jitter as a function of discharge rate (Trontelj et al., 1986). Stimulation single-fiber electromyography reveals that jitter increases with higher rates of stimulation in patients with PPS in relation to the interval from their episode of acute polio (Trojan et al., 1993a; Cashman and Trojan, 1995). This observation implies that these reinnervated motor units may be stressed, with higher rates of discharge resulting in less efficient neuromuscular transmission. Supporting evidence for this theory has also been observed in studies on neuromuscular transmission in frogs. These studies have shown that metabolic support of the motor neuron is essential for the axon to maintain effective neuromuscular transmission, that large reinnervated motor units form less effective neuromuscular synapses, and that synaptic transmission in reinnervated motor units can be improved by reducing the size of the motor unit (Herrera and Grinnell, 1980, 1985). Pathological evidence in support of this theory includes the presence of numerous small, isolated atrophic muscle fibers commonly noted in muscle biopsies from patients with PPS (Cashman et al., 1987; Dalakas, 1988). These numerous observations are consistent with a dropout of muscle fibers as a principal pathophysiological mechanism in PPS. However, it

is essential to note that these electrophysiological findings are seen in polio survivors who are apparently stable as well as in those with features of PPS.

Other theories have focused more specifically on the fatigue seen in patients with PPS. Evidence has been cited that central nervous system mechanisms may be responsible for some components of the severe, debilitating fatigue that is so common in this disorder (Bruno et al., 1995). It has been well documented that the acute polio infection involves not only anterior horn cells but also other central structures, including the midbrain reticular formation, hypothalamus, thalamus, caudate nuclei, putamen, globus pallidus, periaqueductal gray, locus ceruleus, and substantia nigra (Bruno et al., 1994). Involvement of these structures may explain some of the reports of cognitive and extrapyramidal features noted in polio survivors (Bruno et al., 1998). It has been reported that 70% to 96% of polio survivors report symptoms of "brain fatigue," such as problems with concentration, memory, attention, word finding, maintaining wakefulness, and thinking clearly (Bruno et al., 1991). These clinical features may reflect involvement of these central structures. It has also been proposed that the "brain fatigue" noted in PPS is consistent with postviral fatigue syndrome and shares many similarities with chronic fatigue syndrome (Bruno et al., 1998).

The functional deterioration seen in polio survivors may also be attributed to non-neuromuscular mechanisms (Windebank et al., 1991; Windebank, 1995; Kidd et al., 1997; Aurlien et al., 1999). Although it has been difficult to document objective evidence of progressive weakness in PPS (Munsat et al., 1987; Agre et al., 1991; Agre and Rodriquez, 1991c; Ivanyi et al., 1996), there are reports that modest progressive weakness does occur (Dalakas et al., 1986; Klein et al., 2000). Nevertheless, there is evidence that the functional deterioration seen in the vast majority of affected patients stems from underlying orthopedic, neurological, or respiratory disorders (Windebank, 1995; Kidd et al., 1997). The identification of these disorders is key, because they may be managed effectively to help alleviate the chronic functional decline that can occur in PPS (Windebank, 1995; Kidd et al., 1997). Other factors that may be contributory to the symptoms of PPS include disuse atrophy (Agre et al., 1991), overuse weakness (Maynard, 1985; Borg et al., 1988; Peach, 1990; Agre et al., 1991), weight gain and obesity (Agre et al., 1989, 1991), and deconditioning that may follow hospitalization (Agre et al., 1989). Evidence of altered muscle metabolism has also been sought as a possible mechanism of fatigue in PPS. Although there is evidence that creatine phosphate, the primary high-energy store in muscle, is reduced in muscle biopsy samples from patients with PPS, the reduction in creatine phosphate does not correlate with postpolio dysfunction in those individual muscles (Nordgren et al., 1997). Altered high-energy phosphate concentrations assessed with magnetic resonance spectroscopy were not reduced during exercise in patients with PPS

(Sharma et al., 1994), but there was evidence of increased fatigue with delayed recovery consistent with impaired excitation-contraction coupling (Sharma et al., 1994).

DIAGNOSIS AND DIFFERENTIAL DIAGNOSIS

The diagnosis of PPS is made through the recognition of the constellation of typical clinical symptoms and signs of PPS and, at the same time, the exclusion of a wide variety of other disorders that may cause or contribute to these clinical features (Jubelt and Cashman, 1987; Halstead, 1991; Dalakas, 1995b; Windebank, 1995). There are four primary diagnostic criteria for PPS: (1) a credible history of paralytic poliomyelitis, (2) partial recovery of function, (3) a minimum 10-year interval of stabilization, and (4) new onset of weakness or fatigue and pain (Mulder et al., 1972). The most important of these criteria is to confirm the history of remote poliomyelitis (Windebank, 1995). Typically, the interval from poliomyelitis to the onset of PPS is very long, and thus medical records are often not available to assist in confirming the diagnosis of acute poliomyelitis. Many times, it is necessary to pursue a very detailed history regarding the acute illness and to specifically inquire about the essential elements of acute poliomyelitis, including fever, stiff neck, paralysis, and the absence of sensory impairment. It is also important to determine the extent of the acute polio, including whether there was bulbar or respiratory involvement and particularly whether there was a need for ventilatory assistance. It is particularly important to explore the precise nature of the new complaints and to determine whether they are due to new weakness of specific muscle groups, global fatigue, or pain that limits the use of the muscles (Windebank, 1995). This information is very useful to identify the primary mechanisms of the new complaints and to design a rational therapeutic approach (Windebank, 1995).

The differential diagnosis of PPS is quite diverse and includes a wide array of systemic illnesses that may cause fatigue (Jubelt and Cashman, 1987; Windebank, 1995). These illnesses include, but are not limited to, anemia, thyroid disease, and a variety of cardiopulmonary disorders. Certainly, a superimposed neuromuscular disorder such as a myopathy, myasthenic syndrome, or myasthenia gravis could produce significant muscle fatigue that mimics or contributes to PPS. Generalized or focal weakness and fatigue may also be caused by neurological disorders, such as cervical or lumbosacral radiculopathy, entrapment neuropathies, and polyneuropathies, as well as central nervous system disorders, such as stroke, Parkinson's disease, and other neurodegenerative disorders. Although at one time there was concern that patients with remote polio had an increased risk of the development of motor neuron disease or, in particular, amyotrophic lateral

sclerosis (Zilkha, 1962), there is no compelling evidence that substantiates this concern (Armon et al., 1990; Swingler et al., 1992). In addition, the identification of underlying depression is an important component to the differential diagnosis, because depression may also contribute to generalized fatigue (Windebank, 1995). Seeking a history of daytime somnolence and snoring may lead to the recognition of obstructive sleep apnea, which represents an important, treatable cause of hypersomnolence and fatigue in persons with PPS (Steljes et al., 1990; Windebank, 1995). The pain attributed to PPS is often due to underlying musculoskeletal and orthopedic disorders related to instability of and stress on various joints, as well as to inflammatory conditions such as bursitis, tendinitis, and arthritis (Windebank et al., 1995; Kidd et al., 1997; Jubelt and Agre, 2000).

In the vast majority of patients, the diagnosis of PPS is not difficult to make. Nevertheless, it is usually prudent to screen patients with general blood chemistries, including complete blood cell count, chemistry panels, thyroid function tests, erythrocyte sedimentation rate, and serum creatine kinase (Thorsteinsson, 1997). It is often valuable to perform electrodiagnostic studies to confirm the presence of chronic neurogenic changes consistent with remote polio and to exclude a superimposed process of an acquired neuropathic or myopathic disorder (Maynard, 1985; Windebank, 1995; Thorsteinsson, 1997). Localized or regional pain is often evaluated with plain radiographs, although scanning of the spine for foraminal or canal stenosis may be appropriate in certain circumstances. Performance of mean sleep latency tests and polysomnography may be particularly valuable in the assessment of patients for obstructive sleep apnea (Steljes et al., 1990). In patients with respiratory involvement, formal pulmonary function studies are often performed (Bach and Alba, 1991). Patients with dysphagia will require swallowing studies to document and quantify the mechanism of the dysphagia (Sonies and Dalakas, 1995; Sonies, 1996).

TREATMENT

Unfortunately, there is no curative or restorative treatment for PPS. The management of this disorder focuses on general supportive measures designed to promote and preserve function (Jubelt and Cashman, 1987). Commonly embraced guidelines include recommendation to avoid fatigue and exhausting physical activities (Willen and Grimby, 1998; Jubelt and Agre, 2000). In fact, it is essential to educate patients regarding these basic management principles that emphasize energy conservation and pacing of activities (Agre et al., 1989; Thorsteinsson, 1997). In many patients, function and activities may be maintained with the use of strategies that fractionate the activity in numerous sessions separated by rest periods (Agre and Rodriquez, 1991b). Although exercises to improve strength were once believed to be potentially harmful (Mitchell, 1953; Agre et al., 1997), there is compelling evidence that nonfatiguing exercise is beneficial in PPS (Agre, 1995; Agre and Rodriquez, 1997; Thorsteinsson, 1997; Jubelt and Agre, 2000). Numerous studies have reported that mild to moderate weakness can be improved with a nonfatiguing exercise program (Einarsson and Grimby, 1987; Feldman and Soskoline, 1987; Einarsson, 1991b; Fillyaw et al., 1991; Agre et al., 1996, 1997; Jubelt and Agre, 2000). None of these studies have shown evidence of muscle damage as manifested by increased serum creatine kinase concentrations or by electromyographic or muscle biopsy changes (Jubelt and Agre, 2000). The guidelines used for these studies were designed to avoid overuse and typically involved exercise for short intervals, with rest between sessions or sets of exercise. In some cases, exercise was performed on alternate days to avoid overuse and to permit full recovery between exercise sessions. Many patients with PPS are able to engage in nonfatiguing aerobic exercise, which can improve cardiopulmonary condition, fatigue, and endurance (Jones et al., 1989; Kriz et al., 1992; Prins et al., 1994; Ernstoff et al., 1996). However, in patients with more serious residual weakness and functional decline, exercises are to be avoided except for light stretching exercises and range of motion activities. A plan for physical therapy must be individualized for each patient.

The use of bracing and various aids to ambulation may be helpful to avoid the extreme fatigue that accompanies efforts to maintain independent ambulation and routine activities. The maintenance of ideal body weight is helpful, because obesity may provide a magnifying or compounding influence on fatigue and functional decline (Agre et al., 1989; Jubelt and Agre, 2000). Joint pain and muscle pain should be evaluated for underlying musculoskeletal and orthopedic causes. The use of local heat, massage, and anti-inflammatory medications may be beneficial (Jubelt and Cashman, 1987). Decreasing mechanical stress on joints may be achieved with lifestyle changes and with the judicious use of appliances such as orthoses, crutches, wheelchairs, and corsets (Jubelt and Cashman, 1987; Waring et al., 1989; Jubelt and Agre, 2000). On occasion, orthopedic surgery may be valuable in the treatment of refractory and serious musculoskeletal problems (Perry, 1985; Jubelt and Cashman, 1987; Peach and Olejnik, 1991). It is also important to recognize that patients with PPS may acquire other medical disorders that may contribute to the symptoms they experience from PPS. These underlying medical disorders should be aggressively sought and managed.

The management of respiratory insufficiency may often require assistive devices, including rocking beds (Goldstein et al., 1987) and intermittent abdominal pressure ventilators such as the cuirass respirator (Kinnear et al., 1988). These devices provide effective nocturnal ventilatory support and are most useful in patients with relatively mild chronic respiratory failure. In patients with more significant and severe respiratory involvement, especially those with nocturnal sleep-induced hypoxemia or carbon dioxide retention, more aggressive alternatives can be considered, including noninvasive positive pressure ventilation devices such as bilevel positive airway pressure (BiPAP) and continuous positive airway pressure (CPAP) devices (Bach and Alba, 1991). On occasion, progressive respiratory muscle weakness and respiratory failure may necessitate tracheostomy and permanent respiratory support (Fischer, 1985; Bach and Alba, 1991). Patients with sleep apnea should be managed in the same manner as patients without PPS (Bach and Alba, 1991; Dean et al., 1998). Dysphagia can often be managed adequately with conservative measures, including instructions on swallowing techniques (Sonies, 1996).

Several drugs have been investigated as potential therapies for PPS. On the basis of anticholinesterase-responsive neuromuscular transmission abnormalities noted on single-fiber electromyography in PPS (Trojan et al., 1993b), pyridostigmine was investigated as a potential therapy for the fatigue (Trojan et al., 1993b). Although pyridostigmine was effective in a proportion of patients (Trojan et al., 1993b), it was not found to be effective in a multicenter, randomized, double-blind trial (Trojan et al., 1999). A double-blind, placebo-controlled trial of high-dose prednisone was undertaken to determine whether immunosuppression therapy could be beneficial in PPS (Dinsmore et al., 1995). A transient improvement in muscle strength was noted during the high-dose phase of therapy, but this improvement was lost as the prednisone was tapered and discontinued (Dinsmore et al., 1995). Amantadine has shown efficacy in improving fatigue in patients with multiple sclerosis (Murray, 1985), and in a preliminary open-label trial it ameliorated fatigue in eight of nine patients with PPS (Dunn, 1991). However, no efficacy was found in a double-blind, placebo-controlled trial (Stein et al., 1995). The failure of these drugs may in part be related to the inherent difficulty in designing trials for PPS. Factors that need to be considered in the design of future trials include the heterogeneity of patients with PPS, the lengthy course of treatment that may need to be used to demonstrate an effect, and the development of more sensitive methods to detect responses to therapy (Dalakas, 1999).

References

Agre JC: The role of exercise in the patient with post-polio syndrome. Ann N Y Acad Sci 1995;753:321–334.

Agre JC, Rodriquez AA: Neuromuscular function: Comparison of symptomatic and asymptomatic polio subjects to control subjects. Arch Phys Med Rehabil 1990;71:545–551.

Agre JC, Rodriquez AA: Neuromuscular function in polio survivors. Orthopedics 1991a;14:1343–1347.

Agre JC, Rodriquez AA: Intermittent isometric activity: Its effect on muscle fatigue in postpolio subjects. Arch Phys Med Rehabil 1991b;72:971–975.

Agre JC, Rodriquez AA: Neuromuscular function in polio survivors at one-year follow-up. Arch Phys Med Rehabil 1991c;72:7–10.

Agre JC, Rodriquez AA: Muscular function in late polio and the role of exercise in post-polio patients. Neurorehabilitation 1997;8:107–118.

Agre JC, Rodriquez AA, Franke TM: Strength, endurance, and work capacity after muscle strengthening exercise in postpolio subjects. Arch Phys Med Rehabil 1997;78:681–686.

Agre JC, Rodriquez AA, Franke TM, et al: Low-intensity, alternate-day exercise improves muscle performance without apparent adverse effect in postpolio patients. Am J Phys Med Rehabil 1996;75:50–58.

Agre JC, Rodriquez AA, Sperling KB: Symptoms and clinical impressions of patients seen in a postpolio clinic. Arch Phys Med Rehabil 1989;70:367–370.

Agre JC, Rodriquez AA, Tafel JA: Late effects of polio: Critical review of the literature on neuromuscular function. Arch Phys Med Rehabil 1991;72:923–931.

Alter M, Kurland LT, Molgaard CA: Late progressive muscular atrophy and antecedent poliomyelitis. Adv Neurol 1982;36:303–309.

Anderson AD, Levine SA, Gellert H: Loss of ambulatory ability in patients with old anterior poliomyelitis. Lancet 1972;2:1061–1063.

Armon C, Daube JR, Windebank AJ, et al: How frequently does classic amyotrophic lateral sclerosis develop in survivors of poliomyelitis? Neurology 1990;40:172–174.

Aurlien D, Strandjord RE, Hegland O: The postpolio syndrome—a critical comment to the diagnosis. Acta Neurol Scand 1999;100:76–80.

Bach JR, Alba AS: Pulmonary dysfunction and sleep disordered breathing as post-polio sequelae: Evaluation and management. Orthopedics 1991;14:1329–1337.

Bach JR, Alba AS, Bohatiuk G, et al: Mouth intermittent positive pressure ventilation in the management of postpolio respiratory insufficiency. Chest 1987;91:859–864.

Block HS, Wilbourn AJ: Progressive post-polio atrophy: The EMG findings. Neurology 1986;36(suppl 1):137.

Borg K, Borg J, Edstrom L, et al: Effects of excessive use of remaining muscle fibers in prior polio and LV lesion. Muscle Nerve 1988;11:1219–1230.

Bruno RL, Cohen JM, Galski T, et al: The neuroanatomy of post-polio fatigue. Arch Phys Med Rehabil 1994;75:498–504.

Bruno RL, Creange SJ, Frick NM: Parallels between post-polio fatigue and chronic fatigue syndrome: A common pathophysiology? Am J Med 1998;105:66S–73S.

Bruno RL, Frick NM, Cohen J: Polioencephalitis, stress, and the etiology of post-polio sequelae. Orthopedics 1991;14:1269–1276.

Bruno RL, Johnson JC, Berman WS: Vasomotor abnormalities as post-polio sequelae: Functional and clinical implications. Orthopedics 1985;8:865–869.

Bruno RL, Sapolsky R, Zimmerman JR, et al: Pathophysiology of a central cause of post-polio fatigue. Ann N Y Acad Sci 1995;753:257–275.

Buchholz DW, Jones B: Post-polio dysphagia: Alarm or caution? Orthopedics 1991;14:1303–1305.

Campbell AM, Williams ER, Pearce J: Late motor neuron degeneration following poliomyelitis. Neurology 1969;19:1101–1106.

Cashman NR, Maselli R, Wollmann RL, et al: Late denervation in patients with antecedent paralytic poliomyelitis. N Engl J Med 1987;317:7–12.

Cashman NR, Trojan DA: Correlation of electrophysiology with pathology, pathogenesis, and anticholinesterase therapy in post-polio syndrome. Ann N Y Acad Sci 1995;753:138–150.

Codd MB, Mulder DW, Kurland LT, et al: Poliomyelitis in Rochester, Minnesota, 1935–1955: Epidemiology and long-term sequelae. A preliminary report. In Halstead LS, Wiechers DO (eds): Late Effects of Poliomyelitis. Miami, Symposia Foundation, 1985; 121–134.

Cornil V, Lepine R: Sur un cas de paralysie generale spinale anterieure subaigue, suivi d'autopsie. Gaz Med (Paris) 1875;4:127–129.

Cruz Martinez A, Ferrer MT, Perez-Conde MC: Electrophysiological features in patients with non-progressive and late progressive weakness after paralytic poliomyelitis: Conventional E.M.G. au-

tomatic analysis of the electromyogram and single fiber electromyography study. Electromyogr Clin Neurophysiol 1984;24:469–479.

Cruz Martinez A, Perez-Conde MC, Ferrer MT: Chronic partial denervation is more widespread than is suspected clinically in paralytic poliomyelitis: Electrophysiological study. Eur Neurol 1983;22:314–321.

Dalakas M: Oligoclonal bands in the cerebrospinal fluid of post-poliomyelitis muscular atrophy. Ann Neurol 1990;28:196–197.

Dalakas MC: Morphologic changes in the muscles of patients with postpoliomyelitis neuromuscular symptoms. Neurology 1988;38:99–104.

Dalakas MC: Post-polio syndrome 12 years later: How it all started. Ann N Y Acad Sci 1995a;753:11–18.

Dalakas MC: The post-polio syndrome as an evolved clinical entity: Definition and clinical description. Ann N Y Acad Sci 1995b;753:68–80.

Dalakas MC: Pathogenetic mechanisms of post-polio syndrome: Morphological, electrophysiological, virological, and immunological correlations. Ann N Y Acad Sci 1995c;753:167–185.

Dalakas MC: Why drugs fail in postpolio syndrome: Lessons from another clinical trial. Neurology 1999;53:1166–1167.

Dalakas MC, Elder G, Hallett M, et al: A long-term follow-up study of patients with post-poliomyelitis neuromuscular symptoms. N Engl J Med 1986;314:959–963.

Dalakas MC, Sever JL, Fletcher M, et al: Neuromuscular symptoms in patients with old poliomyelitis: Clinical, virological, and immunological studies. In Halstead LS, Wiechers DO (eds): Late Effects of Poliomyelitis. Miami, Symposia Foundation, 1985; 73–90.

Dalakas MC, Sever JL, Madden DL, et al: Late postpoliomyelitis muscular atrophy: Clinical, virologic, and immunologic studies. Rev Infect Dis 1984;6(suppl 2):S562–S567.

Daube JR, Windebank AJ, Litchy WJ: Electrophysiologic changes in neuromuscular function over five years in polio survivors. Ann N Y Acad Sci 1995;753:120–128.

Dean AC, Graham BA, Dalakas M, et al: Sleep apnea in patients with postpolio syndrome. Ann Neurol 1998;43:661–664.

Dean E, Ross J, Road JD, et al: Pulmonary function in individuals with a history of poliomyelitis. Chest 1991;100:118–123.

Dinsmore, S, Drambosia J, Dalakas MC: A double-blind, placebo-controlled trial of high-dose prednisone for the treatment of post-polio syndrome. Ann N Y Acad Sci 1995;753:303–313.

Dowhaniuk M, Schentag CT: Dysphagia in individuals with no history of bulbar polio. Ann N Y Acad Sci 1995;753:87–94.

Drachman DB, Murphy SR, Nigam MP, et al: "Myopathic" changes in chronically denervated muscle. Arch Neurol 1967;16:14–24.

Drory VE, Shapira A, Korczyn AD, et al: Antineurofilament antibodies in postpolio syndrome. Neurology 1998;51:1193–1195.

Dunn MG: Post-polio fatigue treated with amantadine. Arch Neurol 1991;48:570.

Einarsson G: Muscle adaptation and disability in late poliomyelitis. Scand J Rehabil Med Suppl 1991a;25:1–76.

Einarsson G: Muscle conditioning in late poliomyelitis. Arch Phys Med Rehabil 1991b;72:11–14.

Einarsson G, Grimby G: Strengthening exercise program in postpolio subjects. Birth Defects 1987;23:275–283.

Einarsson G, Grimby G, Stalberg E: Electromyographic and morphological functional compensation in late poliomyelitis. Muscle Nerve 1990;13:165–171.

Ernstoff B, Wetterqvist H, Kvist H, et al: Endurance training effect on individuals with postpoliomyelitis. Arch Phys Med Rehabil 1996;77:843–848.

Feldman RM: Late effects of poliomyelitis: Clinical pathophysiology. In Halstead LS, Wiechers DO (eds): Late Effects of Poliomyelitis. Miami, Symposia Foundation, 1985; 109–117.

Feldman RM, Soskoline CL: The use of nonfatiguing strengthening exercises in post-polio syndrome. Birth Defects 1987;23:335–341.

Fetell MR, Smallberg G, Lewis LD, et al: A benign motor neuron disorder: Delayed cramps and fasciculation after poliomyelitis or myelitis. Ann Neurol 1982;11:423–427.

Fillyaw MJ, Badger GJ, Goodwin GD, et al: The effects of long-term non-fatiguing resistance exercise in subjects with post-polio syndrome. Orthopedics 1991;14:1253–1256.

Fischer DA: Poliomyelitis: Late respiratory complications and management. Orthopedics 1985;8:891–894.

Frustace SJ: Poliomyelitis: Late and unusual sequelae. Am J Phys Med 1988;66:328–337.

Goldstein RS, Molotiu N, Skrastins R, et al: Assisting ventilation in respiratory failure by negative pressure ventilation and by rocking bed. Chest 1987;92:470–474.

Guilleminault C, Motta J: Sleep apnea syndrome as a long-term sequela of poliomyelitis. In Guilleminault C (ed): Sleep Apnea Syndromes. New York, KROC Foundation, Ser Vol II, 1978; 309–315.

Halstead LS: Assessment and differential diagnosis for post-polio syndrome. Orthopedics 1991;14:1209–1217.

Halstead LS: Post-polio syndrome. Sci Am 1998;278:42–47.

Halstead LS, Rossi CD: New problems in old polio patients: Results of a survey of 539 polio survivors. Orthopedics 1985; 8:845–850.

Halstead LS, Rossi CD: Post-polio syndrome: Clinical experience with 132 consecutive outpatients. Birth Defects 1987;23:13–26.

Halstead LS, Wiechers DO, Rossi CD: Results of a survey of 201 polio survivors. South Med J 1985;78:1281–1287.

Hayward M, Seaton D: Late sequelae of paralytic poliomyelitis: A clinical and electromyographic study. J Neurol Neurosurg Psychiatr 1979;42:117–122.

Herrera AA, Grinnell AD: Effects of changes in motor unit size on transmitter release at the frog neuromuscular junction. J Neurosci 1985;5:1896–1900.

Herrera AA, Grinnell AD: Transmitter release from frog motor nerve terminals depends on motor unit size. Nature 1980;287:649–651.

Hodes R: Electromyographic study of defects of neuromuscular transmission in human poliomyelitis. Arch Neurol Psychiatr 1948;60:457.

Illa I, Leon-Monzon M, Agboatwalla M, et al: Antiganglioside antibodies in patients with acute polio and post-polio syndrome. Ann N Y Acad Sci 1995;753:374–377.

Ivanyi B, Nelemans PJ, de Jongh R, et al: Muscle strength in postpolio patients: A prospective follow-up study. Muscle Nerve 1996;19:738–742.

Ivanyi B, Nollet F, Redekop WK, et al: Late onset polio sequelae: Disabilities and handicaps in a population-based cohort of the 1956 poliomyelitis outbreak in the Netherlands. Arch Phys Med Rehabil 1999;80:687–690.

Ivanyi B, Ongerboer de Visser BW, Nelemans PJ, de Visser M: Macro EMG follow-up study in post-poliomyelitis patients. J Neurol 1994;242:37–40.

Jones DR, Speier J, Canine K, et al: Cardiorespiratory responses to aerobic training by patients with postpoliomyelitis sequelae. JAMA 1989;261:3255–3258.

Jubelt B, Agre JC: Characteristics and management of postpolio syndrome. JAMA 2000;284:412–414.

Jubelt B, Cashman NR: Neurological manifestations of the postpolio syndrome. Crit Rev Neurobiol 1987;3:199–220.

Jubelt B, Drucker J: Post-polio syndrome: An update. Semin Neurol 1993;13:283–290.

Julien J, Leparc-Goffart I, Lina B, et al: Postpolio syndrome: Poliovirus persistence is involved in the pathogenesis. J Neurol 1999;246:472–476.

Kawamura Y, O'Brien P, Okazaki H, et al: Lumbar motoneurons of man. II: The number and diameter distribution of large- and intermediate-diameter cytons in "motoneuron columns" of spinal cord of man. J Neuropathol Exp Neurol 1977;36:861–870.

Kayser-Gatchalian MC: Late muscular atrophy after poliomyelitis. Eur Neurol 1973;10:371–380.

Kidd D, Howard RS, Williams AJ, et al: Late functional deterioration following paralytic poliomyelitis. Q J Med 1997;90:189–196.

Kinnear W, Petch M, Taylor G, et al: Assisted ventilation using cuirass respirators. Eur Respir J 1988;1:198–203.

Klein MG, Whyte J, Keenan MA, et al: Changes in strength over time among polio survivors. Arch Phys Med Rehabil 2000;81:1059–1064.

Knowlton GC, Bennett RL: Overwork. Arch Phys Med Rehabil 1957;38:18–20.

Kriz JL, Jones DR, Speier JL, et al: Cardiorespiratory responses to upper extremity aerobic training by postpolio subjects. Arch Phys Med Rehabil 1992;73:49–54.

Kurent JE, Brooks BR, Madden DL, et al: CSF viral antibodies: Evaluation in amyotrophic lateral sclerosis and late-onset postpoliomyelitis progressive muscular atrophy. Arch Neurol 1979;36:269–273.

Lane DJ, Hazleman B, Nichols PJ: Late onset respiratory failure in patients with previous poliomyelitis. Q J Med 1974;43:551–568.

Lange DJ: Post-polio muscular atrophy: An electrophysiological study of motor unit architecture. Ann N Y Acad Sci 1995; 753:151–157.

Lange DJ, Smith T, Lovelace RE: Postpolio muscular atrophy. Diagnostic utility of macroelectromyography. Arch Neurol 1989; 46:502–506.

Luciano CA, Sivakumar K, Spector SA, et al: Electrophysiologic and histologic studies in clinically unaffected muscles of patients with prior paralytic poliomyelitis. Muscle Nerve 1996;19:1413–1420.

Lutschg J, Ludin HP: Electromyographic findings in patients after recovery from peripheral nerve lesions and poliomyelitis. J Neurol 1981;225:25–32.

Maselli RA, Cashman NR, Wollman RL, et al: Neuromuscular transmission as a function of motor unit size in patients with prior poliomyelitis. Muscle Nerve 1992;15:648–655.

Maynard FM: Post-polio sequelae—differential diagnosis and management. Orthopedics 1985;8:857–861.

McComas AJ, Upton AR, Sica RE: Motoneurone disease and ageing. Lancet 1973;2:1477–1480.

Mitchell GP: Poliomyelitis and exercise. Lancet 1953;2:90–91.

Mulder DW, Lambert EH, Eaton LM: Myasthenic syndrome in patients with amyotrophic lateral sclerosis. Neurology 1959; 9:627.

Mulder DW, Rosenbaum RA, Layton DD: Late progression of poliomyelitis or forme fruste amyotrophic lateral sclerosis? Mayo Clin Proc 1972;47:756–761.

Munsat TL, Andres P, Thibideau L: Preliminary observations on long-term muscle force changes in the post-polio syndrome. Birth Defects 1987;23:329–334.

Murray TJ: Amantadine therapy for fatigue in multiple sclerosis. Can J Neurol Sci 1985;12:251–254.

Nelson KR: Creatine kinase and fibrillation potentials in patients with late sequelae of polio. Muscle Nerve 1990;13:722–725.

Nordgren B, Falck B, Stalberg E, et al: Postpolio muscular dysfunction: Relationships between muscle energy metabolism, subjective symptoms, magnetic resonance imaging, electromyography, and muscle strength. Muscle Nerve 1997;20:1341–1351.

Palmucci L, Bertolotto A, Doriguzzi C, et al: Motor neuron disease following poliomyelitis: Bioptic study of five cases. Eur Neurol 1980;19:414–418.

Peach PE: Overwork weakness with evidence of muscle damage in a patient with residual paralysis from polio. Arch Phys Med Rehabil 1990;71:248–250.

Peach PE, Olejnik S: Effect of treatment and noncompliance on post-polio sequelae. Orthopedics 1991;14:1199–1203.

Perry J: Orthopedic management of post-polio sequelae. In Halstead LS, Wiechers DO (eds): Late Effects of Poliomyelitis. Miami, Symposia Foundation, 1985; 193–206.

Perry J, Fleming C: Polio: Long-term problems. Orthopedics 1985; 8:877–881.

Pezeshkpour GH, Dalakas MC: Long-term changes in the spinal cords of patients with old poliomyelitis: Signs of continuous disease activity. Arch Neurol 1988;45:505–508.

Plum F, Swanson AG: Central neurogenic hypoventilation in man. Arch Neurol Psychiatry 1959;81:531–560.

Prins JH, Hartung H, Merritt DJ, et al: Effect of aquatic exercise training in persons with poliomyelitis disability. Sports Med Training Rehabil 1994;5:29–39.

Ramlow J, Alexander M, LaPorte R, et al: Epidemiology of the post-polio syndrome. Am J Epidemiol 1992;136:769–786.

Ravits J, Hallett M, Baker M, et al: Clinical and electromyographic studies of postpoliomyelitis muscular atrophy. Muscle Nerve 1990;13:667–674.

Raymond F (with contribution from Charcot JM): Paralysie essentiele de l'enfance: Atrophie musculaire consecutive (Note sur deux cas de paralysie essentiele de l'enfance?) Gaz Med (Paris) 1875;4:225–226.

Robinson LR, Hillel AD, Waugh PF: New laryngeal muscle weakness in post-polio syndrome. Laryngoscope 1998;108:732–734.

Rodriquez AA, Agre JC, Harmon RL, et al: Electromyographic and neuromuscular variables in post-polio subjects. Arch Phys Med Rehabil 1995;76:989–993.

Ryniewicz B, Rowinska-Marcinska K, Emeryk B, et al: Disintegration of the motor unit in post-polio syndrome. Part I. Electrophysiological findings in patients after poliomyelitis. Electromyogr Clin Neurophysiol 1990;30:423–427.

Salazar-Grueso EF, Grimaldi LM, Roos RP, et al: Isoelectric focusing studies of serum and cerebrospinal fluid in patients with antecedent poliomyelitis. Ann Neurol 1989;26:709–713.

Schanke AK: Psychological distress, social support and coping behaviour among polio survivors: A 5-year perspective on 63 polio patients. Disabil Rehabil 1997;19:108–116.

Sharief MK, Hentges R, Ciardi M: Intrathecal immune response in patients with the post-polio syndrome. N Engl J Med 1991;325:749–755.

Sharma KR, Kent-Braun J, Mynhier MA, et al: Excessive muscular fatigue in the postpoliomyelitis syndrome. Neurology 1994;44:642–646.

Smith E, Rosenblatt P, Limauro A: The role of the sympathetic nervous system in acute poliomyelitis. J Pediatr 1949;34:1–11.

Sonies BC: Dysphagia and post-polio syndrome: Past, present, and future. Semin Neurol 1996;16:365–370.

Sonies BC, Dalakas MC: Progression of oral-motor and swallowing symptoms in the post-polio syndrome. Ann N Y Acad Sci 1995;753:87–95.

Stalberg E, Grimby G: Dynamic electromyography and muscle biopsy changes in a 4-year follow-up: Study of patients with a history of polio. Muscle Nerve 1995;18:699–707.

Stein DP, Dambrosia JM, Dalakas MC: A double-blind, placebo-controlled trial of amantadine for the treatment of fatigue in patients with the post-polio syndrome. Ann N Y Acad Sci 1995;753:296–302.

Steljes DG, Kryger MH, Kirk BW, et al: Sleep in postpolio syndrome. Chest 1990;98:133–140.

Swingler RJ, Fraser H, Warlow CP: Motor neuron disease and polio in Scotland. J Neurol Neurosurg Psychiatr 1992;55:1116–1120.

Thorsteinsson G: Management of postpolio syndrome. Mayo Clin Proc 1997;72:627–638.

Tomlinson BE, Irving D: The numbers of limb motor neurons in the human lumbosacral cord throughout life. J Neurol Sci 1977;34:213–219.

Trojan DA, Collet JP, Shapiro S, et al: A multicenter, randomized, double-blinded trial of pyridostigmine in postpolio syndrome. Neurology 1999;53:1225–1233.

Trojan DA, Gendron D, Cashman NR: Electrophysiology and electrodiagnosis of the post-polio motor unit. Orthopedics 1991;14:1353–1361.

Trojan DA, Gendron D, Cashman NR: Anticholinesterase-responsive neuromuscular junction transmission defects in post-poliomyelitis fatigue. J Neurol Sci 1993a;114:170–177.

Trojan DA, Gendron D, Cashman NR: Stimulation frequency-dependent neuromuscular junction transmission defects in patients with prior poliomyelitis. J Neurol Sci 1993b;118:150–157.

Trontelj JV, Mihelin M, Fernandez JM, et al: Axonal stimulation for end-plate jitter studies. J Neurol Neurosurg Psychiatr 1986;49:677–685.

Waring WP, Maynard F, Grady W, et al: Influence of appropriate lower extremity orthotic management on ambulation, pain, and fatigue in a post-polio population. Arch Phys Med Rehabil 1989;70:371–375.

Waring WP, McLaurin TM: Correlation of creatine kinase and gait measurement in the postpolio population. Arch Phys Med Rehabil 1992;73:37–39.

Wekre LL, Stanghelle JK, Lobben B, et al: The Norwegian Polio Study 1994: A nation-wide survey of problems in long-standing poliomyelitis. Spinal Cord 1998;36:280–284.

Wiechers DO: Acute and latent effect of poliomyelitis on the motor unit as revealed by electromyography. Orthopedics 1985;8:870–872.

Wiechers DO, Hubbell SL: Late changes in the motor unit after acute poliomyelitis. Muscle Nerve 1981;4:524–528.

Willen C, Grimby G: Pain, physical activity, and disability in individuals with late effects of polio. Arch Phys Med Rehabil 1998;79:915–919.

Windebank AJ: Differential diagnosis and prognosis. In Halstead LS, Grimby G (eds): Post-Polio Syndrome. Philadelphia, Hanley and Belfus, 1995; 69–88.

Windebank AJ, Litchy WJ, Daube JR: Prospective cohort study of polio survivors in Olmsted County, Minnesota. Ann N Y Acad Sci 1995;753:81–86.

Windebank AJ, Litchy WJ, Daube JR, et al: Late effects of paralytic poliomyelitis in Olmsted County, Minnesota. Neurology 1991;41:501–507.

Zilkha KJ: Discussion on motor neuron disease. Proc R Soc Med 1962;55:1028–1031.

CHAPTER 72

Amyotrophic Lateral Sclerosis

Mark B. Bromberg

Amyotrophic lateral sclerosis (ALS) is a form of motor neuron disease that occurs in adults. It is a neurodegenerative disorder characterized by death of both upper and lower motor neurons. Motor neuron loss is progressive and leads to death from respiratory failure. The pathological factors are incompletely understood, and the efficacy of treatment is limited at this time, but ongoing major research is directed at better understanding and management of the disease.

Clinical neurophysiology has an important role in ALS. Traditionally, neurophysiology has been used to document lower motor neuron loss and has been most valuable in the diagnostic process. Neurophysiological testing provides unique information on the compensatory or secondary changes that occur in muscle with denervation and consequently is a sensitive measure of lower motor neuron loss. Clinical neurophysiology has also provided insight into the pathological changes that occur in muscle with disease progression, and a number of neurophysiological tests can be employed to follow disease progression and are useful in clinical trials. More recently, special neurophysiological methods have been developed to study upper motor neuron loss. This chapter reviews the role of clinical neurophysiology in ALS as it relates to the diagnosis, understanding pathophysiological changes, and monitoring disease progression. Basic features of the disease, including theories of pathogenesis, are presented to enhance the understanding of the use and limitations of clinical neurophysiological tests in ALS. Several aspects of clinical neurophysiological testing related to disease progression are discussed elsewhere.

HISTORY OF AMYOTROPHIC LATERAL SCLEROSIS

The history of ALS is interesting and informative. The clinical and pathological features of ALS were most clearly recognized and annunciated by the French neurologist Jean-Martin Charcot in the 1870s. This was a formative time for modern neurology. Charcot developed the investigative format of longitudinal observation of clear examples of neurological disorders followed by pathological examination at death (Goetz, 2000). He recognized the clinical features of atrophic weakness, fasciculations, and brisk reflexes. He also described the pathological features of pallor of the lateral corticospinal tracts and loss of anterior horn cells, and gave the name "amyotrophic lateral sclerosis" to the disease. Thus, ALS represents one of the seminal diseases in modern neurology. The current diagnostic approach is similar to that of Charcot, with clinical observation for evidence of upper and lower motor neuron involvement combined with clinical neurophysiological testing serving as a sensitive means of assessing anterior horn cell loss.

EPIDEMIOLOGY AND CLINICAL FEATURES

ALS is a disease of adults, and although the most common age at onset is in the sixth decade, symptoms can begin at any adult age, from 20 years into the eighth decade. ALS is classified as a rare disease, but it is not uncommon. The incidence is approximately 0.2 to 2.4 per 100,000 in most parts of the world where formal estimates have been made. A question remains whether the incidence is rising or whether there has been improved ascertainment (Mitsumoto et al., 1998). The male-to-female ratio is approximately 2:1. In 5% to 10% of patients there is a clear family history of inheritance (autosomal dominant), but for the majority the disease is considered sporadic. Although rates of progression vary markedly (Pradas et al., 1993), the progressive loss of motor neurons in ALS is inexorable and leads to death from respiratory failure. Survival statistics indicate that 50% of ALS patients die within 3 to 5 years of symptom onset, but a small proportion of patients survive for many years (Mitsumoto et al., 1998).

ALS begins as a regional disease, with approximately 20% of cases starting in the bulbar region and 80% in a limb (usually asymmetrically) (Brooks et al., 1990). A rough pattern of progression can be discerned. When weakness starts in one limb, the next most likely area to be involved is the contralateral limb, followed by the ipsilateral limb. When weakness starts in the bulbar region, arms and legs are equally likely to be affected next. Respiratory involvement (phrenic nerve) can be predicted on the basis of involvement of limb muscles at the same level of the spinal cord (Brooks et al., 1990). Respiratory failure is rare as the presenting symptom (Parhad et al., 1978). Symptoms of respiratory failure generally appear later in the course of the disease, although signs of failure can be found earlier using pulmonary function testing. This discrepancy can be explained by a reduction in respiratory demands due to reduced levels of physical activity from weak limb and trunk muscles.

The focal onset and insidious progression of weakness can make early recognition and diagnosis challenging (Bromberg, 1999a). ALS is a unique disease, with no other disease truly mimicking its symptoms and signs. The unique features of ALS have been codified by the World Federation of Neurology

(WFN) in a set of research diagnostic criteria that can also be used in the clinic (World Federation of Neurology Research Group on Neuromuscular Diseases, 1994; Brooks et al., 2000). ALS is defined by (1) upper motor neuron loss, (2) lower motor neuron loss, (3) progression within a body region and to other regions, and (4) no other clear cause. ALS may be associated with other diseases, and in such cases it is referred to as ALS-plus. The most common association is with dementia. Approximately 5% of patients have a concomitant dementia, usually with frontal lobe features. However, detailed and serial neuropsychometric testing has been infrequently performed, and some form of cognitive impairment may be more common (Strong et al., 1996). One frontal lobe feature that is fairly common in ALS and is not associated with dementia is labile emotional affect in the form of an ease of crying, laughing, or frequent and forced yawns (Moore et al., 1997).

PATHOLOGY

The primary pathological features recognized by Charcot include degeneration of the lateral columns with gliosis and loss of anterior horn cells (Goetz, 2000). Principal findings on postmortem examination in modern studies are loss of upper and lower motor neurons (Lawyer and Netsky, 1953). Upper motor neuron loss includes the giant cells of Betz and well as smaller pyramidal cells in the motor cortex. This results in myelin loss and gliosis in the pyramidal tracts and anterior and lateral cortical spinal tracts, most commonly in a symmetrical pattern. Degeneration of other central nervous system neurons, including neurons of the spinocerebellar system, can be demonstrated, but these changes are clinically silent (Williams et al., 1990). Lower motor neuron loss in the brainstem occurs to varying degrees in the hypoglossal nucleus and nucleus ambiguus. Anterior horn cell loss is noted throughout the spinal cord. An interesting histological finding in anterior horn cells from patients who died after a relatively short symptomatic period was proximal axonal spheroids and tubular enlargement of axons (Carpenter, 1968). This histological picture may represent an early and acute stage of the disease. Several lower motor neuron nuclei tend to be spared in ALS. These include neurons innervating the external urethral and anal sphincter muscles (nucleus of Onufrowicz, or nucleus X) (Mannen et al., 1977). Neurons dying very late in the course are those innervating the extraocular eye muscles and facial muscles (Mizutani et al., 1990). However, motor neuron vulnerability is not absolute, and ALS patients kept alive by artificial ventilation eventually lose all motor neurons (Hayashi and Kato, 1989).

Ventral roots and peripheral nerves show fiber loss (Lawyer and Netsky, 1953). The phrenic nerve reveals marked axonal loss with some evidence of a dying-back pattern as demonstrated by greater axonal loss distally than proximally in the nerve (Bradley et al., 1983). Distal axonal changes are thought to be secondary to sick nerve cell bodies. Sensory nerve fibers also show morphometric changes, with reductions of 30% reported in the sural nerve, although sensory symptoms are uncommon (Bradley et al., 1983).

Pathologic examination of muscle in ALS shows fiber type atrophy and type grouping (Glasberg and Wiley, 1992). The normal mosaic pattern of different fiber types is altered in ALS by denervation and reinnervation, with reinnervated muscle fibers taking on the same fiber type of the reinnervating motor unit. Fiber type atrophy becomes prominent with continued denervation and reinnervation, leading to consolidation of fibers of the same type into large areas. Fiber type grouping is not unique to ALS but indicates a neuropathic process.

Correlations between clinical and postmortem findings are good, but there are examples of no clinical upper motor neuron signs despite pathological evidence for upper motor loss and pyramidal tract degeneration, and vice versa (Lawyer and Netsky, 1953). Certain families with hereditary ALS may include symptomatic members with no clinical signs or pathological evidence of upper motor neuron loss (Cudkowicz et al., 1998).

PATHOPHYSIOLOGY

The pathophysiology of ALS is proving to be complex, and it is probably a heterogeneous disease with different mechanisms that ultimately cause loss of upper and lower motor neurons, leading to a recognizable ALS phenotype. The disease can be divided into different types (Table 72–1). The first division is into sporadic and familial forms. In the familial form, the majority of families follow an autosomal dominant inheritance pattern, but there are rare recessive forms (Andersen et al., 1996). Dominant familial forms can be divided at this time into those affecting families with known abnormalities in the Cu/Zn superoxide dismutase I (SOD I) gene on chromosome 21 (Rosen et al., 1993), and those in

Table 72–1. Division of ALS into Types Based on Inheritance Patterns

Type	
Sporadic	90%–95%
Autosomal dominant	5%–10%
Chromosome 21 (SOD I)	20%
60 mutations	
Unknown locus	80%
Juvenile onset	Families
Autosomal recessive	Families
Chromosome 2	Families
Chromosome 21	Families
X-linked	Families

SOD I, superoxide dismutase 1 gene.

Table 72–2. Proposed Cascade of Steps or Factors Contributing to Neuronal Death in ALS

Glutamate excitotoxicity
Excess intracellular calcium
Oxidative stress
Mitochondrial energy abnormalities
Neurofilament abnormalities
Necrotic or apoptotic cell death

families with no identified genetic locus. *SOD I* mutations represent approximately 20% of cases of familial ALS (Gaudette et al., 2000). Despite genetic and clinical heterogeneity among ALS patients, there is a feeling that they share common pathophysiological mechanisms in the form of a cascade of steps or factors, ultimately leading to motor neuron death and the recognizable ALS phenotype (Table 72–2). Individuals with different contributing factors may enter the cascade at different points (Rothstein, 1996). It is important to appreciate that no clinical or electrophysiological features distinguish familial from sporadic ALS.

A cause for ALS has not been determined. Initial studies on environmental or epidemiological factors in sporadic ALS have not been rewarding (Mitchell, 2000). Physical trauma, consumption of fresh fish from Lake Michigan, and exposure to welding or soldering materials have been identified as historical factors more common in ALS than in control cohorts (Sienko et al., 1990; Strickland et al., 1996). However, pathophysiological relationships between exposure and disease are not clear, and no practical benefit has occurred with chelation treatment for heavy metals (Conradi et al., 1982).

Research emphasis has shifted from environmental or epidemiological observational studies to genetics-based studies following the discovery of mutations in the Cu/Zn *SOD I* gene. Particular use has been made of transgenic mouse models using *SOD I* mutations and other mutations to perturb various mechanistic systems (Gurney, 1997). Although there is a better understanding of steps in the putative cascade, no clear pattern has emerged to link any one step to cell death in ALS or to link together any steps or factors (Bromberg, 1999b; Xu, 2000). What follows is a brief description of several proposed etiological steps.

Glutamate is the excitatory transmitter for upper and lower motor neurons; however, an excess of glutamate can be neurotoxic (Choi, 1988). An absolute or relative excess of glutamate in ALS patients could occur by a defect in glutamate metabolism by one of the excitatory amino acid transport systems (EAAT 2; also referred to as GLT-1), which is located primarily in the membrane of astrocytes that surround the synapse (Rothstein, 1996). Abnormal EAAT 2 function has been demonstrated in some but not all sporadic and familial (*SOD I* mutations) ALS patients (Rothstein et al., 1995). The abnormal EAAT 2 protein does not represent a gene mutation (Aoki et al., 1998) but is attributed to aberrant RNA processing (Lin et al., 1998). More recent data suggest that EAAT 2 RNA abnormalities are also found in persons with other neurodegenerative diseases and in normal subjects (Honig et al., 2000).

Glutamate neurotoxicity in ALS is felt to be mediated by non-N-methyl-D-aspartate (NMDA) receptors (Rothstein et al., 1993). Non-NMDA receptors are composed of subunits GluR1 through GluR4, and subunit composition determines ionic permeability. In particular, the presence of a GluR2 subunit results in low calcium permeability. However, the regulatory properties of GluR2 are complex, and low calcium permeability requires a post-transcriptional change (RNA editing) in a single amino acid code. Editing efficiency is lower in spinal cord anterior gray regions of ALS subjects, possibly leading to increased calcium permeability and high levels of intracellular calcium (Takuma et al., 1999). The importance of high intracellular calcium lies in its potentiation of the formation of oxygen free radicals (Coyle and Puttfarcken, 1993). Oxygen free radicals are normal by-products of cellular metabolism. There are enzymatic mechanisms to reduce free radical species, and SOD I is one. SOD I catalyzes the reduction of the hydroxyl ion to hydrogen peroxide. A relative excess of free radicals, generated by any mechanism, has been postulated to cause oxidative stress and damage to cellular elements. A potential mechanism is damage to DNA, structural proteins, and lipids (lipid peroxidation), and to neurofilaments (Coyle and Puttfarcken, 1993).

Oxidative stress is highlighted because mutant forms of SOD I are found in 15% to 20% of cases of familial ALS. However, among the 90 different SOD I mutations described, some have reduced enzymatic function, but most mutants have normal or increased function (Brown, 1996). Thus, a gain of function or toxic property is the probable mechanism of mutant SOD I. Gain-of-function mechanisms include reaction with promiscuous substrates such as peroxynitrite to yield nitronium ions that, in turn, yield nitrate tyrosine residues, and reactions with hydrogen peroxide to yield free radical compounds (Brown, 1996; Xu, 2000).

Neurofilaments are cytoskeletal proteins of nerve cells that are composed of heavy, medium, and light chains. Axonal swellings filled with neurofilaments observed in muscle biopsy specimens from early-stage ALS patients suggest that neurofilament disarrangement may be an early pathological step (Carpenter, 1968). The terminal portions of the light chains include a large number of tyrosine residues. Peroxynitrates are a by-product of increased free radical production (Brown, 1996) and can lead to nitration of tyrosine residues. It is postulated that nitration of neurofilaments could lead to cellular dysfunction (Beal et al., 1997). Further support for neurofilament dysfunction in ALS comes from mutations in the gene coding for the terminal region of the heavy chain in a limited number of ALS patients (Al-Chalabi et al., 1999).

Mitochondrial dysfunction may have a role in ALS through several mechanisms (Swerdlow et al., 2000), including increased production of free radicals and impaired electron transport leading to impaired energy production (Cassarino and Bennett, 1999; Beal, 2000). In support are observations in transgenic SOD I mouse models for early structural changes in mitochondria (Wong et al., 1995). A recent trial of creatine in an ALS mouse model showed a marked reduction in the rate of motor neuron loss and an increase in survival of animals feed modest amounts of creatine compared with litter mates on a normal diet (Klivenyi et al., 1999).

Certain lower motor neurons are characteristically spared in ALS, including the external sphincters and the extraocular eye muscles. An explanation for this comes from analysis of levels of the calcium-buffering proteins calbindin and calmodulin in lower motor neurons. These proteins are thought to buffer high levels of intracellular calcium and could prevent or blunt steps in the cascade associated with high calcium. Levels of calbindin and calmodulin are high in extraocular motor nuclei and sphincter motor nuclei and low in other lower motor neurons (Alexianu et al., 1994).

Many pathophysiological steps discussed previously focus on lower motor neurons, although there are no underlying reasons for different mechanisms in the death of upper motor neurons. A hypothesis has been advanced that ALS starts as a disease of upper motor neuron dysfunction and secondarily causes death of lower motor neurons (Eisen et al., 1992). The hypothesis is based in part on dysfunction of cortical inhibitory neurons leading to excess glutamate at synaptic connections onto upper motor neurons, and subsequent overactivity and excess glutamate at the synapse between upper and lower motor neurons (Enterzari-Taher et al., 1997). A supporting factor is the large number of monosynaptic corticospinal connections onto alpha motor neurons in primates, with the greatest number in human primates (Kuypers, 1981).

UPPER MOTOR NEURON LOSS

Motor dysfunction in ALS is caused by loss of both upper and lower motor neurons. However, muscle weakness in ALS is primarily a consequence of lower motor neuron loss. The contribution of upper motor neuron dysfunction to muscle weakness can be assessed by stimulating a motor nerve with a 1-second, 50-Hz stimulus train during the generation of maximum voluntary isometric contraction (MVIC). Any added force generated supports a degree of central activation failure, which in a well-motivated ALS subject represents an upper motor component to weakness. In ALS subjects, the percentage and frequency of added force are low, supporting lower motor neuron loss as the principle determinant of muscle weakness (Kent-Braun et al., 1993, 1998). Upper motor neuron loss causes symp-

Table 72–3. Clinical Signs of Upper and Lower Motor Neuron Involvement in ALS

Signs of upper motor neuron loss
  Labile emotional affect
  Forced yawning
  Exaggerated shout reflex
  Pathological jaw jerk
  Pathological gag reflex
  Spastic tone to passive limb movements
  Pathological tendon reflexes
  Preserved tendon reflexes in weak and atrophic limb
  Clonus
  Hoffmann responses
  Extensor plantar responses
Signs of lower motor neuron loss
  Muscle weakness
  Muscle atrophy
  Fasciculations

Adapted from Brooks B, Miller R, Swash M, et al., for the World Federation of Neurology Research Group on Motor Neuron Diseases: El Escorial Revisited: Revised criteria for the diagnosis of amyotrophic lateral sclerosis. Amyotrophic Lateral Sclerosis 2000;1:293–298.

toms of slower rapid movements and stiff limb movements, and signs of spasticity and pathological tendon reflexes (Table 72–3). Upper motor neuron loss is also likely to have a role in fatigability that is prominent in ALS (Kent-Braun et al., 1993, 1998). A comparison of measures of upper and lower motor neuron loss over time indicates a greater loss of MVIC values than loss of rapid movements, further supporting the prominent role of lower motor neuron loss (Kent-Braun et al., 1993, 1998).

The clinical features of upper motor neuron loss in ALS are complex. Although upper motor neurons may be involved early in the pathological process, upper motor neuron symptoms and signs vary among ALS patients. While most have unequivocal signs, others have equivocal or no upper motor neuron signs. Equivocal upper motor neuron signs are incongruously brisk reflexes, and are regarded as "possible upper motor neuron signs" (Younger et al., 1990). Clinical experience indicates that patients who have incongruously brisk reflexes in weak and atrophic muscles that are fasciculating probably have ALS or at least an inexorably progressive disorder (Gordon et al., 1997). When no upper motor neuron signs are present, patients do not fulfill the criteria for ALS (World Federation of Neurology Research Group on Neuromuscular Diseases, 1994; Brooks et al., 2000). In this regard, some individuals who carry certain SOD I mutations may be symptomatic with lower motor neuron loss but do not have clinical signs or pathological evidence of upper motor neuron loss (Cudkowicz et al., 1998). This leaves open questions about nomenclature of progressive lower motor neuron loss (progressive spinal muscular atrophy). Some forms may represent a separate and potentially treatable entity, such as lower motor syndrome (Pestronk et al., 1994). However, others follow a progressive course and probably represent a lower motor neuron variant. The

more general term "motor neuron disease" would encompass all forms, with a specific designation for ALS-type motor neuron disease (Rowland, 1998).

The physiological effects of upper motor neuron loss can be measured with special clinical neurophysiological techniques, such as transcortical magnetic stimulation. The sensitivity of these techniques is low. Accordingly, clinical neurophysiology in ALS focuses primarily on the lower motor neuron and associated changes with neuron loss.

LOWER MOTOR NEURON LOSS AND COLLATERAL REINNERVATION

Changes in muscle due to lower motor neuron loss can be understood in terms of the motor unit. The concept of a motor unit was put forward by Sir Charles Sherrington to describe the alpha motor neuron, the motor axon, and all muscle fibers innervated by terminal nerve branches. Lower motor neurons innervate variable numbers of muscle fibers, from 20 in finely graded muscles, such as extraocular muscles, to 2,000 in limb muscles (Feinstein et al., 1955). Loss of lower motor neurons initiates a compensatory process of collateral reinnervation (Wohlfart, 1958). In collateral reinnervation, surviving motor neurons sprout terminal processes that establish synaptic contact with orphaned muscle fibers. The reinnervated muscle fibers become electrically and mechanically functional. The clinical effect of collateral reinnervation is to slow the apparent rate of progression of weakness. However, the compensatory process is limited in extent, and surviving motor neurons can increase the number of reinnervated fibers by only 7- to 40-fold (Stålberg, 1982). Furthermore, reinnervating motor units cannot increase their territory within muscle, presumably owing to fascicular boundaries (Kugelberg et al., 1970). When surviving motor neurons succumb to the disease process, compensation fails and greater numbers of muscle fibers remain denervated, leading to muscle atrophy and weakness.

An important clinical variable is the rate of lower motor neuron loss. With a monophasic loss of lower motor neurons, such as with poliomyelitis, there is maximal time for full reinnervation and motor units are very large. In progressive disorders such as ALS, there is less time for surviving motor units to reach their full reinnervation potential before they die. As greater numbers of lower motor neurons die, more muscle fibers remain denervated, leading to decompensation (Stålberg, 1982). It is difficult to determine the degree of lower motor neuron loss in a muscle with clinical or routine electrophysiological testing owing to the dynamic interaction between compensation by collateral reinnervation and decompensation. This issue is important for understanding and measuring the rate of progression. Computer modeling that addresses the relationship between compensation and decompensation provides information about this relationship (Kuether and Lipinski,

1988). When a linear rate of lower motor neuron loss is modeled, strength is unaffected until 50% of lower motor neurons have died, at which time strength falls rapidly. When exponential or sigmoidal rates of lower motor neuron loss are modeled, there are extended periods when strength declines relatively slowly.

The observation in ALS patients when serial quantitative strength measurements (MVIC) are made is that strength falls in a linear pattern (Munsat et al., 1988). However, the effects of the initial compensation and later decompensation of collateral reinnervation support a nonlinear pattern of lower motor neuron loss. Computer modeling suggests that an exponential or sigmoidal pattern of lower motor neuron loss is more likely.

Muscle fibers undergo changes with denervation and reinnervation that are important in interpreting clinical neurophysiological studies. Following denervation, muscle fibers atrophy from an initial diameter of approximately 60 μm to less than half (Dubowitz, 1985). Following reinnervation, muscle fibers increase in diameter and may become hypertrophic. Muscle fiber action potential conduction velocity is proportional to fiber diameter. Conduction velocity in a normal fiber is approximately 4 m/sec; it is lower in atrophic fibers (Stålberg and Trontelj, 1994). As nerve terminals reestablish synaptic contact with denervated muscle fibers, neuromuscular transmission is less secure, but gradually becomes more secure (Lindstrom, 2000). The progressive nature of ALS means that these changes will be present to different degrees in different muscles at different times. An appreciation for the disease process and the clinical state is important in interpreting clinical neurophysiological data.

CLINICAL NEUROPHYSIOLOGY IN THE DIAGNOSIS OF AMYOTROPHIC LATERAL SCLEROSIS

ALS remains a clinical diagnosis based on the history of symptoms and findings on neurological examination and is aided by a limited number of diagnostic tests. The diagnosis can be made actively and should not be made passively as a process of "ruling out" other disorders by a battery of laboratory tests (Bromberg, 1999a). There are few laboratory tests that bear directly on detecting competing diagnoses. Clinical neurophysiological testing is the most important laboratory approach to determining the extent of lower motor neuron loss. Genetic blood testing is informative in only a small percentage of patients in the setting of a clear family history (Gaudette et al., 2000; see Table 72–1).

World Federation of Neurology Diagnostic Criteria

The WFN convened in El Escorial, Spain, in 1994 to formulate a set of research criteria for the diagno-

---

Table 72–4. Levels of Diagnostic Certainty in ALS Based on Clinical Signs of Upper and Lower Motor Neuron Loss

Clinically definite ALS
  Upper and lower motor neuron clinical signs in bulbar plus two spinal regions, or in three spinal regions
Clinically probable ALS
  Upper and lower motor neuron clinical signs in at least two regions with some upper motor neuron signs rostral to lower motor neuron signs
Clinically probable laboratory-supported ALS
  Upper and lower motor neuron clinical signs in one region, or upper motor neuron signs in one region and lower motor neuron signs by electrophysiological criteria in at least two limbs
Clinically possible ALS
  Upper and lower motor neuron clinical signs in one region, or upper motor neuron clinical signs in two or more regions, or lower motor neuron clinical signs rostral to upper motor neuron signs

Adapted from Brooks B, Miller R, Swash M, et al., for the World Federation of Neurology Research Group on Motor Neuron Diseases: El Escorial Revisited: Revised criteria for the diagnosis of amyotrophic lateral sclerosis. Amyotrophic Lateral Sclerosis 2000;1:293–298.

---

sis of ALS (World Federation of Neurology Research Group on Neuromuscular Diseases, 1994). The criteria were designed to ensure enrollment of a uniform set of subjects in clinical trials. They can also be used in the clinic, and serve as a diagnostic algorithm. The criteria were reviewed in 1998 at a subsequent WFN meeting, which led to a revised set of criteria with a limited number of changes (Brooks et al., 2000). The criteria focus on four key features: (1) evidence for upper motor neuron loss; (2) evidence for lower motor neuron loss; (3) evidence for progression within a region and to other regions; and (4) no evidence for an alternative explanation for motor dysfunction. The neuraxis is divided into four regions: head (bulbar), cervical, thoracic, and lumbosacral. The clinical diagnostic signs of upper and lower motor neuron loss are listed in Table 72–3. Clinical neurophysiological testing is an important diagnostic tool because it is an extension of the neurological examination to verify and document the extent of lower motor neuron loss.

At the end of the evaluation process, the distribution of upper and lower motor loss leads to levels of diagnostic certainty: clinically definite, clinically probable, clinically probable–laboratory supported, clinically possible ALS (Table 72–4). The category of clinically suspected ALS, based on lower motor neuron loss only, has been deleted from the revised criteria. The diagnostic levels of probable and possible ALS do not suggest an alternative diagnosis but rather reflect the extent of findings of upper and lower motor neuron loss along the neuraxis. Exclusion of alternative diagnoses by history, imaging studies, and diagnostic tests is implied.

Clinical Neurophysiological Testing

Clinical neurophysiological studies are very helpful in the diagnostic process in suspected ALS be-

---

**Table 72–5. Electrodiagnostic Features of
Lower Motor Neuron Loss in ALS**

Signs of active denervation
  Fibrillation potentials
  Positive sharp waves
  Fasciculation potentials (common in active and chronic
    denervation, but may be absent in some muscles)
Signs of chronic denervation
  Motor unit action potential morphology
    Increased amplitude
    Increased duration
    Increased proportion of polyphasia
  Motor unit instability
  Motor unit recruitment
    Rapid firing rates (usually greater than 10 Hz unless there is
      a significant upper motor neuron component, when rates
      can be less than 10 Hz)
    Reduced interference pattern

Adapted from Brooks B, Miller R, Swash M, et al., for the World Federation of Neurology Research Group on Motor Neuron Diseases: El Escorial Revisited: Revised criteria for the diagnosis of amyotrophic lateral sclerosis. Amyotrophic Lateral Sclerosis 2000;1:293–298.

cause they can exclude other neuromuscular diagnoses, show evidence that clinically affected regions suffer from lower motor neuron loss, and demonstrate that there is lower motor neuron loss in clinically uninvolved regions. The importance of entrusting the electrophysiological study to an electromyographer experienced in interpreting the electromyographic findings in ALS is emphasized in the revised WFN criteria.

Within the WFN diagnostic criteria is a set of electrophysiological criteria designed to identify active and ongoing denervation consistent with a neuropathic process (Table 72–5). The most important electrophysiological test is needle electromyography (EMG). However, there is a spectrum of tests that can be used to exclude other diagnoses and help support the diagnosis of ALS. The full spectrum of tests will be reviewed.

NERVE CONDUCTION STUDIES

The clinical neurophysiological evaluation starts with nerve conduction studies to look for evidence of focal or diffuse neuropathies. A diffuse neuropathy is less likely to be confused with ALS, but there may be concern for predominantly demyelinating motor neuropathies (chronic inflammatory demyelinating polyradiculoneuropathy [CIDP]) that might be treatable. Nerve conduction studies can help identify these neuropathies by recording slowed conduction velocity. Motor nerve conduction values reflect the largest and hence fastest conducting nerve fibers. Consequently, conduction velocity values will fall in ALS with loss of neurons with large-diameter fibers (Feinberg et al., 1999). The limits of slowed conduction velocity in ALS have been determined empirically (Cornblath et al., 1992). Despite very low compound muscle action potential (CMAP) amplitudes in some nerves in ALS, conduc-

tion velocity was never less than 70% of the lower limit of normal, and distal motor latencies and F-wave latencies were rarely greater than 125% of the upper limit of normal. A specific neuropathy characterized by focal conduction block in motor nerves could be confused with ALS and will be discussed below.

A pattern of motor nerve conduction abnormalities in intrinsic hand muscles called the "split hand" pattern has been described in ALS patients (Wilbourn, 2000). The observation is that the CMAP amplitudes recorded from the lateral side of the hand (median nerve–innervated thenar muscles) are frequently lower than from the medial side of the hand (ulnar nerve–innervated hypothenar muscles), which is opposite to the normal pattern of amplitudes. Among ulnar nerve–innervated muscles, the first dorsal interosseous muscle may show the greatest loss of CMAP amplitude. The loss in CMAP amplitude reflects greater denervation as evidenced by lower motor unit estimates in the same pattern (Kuwabara et al., 1999). Speculation as to cause focuses on the relative cortical representation of intrinsic hand muscles.

Sensory nerve conduction studies should be normal in ALS patients. However, sensory nerve action potential amplitudes and conduction velocities are modestly but statistically significantly lower in ALS patients, and show further deterioration over time (Mondelli et al., 1993). The most common sensory abnormality will be focal slowing from entrapment syndromes and reduced or absent distal leg sensory responses in elderly patients. ALS patients can have a peripheral neuropathy from concomitant diseases, such as diabetes. Under these circumstances, it is necessary to assess the pattern and momentum of weakness. Diabetic neuropathies are largely symmetrical and progress slowly, with greater sensory loss than weakness. Diabetic proximal neuropathy (proximal amyotrophy) usually has a sudden onset with pain, and although it can progress in an asymmetrical pattern, there is usually some element of improvement in strength (Barohn et al., 1991). Furthermore, the weakness is usually confined to the lower extremities, and tendon reflexes are reduced or absent.

REPETITIVE NERVE STIMULATION

Clinical neurophysiological tests of neuromuscular junction function may be performed as part of an electrodiagnostic protocol for weakness. The mature acetylcholine receptor is a pentomeric complex composed of α_2, β_1, γ_1, and δ_1 subunits. In contrast, fetal muscle prior to innervation and adult muscle after denervation have an ϵ subunit substituted for the γ subunit (Lindstrom, 2000). The fetal receptor complex has reduced sodium conductance and a lower safety factor for the initiation of a muscle fiber action potential (Lindstrom, 2000). Thus, newly reinnervated muscle fibers mimic a postsynaptic defect in neuromuscular junction transmission. Tests of low-rate repetitive nerve stimulation (2 to 3 Hz) in ALS subjects show decrement in approximately half of proximal (trapezius) muscles and distal (hypothenar) muscles (Denys and Forbes, 1979; Bernstein and Antel, 1981; Killian et al., 1994).

Needle Electromyography

Needle EMG is the most important clinical neurophysiological test for the diagnosis of ALS. The key neurophysiological feature is ongoing neurogenic denervation (Lambert and Mulder, 1957). Needle EMG can show denervation beyond the territory of a single nerve or root. Weakness from chronic myopathies or dystrophies is occasionally recognized in later life and may be in the differential diagnosis of ALS. These disorders will show evidence for myopathic changes on needle EMG. The specific features supporting active and chronic denervation will be discussed.

Abnormal Spontaneous Activity

Fibrillation potentials and positive sharp waves are spontaneous discharges of individual denervated muscle fibers. Denervation may occur in both neurogenic and myopathic diseases (Buchthal and Rosenfalck, 1966; Desmedt and Borenstein, 1975). Although there is controversy as to whether fibrillation potentials and positive sharp waves represent the same phenomena (Dumitru, 1996; Kraft, 1996), the observations that fibrillation potentials can change into positive sharp waves and vice versa supports a common origin (Nandedkar et al., 2000).

Finding fibrillation potentials and positive sharp waves in multiple muscles supports a diffuse process. The full needle EMG study is usually relied on to distinguish between myopathic and neuropathic processes. However, one large study of ALS patients relied only on the presence of fibrillation potentials and positive sharp waves to document diffuse denervation (Ross et al., 1998). The remaining diagnostic criteria for ALS were similar to WFN El Escorial criteria. Patients were followed for several months, and the diagnostic specificity held, with no patient's diagnosis changed. Thus, the presence of fibrillation potentials and positive sharp waves is a supportive diagnostic finding, but abnormal spontaneous activity may not be observed in cranial innervated muscles or early on in limb muscles (de Carvalho et al., 1999).

Fasciculations

Fasciculation potentials have long been observed clinically in ALS, and are included in the electrophysiological criteria (see Table 72–5). The origin of fasciculations is unclear; they may be generated either proximally or, more commonly, distally along the nerve (Wettstein, 1979; Roth, 1982). There are also data indicating that fasciculations in ALS may be activated by cortical magnetic stimulation (de

Carvalho, 2000) and hence represent cortical dysfunction. Fasciculations are common in other disorders and in normal individuals, in whom they are considered to be benign. Several features separate benign fasciculations from those observed in ALS; on needle examination benign fasciculations tend to have normal motor unit configurations for amplitude, duration, and number of phases, are stable from discharge to discharge, and have a higher discharge rate (Trojaborg and Buchthal, 1965; de Carvalho and Swash, 1998). Fasciculations found in ALS differ in that they may have more complex configurations, and the degree of complexity may be greater in weaker muscles. Furthermore, among fasciculations in ALS, less complex examples are more readily activated by voluntary activation. These findings suggest that complex and unstable fasciculations reflect enlarged motor units (de Carvalho and Swash, 1998). In ALS, fasciculations may be observed in clinically strong muscles with no positive waves and fibrillation potentials and whose only signs of denervation is increased fiber density (de Carvalho and Swash, 1998). This implies that fasciculations may constitute one of the earliest signs of lower motor neuron changes in ALS. The WFN criteria emphasize caution in interpreting fasciculations; their absence raises diagnostic doubts, and they may be benign or occur in other denervating disorders.

The remainder of the electrophysiological criteria for ALS focuses on signs of chronic denervation. Important features of the motor unit action potential include reduced recruitment, increased amplitude, and increased complexity of motor unit morphology (see Table 72–5).

Motor Unit Recruitment

Reduced motor unit recruitment reflects the primary pathological process of lower motor neuron loss. Clinical assessment of recruitment is subjective and is based on estimates of the discharge frequency and the number of motor units on the EMG oscilloscope screen. Frequency estimation is commonly carried out at low levels of muscle force because individual units become difficult to discern in a field of many. The number of motor units observed is based on the recording properties of the intramuscular electrode but is similar for concentric and monopolar electrodes (Nandedkar and Sanders, 1991). In general, as the force of muscle contraction slowly increases, there is an orderly increase in the firing rate of a motor unit before the next motor unit is recruited. Newly recruited motor units start at rates of approximately 8 Hz, which increase to approximately 16 Hz before the next motor unit is recruited. In this range, the discharge frequency is not constant (Miller and Sherratt, 1978). Discrimination of discharge frequency is usually aided by the sound of the motor unit discharge over a loudspeaker. Discharge frequency can be estimated semiquantitatively by setting the oscilloscope trace to

10 msec per division on a 10-division oscilloscope screen and observing the number of times an identifiable motor unit occurs per sweep (100 msec per sweep). Under these conditions, a motor unit observed once per sweep at the same position on the screen is discharging at a frequency of 10 Hz, a motor unit moving to the left in successive sweeps is discharging at greater than 10 Hz, and a motor unit discharging twice per sweep has a rate of 20 Hz (Bromberg, 1993a). Lower motor neuron loss in ALS results in higher discharge frequencies and a greater degree of discharge variability (Petajan, 1974; Dorfman et al., 1989). The relationship between lower motor neuron loss and discharge frequency is not linear, and when few lower motor neurons remain, discharge of 40 Hz or more may be encountered (Schulte-Mattler et al., 2000).

Motor unit recruitment is affected by upper motor neuron loss. In clinical examples of upper motor neuron loss without lower motor neuron loss, motor unit discharge frequency and variability are lower than in normal subjects (Andreassen and Rosenfalck, 1978; Shahani and Parker, 1991). It can be appreciated that the degree of upper motor neuron and lower motor neuron loss differs among ALS patients and in different muscles, and the discharge frequency reflects the interaction between these two influences. The WFN electrophysiological criteria (see Table 72–5) recognize the possibility of a lower discharge frequency in ALS due to upper motor neuron loss. Clinical experience indicates that discharge frequencies may be lower in some muscles, but the pattern in most muscles in ALS is higher discharge frequencies.

MOTOR UNIT AMPLITUDE

Motor unit amplitude tends to be higher in ALS owing to the incorporation of more muscle fibers in a motor unit from collateral reinnervation (Nandedkar et al., 1988). Motor unit amplitude is most commonly estimated at low levels of force in conjunction with assessment of recruitment. Amplitude estimation is usually qualitative by viewing the recruitment activity envelope (Nandedkar and Sanders, 1990). When individual motor units are singled out by an amplitude trigger and delay line (Czekajewski et al., 1969), quantitative measures support larger amplitude values even in mildly affected muscles (Partanen and Nousiainen, 1990).

MOTOR UNIT DURATION

Motor unit duration, including the initial part, main spike, and terminal part, but excluding satellite potentials (Stålberg et al., 1986), is increased in ALS. This may be difficult to discern during voluntary recruitment at sweep speeds of 10 msec per division, but increases are statistically significant when individual motor units are measured (Buchthal and Pinelli, 1953; Partanen and Nousiainen, 1990). The complexity of the motor unit waveform is characterized by the number of turns and phases (Stålberg et al., 1986). In ALS, the number of polyphasic (more than four phases) motor units is increased (Buchthal and Pinelli, 1953). In addition, polyphasic and polyturn (more than five turns) motor units show instability from discharge to discharge, reflecting greater variability in neuromuscular junction transmission related to reinnervation and variabilities of conduction along muscle fibers. This variability has been termed "jiggle" (Stålberg and Sonoo, 1994). Motor units in ALS tend to have a greater number of satellite potentials (Partanen and Nousiainen, 1990).

EXAMINATION OF SPECIFIC MUSCLES

The level of WFN diagnostic certainty is based in part on the distribution of lower motor neuron symptoms and signs. Determination of the distribution of lower motor neuron loss in asymptomatic muscles is aided by needle EMG. Accordingly, needle EMG evidence for lower motor neuron loss in bulbar and thoracic paraspinal muscles increases the level of diagnostic certainty (see Table 72–4). Studies of the tongue in ALS show signs of active denervation (fibrillation potentials and positive sharp waves) in a third and chronic denervation (abnormal motor recruitment and increased proportion of polyphasia) in two thirds of patients studied (Preston et al., 1997). Studies of the frontalis, temporalis, mentalis, masseter, and sternocleidomastoid muscles show active denervation in a third and chronic denervation in one half to two thirds (Preston et al., 1997; Finsterer et al., 1998). Needle EMG study of thoracic paraspinal muscles reveals active denervation in up to 75% of ALS patients when two to four spinal segments are examined (Kuncl et al., 1988). Active thoracic paraspinal denervation is observed with almost equivalent frequency in polymyositis, but the clinical circumstances should not present diagnostic confusion. Although the anal sphincter is a muscle that is considered spared in ALS, it is infrequently studied as an aid in the diagnosis. Detailed needle EMG study of the anal sphincter muscles reveals some degree of denervation but less than that found in limb muscles (Carvalho et al., 1995).

Special Electrophysiological Techniques

Special clinical neurophysiological techniques can be used to aid the diagnosis of ALS (Stålberg, 1982). The WFN electrophysiological criteria list several quantitative tests that can detect chronic partial denervation (Table 72–6). Several techniques are based on the single-fiber EMG electrode. The single-fiber EMG electrode provides a detailed view of the motor unit, and can be used to show early signs of denervation and reinnervation by measuring muscle fiber density, neuromuscular jitter, and a view of the whole motor unit with macro-EMG.

Table 72–6. Special Electrophysiological Techniques to Demonstrate Chronic Partial Denervation That Supplement Routine EMG Techniques

Single-fiber electrode:
  Fiber density
  Jitter
  Macro-EMG
Concentric or monopolar electrode:
  Quantitative motor unit analysis
  Analysis of turns and amplitude
Motor unit number estimation:
  A number of techniques available

Adapted from Brooks B, Miller R, Swash M, et al., for the World Federation of Neurology Research Group on Motor Neuron Diseases: El Escorial Revisited: Revised criteria for the diagnosis of amyotrophic lateral sclerosis. Amyotrophic Lateral Sclerosis 2000;1:293–298.

FIBER DENSITY

Fiber density is a relative measurement of the density of muscle fibers in a motor unit. The recording or uptake radius of a single-fiber electrode is about 300 μm (Stålberg and Trontelj, 1994). Accordingly, in normally innervated muscle, when the single-fiber electrode is recording the action potential activity from one muscle fiber, the distribution of muscle fibers in the motor unit is such that activity from more than one fiber can be recorded less than one third of the time. Fiber density values from a muscle represent the average of 20 observations with the electrode at different positions in the muscle (Stålberg and Thiele, 1975). Normal values have been determined empirically and vary between muscles and with subject age, and average 1.15 to 1.80 (Gilchrist and Ad Hoc Committee of the AAEM Special Interest Group on Single Fiber EMG, 1992; Bromberg et al., 1994). Elevated fiber density values are felt to reflect greater numbers of fibers within the motor unit due to collateral reinnervation (Hilton-Brown et al., 1985). In ALS, increased EMG fiber density values are the first sign of denervation, before changes in routine needle EMG are recorded and before changes in muscle strength can be appreciated (Stålberg et al., 1975b). Fiber density values tend to be higher in weaker muscles and increase as muscle weakness increases, but at late stages, fiber density values can fall (Stålberg, 1982; Swash and Schwartz, 1982). The fall is felt to reflect marked loss of motor units.

JITTER

Single-fiber EMG can be used to assess neuromuscular junction transmission across individual junctions and is the most sensitive measure of transmission abnormalities. In practice, the single-fiber EMG electrode is moved close to two muscle fibers of the same motor unit (representing a fiber density of 2.0), and one fiber's action potential is used as the trigger and the variability in timing of the second fiber's action potential is measured as jitter. The jitter of the second fiber's action potential actually represents covariability of two neuromuscular junctions. Normal jitter is thought to represent the variability in the rise time of the end-plate potential (Stålberg et al., 1975a). Jitter variability is measured from 100 consecutive voluntary discharges and expressed as the mean consecutive discharge value. Mean consecutive discharge is calculated, as opposed to the simple mean variability, in order to factor out any systematic changes in jitter variability due to slow trends over the 100 discharges (Ekstedt et al., 1974). Mean consecutive discharge values are obtained from 20 observation sites in a muscle and averaged. Normal jitter values have been determined empirically, and vary among muscles and with age, and average values range from 20 to 35 μsec (Gilchrist and Ad Hoc Committee of the AAEM Special Interest Group on Single Fiber EMG, 1992; Bromberg et al., 1994). In ALS, jitter values are increased in most muscles, including those that are clinically strong (Stålberg, 1982). Jitter in ALS is felt to be abnormal because of a reduced safety factor in neuromuscular junction transmission due to fetal acetylcholine receptor subunits in reinnervated muscle. It is important to note that abnormal jitter in not specific to ALS and can be observed in any neuropathic disorder, many myopathic disorders, and defects of neuromuscular junction disorders such as myasthenia gravis and Lambert-Eaton myasthenic syndrome.

MACROELECTROMYOGRAPHY

Macro-EMG is a technique used to record the summed activity from all muscle fibers in a motor unit. Centric and monopolar EMG needle electrodes have a limited recording or uptake radius of approximately 1500 μm and record action potentials from 7 to 14 muscle fibers of a motor unit (Thiele and Böhle, 1978). To increase the recording or uptake radius, the macro-EMG electrode uses 15 mm of the cannula of a single-fiber electrode as the active electrode (the remaining proximal portion of the cannula is insulated) (Stålberg, 1980). In practice, two amplifiers and display channels are used, and the macro-EMG electrode serves as two electrodes; in one, the single-fiber port is active and the cannula is the reference, and in the other the cannula is active and a separate electrode is the reference. Under weak voluntary muscle activation, the macro-EMG electrode is adjusted to record a single muscle fiber action potential on one channel, which is used to trigger an "averager," which averages activity recorded by the cannula of the macro-EMG electrode on the second channel. The macro-EMG signal is a motor unit potential that has less distinct properties than those of the motor unit potential recorded from concentric and monopolar electrodes, and the measures of interest are macro-motor unit potential amplitude and area. In practice, 20 different macro-EMG potentials are recorded and the median value is used to reduce the influence of extreme values (Stålberg, 1980).

The macro-EMG motor unit potential amplitude is increased in approximately 50% of muscles in ALS (Stålberg, 1982). Amplitude values are normal in subjects with primary upper motor neuron signs and highest in subjects with slow progression. In serial studies, the macro-EMG potential fell in some, attributed to a collapse or decompensation of the motor unit with disease progression (Stålberg, 1982).

QUANTITATIVE ELECTROMYOGRAPHY

The technique of quantitative EMG entails the assessment of motor unit parameters of amplitude, duration, number of phases and turns, and derived parameters, such as area and area-to-amplitude ratio, in a statistically sound manner. This is in contrast to routine needle EMG studies, which rely on qualitative assessment of these parameters. Quantitative EMG relies on isolating individual motor units and accurately measuring specific parameters. Approximately 20 separate motor units are assessed, and the parameters are averaged and compared with similar data from normal subjects. The usefulness of quantitative EMG is that small differences that support chronic partial neurogenic denervation can be gathered. Initial quantitative EMG studies relied on isolating individual motor units with a delay line and manually determining the parameters of interest (Buchthal et al., 1954). The incorporation of computers into modern EMG machines has facilitated the development and use of algorithms to automatically determine and measure the parameters of interest. Algorithms are usually unique to specific EMG machines, and it has been found that automatically measured parameters from identical waveforms may differ among machines (Bromberg et al., 1999). Accordingly, before clinical importance is attributed to quantitative differences in motor unit parameters, it is important that similar data be gathered from normal subjects using the same techniques and that automatically determined parameters be checked manually. In neurogenic disorders, a comparison of many motor unit parameters indicates that amplitude is the most discriminating feature separating neurogenic from normal and myopathic disorders, and that the number of phases and turns is the feature indicating motor unit irregularity (Stewart et al., 1989; Zalewska et al., 1998). Interestingly, motor unit duration is a less sensitive discriminator, but tends to be greater in neurogenic disorders.

The expanded data analysis capability of computers in EMG machines has led to algorithms that can simultaneously identify several different motor unit waveforms from the EMG signal to facilitate acquisition of more data in less time (Stålberg et al., 1996). The process is termed motor unit decomposition or multi-motor unit analysis. Normal reference values have been reported (Bischoff et al., 1994).

INTERFERENCE PATTERN ANALYSIS

The clinical neurophysiological data discussed so far are obtained during weak voluntary muscle contraction. As muscle force increases, more motor units are recruited, and an interference pattern on the oscilloscope screen grows and becomes full. Identification of individual motor units on which to make specific measurements is no longer feasible. However, the interference pattern contains information about the number, amplitude, and complexity of motor units. Analysis of the interference pattern can identify chronic partial neurogenic denervation (Fuglsang-Frederiksen, 2000). As the interference pattern grows, the amplitude of the activity envelope increases, as does the complexity of the pattern. The complexity can be expressed as the number of turns per unit time. This has led to a formal analysis of turns versus amplitude (Stålberg et al., 1983). Turns and amplitude data have been further analyzed in a variety of ways to help distinguish myopathic from neuropathic conditions (Nandedkar et al., 1986a), and other methods of measurement have been developed (Fuglsang-Frederiksen, 2000). As might be expected in ALS, measures of amplitude are increased in many but not all interference patterns, which contrasts with myopathic disorders, in which amplitude measures are reduced or normal (Nandedkar et al., 1986b).

MOTOR UNIT NUMBER ESTIMATION

Motor unit number estimation (MUNE) is a unique electrophysiological method that can assess the number of surviving motor units innervating a muscle or group of muscles (McComas, 1991). MUNE is based on a simple ratio:

$$\frac{\text{Maximal CMAP amplitude or area}}{\text{Average single motor unit amplitude or area}}$$

Although MUNE is based on a straightforward concept, there are several assumptions that have been reviewed (McComas et al., 1971; Brown and Milner-Brown, 1976; Slawnych et al., 1990). The maximal CMAP is obtained by routine percutaneous electrical nerve stimulation. Determination of the average amplitude of a single motor unit is more problematic because single motor units have a range of sizes in both normal and denervated muscle. As a consequence, a number of different MUNE techniques have been developed to address how to obtain a suitable sample of single motor unit values from the motor unit population. Each technique has advantages and disadvantages (Slawnych et al., 1990). Most MUNE techniques are applicable to distal limb muscles, but some can be used to study proximal muscles. MUNE is an estimate, and there is no electrophysiological or anatomical method for counting the number of surviving motor neurons. Accuracy and reproducibility are important issues, and with refinement of techniques, test–retest variability is 10% or less (Shefner et al., 1999; Lomen-Hoerth and Olney, 2000). Several operational principles have emerged. The numerical value defining an abnormal MUNE is best set as a lower limit of normal, similar to CMAP amplitude lower limits of normal. Lower-limit values will differ among muscle and with different MUNE technique. MUNE reproducibility (accuracy) increases when the motor unit count is low, making the technique most appropriate in ALS (Bromberg, 1993b; Felice, 1995).

MUNE is well suited to the study of motor neuron disease because it is the only electrophysiological test unaffected by collateral reinnervation. A number of studies show that MUNE values fall before CMAP amplitude, and performing MUNE in asymptomatic muscles with normal CMAP values can be useful to document diffuse lower motor neuron loss (Felice, 1997; Yuen and Olney, 1997). Accordingly, finding low MUNE values in an asymptomatic and strong muscle can be strongly supportive of diffuse denervation.

ELECTROPHYSIOLOGY OF UPPER MOTOR NEURON LOSS

Most attention has focused on assessing changes due to lower motor neuron loss in ALS, and changes attributed to upper motor neuron loss are not apparent on routine electrophysiological testing. The recent development of techniques to stimulate the motor cortex and corticospinal neurons has provided a means to make direct electrophysiological measurements of upper motor neuron function. Activation of corticospinal neurons was originally accomplished by high-voltage transcranial stimulation (Merton and Morton, 1980), but this was painful and was supplanted by painless magnetic stimulation in which cortical neurons are activated by a collapsing large magnetic field located over the motor cortex (Barker and Jalinous, 1985). Activation of corticospinal motor neurons evokes a response in limb muscles that can be recorded as a CMAP. There are differences between the two techniques; electrical stimulation activates corticospinal neurons directly, whereas magnetic stimulation activates cortical interneurons and corticospinal neurons indirectly (Rothwell, 1991).

Transcranial magnetic stimulation can be used in the study of central conduction time and changes in excitability of both upper and lower motor neurons. The experimental procedure is to record electrical activity from intrinsic hand or distal leg muscles in response to magnetic stimulation of the motor cortex. The evoked response amplitude is enhanced and the latency reduced if the subject generates a low level of tonic voluntary motor activity in the muscles under study (Rothwell et al., 1987). Several latency measurements can be made: (1) motor evoked latency, reflecting the total conduction time from cortex to the muscle, (2) peripheral conduction time from spinal cord to the muscle, measured by stimulating at the appropriate root or derived using F-wave latencies, and (3) central motor delay, calculated by subtracting peripheral time from total time. The amplitude of the cortical evoked response can

be expressed as an absolute value or as a percentage of maximal peripheral evoked CMAP. The stimulation threshold for evoking a motor response can be expressed as a percentage of the maximal magnetic stimulator output.

In ALS, transcranial magnetic stimulation has been used to document upper motor neuron involvement. The yield of finding an abnormal measure depends in part on the number of muscles studied in the arm and leg and the number of measures assessed (Eisen et al., 1990b; Triggs et al., 2000). Abnormal measures include an inability to evoke a response, modest but significantly prolonged motor evoked latencies, low-amplitude evoked responses, and stimulation threshold. Interestingly, central motor delay is not significantly different from that noted in normal subjects. There are technical issues in measuring central and peripheral conduction times, but with these issues in mind, 70% to 100% of ALS subjects have at least one abnormal measure (Eisen et al., 1990a; Triggs et al., 2000). An important group of patients in whom transcranial magnetic stimulation can be helpful is those with equivocal clinical upper motor neuron signs in the form of incongruously brisk tendon reflexes who do not fulfill WFN criteria for definite upper motor neuron signs (see Table 72–3) (Younger et al., 1990). Among 40 patients with equivocal upper motor neuron signs, 75% had abnormalities on transcranial magnetic stimulation and thus could fulfill diagnostic criteria for probable or definite ALS (Triggs et al., 2000).

Transcranial magnetic stimulation can be used to assess synaptic excitability of upper and lower motor neurons. The cortical influence on lower motor neuron excitability can be measured by estimating the change in probability of lower motor neuron firing to voluntary activation following a transcranial conditioning impulse (Day et al., 1989). The experimental procedure is to record voluntary activity from a single motor unit with a needle EMG electrode and then apply transcranial stimulation pulses at random times. An enhanced probability of motor unit discharge occurs approximately 20 msec after the conditioning pulse; it is detected as a peak in the peristimulus histogram. This early level of excitation is felt to reflect a compound monosynaptic excitatory postsynaptic potential from faster conducting corticospinal fibers. Furthermore, the magnitude of the potential is felt to reflect the number of connections between upper motor and lower motor neurons (Eisen et al., 1996). In normal subjects, there is an age-dependent, linear decrease in the potential amplitude thought to reflect upper motor neuron attrition or dysfunction. In most ALS subjects, excitatory potentials are lower than expected for age or are absent. However, in some ALS subjects, the potentials are larger than normal. The reduced amplitude is interpreted as indicating a decrease in the number of functioning upper motor neurons, whereas the increased amplitude is interpreted as possibly reflecting enhanced cortical excitability (Eisen et al., 1996).

The question of enhanced cortical excitability has been studied further by delivering pairs of transcortical magnetic stimuli in a condition-test paradigm (Enterzari-Taher et al., 1997). In normal subjects a condition-test stimulation interval of 30 msec results in marked inhibition of the test excitatory postsynaptic potential by the conditioning stimulus. In ALS subjects, the test excitatory postsynaptic potential is not reduced, and in many subjects is larger than the conditioning excitatory postsynaptic potential (Enterzari-Taher et al., 1997). The observed dysinhibition could be due to a failure of cortical inhibition leading to increased excitation. A mechanism for increased excitability has been advanced based on overactivity of the glutamatergic excitatory system in the cortex (Eisen et al., 1992).

DIFFERENTIAL DIAGNOSIS

The differential diagnosis of ALS is a challenging issue. There is now emphasis on early diagnosis (Bromberg, 1999a), with both advantages and disadvantages (Gelinas, 2000; Smith, 2000), but an accurate diagnosis is essential. When clinical evidence points to ALS, there is the hope of a treatable disorder or an alternative diagnosis with a better prognosis, and this can lead to extensive laboratory tests. The WFN diagnostic criteria provide an algorithm, and although designed for uniformity in clinical trials, the algorithm can be used in the clinic. However, the criteria can be complex in their interpretation and leave a number of clinical situations undiagnosed (Belsh, 2000). The WFN criteria can at least serve as a guideline. Perhaps the most important clinical tool is time, for motor neuron disease, whether classic ALS or another form, is uniquely progressive. If a firm diagnosis is not made and no other diagnosis is apparent from the history, repeating the examination and the electrophysiological studies in 3 to 6 months is the most appropriate approach.

It is important to consider the differential diagnosis from a conservative perspective (Bromberg, 1999a). Many diagnostic tests focus on general medical issues. Other are based on clinical vignettes of patients who appeared to have ALS, but had another disorder. Review of these cases indicates failure to meet WFN criteria. An ever-growing number of laboratory tests leads to the likelihood of finding abnormalities that are more likely to reflect chance associations than a pathological link to ALS (Gudesblatt et al., 1988; Rowland et al., 1992; Jackson et al., 1998). The differential diagnosis is reviewed here from four perspectives. Experience with the WFN criteria has accrued and their diagnostic accuracy can be assessed. There are a number of diseases that superficially resemble ALS that need to be considered during every diagnostic evaluation, and these are also reviewed. Past experience with erroneous diagnoses can be informative and is considered as false initial positive diagnosis (when the diagnosis was changed from ALS to another disease) and false initial negative diagnosis (when the diagnosis was changed from another disease to ALS). While most of the emphasis has been on the former, avoidance of false-negative diagnosis is important because it can lead to unwarranted patient hopes, expensive diagnostic tests, and unnecessary surgery.

Diagnostic Accuracy of World Federation of Neurology Criteria

The WFN criteria appear to provide a high degree of accuracy, although large-scale postmortem reviews have not been performed. In one retrospective study of autopsy-confirmed cases, diagnostic accuracy was complete, and it took an average of 29 months (± 20 months) to reach the El Escorial "definite" level of diagnostic certainty from symptom onset (Gaffney et al., 1992).

In a drug trial in which reduced WFN criteria (possible ALS-laboratory supported, discussed above) were used, no patient among 483 who completed at least 5 months of observation had his or her diagnosis changed (Ross et al., 1998).

Lower Motor Neuropathies

A number of immune-mediated lower motor neuropathies may be treatable with immunosuppressive drugs (Pestronk, 1998). The motor neuropathy most likely to mimic ALS is multifocal motor neuropathy with conduction block because it produces an asymmetrical distribution of weakness and is associated with cramps and fasciculations (Pestronk et al., 1988). Sites of motor conduction block are located away from common entrapment sites. True conduction block is to be distinguished from apparent conduction block due to abnormal temporal dispersion (Cornblath et al., 1991). Criteria have been developed to identify true conduction block, and they include a CMAP amplitude reduction between distal and proximal stimulation sites of 50% or more, and an increase in the negative peak CMAP duration of less than 30% (Lange et al., 1992). Further experience with multifocal motor neuropathy has revealed examples of patients with typical clinical features of multifocal motor neuropathy but without demonstrable conduction block (Pakiam and Parry, 1998). Many patients with multifocal conduction block neuropathy have elevated titers of anti-G_{M1} ganglioside antibodies (Sadiq et al., 1990; Kornberg and Pestronk, 1994). Another disorder with asymmetrical weakness but no conduction block that may mimic ALS is lower motor neuron syndrome (Pestronk et al., 1994). This is a slowly progressive disorder with muscle atrophy and cramps affecting distal limb muscles. These motor neuropathies rarely include sensory symptoms or signs, but exceptions have been reported with multifocal conduction block neuropathy (Valls-Solé et al., 1995). Suspicion for or against motor neuropathies should come from clinical and electrophysiological findings. Multifocal conduction block and lower motor neuron syndromes are very slowly progressive and do not have the momentum of ALS with progression within a region and to other regions. Furthermore, these motor neuropathies produce no upper motor neuron signs, and tendon reflexes are reduced or absent (Pestronk, 1998).

Inflammatory Muscle Disease

Inclusion body myositis is an inflammatory muscle disease that may be confused with ALS. The similarities are that inclusion body myositis, unlike other forms of myositis, has an insidious onset, and asymmetrical distribution of weakness that may begin in distal upper extremity muscles, and is associated with muscle atrophy (Amato et al., 1996). Furthermore, needle EMG shows evidence for active denervation in a diffuse distribution, and motor units may have features suggesting a neurogenic pattern. However, inclusion body myositis does not produce upper motor neuron signs, and the electromyogram includes myopathic motor units (Luciano and Dalakas, 1997; Barkhaus et al., 1999).

False-Positive Diagnoses

Alternative diagnoses focus on treatable disorders. In reviewing the literature on false-positive diagnoses, the clinical descriptions lack upper motor neuron findings, steady progression, and diffuse neurogenic denervation (Caroscio, 1986; Tucker et al., 1991). Immune-mediated motor neuropathies, including multifocal motor conduction block neuropathies and lower motor neuron syndromes, do not produce upper motor neuron symptoms and signs. Kennedy's disease (bulbospinal neuronopathy) is an X-linked form of motor neuron disease (Kennedy et al., 1968). However, it lacks upper motor neuron findings, both on examination and by cortical evoked testing (Weber and Eisen, 1999), and is associated with sensory nerve abnormalities (Ferrante and Wilbourn, 1997). In patients with equivocally brisk tendon reflexes (incongruously brisk reflexes or "possible upper motor neuron signs"), the diagnosis is challenging. However, the diagnostically important issue is progression of weakness within a region and to other regions.

False-Negative Diagnoses

Initial false-negative diagnoses are common, but the clinician making the diagnosis of ALS following an extensive workup by others has the advantage of seeing the disease at a later stage. A review of initial diagnoses frequently reveals that only a narrow differential was entertained (Belch and Schiffman,

1990). For example, slowly progressive hand weakness is mistaken for carpal tunnel syndrome despite atrophy of the first dorsal interosseous muscle, or slowly progressive footdrop is mistaken for an L4-L5 radiculopathy. The missing diagnostic element is accurate anatomical localization and careful clinical examination that would reveal diffuse muscle atrophy and upper motor neuron signs or diffuse denervation on needle EMG.

CLINICAL NEUROPHYSIOLOGICAL MEASUREMENT OF AMYOTROPHIC LATERAL SCLEROSIS PROGRESSION AND PROGNOSIS

Disease Progression

Clinical neurophysiological tests are used primarily to make the diagnosis of ALS. Serial testing is important to document diffuse denervation when the diagnosis is not secure because initial studies show denervation restricted to one or two regions. After the diagnosis is made, progression is usually monitored qualitatively by assessing a patient's functional abilities and measuring muscle strength. Quantitative measurement of disease progression is important in clinical trials in ALS, and is considered in detail elsewhere. The sensitivity of clinical neurophysiological testing for disease progression is an issue. Needle EMG is sensitive to the presence of denervation, and permits a choice of muscles to test to exclude focal lesions. However, needle EMG does not lend itself to quantification of the degree of denervation as a measure of progression. CMAP amplitude is an appropriate measure, but amplitude is influenced by the compensatory effects of collateral reinnervation and the technical issue of reproducible placement of the recording electrodes (Bromberg and Spiegelberg, 1997). Serial CMAP studies show a decline in amplitude over time, but there is a high degree of variability for individual patients, making CMAP measurements less sensitive (Kelly et al., 1990). A combination of electrophysiological measures have been proposed as an "ALS neurophysiological index" (de Carvalho and Swash, 2000).

Few data are available on comparisons between MVIC with clinical neurophysiological test data. Most MVIC data represent megascores from many muscles providing a global assessment, and few studies make comparisons between clinical neurophysiological tests and MVIC from the same muscle. A cross-sectional study comparing a number of clinical neurophysiological tests with MVIC in the biceps brachii muscle shows little correlation among them, attributable to the fact that each test looks at a different aspect of the disease state (Bromberg et al., 1993). A longitudinal study of 68 subjects making similar comparisons over 6 months found changes expected for progression, but changes were mild and not statistically significant over the time period (Bromberg et al., 2001).

MUNE may be the most sensitive clinical neurophysiological test to measure disease progression because it is uninfluenced by collateral reinnervation and measures the primary pathological process of lower motor neuron loss (Bromberg, 1998). MUNE values have been found to fall in a muscle before CMAP amplitude (Felice, 1997). Serial MUNE studies have shown that the rate of lower motor neuron loss is exponential, with an initial rapid loss followed by a slower rate of loss (Brown and Jaatoul, 1974; Galea et al., 1991). This is in distinction to serial MVIC studies plotting megascores that suggest that motor neuron loss is linear, at least over a middle portion of the disease course (Munsat et al., 1988). The compensatory effects of collateral reinnervation preserving strength early in the course of the disease could account for different time courses measured by MUNE and MVIC. Computer models of the effects of collateral reinnervation on strength support an exponential rate of motor neuron loss (Kuether and Lipinski, 1988).

Prognosis

Predicting rates of progression or survival in ALS is challenging because the rate of motor neuron loss varies widely among ALS patients, as reflected in the range of rates of loss of strength and survival times (Pradas et al., 1993; Mitsumoto et al., 1998). There are also external variables related to survival, such as use of gastric feeding tubes and noninvasive ventilation. One effort to predict survival is based on a composite score including age of patient, duration of weakness, and degree of disability. Using data from 194 patients, a table of 25th, 50th, and 75th percentiles was constructed for making predictions (Jablecki, 1989). In another study using MUNE as a measure of lower motor neuron loss, patients whose MUNE values recorded from the hypothenar muscle group fell rapidly over 3 months had life expectancies shorter than those of patients whose values fell slowly (Yuen and Olney, 1997). A further effort incorporates MUNE values into a mathematical model of linear estimates of rates of disease progression to predict survival (Armon and Brandstater, 1999). Clinical drug trial databases are useful to identify predictors of survival but have not included clinical neurophysiological data. Several ongoing clinical trials include clinical neurophysiological tests, and assessment of these measures for prognosis will be available in the future. At this time, each ALS patient must be considered individually to assess disease progression.

SUMMARY

Clinical neurophysiology is a powerful tool for assessing lower motor neuron loss. Since lower motor neuron loss is the principal clinical feature of ALS, electrophysiology has a prominent role in the diagnosis of ALS. The WFN has published a set of criteria for the diagnosis of ALS that includes a subset of electrophysiological criteria. These criteria have been reviewed after several years of experience and have been found to be effective in giving an accurate diagnosis. The electrophysiological criteria focus on the needle EMG study to demonstrate ongoing neurogenic denervation. Other electrophysiological tests are helpful in providing evidence for denervation but are less specific for neurogenic denervation. Measuring progression by clinical neurophysiological testing is difficult because the compensatory effects of collateral reinnervation blunt the changes caused by lower motor neuron loss. MUNE is a unique electrophysiological test that can estimate the number of surviving lower motor neurons innervating a muscle, and it is well suited for following disease progression. Clinical neurophysiological measurement of upper motor neuron loss is challenging. Several techniques can demonstrate the effects of upper motor neuron loss, but they represent indirect measurements and require special magnetic stimulators and data analysis capabilities.

References

Al-Chalabi A,S Andersen P, Nilsson P, et al: Deletions of the heavy neurofilament subunit tail in amyotrophic lateral sclerosis. Hum Mol Genet 1999;8:157–164.

Alexianu M, Ho B-K, Mohamed A, et al: The role of calcium-binding proteins in selective motor neuron vulnerability in amyotrophic lateral sclerosis. Ann Neurol 1994;36:846–858.

Amato A, Gronseth G, Jackson C, et al: Inclusion body myositis: Clinical and pathologic boundaries. Ann Neurol 1996;40:581–586.

Andersen P, Forsgren L, Binzer M, et al: Autosomal recessive adult-onset amyotrophic lateral sclerosis associated with homozygosity for Asp90Ala CuZn-superoxide dismutase mutation. A clinical and genealogical study of 36 patients. Brain 1996;119:1153–1172.

Andreassen S, Rosenfalck A: Impaired regulation of the firing pattern of single motor units. Muscle Nerve 1978;1:416–418.

Aoki M, Lin C, Rothstein J, et al: Mutations in the glutamate transporter EAAT2 gene do not cause abnormal EAAT2 transcripts in amyotrophic lateral sclerosis. Ann Neurol 1998;43:645–653.

Armon C, Brandstater M: Motor unit number estimate–based rates of progression of ALS predict patient survival. Muscle Nerve 1999;22:1572–1575.

Barker A, Jalinous R: Non-invasive magnetic stimulation of human motor cortex. Lancet 1985;1:1106–1107.

Barkhaus P, Periquet M, Nandedkar S: Quantitative electrophysiologic studies in sporadic inclusion body myositis. Muscle Nerve 1999;22:480–487.

Barohn R, Sahenk Z, Warmolts J, Mendell J: The Burns-Garland syndrome (diabetic amyotrophy). Revisited 100 years later. Arch Neurol 1991;48:1130–1135.

Beal M: Mitochondria and the pathogenesis of ALS. Brain 2000; 123:1291–1292.

Beal M, Ferrante R, Browne S, et al: Increased 3-nitrotyrosine in both sporadic and familial amyotrophic lateral sclerosis. Ann Neurol 1997;42:646–654.

Belch J, Schiffman P: Misdiagnosis in patients with amyotrophic lateral sclerosis. Arch Intern Med 1990;150:2301–2305.

Belsh JM: ALS diagnostic criteria of El Escorial Revisited: do they meet the needs of clinicians as well as researchers? Amyotrophic Lateral Sclerosis 2000;1(suppl 1):S57–S60.

Bernstein L, Antel J: Motor neuron disease: Decremental response to repetitive nerve stimulation. Neurology 1981;31:202–204.

Bischoff C, Stålberg E, Falck B, Eeg-Olofsson K: Reference values of motor unit action potentials obtained with multi-MUAP analysis. Muscle Nerve 1994;17:842–851.

Bradley W, Good P, Rasool C, Adelman L: Morphometric and biochemical studies of peripheral nerves in amyotrophic lateral sclerosis. Ann Neurol 1983;14:267–277.

Bromberg M: Electromyographic (EMG) findings in denervation. Crit Rev Phys Rehabil Med 1993a;5:83–127.

Bromberg M: Motor unit estimation: Reproducibility of the spike-triggered averaging technique in normal and ALS subjects. Muscle Nerve 1993b;16:466–471.

Bromberg M: Electrodiagnostic studies in clinical trials for motor neuron disease. J Clin Neurophysiol 1998;15:117–128.

Bromberg M: Accelerating the diagnosis of amyotrophic lateral sclerosis. The Neurologist 1999a;5:63–74.

Bromberg M: Pathogenesis of amyotrophic lateral sclerosis: A critical review. Curr Opin Neurobiol 1999b;12:581–588.

Bromberg M, Scott D, Ad Hoc Committee of the AAEM Single Fiber Special Interest Group: Single fiber EMG reference values: Reformatted in tabular form. Muscle Nerve 1994;17:820–821.

Bromberg M, Spiegelberg T: The influence of active electrode placement on CMAP amplitude. Electroencephalogr Clin Neurophysiol 1997;105:385–389.

Bromberg M, Smith A, Bauerle J: A comparison of two commercial quantitative electromyographic algorithms with manual analysis. Muscle Nerve 1999;22:1244–1248.

Bromberg M, Fries T, Forshew D, Tandan R: Electrophysiologic endpoint measures in a multi-center ALS drug trial. J Neurol Sci 2001;184:51–55.

Bromberg M, Forshew D, Nau K, et al: Unit number estimation, isometric strength, and electromyographic measures in amyotrophic lateral sclerosis. Muscle Nerve 1993;16:1213–1219.

Brooks B, Depaul R, Tan Y, et al: Motor neuron disease. In Porter R, Schoenberg B (eds): Controlled Clinical Trials in Neurological Disease. Norwell, MA, Kluwer Academic, 1990; 249–281.

Brooks B, Miller R, Swash M, Munsat T, for the World Federation of Neurology Research Group on Motor Neuron Diseases: El Escorial revisited: Revised criteria for the diagnosis of amyotrophic lateral sclerosis. Amyotrophic Lateral Sclerosis 2000; 1:293–299.

Brown R: Superoxide dismutase and familial amyotrophic lateral sclerosis: New insights into mechanisms and treatments. Ann Neurol 1996;39:145–146.

Brown W, Jaatoul N: Amyotrophic lateral sclerosis. Electrophysiologic study (number of motor units and rate of decay of motor units). Arch Neurol 1974;30:242–248.

Brown W, Milner-Brown H: Some electrical properties of motor units and their effects on the methods of estimating motor unit numbers. J Neurol Neurosurg Psychiatry 1976;39:249–257.

Buchthal F, Pinelli P: Action potentials in muscular atrophy of neurogenic origin. Neurology 1953;3:591–603.

Buchthal F, Rosenfalck P: Spontaneous electrical activity of human muscle. Electroencephalogr Clin Neurophysiol 1966;20:321–336.

Buchthal F, Guld C, Rosenfalck P: Action potential parameters in normal human muscle and their dependence on physical variables. Acta Physiol Scand 1954;32:200–218.

Caroscio J: Amyotrophic lateral sclerosis: The disease. In Caroscio J (ed): Amyotrophic Lateral Sclerosis. A Guide to Patient Care. New York: Thieme Medical Publishers, Inc, 1986; 2–15.

Carpenter S: Proximal axonal enlargement in motor neuron disease. Neurology 1968;18:841–851.

Carvalho M, Schwartz M, Swash M: Involvement of the external anal sphincter in amyotrophic lateral sclerosis. Muscle Nerve 1995;18:848–853.

Cassarino D, Bennett J: An evaluation of the role of mitochondria in neurodegenerative diseases: Mitochondrial mutations and oxidative pathology, protective nuclear responses, and cell death in neurodegeneration. Brain Research Review 1999;29:1–25.

Choi D: Glutamate neurotoxicity and diseases of the nervous system. Neuron 1988;1:623–634.

Conradi S, Ronnevi L, Norris F: Motor neuron disease and toxic

metals. In Roland L (ed): Advances in Neurology: Human Motor Neuron Disease. Vol 36. New York, Raven Press, 1982; 201–231.

Cornblath D, Kuncl R, Mellits E, et al: Nerve conduction studies in amyotrophic lateral sclerosis. Muscle Nerve 1992;15:1111–1115.

Cornblath D, Sumner A, Daube J, et al: Conduction block in clinical practice. Muscle Nerve 1991;14:869–871.

Coyle J, Puttfarcken P: Oxidative stress, glutamate, and neurodegenerative disorders. Science 1993;262:689–695.

Cudkowicz M, McKenna-Yasek D, Chen C, et al: Limited corticospinal tract involvement in amyotrophic lateral sclerosis subjects with the A4V mutation in the copper/zinc superoxide dismutase gene. Ann Neurol 1998;43:703–710.

Czekajewski J, Ekstedt J, Stålberg E: Oscilloscopic recording of muscle fiber action potentials. The window trigger and the delay unit. Electroencephalogr Clin Neurophyisiol 1969;27:536–539.

Day B, Dressleer D, Maertens de Noordhout A, et al: Electric and magnetic stimulation of human motor cortex: Surface EMG and single motor unit responses. J Physiol 1989;412:449–473.

de Carvalho M: Pathophysiological significance of fasciculation in the early diagnosis of ALS. Amyotrophic Lateral Sclerosis 2000;1(suppl 1):S43–S46.

de Carvalho M, Swash M: Fasciculation potentials: A study of amyotrophic lateral sclerosis and other neurogenic disorders. Muscle Nerve 1998;21:336–344.

de Carvalho M, Swash M: Nerve conduction studies in amyotrophic lateral sclerosis. Muscle Nerve 2000;23:344–352.

de Carvalho M, Bentes C, Evangelista T, Luis M: Fibrillation and sharp-waves: Do we need them to diagnose ALS? Amyotrophic Lateral Sclerosis 1999;1:29–32.

Denys E, Forbes F: Amyotrophic lateral sclerosis: Impairment of neuromuscular transmission. Arch Neurol 1979;36:202–205.

Desmedt J, Borenstein S: Relationship of spontaneous fibrillation potentials to muscle fibre segmentation in human muscular dystrophy. Nature 1975;258:531–534.

Dorfman L, Howard J, McGill K: Motor unit firing rates and firing rate variability in the detection of neuromuscular disorders. Electroencephalogr Clin Neurophyisiol 1989;73:215–224.

Dubowitz V: Muscle Biopsy: A Practical Approach. London, Baillière, 1985.

Dumitru D: Single muscle fiber discharges (insertional activity, end-plate potentials, positive sharp waves, and fibrillation potentials): A unifying proposal. Muscle Nerve 1996;19:221–226.

Eisen A, Enterzari-Taher M, Stewart H: Cortical projections to spinal motoneurons: Changes with aging and amyotrophic lateral sclerosis. Neurology 1996;46:1396–1404.

Eisen A, Kim S, Pant B: Amyotrophic lateral sclerosis (ALS): A phylogenetic disease of the corticomotoneuron? Muscle Nerve 1992;15:219–228.

Eisen A, Shytbel W, Murphy K, Hoirch M: Cortical magnetic stimulation in amyotrophic lateral sclerosis. Muscle Nerve 1990a; 13:146–151.

Eisen A, Shytbel W, Murry K, Hoirch M: Cortical magnetic stimulation in amyotrophic lateral sclerosis. Muscle Nerve 1990b; 13:146–151.

Ekstedt J, Nilsson G, Stålberg E: Calculation of the electromyographic jitter. J Neurol Neurosurg Psychiatry 1974;37:526–539.

Enterzari-Taher M, Eisen A, Stewart H, Nakajima M: Abnormalities of cortical inhibitory neurons in amyotrophic lateral sclerosis. Muscle Nerve 1997;20:65–71.

Feinberg D, Preston D, Shefner J, Logigian E: Amplitude-dependent slowing of conduction in amyotrophic lateral sclerosis and polyneuropathy. Muscle Nerve 1999;22:937–940.

Feinstein B, Lindegård B, Nyman E, Wohlfart G: Morphologic studies of motor units in normal human muscle. Acta Anat 1955;23:127–143.

Felice K: Thenar motor unit number estimates using the multiple point stimulation technique: Reproducibility studies in ALS patients and normal subjects. Muscle Nerve 1995;18:1412–1416.

Felice K: A longitudinal study comparing thenar motor unit number estimates to other quantitative tests in patients with amyotrophic lateral sclerosis. Muscle Nerve 1997;20:179–185.

Ferrante M, Wilbourn A: The characteristic electrodiagnostic features of Kennedy's disease. Muscle Nerve 1997;20:323–329.

Finsterer J, Erdorf M, Mamoli B, Fuglsang-Frederiksen A: Needle electromyography of bulbar muscles in patients. Neurology 1998;51:1417–1422.

Fuglsang-Frederiksen A: The utility of interference pattern analysis. Muscle Nerve 2000;23:18–36.

Gaffney J, Sufit R, Hartman H, et al: Clinical diagnosis of amyotrophic lateral sclerosis (ALS): A clinicopathologic study of "El Escorial" Working Group criteria in 36 autopsied patients. Neurology 1992;42(suppl 3):455.

Galea V, DeBruin H, Cavasin R, McComas A: The numbers and relative sizes of motor units estimated by computer. Muscle Nerve 1991;14:1123–1130.

Gaudette M, Hiranol M, Siddique T: Current status of SOD1 mutations in familial amyotrophic lateral sclerosis. Amyotrophic Lateral Sclerosis 2000;1:83–89.

Gelinas D: Effects of the early diagnosis of amyotrophic lateral sclerosis on the patient: Advantages. Amyotrophic Lateral Sclerosis 2000;1(suppl 1):S73–S74.

Gilchrist JC, Ad Hoc Committee of the AAEM Special Interest Group on Single Fiber EMG: Single fiber EMG reference values: A collaborative effort. Muscle Nerve 1992;15:151–161.

Glasberg M, Wiley C: Pathology-muscle and nerve. In Smith R (ed): Handbook of Amyotrophic Lateral Sclerosis. New York, Marcel Dekker, 1992; 193–208.

Goetz C: Amyotrophic lateral sclerosis: Early contributions of Jean-Martin Charcot. Muscle Nerve 2000;23:336–343.

Gordon P, Rowland L, Younger D, et al: Lymphoproliferative disorders and motor neuron disease: An update. Neurology 1997; 48:1672–1678.

Gudesblatt K, Ludman M, Cohen J, et al: Hexosaminidase A activity and amyotrophic lateral sclerosis. Muscle Nerve 1988;11: 227–230.

Gurney M: The use of transgenic mouse models of amyotrophic lateral sclerosis in preclinical drug studies. J Neurol Sci 1997; 152(suppl 1):S67–S73.

Hayashi H, Kato S: Total manifestations of amyotrophic lateral sclerosis. J Neurol Sci 1989;93:19–35.

Hilton-Brown P, Nandedkar S, Stålberg E: Simulation of fibre density in single-fibre electromyography and its relationship to macro-EMG. Med Biol Eng Comput 1985;23:541–546.

Honig L, Chambliss D, Bigio E, et al: Glutamate transporter EAAT2 splice variants occur not only in ALS, but also in AD and controls. Neurology 2000;55:1082–8.

Jablecki C: Survival prediction in amyotrophic lateral sclerosis. Muscle Nerve 1989;12:833–841.

Jackson C, Amato A, Bryan W, et al: Primary hyperparathyroidism and ALS. Neurology 1998;50:1795–1799.

Kelly J, Thibodeau L, Andres P, Finison L: Use of electrophysiologic tests to measure disease progression in ALS therapeutic trials. Muscle Nerve 1990;13:472–479.

Kennedy W, Alter M, Sung J: Progressive proximal spinal and bulbar muscular atrophy of late onset: A sex-linked recessive trait. Neurology 1968;18:672–80.

Kent-Braun J, Walker C, Weiner M, Miller R: Functional significance of upper and lower motor neuron impairment in amyotrophic lateral sclerosis. Muscle Nerve 1998;21:762–768.

Kent-Braun J, Sharma K, Weiner M, et al: Central basis of muscle fatigue in chronic fatigue syndrome. Neurology 1993;43:125–131.

Killian M, Wilfong A, Burnett L, et al: Decremental motor responses to repetitive nerve stimulation in ALS. Muscle Nerve 1994;17:747–754.

Klivenyi P, Ferrante R, Matthews R, et al: Neuroprotective effects of creatine in a transgenic animal model of amyotrophic lateral sclerosis. Nat Med 1999;5:347–350.

Kornberg A, Pestronk A: The clinical and diagnostic role of anti-GM1 antibody testing. Muscle Nerve 1994;17:100–104.

Kraft G: Are fibrillation potentials and positive sharp waves the same? No. Muscle Nerve 1996;19:216–220.

Kuether G, Lipinski H-G: Computer Simulation of Neuron Degeneration in Motor Neuron Disease. New York, Elsevier, 1988.

Kugelberg E, Edström L, Abbruzzese M: Mapping of motor units in experimentally reinnervated rat muscle. J Neurol Neurosurg Psychiatry 1970;33:319–329.

Kuncl R, Cornblath D, Griffin J: Assessment of thoracic paraspinal muscles in the diagnosis of ALS. Muscle Nerve 1988;11:484–492.

Kuwabara S, Mizobuchi K, Ogawara K, Hattori T: Dissociated hand muscle involvement in amyotrophic lateral sclerosis detected by motor unit number estimates. Muscle Nerve 1999;22:870–873.

Kuypers H: Anatomy of the descending pathways. In Brookhart J, Mountcastle V, Brooks V (eds): Handbook of Physiology, Sect. 1, Vol. 2, Part 1. Bethesda, MD, American Physiological Society, 1981; 597–666.

Lambert E, Mulder D: Electromyographic studies in amyotrophic lateral sclerosis. Mayo Clin Proc 1957;32:441–446.

Lange D, Trojaborg W, Latov N, et al: Multifocal motor neuropathy with conduction block: Is it a distinct clinical entity? Neurology 1992;42:497–505.

Lawyer T, Netsky M: Amyotrophic lateral sclerosis. Arch Neurol Psychiatry 1953;69:172–192.

Lin C-LG, Bristol L, Jin L, et al: Aberrant RNA processing in a neurodegenerative disease: The cause of absent EAAT2, a glutamate transporter, in amyotrophic lateral sclerosis. Neuron 1998;20:589–602.

Lindstrom J: Acetylcholine receptors and myasthenia. Muscle Nerve 2000;23:453–477.

Lomen-Hoerth C, Olney R: Comparison of multiple-point and statistical motor unit number estimation. Muscle Nerve 2000;23: 1525–1533.

Luciano C, Dalakas M: Inclusion body myositis: No evidence for a neurogenic component. Neurology 1997;48:29–33.

Mannen T, Iwata M, Toyokura Y, Nagashima K: Preservation of a certain motoneurone group of the sacral cord in amyotrophic lateral sclerosis: Its clinical significance. J Neurol Neurosurg Psychiatry 1977;40:464–469.

McComas A: Invited review: Motor unit estimation: Methods, results, and present status. Muscle Nerve 1991;14:585–597.

McComas A, Fawcett P, Campbell M, Sica R: Electrophysiological estimation of the number of motor units within a human muscle. J Neurol Neurosurg Psychiatry 1971;34:121–131.

Merton P, Morton H: Stimulation of the cerebral cortex in the intact human subject. Nature 1980;285:227.

Miller R, Sherratt M: Firing rates of human motor units in partially denervated muscle. Neurology 1978;28:1241–1248.

Mitchell J: Amyotrophic lateral sclerosis: Toxins and environment. Amyotrophic Lateral Sclerosis 2000;1:235–250.

Mitsumoto H, Chad D, Pioro E: Amyotrophic Lateral Sclerosis. Philadelphia, FA Davis, 1998.

Mizutani T, Aki M, Shiozawa R, et al: Development of ophthalmoplegia in amyotrophic lateral sclerosis during long-term use of respirators. J Neurol Sci 1990;99:311–319.

Mondelli M, Rossi A, Passero S, Guazzi G: Involvement of peripheral sensory fibers in amyotrophic lateral sclerosis: Electrophysiological study of 64 cases. Muscle Nerve 1993;16:166–172.

Moore S, Gresham L, Bromberg M, et al: A self-report measure of affective lability. J Neurol Neurosurg Psychiatry 1997;63:89–93.

Munsat T, Andres P, Finison L, et al: The natural history of motoneuron loss in amyotrophic lateral sclerosis. Neurology 1988; 38:409–413.

Nandedkar S, Sanders D: Measurement of the amplitude of the EMG envelope. Muscle Nerve 1990;13:933–938.

Nandedkar S, Sanders D: Recording characteristics of monopolar EMG electrodes. Muscle Nerve 1991;14:108–112.

Nandedkar S, Sanders D, Stålberg E: Automatic analysis of the electromyographic interference pattern. Part I: Development of quantitative features. Muscle Nerve 1986a;9:431–439.

Nandedkar S, Sanders D, Stålberg S: Automatic analysis of the electromyographic interference pattern. Part II: Findings in control subjects and in some neuromuscular diseases. Muscle Nerve 1986b;9:491–500.

Nandedkar S, Sanders D, Stålberg E: EMG of reinnervated motor units: A simulation study. Electroencephalogr Clin Neurophysiol 1988;70:177–184.

Nandedkar S, Barkhaus P, Danders D, Stålberg E: Some observations on fibrillations and positive sharp waves. Muscle Nerve 2000;23:888–894.

Pakiam A, Parry G: Multifocal motor neuropathy without overt conduction block. Muscle Nerve 1998;21:243–245.

Parhad I, Clark A, Barron K, Staunton S: Diaphragmatic paralysis in motor neuron disease. Neurology 1978;28:18–22.

Partanen J, Nousiainen U: Motor unit potentials in mildly affected muscle in amyotrophic lateral sclerosis. J Neurol Sci 1990; 95:193–199.

Pestronk A: Multifocal motor neuropathy: Diagnosis and treatment. Neurology 1998;51(suppl 5):S22–S24.

Pestronk A, Cornblath D, Ilyas A, et al: A treatable multifocal motor neuropathy with antibodies to GM1 ganglioside. Neurology 1988;24:73–78.

Pestronk A, Lopate G, Kornberg A, et al: Distal lower motor neuron syndrome with high-titer serum IgM anti-GM1 antibodies: Improvement following immunotherapy with monthly plasma exchange and intravenous cyclophosphamide. Neurology 1994;44:2027–2031.

Petajan J: Clinical electromyographic studies of diseases of the motor unit. Electroencephalogr Clin Neurophyisiol 1974;36: 395–401.

Pradas J, Finison L, Andres P, et al: The natural history of amyotrophic lateral sclerosis and the use of natural history controls in therapeutic trials. Neurology 1993;43:751–755.

Preston D, Shapiro B, Raynor E: The relative value of facial, glossal, and masticatory muscles in the electrodiagnosis of amyotrophic lateral sclerosis. Muscle Nerve 1997;20:370–372.

Rosen D, Siddique T, Patterson D, et al: Mutations in Cu/Zn superoxide dismutase gene are associated with familial amyotrophic lateral sclerosis. Nature 1993;362:59–62.

Ross M, Miller R, Berchert L, et al: Toward earlier diagnosis of amyotrophic lateral sclerosis: Revised criteria. Neurology 1998; 50:768–772.

Roth G: The origin of fasciculations. Ann Neurol 1982;12:542–547.

Rothstein J: Excitotoxicity hypothesis. Neurology 1996;47(suppl 2):S19–S26.

Rothstein J, Jen L, Dykes-Hoberg M, Kuncl R: Chronic inhibition of glutamate uptake produces a model of slow neurotoxicity. Proc Natl Acad Sci USA 1993;90:6591–6595.

Rothstein J, Van Kammen M, Levey A, et al: Selective loss of glial glutamate transporter GLT-1 in amyotrophic lateral sclerosis. Ann Neurol 1995;38:73–84.

Rothwell J: Physiological studies of electrical and magnetic stimulation of the human brain. Electroencephalogr Clin Neurophysiol 1991;43(suppl):29–35.

Rothwell J, Thompson P, Day B, et al: Motor cortex stimulation in intact man. I. General characteristics of EMG responses in different muscles. Brain 1987;110:1173–1190.

Rowland L: What's in a name? Amyotrophic lateral sclerosis, motor neuron disease, and allelic heterogeneity. Ann Neurol 1998;43:691–693.

Rowland L, Sherman W, Latov N, et al: Amyotrophic lateral sclerosis and lymphoma: Bone marrow examination and other diagnostic tests. Neurology 1992;42:1101–1102.

Sadiq S, Thomas F, Kilidireas K, et al: The spectrum of neurologic disease associated with anti-GM1 antibodies. Neurology 1990; 40:1067–1072.

Schulte-Mattler W, Georgiadis C, Tietze K, Zierz S: Relation between maximum discharge rates on electromyography and motor unit number estimates. Muscle Nerve 2000;23:231–238.

Shahani B, Wierzbicka MM, Parker S: Abnormal single motor unit behavior in the upper motor neuron syndrome. Muscle Nerve 1991;14:64–69.

Shefner J, Jillapalli D, Bradshaw D: Reducing intersubject variability in motor unit number estimation. Muscle Nerve 1999;22: 1457–1460.

Sienko D, Davis J, Taylor J, Brooks B: Amyotrophic lateral sclerosis: A case-controlled study following detection of a cluster in a small Wisconsin community. Arch Neurol 1990;47:38–41.

Slawnych M, Laszlo C, Hershler A: A review of techniques employed to estimate the number of motor units in a muscle. Muscle Nerve 1990;13:1050–1064.

Smith R: Effects of the early diagnosis of amyotrophic lateral sclerosis: Disadvantages. Amyotrophic Lateral Sclerosis 2000; 1(suppl 1):S75–S77.

Stålberg E: Macro EMG, a new recording technique. J Neurol Neurosurg Psychiatry 1980;43:475–482.

Stålberg E: Electrophysiological Studies of Reinnervation in ALS. New York, Raven Press, 1982.

Stålberg E, Sonoo M: Assessment of variability in the shape of the motor unit action potential, the "jiggle," at consecutive dishcharges. Muscle Nerve 1994;17:1136–1144.

Stålberg E, Thiele B: Motor unit fibre density in the extensor digitorum communis muscle. J Neurol Neurosurg Psychiatry 1975;38:874–880.

Stålberg E, Trontelj J: Single Fiber Electromyography: Studies in Healthy and Diseased Muscle. New York, Raven Press, 1994.

Stålberg E, Schiller H, Schwartz M: Safety factor in single human motor end-plates studied in vivo with single fibre electromyography. J Neurol Neurosurg Psychiatry 1975a;38:799–804.

Stålberg E, Schwartz M, Trontelj J: Single fibre electromyography in various processes affecting the anterior horn cell. J Neurol Sci 1975b;24:403–415.

Stålberg E, Nandedkar S, Sanders D, Falck B: Quantitative motor unit potential analysis. J Clin Neurophysiol 1996;13:401–422.

Stålberg E, Andreassen S, Falk B, et al: Quantitative analysis of individual motor unit potentials: A proposition for standardized terminology and criteria for measurement. J Clin Neurophysiol 1986;3:313–348.

Stålberg E, Chu J, Bril V, et al: Automatic analysis of the EMG interference pattern. Electroencephalogr Clin Neurophysiol 1983;56:672–681.

Stewart C, Nandedkar S, Massey J, et al: Evaluation of an automatic method of measuring features of motor unit action potentials. Muscle Nerve 1989;12:141–148.

Strickland D, Smith S, Dolliff G, et al: Amyotrophic lateral sclerosis and occupational history: A pilot case-control study. Arch Neurol 1996;53:730–733.

Strong M, Grace G, Orange J, Leeper H: Cognition, language, and speech in amyotrophic lateral sclerosis: A review. J Clin Exp Neuropsychol 1996;18:291–303.

Swash M, Schwartz M: A longitudinal study of changes in motor units in motor neuron disease. J Neurol Sci 1982;56:185–197.

Swerdlow R, Parks J, Pattee G, Parker W: Role of mitochondria in amyotrophic lateral sclerosis. Amyotrophic Lateral Sclerosis 2000;1:185–190.

Takuma H, Kwak S, Yoshizawa T, Kanazawa I: Reduction of GluR2 RNA editing, a molecular change that increases calcium influx through AMPA receptors, selective in spinal ventral gray of patients with amyotrophic lateral sclerosis. Ann Neurol 1999; 46:806–815.

Thiele B, Böhle A: Anzahl der Spike-Komponenten im Motor-Unit Potential. Zeit EEG-EMG 1978;9:125–130.

Triggs W, Menkes D, Onorato J, et al: Transcranial magnetic stimulation identifies upper motor neuron involvement in motor neuron disease. Neurology 2000;53:605–611.

Trojaborg W, Buchthal F: Malignant and benign fasciculations. Acta Neurol Scand 1965;41(suppl 13):251–254.

Tucker T, Layzar R, Miller R, Chad D: Subacute, reversible motor neuron disease. Neurology 1991;41:1541–1544.

Valls-Solé J, Cruz Martinez A, Graus F, et al: Abnormal sensory nerve conduction in multifocal demyelinating neuropathy with persistent conduction block. Neurology 1995;45:2024–2028.

Weber M, Eisen A: Assessment of upper and lower motor neurons in Kennedy's disease: Implications for corticomotoneuronal PSTH studies. Muscle Nerve 1999;22:299–306.

Wettstein A: The origin of fasciculations in motoneuron disease. Ann Neurol 1979;5:295–300.

Wilbourn A: The "split hand syndrome." Muscle Nerve 2000; 23:138.

Williams C, Kozlowski M, Hinton D, Miller C: Degeneration of spinocerebellar neurons in amyotrophic lateral sclerosis. Ann Neurol 1990;27:215–225.

Wohlfart G: Collateral regeneration in partially denervated muscles. Neurology 1958;8:175–180.

Wong P, Pardo C, Borchelt D, et al: An adverse property of a familial ALS-linked SOD1 mutation causes motor neuron disease characterized by vacuolar degeneration of mitochondria. Neuron 1995;14:1105–1116.

World Federation of Neurology Research Group on Neuromuscular Diseases: El Escorial World Federation of Neurology criteria for the diagnosis of amyotrophic lateral sclerosis. J Neurol Sci 1994;124(Suppl):96–107.

Xu Z: Mechanisms of motoneuron degeneration in ALS: What

have SOD1 mutations told us? Amyotrophic Lateral Sclerosis 2000;1:225–244.

Younger D, Rowland L, Latov N, et al: Motor neuron disease and amyotrophic lateral sclerosis: Relation of high CSF protein content to paraproteinemia and clinical syndromes. Neurology 1990;40:595–599.

Yuen E, Olney R: Longitudinal study of fiber density and motor unit number estimate in patients with amyotrophic lateral sclerosis. Neurology 1997;49:573–578.

Zalewska E, Rowinska-Marcinska K, Hausmanowa-Petrusewicz I: Shape irregularity of motor unit potentials in some neuromuscular disorders. Muscle Nerve 1998;21:1181–1187.

Table 74–1. Neuromuscular Complications of HIV and the Stages of HIV Infection

Disease/Syndrome	Stage of HIV Infection		
	Seroconversion	Early	Late
I. Neuropathies			
a. Distal symmetrical polyneuropathy			X
b. Inflammatory demyelinating polyradiculoneuropathy	X	X	X
c. Progressive polyradiculopathy			X
d. Mononeuropathy multiplex	X	X	X
e. Autonomic neuropathy			X
f. Diffuse infiltrative lymphocytosis syndrome		X	
g. Ataxic neuropathy	X	X	
II. Myopathies			
a. HIV-associated myopathy	X	X	X
b. Zidovudine myopathy	X	X	X
c. HIV wasting syndrome			X

central nervous system (CNS) disorders, such as myelopathy, may coexist with DSP. In this setting, patients have the combination of upper and lower motor neuron signs, such as increased knee reflexes and extensor plantar responses, with relatively normal or depressed ankle jerks. Objective muscle weakness is an uncommon sign in DSP (AAN AIDS Task Force, 1991b).

DSP may also be secondary to exposure to neurotoxic antiretroviral medications, such as dideoxyinosine (ddI), dideoxycytidine (ddC), and stavudine (d4T) (Moyle and Sadler, 1998). In early studies, in which patients with advanced HIV infection were treated with these medications, rates of neurotoxic neuropathy were high. More recently, in trials of patients with relatively early HIV infection and higher CD4 counts, DSP is less common. In one such trial, comparing treatment with AZT, ddI, and ddC in subjects with CD4 counts of 200 to 500 cells per millimeter, the incidence of DSP was 3% to 6% in the treatment arms. The highest rate of DSP (6%) was present in the group treated with combination AZT and ddC (Simpson et al., 1997). The risk of developing DSP is increased in groups treated with ddI, d4T, and hydroxyurea compared with ddI and d4T or ddI or d4T alone (Moore et al., 2000). Other causes of toxic or metabolic neuropathies that may occur in the setting of HIV infection include vincristine therapy for Kaposi's sarcoma, isoniazid therapy for tuberculosis, and vitamin B_{12} deficiency (Mulhall and Jennens, 1987; Winer, 1993).

Electrophysiological studies in DSP are consistent with axonal polyneuropathy. Compound muscle action potential amplitudes in the upper and lower extremities are reduced, with relatively normal conduction velocities. F waves are prolonged in latency. Sural sensory responses are the most sensitive feature in DSP, and are reduced in amplitude or absent. Needle electromyography (EMG) examination reveals fibrillation potentials and positive sharp waves

with reduced motor unit recruitment in distal muscles (So et al., 1988; Miller, 1991; Villa et al., 1992; Winer et al., 1992), consistent with axonal neuropathy. There are no distinct electrophysiological changes that differentiate HIV-associated DSP from DSP due to antiretroviral medication.

Treatment for DSP is primarily symptomatic. Correction of metabolic disorders, such as vitamin B_{12} deficiency, diabetes, or thyroid disease, should be attempted. Withdrawal of potential toxins, such as antiretroviral medication, can be considered if clinically feasible. Resolution of painful symptoms after stopping antiretroviral medications may take 8 to 16 weeks, during which time symptoms may intensify before remitting (Berger et al., 1993).

Treatment for painful DSP includes analgesics or prophylactic medications, such as antidepressants or anticonvulsants. Analgesics include nonopioid medications, such as acetaminophen or nonsteroidal anti-inflammatory agents. Escalating pain may require the use of mild opioid combinations with codeine or more potent opioids, such as methadone, morphine, or fentanyl, as necessary. Prophylactic medications include anticonvulsants such as phenytoin, carbamazepine, and gabapentin. Lamotrogine was found to be effective in a small placebo-controlled study (Simpson et al., 2000). A multicenter, double-blind, placebo-controlled study of lamotrigine is currently underway. Other adjuvant medications, such as amitriptyline and mexiletine, were not superior to placebo for painful AIDS-associated DSP (Kieburtz et al., 1998).

A placebo-controlled phase II trial of recombinant human nerve growth factor showed a significant benefit in pain reduction in patients with HIV infection. Phase III trials of nerve growth factor for diabetic neuropathy were negative. However, quantitative measures of nerve regeneration, including quantitative sensory testing and epidermal skin density, were not significantly improved in patients treated with nerve growth factor. Future clinical development of nerve growth factor is uncertain at this time (McArthur et al., 2000).

Inflammatory Demyelinating Polyradiculoneuropathy

Acute inflammatory demyelinating polyradiculoneuropathy (AIDP) often presents at the time of HIV seroconversion or as the first manifestation of HIV infection (AAN AIDS Task Force, 1991b). Chronic inflammatory demyelinating polyradiculoneuropathy (CIDP) can occur at any stage of HIV infection. Of 118 patients with inflammatory neuropathy (39 with AIDP and 79 with CIDP), 9 had HIV infection (Cornblath et al., 1987). Three patients had AIDP and 6 had CIDP. The patients were asymptomatic from the HIV infection except for lymphadenopathy.

Patients with HIV-associated AIDP present with the typical picture of rapidly evolving paresis, mild sensory symptoms, areflexia, and involvement of the respiratory muscles (Scarpini et al., 1991; Ropper, 1992). Patients with CIDP have a slower evolution of chronic, moderate to severe, proximal and distal weakness (AAN AIDS Task Force, 1991a). Sensory symptoms and signs are usually minor, and reflexes are depressed or absent. The average cerebrospinal fluid (CSF) protein concentration in this series was 190 + 52 mg/dL. The average CSF pleocytosis was 23 + 5 cells per millimeter, which is an important differential feature as compared with HIV-seronegative patients with idiopathic demyelinating polyradiculopathy (IDP) (AAN AIDS Task Force, 1991a). Seropositive patients with AIDP frequently have up to 50 mononuclear leukocytes per millimeter, whereas seronegative patients with AIDP rarely have more than 10 mononuclear leukocytes per millimeter (Ropper, 1992).

Electrophysiological studies reveal mixed demyelinative and axonal changes in patients with AIDP, whereas in the patients with CIDP, changes are consistent with primary demyelination with secondary axonal loss (Cornblath et al., 1987). Screening for HIV infection should be considered in all patients with IDP, especially when risk factors are present or when CSF contains a pleocytosis. However, in most studies IDP is uncommon in patients with HIV infection (Snider et al., 1983; Fuller et al., 1993).

Patients with HIV infection may develop bulbar symptoms with cranial nerve involvement (Miller et al., 1988), possibly representing variants of CIDP (Ropper, 1986). Electrophysiological studies in several such patients have revealed motor and sensory conduction velocities less than 60% of normal. Distal latencies and F waves were abnormal. Conduction block was present. In four cases, there was no spontaneous activity on needle examination, suggesting primary demyelination. Other patients had fibrillation potentials, positive sharp waves, and diminished recruitment on needle examination, consistent with axonal degeneration.

All patients with AIDP had some degree of recovery after treatment with plasma exchange. In patients with CIDP, there was spontaneous recovery in two patients while others were treated with prednisone and plasma exchange. There have been no reported controlled treatment trials in HIV-associated IDP.

AIDP has also been reported in children with HIV infection. A 5-year-old HIV-seropositive boy presented with leg pain, developing into asymmetrical weakness with facial diplegia over 72 hours. Compound motor action potentials were unobtainable on the seventh day after onset. Needle examination revealed fibrillation potentials in the deltoid and biceps muscles. He recovered 8 months after treatment with plasma exchange and intravenous immunoglobulin (Raphael et al., 1991).

Progressive Polyradiculopathy

Progressive polyradiculopathy (PP) is an uncommon but characteristic form of neuropathy, occurring in less than 2% of HIV-infected patients (de Gans et al., 1990; Fuller, 1992). PP has been reported under several names, including lumbosacral polyradiculopathy (Fuller, 1992), progressive inflammatory polyradiculopathy presenting as cauda equina syndrome (Dalakas and Pezeshkpour, 1988), myeloradiculitis (Mahieux et al., 1989), polyradiculomyelitis (Mahieux et al., 1989), and subacute ascending polyradiculomyelopathy (Cohen et al., 1993). PP is often associated with systemic cytomegalovirus (CMV) infection, most commonly retinal. In a review of 103 reported cases of progressive polyradiculopathy (Anders and Goebel, 1998), 44% of patients had a history of CMV infection in another organ system, but only 4% of patients were taking the antiviral medication ganciclovir. CMV infection has declined markedly in frequency in the current era of highly active antiretroviral therapy (HAART), as a result of immune reconstitution (Anders and Goebel, 1998). A prospective study of antiretroviral treatment in AIDS-associated CMV nerve disease was suspended due to poor accrual in the current HAART era.

The most common presenting symptom of PP is asymmetrical leg weakness, with rapid progression to flaccid paraparesis. Associated symptoms include lower back pain with radicular features, sacral paresthesias or analgesia, urinary retention, fecal incontinence, variable sensory symptoms, and impotence in males. Examination reveals paraparesis, diminished or absent lower extremity reflexes, and variable sensory loss (Bishopric et al., 1985; Eidelberg et al., 1986; Dalakas and Pezeshkpour, 1988; Mahieux et al., 1989; de Gans et al., 1990; Cohen et al., 1991; Fuller, 1992; Kim and Hollander, 1993). Sixteen percent of cases in one series had a Babinski sign, likely secondary to associated CMV myelitis (Anders and Goebel, 1998). Upper extremity involvement is uncommon in progressive polyradiculopathy (Eidelberg et al., 1986; Behar et al., 1987; Said et al., 1991). In one patient with cervical radicular pain, progressive bilateral arm weakness and areflexia were due to meningeal spread of primary CNS lymphoma (Corral et al., 1997).

PP usually affects patients with late-stage HIV infection and can be the first documented presentation of an opportunistic infection (Mahieux et al., 1989; de Gans et al., 1990; Kim and Hollander, 1993; So and Olney, 1994; Anders and Goebel, 1998). Although PP is most commonly associated with CMV infection, other causes that should be considered include lymphoma, tuberculosis, herpes zoster infection, cryptococcosis, toxoplasmosis, and syphilis (Fuller, 1992; Cohen et al., 1993; Corral et al., 1997).

CSF findings in PP include pleocytosis, elevated protein concentration, and hypoglycorrhachia. CMV is a fastidious organism that is difficult to grow in culture. Positive CMV cultures in CSF have been reported in only 41% of cases of PP (Kim and Hollander, 1993). The diagnostic test of choice for neurological CMV infection is detection of CMV DNA in CSF with polymerase chain reaction, which is present in 65% of cases (Cohen et al., 1993; Miller et al.,

1996). Magnetic resonance imaging (MRI) may reveal leptomeningeal enhancement from the conus to the cauda equina (Fuller, 1992; Kim and Hollander, 1993).

Electrophysiological findings in PP are consistent with acute axonal loss (Miller et al., 1990). Distal compound motor action potential amplitudes are decreased, with variable slowing of conduction velocity. Distal sensory potential amplitudes and conduction velocities are normal or delayed, confounded by the fact that many patients with late-stage HIV infection also have DSP. F waves are prolonged or absent (Miller, 1991). Needle EMG reveals evidence of active denervation, including fibrillation potentials and positive sharp waves, in clinically weak muscles. Denervation is usually present in paraspinal muscles and is consistent with polyradiculopathy (Miller et al., 1990; Cohen et al., 1993). Electrophysiological findings can be difficult to interpret in the setting of concurrent DSP (Dalakas and Pezeshkpour, 1988; So and Olney, 1994). Denervation, out of proportion to a mild to moderate sensorimotor polyneuropathy, is a helpful electrophysiological feature for distinguishing between PP and DSP (Becker et al., 1997).

Although controlled clinical trials have not been performed, case series indicate that treatment with ganciclovir, foscarnet, or cidofovir, singly or in combination, can stabilize symptoms within 2 weeks. However, the overall prognosis of PP is poor. The mean survival time in CMV polyradiculopathy is about 5 weeks without treatment and 14 weeks after treatment with ganciclovir (Morgello and Simpson, 1994).

Mononeuropathy Multiplex

Mononeuritis multiplex (MM), affecting cranial or spinal nerves, may occur at any stage of HIV infection (Parry, 1988). The most common presentation of MM is asymmetrical numbness or painful paresthesias in a patchy distribution, followed by weakness in a nerve root or truncal pattern (Roullet et al., 1994). Sensorimotor symptoms and thoracic hyperesthesia have also been reported. CMV is the most likely cause of MM that occurs in late stages of HIV infection (Roullet et al., 1994), particularly with CD4 lower than 50 cells per millimeter. CMV infection may be diagnosed by CSF polymerase chain reaction or nerve biopsy. Such patients should be treated with ganciclovir, foscarnet, or cidofovir. Other causes of MM include vasculitis (Cornblath et al., 1987; Gherardi et al., 1989), varicella (Mahadeen et al., 1997), and primary HIV infection (Snider et al., 1983). Lymphomatous, cryptococcal, and chronic meningitides have also been implicated in the pathogenesis of MM (Snider et al., 1983).

Two distinct syndromes of mononeuropathy multiplex, based on the patients' CD4 counts, were identified in 21 patients with HIV infection (So and Olney, 1991; So, 1992). Patients with a mean CD4 count of 30 cells per millimeter developed asymmetrical and progressive weakness of three or four limbs. Systemic CMV infection was diagnosed by viral culture or nerve biopsy. Patients treated with ganciclovir had stabilization of their neuropathy, whereas untreated patients died. Patients with a mean CD4 count of 359 cells per millimeter had deficits limited to one or two limbs, and often had spontaneous recovery without treatment.

Electrophysiological studies in MM are consistent with multifocal axonal changes with occasional associated demyelinative features, including conduction block (Miller, 1991; So and Olney, 1991; So, 1992). F waves are absent or delayed. The relative sparing of some nerves on clinical and electrophysiological examination is consistent with the diagnosis of mononeuritis multiplex. Morgello and Simpson have reported one patient with MM who had marked multifocal slowing of sensory and motor nerves with conduction block, consistent with primary demyelination. Autopsy revealed evidence of primary CMV infection of Schwann cells, inducing demyelination (Morgello and Simpson, 1994). As with all other neuropathies that occur with late-stage AIDS, DSP is also present, and should be considered during interpretation of the electrophysiological findings.

Mononeuropathies involving the thoracic, peroneal or lateral femoral cutaneous nerves have been reported with HIV infection (Lange et al., 1988; Miller et al., 1988; Winer et al., 1992). Mononeuropathies may be the initial presentation of CIDP (Miller et al., 1988). Facial palsy is commonly noted in association with HIV seroconversion but can occur at any stage of HIV infection (Lipkin et al., 1985; Wiselka et al., 1987; Brown et al., 1988; Parry, 1988; Belec et al., 1989; Wechsler and Ho, 1989; Raphael et al., 1991; Krasner and Cohen, 1993; Lefaucheur et al., 1996). Unilateral and bilateral facial palsies have been reported in association with lymphoma (Gold et al., 1988; Snider et al., 1983), herpes zoster (Mahadeen et al., 1997), and as part of an IDP (Belec et al., 1989; Ropper, 1994). Electrophysiological studies reveal predominantly axonal changes (Miller, 1991), although demyelinating changes have been reported (Lange, 1994). Other cranial neuropathies include involvement of the third nerve (Lange, 1994), third division of cranial nerve V (Snider et al., 1983), and the superior and recurrent laryngeal nerves (Small et al., 1989).

Case series have shown that early forms of MM and mononeuropathies may respond to immunotherapy, such as corticosteroids, intravenous immunoglobulin, or plasma exchange. Later forms of MM secondary to CMV infection may benefit from treatment with ganciclovir, foscarnet, or cidofovir, singly or in combination (Fuller, 1992).

Autonomic Neuropathy

Autonomic neuropathy is most common in the late stages of HIV infection. The diagnosis of autonomic neuropathy may be difficult in advanced AIDS due to the overlap in symptoms with systemic deterioration and with the development of other neurological disorders, such as myelopathy and dementia (Freeman et al., 1990). In many cases, autonomic neuropathy is also associated with somatic neuropathy (de la Monte et al., 1988; Cohen and Laudenslager, 1989; Freeman, 1997; Veilleux et al., 1995).

Autonomic symptoms are common in HIV-infected patients (Lin-Greenberg and Taneja-Uppal, 1987; Villa and Confalonieri, 1987; Winer et al., 1992). The most common symptoms reported are impotence and decreased libido (Winer et al., 1992). Other symptoms of autonomic neuropathy include orthostatic hypotension, syncope, presyncope, nausea, vomiting, early satiety, gastric fullness with bloating, diarrhea, constipation, rectal incontinence, bladder dysfunction, impotence, and hypohidrosis or hyperhidrosis (Elder et al., 1986; Evenhouse et al., 1987; Lefaucheur et al., 1996; Becker et al., 1997; Floeter et al., 1997; McArthur et al., 2000).

Craddock reported cardiorespiratory arrest in five patients with HIV infection during fine-needle aspiration of the lung (Craddock et al., 1987), an uncommon complication in patients who are not infected with HIV. One case was fatal. Subsequent testing in five additional patients revealed abnormal autonomic testing, suggesting that patients with HIV infection may be at increased risk for complications during invasive procedures because of underlying autonomic nervous system involvement (Craddock et al., 1987; Villa and Confalonieri, 1987; Luginbuhl et al., 1993).

Testing of autonomic function (Lipkin et al., 1985; Low, 1997; McLeod, 1999) includes heart rate variation with deep breathing, heart rate variation with the Valsalva maneuver, blood pressure and heart rate responses to change in posture (standing or tilt), responses to isometric exercise, responses to cold pressor test, quantitative sudomotor axon reflex test, and sympathetic skin responses.

More than 50% of asymptomatic HIV-positive patients have moderate to severe abnormalities in autonomic testing (Villa et al., 1987; Villa et al., 1992). An increased resting heart rate is a common finding in patients with HIV infection, regardless of disease stage (Becker et al., 1997). HIV-infected patients have more severe changes in mean arterial blood pressure falls to tilt and isometric exercise than controls (Cohen and Laudenslager, 1989; Freeman et al., 1990). A prolonged QT interval, which is a predictor for ventricular arrhythmias, is often found in patients with AIDS, suggesting that these patients may be at increased risk for sudden death (Villa et al., 1995). Quantitative sudomotor axon reflex test responses in the arms and legs may be absent in patients with AIDS (Cohen and Laudenslager, 1989), indicating postganglionic sudomotor failure. In patients with orthostatic hypotension, where underlying causes such as medications (tricyclic antidepressants, pain medications, and pentamidine) and dehydration (due to vomiting, diarrhea, and infection) were excluded, tilting from the supine to upright position did not lead to the development of tachycardia, suggesting the presence of generalized autonomic dysfunction (Cohen et al., 1991; Freeman, 1997). Sympathetic skin response was normal in the majority of patients with HIV infection (Veilleux et al., 1995). Pupil cycle time, an infrequently used test of autonomic function, is prolonged in patients with HIV, as compared with age-matched controls subject (Maclean and Dhillon, 1993; Freeman, 1997).

Autonomic test abnormalities can be found in up to 60% of asymptomatic patients with HIV infection (Roullet et al., 1994). Autonomic symptoms and testing worsen with advancing HIV infection or AIDS (Freeman et al., 1990; Scott et al., 1990; Said et al., 1991; Villa et al., 1992; Simpson et al., 1993; Becker et al., 1997). Progression of autonomic dysfunction parallels the progression of disease (Cohen and Laudenslager, 1989; Freeman et al., 1990; Villa et al., 1992; Becker et al., 1997). Previous case series have suggested that significant deterioration in heart rate variation does not occur. However, in these series, many of the older patients with lower CD4$^+$ counts and more abnormal tests compared to the survivors died prior to retesting. Only the younger survivors with higher CD4$^+$ counts were tested serially, and in these survivors a significant deterioration of HRV was not seen (Shahmanesh et al., 1991; Becker et al., 1997). Hemodynamic changes, dysrhythmias (Luginbuhl et al., 1993), and heart rate variation changes on Valsalva maneuver are also commonly seen in children with HIV infection (Ruttimann et al., 1991). Resting tachycardia is common (Ruttimann et al., 1991). Unexpected cardiac arrest and congestive heart failure are also common among children with HIV infection (Plein et al., 1999). These cardiac complications increase as patients progress to AIDS (Ruttimann et al., 1991).

Treatment for autonomic neuropathy is primarily symptomatic, including fluid management and monitoring of cardiac status and blood pressure.

Diffuse Infiltrative Lymphocytosis Syndrome

Diffuse infiltrative lymphocytosis syndrome (DILS) is a Sjögren-like syndrome characterized by multivisceral CD8 T-cell infiltration (Gherardi et al., 1998). Characteristically, patients with DILS have bilateral parotid gland enlargement, sicca, and xerostomia. Other involved organs include the lungs, kidneys, muscles, nerves, and gastrointestinal tract (Moulignier et al., 1997). The prevalence of DILS is approximately 0.8% (Lange, 1994). HIV-positive patients with DILS tend to have higher CD4 counts, fewer opportunistic infections, and longer survival time (Moulignier et al., 1997; Gherardi et al., 1998). Total survival time in one study was 544 months, during which only 1 of 17 patients developed an opportunistic infection (Itescu et al., 1990).

DILS neuropathy is an acute or subacute painful distal symmetrical neuropathy associated with mild to moderate weakness, and can be the first manifestation of HIV infection (Kazi et al., 1996; Moulignier et al., 1997; Berger and Simpson, 1998). It may also present with asymmetrical motor and sensory deficits of focal onset, including unilateral or bilateral facial nerve palsies (Itescu et al., 1990; Kazi et al., 1996; Morgello and Simpson, 1994; Gherardi et al., 1998). Electrophysiological studies in DILS have shown evidence of a predominantly axonal neuropathy (Moulignier et al., 1997; Gherardi et al., 1998). A predominantly demyelinating neuropathy was found in 2 of 12 patients studied (Moulignier et al., 1997). Response to corticosteroids and AZT has been reported (Morgello and Simpson, 1994; Kazi et al., 1996).

Ataxic Neuropathy

Patients with ataxic neuropathy have rarely been reported in association with HIV infection. The development of ataxic neuropathy in two patients was associated with seroconversion to HIV, whereas two patients had the Miller-Fisher Syndrome (Fisher, 1956; Sillevis Smitt and Portegies, 1990; Arranz et al., 1997). Two of the three patients developed symptoms after illnesses, suggesting acute HIV seroconversion with fever, myalgias, headache, and sore throat, whereas the third patient developed symptoms after a case of acute hepatitis. Sensory symptoms, ataxia, and mild weakness began 1 to 3 weeks after the acute illness (Elder et al., 1986; Scarpini et al., 1991; Castellanos et al., 1994).

Nerve conduction studies in one patient with ataxic neuropathy revealed conduction velocities in the demyelinating range (Elder et al., 1986). Autopsy demonstrated inflammation and loss of dorsal root ganglia, consistent with ganglioneuronitis. Electrophysiological testing in another patient revealed denervation in all muscles tested, prolonged F waves, mildly diminished conduction velocities, and prolonged distal latencies (Castellanos et al., 1994). Both of these patients differ from previously reported cases of chronic idiopathic ataxic neuropathy where sensory nerve potentials are usually absent (Dalakas, 1986). EMG findings in the Miller-Fisher syndrome include profound sensory nerve changes with minor motor abnormalities, suggestive of damage to the sensory ganglia or peripheral axons. Mild increases in motor unit potentials and amplitude have also been noted (Fross and Daube, 1987).

MYOPATHIES

Myopathies may occur at any stage of HIV infection (Simpson and Bender, 1988; Chalmers et al., 1991; Manji et al., 1993). The development of myopathy may coincide with HIV seroconversion or may be the presenting or only manifestation of HIV infection. Myopathy can also occur in the presence of other HIV-related neurological complications, such as neuropathy or myelopathy (Dalakas et al., 1990; Cupler et al., 1995), rendering the diagnosis of myopathy more difficult.

Although the incidence of myopathy is unknown, it appears to be an uncommon complication of HIV infection (Simpson et al., 1993). Ninety-six percent of deltoid muscle biopsies in 50 untreated patients with AIDS and the AIDS-related complex, with some degree of muscle wasting, revealed significant histological abnormalities, indicating that subclinical muscle involvement in HIV infection is not uncommon (Gabbai et al., 1990). The diagnosis of myopathy in HIV infection is based on features of proximal muscle weakness, with or without myalgia, an elevated serum creatinine kinase, myopathic changes on EMG, and muscle biopsy histological changes (Robinson, 1991). Myopathies may also occur secondary to opportunistic infections, such as toxoplasmosis, pyomyositis (*Staphylococcus aureus*), cryptococcosis, and *Mycobacterium avium-intracellulare* infection, as well as neoplastic infiltrative diseases such as lymphoma and Kaposi's sarcoma (Tagliati et al., 1998). The three main types of myopathy associated with HIV are HIV-associated myopathy, AZT-related myopathy, and HIV wasting syndrome.

HIV-Associated Myopathy

A polymyositis-like disorder may be the presenting manifestation of HIV infection (Cupler et al., 1995). The primary symptom in HIV-associated myopathy is insidious and progressive proximal weakness, affecting the lower extremities more than the upper extremities (Chalmers et al., 1991). Weakness is typically symmetrical (Simpson and Bender, 1988). Patients have difficulty arising from a low chair or lifting their heads when supine. Fatigue, myalgia, and wasting are also commonly present (Simpson and Bender, 1988; Sillevis Smitt and Portegies, 1990). Serum (creatinine kinase) levels are often elevated, and electrophysiological changes are consistent with a myopathic process (Manji et al., 1993). Muscle biopsy most commonly reveals nonspecific myofiber degeneration, occasionally associated with inflammatory infiltrates. Other reported features include angulated fibers, myofiber necrosis and phagocytosis, internal nuclei, cytoplasmic bodies, and nemaline rods (Simpson et al., 1993). HIV has been detected within the CD4$^+$ cells in the inflammatory infiltrates (Simpson and Bender, 1988; Cupler et al., 1995). Nerve conduction studies are usually normal, unless there is coexisting DSP. Needle EMG reveals short, brief, and polyphasic motor unit action potentials with early recruitment and a full interference pattern. Abnormal spontaneous activity, including fibrillation potentials, positive sharp waves, and chronic repetitive discharges, is often present, seen in 79% of patients (Simpson et al., 1993). The most sensitive muscle for diagnosis of myopathy is the iliopsoas (Tagliati et al., 1998).

DSP is commonly associated with myopathy in patients with HIV infection. Fifty percent of patients with myopathy followed at the Mount Sinai Medical Center in New York from 1984 to 1991 also had a distal polyneuropathy (Simpson et al., 1993). Conversely, among 50 cases of neuropathy, only one case of myopathy was identified (Simpson et al., 1993). In patients with late-stage HIV infection or AIDS, electrophysiological studies often reveal concurrent distal predominantly axonal polyneuropathy. In this setting, nerve conduction studies in patients with myopathy may be abnormal, and late responses may be prolonged. It may be difficult to differentiate small regenerating units from brief and polyphasic motor units. Quantitative analysis of the interference pattern using the on-line turns/amplitude methods may be useful (Lefaucheur et al., 1996). Quantitative motor unit analysis using the mean duration of 20 motor units sampled from one muscle can be compared with normal values (Simpson et al., 1993).

Immunosuppressive therapy, including corticosteroids and intravenous immunoglobulin, can result in improvement (Simpson and Bender, 1988) in patients with HIV-associated myopathy.

Zidovudine-Associated Myopathy

Exposure to AZT has been associated with the development of myopathy. Although myalgias without objective evidence of myopathy are common in patients with HIV (Miller et al., 1991), myalgias or muscle tenderness in thighs and calves may be more common in AZT myopathy (Chalmers et al., 1991; Manji et al., 1993; Simpson et al., 1993; Simpson et al., 1997). Myopathic symptoms have been reported as early as 2 months after initiation of AZT therapy (Cupler et al., 1995). AZT was reported to cause a toxic mitochondrial myopathy, associated with ragged red fibers on histology and mitochondrial abnormalities with paracrystalline inclusions on electron microscopy (Dalakas et al., 1990). These results have not been replicated in other studies (Miller, 1991; Simpson et al., 1993). A prospective study of the frequency of clinical and laboratory markers of myopathy revealed only 6 of 2567 patients with myopathy. One patient received AZT and ddC, whereas four others received ddI, bringing into question the role of AZT in the development of myopathy (Simpson et al., 1998).

As with HIV-associated myopathy, electrophysiologic studies in patients with AZT myopathy reveal normal motor and sensory nerve conductions. Needle EMG can reveal mild to moderate increased fibrillations, positive sharp wave activity, and complex repetitive discharges (Simpson and Bender, 1988; Chalmers et al., 1991). Motor units are brief, small, and polyphasic, with early recruitment and full interference patterns (Chalmers et al., 1991; Simpson et al., 1993). Commonly, proximal muscles, such as quadriceps, deltoids, and paraspinal mus-

cles, are affected. In milder cases, needle EMG may be normal but increased muscle sampling may increase the diagnostic yield (Robinson, 1991). Since HIV-related myopathy and AZT myopathy cannot be distinguished by clinical, electrophysiological, or histological methods, the gold standard of diagnosis is resolution of symptoms following AZT withdrawal.

However, improvement of myopathy after withdrawal of AZT is variable (Chalmers et al., 1991; Simpson et al., 1993). In our experience, the majority of patients do not respond to AZT withdrawal, implying that HIV, rather than AZT, is the cause of myopathy in the majority of these patients. Corticosteroids may be beneficial (Manji et al., 1993). We are currently conducting a study of intravenous immunoglobulin.

HIV Wasting Syndrome

HIV wasting syndrome is characterized by involuntary weight loss of greater than 10% from baseline, chronic diarrhea, chronic weakness, and fever for more than 30 days. Simpson and colleagues (1990) reported five patients with HIV wasting syndrome who had findings similar to patients with HIV-associated myopathy. There was progressive, predominantly proximal lower extremity weakness, neck flexor weakness, and thigh myalgia. Serum creatinine kinase levels were moderately elevated in all five patients. Diarrhea was uncommon in this group. Electrophysiological studies revealed myopathic changes characterized by units with small, brief polyphasic motor unit potentials with full and early recruitment. Four of the five patients had also received AZT (Simpson et al., 1990). In 50 patients with myopathy also followed by our group, 20 had sufficient weight loss for the diagnosis of HIV wasting syndrome (Simpson et al., 1990), suggesting that there may be some overlap in these two syndromes. Histologically, HIV-associated myopathy is characterized by severe type II fiber atrophy (Dalakas et al., 1990).

MOTOR NEURON DISEASE

The incidence of amyotrophic lateral sclerosis (ALS) in the general population is estimated to be 2 per 100,000. The peak age of onset is about 60 years (Eisen and McComas, 1993). In a case series of 50 HIV-infected patients with myopathy, one patient had motor neuron disease (MND) (Simpson et al., 1990). There have been five reported patients with MND associated with HIV infection.

The first three reported patients with HIV-associated MND had electrophysiological changes of widespread denervation (Hoffman et al., 1985; Sher et al., 1988). Histological changes consistent with MND were found in two cases (Hoffman et al., 1985; Sher et al., 1988; Huang et al., 1993). The fourth patient was a 32-year-old man who developed progressive weakness with diffuse fasciculations. Autopsy revealed the coexistence of both myeloradiculopathy and myopathy, indicating the lack of specificity of the diagnosis of MND in the HIV-infected patient (Verma et al., 1990). The fifth patient was a 45-year-old man with progressive limb weakness and EMG findings consistent with MND. Immunoelectrophoresis revealed an IgMκ monoclonal protein with positive anti-asialo GM₁ antibody. Treatment with immunotherapy did not result in clinical improvement. Autopsy revealed profound anterior horn cell loss (Simpson et al., 1994).

Electrophysiological studies in MND reflect the progressive degeneration of anterior horn cells (Eisen and McComas, 1993; Preston and Shapiro, 1998). There are no specific electrophysiological changes in cases of MND with concurrent HIV infection. Compound motor action potentials and conduction velocities are normal until the late stages of MND. Distal latencies are prolonged. Sensory studies are usually not affected, unless there is a coexisting distal sensory neuropathy. Needle examination reveals increased spontaneous activity. Ongoing lower motor neuron degeneration is reflected in denervation on needle EMG. Compensatory reinnervation is a reflection of collateral sprouting from surviving lower motor neurons. Quantitative EMG reveals chronic partial denervation and reinnervation. Motor unit number estimates are reproducible. Electrophysiological studies may be difficult to interpret in the presence of a coexistent DSP.

Although HIV has not been clearly localized within anterior horn cells, by most assays, HIV-like immunoreactivity has rarely been localized in anterior horn cells, suggesting that virus-induced immune mechanisms may play a role in MND (Robert et al., 1989; Simpson et al., 1994). Although it is unlikely that HIV and MND occur together by chance, HIV infection should be considered in the differential diagnosis of progressive motor neuropathy.

CONCLUSION

A variety of peripheral neuropathies may occur at different stages of HIV infection. Electrophysiological studies can differentiate demyelinating and axonal neuropathies and define the presence of a symmetrical or multifocal process. These distinctions are critical in determining the management and predicting outcome of these neuropathies. Autonomic testing can be helpful in detecting the presence of asymptomatic dysfunction, which may be a helpful predictive factor in long-term outcomes, as well as predict the risk of invasive procedures.

Electrophysiological studies, in the context of the clinical pattern of neuromuscular dysfunction and the stage of HIV infection, are useful in distinguishing the different types of neuromuscular disorders. DSP, due either to HIV infection or neurotoxic agents, and other neurologic complications of HIV, such as dementia and myelopathy, must be considered when evaluating the clinical and electrophysiological findings of neuromuscular disorders in patients with HIV infection or AIDS.

As survival time for HIV-infected patients increases, so does the opportunity to develop neurological disorders. It is critical that all clinicians working with such patients be familiar with the diagnosis and management of the neuromuscular complications of HIV infection and AIDS.

References

AAN: Research criteria for diagnosis of chronic inflammatory demyelinating polyneuropathy (CIDP). Report from an Ad Hoc Subcommittee of the American Academy of Neurology AIDS Task Force. Neurology 1991a;41:617–618.

AAN: Nomenclature and research case definitions for neurologic manifestations of human immunodeficiency virus type 1 (HIV-1) infection. Report of a Working Group of the American Academy of Neurology AIDS Task Force. Neurology 1991b;41:778–785.

Anders HJ, Goebel FD: Cytomegalovirus polyradiculopathy in patients with AIDS: Clin Infect Dis 1998;27:345–352.

Arranz Caso JA, Martinez R, Cabrera F, Tejeiro J: Miller Fisher syndrome in a patient with HIV infection. AIDS 1997;11:550–551.

Becker K, Gorlach I, Frieling T, Haussinger D: Characterization and natural course of cardiac autonomic nervous dysfunction in HIV-infected patients. AIDS 1997;11:751–757.

Behar R, Wiley C, McCutchan JA: Cytomegalovirus polyradiculoneuropathy in acquired immune deficiency syndrome. Neurology 1987;37:557–561.

Belec L, Gherardi R, Georges AJ, et al: Peripheral facial paralysis and HIV infection: Report of four African cases and review of the literature. J Neurol 1989;236:411–414.

Berger AR, Arezzo JC, Schaumburg HH, et al: 2',3'-Dideoxycytidine (ddC) toxic neuropathy: A study of 52 patients. Neurology 1993 Feb;43:358–362

Berger JR, Simpson DM: The pathogenesis of diffuse infiltrative lymphocytosis syndrome: An AIDS-related peripheral neuropathy. Neurology 1998;50:855–857.

Bishopric G, Bruner J, Butler J: Guillain-Barre syndrome with cytomegalovirus infection of peripheral nerves. Arch Pathol Lab Med 1985;109:1106–1108.

Brown MM, Thompson A, Goh BT, et al: Bell's palsy and HIV infection. J Neurol Neurosurg Psychiatry 1988;51:425–426.

Castellanos F, Mallada J, Ricart C, Zabala JA: Ataxic neuropathy associated with human immunodeficiency virus seroconversion. Arch Neurol 1994;51:236.

Chalmers AC, Greco CM, Miller RG: Prognosis in AZT myopathy. Neurology 1991;41:1181–1184.

Cohen BA, McArthur JC, Grohman S, et al: Neurologic prognosis of cytomegalovirus polyradiculomyelopathy in AIDS. Neurology 1993;43:493–499.

Cohen JA, Laudenslager M: Autonomic nervous system involvement in patients with human immunodeficiency virus infection. Neurology 1989;39:1111–1112.

Cohen JA, Miller L, Polish L: Orthostatic hypotension in human immunodeficiency virus infection may be the result of generalized autonomic nervous system dysfunction. J Acquir Immune Defic Syndr 1991;4:31–33.

Cornblath DR, McArthur JC, Kennedy PG, et al: Inflammatory demyelinating peripheral neuropathies associated with human T-cell lymphotropic virus type III infection. Ann Neurol 1987;21:32–40.

Cornblath DR, McArthur JC: Predominantly sensory neuropathy in patients with AIDS and AIDS-related complex. Neurology 1988;38:794–796.

Corral I, Quereda C, Casado JL, et al: Acute polyradiculopathies in HIV-infected patients. J Neurol 1997;244:499–504.

Craddock C, Pasvol G, Bull R, et al: Cardiorespiratory arrest and autonomic neuropathy in AIDS. Lancet 1987;2:16–18.

Cupler EJ, Danon MJ, Jay C, et al: Early features of zidovudine-associated myopathy: Histopathological findings and clinical correlations. Acta Neuropathol 1995;90:1–6.

Dalakas MC: Chronic idiopathic ataxic neuropathy. Ann Neurol 1986;19:545–554.

Dalakas MC, Pezeshkpour GH: Neuromuscular diseases associated with human immunodeficiency virus infection. Ann Neurol 1988;23:S38–S48.

Dalakas MC, Illa I, Pezeshkpour GH, et al: Mitochondrial myopathy caused by long-term zidovudine therapy. N Engl J Med 1990;322:1098–1105.

de Gans J, Portegies P, Tiessens G, et al: Therapy for cytomegalovirus polyradiculomyelitis in patients with AIDS: Treatment with ganciclovir. AIDS 1990;4:421–425.

de la Monte SM, Gabuzda DH, Ho DD, et al: Peripheral neuropathy in the acquired immunodeficiency syndrome. Ann Neurol 1988;23:485–492.

Eidelberg D, Sotrel A, Vogel H, et al: Progressive polyradiculopathy in acquired immune deficiency syndrome. Neurology 1986;36:912–916.

Eisen A, McComas AJ: Motor neuron disorders. In Brown WF, Bolton CF (eds): Clinical Electromyography. Boston, Butterworth-Heinemann, 1993; 427–450.

Elder G, Dalakas M, Pezeshkpour G, Sever J: Ataxic neuropathy due to ganglioneuronitis after probable acute human immunodeficiency virus infection. Lancet 1986;2:1275–1276.

Evenhouse M, Haas E, Snell E, et al: Hypotension in infection with the human immunodeficiency virus. Ann Intern Med 1987;107:598–599.

Fisher M: An unusual variant of acute idiopathic polyneuritis (syndrome of ophthalmoplegia, ataxia and areflexia). N Engl J Med 1956;255:57–65.

Floeter MK, Civitello LA, Everett CR, et al: Peripheral neuropathy in children with HIV infection. Neurology 1997;49:207–212.

Freeman R, Roberts MS, Friedman LS, Broadbridge C: Autonomic function and human immunodeficiency virus infection. Neurology 1990;40:575–580.

Freeman R: Autonomic failure and AIDS. In Low PA (ed): Clinical Autonomic Disorders. Philadelphia, Lippincott–Raven Publishers, 1997; 727–735.

Fross RD, Daube JR: Neuropathy in the Miller-Fisher syndrome: Clinical and electrophysiologic findings. Neurology 1987;37:1493–1498.

Fuller GN: Cytomegalovirus and the peripheral nervous system in AIDS. J AIDS 1992;5:S33–S36.

Fuller GN, Jacobs JM, Guiloff RJ: Nature and incidence of peripheral nerve syndromes in HIV infection. J Neurol Neurosurg Psychiatry 1993;56:372–381.

Gabbai AA, Schmidt B, Castelo A, et al: Muscle biopsy in AIDS and ARC: Analysis of 50 patients. Muscle Nerve 1990;13:541–544.

Gherardi R, Lebargy F, Gaulard P, et al: Necrotizing vasculitis and HIV replication in peripheral nerves. N Engl J Med 1989;321:685–686.

Gherardi RK, Chretien F, Delfau-Larue MH, et al: Neuropathy in diffuse infiltrative lymphocytosis syndrome: An HIV neuropathy, not a lymphoma. Neurology 1998;50:1041–1044.

Gold JE, Jimenez E, Zalusky R: Human immunodeficiency virus–related lymphoreticular malignancies and peripheral neurologic disease: A report of four cases. Cancer 1988;61:2318–2324.

Hall CD, Snyder CR, Messenheimer JA, et al: Peripheral neuropathy in a cohort of human immunodeficiency virus–infected patients. Incidence and relationship to other nervous system dysfunction. Arch Neurol 1991;48:1273–1274.

Hoffman PM, Festoff BW, Giron LT, et al: Isolation of LAV/HTLV-III from a patient with amyotrophic lateral sclerosis. N Engl J Med 1985;313:324–325.

Huang PP, Chin R, Song S, Lasoff S: Lower motor neuron dysfunction associated with human immunodeficiency virus infection. Arch Neurol 1993;50:1328–1330.

Itescu S, Brancato LJ, Buxbaum J, et al: A diffuse infiltrative CD8 lymphocytosis syndrome in human immunodeficiency virus (HIV) infection: A host immune response associated with HLA-DR5. Ann Intern Med 1990;112:3–10.

Kazi S, Cohen PR, Williams F, Schempp R, Reveille JD: The diffuse infiltrative lymphocytosis syndrome: Clinical and immunogenetic features in 35 patients. AIDS 1996;10:385–391.

Kieburtz K, Simpson D, Yiannoutsos C, et al: A randomized trial of amitriptyline and mexiletine for painful neuropathy in HIV infection. AIDS Clinical Trial Group 242 Protocol Team. Neurology 1998;51:1682–1688.

Kim YS, Hollander H: Polyradiculopathy due to cytomegalovirus: Report of two cases in which improvement occurred after prolonged therapy and review of the literature. Clin Infect Dis 1993;17:32–37.

Krasner CG, Cohen SH: Bilateral Bell's palsy and aseptic meningitis in a patient with acute human immunodeficiency virus seroconversion. West J Med 1993;159:604–605.

Lange DJ, Britton CB, Younger DS, Hays AP: The neuromuscular manifestations of human immunodeficiency virus infections. Arch Neurol 1988;45:1084–1088.

Lange DJ: AAEM minimonograph no. 41: Neuromuscular diseases associated with HIV-1 infection. Muscle Nerve 1994;17:16–30.

Lefaucheur JP, Verroust J, Gherardi RK: Turns-amplitude analysis assessment of myopathies in HIV-infected patients. J Neurol Sci 1996;136:148–153.

Levy RM, Bredesen DE, Rosenblum ML: Neurological manifestations of the acquired immunodeficiency syndrome (AIDS): Experience at UCSF and review of the literature. J Neurosurg 1985;62:475–495.

Lin-Greenberg A, Taneja-Uppal N: Dysautonomia and infection with the human immunodeficiency virus. Ann Intern Med 1987;106:167.

Lipkin WI, Parry G, Kiprov D, Abrams D: Inflammatory neuropathy in homosexual men with lymphadenopathy. Neurology 1985;35:1479–1483.

Low PA: Laboratory evaluation of autonomic function. In Low PA (ed): Clinical Autonomic Disorders. Philadelphia, Lippincott–Raven Publishers, 1997; 179–208.

Luginbuhl LM, Orav EJ, McIntosh K, Lipshultz SE: Cardiac morbidity and related mortality in children with HIV infection. JAMA 1993;269:2869–2875.

Maclean H, Dhillon B: Pupil cycle time and human immunodeficiency virus (HIV) infection. Eye 1993;7:785–786.

Mahadeen ZI, Brennan RW, Kothari MJ: Bilateral facial palsy secondary to herpes zoster meningoencephalitis in a HIV-positive woman. J Infect 1997;34:261–262.

Mahieux F, Gray F, Fenelon G, et al: Acute myeloradiculitis due to cytomegalovirus as the initial manifestation of AIDS. J Neurol Neurosurg Psychiatry 1989;52:270–274.

Manji H, Harrison MJ, Round JM, et al: Muscle disease, HIV and zidovudine: The spectrum of muscle disease in HIV-infected individuals treated with zidovudine. J Neurol 1993;240:479–488.

McArthur JC, Yiannoutsos C, Simpson DM, et al: A phase II trial of nerve growth factor for sensory neuropathy associated with HIV infection. Neurology 2000;54:1080–1088.

McLeod JG: Evaluation of the autonomic nervous system. In Aminoff MJ (ed): Electrodiagnosis in Clinical Neurology. New York, Churchill Livingstone, 1999; 381–393.

Miller RG, Parry GJ, Pfaeffl W, et al: The spectrum of peripheral neuropathy associated with ARC and AIDS. Muscle Nerve 1988;11:857–863.

Miller RG, Storey JR, Greco CM: Ganciclovir in the treatment of progressive AIDS-related polyradiculopathy. Neurology 1990;40:569–574.

Miller RG: Neuropathies and myopathies complicating HIV infection. J Clin Apheresis 1991;6:110–121.

Miller RG, Carson PJ, Moussavi RS, et al: Fatigue and myalgia in AIDS patients. Neurology 1991;41:1603–1607.

Miller RF, Fox JD, Thomas P, et al: Acute lumbosacral polyradiculopathy due to cytomegalovirus in advanced HIV disease: CSF findings in 17 patients. J Neurol Neurosurg Psychiatry 1996;61:456–460.

Moore RD, Wong WME, Keruly JC, McArthur JC: Incidence of neuropathy in HIV-infected patients on monotherapy versus those on combination therapy with didanosine, stavudine and hydroxyurea. AIDS 2000;14:273–278.

Morgello S, Simpson DM: Multifocal cytomegalovirus demyelinative polyneuropathy associated with AIDS. Muscle Nerve 1994;17:176–182.

Mouligner A, Authier FJ, Baudrimont M, et al: Peripheral neuropathy in human immunodeficiency virus-infected patients with the diffuse infiltrative lymphocytosis syndrome. Ann Neurol 1997;41:438–445.

Moyle GJ, Sadler M: Peripheral neuropathy with nucleoside anti-retrovirals: Risk factors, incidence and management. Drug Safety 1998;19:481–494.

Mulhall BP, Jennens I: Testing for neurological involvement in HIV infection. Lancet 1987;2:1531–1532.

Parry GJ: Peripheral neuropathies associated with human immu-nodeficiency virus infection. Ann Neurol 1988;23:S49–S53.

Piette AM, Tusseau F, Vignon D, et al: Acute neuropathy coinci-dent with seroconversion for anti-LAV/HTLV-III. Lancet 1986; 1:852.

Plein D, Van Camp G, Cosyns B, Alimenti A, Levy J, Vanden-bossche JL: Cardiac and autonomic evaluation in a pediatric population with human immunodeficiency virus. Clin Cardiol 1999;22:33–36.

Raphael SA, Price ML, Lischner HW, et al: Inflammatory demyelin-ating polyneuropathy in a child with symptomatic human im-munodeficiency virus infection. J Pediatr 1991;118:242–245.

Robert ME, Geraghty JJ, Miles SA, et al: Severe neuropathy in a patient with acquired immune deficiency syndrome (AIDS): Evidence for widespread cytomegalovirus infection of periph-eral nerve and human immunodeficiency virus-like immunore-activity of anterior horn cells. Acta Neuropathol 1989;79:255–261.

Robinson LR: AAEM case report #22: Polymyositis. Muscle Nerve 1991;14:310–315.

Ropper AH: Unusual clinical variants and signs in Guillain-Barré syndrome. Arch Neurol 1986;43:1150–1152.

Ropper AH: The Guillain–Barré syndrome. N Engl J Med 1992;326: 1130–1136.

Ropper AH: Further regional variants of acute immune polyneu-ropathy: Bifacial weakness or sixth nerve paresis with pares-thesias, lumbar polyradiculopathy, and ataxia with pharyngeal-cervical-brachial weakness. Arch Neurol 1994;51:671–675.

Roullet E, Assuerus V, Gozlan J, et al: Cytomegalovirus multifocal neuropathy in AIDS: Analysis of 15 consecutive cases. Neurol-ogy 1994;44:2174–2182.

Ruttimann S, Hilti P, Spinas GA, Dubach UC: High frequency of human immunodeficiency virus-associated autonomic neurop-athy and more severe involvement in advanced stages of hu-man immunodeficiency virus disease. Arch Intern Med 1991; 151:2441–2443.

Said G, Lacroix C, Chemouilli P, et al: Cytomegalovirus neuropathy in acquired immunodeficiency syndrome: A clinical and patho-logical study. Ann Neurol 1991;29:139–146.

Scarpini E, Sacilotto G, Lazzarin A, et al: Acute ataxia coincident with seroconversion for anti-HIV. J Neurol 1991;238:356–357.

Scott G, Piaggesi A, Ewing DJ: Sequential autonomic function tests in HIV infection. AIDS 1990;4:1279–1281.

Shahmanesh M, Bradbeer CS, Edwards A, Smith SE: Autonomic dysfunction in patients with human immunodeficiency virus infection. Int J STD AIDS 1991;2:419–423.

Sher JH, Wrzolek MA, Shmuter JB: Motor neuron disease associ-ated with AIDS. J Neuropathol Exp Neurol 1988;47:303.

Sillevis Smitt PA, Portegies P: Fisher's syndrome associated with human immunodeficiency virus infection. Clin Neurol Neuro-surg 1990;92:353–355.

Simpson DM, Bender AN: Human immunodeficiency virus-associ-ated myopathy: Analysis of 11 patients. Ann Neurol 1988;24:79–84.

Simpson DM, Bender AN, Farraye J, et al: Human immunodefi-ciency virus wasting syndrome may represent a treatable my-opathy. Neurology 1990;40:535–538.

Simpson DM, Citak KA, Godfrey E, et al: Myopathies associated

with human immunodeficiency virus and zidovudine: Can their effects be distinguished? Neurology 1993;43:971–976.

Simpson DM, Morgello S, Citak K, et al: Motor neuron disease associated with HIV and anti-asialo GM1 antibody. Muscle Nerve 1994;17:1091.

Simpson DM, Slasor P, Dafni U, et al: Analysis of myopathy in a placebo-controlled zidovudine trial. Muscle Nerve 1997;20:382–385.

Simpson DM, Katzenstein DA, Hughes MD, et al: Neuromuscular function in HIV infection: Analysis of a placebo-controlled com-bination antiretroviral trial. AIDS Clinical Group 175/801 Study Team. AIDS 1998;12:2425–2432.

Simpson DM, Olney R, McArthur J, et al: A placebo-controlled trial of lamotrigine for painful HIV-associated neuropathy. Neu-rology 2000;54:2115–2119.

Small PM, McPhaul LW, Sooy CD, et al: Cytomegalovirus infection of the laryngeal nerve presenting as hoarseness in patients with acquired immunodeficiency syndrome. Am J Med 1989; 86:108–110.

Snider WD, Simpson DM, Nielsen S, et al: Neurological complica-tions of acquired immune deficiency syndrome: Analysis of 50 patients. Ann Neurol 1983;14:403–418.

So YT, Holtzman DM, Abrams DI, Olney RK: Peripheral neuropathy associated with acquired immunodeficiency syndrome. Preva-lence and clinical features from a population-based survey. Arch Neurol 1988;45:945–948.

So Y, Olney RK: Natural history of mononeuropathy multiplex complex or simplex in patients with HIV infection. Neurology 1991;41:375.

So Y: Clinical subdivision of mononeuropathy multiplex in pa-tients with HIV infection. Neurology 1992;42:409.

So YT, Olney RK: Acute lumbosacral polyradiculopathy in ac-quired immunodeficiency syndrome: Experience in 23 patients. Ann Neurol 1994;35:53–58.

Tagliati M, Grinnell J, Godbold J, Simpson DM: Peripheral nerve function in HIV infection: Clinical, electrophysiologic, and labo-ratory findings. Arch Neurol 1999;56:84–89.

Tagliati M, Morgello S, Simpson DM: Myopathy in HIV infection. In Gendelman H, Lipton S, Epstein L, Swindel S (eds): Neurolog-ical and Neuropsychiatric Manifestations of HIV-1 Infection. New York, Chapman and Hall, 1998; 292–302.

Veilleux M, Paltiel O, Falutz J: Sensorimotor neuropathy and ab-normal vitamin B_{12} metabolism in early HIV infection. Can J Neurol Sci 1995;22:43–46.

Verma RK, Ziegler DK, Kepes JJ: HIV-related neuromuscular syn-drome simulating motor neuron disease. Neurology 1990;40: 544–546.

Villa A, Foresti V, Confalonieri F: Autonomic neuropathy and HIV infection. Lancet 1987;2:915.

Villa A, Foresti V, Confalonieri F: Autonomic nervous system dys-function associated with HIV infection in intravenous heroin users. AIDS 1992;6:85–89.

Villa A, Foresti V, Confalonieri F: Autonomic neuropathy and pro-longation of QT interval in human immunodeficiency virus infection. Clin Auton Res 1995;5:48–52.

Wechsler AF, Ho DD: Bilateral Bell's palsy at the time of HIV seroconversion. Neurology 1989;39:747–748.

Winer JB, Bang B, Clarke JR, et al: A study of neuropathy in HIV infection. Q J Med 1992;83:473–488.

Winer JB: Neuropathies and HIV infection. J Neurol Neurosurg Psychiatry 1993;56:739–741.

Wiselka MJ, Nicholson KG, Ward SC, Flower AJ: Acute infection with human immunodeficiency virus associated with facial nerve palsy and neuralgia. J Infect 1987;15:189–190.

NEUROMUSCULAR TRANSMISSION DISORDERS

CHAPTER 75

Diseases Associated with Disorders of Neuromuscular Transmission

Donald B. Sanders

ACQUIRED MYASTHENIA GRAVIS

Acquired myasthenia gravis (MG) is an autoimmune disease in which weakness results from an immunological attack against the neuromuscular junction (Drachman, 1994; Sanders and Howard, 2000). It is not a common disease, affecting approximately 140 people per million in the United States.

Weakness that fluctuates dramatically from time to time is a distinguishing feature of diseases, such as MG, that impair neuromuscular transmission. Weakness typically becomes worse with sustained use and improves after rest. The diagnosis may be elusive, particularly in mild cases, and is frequently delayed for months or even years. Myasthenia

gravis most often begins in the third or fourth decade of life in women and after age 50 in men, but it can affect either sex at any age. As the population has aged, MG now affects more men than women and begins after age 50 in most patients.

Weakness in MG typically varies during the day, usually being least in the morning and becoming worse as the day progresses, especially after prolonged use of affected muscles. Ocular symptoms typically become worse while the patient is reading, watching television, or driving, especially in bright sunlight. Jaw muscle weakness typically becomes worse during prolonged chewing. Clinical worsening in MG has been described following administration of aminoglycoside antibiotics, magnesium, calcium-channel blockers, and iodinated intravenous contrast agents.

In most patients, symptoms fluctuate over the short term but become progressively more severe. Periods of spontaneous improvement are common, especially early in the disease. Weakness becomes maximal during the first year in two thirds of patients. Weakness remains limited to the ocular muscles in about 10% of patients (ocular myasthenia).

The diagnosis of MG is based on finding weakness in the patient, at rest or after activity, that involves certain muscle groups; demonstrating abnormal neuromuscular transmission by electromyography or seeing improvement after administration of cholinesterase inhibitors; and, in most patients, finding antibodies to the acetylcholine receptor (AChR) in the serum.

Pathophysiology

The physiological abnormality in MG results from a reduction in the number of functioning AChRs. Their reduction is due to blockade of the AChR by antibodies, destruction of the receptors, and distortion and simplification of the postsynaptic muscle membrane (Fambrough et al., 1973; Almon et al., 1974; Kao and Drachman, 1976; Drachman et al., 1982). Serum IgG from 90% of patients with MG accelerates the degradation of AChR in tissue cultured muscle (Drachman et al., 1982), which reduces the concentration of AChR on the muscle membrane. Complement-mediated damage to the neuromuscular junction produces the morphological changes in the end-plate. As a consequence of these end-plate changes, acetylcholine, which is released normally from the nerve, has a reduced effect on the muscle. The postjunctional membrane is less sensitive to applied acetylcholine, and there is a reduced probability that a nerve impulse will generate a muscle action potential.

The AChR is a glycoprotein composed of five subunits (two alpha subunits, one beta and one delta subunit, and one gamma or epsilon subunit) arranged circumferentially around a central channel through the muscle membrane (Stroud and Finer-Moore, 1985; Liu et al., 1991). Binding sites for acetylcholine are found on each of the two alpha subunits. These receptors are continuously being metabolized and resynthesized.

The anti-AChR antibodies found in patients with MG are heterogeneous, but it is likely that most are directed against a region on the extracellular side of the alpha subunit of the AChR called the main immunogenic region (MIR). Antibodies developed to the amino acid sequences that characterize the MIR accelerate the destruction of nicotinic AChR in tissue culture (antigenic modulation) and induce neuromuscular blockade in animals. Fragments of antibodies to the MIR that bind to the AChR inhibit binding of antibodies from MG patients, suggesting that the MIR is the target of most myasthenic antibodies.

The initial immunopathological event probably involves a break in tolerance to the MIR and the subsequent production of autoantibodies and complement-mediated lysis of the postsynaptic muscle membrane. The mechanism by which immunological tolerance is broken is not known, and different mechanisms may operate under different conditions.

A total of 10% of patients with MG have a thymic tumor, and 70% have hyperplastic changes in the thymus (germinal centers) that indicate immunological activity. The special relationship between the thymus and MG is unclear, but this gland may contribute to the induction and maintenance of the immunological reaction against the AChR. The thymus contains all the elements necessary for the pathogenesis of MG: myoid cells that express the AChR antigen, antigen presenting cells, and immunocompetent T cells. Thymic lymphocytes from MG patients can produce antibodies to the AChR, and thymic tissue from these patients can stimulate peripheral lymphocytes to produce these antibodies. Thymus tissue from MG patients induces the production of AChR antibodies in severely immunodeficient mice. Surgical removal of the thymus is followed by improvement in most patients, although AChR antibody levels persist or even increase in some patients after thymectomy.

Antibodies that bind to AChR are found in the serum of three-fourths of patients with acquired, generalized MG and one-half of those with ocular myasthenia (Sanders et al., 1992). The relationship between serum antibodies against AChR in the pathophysiology of the disease is not fully understood. Although antibody levels are usually higher in patients with more severe disease, values vary widely and 25% of patients are seronegative (Sanders et al., 1997).

Several observations indicate that seronegative MG is also an antibody-mediated autoimmune disorder: Patients with seronegative MG improve after immunotherapy, such as plasma exchange, immunosuppression, and thymectomy; abnormal neuromuscular transmission can be transferred to animals by injecting immunoglobulin from patients with seronegative MG; and this immunoglobulin has direct blocking effects on neuromuscular transmission when applied in vitro to nerve-muscle preparations (Yamamoto et al., 1991). It is probable that antibodies in these patients are directed against epitopes that are not present in the AChR preparations used in the diagnostic assay or that their affinity is too low for detection. In seronegative patients, the diagnosis is based on the clinical presentation, the response to cholinesterase inhibitors, and the findings on electrophysiological testing. Genetic myasthenia (see the section on genetic myasthenic syndromes, which follows) must be excluded from the differential diagnosis when seronegative MG begins in childhood.

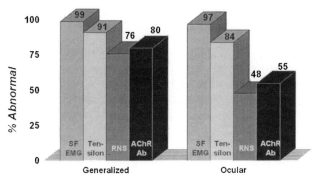

Figure 75–1. Comparison of results of initial diagnostic tests in 550 patients with acquired myasthenia gravis. SF EMG, jitter measurements by single-fiber electromyography in at least one muscle; Tensilon, Tensilon test; RNS, repetitive nerve stimulation tests in a hand and shoulder muscle; AChR Ab, binding assay for serum acetylcholine receptor antibodies. (Sanders DB, Massey JM, Howard JF, unpublished.)

Electrodiagnostic Findings

In MG, an abnormal response to repetitive nerve stimulation is found in a hand or shoulder muscle in 60% of patients with MG (Fig. 75–1). Testing of facial muscles increases the diagnostic sensitivity somewhat, but many patients with MG have normal responses to repetitive nerve stimulation in all tested muscles. Single-fiber electromyography (SFEMG) shows increased jitter in some muscles in almost all patients with MG. Jitter is greatest in weak muscles but may be abnormal even in muscles with normal strength. Patients with mild or purely ocular muscle weakness may have increased jitter only in facial muscles. A suggested strategy in the electrodiagnostic evaluation of a patient with suspected MG is described in Chapter 22.

TRANSIENT NEONATAL MYASTHENIA

A total of 10% of newborns of myasthenic mothers develop a transitory myasthenic reaction due to the transplacental passage of maternal AChR antibodies. The occurrence and severity of neonatal myasthenia are often related to the severity of disease in the mother and her AChR antibody titer, but this is not always true. Newborns with neonatal myasthenia show weak crying and sucking within the first 3 days of life and are often hypotonic. This syndrome resolves spontaneously within a few weeks. Myasthenia does not recur later on. The diagnosis is established by the response to cholinesterase inhibitors and physiological testing.

PENICILLAMINE-INDUCED MYASTHENIA

Patients treated with *d*-penicillamine for rheumatoid arthritis, Wilson's disease, or cystinuria may develop a postsynaptic myasthenic syndrome. Penicillamine-induced myasthenia is usually mild and often restricted to the ocular muscles. The diagnosis is established by the response to cholinesterase inhibitors, characteristic electrophysiological abnormalities, and elevated serum levels of AChR antibodies. It is likely that *d*-penicillamine stimulates or enhances an immunological reaction against the neuromuscular junction. The myasthenic response induced by *d*-penicillamine usually remits within 1 year after the drug is discontinued.

GENETIC MYASTHENIC SYNDROMES

Genetic forms of myasthenia constitute a heterogeneous group of disorders caused by several different abnormalities of neuromuscular transmission and are not immune mediated (Engel et al., 1999). Symptoms are typically present at birth or in early childhood, but they can be delayed until young adulthood. Ocular muscle weakness is usually the most prominent feature, but more widespread weakness is seen in many patients. Abnormal neuromuscular transmission is confirmed by the response to cholinesterase inhibitors and characteristic electrophysiological findings. Cholinesterase inhibitors improve limb muscle weakness in many forms of genetic myasthenia. Ocular muscle weakness is less responsive. Some forms of genetic myasthenia have characteristic clinical features and electrodiagnostic findings.

Congenital myasthenia is a clinical term used to describe patients with one of several genetic neuromuscular defects who have ophthalmoparesis and ptosis at birth or shortly thereafter. Mild facial paresis may also be present and mild generalized weakness sometimes develops as well, but major dysfunction is usually limited to the eye muscles. Microphysiological studies demonstrate reduced miniature end-plate potential (MEPP) amplitude and normal quantal release in some patients, as in acquired MG. In some patients, however, miniature end-plate potential amplitude is not reduced, indicating that the pathophysiology is not the same in all patients with congenital myasthenia (Vincent et al., 1981).

Edrophonium usually produces transient improvement in ocular motility in these patients. The electrodiagnostic findings are similar to those of acquired MG: Repetitive nerve stimulation studies demonstrate a decremental response that is corrected by edrophonium, and SFEMG shows increased jitter. Intracellular recordings of biopsied muscle must be performed to determine the physiological abnormality and thus the specific diagnosis in these patients.

Familial infantile myasthenia has characteristic clinical and electrophysiological features that differ from those of congenital myasthenia. Children with this condition are hypotonic at birth and have severe and repeated bouts of respiratory insufficiency and feeding difficulty (Robertson et al., 1980). They may also have fluctuating ptosis, but other ocular muscle function is usually normal. Edrophonium improves the weakness and the respiratory distress. Infants with this condition become stronger within weeks but have episodes of weakness and life-threatening apnea repeatedly throughout infancy and childhood, sometimes even into adult life (Gieron and Korthals, 1985). Physiological studies in patients with familial infantile myasthenia have demonstrated findings consistent with an abnormality of acetylcholine resynthesis or mobilization (Engel et al., 1981). A specific electrodiagnostic protocol is required to elicit the characteristic abnormalities in this neuromuscular transmission disorder (see Chapter 22) (Figs. 75–2 and 75–3).

The onset of symptoms in *slow channel syndrome* may be delayed until adult life, which makes it difficult to distinguish this condition from acquired MG (Engel et al., 1982; Oosterhuis et al., 1987). The disease is transmitted by autosomal dominant inheritance, and a family history of similar illness is often obtained. Symptoms always begin after infancy, sometimes as late as the third decade. Slowly progressive weakness selectively involves the arm, leg, neck, and facial muscles. Unlike other myasthenic syndromes, symptomatic muscles may be atrophic. Repetitive nerve stimulation studies produce a decremental response. Characteristic repetitive dis-

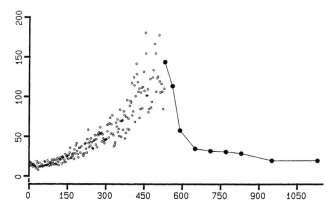

Figure 75–3. Jitter measured in a single end-plate during and after prolonged axonal stimulation in the extensor digitorum communis muscle of a patient with familial infantile myasthenia. Each open circle represents the jitter in 50 consecutive responses during continuous 10-per-second stimulation. Filled circles and solid line indicate jitter in 50 consecutive responses during intermittent stimulation at 10 per second.

charges occur after single-nerve stimulation in most, but not all, muscles and decrease or disappear during repetitive nerve stimulation (Fig. 75–4) (see Chapter 22). The physiological abnormality in this condition is a prolonged open time of the acetylcholine channel.

In *congenital end-plate acetylcholinesterase deficiency*, weakness of facial, oropharyngeal, neck, and limb muscles is noted in the neonatal period or shortly thereafter (Hutchinson et al., 1993). The pupillary light response is sluggish, and there is variable ptosis and ophthalmoparesis. Weakness progresses slowly, and patients develop postural, then fixed, spinal column deformity. There is no response to acetylcholinesterase inhibitors. Repetitive nerve stimulation produces a decrement to 2-Hz stimulation in all muscles. Single-nerve stimulation produces repetitive compound muscle action potentials 6 to 10 ms after the initial response, which fade quickly during repetitive stimulation, even at rates as low as 0.2 Hz, similar to findings in slow channel syndrome. Staining for acetylcholinesterase in the muscle biopsy aids in making the diagnosis.

Limb-girdle myasthenia typically becomes apparent in the teens, with proximal muscle weakness that improves after treatment with ChE inhibitors but slowly progresses otherwise (McQuillen, 1966; Furui et al., 1997). Repetitive nerve stimulation demonstrates a decremental pattern, and there are electromyographic and biopsy findings of a myopathy.

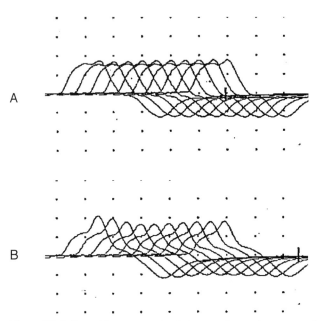

Figure 75–2. Repetitive nerve stimulation studies at 3 per second in the hypothenar muscle of a patient with familial infantile myasthenia. There is no decrement at rest (*A*), but a decremental response typical of myasthenia is seen in a train of stimuli delivered immediately after continuous 3-per-second stimulation for 5 minutes (*B*). Calibration, 5 mV/division. (From Sanders DB: Electrophysiologic study of disorders of neuromuscular transmission. In Aminoff MJ [ed]: Electrodiagnosis in Clinical Neurology. Philadelphia, Churchill Livingstone, 1999;303–321, with permission.)

EATON-LAMBERT SYNDROME

Eaton-Lambert syndrome is a presynaptic abnormality of acetylcholine release that is frequently associated with malignancy, usually small cell lung cancer (SCLC). The probable mechanism is an antibody-mediated attack against the voltage-gated calcium channels (VGCCs) on presynaptic nerve termi-

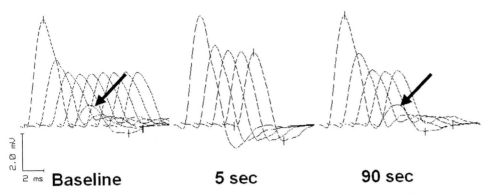

Figure 75–4. Repetitive nerve stimulation studies at 3 per second in the thenar muscle of a patient with slow channel syndrome, before and at indicated intervals after brief maximum voluntary activation of the muscle. There is a pronounced decrement, and the initial response is followed by a repetitive discharge (*arrows*) that undergoes decrements more rapidly than the preceding compound muscle action potential, is virtually absent immediately after activation, and returns thereafter. (From Bedlack RS, Bertorini TE, Sanders DB: Hidden afterdischarges in slow channel congenital myasthenic syndrome. J Clin Neuromusc Dis 2000;1:186–189.)

nals. The syndrome usually begins after age 40 but has been reported in children. Males and females are equally affected. About half the patients with Eaton-Lambert syndrome have an underlying malignancy; most of these have SCLC (Sanders, 1995).

The cancer may be discovered years before or after the symptoms of Eaton-Lambert syndrome begin. Weakness of proximal muscles, especially the legs, is the major symptom. Muscle cramps and tenderness of weak muscles are relatively common. Oropharyngeal and ocular muscles may be mildly affected, but not to the degree seen in MG. The weakness demonstrated on examination is usually relatively mild compared with the severity of symptoms. Strength may improve initially after exercise and then deteriorate with sustained activity. Edrophonium chloride does not improve strength to the degree seen in MG. Tendon reflexes are reduced or absent but are frequently normalized by repeated muscle contraction or tapping the tendon repeatedly. Dry mouth is a common symptom of autonomic dysfunction; other features are impotence and postural hypotension.

Eaton-Lambert syndrome may be first discovered when prolonged paralysis follows the use of neuromuscular blocking agents during surgery. As in MG, clinical worsening in Eaton-Lambert syndrome has been described following administration of aminoglycoside antibiotics, magnesium, calcium channel blockers, and iodinated intravenous contrast agents.

Although both Eaton-Lambert syndrome and MG are immune-mediated disorders of neuromuscular transmission, their clinical features are usually quite distinct. The weakness in Eaton-Lambert syndrome is not usually life-threatening and more closely resembles that of cachexia or polymyositis.

Immunopathology

Patients with Eaton-Lambert syndrome, like those with MG, have an increased risk of other autoim-

mune diseases. Eaton-Lambert syndrome patients who do not have cancer frequently have organ-specific serum autoantibodies, further confirming that the syndrome is immune mediated. In Eaton-Lambert syndrome, the motor nerve terminal active zone particles, which represent the VGCC, have a disorganized appearance and are reduced in number. Similar changes are seen in recipient mice who are injected with IgG from patients with the syndrome. The mechanism is probably based on cross-linking of the VGCC by antibodies.

SCLC cells are of neuroectodermal origin and contain high concentrations of VGCC. Calcium influx into these cells is inhibited by Eaton-Lambert syndrome IgG, and antibodies to the VGCC are found in the sera of most Eaton-Lambert syndrome patients with SCLC, many of those without cancer, and some of those with SCLC who do not have the syndrome (Lennon and Lambert, 1989). VGCC antibody titers do not correlate with disease severity among individuals, but the antibody levels may fall as the disease improves in patients receiving immunosuppression (Leys et al., 1991). These observations suggest that SCLC cells induce VGCC antibodies that react with the VGCC of peripheral nerves and cause Eaton-Lambert syndrome. In Eaton-Lambert syndrome patients who do not have SCLC, the VGCC antibodies may be produced as part of a more general immune-mediated disease.

Diagnostic Procedures

The diagnosis of Eaton-Lambert syndrome is confirmed by electromyography. The characteristic findings are as follows: decreased size of compound muscle action potentials (0.5 to 2 mV in the hand muscles), with further size reduction in response to repetitive nerve stimulation at frequencies between 1 and 5 Hz; doubling of compound muscle action potential size in response to repetitive stimulation at 20 to 50 Hz; and a transitory increase in compound muscle action potential size after brief maximum

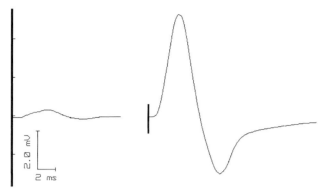

Figure 75–5. Compound muscle action potentials elicited from the thenar muscles at rest (*left*) and immediately after brief maximum voluntary contraction of the muscle. The initial response is about 10% of normal and facilitates almost 1,000% after activation. (From Sanders DB: Electrophysiologic study of disorders of neuromuscular transmission. In Aminoff MJ [ed]: Electrodiagnosis in Clinical Neurology. Philadelphia, Churchill Livingstone, 1999; 303–321, with permission.)

voluntary contraction (Figs. 75–5 and 75–6). Virtually all patients with Eaton-Lambert syndrome have a decrementing response to 3-Hz stimulation in a hand or foot muscle, and almost all have low amplitude compound muscle action potentials in some muscle (Tim et al., 2000). The details of electrophysiological features as well as the suggested electrodiagnostic testing protocol are described in Chapter 22.

The clinical features of Eaton-Lambert syndrome frequently suggest a myopathy; thus, the diagnosis may initially be suspected when needle electromyography performed to assess muscle disease demonstrates markedly unstable motor unit action potentials, a typical finding in the syndrome.

SF-EMG studies in patients with Eaton-Lambert syndrome demonstrate markedly increased jitter with frequent blocking. At many neuromuscular junctions there is a characteristic effect of firing rate, the jitter and blocking decreasing as the firing rate increases (Schwartz and Stålberg, 1975a; Trontelj and Stålberg, 1991; Sanders, 1992), but this is not seen in all end-plates or in all patients with

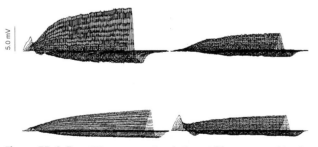

Figure 75–6. Repetitive nerve stimulation at 20 per second in the hypothenar muscles of four patients with Eaton-Lambert syndrome. The initial amplitude, decrement, and subsequent intratetanic facilitation vary considerably among these patients. (From Sanders DB: Electrodiagnosis in Clinical Neurology. Philadelphia, Churchill Livingstone, 1999;303–321, with permission.)

Eaton-Lambert syndrome (Sanders, 1992). Moreover, jitter and blocking may also improve at higher firing rates in some end-plates in patients with MG (Trontelj and Stålberg, 1991).

Overlap Syndrome

There is no single clinical or electromyographic feature that distinguishes between MG and Eaton-Lambert syndrome in all patients. There have been rare cases in which AChR and VGCC antibodies are present, giving evidence of the co-existence of Eaton-Lambert syndrome and MG in the same patient (Newsom-Davis et al., 1991). Facilitation of more than 100% may be seen in certain muscles in patients with clinically typical MG if high stimulation rates are used (Lambert and Rooke, 1965; Simpson, 1966; Brown and Johns, 1974; Dahl and Sato, 1974; Mayer and Williams, 1974; Schwartz and Stålberg, 1975b; Ozdemir and Young, 1976; Singer et al., 1981). Conversely, patients with Eaton-Lambert syndrome may have electromyographic features more characteristic of MG at some time during their illness (Scoppetta et al., 1984). In other patients, mixed clinical and electromyographic features make it impossible to distinguish between the two diseases (Fettel et al., 1978; Boiardi et al., 1979). In patients with such mixed features, the clinical characteristics and the presence of elevated AChR antibodies or lung cancer define the most probable diagnosis (Sanders and Stålberg, 1987).

BOTULISM

Food-borne botulism results from ingestion of a toxin produced by an anaerobic bacterium, *Clostridium botulinum,* which is usually found only in canned foods that have been sterilized incompletely. Neuromuscular symptoms usually begin 12 to 36 hours after ingestion of contaminated food that contains botulinum toxin. The most common form of botulism in the United States is *wound botulism,* which occurs predominantly in drug abusers following subcutaneous injection of heroin (Anonymous, 1995). *Clostridium* bacteria colonize the injection site and release a toxin that produces local and patchy systemic weakness. Major symptoms of food-borne and wound botulism include blurred vision, dysphagia, and dysarthria. Pupillary responses to light are impaired, and tendon reflexes are variably reduced. The weakness progresses for several days and then reaches a plateau. Fatal respiratory paralysis may occur rapidly. Most patients have evidence of autonomic dysfunction, such as dry mouth, constipation, or urinary retention. In patients who survive, recovery may take many months but is usually complete. The edrophonium (Tensilon) test is positive in only about one third of patients and does not distinguish botulism from other causes of neuromuscular blockade (Burningham et al., 1994). The diagnosis of wound botulism is confirmed by wound cultures and serum assay for botulinum toxin (Burningham et al., 1994).

Infantile botulism results from the growth of *C. botulinum* in the infant gastrointestinal tract and the elaboration of small quantities of toxin over a prolonged period. Signs and symptoms of constipation, lethargy, poor sucking, and weak cry usually begin at about 4 months of age. Patients have weakness of the limb and oropharyngeal muscles, poorly reactive pupils, and hypoactive tendon reflexes. Most patients require ventilatory support. The diagnosis of infant botulism is confirmed by demonstrating botulinum toxin in the stool or by isolating *C. botulinum* from stool culture. The details of electrophysiological findings in botulism are described in Chapter 22.

PHARMACEUTICAL AGENTS

Muscle Relaxants

Muscle relaxants block neuromuscular transmission, either by interfering with the interaction of acetylcholine with receptors on the muscle or by directly depolarizing the muscle membrane. Many other medications also have blocking effects on neuromuscular transmission. The most frequently encountered are aminoglycoside and fluoroquinolone antibiotics. For the most part, the neuromuscular blocking effects of these drugs are clinically apparent only when the safety factor of neuromuscular transmission has been lowered by disease or concomitant administration of other drugs. Abnormal neuromuscular transmission may be confirmed in such cases by repetitive nerve stimulation tests or administration of cholinesterase inhibitors, but the diagnosis can usually be made by withdrawing the offending medication and observing improvement in muscle function.

Magnesium

Disturbed neuromuscular transmission from hypermagnesemia occurs in patients with renal insufficiency who receive oral magnesium (e.g., laxatives) and in women who receive magnesium for preeclampsia. Clinically, hypermagnesemia resembles Eaton-Lambert syndrome: There is proximal muscle weakness, which may progress to respiratory insufficiency in severe cases. The ocular muscles are spared, and tendon reflexes are depressed. The diagnosis is made by demonstrating elevated serum magnesium levels and observing the return of tendon reflexes as the serum magnesium level falls. Edrophonium may improve strength in some patients. The response to repetitive nerve stimulation resembles that in Eaton-Lambert syndrome or botulism, with low-amplitude compound muscle action potential responses, a decremental response to low-frequency nerve stimulation, and marked facilitation after muscle activation.

Organophosphates

These agents irreversibly inhibit cholinesterase, producing neuromuscular blockade as well as autonomic and central nervous system dysfunction. Electromyographic studies can be of great value in making a diagnosis and in following the course of intoxication by these agents (Besser et al., 1989). When acetylcholinesterase has been blocked, excess acetylcholine accumulates at the neuromuscular junction and impairs neuromuscular transmission by depolarizing the postjunctional muscle membrane. Receptors on the presynaptic nerve ending are also activated by the excess acetylcholine, producing repetitive discharges when the nerve is activated. Single-nerve stimuli produce repetitive muscle discharges that follow the compound muscle action potential. Repetitive nerve stimulation produces a decrementing pattern. This combination of findings is seen within hours after ingestion of organophosphates (Besser et al., 1989). These electromyographic findings are similar to those seen in congenital end-plate acetylcholinesterase deficiency or slow channel syndrome, and after administration of high doses of acetylcholinesterase inhibitors. Besser and colleagues have described a distinctive "decrement-increment" pattern of response to repetitive nerve stimulation that is seen in the early stages of organophosphate intoxication and, again, later as the intoxication resolves. At the peak of intoxication, the decremental response is so severe that no response is seen after the first few stimuli in a train. The evolution of these electromyographic patterns has been used to assess the severity and progression of the intoxication by these agents.

NERVE AND MUSCLE DISEASES

Neuromuscular transmission is abnormal in many diseases other than those that affect primarily the neuromuscular junction. Patients with amyotrophic lateral sclerosis (ALS) may have fluctuating weakness that responds to cholinesterase inhibitors (Mulder et al., 1959). An abnormal decrement on repetitive nerve stimulation tests has been described in two thirds of patients with ALS so studied (Denys and Norris, 1979). Increased jitter and impulse blocking are seen in most patients with ALS, presumably mainly at immature end-plates resulting from collateral reinnervation; this process also gives rise to clearly increased fiber density. Various manifestations of abnormal neuromuscular transmission have also been reported in syringomyelia, poliomyelitis, peripheral neuropathy, and inflammatory myopathy (Stålberg et al., 1975). In oculocraniosomatic myopathy, the clinical pattern may resemble ocular MG, although the course is usually slowly progressive and the weakness does not fluctuate and usually does not improve after edrophonium. Jitter is increased, especially in facial muscles, in patients with this condition (Krendel et al., 1987), most of whom have myopathic features on EMG of shoulder muscles and characteristic "ragged-red fibers" on muscle biopsy.

ANIMAL VENOMS AND TOXINS

Neuromuscular blockade is the primary effect of envenomation by cobras, kraits, and some other poisonous snakes. Snake toxins that act postsynaptically and bind competitively to the receptor produce patterns of weakness identical to those of MG (Kumar and Usgaonkar, 1968). In such cases, repetitive nerve stimulation demonstrates a decremental response and weakness is reversed by cholinesterase inhibitors. Such toxins include those of cobras and the death adder (*Acanthophis antarcticus*).

References

Almon RR, Andrew CG, Appel SH: Serum globulin in myasthenia gravis: Inhibition of alpha-bungarotoxin binding to acetylcholine receptors. Science 1974;186:55–57.

Anonymous: Wound botulism—California, 1995. MMWR Morb Mortal Wkly Rep 1995;44:889–892.

Besser R, Gutmann L, Dillmann U, et al: End-plate dysfunction in acute organophosphate intoxication. Neurology 1989;39:561–567.

Boiardi A, Bussone G, Negri S: Alternating myasthenia and myastheniform syndrome in the same subject. J Neurol 1979;220:57–64.

Brown JC, Johns RJ: Diagnostic difficulties encountered in the myasthenic syndrome sometimes associated with carcinoma. J Neurol Neurosurg Psychiatry 1974;37:1214–1224.

Burningham MD, Walter FG, Mechem C, et al: Wound botulism. Ann Emerg Med 1994;24:1184–1187.

Dahl DS, Sato S: Unusual myasthenic state in a teen-age boy. Neurology 1974;24:897–901.

Denys EH, Norris FH: Amyotrophic lateral sclerosis impairment of neuromuscular transmission. Arch Neurol 1979;36:202–205.

Drachman DB: Medical Progress: Myasthenia gravis. N Engl J Med 1994;330:1797–1810.

Drachman DB, Adams RN, Josifek LF, Self SG: Functional activities of autoantibodies to acetylcholine receptors and the clinical severity of myasthenia gravis. N Engl J Med 1982;307:769–775.

Engel AG, Ohno K, Sine SM: Congenital myasthenic syndromes: Recent advances. Arch Neurol 1999;56:163–167.

Engel AG, Lambert EH, Mulder DM, et al: Recently recognized congenital myasthenic syndromes: (a) End-plate acetylcholine (ACh) esterase deficiency, (b) putative abnormality of the ACh induced ion channel, (c) putative defect of ACh resynthesis or mobilization—clinical features, ultrastructure and cytochemistry. Ann NY Acad Sci 1981;377:614–639.

Engel AG, Lambert EH, Mulder DM, et al: A newly recognized congenital myasthenic syndrome attributed to a prolonged open time of the acetylcholine-induced ion channel. Ann Neurol 1982;11:553–569.

Fambrough DM, Drachman DB, Satyamurti S: Neuromuscular junction in myasthenia gravis: Decreased acetylcholine receptors. Science 1973;182:293–295.

Fettel MR, Shin HS, Penn AS: Combined Eaton-Lambert syndrome and myasthenia gravis. Neurology 1978;28:398.

Furui E, Fukushima K, Sakashita T, et al: Familial limb-girdle myasthenia with tubular aggregates. Muscle Nerve 1997;20:599–603.

Gieron MA, Korthals JK: Familial infantile myasthenia gravis: Report of three cases with follow-up until adult life. Arch Neurol 1985;42:143–144.

Hutchinson DO, Walls TJ, Nakano S, et al: Congenital endplate acetylcholinesterase deficiency. Brain 1993;116:633–653.

Kao I, Drachman DB: Myasthenic immunoglobulin accelerates acetylcholine receptor degradation. Science 1976;196:527–529.

Krendel DA, Sanders DB, Massey JM: Single fiber electromyography in chronic progressive external ophthalmoplegia. Muscle Nerve 1987;10:299–302.

Kumar SM, Usgaonkar RS: Myasthenia gravis–like picture resulting from snake bite. J Indian Med Assoc 1968;50:428–429.

Lambert EH, Rooke ED: Myasthenic state and lung cancer. In Brain WR, Norris FH (eds): Contemporary Neurology Symposia: The Remote Effects of Cancer on the Nervous System. New York, Grune & Stratton, 1965; 67–80.

Lennon VA, Lambert EH: Autoantibodies bind solubilized calcium channel-omega-conotoxin complexes from small cell lung carcinoma: A diagnostic aid for Lambert-Eaton myasthenic syndrome. Mayo Clin Proc 1989;64:1498–1504.

Leys K, Lang B, Johnston I, Newsom-Davis J: Calcium channel autoantibodies in the Lambert-Eaton myasthenic syndrome. Ann Neurol 1991;29:307–314.

Liu Y, Zheng Y, Camacho P, et al: Functional differences between ACh receptor channels containing gamma and epsilon subunits. Biomed Res 1991;12:83–85.

Mayer RF, Williams IR: Incrementing responses in myasthenia gravis. Arch Neurol 1974;731:24–26.

McQuillen MP: Familial limb-girdle myasthenia. Brain 1966;89:121–132.

Mulder DW, Lambert EH, Eaton LM: Myasthenic syndrome in patients with amyotrophic lateral sclerosis. Neurology 1959;9:627–631.

Newsom-Davis J, Leys K, Vincent A, et al: Immunological evidence for the co-existence of the Lambert-Eaton myasthenic syndrome and myasthenia gravis in two patients. J Neurol Neurosurg Psychiatry 1991;54:452–453.

Oosterhuis HJGH, Newsom-Davis J, Wokke JHJ: The slow channel syndrome: Two new cases. Brain 1987;110:1061–1079.

Ozdemir C, Young RR: The results to be expected from electrical testing in the diagnosis of myasthenia gravis. Ann NY Acad Sci 1976;274:203–222.

Robertson WC, Chun RWM, Kornguth SE: Familial infantile myasthenia. Arch Neurol 1980;37:117–119.

Sanders DB: The effect of firing rate on neuromuscular jitter in Lambert-Eaton myasthenic syndrome. Muscle Nerve 1992;15:256–258.

Sanders DB: Lambert-Eaton myasthenic syndrome: Clinical diagnosis, immune-mediated mechanisms, and update on therapy. Ann Neurol 1995;37(suppl 1):S63–S73.

Sanders DB, Howard FM Jr: Disorders of neuromuscular transmission. In Bradley WG, Daroff RB, Fenichel GM, Marsden CD (eds): Neurology in Clinical Practice. New York, Butterworth Publishers, 2000; 2167–2185.

Sanders DB, Stålberg E: The overlap between myasthenia gravis and Lambert-Eaton myasthenic syndrome. Ann NY Acad Sci 1987;505:864–865.

Sanders DB, Andrews PI, Howard JF Jr, Massey JM: Seronegative myasthenia gravis. Neurology 1997;48(suppl 5):S40–S51.

Sanders DB, Howard JF, Massey JM: Acetylcholine receptor antibody determinations in 724 patients with acquired myasthenia gravis (MG). Annual Scientific Session, Myasthenia Gravis Foundation of America, 1992.

Schwartz MS, Stålberg E: Myasthenic syndrome studied with single fiber electromyography. Arch Neurol 1975a;32:815–817.

Schwartz MS, Stålberg E: Myasthenia gravis with features of the myasthenic syndrome. Neurology 1975b;25:80–84.

Scoppetta C, Casali C, Vaccario ML, Provenzano C: Difficult diagnosis of Eaton-Lambert myasthenic syndrome. Muscle Nerve 1984;7:680–681.

Simpson JA: Disorders of neuromuscular transmission. Proc R Soc Med 1966;59:993–998.

Singer P, Smith L, Ziegler DK, Festoff BW: Posttetanic potentiation in a patient with myasthenia gravis. Neurology 1981;31:1345–1347.

Stålberg E, Schwartz MS, Trontelj JV: Single fibre electromyography in various processes affecting the anterior horn cell. J Neurol Sci 1975;24:403–415.

Stroud RM, Finer-Moore J: Acetylcholine receptor structure, function and evolution. Annu Rev Cell Biol 1985;1:317–351.

Tim RW, Massey JM, Sanders DB: Lambert-Eaton myasthenic syndrome: Electrodiagnostic findings and response to treatment. Neurology 2000;54:2176–2178.

Trontelj JV, Stålberg E: Single motor end-plates in myasthenia gravis and LEMS at different firing rates. Muscle Nerve 1991; 14:226–232.

Vincent A, Cull-Candy SG, Newsom-Davis J, et al: Congenital myasthenia: End-plate acetylcholine receptors and electrophysiology in five cases. Muscle Nerve 1981;4:306–318.

Yamamoto T, Vincent A, Ciulla TA, et al: Seronegative myasthenia gravis: A plasma factor inhibiting agonist-induced acetylcholine receptor function copurifies with IgM. Ann Neurol 1991; 30:550–557.

SECTION XXI

MYOPATHIES

CHAPTER 76

Congenital Myopathies and Muscular Dystrophies

C. Michel Harper

INTRODUCTION

The congenital myopathies and muscular dystrophies are genetic disorders caused by an alteration in the structure and function of skeletal muscle. Although this broad definition could include the myotonic disorders (muscle channelopathies) and metabolic myopathies, with the exception of myotonic dystrophy and proximal myotonic myopathy, these disorders are covered separately in Chapters 79 and 80. The congenital myopathies and muscular dystrophies follow classic mendelian patterns of inheritance. The genetic defects and molecular pathogenic mechanisms are identified in some and are completely unknown in others. The spectrum of clinical manifestations is diverse, ranging from subclinical to lethal disease. Likewise, the age at onset ranges from infancy to adulthood. Although inherited muscle disorders have traditionally been classified by clinical and pathological criteria (Table 76–1), advances in molecular biology permit a more logical classification of these disorders, based on the identification of the affected gene and an understanding of the function of the gene product in both normal and pathological states (Table 76–2).

Role of Electrodiagnostic Studies in the Evaluation of Inherited Myopathy

The evolution of molecular diagnostic testing has put into question the role of electromyography (EMG) and standard muscle biopsy in the diagnosis of many inherited myopathic disorders. Clearly, in some disorders, such as the dystrophinopathies, classic myotonic dystrophy, facioscapulohumeral and oculopharyngeal dystrophies, and some limb-girdle muscular dystrophies, EMG is no longer needed for diagnostic purposes. However, even in these cases, when used judiciously, EMG provides valuable ancillary information regarding the distribution and severity of muscle involvement. When used in conjunction with clinical data, EMG helps differentiate inherited myopathies from either acquired ones or from inherited disorders of the lower motor neuron or peripheral nerve. In addition, the yield of diagnostic information from muscle biopsy is often increased when the EMG is used to help determine the most appropriate muscle to sample.

The findings on EMG in muscle disease complement clinical, genetic, and pathological data but are not disease specific. The physiological alterations of the motor unit produced by muscle disease are outlined in Table 76–3. The EMG is most sensitive in detecting diseases that produce alteration in muscle membrane excitability, or muscle fiber necrosis, splitting, or vacuolation. Alterations in the type of fiber, in muscle fiber diameter or packing density, or in the amount of interstitial tissue are more difficult

---

Table 76–1. Traditional Classification of Inherited Myopathies

Congenital Myopathies
    Central core disease
    Nemaline myopathy
    Myotubular (centronuclear) myopathy
    Myofibrillary myopathy (desmin storage myopathy)
    Congenital fiber type disproportion
    Multicore-minicore disease
    Incompletely characterized congenital myopathies
Muscular Dystrophies
    Dystrophinopathies (Duchenne's, Becker's, Becker variants)
    Facioscapulohumeral dystrophy
    Limb-girdle muscular dystrophy
    Emery-Dreifuss dystrophy
    Congenital muscular dystrophy
    Oculopharyngeal dystrophy
    Distal dystrophy
    Bethlem's myopathy
    Barth's syndrome
    Myotonic dystrophy
Myotonic Disorders and Periodic Paralysis (Channelopathies)
    Chloride channelopathies
        Myotonia congenita
    Sodium channelopathies
        Paramyotonia congenita
        Hyperkalemic periodic paralysis
        Myotonia fluctuans
    Calcium channelopathies
        Hypokalemic periodic paralysis
Metabolic Myopathies
    Glycogenoses
    Disorders of lipid metabolism
    Disorders of the electron transport chain

to detect with EMG unless the changes are severe. This is why some muscle disorders are associated with few, if any, abnormalities on standard EMG testing.

Nerve conduction studies are often normal or mildly abnormal in a nonspecific manner in congenital myopathies and muscular dystrophies. The amplitude of the compound muscle action potential (CMAP) is reduced in some muscle diseases, but such reduction may occur in disorders of the motor neuron, axon, or neuromuscular junction as well. Changes in motor conduction velocity, distal latency, F waves, sensory conduction studies, repetitive stimulation, and needle EMG can usually distinguish myopathy from other disorders of the motor unit. It may be difficult to distinguish myopathic

Table 76–2. Genetic and Molecular Classification of Inherited Myopathies

Congenital Myopathies

Descriptive Classification	Inheritance	Gene	Gene Product
Central core myopathy	AD	RYR1;19q13	Ryanodine
Isolated cardiomyopathy	AD	MYH7;14q	Myosin
Myotubular myopathy	XL	MTMX; Xq28	Myotubularin
	AR	Unknown	Unknown
Nemaline myopathy	AR	NEM2;2q21	Nebulin
	AR>AD	ACTA1;1q24	α-Actin
	AD>AR	TPM3;1q21	Tropomyosin
	AD	TPM2;9p13	Tropomyosin
	AR	Unknown	Unknown
Fiber size disproportion	AR	Unknown	Unknown
Minicore myopathy	AD>AR	Unkown	Unknown

Muscular Dystrophies

Descriptive Classification	Inheritance	Gene	Gene Product
DMD, BMD, Becker variants (dystrophinopathy)	XL	Dystrophin; Xp21	Dystrophin
Emery-Dreifuss	XL	Emerin; Xq28	Emerin
LGMD1A	AD	?Myotilin; 5q22	?Myotilin
LGMD1B	AD	?Laminin A and C 1q11-22	?Laminin A and C
LGMD1C	AD	CAV3; 3p25	Calveolin-3
LGMD1D	AD	7q	Unknown
LGMD2A	AR	CAPN3; 15q15	Calpain-3
LGMD2B (allelic with Miyoshi's myopathy)	AR	Dysferlin; 2p13	Dysferlin
LGMD2C (sarcoglycanopathy)	AR	SGCC; 13q12	γ-Sarcoglycan
LGMD2D (sarcoglycanopathy)	AR	SGCA; 17q	α-Sarcoglycan
LGMD2E (sarcoglycanopathy)	AR	SGCB; 4q12	β-Sarcoglycan
LGMD2F (sarcoglycanopathy)	AR	SGCD; 5q33	δ-Sarcoglycan
LGMD2G	AR	17q11-12	?Telethonin
LGMD2H	AR	9q31-33	Unknown
α2-Laminin congenital MD	AR	α2-Laminin; 6q22	α2-Laminin (merosin)
α7-Integrin congenital MD	AR	α7-Integrin; 12q31	α7-Integrin
Fukuyama's congenital MD	AR	FCMD; 9q31	Fukutin
Walker-Warburg congenital MD	AR	Unknown	Unknown
Muscle-eye-brain congenital MD	AR	Unknown	Unknown
Bethlem's myopathy	AD	COL6A1-2;21q22 COL6A3; 2q37	Collagen VI
Barth's syndrome	XR	G4.5; Xq28	Tafazzin
Emery-Dreifuss MD	XR	EDMD; Xq28	Emerin
Epidermolysis bullosa with late-onset MD	AR	PLEC1; 8q24.13	Plectin
Late-adult-onset 1A distal dystrophy (Welander's)	AD	2p13	?Dysferlin
Late-adult-onset 1B distal dystrophy (Finnish tibial and Markesbery's)	AD	TMD; 2q31-33	Titan
Early-adult-onset 1A distal dystrophy (Nonaka)	AR	9p1-q1	Unknown
Early-adult-onset 1B distal dystrophy (Miyoshi's)	AR	Dysferlin;2p13	Dysferlin
Early-adult-onset 1C distal dystrophy (Laing's)	AD	MPD1; 14q11	Unknown
FSHD	AD	FSHD;4q35	?;Short D4Z4 repeat
Scapuloperoneal dystrophy	AD	12	Unknown
Oculopharyngeal muscular dystrophy	AD	PABP2;13q11	Polyadenyl-binding protein 2
Myotonic dystrophy	AD	DM; 19q13	Myotonin protein kinase
Myotonic dystrophy 2	AD	DM2;3q	Unknown
PROMM	AD	DM2;3q	Unknown

Table continued on following page

Table 76–2. *Continued.*

Muscle Channelopathies

Descriptive Classification	Inheritance	Gene	Gene Product
Chloride channelopathies (myotonia congenita, fluctuans, levior)	MC–AD/AR, MF–AD ML–AD	CLCN-1; 7q35	Chloride channel
Sodium channelopathies (paramyotonia congenita, periodic paralysis, myotonia fluctuans, permaneens, acetazolamide-responsive myotonia)	AD	SCN4A; 17q23	Sodium channel, α-subunit
Hypokalemic periodic paralysis	AD	CACNA1S; 1q32	Calcium channel, α-1S subunit Sodium channel

Mitochondrial Myopathies

Descriptive Classification	Inheritance	Gene	Gene Product
MELAS and MERRF	Maternal	80–90%–point mutations t-RNA	—
KSS	Sporadic, maternal	90%–large single mtDNA deletion, 10%–point mut or duplication	—
CPEO	Sporadic, maternal, AD	50%–large single mtDNA deletion, other single or multiple pt mut in mt or nuc DNA	—

Table 76–3. Alterations of the Motor Unit Produced by Muscle Disease

Primary	EMG Manifestations
Loss of muscle fibers per motor unit	Low CMAP, small polyphasic MUP, rapid recruitment
Fiber necrosis and denervation	Fibrillation potentials
Fiber regeneration and splitting	Small polyphasic MUP, sometimes long-duration MUP, rapid recruitment
Vacuolar change	Fibrillation potentials, Myotonic discharges
Altered membrane excitability	Myotonic discharges, CRDs, or reduced spontaneous and MUP activity
Altered energy utilization	No change or reduced spontaneous and MUP activity
Altered excitation-contraction coupling	No change or reduced spontaneous and MUP activity

Secondary	EMG Manifestations
Altered proportion of fiber typing	No change or large MUP if loss of type I fibers
Reduced diameter of fibers	Small MUP
Increased packing density of muscle fibers	Increased fiber density on SFEMG
Reduced safety factor of NMT	Increased jitter on SFEMG
Increased connective tissue	Increased resistance to needle movement, reduced insertional activity and motor unit recruitment (late)

CMAP, compound muscle action potential; MUP, motor unit potential; CRD, complex repetitive discharges; SFEMG, single-fiber EMG; NMT, neuromuscular transmission.

from neurogenic disorders when the disease is chronic and severe, or when both nerve and muscle are involved. Changes in the size, morphology, and recruitment of motor unit potentials (MUP) that are commonly observed in myopathies are listed in Table 76–3.

CONGENITAL MYOPATHIES

The congenital myopathies were first recognized as a unique inherited clinical syndrome in the 1950s (Shy, 1956). Features that have traditionally been used to distinguish the congenital myopathies from muscular dystrophy, metabolic myopathy, and congenital myasthenic syndromes include the following:

1. Clinical manifestations from birth, including hypotonia, generalized or proximal weakness, and reduced muscle bulk
2. Slow or nonprogressive course with normal or only mild elevation of serum muscle enzymes
3. Association with multiple skeletal deformities, including scoliosis, talipes, congenital hip dislocation, chest anomalies, elongated face, and high-arched palate
4. Relatively distinctive morphological changes on muscle biopsy that allow subclassification into a number of major categories (Table 76–4)

Other histological features important in the diagnosis of congenital myopathy are the absence of inflammation, little or no fiber necrosis, normal glycogen and lipid content, and normal histochemistry, including mitochondrial function.

Molecular studies have led to a better understand-

Table 76–4. Pathological Findings in Congenital Myopathy

Name	Pathological Features
Central core disease	Type I fiber predominance, central cores
Nemaline myopathy	Type I fiber predominance, nemaline rods within sarcomere
Myotubular (centronuclear) myopathy	Type I fiber predominance, central nuclei
Myofibrillar myopathy (desmin storage or related myopathy)	Subsarcolemmal and intermyofibrillar accumulation of desmin
Fiber type disproportion	Reduced number and diameter of type I fibers
Minicore	Multifocal disruption of sarcomeres by multiple small cores
Myopathy with tubular aggregates	Bundles of microtubules in periphery of type I and type II fibers

ing of the pathogenesis of some congenital myopathies. As more information becomes available, it is likely that these disorders, like muscular dystrophy, will be reclassified, based on the abnormal gene and gene product (see Table 76–2).

Electrodiagnostic studies show nonspecific and mild abnormalities in most congenital myopathies. Nerve conduction studies and EMG are often normal or show typical findings of a myopathy with low-amplitude CMAPs and small, polyphasic, rapidly recruited MUPs. Fibrillation potentials are most commonly observed in myotubular myopathy but also occur in nemaline myopathy, congenital fiber-type disproportion myopathy, and myofibrillary myopathy. Myotonic discharges are observed in myotubular and myofibrillary myopathy.

Central Core Disease

GENETICS

Central core disease (CCD) is an autosomal dominant disorder with variable penetrance. Central core disease is caused by mutations in the ryanodine receptor gene (*RYR1*) on chromosome 19q13.1 and is allelic with malignant hyperthermia (Zhang et al., 1993). The mechanism by which mutations in the ryanodine receptor produce CCD is unknown. Presumably, there are alterations of calcium regulation within the sarcoplasmic reticulum or other areas of the muscle fiber. The loss of mitochondria from the central portion of the muscle cell in CCD may result from calcium accumulation within mitochondria secondary to defects in sarcoplasmic calcium regulation (Loke and MacLennan, 1998). Mutations involving the transmembrane-luminal domain of the ryanodine receptor are associated with more severe clinical manifestations in CCD (Lynch et al., 1999). An autosomal dominant form of CCD that produces an isolated cardiomyopathy has been associated with mutations in the myosin gene (*MYH7*) on chromosome 14 (Ko et al., 1996).

CLINICAL MANIFESTATIONS

Central core disease displays variation in the onset and severity of clinical manifestations. CCD usually presents in infancy with hypotonia, proximal weakness, absent deep tendon reflexes, and skeletal deformities (Shy et al., 1963). Congenital dislocation of the hip is the most common skeletal abnormality, but scoliosis, talipes, and finger contractures and high-arched palate also occur (Bethlem et al., 1971). Adolescence or adult-onset cases present with mild proximal weakness and/or exercise intolerance, with myalgias or malignant hyperthermia-like reactions to anesthetics (Bethlem et al., 1966; Loke and MacLennan, 1998). Ocular and other cranial muscles are spared, and respiratory muscle involvement is typically mild. Creatine kinase levels are normal or only slightly elevated. The clinical course of CCD is either slowly progressive or nonprogressive with changes noted only after years of follow-up (Lamont et al., 1998).

PATHOLOGY, ELECTROMYOGRAPHY, AND DIAGNOSIS

The muscle biopsy in CCD reveals type I fiber predominance and characteristic central cores that extend the length of the affected fibers (Fardeau and Tome, 1994). The central region of the muscle fiber stains poorly for oxidative enzymes and demonstrates a deficiency of mitochondria as well as structural alterations of the myofibrils and sarcoplasmic reticulum. Central cores have been described in other congenital myopathies (i.e., nemaline myopathy) and thus are not entirely specific for CCD (Fardeau and Tome, 1994). On electron microscopy, there is alteration of the contractile apparatus as well as depletion of mitochondria and sarcoplasmic reticulum in the region of the core (Hayashi et al., 1989).

In patients with CCD, nerve conduction studies are normal, and the needle EMG shows small, rapidly recruited, polyphasic MUPs with normal spontaneous activity (Bodensteiner, 1994). The EMG is typically normal in mild CCD.

Finding characteristic central cores on routine muscle biopsy in the appropriate clinical setting establishes the diagnosis of CCD. Genetic testing is not routinely available at this time.

Nemaline Myopathy

GENETICS

Nemaline myopathy is genetically and clinically heterogeneous. Autosomal dominant, recessive, and sporadic patterns of inheritance have been described. At least four genes that cause congenital nemaline myopathy have been isolated. The most common form of nemaline myopathy is autosomal recessive, with onset in the infantile period, and is linked to mutations in the nebulin gene on chromosome 2q21-22 (*NEM2*). Nebulin is a large protein found in thin muscle filaments and contributes to the formation of the Z-disk (Pelin et al., 1999). The second most common form of nemaline myopathy is associated with mutations in the skeletal muscle α-actin gene (*ACTA1*) on chromosome 1q42 (Nowak et al., 1999). These may follow either an autosomal recessive or an autosomal dominant pattern. An autosomal dominant form and a few cases of autosomal recessive forms of nemaline myopathy with onset in childhood are caused by mutations in the tropomyosin gene (*TPM2* on 9p13 or *TPM3* on 1q21 (formally known as *NEM1*), which codes for the slow form of α-tropomyosin in the thin filament of the sarcomere (Laing et al., 1995b). When the mutant tropomyosin was expressed in rat muscle, contraction became less sensitive to calcium, but no rod formation was noted (Michele et al., 1999). Other kindreds and isolated cases of nemaline myopathy remain undefined genetically.

CLINICAL MANIFESTATIONS

Autosomal recessive nemaline myopathy most commonly presents in infancy with hypotonia, generalized weakness, feeding difficulties, reduced muscle bulk, and dysmorphic facial features. Extraocular muscles are usually spared, but facial, bulbar, and respiratory muscles are affected. Although the majority of patients follow a relatively nonprogressive course, the development of respiratory insufficiency or cardiomyopathy can lead to death within the first decade of life. In the most severe neonatal autosomal recessive form, there is respiratory distress from birth with hypotonia, feeding difficulties, and a dilated cardiomyopathy, all of which lead to death within the first year of life. The late-onset form is usually autosomal dominant and presents in childhood or adult life with a proximal myopathy that varies considerably in severity and rate of progression. Extraocular, facial, bulbar, and respiratory weakness, cardiomyopathy, and skeletal deformities are usually absent, but respiratory involvement in the absence of generalized muscle weakness has been described (Falga-Tirado et al., 1995). In both autosomal recessive and dominant forms of nemaline myopathy, the weakness can affect distal limb muscles predominantly. The serum creatine kinase is typically normal, even in severely affected patients.

PATHOLOGY

The characteristic pathological finding in nemaline myopathy is the presence of short, granular-appearing rods scattered around the periphery of type I muscle fibers (Fardeau and Tome, 1994). These are best seen on modified Gomori trichrome–stained sections of frozen muscle. Type I fiber pre-

dominance is also observed and correlates with the severity of clinical weakness. The rods are composed of α-actinin and actin and, on electron microscopy, appear to be attached to the Z-disc near the origin of the thin filaments. Rods are also found in some acquired myopathies, for example, inflammatory myopathy and human immunodeficiency virus (HIV)–associated myopathy; thus, they may represent a relatively nonspecific response to thin filament or Z-disc injury.

ELECTROMYOGRAPHY

The EMG in nemaline myopathy shows normal nerve conduction studies and short-duration, low-amplitude, polyphasic MUPs on needle EMG (Shy et al., 1963). The EMG may be normal in mild cases or those with clinical involvement restricted to the respiratory muscles. Some patients develop fibrillation potentials and long-duration, highly polyphasic MUPs, with reduced recruitment as the disease progresses (Karpati et al., 1972; Wallgren-Pettersson et al., 1989). Whether these findings represent involvement of the motor neuron or axon is unclear, as pathologic studies have failed to provide convincing evidence. Similar findings could be caused by a severe chronic myopathy associated with changes in muscle-fiber architecture and a reduced number of motor units (Daube, 1978).

DIAGNOSIS

The diagnosis of congenital nemaline myopathy can be difficult. Nemaline rods are observed in some acquired myopathies and other, congenital myopathies. In addition, the variable age at onset, pattern of inheritance, and clinical course make it difficult to define congenital nemaline myopathy as a single disease entity. It is probable that the formation of nemaline rods represents a fairly nonspecific effect of disruption of various components of the sarcomere. Further advances in the area of molecular genetics are required to refine the classification and diagnosis of nemaline myopathy. Until then, the finding of nemaline rods in the absence of inflammation and in the appropriate clinical setting is sufficient for the diagnosis.

Myotubular Myopathy

GENETICS

Myotubular myopathy is also known as centronuclear myopathy because of the predominance of small type I fibers with central nuclei, which represent immature myotubes, on muscle biopsy. X-linked recessive as well as autosomal recessive and dominant forms of myotubular myopathy have been described (Wallgren-Pettersson et al., 1995). The gene for the X-linked form of myotubular myopathy, *MTMX* (Xq28), codes for a ubiquitous tyrosine phosphatase, myotubularin, which is thought to perform an important function in signal transduction and differentiation (Laporte et al., 1996). The autosomal recessive form has not been linked.

CLINICAL MANIFESTATIONS

The X-linked recessive form begins in early infancy, with severe hypotonia, generalized weakness, and respiratory failure that leads to either death within the first year of life or severe disability, with ophthalmoplegia, generalized hypotonia, and respiratory weakness leading to partial or complete ventilator dependency thereafter (Askansas et al., 1979; Herman et al., 1999). Polyhydramnios and reduced fetal movements are often present during pregnancy. Bilateral ptosis, facial and bulbar weakness, and skeletal deformities are often present. Enlarged head size and hydrocephalus have been associated with myotubular myopathy, but intelligence is usually normal (Joseph et al., 1995). Autosomal dominant centronuclear myopathy can present from early childhood to the third or fourth decade of life (Wallgren-Pettersson et al., 1995). Generalized weakness with reduced muscle bulk, hyporeflexia, and involvement of extraocular and bulbar muscles is common. Elongated facies, high-arched palate, scoliosis, and other skeletal abnormalities are prominent features. The autosomal recessive form is intermediate with regard to both age at onset and clinical severity between the X-linked recessive and autosomal dominant forms. The serum creatine kinase level is typically normal in all forms of myotubular myopathy.

PATHOLOGY AND EMG

Muscle biopsy specimens in all forms of myotubular myopathy show central nuclei in the majority of muscle fibers and type I fiber predominance (Fardeau and Tome, 1994). Interstitial connective tissue is normal.

Nerve conduction studies are normal in both the X-linked and the autosomal dominant forms of myotubular myopathy. In mildly affected cases, the needle examination is normal as well (Serratrice et al., 1978). Otherwise, small, rapidly recruited, polyphasic MUPs are observed. Fibrillation potentials, myotonic discharges, and complex repetitive discharges have also been described, especially in autosomal dominant kindreds (Hawkes and Absolon, 1975).

DIAGNOSIS

The diagnosis of myotubular myopathy continues to rely on the clinical features, EMG, and muscle biopsy. Most *MTMX* gene mutations that produce myotubular myopathy are small point mutations, which has made routine diagnostic screening by genetic testing difficult (Laporte et al., 1997; Buj-Bello et al., 1999). Reports suggest that direct mutational diagnosis of families at risk, in combination with haplotype analysis, can be used to confirm the prenatal diagnosis of X-linked myotubular myopathy (Tanner et al., 1998).

Myofibrillar Myopathy (MFM)

GENETICS

Myofibrillar myopathy comprises a heterogeneous group of disorders that share several important clinical as well as pathological features. The clinical manifestations that occur frequently in MFM include distal as well as proximal weakness, cardiomyopathy, and peripheral neuropathy. In addition, all cases of MFM have focal dissolution of myofibrils, with accumulation of multiple intracellular proteins on muscle biopsy. Since much of the attention has focused on the accumulation of desmin, the MFMs have been referred to as desmin storage or desmin-related myopathies. More than five separate chromosomal loci for MFM have been identified to date (Table 76–5).

All of the MFMs are associated with altered structure and function of desmin or the desmin-associated network of proteins that support the myofibrils at the level of the Z-disk, link myofibrils to the sarcolemma, and protect myofibrils from disruption during active muscle contraction. Desmin is organized into filaments, 10 nm in diameter, that encircle the Z-disk. Desmin filaments are attached to the Z-disk and the sarcolemma. Plectin links adjacent desmin filaments together. αB-Crystallin is a heat-shock protein that is localized to the Z-disk and is upregulated after stress and exercise. It chaperones and protects other proteins, including actin, desmin, tubulin, and a variety of enzymes.

Table 76–5. Chromosomal Loci Associated with Myofibrillary Myopathy

Inheritance	Chromosome/ Gene/Product	Clinical Features
Autosomal dominant (WilhelmsenAN96)	12q, gene unknown	Scapuloperoneal weakness, hearing loss, cardiomyopathy
Autosomal dominant (VicartNG98)	11q21-23, αB-crystallin	Proximal and distal weakness, palatal weakness, cataracts, cardiomyopathy
Autosomal dominant and recessive (GoldfarbNG98)	2q35, desmin	Facial, proximal, and distal limb weakness, hearing loss, cardiomyopathy, gut hypomotility (recessive form)
Autosomal dominant (NicolaoAJHG99)	2q24-31, gene unknown	Proximal and distal limb weakness, early respiratory failure
Autosomal dominant (MelbergAN99)	10q22.3, gene unknown	Proximal and distal limb weakness, cardiomyopathy

CLINICAL MANIFESTATIONS

The clinical features of MFM vary, depending on the type and severity of mutation. The phenotypic features common to most myofibrillar myopathies include distal weakness of equal or greater severity than proximal weakness, pharyngeal and/or respiratory involvement in some, and cardiomyopathy in about 50% of patients (see Table 76–5). As many as 60% of cases have manifestations of a peripheral neuropathy in addition to myopathy (for review see Engel [1999]).

PATHOLOGY

In general, there is focal dissolution of myofibrils and accumulation of multiple intracellular proteins. The accumulated proteins produce granulofilamentous, spheroid, or Mallory body–like inclusions within the muscle fiber (Engel, 1999). Other common but relatively nonspecific findings include variation in fiber size, with increased number of fibers with central nuclei, rimmed vacuoles, minimal if any necrosis, and a mild increase in interstitial connective tissue.

EMG AND DIAGNOSIS (Horowitz and Schmalbruch, 1994; Nakano et al., 1996; Engel, 1999)

Nerve conduction studies in MFM are normal or show features of a mild axonal peripheral neuropathy. Needle EMG shows myopathic or mixed features, with an abundance of abnormal spontaneous activity, including fibrillation potentials, myotonic discharges, and complex repetitive discharges. Fibrillation potentials are frequently observed in the thoracic paraspinal muscles. The diagnosis of MFM is made on the basis of characteristic clinical and pathological features. Routine molecular genetic diagnosis is not available currently.

Congenital Fiber-Type Disproportion Myopathy

GENETICS AND CLINICAL MANIFESTATIONS

There is considerable heterogeneity in the pattern of inheritance and clinical presentation of this disorder, which raises questions about the classification of congenital fiber-type disproportion myopathy (CFTD) as a distinct entity. Most patients present in infancy with hypotonia, generalized muscle weakness with prominent facial involvement but sparing of bulbar and respiratory muscles. Dysmorphic features of the face and other skeletal deformities are common. Other clinical manifestations have been reported, including a progressive limb-girdle myopathy of childhood, rigid spine syndrome, and severe scoliosis with respiratory insufficiency.

PATHOLOGY AND EMG

The only significant pathological alteration in CFTD is a uniform reduction in the diameter of type I fibers compared with type II fibers (Fardeau and Tome, 1994). The EMG has been reported to be normal (Curless and Nelson, 1977), but fibrillation potentials and small polyphasic MUPs have been observed in some cases (Cavanagh et al., 1979).

Incompletely Characterized Syndromes

A number of congenital myopathies do not form distinct nosological entities yet have fairly characteristic findings on muscle biopsy specimens. The histological findings show changes in the sarcomere, cytoplasmic inclusions or other alterations of cellular organelles (see Table 76–4). As with the other congenital myopathies described previously, these disorders usually present in infancy or childhood with a generalized myopathy that is often associated with skeletal deformities. Some cases have prominent facial involvement, while others have only myalgias and cramps with exertion. Cardiomyopathy, ptosis, muscle atrophy, and mental retardation may also occur. The EMG can be normal or shows nonspecific changes in MUP morphology consistent with a myopathy. Spontaneous activity is usually normal, but fibrillation potentials are observed in some cases.

MUSCULAR DYSTROPHIES

Muscular dystrophies are genetic disorders characterized by progressive degeneration of skeletal muscle fibers. Weakness and atrophy of muscles occur when the rate of degeneration outpaces regeneration. Eventually, muscle fibers are replaced with connective tissue. Some muscular dystrophies, such as myotonic dystrophy, are systemic disorders that affect multiple organ systems. In these disorders, the muscle disorder may result from an anabolic defect, rather than a dystrophic process (Rifai et al., 1993). Traditionally, muscular dystrophy has been classified by the pattern of inheritance, clinical features, and findings on muscle biopsy. Individual dystrophies were named after the investigator who first described the disorder or by the distribution of muscle weakness (see Table 76–1). The traditional classification of muscular dystrophy has been modified to reflect advances in the understanding of the molecular pathogenesis, with particular emphasis on abnormalities of the dystrophin-glycoprotein complex (DGC) (Fig. 76–1). The focusing of attention on the DGC began with the identification, localization, and functional characterization of dystrophin (Hoffman et al., 1987). Subsequently, a variety of dystrophin-associated membrane and cytoskeletal proteins were discovered and found to form a transmembranous link between the extracellular matrix and the intracellular cytoskeleton (Lim and Campbell, 1998).

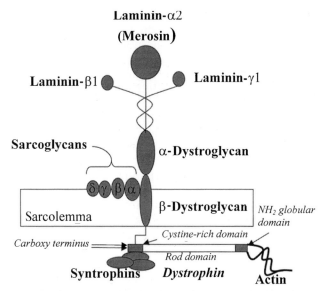

Figure 76–1. Graphic representation of the dystrophin-glycoprotein complex as it transcends the sarcoplasmic membrane linking the extracellular matrix (through merosin) with the intracellular cytoskeleton (through dystrophin and actin).

Alteration of one or more of these proteins may produce muscular dystrophy by changing the signaling or structural properties of the DGC. The muscular dystrophies caused by abnormalities of the DGC include Duchenne's and Becker's dystrophy, so-called Becker variants, many of the limb-girdle dystrophies, some of the congenital muscular dystrophies, and some distal dystrophies (e.g., Miyoshi's myopathy). Advances in understanding the molecular basis of the muscular dystrophies have made it possible to reclassify these disorders, based on the affected structural or regulatory protein (e.g., dystrophinopathies, sarcoglycanopathies, merosin-deficient muscular dystrophy, calpainopathies, dysferlin-deficient myopathy) (Kissel, 1999b) (see Table 76–2). This classification system will certainly expand with further characterization of the DGC.

The rapid evolution of molecular diagnosis has altered the role of EMG in the diagnosis of muscular dystrophies. In the appropriate clinical setting, EMG is no longer needed to establish a diagnosis of a number of disorders (e.g., Duchenne's and Becker's dystrophy; myotonic, facioscapulohumeral, and oculopharyngeal dystrophy; Barth's syndrome; Emery-Dreifuss muscular dystrophy). As molecular testing becomes more routinely available, this list will probably expand. The EMG still plays an important role in the diagnosis of atypical cases, particularly when neurogenic disorders (e.g., spinal muscular atrophy, inherited or acquired neuropathies) or congenital myasthenic syndromes are being considered.

Dystrophinopathies (Duchenne's Dystrophy, Becker's Dystrophy)

GENETICS

The dystrophinopathies are X-linked recessive disorders. The dystrophin gene on Xp21.1 is the largest

in the mammalian genome at 4.2 million base pairs (Hoffman et al., 1987). The gene contains 79 exons and codes for at least six tissue-specific isoforms of dystrophin. The muscle and brain isoforms are full-length transcripts with a molecular weight of 427 kd. The muscle isoform is rod shaped, contains 3,685 amino acids and four functional domains (Koenig et al., 1988). The carboxy terminus is linked to the sarcolemma through an attachment to β-dystroglycan and α-syntrophin (see Fig. 76–1). These proteins are also attached to the cystine-rich domain that has important calcium-binding capabilities. The rod domain consists of a long α-helix containing four hinge regions. The fourth functional domain consists of the NH_2 end of the dystrophin molecule, which binds to the cytoskeletal protein actin.

Dystrophin and the other proteins associated with it function to provide mechanical support and flexibility to the sarcolemma (Lim and Campbell, 1998). Dystrophin may also participate in signal transduction. Without normal dystrophin, the muscle membrane becomes particularly susceptible to damage induced by lengthening contractions. When repair mechanisms fail, necrosis of the fiber is induced by an influx of calcium.

Approximately 65% of the mutations that affect the dystrophin gene are large deletions, 5% are duplications, and the remaining 30% are small deletions or point mutations (Prior, 1995). The 70% with large deletions or duplications of the dystrophin gene are easily detectable by multiplex polymerase chain reaction (PCR) and Southern blot of peripheral blood DNA (Roberts et al., 1991). As many as 30% of cases represent new mutations, with 10% to 20% of these being the result of germline mosaicism (Van Essen et al., 1992). The germline mosaics will escape detection as carriers when mutational analysis is performed on peripheral blood DNA; thus, prenatal testing is still required to determine the status of subsequent male children. Deletions or mutations that alter the reading frame and result in a severe deficiency of dystrophin produce Duchenne's dystrophy. These mutations occur at a frequency of 1 per 3,500 live births. In-frame mutations cause partial deficiency or altered function of dystrophin, leading to milder phenotypic expression (Becker's dystrophy). The frequency of these mutations is only about 10% to 20% of those that produce Duchenne's dystrophy. Female carriers can express the disease when there is disproportionate inactivation of the wild-type X, in the setting of Turner's syndrome (XO) or in the presence of an X-autosomal translocation that involves the Xp21 segment.

CLINICAL MANIFESTATIONS

Duchenne's Dystrophy

Onset of weakness occurs at age 3 to 5 years, with loss of ambulation by 10 years and progression to death over 15 to 30 years. The weakness follows a limb-girdle distribution, with hypertrophy of calf and sometimes other muscles. Axial muscles are affected, producing an exaggerated lumbar lordosis and scoliosis. Respiratory muscle involvement occurs late in the course. Patients may also present with malignant hyperthermia–like reactions to general anesthesia or with an apparently asymptomatic elevation of serum creatine kinase. Creatine kinase is markedly elevated early in the disease and then declines as progressive disease destroys muscle tissue. There is little or no cranial weakness, but cardiomyopathy occurs in all. Some patients have mental retardation. Complications related to progressive weakness include joint contractures and progressive scoliosis, which exacerbates respiratory insufficiency.

Becker's Dystrophy

The clinical distribution of weakness is similar to that in Duchenne's dystrophy, but the disease is less severe and exhibits more variability in the age at onset (age 3 to 20 years), rate of progression (loss of ambulation over 20 to 40 years), and age at which death occurs (30 to 60 years). Molecular diagnostic techniques have led to the recognition of dystrophinopathies, with phenotypes milder than those seen in the classic Duchenne or Becker dystrophy. These include asymptomatic elevation of serum creatine kinase (Bushby et al., 1996), exercise-induced cramps, and myalgias with or without myoglobinuria (Gospe et al., 1989), isolated cardiomyopathy (Ferlini et al., 1999), or isolated quadriceps myopathy (Sunohara et al., 1990).

PATHOLOGY

Segmental muscle necrosis and regeneration of muscle fibers dominate the pathological picture early both in Duchenne's and Becker's dystrophy (Engel et al., 1994). Hypercontracted fibers are a common finding, as is sparse infiltration with inflammatory cells. Later, as the regenerative capacity of the muscle fails, there is progressive muscle fiber loss and replacement with connective tissue. Throughout the course, smaller diameter muscle fibers are relatively resistant to necrosis because of the direct relationship between fiber diameter and surface tension of the plasma membrane (Karpati and Carpenter, 1986). Immunohistochemistry shows an absence of dystrophin in Duchenne's dystrophy and a reduction of dystrophin or altered staining pattern of dystrophin in Becker's dystrophy.

ELECTROMYOGRAPHY

The findings on electrodiagnostic studies in dystrophinopathies depend on the severity and stage of the illness (Bradley et al., 1978; Stålberg and Trontelj, 1994). Nerve conduction studies and EMG usually are normal in patients with asymptomatic elevation of creatine phosphokinase, exertional myalgias and cramps, or isolated cardiomyopathy. In the setting of focal quadriceps myopathy or mild limb-girdle weakness, nerve conduction studies are normal and needle EMG reveals normal insertional activity with small polyphasic MUPs. In Duchenne's or Becker's dystrophy, electrodiagnostic studies are typically performed in childhood when manifestations of weakness and muscle pseudohypertrophy first appear. At this stage, nerve conduction studies are typically normal. Needle EMG shows increased insertional activity with fibrillation potentials and short-duration low-amplitude, polyphasic, rapidly recruited MUPs, particularly in proximal muscles (Kugelberg, 1949). Highly polyphasic MUPs with late satellite potentials are common. Single-fiber EMG shows increased fiber density with a bimodal pattern on jitter analysis (Hilton-Brown and Stålberg, 1983). Some fiber pairs exhibit decreased jitter, owing to fiber splitting, while others show increased jitter secondary to immature, newly reinnervated neuromuscular junctions or changes in conduction along either the nerve terminal or the muscle fiber. As the disease progresses and muscle fibers are replaced with connective tissue, CMAP amplitudes fall, insertional activity diminishes, fibrillation potentials disappear, and MUPs become very small with reduced recruitment. Eventually, the muscle becomes electrically silent.

DIAGNOSIS

Immunostaining of a muscle biopsy specimen for dystrophin is diagnostic for Duchenne's dystrophy but may miss Becker's dystrophy or Becker's variants. Immunoblotting of a small amount of muscle is the most sensitive and specific diagnostic technique and will identify all dystrophinopathies (Hoffman, 1996). A secondary deficiency of sarcoglycans is also detected in dystrophinopathies. Multiplex PCR is a good screening test for deletions and, when combined with Southern analysis, can be used to identify the specific mutation in the 70% of patients with deletions or duplications. Unfortunately, more complicated analytical techniques that are not routinely available are required to detect point mutations or germline mosaics (Mansfield et al., 1993).

Limb-Girdle Muscular Dystrophies

GENETICS

The limb-girdle muscular dystrophies (LGMD) are clinically and genetically heterogeneous. Traditional classification was based on the clinical distribution of weakness and the mendelian pattern of inheritance (LGMD1, autosomal dominant; LGMD2, autosomal recessive). Linkage studies and information related to molecular pathogenesis now permit classification of limb-girdle muscular dystrophy by the affected gene and altered or deficient protein product (Angelini et al., 1999) (Table 76–6). Most of the limb-girdle muscular dystrophy or related syn-

Table 76–6. Genetic Classification of Limb-Girdle Muscular Dystrophy (LGMD)

Type, Inheritance, Gene Locus, Gene Product	Clinical and EMG Features
LGMD1A, autosomal dominant, 5q31, ?myotilin gene	Virginia kindred, juvenile to adult onset, proximal > distal involvement, some have ankle contractures, most have fibrillation potentials
LGMD1B, autosomal dominant, 1pq11–21, ?laminin A and C gene	Proximal > distal involvement, mild elbow and ankle contractures, cardiac conduction defects
LGMD1C, autosomal dominant, 3p25, *CAV3* gene, caveolin-3 deficiency	Proximal > distal involvement, mild to moderate severity, calf muscle hypertrophy
LGMD1D, autosomal dominant, 7q, gene not identified	Juvenile to adult onset, proximal > distal involvement
LGMD2A, autosomal recessive, 15q15–21, *CAPN3* gene, calpain-3 subunit (muscle-specific protease)	First described in Reunion Islands, onset age 2–40 years, proximal weakness, calf muscle hypertrophy, no cardiomyopathy, increased creatine kinase
LGMD2B, autosomal recessive, 2p13, dysferlin gene, dysferlin	Limb-girdle or distal distribution (Miyoshi's myopathy), onset second decade, relatively mild but patient still may lose ability to ambulate after 10–20 years
LGMD2C, autosomal recessive, 13q12, *SGCG* gene, γ-sarcoglycan	Formerly severe childhood autosomal recessive muscular dystrophy (SCARMD), similar to Duchenne's in presentation and course, male: female = 1.
LGMD2D, autosomal recessive, 17q12–21, *SGCA* gene, α-sarcoglycan	Usually SCARMD but more variable age at onset and severity
LGMD2E, autosomal recessive, 4q12, *SGCB* gene, β-sarcoglycan	First described in Indiana Amish kindred, proximal > distal, variable age at onset and severity
LGMD2F, autosomal recessive, chromosome 5q33–34, *SGCD* gene, δ-sarcoglycan	Proximal > distal, variable age at onset and severity
LGMD2G, autosomal recessive, 17q11–12, ?telethonin gene	Distal involvement may predominate, some have rimmed vacuoles on biopsy
LGMD2H, autosomal recessive, 9q31–33, gene unknown	Onset late childhood–early adult, proximal > distal weakness

dromes are caused by defects in the DGC (see Fig. 76–1). Others are related to nuclear or cytoplasmic protein abnormalities, or are as yet undefined.

Limb-Girdle Muscular Dystrophy–Related Sarcoplasmic Proteins

Merosin. This term is used to describe a group of laminins that contain the α2 heavy chain (Pegoraro et al., 1996). Laminins are an integral part of the basal lamina of the muscle fiber, which, in turn, links the muscle fiber to the extracellular matrix. The laminins are heterotrimers consisting of one heavy α chain and two light chains (β and γ). Merosin ($α_2$-laminin) is linked to β-dystroglycan, making it an integral part of the DGC.

Dystroglycans. The dystroglycan complex in muscle consists of two proteins that span the sarcoplasmic membrane, linking dystrophin to the extracellular matrix (Lim and Campbell, 1998). α-Dystroglycan is a 156-kd extracellular protein that binds to merosin and β-dystroglycan, which, in turn, is a 43-kd transmembrane protein that is linked directly to dystrophin, sarcoglycans, dystrobrevins, and the syntrophins.

Sarcoglycans. The sarcoglycan complex is a group of transmembrane proteins that are linked directly to dystrophin and the dystroglycan complex (Lim and Campbell, 1998). There have been five components of the sarcoglycan complex described to date (Table 76–7).

The specific function of the sarcoglycans is unknown, but it is clear that they play an important role in the pathogenesis of muscular dystrophies. The sarcoglycans are absent in dystrophinopathies and in the primary sarcoglycanopathies. Sarcoglycanopathies manifest as congenital muscular dystrophy, distal dystrophy, or classic limb-girdle muscular dystrophy. They have been estimated to account for about 10% of limb-girdle muscular dystrophy in general (Angelini et al., 1999).

Syntrophins. The syntrophin complex consists of three intracellular proteins, each coded by separate genes that bind to the C-terminus of dystrophin (Ahn et al., 1994). The function of syntrophins is unknown, and no cases of muscular dystrophy have been linked to abnormalities of the syntrophin complex.

Dystrobrevin. Dystrobrevin is an intracellular protein that binds to the syntrophin complex and to the C-terminus of dystrophin (Blake et al., 1996). It is thought to be important for the formation and maintenance of the neuromuscular junction. Dystrobrevin is absent in Duchenne's dystrophy and reduced or absent in limb-girdle muscular dystrophy, but a primary deficiency of dystrobrevin has not been described.

Limb-Girdle Muscular Dystrophy–Related Cytoplasmic Proteins

Calpain-3. The calcium-activated neutral protease, calpain-3 (CANP3) is an intracellular soluble protein whose gene is located on chromosome 15. Although the exact function is unknown, mutation of *CANP3* is responsible for LGMD2A (Richard et al., 1995).

Caveolin-3. Caveolin-3 is a membrane-associated protein of skeletal muscle that participates in the formation of small invaginations of the plasma membrane. The *CAV3* gene is located on chromosome 3. Mutations in the *CAV3* gene have been associated with LGMD1C (Minetti et al., 1998) and at least two cases of asymptomatic elevation of serum creatine kinase in children (Carbone et al., 2000).

Dysferlin. Dysferlin is a protein in skeletal muscle that is homologous to the *Caenorhabditis elegans*

Table 76–7. The Sarcoglycans

Protein	Molecular Wt (kd)	Chromosome	Phenotype
α-Sarcoglycan (adhalin)	50	17q	LGMD2D
β-Sarcoglycan	43	4q12	LGMD2E
γ-Sarcoglycan	35	13q12	LGMD2C
δ-Sarcoglycan	35	5q	LGMD2F
Sarcospan	25	12q	?

protein fer-1, which is thought to be important in spermatogenesis (Bashir et al., 1998). The location and function of dysferlin in muscle are unknown. Mutations in the dysferlin gene on chromosome 2p13 are associated with LGMD2B and some distal dystrophies (Miyoshi's myopathy) (Liu et al., 1998).

Collagen VI. Mutations in two genes for type VI collagen, *COL6A1* and *COL6A2* are associated with Bethlem's myopathy (Jobsis et al., 1996). The mechanism of myopathy is unknown but may result from secondary effects on B1-laminin production (Merlini et al., 1994).

CLINICAL MANIFESTATIONS

The clinical pattern of involvement in limb-girdle muscular dystrophy is heterogeneous. Congenital and early childhood onset cases may present with generalized hypotonia and weakness while older children and adults may have proximal weakness, calf hypertrophy, exertional myalgia, lumbar lordosis and ankle contractures. Males are often suspected of having Duchenne's or Becker's dystrophy, but dystrophin is normal. Within this phenotype, α-sarcoglycanopathy is most common, but many other disorders should also be considered (Table 76–8). Autosomal dominant forms typically present later in life with proximal weakness, scapular winging, lumbar lordosis or scoliosis, calf hypertrophy, exertional intolerance, and elevated creatine kinase.

PATHOLOGY

The pathology in limb-girdle muscular dystrophy is nonspecific. Degeneration of muscle fibers with a variable amount of necrosis and regenerating fibers are common, particularly in more severe cases early in the course of the illness. As the disease progresses, the muscle is gradually replaced with connective tissue. Stains and immunoblot for dystrophin are normal. Immunostaining and/or Western blots for sarcoglycans or calpain are used to screen for the known protein deficiencies associated with limb-girdle muscular dystrophy.

ELECTROMYOGRAPHY

The spinal muscular atrophies, chronic inflammatory polyradiculoneuropathies, disorders of neuromuscular transmission, congenital myopathies, met-

abolic myopathies, acquired myopathies, and other muscular dystrophies all may present with clinical manifestations that are very similar to those of limb-girdle dystrophy (see Table 76–8). Electrodiagnostic studies help differentiate myopathies from other disorders of the motor unit that present with proximal weakness, but these studies cannot make a specific diagnosis of limb-girdle dystrophy. The EMG findings in limb-girdle muscular dystrophies typically correlate with the severity of the clinical manifestations and the timing of the study with respect to the course of the disease. More severe forms are associated with fibrillation potentials and small, highly polyphasic MUPs with rapid recruitment. Milder cases have mild myopathic changes or are normal. When EMG is done late in the course of the disease, there may be decreased insertional activity and a mixture of large and small MUPs, owing to extensive remodeling and fibrosis in the muscle.

DIAGNOSIS

The diagnosis of a muscular dystrophy is made in the appropriate clinical setting of proximal weak-

Table 76–8. Differential Diagnosis of Limb-Girdle Myopathy

Infants
Congenital muscular dystrophy
Congenital myotonic dystrophy
Congenital myopathy
Barth's syndrome
Sarcoglycanopathies (LGMD2C–F)
Metabolic myopathy
Toxic myopathy
Congenital myasthenia gravis
Spinal muscular atrophy
Congenital hypomyelinating neuropathy

Children and Adults
Congenital myopathy
Dystrophinopathies
Sarcoglycanopathies
Other LGMD (see Table 76–2)
Facioscapulohumeral dystrophy
Emery-Dreifuss dystrophy
Bethlem's myopathy
Inflammatory myopathy
Metabolic myopathy
Toxic myopathy
Congenital myasthenia gravis
Spinal muscular atrophy
Polyradiculoneuropathy

LGMD, limb-girdle muscular dystrophy.

ness by EMG, serum creatine kinase measurement, and muscle biopsy with standard morphological and histochemical studies. If immunostaining for dystrophin is normal, immunostaining for α-sarcoglycan should be performed. If α-sarcoglycan is deficient, Western blotting will identify the specific subtype of sarcoglycanopathy. If α-sarcoglycan staining is normal, stains for calpain, emerin, merosin, and dysferlin can be performed.

Congenital Muscular Dystrophy

Congenital muscular dystrophy is a heterogeneous group of autosomal recessive disorders that have nonspecific pathological features of a primary myopathy and are clinically manifested at birth by generalized weakness, hypotonia, muscle atrophy, and contractures with or without arthrogryposis multiplex. The dystrophinopathies, congenital myotonic dystrophy, and congenital myopathies with unique pathological features are arbitrarily excluded. Some cases follow a relatively benign course, whereas others progress to death within the first decade and are associated with dysgenesis of the brain (Fukuyama type) and eye (Walker-Warburg type or Santavuori type). Approximately 30% of congenital muscular dystrophies are associated with merosin (α2-laminin) deficiency (Sewry et al., 1995). As discussed in the section on limb-girdle muscular dystrophy, merosin is an integral component of the sarcoplasm protein complex and is coded for by the *LAMA2* gene on 6q22-23 (Pegoraro et al., 1996). Merosin deficiency is frequently associated with white matter signal abnormalities on magnetic resonance imaging of the brain, yet mental retardation is uncommon (Tome and Fardeau, 1994). The Fukuyama type of congenital muscular dystrophy is associated with psychomotor retardation and seizures. The *FCMD* gene is located on chromosome 9q31-33 and codes for the protein fukutin (Kobayashi et al., 1998). The function of fukutin is unknown, but there is evidence to indicate that it is a secretory, rather than a structural, protein. In congenital muscular dystrophy, the serum creatine kinase level is mildly elevated. Nerve conduction studies are normal or, in some cases, show an associated peripheral neuropathy. Needle EMG shows normal spontaneous activity with nonspecific changes consistent with a myopathy.

Emery-Dreifuss Muscular Dystrophy

GENETICS

Emery-Dreifuss muscular dystrophy usually follows an X-linked recessive pattern of inheritance, although autosomal recessive or dominant patterns also occur. The disorder is caused by one or more mutations in the *EDMD* gene on chromosome Xq28 (2.1 kb with six small exons), leading to a truncation of the normal protein product emerin (Bione et al., 1995). Emerin is concentrated in the nuclear membrane, but its function is unknown. Some cases do not have emerin gene mutations. Some cases of rigid spine syndrome that follow an X-linked pattern have mutations in the emerin gene.

CLINICAL MANIFESTATIONS (Meola and Moxley, 1999)

Weakness in Emery-Dreifuss muscular dystrophy follows a scapulohumeroperoneal or limb-girdle distribution. Muscle contractures appear early and may be the most prominent feature of the disease. The cervical spine, elbow, and ankle are most commonly involved, but other joints can also be affected. Cardiac conduction defects are a common and distinguishing feature. Muscle pseudohypertrophy is conspicuously absent. Creatine kinase levels are normal or moderately elevated. The onset is in early to middle childhood, with variable severity and progression. Regular follow-up of affected males and carrier females for cardiac conduction block is indicated, with pacemaker placement as necessary.

PATHOLOGY AND ELECTROMYOGRAPHY

Muscle biopsy findings are nonspecific and consistent with a slowly progressive muscular dystrophy, with variation in fiber diameter, minimal necrosis and regeneration, and an increase in connective tissue (Grimm and Janka, 1994). Electromyography shows nonspecific changes suggestive of a chronic myopathy, including some patients with a mixed population of small and large MUPs. Typically, there is little or no abnormal spontaneous activity (Grimm and Janka, 1994).

DIAGNOSIS

The age at onset, inheritance, contractures, and cardiac involvement all suggest the diagnosis, which can be confirmed by ascertaining the absence of emerin on immunostaining of a muscle biopsy specimen.

Barth's Syndrome

The Barth syndrome is an X-linked recessive disorder linked to the same region (Xq28) as Emery-Dreifuss muscular dystrophy (Barth et al., 1983). Most cases are thought to be caused by mutations in the G4.5 gene, which codes for a family of proteins called tafazzins (Bione et al., 1996). The function of tafazzins is unknown. The clinical manifestations of Barth's syndrome include a limb-girdle myopathy, cardiomyopathy, short stature, and neutropenia (Barth et al., 1983). Onset is usually in infancy, with progression to death in childhood secondary to heart failure or infection. Mitochondrial abnormalities are found in muscle and other tissues. The EMG findings in Barth's syndrome have not been reported.

Bethlem's Myopathy

GENETICS

Bethlem's myopathy is a rare autosomal dominant myopathy with childhood onset caused by a defect in α1 to α3 subunits of type VI collagen (Jobsis et al., 1996). Mutations affecting *COL6A1* or *COL6A2* on chromosome 21q22.3 or COL6A3 on chromosome 2q37 have been described. The mutations disrupt the triple helix motif of collagen, which may affect myoblast differentiation or the organization of extracellular matrix within muscle.

CLINICAL MANIFESTATIONS

Bethlem's myopathy is associated with relatively mild weakness and atrophy of proximal muscles with prominent flexion contractures of elbows, wrists, fingers, knees, and ankles. The weakness preferentially affects extensor muscles. There is no cardiac involvement. Onset is in childhood, with slow or stepwise progression and relatively mild disability. Some adult cases have presented with respiratory muscle involvement. The serum creatine kinase level is only mildly elevated.

PATHOLOGY AND ELECTROMYOGRAPHY

Muscle biopsy in Bethlem's myopathy shows a mild myopathy with little or no necrosis or regeneration. Nerve conduction studies are normal, and needle EMG reveals a mild proximal myopathy with normal spontaneous activity.

DIAGNOSIS

The diagnosis of Bethlem's myopathy should be suspected in patients with a mild autosomal dominant limb-girdle myopathy and flexion contractures. Bethlem's myopathy can be differentiated from X-linked Emery-Deifuss dystrophy by the presence of cardiac involvement and by immunostaining for emerin on muscle biopsy.

Muscular Dystrophy Secondary to Plectin Deficiency

This disorder is also known as epidermolysis bullosa simplex with late-onset muscular dystrophy (EB-MD) because of the frequent occurrence of chronic blistering of the skin that usually precedes the onset of muscular weakness by a number of years. The disorder is caused by mutations in the plectin gene *PLEC1* on chromosome 8q24.13 (Pulkkinen et al., 1996). Plectin is an important cytoskeletal protein that is widely distributed in skin, brain, and muscle. It localizes to the Z-disks of myofibrils.

Chronic skin blisters appear shortly after birth. Ptosis and progressive limb-girdle weakness begin in late childhood to adulthood. Progressive disability with loss of ambulation, and central nervous system involvement with ataxia and dementia, may occur.

In plectin deficiency, there is ultrastructural disorganization of the sarcomere, with absence of staining for plectin. Skin biopsy shows separation of the dermis and epidermis, with an absence of plectin at the junction between the two tissue layers.

Facioscapulohumeral Dystrophy

GENETICS

Facioscapulohumeral dystrophy (FSHD) follows an autosomal dominant pattern of inheritance, with high penetrance but variable expression (prevalence 1 in 20,000). As many as 30% of cases are caused by a spontaneous germline mutation (Kissel, 1999a). Facioscapulohumeral dystrophy is linked to the telomeric portion of chromosome 4 (4q35) in 98% of patients. It has been associated with a reduced number of 3.3-kb tandem repeat segments called D4Z4 in a non–protein-encoding region of the gene (Orrell et al., 1999). The size of the D4Z4 segment correlates inversely with clinical severity, but not with clinical anticipation. The mechanism by which the reduced number of D4Z4 tandem repeats produces disease is unknown.

CLINICAL MANIFESTATIONS

In FSHD, there is slowly progressive asymmetrical weakness of the muscles of facial expression, scapular fixation, proximal upper extremities, and distal extensors of both upper and lower extremities. Facial weakness produces incomplete eye closure, compensatory contraction of the frontalis muscle, and a horizontal smile. Weakness of the trapezius and serratus anterior muscles causes lateral and posterior scapular winging, and pectoral involvement produces flattening of the chest with inverted axillary folds. The biceps and triceps are affected, yet the deltoid is typically spared. Lumbar lordosis is common and weakness in the lower limbs initially affects peroneal muscles, producing bilateral (but often asymmetrical) footdrop. Cardiac muscle is generally spared. Retinal vasculopathy and/or hearing loss is commonly associated; retinal telangiectasia, exudates, and detachment are referred to as Coats' disease.

The onset of FSHD ranges from childhood to adult, but a severe infantile form also exists. The majority of affected patients express signs of the disease by age 20 years. Approximately 20% of patients eventually lose the ability to ambulate, but life expectancy remains unchanged.

PATHOLOGY

Biopsy of mildly affected muscles occasionally shows muscle fiber necrosis, regenerating fibers, variation in fiber diameter, and an increased amount of connective tissue (Munsat et al., 1972). Perivascular or endomysial infiltrates of inflammatory cells are observed in some cases, but findings characteristic of polymyositis are rare.

ELECTROMYOGRAPHY

Nerve conduction studies are usually normal in FSHD. Needle EMG shows short-duration, low-amplitude, polyphasic, rapidly recruited MUPs (Kimura, 1989). The severity of the EMG findings typically varies both between different muscles and between different locations within the same muscle. Fibrillation potentials are generally sparse and reflect the degree of ongoing fiber necrosis within the muscle. Dense fibrillation potentials, particularly in patients with a rapid onset of symptoms, suggests the possibility of an inflammatory myopathy that may present with a similar pattern of involvement (Munsat et al., 1972). Nerve conduction studies and EMG may also help differentiate FSHD from some forms of spinal muscular atrophy that express an FSHD phenotype (Fenichel et al., 1972).

DIAGNOSIS

In 1997, the FSHD consortium established clinical criteria for the diagnosis (Tawil et al., 1998) (Table 76–9). Genetic linkage studies using a variety restriction fragment analysis techniques are now routinely available for diagnostic purposes. Genetic testing has a diagnostic sensitivity of 96% or greater with nearly 100% specificity (Orrell et al., 1999).

Distal Muscular Dystrophy

Distal muscular dystrophy comprises a group of inherited myopathies that are characterized by progressive weakness of distal muscles. Subtypes are classified by the pattern of inheritance, age at onset,

and clinical pattern of muscle weakness, and, in some cases, by molecular genetics. The muscle biopsy shows dystrophic changes, with necrosis and regeneration followed by fiber loss and fibrosis. Many cases have features of inherited inclusion body myopathy, with rimmed vacuoles and eosinophilic inclusions on Gomori trichrome staining. Amyloid stains are positive, and electron microscopy reveals characteristic filamentous inclusions. Unlike sporadic inclusion body myositis, inflammatory infiltrates are conspicuously absent. Similar changes may occur in other dystrophies (e.g., oculopharyngeal dystrophy).

Electrodiagnostic studies help distinguish the distal myopathies from peripheral neuropathy, motor neuron disorders, and lesions of the conus or cauda equina. Nerve conduction studies may show low-amplitude compound muscle action potentials over weak distal muscles, but conduction velocities, distal latencies, and sensory conductions are normal. Needle EMG usually reveals abnormal spontaneous activity with fibrillation potentials and small, polyphasic MUP. As with the clinical manifestations, the EMG changes are more prominent in distal muscles. Some cases have a mixture of large and small MUPs similar to the picture observed in sporadic inclusion body myositis. In this setting, a muscle biopsy may be required to confirm the diagnosis of a distal myopathy.

Nonaka's Myopathy (Early-Adult-Onset Distal Myopathy Type I)

This disorder has been classified by several other names as well, including distal myopathy with rimmed vacuoles (DMRV) and inherited inclusion body myopathy (Sunohara et al., 1989). It has been linked to chromosome 9p1-q1, but the gene has not been isolated (Mitrani-Rosenbaum et al., 1996). The weakness begins in early adulthood and follows a slowly progressive course. Unlike Miyoshi's myopathy (see later), the weakness preferentially affects anterior tibial compartment and small foot muscles (Nonaka et al., 1981).

Miyoshi's Myopathy (Early-Adult-Onset Distal Myopathy Type II)

This is an autosomal recessive disorder that was originally described in Japan, but has a worldwide distribution (Miyoshi et al., 1977). Miyoshi's myopathy has been linked to chromosome 2p13, where it is allelic with LGMD2B (Illarioshkin et al., 1997). The gene and its protein dysferlin have been isolated, but the function is unknown. Dysferlin is homologous to the *Caenorhabditis elegans* protein fer-1, which is thought to be important in spermatogenesis (Bashir et al., 1998).

The disorder typically begins in early adulthood

Table 76–9. Clinical Criteria for Diagnosis Established by FSHD Consortium

Necessary for Diagnosis
Autosomal dominant inheritance, facial weakness, and scapular > hip girdle weakness

Supportive Features
Asymmetry, descending progression, sparing of deltoid and neck flexors, inverted axillary folds and descending clavicles, wrist extensor and abdominal weakness, sparing of calf muscles, high-frequency hearing loss, and retinal vasculopathy

Features That Exclude Diagnosis
Extraocular or pharyngeal muscle weakness, elbow contractures, cardiomyopathy, distal sensory loss, myotonia, or neurogenic findings on EMG

and is characterized by slowly progressive weakness of the distal lower limb muscles. The gastrocnemius and other posterior compartment muscles are affected more than the anterior compartment muscles. Intrinsic foot muscles are typically spared. The weakness and atrophy can be asymmetrical and, with time, may spread to hand muscles as well as quadriceps and proximal upper limb muscles. Reflexes are spared except when muscle weakness and atrophy is severe. Approximately 30% of patients eventually become wheelchair dependent. Creatine kinase is significantly elevated in the majority of patients.

Welander's Distal Myopathy (Late-Adult-Onset Distal Myopathy Type I)

This disorder was originally described by Welander in a large number of Scandinavian families (Welander, 1951) and is also referred to as late-adult-onset autosomal dominant distal dystrophy type I. The clinical manifestations appear after 20 years of age, with progressive weakness involving intrinsic hand muscles (particularly the thumb and index fingers). The weakness typically spreads to involve distal muscles of the lower extremities. Proximal involvement does occur but is relatively uncommon. Some cases have been linked to the dysferlin gene on chromosome 2, others to the *MPD1* locus on 14q11.2-13 (Laing et al., 1995a), but most remain unlinked. As the disease progresses, the weakness spreads from the hands to the distal lower extremity muscles (anterior and posterior compartment) with eventual involvement of proximal muscles in a minority of patients.

Markesbery's Distal Dystrophy (Late-Onset Autosomal Dominant Distal Dystrophy Type II)

This disorder was described by Markesbery and is distinguished from Welander's dystrophy by the predominance of distal leg weakness at the onset (in the fourth or fifth decade) and the occurrence of a cardiomyopathy that can produce congestive heart failure or arrhythmias (Markesbery et al., 1974). From the distal leg, the weakness often spreads to involve the distal upper limb. Proximal weakness is also observed in some cases.

Finnish Tibial Dystrophy

Some classification schemes have grouped this disorder with Markesbery distal dystrophy. It is an autosomal dominant disorder originally described in Finnish kindreds that has been linked to chromosome 2q31-33 (Haravuori et al., 1998). Weakness becomes manifested after age 35 and involves the tibialis anterior as well as other anterior compartment leg muscles preferentially. Intrinsic foot muscles are typically spared. The rate of progression is slow, with little or no spread to proximal muscles. Patients maintain ambulation and have a normal life expectancy.

Oculopharyngeal Dystrophy

GENETICS

Oculopharyngeal muscular dystrophy (OPMD) is an autosomal dominant disorder initially described in French Canadian kindreds (Tome et al., 1994). The frequency of the mutation is approximately 1 in 8,000 in Quebec, but only 1 in 200,000 in France. Most cases are caused by an expanded GCG repeat in the *PABP2* gene (polyadenyl-binding protein 2 gene) on 14q11.2-q13 (Brais et al., 1998). The severity of expression correlates with the number of repeats but the expansions remain stable over time, so anticipation does not occur. A single additional repeat (i.e., GCG7) acts as a recessive mutation, while two or more repeats cause dominant expression.

CLINICAL MANIFESTATIONS

OPMD typically begins after the age of 30 years, with ptosis and dysphagia as the most common presenting symptoms. Extraocular muscles as well as muscles of facial expression and mastication are spared. Proximal and/or distal limb-girdle muscles are involved in most cases. The resting serum lactate level is sometimes elevated (Mirabella et al., 2000).

PATHOLOGY

Nonspecific dystrophic changes are common, but the pathologic hallmark is the finding of 8.5-nm tubulofilamentous intranuclear inclusions on electron microscopy and changes characteristic of inherited inclusion body myopathy (including rimmed vacuoles with eosinophilic inclusions and amyloid deposition) on light microscopy (Tome et al., 1997). Ragged red fibers are observed in some cases, but inflammation is not.

ELECTROMYOGRAPHY

Nerve conduction studies are usually normal; however, some cases have had evidence of an associated length-dependent axonal peripheral neuropathy (Mirabella et al., 2000). Repetitive stimulation studies are normal. Needle EMG shows small, polyphasic, rapidly recruited MUPs and, in some cases, a mixture of small and large motor units in the same muscle.

DIAGNOSIS

Routine genetic testing is very helpful in confirming the diagnosis of OPMD (Mirabella et al., 2000). The disorder can otherwise easily be confused with a defect in neuromuscular transmission or a mitochondrial myopathy.

Myotonic Dystrophy

GENETICS

Classic myotonic dystrophy (type I, or DM1) is an autosomal dominant multisystem disorder caused by an expanded CTG repeat in the myotonin protein kinase (DMPK) gene on chromosome 19q13 (Thornton, 1999). The DMPK is a widely distributed serine/threonine kinase that is involved in phosphorylation-dephosphorylation reactions, but the exact function and role of the enzyme in the pathophysiology of myotonic dystrophy is unknown. The CTG repeat is located in the untranslated 3'-region of the DM gene and contains 5 to 37 repeats in normal subjects. The size of the CTG repeat correlates with the severity of clinical manifestations, and expansion of the repeat accounts for clinical anticipation. Congenital myotonic dystrophy has the largest number of repeats (>1,000) and results exclusively from maternal transmission of the mutation. Traditional epidemiological methods estimate a gene frequency of 1 in 8,000; however, because of variable expression, the actual frequency is probably much greater.

Myotonic dystrophy type II (DM2) encompasses patients with the myotonic dystrophy phenotype but a normal number of CTG repeats in the *DMPK* gene (Day et al., 1999). Likewise, proximal myotonic myopathy (PROMM) shares many clinical features with DM, but it is not linked to abnormalities in the *DMPK* gene (Ricker et al., 1995). Some of the DM2 and PROMM kindreds have recently been linked to chromosome 3q (International Myotonic Dystrophy Consortium, 2000).

CLINICAL MANIFESTATIONS (Meola and Moxley, 1999)

Classic myotonic dystrophy (DM1) is a multisystem disease characterized by myotonia, muscle weakness, and variable involvement of other systems (Table 76–10). Clinical manifestations usually begin in adolescence or early adulthood, with myotonia and weakness that preferentially affects facial, forearm, and peroneal muscle groups. Some cases present later in life with cataracts and minimal neuromuscular manifestations. Myotonia is usually minimized by the patient and described with nonspecific terms, such as arthritis, stiffness, spasms, or cramps. It most frequently affects hand grip but can be demonstrated in other muscles (e.g., facial, tongue, forearm, thenar, quadriceps) by isometric contraction or percussion. The myotonia improves with exercise (i.e., warm-up) and does not worsen

Table 76–10. Systemic Manifestations of Myotonic Dystrophy

Peripheral nerve	Mild distal sensorimotor peripheral neuropathy
Brain	Mild cognitive impairment
Skin	Frontal balding
Eye	Cataracts, retinal pigmentation, ophthalmoparesis
Endocrine	Type II diabetes, hyperparathyroidism, testicular atrophy
Cardiovascular	Cardiac dysrhythmias
Gastrointestinal	Dysmotility

significantly with cold or exercise (i.e., "paradoxical" myotonia). Weakness and atrophy, when present, begin in cranial and distal limb muscles, and progress slowly over time. Symmetrical ptosis and weakness of the muscles of facial expression and mastication produce a characteristic facial appearance. Other cranial muscles, such as the tongue, palate, pharyngeal, sternocleidomastoid, and neck muscles, may also be involved. In the limbs, the weakness first appears in distal muscles (finger and wrist flexors and extensors, ankle dorsiflexors) but may progress to involve proximal muscles as well. Deep tendon reflexes are often reduced or absent in DM, and there may be other signs of a mild length-dependent sensorimotor peripheral neuropathy. DM2 has the same clinical manifestations as DM1, but genetic testing shows normal numbers of CTG repeats. Cases of PROMM differ clinically in the distribution of weakness, which predominantly affects proximal muscles. Clinical myotonia, cataracts, and the other systemic manifestations characteristic of myotonic dystrophy are typically found in PROMM as well. Some patients with PROMM complain of myalgias in addition to weakness.

Congenital myotonic dystrophy is present at birth and is very severe, with hypotonia, respiratory insufficiency, facial weakness, feeding difficulties, mental retardation, and talipes. Clinical myotonia is absent in congenital myotonic dystrophy.

PATHOLOGY

The muscle biopsy may be normal or show mild nonspecific changes in myotonic dystrophy (Harper, 1989). Changes in congenital DM are more severe and distinctive. There are increased numbers of internal nuclei, often arranged in chains along the longitudinal axis of muscle fiber. Ring fibers, sarcoplasmic masses, angulated fibers, and variation in fiber size are common but relatively nonspecific.

ELECTROMYOGRAPHY

Nerve conduction studies are normal or show evidence of a mild length-dependent sensorimotor peripheral neuropathy. Repetitive stimulation produces a variable decrement. The amplitude of the compound muscle action potential is transiently reduced after brief exercise. Needle EMG shows widespread myotonic discharges, fibrillation potentials, and small, polyphasic, rapidly recruited MUPs. Myotonic discharges consist of biphasic spikes or positive waves that fire in bursts of 2 to 20 seconds' duration. They can be triggered by needle movement, by percussion over the muscle, or by muscle contraction. The characteristic "dive-bomber" sound of myotonic discharges is produced by gradual fluctuations in both the frequency (20 to 80 Hz) and the amplitude (20 to 500 μV) of the potentials. Myotonic discharges are not unique to DM but are also observed in other inherited and acquired disorders that enhance sarcolemmal excitability by a variety of mechanisms (see Chapter 80). The discharges tend to be of longer duration in myotonic dystrophy than in myotonia congenita (Daube, 1994). In all inherited myotonic disorders, cooling the muscle initially increases myotonic discharges. In paramyotonia congenita, continued cooling produces a reduction in the myotonic discharges and, eventually, electrical silence. This is associated with reduced MUP recruitment and paralysis of the muscle with slow recovery after warming the muscle. Exercise increases myotonic discharges in paramyotonia but decreases them in all other myotonic disorders.

DIAGNOSIS

Clinical and EMG data can usually distinguish DM1 and DM2 from PROMM and other forms of muscular dystrophy or the channelopathies. Molecular testing is required to confirm the diagnosis of DM1. A combination of PCR and Southern blot techniques will detect CTG expansions in patients and affected family members (Meola and Moxley, 1999). Prenatal molecular genetic testing on amniocytes or chorionic villus cells can reliably identify cases of congenital DM.

References

Ahn A, Yoshida M, Anderson M, et al: A distinct 59kDa dystrophin-associated protein encoded on chromosome 8q23-24. Proc Natl Acad Sci U S A 1994;91:4446–4450.

Angelini C, Fanin M, Freda MP, et al: The clinical spectrum of sarcoglycanopathies. Neurology 1999;52:176–179.

Askansas V, Engel WK, Reddy NB, et al: X-linked recessive congenital muscle fiber hypotrophy with central nuclei: Abnormalities of growth and adenylate cyclase in muscle tissue cultures. Arch Neurol 1979;36:604–609.

Barth PG, Scholte HR, Berden JA, et al: An X-linked mitochondrial disease affecting cardiac muscle, skeletal muscle and neutrophil leucocytes. J Neurol Sci 1983;62:327–355.

Bashir R, Britton S, Strachan T, et al: A gene related to *Caenorhabditis elegans* spermatogenesis factor *fer-1* is mutated in limbgirdle muscular dystrophy type 2B. Nat Genet 1998;20:37–42.

Bethlem J, Van Gool J, Hulsmann WC, et al: Familial nonprogressive myopathy with muscle cramps after exercise: A new disease associated with cores in the muscle fibers. Brain 1966; 89:569–589.

Bethlem J, Van Wijngaarden GK, Meijer AEFH, Fleury P: Observations on central core disease. J Neurol Sci 1971;14:293–299.

Bione S, D'Adamo P, Maestrini E, et al: A novel X-linked gene, G4.5, is responsible for Barth syndrome. Nat Genet 1996;12:385–389.

Bione S, Small K, Aksamonvic VMA, et al: Identification of new mutations in Emery-Dreifuss muscular dystrophy gene and evidence for genetic heterogeneity of the disease. Hum Mol Genet 1995;4:1859.

Blake DJ, Nawrotski R, Peters MF, et al: Isoform diversity of dystrobrevin, the murine 87kd post-synaptic protein. J Biol Chem 1996;27:7802–7810.

Bodensteiner JD: Congenital myopathies. Muscle Nerve 1994;17: 131–144.

Bradley WG, Jones MZ, Mussini JM, Fawcett PRW: Becker type muscular dystrophy. Muscle Nerve 1978;1:111–132.

Brais B, Bouchard JP, Xie YG, et al: Short GCG expansions in the PABP2 gene cause oculopharyngeal muscular dystrophy. Nat Genet 1998;18:164–167.

Buj-Bello A, Biancalana V, Moutou C, et al: Identification of novel mutations in the MTM1 gene causing severe and mild forms of X-linked myotubular myopathy. Hum Mutat 1999;14:320–325.

Bushby K, Goodship J, Haggerty D, et al: Duchenne muscular dystrophy and idiopathic hyperCK-emia in a family causing confusion in genetic counseling. Am J Med Genet 1996;66:237–238.

Carbone I, Bruno C, Sotgia F, et al: Mutation in the CAV3 gene causes partial caveolin-3 deficiency and hyperCKemia. Neurology 2000;54:1373–1376.

Cavanagh NPC, Lake BD, McMeniman P: Congenital fiber type disproportion myopathy: A histological diagnosis with an uncertain clinical outlook. Arch Dis Child 1979;54:735–743.

Curless RG, Nelson MB: Congenital fiber type disproportion in identical twins. Ann Neurol 1977;2:455–459.

Daube JR: The description of motor unit potentials in electromyography. Neurology 1978;28:623–625.

Daube JR: Electrodiagnosis of muscle disorders. In Engel AG, Franzini Armstrong C (eds): Myology, 2nd ed. New York, McGraw-Hill, 1994; 764–794.

Day JW, Roelofs R, Leroy B, et al: Clinical and genetic characteristics of a five-generation family with a novel form of myotonic dystrophy (DM2). Neuromuscul Disord 1999;9:19–27.

Engel AG: Myofibrillar myopathy. Ann Neurol 1999;46:681–684.

Engel AG, Yamamoto M, Fishbeck KH: Dystrophinopathies. In Engel AG, Franzini-Armstrong C (eds): Myology, 2nd ed. New York, McGraw-Hill, 1994; 1133–1187.

Falga-Tirado C, Perez-Peman P, Ordi-Ros J, et al: Adult onset of nemaline myopathy presenting as respiratory insufficiency. Respiration 1995;62:353–354.

Fardeau M, Tome FMS: Congenital myopathies. In Engel AG, Franzini-Armstrong C (eds): Myology, 2nd ed, vol II. New York, McGraw-Hill, 1994; 1487–1532.

Fenichel GM, Emery ES, Hunt P: Neurogenic atrophy simulating facioscapulohumeral dystrophy: A dominant form. Arch Neurol 1967;17:257–260.

Ferlini A, Sewry C, Melis MA, et al: X-linked dilated cardiomyopathy and the dystrophin gene. Neuromuscul Disord 1999;9:339–346.

Goldfarb LG, Park KY, Cervenakova L, et al: Missense mutations in desmin associated with familial cardiac and skeletal myopathy. Nat Genet 1998;19:402–403.

Gospe SM Jr, Lazaro JP, Lava NS, et al: Familial X-linked myalgia and cramps: A nonprogressive myopathy associated with a deletion in the dystrophin gene. Neurology 1989;39:1277–1280.

Grimm T, Janka M: Emery-Dreifuss muscular dystrophy. In Engel AG, Franzini-Armstrong C (eds): Myology, 2nd ed. New York, McGraw-Hill, 1994; 1188–1191.

Haravuori H, Mkela-Bengs P, Figlewicz DA, et al: Tibial muscular dystrophy and late-onset distal myopathy are linked to the same locus on chromosome 2q. Neurology 1998;40:A186.

Harper PS: Myotonic Dystrophy, 2nd ed. Philadelphia, WB Saunders, 1989.

Hawkes CH, Absolon MJ: Myotubular myopathy associated with cataract and electrical myotonia. J Neurol Neurosurg Psychiatry 1975;38:761–764.

Hayashi K, Miller RG, Brownell AK: Central core disease: Ultrastructure of the sarcoplasmic reticulum and T-tubules. Muscle Nerve 1989;12:95–102.

Herman GE, Finegold M, de Gouyon B, et al: Medical complications in long-term survivors with X-linked myotubular myopathy. J Pediatr 1999;134:206–214.

Hilton-Brown P, Stålberg E: The motor unit in muscular dystrophy: A single-fiber EMG and scanning EMG study. J Neurol Neurosurg Psychiatry 1983;46:981–995.

Hoffman EP: Clinical and histopathological features of abnormalities of the dystrophin-based membrane cytoskeleton. Brain Pathol 1996;6:49–61.

Hoffman EP, Brown RH Jr, Kunkel LM: Dystrophin: The protein product of the Duchenne muscular dystrophy locus. Cell 1987; 51:919–928.

Horowitz SH, Schmalbruch H: Autosomal dominant myopathy with desmin storage: A clinicopathologic and electrophysiologic study of a large kinship. Muscle Nerve 1994;17:151–160.

Illarioshkin SN, Ivanova-Smolenskaia IA, Tanaka H, et al: Refined genetic location of the chromosome 2p-linked progressive muscular dystrophy gene. Genomics 1997;42:345–348.

International Myotonic Dystrophy Consortium (IDMC): New nomenclature and DNA testing guidelines for myotonic dystrophy type 1 (DM1). Neurology 2000;54:1218–1221.

Jobsis GJ, Keizers H, Vreijling A, et al: Type VI collagen mutations in Bethlem myopathy, an autosomal dominant myopathy with contractures. Nat Genet 1996;14:113–115.

Joseph M, Pai GS, Holden KR, et al: X-linked myotubular myopathy: Clinical observations in ten additional cases. Am J Med Genet 1995;59:168–173.

Karpati G, Carpenter S, Andermann F: A new concept of childhood nemaline myopathy. Arch Neurol 1972;24:291–304.

Karpati G, Carpenter S: Small-caliber skeletal muscle fibers do not suffer deleterious consequences of dystrophic gene expression. Am J Med Genet 1986;25:653–658.

Kimura J (ed): Myopathies. In Electrodiagnosis in Diseases of Nerve and Muscle: Principles and Practice, 2nd ed. Philadelphia, FA Davis, 1989; 535–557.

Kissel JT: Facioscapulohumeral dystrophy. Semin Neurol 1999a; 19:35–43.

Kissel JT: Muscular dystrophy: Historical overview and classification in the genetic era. Semin Neurol 1999b;19:5–7.

Ko YL, Chen JJ, Tang TK, et al: Malignant familial hypertrophic cardiomyopathy in a family with a 453Arg-to-Cys mutation in the beta-myosin heavy chain gene: Coexistence of sudden death and end-stage heart failure. Hum Genet 1996;97:585–590.

Kobayashi K, Nakahori Y, Miyake M, et al: An ancient retrotransposal insertion causes Fukuyama-type congenital muscular dystrophy. Nature 1998;394:388–392.

Koenig M, Monaco AB, Kunkel LM: The complete sequence of dystrophin predicts a rod-shaped cytoskeletal protein. Cell 1988;53:219–228.

Kugelberg E: Electromyography in muscular dystrophies: Differentiation between dystrophies and chronic lower motor neuron lesions. J Neurol Neurosurg Psychiatry 1949;12:129–136.

Laing NG, Laing BA, Meredith C, et al: Autosomal dominant distal myopathy: Linkage to chromosome 14. Am J Hum Genet 1995a; 56:422–427.

Laing NG, Wilton SD, Akkari PA, et al: A mutation in the alpha-tropomyosin gene TPM3 associated with autosomal dominant nemaline myopathy NEM1. Nat Genet 1995b;9:75–79.

Lamont PJ, Dubowitz V, Landon DN, et al: Fifty-year follow-up of a patient with central core disease shows slow but definite progression. Neuromuscul Disord 1998;8:385–391.

Laporte J, Hu LJ, Kretz C, et al: A gene mutated in X-linked myotubular myopathy defines a new putative tyrosine phosphatase family conserved in yeast. Nat Genet 1996;13:175–182.

Laporte J, Kioschis P, Hu L-J, et al: Cloning and characterization of an alternatively spliced gene in proximal Xq28 deleted in two patients with intersexual genitalia and myotubular myopathy. Genomics 1997;41:458–462.

Lim LE, Campbell KP: The sarcoglycan complex in limb-girdle muscular dystrophy. Curr Opin Neurol 1998;11:443–452.

Liu J, Aoki M, Illa I, et al: Dysferlin, a novel skeletal muscle gene, is mutated in Miyoshi myopathy and limb-girdle muscular dystrophy. Nat Genet 1998;20:31–36.

Loke J, MacLennan DH: Malignant hyperthermia and central core disease: Disorders of Ca^{2+} release channels. Am J Med 1998; 104:470–486.

Lynch PJ, Tong J, Lehane M, et al: A mutation in the transmembrane/luminal domain of the ryanodine receptor is associated with abnormal Ca^{2+} release channel function and severe central core disease. Proc Natl Acad Sci U S A 1999;96:4164–4169.

Mansfield ES, Robertson JM, Lebo RV, et al: Duchenne/Becker muscular dystrophy carrier detection using quantitative PCR and fluorescence-based strategies. Am J Med Genet 1993;48: 200–208.

Markesbery WR, Griggs RC, Leach RP, Lapham LW: Late-onset hereditary distal myopathy. Neurology 1974;24:127.

Melberg A, Oldfors A, Blomstrom-Lundqvist C, et al: Autosomal dominant myofibrillar myopathy with arrhythmogenic right ventricular cardiomyopathy linked to chromosome 10q. Ann Neurol 1999;46:684–693.

Meola G, Moxley RT: Myotonic disorders: Myotonic dystrophy and proximal myotonic myopathy. In Schapira AHV, Griggs RC (eds): Muscle Disorders. Boston, Butterworth-Heinemann, 1999; 115–135.

Merlini L, Morandi L, Granata C, Ballestrazzi A: Bethlem myopathy: Early-onset benign autosomal dominant myopathy with contractures. Description of two new families. Neuromuscul Disord 1994;4:503–511.

Michele DE, Albayya FP, Metzger JM: A nemaline myopathy mutation in alpha-tropomyosin causes defective regulation of striated muscle force production. J Clin Invest 1999;104:1575–1581.

Minetti C, Sotgia F, Bruno C, et al: Mutations in the caveolin-3 gene cause autosomal dominant limb-girdle muscular dystrophy. Nat Genet 1998;18:365–368.

Mirabella M, Silvestri G, de Rosa G, et al: GCG genetic expansions in Italian patients with oculopharyngeal muscular dystrophy. Neurology 2000;54:608–614.

Mitrani-Rosenbaum S, Argov Z, Blumenfeld A, et al: Hereditary inclusion body myopathy maps to chromosome 9p1-q1. Hum Mol Genet 1996;5:159–163.

Miyoshi K, Iwasa M, Kawa H, et al: Autosomal recessive distal muscular dystrophy: A new type of distal muscular dystrophy observed characteristically in Japan. Nippon Rinsho 1977;35: 3922.

Munsat T, Piper D, Cancilla P, et al: Inflammatory myopathy with facioscapulohumeral dystrophy. Neurology 1972;22:335–347.

Nakano S, Engel AG, Waclawik AJ, et al: Myofibrillar myopathy with abnormal foci of desmin positivity. I. Light and electron microscopic analysis. J Neuropathol Exp Neurol 1996;55:549–562.

Nicolao P, Xiang F, Gunnarson LG, et al: Autosomal dominant myopathy with proximal weakness and early respiratory muscle involvement maps to chromosome 2q. Am J Hum Genet 1999;64:788–792.

Nonaka I, Sunohara N, Ishiura S, Satoyoshi E: Familial distal myopathy with rimmed vacuole and lamellar (myeloid) body formation. J Neurol Sci 1981;51:141.

Nowak KJ, Wattanasirichaigoon D, Goebel HH, et al: Mutations in the skeletal muscle alpha-actin gene in patients with actin myopathy and nemaline myopathy. Nat Genet 1999;23:208–212.

Orrell RW, Forrester JD, Tawil R, et al: Definitive molecular diagnosis of facioscapulohumeral muscular dystrophy. Neurology 1999;52:1822–1826.

Pegoraro E, Mancias P, Swerdlow SH, et al: Congenital muscular dystrophy (CMD) with primary laminin α2 deficiency presenting as inflammatory myopathy. Ann Neurol 1996;46:810–814.

Pelin K, Hilpela P, Donner K, et al: Mutations in the nebulin gene associated with autosomal recessive nemaline myopathy. Proc Natl Acad Sci U S A 1999;96:2305–2310.

Prior TW: Perspectives and molecular diagnosis of Duchenne and Becker muscular dystrophies. Clin Lab Med 1995;15:927–941.

Pulkkinen L, Smith FJD, Shimizu, et al: Homozygous deletion mutations in the plectin gene (PLEC1) in patients with epidermolysis bullosa simplex associated with late-onset muscular dystrophy. Hum Mol Genet 1996;5:1539–1546.

Richard I, Broux, O, Allamand V, et al: Mutations in the proteolytic enzyme calpain-3 cause limb-girdle muscular dystrophy type 2A. Cell 1995;81:27–40.

Ricker K, Koch MC, Lehmann-Horn F, et al: Proximal myotonic myopathy: Clinical features of a multisystem disorder similar to myotonic dystrophy. Arch Neurol 1995;52:25–31.

Rifai Z, Kingston WJ, McCraith B, Moxley RT: Forearm 3-methyl-histidine efflux in myotonic dystrophy. Ann Neurol 1993;34:682–686.

Roberts RG, Barby TF, Manners E, et al: Direct detection of dystrophin gene rearrangements by analysis of dystrophin mRNA in peripheral blood lymphocytes. Am J Hum Genet 1991;49:298–310.

Serratrice G, Pellissier JF, Faugere MC, et al: Centronuclear myopathy: Possible central nervous system origin. Muscle Nerve 1978;1:62–69.

Sewry CA, Philot J, Mahoney D, et al: Expression of laminin subunits in congenital muscular dystrophy. Neuromuscul Disord 1995;5:307–316.

Shy GM, Engel WK, Somers JE, Wanko T: Nemaline myopathy: A new congenital myopathy. Brain 1963;86:793–810.

Shy GM, Magee KR: A new congenital non-progressive myopathy. Brain 1956;79:610.

Stålberg E, Trontelj JV: Single Fiber Electromyography: Studies in Healthy and Diseased Muscle, 2nd ed. New York, Raven Press, 1994.

Sunohara N, Arahata K, Hoffman EP: Quadriceps myopathy: A forme fruste of Becker muscular dystrophy. Ann Neurol 1990;28:634–639.

Sunohara N, Nonaka I, Kamei N, Satoyoshi E: Distal myopathy with rimmed vacuole formation: A follow-up study. Brain 1989;112:65.

Tanner SM, Laporte J, Guiraud-Chaumeil C, et al: Confirmation of prenatal diagnosis results of X-linked recessive myotubular myopathy by mutational screening and description of three new mutations in the MTM1 gene. Hum Mutat 1998;11:62–68.

Tawil R, Figlewicz DA, Griggs RC, Weiffenbach B: Facioscapulo-humeral dystrophy: A distinct regional myopathy with a novel molecular pathogenesis. Ann Neurol 1998;43:279–282.

Thornton C: The myotonic dystrophies. Semin Neurol 1999;19:25–33.

Tome FMS, Chateau D, Helbling-Leclerc A, et al: Morphological changes in muscle fibers in oculopharyngeal muscular dystrophy. Neuromuscul Disord 1997;7:63–69.

Tome FMS, Evangelista T, Leclerc A, et al: Congenital muscular dystrophy with merosin deficiency. C R Acad Sci II 1994;317:351–357.

Tome FMS, Fardeau M: Oculopharyngeal muscular dystrophy. In Engel AG, Franzini-Armstrong C (eds): Myology, 2nd ed. New York, McGraw-Hill, 1994; 1233–1245.

Van Essen AJ, Abbs S, Baiget M, et al: Parental and germline mosaicism of deletions and duplications of the dystrophin gene: A European study. Hum Genet 1992;88:249–257.

Vicart P, Cron A, Guicheney P, et al: A missense mutation in the αB-crystallin chaperone gene causes a desmin-related myopathy. Nat Genet 1998;20:92–95.

Wallgren-Pettersson C, Clarke A, Samson F, et al: The myotubular myopathies: Differential diagnosis of the X-linked recessive, autosomal dominant, and autosomal recessive forms and present state of DNA studies. J Med Genet 1995;32:673–679.

Wallgren-Pettersson C, Sainio K, Salmi T: Electromyography in congenital nemaline myopathy. Muscle Nerve 1989;12:587–593.

Welander L: Myopathia distalis tarda hereditaria. Acta Med Scand 1951;141(suppl 265):1.

Wilhelmsen KC, Blake DM, Lynch T, et al: Chromosome 12–linked autosomal dominant scapuloperoneal muscular dystrophy. Ann Neurol 1996;39:507–520.

Zhang Y, Chen HS, Khanna VK, et al: A mutation in the human ryanodine receptor gene associated with central core disease. Nat Genet 1993;5:46–50.

Inflammatory and Infiltrative Myopathies

Devon I. Rubin and Robert C. Hermann

Inflammatory myopathies refers to a heterogeneous group of acquired muscle diseases characterized clinically by muscle weakness and pathologically by inflammatory cell infiltration and necrosis of muscle fibers. This group of disorders has classically been represented by dermatomyositis and polymyositis, although *inclusion body myositis* has become recognized as the most common inflammatory myopathy in older patients. In addition to idiopathic inflammatory myopathies, bacterial, viral, fungal, and parasitic infections can, rarely, involve skeletal muscle and evoke an inflammatory reaction, either in isolation or as part of a systemic infection. Skeletal muscle may also be affected by processes that infiltrate the muscle fibers, with or without a coincident inflammatory response, such as occurs in amyloidosis, sarcoidosis, and carcinomatous infiltration. These different inflammatory and infiltrative myopathies can often be differentiated by their associated extramuscular and systemic manifestations, but in many cases, the clinical and laboratory features may be indistinguishable. Therefore, a systematic approach to these disorders is crucial in establishing a proper diagnosis.

The neuromuscular evaluation of patients with inflammatory and infiltrative myopathies requires the combination of a careful neuromuscular history and examination, a general medical history and physical examination, laboratory studies, and a thorough electrodiagnostic evaluation. The history should consist of the predominant symptomatology, distribution of weakness, temporal profile and course of the symptoms, and associated systemic or non-neurological manifestations. A thorough review of the

---

Unless otherwise indicated, all illustrations in this chapter are copyright by the Mayo Foundation for Medical Education and Research.

family history is helpful to exclude the possibility of a muscular dystrophy, although rarely, inclusion body myositis or myopathy associated with amyloidosis is hereditary. A careful review of medications and toxin exposures is also important to exclude other causes of muscle disease. The general physical and neurological examinations are important, with special attention to the degree, distribution, and symmetry of muscle weakness; muscle size and consistency; muscle stretch reflexes; and sensory findings. Symmetrical, proximal weakness with mildly reduced or preserved reflexes and normal sensation are the most common clinical features on the neurological examination, with few exceptions. In patients with an atypical history or examination, other neuromuscular disorders, such as motoneuron disease, polyradiculopathies, neuromuscular junction disorders, and polyneuropathies, should be considered.

Electrodiagnostic testing is an important step in the evaluation of inflammatory myopathies. However, even for the experienced electromyographer, the evaluation of myopathies can be challenging. Early in the course of the disease, the findings on needle examination may be patchy and subtle, requiring persistence and thoroughness in examining multiple muscles. Furthermore, electromyography is limited in the ability to distinguish between specific inflammatory and infiltrative myopathies, because the findings are similar in the majority of the disorders. This chapter reviews the clinical and electrodiagnostic features of inflammatory and infiltrative myopathies.

CLASSIFICATION

In 1975, Bohan and Peter (1975a, 1975b) presented an initial classification scheme for inflammatory myopathies, which was derived empirically on the basis of clinical presentation and the presence or absence of associated systemic features and malignancies. In this classification, the criteria required to establish the diagnosis of idiopathic polymyositis included (1) progressive proximal weakness, (2) muscle biopsy evidence of muscle fiber necrosis and inflammation, (3) serological elevation of levels of muscle enzymes, and (4) electromyographic abnormalities consistent with a myopathy. In patients who fulfilled these criteria with associated dermatological manifestations, the diagnosis of dermatomyositis could be made. Furthermore, patients were subclassified according to age at onset and the presence or absence of associated neoplasia and systemic connective tissue diseases ("overlap syndromes"). Although this original classification continues to be the most widely referenced in subsequent reports and reviews of inflammatory myopathies, it has limitations. Specifically, as histopathological and immunological advances have emerged, the initial belief that dermatomyositis was simply polymyositis with a rash has been refuted. Muscle biopsy requirements were limited to muscle fiber necrosis, phagocytosis, regeneration, and inflammation; the distinct and different histological features of polymyositis and dermatomyositis had not yet been clearly elucidated. In addition, the absence of inclusion body myositis and other associated infectious disorders in the early classification has led to adaptation of this scheme (Mastalgia and Ojeda, 1985). In this chapter, we separate these disorders into idiopathic inflammatory myopathies with or without associated systemic features, myopathies associated with infectious diseases, and infiltrative myopathies (Table 77–1).

INFLAMMATORY MYOPATHIES

Dermatomyositis and Polymyositis

Polymyositis and dermatomyositis are the prototypical idiopathic inflammatory muscle diseases and are characterized clinically by progressive proximal weakness and histologically by muscle fiber necrosis and inflammatory infiltration. First described by Wagner in 1863, the clinical features and pathogenesis have been further elucidated, and several recent comprehensive reviews have consistently detailed the salient clinical, histopathological, and immunological features of these inflammatory myopathies (Pearson and Bohan, 1977; Whitaker, 1982; Walton, 1983; Mastaglia, 1985b; Kingston and Moxley, 1988; Plotz et al., 1989; Bunch, 1990; Cronin and Plotz,

Table 77–1. Categorization of Inflammatory and Infiltrative Myopathies

Inflammatory myopathies
  Adult dermatomyositis
  Childhood dermatomyositis
  Dermatomyositis associated with malignancy
  Polymyositis
  Polymyositis associated with connective tissue disorders:
    systemic lupus erythematosus, rheumatoid arthritis,
    primary systemic sclerosis, Sjögren's syndrome
  Inclusion body myositis
Infectious myopathies
  Viral: influenza, coxsackievirus, adenovirus, hepatitis B virus,
    human immunodeficiency virus–associated myopathy
  Bacterial: *Staphylococcus, Borrelia burgdorferi*
  Parasitic: toxoplasmosis, trichinosis, cysticercosis,
    echinococcosis, schistosomiasis, trypanosomiasis
Infiltrative myopathies
  Amyloidosis
  Sarcoidosis
  Carcinomatous
Other inflammatory myopathies
  Eosinophilic polymyositis
  Eosinophilia-myalgia syndrome
  Eosinophilic fasciitis
  Graft-versus-host myopathy
  Macrophagic myofasciitis
  Focal myositis
  Polymyalgia rheumatica

1990; Dalakas, 1990, 1991, 1994; Robinson, 1991; Rosenberg, 1991; Amato and Barohn et al., 1997; Callen, 2000). Although early series categorized dermatomyositis and polymyositis as a single disorder, dermatomyositis and polymyositis are now known to be clinically, histologically, and pathologically distinct entities. The annual incidence rate for polymyositis/dermatomyositis is between 0.1 and 2.6 per 100,000 population (Pearson, 1966; Rose and Walton, 1966; Kurland et al., 1969; Medsger et al., 1970; Benbassat et al., 1980). There is a higher frequency in women, with a female-to-male ratio of 2:1. There is a bimodal age at presentation, with peaks of high incidence between ages 5 and 14 and 45 and 64 years. Dermatomyositis occurs in both childhood and adulthood, whereas idiopathic polymyositis occurs predominantly in adults.

Clinical Manifestations

ADULT DERMATOMYOSITIS

Dermatomyositis is characterized by specific dermatological manifestations associated with progressive and symmetrical muscle weakness. The skin abnormalities are present in 90% of affected patients and may precede, coincide with, or follow the muscle weakness. The two most characteristic skin manifestations are a *heliotrope rash* and *Gottron's nodules,* which are virtually pathognomonic for the disease. The heliotrope rash is a violaceous rash, often associated with edema, that involves the periorbital skin. Gottron's nodules are subcutaneous papules that occur most commonly over the extensor surfaces of the metacarpophalangeal and interphalangeal joints but also over the elbow and knee joints. Other cutaneous features that are often seen include an erythematous malar rash and a sun-sensitive flat erythematous rash over the anterior chest (V sign) or shoulders and upper back (shawl sign). Dilated capillary loops in the nailbed may be appreciated with direct magnification. Another, sometimes debilitating manifestation is calcification in the subcutaneous tissues (calcinosis), which occurs in 30% to 70% of cases of childhood dermatomyositis but is rare in adults. In rare instances, patients with typical cutaneous stigmata of dermatomyositis but without clinical or laboratory muscle involvement *(amyopathic dermatomyositis)* have been described (Caproni et al., 1998).

The neuromuscular presentation of dermatomyositis characteristically begins with subacute, progressive proximal weakness that involves the arms and legs. Patients may describe difficulty in rising from a chair, climbing stairs, or lifting objects above the head. Muscle pain and stiffness, particularly in the arms and shoulders, is common and occurs in up to 73% of patients (DeVere and Bradley, 1975). The neurological examination demonstrates symmetrical weakness, most commonly involving muscles of the shoulder and pelvic girdle and neck flex-

ors, although distal muscles may be involved in up to 30% of patients. In rare cases, distal or monomelic weakness is more prominent than symmetrical proximal weakness (Hollinrake, 1969; Stark, 1978; Ledermann, 1984). The weakness may fluctuate in severity from week to week or month to month. In patients experiencing slowly progressive proximal arm and facial weakness, the presentation may be similar to that of facioscapulohumeral dystrophy (Rothstein and Carlson, 1970; Munsat et al., 1972; Bates et al., 1973). Dysphagia due to involvement of the pharyngeal muscles is a common symptom, occurring in up to 40% of cases, and is more common in patients older than 65 (DeVere and Bradley, 1975; Bohan et al., 1977; Lakhanpal et al., 1986; Marie et al., 1999). Muscle bulk is well maintained, although atrophy may occur late in the course of the disease. Without treatment, weakness usually progresses over weeks to months. Myotactic reflexes are either normal or mildly hypoactive, except in patients with severe muscle weakness and atrophy, in whom they may be absent. Flexion contractures at the elbows, hips, knees, and ankles are frequent. In the absence of a superimposed polyneuropathy from a systemic or coincidental connective tissue disorder, the sensory examination findings are invariably normal.

CHILDHOOD DERMATOMYOSITIS

Childhood dermatomyositis is the most common acquired myopathy of childhood. The time of peak incidence is in early adolescence, but children as young as age 2 may be affected. Girls have a slightly higher incidence than that of boys, with a ratio of 3:2. The clinical manifestations of childhood dermatomyositis are similar to those of adult dermatomyositis. Cutaneous manifestations are often prominent and almost always precede the neuromuscular symptoms. As in adult dermatomyositis, periorbital edema, heliotrope malar rash, and a rash on extensor surfaces and light-sensitive regions of the body are common. Once the characteristic rash has developed, progressive muscle weakness follows, involving proximal more often than distal muscles. Shoulder and hip girdle muscles are most frequently involved, although other proximal and distal muscles may also be affected. Muscle pain and cramping are common, particularly early in the course of the disease.

In addition to the neuromuscular and dermatological symptoms, other organ systems may be involved. Gastrointestinal ulceration leading to intestinal hemorrhage or perforation may occur more commonly than in adult dermatomyositis, and subcutaneous calcinosis may lead to skin ulceration (Banker and Victor, 1966). Pulmonary fibrosis may also occur but is less common than in adult dermatomyositis (Crowe et al., 1982).

MALIGNANCY AND DERMATOMYOSITIS

An increased incidence of associated malignancies in dermatomyositis has been suggested by several studies, but the subject remains controversial (Bohan et al., 1977; Callen, 1988; Richardson and Callen, 1989; Dalakas, 1991). The difficulty in establishing an association between malignancies and dermatomyositis has resulted from the retrospective nature of many of the early studies, the lack of control groups, and the difficulty in establishing a causal relationship. The incidence of malignancies in dermatomyositis has been reported as between 7% and 60% but is generally thought to be approximately 25% (DeVere and Bradley, 1975; Bohan et al., 1977; Lakhanpal et al., 1986; Callen, 1988; Callen, 1994; Marie et al., 1999). However, in several population-based studies, no significant association was found between dermatomyositis and malignancies (Medsger et al., 1970; Lakhanpal et al., 1986). In 1994, a meta-analysis of all case-control and cohort studies evaluating the association of dermatomyositis and cancer found that a malignancy was diagnosed within 10 years of the diagnosis in 14% of patients, which was a significantly higher rate than that for a similar number of control subjects (Zantos et al., 1994). Malignancies appear to be much more prevalent in elderly patients than in younger patients (Bohan et al., 1977; Lakhanpal et al., 1986; Marie et al., 1999). In one study, 48% of patients older than 65 had an underlying malignancy, compared with only 9% of patients younger than 65 (Marie et al., 1999). Furthermore, the association with malignancy appears to be stronger in patients with dermatomyositis than in those with polymyositis (Bohan et al., 1977; Manchul et al., 1985; Callen, 1988; Chow et al., 1995; Marie et al., 1999). Many different cancers have been reported in dermatomyositis, including lung, breast, colon, and ovarian cancers (Lakhanpal et al., 1986; Marie et al., 1999). In most cases, the development of an inflammatory myopathy precedes the appearance of a malignancy, although in up to 30% of patients, the malignancy may antedate the myositis by several years (Bohan et al., 1977). It is generally believed that an exhaustive search for cancer in patients with dermatomyositis may not be cost effective or warranted, and a directed approach that is based on a symptom or an abnormal laboratory finding should be used. A careful general medical examination and screening laboratory studies appear to represent the most prudent approach.

POLYMYOSITIS

In the early descriptions of the disorders, polymyositis was, in essence, considered to be "dermatomyositis without a rash." Although later histopathological and immunological studies clearly distinguished dermatomyositis and polymyositis as distinct entities, the clinical neuromuscular presentation of these two entities is indistinguishable. Polymyositis occurs much more commonly in adults than in children, although patients of any age may be affected. The onset is typically between ages 30 and 60. Patients with polymyositis present with subacute, slowly progressive, symmetrical proximal weakness, which usually progresses insidiously over months to years. As in dermatomyositis, the shoulder girdle and pelvic muscles are the most common sites of involvement, although distal and cranial weakness may also occur. Muscle pain may or may not be present.

The age at presentation of polymyositis has certain distinguishing features. In prospectively following 79 consecutive patients with polymyositis, Marie and associates (1999) found that 29% presented after the age of 65. In these patients, there was no significant difference in the clinical presentation, laboratory, or electromyographic findings, but the frequency of dysphagia or underlying malignancies and the mortality rate were higher in the older patients.

Extramuscular Manifestations

Involvement of other organ systems, outside of the neuromuscular and dermatological systems, is not uncommon in dermatomyositis and polymyositis (Bohan et al., 1977; Spiera and Kagen, 1998). Involvement of the lungs is most frequent, is often prominent, and is rarely a presenting feature (Blumbergs et al., 1984). Interstitial lung disease occurs in up to 30% of patients with adult dermatomyositis and polymyositis and may precede the muscular symptoms. Interstitial lung disease is commonly associated with the presence of anti–aminoacyl transfer RNA synthetase antibodies, such as anti–Jo-1 antibodies, in patients with polymyositis but not in those with dermatomyositis (Plotz et al., 1989; Grau et al., 1996). Aspiration pneumonia may occur as a result of weakness in the pharyngeal and esophageal muscles. Symptomatic involvement of the cardiovascular system with arrhythmias, congestive heart failure, pericarditis, and pulmonary hypertension has been described, and subclinical electrocardiographic abnormalities also occur (Bohan et al., 1977; Dalakas, 1991). Raynaud's phenomenon and arthritis frequently occur in patients with dermatomyositis or polymyositis who do not fulfill diagnostic criteria for the "overlap syndrome."

Polymyositis Associated with Connective Tissue Disorders ("Overlap" Syndromes)

Polymyositis may occur in association with clinical and serological features of other systemic connective tissues, such as systemic lupus erythematosus, scleroderma, rheumatoid arthritis, and mixed connective tissue disease (Dalakas, 1991). In the series by Bohan and colleagues (1977) of patients with inflammatory myopathies, progressive systemic sclerosis was the most frequent accompanying disorder, occurring in 36% of patients in the "overlap" group, whereas systemic lupus erythematosus (28%), rheumatoid arthritis (13%), and Sjögren's syndrome (9%) were less frequent. In these "overlap syndromes," there is a significantly higher female preponderance compared with the situation in patients without "overlap" features (Bohan et al., 1977). Muscle involvement may be either a mild or a prominent feature, and other symptoms, such as arthralgias, Raynaud's phenomenon, and myalgias, are frequently coexistent. Muscle involvement in scleroderma has been reported in up to 80% of patients (Medsger et al., 1968, Clements et al., 1978; Olsen et al., 1996). The most common symptom is fatigue, although objective weakness occurs in 30% and is most prominent in proximal muscles (Medsger et al., 1968). Serum creatine kinase levels may be normal or markedly elevated. Electromyography in scleroderma myopathy reveals findings indistinguishable from those in idiopathic polymyositis, with a variable degree of fibrillation potentials and short-duration, low-amplitude motor unit potentials (Hausmanowa-Petrusewica and Kozminska, 1961).

Polymyositis occurs in 4% to 16% of patients with systemic lupus erythematosus (Garton, 1997). Apart from the increased prevalence of antinuclear antibodies and anti–double-stranded DNA antibodies in patients with lupus myositis, there is no difference in the clinical presentation, creatine kinase elevation, or response to treatment compared with patients with "idiopathic" polymyositis (Gartron and Isenberg, 1997). The incidence of myopathy in rheumatoid arthritis is unclear. Several studies have demonstrated electromyographic and histopathological evidence of a myopathy in 6% to 16% of patients, whereas subsequent reports have found no electromyographic evidence of muscle involvement (Rossel, 1963; Miro et al., 1996; Bekklund et al., 1999). An inflammatory myopathy is occasionally seen in patients with Sjögren's syndrome. The incidence of myopathy in Sjögren's syndrome varies from one series to another, but in a study by Cui and colleagues (1997), it appeared to be approximately 6% to 10%. Muscle weakness, myalgias, cramps, and elevation of serum creatine kinase levels may occur. An association between other autoimmune disorders, such as primary biliary cirrhosis, ankylosing spondylitis, and Behçet's syndrome, has also been noted (Arkin et al., 1980; Fuas-Riera, 1991; Miro et al., 1996; Worthmann et al., 1996; Bondeson et al., 1998).

Polymyalgia rheumatica, another rheumatological disorder, is characterized by generalized muscle pain of acute to subacute onset associated with an elevated sedimentation rate and a dramatic response to corticosteroids. Patients with polymyalgia rheumatica are commonly referred for neuromuscular and electrodiagnostic evaluation. There have been only a few studies that evaluated the findings of electromyography in polymyalgia rheumatica. In a review of previous studies in the literature, Trojaberg (1981) identified changes on electromyography in only 7% of patients with polymyalgia rheumatica, and no patient was found to show abnormalities on muscle biopsy. However, in a review of his own patients using quantitative electromyography, the author suggested a much higher incidence (61%) of abnormalities on electromyography. The details of these cases are not reported, and abnormalities on muscle biopsy in 35% suggest that some of these patients may have had polymyositis.

Laboratory Features of Dermatomyositis and Polymyositis

There are no laboratory findings diagnostic of dermatomyositis and polymyositis. Characteristically, muscle enzymes in the serum, including creatine kinase, aldolase, and aminotransferase (aspartate transaminase and alanine transaminase) levels are elevated. Serum creatine kinase and aldolase may be elevated up to 10-fold, although in mild or early cases, muscle enzymes may be normal (DeVere and Bradley, 1977; Bohan et al., 1977). Bohan and colleagues (1977) found normal serum enzyme levels in only 2% of their patients throughout the entire clinical course of the disease. Furthermore, the serum creatine kinase has been shown to parallel the clinical course of the disease, and reduction in creatine kinase usually, but not always, reflects response to treatment. Several isoforms of troponin (troponin T and troponin I) were initially thought to be elevated only with myocardial damage, although some reports have suggested that these so-called cardiac-specific enzymes may be elevated in skeletal muscle diseases as well (Mair, 1997).

Autoantibodies to cellular and nuclear antigens, including antinuclear antibodies, anti-RNP, and anti-Scl, are present in up to 90% of patients with dermatomyositis and polymyositis (Bohan et al., 1977; Targoff, 1994). The most widely recognized myositis-specific antibody is anti-Jo-1 antibody, which is detected in up to 20% of patients with polymyositis or dermatomyositis (Targoff, 1994; Vazquez et al., 1996). A strong association exists between the development of interstitial lung disease and the presence of anti–Jo-1 antibody, which is found in approximately 80% of patients with interstitial lung disease compared with 10% of patients with polymyositis without interstitial lung disease (Targoff, 1994).

Magnetic resonance imaging has been shown to be useful in identifying inflammation, edema, and fibrosis in skeletal muscles involved in inflammatory myopathies (Fujitake et al., 1997; Reimers and Finkenstaedt, 1997). Muscle edema and inflammation result in normal signal intensity on T1-weighted sequences and in increased signal intensity on T2-weighted sequences. The magnetic resonance imaging findings have been shown to correlate with the presence of inflammation on muscle biopsy and with disease activity (Fraser et al., 1991; Reimers and Finkenstaedt, 1997). Serial magnetic resonance imaging findings have also been shown to correlate with clinical course, but at this point, they are not sufficiently sensitive to supersede the clinical, serological, and electromyographic examinations (Fujitaka, 1997).

Histopathological Findings in Dermatomyositis and Polymyositis

The etiology of dermatomyositis and polymyositis is unknown, although an immune-mediated process that causes inflammatory infiltration and fiber necrosis of skeletal muscles fibers is the underlying pathogenetic process in both. Dermatomyositis and polymyositis have different immunological mechanisms and characteristic histopathological changes on muscle biopsy, which clearly define the two disorders as distinct entities. Muscle fiber necrosis with different stages of fiber regeneration and an increase in connective tissue are features common to both dermatomyositis and polymyositis. In neither polymyositis nor dermatomyositis is the mechanism of the activation of the immune system known.

Dermatomyositis

In addition to fiber necrosis, in adult and childhood dermatomyositis, the characteristic finding on muscle biopsy consists of perifascicular inflammatory infiltration consisting of predominantly CD4+ (T-helper) cells, B cells, and macrophages. This inflammatory response is directed at the vascular endothelium, leading to endothelial hyperplasia, obliteration of the capillaries, and disruption of the microcirculation (Dalakas, 1991). This humorally mediated microangiopathy eventually leads to ischemia and microinfarction of muscle fibers and to perifascicular muscle fiber atrophy. The finding of perifascicular atrophy is diagnostic of dermatomyositis and is seen in 90% of children and 50% of adults (Dalakas, 1991) (Fig. 77–1). Furthermore, similar alterations are seen in blood vessels in the skin and gastrointestinal tract.

Polymyositis

In contrast to dermatomyositis, the pathological features of polymyositis consist of endomysial in-

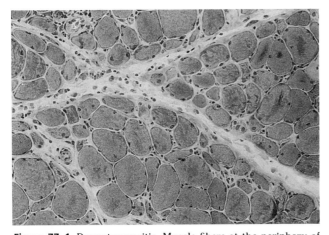

Figure 77–1. Dermatomyositis. Muscle fibers at the periphery of the fascicles have a relatively small diameter and display altered myofibrillar markings. Inflammatory cells are scattered within perimysium, with a lesser number extending into the endomysium (trichrome stain, ×300). (Courtesy of A. G. Engel.)

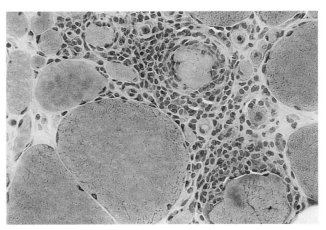

Figure 77–2. Polymyositis. Extensive endomysial inflammatory exudate; some of the inflammatory cells focally surround, invade, and replace non-necrotic muscle fibers (trichrome stain, ×470). (Courtesy of A. G. Engel.)

flammatory cell infiltrates that invade individual non-necrotic muscle fibers, without findings of a microangiopathy or muscle ischemia (Fig. 77–2). The inflammatory cells consist predominantly of CD8+ (cytotoxic) T cells and macrophages, and the expression of major histocompatibility complex (MHC) class I in neighboring or remote muscle fibers suggests an antigen-directed cell-mediated immune response (Dalakas, 1991). Occasional pathological changes, including thinning of myelin sheaths and axonal loss, may occur in a small proportion of intramuscular nerves (Matsubara and Mair, 1979). These morphological changes, along with findings on single-fiber electromyography, suggest that the terminal axons may be involved in the underlying pathological process (Hendriksson, 1978).

Electromyography in Dermatomyositis and Polymyositis

Electrodiagnostic testing is an extension of the neurological examination and is a crucial component of the diagnosis and management of inflammatory myopathies. The most important goal of electromyography is confirmation of the suspected myopathy; other goals are exclusion of neuromuscular diseases such as motoneuron diseases, polyradiculopathies, and neuromuscular junction disorders, which may present with similar symptoms. Furthermore, the distribution of the underlying pathological changes in inflammatory myopathies is often patchy within the same muscle and between different muscles. Needle electromyography provides the means of efficiently assessing multiple regions of a single muscle and sampling of different muscles. The findings on needle examination have been shown to correlate with the pathological changes on muscle biopsy, thereby assisting in the selection of an appropriate muscle for biopsy (Buchthal and Pinelli, 1953). Finally, in patients with inflammatory myopathies who are receiving treatment with corticosteroids, muscle weakness may progressively worsen if the disease is refractory to therapy or, alternatively, as a result of corticosteroid-induced type 2 muscle fiber atrophy. In these cases, the findings on electromyography are often helpful in distinguishing which factor is contributing to progressive clinical symptoms.

Electromyography has definite limitations in the evaluation of inflammatory myopathies. Early in the course of the disease, the findings on needle examination may be subtle and limited to only a few muscles or a single muscle (Streib et al., 1979). The findings are not pathognomonic for a single disease, and the similar abnormalities in the different inflammatory and infiltrative myopathies indicate the importance of obtaining a muscle biopsy sample to establish a definitive diagnosis. Finally, in patients evaluated late in the course of their disease, a mixed pattern of long-duration and short-duration motor unit potentials may be seen on the needle examination, confounding the distinction between a "myopathic" and a "neuropathic" process.

Nerve conduction studies are usually normal in polymyositis and dermatomyositis. Sensory nerve conduction studies demonstrate normal amplitudes and conduction velocities. Motor nerve conduction studies may demonstrate a mild reduction in the compound muscle action potential amplitudes, reflecting a loss or atrophy of individual muscle fibers from motor units, rather than the loss of complete motor units (Barkhaus et al., 1990)

Needle electromyography is the most sensitive electrodiagnostic technique for the evaluation of muscle disease. In 1953, Buchthal and Pinelli first reported reduction in the motor unit potential duration in polymyositis, and they correlated this finding with the presence of inflammation on muscle biopsy. One year later, Lambert and colleagues (1954) described the characteristic triad of findings on electromyography in 80 patients with polymyositis/dermatomyositis. These features were (1) increased insertional activity, with occasional complex repetitive discharges, (2) fibrillation potentials and positive waves, and (3) short-duration, low-amplitude, polyphasic motor unit potentials with rapid recruitment. These findings have been confirmed by numerous other investigators (Trojaberg, 1966; Bohan et al., 1977; DeVere and Bradley, 1977; Mechler, 1974; Streib et al., 1979).

Insertional-Spontaneous Activity

Needle insertion into normal muscle causes a brief burst of electrical activity, lasting less than 500 ms, due to mechanical irritation of individual muscle fibers. In normal resting muscle, no spontaneous discharges occur outside of the end-plate region. In polymyositis and dermatomyositis, inflammation, segmental muscle fiber necrosis, fiber splitting, and changes in regenerating or newly formed muscle fibers may result in separation of portions of the muscle fiber from the neuromuscular junction and possibly instability of the muscle fiber membrane. These pathological changes and others lead to the production of spontaneously occurring positive waves and fibrillation potentials, owing to "functional" denervation of muscle fibers. In the report of Lambert and colleagues (1954), spontaneous activity in the form of fibrillation potentials was seen in 80% of patients. DeVere and Bradley (1977) found electromyographic abnormalities in 89% of patients with polymyositis, although the frequency of fibrillation potentials was only 45%. The identification of fibrillation potentials is probably related to the number of muscles examined. In a study of 40 patients with polymyositis or dermatomyositis, Streib and associates (1979) examined at least eight muscles in each patient and found electromyographic abnormalities in all patients. Fibrillation potentials were most common in the paraspinal muscles (93%). In rare cases, electromyographic findings may be limited to the paraspinal muscles, indicating that in all patients with a suspected inflammatory myopathy who are referred for electrodiagnostic testing, paraspinal muscles should be examined unless there are specific contraindications (Bohan et al., 1977; Albers et al., 1979; Streib et al., 1979; Mitz et al., 1981). The abundance of fibrillation potentials has been shown to correlate inversely with muscle strength and directly with serum creatine kinase elevation, thereby reflecting the extent of the underlying pathological process (Sandstedt et al., 1982). Furthermore, in treated patients, the degree and frequency of fibrillation potentials decrease in up to 40%, reflecting response to therapy (Mechler, 1974; Bohan et al., 1977). In addition to fibrillation potentials, complex repetitive discharges occur in up to 38% of patients, and myotonic discharges may also be identified (Bohan et al., 1977).

Voluntary Motor Unit Potentials

In polymyositis, changes in motor unit potential duration, amplitude, and complexity are the result of complex and changing pathological alterations, including the patchy loss of individual muscle fibers from motor units, and the variation in muscle fiber diameter in split fibers, regenerating muscle fibers, and muscle fibers formed from myotubes, as well as reinnervation of muscle fibers separated from the nerve terminal. In addition, there are changes in connective tissue and changes due to the inflammatory process. There is little evidence to support the idea that some of the pathological changes are due to nerve damage as a result of the inflammation. These pathological changes are reflected on concentric or monopolar needle examination during voluntary activation of the muscle.

The characteristic motor unit potential morphological changes in dermatomyositis and polymyositis are a decrease in duration and amplitude and an increase in the number of phases and turns (Lambert et al., 1954; Bohan et al., 1977; Partanan, 1982). The recruitment pattern of motor unit potentials is abnormally rapid, as an increased number of motor unit potentials are activated relative to the force of muscle contraction. The mean duration of motor unit potentials has been shown to be reduced to nearly 35% of normal (Buchthal and Pinelli, 1953; Lambert et al., 1954). Buchthal and Pinelli (1953) found a correlation between the decrease in mean action potential duration and the presence of inflammation on muscle biopsy. Early studies suggested that a reduction in the number of muscle fibers in a motor unit decreased the duration and amplitude of the motor unit potentials (Kugelberg, 1947). Buchthal and Pinelli expanded on this theory and suggested that it was the *random* loss of muscle fibers that produced asynchrony of firing of individual motor unit potentials, thereby reducing the amplitude and duration and increasing the complexity of the potentials. The degree and distribution of short-duration, low-amplitude, polyphasic motor unit potentials vary and often follow the distribution of fibrillation potentials.

The motor unit potential abnormalities depend on the stage of the disease during which the muscle is examined (Mechler, 1974; Trojaberg, 1981; Partanan, 1982; Sandstedt et al., 1982; Uncini et al., 1990). In the early, or acute, stage, the changes noted earlier are most commonly seen, although in the review by Bohan and colleagues (1977), 10% of patients had completely normal findings on electromyographic examination. In the chronic stage of the disease, motor unit remodeling from muscle fiber splitting or segmental degeneration of individual muscle fibers, followed by reinnervation of regenerating muscle fibers by the same or different motoneuron, may lead to normalization of the motor unit potential duration or an even abnormally increased duration of motor unit potentials (Mechler, 1974; Trojaberg, 1981; Partanen and Lang, 1982; Uncini et al., 1990). Mechler (1974) noted an increased duration of motor unit potentials in 50% of patients in the chronic, treated phase of the disease. Although these findings have led to speculation that a superimposed "neuropathic" process was present, single-fiber electromyographic studies demonstrating increased fiber density and a varying degree of abnormal increased jitter and blocking have suggested that a change in the terminal innervation pattern of muscle fibers due to segmental degeneration and fiber splitting of individual muscle fibers and reinnervation by the same or adjacent motor neuron underlies these findings (Henriksson, 1978).

Since the early reports of electromyographic findings in polymyositis-dermatomyositis, most electrophysiological research has been directed toward quantitative electromyographic techniques, which are more useful in reliably detecting subtle changes early in the course of the disease, as well as in serially and objectively quantifying change and response to treatment (Barkhaus et al., 1990; Trojaberg, 1990; Uncini et al., 1990). Using quantitative electromyographic studies in the biceps brachii, Barkhaus and associates (1990) found abnormalities in 92% of patients and noted that interference pattern analysis was more sensitive than motor unit action potential analysis in demonstrating abnormalities.

Treatment

Dermatomyositis and polymyositis are potentially treatable diseases, and most patients have a favorable response to treatment. Several reviews of the treatment of inflammatory myopathies have described various regimens that used corticosteroids and other immunosuppressant medications (Dalakas, 1994; Villalba and Adams, 1996; Mastalgia et al., 1997). The initial treatment typically begins with corticosteroids at 1 mg/kg per day, with up to 80% of patients demonstrating a complete response. Slow tapering of steroid dosage may begin after normalization of the serum creatine kinase or after a fixed period (e.g., 6 weeks) at the initial dosage (Dalakas, 1994). Alternate-day dosing may be helpful in reducing side effects. One challenging dilemma in patients with inflammatory myopathies who are receiving corticosteroid treatment is the distinction between disease relapse and the development of "steroid-induced myopathy." Electromyography is often useful in distinguishing between the two; both situations may be represented by short-duration, low-amplitude motor unit potentials with voluntary activation, but the absence of fibrillation potentials is more indicative of "steroid myopathy" than of disease relapse. In patients demonstrating prominent abnormal spontaneous activity and fibrillation potentials on needle electromyography, relapse of the inflammatory myopathy must be considered.

In patients whose disease is refractory to corticosteroids, who develop significant steroid-induced side effects, who experience multiple relapses, or in whom the disease is severe and rapidly progressive, alternative immunosuppressant medications are warranted. A controlled study that compared azathioprine and prednisone with prednisone alone revealed no added benefit of azathioprine (Bunch et al., 1980). However, in association with methotrexate, azathioprine has been shown to be of more benefit than methotrexate and leucovorin (Villalba et al., 1995). Methotrexate is also a commonly used second-line agent in inflammatory myopathies and has proved to be of benefit in patients who do not respond to prednisone (Newman and Scott, 1995; Villalba et al., 1996; Villalba and Adams, 1996). Other agents that may be effective include cyclosporine, cyclophosphamide, and chlorambucil (Mastalgia et al., 1998).

In a double-blind randomized, controlled trial of patients administered intravenous immune globulin (1 g/kg per day for 2 days) every 24 days for 3 months, significant but transient improvement was seen clinically and histologically (Dalakas et al., 1993). In these patients, a marked improvement in muscle histology was also noted on serial muscle biopsies. Other prospective, open-labeled trials have demonstrated benefit of intravenous immune globulin as add-on therapy to other immunosuppressants (Mastalgia et al., 1998). Plasmapheresis has also been studied in a randomized controlled trial (Miller et al., 1992), but no significant improvement was seen in patients receiving plasmapheresis compared with those who were administered sham exchange. A non–placebo-controlled study of plasma exchange suggested that 54% of patients with inflammatory myopathies improved, with the best improvement seen in patients with more acute disease (Cherin et al., 1995).

Even with immunosuppressant medications, up to 60% of patients will experience at least one relapse, and between 30% and 60% will have multiple relapses (Phillips et al., 1998). More than half of the relapses occur in within the first 2 years after the diagnosis, and the relapse may occur any time during the course of treatment, including during the initial phase, maintenance phase, or tapering phase. Although the majority of patients respond to treatment, dermatomyositis and polymyositis remain serious disorders, with an overall increased mortality rate. In an early series, DeVere and Bradley (1977) identified an overall mortality rate of 28%, with a higher mortality rate in patients presenting in their 40s through 50s. Compared with the death rate in the general population of the same community, there was a four-fold increase in the death rate in patients with polymyositis. In 69 patients followed for a mean of 11 years, Maugears and associates (1996) found a mortality rate of 43%. As expected, the survival rates decreased from time from diagnosis, with rates of 83% at year 1, 74% at year 2, 67% at year 5, and 55% at year 9. Factors associated with an overall poor prognosis include older age at presentation, the presence of dysphagia, and interstitial fibrosis.

INCLUSION BODY MYOSITIS

In 1967, Chou first described a 66-year-old man with "chronic polymyositis" and histopathological features of nuclear and cytoplasmic inclusions and rimmed vacuoles on muscle biopsy. Four years later, Yunis and Samaha coined the term *inclusion body myositis* after reviewing the cases of several patients with similar histopathological findings. Since then, numerous reports of inclusion body myositis have established this as a distinct clinicopathological entity (Carpenter et al., 1978; Danon et al., 1982; Ringel et al., 1987; Lotz et al., 1989; Sayers et al., 1992; Amato et al., 1996; Oldfors and Lindberg, 1999). Inclusion body myositis is a progressive, acquired inflammatory myopathy of unknown cause that differs from polymyositis and dermatomyositis in the clinical manifestations, electrodiagnostic features, pathology, and response to treatment (Table 77–2). In a review of muscle biopsy samples during a 10-year period at a single institution, Carpenter and colleagues (1978) identified pathological findings consistent with inclusion body myositis in 2%. How-

---

Table 77–2. Characteristics of Inclusion Body Myositis

Clinical features
  Predominance in men older than 50 years
  Slowly progressive weakness
  Distal and proximal weakness with predilection for forearm and quadriceps muscles
  Dysphagia
  Normal or mildly elevated serum creatine kinase
  Refractory to treatment with immunosuppressant agents
Pathological features
  Endomysial inflammation
  Rimmed vacuoles in muscle fibers
  Filamentous cytoplasmic and nuclear inclusions 15 to 18 nm in diameter
  Intracellular amyloid deposition

---

ever, as the features of this disorder have become increasingly recognized, inclusion body myositis has become a more commonly identified inflammatory myopathy in adults, accounting for 15% to 28% of all inflammatory myopathies, and it is widely believed to be the most common inflammatory myopathy in patients older than 59 (Carpenter et al., 1978; Lotz et al., 1989). In a large, retrospective study of 48 patients with biopsy-confirmed inclusion body myositis, Lotz and associates (1989) found a male-to-female ratio of 3:1 and a mean age at onset of symptoms of 56 years, with only 17% of patients presenting before the age of 50. Several other studies have confirmed a male predominance and a mean age at onset in the 50s to 60s (Ringel et al., 1987; Sayers et al., 1992; Amato et al., 1996).

Clinical Manifestations

The most common presenting symptom in inclusion body myositis is slowly progressive, painless muscle weakness, which clinically may resemble that of polymyositis (Calabrese et al., 1987; Lotz et al., 1989). The distribution of weakness is variable, and the arms or legs may be involved, in isolation or in combination. In many cases, proximal muscle involvement is more prominent than is distal involvement (Danon et al., 1982; Calabrese et al., 1987). In the series of Lotz and colleagues (1989), 75% of patients presented with symptoms in the legs only, and proximal leg muscles were more commonly involved than were distal muscles. However, numerous reports have demonstrated that distal weakness is common, may be asymmetrical, and in some patients may be more severe than proximal weakness, a feature that may be helpful in distinguishing inclusion body myositis from polymyositis (Carpenter et al., 1978; Danon et al., 1982; Eisen et al., 1983; Ringel et al., 1987; Lotz et al., 1989; Sayers et al., 1992; Soueidan and Dalakas, 1993; Amato et al., 1996). The most commonly affected muscles that were reported included the biceps, triceps, iliopsoas, quadriceps, and tibialis anterior. However, a finding that some believe is almost pathognomonic for inclusion body myositis is preferential involvement of finger and wrist flexors, knee extensors, and ankle dorsiflexors (Amato et al., 1996; Oldfors and Lindberg, 1999). Furthermore, more severe weakness in the volar forearm muscles compared with the shoulder abductors and in the quadriceps compared with the hip flexors is seen in up to 73% of patients (Amato et al., 1996). In fact, magnetic resonance imaging may aid in the diagnosis of inclusion body myositis by detecting selective atrophy and fibrosis of the forearm muscles (Sekul et al., 1997). Dysphagia due to upper esophageal dysfunction is variable but may be a prominent and presenting symptom, occurring in 40% to 80% of patients (Ringel et al., 1987; Wintzen et al., 1988; Lotz et al., 1989; Sayers et al., 1992; Brannagan et al., 1997; Houser et al., 1998). Severe progressive dysphagia indicates a poor prognosis and in some cases has prompted treatment with cricopharyngeal myotomy. In these cases, the pathological findings of inclusion body myositis have been identified in the omohyoid and cricopharyngeus muscles (Danon and Friedman, 1989; Verma et al., 1991; Houser et al., 1998). In addition, weakness of facial muscles may occur in up to 40% of patients (Brannagan et al., 1997). Sensory symptoms are absent, although some patients have an underlying peripheral neuropathy.

Laboratory and Histopathological Features

The clinical features of inclusion body myositis may differ from those of other inflammatory myopathies but are not pathognomonic. The similarity of symptoms and examination findings to those of dermatomyositis and polymyositis in many patients and the absence of serological markers indicate the necessity of establishing the diagnosis on the basis of morphological changes in the muscle (Carpenter et al., 1978; Lotz et al., 1989). Serum creatine kinase levels are normal or mildly elevated in 80% of patients with inclusion body myositis but rarely are more than 10 times that of normal. The erythrocyte sedimentation rate is mildly elevated in only 18% of patients. In patients with sporadic inclusion body myositis, 13% have been found to have another immune-mediated condition, and 20% have positive autoantibody markers, such as antinuclear antibodies, rheumatoid factor, or anti-SSA antibodies (Leff et al., 1993; Koffman et al., 1998). In addition, 23% of patients have an associated monoclonal gammopathy, without evidence of systemic amyloidosis or myeloma (Dalakas et al., 1997a). Anti-Jo antibodies, which are commonly identified in dermatomyositis, have been found in only 2% of patients with inclusion body myositis (Koffman et al., 1998). Systemic malignancies have been identified in up to 15% of patients, but in only 5% were the malignancies temporally associated with inclusion body myositis.

Histological criteria for probable inclusion body myositis on muscle biopsy have been established (Lotz et al., 1989; Amato et al., 1994) and include (1)

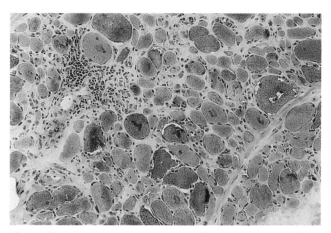

Figure 77–3. Inclusion body myositis. Numerous muscle fibers harbor small vacuoles; other fibers display altered myofibrillar markings. Also note endomysial fibrosis and perivascular and endomysial inflammatory cells (trichrome stain, ×190). (Courtesy of A. G. Engel.)

rimmed vacuoles within muscle fibers, (2) endomysial inflammatory infiltrate with invasion of nonnecrotic fibers, and (3) 15- to 18-nm nonbranching tubulofilamentous inclusions in the cytoplasm or nuclei on electron microscopy, or evidence of amyloid deposition in muscle fibers (Figs. 77–3 and 77–4). When these criteria are met, the predictive value for the diagnosis of inclusion body myositis is greater than 93% (Lotz et al., 1989). Inflammatory cell infiltration is a hallmark of inclusion body myositis, and the cells are predominantly CD8$^+$ T cells and macrophages. The nature of the rimmed vacuoles has been further elucidated. Paired helical filaments consisting of 15- to 21-nm tubulofilaments containing phosphorylated tau protein have been identified within the vacuoles (Askansas et al., 1994). Other findings of presenilin 1 and β-amyloid precursor protein have suggested that inclusion body myositis is a "degenerative" muscle disease, similar to Alzheimer's disease. Deposition of β-amyloid pro-

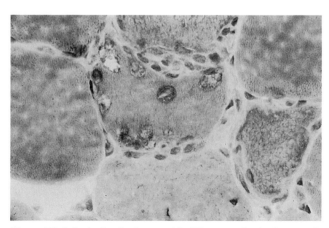

Figure 77–4. Inclusion body myositis. The vacuoles in the muscle fiber are rimmed by membranous material. The fiber is surrounded by inflammatory cells (trichrome stain, ×750). (Courtesy of A. G. Engel.)

tein, localized to 6- to 10-nm filaments, and ubiquitin and hyperphosphorylated tau protein, localized to cytoplasmic tubulofilaments within the vacuoles, has been identified (Askansas et al., 1994).

The pathogenesis of inclusion body myositis remains unknown, but the roles of the inflammatory response and the presence of amyloid in muscle fibers have been questioned. Serial muscle biopsies in eight patients with inclusion body myositis who were treated with corticosteroids demonstrated reduction in the serum creatine kinase level and a decline in the mononuclear inflammatory response, yet all patients continued to worsen clinically (Barohn et al., 1995). Furthermore, an increase in the number of vacuolated muscle fibers and the number of amyloid-positive fibers suggested that the inflammatory response is not the immediate cause of the clinical weakness and may be a secondary reaction to the amyloidogenic material (Barohn et al., 1995). However, the absence of inflammatory infiltrate within amyloid-containing muscle fibers argues against this. The role of autoimmunity has been suggested in response to the high incidence of concomitant immune-mediated disorders in inclusion body myositis, as well as the strong association of the human leukocyte antigen DR3 haplotype with inclusion body myositis (Koffman et al., 1998).

The hereditary inclusion body myopathies compose a clinically and pathogenetically distinct group of disorders that differ from sporadic inclusion body myositis by age at presentation, distribution of weakness, histopathological findings, and genetic predisposition (Askansas and Engel, 1995; Amato et al., 1996). Hereditary inclusion body myopathies consist of autosomal recessive and dominant forms. The onset is usually in the second to third decade, rather than the later onset of sporadic inclusion body myositis. Proximal or distal weakness occurs, although there is relative sparing of the quadriceps muscles. Muscle biopsy samples demonstrate rimmed vacuoles and congophilic amyloid material with 15- to 18-nm tubulofilaments, similar to sporadic inclusion body myositis; however, endomysial inflammation is characteristically absent in the hereditary forms. Linkage to chromosome 9p1-q1 has been identified in some families (Mitrani-Rosenbaum et al., 1996). Electromyographic findings in hereditary inclusion body myopathies do not appear to differ from the findings in sporadic inclusion body myositis. Nerve conduction studies are often normal; needle electromyography demonstrates fibrillation potentials and mixed short-duration, low-amplitude and long-duration, high-amplitude motor unit potentials (Massa et al., 1991; Neville et al., 1992; Argov et al., 1998).

Electromyography in Inclusion Body Myositis

Electromyography is useful in patients with suspected inclusion body myositis, not only to assist in confirming an underlying myopathy but also to exclude other disorders such as spinal muscular

atrophy or chronic inflammatory polyradiculoneuropathy, which may resemble inclusion body myositis clinically. Electromyographic features in inclusion body myositis are similar to those of other myopathies with several exceptions. Nerve conduction studies are usually normal, although mild abnormalities suggesting a peripheral neuropathy or mononeuropathy are seen in 10% to 33% of patients (Calabrese et al., 1987; Lotz et al., 1989; Joy et al., 1990; Brannagan et al., 1997; Barkaus, 1999). The finding of slowed motor and sensory conduction velocities with low amplitudes has raised the possibility of a "neurogenic" component to inclusion body myositis (Eisen et al., 1983). However, given the predilection of the disease to affect distal muscles, the destruction of individual muscle fibers within multiple motor units could lead to a reduction in the compound muscle action potential amplitude. The findings in the patients with inclusion body myositis—the lack of sural and superficial peroneal sensory responses—may not differ from those in normal elderly patients, in whom these sensory responses are often absent.

The characteristic findings on needle examination include (1) increased insertional activity with fibrillation potentials and positive sharp waves, (2) short-duration, low-amplitude, polyphasic motor unit potentials, and (3) a variable number of long-duration, high-amplitude motor unit potentials. Abnormal spontaneous activity, including fibrillation potentials and positive sharp waves, occurs in 93% to 100% of patients (Lotz et al., 1989; Joy et al., 1990; Brannagan et al., 1997). Complex repetitive discharges and occasional myotonic discharges may also be seen (Eisen et al., 1983; Brannagan et al., 1997; Johannes et al., 1998).

Voluntary activation of the muscle demonstrates short-duration, low-amplitude, polyphasic motor unit potentials with rapid recruitment in 77% of muscles, consistent with a myopathic process. However, a distinctive but nonspecific feature of inclusion body myositis is the presence of long-duration, high-amplitude motor unit potentials (Eisen et al., 1983; Dimitru and Newell-Eggert, 1990; Joy et al., 1990; Sayers et al., 1992). In a study of 30 patients with biopsy-proven inclusion body myositis, semiquantitative electromyography revealed a mixed pattern of short- and long-duration motor unit potentials, often occurring within the same muscle in 37% of patients, and other studies have reported this finding in up to 75% of patients (Eisen et al., 1983; Joy et al., 1990). The presence of long-duration motor unit potentials has led to the argument that a concomitant neurogenic process is occurring. However, electrophysiological studies in a group of 17 patients with inclusion body myositis, using a variety of quantitative electromyographic techniques including concentric needle quantitative electromyography, interference pattern analysis, and evaluation of fiber density, failed to find evidence for a neurogenic process (Barkhaus et al., 1999). In this study, all patients demonstrated reduction in the duration or amplitude on concentric needle quantitative electromyography of the biceps muscle, fiber density was normal or borderline increased, and interference pattern analysis demonstrated a full baseline with low amplitude, suggestive of a myopathic process. In other studies, single-fiber electromyography demonstrated an increase in fiber density and jitter, which probably represents reinnervation of newly regenerated muscle fibers by collateral sprouting rather than a primary neurogenic process (Eisen et al., 1983; Dimitru and Newell-Eggert, 1990). It is most likely that the mixed short- and long-duration motor unit potentials reflect the chronicity of the disease rather than an associated neurogenic etiology, because similar findings are seen late in the course of polymyositis (Mechler, 1974; Lotz et al., 1989) and in muscular dystrophies.

Treatment

The successful treatment of inclusion body myositis has remained elusive. Most patients have a slowly progressive and relentless course over years, and the majority are resistant to immunosuppressant medication (Danon and Friedman, 1989; Lotz et al., 1989; Amato et al., 1996). Treatment with corticosteroids has not been demonstrated to be of clinically significant benefit in randomized controlled trials, although in individual patients, a reduction in the creatine kinase level and temporary stabilization or improvement have been reported (Lane et al., 1985; Cohen et al., 1989; Barohn et al., 1995; Levin et al., 1996). A combination of azathioprine and methotrexate demonstrated stabilization of the disease in 63% of patients in a randomized crossover trial with methotrexate and leucovorin, although significant limitations in the study design preclude any firm conclusions (Leff et al., 1993). A small study of four patients treated with intravenous immunoglobulin showed temporary improvement or normalization of muscle strength for 2 to 4 months in three patients (Soueidan and Dalakas, 1993). However, subsequent randomized controlled and open-label noncontrolled trials did not demonstrate significant sustained benefit (Amato et al., 1994; Dalakas et al., 1997b). In one patient, treatment with chlorambucil led to improvement and stabilization of the disease when other immunosuppressants failed, although no long-term trials have been performed to date (Jongen et al., 1995). Other treatments that have been evaluated but have not demonstrated overall benefit include leukocytapheresis and total body irradiation (Kelly et al., 1986; Dau, 1987). The disease invariably progresses and may lead to eventual incapacitation, many years after the onset of symptoms.

INFLAMMATORY MYOPATHIES ASSOCIATED WITH INFECTIOUS DISEASES
Bacterial Myositis

PYOMYOSITIS

Pyomyositis is a localized infectious myopathy caused by bacterial seeding or infiltration of skeletal muscle. The majority of cases are due to *Staphylococcus aureus,* although infection by streptococci and other bacteria may cause an identical syndrome (Adams et al., 1985). Clinically, patients develop localized pain and swelling of a single muscle; multiple muscles are affected in 12% to 60% of patients (Felice et al., 1991). In rare cases, rapidly progressive generalized weakness occurs. Systemic features, such as fever, leukocytosis, or an elevated sedimentation rate, are common. Examination may identify a firm, nodular muscle on palpation. Serum creatine kinase levels may be normal or elevated. Blood cultures are commonly positive and helpful in identifying the causative organism. Treatment is antibiotic therapy and abscess drainage. The etiology of pyomyositis is unknown; pyomyositis often occurs in otherwise healthy subjects. Bacteremia with hematogenous seeding of the muscle appears to be a likely mechanism, although in consideration of the high frequency of bacteremia and the rarity of pyomyositis, other mechanisms most probably contribute.

TUBERCULOSIS

Muscle involvement is uncommon in *Mycobacterium tuberculosis* infection, with an estimated incidence of 0.015%, but it may be increasing in frequency owing to the reemergence of tuberculosis associated with human immunodeficiency virus (HIV) infection. Muscle involvement may occur in one of three forms: (1) extension into the muscle from a primary focus such as retroperitoneal lymph nodes, (2) intramuscular nodular lesions or abscess ("tuberculous pyomyositis"), or (3) a generalized proximal myopathy similar to that in polymyositis. Patients with tuberculous pyomyositis may present with a single mass or with multiple palpable nontender muscle masses in a single muscle (Kim et al., 1997). Alternatively, patients with a more generalized myopathy typically present with progressive proximal weakness over months to years, muscle tenderness and swelling, and other constitutional symptoms such as fever, weight loss, and night sweats. The myopathy may develop in the context of pulmonary or disseminated tuberculosis in 20% to 50% of cases, or in the absence of extramuscular manifestations (Kim et al., 1997).

The serum creatine kinase is often elevated, and abnormal laboratory studies such as erythrocyte sedimentation rate, anemia, and leukocytosis are common. Tuberculin testing is positive in many patients. Short-duration, low-amplitude, polyphasic motor unit potentials and fibrillation potentials on needle examination have been documented in a few reports of tuberculous myopathy (Huang et al., 1999). Histopathological finding on muscle biopsy may show multiple, interstitial nodules with caseating granulomas; varying degrees of fibrosis; and inflammatory infiltration. Isolation of mycobacteria by culture or polymerase chain reaction assay has been reported (Kim et al., 1997; Huang et al., 1999). Improvement may occur with corticosteroid or pyrazinamide therapy (Kim et al., 1997; Huang et al., 1999).

The cause of muscle disease in patients with tuberculosis is unclear. Direct invasion by mycobacteria from hematological dissemination has been proposed. Alternatively, a primary autoimmune myositis, with or without treatment, may decrease cellular immunity and predispose immunocompromised patients to reactivation or primary infection of tuberculosis as a secondary phenomenon (Huang et al., 1999).

Viral Myositis

ACUTE VIRAL MYOSITIS

Muscle involvement related to viral infections has been described in children and adults and may be associated with many different viruses. Although diffuse myalgia is a common symptom in viral infections, often occurring in association with fever and upper respiratory tract features, acute myositis is an uncommon manifestation. Viral myositis has been most commonly reported in children or adults during influenza A and B epidemics (Middleton et al., 1970; Farrell et al., 1980), but the syndrome has been associated with infection by other viruses, including coxsackieviruses, Epstein-Barr virus, parainfluenza virus, echovirus, cytomegalovirus, herpes simplex virus, and adenovirus (Mastaglia, 1985a).

Clinical Manifestations

Viral myositis typically follows the upper respiratory symptoms of influenza. At 1 to 7 days after the convalescent phase of fever, cough, sore throat, and rhinorrhea begins, severe muscle pain in the calves develops, often after a period of inactivity. The pain may persist for several days before improving, and it may limit the person's ability to walk. It is unclear whether objective weakness occurs in children, because the degree of pain often precludes manual muscle examination. In adults, diffuse or proximal weakness occurs in approximately 50% of patients. Muscles, especially calves, are tender and often swollen. The serum creatine kinase level is markedly elevated, and in severe cases, myoglobinuria occurs.

Electromyographic studies are limited. Findings of low-amplitude, polyphasic motor unit potentials have been identified in a few cases. In two cases with the manifestation of severe myoglobinuria, evidence of severe fiber necrosis has been shown on muscle biopsy (Gamboa et al., 1979).

HUMAN IMMUNODEFICIENCY
VIRUS–ASSOCIATED MYOPATHY

Neuromuscular disorders occur in only 10% to 20% of patients infected with HIV; most commonly, these include a distal axonal polyneuropathy, subacute or chronic demyelinating polyradiculopathy,

and multiple mononeuropathies (Dalakas and Pezeshkpour, 1988). Myopathy associated with HIV infection was first described by Snider and associates in 1983. Since then, several more reports of patients with acquired immunodeficiency syndrome (AIDS) with evidence of myopathies have surfaced (Dalakas et al., 1986; Bailey et al., 1987; Simpson and Bender, 1988). The frequency with which a clinical myopathy occurs in HIV-infected patients is not known, but in a retrospective review of 14 patients with neuromuscular disorders and HIV infection, only 2 experienced a myopathy (Lange et al., 1988). In the largest series reported of 11 patients with HIV-associated myopathy, the mean age at onset of muscular symptoms was 35 years (Simpson and Bender, 1988). The majority of patients have had a history of previous opportunistic infections, constituting the AIDS complex, although 36% were infected with HIV but did not have AIDS. Furthermore, myopathy may be the presenting sign of HIV infection (Dalakas et al., 1986).

Clinical Manifestations

In most patients with HIV-associated myopathy, the predominant symptoms include progressive painless weakness, muscle cramps, and occasionally dysphagia (Simpson and Bender, 1988). Weakness is most prominent in proximal arm and leg muscles, although bulbar weakness may also occur. Several patients have been described with recurrent episodes of myoglobinuria (Lange et al., 1988). Symptoms occur at any stage during the course of HIV infection and may be acute, chronic, or episodic (Bailey et al., 1987; Lange et al., 1988; Masanes et al., 1995). Serum creatine kinase levels may be normal or variably elevated.

Electromyography in HIV-associated myopathy demonstrates variable findings. Nerve conduction studies may be normal but often reveal findings consistent with a superimposed peripheral neuropathy (Bailey et al., 1987; Simpson and Bender, 1988). Needle electromyography demonstrates increased insertional activity with fibrillation potentials in 63% of patients, occasional complex repetitive discharges, and short-duration, low-amplitude, polyphasic motor unit potentials in 90% (Bailey et al., 1987; Simpson and Bender, 1988).

The findings on muscle biopsy are not specific for HIV-associated myopathy and are commonly seen in other inflammatory myopathies. Two patterns have been identified: (1) an inflammatory-type pattern with lymphocytic or macrophage infiltrates and muscle fiber necrosis and (2) muscle fiber necrosis with nemaline bodies, without associated inflammation (Dalakas et al., 1986; Stern et al., 1987; Simpson and Bender, 1988). Studies to detect HIV within muscle tissue have been unable to consistently identify the virus, although monoclonal antibodies to p24 antigen and identification of HIV-like viral particles in the endomysial inflammatory infiltrates using electron microscopy of muscle biopsy specimens have been reported (Dalakas et al., 1986; Stern et al., 1987; Simpson and Bender, 1988; Nordstrom et al., 1989). In the series of Simpson and Bender (1988), 5 of 11 patients were treated with immunosuppressant therapy, and all 5 improved within 2 months. Treatment with intravenous immune globulin in a few patients did not demonstrate any significant improvement (Dalakas et al., 1986). Furthermore, some patients improve spontaneously without treatment, leading to the speculation that HIV-associated myopathy has an autoimmune basis rather than being due to direct viral invasion (Snider et al., 1983; Simpson and Bender, 1988). However, it is not known whether the virus directly invades the muscle and causes a cytopathic effect, or triggers an immune-mediated response. The finding of significantly lower plasma selenium levels in HIV-infected patients with muscle involvement compared with HIV-infected patients matched for age and CD4 status without muscle symptoms has suggested a role of selenium in the development of myopathy (Chariot et al., 1997).

Parasitic Myositis

TRICHINOSIS

Trichinosis is a parasitic infection most commonly acquired through the ingestion of undercooked pork. In many cases, infection by the causative protozoan *Trichinosis spiralis* is largely subclinical. In classic trichinosis, there are three stages of the disease. The first stage occurs in the first week after ingestion of the larvae and is due to liberation of the larvae into the small intestine. Symptoms include a prodrome of anorexia, abdominal cramping, nausea, vomiting, diarrhea, fever, and malaise. The second stage occurs after the organism invades the intestinal lymphatics, spreads hematogenously, and is deposited in skeletal muscle, causing muscular weakness and pain. The third stage is the convalescent stage, which begins 5 to 6 weeks after ingestion.

Myopathy due to trichinosis was first described by Marcus and Miller in 1954 in a 30-year-old man with myalgias, muscle weakness and atrophy, and dysphagia. Electromyography demonstrated "the most profuse fibrillation potentials that one of the authors had ever seen" in all muscles examined. Subsequent case reports or small series have suggested a similar clinical picture but a wide spectrum of electromyographic findings (Wayhonis and Johnson, 1964; Davis et al., 1976; Gross and Ochoa, 1979). In most patients, fever and myalgias occur coincident with proximal more often than distal muscle weakness. Several patients have been reported with dysphagia and difficulty in opening the mouth (Marcus and Miller et al., 1954; Wayhonis and Johnson, 1964). Two patients with diplopia from extraocular muscle involvement have also been described (Wayhonis and Johnson, 1964; Davis et al., 1976). Laboratory studies have demonstrated normal or mildly elevated serum creatine kinase levels.

In the few cases in which electromyographic findings have been reported, increased insertional activity with fibrillation potentials and positive waves and short-duration, low-amplitude, polyphasic motor unit potentials were identified (Marcus and Miller et al., 1954; Wayhonis and Johnson, 1964; Gross and Ochoa, 1979). During the convalescent stage, the degree of abnormalities has been shown to diminish (Marcus and Miller et al., 1954; Wayhonis and Johnson, 1964). Muscle biopsy demonstrates perivascular mononuclear and eosinophilic inflammatory infiltration, necrotic fibers, and, in some cases, enlarged fibers containing the nematode larvae (Gross and Ochoa, 1979).

TOXOPLASMOSIS

Toxoplasmosis is a parasitic infection that occurs after ingestion of the cyst or mature oocyte of the protozoan *Toxoplasma gondii*. This protozoan is found in domestic and wild animals, and the cat is the definitive host. Exposure to the protozoan occurs in up to 50% of the general population, and infection is usually subclinical. The most common clinical manifestation is a self-limited syndrome of lymphadenopathy, malaise, fever, and rash. Once ingested, the cyst or oocyte invades the intestine and spreads hematogenously to different organs, forming cysts in the brain, heart, and skeletal muscles.

The incidence of myopathy after *Toxoplasma* infection is unknown, and only rare individual cases have been reported. Patients of all ages, from childhood through adulthood, have been affected. The clinical symptoms include constitutional symptoms such as malaise, fever, and myalgias that last weeks to months. Symmetrical weakness develops in proximal more often than in distal muscles. Patients have been reported with cutaneous manifestations, including periorbital edema, violaceous malar rash, and a scaly erythematous rash over the dorsal aspect of the hands, elbows, and knees (Hendrickx et al., 1979; Topi et al., 1979; Behan et al., 1983). Serum creatine kinase levels may be normal or elevated. The similarity of presentation to dermatomyositis and polymyositis has led to the speculation of a causal relationship between toxoplasmosis and polymyositis-dermatomyositis (Rowland and Breer, 1961; Chandar et al., 1968; Krick and Remington, 1978; Hendrickx et al., 1979; Behan et al., 1983; Cuturic et al., 1997). However, whether toxoplasmosis causes an inflammatory myopathy similar to dermatomyositis or whether an immunosuppressed state in the idiopathic inflammatory myopathies makes patients more susceptible to opportunistic infections remains unclear. Treatment with antiprotozoal therapy has been advocated, and improvement has been reported in isolated cases (Cuturic et al., 1997).

Electromyographic findings in myopathy related to toxoplasmosis are limited to individual case reports and are nonspecific. Increased insertional activity and fibrillation potentials may be present or absent, and short-duration, polyphasic motor unit potentials are common (Samuels and Rietschel, 1976). The diagnosis is made through identification of elevated *Toxoplasma* titers in the serum.

Treatment with pyrimethamine and sulfadiazine leads to resolution of the symptoms.

Myositis is also seen in association with other rare infections, such as disseminated candidiasis, cryptococcosis, *Mycobacterium avium-intracellulare* infection, *Clostridium welchii* infection, Legionnaires' disease, Lyme disease, syphilis, Whipple's disease, leptospirosis, and leprosy. A more detailed discussion of these entities is beyond the scope of this chapter (Banker, 1994).

INFILTRATIVE MYOPATHIES

Amyloid Myopathy

Primary systemic amyloidosis is a disorder of abnormal production of immunoglobulin light chains, producing amyloid fibrils, which infiltrate cardiac, renal, or other organ systems throughout the body. Amyloid myopathy is an uncommon manifestation of primary systemic amyloidosis. In a retrospective review of patients with a diagnosis of systemic amyloidosis at the Mayo Clinic, Gertz and Kyle (1996) identified biopsy-proven amyloid myopathy in 12 of 1,596 patients (0.8%). Similarly, in a review of 3,937 muscle biopsy specimens during a 17-year period at the Cleveland Clinic, 16 cases (0.4%) of amyloid myopathy were identified (Prayson, 1998). However, the recognition of amyloid myopathy has become more frequent with the routine use of Congo red staining of muscle biopsy samples (Spuler et al., 1998).

CLINICAL MANIFESTATIONS

Patients with amyloid myopathy present with proximal more often than distal weakness, pseudohypertrophy, dysphagia, and macroglossia (Prayson, 1998; Spuler et al., 1998; Rubin and Hermann, 1999). Muscle pain occurs in approximately 50% of patients. Enlarged or palpable nodules have been classically described, although studies have identified this finding in less than 25% of patients (Gertz and Kyle, 1996; Spuler et al., 1998; Rubin and Hermann, 1999). A less common manifestation is respiratory failure due to diaphragm involvement (Streeten et al., 1986; Santiago et al., 1987; Ashe et al., 1992). Most patients have been previously diagnosed with systemic amyloidosis and experience multiple organ system complications before the development of muscle weakness, although myopathy may be the presenting feature of amyloidosis (Gertz and Kyle, 1996). Laboratory testing demonstrated a monoclonal gammopathy in the urine or serum in all of the patients in the series of Gertz and Kyle (1996), and bone marrow biopsy reveals evidence of amyloidosis in most patients. Serum creatine kinase lev-

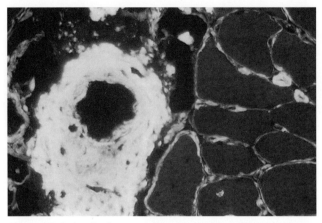

Figure 77–5. Amyloidosis involving skeletal muscles. Heavy amyloid deposits appear in the walls, around the larger blood vessel, and around capillaries. A number of muscle fibers are surrounded by amyloid deposits (Congo red stain viewed under fluorescence optics, ×468). (Courtesy of A. G. Engel.)

els may be normal or mildly elevated but are rarely more than 10 times normal (Spuler et al., 1998; Rubin and Hermann, 1999). Muscle biopsy demonstrates congophilic amyloid deposition in the perivascular, perimysial, or endomysial regions of the muscle, with occasional regions of endomysial and perivascular inflammation and necrotic fibers (Prayson, 1998; Spuler et al., 1998) (Fig. 77–5). In one study, concomitant sural nerve biopsy in 7 of 16 patients with amyloid myopathy demonstrated amyloid deposition within the nerve. This finding suggested the frequent coexistence of amyloid peripheral neuropathy and myopathy, although it may simply have reflected selection bias from the presence of neuropathic symptoms in those selected for nerve biopsy (Prayson, 1998).

The mechanism of myopathy in amyloidosis may be related to mechanical interference with myofiber contraction from amyloid infiltration, interference of electromechanical conduction along the sarcolemma, or ischemia of muscle fibers from infiltration of intramuscular vessels.

ELECTROMYOGRAPHIC FINDINGS

Electrodiagnostic studies in amyloid myopathy are limited owing to the rarity of the disorder (Prayson, 1998; Rubin and Hermann, 1999). In a retrospective study of 17 patients with amyloid myopathy, abnormalities on nerve conduction studies were found in 14 patients and most commonly consisted of peroneal or tibial compound muscle action potentials of low amplitude (Rubin and Hermann, 1999). Not unexpectedly, in keeping with the underlying disorder, patients may have features on nerve conduction studies of a mild underlying peripheral neuropathy or carpal tunnel syndrome (Prayson, 1998; Rubin and Hermann, 1999). Needle examination demonstrates increased insertional activity and fibrillation potentials in all patients and in 69% of muscles examined (Rubin and Hermann, 1999).

These most frequently occur in paraspinals and the gluteus medius. A personal observation by one of the authors (D.I.R.) consisted of prominent fibrillation potentials and short-duration, polyphasic motor unit potentials in the diaphragm and genioglossus, in addition to proximal limb muscles, in a patient with severe systemic amyloidosis and respiratory insufficiency. Myotonic discharges also may be seen, although rarely. Short-duration, low-amplitude, polyphasic motor unit potentials occur in 72% of muscles and, coincident with the distribution of fibrillation potentials, occur more frequently in paraspinals and proximal muscles.

Sarcoid Myopathy

Sarcoidosis is a multisystem disorder of unknown cause characterized by noncaseating granulomatous infiltration of multiple organs. The most common systemic manifestations include hilar adenopathy, pulmonary infiltrates, skin lesions, and uveiitis. Neurological manifestations occur in 5% of patients with sarcoidosis, may involve the central or peripheral nervous system, and are often the presenting or an isolated feature (Goodson, 1960; Stern et al., 1985). In the peripheral nervous system, sarcoidosis may present as unilateral or bilateral cranial neuropathies, a diffuse polyradiculopathy, or myopathy. The incidence of sarcoid myopathy is unknown, but in a review of 2,985 muscle biopsies during a 12-year period at the Cleveland Clinic, 6 (0.02%) demonstrated granulomatous findings consistent with sarcoidosis (Prayson, 1999). Myopathy in sarcoidosis may present in several forms. The most common involvement of muscle in systemic sarcoidosis is asymptomatic infiltration of noncaseating granulomas within the muscles, which have been identified in 50% to 60% of random muscle biopsy samples from patients without clinical weakness (Wallace et al., 1958; Walton, 1983). Symptomatic muscle involvement is much less common and occurs in approximately 0.5% of patients with sarcoidosis (Zisman et al., 1999). This may take the form of asymptomatic palpable nodules or pseudohypertrophy within the muscle or of an acute or a chronic myopathy characterized by progressive myalgias and weakness, similar to other inflammatory myopathies such as polymyositis (Powell, 1953; Silverstein and Siltzbach, 1969).

CLINICAL MANIFESTATIONS

Sarcoid myopathy occurs in 12% of patients with neurological manifestations of sarcoid and rarely is the presenting feature or symptom that leads to the diagnosis of sarcoidosis (Stern et al., 1985; Robberecht et al., 1995). Patients of any age may be affected, although the mean age at presentation in patients with myopathy is 65 years (Gardner-Thorpe, 1972). Among patients with any neurological manifestation of sarcoidosis, black women are more affected than are males or other races; however, a literature review of 59 patients with nodular sarcoid myopathy found a slight male predominance with a mean age at onset of 35 years (Stern et al., 1985; Zisman et al., 1999). The most common presentation is slowly progressive proximal weakness involving the arms and legs (Gardner-Thorpe, 1972; Callen, 1979; Itoh et al., 1980). Distal weakness may predominate or occur with proximal weakness (Gardner-Thorpe, 1972; Robberecht et al., 1995). Rarely, patients may present with dyspnea due to diaphragmatic weakness or ptosis (Gardner-Thorpe, 1972; Dewberry et al., 1993). Myalgias are common, especially in patients with a more acute course. Patients with nodular sarcoidosis demonstrate multiple palpable nodules in 80% and are most common in the lower extremity muscles (Zisman et al., 1999). Patients have also been reported with skin manifestations similar to those of dermatomyositis (Callen, 1979; Itoh et al., 1980). Serum creatine kinase level varies and may be normal or slightly elevated (Callen, 1979; Dewberry et al., 1993). The diagnosis is established on the basis of muscle biopsy, which demonstrates noncaseating granulomas with multinucleated giant cells within the muscle (Gardner-Thorpe, 1972).

ELECTROMYOGRAPHIC FINDINGS

Electrodiagnostic findings in sarcoid myopathy have been reported only in isolated cases or small series (Brun, 1961; Callen, 1972; Gardner-Thorpe, 1972; Dewberry et al., 1993; Robberecht et al., 1995). In most cases, nerve conduction studies are normal. Needle electromyography demonstrates a variable degree of abnormalities. In some patients, the electromyographic findings are normal, whereas in others, fibrillation potentials and positive sharp waves are seen in resting muscle (Gardner-Thorpe, 1972; Dewberry et al., 1993; Robberecht et al., 1995). Abundant myotonic discharges were reported in a single case (Dewberry et al., 1993). Voluntary activation demonstrates short-duration, low-amplitude, polyphasic motor unit potentials in most cases.

Treatment with corticosteroids produces improvement in the degree of weakness in most patients, although some do not respond. No randomized controlled trials of treatment of sarcoid myopathy have been performed. In a review of the literature up to 1972, Gardner-Thorpe found that 20 of 26 patients with sarcoid myopathy who were treated with corticosteroids had a response to treatment, although objective improvement was reported in only 7 patients.

Carcinomatous Myopathy

Infiltration of skeletal muscle by carcinomatous metastases is an exceedingly rare complication of systemic malignancies, having been reported in patients with undifferentiated squamous cell carcinoma and breast carcinoma (Doshi and Fowler, 1983). Progressive weakness may precede or follow the identification of a malignancy. Discrete metastases have been reported in limb muscles, the diaphragm, and the tongue (Brennan, 1971; Zegarelli et al., 1973; Doshi and Fowler, 1983). In the few patients who have been reported, the serum creatine kinase level was normal. Electromyographic studies were not detailed but demonstrated "myopathic" findings. Muscle histology demonstrated carcinomatous infiltration of the muscle with scattered inflammatory cell infiltrates (Doshi and Fowler, 1983).

A subacute necrotizing myopathy, thought to be a paraneoplastic myopathy, has been rarely reported in association with various malignant tumors (Smith, 1969; Swash, 1974; Brownell and Hughes, 1975; Levin et al., 1998; Rini et al., 1999). In these cases, the myopathy often precedes the diagnosis of cancer. Weakness is a prominent manifestation, is rapidly progressive, and involves almost all voluntary muscles within a matter of weeks, with progression to death in less than 3 months. The creatine kinase level is elevated, and electromyography shows "myopathic" changes. The associated malignancies have included gastrointestinal adenocarcinoma, transitional cell carcinoma, prostatic carcinoma, non–small cell carcinoma, and thymoma. Pathologically, the muscles demonstrate prominent necrosis with little inflammation. Treatment with corticosteroids has resulted in improvement in some cases, and rare cases have demonstrated improvement after removal of the primary tumor.

Other Inflammatory Myopathies

EOSINOPHILIC POLYMYOSITIS

Eosinophilic polymyositis is a muscle disorder that occurs as part of the hypereosinophilic syndrome, presenting as weight loss, fatigue, abdominal pain, fever with night sweats, cough with chest pain, rash, and congestive heart failure (Pickering et al., 1998). The findings are diverse but usually include fever, edema, cardiovascular abnormalities, hepatosplenomegaly, and generalized adenopathy with peripheral blood eosinophilia. The disorder occurs between the ages of 20 and 50 and is much more common in men than in women. The neurological manifestations of hypereosinophilic syndrome most commonly consist of a diffuse encephalopathy, focal central nervous system lesions secondary to cerebral infarctions, and peripheral nerve abnormalities, taking the form of a mononeuropathy multiplex or a more diffuse peripheral neuropathy. Muscle involvement, manifested by weak, painful, swollen, and stiff muscles, is less frequent but may be overlooked in the setting of more severe systemic disease. Blood chemistries in hypereosinophilic syndrome demonstrate a marked eosinophilia, with greater than 1,500 eosinophils/mL, that persists for up to 6 months. In addition, there is an eosinophilic infiltration of organs such as the lungs, heart, skin, and peripheral nerves.

Muscle biopsy in eosinophilic polymyositis shows single-fiber necrosis, regeneration, and infiltration by predominantly eosinophilic inflammatory cells. There may be pronounced perivenular eosinophilic cuffing. The creatine kinase level is usually markedly elevated in patients with muscle involvement. The electromyography in eosinophilic polymyositis demonstrates rapid recruitment of low-amplitude, short-duration polyphasic motor unit potentials with fibrillation potentials. Many patients respond to corticosteroids, but long-term treatment may be required because of relapses when corticosteroids are discontinued. The average survival varies in different series, ranging from 9 months to 5 years (Chusid et al., 1975; Fauci et al., 1982). Cardiac and neurological abnormalities are the usual causes of death. The differential diagnosis of eosinophilic polymyositis includes polyarteritis nodosa, hypersensitivity vasculitis, allergic granulomatosis, rheumatoid arthritis with vasculitis, the eosinophilia-myalgia syndrome, toxic oil syndrome, and parasitic infections (Arness et al., 1999).

DIFFUSE FASCIITIS WITH EOSINOPHILIA

Diffuse fasciitis with eosinophilia, or Schulman's syndrome, is a syndrome of subacute evolution of pain, swelling, and tenderness of the hands, forearms, feet, and legs. This is followed by severe induration of the skin and subcutaneous tissues in these areas. There may be low-grade fever, myalgias, cramps, and arthralgias. Carpal tunnel syndrome occurs not infrequently. Vigorous exertion has frequently preceded the onset of the syndrome (Michet et al., 1981). Schulman's syndrome affects adults of age 30 to 60 and occurs equally in men and women. There is generalized pitting edema that most severely involves the arms and legs and spares the face. There is decreased range of motion of the hands, wrist, elbows, and knees. Muscle weakness is not constant and when found is variable in distribution and may be proximal or distal. Laboratory abnormalities in Schulman's syndrome include eosinophilia in 86% of patients, hypergammaglobulinemia in 74%, elevated sedimentation rate in 56%, and positivity for antinuclear antibodies in 25%. The creatine kinase level is mildly increased or normal. Pathologically, there is thickening of the fascia and infiltration by lymphocytes, plasma cells, and eosinophils. Frequently, the infiltrate extends into the muscle, subcutaneous tissue, and dermis. Muscle biopsy in Schulman's syndrome shows perivascular accumulation of lymphocytes, plasma cells, and eosinophils to a mild to moderate degree. The epimysium adjacent to the affected fascia is frequently sclerotic and inflamed. Focal necrosis and regeneration of muscle cells are found in the minority of patients (Barnes et al., 1979). In one study (Lakhanpal et al., 1988), electromyographic results were abnormal in 73% of the patients who were tested.

Fibrillation potentials and low-amplitude, short-duration, polyphasic motor unit potentials have been reported (De Meirsman and Hens, 1983). The treatment of Schulman's syndrome with corticosteroids usually results in improvement, which may be dramatic. Spontaneous remissions occur in the majority of patients, usually after 4 years of disease. Complications include aplastic anemia, thrombocytopenia, and lymphoma and leukemia.

EOSINOPHILIA-MYALGIA SYNDROME

The eosinophilia-myalgia syndrome, associated with L-tryptophan, was first recognized in 1989; it is characterized by the insidious onset of rash and induration of the skin, fever, fatigue, myalgias, paresthesias of the extremities, arthralgias, and alopecia, with peripheral blood eosinophilia (Hertzman et al., 1990). This syndrome occurs predominantly in middle-aged (mean age of 48 years) women and is caused by exposure to contaminated L-tryptophan. The median dosage of L-tryptophan is 1,500 mg/day. There was a total of 1,300 cases in the United States from the spring of 1989 to February 1990. Laboratory abnormalities in eosinophilia-myalgia syndrome consist of eosinophilia with greater than 1,000 cells/mL, elevated liver enzyme levels, and an elevated sedimentation rate in 33%. Eosinophilia-myalgia syndrome has similarities to eosinophilic fasciitis but is a more severe disease with multisystem involvement. It may become chronic even after the exposure to L-tryptophan ceases. Death is uncommon, but it usually occurs as a result of diffuse peripheral nerve and root involvement, primary pulmonary involvement, or primary cardiac involvement.

In 1981, the ingestion of food oils containing a high proportion of denatured rapeseed oil contaminated with an aniline derivative resulted in an epidemic in Spain called the "toxic oil syndrome" (Kilbourne et al., 1983). The toxic oil syndrome has many similarities to the eosinophilia-myalgia syndrome except for a more abrupt onset, often with pneumonitis with fever, cough, dyspnea, and pulmonary infiltrates. Months later, the patients developed a syndrome very similar to the eosinophilia-myalgia syndrome. Neurologically, the patients developed myopathy, multiple mononeuropathies, symmetrical peripheral neuropathy, polyradiculopathy, and multifocal central nervous system lesions that were either inflammatory or ischemic. The signs vary, depending on whether the disease process presents primarily as fasciitis, myositis, or peripheral neuropathy, or a combination of the three. Muscle involvement is usually manifested by muscle pain and tenderness to palpation, atrophy, and weakness that involves proximal more than distal muscles. The muscle pathology consisted of perimyositis, perivasculitis, and fasciitis. Necrosis of muscle fibers was unusual. There was a microangiopathy with inflammatory infiltrates consisting of plasma cells, lymphocytes, and monocytes with occasional eosinophils. Inflammation and fibrosis of the muscle spindle were promi-

nent pathological findings. The electromyographic findings are variable and may show changes in axonal or demyelinating neuropathy or myopathic changes with fibrillations and short-duration, low-amplitude, polyphasic motor unit potentials. Treatment with corticosteroids resulted in some regression of the cutaneous symptoms and reduction in the amount of eosinophils in the blood, but other manifestations were often unresponsive.

MYOSITIS OF CHRONIC GRAFT-VERSUS-HOST DISEASE

The major complication of transplantation is graft-versus-host disease. Graft-versus-host disease results from recognition by the engrafted donor T cells of recipient HLA antigens or a minor non-HLA transplant antigen as foreign. In most patients, acute graft-versus-host disease precedes the more chronic form of the disease. In the acute phase, the principal involvement is of the immune system, skin, liver, and intestine. In the chronic phase, most patients have skin changes, chronic liver disease, severe mucositis, sicca syndrome, and thrombocytopenia. Muscle is affected in a small percentage of patients in the chronic stage of graft-versus-host disease (Anderson et al., 1982; Nelson and McQuillen, 1988; Ferrara and Deeg, 1991). The muscle involvement follows the bone marrow transplantation by 100 days to 54 months and is heralded by proximal weakness with an elevated creatine kinase level. Pathologically, there is an increase in lymphocytes, histiocytes, plasma cells, and eosinophils in the endomysium and perimysium, with variation in muscle fiber diameter and scattered necrotic and vacuolated muscle fibers. The myositis of chronic graft-versus-host disease may be severe and may respond to corticosteroids, azathioprine, or cyclosporine.

EOSINOPHILIC PERIMYOSITIS

Eosinophilic perimyositis is a rare entity characterized by severe myalgias, bronchial asthma, eosinophilia, and normal muscle strength. The erythrocyte sedimentation rate and the serum creatine kinase level are normal. There usually is no evidence of systemic disease. Electromyography reveals fibrillation potentials and short-duration, low-amplitude, polyphasic motor unit potentials. Muscle biopsy demonstrates an inflammatory infiltrate that contains eosinophils, localized primarily to the perimysium. Treatment with corticosteroids usually results in improvement (Serratrice et al., 1980; Fang et al., 1988; Lakhanpal et al., 1988; Trueb et al., 1995).

MACROPHAGIC MYOFASCIITIS

A new type of inflammatory myopathy, called *macrophagic myofasciitis,* has been described in France (Cherin et al., 1999). Patients with this entity have symptoms of myalgias, arthralgias, asthenia, muscle weakness, and fever. The creatine kinase levels and erythrocyte sedimentation rate are elevated, and the electromyography shows "myopathic" findings. The distinctive feature of the illness is the unique pathological picture with infiltration of the epimysium, perimysium, and perifascicular endomysium by inflammatory cells of the monocyte-macrophage lineage. The illness improves with corticosteroid therapy.

FOCAL MYOSITIS

Focal myositis is an uncommon form of localized inflammatory myopathy in which the clinical and histological features are confined to a single limb or even a single muscle. Some believe that this is a form of polymyositis, and patients ultimately develop more diffuse muscle involvement, although reports of patients with monomelic involvement for decades without spread to other muscles suggest that this may be a separate entity (Stark, 1978). The most common presentation in focal myositis is the development of a localized, painful mass within the muscle, although slowly progressive muscle weakness may also occur. Muscles of the lower extremity are most commonly involved, but disease isolated to the upper limb, abdominal muscles, tongue, or neck extensor muscles has been described (Flaisler et al., 1993; Biran et al., 1999). One patient presented with a radial nerve palsy due to compression of the nerve by a nodule of focal myositis within the muscle (Alzagatiti et al., 1999).

Laboratory studies demonstrate normal or mildly elevated serum creatine kinase levels, and the erythrocyte sedimentation rate may be elevated. Electromyographic findings are variable. In some reports, the electromyogram is normal, even in clinically involved muscles (Marie et al., 1998). Other reports have described prominent abnormalities on needle examination, including fibrillation potentials and short-duration, low-amplitude motor unit potentials in all muscles of the symptomatic limb and milder changes scattered in muscles of other limbs and paraspinals (Ledermen, 1984). Magnetic resonance imaging has also been shown to be sensitive in detecting focal myositis, demonstrating gadolinium enhancement and high T2 signal abnormalities within individual muscles.

The etiology of focal myositis is unknown. In a review of 39 cases of focal myositis, Flaisler and associates (1993) noted that approximately one third of patients eventually develop generalized findings, suggesting that this entity is a predecessor to polymyositis. However, cases in which the disease is isolated to a single limb for many years or indefinitely and patients who demonstrate spontaneous resolution of symptoms without specific therapy suggest that this may be a separate disorder.

PROLIFERATIVE FOCAL MYOSITIS

Proliferative focal myositis, or benign pseudosarcomatous mesenchymal lesion, is a discrete, movable, painless mass within muscle that grows rapidly and is of unknown cause. These lesions occur most commonly in the shoulder, thorax, or thigh. There is no recurrence or extension after excision. Pathologically, there is thickening of epimysium, perimysium, and endomysium with proliferation of fibroblasts and histiocytes. Myocytes, myotubules, and muscle giant cells are present. Differentiation from rhabdomyosarcoma may be difficult.

LOCALIZED MYOSITIS OSSIFICANS

Localized myositis ossificans, or traumatic myositis ossificans, is a swelling in traumatized muscles, usually of the arm or thigh (adductors of the thigh in horse riders and arm muscles in throwers). The tender muscle mass becomes hard, and radiographs reveal bone formation. Pathologically, there is a core of highly cellular, pleomorphic histiocytes and fibroblasts surrounded by compact layers of connective tissue. Well-formed bone is found at the periphery. Treatment consists of excision.

MYOSITIS OSSIFICANS PROGRESSIVA

Myositis ossificans progressiva is a progressive widespread ossification of many muscles over a protracted period of time (Munchmeyer's disease). It is associated with congenital anomalies such as microdactyly of the thumb and great toe, exostoses, broad neck of femur, absence of two upper incisors, hypogenitalism, absence of the lobules of the ear, and deafness. In the first decade of life, subcutaneous masses appear, often around the back of the neck and shoulders. These masses gradually shrink, become bony hard, and may distort posture. Myositis ossificans progressiva involves paravertebral, abdominal, chest wall, and extremity muscles. Radiographs reveal bony masses in the shape of the involved muscles. Most patients are confined to a wheelchair by the age of 30. It is inherited as a dominant trait with variable penetrance. Pathologically, there is hemorrhage, inflammation, and proliferation of collagen in connective tissue, followed by new cartilage and bone formation and infiltration.

References

Adams EM, Gudmundsson S, Yocum DE, et al: Streptococcal myositis. Arch Intern Med 1985;145:1020–1023.

Albers JW, Mitz M, Sulaiman AR, Chang GJ: Spontaneous electrical activity and muscle biopsy abnormalities in polymyositis and dermatomyositis. Muscle Nerve 1979;2:503.

Alzagatiti BI, Bertorini TE, Horner LH, et al: Focal myositis presenting with radial nerve palsy. Muscle Nerve 1999;22:956–959.

Amato AA, Barohn RJ, Jackson CE, et al: Inclusion body myositis: Treatment with intravenous immunoglobulin. Neurology 1994; 44:1516–1518.

Amato AA, Gronseth GS, Jackson CE, et al: Inclusion body myositis: Clinical and pathologic boundaries. Ann Neurol 1996;40: 581–586.

Amato AA, Barohn RJ: Idiopathic inflammatory myopathies. Neurol Clin 1997;15:615–648.

Anderson BA, Young V, Kean WF, et al: Polymyositis and chronic graft versus host disease. Arch Neurol 1982;39:188.

Argov Z, Sadeh M, Eisenberg I, et al: Facial weakness in hereditary inclusion body myopathies. Neurology 1998;50:1925–1926.

Arkin CR, Rothschild BM, Florendo NT, Popoff N: Behçet syndrome with myositis: A case report with pathologic findings. Arthritis Rheum 1980;23:600.

Arness MK, Brown JD, Dubey JP, et al: An outbreak of acute eosinophilic myositis attributed to human sarcocystis parasitism. Am J Trop Med Hygiene 1999;61:548–553.

Ashe J, Borel CO, Hart G, et al: Amyloid myopathy presenting with respiratory failure. J Neurol Neurosurg Psychiatr 1992;55:162–165.

Askansas V, Engel WK, Bilak M, et al: Twisted tubulofilaments of inclusion body myositis resemble paired helical filaments of Alzheimer's brain and contain hyperphosphorylated tau. Am J Pathol 1994;144:177–187.

Askansas V, Engel WK: New advances in the understanding of sporadic inclusion-body myositis and hereditary inclusion-body myopathies. Curr Opin Rheumatol 1995;7:486–496.

Bailey RO, Turok DI, Jaufmann BP, Singh JK: Myositis and acquired immunodeficiency syndrome. Hum Pathol 1987;18:749–751.

Banker BQ, Victor M: Dermatomyositis (systemic angiopathy) of childhood. Medicine 1966;45:261–289.

Banker BQ: Other inflammatory myopathies. In Engel AG, Franzini-Armstrong C (eds): Myology: Basic and Clinical, 2nd ed. New York, McGraw-Hill, 1994; 1438–1460.

Barkhaus PE, Nandedkar SD, Sanders DB: Quantitative EMG in inflammatory myopathies. Muscle Nerve 1990;13:247–253.

Barkhaus PE, Periquet MI, Nandedkar SD: Quantitative electrophysiologic studies in sporadic inclusion body myositis. Muscle Nerve 1999;22:480–487.

Barnes L, Rodnan GP, Medsger TA, Short D: Eosinophilic fasciitis: A pathologic study of 20 cases. Am J Pathol 1979;96:493–517.

Barohn RJ, Amato AA, Sahenk Z, et al: Inclusion body myositis: Explanation for poor response to immunosuppressive therapy. Neurology 1995;45:1302–1304.

Bates D, Stevens JC, Hudgson PH: Polymyositis with involvement of facial and distal musculature. J Neurol Sci 1973;19:105–108.

Behan WMH, Behan PO, Draper IT, Williams H: Does Toxoplasma cause polymyositis? Report of a case of polymyositis associated with toxoplasmosis and a critical review of the literature. Acta Neuropathol 1983;61:246–252.

Bekklund SI, Torbergsen T, Husby G, Mellgren SI: Myopathy and neuropathy in rheumatoid arthritis: A quantitative controlled electromyographic study. J Rheumatol 1999;26:2348–2351.

Benbassat J, Geffel D, Zlotnick A: Epidemiology of polymyositis-dermatomyositis in Israel, 1960. Isr J Med Sci 1980;16:197–200.

Biran I, Cohen O, Diment J, et al: Focal, steroid responsive myositis causing dropped head syndrome. Muscle Nerve 1999;22:769–771.

Blumbergs PC, Byrne E, Kakulas BA: Polymyositis presenting with respiratory failure. J Neurol Sci 1984;65:221–229.

Bohan A, Peter JB: Polymyositis and dermatomyositis. N Engl J Med 1975a;292:344–347.

Bohan A, Peter JB: Polymyositis and dermatomyositis. N Engl J Med 1975b;292:403–407.

Bohan A, Peter JB, Bowman RL, Pearson CM: A computer assisted analysis of 153 patients with polymyositis and dermatomyositis. Medicine 1977;56:255–286.

Bondeson J, Veress B, Lindroth Y, Lindgren S: Polymyositis associated with asymptomatic primary biliary cirrhosis. Clin Exp Rheumatol 1998;16:172–174.

Brannagan TH, Hays AP, Lange DJ, Trojaborg W: The role of quantitative electromyography in inclusion body myositis. J Neurol Neurosurg Psychiatr 1997;63:776–779.

Brennan JL: Metastatic tumours of the diaphragm. Br J Surg 1971;58:458–460.

Brownell B, Hughes JT: Degeneration of muscle in association with carcinoma of the bronchus. J Neurol Neurosurg Psychiatr 1975;38:363.

Brun A: Chronic polymyositis on the basis of sarcoidosis. Acta Psychiatr Neurol Scand 1961;36:515–523.

Buchthal F, Pinelli P: Muscle action potentials in polymyositis. Neurology 1953;3:424–436.

Bunch TW, Worthington JW, Combs JJ, et al: Azathioprine with prednisone for polymyositis: A controlled, clinical trial. Ann Intern Med 1980;92:365–369.

Bunch TW: Polymyositis: A case history approach to the differential diagnosis and treatment. Mayo Clin Proc 1990;65:1480–1497.

Calabrese LH, Mitsumoto H, Chou SM: Inclusion body myositis presenting as treatment-resistant polymyositis. Arthritis Rheum 1987;30:397–403.

Callen JP: Sarcoidosis appearing initially as polymyositis. Arch Dermatol 1979;115:1336–1337.

Callen JP: Malignancy in polymyositis/dermatomyositis. Clin Dermatol 1988;6:55–63.

Callen JP: Relationship of cancer to inflammatory muscle diseases: Dermatomyositis, polymyositis, and inclusion body myositis. Rheum Dis Clin North Am 1994;20:943–953.

Callen JP: Dermatomyositis. Lancet 2000;355:53–57.

Caproni M, Salvatore E, Bernacchi E, Fabgri P: Amyotrophic dermatomyositis: Report of three cases. Br J Dermatol 1998;139:1116–1118.

Carpenter S, Karpati G, Heller, Eisen A: Inclusion body myositis: A distinct variety of idiopathic inflammatory myopathy. Neurology 1978;28:8–17.

Chandar K, Mair HJ, Mair NS: Case of toxoplasma polymyositis. Br Med J 1968;1:158–159.

Chariot P, Dubreuil-Lemaire ML, Zhou JY, et al: Muscle involvement in human immunodeficiency virus–infected patients is associated with marked selenium deficiency. Muscle Nerve 1997;20:386–389.

Cherin P, Auperin I, Bussel A, et al: Plasma exchange in polymyositis and dermatomyositis: A multicenter study of 57 cases. Clin Exp Rheumatol 1995;13:270–271.

Cherin P, Laforet P, Gherardi RK, et al: Macrophagic myofasciitis: Description and etiopathogenic hypotheses. Rev Med Interne 1999;20:483–489.

Chou SM: Myxovirus-like structures in a case of human chronic polymyositis. Science 1967;158:1453–1455.

Chow W, Gridley G, Mellemkjaer L, et al: Cancer risk following polymyositis and dermatomyositis: A nationwide cohort study in Denmark. Cancer Causes Control 1995;6:9–13.

Chusid MJ, Dale DC, West BC, Wolff SM: The hypereosinophilic syndrome: Analysis of fourteen cases with review of the literature. Medicine 1975;54:1–27.

Clements PJ, Furst DE, Campion DS, et al: Muscle disease in progressive systemic sclerosis. Arthritis Rheum 1978;21:62–71.

Cohen MR, Sulaiman AR, Garancis JC, Wortmann RL: Clinical heterogeneity and treatment response in inclusion body myositis. Arthritis Rheum 1989;32:734–740.

Cronin ME, Plotz PH: Idiopathic inflammatory myopathies. Rheum Dis Clin North Am 1990;16:655–665.

Crowe WE, Bowe KE, Levinson JE: Clinical and pathogenic implications of histopathology in childhood polydermatomyositis. Arthritis Rheum 1982;25:126.

Cui G, Sugai S, Ogawa Y, et al: (Long-term follow-up of 43 patients with Sjogren's syndrome.) Ryumachi 1997;37:770–780.

Cuturic M, Hayat GR, Vogler CA, Velasques A: Toxoplasmic polymyositis revisited: Case report and review of literature. Neuromusc Dis 1997;7:390–396.

Dalakas MC, Pezeshkpour GH, Gravell M, Sever JL: Polymyositis associated with AIDS retrovirus. JAMA 1986;256:2381–2383.

Dalakas MC, Pezeshkpour GH: Neuromuscular diseases associated with human immunodeficiency virus infection. Ann Neurol 1988;23(suppl):S38–S48.

Dalakas M: Inflammatory myopathies. Curr Opin Neurol Neurosurg 1990;3:689–696.

Dalakas MC: Polymyositis, dermatomyositis, and inclusion-body myositis. N Engl J Med 1991;325:1487–1498.

Dalakas MC, Illa I, Dambrosia JM, et al: A controlled trial of high-dose intravenous immune globulin infusions as treatment for dermatomyositis. N Engl J Med 1993;329:1993–2000.

Dalakas MC: Current treatment of the inflammatory myopathies. Curr Opin Rheumatol 1994;6:595–601.

Dalakas MC, Illa I, Gallardo E, Juarez C: Inclusion body myositis and paraproteinemia: Incidence and immunopathologic correlations. Ann Neurol 1997a;41:100–104.

Dalakas MC, Sonies B, Dambrosia J, et al: Treatment of inclusion body myositis with IVIg: A double-blind, placebo-controlled study. Neurology 1997b;48:712–716.

Danon MJ. Reyes MG, Perurena OH, et al: Inclusion body myositis:

A corticosteroid resistant idiopathic inflammatory myopathy. Arch Neurol 1982;39:760–764.

Danon MJ, Friedman M: Inclusion body myositis associated with progressive dysphagia: Treatment with cricopharyngeal myotomy. Can J Neurol Sci 1989;16:436–438.

Dau PC: Leukocytapheresis in inclusion body myositis. J Clin Apheresis 1987;3:167–170.

Davis MJ, Cilo M, Plaitakis A, Yahr MD: Trichinosis: Severe myopathic involvement with recovery. Neurology 1976;26:37–40.

De Meirsman J, Hens L: Schulman's syndrome: Diffuse fasciitis with eosinophilia: A single fiber electromyography study. Electromyogr Clin Neurophysiol 1983;23:587–591.

DeVere R, Bradley WG: Polymyositis: Its presentation, morbidity, and mortality. Brain 1975;98:637–666.

Dewberry RG, Schneider BF, Cale WF, Phillips LH II: Sarcoid myopathy presenting with diaphragm weakness. Muscle Nerve 1993; 16:832–835.

Dimitru D, Newell-Eggert M: Inclusion body myositis: An electrophysiologic study. Am J Phys Med Rehabil 1990;69:2–5.

Doshi R, Fowler T: Proximal myopathy due to discrete carcinomatous metastases in muscle. J Neurol Neurosurg Psychiatr 1983;46:358–360.

Eaton LM: The perspective of neurology in regard to polymyositis: A study of 41 cases. Neurology 1954;4:245–263.

Eisen A, Berry K, Gibson G: Inclusion body myositis (inclusion body myositis): Myopathy or neuropathy? Neurology 1983;33:1109–1114.

Fang MA, Verity MA, Paulus HE: Subacute perimyositis. J Rheumatol 1988;15:1291–1293.

Farrell MK, Partin JC, Bove KE, et al: Epidemic influenza myopathy in Cincinnati in 1977. J Pediatr 1980;96:545–551.

Fauci AS, Harley JB, Roberts WC, et al: NIH conference: The idiopathic hypereosinophilic syndrome: Clinical, pathophysiologic, and therapeutic considerations. Ann Intern Med 1982; 97:78–92.

Felice K, DeGirolami U, Chad DA: Pyomyositis presenting as rapidly progressive generalized weakness. Neurology 1991;41:944–945.

Ferrara JLM, Deeg HJ: Graft versus host disease. N Engl J Med 1991;324:667.

Flaisler F, Blin D, Asencio G, et al: Focal myositis: A localized form of polymyositis? J Rheumatol 1993;20:1414–1416.

Fraser DD, Frank JA, Dalakas M, et al: Magnetic resonance imaging in the idiopathic inflammatory myopathies. J Rheumatol 1991; 18:1693–1700.

Fuas-Riera S, Martinez-Pardo S, Blanch-Rubio J, et al: Muscle pathology in ankylosing spondylitis: Clinical, enzymatic, electromyographic and histologic correlation. J Rheumatol 1991;18:1368–1371.

Fujitake J, Ishikawa Y, Fujii H, et al: Magnetic resonance imaging of skeletal muscles in the polymyositis. Muscle Nerve 1997;20:1463–1466.

Gamboa ET, Eastwood AB, Hays AP, et al: Isolation of influenza virus from muscle in myoglobinuric polymyositis. Neurology 1979;29:1323–1335.

Gardner-Thorpe C: Muscle weakness due to sarcoid myopathy: Six cases and an evaluation of steroid therapy. Neurology 1972; 22:917–928.

Gartron MJ, Isenberg DA: Clinical features of lupus myositis versus idiopathic myositis: A review of 30 cases. Br J Rheumatol 1997;36:1067–1074.

Gertz MA, Kyle RA: Myopathy in primary systemic amyloidosis. J Neurol Neurosurg Psychiatr 1996;60:655–660.

Goodson WH: Neurologic manifestations of sarcoidosis. South Med J 1960;53:1111–1116.

Grau JM, Miro O, Pedrol E, et al: Interstitial lung disease related to dermatomyositis: Comparative study with patients without lung involvement. J Rheumatol 1996;23:1921–1926.

Gross B, Ochoa J: Trichinosis: Clinical report and histochemistry of muscle. Muscle Nerve 1979;2:394–398.

Hausmanowa-Petrusewica I, Kozminska A: Electromyogrphic findings in scleroderma. Arch Neurol 1961;4:59–65.

Hendrickx GFM, Verhage J, Jennekens FGI, et al: Dermatomyositis and toxoplasmosis. Ann Neurol 1979;5:393–395.

Henriksson KG, Stalberg E: The terminal innervation pattern in polymyositis: A histochemical and SFEMG study. Muscle Nerve 1978;1:3–13.

Hertzman PA, Blevins WL, Mayer J, et al: Association of the eosinophilia-myalgia syndrome with the ingestion of tryptophan. N Engl J Med 1990;322:869–873.

Hollinrake K: Polymyositis presenting as distal muscle weakness: A case report. J Neurol Sci 1969;8:479–484.

Houser SM, Calabrese LH, Strome M: Dysphagia in patients with inclusion body myositis. Laryngoscope 1998;108:1001–1005.

Huang KL, Chang DM, Lu JJ: Tuberculosis of skeletal muscle in a case of polymyositis. Scand J Rheumatol 1999;28:380–382.

Itoh J, Akiguchi I, Midorikawa R, Kameyama M: Sarcoid myopathy with typical rash of dermatomyositis. Neurology 1980;30:1118–1121.

Johannes S, Schubert M, Heidenreich F, et al: Inclusion body myositis: Immune globulins improve muscle strength but not abnormal postures. J Neurol 1998;245:816–818.

Jongen PJH, ter Laak HJ, van de Putte LBA: Inclusion body myositis responding to long term chlorambucil treatment. J Rheumatol 1995;22:576–578.

Joy JL, Oh SJ, Baysal AI: Electrophysiologic spectrum of inclusion body myositis. Muscle Nerve 1990;13:949–951.

Kelly JJ, Madoc-Jones H, Adelman LS, et al: Total body irradiation not effective in inclusion body myositis. Neurology 1986;36:1264–1266.

Kilbourne EM, Rigau-Perez JG, Heath CW Jr, et al: Clinical epidemiology of toxic oil syndrome: Manifestations of a new illness. N Engl J Med 1983;309:1408–1414.

Kim JH, Wallerstein S, Thoe M, et al: Myopathy in tuberculosis: Two presumptive cases and a review of the literature. Milit Med 1997;162:221–224.

Kim JY, Park YH, Choi KH, et al: MRI of tuberculous pyomyositis. J Comput Assist Tomogr 1999;23:454–457.

Kingston WJ, Moxley RT: Inflammatory myopathies. Neurol Clin 1988;6:545–561.

Koffman BM, Rugiero M, Dalakas MC: Immune-mediated conditions and antibodies associated with sporadic inclusion body myositis. Muscle Nerve 1998;21:115–117.

Koffman BM, Sivakumar K, Simonis T, et al: HLA allele distribution distinguishes sporadic inclusion body myositis from hereditary inclusion body myositis. J Neuroimmunol 1998;84:139–142.

Krick JA, Remington JS: Current concepts in parasitology: Toxoplasmosis in the adult—an overview. N Engl J Med 1978;298:550–553.

Kugelberg E: Electromyography in muscular disorders. J Neurol Neurosurg Psychiatr 1947;10:122–136.

Kurland LT, Hauser WA, Ferguson RH, et al: Epidemiologic features of diffuse connective tissue disorders in Rochester, Minn, 1951–1967 with special reference to systemic lupus erythematosis. Mayo Clin Proc 1969;44:649–663.

Lakhanpal S, Bunch TW, Ilstrup DM, Melton LJ III: Polymyositis-dermatomyositis and malignant lesions: Does an association exist? Mayo Clin Proc 1986;645–653.

Lakhanpal S, Duffy J, Engel AG: Eosinophilia associated with perimyositis and pneumonitis. Mayo Clin Proc 1988;63:37–41.

Lakhanpal S, Ginsburg WWW, Michet CJ, et al: Eosinophilic fasciitis: Clinical spectrum and therapeutic responses in 52 cases. Semin Arthritis Rheum 1988;17:221–231.

Lambert EH, Sayre GP, Eaton LM: Electrical activity of muscle in polymyositis. Trans Am Neurol Assoc 1954;79:64–69.

Lane R, Fulthorpe JJ, Hudgson P: Inclusion body myositis: A case with associated collagen vascular disease responding to treatment. J Neurol Neurosurg Psychiatr 1985;48:270–273.

Lange DJ, Britton CB, Younger DS, Hays AP: The neuromuscular manifestations of human immunodeficiency virus infections. Arch Neurol 1988;45:1084–1088.

Lederman RJ, Slanga VD, Wilbourn AJ, et al: Focal inflammatory myopathy. Muscle Nerve 1984;7:142–146.

Leff RL, Miller FW, Hicks J, et al: The treatment of inclusion body myositis: A retrospective review and a randomized, prospective trial of immunosuppressive therapy. Medicine 1993;72:225–235.

Levin K, Mitsumotos H, Agamanolis D: Steroid responsiveness and clinical variability in inclusion body myositis. Muscle Nerve 1986;9:217.

Levin MI, Mozaffar T, Al-Lozi MT, Pestronk A: Paraneoplastic necrotizing myopathy: Clinical and pathological features. Neurology 1998;50:764–767.

Lotz BP, Engel AG, Nishino H, et al: Inclusion body myositis: Observations in 40 patients. Brain 1989;112:727–747.

Mair J: Cardiac troponin I and troponin T: Are enzymes still relevant as cardiac markers? Clin Chim Acta 1997;257:99–115.

Manchul LA, Jin A, Pritchard KI, et al: The frequency of malignant neoplasms in patients with polymyositis-dermatomyositis: A controlled study. Arch Intern Med 1985;145:1835–1839.

Marcus S, Miller RV: An atypical case of trichinosis with report of electromyographic findings. Ann Intern Med 1955;43:615–622.

Marie I, Cardon T, Hachulla E, et al: Magnetic resonance imaging in focal myositis. J Rheumatol 1998;25:378–382.

Marie I, Hatron P, Levesque H, et al: Influence of age on characteristics of polymyositis and dermatomyositis in adults. Medicine 1999;78:139–147.

Masanes F, Pedrol E, Grau JM, et al: Symptomatic myopathies in HIV-1 infected patients untreated with antiretroviral agents: A clinico-pathological study of 30 consecutive patients. Clin Neuropathol 1995;15:221–225.

Massa R, Weller B, Karpati G, et al: Familial inclusion body myositis among Kurdish-Iranian Jews. Arch Neurol 1991;48:519–522.

Mastalgia FL, Ojeda VJ: Inflammatory myopathies: Part I. Ann Neurol 1985a;17:215–227.

Mastalgia FL, Ojeda VJ: Inflammatory myopathies: Part II. Ann Neurol 1985b;17:317–323.

Mastalgia FL, Phillips BA, Zilko P: Treatment of inflammatory myopathies. Muscle Nerve 1997;20:651–664.

Mastalgia FL, Phillips BA, Zilko PJ: Immunoglobulin therapy in inflammatory myopathies. J Neurol Neurosurg Psychiatr 1998; 65:107–110.

Matsubara S, Mair WGP: Ultrastructural changes in polymyositis. Brain 1979;701–725.

Maugears YM, Berthelot JMM, Abbas AA, et al: Long-term prognosis of 69 patients with dermatomyositis or polymyositis. Clin Exp Rheumatol 1996;14:263–274.

Mechler F: Changing electromyographic findings during the chronic course of polymyositis. J Neurol Sci 1974;23:237–242.

Medsger TA, Rodnan GP, Moossy J, et al: Skeletal muscle involvement in progressive systemic sclerosis (scleroderma). Arthritis Rheum 1968;11:554–568.

Medsger TA, Dawson WN, Masi AT: The epidemiology of polymyositis. Am J Med 1970;48:715–723.

Michet CJ, Doyle JA, Ginsburg WW: Eosinophilic fasciitis: Report of 15 cases. Mayo clin Proc 1981;56:27–34.

Middleton PJ, Alexander RM, Szymanski MT: Severe myositis during recovery from influenza. Lancet 1970;2:533–535.

Miller FW, Leitman SF, Cronin ME, et al: Controlled trial of plasma exchange and leukapheresis in polymyositis and dermatomyositis. N Engl J Med 1992;326:1380–1384.

Miro O, Casademont J, Garcia-Carrasco M, et al: Muscle involvement in rheumatoid arthritis: Clinicopathological study of 21 symptomatic cases. Semin Arthritis Rheum 1996;25:421–428.

Mitrani-Rosenbaum S, Argov Z, Blumenfeld A, et al: Hereditary inclusion-body myopathy maps to chromosome 9p1-q1. Hum Mol Genet 1996;5:159–163.

Mitz M, Chang GJ, Albers JW, Sulaiman AR: Electromyographic and histologic paraspinal abnormalities in polymyositis/dermatomyositis. Arch Phys Med Rehabil 1981;62:118–121.

Munsat TL, Piper D, Cancilla P, Mednick J: Inflammatory myopathy with facioscapulohumeral distribution. Neurology 1972;22: 335–347.

Nelson KR, McQuillen MP: Neurologic complications of graft versus host disease. Neurol Clin 1988;6:389.

Neville HE, Baumback LL, Ringel SP, et al: Familial inclusion body myositis: Evidence for autosomal dominant inheritance. Neurology 1992;42:897–902.

Newman Ed, Scott DW: The use of low-dose methotrexate in the treatment of polymyositis and dermatomyositis. J Clin Rheumatol 1995;1:99–102.

Nordstrom DM, Petropolis AA, Giorno R, et al: Inflammatory myopathy and acquired immunodeficiency syndrome. Arthritis Rheum 1989;32:475–479.

Oldfors A, Lindberg C: Inclusion body myositis. Curr Opin Neurol 1999;12:527–533.

Olsen NJ, King LE, Park JH: Muscle abnormalities in scleroderma. Rheum Dis Clin North Am 1996;22:783–796.

Partanen J, Lang H: EMG dynamics in polymyositis. J Neurol Sci 1982;57:221–234.

Pearson CM: Polymyositis. Annu Rev Med 1966;17:63–82.

Pearson CM, Bohan A: The spectrum of polymyositis and dermatomyositis. Med Clin North Am 1977;61:439–457.

Phillips BA, Zilko P, Garlepp MJ, Mastalgia FL: Frequency of relapses in patients with polymyositis and dermatomyositis. Muscle Nerve 1998;21:1668–1672.

Pickering MC, Walport MJ: Eosinophilic myopathy syndromes. Curr Opin Rheumatol 1998;10:504–510.

Plotz PH, Dalakas M, Leff R, et al: Current concepts in the idiopathic inflammatory myopathies: Polymyositis, dermatomyositis, and related disorders. Ann Intern Med 1989;111:143–157.

Pollock JL: Toxoplasmosis appearing to be dermatomyositis. Arch Dermatol 1979;115:736–737.

Powell LW: Sarcoidosis of skeletal muscle: Report of 6 cases and review of the literature. Am J Clin Pathol 1953;23:881–889.

Prayson RA: Amyloid myopathy: Clinicopathologic study of 16 cases. Hum Pathol 1998;29:463–468.

Prayson RA: Granulomatous myositis. Am J Clin Pathol 1999; 112:63–68,

Reimers CD, Finkenstaedt M: Muscle imaging in inflammatory myopathies. Curr Opin Rheumatol 1997;9:475–485.

Richardson JB, Callen JP: Dermatomyositis and malignancy. Med Clin North Am 1989;73:1211–1220.

Ringel SP, Kenny CE, Neville HE, et al: Spectrum of inclusion body myositis. Arch Neurol 1987;44:1154–1157.

Rini BL, Gajewski TF: Polymyositis with respiratory muscle weakness requiring mechanical ventilation in metastatic thymoma treated with octreotide. Ann Oncol 1999;10:973–979.

Robberecht W, Theys P, Lammens M, Leenders J: Distal myopathy as the presenting manifestation of sarcoidosis. J Neurol Neurosurg Psychiatr 1995;59:642–643.

Robinson LR: AAEM Case Report #22: Polymyositis. Muscle Nerve 1991;14:310–315.

Rose AL, Walton JN: Polymyositis: A survey of 89 cases with particular reference to treatment and prognosis. Brain 1966; 89:747–768.

Rosenberg NL: Polymyositis and dermatomyositis, myositis-myalgia, and inclusion body myositis. Curr Opin Neurol Neurosurg 1991;4:693–698.

Rossel I: An electromyographic and histological study of muscles in rheumatoid arthritis. Acta Rheumatol Scand 1963;9:65–78.

Rothstein TL, Carlson CB: Restricted myositis with myoedema simulating facioscapulohumeral muscular dystrophy. Neurology 1970;20:386–387.

Rowland LP, Breer M: Toxoplasmic polymyositis. Neurology 1961; 11:367–370.

Rubin DI, Hermann RC: Electrophysiologic findings in amyloid myopathy. Muscle Nerve 1999;22:355–359.

Samuels BS, Rietschel RL: Polymyositis and toxoplasmosis. JAMA 1976;235:60–61.

Sandstedt PER, Henriksson KG, Larsson LE: Quantitative electromyography in polymyositis and dermatomyositis. Acta Neurol Scand 1982;65:110–121.

Santiago RM, Scharnhorst D, Ratkin G, Crouch EC: Respiratory muscle weakness and ventilatory failure in AL amyloidosis with muscular pseudohypertrophy. Am J Med 1987;83:760–762.

Sayers ME, Chou SM, Calabrese LH: Inclusion body myositis: Analysis of 32 cases. J Rheumatol 1992;19:1385–1389.

Sekul EA, Chow C, Dalakas MC: Magnetic resonance imaging of the forearm as a diagnostic aid in patients with sporadic inclusion body myositis. Neurology 1997;48:863–866.

Serratrice G, Pellissier JF, Cros D, et al: Relapsing eosinophilic perimyositis. J Rheumatol 1980;7:199–205.

Silverstein A, Siltzbach LE: Muscle involvement in sarcoidosis: Asymptomatic, myositis, and myopathy. Arch Neurol 1969;21: 235–241.

Simpson DM, Bender AN: Human immunodeficiency virus–associated myopathy: Analysis of 11 patients. Ann Neurol 1988; 24:79–84.

Smith B: Skeletal muscle necrosis associated with carcinoma. J Pathol 1969;97:207.

Snider WD, Simpson DM, Nielsen S, et al: Neurological complications of acquired immune deficiency syndrome: Analysis of 50 patients. Ann Neurol 1983;14:403–418.

Soueidan SA, Dalakas MC: Treatment of inclusion-body myositis with high-dose intravenous immunoglobulin. Neurology 1993; 43:76–879.

Spiera R, Kagen L: Extramuscular manifestations in idiopathic inflammatory myopathies. Curr Opin Rheumatol 1998;10:556–561.

Spuler S, Emslie-Smith A, Engel AG: Amyloid myopathy: An underdiagnosed entity. Ann Neurol 1998;43:719–728.

Stark RJ: Polymyositis presenting with severe weakness involving only one arm. Aust N Z J Med 1978;8:544–546.

Stern BJ, Krumholz A, Johns C, et al: Sarcoidosis and its neurological manifestations. Arch Neurol 1985;42:909–917.

Stern R, Gold J, Dicarly EF: Myopathy complicating the acquired immune deficiency syndrome. Muscle Nerve 1987;10:318–322.

Streeten EA, de la Monte SM, Kennedy TP: Amyloid infiltration of the diaphragm as a cause of respiratory failure. Chest 1986; 89:790–792.

Streib EW, Wilbourn AJ, Mitsumoto H: Spontaneous electrical muscle fiber activity in polymyositis and dermatomyositis. Muscle Nerve 1979;2:14–18.

Swash M: Acute fatal carcinomatous neuromyopathy. Arch Neurol 1974;30:324.

Targoff IN: Immune manifestations of inflammatory muscle disease. Rheum Dis Clin North Am 1994;20:857–880.

Topi GC, D'Alessandro L, Catricala C, et al: Dermatomyositis-like syndrome due to toxoplasmosis. Br J Dermatol 1979;101:589–591.

Trojaberg W: Electrodiagnosis in the rheumatic diseases. Clin Rheum Dis 1981;7:349–363.

Trojaberg W: Quantitative electromyography in polymyositis: A reappraisal. Muscle Nerve 1990;13:964–971.

Trueb RM, Becker-Wegerich P, Hafner J, et al: Relapsing eosinophilic perimyositis. Br J Dermatol 1995;133:109–114.

Uncini A, Lange DJ, Lovelace RE, et al: Long-duration polyphasic motor unit potentials in myopathies: A quantitative study with pathological correlation. Muscle Nerve 1990;13:263–267.

Vazquez D, Rothfield NF: Sensitivity and specificity of anti-Jo-1 antibodies in autoimmune diseases with myositis. Arthritis Rheum 1996;39:292–296.

Verma A, Bradley WG, Adesina AM, et al: Inclusion body myositis with cricopharyngeus muscle involvement and severe dysphagia. Muscle Nerve 1991;14:470–473.

Villalba L, Adams EM: Update on therapy for refractory dermatomyositis and polymyositis. Curr Opin Rheumatol 1996;8:544–551.

Villalba ML, Hicks JE, Thornton B, et al: A combination of oral methotrexate and azathioprine is more effective than high dose intravenous methotrexate with leucovorin rescue in treatment-resistant myositis (abstract). Arthritis Rheum 1995;38:s307.

Villalba ML, Hicks JE, Thornton B, et al: A combination of oral methotrexate and azathioprine is more effective than high dose intravenous methotrexate with leucovorin rescue in treatment-resistant myositis (abstract). Arthritis Rheum 1996;39:1016–1020.

Wallace SL, Lattes R, Malia JP, et al: Muscle involvement in Boeck's sarcoid. Ann Intern Med 1958;48:497.

Walton J: The inflammatory myopathies. J R Soc Med 1983;76:998–1010.

Walton JN: Disorders of Voluntary Muscle. London, J & A Churchill Ltd, 1969.

Wayhonis GW, Johnson EW: The electromyogram in acute trichinosis: Report of four cases. Arch Phys Med Rehabil 1964;45:177–183.

Whitaker JN: Inflammatory myopathy: A review of etiologic and pathogenetic factors. Muscle Nerve 1982;5:573–592.

Wintzen AR, Bots GAM, Bakker HM, et al: Dysphagia in inclusion body myositis. J Neurol Neurosurg Psychiatr 1988;51:1542–1545.

Worthmann F, Bruns J, Turker T, Gosztonyi G: Muscular involvement in Behcet's disease: Case report and review of the literature. Neuromusc Disord 1996;6:247–253.

Zantos D, Zhang Y, Felson D: The overall and temporal association of cancer with polymyositis and dermatomyositis. J Rheumatol 1994;21:1855–1859.

Zegarelli DJ, Tsukada Y, Pickren, JW, Greene GW: Metastatic tumor to the tongue. Oral Surg 1973;35:202–211.

Zisman DA, Biermann JS, Martinez FJ, et al: Sarcoidosis presenting as a tumorlike muscular lesion: Case report and review of the literature. Medicine 1999;78:112–122.

Endocrine Myopathies and Toxic Myopathies

Anthony A. Amato

ENDOCRINE MYOPATHIES

A variety of endocrine disorders are associated with myopathies. In this section, myopathies associated with thyroid, parathyroid, adrenal, pituitary, and pancreatic dysfunction are discussed. Clinicians must be aware of these disorders because early diagnosis and proper treatment leads to resolution of the myopathy (Kingston, 1983; Kissel and Mendell, 1992; Kaminski and Ruff, 1994; Amato and Dumitru, 2002).

Thyroid Disorders

Both hyperthyroidism and hypothyroidism cause myopathy. Peripheral neuropathy and myasthenia gravis can also be associated with thyroid dysfunction.

THYROTOXIC MYOPATHY

Clinical Features

From 61% to 82% of patients with hyperthyroidism have objective weakness on examination, although subjective weakness is a manifesting complaint in less than 5% of patients (Salick and Pearson, 1967; Puvanendran et al., 1979; Kaminski and Ruff, 1994). The mean age of onset of thyrotoxic myopathy is in the 40s. Hyperthyroidism is more common in women than in men, but thyrotoxic myopathy occurs in similar frequencies in men and women. The longer the patient has been hyperthyroid, the greater is the likelihood of the development of myopathic signs and symptoms. However, the severity of the myopathy does not necessarily relate to the severity of the thyroid dysfunction.

The myopathy usually manifests several months after the onset of other clinical symptoms associated with hyperthyroidism, including nervousness, anxiety, psychosis, tremor, increased perspiration, heat intolerance, palpitations, insomnia, diarrhea, increased appetite, and weight loss. Common goiter, tachycardia, atrial fibrillation, widened pulse pressure, as well as warm, thin, and moist skin can also be seen in patients with hyperthyroidism. Patients with thyrotoxic myopathy present with proximal muscle weakness and atrophy involving the hip girdle more than the shoulder girdle (Puvanendran et al., 1979; Engel, 1988; Kissel and Mendell, 1992; Kaminski and Ruff, 1994). As many as 20% of patients complain of predominantly distal extremity weakness (Puvanendran et al., 1979). Myalgias and fatigue are also common symptoms. Myoglobinuria has been described in rare patients with severe thyrotoxicosis (Bennet and Huston, 1984). Involvement of bulbar, esophagopharyngeal, and respiratory muscles may lead to dysphagia, dysphonia, and respiratory distress (Mier et al., 1989; McElvaney et al., 1990). Ophthalmoparesis and proptosis are well known complications of Graves' disease. Of note, patients can have both Graves' disease and myasthenia gravis, and it can be difficult to distinguish which neuromuscular symptoms are related to the hyperthyroid state from those due to myasthenia gravis. Muscle weakness associated with hyperthyroidism does not fluctuate or significantly improve with anticholinesterase inhibitors.

Clinical examination may also reveal fasciculations and myokymia secondary to thyrotoxicosis-induced irritability of the anterior horn cells or peripheral nerves (Harman and Richardson, 1954; Havard et al., 1963; McCommas et al., 1974; Feibel and Campa, 1976). Peripheral neuropathy is uncommon, but a demyelinating polyneuropathy may rarely occur (Feibel and Campa, 1976). Deep tendon reflexes are typically brisk, but plantar responses are flexor.

Thyrotoxicosis is also associated with a form of hypokalemic periodic paralysis. *Thyrotoxic periodic paralysis* occurs sporadically, although there may be an autosomally dominant inherited susceptibility to the disorder. Thyrotoxic periodic paralysis appears to be more common in Asians but is not restricted to this population (Sataysohi et al., 1963; Kissel and Mendell, 1992). The disorder is more common in men than in women, despite thyrotoxicosis being more prevalent in women. The attacks of weakness are similar to those of familial hypokalemic periodic paralysis. Although most cases of hypokalemic periodic paralysis occur within the first three decades of life, onset of thyrotoxic periodic paralysis may manifest later in adult life. Serum potassium levels tend to be low during the attacks of weakness, but levels can be normal.

Laboratory Features

Primary hyperthyroidism is diagnosed on the basis of elevated thyroxine (T_4) levels and occasionally only the triiodothyronine (T_3) level, while thyroid-stimulating hormone (TSH) level is low. In thyrotoxic periodic paralysis, serum potassium levels are also decreased. The serum creatine kinase levels are usually normal.

Electromyography and Nerve Conduction Studies

Routine motor and sensory nerve conduction studies (NCSs) are usually normal (Buchthal, 1970; Amato and Dumitru, 2002). A single thyrotoxic patient with severe weakness had demyelinating features on NCSs (Feibel and Campa, 1976). Some hyperthyroid patients without concomitant myasthenia gravis have decrementing responses on slow or fast rates of repetitive nerve stimulation (Puvanendran et al., 1979).

Electromyography (EMG) usually shows normal or nonspecific findings (Havard et al., 1963; Ramsay, 1965; Ludin et al., 1969; Puvanendran et al., 1979; Amato and Dumitru, 2002). Fasciculation potentials and, rarely, a focal or generalized myokymia are seen (Harman and Richardson, 1954). Fibrillation potentials and positive sharp waves are not usually seen. Motor unit action potentials (MUAPs) may be reduced in duration, decreased in amplitude, and polyphasic. An early recruitment pattern is not a particularly prominent finding, unless the patient has severe muscle weakness.

Histopathology

Nonspecific myopathic features, including mild fatty infiltrate, muscle fiber atrophy of all types, variability in muscle fiber size, scattered isolated necrotic fibers, decreased glycogen, and increased internal nuclei, may be noted in thyrotoxic myopathy (Waldstein et al., 1958; Havard et al., 1963; Engel, 1972; Hudgson and Kendall-Taylor, 1992; Kaminski and Ruff, 1994). Dilated T-tubules, Z-band streaming, elongated mitochondria, and subsarcolemmal glycogen deposition may be seen on electron microscopy (Engel, 1966).

Muscle biopsy samples in patients with thyrotoxic periodic paralysis demonstrate abnormalities similar to those seen in familial hypokalemic periodic paralysis. Light microscopy may reveal vacuolar changes, whereas sarcolemmal blebs filled with glycogen and dilated terminal cisternae of the sarcoplasmic reticulum may be apparent on electron microscopy.

Pathogenesis

The exact pathogenesis of thyrotoxic myopathy is unknown but may be due to increased catabolism.

There is enhanced glucose uptake and glycolysis in muscle, which is independent of insulin, in the hyperthyroid state (Amato and Dumitru, 2002). In addition, the basal metabolic rate is increased as evidenced by mitochondrial consumption of oxygen, pyruvate, and malate (Janssen et al., 1981). Glycogen is depleted and adenosine triphosphate (ATP) production is reduced secondary to an insulin-resistant state. This leads to fasting hyperglycemia and glucose intolerance. Also, insulin resistance may impair amino acid and protein metabolism (Dubaniewicz et al., 1989). Further, there is accelerated protein catabolism caused by increased lysosomal protease activity (Brown and Millward, 1980; Morrison et al., 1988).

Thyrotoxic periodic paralysis is probably caused by episodic muscle membrane inexcitability. Thyroid hormones increase efflux of potassium from muscle and a subsequent increase in the number and activity of sodium-potassium ATPase pumps (Everts et al., 1990). This results in partial depolarization of the resting membrane potential, which renders the muscle membrane less excitable (Ruff et al., 1988). Depolarization-induced sodium channel inactivation and impaired propagation of the action potential across altered T-tubules may also be responsible for muscle membrane inexcitability (Dulhunty et al., 1986).

Treatment

The myopathy gradually improves over several months after successful treatment of the hyperthyroid state (Kissel and Mendell, 1992). Thyrotoxic periodic paralysis also resolves once the patient becomes euthyroid. Propranolol is useful in preventing and lessening the severity of the attacks of periodic paralysis. Unlike the familial form of hypokalemic periodic paralysis, acetazolamide is ineffective in thyrotoxic periodic paralysis. Unfortunately, extraocular muscle weakness can persist for months or years after treatment of Graves' disease. Corticosteroids and cyclosporine may be beneficial in some patients (Prummel et al., 1989).

HYPOTHYROID MYOPATHY

Clinical Features

One third of patients with hypothyroidism develop proximal upper and lower extremity muscle weakness, myalgias, cramps, and muscle hypertrophy (Salick et al., 1968; Mizusawa et al., 1983; Engel, 1988; Kissel and Mendell, 1992; Kaminski and Ruff, 1994). There are rare reports of rhabdomyolysis (Riggs, 1990) and weakness of the respiratory muscles (Martinez et al., 1989). Some patients may have a superimposed peripheral neuropathy or myasthenia gravis (Takamori et al., 1972). In addition to the proximal weakness and occasional muscle hypertrophy, examination reveals delayed relaxation of the ankle tendon reflex and mounding of the underlying muscles on percussion *(myoedema)*.

Laboratory Features

The serum creatine kinase levels are usually elevated. In primary hypothyroidism, serum T_4 and T_3 levels are decreased, whereas thyroid-stimulating hormone levels are increased.

Histopathology

Muscle biopsies reveal variability in muscle fiber size with atrophy of type 2 and, occasionally, type 1 fibers (Evans et al., 1990; Hudgson and Kendall-Taylor, 1992; Kaminski and Ruff, 1994). Scattered hypertrophic muscle fibers, and necrotic and regenerating muscle fibers may be seen. There may also be increased internal nuclei, ring fibers, glycogen accumulation, and vacuoles. Electron microscopy demonstrates mitochondrial swellings and inclusions, myofibrillar disarray with central core–like changes, autophagic vacuoles, glycogen accumulation, excess lipid, dilated sarcoplasmic reticulum, and T-tubule proliferation (Evans et al., 1990).

Pathogenesis

The pathogenic basis of the hypothyroid myopathy is not known but is likely related to an impaired metabolic state. Hypothyroidism causes reduced metabolism of carbohydrates and fatty acids, leading to decreased ATP production (Schwartz and Oppenheimer, 1978; Ho, 1989). There is reduced protein synthesis, but protein catabolism is also diminished.

Electromyography and Nerve Conduction Studies

Motor and sensory NCSs are usually normal (Buchthal, 1970; Amato and Dumitru, 2002), although some patients with a concomitant peripheral neuropathy may have slow conduction velocities (Moosa and Dubowitz, 1971; Scarpalezos et al., 1973; Shirabe et al., 1975). In addition, patients with hypothyroidism may be at an increased risk for the development of entrapment neuropathies such as carpal and tarsal tunnel syndromes (Rao et al., 1980; Schwartz et al., 1983).

EMG usually reveals normal insertional and spontaneous activity. However, positive sharp waves, fibrillation potentials, and myotonic discharges are seen rarely (Astrom et al., 1961; Scarpalezos et al., 1973; Venables et al., 1978; Amato and Dumitru, 2002). MUAP morphology and recruitment pattern are usually normal, but early recruitment of short-duration, low-amplitude, polyphasic MUAPs may be appreciated in severely affected muscles.

Treatment

The myopathy and electrophysiological abnormalities slowly improve with correction of the hypothyroidism.

Parathyroid Disorders

Myopathies are common in disorders of calcium and phosphate homeostasis. Calcium and phosphate homeostasis requires a complex interaction of intestinal, renal, hepatic, endocrine, skin, and skeletal functions under the regulation of parathyroid hormone and vitamin D (Kissel and Mendell, 1992). There are several forms of vitamin D: (1) vitamin D$_3$, or cholecalciferol, which is derived from the skin; (2) vitamin D$_2$, or ergocalciferol, which is dietary and absorbed through the intestines; and (3) 25-hydroxyvitamin D, which is made in the liver and converted to the more potent metabolite, 1,25-dihydroxyvitamin D, in the kidney. Parathyroid hormone promotes bone resorption, enhances renal calcium absorption and phosphate excretion, and increases 1,25-dihydroxyvitamin D conversion in the kidneys. Serum phosphate levels are dependent on diet, intestinal absorption, and renal excretion. The parathyroid hormone–enhanced synthesis of 1,25-dihydroxyvitamin D results in increased serum calcium and decreased serum phosphate concentrations.

HYPERPARATHYROIDISM AND OSTEOMALACIA

Clinical Features

The vast majority of patients with osteomalacia have muscle weakness (Smith and Stern, 1967; Smith and Stern, 1969; Russell, 1994). However, myopathy occurs in less than 10% of patients with primary hyperparathyroidism (Smith and Stern, 1969; Patten et al., 1974). The myopathy associated with primary hyperparathyroidism and osteomalacia is characterized by symmetrical proximal weakness and atrophy (Vicale, 1949; Bischoff and Esslen, 1965; Smith and Stern, 1967; Smith and Stern, 1969; Patten et al., 1974; Mallette et al., 1975; Turken et al., 1989; Roca et al., 1995). The legs are affected more than the arms. Some patients develop hoarseness and dysphagia (Patten et al., 1974). Rarely, patients have severe neck extensor weakness, the "dropped head syndrome," and severe respiratory muscle involvement (Berenbaum et al., 1993; Gentric and Pennec, 1994). Cramps and paresthesias occur in nearly half of patients (Vicale, 1949). There is stocking-glove loss of pain or vibratory sensation and decreased muscle stretch reflexes suggestive of an underlying peripheral neuropathy in 29% to 57% of patients (Vicale, 1949; Patten et al., 1974). However, some patients have brisk deep tendon reflexes. Nevertheless, plantar responses are flexor. The rare reports of tongue fasciculations, spasticity, and extensor plantar responses in patients with hyperparathyroidism (Patten et al., 1974; Carnevale et al., 1992; Gelinas et al., 1994) probably involved coincidental amyotrophic lateral sclerosis (Jackson et al., 1998).

Secondary hyperparathyroidism usually occurs in patients with chronic renal failure. The myopathy in this condition is similar to that described for primary hyperparathyroidism and osteomalacia (Floyd et al., 1974). In addition, arterial calcification with secondary muscle necrosis and myoglobinuria may complicate secondary hyperparathyroidism (Richardson et al., 1969). Patients with renal failure but without obvious secondary hyperparathyroidism may also develop calciphylaxis (Randall et al., 2000).

Laboratory Features

Serum creatine kinase levels are usually normal in patients with primary and secondary hyperparathyroidism and osteomalacia. In primary hyperparathyroidism, serum calcium levels are usually high, whereas serum phosphate levels are low. There is decreased urinary excretion of calcium and increased excretion of phosphate. In primary hyperparathyroidism, serum parathyroid hormone levels and 1,25-dihydroxyvitamin D levels are elevated. In contrast, 1,25-dihydroxyvitamin D levels are diminished in secondary hyperparathyroidism caused by renal insufficiency. Noninvasive imaging techniques, such as ultrasound, thallium/technetium scintigraphy, computed tomography, and magnetic resonance imaging, may be useful in localizing abnormal parathyroid glands (Norton and Sugg, 1994).

Osteomalacia is characterized by normal or low serum calcium and phosphate levels, depending on the degree of secondary hyperparathyroidism (Russell, 1994). Serum vitamin D levels are also usually diminished in osteomalacia. Urinary excretion of calcium is decreased (except in cases secondary to renal tubular acidosis), whereas excretion of phosphate is increased. In addition, serum alkaline phosphatase levels are usually always elevated. Skeletal survey reveals a decrease in bone density with loss of trabeculae, blurred trabecular margins, and thin cortices (Goldring et al., 1994).

Electromyography and Nerve Conduction Studies

The motor and sensory NCSs are normal, unless the patient has concomitant uremic neuropathy (Skaria et al., 1975; Amato and Dumitru, 2002). EMG usually reveals normal insertional and spontaneous activity, although, rarely, a few fibrillation potentials and positive sharp waves are seen (Mallette et al., 1975). Small-amplitude, short-duration, polyphasic MUAPs may be noted (Prineas et al., 1965; Smith and Stern, 1967; Frame et al., 1968; Patten et al., 1974; Mallette et al., 1975; Schott and Wills, 1975; Irani, 1976). The more severe the disease, the more prominent are the short duration potentials. In long-standing disease, high-amplitude, long-duration MUAPs may be observed. Single-fiber EMG demonstrates increased jitter without significant blocking (Lunghall et al., 1984).

Histopathology

Muscle biopsies reveal type 2 fiber atrophy and, occasionally, atrophy of type 1 fibers (Kaminski and Ruff, 1994).

Pathogenesis

The mechanism of weakness in hyperparathyroidism and osteomalacia is not known. Parathyroid hormone increases muscle proteolysis (Garber, 1983; Baczynski et al., 1985) and, at the same time, impairs energy production and utilization (Hall et al., 1984). In addition, parathyroid hormone may diminish the sensitivity of contractile apparatus to calcium (Kaminski and Ruff, 1994). Importantly, calcium and phosphate levels do not correlate well with the clinical severity of muscle weakness (Frame et al., 1968; Smith and Stern, 1969; Patten et al., 1974). Vitamin D may also have a direct effect on muscle by increasing muscle ATP concentration, accelerating amino acid incorporation into muscle proteins (Birge and Haddad, 1975), and increasing the uptake of calcium by the sarcoplasmic reticulum and mitochondria (Curry et al., 1974; Pointon et al., 1979).

Treatment

Both medical treatment and surgery are effective in the myopathy associated with hyperparathyroidism, and improvement in muscle strength is usually noticeable within a few months (Patten et al., 1974; Kissel and Mendell, 1992; Norton and Sugg, 1994; Nussbaum et al., 1994). Parathyroidectomy is the treatment of choice in symptomatic patients with primary hyperparathyroidism (Norton and Sugg, 1994). Asymptomatic patients or patients with significant perioperative risk may be managed medically (Nussbaum et al., 1994). Patients with secondary hyperparathyroidism usually improve with vitamin D and calcium replacement. Those with end-stage renal failure may respond to renal transplantation. In addition, a subtotal parathyroidectomy can be performed in patients with secondary hyperparathyroidism. Osteomalacic myopathy improves after vitamin D and calcium replacement (Smith and Stern, 1967, 1969; Schott and Wills, 1975; Skaria et al., 1975; Irani, 1976; Goldring et al., 1994; Russell, 1994).

HYPERPARATHYROIDISM AND MOTOR NEURON DISEASE

Rare reports of a condition that mimics amyotrophic lateral sclerosis have been reported in patients with hyperparathyroidism (Patten et al., 1974; Carnevale et al., 1992; Gelinas et al., 1994). Some of these patients improved after resection of parathyroid adenomas. However, close review of the description of these patients suggests that they did not have amyotrophic lateral sclerosis but, instead, hyperparathyroid myopathy (Jackson et al., 1998). In our experience, the presence of hyperparathyroidism in patients who meet clinical and electrophysiological criteria for amyotrophic lateral sclerosis is just coincidental. These patients do not improve with parathyroidectomy and continue to deteriorate, similar to patients with amyotrophic lateral sclerosis (Jackson et al., 1998).

HYPOPARATHYROIDISM

Clinical Features

Myopathy is uncommon in hypoparathyroidism, although tetany secondary to hypocalcemia may occur. Chvostek's and Trousseau's signs can be demonstrated in hypocalcemic patients. Rarely, patients have mild proximal weakness (Wolf et al., 1972; Snowdon et al., 1976; Kruse et al., 1982; Yamaguchi et al., 1987). There is one report of a single patient who developed painless myoglobinuria without objective weakness or tetany (Akmal, 1993).

Laboratory Features

Serum parathyroid hormone and calcium levels are low, whereas serum phosphate levels are high (Hower et al., 1972; Shane et al., 1980). Serum creatine kinase can be normal or mildly elevated.

Electromyography and Nerve Conduction Studies

Motor and sensory NCSs are normal. EMG reveals normal insertional activity and no positive sharp waves or fibrillation potentials. The most striking abnormality noted are fasciculation potentials and doublets, triplets, or multiplets (Kugelberg, 1946; Denslow, 1948; Kugelberg, 1948; Partanen and Lang, 1978; Swash and Schwartz, 1988; Amato and Dumitru, 2002). Hyperventilation increases the frequency of these abnormal potentials. Otherwise, MUAP morphology and recruitment are normal.

Histopathology

Muscle biopsy samples may reveal nonspecific myopathic features (e.g., mild variability in fiber size, increased internal nuclei, and scattered necrotic and regenerating muscle fibers) that may reflect muscle damage secondary to episodes of tetany (Hudgson and Kendall-Taylor, 1992; Kissel and Mendell, 1992; Kaminski and Ruff, 1994). Metabolic analysis can demonstrate decreased glycogen phosphorylase activity (Kaminski and Ruff, 1994).

Pathogenesis

Decreased parathyroid hormone results in diminished synthesis of 1,25-dihydroxyvitamin D, hypocalcemia, and hyperphosphatemia. Osteomalacia can also develop in association with hypoparathyroidism. However, the pathogenic basis of the myopathy associated with hypoparathyroidism is poorly understood. The elevated serum creatine kinase and mild histological abnormalities on muscle biopsy are generally considered to be secondary to tetany. Tetany is caused by the decreased serum calcium concentration that shifts the activation potential of peripheral nerves toward their resting membrane potential (Brink, 1954; Frankenhaeuser, 1957; Frankenhaeuser and Hodgkin, 1957; Akmal, 1993). Thus, the peripheral nerves are hyperexcitable; less current is required to elicit an action potential, which may lead to tetany.

Treatment

Correction of the hypocalcemia and hyperphosphatemia with vitamin D and calcium administration results in the return of muscle strength and resolution of tetany (Wolf et al., 1972; Yamaguchi et al., 1987).

Adrenal Disorders

Increased and decreased corticosteroid levels can result in myopathies. Increased corticosteroid may be endogenous, related to enhanced production, or may be exogenous, caused by iatrogenic administration.

STEROID MYOPATHY

Clinical Features

Endogenous (adrenal or pituitary tumor) or exogenous (corticosteroid medication administration) corticosteroids can result in a myopathy. Steroid myopathy is the most common endocrine-related myopathy. Patients with steroid myopathy present with proximal muscle weakness and atrophy that is worse in the legs than in the arms (Muller and Kugelberg, 1959; Williams, 1959; Golding et al., 1962; Coomes, 1965; Engel, 1988; Kissel and Mendell, 1992; Kaminski and Ruff, 1994). The distal extremities and oculobulbar and facial muscles are normal, as are sensation and the deep tendon reflexes. An increase in truncal adipose tissue and pigmentation of the skin also develop over time (so-called cushingoid appearance).

The incidence of exogenous corticosteroid myopathy is unknown. Women are at greater risk for the development of exogenous steroid myopathy than are men, by approximately 2:1, but the reason is unclear. An increased risk of myopathy is seen with prednisone at dosages of 30 mg/d or more (or equivalent doses of other corticosteroids) (Kissel and Mendell, 1992). Any synthetic corticosteroid can cause the myopathy, but those that are fluorinated (triamcinolone > betamethasone > dexamethasone) are associated with a greater risk than nonfluorinated compounds (Faludi et al., 1967). Importantly, alternate-day dosing and pulsed corticosteroids (e.g., once-a-week or once-a-month dosing) reduces the risk of corticosteroid-induced weakness. Muscle weakness usually develops after the long-term administration of high-dose oral steroids. An acute onset of severe generalized weakness can occur in patients receiving high dosages of intravenous corticosteroids with or without concomitant administration of neuromuscular blocking agents (acute quadriplegic myopathy).

Laboratory Features

The serum creatine kinase level is normal.

Electromyography and Nerve Conduction Studies

Motor and sensory NCSs are normal in steroid myopathy (Buchthal, 1970; Amato and Dumitru, 2002). There is an absence of abnormal insertional or spontaneous activity on EMG. Morphological analysis of the MUAPs is usually normal, but a mild reduction in the maximum peak-to-peak MUAP amplitude during maximal recruitment has been described (Muller and Kugelberg, 1959; Golding et al., 1962; Coomes, 1965; Pleasure et al., 1970; Amato and Dumitru, 2002). The lack of significant abnormalities is understandable given the fact that type 2 muscle fibers are preferentially involved in steroid myopathy (see later). In this regard, type 1 muscle fibers are the first recruited motor units. Because type 1 fibers are not affected as severely as are type 2 fibers, the EMG is normal.

Histopathology

Muscle biopsy samples reveal a preferential atrophy of type 2B fibers, the fast-twitch glycolytic type fibers (Hudgson and Kendall-Taylor, 1992; Kissel and Mendell, 1992; Kaminski and Ruff, 1994) (Fig. 78–1). There may also be a lesser degree of atrophy of type 1 and 2A muscle fibers. Increased lipid droplets may also be seen in type 1 fibers.

Pathogenesis

The exact mechanism of corticosteroid myopathy is unknown but may be related to decreased protein synthesis, increased protein degradation, alterations in carbohydrate metabolism, mitochondrial alterations, or reduced sarcolemmal excitability (Kissel and Mendell, 1992; Kaminski and Ruff, 1994).

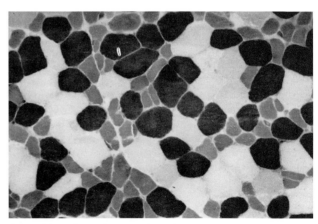

Figure 78–1. Steroid myopathy. Muscle biopsy sample demonstrates type 2B muscle fiber atrophy (intermediate staining fibers are type 2B) (ATPase pH 4.6).

Treatment

Steroid myopathy is treated by stopping the offending medication or by reducing its dose (Faludi et al., 1967; Kissel and Mendell, 1992; Amato and Barohn; 1997b). In many cases, however, corticosteroids are necessary to treat an underlying autoimmune disorder. Tapering to an alternate-day dosing or switching to a weekly or monthly pulsed-regimen steroid may be required in such instances. In addition, patients should be encouraged to exercise to help prevent concomitant disuse atrophy.

A particular problem for clinicians is determining whether progressive or recurrent weakness in a neuromuscular patient being treated with corticosteroids is related to an exacerbation of their underling autoimmune disease (e.g., inflammatory myopathy, myasthenia gravis, chronic inflammatory demyelinating polyneuropathy) versus steroid myopathy (MacLean and Schurr, 1959; Williams, 1959; Afifi et al., 1968; Amato and Barohn, 1997b). After an initial improvement, some patients experience a subsequent decline in muscle function. If the weakness developed while the patient was on tapered steroids, relapse of the underlying disease process is more likely. In contrast, a steroid-induced myopathy needs to be considered when progressive weakness evolves while the patient is on long-term corticosteroids at high doses. Laboratory, radiological, and electrodiagnostic studies may be useful in the case of an inflammatory myopathy. An increasing serum creatine kinase level or signal abnormalities on skeletal muscle magnetic resonance images reflective of edema or inflammation would point to an exacerbation of the myositis (Amato and Barohn, 1997b). In addition, an electromyogram can be useful in that it is usually normal in steroid-induced myopathy, in contrast to the prominent increase in spontaneous activity, myopathic MUAPs, and early recruitment typically seen in inflammatory myopathies. However, in some instances, it is impossible to determine with certainty whether a patient's weakness is related to a relapse of their underlying autoimmune myositis or secondary to a steroid myopathy. In these cases, I taper the steroid medication and closely observe the patient. If the patient deteriorates, the weakness is presumed to be secondary to the underlying neuromuscular disease, and the patient may require increased doses of corticosteroids or the addition of other immunosuppressive medications. If improvement occurs with taper of the corticosteroids, then the weakness is presumed to be steroid myopathy.

ADRENAL INSUFFICIENCY

Adrenal insufficiency can result from intrinsic gland dysfunction or pituitary hypofunction (Prineas et al., 1968; Engel, 1988; Kissel and Mendell, 1992; Kaminski and Ruff, 1994). Subjective weakness and fatigue commonly occur with adrenal insufficiency. Objective weakness is usually related to electrolyte disturbances (e.g., hyperkalemia) or concurrent endocrinopathies associated with panhypopituitarism (e.g., secondary hypothyroidism). The electrodiagnostic evaluation is usually completely normal in patients with adrenal insufficiency. The patients improve with replacement of adrenal hormones.

Pituitary Disorders

ACROMEGALY

Clinical Features

Although most patients with acromegaly have normal strength, some individuals develop insidious proximal muscle weakness over time (Mastaglia et al., 1970; Lewis, 1972; Pickett et al., 1975; Engel, 1988; Kissel and Mendell, 1992; Kaminski and Ruff, 1994). Some weak muscle groups appear hypertrophic. In addition to the myopathy, bony overgrowth related to acromegaly can result in nerve root and spinal cord compression. Patients are also predisposed to the development of entrapment neuropathies such as carpal and tarsal tunnel syndromes.

Laboratory Features

Serum creatine kinase levels may be normal or mildly elevated.

Electromyography and Nerve Conduction Studies

NCSs are normal unless the patient has a related entrapment neuropathy (Stewart, 1966; Lundberg et al., 1970; Mastaglia et al., 1970; Low et al., 1974; Amato and Dumitru, 2002). EMG in patients with the myopathy reveals an absence of abnormal insertional or spontaneous activity. Short-duration, low-amplitude MUAPs may be detected in proximal muscle groups (Mastaglia et al., 1970; Lewis, 1972; Pickett et al., 1975; Amato and Dumitru, 2002). When there is superimposed entrapment of a peripheral nerve or nerve root present, EMG may reveal signs of active denervation (e.g., fibrillation potentials, positive sharp waves) and chronic neurogenic appearing MUAPs.

Histopathology

Muscle biopsy samples reveal scattered necrotic fibers and increased variability in muscle fiber size with hypertrophy and atrophy involving type 1 and type 2 fibers (Mastaglia et al., 1970; Stern et al., 1974). Electron microscopy demonstrates myofibrillar degeneration and increased glycogen deposition.

Pathogenesis

The severity of muscle weakness correlates with the duration of acromegaly rather than with the levels of serum growth hormone (Pickett et al., 1975). Growth hormone increases protein synthesis in muscle, which may lead to muscle fiber hypertrophy (Bigland and Jehring, 1952; Prysor-Jones and Jenkins, 1980). Individuals with acromegaly have lower-than-normal respiratory quotients of their resting muscles (Rabinowitz and Zierler, 1963). In addition, there is an increase in fatty acid oxidation and decreased utilization of glucose in acromegalic patients (Winckler et al., 1964). Therefore, exacerbated growth hormone production leads to preferential utilization of lipids over carbohydrates in muscle. In addition, myofibrillary ATPase activity is reduced (Florini and Ewton, 1989). These factors likely affect the dynamic properties of muscle activity. Further, muscle membranes may be slightly depolarized, rendering them less excitable (Kaminski and Ruff, 1994).

Treatment

Radiation or surgery to remove or reduce the size of the pituitary tumor lowers growth hormone levels and may lead to improved muscle strength (Pickett et al., 1975).

PANHYPOPITUITARISM

Pituitary failure in adults commonly leads to muscle weakness and fatigue due to secondary thyroidism and adrenal insufficiency (Brasel et al., 1965). Growth hormone deficiency may also cause muscle weakness in adults. Deficiency of growth hormone may have a greater role in the myopathy associated with prepubertal panhypopituitarism. Prepubertal panhypopituitarism results in dwarfism and muscle weakness. Patients with prepubertal panhypopituitarism do not significantly improve in regard to muscle strength unless growth hormone is replaced along with adrenal and thyroid hormones (Raben, 1962).

Pancreas Disorders

Peripheral neuropathies are the most common neuromuscular complication associated with diabetes mellitus. The only myopathy associated with diabetes mellitus is muscle infarction.

DIABETIC MUSCLE INFARCTION

Clinical Features

Poorly controlled diabetic patients may develop ischemia and infarction of their muscles. The most common muscles are those in the thigh (quadriceps and hamstrings), but the calf muscles may also be affected (Banker and Chester, 1973; Chester and Banker, 1986; Barohn and Kissel, 1992). Diabetic muscle infarction manifests as an acute onset of pain and swelling, usually in the thigh. The infarct resolves spontaneously over several weeks, although it may recur in the contralateral leg.

Laboratory Features

Serum creatine kinase levels are generally normal but may be elevated if there is significant muscle infarction. Magnetic resonance imaging or computed tomography of the thigh demonstrates signal abnormalities in the affected muscle or muscles.

Electromyography and Nerve Conduction Studies

Motor and sensory NCSs in patients with concomitant diabetic neuropathy may be abnormal. EMG of the involved muscle or muscles demonstrates fibrillation potentials and positive sharp waves as well as small, polyphasic MUAPs with early recruitment (Banker and Chester, 1973).

Histopathology

Biopsy should be avoided, if possible, because it can lead to significant hemorrhage into the infarcted muscle and worsening of symptoms (Barohn and Kissel, 1992). However, when muscle biopsies have been performed, they have demonstrated large areas of necrosis, edema, and inflammatory infiltrate. Also, there is endothelial hyperplasia, and the lumens of small and medium-sized blood vessels may be filled with fibrin, calcium, and lipid debris (Barohn and Kissel, 1992).

Pathogenesis

The ischemic damage results from long-standing, diabetic vasculopathy.

Treatment

Treatment consists of immobilization and pain control.

TOXIC MYOPATHIES

There are numerous drugs and chemicals that are toxic to muscle (Lane and Mastaglia, 1978; Kuncl and Wiggins, 1988; Mastaglia, 1992; Victor and Sieb, 1994; Amato and Dumitru, 2002) (Table 78–1). The various mechanisms of myotoxicity are highly diverse and are directly dependent on the specific toxin in question. Chemicals can directly or indirectly affect muscle tissue. The direct affect can be focal, as might occur secondary to the injection of a drug into tissue, or generalized. Indirect or secondary toxic effects may result from the substance creating an electrolyte imbalance (e.g., diuretics) or inducing an immunological response (e.g., adulterated tryptophan) or from ischemia due to secondary vasculitis or vasospasm (e.g., heroin).

Table 78–1. Toxic Myopathies

Necrotizing myopathies
  Cholesterol-lowering agents (fibric acid derivatives,
    hydroxymethyl glutaryl coenzyme A reductase inhibitors,
    niacin)
  Immunophilins (cyclosporine, tacrolimus)
  Labetalol
  Propofol
  ε-Aminocaproic acid
Amphiphilic agents
  Chloroquine
  Hydroxychloroquine
  Amiodarone
Antimicrotubular agents
  Colchicine
  Vincristine
Mitochondrial myopathies
  Zidovudine (azidothymidine)
Inflammatory myopathies
  Eosinophilia-myalgia syndrome (L-tryptophan)
  Toxic oil syndrome (rapeseed oil)
  D-Penicillamine
  Cimetidine
  Procainamide
  Levodopa
  Phenytoin
  Lamotrigine
Myopathies caused by impaired protein synthesis or catabolism
  Corticosteroids (e.g., steroid myopathy)
  Finasteride
Hypokalemic myopathies
  Genetic disorder (e.g., familial hypokalemic periodic paralysis
    or renal tubular acidosis)
  Diuretics
  Laxatives
  Mineralocorticoids
  Amphotericin
  Lithium
  Alcohol abuse
  Inhalation of toluene
Myopathies caused by multifactorial processes or of unclear
    pathogenesis
  Emetine
  Elinafide
  Omeprazole
  Acute quadriplegic myopathy/critical illness myopathy (high-
    dose corticosteroids, nondepolarizing neuromuscular
    blocking agents, sepsis)
  Alcohol abuse
  Illicit drugs (intramuscular or intravenous injections:
    pentazocine, piritramide, amphetamines, heroin,
    meperidine, cocaine; inhalation of volatile agents: toluene)

A toxic myopathy may manifest with relatively mild myalgias or severe generalized weakness. Obtaining a history and physical examination is obviously crucial to making an accurate diagnosis. Further evaluation, including serum creatine kinase level determination, EMG/NCS, and muscle biopsy, may be necessary. Early diagnosis is essential because most patients recover when the offending agent is withdrawn, provided irreversible muscle damage has not occurred.

This section reviews the clinical, laboratory, and histopathological features and pathogenic mechanisms of toxic myopathies to aid clinicians in making an accurate diagnosis. Further, by understanding the pathophysiology at the cellular level, the electromy-ographer can better appreciate the neurophysiological correlates to muscle injury. Thus, in addressing the toxic myopathies, I have classified the toxic myopathies according to their presumed pathogenic mechanisms (see Table 78–1).

Necrotizing Myopathies

Several drugs can cause a focal or generalized necrotizing myopathy. Focal disorders may be diagnosed on the basis of their highly localized nature within select muscle groups predisposed to muscular injection sites. In these disorders, there is an absence of more widespread complaints or abnormalities. More generalized problems present as diffuse myalgias or weakness that may be accompanied by myoglobinuria.

CHOLESTEROL-LOWERING DRUGS

Cholesterol-lowering agents are widely prescribed and probably are the most common medications implicated in causing toxic myopathy. These cholesterol-lowering agents, which include fibric acid derivatives (Langer and Levy, 1968; Denizot et al., 1973; Pierides et al., 1975; Gabriel and Pearce, 1976; Kwiecinski, 1978; Abourizk et al., 1979; Rush et al., 1986; Marais and Larson, 1990; Pierce et al., 1990; London et al., 1991; Magarian and Lucas, 1991; Shepherd, 1995), 3-hydroxy-3-methyl-glutaryl-coenzyme A reductase (3-HMG-CoA reductase) inhibitors (Corpier et al., 1988; Reaven and Witzum, 1988; Tobert, 1988a, 1988b; Marais and Larson, 1990; Berland et al., 1991; Deslypere and Vermuelen, 1991; Schalke et al., 1992; Bakker-Arema et al., 1997; Davidson et al., 1997) and niacin (Reaven and Witzum, 1988; Litin and Andersone, 1989), can all result in an acute or a more insidiously developing myopathy. Patients may complain of muscle tenderness, cramps, or weakness. When the myopathy is severe, myoglobinuria may occur. The myopathy can present several days to years after beginning the offending agent. On stopping the medication, symptoms tend to completely resolve in several days to months. The following is a discussion regarding necrotizing myopathies in the specific subclasses of cholesterol-lowering agents.

Fibric Acid Derivatives

Clinical Features

Clofibrate and gemfibrozil are branched-chain fatty acid esters and are used for the treatment of hyperlipidemia. A toxic myopathy usually presents within 2 or 3 months after starting the drug but may not manifest until a few years after initiation of the medication (Langer and Levy, 1968; Denizot et al., 1973; Pierides et al., 1975; Gabriel and Pearce, 1976; Abourizk et al., 1979; Rush et al., 1986; Marais and Larson, 1990; Pierce et al., 1990; London et al., 1991; Magarian and Lucas, 1991; Shepherd, 1995; Duell et al., 1998). Generalized weakness, myalgias, cramps, and occasionally myoglobinuria develop. Renal insufficiency and the concurrent administration of an HMG-CoA inhibitor predispose patients to the development of a severe myopathy.

Laboratory Features

Elevated serum creatine kinase levels are usually noted.

Electromyography and Nerve Conduction Studies

Motor and sensory NCSs are completely normal (Langer and Levy, 1968; Pierides et al., 1975; Gabriel and Pearce, 1976; Amato and Dumitru, 2002). Needle EMG demonstrates normal MUAPs in mildly affected individuals. However, fibrillation potentials, positive sharp waves, complex repetitive discharges, and myotonic discharges along with small-amplitude, short-duration MUAPs may be noted in weak muscles (Denizot et al., 1973; Kra, 1974; Abourizk et al., 1979; Rush et al., 1986; Hudgson and Kendall-Taylor, 1992; Amato and Dumitru, 2002). Myotonic discharges have also been demonstrated in animals that were administered clofibrate (Kwiecinski, 1978).

Histopathology

Muscle biopsy samples have demonstrated scattered muscle fiber necrosis (Fig. 78–2). Clofibrate causes noninflammatory necrosis of muscle tissue with fiber size variation and groups of small atrophic muscle fibers in animals (Afifi et al., 1984).

Pathogenesis

The pathogenic mechanism of the myopathy associated with fibric acid derivatives is not known. These medications may destabilize the lipophilic

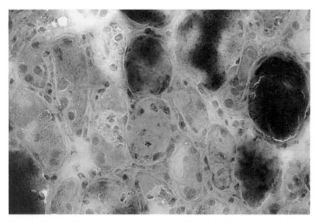

Figure 78–2. Necrotizing myopathy. Muscle biopsy sample from a patient in whom a severe myopathy (generalized weakness, myalgias, elevated serum creatine kinase levels, and myoglobinuria) developed while receiving lovastatin and gemfibrozil reveals widespread necrosis of muscle fibers (hematoxylin and eosin stain).

muscle membrane, resulting in necrosis of muscle fibers (Pierce et al., 1990).

Hydroxymethyl Glutaryl Coenzyme A Reductase Inhibitors

Clinical Features

3-HMG-CoA reductase is a rate-controlling enzyme in cholesterol synthesis. Myalgias, proximal weakness, and, less commonly, myoglobinuria, have been reported with all of the major HMG-CoA reductase inhibitors: lovastatin (Corpier et al., 1988; Reaven and Witzum, 1988; Tobert, 1988a, 1988b; Marais and Larson, 1990; Shepherd, 1995; Jones et al., 1998), simvastatin (Berland et al., 1991; Deslypere and Vermuelen, 1991; Davidson et al., 1997; Galper, 1998; Jones et al., 1998), provastatin (Schalke et al., 1992; Jones et al., 1998), atorvastatin (Bakker-Arema et al., 1997; Duell et al., 1998; Jones et al., 1998), fluvastatin (Jones et al., 1998), and cerivastatin (Jones et al., 1998; von Keutz and Schluter, 1998). The incidence of elevated serum creatine kinase, symptomatic myopathy, or both varies from series to series but is generally considered to be low. In a large study of more than 6,500 patients treated with lovastatin, 35% of patients had an elevated serum creatine kinase level sometime during the study (Dujovne et al., 1991). However, 29% of patients receiving placebo had similar creatine kinase elevations (Dujovne et al., 1991). Approximately 7% to 9% of patients in both the treatment and placebo groups complained of muscle discomfort during the study. Nevertheless, only 0.08% of patients had clinical evidence of myopathy (e.g., objective weakness). Other studies have reported asymptomatic serum creatine kinase elevations in approximately 1% of patients taking lovastatin (Tobert, 1988a, 1988b; Thompson et al., 1991).

Myopathy has also been reported in patients receiving the newer statin medications, although the incidence of myotoxicity may be less with these new agents than that seen with lovastatin. Only 0.08% of 2,361 patients treated with simvastatin developed signs of a toxic myopathy, and the incidence appears to be dose related (Boccuzzi et al., 1991). Similarly, only 0.01% of patients receiving provastatin developed significantly elevated (>10 times normal) serum creatine kinase levels attributable to the drug (Shepherd, 1995). Only a few cases of toxic myopathy have been ascribed to atorvastatin (Bakker-Arema et al., 1997; Duell et al., 1998; Jones et al., 1998). In a review of 337 patients receiving atorvastatin, only 2 individuals had creatine kinase elevations greater than five times normal, and both patients were asymptomatic (Bakker-Arema et al., 1997). Three patients developed muscle pains, but they had normal serum creatine kinase levels. In an 8-week trial that compared the efficacy and safety of lovastatin, simvastatin, provastatin, atorvastatin, and fluvastatin in 518 patients with hypercholesterolemia, myalgias were reported in approximately

1.5% of patients in each treatment group (Jones et al., 1998). No patient had elevated serum creatine kinase levels greater than three times normal. However, interpretation of the study is limited by the short duration of treatment (8 weeks) and the small numbers in each treatment group.

The risk of myotoxicity is markedly increased by the concomitant use of fibric acids (Reaven and Witzum, 1988; Tobert, 1988a, 1988b; Litin and Andersone, 1989; Pierce et al., 1990; Duell et al., 1998), niacin (Reaven and Witzum, 1988), erythromycin (Ayanian et al., 1988), and cyclosporine (Tobert, 1988a, 1988b). In this regard, approximately 5% of patients taking both lovastatin and gemfibrozil developed a severe myopathy (Pierce et al., 1990), whereas a severe myopathy occurred in as many as 30% of patients receiving both lovastatin and cyclosporine (Corpier et al., 1988; Tobert, 1988a, 1988b). Renal and liver dysfunction also increases the risk of statin-induced myotoxicity.

Laboratory Features

Asymptomatic elevations of serum creatine kinase occur in 1% to 35% of patients receiving statin medications, and the levels may be as much as 1,000 times normal in patients with severe myotoxicity.

Electromyography and Nerve Conduction Studies

Routine motor and sensory NCSs are normal. EMG reveals fibrillation potentials, positive sharp waves, and short-duration MUAPs that recruit early significantly weak muscles. Patients with asymptomatic serum creatine kinase elevations usually have normal EMG studies.

Histopathology

Biopsy samples demonstrate muscle fiber necrosis and phagocytosis in severely affected patients (see Fig. 78–2). Subsarcolemmal accumulation of autophagic lysosomes is apparent on electron microscopy. One study reported mild inflammatory infiltrate and membrane attack complex deposition on small blood vessels reminiscent of dermatomyositis in a patient who developed severe proximal weakness, elevated serum creatine kinase levels, and an erythematous rash while being treated with provastatin (Schalke et al., 1992).

Pathogenesis

The pathogenic basis for the toxic myopathy caused by HMG-CoA reductase inhibitors is unknown. Mevalonate is the immediate product of HMG-CoA reductase metabolism (Flint et al., 1997). Subsequently, mevalonate is metabolized to farnesol, which is converted to either squalene or geranylgeraniol. Squalene is the first metabolite committed to the synthesis of cholesterol. In contrast, geranylgeraniol is important in the biosynthesis of

coenzyme Q_{10} (a mitochondrial enzyme important in the production of ATP), dolichol (important in glycoprotein synthesis), isopentyladine (a component of transfer RNA), and in the activation of regulatory proteins (G proteins) (Flint et al., 1997; Galper, 1998). The lipid-lowering affect of HMG-CoA reductase inhibitors may disrupt the cholesterol content in muscle membranes, predisposing the muscle fibers to rhabdomyolysis (London et al., 1991). However, other studies provide evidence that depletion of the metabolites of geranylgeraniol, and not the inhibition of cholesterol synthesis, is the primary cause of myotoxicity (Flint et al., 1997a). In addition, HMG-CoA reductase inhibitors decrease the levels of coenzyme Q, which could impair energy production and result in muscle fiber destruction (Folkers et al., 1990).

Niacin

There are only a few reports of myopathy in patients treated with niacin (Reaven and Witzum, 1988; Litin and Andersone, 1989). Three patients developed myalgias and elevated serum creatine kinase levels (up to 10-fold increase). The symptoms improved and creatine kinase levels normalized after the discontinuation of niacin. Electrodiagnostic studies and muscle biopsies were not performed. In another report, rhabdomyolysis occurred in association with lovastatin and niacin (Reaven and Witzum, 1988). Because niacin can inhibit HMG-CoA reductase, the pathogenic mechanism of the toxic myopathy may be similar to that of the statins.

IMMUNOPHILINS: CYCLOSPORINE AND TACROLIMUS

Clinical Features

The immunophilins (cyclosporine and tacrolimus) are commonly used immunosuppressive agents, especially in transplantation recipients (Amato and Barohn, 1997a). Myalgias and proximal muscle weakness usually develop within a few months after the start of cyclosporine (Noppen et al., 1987; Costigan, 1989; Goy et al., 1989; Grezard et al., 1990; Arellano and Krup, 1991; Amato and Barohn, 1997a). Myoglobinuria may also occur especially in patients also receiving cholesterol-lowering agents or colchicine (Norman et al., 1988; Tobert, 1988a, 1988b; Rieger et al., 1990; Volin et al., 1990). Myoglobinuria and hypertrophic cardiomyopathy with congestive heart failure have also occurred in patients taking tacrolimus (Atkinson et al., 1995; Hibi et al., 1995). Myalgias, muscle strength, and cardiac function improve with reduction or discontinuation of the offending agent.

Laboratory Features

Serum creatine kinase levels are usually elevated.

Electromyography and Nerve Conduction Studies

NCSs are normal. EMG is remarkable for increased muscle membrane instability (e.g., fibrillation potentials, positive sharp waves, and myotonic potentials) and the early recruitment of small-amplitude, short-duration MUAPs (Costigan, 1989).

Histopathology

Muscle biopsy samples demonstrate necrosis, vacuoles, and type 2 muscle fiber atrophy.

Pathogenesis

The pathogenic basis of immunophilin-induced myopathy and cardiomyopathy is not known. The agents may destabilize the lipophilic membranes, causing muscle fiber degeneration, similar to the cholesterol-lowering agents. In this regard, cyclosporine does have a cholesterol-lowering effect. This may explain the increased risk of myotoxicity in patients receiving cyclosporine and the more classic lipid-lowering agents (e.g., fibric acid derivatives, statins).

LABETALOL

Clinical Features

Rare cases of necrotizing myopathy have occurred in patients receiving the antihypertensive medication labetalol (Teicher et al., 1981; Willis et al., 1990). Proximal weakness or myalgias may develop acutely or evolve insidiously. Symptoms resolve after discontinuation of the medication.

Laboratory Features

Serum creatine kinase can be markedly elevated.

Electromyography and Nerve Conduction Studies

EMG demonstrates increased insertional and spontaneous activity with fibrillation potentials and positive sharp waves. Early recruitment of short-duration, small-amplitude, polyphasic MUAPs is seen.

Histopathology

Routine light microscopy may be normal (Teicher et al., 1981) or reveal necrotic and regenerating fibers (Willis et al., 1990). Electron microscopy revealed subsarcolemmal vacuoles in one case (Teicher et al., 1981).

Pathogenesis

The pathogenic etiology for the muscle necrosis seen is not known.

PROPOFOL

Clinical Features

Propofol is an anesthetic agent used for the sedation of mechanically ventilated patients and for the treatment of status epilepticus. Rhabdomyolysis with myoglobinuria, metabolic acidosis, hypoxia, and myocardial arrest occurred in children treated with propofol (Hanna and Ramundo, 1988; Parke et al., 1992; Strickland and Murray, 1995). The syndrome differs from malignant hyperthermia because of the lack of persistent hyperthermia and muscular rigidity. In addition, acute quadriplegic myopathy has occurred in patients treated with propofol and high-dose intravenous corticosteroids in intensive care units (Hanson et al., 1997). The myopathy in these critically ill patients may be due to the high-dose corticosteroids rather than the use of propofol (see acute quadriplegic myopathy later).

Laboratory Features

Serum creatine kinase levels are markedly elevated, and myoglobinuria with renal failure can be seen. Serum chemistries and blood gas analyses demonstrate severe metabolic acidosis and hypoxemia. Hyperkalemia can also develop secondary to massive muscle destruction.

Electromyography and Nerve Conduction Studies

Electrophysiological studies have not been performed or were not reported in the cases associated with rhabdomyolysis in children. Adult patients with acute quadriplegic myopathy had low-amplitude compound muscle action potentials (CMAPs), profuse fibrillation potentials and positive sharp waves, and early recruitment of short-duration, small-amplitude polyphasic MUAPs (Hanson et al., 1997).

Histopathology

Muscle biopsy samples reveal necrosis of skeletal and cardiac muscle (Hanna and Ramundo, 1988; Parke et al., 1992; Strickland and Murray, 1995). The patients who developed acute quadriplegic myopathy had prominent necrosis and loss of thick filaments (Hanson et al., 1997).

Pathogenesis

The mechanism for muscle destruction is unknown.

Treatment

Propofol should be discontinued, and supportive therapy for myoglobinuria, metabolic acidosis, hyperkalemia, and renal failure should be instituted.

∊-Aminocaproic Acid

Clinical Features

∊-Aminocaproic acid, a monoaminocarboxylic acid, is a drug used in the past to reduce the incidence of recurrent hemorrhage after the recent rupture of an intracranial aneurysm. Its mode of action as an antifibrinolytic is believed to be through inhibition of plasminogen activation to plasmin. Some patients receiving the drug for a period of 4 to 7 weeks developed severe muscle pain in the calves or about the shoulder and pelvic girdle regions (MacKay et al., 1978; Lane et al., 1979; Britt et al., 1980; Kennard et al., 1980; Brown et al., 1982; Vanneste and van Wijngaarden, 1982; Morris et al., 1983). Proximal muscle weakness and myoglobinuria also occurred.

Laboratory Features

Serum creatine kinase levels are usually markedly elevated in cases of severe necrotizing myopathy and myoglobinuria.

Electromyography and Nerve Conduction Studies

Motor and sensory NCSs are normal. EMG usually reveals early recruitment of small-amplitude, short-duration MUAPs (MacKay et al., 1978; Vanneste and van Wijngaarden, 1982; Morris et al., 1983; Amato and Dumitru, 2002). Profuse fibrillation potentials, positive sharp waves, complex repetitive discharges, and myotonic discharges are detected in some individuals, although a few patients with mild disease failed to reveal any abnormal spontaneous potentials (MacKay et al., 1978; Lane et al., 1979; Britt et al., 1980; Brown et al., 1982; Vanneste and van Wijngaarden, 1982; Morris et al., 1983).

Histopathology

Muscle biopsy samples reveal significant degrees of segmental myonecrosis and scattered regenerating muscle fibers.

Pathogenesis

The pathogenic mechanism is not known but may be related to ischemia caused by thrombosis of small capillaries (Kennard et al., 1980).

Treatment

After drug cessation, both the myopathy and electrical abnormalities resolve over the course of several months.

Amphiphilic Drug Myopathy (Drug-Induced Autophagic Lysosomal Myopathy)

Amphiphilic drugs contain a hydrophobic region and a hydrophilic region that contains a primary or substituted positively charged amine group. These properties account for the ability of the drugs to interact with the anionic phospholipids of cell membranes and organelles. A toxic neuropathy can also occur with these medications, and the neuropathy may be more severe than the myopathy.

Chloroquine

Clinical Features

Chloroquine is a quinoline derivative used for the treatment of malaria, sarcoidosis, systemic lupus erythematosus, scleroderma, and rheumatoid arthritis (Eadie and Ferrier, 1966; Mastaglia et al., 1977; Estes et al., 1987; Mastaglia, 1992). Slowly progressive, painless, proximal weakness and atrophy can develop in patients on chloroquine. The legs are more severely affected than are the arms. In addition, cardiomyopathy can occur. Further, sensation is often diminished secondary to a superimposed neuropathy. Deep tendon reflexes may be diminished, particularly at the ankle. The "neuromyopathy" appears to be dose related and generally occurs in patients who have taken 500 mg per day for 1 year. However, the neuromyopathy can develop with doses as low as 200 mg per day. The neuromyopathy is reversible after discontinuation of the medication.

Laboratory Features

Serum creatine kinase levels are usually elevated.

Electromyography and Nerve Conduction Studies

Patients with a superimposed neuropathy demonstrate a mild to moderate reduction in the CMAP and sensory nerve action potential (SNAP) amplitudes, along with mild slowing of both motor and sensory NCSs (Mastaglia et al., 1977; Estes et al., 1987; Amato and Dumitru, 2002). Patients with only the myopathy usually have normal NCSs (Eadie and Ferrier, 1966). On EMG, there is an increase in insertional activity with significant amounts of positive sharp waves, fibrillation potentials, and myotonic discharges, primarily in the proximal limb muscles (Eadie and Ferrier, 1966; Mastaglia et al., 1977; Estes et al., 1987; Amato and Dumitru, 2002). Small-amplitude, short-duration, polyphasic MUAPs that recruit early may be noted.

Histopathology

The most prominent abnormality is the presence of acid phosphatase–positive vacuoles in as many as 50% of skeletal and cardiac muscle fibers (Eadie and Ferrier, 1966; Mastaglia et al., 1977; Estes et al., 1987; Mastaglia, 1992; Victor and Sieb, 1994). Type 1 fibers are preferentially affected. On electron microscopy, these vacuoles contain concentric lamellar myeloid debris and curvilinear structures. In addition, autophagic vacuoles may be evident on nerve biopsies.

Pathogenesis

As noted previously, the drug is thought to interact with the lipid membranes. The drug-lipid complexes are resistant to digestion by lysosomal enzymes, which results in the formation of the autophagic vacuoles filled with myeloid debris.

HYDROXYCHLOROQUINE

Hydroxychloroquine is structurally similar to chloroquine and produces a neuromyopathy that is similar but usually not as severe as that seen in chloroquine myopathy (Estes et al., 1987). Vacuoles are typically absent on biopsy, but electron microscopy still may demonstrate abnormal myeloid and curvilinear bodies.

AMIODARONE

Clinical Features

Amiodarone is an antiarrhythmic medication that can cause a neuromyopathy similar to that caused by chloroquine (Meier et al., 1979; Costa-Jussa and Jacobs, 1985; Jacobs and Costa-Jussa, 1985; Alderson, et al., 1987; Roth et al., 1990). Severe proximal and distal weakness develops that affects the legs worse than the arms. In addition, distal sensory loss and reduced deep tendon reflexes are seen. In some patients, tremors and ataxia develop. Amiodarone can cause hypothyroidism, which can cause proximal weakness and myalgias. Patients with renal insufficiency may be more at risk for development of the neuromyopathy. Muscle strength gradually improves after discontinuation of the drug.

Laboratory Features

Serum creatine kinase levels are elevated.

Electromyography and Nerve Conduction Studies

Decreased amplitudes of the CMAPs and SNAPs are evident (Meier et al., 1979). Some studies have reported slow conduction velocities (Roth et al., 1990). EMG demonstrates fibrillation potentials and positive sharp waves in proximal and distal muscles. In weak proximal muscles, the MUAPs are typically polyphasic, short in duration, and small in amplitude and recruit early. Distal muscles are more likely to have large-amplitude, long-duration polyphasic MUAPs with decreased recruitment, reflecting the neurogenic component.

Histopathology

Autophagic vacuoles with myeloid inclusions are evident on muscle biopsy samples. In addition, neu-rogenic atrophy can be appreciated, particularly in distal muscles. Besides myeloid debris, electron microscopy reveals myofibrillar disorganization. Myeloid inclusions are also seen on nerve biopsy samples. The lipid membrane inclusions in muscle and nerve biopsy samples have persisted as long as 2 years after discontinuation of the medication.

Pathogenesis

The pathogenesis is presumably similar to that of other amphiphilic medications, such as chloroquine.

Antimicrotubular Myopathies

COLCHICINE

Clinical Features

Colchicine is commonly prescribed for individuals with gout. The medication is weakly amphiphilic, but its therapeutic and toxic effects are thought to be secondary to its binding with tubulin and prevention of the polymerization of tubulin into microtubular structures (Kuncl and Wiggins, 1988; Mastaglia, 1992; Victor and Sieb, 1994). Colchicine can cause both a generalized peripheral neuropathy and myopathy (Kontos, 1962; Riggs et al., 1986; Kuncl et al., 1987, 1989; Kuncl and Wiggins, 1988; Mastaglia, 1992; Victor and Sieb, 1994; Rutkove et al., 1996). The neuromyopathy usually develops in patients older than 50 years, and it usually occurs after long-term use of the medication, but it can also develop secondary to acute intoxication (Riggs et al., 1986; Kuncl et al., 1987, 1989; Kuncl and Wiggins, 1988). Chronic renal failure appears to be a risk factor for development of the neuromyopathy. Patients present with progressive proximal muscle weakness and distal sensory loss over several months. A loss of fine motor coordination may be noted in the hands. The deep tendon reflexes are diminished. Clinical myotonia may rarely be seen (Rutkove et al., 1996). The neuromyopathy generally resolves within 4 to 6 months after the discontinuation of colchicine.

Laboratory Features

Serum creatine kinase levels may be mildly elevated in asymptomatic patients taking colchicine but are elevated up to 50-fold in symptomatic patients.

Electromyography and Nerve Conduction Studies

NCSs commonly reveal prolonged distal motor and sensory latencies along with reduced CMAP and SNAP amplitudes in the arms and legs (Kontos, 1962; Riggs et al., 1986; Kuncl et al., 1987, 1989; Kuncl and Wiggins, 1988; Amato and Dumitru, 2002). EMG of the distal muscles reveals decreased recruitment of long-duration, high-amplitude, polyphasic MUAPs reflective of the neuropathic process. However, EMG of proximal limb muscles reveals early recruitment of polyphasic MUAPs with short durations and low amplitudes, consistent with a superimposed myopathy. Increased insertional and spontaneous activity (e.g., positive sharp waves, fibrillation potentials, and complex repetitive discharges) are detected in proximal and distal muscle groups as well as the paraspinal muscles. In addition, myotonic discharges may be seen in patients with or without the apparent clinical myotonia (Rutkove et al., 1996).

Histopathology

Muscle biopsy samples demonstrate rare necrotic fibers and scattered fibers with vacuoles containing membranous debris (Kuncl et al., 1987, 1989) (Fig. 78–3). These autophagic vacuoles are acid phosphatase positive. In addition, nerve biopsy samples may reveal axonal degeneration.

Pathogenesis

The neuromyopathy is thought to be due to disruption of the microtubules leading to defective intracellular movement or localization of lysosomes (Kuncl et al., 1987, 1989). This in turn results in the accumulation of autophagic vacuoles.

VINCRISTINE

Clinical Features

Vincristine is a chemotherapeutic agent that primarily acts by disrupting RNA and protein synthesis, as well as the polymerization of tubulin into microtubules. The most frequent adverse effect limiting the use of vincristine is an axonal sensorimotor polyneuropathy characterized by distal muscle weakness and sensory loss (Mastaglia, 1992). The existence of

a toxic myopathy caused by vincristine is less well described. Rarely, patients develop proximal muscle weakness and myalgias, which has been attributed to a toxic myopathy (Bradley et al., 1970).

Laboratory Features

Serum creatine kinase levels have not been reported in patients suspected of having a superimposed myopathy.

Electromyography and Nerve Conduction Studies

The SNAPs and CMAPs have reduced amplitudes, normal or only slightly prolonged distal latencies, and normal or mildly slow conduction velocities (Bradley et al., 1970). EMG demonstrates positive sharp waves, fibrillation potentials, and neurogenic appearing MUAPs in the distally located muscles of the upper and lower extremities.

Histopathology

Biopsy samples of distal muscles demonstrate neurogenic atrophy and occasionally the accumulation of lipofuscin granules, whereas proximal muscle biopsy samples may reveal foci of segmental necrosis (Bradley et al., 1970). On electron microscopy, there is prominent myofibrillar degeneration along with subsarcolemmal accumulation of osmiophilic material. In addition, some myonuclei containing membrane-bound inclusions may be seen. Autophagic vacuoles with spheromembranous debris can also be observed in animals that were administered vincristine (Slotwiner et al., 1966; Anderson et al., 1967), although these vacuoles have not been demonstrated in humans (Bradley et al., 1970).

Pathogenesis

The pathogenic basis of the neuromyopathy is presumably similar to that of colchicine.

Drug-Induced Mitochondrial Myopathy

ZIDOVUDINE (AZIDOTHYMIDINE)

Background

Myopathies related to human immunodeficiency virus (HIV) infection are heterogeneous and include an inflammatory myopathy (polymyositis), microvasculitis, noninflammatory necrotizing myopathy, nemaline rod myopathy, type 2 muscle fiber atrophy secondary to disuse and wasting due to the patient's chronic debilitated state, and a toxic myopathy secondary to azidothymidine (AZT) (Bailey et al., 1987; Richman et al., 1987; Bessen et al., 1988; Simpson and Bender, 1988; Dalakas et al., 1990; Panegyres et

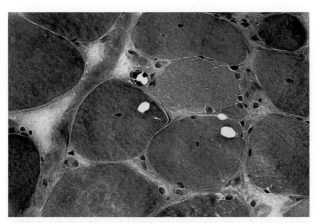

Figure 77–3. Colchicine myopathy. Muscle biopsy reveals variability in muscle fiber size and a few vacuolated muscle fibers (modified Gomori-trichrome stain).

al., 1990; Till and McDonnel, 1990; Chalmers et al., 1991; Espinoza et al., 1991; Mhiri et al., 1991; Mastaglia, 1992; Reyes et al., 1992; Grau et al., 1993; Manji et al., 1993; Peters et al., 1993; Dalakas, 1994; Gherardi and Chariot, 1994; Grau and Casademont, 1994; Simpson et al., 1997). In an HIV-infected patient, one must also consider peripheral neuropathy (e.g., chronic inflammatory demyelinating polyneuropathy) or myasthenia gravis in the differential diagnosis of a weak patient. AZT myopathy and the other myopathic disorders associated with HIV infection are clinically indistinguishable; any of these conditions can manifest as progressive proximal muscle weakness and myalgias. In addition, muscle weakness may be multifactorial, in that an individual patient can have myositis, nemaline rod myopathy, AZT-induced mitochondrial myopathy, and type 2 muscle fiber atrophy (not to mention an HIV-related or drug-induced peripheral neuropathy).

The frequencies of the various types of HIV-associated myopathies, including AZT myopathy, are variable due in part to the retrospective nature of most studies and the different definitions of *myopathy* used in these series of patients. For example, some studies defined *myopathy* as the presence of myalgias or elevated serum creatine kinase. Other studies required objective weakness, electromyographic abnormalities, and abnormal muscle histology. Clearly, more prospective studies are needed to determine the relative frequencies of these neuromuscular disorders in HIV-infected individuals who manifest generalized weakness.

It is apparent from the literature that there is a dose-relationship between AZT and the presence of ragged red fibers on muscle biopsy. However, it remains very controversial as to what causative role this AZT-induced mitochondrial myopathy plays in HIV-infected patients with myalgias, weakness, and elevated serum creatine kinase levels.

Clinical Features

Patients with "AZT myopathy" may present with an insidious onset of progressive myalgias, proximal muscle weakness, and atrophy (Dulhunty et al., 1986; Bailey et al., 1987; Bessen et al., 1988; Simpson and Bender, 1988; Dalakas et al., 1990; Panegyres et al., 1990; Till and McDonnel, 1990; Chalmers et al., 1991; Espinoza et al., 1991; Mhiri et al., 1991; Mastaglia, 1992; Reyes et al., 1992; Grau et al., 1993; Peters et al., 1993; Simpson et al., 1997). However, these clinical features do not help distinguish AZT myopathy from other types of HIV-related myopathies. Further, myalgias, muscle weakness, and elevated serum creatine kinase levels occur in HIV-infected patients who were never treated with AZT.

Laboratory Features

Serum creatine kinase levels may be normal or only mildly elevated. Again, similar elevated creatine kinase levels are evident in other forms of HIV-re-

lated myopathy. If the patient had a markedly elevated serum creatine kinase (e.g., >5 or 10 times the upper limit of normal), I would strongly suspect an inflammatory myopathy as opposed to an AZT-induced mitochondrial myopathy.

Electromyography and Nerve Conduction Studies

NCSs are normal, unless there is a concomitant HIV-related peripheral neuropathy. EMG may demonstrate an increase in needle insertional activity along with positive sharp waves, fibrillation potentials, and complex repetitive discharges (Simpson and Bender, 1988; Panegyres et al., 1990; Chalmers et al., 1991; Simpson et al., 1993; Amato and Dumitru, 2002). Early recruitment of short-duration, small-amplitude, polyphasic MUAPs may be demonstrated, particularly in proximal muscles.

Unfortunately, it is difficult to interpret the electromyograms in most of the reported studies because the abnormalities were not correlated with muscle histopathology. As noted, many patients with ragged red fibers indicative of AZT-induced mitochondrial myopathy also had evidence of necrosis, an inflammatory myopathy, cytoplasmic bodies, or nemaline rods on muscle biopsy samples. It is not clear how often patients with only ragged red fibers on muscle biopsy (a pure AZT myopathy) have muscle membrane instability and myopathic appearing MUAPs on EMG. In this regard, Chalmers and colleagues (1991) reported that fibrillation potentials were common in HIV-infected patients with an inflammatory myopathy on biopsy but were rare in patients without inflammation. Another study reported that patients with acquired immunodeficiency syndrome (AIDS) with ultrastructural mitochondrial abnormalities but no inflammation or nemaline rods on muscle biopsy samples had abnormal spontaneous activity on EMG (Peters et al., 1993). However, the patients did have small polyphasic MUAPs that recruited early.

Histopathology

Muscle biopsy samples are remarkable for the presence of ragged red fibers suggesting mitochondrial abnormalities in AZT myopathy. The number of these ragged red fibers directly correlates with the cumulative dose of AZT received by the patients (Mhiri et al., 1991; Grau et al., 1993). In addition, necrotic fibers, cytoplasmic bodies, nemaline rods, and fibers with microvacuolation may be found on biopsy samples and coexist with the ragged red fibers (Dalakas et al., 1990; Mhiri et al., 1991; Grau et al., 1993). Electron microscopy confirms abnormalities of the mitochondria, myofilaments, and tubules. One would not like to see endomysial inflammation and invasion of non-necrotic fibers in a "pure" AZT myopathy.

Pathogenesis

AZT acts as a false substitute for the viral reverse transcriptase, thereby inhibiting its enzymatic activity and replication of the HIV virus. In addition, AZT inhibits mitochondrial DNA polymerase, which probably accounts for the mitochondrial abnormalities present on muscle biopsy samples. AZT is associated with a decrease in the quantity of mitochondrial DNA and a decline in respiratory chain enzymatic activity (Arnaudo et al., 1991; Mhiri et al., 1991). Although AZT may be responsible for the mitochondrial abnormalities evident on muscle biopsy samples, the contribution of mitochondrial dysfunction to the signs and symptoms of myopathy remains unclear.

Treatment

The percentage of patients with myopathies that improve after AZT withdrawal has varied from 18% to 100% (Simpson and Bender, 1988; Dalakas et al., 1990; Chalmers et al., 1991; Grau et al., 1993; Manji et al., 1993; Peters et al., 1993; Simpson et al., 1997). Discontinuation of AZT is a important consideration, because the withdrawal of AZT may be associated with a deleterious increase in HIV replication. Further, AZT may be beneficial in some patients with HIV-associated inflammatory myopathy (Espinoza et al., 1991). The ideal would be a histological diagnosis before determination of the discontinuation of AZT is made. However, even after a muscle biopsy, the diagnosis may not be clear because both ragged red fibers and inflammation may be present. The presence of abundant abnormal spontaneous activity on EMG or markedly elevated serum creatine kinase levels would lead me to favor an inflammatory myopathy rather than a mitochondrial myopathy as responsible for the patient's symptoms and signs. In such a case, I would recommend a trial of intravenous immune globulin; if this is ineffective, then I recommend nonsteroidal anti-inflammatory drugs or corticosteroids.

In patients with normal or only mildly elevated serum creatine kinase levels and normal or only slightly increased spontaneous activity on EMG, it is impossible to distinguish AZT myopathy from other HIV-associated myopathies. A reasonable approach is a trial of a nonsteroidal anti-inflammatory drug with or without decreasing the dose of AZT (Dalakas et al., 1990). If there is no significant improvement in strength, one should consider discontinuation of AZT and use of one of the other antiviral medications (Jay et al., 1993). Patients should undergo a muscle biopsy if there is still no objective improvement. If the biopsy sample is suggestive of an inflammatory myopathy, immunomodulation of therapy (e.g., intravenous immune globulin or corticosteroids) should be considered. If there are no ragged red fibers on the biopsy sample, the patient can be rechallenged with AZT.

Drug-Induced Inflammatory Myopathies

L-TRYPTOPHAN AND EOSINOPHILIA-MYALGIA SYNDROME

Clinical Features

Eosinophilia-myalgia syndrome was described in the late 1980s and early 1990s and was determined to by caused by a contaminant in the manufacture of L-tryptophan (Belongia et al., 1990; Hertzman et al., 1990; Sagman and Melamed, 1990; Sakimoto, 1990; Smith and Dyck, 1990; Donofrio et al., 1992; Tanhehco et al., 1992). The clinical, laboratory, electrophysiological, and histopathological features were similar to those seen in diffuse fasciitis with eosinophilia (Shulman's syndrome) (Shulman, 1975). The onset of symptoms started within a few weeks or several years from the start of tryptophan ingestion. Patients complained of generalized muscle pain and tenderness along with weakness. Other common symptoms included numbness, paresthesias, arthralgias, lymphadenopathy, dyspnea, abdominal pain, mucocutaneous ulcers, and an erythematous rash. Severe peripheral neuropathies resembling Guillain-Barré syndrome (Heiman-Patterson et al., 1990; Smith and Dyck, 1990) or mononeuropathy multiplex (Selwa et al., 1990) were other important neuromuscular complications.

Laboratory Features

The absolute eosinophil count is elevated ($>1 \times 10^9$ cells/L). The serum creatine kinase level is normal or elevated. Autoantibodies are absent, and the erythrocyte sedimentation rate is usually normal.

Electromyography and Nerve Conduction Studies

NCSs are normal in patients with just the myopathy. However, patients with tryptophan-induced peripheral neuropathy had reduced CMAP and SNAP amplitudes with normal or mildly reduced conduction velocities (Selwa et al., 1990; Smith and Dyck, 1990). In addition, a few patients with a severe Guillain-Barré syndrome–like neuropathy had multifocal conduction block and slow conduction velocities on NCSs (Heiman-Patterson et al., 1990). EMG in patients with the myopathy revealed fibrillation potentials, positive sharp waves, and complex repetitive discharges, along with early recruitment of a mixture of small and large polyphasic MUAPs (Heiman-Patterson et al., 1990; Sagman and Melamed, 1990; Smith and Dyck, 1990). In addition, large polyphasic MUAPs with decreased recruitment were present in patients with a severe neuropathy (Smith and Dyck, 1990). The electrophysiological abnormalities eventually improved on the withdrawal of tryptophan.

Histopathology

Muscle biopsy samples revealed diffuse or perivascular inflammatory infiltrates in the surrounding fascia, perimysium and, to a lesser extent, the endomysium (Emslie-Smith et al., 1991). The inflammatory cells consisted mainly of $CD8^+$ T cells and macrophages, whereas eosinophils and B cells accounted for less than 3% of the inflammatory infiltrate. In contrast to dermatomyositis, deposition of membrane attack complex on blood vessels was not seen. Perivascular inflammatory infiltrate was apparent on nerve biopsy samples in the epineurium, endoneurium, and/or perineurium along with axonal degeneration in patients with the associated polyneuropathy (Heiman-Patterson et al., 1990; Sagman and Melamed, 1990; Selwa et al., 1990; Smith and Dyck, 1990; Turi et al., 1990).

Pathogenesis

Eosinophilia-myalgia syndrome was caused by a contaminant or contaminants in the manufacture of tryptophan. Two trace adulterants have been identified as the possible toxins: 3-phenylaminoalanine (PAA) and 1,1'-ethylidenebis (tryptophan) (EBT) (Mayeno et al., 1992). The mechanism by which this contaminant or contaminants resulted in the disorder is unknown, but the eosinophilia and eosinophilic infiltrate in tissues suggest some form of allergic reaction.

Treatment

Discontinuation of L-tryptophan and treatment with high-dose corticosteroids were usually effective. Some patients experienced relapses on the withdrawal of steroids.

TOXIC OIL SYNDROME

The toxic oil syndrome is quite similar to the eosinophilia-myalgia syndrome associated with tryptophan (Kilbourne et al., 1983). Toxic oil syndrome was restricted to Spain, where it was linked to the ingestion of illegally marked, denatured rapeseed oil as a cooking substitute for olive oil. The disorder has not recurred since 1981, when the use of this oil was halted. Interestingly, the toxic contaminant in the rapeseed oil, 3-phenylamino-1,2-propanediol, is chemically similar to PAA, the adulterant in tryptophan responsible for eosinophilia-myalgia syndrome (Mayeno et al., 1992).

D-PENICILLAMINE

D-Penicillamine is used for the treatment of Wilson's disease, rheumatoid arthritis, and other connective tissue disorders. An inflammatory myopathy occurs in 0.2% to 1.4% of patients treated with D-penicillamine (Schrader et al., 1972; Dawkins et al., 1981; Hall et al., 1984; Takahashi et al., 1986; Taneja

et al., 1990). The clinical, laboratory, histological, and electrodiagnostic findings are essentially the same as those for idiopathic polymyositis or dermatomyositis, both of which have been associated with D-penicillamine. Symptoms resolve after discontinuation of the drug. It is possible for D-penicillamine therapy to be restarted at a lower dosage without recurrence of the inflammatory myopathy.

CIMETIDINE

Cimetidine, a histamine H_2 receptor antagonist, has been associated with rare cases of inflammatory myopathy. One patient developed generalized weakness, myalgias, and interstitial nephritis (Watson et al., 1983). Serum creatine kinase levels were markedly elevated (up to 40,000 IU/L), and EMG was described as being compatible with a myopathy. The muscle biopsy sample revealed mainly perivascular inflammation, predominantly consisting of $CD8^+$ lymphocytes suggestive of a humorally mediated vasculopathy, such as dermatomyositis. However, there were no immunoglobulin or complement deposits noted on small blood vessels. This patient did not have a cutaneous rash, although other cases of cutaneous vasculitis have been reported with cimetidine (Mitchell et al., 1983).

PROCAINAMIDE

Procainamide has been associated with the development of proximal muscle weakness, myalgias, and elevated serum creatine kinase levels (Fontiveros et al., 1980; Lewis et al., 1986). EMG was described as being consistent with a "patchy" myopathy. Perivascular inflammation and rare necrotic muscle fibers may be seen on muscle biopsy samples. The myopathy may be caused by a lupus-like vasculitis that can be seen in patients treated with procainamide. The myopathy resolves after the discontinuation of procainamide.

LEVODOPA

There is a single reported case of proximal muscle weakness and myalgias in a patient with Parkinson's disease with levodopa (L-dopa) therapy (Wolf et al., 1976). In this patient, the muscle symptoms and 10-fold elevation in serum creatine kinase level developed after treatment with levodopa for more than 4 years. NCSs were reported as being "slow," but no data were provided. Interestingly, only rare fasciculation potentials were noted on EMG. Gastrocnemius and quadriceps muscle biopsy samples purportedly showed perivascular inflammation and rare necrotic fibers. Although the authors suggested the patient developed a hypersensitivity vasculitis in response to levodopa, this observation has not been corroborated by other reports.

PHENYTOIN

Hypersensitivity reactions to phenytoin may be responsible for myalgias, muscle weakness, and elevated serum creatine kinase levels in rare patients (Harney and Glasberg, 1983). Muscle biopsy samples may reveal scattered necrotic and regenerating muscle fibers in such cases. EMG demonstrates increased spontaneous activity with fibrillation potentials and positive sharp waves along with small-amplitude, short-duration, polyphasic MUAPs that recruit early. The myopathy improves after discontinuation of the phenytoin and a short course of corticosteroids.

LAMOTRIGINE

Severe myoglobinuria and renal failure associated with a generalized rash, anemia, leukopenia, and thrombocytopenia may occur with lamotrigine (personal observation). The clinical and laboratory features resemble those of thrombocytic thrombocytopenic purpura. The patient improved with plasmapheresis and the discontinuation of lamotrigine.

Myopathies Secondary to Impaired Protein Synthesis or Increased Catabolism

STEROID MYOPATHY

Myopathies related to iatrogenic corticosteroids are discussed in the section on endocrine myopathy.

FINASTERIDE

Clinical Features

Finasteride is used for the treatment of prostatic hypertrophy. It is a 4-azasteroid that inhibits 5α-reductase and thus blocks dihydrotestosterone production in the prostate. One patient treated with finasteride (5 mg q.d.) developed a generalized myopathy characterized by severe proximal greater than distal weakness and atrophy (Haan et al., 1997). Sensation and deep tendon reflexes were normal.

Laboratory Features

Serum creatine kinase levels were normal.

Electromyography and Nerve Conduction Studies

NCSs studies were normal, whereas the EMG revealed small polyphasic MUAPs without abnormal insertional or spontaneous activity.

Histopathology

Muscle biopsy sample demonstrated only mild variability in fiber size, type 2 muscle fiber atrophy, and increased central nuclei.

Pathogenesis

The pathophysiological mechanism for the myopathy is not known. Finasteride has a structure similar to that of corticosteroids; the pathogenic mechanism may be similar to that of steroid myopathy.

Treatment

Discontinuation of finasteride was associated with normalization of strength and improvement in electromyographic abnormalities.

Drug-Induced Hypokalemic Myopathy

CLINICAL FEATURES

Hypokalemia is the most common electrolyte abnormality that results in muscle weakness (Comi et al., 1985). Hypokalemia may be related to an underlying genetic disorder (e.g., familial hypokalemic periodic paralysis or renal tubular acidosis), medications (e.g., diuretics, laxatives, mineralocorticoids, amphotericin, lithium), alcohol abuse, or inhalation of toluene. The clinical, laboratory, histopathological, and electrophysiological features of hypokalemic myopathy are similar regardless of the etiology of the hypokalemia. Patients can present with proximal or generalized weakness. Usually, muscle involvement is symmetrical, although we have seen onset with asymmetrical muscle weakness. Some patients complain of muscle pain and cramps. Severe rhabdomyolysis accompanied by myoglobinuria can also complicate hypokalemia.

Laboratory Features

Potassium levels are usually less than 3 mEq/L. Serum creatine kinase is usually elevated proportional to the severity of muscle weakness. The electrocardiogram may demonstrate bradycardia, flattened T waves, prolonged PR and QT intervals, and notable U waves.

Histopathology

Biopsy samples of very weak muscles may demonstrate vacuoles and scattered necrotic fibers.

Pathogenesis

The mechanism by which muscle weakness develops secondary to hypokalemia is not known. As discussed in regard to primary hypokalemic periodic paralysis, a reduced extracellular potassium concentration may result in an abnormal ratio of gated sodium channels in the active compared with the inactive state. In a partially depolarized state, the number of sodium channels available to be activated would be reduced, making the muscle membrane less excitable. Hypokalemia may also diminish blood flow and suppress the synthesis and storage of glycogen in muscles.

Electromyography and Nerve Conduction Studies

NCSs are usually normal. EMG may demonstrate fibrillation potentials and positive sharp waves as well as early recruitment of small-duration, low-amplitude MUAPs in severely weak muscles.

Treatment

Muscle strength returns with correction of the hypokalemia. The patients need a medical workup to elucidate the underlying cause of the hypokalemia.

Toxic Myopathies with Multifactorial or Unknown Pathogenic Mechanism

EMETINE (IPECAC)

Clinical Features

Emetine (ipecac) is an emetic agent that is also used for the treatment of amebiasis, as well as in aversive conditioning for the treatment of chronic alcoholism. The drug has been abused, particularly in patients with anorexia nervosa and bulimia. Emetine in doses of 500 to 600 mg per day for over 10 days has resulted in a severe proximal myopathy and cardiomyopathy (Bennett et al., 1982; Mateer et al., 1985; Palmer and Guay, 1985). Patients complain of muscle pain, tenderness, and stiffness. Deep tendon reflexes are usually diminished, but the sensory examination is completely normal. The myopathy reverses with withdrawal of the medication.

Laboratory Features

The serum creatine kinase levels may be mildly to moderately elevated.

Electromyography and Nerve Conduction Studies

Sensory and motor NCSs are normal (Bennett et al., 1982; Mateer et al., 1985; Palmer and Guay, 1985). Repetitive nerve stimulation reveals no abnormal decrementing response. EMG demonstrates positive sharp waves and fibrillation potentials as well as early recruitment of small-duration, short-amplitude polyphasic MUAPs in weak muscles.

Histopathology

Muscle biopsy samples reveal generalized muscle fiber atrophy, necrotic fibers, small regenerating fi-

bers, and scattered fibers containing cytoplasmic bodies (Bennett et al., 1982; Mateer et al., 1985; Palmer and Guay, 1985). Targetoid or "moth-eaten" structures are seen on oxidative enzyme stains. On electron microscopy, there is confirmation of cytoplasmic bodies as well as myofibrillar degeneration. The histological appearance of light and electron microscopy is similar to that seen in myofibrillar myopathy (desmin myopathy) (Amato et al., 1998, 1999).

Pathogenesis

Emetine is thought to produce its myotoxic effect by inhibiting muscle protein synthesis, but the exact pathogenic basis for the disorder is not known.

Treatment

The myopathy improves when the emetine use is stopped.

ELINAFIDE

Clinical Features

Elinafide, an experimental chemotherapeutic agent, can cause a toxic myopathy characterized by proximal muscle weakness (Amato et al., 1998, 1999). Cardiomyopathy has also been noted in experimental animals. The myopathy improves after the discontinuation of elinafide.

Laboratory Features

Serum creatine kinase levels are mildly elevated.

Electromyography and Nerve Conduction Studies

EMG reveals increased insertional activity, abundant fibrillation potentials, and positive sharp waves. There is early recruitment of small-amplitude, short-duration, polyphasic MUAPs that are more prominent in the proximal, weaker muscles.

Histopathology

The muscle biopsy samples demonstrate myofibrillar degeneration and cytoplasmic bodies similar to that seen in emetine myopathy. There also is an abnormal accumulation of desmin, dystrophin, gelsolin, neural cell adhesion molecule, β-amyloid precursor protein, and various cell cycle regulatory proteins, as seen in hereditary and sporadic cases of myofibrillar myopathy (desmin myopathy) (Amato et al., 1998, 1999).

Pathogenesis

Elinafide is a DNA intercalator that also inhibits the enzyme topoisomerase II. The pathogenic mechanism of the toxic myopathy is not known. Topoisomerase inhibitors can cause apoptosis, but there has been no evidence of apoptosis by terminal deoxynucleotidyl transferase biotin-dUTP nick end labeling (TUNEL) of the two elinafide-induced myopathies (Amato et al., 1999).

Treatment

The myopathy improves within several weeks after the discontinuation of elinafide treatment.

OMEPRAZOLE

Clinical Features

Omeprazole has been associated with a neuromyopathy (Sellapah, 1990; Garrot et al., 1994; Lacomis et al., 1996; Faucheux et al., 1998). Patients develop proximal weakness and myalgias, predominantly in the lower extremity. In addition, patients complain of distal paresthesias. There is a stocking distribution of sensory loss, and deep tendon reflexes are diminished or absent.

Laboratory Features

Serum creatine kinase levels are normal or mildly elevated.

Electromyography and Nerve Conduction Studies

NCSs are compatible with an axonal sensorimotor polyneuropathy (Faucheux et al., 1998). EMG may reveal small polyphasic MUAPs (Garrot et al., 1994).

Histopathology

Muscle biopsy samples in two patients demonstrated only type 2 muscle fiber atrophy (Garrot et al., 1994; Faucheux et al., 1998). Axonal degeneration was apparent on a superficial peroneal nerve biopsy in one patient (Faucheux et al., 1998).

Pathogenesis

The pathogenic mechanism for the neuromyopathy is unknown.

Treatment

The motor and sensory symptoms improved and serum creatine kinase levels normalized after the withdrawal of omeprazole. However, the neuromyopathy recurred when omeprazole was restarted.

ACUTE QUADRIPLEGIC MYOPATHY AND CRITICAL ILLNESS MYOPATHY

The most common neuromuscular disorders that lead to acute generalized weakness and admission

to an intensive care unit are myasthenia gravis and Guillain-Barré syndrome. However, the differential diagnosis of weakness that develops in a patient who is already in an intensive care unit is quite different and includes critical illness polyneuropathy (Bolton et al., 1984; Zochodne et al., 1987), prolonged neuromuscular blockade (Barohn et al., 1994; Gooch, 1995), and a condition secondary to a myopathic process. This intensive care unit myopathy has been termed *acute quadriplegic myopathy, acute illness myopathy, critical illness myopathy,* and *myopathy associated with thick filament (myosin)* (McFarlane and Rosenthal, 1977; Arellano and Krup, 1991; Danon et al., 1991; Sitwell et al., 1991; Hirano et al., 1992; Lacomis et al., 1993, 1996; Ramsay et al., 1993; Al-Lozi et al., 1994; Zochodne et al., 1994; Gutmann et al., 1996; Rich et al., 1996, 1997; Hanson et al., 1997; Showalter and Engel, 1997; Deconinck et al., 1998; Amato and Dumitru, 2002). For the sake of discussion, I will use the term *acute quadriplegic myopathy* when referring to intensive care unit myopathy. Distinguishing acute quadriplegic myopathy from critical illness neuropathy or from prolonged neuromuscular blockade can be difficult. In addition, patients can have a combination of all three processes, resulting in the generalized weakness. Which of these neuromuscular complications predominates varies from series to series. Some series of intensive care unit weakness have reported critical illness neuropathy to be more common than acute quadriplegic myopathy (Op de Coul et al., 1985; Witt et al., 1991), whereas others (including the author) have found the myopathy to be more frequent (Latronico et al., 1996; Rich et al., 1997; Lacomis et al., 1998). In the largest series to date involving 88 patients, the frequency of acute quadriplegic myopathy (42%) was much more than that of critical illness neuropathy (13%) (Lacomis et al., 1998). Prolonged neuromuscular blockade occurred in only one patient, who also had acute quadriplegic myopathy (Lacomis et al., 1998).

The incidence of the development of acute quadriplegic myopathy in the intensive care unit is not known; there are only a few published prospective series (Douglass et al., 1992; Campellone et al., 1998). Douglass and associates (1992) evaluated 25 consecutive patients who required mechanical ventilation for severe asthma. The patients were treated with dexamethasone 10 mg every 8 hours or hydrocortisone 250 mg every 6 hours. In addition, 22 of the 25 patients also received vecuronium. Weakness developed in 9 of 25 patients (36%), whereas serum creatine kinase levels were elevated in 19 of 25 patients (76%). Patients with acute quadriplegic myopathy required longer mechanical ventilation (12.9 ± 6.6 days) than did patients who did not develop the myopathy (3.1 ± 3.1 days). In a prospective study of 100 consecutive adult patients undergoing liver transplantation, acute quadriplegic myopathy occurred in 7 patients (Campellone et al., 1998). The patients were all treated in the perioperative period with nondepolarizing neuromuscular blocking agents and high-dose corticosteroids. Serum creatine kinase levels were elevated in four of six patients tested. The elevated serum creatine kinase levels remained as high as 10 times the upper limit of normal 25 days after surgery. Muscle biopsy samples in four patients demonstrated scattered muscle fiber necrosis and the selected loss of thick filaments. Three patients later died from sepsis and multiorgan failure. The remaining patients slowly regained strength and the ability to ambulate over 1 to 3 months.

Clinical Features

The first reported case of acute quadriplegic myopathy involved a 24-year-old woman treated with neuromuscular blockade and high doses of intravenous corticosteroids for status asthmaticus (McFarlane and Rosenthal, 1977). Subsequently, there have been numerous reports of acute quadriplegic myopathy, usually developing in patients who received high-dose intravenous corticosteroids, nondepolarizing neuromuscular blockers, or both (Arellano and Krup, 1991; Danon and Carpenter 1991; Sitwell et al., 1991; Hirano et al., 1992; Lacomis et al., 1993, 1996; Ramsay et al., 1993; Al-Lozi et al., 1994; Zochodne et al., 1994; Gutmann et al., 1996; Rich et al., 1996, 1997; Hanson et al., 1997; Showalter and Engel, 1997; Deconinck et al., 1998). Acute quadriplegic myopathy can also occur in critically ill patients with sepsis or multiorgan failure who have not received corticosteroids or nondepolarizing neuromuscular blocking agents (Gutmann et al., 1996; Showalter and Engel, 1997; Deconinck et al., 1998).

Patients with acute quadriplegic myopathy manifest with severe generalized muscle weakness that develops over a period of several days. In addition to extremity and trunkal weakness, facial and, less commonly, extraocular weakness may be seen (Zochodne et al., 1994). The myopathy is often first recognized when the patient is unable to be weaned from the ventilator. Sensory examination is usually normal, although some patients may have superimposed critical illness neuropathy or a peripheral neuropathy from some unrelated etiology (e.g., diabetes mellitus or chronic renal failure). Deep tendon reflexes are decreased or absent.

The morbidity and mortality in acute quadriplegic myopathy and critical illness neuropathy appear to be quite similar (Lacomis et al., 1998). The mortality rate in patients with acute quadriplegic myopathy is high (approximately 30% in one large series) (Lacomis et al., 1998). This increased mortality rate is more related to multiorgan failure and sepsis than to the myopathy. Muscle strength gradually improves over several months in patients who survive the sepsis and multiorgan failure.

Laboratory Features

Serum creatine kinase levels may be normal or moderately elevated in about 50% of patients.

Electromyography and Nerve Conduction Studies

NCSs demonstrate significantly diminished CMAP amplitudes. The distal motor latencies and conduction velocities are normal. Importantly, the SNAP amplitudes are normal or mildly reduced (>80% of the lower limit of normal), which can help distinguish acute quadriplegic myopathy from critical illness myopathy. However, one must remember that an abnormal SNAP does not exclude the diagnosis of acute quadriplegic myopathy, because the patient may have both acute quadriplegic myopathy and critical illness neuropathy or the peripheral neuropathy may be unrelated as noted previously. Repetitive stimulation is usually normal, although decrement in CMAP amplitude on repetitive stimulation (fast and slow rates) has been described (Zochodne et al., 1994; Gooch, 1995; Road et al., 1997). A decrementing response may be demonstrated within 7 days of discontinuation of nondepolarizing neuromuscular agents. This is usually seen in the setting of renal insufficiency resulting in persistently elevated levels of the neuromuscular blocking agent or agents or active metabolites.

Rich and colleagues (1996, 1997) used the technique of direct muscle stimulation to help in distinguishing acute quadriplegic myopathy from critical illness myopathy. Direct muscle stimulation bypasses the distal motor nerve and neuromuscular junction. In critical illness neuropathy or prolonged neuromuscular blockade, one would expect the muscle membrane to retain its excitability. Thus, the direct muscle stimulation CMAP should be near normal despite a low or absent nerve stimulation evoked CMAP. In contrast, if the muscle membrane excitability is reduced (as postulated in acute quadriplegic myopathy; discussion on pathogenesis), both the needle stimulation evoked CMAP and the direct muscle CMAP should be very low. Theoretically, the ratio of needle stimulation evoked CMAP to direct muscle CMAP should be close to 1:1 in a disorder of muscle membrane inexcitability and should approach zero in an acute neuropathy or neuromuscular junction disorder. In this regard, absent or reduced amplitudes of the direct muscle CMAP with needle stimulation evoked CMAP–to–direct muscle CMAP ratios of greater than 0.9 were demonstrated in 11 patients with acute quadriplegic myopathy, whereas needle stimulation evoked CMAP–to–direct muscle CMAP ratios were 0.5 or less in patients with severe neuropathy.

EMG may demonstrate prominent fibrillation potentials and positive sharp waves, but abnormal spontaneous activity is not always present. Myotonic discharges were reported in one patient with acute quadriplegic myopathy, who was also receiving an immunophilin, which is known to cause electrophysiological myotonia (Campellone et al., 1998). There is early recruitment of short-duration, small-amplitude MUAPs. In severe acute quadriplegic myopathy, one may be unable to recruit any MUAP.

Sequential EMG studies reveal profuse spontaneous activity and inability to actively recruit MUAPs early in the course (Road et al., 1997). Over time, small polyphasic MUAPs with early recruitment appear while the patients begin to recover (Road et al., 1997).

Histopathology

Muscle biopsy samples demonstrate a spectrum of histological abnormalities. Type 2 muscle fiber atrophy with or without type 1 fiber atrophy is usually evident (Arellano and Krup, 1991; Sitwell et al., 1991; Hirano et al., 1992; Lacomis et al., 1993, 1996; Al-Lozi et al., 1994; Zochodne et al., 1994; Gooch, 1995; Gutmann et al., 1996; Showalter and Engel, 1997). Scattered necrotic muscle fibers are also frequently seen (Ramsay et al., 1993; Zochodne et al., 1994; Showalter and Engel, 1997; Campellone et al., 1998; Lacomis et al., 1998). There may be more focal or diffuse loss of reactivity for ATPase activity in type 1 fibers than in type 2 fibers. In addition, the loss of thick filaments (myosin) is apparent on electron microscopy and immunohistochemistry (Danon and Carpenter, 1991; Hirano et al., 1992; Lacomis et al., 1993, 1996; Gooch, 1995; Showalter and Engel, 1997; Campellone et al., 1998; Deconinck et al., 1998). Notably, the expression of other structural proteins (e.g., actin, titin, nebulin) are normal or are affected only at an advanced stage of the disease (Showalter and Engel, 1997). Interestingly, calpain expression is markedly enhanced in myosin-deficient acute quadriplegic myopathy muscle biopsy samples (Showalter and Engel, 1997). However, the loss of myosin has not been observed in all cases of acute quadriplegic myopathy. This may be due to sampling bias or the possibility that the pathogenic basis of acute quadriplegic myopathy is multifactorial.

Pathogenesis

The varying laboratory, histological, and electrophysiological features suggest that the pathogenesis may in fact be multifactorial. Although muscle biopsy samples may demonstrate widespread necrosis, the mechanism of muscle fiber necrosis is not known. Importantly, not all patients have significant necrosis on biopsy. Myosin appears to be selectively lost in some patients, as noted previously. The increased expression of calcium-activated proteases (calpains) may be responsible for degradation of myosin (Showalter and Engel, 1997). Perhaps glucocorticoids, nondepolarizing neuromuscular agents, or the milieu of critical illness cause the direct or indirect enhanced expression of calpains. Cytokines released during sepsis can induce a catabolic state in muscle with breakdown of proteins, glycogen, and lipid.

Some electrophysiological studies suggest that there is muscle membrane inexcitability in acute quadriplegic myopathy (see earlier) (Rich et al., 1996, 1997). Three factors may be important in reducing muscle membrane excitability: (1) partial depolarization of the resting membrane potential, (2) reduced muscle membrane resistance, and (3) decreased sodium currents (Rich et al., 1998; Ruff, 1998). In denervated rats treated with corticosteroids, the resting muscle membrane potential is decreased similar to that in denervated, non–steroid-treated control rats (Rich et al., 1998). However, muscle membrane resistance is reduced as a result of increased chloride conductance in denervated rats treated with corticosteroids. The lower membrane resistance decreases the depolarization induced by the opening of sodium channels. The sodium current is diminished either secondary to a reduction in the actual number of sodium channels or an alteration in sodium channel conductance or voltage-dependent gating. Further work is necessary to unravel the pathogenic basis of acute quadriplegic myopathy.

Treatment

Supportive care and treatment of underlying systemic abnormalities (e.g., antibiotics in sepsis, dialysis in renal failure) are the mainstays of treatment. The corticosteroids or nondepolarizing neuromuscular blockers should be stopped, or the doses should be lowered. Patients will require extensive physical therapy to prevent contractures and to help regain muscle strength and functional abilities.

ALCOHOLIC MYOPATHY

Chronic alcohol abuse is more often associated with neuropathy than with myopathy. However, there are three types of alcohol-related myopathy: (1) acute necrotizing myopathy, (2) hypokalemic myopathy, and (3) chronic alcoholic myopathy (Ekbom et al., 1964; Faris et al., 1967; Mayer et al., 1968; Faris and Reyes, 1971; Perkoff, 1971; Curran and Wetmore, 1972; Oh, 1972; Rossouw et al., 1976; Worden, 1976; Rubenstein and Wainapel, 1977; Mastaglia, 1992; Victor and Sieb, 1994; Dumitru, 1995).

Acute necrotizing myopathy is associated with acute muscle pain, swelling, and weakness following or during a recent particularly intense binge of alcohol consumption. Myoglobinuria and acute renal failure may occur. The myalgias and muscle swelling resolve over the course of several days, but muscle weakness may last several weeks. Serum creatine kinase levels are markedly elevated during these attacks. Histological examination of muscle reveals widespread muscle fiber necrosis and intracellular edema. Rare, tubular aggregates also may be seen. Electron microscopy demonstrates myofibrillary disarray and degeneration of mitochondria. Patients require appropriate supportive medical care and nutritional supplementation (many patients are malnourished).

Acute hypokalemic myopathy secondary to alcohol abuse manifests as acute generalized weakness similar to other forms of hypokalemic myopathy. Patients typically do not complain of muscle pain or swelling. Muscle weakness evolves over the time period of 1 or 2 days. Serum potassium levels are very low, usually less than 2.1 mEq/L, whereas the serum creatine kinase level is elevated. Muscle biopsy sample demonstrates vacuoles within muscle fibers during an acute episode. The clinical symptoms and histological abnormalities promptly resolve with correction of the hypokalemia.

Chronic alcoholic myopathy manifests as an insidious onset of primarily proximal limb weakness, especially in the hip girdle. Serum creatine kinase levels may be normal or mildly elevated. Muscle biopsy sample reveals scattered atrophic, necrotic, and regenerating muscle fibers. It is not known if the muscle weakness in this disorder is caused by a direct toxic influence of alcohol on muscle or by malnutrition.

Electromyography and Nerve Conduction Studies

Many patients with a history of chronic excess alcohol abuse often develop symptoms, signs, and electrophysiological features of an axonal, predominantly sensory polyneuropathy (Ekbom et al., 1964; Mayer et al., 1968; Perkoff, 1971; Oh, 1972; Rubenstein and Wainapel, 1977; Amato and Dumitru, 2002). Patients without a superimposed peripheral neuropathy have normal sensory and motor NCSs. During attacks of weakness, EMG of the weak muscles reveals positive sharp waves, fibrillation potentials, and early recruitment of short-duration, low-amplitude MUAPs (Eadie and Ferrier, 1966; Faris et al., 1967; Faris and Reyes, 1971; Perkoff, 1971; Oh, 1972; Rossouw et al., 1976; Worden, 1976). With medical support and correction of any electrolyte disturbances, the membrane instability and MUAP abnormalities resolve.

Pathogenesis

The pathogenic basis for the various forms of alcoholic myopathies is not known. The metabolism of alcohol may lead to the accumulation of toxic metabolites (e.g., acetaldehyde) or of free radicals that may be toxic to sarcolemmal, mitochondrial, and peroxisomal lipid membranes (Victor and Sieb, 1994). In addition, alcohol may have a direct toxic effect on ion channels. Chronic alcohol abuse may also impair glycolysis and glycogenolysis (Bollaert et al., 1989; Trounce et al., 1990). However, defects in oxidative metabolism were not demonstrated in other detailed biochemical studies (Cardellach et al., 1992). Further work is required to fully elucidate the pathogenic role of alcohol in myopathies.

MYOPATHIES SECONDARY TO ILLICIT DRUGS

Illicit drugs and controlled medications (e.g., heroin, meperidine, cocaine, pentazocine, piritramide, amphetamines) may cause a necrotizing myopathy

(Norman et al., 1970; Richter et al., 1971; Levin and Engel, 1975; Oh et al., 1975; Johnson et al., 1976; Cogen et al., 1978; Partanen and Danner, 1982; Choucair and Ziter, 1984; Mastaglia, 1992; Amato and Dumitru, 2002; Van den Bergh et al., 1997). Muscle tissue can be injured as a direct result of trauma due to needle insertions, rhabdomyolysis secondary to pressure or ischemia (as can occur with prolonged loss of consciousness), ischemia caused by vasoconstriction, or the direct toxic effects of the drugs (or adulterants) on muscle tissue. Serum creatine kinase levels may be elevated, and biopsy samples demonstrate necrotic muscle fibers. Motor and sensory NCSs are normal, whereas EMG reveals fibrillation potentials, positive sharp waves, and myopathic MUAPs.

Inhalation of volatile agents (e.g., toluene) also causes generalized muscle weakness and, occasionally, myoglobinuria. Toluene causes distal renal tubular acidosis with associated severe hypokalemia, hypophosphatemia, and mild hypocalcemia. Muscle strength returns after correction of the electrolyte abnormalities and abstinence from inhaling volatile agents.

References

Abourizk N, Khalil BA, Bahuth N, et al: Clofibrate-induced muscular syndrome. J Neurol Sci 1979;42:1–9.
Afifi AK, Bergman RA, Harvey JC: Steroid myopathy. Johns Hopkins Med J 1968;123:158–174.
Afifi AK, Hajj SS, Tekian A, et al: Clofibrate-induced myotoxicity in rats. Eur Neurol 1984;23:182–197.
Akmal M: Rhabdomyolysis in a patient with hypocalcemia due to hypoparathyroidism. Am J Nephrol 1993;13:61–63.
Alderson K, Griffin JW, Cornblath DR, et al: Neuromuscular complications of amiodarone therapy. Neurology 1987;37(suppl):355.
Al-Lozi MT, Pestronk A, Yee WC, et al: Rapidly evolving myopathy with myosin-deficient fibers. Ann Neurol 1994;35:273–279.
Amato AA, Barohn RJ: Idiopathic inflammatory myopathies. Neurol Clin 1997b;15:615–648.
Amato AA, Barohn RJ: Neurological complications of transplantations. In Harati Y, Rolack LA (eds): Practical Neuroimmunology. Boston, Butterworth-Heineman, 1997a; 341–375.
Amato AA, Dumitru D: Acquired myopathies. In Dumitru D, Amato AA, Zwartz MJ (eds): Electrodiagnostic Medicine, 2nd ed. Philadelphia, Hanley & Belfas, 2002; 937–1041.
Amato AA, Jackson CE, Lampin S, Kagan-Hallet K: Myofibrillar myopathy: No evidence of apoptosis by TUNEL. Neurology 1999;52:861–863.
Amato AA, Kagan-Hallet K, Jackson CE, et al: The wide spectrum of myofibrillar myopathy suggests a multifactorial etiology and pathogenesis. Neurology 1998;51:1646–1655.
Anderson P, Song S, Slotwiner P: The fine structure of spheromembranous degeneration of skeletal muscle induced by vincristine. J Neuropathol Exp Neurol 1967;26:15–24.
Arellano F, Krup P: Muscular disorders associated with cyclosporine [letter]. Lancet 1991;337:915.
Arnaudo E, Dalakas M, Shanske S, et al: Depletion of mitochondrial DNA in AIDS patients with zidovudine-induced myopathy. Lancet 1991;1:508–510.
Astrom K-E, Kugelberg E, Muller R: Hypothyroid myopathy. Arch Neurol 1961;5:472–482.
Atkinson P, Joubert G, Barron A, et al: Hypertrophic cardiomyopathy with tacrolimus in paediatric transplant patient. Lancet 1995;345:894–896.
Ayanian JZ, Fuch CS, Stone RM: Lovastatin and rhabdomyolysis. Ann Intern Med 1988;109:682–683.

Baczynski R, Massry SG, Magott M, et al: Effect of parathyroid hormone on energy metabolism of skeletal muscle. Kidney Int 1985;28:722–727.

Bailey RO, Turok DI, Jaufmann BP, et al: Myositis and acquired immunodeficiency syndrome. Hum Pathol 1987;18:749–751.

Bakker-Arema RG, Best J, Fayad R, et al: A brief review paper on the efficacy and safety of atorvastatin in early clinical trials. Atherosclerosis 1997;131:17–23.

Banker BQ, Chester CS: Infarction of thigh muscle in the diabetic patient. Neurology 1973;23:667–677.

Barohn RJ, Jackson CE, Rogers SJ, et al: Prolonged paralysis due to nondepolarizing neuromuscular blocking agents and corticosteroids. Muscle Nerve 1994;17:647–654.

Barohn RJ, Kissel JT: Painful thigh mass in a young woman: Diabetic thigh infarction. Muscle Nerve 1992;15:850–855.

Belongia EA, Hedberg CW, Gleich GJ, et al: An investigation of the case of the eosinophilia myalgia syndrome associated with tryptophan use. N Engl J Med 1990;323:357–365.

Bennet WR, Huston DP: Rhabdomyolysis in thyroid storm. Am J Med 1984;77:733–735.

Bennett HS, Spiro AJ, Pollack MA, et al: Ipecac-induced myopathy simulating dermatomyositis. Neurology 1982;32:91–94.

Berenbaum F, Rajzbaum G, Bonnchon P, Amor B: Une hyperparathyroide revelee une chute de la tete. Rev Rhum Mal Osteoartic 1993;60:467–469.

Berland Y, Coponat H, Durand C, et al: Rhabdomyolysis and simvastatin use. Nephron 1991;57:365–366.

Bessen LJ, Green JB, Louie E, et al: Severe polymyositis-like syndrome associated with zidovudine therapy of AIDS and ARC. N Engl J Med 1988;318:708.

Bigland B, Jehring B: Muscle performance in rats, normal and treated with growth hormone. J Physiol 1952;116:129–136.

Birge SG, Haddad JG: 25-Hydroxycholecalciferol stimulation of muscle metabolism. J Clin Invest 1975;56:1100–1107.

Bischoff A, Esslen E: Myopathy with primary hyperparathyroidism. Neurology 1965;15:64–68.

Boccuzzi SJ, Bocanegra TS, Walker JF, et al: Long-term safety and efficacy profile of simvastatin. Am J Cardiol 1991;68;1127–1131.

Bollaert PE, Robin-Lherbier B, Escanye JM, et al: Phosphorus nuclear magnetic resonance evidence of abnormal skeletal muscle metabolism in chronic alcoholics. Neurology 1989;39:821–824.

Bolton CF, Gilbert JJ, Hahn AF, Sibbald WJ: Polyneuropathy in critically ill patients. J Neurol Neurosurg Psychiatry 1984;47:1223–1231.

Bradley WG, Lassman LP, Pearce GW, et al: The neuromyopathy of vincristine in man: Clinical, electrophysiological and pathological studies. J Neurol Sci 1970;10:107–131.

Brasel JA, Wright JC, Wilkins L, Blizzard RM: An evaluation of seventy five patients with hypopituitarism. Am J Med 1965;38:484–498.

Brink F: The role of calcium ion in neural processes. Pharmacol Rev 1954;6:245–298.

Britt CW, Light RR, Peters BH, et al: Rhabdomyolysis during treatment with epsilon-aminocaproic acid. Arch Neurol 1980;37:187–188.

Brown JA, Wollmann RL, Mullan S: Myopathy induced by epsilon-aminocaproic acid. J Neurosurg 1982;57:130–134.

Brown JG, Millward DJ: The influence of thyroid status on skeletal muscle protein metabolism. Biochem Soc Trans 1980;8:366–367.

Buchthal F: Electrophysiological abnormalities in metabolic myopathies and neuropathies. Acta Neurol Scand 1970(suppl 43):129–176.

Campellone JV, Lacomis D, Kramer DJ, et al: Acute myopathy after liver transplantation. Neurology 1998;50:46–53.

Cardellach F, Galpfre J, Grau JM, et al: Oxidative metabolism in muscle from patients with chronic alcoholism. Ann Neurol 1992;312:515–518.

Carnevale V, Minisola S, Romagnoli E, et al: Concurrent improvement of neuromuscular and skeletal involvement following surgery for primary hyperparathyroidism. J Neurol 1992;239:57.

Chalmers AC, Greco CM, Miller RG: Prognosis in AZT myopathy. Neurology 1991;41:1181–1184.

Chester C, Banker B: Focal infarctions of muscle in diabetics. Diabetic Care 1986;9:623–630.

Choucair AK, Ziter FA: Pentazocine abuse masquerading as familial myopathy. Neurology 1984;34:524–527.

Cogen FC, Rigg G, Simmons JL, et al: Phencyclidine-associated acute rhabdomyolysis. Ann Intern Med 1978;88:210–212.

Comi G, Testa D, Cornelio F, Canal M: Potassium depletion myopathy: A clinical and morphological study of six cases. Muscle Nerve 1985;8:17–21.

Coomes EN: The rate of recovery of reversible myopathies and the effects of anabolic agents in steroid myopathy. Neurology 1965;18:523–530.

Corpier C, Jones P, Suki W, et al: Rhabdomyolysis and renal injury with lovastatin use. JAMA 1988;260:239–241.

Costa-Jussa FR, Jacobs JM: The pathology of amiodarone neurotoxicity. I. Experimental changes with reference to changes in other tissues. Brain 1985;108:735–752.

Costigan DA: Acquired myotonia, weakness and vacuolar myopathy secondary to cyclosporine. Muscle Nerve 1989;12:761.

Curran JR, Wetmore SJ: Alcoholic myopathy. Dis Nerv Syst 1972;33:19–22.

Curry OB, Basten JF, Francis MJO, Smith R: Calcium uptake by the sarcoplasmic reticulum of muscle from vitamin D deficiency in rabbits. Nature 1974;249:83–84.

Dalakas M: HIV or zidovudine myopathy? Neurology 1994;44:360–361.

Dalakas MC, Illa I, Pezeshkpour GH, et al: Mitochondrial myopathy caused by long-term zidovudine therapy. N Engl J Med 1990;322:1098–1105.

Danon MJ, Carpenter S: Myopathy with thick filament (myosin) loss following prolonged paralysis with vecuronium during steroid treatment. Muscle Nerve 1991;14:1131–1139.

Davidson MH, Stein EA, Dujoven CA, et al: The efficacy and six week tolerability of simvastatin 80 and 160 mg/day. Am J Cardiol 1997;79:38–42.

Dawkins RL, Zilko PJ, Carrano J, et al: Immunobiology of D-penicillamine. J Rheumatol 1981;8(suppl):56–61.

Deconinck N, Van Parijs V, Beckers-Bleukx G, Van den Bergh P: Critical illness myopathy unrelated to corticosteroids or neuromuscular blocking agents. Neuromusc Disord 1998;8:186–192.

Denizot M, Fabre J, Pometa D, et al: Clofibrate, nephrotic syndrome, and histological changes in muscle. Lancet 1973;1:1326.

Denslow JS: Double discharge in human motor units. J Neurophysiol 1948;11:209–215.

Deslypere J, Vermuelen A: Rhabdomyolysis and simvastatin. Ann Intern Med 1991;114:342.

Donofrio PD, Stanton C, Miller VS, et al: Demyelinating polyneuropathy in eosinophilia-myalgia syndrome. Muscle Nerve 1992;15:796–805.

Douglass JA, Tuxen DV, Horne M, et al: Myopathy in severe asthma. Am Rev Respir Dis 1992;146:517–519.

Dubaniewicz A, Kaciuba-Uscilko H, Nazar K, Budohoski L: Sensitivity of the soleus to insulin in resting and exercising with experimental hypo- and hyperthyroidism. Biochem J 1989;263:243–247.

Duell PB, Connor WE, Illingsworth DR: Rhabdomyolysis after taking atorvastatin with gemfibrozil. Am J Cardiol 1998;81:368–369.

Dujovne CA, Chremos AN, Pool JL, et al: Expanded Clinical Evaluation of Lovastatin (EXCEL) study results. IV. Additional perspectives on the tolerability of lovastatin. Am J Med 1991;91(suppl 1B):25–30.

Dulhunty AF, Gage PW, Lamb GD: Differential effects of thyroid hormone on T-tubules and terminal cisternae in rat muscles. J Muscle Res Cell Motil 1986;7:225–236.

Dumitru D: Electrodiagnostic Medicine. Philadelphia: Hanley & Belfus, 1995; 1031–1129.

Eadie MJ, Ferrier TM: Chloroquine myopathy. J Neurol Neurosurg Psychiatry 1966;29:331–337.

Ekbom K, Hed R, Kirstein L, et al: Muscular affections in chronic alcoholism. Arch Neurol 1964;10:449–458.

Emslie-Smith AM, Engel AG, Duffy J, Bowles CA: Eosinophilia myalgia syndrome: I. Immunocytochemical evidence for a T-cell-mediated immune effector response. Ann Neurol 1991;29:524–528.

Engel AG: Electron microscopic observations in thyrotoxic and corticosteroid-induced myopathies. Mayo Clin Proc 1966;41:785–796.

Engel AG: Metabolic and endocrine myopathies. In Walton JN (ed): Disorders of Voluntary Muscle, 5th ed. Edinburgh, Churchill-Livingstone, 1988; 811–868.

Engel AG: Neuromuscular manifestations of Graves' disease. Mayo Clin Proc 1972;47:919–925.

Espinoza LR, Aguilar JL, Espinoza CG, et al: Characteristics and pathogenesis of myositis in human immunodeficiency virus infection: Distinction form azidothymidine myopathy. Rheum Dis Clin North Am 1991;17:117–129.

Estes ML, Ewing-Wilson D, Chou SM, et al: Chloroquine neuromyotoxicity: Clinical and pathological perspective. Am J Med 1987; 82:447–455.

Evans RM, Watanabe I, Singer PA: Central changes in hypothyroid myopathy: A case report. Muscle Nerve 1990;13:952–956.

Everts ME, Dorup I, Flyvberg A, et al: Na(+)-K(+) pump in rat muscle: Effects of hypophysectomy, growth hormone, and thyroid hormone. Am J Physiol 1990;259:E278–E283.

Faludi G, Gotlieb J, Meyers J: Factors influencing the development of steroid-induced myopathy. Ann N Y Acad Sci 1967;138:61–72.

Faris AA, Reyes MG, Arbrams RM: Subclinical alcoholic myopathy: Electromyographic and biopsy study. Trans Am Neurol Assoc 1967;92:102–106.

Faris AA, Reyes MG: Reappraisal of alcoholic myopathy. J Neurol Neurosurg Psychiatry 1971;34:86–92.

Faucheux JM, Tourneize P, Viguier A, et al: Neuromyopathy secondary to omeprazole treatment. Muscle Nerve 1998;21:261–262.

Feibel JH, Campa JF: Thyrotoxic neuropathy (Basedow's paraplegia). J Neurol Neurosurg Psychiatry 1976;39:491–497.

Flint OP, Masters BA, Gregg RE, Durham SK: Inhibition of cholesterol synthesis by squalene synthase inhibitors does not induce myotoxicity in vitro. Toxicol Appl Pharmacol 1997;145:91–98.

Florini JR, Ewton DZ: Skeletal muscle fiber types and myosin ATPase activity do not change with age or growth hormone administration. J Gerontol 1989;44:B110–B117.

Floyd M, Ayar DR, Barwick DD, et al: Myopathy in chronic renal failure. Q J Med 1974;53:509–524.

Folkers K, Langsjoen P, Willis R, et al: Lovastatin decreases coenzyme Q levels in humans. Proc Natl Acad Sci U S A 1990;87: 8931–8934.

Fontiveros ES, Cumming WJK, Hudgson P: Procainamide-induced myositis. J Neurol Sci 1980;45:143–147.

Frame B, Heinze EG, Block MA, Manson GA: Myopathy in primary hyperparathyroidism: Observations in three patients. Ann Intern Med 1968:1022–1027.

Frankenhaeuser B, Hodgkin AL: The action of calcium on the electric properties of squid axons. J Physiol 1957;137:218–244.

Frankenhaeuser B: The effect of calcium on the myelinated nerve fiber. J Physiol 1957;137:245–260.

Gabriel R, Pearce JMS: Clofibrate-induced myopathy and neuropathy. Lancet 1976;2:906.

Galper JB: Increased incidence of myositis in patients treated with high-dose simvastatin. Am J Cardiol 1998;81:259.

Garber AJ: Effects of parathyroid hormone on skeletal muscle protein and amino acid metabolism in the rat. J Clin Invest 1983;71:1806–1821.

Garrot FJ, Lacambrac D, Del Sert T, et al: Subacute myopathy during omeprazole therapy. Lancet 1994;340:672.

Gelinas DF, Miller RG, McVey AL: Reversible neuromuscular dysfunction associated with hyperparathyroidism [abstract]. Neurology 1994;44(suppl 2):A348.

Gentric A, Pennec YL: Fatal primary hyperparathyroidism with myopathy involving respiratory muscles. J Am Geriatr Soc 1994;42:1306.

Gherardi R, Chariot P: HIV or zidovudine myopathy? Neurology 1994;44:361–362.

Golding DN, Murray SM, Pearce GW, et al: Corticosteroid myopathy. Ann Phys Med 1962;6:171–177.

Goldring SR, Krane SM, Avioli LV: Disorders of calcification: Osteomalacia and rickets. In De Groot (ed): Endocrinology, 3rd ed. Philadelphia, WB Saunders, 1994; 1204–1227.

Gooch JL: AAEM case report #29: Prolonged paralysis after neuromuscular blockade. Muscle Nerve 1995;18:937–942.

Goy JJ, Stauffer JC, Deruaz JP, et al: Myopathy as a possible side effect cyclosporine. Lancet 1989;1:1446–1449.

Grau JM, Casademont J: HIV or zidovudine myopathy [letter]? Neurology 1994;44:361.

Grau JM, Masanes F, Pedreo E, et al: Human immunodeficiency virus type 1 infection and myopathy: Clinical relevance of zidovudine therapy. Ann Neurol 1993;34:206–211.

Grezard O, Lebranchu Y, Birmele B, et al: Cyclosporine-induced muscular toxicity. Lancet 1990;1:177.

Gutmann L, Blumenthal D, Schochet SS: Acute type II myofiber atrophy in critical illness. Neurology 1996;46:819–821.

Haan J, Hollander JMR, van Duinin SG, et al: Reversible severe myopathy during treatment with finasteride. Muscle Nerve 1997;20:502–504.

Hall JT, Fallahi S, Koopman WJ: Penicillamine-induced myositis: Observations and unique features in two patients and review of the literature. Am J Med 1984;77:719.

Hanna JP, Ramundo ML: Rhabdomyolysis and hypoxia associated with prolonged propofol infusion in children. Neurology 1988; 50:301–303.

Hanson P, Dive A, Brucher J-M, et al: Acute corticosteroid myopathy in intensive care patients. Muscle Nerve 1997;20:1371–1380.

Harman JB, Richardson AT: Generalized myokymia in thyrotoxicosis. Lancet 1954;267:473–474.

Harney J, Glasberg MR: Myopathy and hypersensitivity to phenytoin. Neurology 1983;33:790–791.

Havard CWH, Campbell EDR, Ross HB, et al: Electromyographic and histologic findings in the muscles of patients with thyrotoxicosis. Q J Med 1963;32:145–163.

Heiman-Patterson TD, Bird SJ, Parry GJ, et al: Peripheral neuropathy associated with eosinophilia-myalgia syndrome. Ann Neurol 1990;28:522–528.

Hertzman PA, Blevins WL, Mayer J, et al: Association of the eosinophilia-myalgia syndrome with the ingestion of tryptophan. N Engl J Med 1990;322:869–873.

Hibi S, Hisawa A, Tamai M, et al: Severe rhabdomyolysis with tacrolimus [letter]. Lancet 1995;346:702.

Hirano M, Ott BR, Rapps EC, et al: Acute quadriplegic myopathy: A complication of treatment with steroids, nondepolarizing blocking agents, or both. Neurology 1992;42:2082–2087.

Ho K-L: Basophilic bodies of skeletal muscle in hypothyroidism: Enzyme histochemical and ultrastructural studies. Hum Pathol 1989;20:1119–1124.

Hower J, Struck H, Tackman W, Stolecke H: CPK activity in hypoparathyroidism. N Engl J Med 1972;287:1098.

Hudgson P, Kendall-Taylor P: Endocrine myopathies. In Mastaglia FL, Walton JN (eds): Skeletal Muscle Pathology. Edinburgh, Churchill Livingstone, 1992; 493–509.

Irani PF: Electromyography in nutritional osteomalacic myopathy. J Neurol Neurosurg Psychiatry 1976;39:686–693.

Jackson CE, Amato AA, Bryan WW, et al: Primary hyperparathyroidism and ALS: Is there a relation? Neurology 1998;50:1795–1799.

Jacobs JM, Costa-Jussa FR: The pathology of amiodarone neurotoxicity. II. Peripheral neuropathy in man. Brain 1985;108:753–769.

Janssen JW, Delange-Berkout IW, Van Hardeveld C, Kassenaar AA: The disappearance of L-thyroxine and triiodothyronine from plasma, red and white skeletal muscle after administration of one subcutaneous dose of L-thyroxin to hyperthyroid and euthyroid rats. Acta Endocrinol 1981;97:226–230.

Jay CA, Hench K, Ropka M: Improvement of AZT myopathy after change to dideoxyinsine (ddI) or dideoxycytosine (ddC) [abstract]. Neurology 1993;43(suppl 2):A373–A374.

Johnson KR, Hseueh WA, Glusman SM, et al: Fibrous myopathy: A rheumatic complication of drug abuse. Arthritis Rheum 1976; 19:923–926.

Jones P, Kafonek S, Laurora I, Hunningshake D, and the CURVES Investigators: Comparative dose efficacy study of atorvastatin versus simvastatin, provastatin, lovastatin, and fluvastatin in patients with hypercholesterolemia (The CURVES Study). Am J Cardiol 1998;81:582–587.

Kaminski HJ, Ruff RL: Endocrine myopathies (hyper- and hypofunction of adrenal, thyroid, pituitary, and parathyroid glands and iatrogenic corticosteroid myopathy). In Engel AG, Franzini-Armstrong C (eds): Myology, 2nd ed. New York, McGraw-Hill, 1994; 1726–1753.

Kennard C, Swash M, Henson RA: Myopathy due to epsilon amino-caproic acid. Muscle Nerve 1980;3:202–206.

Kilbourne EM, Rigau-Perez JG, Heath CW, et al: Clinical epidemiology of toxic-oil syndrome. N Engl J Med 1983;309:1408–1414.

Kingston WJ: Endocrine myopathies. Semin Neurol 1983;3:258–264.

Kissel JT, Mendell JR: The endocrine myopathies. In Rowland LP, DiMauro S (eds): Handbook of Clinical Neurology, Vol 18 (62): Myopathies. Amsterdam, Elsevier Science Publishers BV, 1992; 527–551.

Knochel JP: The clinical status of hypophosphatemia: An update. N Engl J Med 1985;313:447–449.

Kontos HA: Myopathy associated with chronic colchicine toxicity. N Engl J Med 1962;266:38–39.

Kra SJ: Muscle syndrome with clofibrate usage. Conn Med 1974; 38:348–349.

Kruse K, Scheunemann W, Baier W, Schaub J: Hypocalcemic myopathy in idiopathic hypoparathyroidism. Eur J Pediatr 1982;138:280–282.

Kugelberg E: Activation of human nerves by hyperventilation and hypocalcemia. Arch Neurol Psychiatry 1948;60:153–164.

Kugelberg E: Neurologic mechanism for certain phenomena in tetany. Arch Neurol Psychiatry 1946;56:507–521.

Kuncl RW, Cornblath DR, Avila O, et al: Electrodiagnosis of human colchicine myoneuropathy. Muscle Nerve 1989;12:360–364.

Kuncl RW, Duncan G, Watson D, et al: Colchicine myopathy and neuropathy. N Engl J Med 1987;316:1562–1568.

Kuncl RW, Wiggins WW: Toxic myopathies. Neurol Clin 1988;6:593–619.

Kwiecinski H: Myotonia induced with clofibrate in rats. J Neurol 1978;219:107–116.

Lacomis D, Giuliani MJ, Van Cott A, Kramer DJ: Acute myopathy of the intensive care: Clinical, electromyographic, and pathological aspects. Ann Neurol 1996;40:645–654.

Lacomis D, Petrella JT, Giuliani MJ: Causes of neuromuscular weakness in the intensive care unit: A study of ninety-two patients. Muscle Nerve 1998;21:610–617.

Lacomis D, Smith TW, Chad DA: Acute myopathy and neuropathy in status asthmaticus: Case report and literature review. Muscle Nerve 1993;16:84–90.

Lane RJM, Mastaglia FL: Drug-induced myopathies in man. Lancet 1978;2:562–565.

Lane RJM, McLelland NJ, Martin AM, et al: Epsilon aminocaproic acid (EACA) myopathy. Postgrad Med J 1979;55:282–285.

Langer T, Levy RI: Acute muscular syndrome associated with administration of clofibrate. N Engl J Med 1968;279:856–858.

Latronico N, Fenzi F, Recupero D, et al: Critical illness myopathy and neuropathy. Lancet 1996;347:1579–1582.

Levin BE, Engel WK: Iatrogenic muscle fibrosis: Arm levitation as an initial sign. JAMA 1975;234:621–624.

Lewis CA, Boheimer N, Rose P, Jackson G: Myopathy after short-term administration of procainamide. Br Med J 1986;292:593–597.

Lewis PD: Neuromuscular involvement in pituitary gigantism. Br Med J 1972;2:499–500.

Litin SC, Andersone CF: Nicotinic acid–associated myopathy: A report of three cases. Am J Med 1989;86:481–483.

London F, Gross KF, Ringel SP: Cholesterol-lowering agent myopathy (CLAM). Neurology 1991;41:1159–1160.

Low PA, McLeod JG, Turtle JR, et al: Peripheral neuropathy in acromegaly. Brain 1974;97:139–153.

Ludin HP, Spiess H, Koenig MP: Neuromuscular dysfunction associated with thyrotoxicosis. Eur Neurol 1969;2:269–278.

Lundberg PO, Osterman PO, Stalberg E: Neuromuscular signs and symptoms in acromegaly. In Walton JN, Canal N, Scarlato G (eds): Muscle Diseases. Proceedings of an International Congress, Milan, May 19–21, 1969. Amsterdam, Excerpta Medica, 1970; 531–534.

Lunghall S, Akerstrom G, Johansson G, et al: Neuromuscular involvement in primary hyperparathyroidism. J Neurol 1984;231:263–265.

MacKay AR, Sang UH, Weinstein PR: Myopathy associated with epsilon amino-caproic acid (EACA) therapy: Report of two cases. J Neurosurg 1978;49:597–601.

MacLean D, Schurr PH: Reversible amyotrophy complicating treatment with fluodrocortisone. Lancet 1959;516:701–702.

Magarian GJ, Lucas LM: Gemfibrozil-induced myopathy. Arch Intern Med 1991;154:1873–1874.

Mallette LE, Patten BM, Engel WK: Neuromuscular disease in secondary hyperparathyroidism. Ann Intern Med 1975;82:474–483.

Manji H, Harrison MJG, Round JM, et al: Muscle disease, HIV and zidovudine: The spectrum of muscle disease in HIV-infected individuals treated with zidovudine. J Neurol 1993;240:479–488.

Marais GE, Larson KK: Rhabdomyolysis and acute renal failure induced by combination lovastatin and gemfibrozil therapy. Ann Intern Med 1990;112:228–230.

Martinez FJ, Bermudez-Gomez M, Celli BR: Hypothyroidism: A reversible cause of diaphragmatic dysfunction. Chest 1989;96:1059–1063.

Mastaglia FL: Toxic myopathies. In Rowland LP, DiMauro S (eds): Handbook of Clinical Neurology, vol 18: Myopathies. Amsterdam, Elsevier Science Publishers BV, 1992; 595–622.

Mastaglia FL, Barwick DB, Hall R: Myopathy in acromegaly. Lancet 1970;2:907–909.

Mastaglia FL, Papadimitriou JM, Dawkins RL, et al: Vacuolar myopathy associated with chloroquine, lupus erythematosus and thymoma. J Neurol Sci 1977;34:315–328.

Mateer JE, Farrell BJ, Chou SSM, et al: Reversible ipecac myopathy. Arch Neurol 1985;42:188–190.

Mayeno AN, Belongia EA, Lin F, et al: 3-(Phenylamino)alanine: A novel aniline-derived amino acid associated with the eosinophilic-myalgia syndrome: A link to the toxic oil syndrome. Mayo Clin Proc 1992;67:1134.

Mayer RF, Garcia-Mullin R, Eckholdt JW: Acute "alcoholic" myopathy. Neurology 1968;18:275.

McCommas AJ, Sica REP, McNabb AR, et al: Evidence for reversible motoneurone dysfunction in thyrotoxicosis. J Neurol Neurosurg Psychiatry 1974;37:548–558.

McElvaney GN, Wilcox PG, Fairborn MS, et al: Respiratory muscle weakness and dyspnea in thyrotoxic patients. Am Rev Respir Dis 1990;141:1221–1227.

McFarlane IA, Rosenthal FD: Severe myopathy after status asthmaticus. Lancet 1977;1:615.

Meier C, Kauer B, Muller U, Ludin HP: Neuromyopathy during amiodarone treatment: A case report. J Neurol 1979;220:231–239.

Mhiri C, Baudrimont M, Bonne G, et al: Zidovudine myopathy: A distinctive disorder associated with mitochondrial dysfunction. Ann Neurol 1991;29:606–614.

Mier A, Brophy C, Wass JA, et al: Reversible muscle weakness in hyperthyroidism. Am Rev Respir Dis 1989;139:529–533.

Mitchell CG, Magnussen AR, Weiler JM: Cimetidine-induced cutaneous vasculitis. Am J Med 1983;75:875.

Mizusawa H, Takagi A, Sugita H, et al: Mounding phenomena: An experimental study in vitro. Neurology 1983;33:90–93.

Moosa A, Dubowitz V: Slow nerve conduction velocity in cretins. Arch Dis Child 1971;46:852–854.

Morris CDW, Jacobs P, Berman PA, et al: Epsilon-aminocaproic acid–induced myopathy. S Afr Med J 1983;64:363–366.

Morrison WL, Gibson JN, Jung RT, Rennie MJ: Skeletal muscle and whole body protein turnover in thyroid disease. Eur J Clin Invest 1988;18:62–68.

Muller R, Kugelberg E: Myopathy in Cushing's syndrome. J Neurol Neurosurg Psychiatry 1959;22:314–319.

Noppen D, Verlkeriers B, Dierckx R, et al: Cyclosporine and myopathy. Ann Intern Med 1987;107:945–946.

Norman D, Illingworth DR, Munson J, Hosenpud J: Myolysis and acute renal failure in heart transplant recipient receiving lovastatin. N Engl J Med 1988;318:46–47.

Norman MG, Temple AR, Murphy JV: Infantile quadriceps-femoris contracture resulting from intramuscular injections. N Engl J Med 1970;282:964–966.

Norton JA, Sugg SL: Surgical management of hyperparathyroidism. In De Groot (ed): Endocrinology, 3rd ed. Philadelphia, WB Saunders, 1994; 1106–1122.

Nussbaum SR, Neer RM, Potts JT Jr: Medical management of hyperparathyroidism and hypercalcemia. In De Groot (ed): Endocrinology, 3rd ed. Philadelphia, WB Saunders, 1994; 1094–1105.

Oh SJ, Rollins JL, Lewis I: Pentazocine-induced fibrous myopathy. JAMA 1975;231:271–273.

Oh SJ: Chronic alcoholic myopathy: An entity difficult to diagnose. South Med J 1972;65:449–452.

Op de Coul AAW, Lambregts PC, Koeman J, et al: Neuromuscular complications in patients given Pavulon (pancuronium bromide) during artificial ventilation. Clin Neurol Neurosurg 1985;87:17–22.

Palmer EP, Guay AT: Reversible myopathy secondary to abuse of ipecac in patients with major eating disorders. N Engl J Med 1985;313:1457–1459.

Panegyres PK, Papadimitriou JM, Hollingsworth PN, et al: Vesicular changes in the myopathies of AIDS: Ultrastructural observations and their relationship to zidovudine treatment. J Neurol Neurosurg Psychiatry 1990;53:649–655.

Parke TJ, Steven JE, Rice ASC, et al: Metabolic acidosis and myocardial failure after propofol infusion in children: Five case reports. Br Med J 1992;305:613–616.

Partanen JV, Danner R: Fibrillation potentials after muscle injury in humans. Muscle Nerve 1982;5:S70–S73.

Partanen JV, Lang AH: An analysis of double discharges in the human electromyogram. J Neurol Sci 1978;36:363–375.

Patten BM, Bilezikian JP, Mallette LE, et al: Neuromuscular disease in primary hyperparathyroidism. Ann Intern Med 1974;80:182–193.

Perkoff GT: Alcoholic myopathy. Annu Rev Med 1971;22:125–132.

Peters BS, Winer J, Landon DN, et al: Mitochondrial myopathy associated with chronic zidovudine therapy in AIDS. Q J Med 1993;86:5–15.

Pickett JBE, Layzer RB, Levin SR, et al: Neuromuscular complications of acromegaly. Neurology 1975;25:638–645.

Pierce LR, Wysowski DK, Gross TP: Myopathy and rhabdomyolysis associated with lovastatin-gemfibrozil combination therapy. JAMA 1990;264:71–75.

Pierides AM, Alvarez-Ude F, Kerr DNS, et al: Clofibrate-induced muscle damage in patients with chronic renal failure. Lancet 1975;2:1279–1282.

Pleasure DE, Walsh GO, Engel WK: Atrophy of skeletal muscle in patients with Cushing's syndrome. Arch Neurol 1970;22:118–125.

Pointon JJ, Francis MJO, Smith R: Effect of vitamin D deficiency on sarcoplasmic reticulum and troponin C concentration of rabbit skeletal muscle. Clin Sci 1979;57:257–263.

Prineas JW, Hall R, Barwick DD, et al: Myopathy associated with pigmentation following adrenalectomy for Cushing's syndrome. Q J Med 1968;37:63–77.

Prineas JW, Mason AS, Henson RA: Myopathy in metabolic bone disease. Br Med J 1965;1:1034–1036.

Prummel MF, Mourits MP, Berout A, et al: Prednisone and cyclosporine in the treatment of severe Graves' disease. N Engl J Med 1989;321:1353.

Prysor-Jones RA, Jenkins JS: Effect of excessive secretion of growth hormone on tissues of the rat, with particular reference to the heart and skeletal muscle. J Endocrinol 1980;85:75–82.

Puvanendran K, Cheah JS, Naganathan N, et al: Neuromuscular transmission in thyrotoxicosis. J Neurol Sci 1979;43:47–57.

Raben MS: Growth hormone: Clinical use of growth hormone. N Engl J Med 1962;266:86.

Rabinowitz D, Zierler KL: Differentiation of active from inactive acromegaly by studies of forearm metabolism and response to intra-arterial insulin. Bull Johns Hopkins Hosp 1963;113:211–224.

Ramsay DA, Zochodne DW, Robertson DM, et al: A syndrome of acute severe muscle necrosis in intensive care unit patients. J Neuropathol Exp Neurol 1993;52:387–398.

Ramsay ID: Electromyography in thyrotoxicosis. Q J Med 1965;34:255–267.

Randall DP, Fisher MA, Thomas C: Rhabdomyolysis as the presenting manifestation of calciphylaxis. Muscle Nerve 2000;23:289–293.

Rao SN, Katiyar BC, Nair KRP, et al: Neuromuscular status in hypothyroidism. Acta Neurol Scand 1980;61:167–177.

Reaven P, Witzum J: Lovastatin, nicotinic acid and rhabdomyolysis. Ann Intern Med 1988;109:597–598.

Reyes MG, Casanova J, Varricchio F, et al: Zidovudine myopathy. Neurology 1992;42:1252.

Rich MM, Bird SJ, Raps EC, et al: Direct muscle stimulation in acute quadriplegic myopathy. Muscle Nerve 1997;20:665–673.

Rich MM, Pinter MJ, Kraner SD, Barchi RL: Loss of electrical excitability in an animal model of acute quadriplegic myopathy. Ann Neurol 1998;43:171–179.

Rich MM, Teener JW, Raps EC, et al: Muscle is electrically inexcitable in acute quadriplegic myopathy. Neurology 1996;46:731–736.

Richardson JA, Herron G, Reitz R, Layzer R: Ischemic ulcerations of the skin and necrosis of muscle in azotemic hyperparathyroidism. Ann Intern Med 1969;71:129–138.

Richman DD, Fischl MA, Grieco HM, et al: The toxicity of azidothymidine (AZT) in the treatment of patients with AIDS and AIDS-related complex. N Engl J Med 1987;317:192–197.

Richter RW, Challenor YB, Pearson J, et al: Acute myoglobinuria associated with heroin addiction. JAMA 1971;216:1172–1176.

Rieger EH, Halasz NA, Wahlstrom HE: Colchicine neuromyopathy after renal transplantation. Transplantation 1990;49;1196–1198.

Riggs JE, Schochet SS, Gutmann L, et al: Chronic colchicine neuropathy and myopathy. Arch Neurol 1986;43:521–523.

Riggs JE: Acute exertional rhabdomyolysis in hypothyroidism: The result of a reversible defect in glycogenolysis? Milit Med 1990;155:171–172.

Road J, Mackie G, Jiang T-X, et al: Reversible paralysis with status asthmaticus, steroids, and pancuronium: Clinical electrophysiological correlates. Muscle Nerve 1997;20:1587–1590.

Roca B, Minguez C, Saez-Royuela A, Simon E: Dementia, myopathy, and idiopathic hyperparathyroidism. Postgrad Med J 1995;71:702.

Rossouw JE, Keeton RG, Hewlett RH: Chronic proximal muscular weakness in alcoholics. S Afr Med J 1976;50:2095–2098.

Roth R, Itabashi H, Louie J, et al: Amiodarone toxicity: Myopathy and neuropathy. Am Heart J 1990;119:1223–1225.

Rubenstein AE, Wainapel SF: Acute hypokalemic myopathy in alcoholism: A clinical entity. Arch Neurol 1977;34:553–555.

Ruff RL, Simoncini L, Stuhmer W: Slow channel inactivation in mammalian muscle: A possible role in regulating excitability. Muscle Nerve 1988;11:502–510.

Ruff RL. Why do ICU patients become paralyzed? Ann Neurol 1998;43:154–155.

Rush P, Baron M, Kapusta M: Clofibrate myopathy: A case report and a review of the literature. Semin Arthritis Rheum 1986;15:226–229.

Russell JA: Osteomalacic myopathy. Muscle Nerve 1994;17:578–580.

Rutkove SB, De Girolami U, Preston DC, et al: Myotonia in colchicine myoneuropathy. Muscle Nerve 1996;19:870–875.

Sagman DL, Melamed JC: L-Tryptophan induced eosinophilia-myalgia syndrome and myopathy. Neurology 1990;40:1629–1630.

Sakimoto K: The cause of the eosinophilia-myalgia syndrome associated with tryptophan use. N Engl J Med 1990;323:992.

Salick AI, Colachis SC, Pearson CM: Myxedema myopathy: Clinical, electrodiagnostic, and pathologic findings in advanced case. Arch Phys Med Rehabil 1968;49:230–237.

Salick AI, Pearson CM: Electrical silence of myoedema. Neurology 1967;17:899–901.

Sataysohi E, Murakami K, Kowa H, et al: Periodic paralysis in hyperthyroidism. Neurology 1963;13:746–752.

Scarpalezos S, Lygidakis C, Papageorgiou C, et al: Neural and muscular manifestations of hypothyroidism. Arch Neurol 1973;29:140–144.

Schalke BB, Schmidt B, Toyka K, Hartung H-P: Provastatin-associated inflammatory myopathy. N Engl J Med 1992;327:649–650.

Schott GD, Wills MR: Myopathy in hypophosphatemic osteomalacia presenting in adult life. J Neurol Neurosurg Psychiatry 1975;38:297–304.

Schrader PL, Peters HA, Dahl DS: Polymyositis and penicillamine. Arch Neurol 1972;27:456–457.

Schwartz HL, Oppenheimer JH: Physiologic and biochemical actions of thyroid hormone. Pharmacol Ther (B) 1978;3:349–376.

Schwartz MS, Mackworth-Young CG, McKeran RO: The tarsal tunnel syndrome in hypothyroidism. J Neurol Neurosurg Psychiatry 1983;46:440–442.

Sellapah S: An unusual side effect of omeprazole therapy: A case report. Br J Gen Pract 1990;40:389.

Selwa JF, Feldman EL, Blaivas M: Mononeuropathy multiplex in tryptophan-associated eosinophilia-myalgia syndrome. Neurology 1990;40:1632–1633.

Shane E, McClane KA, Olarte MR, Bilezikian JP: Hypoparathyroidism and elevated serum enzymes. Neurology 1980;30:192–195.

Shepherd J: Fibrates and statins in the treatment of hyperlipidemia: An appraisal of their efficacy and safety. Eur Heart J 1995;16:5–13.

Shirabe T, Tawara S, Terao A, et al: Myxoedematous polyneuropathy: A light and electron microscopic study of the peripheral nerve and muscle. J Neurol Neurosurg Psychiatry 1975;38:241–247.

Showalter CJ, Engel AG: Acute quadriplegic myopathy: Analysis of myosin isoforms and evidence for calpain-mediated proteolysis. Muscle Nerve 1997;20:316–322.

Shulman LE: Diffuse fasciitis with eosinophilia: A new syndrome? Trans Assoc Am Physicians 1975;88:70–86.

Simpson DM, Bender AN: Human immunodeficiency virus-associated myopathy: Analysis of 11 patients. Ann Neurol 1988;24:79–84.

Simpson DM, Bender AN, Farraye J, et al: Human immunodeficiency virus wasting syndrome represents a treatable myopathy. Neurology 1990;40:535–538.

Simpson DM, Citak KA, Godfrey E, et al: Myopathies associated with human immunodeficiency virus and zidovudine: Can their effects be distinguished? Neurology 1993;43:971–976.

Simpson DM, Slasor P, Dafni U, et al: Analysis of myopathy in a placebo-controlled zidovudine trial. Muscle Nerve 1997;20:382–385.

Sitwell LD, Weishenker BG, Monipetit V, Reid D: Complete ophthalmoplegia as a complication of acute corticosteroid- and pancuronium-associated myopathy. Neurology 1991;41:921–922.

Skaria J, Kattyar BC, Srivastava TP, Dube B: Myopathy and neuropathy associated with osteomalacia. Acta Neurol Scand 1975;51:37–58.

Slotwiner P, Song S, Andersone P: Spheromembranous degeneration of muscle induced by vincristine. Arch Neurol 1966;15:172–176.

Smith BE, Dyck PJ: Peripheral neuropathy in the eosinophilic-myalgia syndrome associated with L-tryptophan ingestion. Neurology 1990;40:1035–1040.

Smith R, Stern G: Muscular weakness in osteomalacia and hyperparathyroidism. J Neurol Sci 1969;8:511–520.

Smith R, Stern G: Myopathy, osteomalacia and hyperparathyroidism. Brain 1967;90:593–602.

Snowdon JA, Macfie AC, Pearce JB: Hypocalcemic myopathy and parathyroid psychosis. J Neurol Neurosurg Psychiatry 1976;38:48–52.

Stern LZ, Payne CM, Hannapel LK: Acromegaly: Histochemical and electron microscopic changes in deltoid and intercostal muscle. Neurology 1974;24:589–593.

Stewart BM: The hypertrophic neuropathy of acromegaly. Arch Neurol 1966;14:107–110.

Strickland RA, Murray MJ: Fatal metabolic acidosis in pediatric patient receiving an infusion of propofol in the intensive care unit: Is there a relationship? Crit Care Med 1995;23:405–409.

Swash M, Schwartz MS: Neuromuscular Diseases: A Practical Approach to Diagnosis and Management. London, Springer-Verlag, 1988.

Takahashi K, Ogita T, Okudaira H, et al: D-Penicillamine–induced polymyositis in patients with rheumatoid arthritis. Arthritis Rheum 1986;29:560–564.

Takamori M, Gutman L, Crosby TW, et al: Myasthenic syndromes in hypothyroidism. Arch Neurol 1972;26:326–335.

Taneja V, Mehra N, Singh YN, et al: HLA-D region genes and susceptibility to D-penicillamine-induced polymyositis. Arthritis Rheum 1990;33:1445–1447.

Tanhehco JL, Wiechers DO, Golbus J, et al: Eosinophilia-myalgia syndrome: Myopathic electrodiagnostic characteristics. Muscle Nerve 1992;15:561–567.

Teicher A, Rosenthal T, Kissen E, Sarova I: Labetolol-induced toxic myopathy. Br Med J 1981;282:1824–1825.

Thompson PD, Gadaleta PA, Yurgalevitch S, et al: Effects of exercise and lovastatin on serum creatine kinase activity. Metabolism 1991;40:1333–1336.

Till M, McDonnel KB: Myopathy with human immunodeficiency virus type 1 (HIV) infection: HIV-1 or zidovudine? Ann Intern Med 1990;113:492–494.

Tobert J: Efficacy and long-term adverse effect pattern of lovastatin. Am J Cardiol 1988a;62:28J–33J.

Tobert J: Rhabdomyolysis in patients receiving lovastatin after cardiac transplantation. N Engl J Med 1988b;318:48.

Trounce I, Byrne E, Dennett X: Biochemical and morphological studies of skeletal muscle in experimental chronic alcoholic myopathy. Acta Neurol Scand 1990;82:386–391.

Turi GK, Solitaire GB, James N, Dicker R: Eosinophilia-myalgia syndrome (L-tryptophan-associated neuromyopathy). Neurology 1990;40:1793–1796.

Turken SA, Cafferty M, Silverberg SJ, et al: Neuromuscular involvement in mild, asymptomatic, primary hyperparathyroidism. Am J Med 1989;87:553–557.

Van den Bergh PYK, Guettat L, Berg BCV, Martine J-J: Focal myopathy associated with chronic intramuscular injection of piritramide. Muscle Nerve 1997;29:1598–1600.

Vanneste JAL, van Wijngaarden GK: Epsilon-aminocaproic acid myopathy. Eur Neurol 1982;21:242–248.

Venables GS, Bates D, Shaw DA: Hypothyroidism with true myotonia. J Neurol Neurosurg Psychiatry 1978;41:1013–1015.

Vicale CT: The diagnostic features of a muscular syndrome resulting from hyperparathyroidism, osteomalacia, owing to renal tubular acidosis, and perhaps to related disorders of calcium metabolism. Trans Am Neurol Assoc 1949;74:143–147.

Victor M, Sieb JP: Myopathies due to drugs, toxins, and nutritional deficiency. In Engel AG, Franzini-Armstrong C (eds): Myology, 2nd ed. New York, McGraw-Hill, 1994; 1697–1725.

Volin L, Jarventie, Ruut U: Fatal rhabdomyolysis as a complication of bone marrow transplantation. Bone Marrow Transplant 1990;6:59–60.

von Keutz E, Schluter G: Preclinical safety evaluation of cerivastatin, a novel HMG-CoA reductase inhibitor. Am J Cardiol 1998;82:11J–17J.

Waldstein SS, Bronsky D, Shrifter HB, et al: The electromyogram in myxedema. Arch Intern Med 1958;101:97–102.

Watson AJS, Dalbow MH, Stachura I, et al: Immunologic studies in cimetidine-induced nephropathy and polymyositis. N Engl J Med 1983;308:142–145.

Williams RS: Triamcinolone myopathy. Lancet 1959;516:698–700.

Willis JK, Tilton AH, Harkin JC, Boineau FG: Reversible myopathy due to labetalol. Pediatr Neurol 1990;6:275–276.

Winckler B, Steele R, Altszuller N, et al: Effect of growth hormone on free fatty acid metabolism. Am J Physiol 1964;206:174–178.

Witt NJ, Zochodne DW, Bolton CF, et al: Peripheral nerve function in sepsis and multiorgan failure. Chest 1991;99:176–184.

Wolf S, Goldberg LS, Verity MA: Neuromyopathy and periarteriolitis in a patient receiving levodopa. Arch Intern Med 1976;136:1055–1057.

Wolf SM, Lusk W, Weisberg L: Hypocalcemia myopathy. Bull Los Angeles Neurol Soc 1972;37:167.

Worden RE: Pattern of muscle and nerve pathology in alcoholism. Ann N Y Acad Sci 1976;273:351–359.

Yamaguchi H, Okamoto K, Shooji M, et al: Muscle histology of hypocalcemic myopathy in hypoparathyroidism [letter]. J Neurol Neurosurg Psychiatry 1987;50:817–818.

Zochodne DW, Bolton CF, Wells GF, et al: Critical illness polyneuropathy: A complication of sepsis and multiorgan failure. Brain 1987;110:819–842.

Zochodne DW, Ramsey DA, Saly V, et al: Acute necrotizing myopathy of the intensive care: Electrophysiological studies. Muscle Nerve 1994;17:285–292.

C H A P T E R 79

Metabolic Myopathies

Barend P. Lotz

The metabolic myopathies are either acquired or hereditary. Free fatty acids are the dominant source of energy (adenosine triphosphate [ATP]) for muscle during rest, light aerobic exercise, and prolonged low-intensity endurance exercise. At exercise levels of around 75% of maximum oxygen uptake, glycogen is the main source of energy, provided via aerobic glycolysis. During dynamic exercise close to maximal oxygen uptake and during isometric exercise, the energy is supplied via anaerobic glycolysis. Fatigue sets in once glycogen stores are depleted, and the muscle is then totally dependent on free fatty acids for its energy needs. A history of cramping, stiffness, or muscle pain shortly after maximal exertion, such as lifting heavy weights, would be suggestive of a glycogen storage disease. These symptoms, precipitated by prolonged exercise, are most likely due to a lipid storage disorder. However, because of partial enzyme deficiencies, clinical overlap is common, and a clinical distinction cannot be made reliably. Also, mitochondria are central to energy production in general, and pyruvate and nonesterified free fatty acids are the major substrates oxidized in the mitochondria. Most of the mitochondrial disorders, however, are recognized on the basis of other distinctive clinical features. Both muscle contraction and relaxation are energy dependent, and muscle cramps, stiffness, or myalgia are thus early and unifying clinical features in most of the metabolic myopathies. If the energy failure becomes critical, rhabdomyolysis with secondary myoglobinuria ensues.

DISORDERS OF GLYCOGEN METABOLISM

The biochemical pathways involved in glycogenosis and glycogenolysis are shown in Figure 79–1. The specific enzyme defects described are indicated by

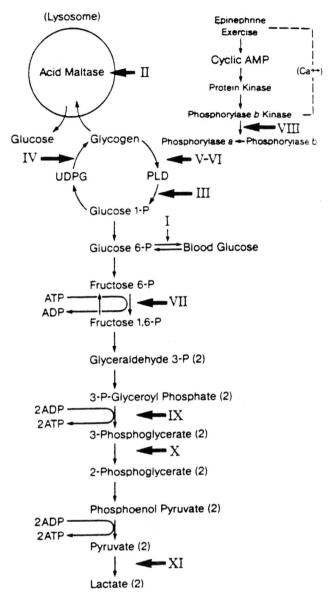

Figure 79–1. The metabolic pathways involved in glycogen metabolism. Roman numerals indicate enzyme defects in glycogenolysis and glycolysis. See text for details. (From Di Mauro S, Miranda AF, Sokoda S, et al: Metabolic myopathies. Am J Med Genet 25:635, 1986, with permission.)

Table 79–1. Glycogen Storage Diseases

Roman Numeral	Enzyme Defect	Subunit or Isozyme	Chromosome Location
II	Acid maltase	—	17q23
III	Debrancher	—	1p21
IV	Branching	—	3p12
V	Muscle phosphorylase	Muscle	11q13
VI	Liver phosphorylase	Liver	14
VII	Phosphofructokinase	Muscle	12q13
		Platelet	10(p)
		Liver	21(q22.3)
VIII	Phosphorylase *b* kinase	α Muscle	Xq12-q13
		α Liver	Xp22.2-p22.1
		β Liver at muscle	16q12-q13
		γ	7p12-q21
IX	Phosphoglycerate kinase	A	X(q13)
X	Phosphoglycerate mutase	Muscle	7
		Brain	10
XI	Lactate dehydrogenase	Muscle	11p15.1-p14.1
		Heart	12

the roman numeral assigned to each disorder. The numerals were assigned in order of discovery, but there is disagreement in naming after phosphofructokinase deficiency (glycogenosis VII) (Di Mauro and Tsujino, 1994). The roman numeral, the enzyme defect, the specific enzyme subunit or the tissues in which the enzyme is found, and the chromosomal location of the genetic defects are listed in Table 79–1. Glycogenosis type I (von Gierke's disease) does not affect muscle and is not discussed. The standard screening procedure for most of these disorders is the ischemic exercise test. Many variants of this test have been described. In principle, venous lactate levels are obtained at rest and compared with samples obtained for up to 10 minutes after 1 minute of ischemic exercise. The standard technique is to place a sphygmomanometer cuff over the upper arm and to inflate this to a level above the systolic blood pressure. The patient is then instructed to squeeze the hand once every second, with a force of about 30% of maximal hand grip strength, for 1 minute. Next, the cuff is deflated, and further blood specimens are collected for lactate estimation at 1, 3, 5, and 10 minutes after exercise. A normal result is a rise in venous blood lactate of 2.5 to 3 times above the baseline level, with a maximum rise recorded after 3 to 5 minutes. False normal values can be obtained if the patient does not fully cooperate, and the blood specimens for venous lactate estimation should be kept on ice before analysis. A potential complication of the test is the induction of myonecrosis in the forearm muscles that are examined, but this appears to be a very rare complication.

Electromyographic Studies in Glycogen Storage Diseases

As a rule, these disorders have normal motor and sensory nerve conduction velocities, but low compound muscle action potential amplitudes may be recorded from atrophic muscles. In patients afflicted with these disorders, branching and debranching enzyme deficiencies may be associated with sensorimotor axonal neuropathies, in which case the sensory nerve action potentials may also be low or absent. The electromyographic examination is characterized by myopathic motor unit potentials in clinically affected muscles, and most of these disorders also show increased insertional activity in clinically affected muscles. Glycogen storage disorders are characterized in particular by the presence of myo-

Table 79–2. The Electromyographic Findings in the Different Glycogen Storage Disorders

Deficiency	Conduction Studies	Needle Electromyography	
		Insertional Activity	*Motor Unit Potentials*
Acid maltase	Usually normal	Myotonia, fibrillation potentials, and chronic repetitive discharges in proximal muscles	Normal or myopathic
Phosphyorylase *b* kinase	Usually normal	Fibrillation potentials after rhabdomyolysis	Myopathic
Myophosphorylase	Low CMAPs, decremental response	Fibrillation potentials and myotonia after rhabdomyolysis	Myopathic
Debranching enzyme	Sensorimotor axonal neuropathy	Fibrillation potentials, myotonia, and chronic repetitive discharges in affected muscles	Neurogenic and myopathic
Phosphofructokinase	Low CMAPs, decremental response	Fibrillation potentials and myotonia after rhabdomyolysis	Myopathic
Phosphoglycerate kinase	Normal	Normal	Normal
Phosphoglycerate mutase	Normal between attacks	Normal between attacks	Normal between attacks
Lactate dehydrogenase	Normal between attacks	Normal	Normal
Branching enzyme	Sensorimotor axonal neuropathy	Unknown	Unknown

CMAPs, compound muscle action potential amplitudes.

tonic discharges and chronic repetitive discharges in affected muscles. As in any active myopathy, fibrillation potentials are common, especially after rhabdomyolysis. A unique feature of the cramps associated with glycogen storage disorders is that they are electrically silent. This was first reported in McArdle's disease and has also been well documented in phosphofructokinase deficiency. In theory, electrically silent cramps should be present in all glycogen storage disorders characterized by muscle cramping. Prolonged repetitive discharges at rapid rates may also induce a decremental response in all patients with electrically silent muscle cramping (Table 79–2).

Acid Maltase Deficiency (Glycogenosis Type II)

Acid maltase is a lysosomal α-glucosidase and the only glycolytic enzyme that is also a lysosomal enzyme. It is interesting that acid maltase deficiency was also the first lysosomal storage disease to be recognized (Lejeune et al., 1963). The enzyme is unique in that it hydrolyzes both α-1,4-glucoside and α-1,6-glucoside linkages and thus releases glucose from glycogen, oligosaccharides, and maltose (Brown et al., 1970). The acid maltase isozymes in skeletal muscle, heart muscle, and liver are identical, but renal acid maltase has different antigenic properties and thermostability. Patients with acid maltase deficiency can be expected to have involvement of skeletal muscle, heart muscle, and liver. However, glycogenolysis is not completely compromised by the absence of acid maltase, because alternate pathways for glycogenolysis are available. Acid maltase deficiency is inherited as an autosomal recessive trait.

CLINICAL SPECTRUM OF ACID MALTASE DEFICIENCY

Infantile Acid Maltase Deficiency

Disease onset is within the first few months of life, and it is characterized by muscle weakness and enlargement of the heart, tongue, and liver. Patients usually die from cardiorespiratory failure within the first 2 years of life. Glycogen accumulation is also present in smooth muscle, endothelial cells, lymphocytes, the eye (except the pigmentary epithelium), renal glomeruli, renal interstitial cells, the brain (except the cerebellum), spinal cord, and Schwann cells.

Childhood Acid Maltase Deficiency

Onset is in early childhood, and proximal muscle weakness, weakness of the respiratory muscles, and calf hypertrophy are typical features. Some patients have a rigid spine syndrome phenotype (Fadic et al., 1997). Liver, heart, or tongue involvement occurs infrequently. An association with basilar artery aneurysms secondary to glycogen deposition in arterial smooth muscle have been reported in some families (Makos et al., 1987). Survival beyond the second decade of life is rare.

Adult Acid Maltase Deficiency

Onset is after age 20 with slowly progressive proximal muscle weakness. The hip adductors and the sternal head of the pectoralis major muscle selectively may be affected more severely, resulting in a phenotype similar to that seen in limb-girdle muscle dystrophy. One third of the patients present with respiratory failure, and respiratory weakness is eventually noted in all patients. There is no enlargement of the liver or heart. Complaints of myalgia, muscle stiffness, or muscle cramps are not present. The enzyme is only partially deficient, and utilization of glycogen for energy production is not impaired. The reasons for the muscle breakdown are thus poorly understood, but it may result from excessive glycogen storage or the release of lysosomal enzymes from the secondary lysosomes (Griffin, 1984).

LABORATORY TESTS

Serum Enzymes

In adults, moderate creatine kinase elevations (<2000 IU/L) are found. In children, both creatine kinase and liver enzymes (aspartate aminotransferase and lactate dehydrogenase) levels are elevated (Engel et al., 1973).

Electromyographic Studies

The motor and sensory nerve conduction studies are usually normal, but low compound muscle action potentials may be recorded from atrophic muscles. The changes are more severe in the infantile and childhood forms of the disease, and the electrophysiological findings may be normal in the early stages of adult-onset acid maltase deficiency. The typical electromyographic findings are those of a myopathy with short-duration, low-amplitude, polyphasic motor unit potentials present in weak muscles. A characteristic finding in these disorders is the presence of increased insertional activity in proximal muscles—in particular, the paraspinal and abdominal muscles. The increased insertional activity consists of fibrillation potentials (positive waves and spikes), complex repetitive discharges, and myotonic discharges (Engel et al., 1973). Clinical myotonia is absent.

Muscle Histology

The histological findings are those of a vacuolar myopathy (Fig. 79–2A) with nearly all the muscle fibers affected in clinically weak muscles. The vacuoles are strongly acid phosphatase positive, indicating their autophagic origin. The intrafusal muscle fibers are also affected. Denervation atrophy and single muscle fibers with increased numbers of small lipid droplets have been reported. Ultrastructural examination shows the accumulation of glycogen in large lakes, either free between the myofibrils or bound by a limiting membrane (see Fig. 79–2B).

CLINICAL-GENETIC CORRELATIONS

The gene coding for acid maltase (*GAA* gene) is located on chromosome 17. Previously attributed to the 17q23 region, it has been linked by fluorescence hybridization to 17q25.2→q25.3, just distal to the thymidine kinase gene (Kuo et al., 1997). α-Glucosidase exhibits genetic polymorphism in the normal

population with three alleles (*GAA1, GAA2,* and *GAA4*) segregating with genetic frequencies of 0.9, 0.03, and 0.06, respectively. These alleles result from different nucleotide transitions (Huie et al., 1996). The *GAA* gene is approximately 20 kb long, consisting of 20 exons, with the first exon noncoding (Hoefsloot et al., 1990). The coding sequence of the catalytic site domain is interrupted by an intron of 101 bp. Deletions, missense mutations, or nucleotide transversions in the exons and introns have been described to cause clinical disease. About 30% of patients have one of seven common mutations, and it was estimated that the mutant gene frequency was 0.005, giving an expected number of individuals born with acid maltase deficiency to be 1 in 40,000 births (Martiniuk et al., 1998). Depending on the genetic defect, the enzyme may be absent, present but functionally inactive, or partially deficient with reduced activity (Ninomiya et al., 1984; Di Mauro and Tsujino, 1994). Defects in the synthesis, glycosylation, phosphorylation, maturation, intracellular transport, and abnormal degradation of the enzyme have been documented (Reuser et al., 1985). A correlation between the biochemical defect, the genetic defect, and the clinical phenotype has become apparent (Wokke et al., 1995). Early-onset cases appear to have deficiencies of catalytic activity (Reuser et al., 1985). Most adult-onset cases carry a T-to-G transversion at position −13 of intron 1 (Huie et al., 1996). In an elegant study that included three generations, it was shown that the grandfather, with adult-onset disease, was a compound heterozygote for the T-to-G transversion in intron 1 and had a deletion of a single base-pair, 525T, thus reducing acid α-glucosidase activity by 70%. His grandchild had neonatal disease onset because of a homozygous 1-bp 525T deletion, resulting in complete absence of the catalytic enzyme (Kroos et al., 1995). Both the structural gene and the DNA copy (complementary DNA [cDNA]) of the messenger RNA (mRNA) needed for enzyme synthesis have been isolated and analyzed. At this point, it appears that lack of GAA mRNA is common in infantile-onset cases.

DIAGNOSIS OF ACID MALTASE DEFICIENCY

Elevated creatine kinase levels are a sensitive marker of acid maltase deficiency and are found in nearly all patients (Ausems et al., 1999). A definitive diagnosis can be made by measuring acid maltase activity in muscle, cultured fibroblasts, lymphocytes, and urine. Urinary assays, however, are complicated by the presence of the urinary acid maltase isozyme that has normal activity in acid maltase deficiency. To rule out the pseudodeficiency state in carriers of the *GAA2* allele, patients with low leukocyte activity should have a repeat assay performed on cultured fibroblasts, using artificial substrate. A prenatal diagnosis can be made by measuring enzyme activity on cultured amniotic fluid cells or by ultrastructural examination of amniotic fluid cells

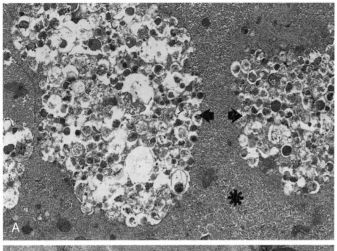

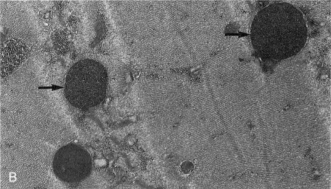

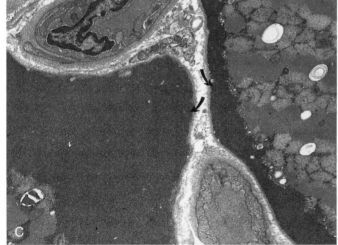

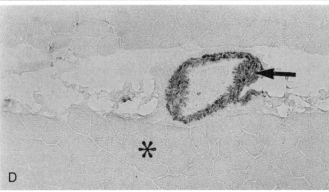

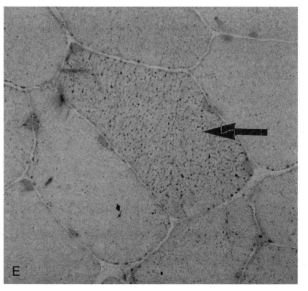

Figure 79–2. Muscle histology in metabolic disorders. *A,* Acid maltase deficiency, electron micrograph. The autophagic vacuoles are indicated by *arrows,* and free glycogen accumulation is indicated by the *asterisk* (original magnification, ×15,000). *B,* Acid maltase deficiency, electron micrograph. The *arrows* point to large, densely packed accumulations of membrane-bound glycogen granules (original magnification, ×26,000). *C,* Glycogen storage myopathy, electron micrograph. Subsarcolemmal accumulations of glycogen granules are indicated by *arrows;* also known as "blebs" (original magnification, ×16,800). *D,* Myophosphorylase deficiency: normal reaction in blood vessel (*arrow*), with absence of any reaction in muscle fibers (*asterisk*) (myophosphorylase-reacted sections; original magnification, ×200). *E,* Excess accumulation of small lipid droplets in type 1 muscle fibers (*arrow*). (Oil red O–stained section; original magnification, ×800.)

obtained during the second trimester of pregnancy. Also, genetic testing is available for family members once a specific genetic defect has been identified in one other affected family member (Tzall et al., 1991).

TREATMENT

No effective therapy is available at the present. A high-protein diet (25% to 30% of daily calorie intake) has been used, but the results have been disappointing, particularly in children. In adults, some improvement in respiratory status may occur.

Phosphorylase *b* Kinase Deficiency (Glycogenosis Type VIII)

Phosphorylase *b* kinase regulates glycogen metabolism via an inhibitory action on glycogen synthetase and the conversion of less active *b* phosphorylase to more active *a* phosphorylase. Thus, activation of phosphorylase *b* kinase turns off glycogen synthesis and stimulates glycogenolysis. Phosphorylase *b* kinase is activated by an epinephrine-sensitive cyclic AMP–activated protein kinase or directly by increased cytoplasmic calcium concentration, conditions that are present during exercise. The enzyme is composed of four different subunits: α, β, γ, and δ. Each subunit is coded for by one or more genes (see Table 79–1). Depending on how severely the subunits are affected, different clinical syndromes have been reported.

CLINICAL FEATURES

In humans, the best-studied syndrome is that of an X-linked recessive disorder with onset in middle age. Distal muscle weakness, with or without muscle cramping on exertion, are typical clinical features (Clemens et al., 1990). The genetic defect in at least some patients is a nonsense mutation in the muscle α subunit (Wehner et al., 1994). An autosomal recessive syndrome secondary to abnormality of the β subunit has also been described. This subunit is present both in muscle and in liver. Onset was in childhood or adolescence, and myalgia, muscle cramps, weakness induced by exercise, and myoglobinuria were the salient clinical findings. Some patients also have hepatomegaly or fatal cardiomyopathy (Bashan et al., 1981).

LABORATORY INVESTIGATIONS

In patients with myopathy, creatine kinase levels are increased. The ischemic exercise test is usually normal because of incomplete phosphorylase *b* kinase deficiency or because of direct activation of phosphorylase *b* via metabolites that accumulate with exercise. Muscle biopsy specimens may be normal but typically show subsarcolemmal accumulations of glycogen (see Fig. 79–2C). A definitive diagnosis is made on muscle by demonstrating a severe or total lack of phosphorylase *b* kinase activity, even though total phosphorylase activity may be normal.

Electromyographic Studies

The nerve conduction studies and the needle examination may be completely normal. In severely affected individuals, nonspecific myopathic features (short-duration, low-amplitude, polyphasic motor unit potentials) may be present in weak muscles. After an episode of rhabdomyolysis, increased insertional activity consisting of fibrillation potentials (positive wave and spikes) may be present for some time.

TREATMENT

There is no specific therapy. Prednisone therapy was ineffective in one patient. A high-protein diet (25% to 30% of daily calorie intake) may be helpful.

Phosphorylase Deficiency (McArdle's Disease; Glycogenosis Type V)

Phosphorylase initiates glycogen breakdown by removing 1,4-glycosyl residues from the outer branches of the glycogen molecule, each time liberating a glucose-1-phosphate molecule. This process continues until the outer chains are shortened to about four glycosyl units, and this "truncated" form of glycogen is known as *phosphorylase limit dextrin.* Phosphorylase limit dextrin can be degraded completely by debranching enzyme, and the combined action of these two enzymes on glycogen is to produce glucose-1-phosphate (93%) and glucose (7%). Phosphorylase isozymes are present in numerous tissues of the body, but human muscle has only one isozyme. Patients who lack normal activity of this isozyme have myophosphorylase deficiency (McArdle's disease). The gene coding for this isozyme is located on chromosome 11 (Lebo et al., 1990) (see Table 79–1). This isozyme is also present in heart muscle and in the brain, but the muscle isozyme accounts for less than 50% of the phosphorylase activity in these organs. Thus, patients with McArdle's disease have partial phosphorylase deficiencies in the brain and heart muscle, but clinical evidence for cardiomyopathy or encephalopathy is lacking.

CLINICAL FINDINGS

The salient feature of this disorder is high-intensity exercise intolerance with myalgia, muscle stiffness, and cramps. With low-intensity exercise, patients usually experience a "second wind" with improved endurance. Severe rhabdomyolysis with renal failure is relatively common and may be life threatening. There is a male predominance, and most of the patients present before the age of 15 years. Rare presentations include onset late in life with mild proximal weakness, mild fatigability in adults, infants with mild congenital weakness, and infants with severe weakness and respiratory failure (Di Mauro and Tsujino, 1994).

LABORATORY FINDINGS

Resting creatine kinase values are elevated in nearly all patients. There is a flat venous lactate response after the ischemic exercise test. The electrocardiographic changes are nonspecific, and the incidence of electroencephalographic abnormalities is unknown.

Electromyographic Studies

The motor and sensory nerve conduction studies are usually normal between attacks. Once permanent muscle weakness develops, the compound muscle action potentials may be low when recorded from weak muscles. Even between attacks, motor unit potential analysis shows typical myopathic abnormalities. In some patients, especially after an episode of rhabdomyolysis, there is increased insertional activity with fibrillation potentials and myotonic discharges in affected muscles. A characteristic finding is the electrical silence of the muscle cramps. This finding differentiates these cramps from other causes of cramping, where the cramps usually consist of excessive electromyographic activity (McArdle, 1951). Prolonged and rapid stimulation (20-Hz stimulation for 50 seconds) has been described as resulting in a greater than 25% decrement in hypothenar muscles. The decrement is the result of energy failure and electrical silence in some of the muscle fibers after excessive exercise.

Muscle Histology

Light microscopy shows a vacuolar myopathy with glycogen accumulation (blebs) in subsarcolemmal and intermyofibrillar locations (see Fig. 79–2C). The histochemical reaction for myophosphorylase is usually absent in muscle fibers but present in blood vessels (see Fig. 79–2D). Rarely, some enzyme activity is still present in a few muscle fibers, either because of residual enzyme activity or because of the presence of regenerating muscle fibers that express a different isozyme from mature muscle fibers.

Clinical-Genetic Correlations

The three genes that code for the muscle, heart, and brain isozymes have been localized, cloned, and sequenced. More than 21 different point mutations have been identified, including missense and stop mutations or destruction of the start codon (Tsujino et al., 1993a). In whites, the most common mutation is the substitution of thymine for cytosine on codon 49, in exon 1, changing an encoded arginine to a stop codon (Vorgerd et al., 1998). In Japan, a single-codon 708/709 deletion is the most common genetic abnormality. Inheritance of McArdle's disease is autosomal recessive, but pseudodominant transmission has been found because of manifesting heterozygotes or mating of homozygotes with heterozygotes.

TREATMENT

A high-protein diet is beneficial for most patients (Slonim and Goans, 1985). Other attempts at bypassing the metabolic block, such as oral glucose and fructose administration, glucagon injections, infusions of emulsified fat, and the administration of norepinephrine and heparin, may increase exercise tolerance but are impractical for routine clinical use.

Debrancher Deficiency (Cori-Forbes Disease; Glycogenosis Type III)

Debrancher enzyme has oligo-1,4-1,4-glucantransferase and amylo-1,6-glucosidase activities, which allow for the degradation of phosphorylase limit dextrin. Defects of transferase and/or glucosidase activities have been described in the liver, skeletal muscle, and heart muscle. Debrancher deficiency has been classified biochemically into three groups: *type IIIA*, with lack of both transferase and glucosidase activity in muscle and liver; *type IIIB*, with lack of both activities in liver but not in muscle or heart; and *type IIIC*, with loss of only transferase activity in liver and muscle (Chen et al., 1987; Ding et al., 1990).

CLINICAL SPECTRUM OF DEBRANCHER DEFICIENCY

There is a 3:1 male predominance, and inheritance is autosomal recessive.

Infantile Debrancher Deficiency

Glycogen storage is present in the liver (hepatomegaly) and muscle (cardiomegaly), but liver dysfunction predominates with recurrent episodes of hypoglycemia, resulting in seizures. Death occurs before the age of 5 years.

Childhood Debrancher Deficiency

All patients have hepatomegaly with liver dysfunction that results in growth retardation and episodes of hypoglycemia that may cause seizures. Muscle weakness is transient and resolves spontaneously by puberty.

Adult Debrancher Deficiency

Onset occurs after the third decade. Muscle weakness is common and slowly progressive and usually predominates in distal extremity muscles (Cornelio et al., 1984). The distal muscle wasting was associated with hypertrophy of proximal muscles in two brothers (Marbini et al., 1989). Muscle cramps, myalgia, and stiffness are noted by half of patients; rhabdomyolysis is rare; and clinical cardiopathy is uncommon. A distal polyneuropathy was present and confirmed by electromyographic studies and nerve pathology in a few patients (Powell et al., 1985; Moses et al., 1986).

LABORATORY FINDINGS

The ischemic exercise test fails to show the expected increase in venous lactate levels (Cornelio et al., 1984). The metabolic block in the liver is demonstrated by a failure of blood glucose levels to increase after the administration of glucagon or epinephrine. Echocardiography demonstrates ventricular hypertrophy in nearly all patients, despite the lack of clinical or radiological evidence of cardiomegaly or congestive heart failure (Moses et al., 1989). Muscle histology shows an accumulation of glycogen between muscle fibrils and in lysosomes; vacuolization may be severe, and these findings are very similar to those found in acid maltase deficiency (see Fig. 79–2B). Glycogen also accumulates in skin, intramuscular nerves, Schwann cells and axons of sural nerves, the brain, endomyocardium, and cultured muscle cells.

Electromyographic Studies

Motor and sensory nerve conduction studies may be characterized by low motor and sensory nerve action potentials and moderate slowing of conduction velocities, findings consistent with an axonal neuropathy. The neuropathy is caused by glycogen accumulation in peripheral nerve. The needle examination typically shows myopathic features with fibrillation potentials (positive waves and spikes), complex repetitive discharges, and myotonic discharges in distal muscles. The combination of denervation and myopathic features in distal muscles (long-duration, high-amplitude motor units potentials and short-duration, low-amplitude polyphasic motor unit potentials) may be confused with motor neuron disease or inclusion body myositis, which are common pitfalls.

Clinical-Genetic Correlations

The overall incidence of debrancher deficiency in the United States is about 1 in 100,000 live births. The debrancher gene maps to chromosome 1 (see Table 79–1). The complete cDNA of the enzyme contains 7,072 bp with a 4,596-bp coding region (Yang et al., 1992). The liver isozyme mRNA sequence is identical to the muscle isozyme sequence except for the 5′ end. Thus, the muscle and liver isoforms are generated via different RNA transcriptions from a single gene, explaining why patients have defects in

one or both isozymes. Mutations in the gene described to date include insertion mutations; deletions in exons 3, 4, 21, and 26 and nucleotide 4455T; nonsense mutations in the 3′ coding region; and compound heterozygotes for two different mutations (Shen et al., 1996; Hadjigoergiou et al., 1999). The exon 3 deletion apparently prevents the expression of the liver isozyme, so debrancher type IIIb can now be distinguished from debrancher type IIIa with the use of a blood test (Shen et al., 1996). The 4455T nucleotide deletion is ethnic specific, affecting North African Jews with a carrier prevalence of 1 in 35 and a clinical prevalence of 1 in 5,400 (Parvari et al., 1996). Using three polymorphic markers within the debrancher gene for linkage analysis, carrier detection and prenatal diagnosis are possible (Shen et al., 1997).

TREATMENT

A high-protein diet may be of some benefit. Children should be protected from hypoglycemia with frequent meals and nocturnal gastric infusions of glucose.

Phosphofructokinase Deficiency (Tarui's Disease, Glycogenosis Type VII)

Phosphofructokinase catalyses the irreversible conversion of fructose-6-phosphate to fructose-1,6-diphosphate. The enzyme consists of three subunits: M (muscle), L (liver), and P (platelet), each encoded by a different gene (see Table 79–1). Phosphofructokinase is also present in other tissues; erythrocytes contain subunits M and L, but only the M subunit is expressed in mature muscle. The M subunit accounts for more than 90% of heart and more than 50% of brain phosphofructokinase activity.

CLINICAL SPECTRUM OF PHOSPHOFRUCTOKINASE DEFICIENCY

This disorder has a 9:1 male predominance and a high prevalence in Ashkenazi Jews and Italians. The salient clinical findings in adults are those of a myopathy and red blood cell hemolysis. For unknown reasons, heart or brain abnormalities appear to be rare. The muscle symptoms and findings are similar to those noted in McArdle's disease, and muscle cramps, stiffness, and myalgia are usually present. The clinical findings are summarized in Table 79–3 (Rowland et al., 1986). Additional, but rare, features include jaundice secondary to red blood cell hemolysis, gout, hepatomegaly, and gastric ulcers. In a few families, infants were noted to have a multisystem disorder with severe myopathy, resulting in respiratory failure and death in the first few years of life. Some of these infants also had multiple joint contractures, seizures, cortical blindness, corneal

Table 79–3. Clinical Features of 25 Patients (21 Men, 4 Women) Who Lack the M Subunit of Phosphofructokinase

Clinical Findings	Present	Absent	Not Recorded
Country of Residence			
United States	14/25	—	—
Ashkenazi Jews	11/14	—	—
Japan	6/25	—	—
Europe	5/25	—	—
Families with multiple affected siblings	4/29	—	—
Exercise intolerance	25/25	0/25	0/25
Myoglobinuria	10/25	6/25	9/25
Renal failure	1/13	5/13	7/13
Second wind	7	2	16
Fixed limb weakness	3/25	—	—
Contractures	5	0	15

Modified from Rowland LP, Di Mauro S, Layzer RB: Phosphofructokinase deficiency. In Engle AG, Banker BQ (eds): Myology. New York, McGraw-Hill, 1986, with permission.

clouding, and cardiomyopathy. Hemolysis, however, was absent (Amit et al., 1992). Presumably, this multisystem disorder is related to the absence of an unknown activator common to all phosphofructokinase isozymes. As can be expected, a few patients with hemolytic anemia with no or minimal myopathic findings have also been recognized (Etiemble and Kahn, 1976). In one family, an association was noted between phosphofructokinase deficiency and non–insulin-dependent diabetes mellitus (Ristow et al., 1997).

LABORATORY INVESTIGATIONS

Creatine kinase levels are usually increased, the ischemic exercise test shows no increase in venous lactate, and the hemolysis is reflected in increased reticulocyte counts, high unconjugated bilirubin serum levels, and increased uric acid serum levels. The hyperuricemia is the result of a net degradation of ATP to adenosine diphosphate (ADP) or adenosine monophosphate (AMP), which are rapidly metabolized to several purine metabolites, including uric acid.

Electromyographic Studies

The electromyographic findings are similar to those described for McArdle's disease. The nerve conduction studies usually are normal except for low compound motor unit potential amplitudes recorded from clinically weak muscles. The needle examination demonstrates myopathic motor unit potentials, and fibrillation potentials and myotonic discharges may be seen with insertional activity. As in McArdle's disease, prolonged rapid stimulation results in a decremental response of the compound muscle action potential amplitudes, and the muscle cramps are electrically silent.

Muscle Histology

There is accumulation of glycogen between muscle fibers and at subsarcolemmal locations (see Fig. 79–2C). In addition, some adult cases have accumulations of periodic acid–Schiff (PAS)-positive polysaccharides, noted as finely granular filamentous material on electron microscopy, similar to those seen in polyglucosan body disease.

Clinical-Genetic Correlations

Inheritance is autosomal recessive. cDNA of the M subunit has been sequenced, and the full genomic organization of the gene is known. The phosphofructokinase gene maps proximal to the locus of *MODY3*, one of the genetic defects that causes maturity-onset diabetes of the young (Howard et al., 1996). Thus, phosphofructokinase was excluded as a candidate for the *MODY3* gene. Phosphofructokinase M deficiency per se, however, causes impaired insulin secretion in response to glucose and as such is a candidate gene predisposing to non–insulin-dependent diabetes mellitus. More than 15 deletions or point mutations that cause this disorder have been described (Raben and Sherman, 1995).

THERAPY

Glucose loading is ineffective. A high-protein diet may be beneficial.

Phosphoglycerate Kinase Deficiency (Glycogenosis Type IX)

Phosphoglycerate kinase 1 converts 3-P-glyceryol phosphate to 3-phosphoglycerate. It is a monomeric enzyme with no tissue-specific isoforms except for phosphoglycerate kinase 2, which is present only in spermatogenic cells. The defect is expressed in all tissues.

CLINICAL FEATURES

Typical findings include nonspherocytic hemolytic anemia and central nervous system abnormalities such as mental retardation, behavioral abnormalities, seizures, and strokelike episodes. Muscle involvement is rare, but patients may present with slowly progressive exercise intolerance, cramps, and myoglobinuria (Di Mauro et al., 1983). Some "muscle patients" also have central nervous system abnormalities but curiously appear not to have hemolytic anemia. Hemizygous males present shortly after birth with severe hemolytic anemia, jaundice, and splenomegaly. Heterozygous females may be normal or have only mild hemolytic anemia.

LABORATORY INVESTIGATIONS

Blood creatine kinase levels may be elevated. The ischemic muscle exercise test shows minimal or no rise in venous lactate.

Electromyographic Studies

All electrophysiological studies to date have been reported to be normal.

Muscle Histology

Convincing evidence of glycogen accumulation is usually present only on ultrastructural examination.

Clinical-Genetic Correlation

The gene for phosphoglycerate kinase 1 is encoded on the X chromosome (see Table 79–1) and has been cloned. Heterozygous woman may be symptomatic as described. The varying clinical expression of the disease is thought to be the consequence of the unique biochemical properties of the individual phosphoglycerate kinase mutants, which include missense and splice site mutations, as well as small deletions. One mutation that results in muscle weakness is an 837T-to-C transversion in codon 252 (Sugie et al., 1994).

Phosphoglycerate Mutase Deficiency (Glycogenosis Type X)

Phosphoglycerate mutase catalyzes the conversion of 3-phosphoglycerate to 2-phosphoglycerate. It is a dimeric enzyme, and different proportions of muscle (MM), brain (BB), or hybrid (MB) isozymes are expressed in different tissues. A primary muscle disease with a defect of only the MM isozyme has been identified.

CLINICAL FEATURES

This is a rare disease. Except for one Italian, all the patients diagnosed with this disorder have been African Americans. The presenting complaints in all patients are myalgia, muscle cramps, and muscle stiffness, induced by strenuous exercise. The majority of the patients report attacks of exercise-induced rhabdomyolysis.

LABORATORY FINDINGS

Increased creatine kinase levels are found even between attacks. The forearm ischemic exercise test shows a lower-than-expected increase in venous lactate levels. Because the BB isozyme accounts for about 5% of the phosphoglycerate mutase activity in muscle, the metabolic block is not complete.

Electromyographic Studies

All electrophysiological studies have been reported as normal.

Muscle Histology

Some accumulations of glycogen may be demonstrable, but in the majority of cases, the total glycogen content is normal.

Clinical-Genetic Correlation

The gene for phosphoglycerate mutase localizes to chromosome 7 (see Table 79–1), and the inheritance pattern is autosomal recessive. Complete cDNA of the gene has been sequenced. The gene spans 2.83 kb and has a 3-exon/2-intron structure. In five patients with this disorder, three different point mutations that cause this disease were identified (Tsujino et al., 1993b).

Lactate Dehydrogenase Deficiency (Glycogenosis Type XI)

Lactate dehydrogenase is a tetrameric enzyme composed of M and H subunits that combine in different ratios to form five isozymes. The M subunit is expressed in skeletal muscle, and the H subunit is expressed in heart muscle. Lactate dehydrogenase converts pyruvate to lactate under anaerobic conditions.

CLINICAL FEATURES

The presenting complaints in most patients are myalgia, muscle cramps, and muscle stiffness induced by strenuous exercise, as well as exercise-induced rhabdomyolysis. Some patients have an erythematous rush over the extensor surface of the extremities (Takayasu et al., 1991), and one patient had unusual "uterine stiffness" during pregnancy and delivery, necessitating a cesarean section (Maekawa et al., 1990). At least one female patient with the enzyme deficiency was asymptomatic at the time of testing (Maekawa et al., 1984).

LABORATORY FINDINGS

The ischemic forearm exercise test showed a lower than expected increase in venous lactate and a disproportionate increase in blood pyruvate levels.

Electromyographic Studies

Electrophysiological studies are largely lacking but were reported to be normal between attacks.

Muscle Histology

Results are normal.

Molecular Genetics

Disease inheritance is autosomal recessive. Frame-shift deletions and nonsense mutations were found in the lactate dehydrogenase gene.

Branching Enzyme Deficiency (Andersen's Disease, Glycogenosis Type IV)

This enzyme catalyzes the addition of a short glucosyl branching chain (about seven glucosyl units) to the naked peripheral chain of nascent glycogen during glycogen synthesis. It is presumed that the enzyme is a monomer, and thus defects should be present in all tissues in which glycogen is stored. Clinically, however, liver disease predominates for unknown reasons. Adult polyglucosan body disease also appears to result from branching enzyme deficiency, but branching enzyme activity is normal in the muscle of most patients with this disorder.

CLINICAL FEATURES

Typically, branching enzyme disease is a rapidly progressive disease of infancy with liver failure as the dominant clinical finding. Patients usually die before the age of 4 years from liver cirrhosis or its complications. The liver disease, however, is not always progressive. Hydrops fetalis, cardiomyopathy, and hypotonia secondary to muscle weakness are present in some patients (Alegria et al., 1999). Adults with polyglucosan body disease may have muscle weakness secondary to upper and lower motor neuron disease but also have other clinical findings, including glove and stocking sensory loss, neurogenic bladder, or dementia (Bruno et al., 1993).

LABORATORY FINDINGS

Serum creatine kinase levels are inconsistently elevated. There is a normal increase in blood glucose levels after glucagon or epinephrine administration. Cardiomegaly is present in some patients.

Electromyographic Studies

The results of nerve conduction studies are consistent with an axonal sensorimotor neuropathy, characterized by low motor and sensory compound action potentials and minimal slowing of nerve conduction velocities. Detailed electromyographic findings have not yet been reported.

Muscle Histology

Deposits of both glycogen and polysaccharides are found in muscle fibers as well as in the skin, liver, heart, and gray and white matter of the central nervous system. In sural nerve biopsy specimens from patients with adult polyglucosan body disease, the bodies are present in Schwann cell cytoplasm and in the axoplasm of myelinated fibers.

Clinical-Genetic Correlation

Inheritance is autosomal recessive, and the gene, encoding 2,106 bp, has been copied and mapped to chromosome 3 (see Table 79–1). Missense mutations and deletions of the gene have been reported (Bao et al., 1996). These studies indicated that milder forms of the disease result from mutations with retained branching enzyme activity.

THERAPY

Liver transplantation has been of benefit in some patients. Unfortunately, it does not appear that the enzyme is transferred to other enzyme-deficient tissues after liver transplantation, as one patient developed intractable cardiomyopathy 2 years after surgery (Sokal et al., 1992). However, some patients actually improved with decreased amounts of glycogen accumulations in the heart and muscle after transplantation (Selby et al., 1991). To explain this, it has been postulated that systemic microchimerism occurs after liver transplantation, which may ameliorate pancellular enzyme deficiencies.

DISORDERS OF LIPID METABOLISM

Lipid Metabolism and Basic Concepts

During fasting, free fatty acids are oxidized in the muscle as an energy source. They are derived mostly from dietary triglycerides esterified in the liver but also from circulating lipoprotein complexes and from neutral lipid droplets stored in muscle fibers. The movement of free fatty acids from the plasma into the muscle fiber cytosol occurs via simple diffusion. Short- and medium-chain fatty acids are able to cross the outer and inner mitochondrial membranes as free esters, to enter the mitochondrial matrix.

After activation to their coenzyme A (CoA) esters, the free fatty acids are available for β-oxidation. The mitochondrial membranes are impermeable to long-chain fatty acids. Thus, they are transported from the cytosol to the matrix of the mitochondria via a transport system involving carnitine palmitoyltransferase (CPT) and carnitine (Fig. 79–3). Free fatty acids are first activated to become long-chain acyl-CoA by long-chain acyl-CoA synthetase, located in the mitochondrial outer membrane. Long-chain acyl-CoA is transported across the outer mitochondrial membrane in exchange for a CoA thioester and is then converted to acylcarnitine by CPTI, which is bound to the outer mitochondrial membrane. The long-chain acylcarnitine is then translocated across the mitochondrial inner membrane by carnitine: acylcarnitine translocase, in exchange for free carnitine. CPTII, bound to the inner mitochondrial membrane, now reverses the reaction and converts acylcarnitine back to free carnitine and long-chain free fatty acids. The free fatty acids are then available for β-oxidation in the mitochondrial matrix. Metabolism of free fatty acids occurs only aerobically, and carnitine is crucial in control of the influx

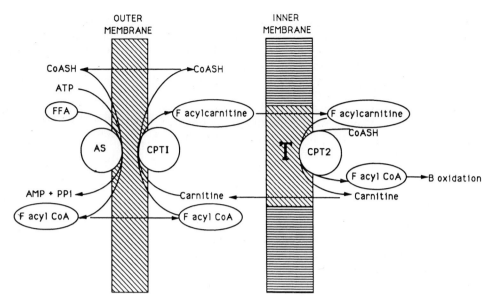

Figure 79–3. The metabolic pathways involved in the uptake of long-chain free fatty acids into mitochondria. (From Frank L. Mastaglia, Lord Walton of Detchant: Skeletal Muscle Pathology. London, Churchill Livingstone, 1992.)

of long-chain fatty acids into mitochondria. Carnitine can also combine with short- and medium-chain acyl-CoAs in the mitochondrial matrix (carnitine acyltransferase mediated) to produce acylcarnitines, which are shuttled out of the mitochondria. Mitochondrial β-oxidation involves a repeat of four reactions (Fig. 79–4). The end result of β-oxidation is the shortening of a fatty acid molecule by two carbon atoms. In the process, electrons are carried

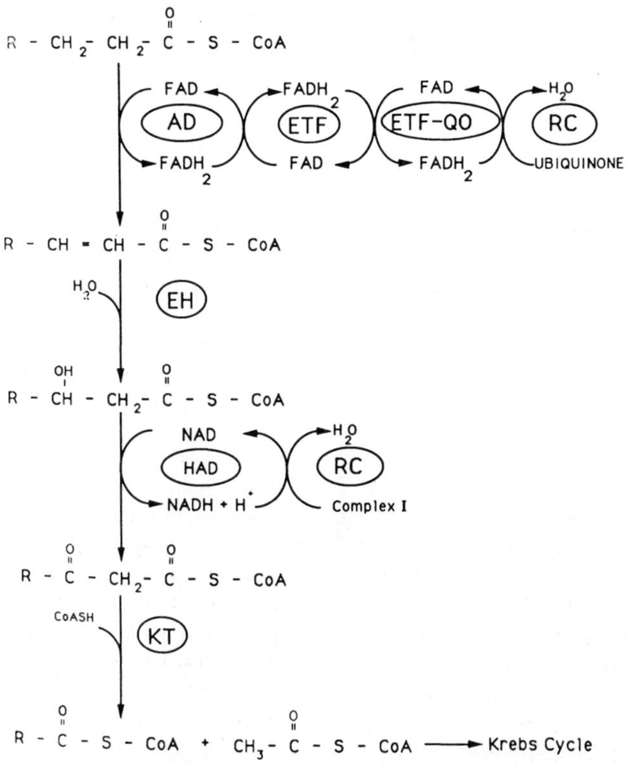

via electron transfer flavoprotein and electron transfer flavoprotein ubiquinone oxidoreductase to coenzyme Q and then via nicotinamide adenine dinucleotide (NAD) to complex I of the respiratory chain.

REGULATION OF FATTY ACID METABOLISM IN MUSCLE

Malonyl-CoA, an intermediary of fatty acid synthesis, is a potent inhibitor of CPTI. During prolonged exercise, malonyl-CoA levels decease in muscle, and thus CPT activity increases. This is an important mechanism for the short-term regulation of fatty acid metabolism. The controversy as to whether there are selective CPTI and CPTII deficiencies was settled when it was shown that these two enzymes map to different genes on different chromosomes (Britton et al., 1995).

Disorders of lipid metabolism that affect skeletal muscle include the following:

- Defective transport of free fatty acids into mitochondria (e.g., CPT and carnitine deficiency)
- Defects in the oxidation of fatty acids (e.g., long-, medium-, or short-chain acyl-CoA dehydrogenase deficiency and 3-hydroxy acyl-CoA dehydrogenase deficiency)
- Defects in the respiratory chain, including mitochondrial cytopathies
- Defects in utilization of endogenously synthesized triglycerides (e.g., multisystem triglyceride storage disease)

Carnitine Palmitoyltransferase Deficiency

CLINICAL FEATURES OF CARNITINE PALMITOYLTRANSFERASE I DEFICIENCY

The typical clinical presentation is that of a Reye's-like syndrome with coma, nonketotic hypo-

Figure 79–4. Mitochondrial β-oxidation; one run of a repeat of four reactions. (From Frank L. Mastaglia, Lord Walton of Detchant: Skeletal Muscle Pathology. London, Churchill Livingstone, 1992.)

glycemia, hepatomegaly, hyperammonemia, and increased levels of serum transaminases and free fatty acids (Roe and Coates, 1995). These attacks are usually induced by fasting secondary to a viral infection or diarrhea. Renal tubular acidosis may be present as well (Falik-Borenstein et al., 1992). Unfortunately, persistent neurological deficits are common. Chronic muscle weakness and cardiomyopathy have not been reported in CPT I deficiency, because the enzyme deficiency is present in liver and fibroblasts but not in muscle (Britton et al., 1995).

Molecular Genetics

Inheritance is autosomal recessive, and the gene has been mapped to chromosome 11q13. The expression of CPT I in liver and fibroblasts, but not in muscle, allows for the use of fibroblast assays to differentiate the "muscle" and "liver" forms of CPT deficiency.

Treatment

Recurrent episodes of Reye's syndrome have been treated successfully with glucose infusion, and attacks can be prevented if fasting is avoided. Frequent feeding and replacement of dietary long-chain fatty acids with medium-chain triglycerides are beneficial.

CLINICAL FEATURES OF CARNITINE PALMITOYLTRANSFERASE II DEFICIENCY

Adult Form

This is the most common type of presentation, and it is characterized by recurrent attacks of myalgia and rhabdomyolysis, precipitated by prolonged exercise. Weakness is transient and present only during the acute attacks. The ability to perform short-duration, high-intensity exercise is not impaired, and the first attacks are usually documented before the age of 20 years. Contrary to findings in the glycogen storage diseases, there is no "second wind" phenomenon, and the patient does not experience warning signs such as myalgia or muscle stiffness before rhabdomyolysis. The attacks usually start a few hours after exercise, and any muscle that was overworked can be affected, including cranial muscles. Attacks can also be precipitated by fasting, exposure to cold, a high fat intake, viral infections, fever, severe emotional stress, pregnancy, general anesthesia, and the use of ibuprofen or high doses of diazepam.

Infantile Form

These patients die young and present with hypoketotic hypoglycemia and congenital and cardiac abnormalities (Roe and Coates, 1995). Clinically, these patients can be distinguished from those with the severe form of hypoketotic hypoglycemia secondary to CPT I deficiency on the bases of cardiac involvement and their poor prognosis.

Atypical clinical presentations include the following:

- Heterogeneous carriers with persistent muscle weakness (Kieval et al., 1989)
- Patients with external ophthalmoplegia and ragged red fibers on muscle histology (Gieron and Korthals, 1987)
- Purely hepatic CPT deficiency without muscle symptoms or signs (Tein et al., 1989)
- Muscle CPT deficiency in association with liver CPT deficiency, as noted by delayed ketogenesis on fasting and increased lipid storage in the liver
- CPT deficiency and carnitine deficiency with multiorgan involvement (Hug et al., 1991)

LABORATORY FINDINGS

Creatine kinase levels and muscle histology are normal between attacks of rhabdomyolysis. With rare exception, the mitochondria are structurally normal. CPT II activity is reduced by 80% to 90% in homozygotes and by 50% in symptomatic heterozygotes.

Electromyographic Studies

The nerve conduction and electromyographic studies are usually normal between attacks. Myopathic motor unit potentials and fibrillation potentials (positive waves and spikes) are present in affected muscles for a limited time after an attack of rhabdomyolysis. After repeated attacks, however, myopathic motor unit potentials may be present, even between attacks.

Molecular Genetics

Inheritance is autosomal recessive. The gene is located on chromosome 1p32; it spans approximately 20 kb and is composed of five exons (Gallera et al., 1994). At least three polymorphisms of the gene have been recognized in the normal population. Interestingly, although these polymorphisms do not affect enzyme activity alone, they do exacerbate defects produced by other mutations that disrupt enzyme activity (Taroni et al., 1992). The most frequent mutation resulting in the adult form of the disease was a C-to-T transposition at nucleotide 439, resulting in an S133-to-L substitution. This mutation accounts for about 60% of all adult cases reported worldwide (Martin et al., 1999). Different mutations, including compound heterozygosity and small deletions, have been reported in the infantile and adult forms of the disease. The 413 AG deletion is particularly common in Ashkenazi Jews. The genetic defects typically result in some residual enzyme production, consistent with the biochemical findings, which indicate that total enzyme deficiency does not occur.

PATHOGENESIS OF ATTACKS OF RHABDOMYOLYSIS AND VARYING EXPRESSION OF CARNITINE PALMITOYLTRANSFERASE II DEFICIENCY

In muscle CPT II deficiency, the total muscle CPT activity is normal, but the enzyme is abnormally inhibited by its substrate and product. Thus, it appears that the mutant enzyme functions well under normal conditions but is vulnerable when fatty acid metabolism is stressed. The difference in the severity of the clinical findings in adults and infants is not determined by the degree of CPT II tissue reduction, because the reductions are similar (80% to 90%) for both age groups. Also, the differences are not attributable to differences in tissue distribution of the enzyme deficiency, because isoforms of the enzyme do not exist. However, because CPT I activity is normal in fetal tissue, long-chain acylcarnitines can still be produced in infants. These long-chain acylcarnitines are arrhythmogenic to heart muscle, and this contributes to the high mortality rate in this age group (Hug et al., 1991).

TREATMENT

Patients must avoid situations known to precipitate attacks. A high-carbohydrate, low-fat diet; frequent meals; and carbohydrate supplementation before and during sustained exercise are recommended. Children with symptomatic CPT II deficiency may benefit from dietary changes or from pharmacological inhibition of CPT I in an attempt to reduce production of the cardiotoxic long-chain acylcarnitines.

Carnitine Deficiency

Carnitine is derived mostly from dietary sources (75%), but it is also synthesized from lysine and methionine in the liver and kidney. Carnitine synthesized in hepatocytes is released into the blood, from which it is taken up by peripheral tissues, against a concentration gradient, so that tissue carnitine levels are 20 to 40 times higher than blood levels. The transport system responsible for this gradient is a sodium-dependent carnitine transporter, and defects in this system were linked to chromosome 5q31 (Shoji et al., 1998). More specifically, a full-length cDNA was cloned for OCTN2 (Wu et al., 1998), a member of the organic cation transporter family, and the gene encoding OCTN2 was designated *SLC22A5*. This gene is now believed to control the sodium-dependent carnitine transporter system. Carnitine is present in free and esterified forms. The esters are short-, medium-, and long-chain acylcarnitines and account for about 25% of total carnitine in serum and 15% in liver and skeletal muscle. The free-to-esterified ratios change with fasting, when up to 60% of the total carnitine in urine may be esterified. Of total body carnitine, 95% is stored in muscle.

CLINICAL FEATURES OF CARNITINE DEFICIENCY

Primary Carnitine Myopathy

Inheritance is probably autosomal recessive; decreased levels of muscle carnitine have been reported in the muscle of both asymptomatic parents of a symptomatic 8-year-old boy (VanDyke et al., 1975). The time of disease onset varies from childhood to early adulthood (Caravaglia et al., 1991). Patients develop symmetrical, slowly progressive, proximal muscle weakness in the extremities; rarely, the face and tongue muscles also are affected. There is no history of myalgia, muscle cramping, or exercise-induced rhabdomyolysis. Stress, such as pregnancy, may exacerbate the muscle weakness, and cardiomyopathy with congestive cardiac failure may develop in a few patients. Muscle carnitine levels are low, serum carnitine levels are variable, and liver and heart carnitine levels are normal. Presumably, there is a defect in carnitine transport to muscle (Treem et al., 1988), but this could not be confirmed in all the reported patients, suggesting genetic heterogeneity (Willner et al., 1979). New discoveries in the genetic control of carnitine transport should clarify the exact cause of this disorder in the near future.

Systemic Carnitine Deficiency

After initial confusion in which patients with primary systemic carnitine deficiency were thought to have secondary carnitine deficiency (Engel et al., 1981), genetic discoveries have begun to more accurately distinguish the different clinical syndromes. Shortly after this disorder was described for the first time, it was postulated that the disease was caused by carnitine deficiency secondary to an inherited deficiency of an enzyme responsible for carnitine biosynthesis (Chapoy et al., 1980). It has now become apparent that the primary defect is one of carnitine transport, specifically of establishing a concentration gradient across cell membranes. This results in low tissue carnitine levels in the liver, heart, skeletal muscle, kidney, and fibroblasts but also impedes the reabsorption of carnitine in the kidney with excessive loss of carnitine in the urine (Waber et al., 1982). Inheritance of this defect is autosomal recessive, and in unrelated families with systemic carnitine deficiencies, different mutations have been reported in the *SLC22A5* gene (Nezu et al., 1999). The systemic deficiency is differentiated from the myopathic form on the basis of low carnitine concentrations in tissues other than muscle (Karpati et al., 1975; Tripp et al., 1981). The salient clinical findings are those of a hypertrophic cardiomyopathy and/or attacks of hypoketotic hypoglycemia (Reye's syndrome), associated with muscle weakness. Exercise-induced fatigue, vomiting, abdominal pain, and hepatomegaly were also presenting symptoms is some families. Total and esterified carnitine levels are low in all tissues and in serum.

Treatment. It appears that the transport defect can be corrected partially with high carnitine serum concentrations (Hug et al., 1991). After treatment with oral L-carnitine (100 to 150 mg/kg per day), many patients experience a dramatic improvement in muscle strength, a reduction in cardiac size, and complete or partial repletion of carnitine levels. For the attacks of Reye's syndrome, glucose should be infused intravenously. In general, patients should avoid fasting and stay on a low-fat diet.

Secondary Carnitine Deficiency

This deficiency is seen in patients with an organic aciduria such as proprionic acidemia (Di Donato et al., 1984), a mitochondrial respiratory chain defect, or renal Fanconi's syndrome or in patients receiving hemodialysis or valproate therapy. The common denominator that results in carnitine deficiency in these syndromes is the accumulation of acyl-CoAs in the mitochondrial matrix. The acyl-CoAs combine with carnitine to form acylcarnitine, which leaks from the muscle cells into the blood and then is excreted in the urine. The clinical picture is similar to that seen in systemic carnitine deficiency.

LABORATORY INVESTIGATIONS

Creatine kinase levels are variably elevated. Muscle histology reveals lipid accumulation in type 1 muscle fibers (see Fig. 79–2E), and there are low, total muscle carnitine levels.

Electromyographic Studies

The motor and sensory nerve conduction studies are usually normal, although low-amplitude compound muscle action potentials may be recorded from atrophic muscles. The needle examination typically shows myopathic motor unit potentials (low-amplitude, short-duration, polyphasic motor unit potentials), and insertional activity may be abnormal with fibrillation potentials in clinically weak muscles.

THERAPY

Carnitine supplementation (2 to 4 g/day) can be beneficial in primary and secondary carnitine deficiency. A low–total fat diet is recommended. The benefits of riboflavin or prednisone therapy are questionable.

Disorders of β-Oxidation

LONG-CHAIN ACYL-COENZYME A DEHYDROGENASE, MEDIUM-CHAIN ACYL-COENZYME A DEHYDROGENASE, AND SHORT-CHAIN ACYL-COENZYME A DEHYDROGENASE DEFICIENCIES

These enzymes belong to the acyl-CoA dehydrogenase family of enzymes, and all are tetrameric mitochondrial flavoproteins, which probably evolved from a common ancestral gene. Acyl-CoA dehydrogenases act on free fatty acids of specific lengths; long-chain acyl-CoA dehydrogenase acts on substrates with 12 or more carbon atoms, medium-chain acyl-CoA dehydrogenase acts on substrates with 4 to 14 carbon atoms, and short-chain acyl-CoA dehydrogenase on substrates with 4 to 6 carbon atoms.

Clinical Features

The clinical findings in all these deficiencies are fairly similar. Typically, infants present with failure to thrive, metabolic crises secondary to nonketotic hypoglycemia, hypotonia, and variable findings of hepatomegaly, seizures, and cardiomegaly. In its most severe form, this is a cause for sudden infant death syndrome. Most patients die in childhood, but in those with a milder form of the disease, the metabolic attacks cease in adulthood. In adults, the salient features are those of proximal limb myopathy, usually with neck extensor weakness, and lipid excess on muscle histochemistry (see Fig. 79–4). Many patients have permanent neurological deficits as a consequence of the recurrent metabolic attacks. Viral infections are the precipitating event in the majority of patients who present with nonketotic hypoglycemia (Iafolla et al., 1994). One patient who presented with ophthalmoplegia and multicores on muscle biopsy was found to have a short-chain acyl-CoA dehydrogenase deficiency (Tein et al., 1999). All patients with "authentic cases" of short-chain acyl-CoA dehydrogenase deficiency had neurological deficits, including hypotonia/hypertonia, hyperactivity, and/or developmental delay, but hypoglycemia was not a prominent clinical finding. The muscle and metabolic findings can occur separately, and at least some adults have exercise-induced episodes of myoglobinuria, muscle cramping, myalgia, and stiffness.

Laboratory Findings

Urinary analysis of metabolic breakdown products reveals the following findings:

- Long-chain acyl-coenzyme A dehydrogenase deficiency: Excess of C12-C14 dicarboxylic acids
- Medium-chain acyl-coenzyme A dehydrogenase deficiency: Excess of three glycine conjugates (hexanoylglycine, suberylglycine, and phenylpropionylglycine) and shorter-length dicarboxylic acids
- Short-chain acyl-coenzyme A dehydrogenase deficiency: Excess of short-chain metabolites such as ethylmalonate and methylsuccinate

Electromyographic Studies

Results of detailed electromyographic studies are lacking.

Diagnosis

Secondary carnitine deficiency may be a feature in all of these patients, except for those with short-chain acyl-CoA dehydrogenase, who have normal carnitine levels (Bhala et al., 1995) The urinary findings can be misleading, and patients with celiac disease have been shown to have excess excretion of dicarboxylic acids in urine, which normalized completely with a gluten-free diet (Costa et al., 1996). Thus, a definitive diagnosis is made by demonstrating the specific enzyme defect in fibroblasts or muscle. For middle-chain acyl-CoA dehydrogenase deficiency, an accurate diagnosis can be made by analyzing acylcarnitine in blood with tandem mass spectrometry (Van Hove et al., 1993). Using this method in a prospective neonatal screening program in Pennsylvania, 9 cases were identified among the first 80,371 infants screened (Ziadeh et al., 1995). The definitive assay for short-chain acyl-CoA dehydrogenase deficiency is an electron transfer flavoprotein–linked enzyme assay with butyryl-CoA as substrate, performed after immunoactivation of medium-chain acyl-CoA dehydrogenase (Bhala et al., 1995).

Genetic-Clinical Correlation

The defective gene for long-chain acyl-CoA dehydrogenase has been mapped to chromosome 2q34-q35 (Yang-Feng et al., 1991), and a mouse model of the disease has been produced (Kurtz et al., 1998). Medium-chain acyl-CoA dehydrogenase has been mapped to chromosome 1p31, and the majority of patients were compound heterozygotes for the 985A-G mutation, in addition to a second mutation (Ziadeh et al., 1995). Deletions and many other mutations with nucleotide substitutions have been described in patients, but it has not been possible to draw a direct correlation between the genotypic and phenotypic expressions (Andresen et al., 1997). Short-chain acyl-CoA dehydrogenase maps to chromosome 12q22-ater (Corydon et al., 1997). Of the first four patients with short-chain acyl-CoA dehydrogenase deficiency in which genetic studies were performed, all displayed compound heterozygosity (Gregersen et al., 1998).

Treatment

Carnitine supplementation is beneficial in preventing metabolic attacks. Supplementation also improves liver or heart function but not muscle weakness. Low-fat high-carbohydrate feedings and riboflavin supplementation reduce the frequency and the severity of the metabolic crisis but do not prevent progression of the disease (Ribes et al., 1992).

CARNITINE-ACYLCARNITINE TRANSLOCASE DEFICIENCY

These patients present with Reye's syndrome–like attacks, including hypoketotic hypoglycemia, hyperammonemia, seizures, and apneic episodes. They have cardiomyopathy with ventricular hypertrophy, bradycardia, hepatomegaly, muscle weakness, and systemic carnitine deficiency, and they excrete large amounts of dicarboxyl acids in the urine. The majority of these patients have low or undetectable enzyme activity in body tissues and die within months of birth. Patients with as little as 5% residual enzyme activity may have a relatively benign clinical course (Morris et al., 1998). To date, 12 cases with this disorder have been described worldwide. The gene that controls carnitine-acylcarnitine translocase has been mapped to chromosome 3p21.31 (Viggiano et al., 1997), and the gene has been cloned and sequenced.

Treatment

One patient responded favorably to peritoneal dialysis and a high-calorie, low-protein diet that was high in long-chain fatty acids and medium-chain triglyceride oils (Al Aqeel et al., 1999).

3-HYDROXY ACYL-COENZYME A DEHYDROGENASE DEFICIENCY

The defect presents in infancy with metabolic encephalopathy, cardiomyopathy, myopathy, or a combination of these.

Electromyographic Studies

This disorder has not been well studied. In one infant, a progressive sensorimotor distal polyneuropathy was described, with slowing of nerve conduction velocities and electromyographic evidence of denervation in distal muscles.

Defects of the Respiratory Chain

ELECTRON TRANSFER FLAVOPROTEIN AND ELECTRON TRANSFER FLAVOPROTEIN–COENZYME Q OXIDOREDUCTASE DEFICIENCIES

Patients with these defects are unable to oxidize the products of the following dehydrogenase reactions, as well as others: short-chain acyl-CoA dehydrogenase, medium-chain acyl-CoA dehydrogenase, long-chain acyl-CoA dehydrogenase, glutaryl-CoA, dimethylglycine, and isovaleryl-CoA. Thus, the disorder is also known as *multiple acyl-CoA dehydrogenase deficiency* or, because of the increased urinary excretion of glutaric acid, *glutaric aciduria type II.*

Two clinical presentations are recognized.

1. *Neonatal onset with severe metabolic encephalopathy (Reye's-like syndrome):* Some patients have associated congenital abnormalities. A peculiar "sweaty feet" odor and early death are typical.
2. *Childhood onset with proximal muscle weakness and excess lipid storage in muscle:* This group has very high urinary levels of ethylmalonic and adipic acids (see Fig. 79–4).

In all cases, secondary carnitine deficiency is present.

Riboflavin-Responsive Glutaric Aciduria Type II

This is a defect of multiple flavin-dependent acyl-CoA dehydrogenases. This defect results in abnormalities involving the metabolism of medium- and short-chain acyl-CoA dehydrogenase and of respiratory complex I, a flavin-dependent enzyme. Clinically, the patients present in infancy with a Reye's-like syndrome or as adults with a progressive lipid storage myopathy. Both groups respond well to riboflavin therapy. The urinary acid excretion profile is similar to that of glutaric aciduria type II.

Multisystem Triglyceride Storage Disease (Chanarin's Disease)

The specific enzyme defects responsible for this disorder are unknown, but it appears that it results from an inability to degrade endogenously synthesized triglycerides (Radom et al., 1987). Neutral lipid accumulates in muscle fibers (see Fig. 79–4) and also in hepatocytes, gastrointestinal epithelium, the endometrium, epidermal basal and granular cells, and bone marrow cells. A proximal myopathy and central nervous system defects can be present.

MITOCHONDRIAL CYTOPATHIES

It is generally accepted that mitochondria originated about 1.5 billion years ago from bacteria-like organisms that incorporated into larger, anaerobic cells to support their energy demands. Mitochondria contain genetic material known as mitochondrial DNA (mtDNA) that translates for 13 translation products, which are part of complexes I, III, IV, and V of the mitochondrial respiratory chain. mtDNA also encodes the 12S and 16S ribosomal RNA (rRNA) and the 22 transfer RNA (tRNA) genes required for mitochondrial protein synthesis (Wallace, 1999). The mtDNA codes for only a small portion of the proteins in each complex. The remaining mitochondrial oxidative phosphorylation proteins, the metabolic enzymes, the DNA and RNA polymerases, the ribosomal proteins, and the mtDNA regulatory factors, such as mitochondrial transcription factor A, are all encoded by nuclear genes (Shoffner and Wallace, 1992). Because spermatozoa are devoid of mitochondria, humans inherit their full complement of mtDNA from the mother. Thus, only genetic disorders resulting from a selective defect in mtDNA are inherited maternally.

Principles Concerning Mitochondrial Function and Evaluation

Mitochondrial Function

Mitochondria generate cellular energy in the form of ATP through oxidative phosphorylation. The major substrates oxidized are pyruvate and free fatty acids. The mitochondrial metabolism of free fatty acids has been discussed. Pyruvate is the end product of glycolysis and can be metabolized as follows:

1. Transamination to alanine
2. Reduction to lactate under anaerobic conditions
3. Oxidization to acetyl-CoA, via the pyruvate dehydrogenase complex, under aerobic conditions

Acyl-CoA transport across the mitochondrial inner membrane occurs in exchange for hydroxyl ions and is mediated by monocarboxylate translocase. The pyruvate dehydrogenase complex is shown in Fig. 79–5. It consists of three catalytic enzymes: pyruvate dehydrogenase (E1), dihydrolipoamide acetyltransferase (E2), and dihydrolipoamide dehydrogenase (E3). The nuclear genes that encode for the different subunits of each enzyme are known. Acetyl-CoA is oxidized via the Krebs cycle, and the hydrogen atoms released via this process are supplied to the

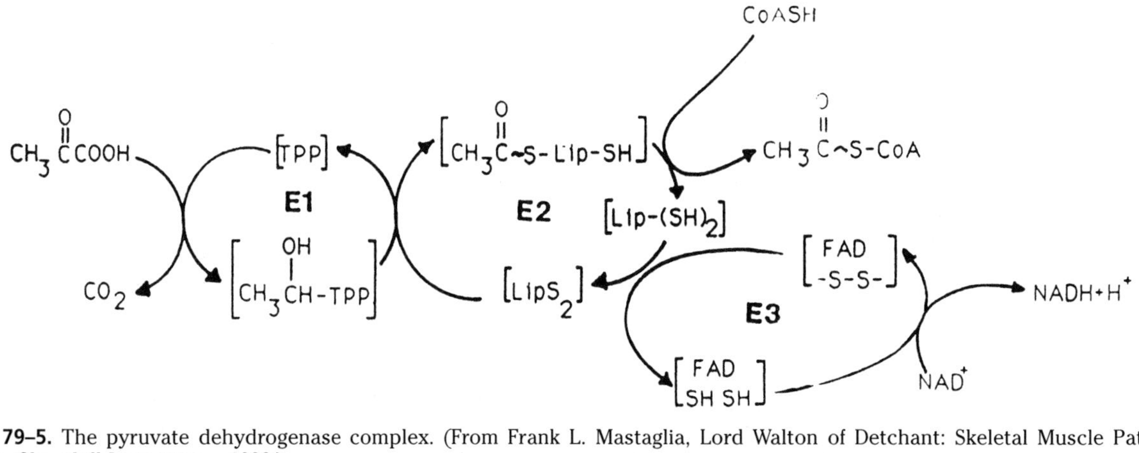

Figure 79–5. The pyruvate dehydrogenase complex. (From Frank L. Mastaglia, Lord Walton of Detchant: Skeletal Muscle Pathology. London, Churchill Livingstone, 1992.)

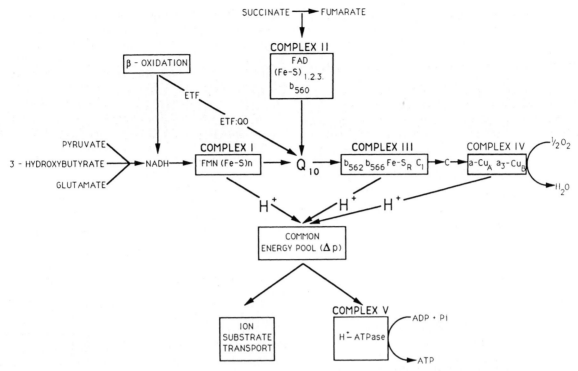

Figure 79–6. The mitochondrial respiratory chain. (From Morgan-Hughes JA: Mitochondrial diseases. In Engel AG, Franzini-Armstrong C [eds]: Myology. New York, McGraw-Hill, 1994; 1554, with permission.)

mitochondrial respiratory chain (Fig. 79–6). The chain consists of five multisubunit complexes (I–V), linked by the electron carriers coenzyme Q10 (ubiquinone) and cytochrome C. (Note that other cytochromes [e.g., cytochrome b_{560}, c_1, a, or a_3] are subunits of the respiratory complexes and should not be confused with cytochrome C.) According to the chemiosmotic theory (Mitchell, 1961), the free energy derived from electron transport is coupled to translocation of protons across the mitochondrial inner membrane. The inner membrane is impermeable to ions. Thus, proton translocation generates a transmembrane electrical potential and pH difference, which provide the energy to drive ATP synthesis.

MITOCHONDRIAL GENOME

Human mtDNA is a closed, circular, double-stranded 16.5-kb molecule. The guanine-rich heavy strand codes for subunits in complexes I, III, IV, and V. The cytosine-rich light strand codes for one subunit on complex I and for eight tRNAs. The genes are so tightly packed that some open reading frames for genes may overlap with introns. Mitochondria are thus at a special risk for genetic "accidents" such as deletions or point mutations.

Laboratory Findings Common to Mitochondrial Defects

MUSCLE HISTOLOGY

Most mitochondrial disorders show histological abnormalities in muscle, even if there is no evidence

for muscle disease on clinical or electromyographic examination. Respiratory chain defects are typically associated with mitochondrial proliferation (ragged red fibers) and ultrastructural mitochondrial abnormalities (Fig. 79–7A, B). These defects include enlarged mitochondria; distorted, circular, or branching cristae; osmiophilic dense bodies; and an array of crystalloid inclusions. The term *ragged red fibers* refers to the predominantly subsarcolemmal accumulation of red material (collections of mitochondria) on trichrome-stained sections. Succinate dehydrogenase is the most specific stain for mitochondrial proliferation and shows the ragged red fibers as "ragged blue fibers" (see Fig. 79–7C). Ragged blue fibers in association with strongly reactive blood vessels for succinate dehydrogenase is strongly suggestive of MELAS (myopathy, encephalopathy, lactic acidosis, and strokelike episodes). These fibers are usually cytochrome oxidase negative (see Fig. 79–7D) and may contain increased numbers of small lipid droplets or excess glycogen. Cytochrome oxidase–reacted sections may also reveal nonreactive fibers in the absence of mitochondrial proliferation, identifying additional cases of mitochondrial disease, especially those secondary to mtDNA mutations. It should be noted that morphological abnormalities in isolated mitochondria are nonspecific findings and that these abnormalities can occur secondary to metabolic stress in any muscle, as seen in muscle dystrophies, inflammatory myopathies, and muscle storage diseases. The morphological changes in primary mitochondrial diseases, however, are more severe and generalized.

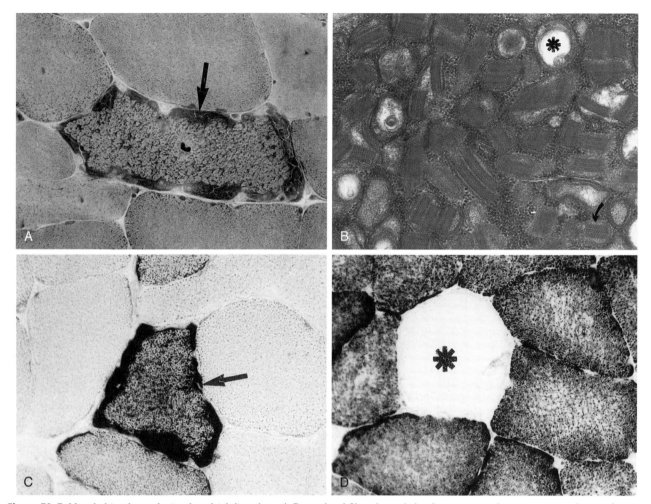

Figure 79–7. Muscle histology of mitochondrial disorders. *A,* Ragged red fiber (*arrow*) (trichrome-stained section; original magnification, ×800). *B,* Electron micrograph of a large subsarcolemmal accumulation of structurally abnormal mitochondria (original magnification, ×56,000). Note the paracrystalloid inclusions (*arrow*) and disorganized mitochondrial cristae (*asterisk*). *C,* Ragged blue fiber indicated by *arrow* (succinate dehydrogenase–reacted sections; original magnification, ×800). *D,* Cytochrome C oxidase–negative fiber indicated by the *asterisk* (cytochrome C oxidase–reacted sections, original magnification, ×800).

ELECTROMYOGRAPHIC EXAMINATION

In many of these disorders, there is clinical evidence for a myopathy and an associated distal polyneuropathy. The neuropathy is predominantly axonal in MERRF (myoclonic epilepsy and ragged red fibers), NARP (neurogenic weakness, ataxia, and retinitis pigmentosa), and Kearns-Sayre syndrome, and thus the motor and sensory conduction velocities are relatively normal in these disorders. The compound muscle action potentials and the sensory nerve action potential amplitudes may therefore be low or absent. The neuropathy associated with MNGIE (myoneurogastrointestinal encephalopathy) is demyelinating and axonal and thus the nerve conduction velocities may be slower than in the above-mentioned disorders. In mitochondrial disorders with myopathy, the electromyogram may show evidence of a chronic myopathy. Increased insertional activity, however, is absent in these disorders, unless there has been a recent episode of rhabdomyolysis. The typical electromyographic findings in the mitochondrial syndromes are listed in Table 79–4.

Table 79–4. Electromyographic Findings in Common Mitochondrial Syndromes

Syndrome	Nerve Conduction Studies	Needle Examination	
		Motor Unit Potentials	*Insertional Activity*
MERRF	Rarely, sensorimotor axonal polyneuropathy*	Myopathic	Normal
MELAS	Normal	Myopathic, mild	Normal
NARP	Sensory axonal polyneuropathy*	Normal	Normal
MNGIE	Demyelinating and axonal polyneuropathy*	Myopathic	Normal
Kearns-Sayre syndrome	Sensorimotor axonal polyneuropathy*	Myopathic	Normal

*Polyneuropathy may be present, in which case neurogenic motor unit potentials may be present distally in the extremities.

MERRF, myoclonic epilepsy with ragged red fibers, ataxia, and muscle weakness; MELAS, mitochondrial myopathy, encephalopathy, lactic acidosis, and strokes; NARP, neurogenic weakness, ataxia, and retinitis pigmentosa; MNGIE, myoneurogastrointestinal encephalopathy.

ISCHEMIC MUSCLE EXERCISE TEST

There is an abnormally high increase in venous lactate levels in most patients.

Biochemical Classification of Mitochondrial Diseases

A simplified classification of mitochondrial diseases is given in Table 79–5; only the more common disorders are listed, with an emphasis on those that result in muscle weakness.

Clinical Phenotypes of Mitochondrial Dysfunction

Unexplained attacks of lactic acidosis and certain clinical syndromes are highly suspicious of mitochondrial defects. These syndromes and their associated clinical findings are listed in Table 79–6. This syndromic classification is clinically valuable because it alerts the clinician to a possible underlying mitochondrial defect in patients with the appropriate clinical findings.

Table 79–5. Biochemical Classification of Mitochondrial Diseases

Site of Defect	Deficiency
Mitochondrial substrate transport	Primary muscle carnitine
	Primary systemic carnitine
	Carnitine palmitoyltransferase
Mitochondrial substrate utilization	Fatty acid oxidation
	Long-chain acyl-CoA dehydrogenase
	Medium-chain acyl-CoA dehydrogenase
	Short-chain acyl-CoA dehydrogenase
	Multiple acyl-CoA dehydrogenase (MAD)
	Riboflavin responsive MAD
	Pyruvate oxidation
	Pyruvate dehydrogenase (E1)
	Dihydrolipoamide acetyltransferase (E2)
	Dihydrolipoamide dehydrogenase (E3)
	Krebs cycle enzymes
	Fumarase
	Aconitase
Mitochondrial respiratory chain	NADH-CoQ reductase (complex I)
	Succinate-CoQ reductase (complex II)
	CoQ10
	CoQ-cytochrome C reductase (complex III)
	Cytochrome C oxidase (complex IV) deficiency
	Multiple respiratory enzyme
	Complex V
	Luft's disease

CoA, coenzyme A; CoQ, coenzyme Q.
Modified from Morgan-Hughes JA: Mitochondrial diseases. In Engle AG, Franzini-Armstrong C (eds): Myology. New York, McGraw-Hill, 1994, with permission.

Table 79–6. Syndromes Commonly Present in Mitochondrial Diseases

Syndrome	Clinical Features
Kearns-Sayre	External ophthalmoplegia, retinitis pigmentosa, sensorineural hearing loss, conduction defects, short stature, ataxia, increased cerebrospinal fluid protein
MELAS	Mitochondrial myopathy, encephalopathy, lactic acidosis, strokes
MERRF	Myoclonic epilepsy with ragged red fibers; ataxia, muscle weakness
MNGIE	Myoneurogastrointestinal encephalopathy
NARP	Neurogenic weakness, ataxia, retinitis pigmentosa
MSL	Multiple symmetrical lipomatosis
May-White	Myoclonus, ataxia, deafness
Alpers'	Progressive infantile poliodystrophy with cortical and subcortical spongiform degeneration and hepatocellular dysfunction
Leigh's	Subacute necrotizing encephalopathy with cystic necrosis and spongiform degeneration in subcortical brain structures
Pearson's	Bone marrow/pancreatic disease

Defects of Mitochondrial Metabolism

DEFECTS OF THE PYRUVATE DEHYDROGENASE COMPLEX

Most commonly, these defects affect only the E1 subunit. Pyruvate dehydrogenase complex defects affect most tissues in the body and have been documented in the liver, brain, kidney, muscle, heart, lymphocytes, and fibroblasts. Defects of this complex are some of the most common causes of primary lactic acidosis in humans.

Clinical Features

- *Severe phenotype:* Patients present during the neonatal period with lactic acidosis, elevated pyruvate levels, hypotonia, dysmorphic features, and feeding and breathing difficulties (Robinson et al., 1989).
- *Intermediate phenotype:* These patients present in late infancy with severe or episodic lactic acidosis and the clinical features of Leigh's subacute necrotizing encephalomyelitis (Kretzschmer et al., 1987).
- *Mild phenotype:* The clinical findings develop during infancy or childhood and consist of intermittent ataxia, dysarthria, and choreoathetoid movements (Blass et al., 1971).

Neuropathology

Cerebral atrophy and cystic necrosis are present in the cerebral hemispheres, basal ganglia, brainstem, and spinal cord.

Clinical-Genetic Correlation

The E1 subunit of the pyruvate dehydrogenase complex is located on the Xp22.2-p22.1 region (Borglum et al., 1997). It is one of the few X-linked diseases in which a high proportion of heterozygous females manifest severe clinical signs and symptoms. More than 50 different mutations, including deletions, insertions, and point mutations, are known, and exons 10 and 11 are commonly involved (Dahl, 1995). It appears that heterozygous females with missense mutations may have a milder phenotype and that insertions and deletions in hemizygous males could result in a very severe metabolic disorder that results in intrauterine death (Matthews et al., 1994).

Treatment

Very rarely, patients are thiamin responsive, and at least one patient had a temporary, favorable response to acetazolamide.

DEFECTS OF THE KREBS CYCLE

Fumarase Deficiency

This disease presents in infants with the clinical findings of diffuse encephalopathy, hypotonia, microcephaly, facial dysmorphism, seizures, and structural brain abnormalities. Fumaric aciduria and mild hyperammonemia are usually present. The genetic defect has been localized to chromosome 1q42.1, and mutations were confirmed in this gene (Bourgeron et al., 1994).

Aconitase Deficiency

This deficiency has been described in association with skeletal muscle succinate dehydrogenase deficiency in a young man with exercise intolerance, myalgia, muscle cramps, and rhabdomyolysis (Haller et al., 1989).

DEFECTS OF THE RESPIRATORY CHAIN

Complex I (NADH Ubiquinone Oxidoreductase)

Of the approximately 41 polypeptides of respiratory complex I, seven subunits are encoded by mtDNA; these are designated MTND1, MTND2, MTND3, MTND4, MTND4L, MTND5, and MTND6. The genetic localization for most of these subunits is known; for example, MTND1 is encoded by the guanine-rich heavy strand between nucleotide pairs 3307 and 4262 (Wallace et al., 1994). Different mitochondrial mutations have been described in patients with maternal inheritance, but the majority of clinically symptomatic mutations are located on different chromosomes of the nuclear genome. The mutations described until 1999 were reviewed by Smeitink and van den Heuvel (1999). The clinical disorders associated with complex I defects are

Table 79–7. Association Between Mitochondrial Encephalomyopathies and Specific Mitochondrial Defects

Syndrome	Complex Defects
Early onset	
Lethal infantile encephalomyopathies with lactic acidosis and spongiform degeneration	I, III, I + IV
Hypotonia, growth retardation, cardiomyopathy, encephalopathy, and liver failure	I, IV, I + IV, II, III
Alpers' syndrome	I, IV, PDC, Krebs cycle
Leigh's syndrome	I, II, IV, V, PDC
Pearson's syndrome	I
Progressive encephalopathy, myoclonic seizures, and short stature	II
de Toni-Fanconi-Debré syndrome	IV
Childhood or adult onset	
Kearns-Sayre syndrome	I, II, III, IV, I + IV, I–IV, V
MELAS	I, I–III, III, I + IV, I–IV
MERRF	IV, I + IV
MERRF + MELAS	I, IV
MNGIE	IV
Dementia, ataxia, deafness, myoclonus, and retinopathy	I, IV
Dementia, ataxia, deafness, and myopathy	I, I–III
Progressive macrocephalic encephalopathy, hypertrophic cardiopathy, and ketoacidosis	I
Leber's hereditary optic neuropathy	I, III, IV
Mild myopathy, cramps, and rhabdomyolysis	II
Isolated cardiomyopathy or myopathy and cardiomyopathy	II
Optic atrophy and cerebellar ataxia	II
Encephalopathy, ophthalmoplegia, and tubulopathy	III
Myopathy, exercise intolerance, and myoglobinuria	III
NARP	V
Multiple symmetrical lipomatosis	IV
Myopathy, encephalopathy, lactic acidosis, myoglobinuria	Coenzyme Q10

PDC, pyruvate dehydrogenase complex; MELAS, mitochondrial myopathy, encephalopathy, lactic acidosis, and strokes; MERRF, myoclonic epilepsy with ragged red fibers, ataxia, and muscle weakness; MNGIE, myoneurogastrointestinal encephalopathy; NARP, neurogenic weakness, ataxia, and retinitis pigmentosa.

listed in Table 79–7. Defects of this complex have also been described in Leber's hereditary optic neuropathy, Parkinson's disease, and idiopathic dystonia. However, the most common clinical presentation in this group is with a MELAS-like syndrome (Morgan-Hughes et al., 1990). Patients may also present with a myopathy characterized by limb weakness and exercise intolerance, without muscle cramping or rhabdomyolysis. Careful examination of these patients usually reveals additional clinical findings commonly associated with mitochondrial diseases. Most patients with complex I deficiencies also have abnormalities of the other respiratory chain complexes (see Table 79–7). The combination of defects in complexes I, III, and IV, but not complex II, is particularly common in patients with severe depletion of mtDNA. A distinctive phenotype of isolated complex I deficiency in children has been recognized; it is characterized by fatal progressive macrocephaly, hypertrophic cardiomyopathy, and lactic acidosis (Slepetz et al., 1991). Pearson's syndrome and some cases of Leber's hereditary optic neuropathy also localize selectively to defects in complex I.

Complex II (Succinate Ubiquinone Oxidoreductase)

None of the four polypeptides (flavoprotein, iron sulfur protein, SDHC, and SDHD) that make up this complex are encoded by mtDNA. All genetic defects are located on the nuclear genome. The flavoprotein subunit of the complex has been mapped to chromosome 5p15, and a mutation of this gene was the first report of a nuclear gene mutation that causes a mitochondrial respiratory chain deficiency (Bourgeron et al., 1995). The major clinical groups associate with complex II deficiency are listed in Table 79–7. Hypertrophic cardiomyopathy is commonly seen as part of the clinical expression of this defect (Reichmann and Angelini, 1993).

Complex III (Ubiquinone Cytochrome C Oxidoreductase)

This complex consists of 9 or 10 polypeptides, one of which, the cytochrome *b* subunit, is encoded by the guanine-rich heavy strand of mtDNA between nucleotide pairs 14747 and 15887. The major clinical groups associate with complex III deficiency are listed in Table 79–7. Mutations in the cytochrome *b* gene have been found in patients with proximal myopathy, exercise intolerance, rhabdomyolysis, and ragged red fibers in muscle biopsy specimens (Andreu et al., 1999). Because there was no evidence of maternal inheritance in these patients, it was suggested that the disorder results from somatic mutations in myogenic stem cells, after germ-layer differentiation.

Complex IV (Cytochrome C Oxidase)

This complex has 13 subunits, of which 3 are encoded by mtDNA, and they are the actual catalytic subunits that carry out the electron transfer function. Surprisingly, it appears that most of the diseases that cause mutations are encoded by nuclear, rather than mitochondrial, genes. Thus, a recurrence rate of 25% (autosomal recessive inheritance) can be used as a rule of thumb for genetic counseling in cytochrome oxidase deficiencies (Parfait et al., 1997). However, specific mutations have been described in all three of the mitochondrial genes (*MTCO1, MTCO2,* and *MTCO3*) that code for these subunits. *MTCO1* mutations result in cataracts, sensorineural hearing loss, myoclonic epilepsy, cerebel-

lar ataxia, optic atrophy, and myopathy (Bruno et al., 1999). *MTCO2* mutations cause myopathy and lactic acidosis (Rahman et al., 1999), ataxia, distal myopathy, optic atrophy, retinitis pigmentosa, and dementia (Clark et al., 1999). *MTCO3* mutations induce muscle cramps and myoglobinuria (Keightley et al., 1996), exercise intolerance, and proximal myopathy (Hanna et al., 1998b). The spectrum of clinical disorders associated with complex IV deficiency is listed in Table 79–7. Cytochrome C oxidase deficiencies are usually associated with other complex deficiencies. Most of the patients with nuclear gene mutations present with Leigh's syndrome, but neonatal-onset lactic acidosis and generalized muscle weakness, with death before 1 year of age, are also common (Van Biervliet et al., 1977). Some of the early-onset cases have renal involvement as well (de Toni-Fanconi-Debré syndrome). A single patient with only proximal muscle weakness and exercise intolerance has also been reported. Ragged red fibers were absent in this patient's muscle biopsy specimen, but there was evidence for lipid and glycogen storage. The diagnosis can usually be made on the basis of muscle histochemistry, which shows the absence of cytochrome oxidase activity in extrafusal muscle fibers but normal cytochrome oxidase activity in intrafusal muscle fibers. In a few infants, cytochrome oxidase activity is absent at birth but normalizes over the next few years; this is called "benign infantile myopathy" (Zeviani et al., 1987). In these patients, the episodes of lactic acidosis and the muscle weakness abate spontaneously as cytochrome oxidase activity normalizes.

Complex V (Adenosine Triphosphate Synthetase)

The complex has 12 to 18 subunits, of which 1 (ATPase 6 and ATPase 8) are encoded by mtDNA. ATPase 6 is encoded by nucleotides 8527 to 9207. Most of the complex V abnormalities were the result of an mtDNA mutation that involved the ATPase 6 gene, and these patients presented in infancy with Leigh's syndrome. In a comparison of 9 Leigh's syndrome patients secondary to an mtDNA 8993T-C mutation, with 18 Leigh syndrome patients with an 8993T-G mutation, it was found that the 8993T-C group did not develop retinitis pigmentosa and that in general, these patients had a milder form of the disease (Fujii et al., 1998). The percentage of abnormal mitochondria correlated with the clinical severity; in patients with 70% to 80% abnormal mitochondria, NARP syndrome developed, and in those with more than 90% abnormal mitochondria, Leigh's syndrome developed (Holt et al., 1990). At least two patients have been described with muscle weakness (Clark et al., 1982), and two patients had euthyroid hypermetabolism—Luft's disease (Luft et al., 1962). These patients had severe heat intolerance, hyperhidrosis, polyphagia, and relatively mild muscle weakness. Muscle biopsy findings included structurally abnormal mitochondria but no ragged red fibers.

Coenzyme Q10 Deficiency

Encephalopathy with exercise intolerance and recurrent bouts of rhabdomyolysis are typical clinical findings (Ogasahara et al., 1989). The encephalopathy includes seizures and progressive cerebellar dysfunction.

Clinical-Genetic Correlation in Mitochondrial Syndromes

It was expected that a rational classification of the mitochondrial diseases would be possible as soon as the specific genetic defects were established. Unfortunately, the experience up to this point has been rather disappointing, as it has become clear that there is poor correlation between the specific DNA abnormalities and the clinical phenotype. For example, patients with large single mutations can present with Kearns-Sayre syndrome, Leigh's disease, or adult-onset diabetes or only with benign nonprogressive ptosis in adult life. Similarly, diverse clinical syndromes have been reported with multiple deletions or single–base-pair substitutions in the mitochondrial genome. Some of the confusion can be explained by mitochondrial heteroplasmy—that is, the coexistence in varying proportions of wild-type and mutated mitochondria and the varying expression of mitochondrial abnormalities in different tissues of the same patient. It has also become clear that disease will be expressed in specific tissues only if the proportion of mutant genes exceeds a specific percentage of the total number of mitochondrial genes in that tissue. Thus, many asymptomatic members in a given family may have the same genetic defect but exhibit no clinical evidence of disease. Deletions of mtDNA in skeletal muscle can be detected with Southern blot hybridization. Pooled data from four laboratories showed deletions in 38% of patients with histologically defined mitochondrial myopathies; 50% of patients with oculoskeletal myopathy; 89% of patients with progressive external ophthalmoplegia, retinitis pigmentosa, or deafness, or a combination of these; and 87% of patients with Kearns-Sayre syndrome (Morgan-Hughes, 1994). Of note was the absence of deletions in patients with limb weakness alone, MELAS, MERRF, MNGIE, muscle cytochrome oxidase deficiency, Luft's disease, muscle coenzyme Q10 deficiency, and deficiency of mitochondrial ATP synthase. Because of the low concentration of mtDNA deletions in blood products, Southern blot hybridization is not reliable in detecting these, but deletions can usually be detected with selective polymerase chain reaction amplification. These results should be interpreted with caution, because deletions are also detectable in otherwise normal persons. At this point, it appears that the risk of inheriting large deletions is about

4%, an important fact for genetic counseling (Ozawa et al., 1988). Also, in many families, multiple mtDNA deletions have been reported that can result in the clinical expression of disease in compound heterozygotes as outlined previously. Duplications of mtDNA are rare, but in at least one family in which such a duplication was found, disease transmission occurred from mother to daughter (Rotig et al., 1992).

SELECTED MITOCHONDRIAL SYNDROMES

The following is not an exhaustive list of mitochondrion-related syndromes, and only the syndromes in which muscle weakness or neuropathy are salient features are discussed. Relatively common mitochondrial diseases such as Leber's hereditary optic neuropathy and Leigh's syndrome are not discussed.

MELAS

The mitochondrial tRNA for leucine is encoded by nucleotides 3230 to 3304. In 93 of 110 patients presenting with this syndrome, an A-to-G transitional mutation was found at nucleotide position 3243 in the mitochondrial gene (Goto et al., 1990). However, the same mutation may also result in other syndromes, including a combination of MELAS and MERRF (Chinnery et al., 1998), Leigh's syndrome (Sue et al., 1999), and non–insulin-dependent diabetes mellitus with sensorineural hearing loss. In some populations, this mutation may account for 1% to 3% of all cases of maternally inherited non–insulin-dependent diabetes mellitus (Velho et al., 1996). Other mutations that may also result in a MELAS syndrome include T-to-C transition at position 3271 in the tRNA$^{eu(UUR)}$ gene (Goto et al., 1991) or a G-to-A transition at position 583 in the mitochondrial phenylalanine tRNA gene (Hanna et al., 1998a). Thus, the majority of patients display maternal inheritance, and 56% to 95% of mitochondria in a specific organ need to be mutated to result in clinical disease. The disease onset is between 2 and 40 years of age. The attacks are migraine-like, with headache and vomiting. Loss of consciousness, seizures, and eventually dementia may follow. Other clinical findings include hemiplegia, cortical blindness, pigmentary retinopathy, cardiomyopathy, and short stature. Death may result from cardiopulmonary failure or status epilepticus, usually two to four decades after onset of the clinical findings. Investigations have shown the presence of basal ganglia calcifications, lactic acidosis in blood and cerebrospinal fluid, and ragged red, ragged blue, and cytochrome oxidase–negative fibers on muscle histology. The strokelike events may result from endothelial pathology and subsequent ischemia secondary to mitochondrial proliferation in the blood vessels or as a consequence of a focal cytopathy secondary to mitochondrial dysfunction.

Electromyographic Studies

The findings are usually normal. Mild myopathic motor unit potentials may be present on the needle examination. In patients with diabetes, all the usual diabetic neuropathies may develop over time.

MERRF

The mitochondrial tRNA for lysine is encoded by nucleotides 8295 to 8364. About 80% to 90% of all patients with MERRF have an A-to-G transition at nucleotide 8344 of the tRNA lysine gene (Shoffner and Wallace, 1992). Other mutations described were a T-to-C transition at position 8356 and a G-to-A transition in position 8363 of the same gene (Santorelli et al., 1996). A T7512C transmutation in the mitochondrial tRNA serine gene has been documented in patients with a MERRF/MELAS overlap syndrome (Jaksch et al., 1998). Thus, MERRF has a maternal pattern of inheritance. In clinically affected patients, the proportion of mutant mtDNA genomes in muscle was more than 80%. The clinical syndrome consists of myoclonus (60%), epilepsy (45%), hearing loss (40%), and polyneuropathy (20%). Other features include cerebellar dysfunction, dementia, optic atrophy, short stature, and multiple lipoma. Ragged red fibers and COX-negative fibers are present on muscle biopsy specimens.

Electromyographic Studies

The nerve conduction studies are usually normal, but in the small number of patients with a polyneuropathy, the findings are those of an axonal sensorimotor neuropathy. This consists of low sensory and motor compound action potentials with relatively normal nerve conduction studies. Motor unit potential analysis may reveal myopathic motor unit potentials.

NARP

The genetic mutations involved in this disorder were covered in the discussion of complex V deficiency (ATPase 6 gene mutation). The same mutation can also result in Leigh's syndrome and sometimes Kearns-Sayre syndrome. Inheritance is maternal, and the common clinical findings are sensory neuropathy, cerebellar ataxia, and retinitis pigmentosa. Other clinical features may include dementia, seizures, and proximal muscle weakness. Serum lactate levels are normal, and ragged red fibers are absent on muscle histology.

Electromyographic Studies

Nerve conduction studies reveal low or absent sensory nerve action potentials, consistent with a sensory axonal neuropathy. The needle examination is normal.

MNGIE

This syndrome is caused by a mutation in the thymidine phosphorylase gene. The gene is localized on chromosome 22q13.32-qter (Hirano et al., 1998). The thymidine phosphorylase enzyme has angiogenic effects, because it is an endothelial cell growth factor, catalyzes conversion between thymine and thymidine, and plays a role in the homeostasis of cellular nucleotide pools. Disease onset is usually before age 20. Typically, the patients present with a proximal myopathy and progressive external ophthalmoplegia, a mixed axonal and demyelinating distal polyneuropathy, gastrointestinal dysfunction with malabsorption, diarrhea and pseudo-obstruction, and a progressive leukoencephalopathy. Other findings include neurosensory hearing loss, retinal degeneration, and a thin body habitus. Brain imaging studies may reveal diffuse white matter disease with basal ganglia calcifications in about 25% of cases. The distal polyneuropathy has been interpreted as primarily demyelinating with secondary axonal loss, or vice versa (Simon et al., 1990). Ragged red and ragged blue fibers, cytochrome oxidase–negative fibers, and evidence of denervation atrophy were present on muscle histology. The gastrointestinal dysfunction is secondary to a severe visceral neuropathy. About two thirds of the patients have lactic acidosis. Inheritance is probably autosomal recessive, even though multiple deletions have been found in mtDNA. It is hypothesized that the mitochondrial defects are caused by disrupted intergenomic communications secondary to the genomic mutation (Nishino et al., 1999).

Electromyographic Studies

Nerve conduction studies show low sensory and motor compound muscle action potentials with mild to moderate slowing of nerve conduction velocities. In patients with proximal muscle weakness, myopathic motor unit potentials may be present in the weak muscles.

Kearns-Sayre Syndrome

This syndrome usually results from a single large mtDNA deletion. The most common of these is a 4,977-bp deletion between mitochondrial nucleotides 8488 and 13460. Thai patients with this syndrome have a unique 3,558-bp deletion between mitochondrial nucleotides 10204 to 13761 or 10208 to 13765 (Lertrit et al., 1999). Most deletions preserve the promoters of transcription of heavy and light strands, the 12S and 16S rRNA genes, and the origin of heavy-strand replication. The majority of patients present sporadically, but sometimes this is a familial disorder. The cardinal clinical features are progressive external ophthalmoplegia, retinitis pigmentosa, cardiac conduction block, and a proximal myopathy. Other clinical features may include a sensorimotor distal polyneuropathy, hearing loss, cerebellar ataxia, impaired cognition, central sleep apnea, and a short stature. Rarely, patients may also present with strokelike symptoms, malabsorption, diabetes, hypothyroidism, and hypoparathyroidism. Laboratory tests confirm lactic acidosis and high cerebrospinal fluid protein levels in most patients and basal ganglia calcification in about 5%. Ragged red fibers and cytochrome oxidase–negative fibers are typically found on muscle histology.

Electromyographic Studies

In patients with this clinical finding, the neuropathy is predominantly axonal, and thus motor nerve conduction studies may show normal or slightly reduced conduction velocities. The sensory nerve conduction studies are characterized by reduced sensory nerve action potential amplitudes and slight reductions in conduction velocities. The needle examination may be normal or reveal mild myopathic motor unit potentials.

Progressive External Ophthalmoplegia

Impaired eye movements are common in mitochondrial disorders such as Kearns-Sayre and MNGIE syndromes. A clearly defined subgroup of patients with progressive external ophthalmoplegia (PEO) were identified in kindreds in which many members were affected in an autosomal dominant pattern of inheritance. These patients are now classified as PEO1 (gene locus 10q23.3-q24.3), PEO2 (gene locus 3p14.1-p21.2), PEO3 (gene locus 4q35), and PEO4 (all families not yet mapped). Disease onset in these patients is usually after 20 years of age; patients with PEO1, PEO2, and PEO3 have the additional features of proximal muscle weakness and cataracts (Suomalainen et al., 1992; Kaukonen et al., 1996, 1999) beyond external ophthalmoplegia. Some patients with PEO1 also have psychiatric disorders and patients with PEO3 usually have minimal extremity weakness but may have sensorineural deafness, dementia, or thyroid disease. Patients with PEO4 form a heterogeneous group that will be classified more accurately in the future. A large Swedish family in whom autosomal dominant PEO occurred in association with hypogonadism, cataracts, and proximal limb weakness may fall into this group, but the known genetic mutations have not yet been excluded in this kindred (Melberg et al., 1996). In all of these groups, multiple DNA deletions are found, presumably because the nuclear mutations disrupt mechanisms that normally prevent mtDNA deletions or facilitate their repair. Ragged red fibers are usually present on histological examination.

Electromyographic Studies

Only a few electrophysiological studies have been reported, but these generally showed myopathic changes on needle examination with normal nerve conduction studies.

References

Al Aqeel A I, Rashed MS, Wanders RJA: Carnitine-acylcarnitine translocase deficiency is a treatable disease. J Inherit Metab Dis 1999;22:271.

Alegria A, Martins E, Dias M, et al: Glycogen storage disease type IV presenting as hydrops fetalis. J Inherit Metab Dis 1999; 22:330.

Amit R, Bashan N, Abarbanel JM, et al: Fatal familial infantile glycogen storage disease: Multisystem phosphofructokinase deficiency. Muscle Nerve 1992;15:455.

Andresen BS, Bross P, Udvari S, et al: The molecular basis of medium-chain acyl-CoA dehydrogenase (MCAD) deficiency in compound heterozygous patients: Is there correlation between genotype and phenotype? Hum Mol Genet 1997;6:695.

Andreu AL, Hanna MG, Reichmann H, et al: Exercise intolerance due to mutations in the cytochrome b gene of mitochondrial DNA. N Engl J Med 1999;341:1037.

Ausems MGEM, Lochman P, van Diggelen, et al: A diagnostic protocol for adult-onset glycogen storage disease type II. Neurology 1999;52:851.

Bao Y, Kishnani P, Wu J-W, et al: Hepatic and neuromuscular forms of glycogen storage disease type IV caused by mutations in the same glycogen-branching enzyme gene. J Clin Invest 1996;97:941.

Bashan N, Iancu TC, Lerner A, et al: Glycogenosis due to liver and muscle phosphorylase kinase deficiency. Pediatr Res 1981; 15:299.

Bhala A, Willi SM, Rinaldo P, et al: Clinical and biochemical characterization of short-chain acyl-coenzyme A dehydrogenase deficiency. J Pediatr 1995;126:910.

Blass JP, Kark RAP, Engel WK: Clinical studies of a patient with pyruvate decarboxylase deficiency. Arch Neurol 1971;25:449.

Borglum AD, Flint T, Hansen LL, et al: Refined localization of the pyruvate dehydrogenase E11-alpha gene (PDHA1) by linkage analysis. Hum Genet 1997;99:80.

Bourgeron T, Chretien D, Poggi-Bach J, et al: Mutation of the fumarase gene in two siblings with progressive encephalopathy and fumarase deficiency. J Clin Invest 1994;93:5214.

Bourgeron T, Rustin P, Chretien D, et al: Mutation of a nuclear succinate dehydrogenase gene results in mitochondrial respiratory chain deficiency. Nat Genet 1995;11:144.

Britton CH, Schultz RA, Zhang B, et al: Human liver mitochondrial carnitine palmitoyltransferase I: Characterization of its cDNA and chromosomal localization and partial analysis of the gene. Proc Natl Acad Sci U S A 92:1995;1984.

Brown BI, Brown DH, Jeffrey PL: Simultaneous absence of α-1,4-glucosidase and α-1,6-glucosidase activities (pH 4) in tissues of children with type II glycogen storage disease. Biochemistry 1970;9:1416.

Bruno C, Martinuzzi A, Tang Y, et al: A stop-codon mutation in the human mtDNA cytochrome c oxidase I gene disrupts the functional structure of complex IV. Am J Hum Genet 1999; 65:611.

Bruno C, Servidei S, Shanske S, et al: Glycogen branching enzyme deficiency in adult polyglucosan body disease. Ann Neurol 1993;33:88.

Caravaglia B, Uziel G, Dworzak F: Primary carnitine deficiency: Heterozygote and intrafamilial phenotypic variation. Neurology 1991;41:1691.

Chen YT, He JK, Ding JH, et al: Glycogen debranching enzyme: Purification, antibody characterization, and immunoblot analysis of type III glycogen storage disease. Am J Hum Genet 1987; 41:1002.

Chapoy PR, Angelini C, Brown WJ, et al: Systemic carnitine deficiency—a treatable inherited lipid-storage disease presenting as Reye's syndrome. N Engl J Med 1980;303:1389.

Chinnery PF, Howell N, Lightowlers RN, et al: MELAS and MERRF: The relationship between maternal mutation load and the frequency of clinically affected offspring. Brain 1998;121:1889.

Clark JB, Hayes DJ, Morgan-Hughes JA, et al: Mitochondrial myopathies: Disorders of the respiratory chain and oxidative phosphorylation system. J Inherit Metab Dis 1982;7:62.

Clark KM, Taylor RW, Johnson MA, et al: An mtDNA mutation in the initiation codon of the cytochrome c oxidase subunit II gene results in lower levels of the protein and a mitochondrial encephalopathy. Am J Hum Genet 1999;64:1330.

Clemens PR, Yamamoto M, Engel AG: Adult phosphorylase b kinase deficiency. Ann Neurol 1990;28:529.

Cornelio F, Gresolin N, Singer PA: Clinical varieties of neuromuscular disease in debrancher deficiency. Arch Neurol 1984;41:1027.

Corydon MJ, Andresen BS, Bross P, et al: Structural organization of the human short-chain acyl-CoA dehydrogenase gene. Mamm Genome 1997;8:922.

Costa CG, Verhoeven NM, Kneepkens CMF, et al: Organic acid profiles resembling a beta-oxidation defect in two patients with coeliac disease. J Inherit Metab Dis 1996;19:177.

Dahl HH: Pyruvate dehydrogenase E1alpha deficiency: Males and females differ yet again. Am J Hum Genet 1995;56:553.

Di Donato S, Rimodi M, Garavaglia B, et al: Propionylcarnitine excretion in propionic and methylmalonic acidurias: A cause of carnitine deficiency. Clin Chim Acta 1984;139:13.

Di Mauro S, Dalakas M, Miranda AF: Phosphoglycerate kinase deficiency: Another cause of recurrent myoglobniuria. Ann Neurol 1983;13:11.

Di Mauro S, Miranda AF, Sokoda S, et al: Metabolic myopathies. Am J Med Genet 1986;25:635.

Di Mauro S, Tsujino S: Nonlysosomal glycogenosis. In Engel AG, Franzini-Armstrong C (eds): Myology. New York, McGraw-Hill, 1994.

Ding JH, DeBarsy TH, Brown BI: Immunoblot analysis of glycogen debranching enzyme in different subtypes of glycogen storage disease type III. J Pediatr 1990;116:95.

Engel AG, Gomez MR, Seybold ME, et al: The spectrum and diagnosis of acid maltase deficiency. Neurology 1973;13:95.

Engel AG, Rebouch CJ, Wilson D, et al: Primary systemic carnitine deficiency. II. Renal handling of carnitine. Neurology 1981;31:819.

Etiemble J, Kahn APB: Hereditary hemolytic anemia with erythrocyte phosphofructokinase deficiency. Hum Genet 1976;31:83.

Fadic R, Waclawik AJ, Brooks BR, et al: The rigid spine syndrome due to acid maltase deficiency. Muscle Nerve 1997;20:364.

Falik-Borenstein ZC, Jordan SC, Saudubray JM, et al: Renal tubular acidosis in carnitine palmitoyltransferase type I deficiency. N Engl J Med 1992;327:24.

Fujii T, Hattori H, Higuchi Y, et al: Phenotypic differences between T-C and T-G mutations at nt8993 of mitochondrial DNA in Leigh syndrome. Pediatr Neurol 1998;18:275.

Gallera C, Verderio E, Floridia G, et al: Assignment of the human carnitine palmitoyltransferase II gene (CPT I) to chromosome 1p. Genomics 1994;24:195.

Gieron MA, Korthals JK: Carnitine palmitoyltransferase deficiency with permanent weakness. Pediatr Neurol 1987;3:51.

Goto Y, Nonaka I, Horai S: A mutation in the tRNA^Leu(UUR) associated with the MELAS subgroup of mitochondrial encephalomyopathies. Nature 1990;348:651.

Goto Y, Nonaka I, Horai S: A new mtDNA mutation associated with mitochondrial myopathy, encephalopathy, lactic acidosis and stroke-like episodes (MELAS). Biochim Biophys Acta 1991;1097:238.

Gregersen N, Winter VS, Corydon MJ, et al: Identification of four new mutations in the short-chain acyl-CoA dehydrogenase (SCAD) gene in two patients: One of the variant alleles, 511C-T, is present at an unexpected high frequency in the general population, as was the case for 625G-A, together conferring susceptibility to ethylmalonic aciduria. Hum Mol Genet 1998;7:619.

Griffin JL: Infantile acid maltase deficiency: I. Muscle fiber destruction after lysosomal rupture. Virchows Arch 1984;45:23.

Hadjigeorgiou GM, Comi GP, Bordoni A, et al: Novel donor splice site mutations of AGL gene in glycogen storage disease type IIIa. J Inherit Metab Dis 1999;22:762.

Haller RG, Henriksson KG, Jorfeldt L: Deficiency of skeletal muscle succinate dehydrogenase and aconitase. J Clin Invest 1991;88:1197.

Hanna MG, Nelson IP, Morgan-Hughes JA, et al: MELAS: A new disease associated mitochondrial DNA mutation and evidence for further genetic heterogeneity. J Neurol Neurosurg Psychiatry 1998a;65:512.

Hanna MG, Nelson IP, Rahman S, et al: Cytochrome c oxidase

deficiency associated with the first stop-codon point mutation in human mtDNA. Am J Hum Genet 1998b;63:29.

Hirano M, Garcia-de-Yebenes J, Jones J, et al: Mitochondrial neurogastrointestinal encephalopathy syndrome maps to chromosome 22q13.32-qter. Am J Genet 1998;63:526.

Hoefsloot LH, Koogeveen-Westerveld M, Kroos MA, et al: Characterization of the human alpha-glucosidase gene. Biochem J 1990;272:493.

Holt IJ, Harding AE, Petty RKH, et al: A new mitochondrial disease associated with mitochondrial DNA heteroplasmy. Am J Hum Genet 1990;46:428.

Howard TD, Akots G, Gowden DW: Physical and genetic mapping of the muscle phosphofructokinase gene (PFKM): Reassignment to human chromosome 12q. Genomics 1996;34:122.

Hug G, Bove KE, Soukup S: Lethal neonatal multiorgan deficiency of carnitine palmitoyltransferase II. N Engl J Med 1991;325:1862.

Huie ML, Menaker M, McAlpine, et al: Identification of an E689K substitution as the molecular basis of the human acid alpha-glucosidase type 4 allozyme (GAA4). Ann Hum Genet 1996;60:365.

Iafolla AK, Thompson RJ Jr, Roe CR: Medium-chain acyl-coenzyme A dehydrogenase deficiency: Clinical course in 120 affected children. J Pediatr 1994;124:409.

Jaksch M, Hofmann S, Kleinle S, et al: A systematic mutation screen of 10 nuclear and 25 mitochondrial candidate genes in 21 patients with cytochrome c oxidase (COX) deficiency shows tRNA-ser(UCN) mutations in a subgroup with syndromal encephalopathy. J Med Genet 1998;35:895.

Karpati F, Carpenter S, Engel AG: The syndrome of systemic carnitine deficiency: Clinical, morphological, biochemical and pathophysiological features. Neurology 1975;25:16.

Kaukonen JA, Amati P, Suomalainen A, et al: An autosomal locus predisposing to multiple deletions of mtDNA on chromosome 3p. Am J Genet 1996;58:763.

Kaukonen J, Seviani M, Comi GP, et al: A third locus predisposing to multiple deletions of mtDNA in autosomal dominant progressive external ophthalmoplegia (letter). Am J Hum Genet 1999;65:256.

Keightley JA, Hoffbuhr KC, Burton MD, et al: A microdeletion in cytochrome c oxidase (COX) subunit III associated with COX deficiency and recurrent myoglobinuria. Nat Genet 1996;12:410.

Kieval RI, Sotrel A, Weinblatt ME: Chronic myopathy with a partial deficiency of the carnitine palmitoyltransferase enzyme. Arch Neurol 1989;46:575.

Kretzschmer HA, Dearmond SJ, Koch TC: Pyruvate dehydrogenase deficiency as a cause of subacute necrotizing encephalopathy (Leigh disease). Pediatrics 1987;79:370.

Kroos MA, Van der Kraan M, Van Diggelen OP, et al: Glycogen storage disease type II: Frequency of three common mutant alleles and their associated clinical phenotypes studied in 121 patients. J Med Genet 1995;32:836.

Kuo W-L, Hirschhorn R, Huie M, et al: Localization and ordering of acid alpha-glucosidase (GAA) and thymidine kinase (TK1) by fluorescence in situ hybridization. Hum Genet 1997;97:404.

Kurtz DM, Rinaldo P, Rhead WJ, et al: Targeted disruption of mouse long-chain acyl-CoA dehydrogenase gene reveals crucial roles for fatty acid oxidation. Proc Natl Acad Sci U S A 1998;95:15592.

Lebo RV, Anderson LA, Di Mauro S, et al: Rare McArdle disease locus polymorphic site on 11q13 contains CpG sequence. Hum Genet 1990;86:17.

Lejeune N, Thinès-Sempoux D, Hers HG: Tissue fractionation studies: Intracellular distribution and properties of α-glucosidases in rat liver. Biochem J 1963;86:16.

Lertrit P, Imsumran A, Karnkirawattana P, et al: A unique 3.5-kb deletion of the mitochondrial genome in Thai patients with Kearns-Sayre syndrome. Hum Genet 1999;105:127.

Luft R, Ikkos D, Palmieri G: A case of severe hypermetabolism of nonthyroid origin with a defect in the maintenance of mitochondrial respiratory chain control: A correlated clinical, biochemical and morphological study. J Clin Invest 1962;41:1776.

Maekawa M, Kanda S, Sudo K, et al: Estimation of the gene frequency of lactate dehydrogenase subunit deficiencies. Am J Hum Genet 1984;36:1204.

Maekawa M, Sudo K, Kanno T, et al: Molecular characterization of genetic mutation in human lactate dehydrogenase-A (M) deficiency. Biochem Biophys Res Commun 1990;168:677.

Makos MM, McComb RD, Hart MN, et al: Alpha-glucosidase deficiency and basilar artery aneurysms. Ann Neurol 1987;22:629.

Marbini A, Gemignani F, Saccardi F, et al: Debrancher deficiency neuromuscular disorder with pseudohypertrophy in two brothers. J Neurol 1989;236:418.

Martin MA, Rubio JC, De Bustos F, et al: Molecular analysis in Spanish patients with muscle carnitine palmitoyltransferase deficiency. Muscle Nerve 1999;22:941.

Martiniuk F, Chen A, Mack A, et al: Carrier frequency for glycogen storage disease type II in New York and estimates of affected individuals born with the disease. Am J Genet 1998;79:69.

Mathews PM, Brown RM, Otero LJ, et al: Pyruvate dehydrogenase deficiency: Clinical presentation and molecular genetic characterization of five new patients. Brain 1994;117:435.

McArdle B: Myopathy due to a defect in muscle glycogen breakdown. Clin Sci 1951;10:13.

Melberg A, Lundberg PO, Henriksson KG, et al: Muscle-nerve involvement in autosomal dominant progressive external ophthalmoplegia with hypogonadism. Muscle Nerve 1996;19:751.

Mitchell P: Coupling of phosphorylation to electron and hydrogen transfer by a chemiosmotic type of mechanism. Nature 1961; 191:144.

Morgan-Hughes JA: Mitochondrial diseases. In Engel AG, Franzini-Armstrong C (eds): Myology. New York, McGraw-Hill, 1994.

Morgan-Hughes JA, Hayes KJ, Cooper JM, et al: Mitochondrial myopathies: Deficiencies localized to complex I and complex II of the mitochondrial respiratory chain. Biochem Soc Trans 1990;113:648.

Morris AAM, Olpin SE, Brivet M, et al: A patient with carnitine-acylcarnitine translocase deficiency with a mild phenotype. J Pediatr 1998;132:514.

Moses SW, Gadoth N, Bashan N, et al: Neuromuscular involvement in glycogen storage disease type III. Acta Paediatr Scand 1986; 75:289.

Moses SW, Wanderman KL, Myroz A, et al: Cardiac involvement in glycogen storage disease type III. Eur J Pediatr 1989;148:764.

Nezu J, Tamai I, Oku A, et al: Primary systemic carnitine deficiency is caused by mutations in a gene encoding sodium ion–dependent carnitine transporter. Nat Genet 1999;1:91.

Ninomiya N, Matsuda I, Matsuoka T: Demonstration of acid α-glucosidase in different types of Pompe disease by use of an immunochemical method. J Neurol Sci 1984;66:129.

Nishino I, Spinazzola A, Hirano M: Thymidine phosphorylase gene mutations in MNGIE, a human mitochondrial disorder. Science 1999;283:689.

Ogasahara S, Engel AG, Frens D, et al: Muscle coenzyme Q deficiency in familial mitochondrial encephalomyopathy. Proc Natl Acad Sci U S A 1989;86:2379.

Ozawa T, Yoneda M, Tanaka M: Maternal inheritance of deleted mitochondrial DNA in a family with mitochondrial myopathy. Biochem Biophys Res Commun 1988;154:1240.

Parfait B, Percheron A, Chretien D: No mitochondrial cytochrome oxidase (COX) gene mutations in 18 cases of COX deficiency. Hum Genet 1997;247.

Parvari R, Moses S, Shen J, et al: A single-base deletion in the 3-prime coding region of glycogen-debranching enzyme is prevalent in glycogen storage disease type IIIA in a population of North African Jewish patients. Eur J Hum Genet 1996;5:266.

Powell HC, Haas R, Hall CL, et al: Peripheral nerve in type III glycogenosis: Selective involvement of unmyelinated fiber Schwann cells. Muscle Nerve 1985;8:667.

Raben N, Sherman JB: Mutations in muscle phosphofructokinase gene. Hum Mutat 1995;6:1.

Radom J, Salvayre R, Negrè A: Metabolism of neutral lipids in cultured fibroblasts from multisystem (or type 3) lipid storage myopathy. Eur J Biochem 1987;164:703.

Rahman S, Taanman J-W, Cooper JM, et al: A missense mutation of cytochrome oxidase subunit II causes defective assembly and myopathy. Am J Hum Genet 1999;65:1030.

Reichmann H, Angelini C: Single muscle fibre analyses in 2 brothers with succinate dehydrogenase deficiency. Eur Neurol 1993; 34:95.

Reuser AJJ, Kroos M, Oude Elferink RPJ, et al: Defects in synthe-

sis, phosphorylation, and maturation of acid α-glucosidase in glycogenosis type II. J Biol Chem 1985;260:8336.

Ribes E, Riudor E, Navarro C, et al: Fatal outcome in a patient with long-chain 3-hydroxyacyl-CoA dehydrogenase deficiency. J Inherit Metab Dis 1992;15:278.

Ristow M, Vorgerd M, Mohlig M, et al: Deficiency of phospho-fructo-1-kinase/muscle subtype in humans impairs insulin secretion and causes insulin resistance. J Clin Invest 1997;100: 2833.

Robinson BH, Chun K, Mackay N: Isolated and combined deficiencies of the α-keto acid dehydrogenase complexes. Ann N Y Acad Sci 1989;573:337.

Roe CR, Coates PM: Mitochondrial fatty acid oxidation. In Scriver CR, Sly WS, Valle D (eds): The Metabolic and Molecular Bases of Inherited Disease, ed 7. New York, McGraw-Hill, 1995.

Rotig A, Bessis J-L, Romero N: Maternally inherited duplication of the mitochondrial genome in a syndrome of proximal tubulo-pathy, diabetes mellitus and cerebellar ataxia. Am J Hum Genet 1992;50:364.

Rowland LP, Di Mauro S, Layzer RB: Phosphofructokinase deficiency. In Engel AG, Banker BQ (eds): Myology. New York, McGraw-Hill, 1986.

Santorelli FM, Mak S-C, El-Schahawi M, et al: Maternally inherited cardiomyopathy and hearing loss associated with a novel mutation in the mitochondrial tRNA(lys) gene (G8363A). Am J Hum Genet 1996;58:933.

Selby R, Starzl TE, Unis E, et al: Liver transplantation for type IV glycogen storage disease with complete branching enzyme deficiency (type IV glycogenosis). N Engl J Med 1991;324:39.

Shen J, Bao Y, Liu H-M, et al: Mutations in exon 3 of the glycogen debranching enzyme gene are associated with glycogen storage disease type III that is differentially expressed in liver and muscle. J Clin Invest 1996;98:352.

Shen J, Liu M-H, Bao Y, et al: Polymorphic markers of the glycogen debranching enzyme gene allowing linkage analysis in families with glycogen storage disease type III. J Med Genet 1997;34:38.

Shoffner JM, Wallace DC: Mitochondrial genetics: Principles and practice (editorial). Am J Hum Genet 1992;51:1179.

Shoji Y, Koizumi A, Kayo T, et al: Evidence for linkage of human primary systemic carnitine deficiency with D5S436: A novel gene locus on chromosome 5q. Am J Hum Genet 1998;63:101.

Simon LT, Horoupian DS, Dorfman LJ, et al: Polyneuropathy, ophthalmology, leukoencephalopathy, and intestinal pseudo-obstruction: POLIP syndrome. Ann Neurol 1990;28:349.

Slepetz DM, Goodyer PR, Rozen R: Congenital deficiency of a 20-kD subunit of mitochondrial complex I in fibroblasts. Am J Hum Genet 1991;48:1121.

Slonim AE, Goans PJ: McArdle's syndrome: Improvement with a high protein diet. N Engl J Med 1985;312:355.

Smeitink J, van den Heuvel L: Human mitochondrial complex I in health and disease. Am J Hum Genet 1999;64:1505.

Sokal EM, Van Hoof F, Alberti D, et al: Progressive cardiac failure following orthotopic liver transplantation for type IV glycogen storage disease. Eur J Pediatr 1992;151:200.

Sue CM, Bruno C, Andreu AL, et al: Infantile encephalopathy associated with the MELAS A3243G mutation. J Pediatr 1999; 134:696.

Sugie H, Sugie Y, Ito M, et al: A novel missense mutation (837T-C) in the phosphoglycerate kinase gene of a patient with a myopathic form of phosphoglycerate kinase deficiency. J Child Neurol 1994;13:95.

Suomalainen A, Majander A, Haltia M, et al: Multiple deletions of mitochondrial DNA in several tissues of a patient with severe retarded depression and familial progressive external ophthalmoplegia. J Clin Invest 1992;90:61.

Takayasu S, Fujiwara S, Waki T: Hereditary lactate dehydrogenase M-subunit deficiency: Lactate dehydrogenase activity in skin lesions and in hair follicles. J Am Acad Dermatol 1991;24:339.

Taroni F, Verderio E, Fiorucci S, et al: Molecular characterization of inherited carnitine palmitoyltransferase II deficiency. Proc Natl Acad Sci U S A 1992;89:8429.

Tein I, Demaugre F, Bonnefont JP, et al: Normal muscle CPT 1 and CPT2 activities in hepatic presentation patients with CPT1 deficiency in fibroblasts. J Neurol Sci 1989;92:229.

Tein I, Haslam RHA, Rhead WJ, et al: Short-chain acyl-CoA dehydrogenase deficiency: A cause of ophthalmoplegia and multicore myopathy. Neurology 1999;52:366.

Treem WR, Stanley CA, Finegold DN, et al: Primary carnitine deficiency due to a failure of carnitine transport in kidney, muscle, and fibroblasts. N Engl J Med 1988;319:1331.

Tripp ME, Katcher ML, Peters HA: Systemic carnitine deficiency presenting as familial endocardial fibroelastosis: A treatable cardiomyopathy. N Engl J Med 1981;305:385.

Tsujino S, Shanske S, Di Mauro S: Molecular genetic heterogeneity of myophosphorylase deficiency (McArdle disease). N Engl J Med 1993a;329:241.

Tsujino S, Shanske S, Sakoda S, et al: The molecular genetic basis of muscle phosphoglycerate mutase (PGAM) deficiency. Am J Hum Genet 1993b;52:472.

Tzall S, Martiniuk F, Hirschhorn R: Identification of *Taq*I and *Hind*II RFPLs at the acid alpha glucosidase (GAA) locus. Nucleic Acids Res 1991;19:1727.

Tzall S, Martiniuk F, Ozelius L, et al.: Further characterization of *Pst*I RFLPs at the acid alpha glucosidase (GAA) locus. Nucleic Acids Res 1991;19:1727.

Van Biervliet JPGM, Bruinvis I, Ketting D: Hereditary mitochondrial myopathy with lactic acidaemia, a De-Toni-Fanconi-Debrè syndrome, and a defective respiratory chain in voluntary striated muscle. Pediatr Res 1977;11:1088.

VanDyke DH, Griggs RC, Markesbury WR, et al: Hereditary carnitine deficiency of muscle. Neurology 1975;25:154.

Van Hove JLK, Zhang W, Kahler SG, et al: Medium-chain acyl-CoA dehydrogenase (MCAD) deficiency: Diagnosis by acylcarnitine analysis in blood. Am J Hum Genet 1993;52:958.

Velho G, Byrne MM, Clement K, et al: Clinical phenotypes, insulin secretion, and insulin sensitivity in kindreds with maternally inherited diabetes and deafness due to mitochondrial tRNA Leu(UUR) gene mutation. Diabetes 1996;45:478.

Viggiano L, Iacobazzi V, Marzella R, et al: Assignment of the carnitine-acylcarnitine translocase gene (CACT) to human chromosome band 3p21.31 by in situ hybridization. Cytogenet Cell Genet 1997;79:62.

Vorgerd M, Kubisch C, Burwinkel B, et al: Mutation analysis in myophosphorylase deficiency (McArdle disease). Ann Neurol 1998;43:326.

Waber LJ, Valle D, Neill C: Carnitine deficiency presenting as familial cardiomyopathy: A treatable defect in carnitine transport. J Pediatr 1982;101:700.

Wallace DC: Mitochondrial disease in man and mouse. Science 1999;283:1482.

Wallace DC, Lott MT, Torroni A, et al: Report of the committee on human mitochondrial DNA. In Cuticchia AJ, Pearson PL (eds): Human Gene Mapping, 1993: A Compendium. Baltimore, Johns Hopkins University Press, 1994.

Wehner M, Clemens PR, Engel AG, et al: Human muscle glycogenosis due to phosphorylase kinase deficiency associated with a nonsense mutation in the muscle isoform of the alpha subunit. Hum Mol Genet 1994;3:1983.

Wokke JHJ, Ausems MGEM, van den Boogaard M-J, et al: Genotype-phenotype correlation in adult-onset acid maltase deficiency. Ann Neurol 1995;38:450.

Willner J, Di Mauro S, Eastwood A, et al: Muscle carnitine deficiency: Genetic heterogeneity. J Neurol Sci 1979;41:235.

Wu X, Prasad PD, Leibach FH, et al: cDNA sequence, transport function, and genomic organization of human OCTN2, a new member of the organic cation transporter family. Biochem Biophys Res Commun 1998;246:589.

Yang B-Z, Ding JH, Bao Y, et al: Molecular basis of the enzymatic variability in type III glycogen storage disease (GSD-III). Am J Hum Genet 1992;51(suppl):A28.

Yang-Feng TL, Indo Y, Glassberg, et al: Chromosomal assignment of the gene encoding human long chain acyl-CoA dehydrogenase (abstract). Cytogenet Cell Genet 1991;58:1874.

Zeviani M, Peterson P, Servidei S: Benign reversible muscle cytochrome c oxidase deficiency: A second case. Neurology 1987;37:64.

Ziadeh R, Hoffman EP, Finegold DN, et al: Medium chain-CoA dehydrogenase deficiency in Pennsylvania: Neonatal screening shows high incidence and unexpected mutation frequencies. Pediatr Res 1995;37:675.

Channelopathies

Philip G. McManis

INTRODUCTION

The application of molecular biology to neurological disorders has led to an explosion of knowledge about mechanisms of diseases that had been poorly understood. The secrets of many seemingly bizarre conditions have been unlocked by the analysis of alterations in the genetic code, showing that trivial changes in the sequence of nucleic acids coding for various proteins cause major changes in function, and a library of mutations is now accumulating to aid in the diagnosis of these conditions.

We now know that many neuromuscular disorders, particularly those with fluctuating or episodic symptoms, are due to alterations in the function of ion channels on cell membranes. These channels, or pores, control the flow of ionized species, particularly sodium, potassium, calcium, and chloride ions. In general, the opening and closing of these channels are controlled by voltages applied to cell membranes, such as when an action potential travels along a peripheral nerve and crosses the neuromuscular junction to reach a muscle membrane. This sequence of events is entirely dependent on the function of a series of ion channels. The wave of depolarization is propagated along the nerve by ion fluxes controlled by ionic channels on the axolemma. The release of acetylcholine into the neuromuscular junction is mediated by the opening of voltage-gated calcium channels. The contraction of muscle fibers is controlled by sodium, potassium, and chloride channels on the sarcolemma, and excitation-contraction coupling in the muscle fiber is determined by calcium channels (dihydropyridine and ryanodine receptors).

Ion channels have been implicated as targets of genetic neurological diseases. Abnormalities of the amino acid sequences of the proteins that constitute these channels cause the channels to pass too few

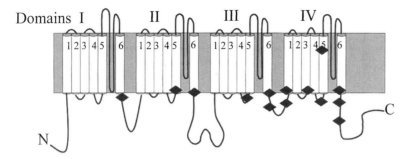

Domains I   II   III   IV

Figure 80–1. Alpha subunit of the skeletal muscle sodium channel (SCN4A). Each subunit consists of four homologous domains. Each domain contains six transmembrane segments. The S4 segment contains the voltage sensor, and the loops between segments 5 and 6 form the ion pore of the channel. The diamond symbols indicate the site of major mutations resulting in skeletal muscle sodium channelopathies (e.g., periodic paralysis, paramyotonia congenita, and potassium-aggravated myotonia).

(failure to open adequately or for a sufficient time) or too many (leaky channels or channels with a prolonged open time) ions. These abnormalities of ion channel function are grouped under the rubric "channelopathies."

The largest number of known genetic mutations affecting ion channels involves the human skeletal muscle sodium channel (SCN4A) (Fig. 80–1). Abnormalities of this gene are implicated in paramyotonia congenita, hyperkalemic periodic paralysis, an overlap syndrome linking these two disorders, and myotonia fluctuans. A number of autoimmune or genetic disorders that affect calcium channels have been identified, including several that affect neuromuscular function. The L-type voltage-gated calcium channel of skeletal muscle (dihydropyridine receptor) is affected in hypokalemic periodic paralysis. The ryanodine receptor on skeletal muscle is abnormal in malignant hyperthermia and central core disease (Greenberg, 1997). Calcium channel dysfunction may occur as the result of a nongenetic autoimmune disease, such as the presynaptic neuromuscular junction defect in Lambert-Eaton myasthenic syndrome. Inherited chloride channel disorders cause myotonia congenita (Koch et al., 1992; Koty et al., 1996; Brugnoni et al., 1999), and antibody-mediated potassium channel dysfunction is implicated in at least some cases of Isaac's neuromyotonia (Shillito et al., 1995).

Abnormal ion channel function characterizes paroxysmal disorders of the central nervous system as well as neuromuscular diseases. Genetic defects affecting the nicotinic acetylcholine receptor within the brain are implicated in autosomal dominant frontal lobe epilepsy (Steinlein et al., 1995), and a potassium channel mutation is associated with benign familial neonatal convulsions (Biervert et al., 1998). Calcium channel (neuronal P/Q type) alterations in the brain have been implicated in some forms of familial hemiplegic migraine (Spranger et al., 1999), in hereditary episodic ataxia type 2, and in hereditary spinocerebellar ataxia type 6 (SCA-6). Episodic ataxia type 1 with myokymia is thought to result from a potassium channel mutation (Browne et al., 1994). Some paroxysmal movement disorders are familial, and some of these may be due to ion channel mutations. It is not yet understood how channelopathies produce these protean clinical manifestations (Greenberg, 1999).

Among non-neurological conditions, paroxysmal cardiac arrhythmias occur in the "long QT interval" syndrome, a cardiac muscle channelopathy (Ackerman and Clapham, 1997; Jervell and Lange-Nielsen, 1957), and mutations at multiple genes are known to produce this clinical syndrome. More than 35 different mutations in four different genes (three potassium channel genes and a sodium channel gene) may produce the common end result of a prolongation of the QT interval on the electrocardiogram, and a predisposition to cardiac arrhythmias and sudden death (Ackerman, 1998). Patients with hyperkalemic periodic paralysis known to be due to sodium channel mutations may also have the long QT interval syndrome (Andersen et al., 1971; Sansone et al., 1997).

In many of these disorders, the precise link between the genetic mutation and the clinical manifestations of the disorder remains to be elucidated. However, identification of the responsible genetic mutation eventually leads to a better understanding of the mechanisms of the membrane malfunctions that produce the symptoms of the disease, and better treatments should be forthcoming.

The common theme in the ion channel disorders is the episodic or paroxysmal nature of the symptoms. People who often are otherwise normal experience the sudden onset of transient symptoms lasting seconds to hours, with complete resolution and a return to normal between the episodes. For many of these syndromes, there are recognized triggers (e.g., adrenergic stimulation in long QT interval syndrome, and exercise or dietary changes in the periodic paralyses). For many of these conditions, a particular syndrome due to malfunction of a single type of ion channel can be produced by any of a large number of different mutations affecting the function of that channel.

Another characteristic of the channelopathies is the lack of a close relationship between specific clinical phenotypes and genetic mutations. A single clinical symptom can result from many different genetic abnormalities. For instance, myotonia may occur when there are alterations in the sodium channels, chloride channels, or potassium channels. Second, different point mutations at various sites on the proteins that constitute ion channels can cause identical clinical conditions. Third, genetic mutations on a single channel gene may cause different clinical syndromes; mutations of the sodium channel gene on chromosome 17 (SCN4A) can cause hyperkalemic periodic paralysis, paramyotonia congenita, or myotonia.

CHANNELOPATHIES AND MUSCLE DISEASE

Most of the ion channel disorders thus far recognized affect skeletal muscle. There are two broad groups of muscle disease caused by ion channel dysfunction: the myotonias and the periodic paralyses. Although the genetic mutations that cause these diseases have been discovered only in the last decade, there has been evidence of abnormalities of the function of ion channels for much longer (Bryant, 1962). The inherited myotonic muscle disorders are the most common of these channelopathies. These myotonias are different from other ion channel disorders in that some of the symptoms are present constantly, while others are episodic. All of these disorders cause muscle stiffness that is present throughout the day, although the intensity of the myotonia and the degree of weakness vary with factors such as temperature and exercise. Weakness and poor muscle development are constant in proximal upper limb muscles in Becker's recessive generalized myotonia, but paroxysmal weakness occurs in paramyotonia congenita. The prototypical muscle channelopathies are the periodic paralysis variants. These hereditary disorders cause attacks of weakness at variable intervals, can be provoked by external factors, and produce few or no symptoms between attacks.

Muscle ion channelopathies can be classified according to the type of ion channel affected (Table 80–1). These are almost always inherited disorders, but neuromyotonia is an acquired condition that is generally autoimmune or paraneoplastic in origin.

Clinical Features

MYOTONIA

The term *myotonia* (literally, an increase in muscle tone or stiffness generated by the muscle itself) refers to delayed relaxation of muscle after a strong

---

Table 80–1. Known Muscle Ion Channel Disorders

Sodium Channel
  Hyperkalemic periodic paralysis
  Paramyotonia congenita
  Myotonia fluctuans
  Myotonia permanens
  Hypokalemic periodic paralysis
Calcium Channel
  Hypokalemic periodic paralysis
  Malignant hyperthermia (ryanodine receptor)
Chloride Channel
  Recessive generalized myotonia
  Myotonia congenita
Potassium Channel
  Neuromyotonia

Table 80–2. Characteristics of Clinical and "Electrical" Myotonia

Clinical myotonia	Delayed relaxation of muscle ("grip" myotonia)
	Muscle contracts when irritated ("percussion" myotonia)
	Occurs in
	Inherited myotonic syndromes
	Neuromyotonia
	Always associated with "electrical" myotonia
Electrical myotonia	Discharges recorded on needle examination of muscle
	Repetitive, involuntary firing of muscle fibers
	Waxes and wanes in amplitude and frequency
	Occurs in
	Inherited myotonic syndromes
	Acute neurogenic or myopathic processes
	Other neuromuscular diseases, such as acid maltase deficiency
	Sometimes associated with clinical myotonia

---

contraction ("grip" myotonia), or to a localized contraction of muscle after percussion of the muscle. Muscles may contract spontaneously when they are stretched. Thus, myotonia is a clinical phenomenon (Table 80–2). The prolonged contraction or delay in relaxation is the result of muscle membrane instability and consequent hyperexcitability of muscle fibers. The membrane is depolarized more easily than normally is the case, and repeated depolarizations may occur for several seconds after muscle stimulation or activation. Myotonia results from abnormalities of muscle membrane ion channels that alter the resting membrane potential and affect ion fluxes during depolarization and/or repolarization. The delay in relaxation of flexor muscles after an object is grasped forcefully causes difficulty in letting go. When the person attempts to relax the finger muscles after the strong squeeze, the flexor muscles fail to relax and the hand is slow to open. The wrist usually flexes to aid in straightening the fingers. Flexing the wrist shortens the long finger flexors, thereby preventing them from contracting forcefully and allowing the finger extensors to overcome the flexor myotonia.

"Percussion" myotonia can be elicited most easily in the tongue, forearm extensor, and thenar muscles. When a sharp tap is applied, there is a localized contraction of the muscle, which causes mounding around a dimple in the tapped area. Often, there is shortening of the muscle, with resulting joint movement; this can be readily observed in the abductor pollicis brevis and extensor digitorum communis muscles.

Clinically evident myotonia occurs almost exclusively in the inherited myotonic syndromes. However, electrical myotonia, the electrical discharges recorded during needle electrode examination, may occur in clinical settings in which there is no clinical evidence of myotonia (see Table 80–2). Myotonic discharges may be found on needle examination of the muscles of patients who do not have a familial myotonic disorder, but these are rarely associated with clinical myotonia. Acute muscle inflammation and acute denervation as well as certain drugs may cause myotonic discharges with needle movement in the muscles, but there are no afterdischarges or clinical correlates of these discharges.

In most of the myotonic disorders, clinical and electrical myotonia are lessened or transiently abolished by exercising the affected muscles with repeated voluntary contractions, and are aggravated by cooling. Exceptions to this pattern include paramyotonia congenita, in which the myotonia worsens (and sometimes is only present) after exercise, and proximal myotonic myopathy, in which the myotonia may be relieved by cooling.

Pain is uncommon in myotonia. However, painful muscle stiffness may occur in the rare sodium channel myotonic disorders known as myotonia fluctuans and myotonia permanens (see following sections). Painful myotonia may also occur in proximal myotonic myopathy, although this is not an ion channel disorder. Some patients with myotonia congenita have painful cramps, although the myotonia itself does not appear to be painful. Neuromyotonia may also cause painful muscle contractions.

WEAKNESS

The other hallmark of the muscle ion channel disorders is weakness. Typically, this is episodic, as occurs in the periodic paralyses, but there may be permanent proximal muscle weakness late in the course of periodic paralysis, and mild permanent weakness is a feature in some of the hereditary myotonic disorders.

Episodes of weakness are characteristic of periodic paralysis. They may be mild and brief, especially in hyperkalemic periodic paralysis, or prolonged and severe, especially in hypokalemic periodic paralysis. Patients with primary hyperkalemic periodic paralysis usually begin having attacks in the first decade of life, and have very labile muscle strength. Attacks of weakness are brief (usually minutes, up to 1 hour) but may occur many times a day. In contrast, patients with hypokalemic periodic paralysis begin having attacks in the second or third decade and have attacks that last hours to days, but the attacks are generally infrequent (less than one per week). The weakness may be precipitated by dietary changes, especially in the hypokalemic form, and is strongly associated with rest after exercise. Often, the attacks begin during sleep.

Muscles are often weaker after a period of rest in patients with myotonia congenita and recessive generalized myotonia. There is generally an increase in strength on warming up the muscles with repeated contractions.

ELECTROPHYSIOLOGY OF MYOTONIC DISORDERS: GENERAL PRINCIPLES
Nerve Conduction Studies

Motor and sensory nerve conduction velocities are generally normal in the inherited myotonic dis-

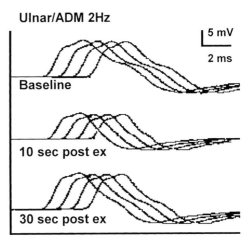

Figure 80–2. Repetitive stimulation in a patient with myotonia congenita illustrating the characteristic transient drop in the amplitude of the compound muscle action potential immediately after brief isometric exercise, with a rapid return to baseline.

orders. Some patients with myotonic dystrophy, which is not due to an ion channelopathy, have an associated peripheral neuropathy with mild slowing of conduction, and motor nerve conduction velocities may be abnormal in neuromyotonia.

Compound muscle action potentials are normal in amplitude in resting muscle unless there is muscle wasting distally, such as that which may occur in myotonic dystrophy and in recessive generalized myotonia. The compound muscle action potentials may also be low in amplitude in muscles that are weakened by an attack of periodic paralysis or paramyotonia congenita.

Repetitive motor nerve stimulation often produces a characteristic change in patients with the myotonic disorders, particularly myotonia congenita and most prominently in recessive generalized myotonia (Fig. 80–2). There is a small decrement (decrease in amplitude) in the compound muscle action potential when the nerve supplying the muscle being studied is stimulated supramaximally and repetitively at low rates (2 to 5 Hz); this decrement is greatest with the first few stimuli. The decrement is generally between 10% and 20% but may range from 5% to 50%. If the muscle is exercised briefly by having the subject contract the muscle forcefully for 5 seconds three or four times, the amplitude of the compound muscle action potential becomes smaller but the decrement is abolished. The amplitude then returns to baseline, and the decrement reappears over the following 30 to 60 seconds. This is a pattern of responses that does not occur in disorders other than the congenital myotonias. It may be seen in myotonic dystrophy as well as the ion channel myotonias, but not in the periodic paralyses.

Rapid repetitive stimulation (more than 10 Hz) may also produce a decremental response in myotonic syndromes. Unlike the neuromuscular transmission defect disorders, the decrement continues to worsen after the first few stimuli (Streib, 1987), and the decrement is more pronounced with higher frequencies of stimulation. Sometimes, the decrement does not appear unless the stimulation rate is 25 Hz or greater.

Needle Examination

Myotonic discharges can be recorded from muscles in several settings.

WITH NEEDLE MOVEMENT (INSERTIONAL ACTIVITY)

When the muscles of patients affected by familial myotonic disorders are examined with an electromyographic needle electrode, there are characteristic electrical abnormalities termed *myotonic discharges*. The discharges are of several types, and the form of the discharge depends on whether the muscle is relaxed or contracting. The abnormal electrical activity consists of repetitively firing muscle fiber potentials discharging spontaneously at moderate to high frequencies (Fig. 80–3). These discharges are the hallmark of the myotonic disorders. They are induced in resting muscle by the needle electrode irritating muscle membranes and consist predominantly of positive waves, although spike waveforms also occur at rest. Both the amplitude and the frequency of the discharge must increase and then decrease, for the electrical activity to be classified as a myotonic discharge. The sound is easily recognized over the loudspeaker and is said to resemble the noise of a World War II dive-bomber. Since many have never heard the rising and falling note of a divebomber (which results from frequency shifts related to the Doppler effect), one may compare the sound of myotonic discharges to the lowing of cattle.

The feature that distinguishes myotonic discharges from trains of positive waves or other forms of spontaneous activity is that the potentials wax and wane (increase and decrease) in amplitude and frequency. Fibrillation potentials and positive waves may gradually decrease in amplitude and frequency but never increase before decreasing. Complex repetitive discharges are sometimes mistaken for myotonic discharges, but the distinction should be easy; complex repetitive discharges fire with unvarying amplitude and frequency, sounding like a motor running at a constant speed.

Figure 80–3. Characteristic myotonic discharge recorded from a patient with myotonic dystrophy. The frequencies of the potentials within the discharge typically range from 20 to 100 Hz. The distinguishing sound of the myotonic discharge is produced by the waxing and waning of both the amplitude and the frequency of the individual components.

These discharges are generally profuse in the primary myotonic disorders. The firing frequency of the discharges varies greatly; the rate may be as low as 1 Hz or as high as 150 Hz, but it is generally between 30 and 80 Hz. When multiple myotonic discharges fire together, they may obscure the motor unit potentials, making it difficult to evaluate the motor units for myopathic changes. The frequency is lower and the discharges last longer in myotonic dystrophy than in the ion channel myotonias. In other conditions in which myotonic discharges occur without clinical myotonia, the discharges are sparse and often fire singly.

AFTER VOLUNTARY CONTRACTION ("AFTERDISCHARGES")

After a strong contraction, the myotonic discharges are predominantly spike waveforms, in contrast with the positive waves seen in resting muscles. When the subject contracts the muscle forcefully with a needle electrode in place, there are motor unit potentials that swamp the myotonic discharges. When the subject relaxes the effort, the muscle fails to relax; the motor unit potentials cease firing, but there are showers of spike waveforms ("afterdischarges") that correlate with the failure of relaxation. These discharges gradually wane and eventually stop, allowing the muscle to relax fully. They correlate with clinical grip myotonia and are present only in the primary myotonic disorders. They are not seen in other conditions that cause myotonic discharges in resting muscle without clinical myotonia.

WITH MUSCLE PERCUSSION

Brief bursts of myotonic discharges can be elicited in resting muscle by tapping over the muscle, adjacent to the needle insertion site. The bursts of electrical potentials fire with a waxing and waning pattern.

Fibrillation Potentials

Fibrillation potentials are uncommon in the myotonic disorders. They are most often seen in myotonic dystrophy; in the ion channelopathies they occur only as paramyotonia congenita as the muscle is cooled. Care needs to be taken not to confuse slow-firing myotonic discharges with fibrillation potentials, as mentioned previously.

Motor Unit Potentials

The motor unit potentials are usually normal in the ion channelopathies. Motor unit potentials may be low in amplitude and short in duration, with an increase in the percentage of polyphasic motor unit potentials (changes characteristic of myopathies) in the muscles of patients with severe weakness from recessive generalized myotonia. There are abnormalities of motor unit potential firing in muscles weakened by attacks of periodic paralysis. The weakness correlates with muscle membrane inexcitability, so motor unit potentials fire in reduced numbers, producing a reduced recruitment rate and a reduced density of the interference pattern. Patients with the late-life myopathy of periodic paralysis also have myopathic alterations to the motor unit potentials and may have fibrillation potentials.

It may be difficult to evaluate the motor unit potentials in myotonic disorders in which there are profuse myotonic discharges obscuring the voluntarily activated potentials. However, if the needle is held still in the muscle, the discharges slowly decrease in number and firing rate and the voluntary motor unit potentials are easier to distinguish. When examining motor unit potentials, the movements of the needle must be small in order to minimize the myotonic discharges, and the level of muscle activation must be low and held constant. With patience, motor unit potentials can be studied in all these disorders.

INHERITED MYOTONIC SYNDROMES

The vast majority of patients with clinical myotonia or myotonic discharges on electromyography have inherited disorders. Of these, the most common (incidence, 5 per 100,000 of the population) is myotonic dystrophy (Steinert's disease). This is an autosomal dominant inherited disorder associated with an expansion of trinucleotide repeats on chromosome 19, and it is not an ion channel disorder. However, it may be confused with some of the channelopathies, particularly myotonia congenita, and

---

Table 80–3. Muscle Disorders Causing Stiffness

Hereditary
  Myotonic dystrophy (Steinert's disease)
  Proximal myotonic myopathy
  Nondystrophic myotonias
    Myotonia congenita
      Autosomal dominant (Thomsen's disease)
      Autosomal dominant with recurrent cramps
      Autosomal recessive (Becker's recessive generalized
        myotonia)
    Paramyotonia congenita
    Myotonia fluctuans or permanens
    Periodic paralysis, hyperkalemic form
  Chondrodystrophic myotonia (Schwartz-Jampel syndrome)
  Rippling muscle disease
  Neuromyotonia (usually acquired)
  Rigid spine syndrome
Acquired
  Neuromyotonia
  Hypothyroid myopathy

Table 80–4. Clinical Features of Channelopathies

Channelopathies with predominant weakness
  Hyperkalemic periodic paralysis
  Hypokalemic periodic paralysis
  Normokalemic periodic paralysis
  Paramyotonia congenita
Channelopathies with predominant myotonia
  Myotonia congenita
    Autosomal dominant (Thomsen's disease)
    Autosomal recessive (Becker's disease)
  Paramyotonia congenita
  Myotonia fluctuans
  Myotonia permanens
  Neuromyotonia

---

the characteristic clinical muscular abnormalities and systemic manifestations and the electrophysiological features should be recognized. It is discussed at the end of this section.

The nondystrophic hereditary myotonias are divided into the chloride channel disorders (myotonia congenita) and the sodium channel disorders (paramyotonia congenita, myotonia fluctuans or permanens, and hyperkalemic periodic paralysis) (Tables 80–3 and 80–4). Unlike myotonic dystrophy, all these are due to ion channel dysfunction. These conditions cause clinical myotonia and weakness in differing degrees. Muscle stiffness predominates over weakness in myotonia congenita. Myotonia occurs in some patients with hyperkalemic periodic paralysis, although it is never the dominant symptom. Paramyotonia congenita causes both myotonia and weakness, but the distinctive responses to cold and exercise distinguish it from the other nondystrophic myotonias.

Channelopathies Associated with Myotonia

NONDYSTROPHIC HEREDITARY MYOTONIC DISORDERS

Myotonia Congenita

There are three forms of myotonia congenita that share many clinical features. The first to be described was autosomal dominant myotonia congenita (Thomsen's disease). Symptoms, predominantly myotonia, are present from birth. In some families with myotonia congenita, the affected individuals suffer from frequent, painful muscle cramps. Although the clinical features are otherwise similar, this appears to be a genetically distinct variant. The third and most common type of myotonia "congenita" is Becker's recessive generalized myotonia. In this disorder, the symptoms are not congenital but begin at age 5 to 15 years. The myotonia is more severe than in Thomsen's disease, and proximal upper limb weakness is a frequent feature (Franke et al., 1991).

Clinical Features. In these three conditions, the major symptom is the myotonic muscle stiffness, which tends to be most apparent in forearm flexor and facial muscles. Patients with the autosomal dominant inherited form (Thomsen's) have nearly normal strength, which distinguishes them from the dystrophic myotonic disorders (e.g., myotonic dystrophy) and patients with severe forms of Becker's recessive generalized myotonia. The muscle stiffness is most pronounced after rest and subsides transiently after exercise. The myotonia is painless, but some families with myotonia congenita have frequent, painful muscle cramps. Myotonia may be very severe, and the intensity of the myotonic contractions may be sufficient to "bulk up" the muscles, but the muscle strength is much less than the physique would suggest.

Weakness is often present in rested muscles but is mild in degree and rarely a prominent feature. Patients do not complain of weakness. Typically, the muscles become weaker during a period of rest, and repeated contractions are necessary to work off the weakness and "warm up" the muscles to normal or near-normal strength. Repeated voluntary contractions of muscles affected by myotonia decrease the intensity of the delay in muscle relaxation for a short time. Patients may learn to warm their muscles up by performing several strong contractions prior to attempting a task requiring maximal strength or if they wish to minimize the myotonia. This effect is seen in all the myotonic disorders except paramyotonia congenita, where exercise paradoxically worsens the myotonia and weakens the muscles. Prolonged episodes of weakness (periodic paralysis) do not occur. The extramuscular features of myotonic dystrophy are absent. Muscles are usually well developed despite the weakness, probably because of work hypertrophy from the myotonia. Some patients have a herculean appearance, with massive enlargement of muscles in unusual sites, such as the feet. In all the myotonic disorders, the myotonia is aggravated by cooling, and this can be used in the clinical setting to elicit myotonia when it is not apparent at rest in warm muscles.

Percussion myotonia may be elicited by tapping the forearm or facial muscles. This phenomenon is most easily elicited by a sharp tap over the abductor pollicis brevis muscle in the hand or the extensor digitorum communis muscle in the forearm extensor mass. The resulting prolonged involuntary contraction of the percussed muscle is one of the most reliable and diagnostic signs of muscle disease. The percussion myotonia will subside with repeated taps or if the muscle is exercised before percussion.

Patients with Becker's recessive generalized myotonia, which is more common than Thomsen's syndrome, may have muscle wasting and weakness, especially in proximal upper limb muscles. This may cause some difficulty in distinguishing these patients from patients with myotonic dystrophy, but the distribution of muscle atrophy and weakness is different. Like patients with autosomal dominant myotonia congenita, the muscles often are weaker after a period of rest and require several contrac-

tions in order to "warm up." Myotonia is aggravated by exposure to cold. Repeated contraction of the muscle decreases the myotonia for a short time.

Although these clinical features are often striking in their presentation, the intensity of symptoms varies remarkably between individuals, even within the same family and in patients with identical mutations (Koty et al., 1996). Some patients known to be positive for the genetic mutations are asymptomatic or minimally symptomatic, and there are occasional affected individuals who have no myotonic discharges on muscle needle examination. This suggests the possibility that other abnormalities of ion channel function may modulate the effects of the chloride channel mutations.

The responses to exercise and cooling in the various myotonic syndromes can be used to good effect to help establish the diagnosis, especially in mild cases, and to distinguish one from another.

Electrophysiology

Nerve Conduction Studies. Standard motor and sensory nerve conduction studies show normal amplitudes and conduction velocities. Slow (2 to 5 Hz) repetitive stimulation of motor nerves often causes a small decrement in amplitude and area of the compound muscle action potential (see Fig. 80–2). The decrement in amplitude is around 15% but rarely is as much as 50%. The appearance of the decremental response is similar to the neuromuscular junction disorders. After brief (10 to 20 seconds), forceful contraction of the muscle being studied, the decrement is repaired (disappears), but the amplitude and area of the compound muscle action potential diminish by 10% to 15%. Over the next 30 seconds, the decrement reappears progressively and the amplitude returns to baseline. These responses to slow repetitive stimulation and brief exercise are characteristic of the congenital myotonias and do not occur in other conditions. Prolonged exercise does not induce a long-lasting change in the motor responses, nor does it produce weakness.

Rapid repetitive stimulation at rates of 10 Hz or more for 10 seconds causes a decrement of at least 25% and usually more than 50% in patients with recessive generalized myotonia (Deymeer et al., 1998). Patients with other nondystrophic myotonias have a decrement of less than 25%. This testing appears to distinguish patients with transient weakness from other patients, and is more likely to be abnormal in patients with recessive myotonia than in those with the milder, dominant form of myotonia congenita.

Needle Electrode Examination. Insertion of a needle recording electrode into the muscles induces the myotonic discharges described previously. In myotonia congenita, the discharges are briefer and fire at higher frequencies than the discharges seen in myotonic dystrophy. Myotonic discharges are provoked by movement of the electrode in the muscle or by tapping the muscle adjacent to the needle. The motor unit potentials produced by voluntary contraction of the muscle are normal in amplitude, duration, configuration, and recruitment pattern, but it can be difficult to evaluate the voluntary potentials when the myotonia is profuse. When a patient relaxes the voluntary effort after a strong contraction, there are prolonged trains of electrical potentials that fire spontaneously for several seconds. These correlate with the inability to relax the muscle quickly. These "after-discharges" are lower in amplitude and shorter in duration than the voluntary motor unit potentials. Thus, attempted relaxation is associated with ongoing electrical activity instead of electrical silence, although there is an abrupt change in electrical activity.

Response to Exercise. Brief exercise abolishes the decremental response to repetitive stimulation and reduces the myotonia produced by needle movement, muscle percussion, and muscle contractions. Prolonged exercise also diminishes the myotonia, but there is no progressive loss of compound muscle action potential amplitude like the one that occurs in paramyotonia congenita and the periodic paralyses.

Response to Cooling. Cooling the limb increases the myotonia but does not change the amplitude of the CMAP or cause a loss of voluntary motor unit potentials.

Genetic Abnormalities. Linkage analysis studies show that both Thomsen's autosomal dominant myotonia congenita and Becker's recessive myotonia congenita map to the long arm of chromosome 7, where a chloride channel gene is situated (7q35) (Koch et al., 1992). A specific mutation in the chloride channel coding region has been shown to be common to both disorders (Koch et al., 1992). Subsequently, point mutations at a number of different sites in the chloride channel gene (*CLCN1*) have been shown to cause myotonia congenita (Brugnoni et al., 1999).

Paramyotonia Congenita

This is an uncommon condition with features of both the myotonic disorders and the periodic paralyses, although the clinical features distinguish it from the other myotonias, and the electrophysiological findings are unique.

Clinical Features. Paramyotonia congenita is inherited in an autosomal dominant fashion with full penetrance and, in common with hyperkalemic periodic paralysis, is due to mutations in the alpha subunit of the human skeletal muscle sodium channel gene on the long arm of chromosome 17. The disorder has more in common with hyperkalemic periodic paralysis than the other nondystrophic myotonias, but myotonia is more prominent than in periodic paralysis and attacks of weakness are less frequent and less severe.

The hallmark of the condition is the muscle stiffness and weakness induced by exercise and exposure to cold. Like other myotonic syndromes, the myotonia increases with cooling of the muscles. Unlike the other disorders, the myotonia worsens with exercise instead of improving ("paradoxical" myotonia). Myotonia may be difficult to detect until repeated muscle contractions are performed. During rest after the exercise-induced increase in myotonia, there is an abrupt loss of muscle power that lasts for some minutes, sometimes as long as 90 minutes (Streib, 1987). This postexercise weakness is reminiscent of the periodic paralyses, but the weakness is of rapid onset in paramyotonia, whereas the weakness progresses slowly over 10 to 30 minutes in the periodic paralyses (McManis et al., 1986; Streib, 1987).

In muscles that are cooled, there is an early increase in muscle stiffness and myotonia, followed by progressive weakness, eventually leading to marked loss of strength or paralysis that may last for minutes or hours. Patients with this condition can ease the severity of their symptoms by living in a warm climate. Exposure to cold causes the rapid onset of myotonia in the facial muscles, especially the periorbital and chin muscles, producing difficulty in opening the eyes and in talking. Further cooling results in muscle paralysis, especially if the muscles are exercised when cold. The paralysis is associated with muscle stiffness.

Some patients with paramyotonia also have attacks of weakness not associated with cold or exercise, and these can be precipitated by potassium loading. The similarities to hyperkalemic periodic paralysis are sometimes striking, and it comes as no surprise that both conditions are due to mutations in the alpha subunit of the human muscle sodium channel gene (*SCN4A*) on chromosome 17q (Ebers et al., 1991; Ptacek et al., 1991, 1992; Wagner et al., 1997). The clinical manifestations depend on the mutation in the sodium channel gene, so that some mutations cause only attacks of paralysis (hyperkalemic periodic paralysis), some cause the paradoxical myotonia and cold-induced symptoms (paramyotonia congenita), and some cause affected individuals to have both of these symptoms. In both paramyotonia and in all forms of periodic paralysis, patients may develop permanent weakness caused by a proximal myopathy in middle or late life.

Electrophysiology

Nerve Conduction Studies. Like the other nondystrophic myotonias, the motor and sensory nerve conduction studies are normal. It is uncommon to find a decrement at rest with slow repetitive stimulation of warm muscles. If the muscles are cooled, a decrement to slow repetitive stimulation appears or worsens.

Needle Examination. The motor unit potentials are normal in size and configuration. Needle examination of warm muscles shows only rare myotonic discharges, most easily elicited in periorbital muscles. In a muscle weakened by cold or exercise, there is a loss of motor units under voluntary control, producing a marked loss of recruitment (reduced interference pattern) and a pseudoneurogenic

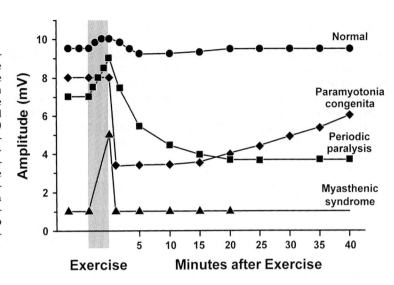

Figure 80–4. Changes in compound muscle action potential amplitude in response to 5 minutes of exercise of the tested muscle. There is a small rise in amplitude with exercise in normal subjects, with a rapid return to baseline levels. In paramyotonia congenita, there is an abrupt fall in amplitude with exercise followed by a gradual return to the initial amplitude over 90 minutes or more. In the periodic paralyses, the amplitude may be low at rest, especially in the hyperkalemic form, and there is a gradual decrease in amplitude over the 15 to 30 minutes after exercise. The amplitude recovers slowly over several hours. In contrast, Lambert-Eaton myasthenic syndrome shows a low amplitude at rest, with a striking increase in amplitude in response to exercise, and a rapid return to baseline amplitudes within 30 seconds of the termination of exercise.

pattern of motor unit firing. If a late-life myopathy has developed, there may be small motor unit potentials and spontaneous firing of muscle fibers (fibrillation potentials) related to a vacuolar change in the muscle fibers.

Response to Exercise. Immediately after 30 seconds to 5 minutes of forceful contraction of the muscle under testing, there is a rapid fall in the amplitude of the compound muscle action potential. The amplitude gradually recovers over the next 30 to 90 minutes (Streib, 1987). The fall in amplitude correlates with the reduction in muscle strength and with the loss of the ability to activate motor units.

The sudden fall in compound muscle action potential amplitude with slow subsequent recovery distinguishes paramyotonia congenita from other myotonic syndromes and the periodic paralyses (Fig. 80–4).

Response to Cooling. There is a characteristic sequence of electrical events that occurs with muscle cooling. As the muscle temperature falls toward 32°C, there is an increase in the myotonic discharges produced by needle movement and by muscle contraction. With further cooling, there is intense fibrillation-like spontaneous firing of muscle fibers as the muscle depolarizes. When the muscle is very cold, there is electrical silence and the patient is unable to activate more than a few motor unit potentials, if any. A few motor unit potentials may fire if the patient attempts to contract rested, cold muscles, but exercising the muscle causes all electrical activity to cease. At this stage, no compound muscle action potential can be evoked, and there is no insertional activity on needle examination. As muscle warming occurs, there is a slow return of voluntarily activated motor units and a reduction in myotonia.

Nerve conduction studies performed on these cooled muscles show a progressive loss of compound muscle action potential amplitude with return of amplitude on warming.

Other Channelopathies Associated with Myotonia

Hyperkalemic periodic paralysis is a sodium channelopathy associated with recurrent attacks of weakness as well as mild myotonia. It is discussed in detail in the section on periodic paralysis to follow.

Myotonia Fluctuans (Potassium-Sensitive Myotonia Congenita). In 1990, Ricker and colleagues described a previously unrecognized type of myotonic disorder that has subsequently been shown to be due to a mutation on the muscle sodium channel gene (Ricker et al., 1994). Patients with myotonia fluctuans show remarkable variation in the intensity of myotonia. Symptoms appear after a period of rest following muscular exercise. This pattern is the same as that seen in patients with hyperkalemic periodic paralysis, but there is myotonia instead of weakness. In addition, patients with myotonia fluctuans show a marked aggravation of myotonia when administered potassium and an improvement in symptoms when treated with carbonic anhydrase inhibitors.

Patients with this autosomal dominant condition describe progressive stiffness and clumsiness of limb movement while exercising, and the symptoms become much worse during rest after prolonged exercise. The muscle stiffness is often painful, especially in chest muscles (Rosenfeld et al., 1997), and may be so severe that patients fall to the ground or are unable to rise from a position of rest, even though there is no weakness. The severe symptoms last for several minutes, then slowly resolve. Momentary muscle stiffness may occur in rested muscles with quick movements, such as forceful biting or rapid eye movements (Ricker et al., 1990), but the severity of muscle stiffness varies from day to day.

Laboratory testing shows myotonic discharges on needle examination of muscles. There is no weakness or aggravation of myotonia with cooling of muscles, but oral potassium loading causes marked worsening of stiffness (without weakness) within 30 minutes. When myotonia is present, the patients can lessen the muscle stiffness by "warming up" the muscles with repeated contractions, but the myotonia returns during rest after exercise. There is improvement in myotonic symptoms with acetazolamide treatment.

Myotonia Permanens. A family with persistent, severe myotonia and a muscle sodium channel mutation has been described (Lerche et al., 1993). The symptoms are like those of myotonia fluctuans but are persistent, rather than episodic. Weakness does not occur, although the myotonia can be severe enough to impair respiration.

Sodium Channel Structure and Function

The adult muscle sodium channel gene consists of four sections called domains. Each of these domains contains six segments that cross the muscle membrane and are connected to form a single continuous protein. Thus, the sodium channel consists of a single protein sequence that zigzags in and out of the muscle fiber cell across the muscle membrane. The proteins are held together, producing a cylinder, which is a channel through the membrane. Changes in the conformation of the channel allow or prevent the passage of ions, and the conformation changes in response to applied voltages ("voltage gating").

Mutations in the protein sequence generally affect a single amino acid at a point in the sequence that is critical for the sensing of applied voltages or for the changes in channel conformation that open or close the channel.

Thus, mutations of the *SCN4A* gene can produce episodic weakness (hyperkalemic periodic paralysis), paradoxical myotonia (paramyotonia congenita), a combination of the two (paralysis periodica paramyotonica), or myotonia in isolation (myotonia fluctuans and myotonia permanens). All these allelic disorders show sensitivity to potassium and a symptomatic relationship to rest after exercise.

Chondrodystrophic Myotonia (Schwartz-Jampel Syndrome)

This is a rare autosomal recessive disorder in which multiple skeletal and facial deformities are combined with muscle myotonia. In addition to the myotonic myopathy, the patients have very narrow palpebral fissures (blepharophimosis), joint contractures, myopia, epiphyseal cartilage abnormalities, pectus carinatum, kyphoscoliosis, and dwarfism. Muscles are stiff and firm to palpation, and generalized weakness is present (Ishpekova et al., 1996). Myotonia can be elicited clinically as well as on needle examination. The myotonia may be generated in peripheral nerves, as much of the myotonia disappears with neuromuscular blockade (Cadilhac et al., 1975). Unlike other myotonic disorders, there is no warming-up phenomenon with repeated muscle contractions (Lehmann-Horn et al.,

1990). The motor and sensory nerve conduction studies are normal (Ishpekova et al., 1996).

The myotonia may be due to a sodium channel defect, perhaps in concert with abnormalities of other ion channels (Lehmann-Horn et al., 1990). The mutations causing this disorder are unknown at present.

ACQUIRED MYOTONIA

Neuromyotonia

In 1961, Isaacs described a disorder characterized by muscle stiffness owing to spontaneous and continuous firing of muscle fibers. His patients also had muscle twitching described as fasciculation, although some of the movements may have been myokymia. This disorder is often termed *Isaacs' syndrome*, although others described similar clinical findings before him (De Jong et al., 1951; Gamstorp and Wohlfart, 1959). Subsequently, small numbers of patients with this disorder have been reported, and the syndrome has been delineated more precisely. The clinical and electrophysiological features are the result of ion channel abnormalities of peripheral nerves, unlike the myotonic disorders that are due to muscle membrane abnormalities. "Neuromyotonia" is the preferred term, since all patients with variants of this syndrome have the diagnostic high-frequency discharges. Other terms applied to this syndrome include continuous muscle fiber activity, neurotonia, continuous motor neuron discharges, acquired myotonia, generalized myokymia, and undulating myokymia. Some patients lack the fasciculations and myokymia or the sweating or painful cramps that occur in Isaacs' syndrome. The disorder is probably identical to Morvan's fibrillary chorea, although some of the patients with that condition have central nervous system abnormalities, including confusion, insomnia, and hallucinations (Serratrice and Azulay, 1994).

CLINICAL FEATURES

The most conspicuous clinical features are muscle stiffness and weakness. There are frequent cramps, generally precipitated by movement, and muscles fail to relax normally after voluntary activation in a manner similar to the myotonic disorders. This myotonia affects face and limb muscles; laryngeal muscles may be affected and cause stridor. Myotonia of the tongue and face cause a characteristic dysarthria, with slow and imprecise oral-lingual movements. In the limbs, the myotonia and weakness affect the distal muscles more than the proximal ones. Weakness is most pronounced in wrist and finger extensors and in ankle and toe dorsiflexors, while myotonia is most easily elicited in wrist and finger flexor muscles. Patients tend to keep the wrists and interphalangeal joints flexed, while the metacarpophalangeal joints are hyperextended. The feet are held in a plantar-flexed posture.

Muscle fasciculation is sometimes present, and some patients have striking myokymia, which is a visible repetitive movement of muscle often having a vermiform or undulating appearance but sometimes resembling a small, repetitive twitch. Myokymia may be seen in a single area but is more commonly a widespread phenomenon (Gamstorp and Wohlfart, 1959).

One of the most remarkable features is the bizarre slowness of movement exhibited by patients with this disorder, sometimes mistaken for a psychogenic process. This false impression may be reinforced by the breathy voice produced by myotonia of the vocal cords.

The ailment is now known to be due to antibodies directed against potassium channels in the majority of cases (Shillito et al., 1995; Hart et al., 1997). A small proportion of patients have the neuromyotonia as the result of an inherited or acquired peripheral neuropathy (Newsom-Davis and Mills, 1993; Maddison et al., 1999). In a few cases, the neuromyotonia appears to have been a paraneoplastic phenomenon, associated with small cell lung cancer (Partanen et al., 1980) or mediastinal neoplasms (Walsh, 1976).

This is one of only three conditions known to be due to autoantibodies directed against ion channel proteins, the others being myasthenia gravis (postsynaptic acetylcholine receptor proteins) and the Lambert-Eaton myasthenic syndrome (presynaptic voltage-gated calcium channels).

ELECTROPHYSIOLOGY

Motor and sensory amplitudes and distal latencies are normal, and there is no slowing of motor conduction velocities (Maddison et al., 1999). Motor—but not sensory—axonal time constants are prolonged in distal peripheral nerve segments, suggesting abnormalities of the membrane properties at nodes of Ranvier (Maddison et al., 1999). These axonal membrane abnormalities may be the result of the antibodies directed against voltage-gated potassium channels, which are known to be present in acquired forms of neuromyotonia (Shillito et al., 1995; Hart et al., 1997). Sometimes, repetitive firing of compound muscle action potentials occurs after single stimuli ("stimulus-induced repetitive discharges"). Repetitive nerve stimulation may elicit prolonged neuromyotonic discharges.

Needle examination reveals very high frequency (200 to 300 Hz) discharges related to needle movement or muscle contraction. These are called neurotonic or neuromyotonic discharges. As often happens in the myotonic disorders, it is difficult to obtain electrical silence at rest. In resting muscles, there may be fibrillation and fasciculation potentials as well as myokymic discharges (spontaneous, repetitive, high-frequency bursts of muscle potentials; bursts recur at frequencies between 0.5 and 5 Hz,

while the potentials within each burst fire at up to 300 Hz). Voluntarily activated single motor units often fire erratically in doublets, triplets, or multiplets at high frequencies (Newsom-Davis and Mills, 1993). The myotonic discharges typical of the muscle channelopathies do not occur. Motor unit potentials are generally normal in size and morphology but may be short in duration, and they are sometimes large distally when the neuromyotonia is due to a neuropathic process.

The neuromyotonia persists during sleep and anesthesia and after peripheral nerve block, but disappears with curarization, indicating that the discharges originate in peripheral nerves distally.

TREATMENT

Symptoms are generally improved by oral carbamazepine or phenytoin. Symptomatic relief with acetazolamide may occur in the absence of a response to the anticonvulsant drugs. Other sodium-channel blocking drugs, such as mexiletine or tocainide, may be helpful in relieving the myotonic symptoms. Several patients have responded to immune suppression or to plasmapheresis.

PERIODIC PARALYSIS

The term *periodic paralysis* refers to a group of muscle disorders with episodes of weakness. The primary or inherited periodic paralyses are associated with muscle ion channel abnormalities and changes in serum potassium levels (Table 80–5). These are rare inherited conditions, although there are certain geographic areas where there are clusters of patients owing to the autosomal dominant inheritance pattern. Many clinicians have never encountered an affected patient; this is partly related to the fact that affected families are more familiar with the manifestations and management of the condition than are their doctors, and do not come to medical attention unless the symptoms are difficult to control.

Periodic paralysis may also occur in patients with secondary causes of hyperkalemia or hypokalemia, most commonly with low serum potassium in patients with thyrotoxicosis. Patients with hypokalemic periodic paralysis secondary to thyrotoxicosis are usually male and often Asians, although the condition certainly occurs in females and whites. Pa-

---

Table 80–5. Inherited Periodic Paralysis Syndromes

Sodium channel
    Hyperkalemic periodic paralysis
    Paramyotonia congenita
    Normokalemic periodic paralysis
    Hypokalemic periodic paralysis (occasionally)
Calcium channel
    Hypokalemic periodic paralysis (most)

tients with high or low potassium levels from the use of diuretics, potassium-wasting colonic lesions, or renal disease occasionally develop periodic paralysis, but the change in serum potassium necessary to cause weakness is much greater than in the familial periodic paralysis syndromes, where the serum potassium level may rise or fall but remain within the range of normal. These secondary forms of periodic paralysis are not due to ion channelopathies and are not discussed further.

In all forms of periodic paralysis, there is episodic weakness that most commonly begins during a period of rest after exercise. In hyperkalemic periodic paralysis, the weakness may be restricted to a single limb or even to a single muscle, and attacks may come and go over the course of an hour or so. Attacks in the hypokalemic form tend to last longer and to be generalized, but they are more frequent and more severe in the lower limbs. In all forms of periodic paralysis, the respiratory muscles are relatively spared and cranial muscles are not affected by weakness, although some hyperkalemic patients have facial muscle myotonia. The respiratory sparing may be more illusion than reality, as patients could lose a substantial proportion of respiratory muscle strength without being aware of it when they are lying immobile in bed.

The attacks are often associated with mild to moderate muscle pain in the affected limbs. If a patient is aware that an attack is beginning, he or she may be able to work off the symptoms by gently exercising the affected muscles, such as by walking around instead of resting. Sometimes, this aborts the attack, but at other times the attack is simply delayed until the patient rests. The attacks become less frequent in middle age and generally cease as the patient ages, but a late-life myopathy is a frequent if not universal occurrence (Bradley et al., 1990; Links et al., 1990). The incidence and severity of the myopathy are not related to the frequency or severity of episodic weakness in youth (Bradley et al., 1990); some patients never have paralytic attacks but still develop a myopathy. Muscle biopsy shows that the myopathy is associated with vacuolar changes in the myofibrils.

Episodes of weakness may be related to diet. In hyperkalemic periodic paralysis, the attacks are more frequent during periods of fasting, and frequent small meals may reduce the attack rate. A high-carbohydrate, salty meal (e.g., pasta or pizza) may provoke an attack in patients with hypokalemic periodic paralysis.

Dietary manipulations often help reduce the frequency of attacks, and carbonic anhydrase–inhibiting drugs are beneficial for most patients. Traditionally, acetazolamide has been used to reduce the frequency and severity of attacks, but recent studies suggest that dichlorphenamide may be more effective (Tawil, 2000). Potassium-wasting diuretics may help patients with hyperkalemic periodic paralysis and potassium supplements help those with the hypokalemic form, especially during attacks.

Myotonia may be found in patients with hyperkalemic periodic paralysis, but it is very unusual in the hypokalemic form. When present, the myotonia is very mild and is most easily found in the orbicularis oculi muscles. It is very easily suppressed by exercise and consequently may be difficult to identify. Like all myotonic disorders, the myotonia is made worse by exposure to cold.

All the periodic paralyses are inherited in an autosomal dominant fashion. The penetrance in men approaches 100% but is substantially less in females (about 50%). Among affected males, sodium channel mutations (hyperkalemic and normokalemic periodic paralysis, myotonia fluctuans, and paramyotonia congenita) are more likely to occur without clinical symptoms than are calcium channel mutations (hypokalemic periodic paralysis). There are female calcium channel mutation carriers without symptoms, but male patients with calcium channel mutations appear to be universally affected.

Hyperkalemic Periodic Paralysis

CLINICAL FEATURES

The hyperkalemic form of periodic paralysis is an autosomal dominant condition with high penetrance in both sexes. However, the symptoms may be minimal and ignored, giving the misleading impression that penetrance is low or that the disease is often sporadic. Symptomatic patients develop signs and symptoms early in life, often in the first year. Episodes of paralysis tend to be frequent, focal, and short-lived (1 or 2 hours), and they may recur several times in the course of a single day. The attacks of weakness begin during rest, usually after exertion. The weakness is sometimes restricted to the muscles used during exercise. Most often, the attacks begin during sleep and are worst in the lower limbs, but they may affect trunk and upper limb muscles. Cranial muscles are spared. Episodes are more frequent with fasting and with a high-potassium diet. Some patients with hyperkalemic periodic paralysis have clinically evident myotonia, although this is never a prominent symptom and is generally restricted to the facial muscles, as discussed previously.

In middle age and late life, patients develop a proximal myopathy. Biopsy of muscles shows vacuolation of the muscle fibers. It was thought that this proximal myopathy was less common in the hyperkalemic than in the hypokalemic form, but recent studies suggest that the incidence is very high (probably universal) in all patients with periodic paralysis (Bradley et al., 1990; Links et al., 1990).

GENETICS

In a 1999 paper, Bulman and colleagues noted that 23 different missense mutations in the alpha-1 subunit of the adult muscle sodium channel gene had been published. These mutations cause hyperkalemic periodic paralysis or paramyotonia congenita, or both. The type and position of the mutation determine whether the dominant symptom is weakness (periodic paralysis) or myotonia (paramyotonia or myotonia fluctuans or permanens).

ANDERSEN'S SYNDROME

Some patients with periodic paralysis have cardiac ventricular dysrhythmias and dysmorphic features, a triad described by Andersen and associates in 1971. It is important to recognize this variant because of the potential for patients to develop fatal arrhythmias (Sansone et al., 1997). This form of periodic paralysis is probably part of the hyperkalemic periodic paralysis spectrum, but a recent report suggested that affected patients may have increased, decreased, or unchanged serum potassium in spontaneous attacks (Sansone et al., 1997). Andersen's syndrome is genetically distinct from the other periodic paralyses and does not show linkage to the calcium or sodium channel mutations demonstrated to cause the more common forms of periodic paralysis. It is thought that Andersen's syndrome is the result of multiple genetic defects combining to produce the clinical features. This is made more probable by the presence of distinctive facial dysmorphism and short index fingers, as shown in Figure 80–5.

NORMOKALEMIC PERIODIC PARALYSIS

There are patients with frequent, mild episodes of muscle weakness resembling hyperkalemic periodic paralysis whose serum potassium level does not change during the attack. These patients are usually sensitive to potassium ingestion and have exercise-induced weakness. At least some families have so-

dium channel mutations (Lehmann-Horn et al., submitted for publication).

Hypokalemic Periodic Paralysis

CLINICAL FEATURES

This is probably the most frequent type of periodic paralysis, although precise prevalence rates are not available. There are several features that distinguish this form of periodic paralysis from the hyperkalemic form. Most obvious is the change in serum potassium level, which decreases in the attack rather than increasing. Unlike hyperkalemic periodic paralysis, which starts at a very young age, the attacks generally do not begin until the end of the first decade of life, and sometimes not until the late teens (usually between the ages of 7 and 18 years). Episodes of weakness are more severe, last longer, and affect more of the body than the hyperkalemic form but occur less frequently, typically once or twice weekly (Table 80–6). With increasing

Table 80–6. Clinical Features of the Major Types of Periodic Paralysis

	Hyperkalemic	Hypokalemic
Age at onset	<5 yr	8–20 yr
Duration of attack	Minutes to hours	Hours to days
Frequency of attacks	Very frequent	Infrequent
Distribution of weakness	Focal	Widespread
Dietary precipitants	Fasting	Carbohydrates
Myotonia	Face	Usually absent
Ion channel affected (gene)	Sodium (*SCN4A*)	Calcium (*CACNA1S*)

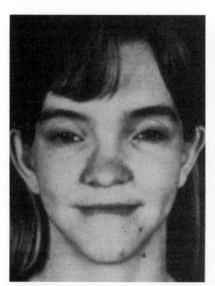
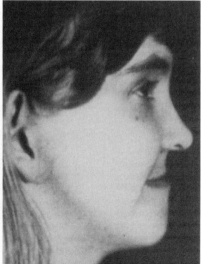
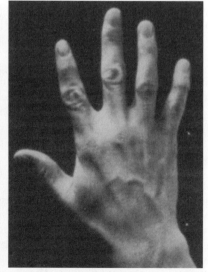

Figure 80–5. Typical dysmorphic facial characteristics of patients with Andersen's syndrome. Note the widely spaced eyes, low ears, and short index finger. (From Sansone V, Griggs RC, Meola G, et al: Andersen's syndrome: A distinct periodic paralysis. Ann Neurol 1997;42:308, with permission. Copyright 1997. Reprinted by permission of John Wiley & Sons.)

age the attacks of weakness become less frequent, but eventually the majority of patients develop a proximal myopathy with permanent weakness of variable severity. Careful examination or muscle biopsy shows this myopathy in most, if not all, patients.

Although hypokalemic periodic paralysis is inherited in an autosomal dominant way, the male-to-female ratio is 3 or 4 to 1. The explanation for this discrepancy is that many women carry the genetic mutation but have few or no symptoms. We have observed families in which obligate carrier females have never had paralytic attacks but have developed proximal weakness late in life, and other women with only one or two attacks in their lives. The reason for the reduced penetrance in women is unknown.

GENETICS

Bulman and colleagues identified a sodium channel (*SCN4A*) mutation in patients with hypokalemic periodic paralysis (Bulman et al., 1999). However, most hypokalemic periodic paralysis patients with identified mutations have calcium channel gene abnormalities. These mutations affect the dihydropyridine-sensitive (L-type) calcium channel receptor on chromosome 1 (alpha-1 subunit of CACNA1S) (Ptacek et al., 1994).

Electrophysiology in Periodic Paralysis

NERVE CONDUCTION STUDIES

Between attacks of weakness, the nerve conduction studies are normal in patients with periodic paralysis. During the attacks, the compound muscle action potential decreases in amplitude and duration in parallel with the severity of weakness. In a severe attack, the muscle may be completely inexcitable, and even direct stimulation, of the muscle itself fails to elicit a response, indicating that the source of the weakness is the muscle, rather than the nerve or the neuromuscular junction. The decrease of the compound muscle action potential in weak muscles forms the basis of the prolonged exercise test used in the diagnosis of periodic paralysis (McManis et al., 1986).

BRIEF EXERCISE

In hypokalemic periodic paralysis, the compound muscle action potential is stable at rest. There is no decrement to slow repetitive stimulation, and brief (10 to 30 seconds) exercise produces no change in the amplitude or a decrement. In hyperkalemic periodic paralysis, paralytic attacks occur frequently. As a consequence, the compound muscle action potential is often unstable, and it is difficult to establish a baseline amplitude for comparison.

There is no decrement at rest or after brief exercise, but progressive weakness and diminishing amplitudes may begin after even 30 seconds of exercise.

PROLONGED EXERCISE

Prolonged exercise (5 minutes of strong, repeated contractions) often induces weakness and a fall in the compound muscle action potential amplitude in all forms of periodic paralysis (McManis et al., 1986). This effect occurs in patients with secondary forms of periodic paralysis as well as with the inherited forms. The amplitude of the compound muscle action potential falls progressively, beginning within 1 or 2 minutes of the exercise. The decrease in amplitude is gradual, rather than abrupt, usually taking 10 to 30 minutes to reach the nadir. There is a gradual recovery beginning after 30 to 60 minutes, although full recovery may take several hours. In contrast, exercise causes a sudden fall in compound muscle action potential amplitude in paramyotonia congenita beginning immediately after exercise, followed by a gradual return to baseline (see Fig. 80–3).

The exercise test is a safe and effective method of screening patients for periodic paralysis, as it may be abnormal in all forms, both primary and secondary. It may be necessary to repeat the test if weakness does not occur after exercise, especially in patients with hypokalemic periodic paralysis. The diagnostic yield can be increased if patients are instructed to eat salty, high-carbohydrate food before the test if they are suspected of having the hypokalemic form, or to fast if the hyperkalemic form is suspected.

INTRA-ARTERIAL EPINEPHRINE

If the exercise test is abnormal, it is helpful to know whether the patient has hypokalemic or hyperkalemic periodic paralysis. This can be determined by measuring the changes in serum potassium during a spontaneous or induced attack, although this information is not always available. In patients with positive exercise tests and known hypokalemia, the secondary forms of the disease need to be recognized and treated appropriately. One method of distinguishing primary hypokalemic periodic paralysis from all other types of periodic paralysis is to infuse dilute epinephrine into the radial artery at the wrist and record the median/thenar compound muscle action potential. In primary hypokalemic periodic paralysis, the response will decrease in amplitude after the infusion but the amplitude will remain unaffected in all other patients. This testing requires specialized equipment and technical assistance and should not be attempted in laboratories unfamiliar with the technique.

NEEDLE ELECTROMYOGRAPHY

Between attacks of paralysis, the needle examination of muscles is normal in most periodic paralysis patients. In the hyperkalemic form, there may be myotonic discharges in proximal muscles, especially facial muscles, in some patients, but this can be hard to find because contraction of muscles rapidly abolishes the myotonia. Myotonia is rarely seen in hypokalemic periodic paralysis. Muscles weakened by periodic paralysis show reduced or absent insertional activity and motor unit potential recruitment. Late in life, a progressive proximal myopathy develops in all forms of familial periodic paralysis. This myopathy causes the motor unit potentials to become smaller in amplitude and duration, and rapid recruitment of motor units may occur, with low effort levels. Fibrillation potentials occur, and these correlate with the presence of vacuolar changes.

During an attack of paralysis, the muscle becomes electrically silent. Insertional and spontaneous activities are absent, and the patient can activities few or no motor units. With recovering strength, the motor units become progressively more easily activated until a full recruitment pattern returns. This process is associated with a progressive return of the insertional activity.

Distinguishing the Myotonic Disorders and Periodic Paralyses

The characteristic electrophysiological features of the various ion channel disorders are described in the aforementioned sections. It is sometimes difficult to distinguish the various forms of myotonia or periodic paralysis, but testing in the electromyography laboratory may provide sufficient information to classify these conditions accurately prior to obtaining molecular testing. The number of genetic tests should be reduced if the diagnosis can be established with clinical and electrophysiological means. Molecular testing may then be used to confirm a diagnosis or to distinguish between small numbers of conditions in which the genetic mutations are known. The failure to find a known mutation in suspected ion channel disease does not exclude that disease, as not all mutations are known and new mutations are still being identified.

As shown in Table 80–7, there are several electrophysiological techniques that can be used to help distinguish the myotonias and periodic paralyses. Standard nerve conduction studies are generally normal, although there is a small decrement with slow repetitive stimulation, of motor nerves in myotonia congenita. As described previously, there is a typical sequence of events in response to brief exercise in myotonia congenita, and a dramatic fall in motor response amplitude often occurs in paramyotonia congenita, especially if the muscle is cool. Prolonged exercise (5 minutes of strong, sustained contractions with short rest periods every 15 to 20 seconds) causes no change in most conditions, but there is an immediate fall in amplitude in paramyotonia congenita with a slow recovery over 60 to 90 minutes.

In all forms of periodic paralysis, there is a progressive fall in compound muscle action potential amplitude after prolonged exercise in most patients. The reduction in amplitude reaches its nadir after about 20 minutes, followed by a slow recovery to baseline. This response occurs in both primary and secondary forms of periodic paralysis, but not in any other condition. The response to exercise in various neuromuscular diseases is illustrated in Figure 80–4.

Cooling induces weakness in paramyotonia congenita, and the compound muscle action potential falls in proportion to the degree of weakness. Cooling may also induce changes on needle examination of muscles in these disorders. There is an increase in myotonia except with myotonia fluctuans. In paramyotonia congenita, the cold-induced weakness is associated with an inability to activate voluntary motor unit potentials, causing a reduction in recruitment. Exercise reduces myotonic discharges except in paramyotonia, where exercise paradoxically increases the myotonia. There is a reduction in motor unit recruitment after strong exercise in paramyo-

Table 80–7. Electrophysiological Findings in Channelopathies

	MC	PMC	MF	PP	NeuroMy
Nerve Conduction Studies					
Decrement (2 Hz)	Yes	No	No	No	No
Brief exercise	Repair	Fall	NC	NC	NC
Prolonged exercise	NC	Fall	NC	Fall	NC
Cooling	NC	Fall	NC	NC	NC
Needle Examination					
Myotonic discharges					
Cooling	Incr	Incr	NC	Incr	—
Exercise	Decr	Incr	Decr	Decr	NC
Recruitment					
Cooling	NC	Decr	NC	NC	—
Exercise	NC	Decr	NC	Decr	NC

MC, myotonia congenita; PMC, paramyotonia congenita; MF, myotonia fluctuans; PP, periodic paralysis; NeuroMy, neuromyotonia; Repair, repair of decrement to slow repetitive stimulation; NC, no change; Fall, reduction in compound muscle action potential amplitude; Incr, increased; Decr, decreased; —, no information.

tonia congenita and the periodic paralyses, in keeping with clinical weakness.

Potassium loading is sometimes used to distinguish the hyperkalemic and hypokalemic forms of periodic paralysis. Oral potassium administration brings on an episode of weakness in hyperkalemic periodic paralysis and worsens myotonia in myotonia fluctuans. Potassium loading carries a risk of cardiac arrhythmias, especially in Andersen's syndrome, so electrocardiographic monitoring and the availability of resuscitation equipment are mandatory. Alternative ways of distinguishing the forms of periodic paralysis are to monitor the serum potassium in spontaneous attacks (which can be provoked by dietary manipulations of carbohydrate and salt intake), to administer glucose and insulin, or to perform the intra-arterial epinephrine test discussed previously.

This type of physiological testing is still useful despite the availability of genetic mutational analysis. In addition, there are some families or individuals in whom the mutations have not been identified, so the precise diagnosis cannot always be determined with genetic testing.

CONDITIONS CAUSING SYMPTOMS AND SIGNS RESEMBLING THE CHANNELOPATHIES

Myotonic Dystrophy

A discussion of myotonic dystrophy and the related disorder, proximal myotonic myopathy, is important in this context, even though they are not the result of primary ion channel mutations. The neuromuscular features may be confused with channelopathies, particularly Becker's recessive generalized myotonia. Myotonic dystrophy (Steinert's disease) and recessive generalized myotonia both cause muscle weakness and wasting as well as myotonia, but there are clinical, electrophysiological, and genetic differences that should make it possible to distinguish the two conditions. In myotonic dystrophy, the distribution of muscle wasting is characteristic and progressive and, when fully developed, permits the immediate recognition of the disorder (Harper, 1989). The temporal and masseter muscles are weak and often markedly atrophic, producing a long, narrow facial appearance, which is emphasized by the frequent presence of frontal balding ("hatchet" facies), and bilateral partial ptosis. The sternocleidomastoid muscles are typically very wasted, and the neck looks thin. Limb muscle weakness is most pronounced in forearm, hand, and distal lower limb muscles, whereas proximal limb girdle muscles are relatively spared. In contrast, recessive generalized myotonia causes weakness predominantly in proximal upper limb muscles. Proximal myotonic myopathy may also be confused with these two disorders (see the following).

The myotonia of myotonic dystrophy is relatively mild except in hand and forearm muscles, which cause grip myotonia, producing the well-known difficulty in releasing the grip after shaking hands or holding an object tightly. This myotonia diminishes with repeated contractions, the so-called "warming-up" phenomenon. There is percussion myotonia in tongue and thenar muscles after a sharp tap on these muscles, and other skeletal muscles may contract in the region of percussion of the muscle, causing a dimpling or mounding of the muscle in the tapped area. There is often clinical and/or nerve conduction evidence of an axonal peripheral neuropathy.

However, it is often the systemic features that most easily distinguish this condition from other myotonic disorders. These include frontal balding; glucose intolerance with hyperinsulinism (or frank diabetes); other endocrine disturbances, including testicular atrophy, reduced fertility, and gynecomastia; and lens opacities or cataracts, which have a pathognomonic appearance on slit-lamp examination. They are in the posterior subcapsular region and are multicolored or iridescent. Intracardiac conduction defects occur in 90% of patients with this condition. There may be a mild cardiomyopathy, although severe cardiac failure is rare. Mild mental retardation is seen in one third to one half of patients, and IgG deficiency is frequent. Unlike other muscle diseases, smooth muscle (e.g., gastrointestinal and uterine) is sometimes affected.

ELECTRODIAGNOSTIC STUDIES

Electrodiagnostic studies may show a mild axonal peripheral neuropathy. Slow (2 to 5 Hz) repetitive stimulation of motor nerves causes a 10% to 15% decrement at rest. Brief exercise (e.g., a strong contraction for 15 seconds) repairs the decrement, but transiently reduces the compound muscle action potential amplitude. The amplitude returns to baseline, and the decrement recurs with 30 seconds of rest. Prolonged exercise (5 minutes) provokes no additional abnormality.

On needle examination, there are myotonic discharges in most muscles, although these are present in only a few muscles in mild cases. When they are sparse, they are most frequent in hand and forearm muscles. The myotonic discharges themselves are long-lasting and slow-firing. At times, the myotonic discharges may fire so slowly that they resemble fibrillation potentials.

Motor unit potentials tend to be short in duration, low in amplitude, and polyphasic, especially in muscles that are weak.

Children of mothers with myotonic dystrophy may have a very severe form of the disorder, with symptoms present from birth (Harper, 1975). Mothers may even note reduced fetal movements during pregnancy. Some infants die within hours of birth. The respiratory muscles may be weak (the usual cause of death in affected infants); the diaphragm is more affected than the intercostal muscles.

Patients with myotonic dystrophy may experience shortness of breath during the day and hypoventilation at night. The precise cause can be further investigated by pulmonary function studies and sleep studies. Electrophysiological studies including transcranial magnetic stimulation and phrenic stimulation, with recording from the diaphragm, as well as needle electromyography of the diaphragm, may also be useful in evaluating these patients (see Chapters 11 and 32).

Myotonic dystrophy is due to a trinucleotide expansion (CTG repeats) in the *DMPK* gene on chromosome 19 (Harley et al., 1992). There is a 98% concordance between the classic clinical syndrome and the genetic abnormality (Thornton and Ashizawa, 1999), indicating the accuracy of clinical diagnosis. Some of the patients with typical clinical findings who lack the expansion might have point mutations, but there is clinical overlap with a similar but only recently recognized disorder, proximal myotonic myopathy (PROMM), and some patients with PROMM may be misdiagnosed as having myotonic dystrophy. In addition, there are patients with what appears to be typical myotonic dystrophy who have no *DMPK* gene expansion and who have genetic linkage to chromosome 3, like families with PROMM.

In myotonic dystrophy, clinical myotonia is often reduced by treatment with phenytoin. Many patients respond to low doses of this medication, such as 100 mg daily, but larger doses are needed in some patients (up to 400 mg per day). This treatment is beneficial in those whose main complaint is muscle stiffness, but the weakness is often more troublesome and phenytoin does not help this symptom.

Proximal Myotonic Myopathy

In 1994 and 1995, a series of papers appeared, describing a muscular disorder resembling myotonic dystrophy, but without an expansion of the CTG triplet sequence on chromosome 19 (Ricker et al., 1994a, 1995; Tawil et al., 1994). It is inherited in an autosomal dominant fashion and is characterized by myotonia and weakness in proximal muscles, and cataracts. Patients with this disorder show many of the systemic features of myotonic dystrophy, including clinical myotonia, cataracts, frontal balding, cardiac conduction defects, and testicular atrophy in males, but they have a distribution of muscle involvement different from myotonic dystrophy. Because of the predominant involvement of the limb girdle muscles and relative sparing of the forearm and leg muscles, which are typically weak and atrophic in myotonic dystrophy, this condition has been called proximal myotonic myopathy. In Germany, the frequencies of PROMM and myotonic dystrophy appear to be similar (Thornton and Ashizawa, 1999).

One interesting aspect of this disorder is that the myotonia is aggravated by heat and reduced by cooling, at least in some patients (Sander et al.,

1996). This is a distinguishing point from other myotonic disorders that exhibit the opposite pattern.

Some families with "proximal" myotonic myopathy have predominantly distal, rather than proximal, muscle atrophy and weakness, like myotonic dystrophy patients, but they do not have a trinucleotide repeat in the *DMPK* gene. Because the clinical findings are different from PROMM and more like myotonic dystrophy while the genetic abnormalities are similar to (or possibly the same as) PROMM, these patients are classified separately as having myotonic dystrophy type 2 (or DM2). The genetic defect is unknown at this point, but there is evidence linking both PROMM and DM2 to the long arm of chromosome 3 (Ranum et al., 1998; Ricker et al., 1999).

Rippling Muscle Disease

Rippling muscle disease is an autosomal dominant inherited disorder in which the main symptoms are cramping and myalgia associated with muscle stiffness (Ricker et al., 1989). These symptoms are most prominent during or immediately after exercise. Affected individuals can produce pathognomonic waves of muscle contraction passing through a muscle that is stretched after a contraction. These waves ("ripples") are electrically silent. Another feature is that percussion of a muscle causes a localized mounding similar to that seen in the myotonic disorders. Serum creatine kinase is often mildly increased. The condition is inherited in an autosomal dominant fashion, and genetic linkage studies suggest that the phenotype may be produced by multiple different genetic mutations; one of the gene mutations is on the long arm of chromosome 1 (Stephen et al., 1994).

This condition is not due to abnormalities of ion channel function and does not cause electrical discharges on the needle examination of muscles. However, the clinical features of muscle stiffness and percussion-induced muscle contraction are similar to those seen in the myotonic disorders, and rippling muscle disease should be considered in the differential diagnosis of the myotonic syndromes, especially when the muscle contractions are electrically silent.

Cramp-Fasciculation Syndrome

Patients with this condition complain of frequent cramps and muscle stiffness, and examination of the muscles often reveals the twitching of fasciculation, especially in calf and foot muscles (Tahmoush et al., 1991). The symptoms are aggravated by exercise. Clinical examination is otherwise unremarkable; there is no myotonia with muscle percussion, and forceful contractions may precipitate a cramp, but not myotonia. Patients can often induce cramps by strong contractions, especially in calf and foot muscles. The most troublesome symptom is the painful cramping, which can occur in any limb muscle and even in trunk muscles. Cramps are often triggered by sudden movements or simple maneuvers, such as turning in bed, making the patients move very cautiously.

The electromyographic findings are diagnostic. Routine nerve conduction studies are normal, but there are large numbers of fasciculation potentials in resting muscles studied with surface electrodes. Repetitive nerve stimulation at rates between 2 and 10 Hz induces prolonged trains of spontaneously firing motor unit potentials and frank cramp discharges. Needle examination shows the fasciculation potentials and cramp discharges in symptomatic muscles, but no other abnormality. There are no myotonic discharges and motor unit potentials are normal. Carbamazepine therapy may be helpful (Tahmoush et al. 1991).

Hypothyroid Myopathy

Muscle weakness and stiffness are prominent features of hypothyroidism. Muscles feel firm and tendon reflexes are slow to relax, causing "hung-up" ankle jerks. This delay in relaxation is due to prolonged activity in muscle activated by stretch. Muscles that are percussed show a localized contraction or mounding sometimes called myoedema. The mounding of the muscle persists for several seconds after percussion. The delayed relaxation after stretch or contraction and the effect of percussion on muscle resemble the findings in myotonia. Patients with hypothyroidism often have slowed nerve conduction velocities and low-amplitude motor and sensory responses as well as the myopathy, and needle examination of muscle shows that the slow relaxation is due to motor unit activity, rather than waxing and waning myotonic discharges. Symptoms are often very slow to improve with thyroid hormone replacement.

TREATMENT OF ION CHANNEL DISORDERS

The treatment of myotonia varies with the clinical syndrome and the nature of the muscle membrane abnormality. Myotonia congenita is due to an abnormality of the chloride channels and is best treated with sodium channel–blocking drugs, such as mexiletine (150 mg twice daily, up to 300 mg three times daily). Tocainide can also be used. Patients with myotonia fluctuans may be resistant to mexiletine and tocainide but respond to flecainide, another sodium channel–blocking agent. The differential effects of these channel blockers may relate to the fact that mexiletine and tocainide block channels in the closed (inactivated) state, while flecainide blocks the channels in the open state (Rosenfeld et al., 1997). It is important to exclude cardiac conduc-

tion defects prior to beginning to treat patients with these drugs. Unlike myotonic dystrophy, myotonia congenita rarely responds to carbamazepine or phenytoin.

The sodium channelopathies respond to the carbonic anhydrase drugs. Traditionally, acetazolamide is used, but recent evidence points to greater benefits from dichlorphenamide (Tawil et al., 2000). How the carbonic anhydrase inhibitors improve the symptoms in sodium channelopathies is not understood, but both the myotonia and the episodic weakness improve with this treatment. Acetazolamide and dichlorphenamide also reduce the frequency and severity of attacks in hypokalemic periodic paralysis, even though this condition is caused by a calcium channel abnormality in the majority of families. There is some evidence to suggest that the myopathy that develops in late life in patients with all forms of periodic paralysis also improves with, and may be prevented by, dichlorphenamide.

Both acetazolamide and dichlorphenamide can cause a metabolic acidosis with high chloride levels and depletion of sodium and potassium. Common side effects include hand and perioral tingling and a metallic taste to carbonated beverages. Patients may develop renal calculi, and patients with a history of renal tract stones should not be treated with the carbonic anhydrase inhibitors. The maintenance dose of acetazolamide varies from 125 mg a day to 250 mg three times a day, while effective dichlorphenamide doses range between 25 mg a day and 50 mg three times a day.

Diet plays an important role in the management of symptoms in the periodic paralyses. Avoidance of high-sodium, high-carbohydrate foods reduces the attack frequency in the hypokalemic form, and potassium supplements in the form of potassium-rich foods or tablets are beneficial. Potassium taken orally usually aborts attacks. Some patients benefit from treatment with diuretics. One report suggests that verapamil helps in hypokalemic periodic paralysis (Berwick, 1988).

Patients with the hyperkalemic form should avoid fasting, and frequent small meals may be helpful in reducing attacks. Diuretic therapy is sometimes beneficial, but some patients are made worse by or are intolerant of diuretics. Salbutamol tablets or inhaled salbutamol may abort or prevent attacks in this form (Hanna et al., 1998).

As mentioned previously, anticonvulsants reduce symptoms in neuromyotonia, but the autoimmune forms are best treated with plasmapheresis or immunosuppression.

References

Ackerman MJ: The long QT syndrome: Ion channel diseases of the heart. Mayo Clin Proc 1998;73:250–269.

Ackerman MJ, Clapham DE: Ion channels: Basic science and clinical disease. N Engl J Med 1997;336:1575–1586.

Andersen ED, Krasilnikoff PA, Overvad H: Intermittent muscular weakness, extrasystoles, and multiple developmental abnormalities: A new syndrome? Acta Pediatr Scand 1971;60:559–564.

Berwick C: Familial hypokalemic periodic paralysis. Muscle Nerve 1988;11:1092–1093.

Biervert C, Schroeder BC, Kubisch C, et al: A potassium channel mutation in neonatal human epilepsy. Science 1998;279:403–406.

Bradley WG, Taylor R, Rice DR, et al: Progressive myopathy in hypokalemic periodic paralysis. Arch Neurol 1990;47:1013–1017.

Browne DL, Gancher ST, Nutt JG, et al: Episodic ataxia/myokymia syndrome is associated with point mutations in the human potassium channel gene, *KCNA1*. Nat Genet 1994;8:136–140.

Brugnoni R, Galantini S, Confalonieri P, et al: Identification of three novel mutations in the major human skeletal muscle chloride channel gene (*CLCN1*), causing myotonia congenita. Hum Mutat 1999;14:447.

Bryant SH: Muscle membrane of normal and myotonic goats in normal and low external chloride. Fed Proc 1962;21:312.

Bulman DE, Scoggan KA, van Oene MD, et al: A novel sodium channel mutation in a family with hypokalemic periodic paralysis. Neurology 1999;53:1932–1936.

Burns RJ, Bretag AH, Blumbergs PC, et al: Benign familial disease with muscle mounding and rippling. J Neurol Neurosurg Psychiatry 1994;57:344–347.

Cadilhac J, Baldet P, Greze J, et al: EMG studies of two family cases of the Schwartz and Jampel syndrome (osteo-chondromuscular dystrophy with myotonia). Electromyogr Clin Neurophysiol 1975;15:5–12.

Caughey JE, Pachomov N: The diaphragm in dystrophia myotonica. J Neurol Neurosurg Psychiatry 1959;22:311.

Church SC: The heart in myotonia atrophica. Arch Intern Med 1967;119:176.

De Jong HH, Matzner IA, Unger AA: Clinical and physiological studies in a case of myotonia. Arch Neurol Psychiatry 1951;65:181–188.

Deymeer F, Cakirkaya S, Serdaroglu P, et al: Transient weakness and compound muscle action potential decrement in myotonia congenita. Muscle Nerve 1998;21:1334–1337.

Ebers GC, George AL, Barchi RL, et al: Paramyotonia congenita and hyperkalemic periodic paralysis are linked to the adult muscle sodium channel gene. Ann Neurol 1991;30:810–816.

Franke C, Iazzio PA, Hatt H, et al: Altered Na$^+$ channel activity and reduced Cl$^-$ conductance cause hyperexcitability in recessive generalized myotonia (Becker). Muscle Nerve 1991;14:762–770.

Gamstorp I, Wohlfart G: A syndrome characterized by myokymia, myotonia, muscle wasting, and increased perspiration. Acta Psychiatr Neur Scand 1959;34:181–194.

Greenberg DA: Calcium channels in neurological disease. Ann Neurol 1997;42:275–282.

Greenberg DA: Neuromuscular disease and calcium channels. Muscle Nerve 1999;22:1341–1349.

Griggs RC, Davies RJ, Anderson DC, et al: Cardiac conduction in myotonic dystrophy. Am J Med 1975;59:37.

Hanna MG, Stewart J, Schapira AHV, et al: Salbutamol treatment in a patient with hyperkalemic periodic paralysis due to a mutation in the skeletal muscle sodium channel gene (*SCN4A*). J Neurol Neurosurg Psychiatry 1998;65:248–250.

Harley HG, Brook JD, Rundle SA, et al: Expansion of an unstable DNA region and phenotypic variation in myotonic dystrophy. Nature 1992;355:545–546.

Harper PS: Congenital myotonic dystrophy in Britain. I. Clinical aspects. Arch Dis Child 1975;50:505.

Harper PS: Myotonic Dystrophy, 2nd ed. Philadelphia, WB Saunders, 1989.

Hart IK, Waters C, Vincent A, et al: Autoantibodies detected to expressed K$^+$ channels are implicated in neuromyotonia. Ann Neurol 1997;41:238–246.

Isaacs H: A syndrome of continuous muscle-fibre activity. J Neurol Neurosurg Psychiatry 1961;24:319–325.

Ishpekova B, Rasheva M, Moskov M: Schwartz-Jampel syndrome: Clinical, electromyographic and genetic studies. Electromyogr Clin Neurophysiol 1996;36:151–155.

Jervell A, Lange-Nielsen F: Congenital deaf-mutism, functional heart disease with prolongation of the Q-T interval, and sudden death. Am Heart J 1957;54:59–68.

Koch MC, Steinmeyer K, Lorenz C, et al: The skeletal muscle chloride channel in dominant and recessive human myotonia. Science 1992;257:797–800.

Koty PP, Pegoraro E, Hobson G, et al: Myotonia and the muscle chloride channel: Dominant mutations show variable penetrance and founder effect. Neurology 1996;47:963–968.

Lehmann-Horn F, Heine R, Pica U, et al: The clinical spectrum of the T704M sodium channel mutation (submitted for publication).

Lehmann-Horn F, Iaizzo PA, Franke C, et al: Schwartz-Jampel syndrome: II. Na$^+$ channel defect causes myotonia. Muscle Nerve 1990;13:528–535.

Lerche H, Heine R, Pica U, et al: Human sodium channel myotonia: Slowed channel inactivation due to substitutions for glycine within the III/IV linker. J Physiol (Lond) 1993;470:13.

Links TP, Zwarts MJ, Oosterhuis HJGH: Improvement of muscle strength in familial hypokalaemic periodic paralysis with acetazolamide. J Neurol Neurosurg Psychiatry 1988;51:1142–1145.

Links TP, Zwarts MJ, Wilmink JT, et al: Permanent muscle weakness in familial hypokalaemic periodic paralysis. Brain 1990;113:1873–1889.

Maddison P, Newsom-Davis J, Mills KR: Strength-duration properties of peripheral nerve in acquired neuromyotonia. Muscle Nerve 1999;22:823–830.

McManis PG, Lambert EH, Daube JR: The exercise test in periodic paralysis. Muscle Nerve 1986;9:704–710.

Newsom-Davis J, Mills KR: Immunological associations of acquired neuromyotonia (Isaacs' syndrome): Report of five cases and literature review. Brain 1993;116:453–469.

Partanen VS, Soininen H, Saksa M, et al: Electromyographic and nerve conduction findings in a patient with neuromyotonia, normocalcemic tetany and small-cell lung cancer. Acta Neurol Scand 1980;61:216–226.

Ptacek LJ, George AL, Barchi RL, et al: Mutations in an S4 segment of the adult skeletal muscle sodium channel cause paramyotonia congenita. Neuron 1992;8:891–897.

Ptacek LJ, George AL, Griggs RC, et al: Identification of a mutation in the gene causing hyperkalemic periodic paralysis. Cell 1991;67:1021–1027.

Ptacek LJ, Gouw L, Kwiecinski H, et al: Sodium channel mutations in paramyotonia congenita and hyperkalemic periodic paralysis. Ann Neurol 1993;33:300–307.

Ptacek LJ, Tawil R, Griggs RC, et al: Dihydropyridine receptor mutations cause hypokalemic periodic paralysis. Cell 1994;77:863–868.

Ptacek LJ, Trimmer JS, Agnew WS, et al: Paramyotonia congenita and hyperkalemic periodic paralysis map to the same sodium-channel gene locus. Am J Hum Genet 1991;49:851–854.

Ranum LP, Rasmussen PF, Benzow KA, et al: Genetic mapping of a second myotonic dystrophy locus. Nat Genet 1998;19:196–198.

Ricker K, Lehmann-Horn F, Moxley RT: Myotonia fluctuans. Arch Neurol 1990;47:268–272.

Ricker K, Moxley RT, Rohkamm R: Rippling muscle disease. Arch Neurol 1989;46:405–408.

Ricker K, Grimm T, Koch MC, et al: Linkage of proximal myotonic myopathy to chromosome 3q. Neurology 1999;52:170–171.

Ricker K, Koch MC, Lehmann-Horn F, et al: Proximal myotonic myopathy: A new dominant disorder with myotonia, muscle weakness, and cataracts. Neurology 1994a;44:1448–1452.

Ricker K, Koch MC, Lehmann-Horn F, et al: Proximal myotonic myopathy: Clinical features of a multisystem disorder similar to myotonic dystrophy. Arch Neurol 1995;52:25–31.

Ricker K, Moxley RT, Heine R, et al: Myotonia fluctuans: A third type of muscle sodium channel disease. Arch Neurol 1994b;51:1095–1102.

Rosenfeld J, Sloan-Brown K, George AL Jr: A novel muscle sodium channel mutation causes painful congenital myotonia. Ann Neurol 1997;42:811–814.

Sander HW, Tavoulareas GP, Chokroverty S: Heat-sensitive myotonia in proximal myotonic myopathy. Neurology 1996;47:956–962.

Sangiuolo F, Botta A, Mescoraca A, et al: Identification of five new mutations and three novel polymorphisms in the muscle chloride channel gene (*CLCN1*) in 20 Italian patients with dominant and recessive myotonia congenita. Hum Mutat 1998;11:331.

Sansone V, Griggs RC, Meola G, et al: Andersen's syndrome: A distinct periodic paralysis. Ann Neurol 1997;42:305–312.

Serratrice G, Azulay JP: [What is left of Morvan's fibrillary chorea]? Rev Neurol 1994;150:257–265.

Shillito P, Molenaar PC, Vincent A, et al: Acquired neuromyotonia: Evidence for autoantibodies directed against K$^+$ channels of peripheral nerves. Ann Neurol 1995;38:714–722.

Spranger M, Spranger S, Schwab S, et al: Familial hemiplegic migraine with cerebellar ataxia and paroxysmal psychosis. Eur Neurol 1999;41:150–152.

Steinlein OK, Mulley JC, Propping P, et al: A missense mutation in the neuronal nicotinic acetylcholine receptor alpha 4 subunit is associated with autosomal dominant nocturnal frontal lobe epilepsy. Nat Genet 1995;11:201–203.

Stephen DA, Buist NRM, Chittenden AB, et al: A rippling muscle disease gene is localised to 1q41: Evidence for multiple genes. Neurology 1994;44:1915–1920.

Streib EW: Differential diagnosis of myotonic syndromes. Muscle Nerve 1987;10:603–615.

Tahmoush AJ, Alonso RJ, Tahmoush GP, et al: Cramp-fasciculation syndrome: A treatable hyperexcitable peripheral nerve disorder. Neurology 1991;41:1021–1024.

Tawil R, McDermott MP, Brown R Jr, et al: Randomized trials of dichlorphenamide in the periodic paralyses. Ann Neurol 2000;47:46–53.

Tawil R, Ptacek LJ, Pavlakis SG, et al: Andersen's syndrome: Potassium-sensitive periodic paralysis, ventricular ectopy, and dysmorphic features. Ann Neurol 1994;35:326–330.

Thornton CA, Ashizawa T: Getting a grip on the myotonic dystrophies. Neurology 1999;52:12–13.

Thornton CA, Griggs R, Moxley RT: Myotonic dystrophy with no trinucleotide repeat expansion. Ann Neurol 1994;35:269–272.

Wagner S, Lerche H, Mitrovic N, et al: A novel sodium channel mutation causing a hyperkalemic paralytic and paramyotonic syndrome with variable expressivity. Neurology 1997;49:1018–1025.

Walsh JC: Neuromyotonia: An unusual presentation of intrathoracic malignancy. J Neurol Neurosurg Psychiatry 1976;39:1086–1091.

INTENSIVE CARE– AND CRITICAL ILLNESS–RELATED NEUROMUSCULAR DISORDERS

C H A P T E R 81

Assessment of Patients in the Intensive Care Unit

Charles F. Bolton

Intensive care specialists in medical-surgical intensive care units (ICUs) concentrate mainly on dealing with disorders of the heart and lungs and the frequent complications of sepsis and multiple organ failure. High cost always looms, and thus early weaning of the patient from the ventilator and dismissal to a general hospital ward are primary objectives. Neurologists typically find the environment of the ICU intimidating, partly because of the difficulty in conducting a clinical examination: a comatose and intubated patient cannot give a history, and splints, bandages, and other devices prevent access to limbs for adequate assessment. In addition, electrophysiologists are concerned that the recording will be difficult to perform and will be contaminated by artifact. Thus, neurologists and, particularly, electrophysiologists appear only occasionally in medical-surgical ICUs. The result of this is continuing uncertainty about the reasons for difficulty in weaning patients from the ventilator. Another result is that the patient may never be weaned or may remain ventilator dependent, or the cause of ventilator dependency may not be identified. If weaning from the ventilator is ultimately successful, nurses and doctors, in general, or rehabilitation ward staff members may be puzzled by the patient's difficulty in sitting, inability to walk, and trouble with using the upper limbs for daily tasks, such as shaving, combing the hair, eating, and drinking.

Investigators have shown that, in the last 15 years, in view of the limitation of neurological assessment in the ICU, electrophysiological studies are especially valuable (Bolton, 1987, 1996a; Lacomis et al., 1998), and they may be conducted in patients of all ages (Bolton, 1996a). Electrophysiological studies localize the disorder to the brain, spinal cord, peripheral nerve, neuromuscular junction, or muscle. The prevalence of these various disorders may vary according to the type of patient admitted to the ICU, as reported in a detailed study by Lacomis and colleagues (1998) (Table 81–1)

With attention to certain details, artifact-free records can be obtained regularly when tests are supplemented by other studies, such as magnetic resonance imaging, measurement of creatine phosphokinase level, and muscle biopsy. An accurate diagnosis of the neuromuscular condition can almost always be achieved.

The following discussion applies chiefly to adults, but the principles apply to children.

HISTORY

If the patient is alert and able to write, an adequate history can be taken by having the patient respond in writing. If limb paralysis precludes this approach, the patient may respond by nodding or shaking the head for "yes" or "no" answers. If the patient is stuporous, confused, or comatose or if the patient is a child, the history must be obtained from the referring physician, emergency physician, or intensive care specialist or from the hospital record. If relatives are present, they often can give valuable information. Information also may be obtained from a telephone interview of a friend or employer.

With regard to the neuromuscular system, it is important to elicit the presence of symptoms in the hours, days, or weeks preceding the final event. These symptoms include spinal or radicular pain, bulbar or limb weakness, cramps or twitches, and fatigability of muscles. If the patient was admitted to the ICU after a major surgical procedure, complications from the operation may explain the neuromuscular problem; for example, an operation on the thoracic aorta may be accompanied by spinal cord ischemia that results in paraplegia. One should note any medications that have been administered. Neuromuscular blocking agents, even short-acting ones such as vecuronium, may have a prolonged action (more than a few hours) if the patient has renal or liver failure.

One should note the reasons for intubation and mechanical ventilation. Is it because of airway protection or weakness of the respiratory muscles? Next, one should note the type of mechanical ventilation, the frequency of intermittent mandatory ventilation, the degree of pressure support, and so forth, and the pertinent blood gas levels. Has an attempt been made to assess the patient's ability to breathe while off the ventilator?

PHYSICAL EXAMINATION

A general inspection of the skin may reveal localized edema and redness at a site of prolonged compression. This is particularly likely to occur in a patient who has been in a drug-induced coma for several hours. If pressure occurs at the site of an underlying peripheral nerve, it will cause mononeuropathy. The clinician should compare a paretic lower limb with the opposite one and look for increased temperature, redness, and dry skin in the paretic limb. These signs of sympathetic insufficiency suggest that the paresis is the result of a lesion of the lumbosacral plexus, because sympathetic fibers bypass the caudal nerve roots and join the lumbosacral plexus.

Table 81–1. Electromyographic Diagnoses in 92 Patients

Diagnosis	No.	Total (%)
Myopathy		43 (46)
Myopathy (acquired in the ICU)	39*	
Myopathy (pre-ICU)	4	
Peripheral neuropathy (sensorimotor)		26 (28)
Demyelinating polyneuropathy (AIDP or CIDP)	13	
Axonal polyneuropathy (acquired in the ICU)	12	
Axonal polyneuropathy (pre-ICU)	1	
Neuromuscular junction defect		3 (3)
Myasthenia gravis	1	
Post-NMBA	2*	
Motor neuron disease		7 (7)
Brachial plexopathy		7 (7)
Ischemic mononeuropathies		3 (3)
Other		2 (2)
Normal limb study		3 (3)
Total (number of diagnoses)		94

*Two also had neuromuscular junction defects and myopathy and are included in both groups.

AIDP, acute inflammatory demyelinating polyneuropathy; CIDP, chronic inflammatory demyelinating polyneuropathy; ICU, intensive care unit; NMBA, neuromuscular junction blocking agent.

From Lacomis D, Petrella JT, Giuliani MJ: Causes of neuromuscular weakness in the intensive care unit: A study of ninety-two patients. Muscle Nerve 1998;21:577–583.

The presence of ptosis, asymmetrical ocular palsies, and facial weakness, particularly if variable, suggests a neuromuscular transmission defect. The response to a tug on the endotracheal tube assesses the patient's ability to swallow and to cough. An abnormality of swallowing or coughing may indicate motor neuron disease, severe Guillain-Barré syndrome, or a neuromuscular transmission defect.

The respiratory system should be assessed in the presence of the intensive care specialist and, if necessary, with the assistance of the respiratory technologist. One should assess the patient's ability to breathe by either entirely discontinuing mechanical ventilation or altering mechanical ventilation by stopping intermittent mandatory ventilation but keeping the patient on pressure support or continuous positive airway pressure (to overcome airway/ventilator resistance) to a maximum of 15 minutes, to maintain reasonable oxygenation. Mechanical ventilation is restored if the patient shows evidence of respiratory distress, arterial oxygen saturation less than 90% (based on an oximeter reading), or a marked increase in breathing rate or blood pressure. In the ICU, I have made these observations during needle electromyography (EMG) of the diaphragm, wherein the pattern of respiration is accurately assessed by observing the bursts of motor unit potentials with each inspiration. This pattern may be of localizing value (Fig. 81–1). One should look for the overall strength and rate of respiratory effort. If the patient has predominant weakness of the chest wall muscles, there will be little movement of these muscles on attempted inspiration but forceful outward movement of the abdominal muscles as the diaphragm descends. Alternatively, if there is predominant weakness of the diaphragm (both hemidiaphragms have to be substantially weak for this sign to appear), the chest wall muscles will move outward on inspiration, but the abdominal muscles will not move or, paradoxically, may move inward. These are important clinical signs that, in my experience, are often missed.

The presence or absence of generalized or local wasting of muscle is often difficult to determine, because tissue edema may have developed. However, if the patient has voluntary or semivoluntary movements, one should notice the pattern of these movements in the bulbar and limb muscles. From this pattern, it may be possible to determine the presence of hemiplegia, quadriplegia, or paraplegia. If no such movements are present, one should compress the patient's nail bed with a pencil to produce a painful stimulus and note carefully the pattern of response. A single flexion movement of the stimulated limb, or even of the ipsilateral or contralateral limbs, may be explained entirely by a reflex response at the spinal cord level and may occur even in brain death. However, a more complex, voluntary-type movement indicates a degree of cerebral function. If the patient's opposite hand accurately moves in a coordinated way to attempt to remove the painful stimulus, reasonable function can be anticipated in that limb.

The pattern of limb movement may give additional clues about the presence or absence of neuromuscular disease. For example, a painful stimulus that does not cause limb movement but causes vigorous facial grimacing implies normal afferent conduction of pain sensation through peripheral nerves and the spinal cord to the thalamus and an efferent response

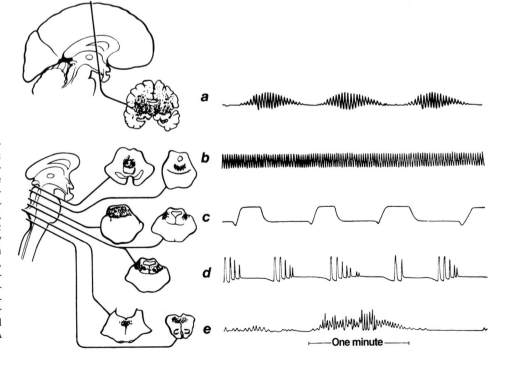

Figure 81–1. Abnormal respiratory patterns associated with pathologic lesions *(shaded areas)* at various locations in the brain. *a*, Cheyne-Stokes respirations; *b*, central neurogenic hyperventilation; *c*, apneusis; *d*, cluster breathing; and *e*, ataxic breathing. Here, respiratory movements were recorded with a chest-abdomen pneumograph, but such patterns can be detected from needle electromyographic recordings of the diaphragm. (From Plum F, Posner JB: The Diagnosis of Stupor and Coma, 3rd ed. Philadelphia, FA Davis, 1980.)

——One minute——

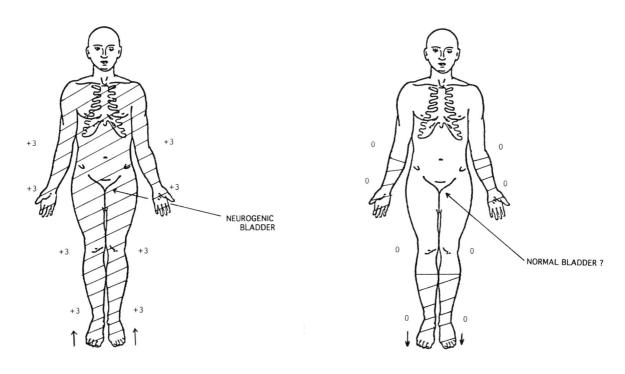

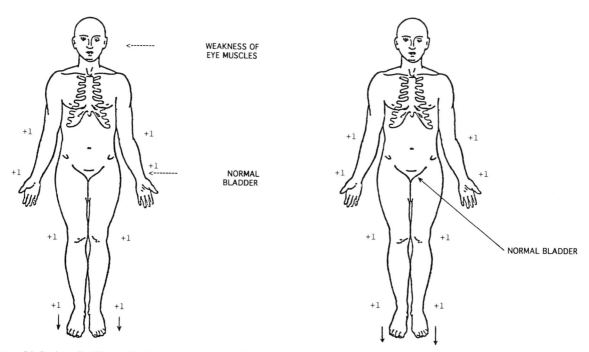

Figure 81–2. *A* to *D,* "Typical" physical findings in sites of nervous system dysfunction that may cause the syndrome of acute limb and respiratory weakness. (The *numbers* indicate briskness of deep tendon reflexes, the *arrows* indicate plantar responses, and the *lateral lines* indicate areas of sensory loss.)

E. PROBLEM CASE

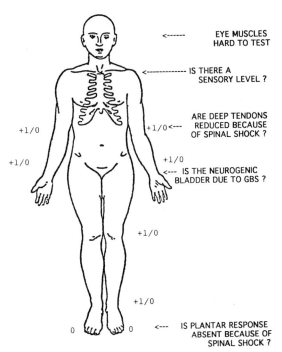

EYE MUSCLES
HARD TO TEST

IS THERE A
SENSORY LEVEL ?

ARE DEEP TENDONS
REDUCED BECAUSE
OF SPINAL SHOCK ?

IS THE NEUROGENIC
BLADDER DUE TO GBS ?

IS PLANTAR RESPONSE
ABSENT BECAUSE OF
SPINAL SHOCK ?

Figure 81–2 *(Continued)*. *E*, The problem case illustrates that these "typical" signs may be absent or difficult to interpret. Electrophysiologic studies (at times, magnetic resonance imaging of the cervical spinal cord) are often necessary. (From Bolton CF, Young GB: The neurological consultation and neurological syndromes in the intensive care unit. Ballieres Clin Neurol 1996; 5:447–475.)

through motor pathways and peripheral nerves to cranial muscles, but not to limb muscles. This pattern is often seen in severe forms of critical illness polyneuropathy. A similar pattern may be seen in cases of high cervical spinal cord dysfunction, except, in severe cases, the facial grimacing is absent because the pain pathways are interrupted by the spinal cord lesion.

The reflexive responses of the limbs to somatic stimulation may show local areas of weakness. For example, a vigorous upward movement of the great toe in response to plantar stimulation on one side may not occur on the other side because of localized peroneal nerve palsy. In addition, the unilateral absence of a knee jerk may suggest lumbosacral plexopathy, with particular involvement of the femoral nerve.

In cases of acute spinal cord dysfunction, trauma, ischemia, or infection, spinal shock often causes flaccidity and areflexia, simulating a lower motor neuron disorder such as polyneuropathy. Thus, from the clinical examination alone, it may be difficult to determine whether quadriplegia results from polyneuropathy or spinal cord dysfunction. Hence, magnetic resonance imaging is often necessary on an emergency basis. Electrophysiological studies may be necessary within 3 days after admission to the

ICU. The results of these studies provide evidence about whether the patient has polyneuropathy. The level of dysfunction can be determined accurately with careful testing with a pin to determine a sensory level. (After the test, the pin must immediately be placed in the "sharp" container for disposal.) However, if the patient is heavily sedated, this sign may be eliminated. Moreover, I have found it difficult to determine a sensory level in patients with lesions of the high cervical spinal cord. The typical findings on neurological examination of patients with lesions at these various sites in the nervous system and the confusion that often arises in "a problem case" are shown in Figure 81–2.

After the foregoing clinical assessment has been made, the syndrome of rapidly developing limb and respiratory weakness presenting before or after admission to the ICU should be systematically investigated pathophysiologically (Table 81-2 and Fig.

Table 81–2. Differential Diagnosis in the Intensive Care Unit of the Syndrome of Rapidly Developing Limb and Respiratory Muscle Weakness

Weakness Before Admission	Weakness After Admission
Disorders of Spinal Cord	
Traumatic myelopathy	Acute transverse myelitis
Acute epidural compression from neoplasm, infection	Acute ischemia
Motor Neuron Disease	
Acute Polyneuropathies	
Guillain-Barré syndrome	Critical illness polyneuropathy
Axonal forms of Guillain-Barré syndrome	Motor neuropathy (neuromuscular blockers)
Acute motor and sensory neuropathy	
Acute motor axonal neuropathy	
Miller-Fisher syndrome	
Chronic Polyneuropathies	
Chronic inflammatory demyelinating polyneuropathy	Chronic polyneuropathies plus sepsis
Diabetic polyneuropathy	
Neuromuscular Transmission Defects	
Myasthenia gravis	Neuromuscular blocker
Lambert-Eaton myasthenic syndrome	
Hypocalcemia	
Hypermagnesemia	
Organophosphate poisoning	
Wound botulism	
Tick-bite paralysis	
Myopathy	
Muscular dystrophy: e.g., Duchenne's, myotonic	Cachectic myopathy
Acute necrotizing myopathy: myoglobinuria	Necrotizing myopathy of intensive care
	Critical illness myopathy

From Bolton CF, Young GB: The neurological consultation and neurological syndromes in the intensive care unit. Baillieres Clin Neurol 1996; 5:447-475.

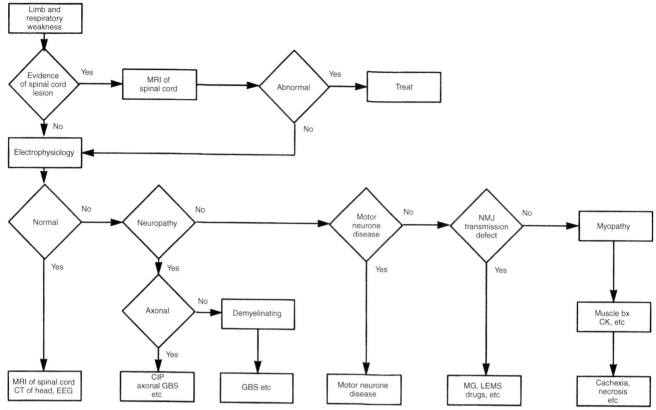

Figure 81–3. An algorithm to guide the approach to the investigation of patients in an intensive care unit who have weakness of limb and respiratory muscles. Positive findings on serologic testing or stool culture for *Campylobacter jejuni* may be the earliest warning of the axonal form of Guillain-Barré syndrome (GBS). bx, biopsy; CIP, critical illness polyneuropathy; CK, creatine phosphokinase; CT, computed tomography; EEG, electroencephalography; LEMS, Lambert-Eaton myasthenic syndrome; MG, myasthenia gravis; MRI, magnetic resonance imaging; NMJ, neuromuscular junction. (From Bolton CF, Young GB: The neurological consultation and neurological syndromes in the intensive care unit. Ballieres Clin Neurol 1996;5:447–475.)

81–3), that is, spinal cord, peripheral nerve, neuromuscular junction, and muscle.

ELECTROPHYSIOLOGICAL EVALUATION

Clinical neurophysiologists are often concerned that technical problems will prevent effective studies from being conducted in the ICU. However, when attention is paid to certain details, all studies usually performed in outpatient EMG laboratories can be performed in both adult and pediatric ICUs (Table 81–3). The value of some of these tests—automated interference pattern analysis and power spectral analysis of the diaphragm, somatosensory evoked potentials of the phrenic nerve, and measurement of muscle force and "sound"—has yet to be fully tested in the ICU.

The clinical examination may be especially difficult in children because of their small size, the confined space of the incubator, endotracheal tubes, vascular catheters, and splints and bandages applied to parts of the body. Electrophysiological studies are valuable in investigating unexplained limb weakness, hypotonia, increased creatinine phosphokinase levels, or difficulty in weaning from the ventilator. The results are important for establishing a diagnosis and for following the course of the illness. No complications result from these investigations.

Studies can readily be performed in the ICU with a portable EMG instrument. Newer EMG instruments with improved front-end hardware and software have decreased the incidence of artifact. Personnel in the ICU should be consulted to obtain the information needed about the history and physical examination and to decide which tests can be performed safely, with the patient's condition and the necessity of maintaining treatment and monitoring devices taken into account. To avoid 60-Hz artifact, all devices attached to the patient should be unplugged from the wall unless they are absolutely necessary. While one applies surface electrodes or stimulates peripheral nerves, the attending nurse should be consulted and, if necessary, should assist with proper positioning of the patient and with adjusting the position of the endotracheal tubes and vascular catheters. Sedation (dosage and timing) should be given under the direction of the intensive care specialist to avoid the pain of needle EMG but still to permit the evaluation of voluntary muscle activity.

Applying an electrical stimulus near an intravascular catheter that leads to the heart is of theoretical concern because of possible induction of arrhyth-

Table 81–3. Electrophysiological Tests That May Be Used in the Intensive Care Unit

Condition	Site of Dysfunction	Test	Reference
Severe encephalopathy	Brain	Somatosensory evoked potential	Aminoff and Eisen, 1998
		Brainstem auditory evoked potential	Picton et al., 1999
Neurologic respiratory insufficiency	Brain, spinal cord, phrenic nerves, neuromuscular junction, diaphragm	Transcranial and cervical magnetic stimulation	Zifko et al., 1996b
		Phrenic nerve somatosensory evoked potential	Zifko et al., 1995
		Phrenic nerve conduction study	Chen et al., 1995
		Repetitive phrenic nerve stimulation	Zifko et al., 1997
		Needle EMG of diaphragm	Bolton et al., 1992
		Automated interference pattern analysis of diaphragm	Collins, et al., 1997
		Power spectral analysis of diaphragm	Chen et al., 1996
Polyneuropathies	Peripheral nerves	Motor and sensory nerve conduction needle EMG	Bolton et al., 1986
Neuromuscular transmission defects	Neuromuscular junction	Repetitive limb nerve stimulation	Kimura, 1989
		Stimulated single-fiber EMG	Schwarz et al., 1997
Myopathies	Skeletal muscle	Motor and sensory nerve conduction needle EMG	Bolton et al., 1986
		Direct muscle stimulation	Rich et al., 1997
Other tests		Measurement of muscle force and "sound"	Bolton et al., 1989

EMG, electromyography.

mias or asystole. However, I often have stimulated near these sites in adults and children and have not had such complications. In the opinion of cardiology experts, the electrical stimuli are too small to cause an arrhythmia or asystole.

Patients with sepsis frequently have increased body temperature, which may spuriously decrease the latency and amplitude of compound muscle action potentials. Hence, the skin temperature of the limb should routinely be recorded. The use of near-nerve recordings may partially overcome recording difficulties in patients with edema. Repetitive nerve stimulation with recording of the compound muscle action potential may help to uncover neurotransmission defects.

In applying electrodes, it may be necessary to splint the patient's limb to avoid excessive movement that may loosen electrode contact. One should prepare the skin adequately to decrease resistance. One should clean the skin with alcohol, and then dry and rub it. Effective electrode paste, gel, or adhesive contacts should be used during needle EMG. If 60-Hz artifact cannot be eliminated, one should use the notch filter. Keep in mind that, in children, the underlying nerve, muscle, and bone may be near the skin surface. Hence, short needle electrodes should be used. The needle should be advanced through the tissues carefully, with one constantly monitoring the presence or absence of insertional activity to ensure that the needle is always in muscle. This caution is particularly relevant to needle EMG of the chest wall of children, in whom underlying muscle, including the diaphragm, may be near the skin surface.

During needle EMG of the diaphragm, it may be necessary to discontinue intermittent mandatory ventilation briefly, to observe the type of voluntary respirations, as reflected in the electrical activity from the diaphragm during inspiration. At this time, the patient should receive sufficient pressure support to supply oxygen, and the patient's condition should be monitored by observing the heart rate, respiration, and blood gas values. Mechanical ventilation should be resumed immediately if the patient appears to be in respiratory or cardiac distress.

If needle EMG of the diaphragm has been performed, it is wise to counsel the attending nurse that the patient's heart rate and respirations should be watched closely. If the patient seems in distress, the chest wall should be auscultated to determine whether the breath sounds are decreased on the side on which the procedure was performed. In the event of possible pneumothorax, emergency chest radiography should be performed. If pneumothorax occurs, one should insert a chest tube. This complication has occurred in only 2 of the 400 procedures that I have performed. Patients who appear to be at risk of this rare complication have asthma or chronic obstructive lung disease and are on a ventilator.

The series of steps I have taken in performing electrophysiological tests in the ICU are described in Table 81–4. The sympathetic skin response is tested before any other stimuli are applied, to avoid habituation. Needle EMG of the diaphragm is performed early, without sedation, so observations of motor unit potentials during inspiratory bursts will give an accurate idea of central drive, with a pressure support of 10 cm H_2O to overcome ventilator airway resistance. Next, a narcotic agent is given intravenously to make subsequent testing more comfortable; this is especially important for patients with Guillain-Barré syndrome, who find such testing uncomfortable.

The main conditions that are detected with this systematic approach are described briefly in the

Table 81–4. Order of Procedures for Electrophysiological Investigation of Neuromuscular Disorders in an Intensive Care Unit

1. Record skin temperature
2. Measure cardiac RR interval and sympathetic skin response
3. Needle electromyography of chest wall muscles or diaphragm (without sedative, on pressure support of 10 cm H_2O)
4. Intravenous administration of narcotic agent
5. Phrenic nerve conduction
6. Motor and sensory nerve conduction
7. Repetitive nerve stimulation: 3 and 20/s
8. Needle electromyography of limb muscles

next sections. These conditions, including ventilator disorders, are described in detail in other chapters.

SYNDROME OF ACUTE LIMB AND RESPIRATORY WEAKNESS DEVELOPING BEFORE ADMISSION TO THE INTENSIVE CARE UNIT

This category (see Table 81–2) involves patients who present with rapidly developing paralysis that includes the respiratory muscles; thus, endotracheal intubation and mechanical ventilation are necessary. The course may be so rapid that there is not sufficient time to make an accurate diagnosis. Thus, investigations must proceed after the patient is admitted to the ICU. In this acutely developing situation, clinical signs may be confusing. The differential diagnosis should be approached systematically, and the relevant conditions should be eliminated (see Fig. 81–3).

Brain

In my experience, somatosensory evoked potentials are valuable in determining the severity of *encephalopathy*, particularly anoxic-ischemic encephalopathy. Severe trauma or metabolic toxic illnesses affecting the brain may interfere with respiration through a lack of central drive to the extent that endotracheal intubation and mechanical ventilation are required. The results of limb conduction studies and phrenic nerve conduction studies are normal. Needle EMG of limb muscles shows an absence of or a decrease in the number of motor unit potentials. The pattern of firing of motor unit potentials in the diaphragm is abnormal, and this is of localizing value (see Fig. 81–1).

Spinal Cord Compression

In acute disorders of the high cervical spinal cord (see Fig. 81–2), for example, *compression* resulting from neoplasm or infection or acute transverse myelitis, the traditional signs of localized spinal cord

disease may be absent. Hyperreflexia is usually abolished by spinal shock, and the sensory level may be difficult to determine, particularly in high cervical lesions. Thus, magnetic resonance imaging of the spinal cord on an emergency basis is often necessary.

In motor conduction studies, the amplitude of compound muscle action potentials is decreased because of anterior horn cell disease when the injury occurred at least 5 days earlier. When sensory conduction is normal and clinical sensory loss is present, the lesion is proximal to the dorsal root ganglion, usually indicating myelopathy. Needle EMG abnormalities appear after a 10- to 20-day interval, depending on the distance between the muscle and the site of injury along the nerve. The pattern of needle EMG signs of denervation should assist in localizing the segmental level, in determining whether it is unilateral or bilateral, and in roughly estimating the number of segments involved, although the results may not be precise because of the considerable overlap of innervation, particularly of the paraspinal muscles. In somatosensory evoked potential studies, scalp recordings show delayed or absent potentials. Normal peripheral nerve and delayed or absent T12 responses suggest that the lesion is in the region of the cauda equina or lumbosacral plexus. Unless the spinal cord lesion clearly involves the somesthetic pathways, the results of somatosensory evoked potential studies may be normal even in the presence of a large spinal cord lesion.

Spinal Cord

If the high cervical *spinal cord* is damaged, endotracheal intubation and ventilation may be required. Conditions that may produce such lesions are trauma at birth, compression by neoplasm, hemorrhage, or infection, and acute transverse myelitis. The results of motor and sensory conduction studies of limb nerves are normal. Because the phrenic nerves arise from spinal segments C3-5, the amplitude of compound muscle action potentials from the diaphragm may be considerably reduced or absent, although latency is relatively preserved. Needle EMG shows an absence of or a decreased number of motor unit potentials. Muscles innervated by the involved high cervical segments demonstrate fibrillation potentials and positive sharp waves 2 weeks after the lesion occurs. To confirm the localization further, needle EMG of the cervical paraspinal and the shoulder muscles supplied predominantly by C4 (i.e., the upper border of the trapezius and the levator scapulae) should also show evidence of denervation.

In lesions of the lower cervical spinal cord, often caused by traumatic hyperextension injuries of the neck resulting in quadriplegia, respiratory difficulty is the result of upper motor neuron weakness of chest wall muscles. Thus, the findings of phrenic nerve conduction studies and needle EMG of the diaphragm are normal. However, there is a relative lack of firing of motor unit potentials from chest wall muscles, and fibrillation potentials and positive sharp waves are not present.

Motor Neuron Disease

Motor neuron disease may present—for the first time and initially undiagnosed—as severe respiratory insufficiency (Chen et al., 1996). The typical combined upper and lower motor neuron signs of hyporeflexia or hyperreflexia, muscle wasting and fasciculations, atrophy, and fasciculations of the tongue may not be obvious. Electrophysiological studies, including phrenic nerve conduction and needle EMG of the chest wall and diaphragm and comprehensive needle EMG of limb muscles, often suggest the diagnosis. However, it still may be necessary to proceed with magnetic resonance imaging studies. Atypical motor neuron disease, such as motor neuropathy with multifocal conduction block, should be excluded (Preston and Kelly, 1993).

Acute Polyneuropathy

Polyneuropathy is suspected (see Fig. 81–2) in the presence of muscle weakness, hyporeflexia, distal sensory loss, and the absence of upper motor neuron signs or bladder dysfunction, but these signs may not always be obvious. For example, bladder dysfunction and extensor plantar responses are seen occasionally in Guillain-Barré syndrome. Thus, electrophysiological studies are of great value.

In acute inflammatory demyelinating polyneuropathy (Guillain-Barré syndrome), the electrophysiological features are those of demyelination of peripheral nerve. In the initial stages, conduction velocities may be decreased only mildly, but the diagnosis is suggested by the prolongation or absence of F waves (Kimura, 1978), evidence of conduction block, and absence of abnormal spontaneous activity in muscle, with the remaining motor unit potentials firing rapidly. Thus, even within hours after onset, the findings often strongly suggest Guillain-Barré syndrome. Phrenic nerve conduction studies and needle EMG of the diaphragm are particularly valuable in establishing the type and severity of the involvement of the phrenic nerve and diaphragm (Markand et al., 1984; Zifko et al., 1996a). Serial electrophysiological studies to follow the course of treatment, such as plasmapheresis, hyperimmune globulin, or corticosteroids, are valuable. However, in my experience, symptomatic improvement may precede electrophysiological improvement.

Several variants of Guillain-Barré syndrome are primarily axonal, rather than demyelinating. All of them are likely to have (but not in every case) *Campylobacter jejuni* as the factor precipitating the immune-mediated polyneuropathy. These variants

are discussed later (except the Miller Fisher variant—ophthalmoplegia, ataxia, and areflexia—which rarely requires admission to the ICU). Positive results on serological testing or stool culture for *C. jejuni* may be the earliest evidence of these axonal variants (Bolton, 1995).

The acute axonal form of Guillain-Barré syndrome, now called *acute motor and sensory axonal neuropathy* (Feasby et al., 1986), usually presents with a rapidly developing paralysis that reaches completion within hours and requires early admission to the ICU and full ventilatory assistance. Although the severity of the condition varies, all muscles of the body, including cranial, eye, and pupillary muscles, may be completely paralyzed. Thus, clinically, acute motor and sensory axonal neuropathy simulates the syndrome of brain death, but the electroencephalogram is relatively normal. All peripheral nerves, including cranial nerves, may be unresponsive to electrical stimulation, even with stimuli of high voltage and long duration. Often, sensory and muscle compound action potentials are reduced or absent.

In acute paralytic syndromes of children and young adults (McKhann et al., 1991), now called *acute motor axonal neuropathy,* a symmetrical ascending weakness develops over days, sensation is normal, deep tendon reflexes are often preserved, and the concentration of protein in the cerebrospinal fluid is increased. The electrophysiological features are consistent with a pure motor dysfunction, a primary dysfunction of anterior horn cells or proximal axons. The amplitude of muscle compound action potentials is reduced, but the latency is normal. Sensory conduction is normal. There are various degrees of muscle denervation. Respiratory paralysis may be significant. Good recovery eventually occurs. This is a variant of Guillain-Barré syndrome and can be related to *C. jejuni* enteritis and G_{M1} antibodies (Hartung et al., 1995).

Other polyneuropathies, such as acute porphyria, should also be considered and excluded when necessary. If there is any suspicion of Lyme disease or human immunodeficiency virus (HIV) infection, the appropriate antibody tests should be performed.

Chronic Polyneuropathies

Occasionally, *chronic polyneuropathies* evolve as rapidly developing respiratory insufficiency. Although rare, this situation may occur in chronic inflammatory demyelinating polyneuropathy and diabetic polyneuropathy. In addition to noting the more typical clinical and electrophysiological signs of these polyneuropathies, it is worthwhile to perform phrenic nerve conduction studies and needle EMG of the diaphragm to demonstrate that the respiratory insufficiency results from the neuropathy.

Neuromuscular Transmission Defects

Defects in neuromuscular transmission (see Fig. 81–2) are rare but present particular challenges in diagnosis. Both myasthenia gravis (Maher et al., 1998) and Lambert-Eaton myasthenic syndrome (Nicolle et al., 1996) may present, for the first time with respiratory insufficiency. Rarely, patients with *myasthenia gravis* may present for the first time in respiratory failure, in which weakness tends to involve particularly the muscles of swallowing and breathing. This appears to be a syndrome. Levels of acetylcholine antibodies are normal, a rare variant of myasthenia gravis (Burges et al., 1994), and the results of repetitive nerve stimulation studies are often normal. The diagnosis of myasthenia gravis rests on the variability in the weakness of the eye and facial muscles and positive findings on the edrophonium (Tensilon) test and single-fiber EMG. Phrenic nerve conduction and needle EMG studies of the diaphragm may demonstrate partial denervation of the diaphragm. The condition of the patient improves with immunosuppressive therapy. The respiratory muscles strengthen, and the patient is successfully weaned from the ventilator.

Other types of presynaptic neuromuscular transmission defects—Lambert-Eaton myasthenic syndrome, hypocalcemia, hypermagnesemia, and wound botulism—may also be identified electrophysiologically. In organophosphate poisoning, a repetitive discharge appearing after a single electrical shock to a peripheral nerve is diagnostic. The effective maneuver in diagnosing tick-bite paralysis is to search carefully for the tick and to remove it.

Myopathies

Myopathies usually do not pose a difficult diagnostic problem (see Fig. 81–2), because the diagnosis is usually evident, having been established previously in chronic cases such as muscular dystrophy. However, respiratory muscles occasionally are involved, and these patients require intubation and admission to the ICU. In acute myopathies, such as necrotizing myopathy with myoglobinuria, the diagnosis is evident because of the high levels of creatinine phosphokinase and, at times, myoglobinuria and evidence of muscle necrosis on muscle biopsy.

SYNDROME OF ACUTE LIMB AND RESPIRATORY WEAKNESS DEVELOPING AFTER ADMISSION TO THE INTENSIVE CARE UNIT

In large medical and surgical ICUs, I have estimated that at least 50% of patients have significant involvement of the nervous system. Neuromuscular problems are more frequent than generally recognized. Sepsis and multiple organ failure now occur in 20% to 50% of patients in a medical ICU (Tran et al., 1990), and 70% of these patients have critical illness polyneuropathy (Witt et al., 1991). Neuromuscular blocking agents and corticosteroids may cause

other distinctive neuromuscular syndromes (Bolton et al., 1994). Because of the difficulty in clinically evaluating these patients, neuromuscular problems can be identified only through electrophysiological testing (Bolton, 1987), at times supplemented by muscle and, rarely, nerve biopsy. These investigations aid in managing problems such as difficulty in weaning from the ventilator and limb weakness during recovery. The subject has been reviewed in the literature (Leijten and de Weerd, 1994; Bolton, 1996b; Hund, 1996).

Myelopathy

Myelopathies seen in the ICU are classified as follows: traumatic; compressive from neoplasm, hemorrhage, or infection in the epidural space; and vascular, such as spinal cord infarction resulting from surgical procedures on the aorta. However, in almost all cases, the myelopathy will have occurred before admission to the ICU and will have been managed as described earlier. If not, magnetic resonance imaging is of great diagnostic value.

Critical Illness Polyneuropathies

Critical illness polyneuropathy is the most common polyneuropathy seen in the ICU and is a regular complication of the syndrome of sepsis and multiple organ failure (Bolton et al., 1984; Couturier et al., 1984; Zochodne et al., 1987). It is manifested as difficulty in weaning from the ventilator and various degrees of limb weakness, just at the time the patient seems to be recovering from the sepsis syndrome. It may be the most common cause of long-term ventilator dependence (Spitzer et al., 1992). Only severe polyneuropathies cause obvious clinical signs, but electrophysiological studies demonstrate the presence of pure axonal (predominantly motor) and sensory polyneuropathy. Phrenic nerve conduction studies and needle EMG of the diaphragm (Bolton, 1993b) and chest wall muscles provide additional and more direct evidence of involvement of the neuromuscular respiratory system. In mild cases, recovery occurs in a matter of weeks and, in severe cases, in a matter of months. Serial electrophysiological studies are often valuable in determining the ultimate prognosis and in gauging the rate of recovery. However, patients with particularly severe polyneuropathies may not recover.

Neuromuscular Transmission Defects

The most common type of *neuromuscular transmission defect* seen in the ICU results from the use of neuromuscular blocking agents. The frequency of the use of these agents in ICUs varies considerably.

These drugs are used to decrease metabolic demands, to prevent shivering or "fighting" with the ventilator, to decrease intracranial pressure, and to improve chest compliance (Partridge et al., 1990). In the ICU at Victoria Hospital, London, Canada, neuromuscular blocking agents have been used infrequently, and systematic studies of critically ill patients by repetitive nerve stimulation have failed to demonstrate a defect in neuromuscular transmission, aside from the phenomenon of pseudofacilitation, a normal variation (Bolton et al., 1986). Instead, in critically ill patients, the limb weakness and difficulty in weaning from the ventilator are usually shown to have resulted from critical illness polyneuropathy or myopathy (Zochodne et al., 1987).

Reports have delineated three relatively distinct syndromes associated with the use of neuromuscular blocking agents. In the first syndrome (Gooch et al., 1991), a critically ill patient in the ICU is given neuromuscular blocking agents, either vecuronium or pancuronium bromide, for longer than 48 hours to ease ventilation, and when this treatment is stopped the patient develops quadriplegia and, later, cannot be weaned from the ventilator. Electrophysiological studies have shown a relatively pure axonal degeneration, varying increases in the creatinine phosphokinase level, and, on muscle biopsy, mixed features of denervation and muscle fiber necrosis. Recovery usually occurs over a matter of weeks or a few months, depending on the severity. This syndrome probably is a variant of critical illness polyneuropathy. The predominant involvement of distal motor axons causes motor unit potentials to appear "myopathic" on needle EMG.

In the second syndrome (Danon and Carpenter, 1991; Hirano et al., 1992; Lacomis et al., 1993), a previously healthy, usually young person or child develops severe asthma that requires large doses of corticosteroids, neuromuscular blocking agents, and full mechanical ventilation for several days. This syndrome may also be seen after an organ transplantation operation, in which neuromuscular blocking agents and corticosteroids are regularly used (Lacomis et al., 1996). These two syndromes, which have been called *acute quadriplegic myopathy* (Hirano et al., 1992), should be called *critical illness myopathy* (see Chapters 82 and 83). After discontinuation of this therapy, the patient has quadriplegia and cannot be weaned from the ventilator. Electrophysiological studies often point to primary myopathy. Creatinine phosphokinase levels may be variably increased. However, the distinctive feature appears on muscle biopsy. Certain stains show a loss of structure of muscle fibers centrally. Electron microscopy shows that this results from a loss of thick filaments. Various amounts of muscle necrosis may also be seen. Spontaneous and relatively satisfactory recovery occurs.

In the third syndrome, pancuronium bromide or vecuronium is given to a patient with renal failure. Because of renal failure, the neuromuscular blockade may be prolonged for several weeks after the treatment has been discontinued. In this syndrome, repetitive nerve stimulation studies demonstrate typical postsynaptic neuromuscular transmission. Prompt recovery should occur (Segredo et al., 1992). These three syndromes may occur in various combinations and, in many patients, sepsis or systemic inflammatory response syndrome and critical illness polyneuropathy may be key underlying factors.

Myopathies

Traditionally, generalized *wasting of muscle* has been attributed to disuse atrophy or catabolic myopathy (Roussos and Macklem, 1982; Penn, 1986). Although wasting of muscle clearly causes muscle weakness, it is accompanied by normal electrophysiological results and normal levels of creatinine phosphokinase. Muscle biopsy findings may be normal or may show type II muscle fiber atrophy. In my experience, the most common cause of muscle wasting has been critical illness polyneuropathy. In addition to denervation atrophy, occasional scattered necrotic muscle fibers have been noted, and this may explain the mild increase in the creatinine phosphokinase level in a few of our patients who had sepsis and multiple organ failure.

Panfascicular muscle fiber necrosis occurs acutely with various precipitating factors, including infection, drugs, and fever (Penn, 1986). Because of the high incidence of infection and various medications in the ICU, this condition would be expected to be more common than it is. Ramsay et al. called this "necrotizing myopathy of intensive care" (Ramsay et al., 1993). Patients develop severe muscle weakness and tenderness. Creatinine phosphokinase levels are high, and myoglobinuria may develop. Electrophysiological studies may be normal or may show some abnormal spontaneous activity. The diagnosis is made on the basis of biopsy findings, which demonstrate diffuse necrosis, possibly with some inflammatory reaction. Recovery usually occurs promptly, but four of the five patients reported by Ramsay et al. did not show recovery (Ramsay et al., 1993).

The prevalence of myopathy may vary according to the type of patient admitted to the ICU. It was especially high in the study by Lacomis et al. (Lacomis et al., 1998), in 39 of 92 patients studied electrophysiologically. The high prevalence may result from the frequent administration of neuromuscular blocking agents and corticosteroids.

DIFFICULTY IN WEANING FROM THE VENTILATOR AND ELECTROPHYSIOLOGICAL STUDIES OF THE RESPIRATORY SYSTEM

The techniques of phrenic nerve conduction and needle EMG of the diaphragm (Bolton, 1993a; Bolton,

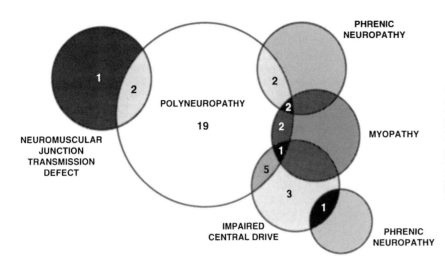

Figure 81–4. The types of neuromuscular disorders among 40 patients who could not be weaned from ventilation. Thirty-eight (95%) had a neuromuscular disorder, and 15 (38%) had a combination of disorders. (From Maher J, Rutledge F, Remtulla H, et al: Neuromuscular disorders associated with failure to wean from the ventilator. Intensive Care Med 1995; 21:737–743. By permission of Springer-Verlag, Berlin, 1995.)

1993b) have proved valuable in establishing that respiratory insufficiency is caused by a neuromuscular disorder. The techniques determine impairment of "central drive": a disturbance of the voluntary or automatic centers of respiration or disorders of the phrenic nerves, neuromuscular junction, or muscle. For example, in patients with Guillain-Barré syndrome, the degree of involvement of the phrenic nerves can be determined, and this supplements measurements, including vital capacity, in determining the need for respiratory assistance (Zifko et al., 1996a). Documenting the degree of axonal degeneration or demyelination of phrenic nerves helps with long-term prognostication. In a study of 40 patients with difficulty in being weaned from the ventilator when a neuromuscular cause was suspected, 38 were shown to have a neuromuscular cause (Fig. 81–4) (Maher et al., 1995). Most of these patients had critical illness polyneuropathy, but there were various combinations of unilateral phrenic nerve damage, neuromuscular transmission defects, and primary myopathies. Combined electrophysiological studies of limbs and the respiratory system greatly assisted in identifying these conditions and in rendering a prognosis. For a detailed discussion of neuromuscular respiratory insufficiency in the ICU, see Chapter 84.

Mononeuropathies

Damage to the brachial or lumbosacral plexus or to peripheral nerves may occur by various mechanisms before or after admission to the ICU. *Mononeuropathies* are often difficult to evaluate clinically, and electrophysiological or imaging studies are often necessary to establish the diagnosis. In the study by Lacomis et al., the incidence was 11% (Lacomis et al., 1998).

Mononeuropathy Syndromes

Lumbosacral or brachial plexopathies may result from direct trauma, usually from a motor vehicle

accident or surgical procedure. Insertion of catheters into the iliac arteries or aorta may dislodge thrombi, and the embolization that results will impair the vascular supply of nerves and thus will produce focal ischemic plexopathy (Wilbourn et al., 1983). Direct surgical trauma to vessels may also produce vascular insufficiency.

Motorcycle accidents commonly traumatize the brachial plexus. Proximal lesions are suggested by Horner's syndrome, winging of the scapula, and paralysis of the diaphragm. Electrophysiological studies, ideally performed at least 3 weeks after the event, further help to localize the lesion. Myelography, computed tomographic myelography, or magnetic resonance imaging may provide more positive evidence of root avulsion that would preclude attempts at operative nerve repair.

Fractures of the pelvis may cause various patterns of damage to the lumbosacral plexus. Observations of focal weakness on reflex or voluntarily induced movement in combination with abnormalities of the deep tendon reflexes may provide an initial clue to the presence of plexopathy. Thus, weakness of hip adduction and flexion and knee extension and the absence of the knee jerk suggest damage to L2-4 roots of the lumbosacral plexus. Electrophysiological studies should demonstrate abnormalities on motor and sensory nerve conduction and, in particular, on needle EMG, which would localize the lesion to the brachial or lumbosacral plexus.

There are several types of *mononeuropathies.* If the primary reason for admitting the patient to the ICU is the postoperative state, the surgical procedure may have produced mononeuropathy when operating room equipment or perhaps the operation itself directly damaged peripheral nerves. Various limb nerves can be damaged by trauma. For example, weakness of dorsiflexion of the wrist and digits and the absence of a brachioradialis reflex suggest damage of the radial nerve in the spiral groove of the humerus by fracture or direct compression. Phrenic nerves, either bilaterally or unilaterally, may be damaged at operation by direct trauma or the application of cold (e.g., the hypothermia associated with cardiac surgery) (Abd et al., 1989).

More distal nerves may be damaged from impaired nutrient blood supply through distal embolization. Thus, after cardiac or vascular surgery, patients may have different combinations of femoral or sciatic nerve (or both) damage. Electrophysiological studies demonstrate axonal degeneration of motor and sensory fibers.

Patients receiving anticoagulation are at risk of hemorrhage. A sudden increase in tissue pressure from local bleeding may produce a *compartment syndrome,* resulting in ischemia to nerve as well as muscle. The compartments most commonly involved are the iliopsoas and gluteal, and the condition produces acute femoral or sciatic nerve damage (Matsen, 1980). Fractures and soft tissue trauma may also produce compartment syndromes. Urgent computed tomography should be performed to identify the location of the hemorrhage and to allow surgical decompression of the nerve. Electrophysiological studies may be less helpful in this emergency situation.

References

Abd AG, Braun NM, Baskin MI, et al: Diaphragmatic dysfunction after open heart surgery: Treatment with a rocking bed. Ann Intern Med 1989;111:881–886.

Aminoff MJ, Eisen AA: AAEM minimonograph 19: Somatosensory evoked potentials. Muscle Nerve 1998;21:277–290.

Bolton CF: Electrophysiologic studies of critically ill patients. Muscle Nerve 1987;10:129–135.

Bolton CF: AAEM minimonograph 40: Clinical neurophysiology of the respiratory system. Muscle Nerve 1993a;16:809–818.

Bolton CF: EMG in the critical care unit. In Brown WF, Bolton CF (eds): Clinical Electromyography, 2nd ed. Boston, Butterworth-Heinemann, 1993b;759–773.

Bolton CF: The changing concepts of Guillain-Barré syndrome. N Engl J Med 1995;333:1415–1417.

Bolton CF: Electromyography in the critical care unit. In Jones HR Jr, Bolton CF, Harper CM Jr (eds): Pediatric Clinical Electromyography. Philadelphia, Lippincott—Raven, 1996a;445–466.

Bolton CF: Sepsis and the systemic inflammatory response syndrome: Neuromuscular manifestations. Crit Care Med 1996b;24: 1408–1416.

Bolton CF, Gilbert JJ, Hahn AF, Sibbald WJ: Polyneuropathy in critically ill patients. J Neurol Neurosurg Psychiatry 1984;47: 1223–1231.

Bolton CF, Grand'Maison F, Parkes A, Shkrum M: Needle electromyography of the diaphragm. Muscle Nerve 1992;15:678–681.

Bolton CF, Laverty DA, Brown JD, et al: Critically ill polyneuropathy: Electrophysiological studies and differentiation from Guillain-Barré syndrome. J Neurol Neurosurg Psychiatry 1986;49: 563–573.

Bolton CF, Parkes A, Thompson TR, et al: Recording sound from human skeletal muscle: Technical and physiological aspects. Muscle Nerve 1989;12:126–134.

Bolton CF, Young GB: Neurological changes during severe sepsis. In Dobb GJ, Bion J, Burchardi H, Dellinger RP (eds): Current Topics in Intensive Care. London, WB Saunders, 1994;180–217.

Burges J, Vincent A, Molenaar PC, et al: Passive transfer of seronegative myasthenia gravis to mice. Muscle Nerve 1994;17: 1393–1400.

Chen R, Collins S, Remtulla H, et al: Phrenic nerve conduction study in normal subjects. Muscle Nerve 1995;18:330–335.

Chen R, Collins SJ, Remtulla H, et al: Needle EMG of the human diaphragm: Power spectral analysis in normal subjects. Muscle Nerve 1996;19:324–330.

Collins SJ, Chen RE, Remtulla H, et al: Novel measurement for automated interference pattern analysis of the diaphragm. Muscle Nerve 1997;20:1038–1040.

Couturier JC, Robert D, Monier P: Polyneurites compliquant des séjours prolongés en réanimation: À propos de 1 cas d'étiologie encore enconnue. Lyon Med 1984;252:247–249.

Danon MJ, Carpenter S: Myopathy with thick filament (myosin) loss following prolonged paralysis with vecuronium during steroid treatment. Muscle Nerve 1991;14:1131–1139.

Feasby TE, Gilbert JJ, Brown WF, et al: An acute axonal form of Guillain-Barré polyneuropathy. Brain 1986;109:1115–1126.

Gooch JL, Suchyta MR, Balbierz JM, et al: Prolonged paralysis after treatment with neuromuscular junction blocking agents. Crit Care Med 1991;19:1125–1131.

Hartung HP, Pollard JD, Harvey GK, Toyka KV: Immunopathogenesis and treatment of the Guillain-Barré syndrome. Part II. Muscle Nerve 1995;18:154–164.

Hirano M, Ott BR, Raps EC, et al: Acute quadriplegic myopathy: A complication of treatment with steroids, nondepolarizing blocking agents, or both. Neurology 1992;42:2082–2087.

Hund EF: Neuromuscular complications in the ICU: The spectrum of critical illness-related conditions causing muscular weakness and weaning failure. J Neurol Sci 1996;136:10–16.

Kimura J: Proximal versus distal slowing of motor nerve conduction velocity in the Guillain-Barré syndrome. Ann Neurol 1978; 3:344–350.

Kimura J: Electrodiagnosis in Diseases of Nerve and Muscle: Principles and Practice, 2nd ed. Philadelphia, FA Davis, 1989;184–200.

Lacomis D, Giuliani MJ, Van Cott A, Kramer DJ: Acute myopathy of intensive care: Clinical, electromyographic, and pathological aspects. Ann Neurol 1996;40:645–654.

Lacomis D, Petrella JT, Giuliani MJ: Causes of neuromuscular weakness in the intensive care unit: A study of ninety-two patients. Muscle Nerve 1998;21:610–617.

Lacomis D, Smith TW, Chad DA: Acute myopathy and neuropathy in status asthmaticus: Case report and literature review. Muscle Nerve 1993;16:84–90.

Leijten FS, de Weerd AW: Critical illness polyneuropathy: A review of the literature, definition and pathophysiology. Clin Neurol Neurosurg 1994;96:10–19.

Maher J, Grand'Maison F, Nicolle MW, et al: Diagnostic difficulties in myasthenia gravis. Muscle Nerve 1998;21:577–583.

Maher J, Rutledge F, Remtulla H, et al: Neuromuscular disorders associated with failure to wean from the ventilator. Intensive Care Med 1995;21:737–743.

Markand ON, Kincaid JC, Pourmand RA, et al: Electrophysiologic evaluation of diaphragm by transcutaneous phrenic nerve stimulation. Neurology 1984;34:604–614.

Matsen FA III: Compartmental Syndromes. New York, Grune & Stratton, 1980.

McKhann GM, Cornblath DR, Ho T, et al: Clinical and electrophysiological aspects of acute paralytic disease of children and young adults in northern China. Lancet 1991;338:593–597.

Nicolle MW, Stewart DJ, Remtulla H, et al: Lambert-Eaton myasthenic syndrome presenting with severe respiratory failure. Muscle Nerve 1996;19:1328–1333.

Partridge BL, Abrams JH, Bazemore C, Rubin R: Prolonged neuromuscular blockade after long-term infusion of vecuronium bromide in the intensive care unit. Crit Care Med 1990;18:1177–1179.

Penn A: Myoglobinuria. In Engel AG, Banker BQ (eds): Myology: Basic and Clinical, vol 2. New York, McGraw-Hill, 1986;1792–1793.

Picton TW, Taylor MJ, Durieux-Smith A: Brainstem auditory evoked potentials in infants and children. In Aminoff MJ (ed): Electrodiagnosis in Clinical Neurology, 4th ed. New York, Churchill-Livingstone, 1999;485–511.

Preston DC, Kelly JJ Jr: Atypical motor neuron disease. In Brown WF, Bolton CF (eds): Clinical Electromyography, 2nd ed. Boston, Butterworth-Heinemann, 1993;451–476.

Ramsay DA, Zochodne DW, Robertson DM, et al: A syndrome of acute severe muscle necrosis in intensive care unit patients. J Neuropathol Exp Neurol 1993;52:387–398.

Rich MM, Bird SJ, Raps EC, et al: Direct muscle stimulation in acute quadriplegic myopathy. Muscle Nerve 1997;20:665–673.

Roussos C, Macklem PT: The respiratory muscles. N Engl J Med 1982;307:786–797.

Schwarz J, Planck J, Briegel J, Straube A: Single-fiber electromyography, nerve conduction studies, and conventional electromyography in patients with critical-illness polyneuropathy: Evidence for a lesion of terminal motor axons. Muscle Nerve 1997; 20:696–701.

Segredo V, Caldwell JE, Matthay MA, et al: Persistent paralysis in critically ill patients after long-term administration of vecuronium. N Engl J Med 1992;327:524–528.

Spitzer AR, Giancarlo T, Maher L, et al: Neuromuscular causes of prolonged ventilator dependency. Muscle Nerve 1992;15:682–686.

Tran DD, Groeneveld AB, van der Meulen J, et al: Age, chronic disease, sepsis, organ system failure, and mortality in a medical intensive care unit. Crit Care Med 1990;18:474–479.

Wilbourn AJ, Furlan AJ, Hulley W, Ruschhaupt W: Ischemic monomelic neuropathy. Neurology 1983;33:447–451.

Witt NJ, Zochodne DW, Bolton CF, et al: Peripheral nerve function in sepsis and multiple organ failure. Chest 1991;99:176–184.

Zifko U, Chen R, Remtulla H, et al: Respiratory electrophysiological studies in Guillain-Barré syndrome. J Neurol Neurosurg Psychiatry 1996a;60:191–194.

Zifko U, Nicolle MW, Remtulla H, Bolton CF: Repetitive phrenic nerve stimulation study in normal subjects. J Clin Neurophysiol 1997;14:235–241.

Zifko U, Remtulla H, Power K, et al: Transcortical and cervical magnetic stimulation with recording of the diaphragm. Muscle Nerve 1996b;19:614–620.

Zifko UA, Young BG, Remtulla H, Bolton CF: Somatosensory evoked potentials of the phrenic nerve. Muscle Nerve 1995;18: 1487–1489.

Zochodne DW, Bolton CF, Wells GA, et al: Critical illness polyneuropathy: A complication of sepsis and multiple organ failure. Brain 1987;110:819–841.

Acute Polyneuropathies Encountered in the Intensive Care Unit

Marie-An C. J. de Letter and Leo H. Visser

MUSCLE WEAKNESS IN THE INTENSIVE CARE UNIT

Neuromuscular disorders are said to be encountered in approximately 1.5% of the patients in the intensive care unit. These disorders can be divided into two categories of patients (see Chapter 81). One category of patients is admitted to the intensive care unit due to an underlying neuromuscular disorder, mainly Guillain-Barré syndrome and myasthenia gravis. In the other category of patients, a so-called acquired neuromuscular disorder develops during their stay in the intensive care unit after admission for other reasons (e.g., multitrauma, severe infections, [multiple] organ dysfunction, and so on). In this second group of patients, the symptoms mainly consist of muscle weakness, wasting, and difficulties in weaning from the artificial respirator. The acquired muscle weakness after admission to the intensive care unit can be due to the following.

- A polyneuropathy such as critical illness polyneuropathy (CIP), which is an axonal motor or a sensorimotor polyneuropathy; however, the histopathology shows myopathic changes in a notable proportion of the patients
- A neuromuscular transmission defect due to a transient neuromuscular blockade related to the use of neuromuscular blocking agents
- A myopathy consisting of (1) critical illness myopathy (Gutmann, 1999; Hund, 1999), in which both

electrophysiological and histopathological features are consistent with a myopathy—frequently not the case, so we consider them part of CIP; (2) myopathy with thick filament loss, critical illness myopathy, or acute quadriplegic myopathy (Danon and Carpenter, 1991; Douglas et al., 1992; Hirano et al., 1992; Lacomis et al., 1996); and (3) acute necrotizing myopathy of intensive care (Ramsay et al., 1993; Bolton, 1994; Zochodne et al., 1994).

The clinical assessment of patients with muscle weakness is described in Chapter 81. In this chapter, CIP is discussed. Both neuromuscular transmission defects and the myopathies encountered in the intensive care unit are discussed in Chapter 83.

CRITICAL ILLNESS POLYNEUROPATHY

History

The most frequent cause of the acquired neuromuscular disorders in the intensive care unit is CIP. The first detailed reports of CIP were published in the early 1980s by Bolton and associates (1984, 1986), Op de Coul and colleagues (1985), Roelofs and associates (1983), and Couturier and colleagues (1984). All of the reported patients were admitted to the intensive care unit, requiring artificial respiration and multiple drugs, such as sedatives, neuro-muscular blocking agents (Op de Coul et al., 1985, 1991; Gooch et al., 1991; Kupfer et al., 1991; Rossiter et al., 1991; Subramony et al., 1991), steroids (Mac-Farlane and Rosenthal, 1977; Lacomis et al., 1996), and antibiotics. The relationship of CIP with sepsis was established in important prospective studies (Witt et al., 1991; Berek et al., 1996; Hund et al., 1996; Zifko et al., 1998).

Clinical Features

The clinical features of CIP are muscle weakness, wasting, decreased or absent tendon reflexes, and difficulties in weaning from the artificial respirator. Due to the variability of its clinical features, CIP can be easily overlooked after a patient has had a prolonged stay in the intensive care unit (Coakley et al., 1992). The muscle weakness is most promi-nent in the lower extremities and located more distal than proximal. The exact onset of these symptoms can be difficult to determine due to the use of neuro-muscular blocking agents or sedatives. Approxi-mately 3 days after the discontinuation of neuro-muscular blocking agents, both clinical and electrophysiological testing of the motor functions is reliable and the motor symptoms become evident. In many instances, difficulty in weaning from the artificial respirator is the prevailing symptom of CIP and a reason to consult the neurologist. Muscle wasting is observed in one third of the patients (Zifko et al., 1998). Reflexes are usually absent, but this is not a prerequisite for the diagnosis (Hund et al., 1996). Sensory symptoms are often difficult to test in the sedated or intubated patients in the inten-sive care unit. The presence of pain or paresthesias, however, mostly suggests a polyneuropathy second-ary to the use of metronidazole; this primarily af-fects the sensory nerve fibers (Witt et al., 1991). Zifko and colleagues (1998) found that reliable infor-mation on sensation could be obtained in 17 of the 62 patients with CIP (27%). Ten of the patients had distal, symmetrical hypesthesia. Impaired con-sciousness, suggestive of an encephalopathy, is of-ten present, which makes clinical testing even more unreliable. Leijten and associates (1997) found that the sensitivity of the clinical judgment of CIP was 60% compared with concurrent polyneuropathy di-agnosed with electromyography.

CIP is often preceded by critical illness encepha-lopathy, which is a poorly recognized illness. The clinical features of the encephalopathy are impaired attention, concentration, orientation, and writing (Jackson et al., 1985; Young et al., 1990). The pres-ence of excessive theta activity on the electroen-cephalogram may be helpful in the diagnostic pro-cess (Young et al., 1992).

Electrophysiological Features

Electrophysiological testing demonstrates depres-sion of the amplitudes of the compound muscle action potentials within 1 week of the onset of CIP. Conduction velocities, distal motor latencies, and responses to repetitive nerve stimulation are nor-mal. A sensory conduction examination can show decreased sensory nerve action potential ampli-tudes, which confirms the presence of a polyneurop-athy. Such information is usually obtained by serial monitoring.

Needle electromyography reveals the spontane-ous activity of muscle fibers at rest and is more abundant in distal than in proximal muscles. Sponta-neous activity is usually present 3 weeks after the start of artificial respiration (Bolton, 1996); however, it can be found within the first 2 weeks (Op de Coul et al., 1991). Sometimes there are signs of myopathic changes in the motor unit potentials, with a short duration and low amplitudes on voluntary activa-tion.

Dysfunction of the neuromuscular junction in in-tensive care unit patients due to a preexisting disor-der or the toxic effect of neuromuscular blocking agents or aminoglycosides can be excluded by re-petitive nerve stimulation (Segredo et al., 1992). The somatosensory evoked potentials can be tested for disturbances of the spinal dorsal columns.

Diaphragm and chest wall needle electromyogra-phy, especially when performed on patients who fail to wean from the ventilator, shows spontaneous activity of the diaphragm (Bolton, 1993a; Zifko et al., 1998) (see Chapter 96).

Proposed Diagnostic Criteria

There are no uniform diagnostic criteria for CIP. To diagnose CIP, the clinical and electrophysiologi-cal features should be present. The criteria that we used in a prospective study are listed in Table 82–1.

Incidence and Characteristics

In a prospective study, Lacomis and associates (1998) monitored the incidence of neuromuscular disorders in 92 patients in the intensive care unit. This revealed a myopathy in 39 (42%) and a polyneu-ropathy in 26 (28%) of the patients with neuromus-cular disorders. The polyneuropathies were of the demyelinating type (Guillain-Barré syndrome) in 13 patients, acquired (in the intensive care unit) axonal type in 12 patients, and preexistent axonal type in 1 patient. The relatively high incidence of myopathies could be related to the high percentage of organ transplantations and the use of high-dose steroids in this study group. Prospective studies on CIP re-vealed an incidence of 33% to 44% of CIP in patients who were on an artificial respirator for at least 1 week (Coakley et al., 1993; Leijten et al., 1995; De Letter et al., 2000a). In patients with sepsis, the incidence increased to 70% (Witt et al., 1991; Hund et al., 1997).

All age groups are involved, but CIP is rare in

Table 82-1. Diagnostic Criteria of Critical Illness Polyneuropathy

Clinical
  No use of neuromuscular blocking agents for at least 3 d
  Motor sum score <26 (see Natural History)
  Decreased or absent tendon reflexes
  Findings present on at least two subsequent visits, which were performed two times weekly
AND
Electrophysiological
  1. CMAP amplitude in ulnar nerve absent or decreased below
    Wrist stimulation <4.2 mV
    Below elbow stimulation <3.7 mV
    Above elbow stimulation <4.0 mV
  AND
  CMAP amplitude in peroneal nerve absent or decreased below
    Ankle stimulation <2.6 mV
    Below knee stimulation <2.6 mV
    Above knee stimulation <2.6 mV
  2. CMAP amplitude in ulnar or peroneal nerve absent or decreased (as mentioned above)
AND
  At least one of the following criteria
    1. Spontaneous muscle fiber activity at rest (fibrillations or positive waves) in at least two of the examined muscles.
    2. Ratio of the area of the proximal CMAP versus the distal CMAP >0.89 in the nerve with decreased CMAP amplitude.
    3. SNAP amplitude in ulnar nerve <18 μV or SNAP amplitude in sural nerve <10 μV

CMAP, compound motor action potential; SNAP, sensory nerve action potential.

children (Gooch, 1995), and most patients are older than 50 years. Males predominate in CIP, with an approximate ratio of 2:1 (Bolton and Breuer, 1999). The main reasons for admission to the intensive care unit of the patients who develop CIP are severe trauma, infections, and major surgery.

Risk Factors

Factors that contribute to the development of CIP, the so-called risk factors, were determined in our prospective study. During a follow-up period of 1.5 years, all patients in the intensive care unit were monitored clinically and electrophysiologically from day 4 of the start of artificial respiration. The occurrence of CIP was related to the Acute Physiology, Age and Chronic Health Evaluation (APACHE)-III score and the presence of systemic inflammatory response syndrome (De Letter et al., 1999). The APACHE-III score is a methodology that is used to predict hospital mortality risk for critically ill hospitalized adults (Knaus et al., 1991; Friedland et al., 1996). The score is the sum for three groups of variables that concern physiology, age, and long-term health. The physiology is represented in weighted laboratory abnormalities and vital signs (pulse, mean blood pressure, temperature, respiratory rate, PaO_2, hematocrit, white blood cell count, creatinine, urine output, blood urea nitrogen, sodium, serum albumin, bilirubin, and glucose) (Knaus

et al., 1991). The presence of systemic inflammatory response syndrome includes two or more of the following clinical manifestations: (1) body temperature greater than 38°C or less than 36°C; (2) heart rate greater than 90 beats per minute; (3) tachypnea, manifested by a respiratory rate greater than 20 breaths per minute, or hyperventilation as indicated by $PaCO_2$ of less than 32 mm Hg; and (4) alteration in the white blood cell count, such as a count greater than 12,000/mm^3, a count less than 4,000/mm^3, or the presence of more than 10% immature neutrophils (Bone et al., 1992).

The risk of the development of CIP in the study was 72% whenever the APACHE-III score was greater than 85 and systemic inflammatory response syndrome was present. These patients belong to the high-risk group ($n = 22$) for the development of CIP (Fig. 82-1). In the low-risk group ($n = 16$), the APACHE-III score was less than 70 and systemic inflammatory response syndrome was not present. All other patients belonged to the medium-risk group ($n = 62$).

Natural History

The electrophysiological changes of CIP show both motor and sensory axonal dysfunctions of upper and lower extremities (Zochodne et al., 1987; Witt et al., 1991; Coakley et al., 1993; Latronico et al., 1996); however, Hund and colleagues (1997) showed normal sensory nerve action potential amplitudes.

In the prospective study by Berek and associates (1996) of 22 patients with sepsis, systemic inflammatory response syndrome, or multiple organ dysfunction syndrome, 9 patients (41%) had clinical signs of a polyneuropathy during their stay in the intensive care unit and 7 patients (32%) showed these features 2 to 3 months later. In an electrophysiological examination, 16 patients (72.7%) had signs of pure axonal polyneuropathy. The authors stated that electrophysiological investigation is superior to clinical neurological examination in the detection of polyneuropathies and noted the difficulties in clinically confirming sensory symptoms, often due to sedation and prolonged intubation.

If no sensory symptoms are present, a myopathic form, an axonal motor polyneuropathy, or a combination of these two could underlie CIP. The electrophysiological changes of CIP show both motor and sensory axonal dysfunctions of upper and lower extremities (Zochodne et al., 1987; Witt et al., 1991; Coakley et al., 1993; Latronico et al., 1996); however, the findings of Hund and colleagues (1997) revealed normal sensory nerve action potential amplitudes. The follow-up of the electrophysiological changes in the lower extremities is often difficult and unreliable due to edema. Electrophysiological registrations of the upper extremities and needle electromyography therefore appear (technical) to be more reliable in diagnosing CIP or monitoring patients who are at risk for the development of CIP in the intensive care

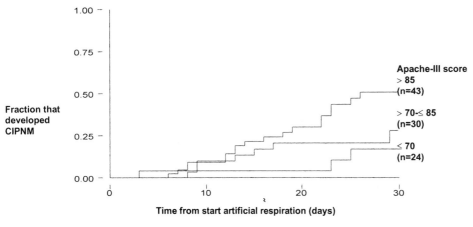

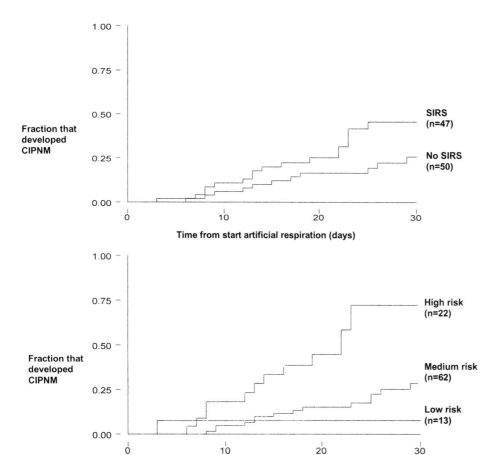

Figure 82–1. Kaplan-Meier curves showing the proportion of patients in whom critical illness polyneuropathy develops within 30 days after the start of artificial respiration. The low-risk group consisted of patients with an Acute Physiology Age and Chronic Health Evaluation (APACHE)-III score of ≤70 and no systemic inflammatory response syndrome. The high-risk group consisted of patients with an APACHE-III score of >85 and the presence of systemic inflammatory response syndrome. The medium-risk group consisted of all other patients. (From De Letter MACJ, Schmitz PIM, Visser LH, et al: Risk factors for the development of polyneuropathy or myopathy in critically ill patients. Neurology 1999;Suppl 2:A131.)

unit. Electromyography of patients with CIP contains the denervation potentials that are most abundant in the distal muscles, with a proximal-to-distal gradient during recovery of the clinical and electrophysiological disturbances. This fits with the changes in the conduction study, which mainly shows features of a polyneuropathy. Needle electromyography shows signs of acute denervation, which is one of the features of CIP (Berek et al., 1996; Hund et al., 1996). If the conduction study is influenced by neuromuscular blocking agents, which are often administered in the early phase of the artificial respiration,

needle electromyography can confirm early signs of CIP, showing denervation potentials or myopathic alterations of the motor unit potentials. For correct testing of the motor unit potential, however, problems often lie in the inability to perform voluntary activation in severely affected patients. Spitzer and associates (1992) expressed the importance of needle electromyography in the intensive care unit in general. If the diagnosis of neuromuscular problems remains unclear, the decision can be made to perform a muscle biopsy and to assess the mechanism of weakness in patients with proximal involvement.

In critical illness polyneuropathy and myopathy (CIPNM), the muscle biopsy samples reveal a considerable contribution of myopathic changes that did not correlate with the electrophysiological changes showing mainly signs of (sensori)motor axonal polyneuropathy (Latronico et al., 1996; De Letter et al., 2000a).

Histopathology

Postmortem analysis shows widespread axonal degeneration of both motor and sensory nerve fibers, with extensive denervation atrophy of limb and respiratory muscles (Zochodne et al., 1987). In case of acute denervation, some angular atrophy of isolated scattered muscle fibers is present; however, chronic denervation shows type grouping of angular atrophic muscle fibers. Evidence for the more myopathic form of CIP lies in the presence of round atrophic muscle fibers, which are scattered with some necrotic muscle fibers. Op de Coul and associates (1991) performed muscle biopsies in 7 of 22 patients with CIP. Myopathic and neuropathic changes were found in four (57%) and two (29%) patients, respectively. In two patients, a biopsy sample of the sural nerve was taken, revealing loss of myelin in one sample and no abnormalities in the other. Latronico and colleagues (1996) examined 24 patients with clinical and electrophysiological signs of CIP. Muscle biopsy demonstrated a primary myopathy in 14 patients (60%), neuropathic changes in 4 patients (17%), and features of both myopathy and neuropathy in 5 patients (22%). In 11 patients (46%), standard light microscopy showed scattered necrosis of muscle fibers without evidence of vascular occlusion or inflammatory infiltrates. In our prospective study, we performed open biopsy of the quadriceps femoral muscle in 30 patients with CIP (De Letter et al., 2000a). Standard light microscopic examination showed neuropathic changes in 11 patients (37%), myopathic changes in 12 patients (40%), and both neuropathic and myopathic changes in 7 patients (23%). Muscle fiber necrosis was present in only 9 of the muscle biopsy sample (30%), showing a sparse and scattered pattern. The myopathic features mainly evident in the standard light microscopic examination of muscle biopsies result in the use of the preferable term *critical illness polyneuropathy and myopathy* (De Letter et al., 2000a). There was no relation between the presence of muscle fiber necrosis and the level of creatine phosphokinase in the serum.

Immunohistochemistry

Bazzi and associates (1996) studied the expression of HLA-I, T-helper 1 cells, T-cytotoxic cells, B cells, and membrane attack complex in two patients with critical illness myopathy and could not find cellular infiltrates. In one patient, T-helper 1 cells, T-cytotoxic cells, and B cells were present. Both cases, however, also showed HLA-I upregulation and scattered microvascular deposits of membrane attack complex, suggesting that at least some patients with CIPNM may be affected with an autoimmune-inflammatory myopathy.

Our immunohistochemical examination of 30 muscle biopsy samples from patients with CIPNM also showed evidence of immune activation (De Letter et al., 2000a). Evidence of immune activation was indicated either as small, clustered infiltrates or by the presence of isolated inflammatory cells. These cells consisted of macrophages (Fig. 82–2A) and T-helper 1 cells, not of T-cytotoxic cells or B cells. The vascular endothelium (see Fig. 82–2B) macrophages and T-helper 1 cells showed an activated phenotype (HLA-DR positive), and in the same muscle biopsy sample, there was expression of several adhesion molecules on the vascular endothelium (see Fig. 82–2C). Moreover, membrane attack complex–positive staining was seen on the endothelium and on necrotic muscle fibers (see Fig. 82–2D), when present. The expression of membrane attack complex initiates capillary destruction and increases vascular permeability to allow extravasation of inflammatory cells (Hohlfeld and Engel, 1994).

The site and size of the inflammation do not reflect a strong pathological stimulus leading to heterogeneity in the standard light microscopic changes (Zochodne et al., 1987; Wokke et al., 1988; Danon and Carpenter, 1991; Op de Coul et al., 1991; Subramony et al., 1991; Coakley et al., 1993; Al-Lozi et al., 1994; Hohlfeld and Engel, 1994; Gutmann et al., 1996; Latronico et al., 1996).

The weak, but persistent, inflammatory response is accompanied by the release of proinflammatory (see Fig. 82–2E and F) and anti-inflammatory (see Fig. 82–2G) mediators. Interleukin 1β, tumor necrosis factor αR75, and, surprisingly, interferon γ were expressed by muscle fibers. Tews and colleagues (1996) postulated that the expression of cytokines (interleukin 1α, 1β, and 2 and tumor necrosis factor α) by muscles fibers in inflammatory myopathies may induce and mediate the process of autoimmunization and antigen expression without the primary presence of inflammatory cells.

The production of interleukin 12 by monocytes as recognized histomorphologically (see Fig. 82–2H) could be considered a powerful activator of the immune cascade and as inducing the proliferation of T cells. The best-documented activity for interferon γ is the increased expression of HLA-DR molecules on muscle fibers, neighboring endothelial cells, and macrophages. Subsequently, the increased expression of HLA-DR molecules by muscle fibers will enhance the presentation of potential (auto)antigens. Interferon γ also sustains the activation of macrophages and the production of proinflammatory cytokines. This leads to an upregulation of adhesion molecules on the vascular endothelium (Debets and Savelkoul, 1996).

In the muscle biopsy samples of patients with

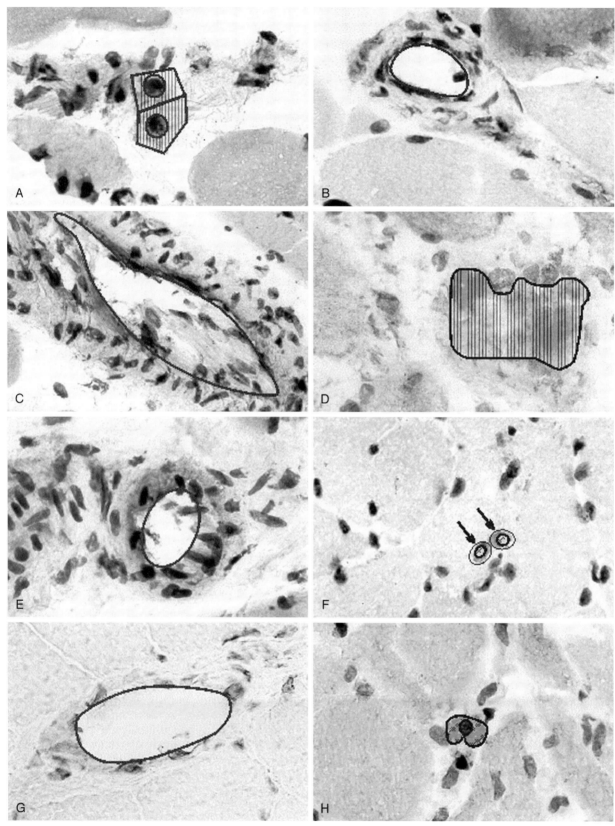

Figure 82–2. *A* to *H*, Immunohistochemical analysis of muscle biopsy samples from patients with critical illness polyneuropathy and myopathy. Positive staining is indicated with black lining. *A*, Macrophages (CD68) near a necrotic muscle fiber. *B*, HLA-DR staining on the vascular endothelium. *C*, Vascular cell adhesion molecule present on the endothelium of a blood vessel. *D*, Membrane attack complex (C5b-9) staining in a necrotic muscle fiber. *E*, TNFαR75 present on the endothelium of a blood vessel in the perimysium. *F*, Interferon-γ staining juxtanuclear in the cytoplasm of a muscle fiber (*arrows*). The juxtanuclear production of this cytokine makes it look like nuclear staining. *G*, Interleukin-10 present on the vascular endothelium. *H*, Interleukin-12 staining positive in the cytoplasm of a cell with a horseshoe-like nucleus containing a basophilic spot, histomorphological characteristics of a monocyte.

CIPNM, the presence of tissue damage is possibly related to increased vascular permeability. This is due to the expression of adhesion molecules (vascular cell adhesion molecule, intercellular adhesion molecule-1) and membrane attack complex–induced capillary destruction and occasionally by necrotic muscle fibers, which may result in an increased number of HLA-DR–positive cells. We speculate that these endothelial cells and scattered macrophages could present the potential autoantigens to the migrating $CD4^+$ T cells. Eventually, the immune activation in the muscle tissue revealed minor infiltrates with some inflammatory cells in only 27% of the biopsy samples. The size and relatively low percentage of inflammatory cells are unlikely due to a sampling error, as no biopsy samples showed larger infiltrates or infiltrates with cell types other than CD68-, CD4-, and, less frequently, CD8-positive cells. On the other hand, anti-inflammatory cytokines, as demonstrated by the abundant expression of interleukin 10, seem to play a part. These can be regarded as preventing severe inflammation in the muscle tissue and eventually leading to convalescence.

Support for the hypothesis that the presence of immune activation in the muscle tissue is due to CIPNM and not to an inflammatory process elsewhere in the body is shown in the role of HLA-DR, tumor necrosis factor αR75, and interleukin 10, which differ with statistical significance from control biopsies. Further support was obtained from a serum examination on the presence of soluble adhesion molecules as soluble intercellular adhesion molecule, soluble vascular cell adhesion molecule, and soluble E-selectin in eight patients with CIPNM and two critically ill patients without CIPNM. The preliminary data reveal the role of soluble intercellular adhesion molecule in patients with CIPNM, which suggests the presence of a specific inflammatory process. This was not found in the two control patients. Other arguments against nonspecific changes in the muscle tissue of patients with CIPNM resulted from the fact that the distribution of the erythrocyte sedimentation rate and the severity of sepsis did not differ between the patients with CIPNM and the patients in the intensive care unit without CIPNM ($n = 66$). Also, the level of the erythrocyte sedimentation rate did not correlate with the standard light microscopic changes in the muscle biopsy samples of the patients with CIPNM.

Pathogenetic Model

Previous, mainly retrospective studies postulated that the combinations of sepsis–systemic inflammatory response syndrome, multiple-organ dysfunction syndrome, and drugs (neuromuscular blocking agents, steroids, a combination of both, or aminoglycosides) represented possible causes of CIP. The causative descriptions of the mainly retrospective series of prolonged neuromuscular blockade can be divided into those that are based on pharmacokinetics (Fahey et al., 1981; Smith et al., 1987; Lynam et al., 1988; Segredo et al., 1990; Shearer et al., 1991; Hoyt, 1994) and those that are based on neuromuscular function (Shanks et al., 1985; Wokke et al., 1988; Darrah et al., 1989; Partridge et al., 1990; Vanderheyden et al., 1992). The pharmacokinetically based blockade is attributed to decreased renal clearance of active metabolites of vecuronium. Although Op de Coul and associates (1985) suggested that neuromuscular blocking agents could cause CIP, this was not found in further prospective studies and especially not in our latest study with a large control group. The amount of vecuronium that was administered during the first week of the artificial respiration, with or without disturbed kidney functions, steroids, or aminoglycosides, was not a risk factor for the development of CIP, nor are all possible combinations of these drugs identified as such. Concomitant use of several drugs alters the duration of action of neuromuscular blocking agents. Drugs that were investigated, which can potentiate blockade, were aminoglycosides and midazolam. No differences were shown between the patients in whom CIP developed and those in whom it did not. A neurotoxic effect on the neuromuscular junction from aminoglycosides is known (Sokoll and Gergis, 1981); repetitive nerve stimulation, however, in the electrophysiological monitoring of patients did not show such dysfunction. In summary, prospective studies report that drugs do not play a part in the development of neuromuscular disorders in patients in the intensive care unit (Witt et al., 1991; Coakley et al., 1993; Leijten et al., 1995; Berek et al., 1996; Latronico et al., 1996; De Letter et al., 1999).

In patients who are critically ill, which is reflected in a high APACHE-III score, the host response seems to lead to dysfunction of the neuromuscular system. On the other hand, the proinflammatory cytokines tumor necrosis factor α and interleukin 1 are known to play a pivotal role in systemic inflammatory response syndrome. Severe organ dysfunction, trauma, or major surgery may serve as a trigger that induces antigen-presenting cells to produce interleukins 1, 6, 8, 10, and 12 and tumor necrosis factor α. This results in activation and influx of mainly T-helper 1 cells, monocytes, macrophages, and neutrophils. As a result of this immune activation, adhesion molecules are also produced, leading to an increased vascular permeability (Nieuwenhuijzen et al., 1997). Extravasation of (inflammatory) cells, edema, and therefore tissue damage result in various systems, including the neuromuscular system. A disturbed microcirculation with resulting endoneurial edema and hypoxia may be responsible for primary axonal degeneration (Zochodne et al., 1987; Bolton and Breuer, 1999).

Thus far, data indicate that critically ill patients with both a high APACHE-III score and the presence of systemic inflammatory response syndrome are most prone to the development of CIP, which fits with the categories of patients who are mentioned

Pathogenesis of CIP

MODS
SIRS

Excessive, destructive, generalized immune activation

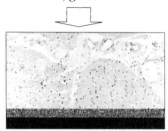

Muscle and/or nerve damage (CIP)

Figure 82–3. Hypothetical representation of possible interactions in the immunopathology of critical illness polyneuropathy. An as-yet-unidentified trigger induces local immune activation in patients with multiple organ dysfunction syndrome, systemic inflammatory response syndrome, or both. This consists of the activity of antigen-presenting cells, including the presentation of (auto)antigens to specific T-cells and cytokine production. Eventually, the effects of intercellular adhesion molecule, vascular cell adhesion molecule, and membrane attack complex, or complement 5b-9, on the vascular endothelium in the muscle tissue cause an increased vascular permeability with extravasation of inflammatory cells and their products, leading to damage of the muscle or nerve tissue.

in the pathogenetic model (Fig. 82–3). The high incidence of CIP (approximately 70%) in patients with sepsis or systemic inflammatory response syndrome, as found in previous studies, supports the model.

Variants

Because critical illness is not necessarily associated with artificial respiration, this should mean that CIP also occurs outside the intensive care unit. Reports of polyneuropathy in patients with severe burns and systemic inflammatory response syndrome were described by de Saint-Victor and associates (1994). Gorson and Ropper (1993) reported the development of CIP in five patients with severe respiratory problems who later required artificial respiration. The severe subacute, mainly motor axonal polyneuropathy that occurs in end-stage renal disease with trauma or sepsis may also be considered a variant of CIP (Bolton and Young, 1990).

Prognosis and Treatment

The prognosis of the polyneuropathy is directly related to the prognosis of the underlying critical illness. Because multiple organ failure is fatal for about 50% to 60% of patients, a significant number of patients will die as a result of the underlying critical illness. Previous reports on the prognosis of CIP have been rather optimistic (Hund et al., 1996), the overall mortality rates vary in prospective studies from 36% (Leijten et al., 1995) to 55% (M. A. C. J. De Letter, unpublished data). We hypothesize that in some patients, CIP is an additional factor in the organ failure and a factor contributing to the persistent, severe illness, resulting in death. The patients who survive usually recover from CIP, and in general the long-term outcome is good. We believe that the residual findings in CIP are underestimated. The presence of critical illness is associated with a higher mortality rate and a prolonged rehabilitation. Leijten and colleagues (1995) found that five of eight patients (63%) with delayed recovery beyond 4 weeks after discharge from the intensive care unit still had a persistent motor handicap after 1 year. Regarding long-term follow-up, very few data are available. However, Zifko (2000) studied CIP in 11 of 13 surviving patients 1 to 2 years after the onset of the disease. Five of them had signs of mononeuropathy; further quality of life was seriously impaired. The patients' electrophysiological features revealed abnormalities in the motor, sensory, and phrenic conduction studies.

Thus far, no prognostic factors with a significant influence on the natural history of CIP have been identified. Data from prospective studies only have provided the determination of risk factors for the development of CIP (De Letter et al., 1999). Because it is technically possible to monitor patients who are defined as being at (high) risk for the development of CIP, early detection of CIP should be possible with an early start of the rehabilitation therapy; the importance of this was described earlier (Leijten et al., 1995). Furthermore, there may be therapeutic strategies for CIP. Because local (muscle tissue), low-level immune activation was demonstrated to play a role in CIP, immunomodulating therapy could be considered. Previous results of patient treatment in the early phase of sepsis with intravenous immunoglobulin were promising; the incidence of CIP decreased dramatically (Mohr et al., 1997). Patients at risk for the development of CIP might be treated successfully using immune therapy; however, the clinician should not wait until CIP has developed (Wijdicks and Fulgham, 1994). This still must be tested in a prospective, randomized, placebo-controlled trial.

DIFFERENTIAL DIAGNOSIS

Critical Illness Myopathy

There has been much debate as to the incidence of a myopathy, which may occur independently or in association with a polyneuropathy in critically ill patients (Hund, 1999). The distinction between axonal motor polyneuropathy and myopathy in CIP is often difficult. Often, clinical testing of the sensory functions is neither reliable nor helpful in the determination. Theoretically, predominant proximal weakness, neck flexor weakness, and facial weakness occur more often in patients with myopathy. On needle electromyography, low amplitudes and short duration of the motor unit potentials suggest a myopathy. Normal sensory nerve action potential amplitudes and decreased compound motor action potential (CMAP) amplitudes are usually present in the conduction study. However, absent or decreased sensory nerve action potential amplitudes do not exclude a myopathy. Because of tissue edema, sensory nerve action potential amplitudes may be spuriously low. If serious edema is absent, serial examinations may reveal a significant fall in sensory nerve action potential amplitudes in CIP. Reliable examination of the motor unit potentials on voluntary activation is also difficult in patients with severe muscle weakness. Rich and associates (1997) described in neuropathy or end-plate dysfunction that the excitability of the muscle remains normal, which appeared not to be the case in acute quadriplegic myopathy. We postulate that direct muscle stimulation can be helpful in the distinction of polyneuropathy and myopathy in the spectrum of CIP. Determination of the creatinine phosphokinase serum concentration is also helpful in revealing myopathic changes. Elevated levels of creatine phosphokinase suggest a necrotizing myopathy; furthermore, severe myopathy is associated with myoglobinurea. The best method to differentiate between underlying polyneuropathy or myopathy is a muscle biopsy using standard light microscopic examination of the muscle tissue. As mentioned in the introductory paragraphs, we prefer to consider critical illness myopathy as part of CIPNM.

Guillain-Barré Syndrome

Guillain-Barré syndrome is a (sub)acute, immune-mediated polyneuropathy. Clinical features that are required for diagnosis are (1) progressive motor weakness of more than one limb (degree ranges from minimal ataxia, to total paralysis of the legs, to total paralysis of the muscles of all four extremities and the trunk, to bulbar and facial paralysis, and to external ophthalmoplegia) and (2) areflexia (universal areflexia is the rule, although distal areflexia with definite hyporeflexia of the biceps and knee jerks will suffice if other features are consistent).

The diagnostic criteria are based on clinical, laboratory, and electrodiagnostic criteria and are defined by Asbury and Cornblath (1990).

The clinical spectrum of Guillain-Barré syndrome consists of acute inflammatory demyelinating polyradiculoneuropathy, acute motor axonal neuropathy, acute motor sensory axonal neuropathy, and Miller-Fisher syndrome. These heterogeneous groups of pathological entities most likely have their own

pathogenesis. In about two thirds of all patients, Guillain-Barré syndrome is preceded by infections. We pointed out that motor Guillain-Barré syndrome without sensory loss is characterized by rapid onset of weakness, early nadir, distal-dominant weakness, sparing of the cranial nerves, and a preceding gastrointestinal infection, often subsequent to *Campylobacter jejuni* infection (Visser et al., 1995). The electrodiagnostic findings of the axonal types of Guillain-Barré syndrome show little evidence of demyelination; low distal CMAP amplitudes usually characterize signs of axonal damage. The presence of spontaneous activity in the remainder of the muscle fibers on needle electromyography also confirms this. The clinical picture may show many similarities with CIP. Many patients with acute motor neuropathy have high IgG anti-GM1 titers or IgG antibodies to anti–GalNac-GD1a (Kaida et al., 2000). These antibodies are not found in CIP (De Letter et al., 2000b).

A *C. jejuni* infection has been postulated to induce both acute motor neuropathy and acute motor sensory neuropathy, as well as Miller-Fisher syndrome. An acute motor neuropathy in the Dutch Guillain-Barré syndrome study population was never caused by a cytomegalovirus infection. Cytomegalovirus-related Guillain-Barré syndrome patients have a different clinical pattern. They are significantly younger; have a severe initial course, indicated by a high frequency of artificial respiration; and often develop cranial nerve involvement and severe sensory loss (Visser et al., 1996). It is possible that anti-GM2 antibodies are important in cytomegalovirus-associated Guillain-Barré syndrome.

ELECTROPHYSIOLOGICAL EVALUATION AND FINDINGS

The electrophysiological characteristics of Guillain-Barré syndrome point to a demyelinating polyneuropathy with an occasional and variable axonal component. Disturbance of the Schwann cells causes segmental demyelination, which results in significant reduction in conduction velocity. Conduction block clinically results in weakness and sensory loss. Increased desynchronization and temporal dispersion cause loss of reflexes. A prolonged refractory period with blocking at high frequency possibly accounts for reduced strength despite maximal voluntary effort.

Sensory Conduction Studies

This study should include multiple sensory nerves in both the upper and lower limbs, such as the sural, superficial peroneal, median, and ulnar nerves. The more distal nerves are affected earlier in the course of the disease than are the proximal nerves. This can be explained by the less protective myelin coating of this part of the nervous system, predisposing it to damage. Nerves that traverse entrapment sites are even more prone to involvement.

In axonal-type Guillain-Barré syndrome, the sensory nerve action potential amplitudes become significantly lowered after about 4 to 6 weeks. The sensory nerve action potential amplitude drops to 20% or less of normal values and commonly disappears between 3 to 4 weeks after onset of the disease. The conduction velocity and latency do not drop below 80% to 90% of the normal mean value. Conduction block or axonal loss is suspected when the alteration in sensory nerve action potential amplitude is larger than in conduction velocity.

Somatosensory Evoked Potential Conduction Studies

To study the proximal aspects of the sensory conduction system in Guillain-Barré syndrome, somatosensory evoked potential techniques are useful. Segmental conduction times, using Erb's point (N9) and cervical (N11) potentials (upper extremity), lumbar (N20) potential, and the central conduction, can be calculated. Central conduction times are essentially normal.

In Guillain-Barré syndrome, there seems to be a predisposition toward the proximal or nerve root regions. These features explain why patients have complaints of sensation and clinical abnormalities and only a few distal electrophysiological sensory nerve action potential abnormalities. Somatosensory evoked potential studies of both the upper and lower limbs should be performed, but because the neural pathway of the lower limbs is considerably longer, it is more beneficial to study them first.

Motor Conduction Studies

To establish the diagnosis and monitoring of Guillain-Barré syndrome, distal motor latencies, conduction velocities, F waves, H reflexes, and CMAP amplitudes, duration, and morphology are used. In 80% to 90% of the patients, at least one of these motor nerve parameters is disturbed. The distal motor latency and CMAP conduction velocity measurements reach a peak reduction of 60% to 80% of the normal mean values about 3 weeks after the onset of the clinical symptoms. After 4 weeks, the values begin to increase to normal over several weeks to months, although 1 year or longer can be required. In general, there is little correlation between the clinical presentation and nerve conduction velocity or distal motor latency.

To perform an examination of the F waves in Guillain-Barré syndrome, high amplifier gains (100 to 200 μV/cm), prolonged pulse duration, and increased current intensities should be used to conclude that F waves are reduced in number. Some type of abnormality can be expected in 80% to 90% of the patients, and the absence of F waves should be considered a definite abnormality. H reflexes should also be tested in the lower limbs to assess possible disturbed proximal neural conduction.

The most frequently encountered abnormality early in Guillain-Barré syndrome is conduction block. Such a block is present if there is a reduction in the peak-to-peak CMAP amplitude of more than 20% (a drop in proximal compared with distal CMAP), as defined by Asbury and Cornblath (1990), in the following nerves: (1) median (proximal arm compared with wrist, recording from thenar muscles), (2) ulnar (Erb's point compared with wrist, recording from hypothenar muscles), and (3) peroneal (popliteal fossa to ankle, recording from extensor digitorum brevis). Due to the lack of unanimity on the percentage of amplitude reduction, a range of 20% to 40% is used. In pseudo–conduction block, a reduction in amplitude is a result of excessive temporal dispersion, which may increase the duration of the potential, with a concomitant and compensatory reduction in amplitude. To distinguish between conduction block and temporal dispersive effects, small-segment stimulation can be used to localize focal reduction in amplitude. The conduction block is pathophysiologically caused by the loss of myelin, leading to conduction failure and symptoms of weakness and sensory loss. Permanent reduction of function is secondary to axonal loss.

Abnormalities with regard to the phrenic nerve are frequently noted, although reduced ventilatory capacity is not due to reduced conduction velocity in the phrenic nerve. If present, axonal damage of this nerve can be diagnosed with needle electromyography of the diaphragm.

In addition, abnormalities of the facial nerve can be tested in Guillain-Barré syndrome, as well as those of the supraorbital nerve. Direct facial nerve stimulation and the blink reflex reveal abnormalities in either or both pathways.

Needle Electromyography Examination

Positive sharp waves and fibrillation potentials at rest appear between 2 to 4 weeks, peaking about 6 to 15 weeks (earlier in the proximal than in the distal muscles). Within the first 3 weeks, myokymia (complex bursts of repetitive discharges that cause vermicular movements of the skin) are detected, especially in the facial muscles.

This examination is mainly adjunctive to explore other disease entities.

In Guillain-Barré syndrome, a reduced recruitment for motor unit potentials is one of the earliest findings. After about 6 to 16 weeks, voluntary motor unit potential amplitude, duration, and number of phases increase. These findings imply (1) axonal loss with motor unit remodeling and (2) reverse motor unit remodeling during axonal regrowth.

Single-fiber electromyography shows mild-to-moderate increase in fiber density later in the course of Guillain-Barré syndrome, substantiating the initial phases of motor unit remodeling in patients with axonal loss.

ELECTRODIAGNOSTIC CRITERIA OF GUILLAIN-BARRÉ SYNDROME AND THEIR VALIDATION

Most electrodiagnostic criteria have been defined on the basis of demyelination. Alam (1998) studied the six different sets of criteria that have been used in previous studies and applied them to 43 patients with the clinical diagnosis of Guillain-Barré syndrome. This resulted in 21% to 72% of the patients having the diagnosis of acute inflammatory demyelinating polyradiculoneuropathy. The sets were defined by Albers and colleagues (1985), Albers and Kelly (1989), Cornblath (1990), Ho and associates (1997), and Meulstee and van der Meché (1995). Although the criteria of Albers (Albers et al., 1985; Albers and Kelly, 1989) identified most cases as acute inflammatory demyelinating polyradiculoneuropathy, the importance of performing analyses on the criteria to achieve consensus and to reduce the variability in diagnosing the acute inflammatory demyelinating polyradiculoneuropathy variant of Guillain-Barré syndrome was emphasized.

In acute inflammatory demyelinating polyradiculoneuropathy, most distal sites, roots, and physiological entrapment sites are fragile, and early demyelination and secondary axonal degeneration occur there. Axonal degeneration easily masks demyelinating conduction changes. However, with careful follow-up, the presence of delayed F waves or increased distal motor latencies definitely mitigates against primary axonal pathology, as in acute motor axonal neuropathy or acute motor sensory axonal neuropathy.

Electrodiagnostic primary axonal Guillain-Barré syndrome was defined by Hadden and associates (1998) and Ho and colleagues (1997) as (1) no evidence of demyelination and (2) CMAP amplitude less than 80% of the lower limit of normal.

TREATMENT AND PROGNOSIS

The treatment of Guillain-Barré syndrome with intravenous immunoglobulin or plasma exchange results in earlier recovery, but morbidity rates remain considerable. Trials may lead to other methods of improving outcome.

The time of recovery depends on the extent of demyelination and axonal degeneration. Patients with severe axonal loss may not regain motor function for 1 to 2 years, implying a poor prognosis. Axonal regeneration takes considerably longer than remyelination. The Dutch multicenter study on prognostic factors that influence Guillain-Barré syndrome revealed that a preceding gastrointestinal illness, older age ($\geq$50 years), severe weakness (a Medical Research Council sum score of <40 at the start of the treatment), and rapid progression of weakness within 4 days of onset of weakness were important independent, significant prognostic factors at 6 months of follow-up (Visser, 1999). Others found that the electrodiagnostic finding of a low CMAP amplitude (<4 mV) is an important prognostic factor.

To distinguish CIP from the acute motor axonal variant of Guillain-Barré syndrome, the following characteristics may be useful (De Letter et al., 2000b).

- Guillain-Barré syndrome is the primary neurological reason for admission to the intensive care unit. On the other hand, CIP develops during a patient's stay in the intensive care unit for another reason.
- Infectious symptoms like fever and diarrhea usually subside before the clinical features of Guillain-Barré syndrome appear.
- The characteristic alterations in the cerebrospinal fluid of Guillain-Barré syndrome patients include a raised protein level and a normal to slightly elevated cell count.
- There is a possibility of detecting IgG antibodies against GM1, GM1b, GD1a, and GalNac-GD1a in the serum of axonal Guillain-Barré syndrome patients.
- Electrodiagnostic changes in Guillain-Barré syndrome occur in both sensory and motor nerves in about 80% of the patients in the Western world. In CIP, there is clinically a predominantly motor dysfunction. Both CIP and axonal-type Guillain-Barré syndrome show sensorimotor or pure motor axonal features. Critical illness polyneuropathy and myopathy can sometimes be distinguished from Guillain-Barré syndrome by the presence of myopathic motor unit potentials on voluntary activation.
- During the progression of Guillain-Barré syndrome, the demyelinating features of the nerve conduction study may change into a secondary axonal pattern. In the latter, slow nerve conduction velocity remains in some patients and the initial needle electromyography study lacks spontaneous activity (Chen, 1998). In CIP, spontaneous activity of the muscle fibers is an early feature. Further phrenic nerve conduction studies usually show no significantly prolonged latencies in CIP (Bolton et al., 1986).
- Severe autonomic disturbances are more common in the patient with Guillain-Barré syndrome after the polyneuropathy has developed than in patients with CIP (Bolton et al., 1986).
- Septic encephalopathy may be present before the onset of CIP. Patients with Guillain-Barré syndrome do not have a disturbed consciousness.

Porphyric Neuropathy

Porphyric neuropathy is an acute or subacute, predominantly motor neuropathy. Disturbances of porphyrin metabolism are associated with acute attacks of neurological disease in cases of hepatic porphyrias. These porphyrias, consisting of acute intermittent porphyria, hereditary coproporphyria, and variegate porphyria, are caused by enzyme defects (uroporphyrinogen-1-synthetase, coproporphyrinogen oxidase, or protoporphyrinogen oxidase, respectively). Acute intermittent porphyria (Stein and Tschudy, 1970; Kappas et al., 1993), hereditary coproporphyria (Magnussen et al., 1975), and variegate porphyria (Eales et al., 1980) all occur on a genetic basis. The attacks of acute hepatic porphyrias may be precipitated by drugs (most often barbiturates, estrogens, ethanol excess, griseofulvin, hydantoins, meprobamate, oral contraceptives, and sulfonamides), hypoglycemia, and hormonal influences. The last results in the occurrence of acute intermittent porphyria in the luteal phase of the menstrual cycle and not before puberty in either sex. The excess of heme precursors that is being produced during the attacks is detectable in urine, feces, and blood. Therefore, they serve as diagnostic tools for the specific types of porphyria (Windebank and Bonkovsky, 1993).

The change in color of the urine is due to the oxidation of the porphyrinogens. The conversion to the corresponding porphyrin causes the urine to turn red or purple. Porphobilinogen may polymerize to porphobilin, which has a black color.

The clinical features are as follows.

- Acute, colicky abdominal pain occurs; it is not known whether the pain is caused by local effects of heme precursors or heme deficiency on muscles and nerves of the gastrointestinal tract or by acute autonomic neuropathy with sympathetic hyperreactivity. The latter is a prominent feature during porphyric attacks.
- Psychiatric disturbances vary from restlessness and agitation to psychosis, coma, and seizure.
- Acute neuropathy develops within 2 to 3 days of the onset of abdominal and psychiatric symptoms and may mimic Guillain-Barré syndrome.

The first symptoms may be back or limb pain. Motor symptoms are the earliest and most prominent clinical features. The weakness is occasionally asymmetrical or patchy and may begin in the upper limbs or cranial nerves (commonly, facial weakness and swallowing difficulty), and proximal muscles are as likely to be affected as are the distal ones. Atrophy is seen early, may be severe, and is probably due to axonal degeneration and generalized weight loss. Sensory symptoms are less prominent but may involve patchy or migratory painful paresthesias. Progression to maximal deficit, with possible respiratory insufficiency, usually occurs in a few days but may be stepwise for several weeks.

ELECTROPHYSIOLOGICAL EVALUATION AND FINDINGS

Electrophysiological examination of acute neuropathy may show normal nerve conduction studies and needle electromyography during the first few days of the illness. The primary process involves an axonal degeneration that results in a decrease in the compound action potentials, which is usually related to the severity of muscle weakness. There is no prominent sensory involvement. Slowing of the conduction velocity is present only if degeneration of the majority of motor axons occurs or during the regeneration phase. Somatosensory evoked potentials and spinal motor evoked potentials are useful because proximal and cranial innervated muscles are mostly involved. Needle electromyography of clinically involved muscles reveals denervation po-

tentials in 5 to 10 days and features of reinnervation during recovery (Windebank and Bonkovsky, 1993).

TREATMENT AND PROGNOSIS

The most important strategy in neuropathic porphyria is to avoid acute attacks. The so-called porphyrogenic drugs, which induce cytochrome P-450, should not be used, and situations that lead to hypoglycemia should be avoided. For the administration of carbohydrate nutrition, glucose should be used. For treatment of the underlying defect, intravenous heme is effective and the therapy of choice (Watson, 1975; Lamon et al., 1979).

Psychiatric symptoms such as agitation and anxiety can be treated with chlorpromazine. In the case of seizures, bromides are thus far the therapy of choice. Most anticonvulsants are, however, inducers of porphyric attacks. Pain can be treated with meperidine and morphine.

The prognosis for recovery from the neuropathic damage depends on the severity of axonal and neuronal loss (Bosch et al., 1977). Good functional recovery is the rule. The mortality rate for acute attacks is less than 10% (Lamon et al., 1979). Recovery from the psychiatric and autonomic features is usually rapid. Finally, screening should be performed for latent disease in all at-risk relatives.

References

Alam TA: Electrodiagnostic studies in Guillain-Barré syndrome: Distinguishing subtypes by published criteria. Muscle Nerve 1998;21:1275–1279.

Albers JW, Donofrio PD, McGonagle TK: Sequential electrodiagnostic abnormalities in acute inflammatory demyelinating polyradiculoneuropathy. Muscle Nerve 1985;8:528–539.

Albers JW, Kelly JJ: Acquired inflammatory demyelinating polyneuropathies: Clinical and electrodiagnostic features. Muscle Nerve 1989;12:435–451.

Al-Lozi MT, Pestronk A, Yee WC: Rapidly evolving myopathy with myosin-deficient muscle fibers. Ann Neurol 1994;35:273–279.

Asbury AK, Cornblath DR: Assessment of current diagnostic criteria for Guillain-Barré syndrome. Ann Neurol 1990;27(suppl):S21–S24.

Bazzi P, Moggio M, Prelle A: Inflammatory myopathy in intensive care patients. J Neurol 1996;243(suppl 2):S111.

Berek K, Margreiter J, Willeit J, et al: Polyneuropathies in critically ill patients: A prospective evaluation. Intensive Care Med 1996; 22:849–855.

Bolton CF, Gilbert JJ, Hahn AF: Polyneuropathy in critically ill patients. J Neurol Neurosurg Psychiatry 1984;47:1223–1231.

Bolton CF, Laverty DA, Brown JD, et al: Critically ill polyneuropathy: Electrophysiological studies and differentiation from Guillain-Barré syndrome. J Neurol Neurosurg Psychiatry 1986;49:563–573.

Bolton CF, Young GB: Neurological Complications of Renal Disease. London, Butterworths, 1990.

Bolton CF: Clinical neurophysiology of the respiratory system. Muscle Nerve 1993a;16:809–818.

Bolton CF: Neuromuscular complications of sepsis. Intensive Care Med 1993b;19:558–563.

Bolton CF: Muscle weakness and difficulty in weaning from the ventilator in the critical care unit. Chest 1994;106:1–2.

Bolton CF: Critical illness polyneuropathy. In Thomas PK, Asbury A (eds): Peripheral Nerve Disorders II. Oxford, Butterworth-Heinemann, 1995; 262–270.

Bolton CF: Sepsis and the systemic inflammatory response syndrome: Neuromuscular manifestations. Crit Care Med 1996;24: 1408–1416.

Bolton CF, Breuer AC: Critical illness polyneuropathy: A useful concept. Muscle Nerve 1999;22:419–422.

Bone RC, Balk RA, Cerra FB, et al: Definitions for sepsis and organ failure and guidelines for the use of innovative therapies in sepsis. Chest 1992;101:1644–1655.

Bosch EP, Pierach CA, Bossenmaier IA, et al: Effect of hematin in porphyric neuropathy. Neurology 1977;27:1053.

Chen R: Electrophysiological studies in the critical care unit: Investigating polyneuropathies. Can J Neurol Sci 1998;25:32–35.

Coakley JH, Nagendran K, Ormerod IE, et al: Prolonged neurogenic weakness in patients requiring mechanical ventilation for acute airflow limitation. Chest 1992;101:1413–1416.

Coakley JH, Nagendran K, Honovar M, et al: Preliminary observations on the neuromuscular abnormalities in patients with organ failure and sepsis. Intensive Care Med 1993;19:323–328.

Cornblath DR: Electrophysiology in Guillain-Barré syndrome. Ann Neurol 1990;27(suppl):S17–S20.

Couturier JC, Robert D, Monier P: Polynévrites compliquant des sejours prolongés en réanimation: A propos de 11 cas d'étiologie encore inconnue. Lyon Med 1984;252:247–249.

Danon MJ, Carpenter S: Myopathy with thick filament (myosin) loss following prolonged paralysis with vecuronium during steroid treatment. Muscle Nerve 1991;4:1131–1139.

Darrah W, Johnston J, Mirakhur R: Vecuronium infusions for prolonged muscle relaxation in the intensive care. Crit Care Med 1989;17:1297–1300.

De Letter MACJ, Schmitz PIM, Visser LH, et al: Risk factors for the development of polyneuropathy or myopathy in critically ill patients. Neurology 1999;Suppl 2:A131.

De Letter MACJ, van Doorn PA, Savelkoul HFJ, et al: Critical illness polyneuropathy and myopathy (critical illness polyneuropathy and myopathy): Evidence for local immune activation by cytokine expression in the muscle tissue. J Neuroimmunol 2000a; 106:206–213.

De Letter MACJ, Visser LH, Ang W, et al: Distinctions between critical illness polyneuropathy and axonal Guillain-Barré syndrome. J Neurol Neurosurg Psychiatry 2000b;68:397–398.

De Saint-Victor JF, Durand G, Le Gulluche Y, et al: Neuropathies du syndrome de sepsis avec defaillance multiviscerale chez les brules: 2 Cas avec revue de la literature. Rev Neurol (Paris) 1994;150:149–154.

Debets R, Savelkoul HFJ: Cytokines as cellular communicators: Mediators of inflammation. 1996;5:417–423.

Douglas JA, Tuxen DV, Horne M, et al: Myopathy in severe asthma. Am Rev Respir Dis 1992;146:517–519.

Dumitru D: Generalized peripheral neuropathies. In Dumitru D (ed): Electrodiagnostic Medicine. Philadelphia, Hanley & Belbus, 1994; 741–850.

Eales L, Day RS, Blekkenhorst GH: The clinical and biochemical features of variegate porphyria: An analysis of 300 cases studied at Groote Schuurr Hospital, Cape Town. Int J Biochem 1980; 12:837.

Fahey M, Morris RB, Miller R, et al: Pharmacokinetics of Org NC45 (Norcuron) in patients with and without renal failure. Br J Anaesth 1981;53:1049–1053.

Friedland JS, Porter JC, Daryanani S, et al: Plasma proinflammatory cytokine concentrations, Acute Physiology and Chronic Health Evaluation (APACHE) III scores and survival in patients in an intensive care unit. Intensive Care Med 1996;24:1775–1781.

Gooch JL, Suchyta MR, Balbierz JM, et al: Prolonged paralysis after treatment with neuromuscular junction blocking agents. Crit Care Med 1991;19:1125–1131.

Gooch JL: Prolonged paralysis after neuromuscular blockade. Muscle Nerve 1995;18:937–942.

Gorson KC, Ropper AH: Acute respiratory failure neuropathy: A variant of critical illness polyneuropathy. Crit Care Med 1993; 21:267–271.

Gutmann L, Blumenthal D, Gutmann L, et al: Acute type-II myofiber atrophy in critical illness. Neurology 1996;46:819–821.

Gutmann L, Gutmann L: Critical illness neuropathy and myopathy. Arch Neurol 1999;56:527–528.

Hadden RD, Cornblath DR, Hughes RA, et al: Electrophysiological classification of Guillain-Barré syndrome: Clinical associations and outcome. Ann Neurol 1998;44:780–788.

Hirano M, Ott BR, Raps EC, et al: Acute quadriplegic myopathy: A complication of treatment with steroids, nondepolarizing agents, or both. Neurology 1992;42:2082–2087.

Ho TW, Li CY, Cornblath DR, et al: Patterns of recovery in the Guillain-Barré syndromes. Neurology 1997;48:695–700.

Hohlfeld R, Engel AG: The immunobiology of muscle. Immunol Today 1994;15:269–274.

Hoyt JW: Persistent paralysis in critically ill patients after the use of neuromuscular blocking agents. New Horizons 1994;2:48–55.

Hund EF, Fogel W, Krieger D, et al: Critical illness polyneuropathy: Clinical findings and outcomes of a frequent cause of neuromuscular weaning failure. Crit Care Med 1996;24:1328–1333.

Hund E, Genzwürker H, Böhrer H, et al: Predominant involvement of motor fibers in patients with critical illness polyneuropathy. Br J Anaesth 1997;78:274–278.

Hund E: Myopathy in critically ill patients. Crit Care Med 1999; 27:2544–2547.

Jackson AC, Gilbert JJ, Young GB, et al: The encephalopathy of sepsis. Can J Neurol Sci 1985;12:303–307.

Kaida K, Kusunoki S, Kamakura K, et al: Guillain-Barré syndrome with antibody to a ganglioside, N-acetylgalactosaminyl GD1a. Brain 2000;123:116–124.

Kappas A, Sassa S, Anderson KE: The porphyrias: In Stanbury JB, Wyngaarden JB, Fredrickson DS, et al (eds): The Metabolic Basis of Inherited Disease, 5th ed. New York, McGraw-Hill, 1993; 1301.

Knaus WA, Wagner DP, Draper EA, et al: The APACHE III prognostic system. Chest 1991;100:1619–1636.

Kupfer Y, Namba T, Kaldawi E, et al: Prolonged weakness after long-term infusion of vecuronium bromide. Ann Intern Med 1991;117:484–486.

Lacomis D, Giuliani MJ, Van Cott A, et al: Acute myopathy of intensive care: Clinical, electromyographic, and pathological aspects. Ann Neurol 1996;40:645–654.

Lacomis D, Petrella JT, Giuliani MJ: Causes of neuromuscular weakness in the intensive care unit: A study of ninety-two patients. Muscle Nerve 1998;21:610–617.

Lamon JM, Frykholm BC, Hess RA, et al: Hematin therapy for acute porphyria. Medicine 1979;58:252–269.

Latronico N, Fenzi F, Recupero D, et al: Critical illness myopathy and neuropathy. Lancet 1996;347:1579–1582.

Leijten FSS, Harinck-De Weerd JE, Poortvliet DCJ, et al: The role of polyneuropathy in motor convalescence after prolonged mechanical ventilation. JAMA 1995;274:1221–1225.

Leijten FSS, Poortvliet DCJ, De Weerd AW: The neurological examination in the assessment of polyneuropathy in mechanically ventilated patients. Eur J Neurol 1997;4:124–129.

Lynam DP, Cronnelly R, Castagnoli KP, et al: The pharmacodynamics and pharmacokinetics of vecuronium in patients anesthetized with isoflurane with normal renal function or with renal failure. Anesthesiology 1988;69:227–231.

MacFarlane IA, Rosenthal FD: Severe myopathy after status asthmaticus. Lancet 1977;2:615.

Magnussen CR, Doherty JM, Hess RA, et al: Grand mal seizures and acute intermittent porphyria: The problem of differential diagnosis and treatment. Neurology 1975;25:121–125.

Meulstee J, van der Meché FGA: Electrodiagnostic criteria for polyneuropathy and demyelination: Application in 135 patients with Guillain-Barré syndrome. Dutch Guillain-Barré Study Group. J Neurol Neurosurg Psychiatry 1995;59:482–486.

Mohr M, Englisch L, Roth A, et al: Effects of early treatment with immunoglobulin on critical illness polyneuropathy following multiple organ failure and gram-negative sepsis. Intensive Care Med 1997;23:1144–1149.

Nates JL, Cooper DJ, Day B, et al: Acute weakness syndromes in critically ill patients: A reappraisal. Anaesth Intens Care 1997; 25:502–513.

Nieuwenhuijzen GAP, Knapen MFCM, Oyen WJG, et al: Organ damage is preceded by changes in protein extravasation in an experimental model of the multiple organ dysfunction syndrome. Shock 1997;7:98–104.

Op de Coul AAW abstract 1983.

Op de Coul AAW, Lambregts PC, Koeman J, et al: Neuromuscular complications in patients given Pavulon (pancuronium bromide) during artificial respiration. Clin Neurol Neurosurg 1985; 87:17–22.

Op de Coul AAW, Verheul GAM, Leyten ACM, et al: Critical illness polyneuromyopathy after artificial respiration. Clin Neurol Neurosurg 1991;93:27–33.

Partridge BL, Abrams J, Basemore C, et al: Prolonged neuromuscular blockade after long-term vecuronium infusion in the intensive care unit. Crit Care Med 1990;18:1177–1179.

Ramsay DA, Zochodne DW, Robertson DM, et al: A syndrome of acute severe muscle necrosis in intensive care unit patients. J Neuropathol Exp Neurol 1993;52;387–398.

Rich MM, Bird SJ, Raps EC, et al: Direct muscle stimulation in acute quadriplegic myopathy. Muscle Nerve 1997;20:665–673.

Roelofs RI, Cerra F, Bielka N, et al: Prolonged respiratory insufficiency due to acute motor neuropathy: A new syndrome. Neurology 1983;33:240.

Rossiter A, Souney PF, McGowan S, et al: Pancuronium-induced prolonged neuromuscular blockade. Crit Care Med 1991;19: 1583–1587.

Segredo V, Matthay MA, Sharma ML: Prolonged neuromuscular blockade after long-term administration of vecuronium in two critically ill patients. Anesthesiology 1990;72:566–570.

Segredo V, Caldwell JE, Matthay MS, et al: Persistent paralysis in critically ill patients after long-term administration of vecuronium. N Engl J Med 1992;20:524–528.

Shanks A, Long T, Aitkenhead A: Prolonged neuromuscular blockade following vecuronium. Br J Anaesth 1985;57:807–810.

Shearer ES, O'Sullivan EP, Hunter JM: Clearance of atracurium and laudanosine in the urine and by continuous venovenous haemofiltration. Br J Anaesth 1991;67:569–573.

Smith C, Hunter J, Jones R: Vecuronium infusions in patients with renal failure in an ICU. Anesthesiology 1987;42:387–393.

Sokoll MD, Gergis SD: Antibiotics and neuromuscular function. Anesthesiology 1981;55:148–159.

Spitzer AR, Giancarlo T, Maher L, et al: Neuromuscular causes of prolonged ventilator dependency. Muscle Nerve 1992;15:682–686.

Stein JA, Tschudy DP: Acute intermittent porphyria: A clinical and biochemical study of 46 patients. Medicine 1970;49:1.

Subramony SH, Carpenter DE, Raju S, et al: Myopathy and prolonged neuromuscular blockade after lung transplant. Crit Care Med 1991;19:1580–1582.

Tews DS, Goebel HH: Cytokine expression profile in idiopathic inflammatory myopathies. J Neuropathol Exp Neurol 1996;55: 342–347.

Vanderheyden BA, Reynolds HN, Gerold KB, Emanuele T: Prolonged paralysis after long-term vecuronium infusion. Crit Care Med 1992;20:304–307.

Visser LH, van der Meché FGA, Van Doorn PA, et al: Guillain-Barré syndrome without sensory loss (acute motor neuropathy): A subgroup with specific clinical, electrodiagnostic and laboratory features. Brain 1995;118:841–847.

Visser LH, van der Meché FGA, Meulstee J, et al: Cytomegalovirus infection and Guillain-Barré syndrome: The clinical, electrophysiologic and prognostic features. Neurology 1996;47:668–673.

Watson CJ: Hematin and porphyrin. N Engl J Med 1975;293:605–607.

Wijdicks EF, Fulgham JR: Failure of high dose intravenous immunoglobulins to alter the clinical course of critical illness polyneuropathy. Muscle Nerve 1994;17:1494–1495.

Windebank AJ, Bonkovsky HL: Porphyric neuropathy. In Dyck PJ, Thomas PK (eds): Peripheral Neuropathy, Vol II, 3rd ed. Philadelphia, WB Saunders, 1993; 1161–1168.

Witt NJ, Zochodne DW, Bolton CF, et al: Peripheral nerve function in sepsis and multiple organ failure. Chest 1991;99:176–184.

Wokke JHJ, Jennekens FGI, van den Oord CJM, et al: Histological investigations of muscle atrophy and end plates in two critically ill patients with generalized weakness. J Neurol Sci 1988; 88:95–106.

Young GB, Bolton CF, Austin TW, et al: The encephalopathy associated with septic illness. Clin Invest Med 1990;13:297–304.

Young GB, Bolton CF, Archibald YM, et al: The electroencephalogram in sepsis-associated encephalopathy. J Clin Neurophysiol 1992;9:145–152.

Zifko UA, Zipko HT, Bolton CF: Clinical and electrophysiological findings in critical illness polyneuropathy. J Neurol Sci 1998; 159:186–193.

Zifko UA: Long-term outcome of critical illness polyneuropathy. Muscle Nerve 2000;Suppl 9:S49–S52.

Zochodne DW, Bolton CF, Wells GA, et al: Critical illness polyneuropathy: A complication of sepsis and multiple organ failure. Brain 1987;110:819–842.

Zochodne DW, Ramsay DA, Saly V, et al: Acute necrotizing myopathy of intensive care: Electrophysiological studies. Muscle Nerve 1994;17:285–292.

Myopathies and Disorders of Neuromuscular Transmission

Shawn J. Bird

During the past two decades, it has been increasingly recognized that the development of neuromuscular weakness in the intensive care unit frequently contributes to prolonged ventilator dependence and intensive care unit stays, with increased morbidity and costs. In a prospective study of 21 patients, Spitzer and associates (1992) found a neuromuscular cause of weakness in 62% of intensive care unit patients who had difficulty in being weaned from mechanical ventilation. The majority of these patients did not have a pre-existing neuromuscular disorder but rather developed one as a consequence of critical illness.

The list of neuromuscular disorders that may develop in the intensive care unit is extensive. A useful way to organize the differential diagnostic approach is to separate conditions that produce weakness severe enough to warrant intensive care unit care from those that develop as a consequence of critical illness or treatment in the intensive care unit. Myasthenia gravis and the Guillain-Barré syndrome are examples of disorders that commonly produce profound weakness and respiratory failure that necessitate intensive care unit admission. Three distinct syndromes develop as a consequence of critical illness and its treatment: an axonal sensory-motor polyneuropathy termed *critical illness polyneuropathy,* an acute myopathy predominantly associated with the use of neuromuscular blocking agents and high-dose corticosteroids, and prolonged pharmacological neuromuscular blockade.

The success of critical care medicine and prolonged survival, often in the setting of sepsis, has resulted in an increased incidence of these disorders. The widespread use of neuromuscular blocking agents and corticosteroids and the larger number of organ transplantations have also resulted in more patients with these disorders, especially acute myopathy. Although these disorders are common, there is a disparity in the reported incidence of critical illness polyneuropathy and myopathy. Recognition of even severe neuromuscular weakness may be limited by the presence of encephalopathy or sedation. There also are differences in the definitions used to identify these disorders and in the extent of electrophysiological and histopathological evaluations. In many patients, myopathy and neuropathy likely coexist. There may be differences in the patient populations at different centers, with populations of predominantly septic patients having a predominance of neuropathy (Zifko et al., 1998) and populations of transplant recipients who receive corticosteroids (Rich et al., 1997; Campellone et al., 1998; Lacomis et al., 1998) or those who use more neuromuscular blocking agents having a predominance of myopathy.

Despite the difficulties in defining the precise disorder in some patients, recognition of significant weakness or the inability to be weaned from mechanical ventilation due to a neuromuscular cause is helpful. This may prevent unnecessary investigative studies, such as central nervous system imaging, and may suggest delayed extubation until respiratory muscle strength is adequate. Information on axonal loss or myopathy may provide data to predict a realistic timeline for the recovery of strength and ambulation. There may be specific pharmacological interventions in the future.

MYOPATHIES

Critical Illness Myopathy

An acute myopathy may develop as a complication of critical illness, most often in association with the use of corticosteroids and neuromuscular blocking agents. In addition to *critical illness myopathy* (CIM), other names given to this syndrome have included *acute quadriplegic myopathy, thick filament myopathy, acute (necrotizing) myopathy of intensive care, rapidly evolving myopathy with myosin-deficient fibers,* and *critical care myopathy.* For consistency, a single term is preferred, and CIM has been proposed (Lacomis et al., 2000).

This myopathy was first reported in 1977 in a woman with asthma treated with both corticosteroids and neuromuscular blocking agents (MacFarlane and Rosenthal, 1977). There have been numerous other reports in status asthmaticus (Van Marle and Woods, 1980; Kaplan et al., 1986; Knox et al., 1986; Bachmann et al., 1987; Kupfer et al., 1987; Picado et al., 1988; Williams et al., 1988; Shee, 1990; Danon and Carpenter, 1991; De Smet et al., 1991; Sitwell et al., 1991; Douglass et al., 1992; Griffin et al., 1992; Waclawik et al., 1992; Lacomis et al., 1993; Leatherman et al., 1996; Road et al., 1997). In a prospective trial, one third of patients with status asthmaticus who received these agents developed clinical myopathy (Douglass et al., 1992). Shortly after the initial report in asthmatics, Sher and colleagues (1979) reported a patient with sepsis, multiorgan failure, and exposure to corticosteroids and neuromuscular blocking agents who developed an acute myopathy. Subsequently, this myopathy has been reported in numerous types of critical illness (Op de Coul et al., 1985; Gooch et al., 1991; Bird et al., 1992; Hirano et al., 1992; Gooch et al., 1993; Ramsay et al., 1993; Barohn et al., 1994; Zochodne, 1994; Rich et al., 1997), particularly in patients with acute respiratory distress syndrome and after organ transplantation (Subramony et al., 1991; Faragher et al., 1996; Lacomis et al., 1996; Wijdicks et al., 1996; Campellone et al., 1998). It has also become apparent that patients with critical illness and sepsis can develop CIM even though they have not been treated with either neuromuscular blocking agents or corticosteroids (Hirano et al., 1992; Latronico et al., 1996; Rich et al., 1997; Showalter and Engel, 1997; Deconinck et al., 1998). This acute myopathy also can occur in children (Benzing et al., 1990; Pascucci, 1990; Gooch, 1995; Bird et al., 1999).

Risk Factors and Clinical Features

It appears from the numerous case reports that the most potent risk factors are the use of high-dose corticosteroids, usually a total dose of 1000 mg methylprednisolone or the equivalent (Lacomis et al., 2000), and neuromuscular blocking agents, regardless of the underlying cause of critical illness. In general, the higher the total dose of neuromuscular blocking agents and corticosteroids, the more likely it is CIM will develop (Douglass et al., 1992). In one of few prospective studies, CIM developed in 7% of patients after liver transplantation (Campellone et al., 1998). The risk factors for the development of CIM included higher corticosteroid doses

and a greater severity of critical illness, as measured with the Acute Physiology and Chronic Health Evaluation (APACHE-II) score. Sedative drugs, such as propofol, which are widely used in the intensive care unit, may also be risk factors for CIM; they produce prolonged immobility, which may have similar effects to denervation (Berg, 1975). Sepsis and the systemic inflammatory response syndrome alone also appear to be the sole risk factor in some patients. Bolton and colleagues (Bolton et al., 1993; Bolton, 1993, 1996) detailed the widespread effects of sepsis on the central nervous system, peripheral nerve, and muscle. Although they emphasized the common association of encephalopathy and critical illness polyneuropathy, they speculated that the underlying poorly understood pathophysiology of those disorders would also likely affect muscle.

The prototypical clinical presentation of CIM is that of a critically ill patient on mechanical ventilation who is treated with corticosteroids and neuromuscular blocking agents and, often, is septic. The myopathy develops acutely but is often difficult to recognize early due to coexistent encephalopathy, sedation, or both. As the encephalopathy or sedation resolves days to weeks later, it becomes apparent that there is an underlying quadriparesis. It may be noted that the newly alert patient only grimaces to painful stimuli, indicating a profound quadriparesis. Some patients have only mild weakness, but many are severely affected, and weaning from the ventilator is often delayed secondary to diaphragm weakness. Failure to be weaned from the ventilator may be the first recognized manifestation. The weakness is not usually length related, distally predominant as is critical illness polyneuropathy. There is proximal as well as distal quadriparesis. Neck flexors and facial muscles may be involved. Extraocular movements are usually spared but have been involved in a few patients (Sitwell et al., 1991). Sensation is spared, if it can be evaluated, and reflexes are decreased in parallel with the decrease in strength.

Patients who survive the period of critical illness normally recover within 1 to 3 months (Lacomis et al., 1998). Other than those with only status asthmaticus, there is a high mortality rate in these patients due to the underlying disease. In a prospective study of liver transplant recipients with CIM, the mean time in the intensive care unit was 49 days for those with CIM but only 14 days for those without CIM (Campellone et al., 1998). Failure to be weaned from mechanical ventilatory support is a major contributor to longer stays and greater morbidity.

There is no specific pharmacological treatment for CIM. Limiting the use of neuromuscular blocking agents, especially continuous infusions for long periods, seems prudent. Awareness of this disorder has resulted in attempts to restrain excessive use and to develop guidelines for their use in the intensive care unit (Hansen-Flaschen et al., 1993; Sladen, 1995). Recognition of this disorder in a particular patient may suggest that high-dose corticosteroids be reduced or discontinued. Avoidance of corticosteroids may also be wise in those who have had this myopathy, because recurrent CIM has been reported with neuromuscular blocking agents and steroids (Kohler et al., 1998) or with steroids alone (Lindenbaum et al., 2000).

ELECTRODIAGNOSTIC STUDIES

The clinical presentations of this myopathy, critical illness polyneuropathy, and prolonged pharmacological neuromuscular blockade are similar. Each is manifest by flaccid quadriparesis with diaphragmatic involvement; therefore, electrophysiological studies (nerve conduction studies and electromyography) are essential in the evaluation of the weak, critically ill patient (Bolton, 1987; Raps et al., 1994; Bird and Rich, 2000). The work of Bolton has emphasized the importance of careful electrophysiological studies in the intensive care unit setting (Bolton, 1987). Not only do these studies confirm the presence of a neuromuscular disorder, but in most circumstances, they allow one to differentiate among polyneuropathy, myopathy, and a disorder of neuromuscular transmission (Table 83–1). They also may demonstrate substantial sensory involvement when none is apparent on the clinical examination. However, electrodiagnostic studies are often difficult to conduct in the intensive care unit setting. Electrical noise from the intensive care unit equipment, local edema, and lines over recording and stimulating sites make it troublesome to confidently record small potentials, particularly sensory responses. Sedated or encephalopathic patients or those with profound weakness cannot cooperate with the needle electromyographic examination, which requires voluntary muscle activation. It is often necessary to repeat the studies when the sedation or encephalopathy is resolving or when the quadriparesis is less profound.

Nerve conduction studies in CIM are generally normal except for diminished compound muscle action potential (CMAP) amplitudes with relatively preserved sensory nerve action potential (SNAP) amplitudes (Op de Coul et al., 1985; Zochodne et al., 1994; Lacomis et al., 1996; Rich et al., 1997). Patients with low SNAP amplitudes may have coexistent critical illness polyneuropathy, a pre-existing neuropathy, or substantial limb edema (precluding an adequate SNAP recording). Sensory and motor response conduction velocities are normal, as are distal motor and F-wave latencies. Low-amplitude or absent phrenic CMAPs may be seen in those with diaphragmatic weakness. Repetitive nerve stimulation studies at low frequencies (2 to 3 Hz) are normal. Occasionally, a decremental response is seen with repetitive stimulation if there is superimposed pharmacological neuromuscular blockade. However, this occurs only during the administration or shortly after the discontinuation of neuromuscular blocking agents (see later).

The motor response amplitudes increase during clinical recovery (Zochodne, 1998). This reappearance of or increase in the motor amplitudes often parallels the clinical recovery of muscle contractile force (Bird et al., 1992). Several other interesting observations have been made in this disorder. The duration of the CMAP appears to be significantly increased, concomitant with a drop in amplitude, in many patients (Bolton et al., 1994). The duration returns to normal as the amplitude recovers, suggestive of a muscle membrane conduction abnormality. It has also been noted that the sensory response amplitudes, although relatively spared, may increase in amplitude during recovery. Whether this is due to resolving limb edema, improvement of a superimposed neuropathy, or another process entirely is unknown. It has been proposed that in the setting of sepsis, there is a generalized abnormality of membrane excitability that affects muscle, nerve, and brain, producing weakness, reduced SNAP amplitudes, and encephalopathy, respectively (Bolton, 1993; Teener et al., 1999).

Needle electromyography may demonstrate fibrillation potentials and positive sharp waves in half or

Table 83–1. Electrophysiological Features Typical of the Neuromuscular Disorders That Develop in the Setting of Critical Illness

	Critical Illness Myopathy	Persistent Pharmacological Paralysis	Critical Illness Polyneuropathy
Nerve conduction studies			
SNAP amplitude	NL (occasionally ↓)	NL	↓ To absent
CMAP amplitude	↓ To absent	↓ To absent	↓ To absent
Repetitive nerve stimulation studies	NL	Decremental CMAP response	NL
Needle electromyographic studies			
Spontaneous activity	None to prominent	None	Usually; often prominent
MUP morphology	↓ Amplitude and duration	↓ Amplitude and duration	Normal (early); ↑ amplitude, duration, and polyphasia (later, after collateral sprouting)
MUP recruitment	Early full	Early full	Decreased
Direct muscle stimulation	Absent or ↓ ↓	Normal	Normal

CMAP, compound muscle action potential; MUP, motor unit potential; NL, normal; SNAP, sensory nerve action potential; ↑, increased; ↓, decreased.

more of those studied (Zochodne et al., 1994; Lacomis et al., 1996; Rich et al., 1997; Road et al., 1997; Campellone et al., 1998). The spontaneous activity is often quite sparse, but in some patients the fibrillation potentials are more pronounced, particularly in the minority with significantly elevated serum creatine kinase levels. Lack of spontaneous activity and reduced insertional activity may be seen in severely weak patients with markedly reduced or absent CMAP amplitudes (Bird and Rich, 2000). This could reflect muscle membrane inexcitability in these individuals (see later). Complex repetitive discharges have also been reported on occasion (Road et al., 1997). With voluntary muscle activation, low-amplitude, short-duration motor unit potentials are seen with early full recruitment. Serial quantitative needle electromyographic motor unit potential analysis may reveal low-amplitude motor unit potentials that increase in amplitude during recovery (Hoke et al., 1999). However, many patients are unable to voluntarily contract muscle due to encephalopathy or sedation. Repeating the study as the encephalopathy resolves often allows an adequate needle electromyographic examination and demonstration of these myopathic features. Some are so severely affected that they are unable to generate any voluntary activity. As a consequence, it may be extremely difficult to differentiate CIM from critical illness polyneuropathy on the needle examination. In these patients, there may be a role for the technique of direct muscle stimulation.

Muscle membrane inexcitability can be demonstrated by direct needle electrical stimulation in patients with severe CIM manifest by absent or markedly reduced CMAPs (Rich et al., 1996, 1997). Paralyzed muscle in some patients with CIM will not produce action potentials, even when directly stimulated. In contrast, muscle is easily excitable in patients with acute and chronic neuropathies (Rich et al., 1996). Serial studies have shown recovery of muscle membrane excitability as strength improves and the CMAP amplitudes rise. The importance of this technique is twofold. First, this phenomenon of muscle membrane inexcitability, in conjunction with similar physiological findings in an animal model of this disorder (Rich et al., 1998), suggests that it may play an important role in the pathogenesis of the weakness. Second, it may prove to be helpful in distinguishing CIM from critical illness polyneuropathy when the weakness is severe. Its usefulness is otherwise limited at this time in less severely affected patients. The lack of normative data and the limits of the technique are such that modest reductions in excitability cannot be reliably identified.

Historically, the technique of direct muscle stimulation was used to differentiate denervated from innervated muscle (Rogoff, 1980). In the setting of possible CIM, direct muscle stimulation is used to determine muscle membrane excitability rather than chronaxie or rheobase as previously measured in the historical studies of denervation. Lack of muscle

membrane excitability with direct muscle stimulation had previously been demonstrated only in periodic paralysis (Mitchell, 1899; Rich et al., 1997). Direct muscle stimulation can be performed using a monopolar electromyographic needle electrode as the cathode and a subdermal needle placed 1 to 2 cm laterally as the anode, similar to the technique of stimulation single-fiber electromyography. However, as opposed to stimulation single-fiber electromyography, the stimulating electrodes are placed in the distal third of the muscle, away from the end-plate band. The muscle is stimulated with gradually increasing current until a clear twitch is palpable. Guided by the twitch, a subdermal needle electrode (12 mm long, 0.4-mm diameter, stainless steel) is placed as the recording electrode 1 to 5 cm away from the stimulation electrode. Shorter distances are used for small hand muscles, such as the abductor pollicis brevis, and the longer separation is used for muscles such as tibialis anterior and extensor digitorum communis. A second subdermal needle electrode or surface electrode is placed just off the muscle distally as a reference. The active recording

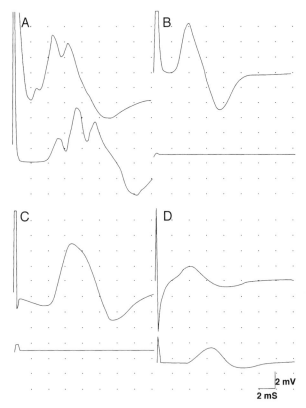

Figure 83–1. Direct muscle stimulation in various neuromuscular disorders. *Top trace,* compound muscle action potentials (CMAPs) obtained with direct muscle stimulation (dmCMAP). *Bottom trace,* CMAPs obtained with nerve stimulation (neCMAP) using the same recording electrodes. *A,* Anterior tibial muscle from a normal subject. *B,* Severe chronic denervation (>12 months), from abductor pollicis brevis. *C,* Anterior tibial muscle during pharmacological neuromuscular blockade. *D,* Abductor pollicis brevis during an acute attack of periodic paralysis. (In *A–D,* 2 mV and 2 ms per division.) (Reprinted with permission from Rich MM, Bird SJ, Raps EC, et al: Direct muscle stimulation in acute quadriplegic myopathy. Muscle Nerve 1997;20:665–673.)

electrode is moved to maximize the amplitude of the direct muscle response—direct muscle CMAP. If no twitch is palpable, the recording electrode should be moved to several positions to ensure that small responses are not missed. Stimulation is then performed over a range of currents from 5 to 75 mA. A maximal response is usually obtained with stimulus intensities between 30 and 75 mA. At high current intensities, there is no further increase in the direct muscle CMAP, and it is obscured by increasing stimulus artifact. After the direct muscle CMAP is obtained, supramaximal stimulation is applied over the nerve innervating that muscle, and the standard nerve-evoked motor response (nerve-evoked CMAP) is recorded from the same recording electrode array. For the tibialis anterior, the peroneal nerve would be stimulated over the fibular head to produce the nerve-evoked CMAP.

With this technique, a large direct muscle CMAP can be easily obtained from normal individuals, typically close to the standard CMAP amplitudes (Rich et al., 1996) (Fig. 83–1A). Normal direct muscle CMAP responses can also be obtained from completely denervated muscle, whether acute, as in the Guillain-Barré syndrome, or chronic with significant atrophy (Rich et al., 1996, 1997) (see Fig. 83–1B). The direct muscle CMAP is also normal during pharmacological neuromuscular blockade, with an absent nerve-evoked CMAP (see Fig. 83–1C). The nerve-evoked CMAP amplitudes may be profoundly reduced or absent in either CIM or critical illness polyneuropathy. However, the direct muscle CMAP

amplitude is near normal in neuropathy but reduced or absent in CIM (Fig. 83–2). A comparison of the nerve and muscle stimulation response (nerve-evoked CMAP/direct muscle CMAP) has the potential to help separate these two disorders in severely affected individuals. In the setting of polyneuropathy, the nerve-evoked CMAP/direct muscle CMAP ratio is near 0. If the patient has severe CIM, both responses are absent, or if the responses are very small, the nerve-evoked CMAP/direct muscle CMAP ratio is near 1.

Clinical recovery of patients parallels recovery of muscle membrane excitability and an increase in both the nerve-evoked CMAP and the direct muscle CMAP (Rich et al., 1997) (Fig. 83–3). This may suggest that weakness in CIM is in part the result of muscle membrane inexcitability. This may also account for patients with myopathy who have markedly reduced CMAP amplitudes despite relatively normal muscle morphology. This mechanism of weakness is analogous to that of periodic paralysis, where there is profound weakness, markedly decreased CMAP amplitudes, and relatively normal muscle morphology. Direct muscle stimulation has also been performed in patients with periodic paralysis. The direct muscle response amplitudes are markedly reduced during the attack, just as they are in severe CIM (Rich et al., 1997) (see Fig. 83–1D). The direct muscle stimulation CMAP amplitudes return to normal as the patient with periodic paralysis regains strength, just as the CMAP amplitudes rise during recovery from CIM.

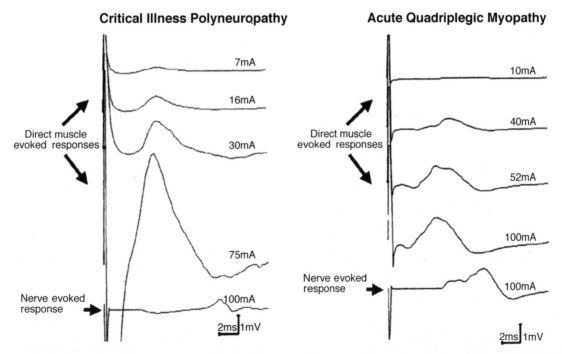

Figure 83–2. Muscle is electrically inexcitable in critical illness myopathy. Compound muscle action potentials (CMAPs) from the anterior tibial muscles of a patient with critical illness polyneuropathy *(left)* and critical illness myopathy *(right)*. *Top four traces,* obtained with direct muscle stimulation (dmCMAP). *Bottom trace,* recorded with supramaximal nerve stimulation (neCMAP). *Shown at the right of each tracing:* stimulation current intensity. (Adapted with permission from Rich MM, Bird SJ, Raps EC, et al: Direct muscle stimulation in acute quadriplegic myopathy. Muscle Nerve 1997;20:665–673.)

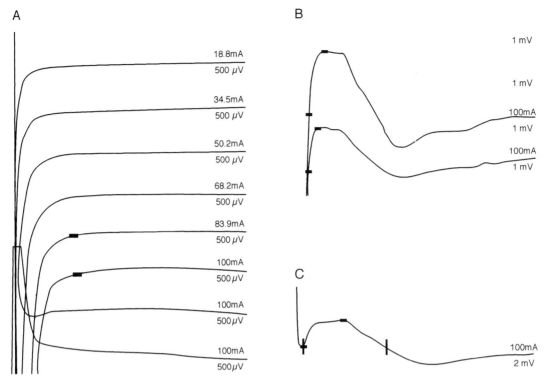

Figure 83–3. Recovery of muscle excitability in critical illness myopathy. Anterior tibial muscle compound muscle action potentials (CMAPs) from a 10-month-old boy with critical illness myopathy. *A,* Direct muscle stimulation *(top six traces)* and peroneal nerve stimulation at the knee *(bottom two traces).* No responses are obtained at a time of severe quadriplegia. *B* and *C,* During clinical recovery of strength 18 days later, CMAPs returned. *B,* direct muscle stimulation (large stimulus artifact at high current intensities and small interelectrode distances). *C,* peroneal nerve stimulation at the knee. (In *A–C,* the stimulation current intensity and vertical sensitivity is shown at the right of each tracing; horizontal axis is 2 ms per division.)

LABORATORY AND PATHOLOGICAL FEATURES

Serum creatine kinase levels are elevated in a minority of reported patients. In a retrospective series of 39 patients with CIM, the creatine kinase level was elevated in 27%. The majority of values were less than 1000 IU/L (normal, <200 IU/L), but a few were higher. The limited number of reports of higher or more consistently elevated creatine kinase levels likely relates to the timing of the serum studies. In a prospective study of patients with status asthmaticus and CIM, all had serum creatine kinase elevations that peaked at 2 to 5 days after intravenous corticosteroid exposure and normalized by 16 days (Douglass et al., 1992). The underlying critical illness and encephalopathy generally delay the awareness that neuromuscular weakness is present. When the neurological investigation is performed, it is often beyond the period at which the creatine kinase level is elevated. Therefore, a normal serum creatine kinase level obtained a few weeks after the probable onset of weakness does not weigh against the diagnosis of CIM.

Pathological studies of muscle in CIM reveal a spectrum of abnormalities (Chad and Lacomis, 1994; Zochodne et al., 1994; Lacomis et al., 1996). A number of nonspecific abnormalities are common, such as myofiber size variability or atrophy (especially of type 2 fibers). In many biopsy samples, the only significant abnormality is muscle fiber atrophy. There is no lymphocytic inflammation. A varying degree of myofiber necrosis and regeneration is seen in 0% to 65% of fibers (Lacomis et al., 2000). In a few patients, muscle fiber necrosis is the predominant finding, and in these cases, serum creatine kinase levels may be markedly elevated. Features of a disrupted intramyofibrillar network with oxidative reagents (NADH-TR) are often seen. A variety of other abnormalities have been reported in a few cases, such as selective type 2 atrophy (Al-Lozi et al., 1994; Gutmann et al., 1996), glycogen accumulation (Hirano et al., 1992), and rimmed vacuoles (Danon and Carpenter, 1991).

The characteristic pathological finding of CIM, however, is the loss of myosin thick filaments, leading some to call this disorder "thick-filament myopathy." This is seen as a patchy loss of myofiber staining with ATPase (at alkaline or acid pH) in nonnecrotic fibers (Fig. 83–4). Electron microscopy of the muscle confirms the loss of myosin thick filament (Danon and Carpenter, 1991; Lacomis et al., 1996, 1998), with disruption of myosin (A bands) with otherwise normal cellular architecture (Fig. 83–5). Loss of myosin can also be confirmed immunohistochemically (Lacomis et al., 1996). Evidence of this pattern of myosin loss can be seen in up to 78% of those with CIM (Lacomis et al., 1996). Myosin loss can also be seen focally in other disorders

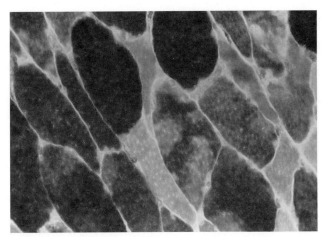

Figure 83–4. Muscle biopsy from a patient with critical illness myopathy. A myosin-ATPase (pH 4.3)–reacted section demonstrates the characteristic patchy pallor, or lack of reactivity, indicative of myosin loss. (Courtesy of Dr. David Lacomis.)

such as dermatomyositis, but the widespread loss of myosin is quite unique to CIM.

It is possible that these various pathological patterns represent a spectrum of severity due to the same pathophysiological mechanism or are due to different effects at different periods of the disease. Myosin loss and muscle fiber necrosis probably contribute significantly to persistent weakness, but it is likely that muscle membrane inexcitability also accounts for some of the weakness seen early in the disorder. This is especially the case in patients with marked weakness who have low-amplitude or absent CMAPs and unimpressive muscle biopsies.

CONTROVERSIES REGARDING CRITICAL ILLNESS MYOPATHY

When an intensive care unit patient who has received neuromuscular blocking agents and intravenous corticosteroids develops a flaccid quadripar-

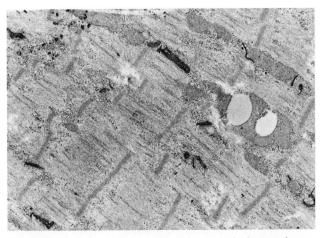

Figure 83–5. Electron microscopy of a muscle biopsy from a patient with critical illness myopathy. This demonstrates the preservation of Z-bands and lack of interconnecting myosin thick filaments.

esis with all the electrophysiological hallmarks of this myopathy (see Table 83–1), there is little difficulty in making a differentiation from critical illness polyneuropathy. However, there is a large heterogeneous group of patients who have clinical and electrodiagnostic features common to both disorders and are not as easy to classify (Breuer, 1999; Teener et al., 1999). The clinical presentation (quadriparesis) and risk factors (sepsis) of these two disorders may overlap, such that it is not possible to determine the cause of generalized weakness based on the clinical setting alone. Although critical illness polyneuropathy has been most closely linked to sepsis (Bolton, 1996), CIM has developed in patients affected by sepsis who did not receive either neuromuscular blocking agents or corticosteroids (Latonico et al., 1996; Rich et al., 1997; Showalter and Engel, 1997).

The electrophysiological studies that are most easily performed in the intensive care unit—motor nerve conduction studies and evaluation of spontaneous activity during needle electromyographic examination—do not allow a reliable distinction between CIM and critical illness polyneuropathy, because the presence of fibrillation potentials and reduced CMAP amplitudes are electrophysiological findings common to both disorders. Sensory nerve conduction studies are often hampered by technical factors, or SNAPs may be low due to coexisting critical illness polyneuropathy. The assessment of motor unit potential morphology and recruitment is often limited by inadequate patient cooperation. In these circumstances, myopathic features on the needle electromyographic examination may become apparent in CIM only during recovery (Bird et al., 1992; Rich et al., 1997; Road et al., 1997). Muscle biopsy can help differentiate CIM from a neurogenic disorder in many, but often a confident pathological diagnosis cannot be made. Direct muscle stimulation may overcome some of these limitations and allow the identification of those with severe CIM (see Fig. 83–2).

Critical illness polyneuropathy as an axonal sensory-motor polyneuropathy is well established. Whether a purely motor form of critical illness polyneuropathy exists is controversial. A purely motor form of critical illness polyneuropathy has been proposed in reports of patients with severe weakness, reduced CMAP amplitudes, and relatively preserved sensory function (Hund et al., 1997; Schwarz et al., 1997). A distal motor axonopathy has been offered as the possible explanation of these clinical and electrophysiological features. However, CIM also produces reduced CMAP amplitudes and spontaneous activity (fibrillation potentials), and these two features alone are insufficient to distinguish reliably between myopathy and motor neuropathy, especially when needle electromyographic evaluation is limited. Given the controversy in the differentiation of CIM from a putative motor form of critical illness polyneuropathy, diagnostic criteria for CIM for re-

Table 83–2. Proposed Diagnostic Criteria for Critical Illness Myopathy for Research Studies

Major Features	Supportive Features	Classification
1. SNAP amplitudes >80% LLN in two or more nerves 2. Needle EMG with short-duration, low-amplitude MUPs with early full recruitment, with or without fibrillation potentials* 3. Absence of a decremental response on repetitive nerve stimulation 4. Muscle histopathological findings of myopathy with myosin loss	1. CMAP amplitudes <80% LLN without conduction block 2. Elevated CK† 3. Demonstration of electrical inexcitability	Definite CIM: presence of all four major features Probable CIM: presence of any three major features and one or more supportive features Possible CIM: presence of major features 1 and 3 or of 2 and 3, and one or more supportive features‡

*May not be apparent until recovery begins or encephalopathy/sedation remits.
†Best assessed in first week of illness.
‡May have pre-existing polyneuropathy or coexisting critical illness polyneuropathy causing low SNAP amplitudes.
CIM, critical illness myopathy; CK, creatine kinase; CMAP, compound muscle action potential; EMG, electromyography; LLN, lower limit of normal; MUP, motor unit potential; SNAP, sensory nerve action potential.
From Lacomis D, Zochodne DW, Bird SJ: Critical illness myopathy: What's in a name? Muscle Nerve 2000;23:1785–1788.

search studies have been proposed (Lacomis et al., 2000) (Table 83–2).

ANIMAL MODELS AND PATHOGENESIS

The pathogenetic mechanisms involved in the development of CIM are likely multifactorial (Fig. 83–6). They must, however, account for the unique features seen in many patients, including rapidly developing severe quadriparesis and markedly reduced or absent CMAPs despite a lack of significant myonecrosis, the distinctive patchy loss of myosin thick filaments, and the lack of muscle membrane electrical excitability.

Concurrent denervation of muscle and corticosteroid treatment in rats is a useful model of human CIM. This model produces all of the unique features of CIM that were noted. Nerve section, producing

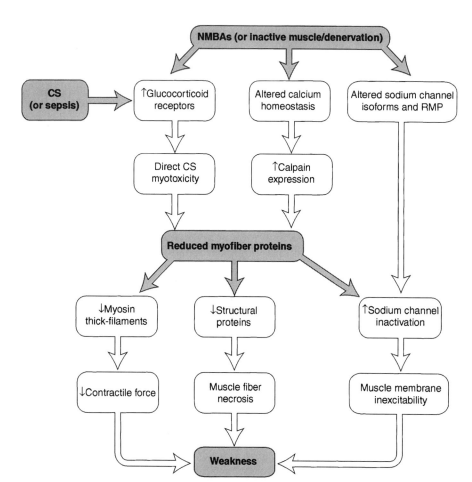

Figure 83–6. Proposed factors involved in the pathogenesis of critical illness myopathy. CS, Corticosteroids; NMBAs, neuromuscular blocking agents; RMP, resting membrane potential.

denervation of muscle, probably is a reasonable simulation of the changes seen with neuromuscular blocking agents. Neuromuscular blocking agents produce all of the changes in muscle fiber properties seen after denervation (Rich et al., 1998a), including a decrease in resting membrane potential, an increase in specific membrane resistance, reappearance of tetrodotoxin-resistant sodium channels, and spread of acetylcholine sensitivity over the surface of the fiber (Berg and Hall, 1975; Cangiano et al., 1977). Rouleau and colleagues (1987) sectioned rat sciatic nerve, producing denervation, and concurrently treated with corticosteroids. The pathological hallmark of marked myosin depletion was seen at 7 and 13 days but not in those rats treated with corticosteroids or denervation alone. The same pathological features have been confirmed by others using this model (Massa et al., 1992; Rich et al., 1998a). If the nerve is instead crushed, the myopathy and loss of myosin thick filaments rapidly reverse within 1 week of reinnervation (Massa et al., 1992).

This model of CIM, in which rats are treated with high-dose corticosteroids and muscle is denervated in vivo by transection of nerve, produces not only the unique pathological features of myosin loss in this disorder but also the electrophysiological features (Rich et al., 1998a). The study of affected muscle in vitro by intracellular recording of individual muscle fibers demonstrated loss of excitability (Fig. 83–7). The loss of excitability was not due solely to changes in resting membrane potential or to decreases in specific membrane resistance. Although most muscle fibers lacked the ability to generate action potentials when directly stimulated, in some of the mildly affected fibers, a small-amplitude action potential was obtained (Fig. 83–8). The small-amplitude action potentials and the decreased rate

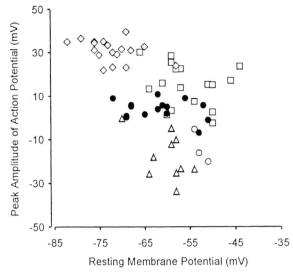

Figure 83–8. Sodium current is significantly reduced in individual muscle fibers in an animal model of critical illness myopathy: action potential (AP) peak amplitude versus resting membrane potential (RMP). Control fibers *(diamonds)*: RMP around −75 mV and peak APs around +30 mV. Denervated muscle fibers *(squares)*: RMP around −55 mV and APs that peak lower at +10 to +30 mV but still reach threshold to produce APs. Steroid-treated, denervated fibers (RMP around −55mV) failed to generate an AP in 83% of those studied. In those that did *(solid and open circles)*, the peak AP was −10 to +10 mV; this is consistent with a severe reduction in sodium current. (Adapted with permission from Rich et al., 1998a.)

of rise to threshold suggested that there was a marked reduction in sodium current.

Sodium current could be reduced if the number of sodium channels in the muscle fiber membrane is reduced, if sodium channels inactivate abnormally, or both. The inexcitable muscle fibers have only one third the number of adult sodium channel isoforms. However, the embryonic isoform is increased. This isoform cannot be measured by toxin binding assays, but RNA levels for this isoform were found at high levels (Rich et al., 1998b). The total number of sodium channels may not be significantly reduced in the animal model of CIM. Alternatively, sodium current could be reduced if sodium channels are present but are inactivating abnormally. This is what occurs in hyperkalemic periodic paralysis when genetically abnormal sodium channels lead to a depolarization of the membrane that results in inactivation of the majority of sodium channels. Inactivated sodium channels cannot open to carry current during an action potential, and the muscle becomes inexcitable. Sodium channel inactivation in CIM might be increased due to an elevation in the numbers of embryonic (SkM2) isoforms (Rich et al., 1998b). This channel isoform inactivates at a more negative membrane potential level than the adult (SkM1) isoform. A further hit, such as treatment with high-dose corticosteroids or changes in the cellular milieu during sepsis, may further increase the propensity of sodium channels to inactivate. Most of these channels would then be inactivated

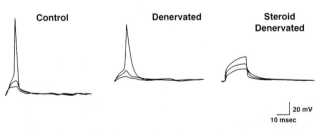

Figure 83–7. Individual muscle fibers become inexcitable in an animal model of critical illness myopathy. Intracellular recordings are from three individual muscle fibers demonstrating the action potential elicited by intracellular injection of depolarizing current. *Left,* a control muscle fiber (resting membrane potential [RMP], −79 mV). Superimposed are two subthreshold stimuli that elicit no action potential; the third stimulus is suprathreshold producing a large action potential. *Middle,* from a denervated muscle fiber. The RMP of −57 mV contributes to inactivation of sodium channels, so the action potential is not as sharp and peaks at a lower potential than in the normal fiber. *Right,* three superimposed traces from an inexcitable fiber with an RMP of −57 mV (treated with steroids and denervated). Despite long, large pulses of depolarizing current, no action potential can be elicited. (Adapted with permission from Rich et al., 1998a.)

at the altered membrane potential of denervated, corticosteroid-treated muscle and would not be available to carry current during initiation of an action potential, resulting in reduced or absent excitability.

Myosin depletion is commonly seen in CIM and the animal model, but the exact mechanism is not clear. In a study of seven patients with CIM, other structural proteins (titin, nebulin, and actin) were found to also be reduced early in the disorder but to a lesser degree than myosin (Showalter and Engel, 1997). There was evidence of significantly enhanced expression of calpain, a calcium-activated protease, in atrophic myofibers. Other proteolytic pathways, as measured by ubiquitin and cathepsin B, were not increased. This suggested that altered cellular calcium homeostasis may play a role in the degradation of myosin. This mechanism could affect other proteins as well, including those associated with the sodium channel.

Inactive muscle, such as occurs in critically ill patients who are not moving due to neuromuscular blocking agents or who are sedated, develops a partial loss of resting potential that tends to inactivate sodium channels (Berg and Hall, 1975) in a similar manner as those that have been denervated. There also is an up-regulation of glucocorticoid receptors (DuBois and Almon, 1981). These factors may particularly render the muscle vulnerable to corticosteroid myotoxicity. Corticosteroids may then trigger an intracellular catabolic process, perhaps related to altered calcium homeostasis. The deleterious effect of sepsis and the systemic inflammatory response syndrome on muscle has also been suggested by the work of Bolton and others (Zochodne et al., 1986; Bolton, 1993, 1996). They observed electrophysiological and morphological findings of myopathy, often coexistent with polyneuropathy, that they termed *myopathy in critical illness.* They suggested that this may be due to a reduction in the bioenergetic reserves, as measured by phosphorus-31 nuclear magnetic resonance imaging of affected muscle (Zochodne et al., 1987). Bolton (1996) also proposed that there is denervation secondary to critical illness polyneuropathy in some patients and that the concomitant use of corticosteroids may induce myopathy, much like the animal models of CIM as described. All of these factors may result in a loss of myosin and other structural proteins, resulting in a spectrum of effects that produce weakness (see Fig. 83–6).

Other Myopathies

Other than CIM, few myopathic disorders develop de novo in the setting of the intensive care unit. These disorders include rhabdomyolysis, or acute necrotizing myopathy, and cachectic myopathy. Most other acquired myopathies, such as polymyositis, are gradually progressive and do not typically produce acute weakness. One must always keep in mind the possibility of a pre-existent disorder, particularly when limb weakness is one of the presenting complaints. Rarely, disorders such as polymyositis, dermatomyositis, and human immunodeficiency virus–associated myositis may result in intensive care unit admission due to respiratory failure or marked dysphagia (Zochodne, 1998). Acid maltase deficiency may result in respiratory failure in adults early in the course of the disease (Rosenow and Engel, 1978; Keunen et al., 1984). Some mitochondrial myopathies may have recurrent respiratory insufficiency as a major feature (Barohn et al., 1990). Patients with myotonic dystrophy may be more susceptible to respiratory failure after anesthesia for surgical procedures (Kohn et al., 1964). However, in most of these disorders, the features that necessitate intensive care unit care usually develop subacutely in the setting of a more long-standing illness.

Muscle weakness may develop acutely in the intensive care unit due to rhabdomyolysis rather than to CIM. Some have used the term *acute necrotizing myopathy* when rhabdomyolysis occurs in the setting of critical illness and with the use of neuromuscular blocking agents and corticosteroids (Ramsay et al., 1993; Zochodne et al., 1994). However, as noted earlier, this is a relatively uncommon end of the pathological spectrum of CIM in which muscle fiber necrosis is prominent.

Rhabdomyolysis may be due to a variety of infections or physical trauma (Singh and Scheld, 1996; Zager, 1996; David, 2000) encountered in the intensive care unit setting. Rhabdomyolysis has been linked with some specific bacterial agents, most frequently *Legionella* (Posner et al., 1980; Malvy et al., 1992; Byrd and Roy, 1998). It has also been reported with *Staphylococcus aureus, Streptococccus,* salmonella, *Haemophilus influenzae,* and *Escherichia coli* (David, 2000). Viral infections, particularly influenza virus, may cause muscle necrosis but are not likely to develop in the intensive care unit. Rhabdomyolysis may also be seen in the intensive care unit after trauma, surgery, or limb ischemia as part of a compartment syndrome (Slater and Mullins, 1998; Szewczyk et al., 1998; David, 2000). In these circumstances of physical injury, there is localized weakness, and generalized weakness with respiratory failure is less of a concern.

Pharmacological agents may cause muscle necrosis via a variety of mechanisms, including direct myotoxicity, hypokalemia, or fever and excessive muscle activity. The list of legal and illicit drugs that may cause rhabdomyolysis is extensive (David, 2000), but only a few are seen commonly in the intensive care unit. In organ recipients, the combination of cholesterol-reducing agents and cyclosporine, or certain antibiotics, may result in muscle fiber necrosis (Grunden, 1997). The hydroxymethyl glutaryl coenzyme A reductase inhibitors (e.g., simvastatin, lovastatin, atorvastatin) may also cause rhabdomyolysis in the setting of renal failure (Biesenbach et al., 1996) and with the concomitant use of colchicine (Rana et al., 1997) or gemfibrozil (Duell et al., 1998). Colchicine is also myotoxic in the setting of renal failure. Illicit drugs such as cocaine, amphetamines, and Ecstasy may produce acute rhabdomyolysis (David, 2000), but this is generally accompanied by signs of central nervous system involvement similar to the hypermetabolic states described later.

Acute muscle fiber necrosis may also be seen as part of a spectrum of abnormalities associated with certain hypermetabolic states, such as the serotonergic syndrome or the neuroleptic malignant syndrome. The serotonergic syndrome is associated with the use of selective serotonin reuptake inhibitors. It is generally manifest by varying degrees of hyperthermia, leukocytosis, autonomic instability, agitation, and encephalopathy, even to the point of coma (Bertorini, 1997). Antipsychotic medications can produce the neuroleptic malignant syndrome. In some instances, these drugs may cause rhabdomyolysis in the absence of the other features of neuroleptic malignant syndrome (Marinella, 1997; Koren et al., 1998). Neuroleptic malignant syndrome presents with features similar to those of the serotonergic syndrome, although in general, there is more muscle rigidity. These states present with features such as fever, leukocytosis, and encephalopathy that may mimic sepsis, and when associated with rhabdomyolysis, they could easily be confused with CIM.

Muscle weakness due to profound hypokalemia and hypophosphatemia may develop in the intensive care unit. Severe hypokalemia may develop secondary to diuretics, amphotericin B use, or renal tubular acidosis and produce rhabdomyolysis (Zager, 1996). Hypophosphatemia may produce a similar disorder (Gravelyn et al., 1988; Singhal et al., 1992).

Patients with rhabdomyolysis typically present with weakness that may be proximal or generalized. Myalgias and swelling in the affected muscles are common. Cranial nerve function, sensation, and tendon reflexes are normal. Persistent weakness after recovery is unusual, but the immediate complications warrant more concern. Massive muscle necrosis results in the release of potassium and initially sequesters calcium. The resultant hyperkalemia and hypocalcemia can produce life-threatening cardiac arrhythmias. The most serious complication is that of acute renal failure; this develops in about 17% of those who have myoglobinuria (Ward, 1988) and is manifest by oliguria or anuria. Muscle and nerve may be irreversibly damaged by the ischemia produced locally in compartment syndromes.

The serum creatine kinase level is elevated in rhabdomyolysis, often to greater than 10,000 IU/L. Myoglobinuria is frequently present, resulting in a brownish discoloration of the urine. This can be confirmed by the laboratory measurement of myoglobin in the urine. There are no characteristic histopathological features of rhabdomyolysis. The muscle biopsy demonstrates varying degrees of myofiber necrosis, without inflammation, myosin loss, or other specific features.

The electrophysiological features of rhabdomyolysis are those of an acute myopathy. Nerve conduction studies demonstrate normal sensory and motor responses. The CMAPs may be reduced when recording from muscles where there is severe myonecrosis, but this is unusual. Repetitive nerve stimulation studies are normal, reflecting normal neuromuscular transmission. Fibrillation potentials are often seen on needle electromyographic examination. Short-duration, small-amplitude motor unit potentials with early full recruitment are seen in affected muscles that are significantly weak. Muscles that are strong have no clear abnormalities of motor unit potential morphology or recruitment.

Differentiation of rhabdomyolysis due to drugs or infectious agents from CIM may be difficult in the absence of historical, clinical, or toxicological clues to one of the causes of rhabdomyolysis. In general, there is much less myonecrosis in most cases of CIM, and as a result, the creatine kinase levels are higher in rhabdomyolysis. The electrophysiological features of an acute myopathy are common to both. Even the muscle biopsy features may overlap, although the demonstration of selective myosin loss is seen only in CIM.

Cachectic myopathy, also termed *disuse,* or *catabolic myopathy,* is an ill-defined entity that may be seen as a complication of critical illness. In the setting of prolonged critical illness, mild atrophy and weakness may be noted. This weakness never is severe or results in prolonged ventilatory support. It may contribute to slower-than-expected recovery of ambulatory independence. The electrophysiological studies invariably show normal sensory and motor nerve responses, repetitive nerve stimulation, and needle electromyography. Serum creatine kinase levels are normal, and muscle biopsy results are usually normal. On occasion, type 2 muscle fiber atrophy, a nonspecific finding, is seen. The clinical, electrophysiological, and pathological features allow a ready differentiation from those with CIM. The pathogenesis of cachectic myopathy is uncertain. It may be related to the undetermined processes that produce cachectic states in advanced cancer or severe congestive heart failure.

DISORDERS OF NEUROMUSCULAR TRANSMISSION

Prolonged Pharmacological Neuromuscular Blockade

Nondepolarizing neuromuscular blocking agents are quaternary ammonium compounds that bind to the α subunit of the acetylcholine receptor (Hunter, 1995). The postsynaptic ion channel thus will not open, and the membrane will not depolarize, rendering the muscle paralyzed. These agents have been used to allow more efficient mechanical ventilation in a variety of disorders that produce severe respiratory failure (Hansen-Flaschen et al., 1993; Sladen, 1995). In addition to being linked to the development of CIM, the effects of neuromuscular blocking agents can persist in individual patients, creating unexpected weakness and inability to wean from mechanical ventilation. This is particularly the case in patients with impaired hepatic or renal function. Although these drugs are metabolized in the liver, they are secreted in the urine, and pharmacologically active deacetylated metabolites accumulate in the setting of renal failure (Hunter, 1995).

Prolonged pharmacological blockade has been reported with all neuromuscular blocking agents, particularly with the aminosteroid forms, vecuronium and pancuronium (O'Connor and Russell, 1988; Partridge et al., 1990; Segredo et al., 1990, 1992; Kupfer et al., 1992; Vanderheyden et al., 1992). It has also been reported with the benzylisoquinolone form, atracurium (Bizzard-Scmid and Desai, 1986). Segredo and coworkers (1992) studied 16 consecutive patients in the intensive care unit who received vecuronium for at least 2 consecutive days. Neuromuscular blockade and weakness were prolonged in seven patients and persisted for up to 7 days after the cessation of the drug. All of the seven patients had renal failure (creatinine clearance <30 mL/min) and elevated plasma levels of the 3-desacetyl metabolite of vecuronium. Although this drug is primarily metabolized by the liver, the underlying renal failure allows accumulation of active metabolites (3-desacetyl-vecuronium), which can also produce neuromuscular blockade and prolonged weakness.

Electrophysiological studies can readily demonstrate prolonged neuromuscular blockade as the underlying cause of persistent weakness in most circumstances when it occurs due to the prolonged effects of neuromuscular blocking agents. Repetitive nerve stimulation studies show a decremental response in the compound muscle action potential, confirming the physiological abnormality of neuromuscular transmission (Segredo et al., 1992; Barohn et al., 1994; Raps et al., 1994) (Fig. 83–9). Needle electromyographic examination may show fibrillation potentials and short-duration motor unit potentials, much like those seen in botulism. One must be aware that there may be those with severe blockade in whom no motor response is obtained (see Fig. 83–1C), and as such, no decremental response can be demonstrated. This may be due to severe prolonged pharmacological blockade or the development of acute myopathy (CIM). The electrophysiological studies, including repetitive nerve stimulation, should be repeated approximately 1 week after cessation of the drug if weakness persists. The effects of prolonged pharmacological neuromuscular blockade would no longer be a likely consideration at that point.

These agents are used more sparingly with the awareness of the potential problem of prolonged pharmacological blockade, as well as CIM (Hansen-Flaschen et al., 1991; Raps et al., 1994). When neuro-

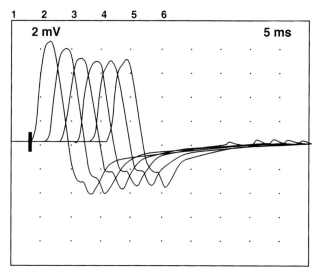

Figure 83–9. Abnormal neuromuscular transmission caused by pharmacological blockade by vecuronium. This can be demonstrated by two per second repetitive nerve stimulation, as shown here from the median nerve. A decremental response is obtained that is characteristic of a defect in neuromuscular transmission. This typically will disappear within a few hours of drug discontinuation but may persist for days to 1 week in those with hepatic or renal failure. Vertical axis is 2 mV per division, and the horizontal axis is 5 ms per division.

muscular blocking agents are used and weakness persists due to prolonged neuromuscular blockade, it should not persist beyond 1 week after cessation of the blocking agent, and it typically lasts for only a few hours. If weakness persists longer than 1 week, other etiologies, such as CIM, need to be considered.

References

Al-Lozi MT, Pestronk A, Yee WC, et al: Rapidly evolving myopathy with myosin-deficient fibers. Ann Neurol 1994;35:273–279.

Bachmann P, Gaussorgues P, Piperno D, et al: Acute myopathy after status asthmaticus. Presse Med 1987;16:1486–1488.

Barohn RJ, Clanton T, Sahenk Z, Mendell JR: Recurrent respiratory insufficiency and depressed ventilatory drive complicating mitochondrial myopathies. Neurology 1990;40:103–106.

Barohn RJ, Jackson CE, Rogers SJ, et al: Prolonged paralysis due to nondepolarizing blocking agents and corticosteroids. Muscle Nerve 1994;17:647–652.

Benzing G, Iannaccone ST, Bove KE, et al: Prolonged myasthenic syndrome after one week of muscle relaxants. Pediatr Neurol 1990;6:190–196.

Berg DK, Hall ZW: Increased extrajunctional acetylcholine sensitivity produced by chronic acetylcholine sensitivity produced by chronic post-synaptic neuromuscular blockade. J Physiol 1975;244:659–676.

Bertorini TE: Myoglobinuria, malignant hyperthermia, neuromalignant malignant syndrome and serotonin syndrome. Neurol Clin 1997;15:649–671.

Biesenbach G, Janko O, Stuby U, et al: Myoglobinuric renal failure due to long-standing lovastatin therapy in a patient with renal insufficiency. Nephrol Dial Transplant 1996;11:2059–2060.

Bird SJ, Mackin GA, Schotland DL, Raps EC: Acute myopathic quadriplegia: A unique syndrome associated with vecuronium and steroid treatment. Muscle Nerve 1992;15:1208.

Bird SJ, Rich MM: Neuromuscular complications of critical illness. Neurologist 2000;6:2–11.

Bird SJ, Taylor PJ, Haplea S, et al: Myopathy in critically ill children with loss of electrical muscle excitability. Muscle Nerve 1999;22:1318.

Bizzard-Scmid MD, Desai SP: Prolonged neuromuscular blockade with atracurium. Can Anaesth Soc J 1986;33:209–212.

Bolton CF: Electrophysiologic studies of critically ill patients. Muscle Nerve 1987;10:129–135.

Bolton CF: Neuromuscular complications of sepsis. Intensive Care Med 1993;19:S58–S63.

Bolton CF: Sepsis and the systemic inflammatory response syndrome: Neuromuscular manifestations. Crit Care Med 1996;24:1408–1416.

Bolton CF, Young GB, Zochodne DW: The neurologic complications of sepsis. Ann Neurol 1993;33:94–100.

Bolton CF, Young GB, Zochodne DW: Neurologic changes during severe sepsis. In Dobb GJ, Brim J, Burehardi H, Dellinger RP (eds): Current Topics in Intensive Care. Philadelphia, WB Saunders, 1994; 180–217.

Breuer AC: Critical illness polyneuropathy: An outdated concept. Muscle Nerve 1999;22:422–424.

Byrd RP, Roy TM: Rhabdomyolysis and bacterial pneumonia. Respir Med 1998;92:359–362.

Campellone JV, Lacomis D, Kramer DJ, et al: Acute myopathy after liver transplantation. Neurology 1998;50:46–53.

Cangiano A, Lutzemberger L, Nicotra L: Non-equivalence of impulse blockade and denervation in the production of membrane changes in rat skeletal muscle. J Physiol 1977;273:691–706.

Chad DA, Lacomis D: Critically ill patients with newly acquired weakness: The clinicopathologic spectrum. Ann Neurol 1994;35:257–259.

Danon MJ, Carpenter S: Myopathy with thick filament (myosin) loss following prolonged paralysis with vecuronium during steroid treatment. Muscle Nerve 1991;14:1131–1139.

David WS: Myoglobinuria. Neurol Clin 2000;18:215–243.

Deconinck N, Van Parijs V, Beckers-Bleukx G, et al: Critical illness myopathy unrelated to corticosteroids or neuromuscular blocking agents. Neuromuscul Disord 1998;8:186–192.

De Smet Y, Jaminet M, Jaeger U, et al: Myopathie aigue cortisonique de l'asthmatique. Rev Neurol 1991;147:682–685.

Douglass JA, Truxen DV, Horne M, et al: Myopathy in severe asthma. Am Rev Respir Dis 1992;146:517–519.

DuBois D, Almon RR: A possible role for glucocorticoids in denervation atrophy. Muscle Nerve 1981;4:370–373.

Duell PB, Connor WE, Illingworth DR: Rhabdomyolysis after taking atorvastatin with gemfibrozil. Am J Cardiol 1998;81:368–370.

Faragher MW, Day BJ, Dennett X: Critical care myopathy: An electrophysiological and histologic study. Muscle Nerve 1996; 19:516–518.

Gooch JL: Prolonged paralysis after neuromuscular blockade. Muscle Nerve 1995;18:937–942.

Gooch JL, Moore MH, Ryser DK: Prolonged paralysis after neuromuscular junction blockade: Case reports and electrodiagnostic findings. Arch Phys Med Rehabil 1993;74:1007–1011.

Gooch JL, Suchyta MR, Balbierz JM, Petajan JH: Prolonged paralysis after treatment with neuromuscular junction blocking agents. Crit Care Med 1991;19:1125–1131.

Griffin D, Fairman N, Coursin D, et al: Acute myopathy during treatment of status asthmaticus with corticosteroids and steroidal muscle relaxants. Chest 1992;102:510–514.

Gravelyn TR, Brophy N, Siegert C, Peters-Golden M: Hypophosphatemia associated respiratory muscle weakness in a general inpatient population. Am J Med 1988;84:870–876.

Grunden JW, Fisher KA: Lovastatin-induced rhabdomyolysis possibly associated with clarithromycin and azithromycin. Ann Pharmacother 1997;859–861.

Gutmann L, Blumenthal D, Gutmann L, Schochet SS: Acute type II myofiber atrophy in critical illness. Neurology 1996;46:819–821.

Hansen-Flaschen JH, Brazinsky S, Basile C, et al: Use of sedating drugs and neuromuscular blocking agents in patients requiring mechanical ventilation for respiratory failure: A national survey. JAMA 1991; 266:2870–2875.

Hansen-Flaschen JH, Cowen J, Raps EC: Neuromuscular blockade in the intensive care unit: More than we bargained for. Am Rev Respir Dis 1993;147:234–236.

Hirano M, Ott BR, Raps EC, Minetti C, et al: Acute quadriplegic myopathy: A complication of treatment with steroids, nondepolarizing blocking agents, or both. Neurology 1992;42:2082–2087.

Hoke A, Rewcastle NB, Zochodne DW: Acute quadriplegic myopathy unrelated to steroids or paralyzing agents: Quantitative electromyography studies. Can J Neurol Sci 1999;26:325–329.

Hund E, Genzwurker H, Bohrer H, et al: Predominant involvement of motor fibres in patients with critical illness polyneuropathy. Br J Anaesth 1997;78:274–278.

Hunter JM: New neuromuscular blocking drugs. N Engl J Med 1995;332:1691–1699.

Kaplan PW, Rocha W, Sanders DB, et al: Acute steroid-induced tetraplegia following status asthmaticus. Pediatrics 1986;78: 121–123.

Keunen RW, Lambregts PC, Op De Coul AA, Joosten EM: Respiratory failure as an initial symptom of acid maltase deficiency. J Neurol Neurosurg Psychiatr 1984;47:549–552.

Knox AJ, Mascie-Taylor BH, Muers MF: Acute hydrocortisone myopathy in acute severe asthma. Thorax 1986;41:411–412.

Kohler A, Jolliet P, Schnorf A, et al: Two identical episodes of acute quadriparesis in an intensive care unit patient. Intensive Care Med 1998;24:891–892.

Kohn NN, Faires JS, Rodman T: Unusual manifestations due to involvement of involuntary muscle in dystrophica myotonia. N Engl J Med 1964;271:1179–1183.

Koren W, Koren E, Nacasch N, et al: Rhabdomyolysis associated with clozapine treatment in a patient with decreased calcium-dependent potassium permeability of cell membranes. Clin Neuropharmacol 1998;21:262–264.

Kupfer Y, Namba T, Kaldawi E, Tessler S: Prolonged weakness after long-term administration of vecuronium bromide. Ann Intern Med 1992;117:484–486.

Kupfer Y, Okrent DG, Twersky RA, Tessler S: Disuse atrophy in a ventilated patient with status asthmaticus receiving neuromuscular blocking blockade. Crit Care Med 1987;15:795–796.

Lacomis D, Giuliani MJ, Van Cott A, Kramer DJ: Acute myopathy of intensive care: Clinical, electromyographic, and pathological aspects. Ann Neurol 1996;40:645–654.

Lacomis D, Petrella JT, Giuliani MJ: Causes of neuromuscular weakness in the intensive care unit: A study of ninety-two patients. Muscle Nerve 1998;21:610–617.

Lacomis D, Smith TW, Chad DA: Acute myopathy and neuropathy in status asthmaticus: Case report and literature review. Muscle Nerve 1993;16:84–90.

Lacomis D, Zochodne DW, Bird SJ: Critical illness myopathy: What's in a name? Muscle Nerve 2000;23:1785–1788.

Latronico N, Fenzi F, Recupero D, et al: Critical illness myopathy and neuropathy. Lancet 1996;347:1570–1582.

Leatherman JW, Fluegel WL, David WS, et al: Muscle weakness in mechanically ventilated patients with severe asthma. Am J Respir Crit Care Med 1996;153:1686–1690.

Lindenbaum Y, Nations SP, Barohn RJ, Wolfe GI: Recurrent critical illness myopathy in an asthmatic patient treated with corticosteroids. J Clin Neuromuscul Dis 2000;1:145–146.

MacFarlane IA, Rosenthal FD: Severe myopathy after status asthmaticus. Lancet 1977;2:615.

Malvy D, Dessailles PH, Monseau Y, et al: Legionnaire's disease and rhabdomyolysis. Intensive Care Med 1992;18:132–135.

Marinella MA: Rhabdomyolysis associated with haloperidol without evidence of NMS. Ann Pharmacother 1997;31:927.

Massa R, Carpenter S, Holland P, Karpati G: Loss and renewal of thick myofilaments in glucocorticoid-treated rat soleus after denervation and reinnervation. Muscle Nerve 1992;15:1290–1298.

Mitchell JK: A study of a case of family periodic paralysis. Am J Med Sci 1899;145:513–518.

O'Connor M, Russell WJ: Muscle strength following anaesthesia with atracurium and pancuronium. Anaesth Intensive Care 1988;16:255–259.

Op de Coul AAW, Lambregts PCLA, Koeman J, et al: Neuromuscular complications in patients given Pavulon (pancuronium bromide) during artificial ventilation. Clin Neurol Neurosurg 1985; 87:17–22.

Partridge BL, Abrams JH, Bazemore C, et al: Prolonged neuromuscular blockade after long-term infusion of vecuronium bromide in the intensive care unit. Crit Care Med 1990;18:1177–1180.

Pascucci RC: Prolonged weakness after extended mechanical ventilation in a child. Crit Care Med 1990;18:1181–1182.

Picado C, Montserrat J, Agusti-Vidal A: Muscle atrophy in severe exacerbation of asthma requiring mechanical ventilation. Respiration 1988;53:201–203.

Posner MR, Caudill MA, Brass R, Ellis E: Legionnaire's disease associated with rhabdomyolysis and myoglobinuria. Arch Intern Med 1980;140:848–850.

Ramsay DA, Zochodne DW, Robertson DM, et al: A syndrome of acute severe muscle necrosis in intensive care unit patients. J Neuropathol Exp Neurol 1993;52:387–398.

Rana SS, Giuliani MJ, Oddis CV, Lacomis D: Acute onset of colchicine myoneuropathy in cardiac transplant recipients: Case studies of three patients. Clin Neurol Neurosurg 1997;99:266–270.

Raps EC, Bird SJ, Hansen-Flaschen J: Prolonged muscle weakness after neuromuscular blockade in the intensive care unit. Crit Care Clin 1994;10:799–813.

Rich MM, Bird SJ, Raps EC, et al: Direct muscle stimulation in acute quadriplegic myopathy. Muscle Nerve 1997;20:665–673.

Rich MM, Kramer SD, Barchi RL: Altered gene expression in an animal model of acute quadriplegic myopathy. Ann Neurol 1998b;43:461.

Rich MM, Pinter MJ, Kraner SD, Barchi RL: Loss of electrical excitability in an animal model of acute quadriplegic myopathy. Ann Neurol 1998a;43:171–179.

Rich MM, Teener JW, Raps EC, et al: Muscle is electrically inexcitable in acute quadriplegic myopathy. Neurology 1996;46:731–736.

Road J, Mackie G, Jiang T, et al: Reversible paralysis with status asthmaticus, steroids, and pancuronium: Clinical electrophysiological correlates. Muscle Nerve 1997;20:1587–1590.

Rogoff JB: Traditional electrodiagnosis. In Johnson EW (ed): Practical Electromyography, Baltimore, Williams & Wilkins, 1980; 326–337.

Rosenow EC, Engel AG: Acid maltase deficiency in adults presenting as respiratory failure. Am J Med 1978;64:485–491.

Rouleau G, Karpati G, Carpenter S, et al: Glucocorticoid excess induces preferential depletion of myosin in denervated skeletal muscle fibers. Muscle Nerve 1987;10:428–438.

Schwarz J, Planck J, Briegel J, Straube A: Single-fiber electromyography, nerve conduction studies, and conventional electromyography in patients with critical-illness polyneuropathy: Evidence for a lesion of terminal motor axons. Muscle Nerve 1997; 20:696–701.

Segredo V, Caldwell JE, Matthay MA, et al: Persistent paralysis in critically ill patients after long-term administration of vecuronium. N Engl J Med 1992;327:524–525.

Segredo V, Matthay MA, Sharma ML, et al: Prolonged neuromuscular blockade after long-term administration of vecuronium in two critically-ill patients. Anesthesiology 1990;72:566–570.

Shee CD: Risk factors for hydrocortisone myopathy in acute severe asthma. Respir Med 1990;84:229–233.

Sher JH, Shafiq SA, Schutta HS: Acute myopathy with selective lysis of myosin filaments. Neurology 1979;29:100–106.

Showalter CJ, Engel AG: Acute quadriplegic myopathy: Analysis of myosin isoforms and evidence for calpain-mediated proteolysis. Muscle Nerve 1997;20:316–322.

Singh U, Scheld WM: Infectious etiologies of rhabdomyolysis: Three case reports and review. Clin Infect Dis 1996;22:642–649.

Singhal PC, Kumar A, Desroches L, et al: Prevalence and predictors of rhabdomyolysis in patients with hypophosphatemia. Am J Med 1992;92:458–461.

Sitwell LD, Weinhenker BG, Monpetit V, Reid D: Complete ophthalmoplegia as a complication of acute corticosteroid- and pancuronium-associated myopathy. Neurology 1991;41:921–922.

Sladen RN: Neuromuscular blocking agents in the intensive care unit: A two-edged sword. Crit Care Med 1995;23:423–428.

Slater MS, Mullins RJ: Rhabdomyolysis and myoglobinuric renal failure in trauma and surgical patients: A review. J Am Coll Surg 1998;186:693–716.

Spitzer AR, Giancarlo T, Maher L, et al: Neuromuscular causes of prolonged ventilator dependency. Muscle Nerve 1992;15:682–686.

Subramony SH, Carpenter DE, Raju S, et al: Myopathy and prolonged neuromuscular blockade after liver transplantation. Crit Care Med 1991;19:1580–1582.

Szewczyk D, Ovadia P, Abdullah F, Rabinovici R: Pressure-induced rhabdomyolysis and acute renal failure. J Trauma 1998;44:384–388.

Teener JW, Rich MM, Bird SJ: Other causes of acute weakness in the intensive care unit. In Miller DH, Raps EC (eds): Critical Care Neurology. Boston, Butterworth-Heinemann, 1999; 69–89.

Vanderheyden BA, Reynolds HN, Gerold KB, et al: Prolonged paralysis after long-term vecuronium infusion. Crit Care Med 1992; 20:304–306.

Van Marle W, Woods KL: Acute hydrocortisone myopathy. Br Med J 1980;281:271–272.

Waclawik AJ, Sufit RL, Beinlich BR, Schutta HS: Acute myopathy with selective degeneration of myosin thick filaments following status asthmaticus treated with methylprednisolone and vecuronium. Neuromuscul Disord 1992;2:19–26.

Ward MH: Factors predictive of acute renal failure in rhabdomyolysis. Arch Intern Med 1988;148:1553–1556.

Wijdicks EFM, Litchy WJ, Wiesner RH, et al: Neuromuscular complications associated with liver transplantation. Muscle Nerve 1996;19:696–700.

Williams TJ, O'Hehir RE, Czarny D, et al: Acute myopathy in severe acute asthma treated with intravenously administered corticosteroids. Am Rev Respir Dis 1988;137:460–463.

Zager RA: Rhabdomyolysis and myohemoglobinuric acute renal failure. Kidney Int 1996;49:314–326.

Zifko U, Zipko H, Bolton CF: Clinical and electrophysiological findings in critical illness polyneuropathy. J Neurol Sci 1998; 159:186–198.

Zochodne DW, Bolton CF, Thompson RT, et al: Myopathy in critical illness. Muscle Nerve 1986;9:652.

Zochodne DW, Bolton CF, Laverty D, et al: The effects of sepsis on muscle function: An electrophysiologic and P-31 NMR study. Electroencephalogr Clin Neurophysiol 1987;66:S115–S116.

Zochodne DW, Ramsay DA, Saly V, et al: Acute necrotizing myopathy of intensive care: Electrophysiological studies. Muscle Nerve 1994;17:285–292.

Zochodne DW: Myopathies in the intensive care unit. Can J Neurol Sci 1998;25:S40–S42.

Intensive Care– and Critical Illness–Related Neuromuscular Disorders: Ventilator Disorders

Udo A. Zifko

Neuromuscular diseases associated with ventilatory disorders requiring admission to an intensive care unit (ICU) are not uncommon. Among them, Guillain-Barré syndrome (GBS) and myasthenia gravis (MG) are most frequently encountered. Of the neuromuscular diseases that develop in the ICU setting and may cause respiratory muscle weakness with the need for prolonged ventilation, critical illness polyneuropathy (CIP) and critical care myopathy are most often seen. But other, less common neuromuscular diseases may occasionally also cause acute respiratory failure requiring critical care monitoring or intubation and ventilation of the patient. By contrast, other neuromuscular diseases such as amyotrophic lateral sclerosis, which are consistently associated with respiratory muscle weakness, are treated only in the ICU setting with assisted ventilation, if the patient so desires or, in emergencies, if the etiology is still unclear.

The neurologist's and the neurophysiologist's task is to diagnose the underlying disease, to predict the course of the condition, and to provide for patient management and treatment. Achieving this task requires extensive clinical experience and close interdisciplinary cooperation with pulmonologists and intensive care physicians.

In this chapter, the diagnosis and management of neuromuscular diseases with respiratory muscle involvement are reviewed and the diagnostic steps needed to clarify neuromuscular respiratory failure of unclear origin are described.

MOTOR NEURON DISORDERS

Respiratory failure is quite common in advanced motor neuron disease (MND). In fact, it is the leading cause of death. A neurophysiological diagnostic evaluation provided evidence of respiratory muscle involvement in 86% of 36 patients at the time the diagnosis of MND was made, although 81% of the patients did not report any respiratory problems (Schiffmann and Belsh, 1993). This discrepancy can be explained, at least in part, by the considerable physiological pulmonary functional reserve, which ensures that minor respiratory muscle weakness remains asymptomatic for some time. Rarely, involvement of the respiratory motor neurons is the initial abnormality of MND, resulting in severe neuromuscular respiratory failure of unclear origin (Chen et al., 1996). On account of the variable onset and extent of respiratory muscle involvement in the different stages of the condition, a meticulous neurophysiological examination and pulmonological evaluation are indispensable for appropriate symptomatic management of the patients.

Early Clinical Signs of Respiratory Muscle Weakness

Often missed, the early signs and symptoms of respiratory muscle weakness are recognized only from the patient's history and careful physical examination when the clinician has them in mind. They include increased fatigability, poor sleep with frequent waking spells at night, and headache in the mornings as well as use of an additional pillow at night. These early symptoms are later followed by an appreciable shortness of breath when the patient is lying flat and by shortness of breath and dyspnea on exertion (Fallat et al., 1979; Rochester and Esau, 1994; Vitacca et al., 1997). Advanced respiratory muscle involvement is associated with an increased

respiratory rate and shallow breathing. Patients tend to keep their verbal utterances brief, make more frequent use of the accessory respiratory muscles, and develop a paradoxical breathing pattern (inward abdominal wall movement on inspiration). In addition, they cough and sniff less vigorously. Poor appetite and weight loss are frequent accompanying signs.

Diagnosis

Neurophysiological studies are critically important both for the diagnosis of MND and for an evaluation of potential respiratory muscle involvement. They play a special role in patients with primary respiratory muscle weakness, because limb involvement is usually quite discrete or altogether absent in such cases. In a multicenter study by the author, all patients with recently diagnosed MND were subjected to phrenic nerve conduction studies and needle electromyography (EMG) of the diaphragm. Preliminary data showed these studies to be important predictors of the long-term course and a sound basis of patient management (Lahrmann et al., 2000). Since the diaphragmatic compound muscle action potential (DCMAP) varies considerably, as already described in Chapter 35, baseline DCMAPs and latencies should be recorded in all cases during the early stages of the condition, whether patients present with clinical symptoms of respiratory muscle weakness or not. They proved to be the most specific studies in showing whether respiratory insufficiency is attributable to progressive neuromuscular weakness and were particularly helpful in excluding other causes of dyspnea. Variations in DCMAP amplitude mean that care should be taken

Figure 84–1. Phrenic nerve conduction study and needle electromyogram of the diaphragm in a patient with amyotrophic lateral sclerosis. The latency is prolonged, and the amplitude is reduced. The number of motor unit potentials is reduced, and the motor units are large, prolonged and polyphasic (trace 4 on electromyogram).

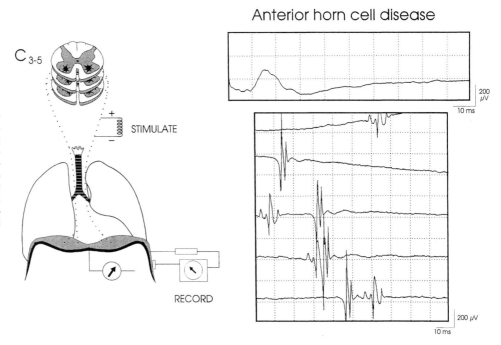

to stimulate the phrenic nerve during the same respiratory cycle (expiration-inspiration). In the author's laboratory, a point is made to obtain recordings at the beginning of quiet, nonforced inspiration, as determined by observation of the abdominal wall. Typical findings of phrenic nerve neurography include an increasing reduction of the DCMAP amplitude. Latency is often also moderately prolonged and resembles that of limb motor nerves. On needle electromyography of the diaphragm, direct evidence of a potential involvement of the C3-5 motor neurons is seen earlier in the initial stages than on phrenic nerve neurography. Fibrillation potentials and positive sharp waves may be observed between inspiratory bursts and indicate recent denervation. However, there is often evidence of denervation and reinnervation. Thus, motor unit potentials during inspiratory bursts are decreased in number, and the remaining ones are large and polyphasic (Fig. 84–1). These motor unit potentials are easily distinguished from the low-amplitude short-duration motor unit potentials that are a normal feature of the human diaphragm. If motor unit potentials are significantly decreased in number and diaphragm CMAPs are low bilaterally, neuromuscular respiratory insufficiency is likely. Thus, some amyotrophic lateral sclerosis (ALS) clinics utilize these studies routinely.

Future investigations may show that the technique of magnetic stimulation of the cerebral cortex and cervical spinal cord (Zifko et al., 1996a) may prove valuable in determining upper motor neuron weakness of the diaphragm.

Together with these neurophysiological studies, some lung function parameters give valuable and indispensable diagnostic information (Brooks, 1996). Forced vital capacity (FVC) is considered to be a reliable predictor (Nakono et al., 1976; Fallat et al., 1979; Ringel et al., 1993). It should always be measured with the patient seated and reclining, lest diaphragmatic weakness be missed. FVC is important for the patient's respiratory management (Fig. 84–2). But it also plays a major role in deciding about the need for other measures, particularly those of an invasive nature, such as insertion of a percutaneous enterogastrostomy (PEG) tube. In

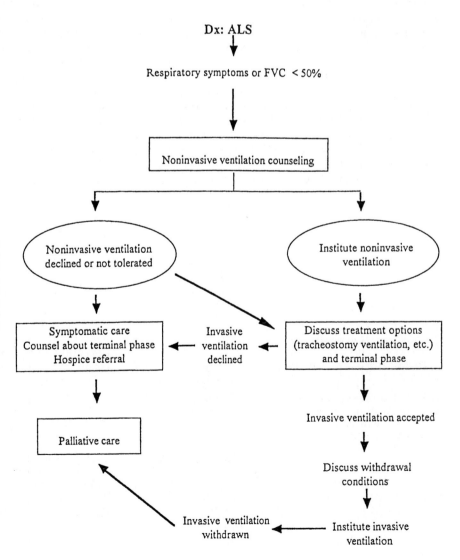

Figure 84–2. Algorithm for respiratory management in amyotrophic lateral sclerosis (ALS). Dx, diagnosis; FVC, forced vital capacity. (With permission from Miller MG, Rosenberg JA, Gelinas DF, et al: Practice parameter: The care of the patient with amyotrophic lateral sclerosis [an evidence-based review]. Neurology 1999;52: 1311–1323.)

patients with an FVC below 30%, the risk of complications following gastrostomy was found to be higher than in those with an FVC above 50%.

Maximal inspiratory pressure is a particularly sensitive parameter for inspiratory muscle weakness (Fallat et al., 1979). But its accuracy in MND has not yet been documented. The author's experience in other neuromuscular diseases with concomitant weakness of the facial muscles such as myotonic dystrophy or MG (Zifko et al., 1996b; Zifko et al., 1999) is that it did not correlate with neurophysiological and clinical findings.

Nocturnal pulse oximetry is helpful in identifying hypoventilation. In its early and moderately advanced stages, nocturnal hypoventilation is easily treated with noninvasive measures so that the patient's well-being can often be significantly improved, and the sequelae of nocturnal desaturation can be prevented. In the author's experience, complete polysomnography is unnecessary in most cases, but it should always be added to the battery of diagnostic studies if other sleep-associated conditions such as upper airways disease or episodes of central sleep apnea are suspected clinically or on the basis of the patient's history.

POLYNEUROPATHIES

Guillain-Barré Syndrome

Dramatic advances in the treatment of GBS (Hahn, 1996) and considerable improvements in intensive care management have resulted in a significant fall in the mortality rate (Bolton, 1995). However, GBS is still associated with a mortality rate of 3% to 5% in general and of 5% to 8% in ventilated patients. Mortality rates are no lower in highly specialized and experienced intensive care units (Wijdicks, 1997). About one third of all GBS patients (14% to 44%) need ventilatory support. The percentage is even higher in patients transferred to ICUs for monitoring because of the threat of respiratory failure (65% to 70%). Clinical symptoms, differential diagnosis, electrophysiological findings, and management are described in Chapter 35.

CAUSES OF UNDERLYING RESPIRATORY FAILURE

Respiratory muscle weakness in GBS is caused mainly by phrenic nerve involvement with secondary diaphragmatic weakness. Other factors include weakness of the intercostal, abdominal, and accessory respiratory muscles as well as retained airway secretions, atelectasis, the position of lying flat, concomitant autonomic nervous dysfunction, and secondary infections such as bronchitis or pneumonia. Seventy percent to 80% of all ventilated GBS patients present with clinical signs of autonomic nervous system involvement (Singh et al., 1987; Zochodne, 1994). Among these, cardiac dysrhythmias such as tachycardia, bradycardia, or even asystole carry

particular risks and often need temporary pacing. Marked hemodynamic instability reflecting autonomic dysregulation is a major therapeutic challenge and requires meticulous hemodynamic monitoring. Autonomic nervous system complications are the leading causes of death in GBS patients (Winer and Hughes, 1988; Ng et al., 1995).

DIAGNOSIS

It is important to detect the potential for developing respiratory nerve involvement early in the course of the disease. In a retrospective study of 40 patients, respiratory electrophysiological studies during the first 3 days following admission showed the need for ventilation to be closely correlated with the DCMAP amplitude and area as well as with abnormalities in the diaphragmatic needle electromyographic tracing (Zifko et al., 1996c). In addition, all patients who were in need of ventilatory support at any time during their disease had abnormal phrenic nerve conduction studies and/or diaphragmatic electromyograms. At the time of the examination, FVC was abnormal in no more than 80% of cases. These data suggest that when the GBS patient presents for their first neurophysiological evaluation additional electrophysiological studies of the phrenic nerve and the diaphragm will be helpful in improving management of the patient (Fig. 84–3). Fibrillation potentials and positive sharp waves in the diaphragm and chest wall muscles indicate axonal degeneration of phrenic and intercostal nerves. In proximal demyelination of the phrenic nerve, abnormal spontaneous activity may be absent, but motor unit potentials are decreased in number. The diaphragm CMAPs may have normal amplitude and latency, indicating normal phrenic nerve pathology distally. Similar conclusions can be drawn from the data of Gourie-Devi and Ganapathy (1985). Putting aside DCMAP and diaphragmatic EMG data, they found phrenic nerve latency to correlate with the severity of the disease, its morbidity and mortality (Gourie-Devi and Ganapathy, 1985).

Later in the course of the disease, clinical signs such as increased respiratory rate, shortness of breath while speaking, paradoxical movements of the diaphragm and poor coughing, and oropharyngeal muscle involvement are important clues for detecting impending respiratory failure. FVC monitoring with spirometry at intervals of 4 to 8 hours and pulse oximetry, particularly at night, are simple noninvasive bedside tests. Depending on the clinical picture, chest radiographs and capillary blood gas analyses should also be ordered.

VENTILATION

Mechanical ventilation is indicated whenever the patient deteriorates clinically and the VC drops to 15 mL/kg or less. Maximal inspiratory pressure readings of less than 25 cm H_2O are critical. Clinically, a respiratory rate above 30 per minute should prompt

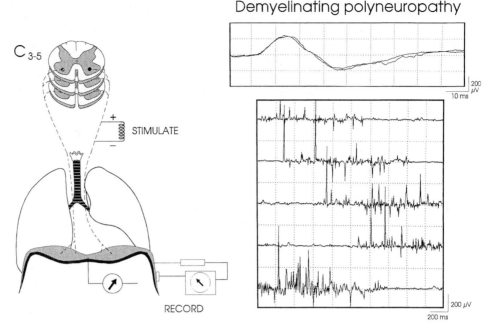

Figure 84–3. Phrenic nerve conduction study and needle electromyogram of the diaphragm in a patient with Guillain-Barré syndrome. The latency is markedly prolonged, and the amplitude is reduced. The motor units are not clearly abnormal in morphology, consistent with demyelination in the phrenic nerve.

intubation. The critical maximal expiratory pressure is 40 cm H_2O. If the FVC drops to 50% of baseline, patients probably need mechanical ventilation within the next 36 hours (Chevrolet and Deleamont, 1991). Many GBS patients accept endotracheal intubation with intermittent mandatory ventilation. In view of the prolonged ventilation needs, however, orotracheal tubes are preferred over the nasotracheal route (Pendersen, 1991). Ventilation is designed to restore blood gases to normal. As a rule, this is no problem, provided that pulmonary infections are absent. Two to three weeks after the commencement of mechanical ventilation, patients tend to respond to immunomodulatory therapy. At this time, electrophysiological studies may give a clue to axonal involvement, allowing more precise predictions to be made. Approximately one third of all GBS patients are ready for weaning within 2 weeks (Ropper and Kehne, 1985; Borel et al., 1991). Patients presenting with a primary axonal variant of GBS, which carries a poorer prognosis, should undergo tracheostomy earlier. If well tolerated at a pressure of 5 cm H_2O, mechanical ventilation can be terminated between days 20 and 30, on average. Weaning is best timed in accordance with the FVC, which should be above 15 mL/kg. Children with GBS usually need shorter ventilation times (17 days, on average) (Bos et al., 1987). In patients with extensive axonal degeneration of the phrenic nerve, prolonged ventilation for as long as 1 year is often inevitable (Sunderrajan and Davenport, 1985; Ropper, 1986; Chalmers et al., 1996). Patients should not be weaned from the ventilator if they still show major signs of autonomic nervous system dysfunction, because the stress of weaning may aggravate blood pressure peaks and tachycardias.

SUPPORTIVE MEASURES

Conservative measures for expanding the lung volume carry particular weight. If respiratory muscle failure threatens to develop, these measures help to avoid intubation, as they prevent progressive respiratory insufficiency by their positive effect on atelectases. Ideally, GBS patients should train on an incentive spirometer every hour. In addition, they should be prompted by their physiotherapist to breathe in and cough vigorously at short intervals. These exercises should be repeated every 10 minutes. Tapping massage, trunk-up positioning, and whatever prevents aspiration or pulmonary infections are other important supportive measures.

Critical Illness Neuropathy

Respiratory paralysis in critically ill patients was first described in 1983 (Bolton et al., 1983; Rivner et al., 1983; Roelofs et al., 1983). Clinical and electrophysiological findings in CIP are described at length in Chapter 35. CIP is the most common neuromuscular cause of failure to wean, which is seen as an increasingly more frequent neuromuscular complication in the ICU setting (Zochodne and Bolton, 1996; Zifko et al., 1998a). The muscles of respiration are frequently involved in CIP. Characteristic electrophysiological findings are decreased or absent diaphragmatic CMAPs, denervation potentials in diaphragm and chest wall muscles, and a decreased number of motor unit potentials. These abnormalities gradually disappear as recovery from CIP occurs. While it has been difficult to statistically prove the relationship between electrophysiological findings and the length of ventilation because so many other clinical factors, such as underlying diseases or associated cardiopulmonary disorders, are important parameters in difficulty in weaning from the ventilator and prolonged stay in the ICU, the author has seen the importance of phrenic nerve conduction studies and needle electromyographic studies of the diaphragm in the individual management of such patients (Zifko et al., 1998a).

Other Polyneuropathies

Phrenic nerve involvement is present in numerous neuropathies, among them hereditary motor and sensory neuropathy (HMSN) types I and II (Laroche et al., 1988; Gilchrist et al., 1989; Hardie et al. 1990; Carter et al., 1992;), diabetes mellitus (White et al., 1992; Fisher et al., 1997), sarcoidosis, diphtherial neuropathy, leprosy, lead- and arsenic-induced neuropathies (Bansal et al., 1991), porphyria, uremia (Zifko et al., 1995a), and alcoholic and multifocal neuropathy (Cavaletti et al., 1998). Unless associated with other neuromuscular or cardiopulmonary diseases, it does usually not necessitate ventilation. However, if sepsis occurs in the course of these polyneuropathies (i.e., diabetic or uremic), CIP may be superimposed, causing limb and respiratory weakness before or after admission to the ICU. Successful treatment of sepsis results in gradual resolution of the superimposed CIP (Bolton, 1996).

Mononeuropathies

In the author's experience, mononeuropathies of the phrenic nerve are not uncommon, even though the true incidences are still poorly documented. They often go undiagnosed, as phrenic nerve lesions may be asymptomatic and the elevation of the diaphragm seen on radiographs is frequently thought to be preexistent or idiopathic. Phrenic nerve mononeuropathies may occur at any age. They have multiple causes and may be associated with a variety of symptoms.

SYMPTOMS

The many anatomical variants of phrenic innervation (see Chapter 35) and the variable severity of the underlying lesion explain the tremendous variability of symptoms. In many cases, phrenic nerve lesions cause short-lived symptoms or are altogether asymptomatic. Such mild symptoms as may be present are, at times, masked by the severity of associated conditions such as injuries or tumors. Patients are often asymptomatic for years or even a lifetime, and the elevated diaphragm incidentally seen on chest radiographs is misdiagnosed as congenital (nonparalytic). Thomas (1970) pointed out that in congenital eventration, true paradoxical motion of the diaphragm is absent. The initial passive upward movement of the redundant portion of the diaphragm, until the slack is taken up, is sometimes confused with paradoxical motion. The muscular portion contracts simultaneously with the opposite diaphragm (Iverson et al., 1976).

Dyspnea on strenuous physical exertion is one of the major symptoms of phrenic nerve lesions. But the respiratory rate may also be increased at rest, with the patient lying flat on his or her back. Atelectasis on the paralyzed side, due to diaphragmatic elevation in combination with a mediastinal shift toward the normal side during inspiration, is the underlying pathophysiological mechanism. Abdominal symptoms may also be present. These depend on the side affected. In right diaphragmatic paralysis, the patient may develop symptoms of gallbladder dysfunction. In left-sided paralyses, the symptoms may be those of gastric outlet obstruction; that is, nausea, vomiting, bloating, and pain. Gastric symptoms can be relieved by having the patient lie on the left or the right side, depending on which position is necessary to improve gastric drainage (Chin and Lynn, 1956). Volvulus of the stomach has been reported in instances with a very high left hemidiaphragm (Kirklin and Hidgson, 1947). Gastric and gallbladder symptoms are due to elevation of the ipsilateral hemidiaphragm and consequent displacement of the intra-abdominal organs. Cardiac signs and symptoms include palpitations, tachycardia, and extrasystoles (Iverson et al., 1976).

CLINICAL FINDINGS

Speaking or minor exertion such as undressing may often be enough to cause labored, accelerated, or shallow breathing. On the affected side, respiratory sounds may be weak or altogether absent and the lung may be dull to percussion. The clinician may also detect Hoover's sign—that is, an uninhibited movement of the costal margin away from the midline on the side of the injury may be present (Hoover, 1913). This is due to intercostal muscle contraction, which is no longer opposed by the paralyzed ipsilateral hemidiaphragm. Potential associated abnormalities should be sought. These may include injuries of other brachial and/or cervical plexus nerves. Skeletal injuries of the shoulder girdle, the scapula, the neck, or the trunk as well as extensive hematomas in the distal neck may give an indirect clue.

DIAGNOSIS

In the diagnosis and differential diagnosis of phrenic nerve paresis, phrenic nerve neurography and needle EMG of the diaphragm are the most important studies (Bolton, 1993). Their outcome mimics the neurophysiological findings to be expected in traumatic nerve lesions and, depending on the stage during which the tests are made, provides reliable evidence of the severity of the lesion. When evaluating potential phrenic nerve lesions, the clinician should remember that the nerve can be stimulated only at a single site so that conduction blocks will go unnoticed. In the thoracic region, iatrogenic phrenic nerve injuries are quite common and an early assessment of their severity is helpful in their treatment (see following discussion). Unlike the case in the limb muscles, only a few motor units are accessible for examination in the diaphragm; thus, incomplete lesions of the bulky multifidus muscle may be missed on EMG, even if the examination is properly done. This should be considered when one interprets neurophysiological findings. Reduced CMAPs and evidence of denervation on needle EMG may be due to a lesion anywhere along the course of the phrenic motor neurons. Denervation in cervical paraspinal muscles will localize the lesion to an intraspinal location, and in that in C4-5–innervated muscles, such as the upper border of trapezius or the levator scapulae, to a brachial plexus location (if the paraspinal muscles are normal). Normal needle EMG studies of these muscles localize the lesion to the neck or thorax distal to the point of electrical phrenic nerve stimulation.

Results of both radiological studies and fluoroscopy may be either false positive or false negative during the early stage of the condition. On chest radiographs, atelectases on the affected side and a mediastinal shift toward the normal side provide an indirect clue. Kienböck's sign is positive on fluoroscopy, if the affected diaphragm moves paradoxically after slow expiration and a vigorous sniff. Sonography for evaluating diaphragmatic motility is of particular importance in the diagnosis of birth injuries of the phrenic nerve (Zifko et al., 1995b). Lung function parameters may be normal. But they may also show a restrictive pattern, depending on the severity of the lesion. The importance of measuring the FVC with the patient seated and reclining, and the transdiaphragmatic pressure, has already been stressed in Chapter 35.

CAUSES

Table 84–1 lists the potential causes of phrenic nerve paresis. Phrenic nerve lesions may be localized along the entire course of the nerve from the nerve root to the cervical and thoracic segments and the distal ends in pleural adhesions. Among the causes of phrenic nerve paresis are trauma, tumors, compression, and displacement by other structures, iatrogenic injuries, and inflammatory diseases.

Tumors

Intrathoracic compression of the phrenic nerve by a tumor is the most common cause of phrenic

nerve paresis (Malin, 1979). In most cases, the nerve is compressed by a malignant lung tumor. Among malignant tumors, squamous cell carcinoma ranks first, followed by small cell and adenoid bronchial carcinoma. Metastases of lung tumors may also cause phrenic nerve paresis, either on the same side or on the opposite side. Lymphomas, thymomas, and Recklinghausen's neurofibromatosis are other causes.

Trauma

Complete traumatic spinal cord injuries at the level of C4 or above result in respiratory insufficiency requiring mechanical ventilation. The development of phrenic nerve pacemakers and the advanced techniques of ventilation at home (see following discussion) has allowed outpatient management of affected patients. A full neurological and neurophysiological evaluation is required in these patients (Girsch et al., 1996). If phrenic nerve conduction and needle EMG of the diaphragm show significant axonal degeneration, phrenic nerve pacing is not indicated. If the respiratory paralysis is entirely upper motor neuron (normal phrenic nerve conduction and absent motor units on needle electromyography of the diaphragm), phrenic nerve pacing may be indicated. Owing to corticospinal tract involvement at the level of the spinal cord injury, needle EMG of the intercostal muscles will show no denervation potentials or motor units. Additionally, transcortical magnetic stimulation studies are valuable in the diagnosis of spinal cord injuries, and particularly in the prognosis of incomplete spinal cord injuries, such as vascular lesions of the spinal cord (Zifko et al., 1997a).

Traumatic lesions of the phrenic nerve most often result from radicular avulsion at the level of C4 (Rohr and Lenz, 1960a, 1960b). Along the farther course of the neural system, any traumatic lesion of the cervical and brachial plexuses may cause phrenic nerve paresis. More distal phrenic nerve lesions may be due to chest trauma, including both contusions and penetrating injuries such as shotgun wounds or stabbings (Nelson et al., 1968).

Iatrogenic injuries of the phrenic nerve are common causes of phrenic nerve lesions. Most of them occur during open chest surgery (Mok et al., 1991; Tripp and Bolton, 1998). The nerve may be directly damaged when a mass invading the nerval tissue is resected. Inadvertent manipulation of the nerve with surgical instruments may cause reversible incomplete compression, or even complete bisection. Hypothermia is a very frequent causal factor during open chest surgery. It may result in unilateral—and rarely bilateral—phrenic nerve lesions (Laub et al., 1991). The severity of hypothermic lesions sustained during cardiac surgery varies. It may range from short-lived incomplete paresis to complete paresis (Wilcox et al., 1988). Even if unilateral, complete paresis may be fatal for newborns and infants (Wilcox et al., 1988). But deaths from hypothermic

---

Table 84–1. Causes of Phrenic Nerve Mononeuropathies

Tumors	Infections
Trauma	Neuralgic amyotrophy
Iatrogenic	Idiopathic
Compression	

bilateral phrenic nerve lesions after heart surgery have also been reported in adults (Raffa et al., 1994). This explains the need for early neurophysiological, pulmonological, and radiological evaluation to establish the severity of the lesion and to institute proper management in good time (Mok et al., 1991; Zifko et al., 1995b). Phrenic nerve lesions secondary to ligation of the ductus arteriosus in newborns and to high cervical chordotomy have been described (Hill and Polk, 1976; Yeh et al., 1977). But the nerve may also be injured during subclavian vein catheterization and brachial plexus blockade (Epstein et al., 1976; Obel, 1976). Radiation-induced induration is another rare iatrogenic cause (Malin, 1979).

Birth trauma is a frequent special variant of iatrogenic phrenic nerve lesions (Zifko et al., 1995b). In 1902, Naunyn reported the first birth palsy of the phrenic nerve associated with a brachial plexus injury. His description was followed by a number of case reports of diaphragmatic paralysis in newborns. The incidence varies from 0.03% in the author's series to 0.5% of all newborns in a pediatric intensive care unit (Greene et al., 1975; Zifko et al., 1995b). Birth palsies of the phrenic nerve are usually associated with unilateral lesions of other nerves of the brachiocervical plexus. But isolated and bilateral lesions have also been seen. Diaphragmatic paralysis caused during deliveries usually occurs in association with breech positions (Schiffrin, 1952; Iverson et al., 1976). Hyperextension of the nerve on stretching and turning the head and neck during delivery is the underlying mechanism. The severity of hyperextension varies, depending on how often this mechanism comes into play. Both spontaneous remission within days and persistent complete lesions have been reported. Associated birth injuries, such as extensive brachial plexus lesions and fractures of the clavicle or arm, herald a poor prognosis (Zifko et al., 1995b).

Compression

Phrenic nerve compression may be caused by a mass, but cervical radicular lesions due to a disk slipping laterally are not uncommon. Large goiters, aortic aneurysms, subphrenic or liver abscesses, and malformations of the hyoid bones may also compress the phrenic nerve (Malin, 1979).

Infections

Infectious diseases are a rather rare cause of phrenic nerve mononeuropathy. Pneumonia, tuberculosis, serum neuritis caused by tetanus toxin, herpes zoster, diphtheria, spinal cervical arachnoiditis, syphilitic meningomyelitis, and poliomyelitis are likely culprits (Malin, 1979).

Neuralgic Amyotrophy of the Shoulder—Idiopathic Brachial Plexus Neuropathy

Phrenic nerve involvement is one of the less well known variants of idiopathic brachial plexus neuropathy or Parsonage-Turner syndrome. It may occur alone in the course of neuralgic amyotrophy or in association with other nerve lesions, may be unilateral or bilateral, and may recur on alternating sides (Comroe et al., 1951; Tsairis et al., 1972; Walsh et al., 1987; Lahrmann et al., 1999).

Phrenic nerve involvement in neuralgic amyotrophy of the shoulder is diagnosed on the basis of a typical history of pain in the C4 dermatome, followed by dyspnea. To confirm the diagnosis, the neurogenic cause of the dyspnea must be established by phrenic nerve conduction studies and EMG of the diaphragm and other potential causes must be ruled out by appropriate diagnostic studies. These include magnetic resonance imaging of the cervical spine to exclude cervical root lesions, chest radiography to rule out intrathoracic phrenic nerve compression, and serologic tests. What course the condition takes essentially depends on whether involvement is unilateral or bilateral. If the nerve is affected bilaterally, severe respiratory disorders requiring transitory ventilatory support may occur. Unilateral involvement may be asymptomatic or cause symptoms (see previous discussion). Recovery of phrenic nerve function after neuralgic amyotrophy of the shoulder appears to be less rapid than that in the limbs (Mulvey et al., 1993; Hughes et al., 1999).

Idiopathic

In some cases, the factors underlying phrenic nerve lesions cannot be identified. A closer look at the older literature shows, however, that what was described as idiopathic may, in fact, have been an isolated lesion of the phrenic nerve in association with neuralgic amyotrophy (Lagueny et al., 1992; Mulvey et al., 1993). Stretch injuries to the phrenic nerve are another unusual cause of unilateral diaphragmatic paralysis (Tiede et al., 1994). Some authors attributed phrenic nerve paresis to whiplash injuries sustained in road accidents (Iverson et al., 1976).

TREATMENT

Initially, symptomatic relief should be provided by placing the patient in the trunk-up position, delivering oxygen, having the patient undergo active and passive respiratory exercises, and preventing bronchitis or pneumonia or treating them aggressively at an early stage. Negative-pressure ventilation in children with phrenic nerve lesions following heart surgery was found to be a useful alternative to positive airway pressure ventilation (Raine et al., 1992). Children with complete phrenic nerve lesions benefited from plication of the diaphragm, which improves ventilation on the normal side and provides symptomatic relief by preventing recurrent pneumonia due to atelectasis (Glassman et al., 1994). Nerve autografting proved to be an excellent treatment of the root cause of complete phrenic nerve lesions

(Zifko et al., 1995b). To prevent complete inactivation of the diaphragm in a patient with a high spinal lesion who underwent positive-pressure ventilation for 8 months, the phrenic nerve on one side was challenged with a short series of electrical stimuli for 30 minutes every day. Measurements of diaphragmatic thickness with ultrasound and lung studies showed that electrical stimulation delayed disuse atrophy of the diaphragm (Ayas et al., 1999).

ABNORMALITIES OF NEUROMUSCULAR TRANSMISSION

In patients with muscle weakness of unclear origin, abnormalities of neuromuscular transmission should always be suspected. These may be presynaptic or postsynaptic; they may occur at any age and span a wide spectrum of hereditary, autoimmune, and paraneoplastic syndromes as well as intoxications. All of them may cause respiratory failure requiring ventilatory support and intensive care.

Myasthenia Gravis

Myasthenia gravis (MG) is by far the most common neuromuscular transmission disorder, with a reported prevalence of 1 in 10,000 to 1 in 50,000 (Simpson, 1978; Havard and Scadding, 1983). At some time during the course of the autoimmune disease, 15% to 20% of the patients develop a myasthenic crisis, which is characterized by respiratory failure necessitating mechanical ventilation. Although mortality rates dropped dramatically from 80% (Tether, 1958; Osserman and Genkins, 1963) to 4% to 5% (Cohen and Younger, 1981; Thomas et al., 1997) in the past 50 years, episodes of myasthenic crisis continue to be a potential threat to life. Mimicking that of the disease in general, the age and sex distribution of patients suffering from myasthenic crises shows a bimodal pattern with an early peak (below age 55 years), mainly in women, and a later peak (older than age 55 years) for both sexes alike. The mean age at the time of the first crisis is 55 years, with a male-to-female ratio of 2:1 (Cohen and Younger, 1981; Ferguson et al., 1982; Thomas et al., 1997).

Precipitating Factors

One third of all patients develop myasthenic crises without any obvious cause or preceding illness. Often described as a cause of respiratory muscle weakness in the past (Tether, 1958; Osserman and Genkins, 1963), "cholinergic crises" are hardly mentioned any more in more recent reports (Ferguson et al., 1982; Thomas et al., 1997). Infections are the most common precipitants. Thomas and colleagues recorded them in 38% of all cases, followed by aspiration pneumonia in 10% (Thomas et al., 1997). Myasthenic crises may also be drug related. Drugs

known to aggravate myasthenia (e.g., aminoglycosides) are major precipitants. But caution should also be exercised before administering steroids and shortly before discontinuing them. Patients receiving steroids should invariably be alerted to the risk of episodes of crisis, just as they should be told about other potential causes. In addition, they should be provided with a patient identification (ID) card listing all drugs to be avoided. Ideally, they should also be given a list of addresses of myasthenia emergency units when traveling abroad. Operations, pregnancies (particularly early pregnancy), deliveries, and other major physical and emotional stressors may also precipitate episodes of crisis.

Symptoms

Progressive respiratory muscle weakness is most commonly encountered in generalized MG. But acute myasthenic crises may also occur in isolated oculobulbar variants. Limb muscle involvement was, for instance, absent in no fewer than 20% of the patients seen by Thomas and associates (1997). Isolated respiratory muscle involvement is a special feature and represents a major diagnostic challenge (Davis et al., 1976; Mier et al., 1990). It may be the first manifestation of the disease and brings patients to the ICU for the treatment of respiratory muscle weakness of unclear origin (Maher et al., 1998). Aside from isolated bulbar and/or respiratory muscle involvement, anti-acetylcholine receptor antibody (anti-AChR) negativity is another frequent special feature of the condition. Both Maher and colleagues (1998) and Evoli and associates (1996) found anti-AChR antibody titers to be frequently negative in MG patients with predominant respiratory muscle involvement. This fact and the intervals between blood sampling and the availability of the antibody titers underscore the importance of neurophysiological studies mainly of the respiratory tract (Zifko et al., 1999) and of the edrophonium test (see later sections).

Clinical signs of a cholinergic crisis (miosis, sweating, excessive inspissated sputum, muscle fasciculations, abdominal cramps, and diarrhea) with respiratory abnormalities caused by bronchospasm, aspiration, and difficulties in expectorating the inspissated mucus should prompt drug withdrawal, intubation and ventilation, antibiotic coverage, and, if necessary, the aspiration of secretions by bronchoscopy.

Course

The reported mean time to the first crisis varies considerably, ranging from 8 months (Thomas et al., 1997) to 5 to 6 years (Gracey et al., 1983; Sellman and Mayer, 1985). The mean time on the ventilator is 14 days, and the mean length of stay in hospital is 35 days. However, more protracted crises are not uncommon. In the series of Thomas and colleagues (1997), 25% of all patients needed ventilatory support for more than 1 month. The longest crisis was reported to last for 22 months (Selecky and Ziment, 1974). Ventilation for more than 2 weeks was associated with a three-fold increase in length of stay and a two-fold increase in the likelihood of functional dependence (Thomas et al., 1997). Patients with fatal outcomes usually present with extensive comorbidity. Sepsis-related complications and cardiopulmonary conditions were the most common causes of death.

DIAGNOSIS

After the diagnosis of MG has been confirmed, FVC, transdiaphragmatic pressure, and the alveo-alveolar gradient should be measured, and chest radiographs as well as other studies dictated by whatever associated diseases the patient has should be ordered. Respiratory muscle weakness of unclear origin is a particular challenge. The patient's history and clinical findings (see Chapter 35) will guide the subsequent neurophysiological evaluation. Motor and sensory neurography of the limb nerves should always be combined with repetitive stimulation at both low (3 Hz) and high frequencies (30 or 40 Hz). Depending on the patient's clinical status, low-frequency stimulation after brief 10-second muscle activation (post-tetanic potentiation) and after 90-second activation (post-tetanic exhaustion) should be added to the testing regimen. What nerve is to be examined is decided by the clinical manifestations. In general, proximal nerves (accessory nerve or facial nerve) are more sensitive than distal nerves. In patients with isolated or predominant respiratory muscle involvement, repetitive phrenic nerve stimulation is essential (Zifko et al., 1997b; Zifko et al., 1998a). Its distinctive features are described in Chapter 35. In dyspneic MG patients, repetitive accessory nerve stimulation may be negative, while repetitive phrenic nerve stimulation is clearly positive (Zifko et al., 1999). Although quite complex and time-consuming, repetitive stimulation of the phrenic nerve should be an integral element in the diagnostic evaluation of unclear respiratory disorders. This also applies to single-fiber EMG, which should invariably be done in the ICU when respiratory disorders are suspected to be due to abnormalities of neuromuscular transmission and the results of repetitive stimulation are noncontributory (Maher et al., 1998).

Results of the application of a single electrical stimulus to the phrenic nerve may also be abnormal in MG patients with diaphragmatic involvement. Both a low DCMAP and a slightly prolonged latency have been described (Zifko et al., 1999). Phrenic nerve conduction studies may be important in patients with MG crises following thymectomy, because the phrenic nerve may be injured during the procedure, particularly along the transsternal route.

Needle EMG also plays an important role in these patients (Maher et al., 1998). In four patients with predominant or isolated respiratory muscle involve-

ment, Maher and colleagues quoted recorded abnormal spontaneous activities in terms of fibrillation potentials and positive sharp waves from the diaphragm, which they related to functional denervation. In about 10% of all MG patients, functional denervation may also be present in the limb muscles (Klein et al., 1964; Oosterhuis and Bethlem, 1973; Barbieri et al., 1982; Witt and Bolton, 1988).

Sleep studies in 20 MG patients often showed sleep-associated symptoms such as waking up at night, headaches in the morning, and a feeling of shortness of breath (Quera-Salva et al., 1992). In addition, they consistently showed abnormalities of rapid eye movement (REM) sleep as well as diaphragmatic weakness during the daytime confirmed by transdiaphragmatic pressure measurements.

Like the results of the comprehensive neurophysiological evaluation, the response to the edrophonium test is highly accurate diagnostically in about 90% to 95% of cases. But a negative outcome does not exclude MG as the factor underlying the respiratory disorder in the individual case, and a positive outcome is not specific for MG.

MANAGEMENT

Ventilation is planned and implemented as in other neuromuscular diseases. Its details are described in the section on ventilation of GBS patients and the method is discussed at length in Wijdicks' work (1997). Measures specific for patients with suspected or confirmed MG include plasmapheresis, which should be done five times on two consecutive days, followed by three exchanges on alternating days. Nonresponders to plasmapheresis should be given corticosteroids, 60 mg daily. This dose should be continued for one month and then slowly reduced. Immunoadsorptive therapy (Shibuya et al., 1994; Grob et al., 1995) is more effective than plasmapheresis. It should be administered on five consecutive days, and it reduces circulating anti-AChR titers by 60%. Patients can be expected to respond to it within 2 (1 to 4) days (Shibuya et al., 1994). High-dose intravenous immunoglobulins have also been reported to be helpful in exacerbations. But as their usefulness in myasthenic crises is still controversial, they cannot be recommended as the drug of first choice at this point in time. Immunosuppression with cyclosporins, 5 mg/kg body weight divided in 2 doses daily, has been found to be equally as useful. Improvements are usually seen about 2 weeks after instituting treatment (Tindall et al., 1987).

Oral pyridostigmine should be stopped in the ICU because of increased pulmonary secretions, bradycardia, and other side effects. This agent should be reintroduced only when the patient is stable and renal function is normal. Depending on the patient's clinical response, the dose should be slowly increased (Saltis et al., 1993; Rieder et al., 1995).

Lambert-Eaton Myasthenic Syndrome

The Lambert-Eaton myasthenic syndrome (LEMS) is a rare abnormality of neuromuscular transmission. Its typical clinical signs and symptoms include fluctuating proximal muscle weakness, reduced or nonelicitable tendon reflexes, and cholinergic autonomic symptoms, such as constipation, dryness of the mouth, dry eyes, impotence, and pupillary abnormalities. The diagnosis of LEMS is clinched by electrophysiological studies—that is, by repetitive high-frequency nerve stimulation. Isolated or predominant involvement of the respiratory muscles is a constant finding in LEMS patients (Gracey and Southern, 1987; O'Neill et al., 1988; Wilcox et al., 1988; Laroche et al., 1989; Anderson et al., 1990; Barr et al., 1993; Beydoun, 1994; Nicolle et al., 1996; Zifko et al., 1998a). Relatively frequent reports of respiratory muscle involvement in LEMS suggest that the condition may often go undiagnosed in patients with respiratory disorders of unclear origin. But even patients known to suffer from LEMS may develop rapidly progressive respiratory muscle weakness. The prognosis depends mainly on whether LEMS is associated with neoplastic disease.

Neonatal Myasthenia Gravis

This condition is caused by the diaplacental transport of maternal antibodies to the fetus (Fenichel, 1978; Ohta et al., 1981; Engel, 1984). Affected infants show general weakness and hypertension and have difficulties in feeding within the first 4 days. But they usually recover within 2 to 4 weeks. Neonatal MG is easily diagnosed with electrodiagnostic techniques. Phrenic nerve conduction studies and needle EMG studies of the diaphragm are valuable in children with undiagnosed respiratory insufficiency.

Congenital Myasthenia Gravis

This hereditary abnormality of neuromuscular transmission is an autosomal recessive disease with both presynaptic and postsynaptic changes. It is characterized by hypotension, poor feeding, and respiratory disorders. Affected children often experience repeated apneic episodes, which may be fatal. As a rule, the condition improves within the first 2 years of life. But minor muscle weakness or increased fatigability may persist. The diagnosis is made by repetitive low-frequency stimulation studies (2 to 10 cycles per second). Treatment is symptomatic.

Juvenile Myasthenia Gravis

Juvenile MG is an autoimmune disease of neuromuscular synapses. Its course mimics that of adult MG. Neonatal, congenital, and juvenile MG are described in detail by Harper (1995).

Botulism

Of the eight botulinum toxin types, five may be pathogenic in humans. Among these subtypes A, B, and E are most common.

Contaminated food is the most frequent source of botulism. Patients develop characteristic autonomic symptoms and muscle weakness, which is usually generalized, with accentuation in the bulbar and ocular muscles. But respiratory muscle weakness necessitating ventilation may also occur. Electrophysiological studies using repetitive low-frequency stimulation (2 to 5 cycles per second) show no decrements or, at best, slow decrements. An incremental response may be seen after muscle contraction. Increments of 125% to 200% are elicited by repetitive high-frequency stimulation (20 to 50 cycles per second) (Gutmann and Pratt, 1976). Single-fiber EMG shows increased jitter and blocking of motor units. On needle EMG, brief, low, irregular muscle potentials are usually recorded. The diagnosis is confirmed by the presence of toxin in serum or feces.

In patients with wound botulism, muscle weakness is usually less severe and develops less rapidly than that in food-borne botulism. As a result, respiratory muscle involvement is less common. Electrophysiological findings are similar to those in food-borne botulism. But unlike the case in food-borne botulism, toxin is present only in serum, while the feces are sterile (Hikes and Manoli, 1981; Rapoport and Watkins, 1984).

Infantile botulism is characterized by severe constipation, hypotension, difficult feeding, and ophthalmoplegia. Botulinum toxin has also been detected in some cases of sudden crib death (Arnon et al., 1978).

Other Neuromuscular Toxins and Drugs

Neuromuscular transmission may be acutely blocked by a variety of toxic substances, among them snake, spider, and scorpion venom (see Chapter 75).

MYOPATHIES

Myopathies may result in respiratory muscle weakness necessitating ventilation or may occur in the intensive care setting. The latter variant is described at length in Chapters 81 and 82. Respiratory muscle involvement is often associated with myopathies. Hence, respiratory electrophysiological studies are valuable in diagnosing diaphragmatic weak-

Table 84–2. Myopathic Causes of Respiratory Failure

Myotonic dystrophy
Muscular dystrophy
Polymyositis, dermatomyositis
Thick filament myopathy
Glycogen storage diseases
  Pompe's disease
  McArdle's disease
  Tarui's disease
Acute rhabdomyolysis
Hypokalemia
Hypophosphatemia
Mitochondrial myopathy
Nemaline body myopathy

ness in these patients. It is rarely an initial symptom, however. Table 84–2 lists myopathies in adults that may cause respiratory muscle weakness. Infantile myopathies are reviewed in Chapters 86 and 95.

Inflammatory Myopathies

Dermatomyositis and polymyositis are rare causes of admission to the ICU (DeVere and Bradley, 1975; Howard et al., 1993). But respiratory muscle involvement has repeatedly been reported (Lahrmann et al., 1997).

Myopathies Associated with Other Diseases

Respiratory muscle involvement in myopathies associated with systemic diseases such as sarcoidosis (Dewberry et al., 1993; Ost et al., 1995; Pringle and Dewar, 1997), hypophosphatemia (Gravelyn et al., 1988; Wijdicks, 1994), hypokalemia, trichinosis (Davis et al., 1976), or alcoholic rhabdomyolysis has been described.

Myotonic Dystrophy

Respiratory disorders are a common finding in myotonic dystrophy. They have many causes, including abnormalities of central respiratory regulation and abnormalities of the corticospinal pathways to the phrenic motor neurons as well as direct diaphragmatic weakness (Zifko et al., 1996a). So, testing the central respiratory pathway using transcortical and cervical magnetic stimulation with recording from the diaphragm, and testing the peripheral respiratory system using phrenic nerve conduction and needle EMG of the diaphragm and chest wall muscles, are important in the differential diagnosis for respiratory insufficiency. This differentiation is necessary for therapeutic decisions. Respiratory insufficiency may be a problem in the wake of anesthesia because of difficulties in weaning. Postoperatively, there should be careful use of opi-

oids and sedatives and vigorous monitoring with aggressive bronchopulmonary toilet. The long-term prognosis of temporary respiratory insufficiency in patients with myotonic dystrophy in general is quite good, even if they require ventilatory assistance in the ICU.

Acid Maltase Deficiency

This rare, autosomal recessive disease may occasionally be associated with severe respiratory muscle weakness of rapid onset, which may be a problem diagnostically. Mechanical ventilation and optimal intensive care are of primary importance, because patients may recover spontaneously even after prolonged ventilation or may at least be switched to permanent home-care ventilatory support.

Other Myopathies with Respiratory Muscle Weakness

Respiratory muscle involvement has been described in a variety of other myopathies. These include Bethlem myopathy (Haq et al., 1999), multicore myopathy (Zeman et al., 1997), localized muscular dystrophy (Bosman et al., 1988), human immunodeficiency virus (HIV) myopathy (Altobellis et al., 1992; Wijdicks, 1994), mitochondrial myopathies (Barohn et al., 1990; Kim et al., 1991), carnitine palmitoyl transferase deficiency myopathy (Joutel et al., 1993), and limb-girdle muscular dystrophy (Robertson and Roloff, 1994).

FAILURE TO WEAN

Sepsis and multiple organ failure occur in 20% to 50% of patients in a medical ICU (Train et al., 1990), and 70% of the patients have CIP (Witt et al., 1991). Neuromuscular blocking agents and steroids may cause further distinctive neuromuscular syndromes (Bolton et al., 1994). In addition, impaired central respiratory drive may cause or contribute to prolonged mechanical ventilation. Consequently, patients with central or peripheral neurological diseases requiring prolonged mechanical ventilation should invariable be seen by a neurologist for a comprehensive clinical evaluation and for neurophysiological studies of the respiratory system (see Chapter 35).

In the ICU, neurophysiological studies in respiratory disorders of unclear origin should be started with measurements of motor and sensory nerve conduction velocities in the lower and upper extremities. Often, these studies establish the presence of neuropathy and its underlying pathophysiological mechanisms (axonal versus demyelinating). Neurography of the phrenic nerve can easily be done in the intensive care setting. Very rarely, subclavian vein catheters or open chest injuries may be a problem. If neurography is noncontributory and/or if an abnormality of neuromuscular transmission is suspected clinically, repetitive nerve stimulation at 3 Hz and 30 or 40 Hz should be added. What nerve should be stimulated depends on the clinical findings. If isolated diaphragmatic involvement is suspected, the phrenic nerve is the best choice. Rarely, single-fiber EMG, preferably stimulated, will be needed in the intensive care setting. Neurophysiological studies should also include limb muscle electromyograms. These should be recorded from proximal and distal muscles of both the upper and the lower limbs. Intercostal and diaphragmatic electromyograms provide important information on the type and extent of respiratory muscle involvement.

If autonomic nervous system involvement is suspected, assessment of sympathetic skin responses and heart rate variability should be the first step in the diagnostic evaluation.

If abnormalities of central respiratory regulation are suspected, transcortical magnetic stimulation with signals picked up from the diaphragm are particularly helpful. In suspicious cases, this procedure should invariably be added to the battery of tests, because many patients with confirmed peripheral respiratory muscle weakness also show signs of central respiratory muscle failure.

HOME CARE VENTILATION

The management of patients with neuromuscular disorders with mechanical ventilation at home requires special expertise. In 1996, "Consensus on Treatment of Respiratory Insufficiency and Ventilatory Support" was published by the European Neuromuscular Group in Netherlands (39th ENMC International Workshop, 1996).

PHASE I: START OF CHECK-UPS
A. Information and education have to be provided to patients and patient organizations and doctors about the possibility of respiratory insufficiency and the opportunity to obtain home mechanical ventilation to facilitate interaction between patients and physicians experienced in home mechanical ventilation.
B. Patients should preferably be treated by the medical staff of an organization for home mechanical ventilation for their respiratory insufficiency. The organization should preferably be part of a network including, among others, other organizations for home mechanical ventilation, centers for neuromuscular diseases, and rehabilitation centers so that a multidisciplinary approach is possible.
C. Annual check-ups of patients for the potential to develop respiratory insufficiency should start when vital capacity is less than 50% of expected value. This is normally about 1 year

after the end of ambulation in patients with Duchenne's muscular dystrophy. Validation of the neurological diagnosis is indicated. Physical examination for mobility, activities of daily life (ADL), and scoliosis should be performed regularly. Exercises for maintaining mobility of the thorax and the quality of pulmonary tissue should be continued. The basic parameters to be examined during the checks-ups are as follows:
1. complaints and/or symptoms of the patient
2. vital capacity with the patient in the supine and sitting positions
3. blood gas analysis
Consultation with the patient's neurologist, general practitioner, or other physician is advisable.
D. Hospitalization of the patient when vital capacity is less than 1 L and/or daytime partial pressure of carbon dioxide (PCO_2) is greater than 45 mm Hg and/or symptoms or complaints are present. Perform measurement of nocturnal blood gases (PCO_2 and PO_2) during sleep (various methods can be used).
E. Prepare patient and family to enable them to make a choice regarding ventilation through adequate education. Contact with other patients and patient organizations is advisable. Adequate contact between patient, general practitioner, and a center for home ventilation is necessary.
When respiratory insufficiency is apparent and the patient indicates a positive choice regarding mechanical ventilation, the practitioner should prepare and arrange a care system at home within an adequate amount of time.
Closely monitor and attempt to fulfill the needs of the patient with regard to vocation (work), hobby, travel, and social life.
F. Information and education has to be provided to the patient, family members, and caregivers about respiratory symptoms and the techniques of assisted ventilation through an uncuffed tracheostomy tube.

PHASE II: START OF MECHANICAL VENTILATION
A. Explain to the patient, well in advance, the different therapeutic strategies of home mechanical ventilation, including noninvasive methods.
B. Consider the present state, rate, evolution (progressiveness), and natural history of the disease before advising the patient on the preferred method of home mechanical ventilation.
C. Noninvasive (nasal) ventilation is often the first choice that is taken into consideration. The following factors have to be assessed in the decision to utilize this type of ventilation:
1. safety of the modality (hours of unassisted ventilation)
2. state of glottic function, the risk of aspiration or swallowing disorders

3. effect of the modality on survival

Information and education must be provided to the patient about the technique of assisted coughing.

D. Tracheostomal ventilation through an uncuffed tube (cannula) is considered when noninvasive means are not feasible. In the case of glottic dysfunction, recurrent desaturation (leakage of air during the night), or recurrent atelectasis, use of cuffed or customized tubes should be considered, sometimes in conjunction with a PEG (percutaneous enterogastrotomy).

E. The choice of ventilator depends on safety, portability, service, reliability, and availability. Use of volume-cycled ventilators is the preferred method for ventilation via tracheostoma. It is not recommended to use pressure-targeted ventilators without alarms and batteries for users without considerable ability to breathe on their own.

F. Oxygen is rarely indicated; it is used only when hypoventilation is corrected and Sao_2 is less than 90%.

G. In conjunction with the organization of home mechanical ventilation, efficiency of ventilation should be ensured, including Sao_2 and arterial blood gases (ABGs). The goal is normal ABGs.

H. The following aspects should be arranged: preparation of home situation, caregivers, possible alternatives, and financial implications including insurance coverage—all in conjunction with the staff involved in the mechanical ventilation program.

I. Education of all persons (patient, family members, caretakers, general practitioners, etc.) is essential. The home mechanical ventilation organization is responsible for this education.

PHASE III: START OF HOME MECHANICAL VENTILATION (HMV)

A. Home mechanical ventilation should preferably take place in the home of the patient. Home is defined as the place where the patient lived before he/she used mechanical ventilation. If this is not possible, alternatives can be considered.

B. Assistance has to be arranged in the home situation with regard to respiratory and non-respiratory problems.

C. Support and educate persons involved in care system at home. The basic education has to be completed before the patient can be discharged from the hospital.

D. A 24-hour support service should be available to manage device breakdown and technical problems. The person responsible for the home care program in mechanical ventilation has to prepare a list of contacts to solve medical problems and/or emergencies.

E. Regular check-ups during the HMV program are necessary to ensure that the home mechanical ventilation apparatus is working properly. The program should be supervised by a physician with specific skill in mechanically-ventilation, who will decide the frequency and modalities of the check-ups, the change of accessories (canula, nasal masks, etc.), and other measures aimed at the safety of the patient.

F. Continue consideration and support for education, vocation (work), hobby, travel, social life, mainly through patient associations.

G. When patients intend to travel, provide address of a specialist center and name of physician in the region/country of destination. The patient should be provided with the phone number of a physician responsible for the home mechanical ventilation in case the physician of the specialist center in another country needs information.

Acknowledgment

The author wishes to thank Miss Ingeborg Haigner for expert secretarial assistance, and C. F. Bolton, W. Wihlidal, and H. Remtulla, EMG Laboratory, Victoria Hospital, London, Canada, for their help in preparing several of the figures.

References

Altobellis SS, Roy TM, Joyce BW, et al: Respiratory failure and death from HIV-associated myopathy. J Kent Med Assoc 1992; 90:174–177.

Anderson TJ, Carroll GJ, Avery SF, et al: Eaton-Lambert myasthenic syndrome: Two cases with typical and atypical features. NZ Med J 1990;103:240–242.

Arnon S, Midura T, Damus K, et al: Intestinal infection and toxin production by *Clostridium botulinum* as one cause of sudden infant death syndrome. Lancet 1978;1:1273–1277.

Ayas NT, McCool FD, Gore R, et al: Prevention of human diaphragm atrophy with short periods of electrical stimulation. Am J Respir Crit Care Med 1999;159:2018–2020.

Bansal SK, Haldar N, Dhand UK, et al: Phrenic neuropathy in arsenic poisoning. Chest 1991;100:878–880.

Barbieri S, Weiss GM, Daube JR: Fibrillation potentials in myasthenia gravis. Muscle Nerve 1982;5:50.

Barohn RJ, Clanton T, Sahenk Z, et al: Recurrent respiratory insufficiency and depressed ventilatory drive complicating mitochondrial myopathies. Neurology 1990;40:103–106.

Barr CW, Claussen G, Thomas D, et al: Primary respiratory failure as the presenting symptom in Lambert-Eaton myasthenic syndrome. Muscle Nerve 1993;16:712–715.

Beydoun SR: Delayed diagnosis of Lambert-Eaton myasthenic syndrome in a patient presenting with recurrent refractory respiratory failure. Muscle Nerve 1994;17:689–690.

Bolton CF, Brown JD, Sibbald WJ: The electrophysiologic investigation of respiratory paralysis in critically ill patients. Neurology 1983;33:186.

Bolton CF, Young GB, Zochodne DW: Neurological changes during severe sepsis. Curr Top Intensive Care 1994;1:759–773.

Bolton CF: Clinical neurophysiology of the respiratory system. Muscle Nerve 1993;16:809–818.

Bolton CF: The changing concepts of Guillain-Barré syndrome. N Engl J Med 1995;333:1415–1417.

Bolton CF: Neuromuscular conditions in the intensive care unit. Intensive Care Med 1996;22:841–843.

Borel CO, Tilford C, Nichols DG: Diaphragmatic performance during recovery from acute ventilatory failure in Guillain-Barré syndrome and myasthenia gravis. Chest 1991;99:444–451.

Bos AP, van der Meché FGA, Witsenburg M, et al: Experiences with Guillain-Barré syndrome in a pediatric intensive care unit. Intensive Care Med 1987;13:328–331.

Bosman C, Bachelet V, Boldrini R, et al: Diaphragmatic paralysis due to partial diaphragmatic hypoplasia mimicking a localized muscular dystrophy: A case report. Clin Neuropathol 1988; 7:33–38.

Brooks BR: Natural history of ALS: Symptoms, strength, pulmonary function, and disability. Neurology 1996;47(suppl 2):71–82.

Carter GT, Kilmer DD, Bonekat HW, et al: Evaluation of phrenic nerve and pulmonary function in hereditary motor and sensory neuropathy, type I. Muscle Nerve 1992;15:459–462.

Cavaletti G, Zincone A, Marzorati L, et al: Rapidly progressive multifocal motor neuropathy with phrenic nerve paralysis: Effect of nocturnal assisted ventilation. J Neurol 1998;245:613–616.

Chalmers RM, Howard RS, Wiles CM, et al: Respiratory insufficiency in neuronopathic and neuropathic disorders. Q J Med 1996;89:477–482.

Chen R, Grand'Maison F, Strong MJ, et al: Motor neuron disease presenting as acute respiratory failure: A clinical and pathological study. J Neurol Neurosurg Psychiatry 1996;60:455–458.

Chevrolet JC, Deleamont P: Repeated vital capacity measurements as predictive parameters for mechanical ventilation need and weaning success in the Guillain-Barré syndrome. Am Rev Respir 1991;144:814–818.

Chin EF, Lynn RB: Surgery of eventration of the diaphragm. J Thorac Cardiovasc Surg 1956;32:6.

Cohen MA, Younger D: Aspects of the natural history of myasthenia gravis: Crisis and death. Ann N Y Acad Sci 1981;377:670–677.

Comroe JHJR, Wood FC, Kay CF, et al: Motor neuritis after tetanus antitoxin with involvement of muscles of respiration. Am J Med 1951;10:786–789.

Davis J, Goldman M, Loh L, et al: Diaphragm function and alveolar hypoventilation. Q J Med 1976;45:87–100.

Davis MJ, Cilo M, Plaitakis A, et al: Trichinosis: Severe myopathic involvement with recovery. Neurology 1976;26:37–40.

DeVere R, Bradley WG: Polymyositis: Its presentation, morbidity and mortality. Brain 1975;98:637–666.

Dewberry RG, Schneider BF, Cale WF, et al: Sarcoid myopathy presenting with diaphragm weakness. Muscle Nerve 1993;16: 832–835.

Engel A: Myasthenia gravis and myasthenic syndromes. Ann Neurol 1984;10:519–534.

Epstein EJ, Quereshi MSA, Wright JS: Diaphragmatic paralysis after supraclavicular puncture of subclavian vein. Br Med J 1976;2:693–694.

Evoli A, Batocchi AP, LO Monaco M, et al: Clinical heterogeneity of seronegative myasthenia gravis. Neuromuscul Disord 1996; 6:155–161.

Fallat RJ, Jewitt B, Bass M, et al: Spirometry in amyotrophic lateral sclerosis. Arch Neurol 1979;36:74–80.

Fenichel G: Clinical syndromes of myasthenia in infancy and childhood: A review. Arch Neurol 1978;35:97–103.

Ferguson JT, Murphy RP, Lascelles RG: Ventilatory failure in myasthenia gravis. J Neurol Neurosurg Psychiatry 1982;45:217–222.

Fisher MA, Leehey DJ, Gandhi V, et al: Phrenic nerve palsies and persistent respiratory acidosis in a patient with diabetes mellitus. Muscle Nerve 1997;20:900–902.

Gilchrist D, Chan CK, Deck JH: Phrenic involvement in Charcot-Marie-Tooth disease: Pathologic documentation. Chest 1989;96: 1197–1199.

Girsch W, Deutinger M, Bayer GS, et al: Vienna phrenic pacemaker—experience with diaphragm pacing in children. Eur J Pediatr Surg 1996;6:140–143.

Glassman LR, Spencer FC, Baumann G, et al: Successful plication for postoperative diaphragmatic paralysis in an adult. Ann Thorac Surg 1994;58:1754–1755.

Gourie-Devi M, Ganapathy GR: Phrenic nerve conduction time in Guillain-Barré syndrome. J Neurol Neurosurg Psychiatry 1985; 48:245–249.

Gracey DR, Divertic MB, Howard FM: Mechanical ventilation for respiratory failure in myasthenia gravis: Two-year experience with 22 patients. Mayo Clin Proc 1983;58:597–602.

Gracey DR, Southern PA: Respiratory failure in Lambert-Eaton myasthenic syndrome. Chest 1987;91:716–718.

Gravelyn TR, Brophy N, Siegert C, et al: Hypophosphatemia-associated respiratory muscle weakness in a general inpatient population. Am J Med 1988;84:870–876.

Greene W, L'Heureux PL, Hunt CE: Paralysis of the diaphragm. Am J Dis Child 1975;1402–1405.

Grob D, Simpson D, Mitsumoto H, et al: Treatment of myasthenia gravis by immunoadsorption of plasma. Neurology 1995;45:338–344.

Gutmann L, Pratt L: Pathophysiologic aspects of human botulism. Arch Neurol 1976;33:175–179.

Hahn AF: Management of Guillain-Barré syndrome (GBS). Bailliere's Clin Neurol 1996;9:627–644.

Haq RU, Speer MC, Chu ML, et al: Respiratory muscle involvement in Bethlem myopathy. Neurology 1999;52:174–176.

Hardie R, Harding AE, Hirsch N, et al: Diaphragmatic weakness in hereditary motor and sensory neuropathy. J Neurol Neurosurg Psychiatry 1990;53:348–350.

Harper CM: Neuromuscular transmission disorder in childhood. In Jones HR, et al (eds): Pediatric Clinical Electromyography. Lippincott-Raven 1996; 353–386.

Havard C, Scadding G: Myasthenia gravis: Pathogenesis and current concepts in management. Drugs 1983;26:174–184.

Hikes D, Manoli A: Wound botulism. J Trauma 1981;21:68–71.

Hill GE, Polk SL: Hypoventilation after high unilateral cervical chordotomy in a patient with preexisting injury of the phrenic nerve. South Med J 1976;69:718–746.

Hoover CF: Functions of the diaphragm and their diagnostic importance. Arch Intern Med 1913;12:214.

Howard RS, Wiles CM, Hirsch NP, et al: Respiratory involvement in primary muscle disorders: Assessment and management. Q J Med 1993;86:175–189.

Hughes PD, Polkey MI, Moxham J, et al: Long-term recovery of diaphragm strength in neuralgic amyotrophy. Eur Respir J 1999; 13:379–384.

Iverson LI, Mittal A, Dugan DJ, et al: Injuries to the phrenic nerve resulting in diaphragmatic paralysis with special reference to stretch trauma. Am J Surg 1976;132:263–269.

Joutel A, Moulonguet A, Demaugre F, et al: Type II carnitine palmitoyl transferase deficiency complicated by acute respiratory failure. Rev Neurol 1993;149:797–799.

Kim GW, Kim SM, Sunwoo IN, et al: Two cases of mitochondrial myopathy with predominant respiratory dysfunction. Yonsei Med J 1991;32:184–189.

Kirklin BR, Hidgson JR: Roentgenographic characteristics of diaphragmatic hernia. Am J Roentgenol 1947;58:77.

Klein JJ, Gottlieb AJ, Mones RJ, et al: Thymoma and polymyositis. Onset of M.G. after thymectomy: Report of 2 cases. Arch Intern Med 1964;113:142–152.

Lagueny A, Ellie E, Saintarailles J, et al: Unilateral diaphragmatic paralysis: An electrophysiological study. J Neurol Neurosurg Psychiatry 1992;55:316–318.

Lahrmann H, Grisold W, Authier FJ, et al: Neuralgic amyotrophy with phrenic nerve involvement. Muscle Nerve 1999;22:437–442.

Lahrmann H, Grisold W, Zifko UA: Respiratory muscle involvement in dermatomyositis. Neuromuscul Disord 1997;7(6):453.

Lahrmann H, Albrecht G, Hitzenberger P, et al: Value of electrophysiologic studies of the diaphragm in ALS. J Neurol 2000; 247:25.

Laroche CM, Carroll N, Moxham J, et al: Diaphragm weakness in Charcot-Marie-Tooth disease. Thorax 1988;43:478–479.

Laroche M, Mier AK, Spiro SG, et al: Respiratory muscle weakness in the Lambert-Eaton myasthenic syndrome. Thorax 1989;44: 913–918.

Laub GW, Muralidharan S, Chen C, et al: Phrenic nerve injury: A prospective study. Chest 1991;100:376–379.

Maher J, Grand'Maison F, Nicolle MW, et al: Diagnostic difficulties in myasthenia gravis. Muscle Nerve 1998;21:577–583.

Malin JP: Zur Ätiologie der Phrenicusparese. Nervenarzt 1979; 50:448–456.

Mier A, Laroche C, Geen M: Unsuspected myasthenia gravis presenting as respiratory failure. Thorax 1990;45:422–423.

Miller RG, Rosenberg JA, Gelinas DF, et al: Practice parameter: The care of the patient with amyotrophic lateral sclerosis (an evidence-based review). Neurology 1999;52:1311–1323.

Mok Q, Ross-Russell R, Mulvey D, et al: Phrenic nerve injury in infants and children undergoing cardiac surgery. Br Heart J 1991;65:287–292.

Mulvey DA, Aquilina RJ, Elliott MW, et al: Diaphragmatic dysfunction in neuralgic amyotrophy: An electrophysiologic evaluation of 16 patients presenting with dyspnea. Am Rev Respir Dis 1993;147:67–71.

Nakano KK, Bass H, Tyler HR, et al: Amyotrophic lateral sclerosis: A study of plulmonary function. Dis Nerv Syst 1976;37:32–35.

Naunyn B: Ein Fall von Erbscher Plexuslähmung mit gleichseitiger Sympathicuslähmung. Dtsch Med Wochenschr 1902;28:52–55.

Nelson KG, Jolly PC, Thomas PA: Brachial plexus injuries associated with missile wounds of the chest. J Trauma 1968;8:268–275.

Ng KKP, Howard RS, Fish DR, et al: Management and outcome of severe Guillain-Barré syndrome. Q J Med 1995;88:243–250.

Nicolle MW, Stewart DJ, Remtulla H, et al: Lambert-Eaton myasthenic syndrome presenting with severe respiratory failure. Muscle Nerve 1996;19:1328–1333.

Obel IWP: Transient phrenic-nerve paralysis following subclavian veinpuncture. Anesthesiology 1976;33:369–370.

Ohta M, Matsubara F, Hayashi K, et al: Acetylcholine receptor antibodies in infants and mothers with myasthenia gravis. Neurology 1981;31:1019–1022.

O'Neill JH, Murray NMF, Newsom-Davis J: The Lambert-Eaton myasthenic syndrome: A review of 50 cases. Brain 1988;111:577–596.

Oosterhuis H, Bethlem J: Neurogenic muscle involvement in myasthenia gravis: A clinical and histopathological study. J Neurol Neurosurg Psychiatry 1973;36:244–254.

Osserman KE, Genkins G: Studies in myasthenia gravis: Reduction in mortality rate after crisis. JAMA 1963;183:97–101.

Ost D, Yeldandi A, Cugell D: Acute sarcoid myositis with respiratory muscle involvement: Case report and review of the literature. Chest 1995;107:879–882.

Pendersen J: The effect of nasotracheal intubation on the paranasal sinuses. Acta Anaesthesiol Scand 1991;35:11–13.

Pringle CE, Dewar CL: Respiratory muscle involvement in severe sarcoid myositis. Muscle Nerve 1997;20:379–381.

Quera-Salva MA, Guilleminault C, Chevret S, et al: Breathing disorders during sleep in myasthenia gravis. Ann Neurol 1992;31:86–92.

Raffa H, Kayali MT, Al-Ibrahim K, et al: Fatal bilateral phrenic nerve injury following hypothermic open heart surgery. Chest 1994;105:1268–1269.

Raine J, Samuels MP, Mok Q, et al: Negative extrathoracic pressure ventilation for phrenic nerve palsy after paediatric cardiac surgery. Br Heart J 1992;67:308–311.

Rapoport S, Watkins P: Descending paralysis resulting from occult wound botulism. Ann Neurol 1984;16:359–361.

Rieder P, Louis M, Jolliet P, et al: The repeated measurement of vital capacity is a poor predictor of the need for mechanical ventilation in myasthenia gravis. Intensive Care Med 1995;21:663–668.

Ringel SP, Murphy JR, Alderson MK, et al: The natural history of amyotrophic lateral sclerosis. Neurology 1993;43:1316–1322.

Rivner MH, Kim S, Greenberg M, et al: Reversible generalized paresis following hypotension: A new neurological entity. Neurology 1983;33:164.

Robertson PL, Roloff DW: Chronic respiratory failure in limb-girdle muscular dystrophy: Successful long-term therapy with nasal bilevel positive airway pressure. Pediatr Neurol 1994;10:328–331.

Rochester DF, Esau SA: Assessment of ventilatory function in patients with neuromuscular disease. Clin Chest Med 1994;14:751–763.

Roelofs RJ, Cerra F, Bielka N, et al: Prolonged respiratory insufficiency due to acute motor neuropathy: A new syndrome? Neurology 1983;33:240.

Rohr H, Lenz H: Störungen der Zwerchfellmotorik bei cervikalen Wurzelschädigungen. Nervenarzt 1960a;31:359–365.

Rohr H, Lenz H: Zwerchfellähmungen nach traumatischer Schädigung der cervikalen Spinalwurzeln. Acta Neurochir 1960b;8:44–69.

Ropper AH, Kehne SM: Guillain-Barré syndrome: Management of respiratory failure. Neurology 1985;35:1662–1665.

Ropper AH: Severe acute Guillain-Barré syndrome. Neurology 1986;36:429–432.

Saltis LM, Martin BR, Traeger SM, et al: Continuous infusion of pyridostigmine in the management of myasthenic crisis. Crit Care Med 1993;21:938–940.

Schiffman PL, Belsh JM: Pulmonary function at diagnosis of amyotrophic lateral sclerosis. Chest 1993;103:2.

Schiffrin N: Unilateral paralysis of the diaphragm in the newborn infant due to phrenic nerve injury, with and without associated brachial palsy. Pediatrics 1952;9:69–76.

Selecky PA, Ziment I: Prolonged respirator support for the treatment of intractable MG. Chest 1974;65:207–209.

Sellman MS, Mayer RF: Treatment of myasthenic crisis in late life. South Med J 1985;78:1208–1210.

Shibuya N, Sato T, Osame M, et al: Immunoadsorption therapy for myasthenia gravis. J Neurol Neurosurg Psychiatry 1994;57:578–581.

Simpson J: Myasthenia gravis: A personal view of pathogenesis and mechanism, part I. Muscle Nerve 1978;1:45–56.

Singh NK, Jaiswal AK, Misra S, et al: Assessment of autonomic dysfunction in Guillain-Barré syndrome and its prognostic implications. Acta Neurol Scand 1987;75:101–105.

Sunderrajan EV, Davenport J: The Guillain-Barré syndrome: Pulmonary-neurologic correlations. Medicine 1985;64:333–341.

Tether JE: Management of myasthenic and cholinergic crises. Am J Med 1958;19:740–742.

Thomas CE, Mayer SA, Gungor Y, et al: Myasthenic crisis: Clinical features, mortality, complications, and risk factors for prolonged intubation. Neurology 1997;48:1253–1260.

Thomas TV: Congenital eventration of the diaphragm: A collective review. Ann Thorac Surg 1970;10:18.

Tiede RH, Hover JR, Davies SF: Unilateral phrenic nerve paralysis from cutting down a christmas tree. South Med J 1994;87:1161–1163.

Tindall RS, Rolins JA, Phillips JT, et al: Preliminary results of a double-blind, randomized, placebo-controlled trial of cyclosporine in myasthenia gravis. N Engl J Med 1987;316:719–724.

Train DD, Groeneveld ABJ, van der Meuien J, et al: Age, chronic disease, sepsis, organ system failure, and mortality in a medical intensive care unit. Criti Care Med 1990;18:474–479.

Tripp HF, Bolton JW: Phrenic nerve injury following cardiac surgery: A review. J Card Surg 1998;13:218–223.

Tsairis P, Dyck PJ, Mulder DW: Natural history of brachial plexus neuropathy. Arch Neurol 1972;27:109–117.

Vitacca M, Clini E, Facchetti D, et al: Breathing pattern and respiratory mechanics in patients with amyotrophic lateral sclerosis. Eur Respir J 1997;10:1614–1621.

Walsh NE, Dumitru D, Kalantri A, et al: Brachial neuritis involving the bilateral phrenic nerves. Arch Phys Med Rehabil 1987;68:46–48.

White JE, Bullock RE, Hudgson P, et al: Phrenic neuropathy in association with diabetes. Diabet Med 1992;9:954–956.

Wijdicks EFM: Neurology of Critical Illness. Philadelphia, FA Davis, 1994.

Wijdicks EF: Management of pulmonary complications. In Wijdicks EF (ed): Clinical Practice of Critical Care Neurology. Philadelphia, Lippincott-Raven, 1997.

Wilcox P, Baile EM, Hards J, et al: Phrenic nerve function and its relationship to atelectasis after coronary artery bypass surgery. Chest 1988;93:693–698.

Wilcox PG, Morrison NJ, Anzarut ARA, et al: Lambert-Eaton myasthenic syndrome involving the diaphragm. Chest 1988;93:604–606.

Winer JB, Hughes RA: Identification of patients at risk of arrhythmia in the Guillain-Barré syndrome. Q J Med 1988;68:735–739.

Witt NJ, Bolton CF: Neuromuscular disorders and thymoma. Muscle Nerve 1988;11:398–405.

Witt NJ, Zochodne DW, Bolton CF, et al: Peripheral nerve function in sepsis and multiple organ failure. Chest 1991;99:176–184.

Yeh TF, Amka P, Pildes RS, et al: Diaphragmatic paralysis after surgical ligation of patent ductus arteriosus. Lancet 1977;2:461.

Zeman AZJ, Dick DJ, Anderson JR, et al: Multicore myopathy presenting in adulthood with respiratory failure. Muscle Nerve 1997;20:367–369.

Zifko UA, Auinger M, Albrecht G, et al: Phrenic neuropathy in chronic renal failure. Thorax 1995a;50:793–794.

Zifko UA, Hartmann M, Girsch W, et al: Diaphragmatic paresis in newborns due to phrenic nerve injury. Neuropediatrics 1995b; 26:281–284.

Zifko UA, Remtulla H, Power K, et al: Transcortical and cervical magnetic stimulation with recording of the diaphragm. Muscle Nerve 1996a;19:614–620.

Zifko UA, Hahn AF, Remtulla H, et al: Central and peripheral respiratory electrophysiological studies in myotonic dystrophy. Brain 1996b;119:1911–1922.

Zifko UA, Chen R, Remtulla H, et al: Respiratory electrophysiological studies in Guillain-Barré syndrome. J Neurol Neurosurg Psychiatry 1996c;60:191–194.

Zifko UA, Young BG, Bolton CF: Electrophysiologic monitoring in neurological respiratory insufficiency. J Neurol Neurosurg Psychiatry 1997a;62:299–300.

Zifko UA, Nicolle MW, Remtulla H, et al: Repetitive phrenic nerve stimulation study in normal subjects. J Clin Neurophysiol 1997b;14:235–241.

Zifko UA, Bolton CF, Nicolle MW: Repetitive nerve stimulation in studies of respiratory involvement in myasthenia gravis. Ann N Y Acad Sci 1998a;841:716–719.

Zifko UA, Zipko HT, Bolton CF: Clinical and electrophysiological findings in critical illness polyneuropathy. J Neurol Sci 1998b; 159:186–193.

Zifko UA, Nicolle MW, Grisold W, et al: Repetitive phrenic nerve stimulation in myasthenia gravis. Neurology 1999;53:1083–1087.

Zochodne DW: Autonomic involvement in Guillain-Barré syndrome: A review. Muscle Nerve 1994;17:1145–1155.

Zochodne DW, Bolton CF: Neuromuscular disorders in critical illness. Baillieres Clin Neurol 1996;5:645–671.

C H A P T E R 85

Pediatric Electromyography: Clinical Indications and Methodology

H. Royden Jones, Jr., and Basil T. Darras

The diagnostic role of pediatric electromyography (EMG) changed significantly during the last decades of the 20th century. Major scientific advances occurred in the identification of the specific molecular pathogenesis for many peripheral nerve and muscle disorders. These significant breakthroughs in DNA analysis are providing a continually evolving list of new laboratory methods capable of providing a precise explanation for a child's symptoms. The ability to use these very specific DNA Southern blot analyses depends on the pediatric neurologist's ability to reach a reasonable clinical diagnosis. These studies are relatively expensive, and no broad laboratory "profile" exists that economically screens all children evaluated with a specific clinical presentation such as proximal weakness. In 1979, when one of the authors (H.R.J.) developed the Children's Hospital Boston EMG laboratory, boys with Duchenne or Becker muscular dystrophy were frequently evaluated. In the 1980s, at the Children's Hospital Boston, Kunkel (1986) identified the dystrophin gene. This seminal event has been increasingly recapitulated with the identification of specific DNA testing parameters for disorders such as the spinal muscular atrophies, Charcot-Marie-Tooth type I peripheral neuropathies, and other myopathies, including myotonic dystrophy. Subsequently, we no longer perform EMG when boys present with a clinical phenotype typical of a dystrophinopathy.

Additional new testing modalities are available that limit the need for EMG in certain clinical settings. Examples include antibody-specific testing for myasthenia gravis, providing a very accurate means to study the subacute forms of this neuromuscular transmission disorder. However, in the acute clinical setting, EMG still offers the opportunity to make a rapid neurophysiological diagnosis. The Children's Hospital Boston colleagues have been evaluating the possible role of magnetic resonance imaging in the diagnosis of children who present with both Guillain-Barré syndrome and polymyositis. There is an increasing clinical spectrum of neuromuscular disorders for which traditional EMG is no longer routinely indicated. However, personnel in our EMG laboratory keep reasonably busy evaluating various disorders of the peripheral motor unit (Darras and Jones, 2000). We also are commonly consulted for an evolving spectrum of acute pediatric neuromuscular illnesses for which EMG provides specific diagnostic assistance; this is particularly true in the intensive care unit (Jones and Darras, 2000).

Because of the uncomfortable nature of this testing method, some highly respected colleagues advocate the use of anesthesia for all children under age 12 who require any type of invasive procedure, including EMG. We have used this technique for a number of years for any child who requires repetitive motor nerve stimulation, some toddlers who require extensive testing, and mentally compromised children to whom one is not able to explain the purposes and nature of electromyographic testing. The issue that continues to concern us, in reference to the routine or required use of anesthesia, is the very rare but definite chance of a serious anesthesia complication. In addition, because the evaluation of motor unit potentials (MUPs) is particularly essential in many instances, we find that we are best able to evaluate the child's motor unit size and recruitment pattern when the child is not anesthetized, in comparison with careful attempts to have the anesthesiologist partially awaken the youngster by diminishing the anesthetic concentration. Therefore, we strive to reassure the child and his or her parents that we are making this study both practical to the clinical question and friendly to the child by getting the child interested in the sound of the MUPs

(Jones et al., 1987). It is heartwarming to see how often one is able to develop a rapport with the cooperative child and subsequently achieve a clinically successful study.

The basic value of nerve conduction studies (NCSs) and electromyographic assessment is that these studies provide an important extension to the neurological examination. Our diagnostic approach with children is similar to that with adults: a careful clinical evaluation, various blood studies that increasingly include genetic analyses (Darras and Jones, 2000), and sometimes NCS/EMG (Thomas and Lambert, 1960; Gamstorp, 1963; Baer and Johnson, 1965; Gamstorp and Shelburne, 1965; Shahani and Young, 1981; Cruz Martinez et al., 1983; Miller and Kuntz, 1986; Parano et al., 1993). Muscle or nerve biopsy or both may be later indicated based on the results of EMG. However, the very significant breakthrough with DNA analyses makes these histopathological methods less commonly indicated, just as with EMG.

Although pediatric neurologists and physiatrists are occasionally on staff in electromyography laboratories in children's hospitals, typically, adult clinical neurophysiologists or physiatrists are primarily responsible for performing these studies. Often, such physicians have had relatively little experience during their training in EMG with evaluation of the broad spectrum of childhood neuromuscular illnesses, particularly those that affect infants. Even at major academic centers with reputations for expertise in the diagnosis and treatment of these disorders, the number of children evaluated in an EMG laboratory is relatively small compared with the number of adults. At the EMG laboratory at the Children's Hospital Boston, we perform approximately 125 to 150 studies annually (Darras and Jones, 2000). This is about 10% of the total adult volume of electromyographic examinations performed at the Lahey Clinic. In many North American hospitals, a significant number of years are required to gain a broad clinical electromyographic perspective on a number of the pediatric neuromuscular disorders. However, in some countries, clinical neurophysiologists such as Matthew Pitt at London's Great Ormond Street Hospital have rapidly acquired a broad experience; Pitt evaluates 350 to 400 children annually. Although a number of pediatric neuromuscular diseases are analogous to the adult, the relative frequency of these illnesses varies greatly when populations of different ages are compared. Two common clinical indications for an adult EMG infrequently occur in childhood: carpal tunnel syndrome and nerve root lesions. In contrast, more infants are referred to the Children's Hospital Boston EMG laboratory for evaluation of the floppy infant syndrome than those referred for mononeuropathies.

In this introductory chapter to the section on pediatric neuromuscular disorders, we provide a clinically relevant, practical approach to the indications for and performance of EMG in children. Initially, we present a broad set of general neurophysiological guidelines, followed by more specific electromyographic concepts and recommendations. A few tables in Section XXXI provide various normative data for NCS/EMG in infants and children of different ages (Jablecki, 1986; Harmon et al., 1992). Ideally, normative data for NCS and MUP parameters have to be independently established. When the EMG laboratory at the Children's Hospital Boston opened in 1979, we considered collecting our own normal values for pediatric sensory and motor NCSs as well as for needle EMG; however, given the ethical considerations involved in the collection of such normative data for both infants and children, we did not feel able to pursue this. Rather, we extrapolated our initial normative data from various earlier and somewhat limited evaluations (Thomas and Lambert, 1960; Gamstorp, 1963; Baer and Johnson, 1965; Gamstorp and Shelburne, 1965; Shahani and Young, 1981; Cruz Martinez et al., 1983) and later added other normative data (Miller and Kuntz, 1986; Parano et al., 1993). Each of these studies varied as to the numbers of children examined and the specific techniques that were used. The 1986 report of Miller and Kuntz, primarily from the Mayo Clinic, is frequently cited. Unfortunately, this report was based on relatively small numbers of children and included only 23 infants: 4 neonates, 6 infants aged 1 to 6 months, and 13 children aged 7 to 12 months. In 1993, another larger series was published from the Babies Hospital at Columbia Presbyterian in New York. This provided normative nerve conduction values for 155 healthy children aged 7 days to 14 years, including 20 neonates, 23 infants aged 1 to 6 months, and 25 children aged 7 to 12 months (Parano et al., 1993). The various studies attempting to establish normal pediatric values are carefully collated by Harmon and his colleagues (Harmon et al., 1992; Jones et al., 1996).

GENERAL APPROACH TO PEDIATRIC ELECTROMYOGRAPHY

Before the EMG, we review the child's history with the child and the parents and perform a relevant neurological examination. The performance of a pediatric EMG always provides an extension to the clinical evaluation as well as an added challenge to an electromyographer, especially the study of a neonate or toddler (Jablecki, 1986; Jones et al., 1987, 1996; Turk, 1989). Before the examination is begun, the purpose of the EMG must be explained to both the parents and the child if he or she is old enough to comprehend. In this setting, it is very important to gain the parents' and child's confidence as well as appreciate that the pediatric electromyographer is empathic to their various concerns. We tell the parents that we will treat their child as we would our own, and this is always reassuring to them. The time taken to ensure that both the child and the parents are comfortable with the need for the EMG

is repaid in both the ease of performance of the EMG and the reliability of the derived data. With older children, we are always forthright in explaining that the EMG has variable levels of discomfort. However, we conclude by stating that we try to minimize this in every possible way. It is important to provide a quiet environment, encouraging the child to relax (Jablecki, 1986; Jones et al., 1987, 1996; Turk, 1989). We also use a variety of toys such as a "TV" music box, stuffed animals, and books, so parents can interact with their child and make the environment of the laboratory more friendly.

One survey of pediatric EMG practice patterns reported that 32% of laboratory directors discouraged or prohibited parental presence (Hays et al., 1993), although a number of our colleagues are comfortable with having parents remain with their child during the study, and it is difficult for us to imagine that any physician would prohibit a parent from being present during a pediatric EMG. In the same study, an even more profound lack of parental presence during EMG in older children was reported; only 30% were in attendance with school-aged children, and just 14% were in attendance with adolescents (Hays et al., 1993). In our practice, all parents are asked to accompany their children. Good rapport with the parents, permitting them to interact with their child while providing the child with a secure environment, helps the electromyographer obtain a better-than-adequate examination. Having a parent sit on the edge of the examining table or comfortably in a lounge chair while holding an infant reassures the child and often enables the electromyographer to complete the examination. When the parents recognize that the physician performing the study shares their concern for the well-being of their child, they are almost always very cooperative. On occasion, the demonstration of a sensory NCS on the parent may relieve a child's or a parent's anxieties. Older children are encouraged to participate in the process. Initially, we perform sensory NCSs, because these studies generally require a very mild stimulus shock. This often helps the child to become comfortable with the electromyographer. It is then easier to proceed to motor conduction studies, for which we have the child observe "the mountains" build up on the electromyographic screen. Last, many children can get through the needle portion of the examination by listening to the loudspeaker and concomitantly offering opinions as to what the sounds they make can be likened to. At times, their responses are quite humorous: "out of the mouths of babes!"

Toddlers and preschoolers obviously do not appreciate the purpose for which they are being evaluated. Often, one can study the young child without sedation by having the parent hold the child on his or her lap. At times, an assistant, such as a fellow, resident, or nurse, is extremely helpful if the infant's extremities must occasionally be restrained, However, we do not proceed past this stage; we do not use multiple restraints. If necessary, we reschedule the EMG and perform the study with the child under general anesthesia with nitrous oxide and propofol (Diprivan; Stuart Pharmaceuticals, Wilmington, DE). Infants younger than 1 year usually do not require anesthesia unless it is necessary to perform repetitive motor nerve stimulation to evaluate a potential neuromuscular transmission defect or unless the infant is pathologically irritable, such as may occur in a child with Krabbe's disease, although due to DNA testing, we do not often see this type of child.

Our anesthesiologists premedicate the child with midazolam (Versed; Roche Laboratories, Nutley, NJ), followed by induction with nitrous oxide and anesthesia maintenance with propofol. Both agents have a short duration of action and permit the child to be brought out of anesthesia rapidly. Midazolam is rapidly reversed with the benzodiazepine antagonist flumazenil. One is able to successfully evaluate insertional rest activity soon after the child falls asleep and to complete the MUP evaluation at the end of the study, when the child is more aroused. Anesthesia is also valuable for the evaluation of neuromuscular transmission defects by performing repetitive motor nerve stimulation at rapid and uncomfortable rates of 10 to 50 Hz. Stimulation of this intensity is often not well tolerated by the unsedated younger child, who is too young to understand the purpose of the study. Our physicians follow the American Academy of Pediatrics guidelines for monitoring infants and children after sedation (Committee on Drugs, 1992). The recently sedated child must not be permitted to walk alone because he or she could fall, resulting in serious injury, and the child must not leave the nurse's supervision until he or she has satisfactorily recovered from the sedation.

The tiny extremities of the newborn present logistical challenges that make it technically difficult to perform NCSs and EMG as outlined in detail by Jones and colleagues (1996). The peripheral nerves are relatively close to the surface in most children. It is important to keep the infant warm. With newborns, the EMG is now almost always performed in the neonatal intensive care unit and usually under infrared lamps. In general, NCSs require relatively minimal to modest stimuli compared with the degree required for the average adult study.

Although the needle EMG portion of the study is usually not as well tolerated as NCSs, on most occasions we are able to obtain an adequate examination without sedation. Older children, with whom you can gain good rapport, need to have a reasonable discussion on what to expect. Their concerns need to be assuaged about the anticipated discomfort before insertion of the first electrode. We attempt not to mention the word "needle" but simply state that we are putting tiny wire microphones or electrodes into the muscle. The feeling of discomfort is likened to that of a mosquito bite or a pinch. It is important to avoid having the child see any blood whenever possible by being certain hemostasis is achieved before moving on to the next site.

Overall, the pediatric electromyographer formu-

lates the study similar to that of an adult. With processes that are diffuse, such as generalized peripheral neuropathies or myopathies, but predominantly affect the legs, we often examine one leg, and if the results are normal, we do not find value in the examination of the other extremities. However, when there is the possibility of multifocal or diffuse lesions, which occurs with Guillain-Barré syndrome, or of a potentially serious diagnosis such as spinal muscular atrophy, we usually examine one or two other extremities to demonstrate a diffuse or multifocal process. When the clinical issue involves a mononeuropathy versus a plexus level lesion in a single extremity, several motor and sensory nerves and multiple muscles have to be examined. At least 50% of the children seen in this setting at the Children's Hospital Boston have a traumatic etiology, so only a single extremity needs to be evaluated. However, when specific abnormalities are demonstrated without evidence of a traumatic cause, the similarly affected homologous area in the contralateral extremity is examined for comparison to look for concomitant "asymptomatic" similar lesions.

EVOLUTIONARY MATURATIONAL CHANGES AFFECT THE RESULTS OF PEDIATRIC NERVE CONDUCTION STUDIES

Electromyographers who evaluate infants and children must become familiar with an evolving neurophysiological database related to the maturation of peripheral nerves and muscle (Harmon et al., 1992; Jones et al., 1996). The evaluation of an infant or a toddler relies on knowledge of the normal reference scale for changes that occur during the first 3 to 5 years of life. These must be appreciated to appropriately interpret the results of a pediatric EMG. Myelination of peripheral nerves begins during the fourth gestational month (Gamble and Breathnach, 1965). A direct relationship exists between the axonal diameter and the eventual thickness of the myelin sheath. Conduction velocity increases in proportion to the diameter of the nerve fibers, with the ratio being about 6:1 (Carpenter and Bergland, 1957). In the anterior cervical nerve roots of newborns and infants, the fiber reaches its maximum diameter—200% of the initial values at 2 to 5 years (Cottrell, 1940; Thomas and Lambert, 1960). No unusual acceleration of myelination occurs just after birth (Thomas and Lambert, 1960). The nodes of Ranvier are remodeled, with internodal distances obtaining a peak number at the age of 5 years (Gutrecht and Dyck, 1970). Nerve conduction evaluations in premature infants indicate that the maturation of peripheral nerves is primarily related to age from conception rather than to age from birth (Dubowitz et al., 1968). Changes in nerve conduction velocity (NCV) may permit an estimation of fetal development and a distinction between infants with small birth weight and those with low gestational age (Bhatia et al., 1991; Bhatia and Prakash, 1993).

EFFECTS OF FETAL NUTRITION AND MATERNAL DRUG ABUSE

Fetal nutrition is an important factor that influences peripheral nerve myelination. Infants who have been malnourished in utero will have NCSs that reflect these adverse effects (Robinson and Robertson, 1981).

In contrast, in a study of 25 infants born to drug-dependent mothers, leading to infantile passive drug addiction and subsequent neonatal abstinence syndrome, normal motor conduction velocities (MCVs) were demonstrated in all (Doberczak et al., 1986). The EMG was normal in 21 of 23 infants; 2 infants had signs of minimal partial denervation. Six infants were in the 10th percentile size for gestational age but had normal NCVs that were consistent with infants of equal gestational age (Cruz Martinez et al., 1983).

NORMAL PEDIATRIC NERVE CONDUCTION AND ELECTROMYOGRAPHIC PARAMETERS

A relatively small number of studies have been published that define the normal range of nerve conduction values for both motor and sensory nerve conduction parameters as well as for needle EMG. The infant and toddler demonstrate the greatest degree of maturation during the first 3 years of life. Unfortunately, because these data apply to an invasive and uncomfortable procedure, the various studies have had relatively few subjects with less than ideal controls vis-à-vis what one can obtain in a mature adult. Some generalizations are available. Nerve conduction parameters for a neonate are about one half those of a 3-year-old child, whose values are close to those of a fully mature adult. Certainly, by the age of 5 years, there are no significant differences in values compared with those of an adolescent or adult. Similar to those with needle EMG, the neonate's MUPs are smaller in both amplitude and duration and actually are easily compared with those that one normally typifies as "myopathic" in the older child. The subsequent paragraphs in this section expand somewhat on these general concepts.

MOTOR NERVE CONDUCTION PARAMETERS

Maturation of myelinated nerve fibers is equivalent whether the child is delivered at term or born prematurely but otherwise healthy (Wagner and Buchthal, 1972). NCV findings in premature infants of 23 to 27 weeks' gestation generally have values between 8 to 15 m per second for median motor fibers (Cruz Martinez et al., 1983). Gestational age is the important factor in determining the level for normal values. Infants of similar age but different weights had similar NCV results. Birth weight per se did not affect the results. Nerve conduction parameters are approximately half those of adult values and average 27 m per second for motor conduction velocity at birth, approaching 36 m per second at 6 months. Full-term newborns have equivalent motor conduction velocities (i.e., 20 to 30 m per second) in the upper and lower extremities. This contrasts with older children and adults, in whom the NCVs for motor nerves in the arm are 7 to 10 m per second faster than the legs. Compound muscle action potentials (CMAPs) triple in size for the upper extremity and double in amplitude for the lower extremity as the child matures (Thomas and Lambert, 1960; Wagner and Buchthal, 1972). Nerve conduction parameters equivalent to adult values are reached by age 3 to 5 years (Baer and Johnson, 1965; Cruz Martinez et al., 1978). (See the tables in Section XXXI.)

SENSORY CONDUCTION

It is possible to routinely obtain sensory nerve action potentials (SNAPS) in normal newborns; maturational changes are similar to those of motor fibers. In the full-term infant, sensory NCV is 50% that of the adult; it gradually increases to the adult sensory NCV value by age 4 years. In the child aged 2 to 4 months, the sensory NCV has reached 50%, and by 12 months, the sensory NCV is 75% of adult values (Cruz Martinez et al., 1978; Hays et al., 1993). The values for mixed NCS and pure sensory conduction are similar. SNAP amplitudes in the newborn are slightly below those in the adult for the median and ulnar nerves. These amplitudes attain adult values by age 6 to 12 months and surpass them by age 1 to 6 years (Cruz Martinez et al., 1978). With proximal sensory nerve stimulation, two distinct peaks may be recorded in an infant's SNAP. This bifid response may first appear at age 3 months (Jablecki, 1986) and persist until age 4 to 6 years (Oh, 1984). These findings are attributed to maturational differences in two groups of sensory fibers (Cruz Martinez et al., 1983). The evaluation of SNAPs is very important in floppy infants to differentiate spinal muscular apathy from a rare congenital neuropathy. (See the tables in Section XXXI.)

LONG LATENCY WAVES: H REFLEXES AND F WAVES

In contrast to adults, infants normally have an ulnar nerve H reflex. The ulnar conduction velocity for H reflex afferent fibers in newborns is 10% faster than that for motor fibers (Thomas and Lambert, 1960). The presence of the H reflex in the upper extremities represents the lack of central nervous system myelination in the newborn and young infant. An H reflex was present with ulnar nerve stimulation in 34 of 39 full-term infants (Thomas and Lambert, 1960). This response disappeared by age 1 year. H reflexes may also be defined in median (Cruz Martinez et al., 1977) and tibial (Mayer and Mosser, 1969; Bryant and Eng, 1991) nerves in similar-age children, including premature (Cruz Martinez et al., 1977) and full-term (Doberczak et al., 1986) infants. With the opposing influences of progressive axonal myelination and increasing limb length, H-reflex and F-wave latencies initially decrease and later increase with age when recorded from the triceps surae (Cruz Martinez et al., 1977) and the abductor pollicis brevis (Parano et al., 1993) muscles, respectively. The latency of the H reflex, recorded from the intrinsic muscles of the hand, correlates with the child's body length until age 1 year (Jablecki, 1986).

In newborns, F waves can be recorded from most limb nerves. Median nerve F-wave values are 16 ± 1.5 ms for infants younger than 3 months and 14.4 ± 1.6 ms for older infants (Shahani and Young, 1981; Kwast et al., 1984; Parano et al., 1993). Peroneal F-wave latencies range from 20 to 25 m per second for infants 0 to 12 months old (Parano et al., 1993).

NEUROMUSCULAR TRANSMISSION

The neuromuscular junction is not fully mature at birth. Furthermore, the basis of normal values in the adult depends on a cooperative patient who is able to voluntarily exercise muscle for 10 to 60 seconds, allowing for the assessment of post-tetanic facilitation or exhaustion. Only a few attempts have been made to establish the range of normal neonatal neuromuscular junction function and physiology. One study of 17 newborns included 6 premature infants of gestational ages 34 and 42 weeks (Koenigsberger et al., 1973). The methodology that was used differed from that typically applied to adults. A continuous stimulation of 1 to 50 Hz was performed for 15 seconds in these infants. The discomfort of this procedure precludes this methodology from being applied to a cooperative, alert adult for longer than 0.3 to 1.0 second. The only way to ethically recapitulate this method would be to perform it with the aid of anesthesia. That, of course, cannot be justified today in a healthy baby.

In normal newborns, no change in CMAP amplitude was observed at a rate of 1 to 2 Hz (Koenigsberger et al., 1973). However, at 5 to 10 Hz, five of the eight infants demonstrated a 10% or more facilitation. The first signs of a decremental response were found at repetitive motor nerve stimulation rates of 20 Hz. These averaged 24% in 12 of 17 normal newborn infants. The degree of decrement was greatest in the most premature infants studied, those born at 34 weeks' gestation (Koenigs-

berger et al., 1973). The normal newborn's neuromuscular junction was very sensitive to 50-Hz stimulation. All 17 infants had an average decrement of 51% at this rapid stimulation rate. Confirmatory studies have not been conducted because it is difficult to study normal newborns with this uncomfortable procedure. Therefore, the rapid and most uncomfortable forms of repetitive stimulation are not as helpful in evaluating postsynaptic infantile neuromuscular transmission defect because of the poor safety factor present in the immature neuromuscular junction. In a study of infantile botulism, infantile neuromuscular transmission function was evaluated by more standard techniques. Decremental changes of greater than 10% at the rates of 2 to 5 Hz are considered to be abnormal, as are facilitative increases of more than 23% with 20 to 50 Hz (Cornblath, 1986).

The electrodiagnostic evaluation of neuromuscular transmission defects in infancy and early childhood can be difficult for the electromyographer who is inexperienced or unfamiliar with pediatric EMG. There are no well-defined, repetitive motor nerve stimulation norms for the immature neuromuscular junction of the newborn. Also, the multiple technical difficulties encountered during the performance of pediatric electromyographic studies, the maturational changes in the size of MUPs and the parameters of nerve conduction studies, and even the plethora of pitfalls in the interpretation of electromyographic data in infancy may on occasion lead to inconclusive results or erroneous electromyographic clinical correlations. Despite these variables, if a pediatric EMG is designed, performed, and interpreted carefully, the electromyographic study of a floppy infant can offer valuable differential diagnostic information and/or help the clinician determine the need for a muscle biopsy or DNA analysis or both.

INFANTILE NERVE CONDUCTION STUDIES

Measurements

When NCSs are performed, the pediatric electromyographer has to be fastidious in obtaining accurate measurements because of an infant's inherently small size. In the first year of life, the average distance available for performing conduction velocities over a specific nerve is no more than 8 to 10 cm. If the electromyographer is not fastidious recording the precise distances, minor errors in measurement may lead to major changes in results. For example, if just a 1-cm error is made, the calculation of a conduction velocity will have at least a 12% error.

Stimulating Electrodes

The electrodes used in our laboratory are similar in type to those traditionally found in adult EMG laboratories. When evaluating infants and toddlers, it is best to use stimulating cathode-anode electrodes with an interelectrode distance of 1.5 to 2.0 cm. Some manufacturers of electromyographic equipment provide an adaptor that allows for shorter distances between the cathode-anode, especially for use in pediatric EMG laboratories. These are particularly useful when studying infants and toddlers. We find it both useful and important to initially study sensory function in each child. Traditional spring electrodes are very effective for median nerve orthodromic stimulation from the third finger, which provides the best opportunity for a reasonable interelectrode distance. Sensory conduction studies require just a few milliamps of current to define a reproducible SNAP in most children with intact sensory function. The newer styled self-adhesive electrodes may be sized individually with scissors. These are primarily used as stimulating sources for orthodromic studies by attaching alligator clips from wires connected to the primary stimulator. In contrast, if one uses antidromic techniques, these adhesive electrodes serve equally well as recording electrodes.

Recording Electrodes

The standard adult-size surface electrodes are usually effective. With premature infants and neonates, we also use a set of similar but somewhat smaller surface electrodes.

Sensory Nerve Conduction

The low degree of discomfort experienced by the child during the recording of SNAPs leads us to usually begin our pediatric electromyographic examination with sensory conduction studies. A relatively minimal stimulus is required; this provides a well-tolerated introduction to the electromyographic procedure for the child. When studying the older child, sometimes we print a copy of the initial response and give it to the child. This seems to break the ice and provides better rapport between the examining physician and the patient. Sensory NCSs are obtained by either orthodromic or antidromic techniques. Technical problems may occur while performing sensory NCSs. The relatively short fingers of the infant do not offer much latitude for the traditional 2- to 3-cm difference between G1 and G2. The third digit is the longest and is the one best suited to study median antidromic or orthodromic SNAPS. Some authors, such as Charles F. Bolton, find the antidromic median stimulation better tolerated (Jones et al., 1996). Antidromic ulnar and musculocutaneous SNAPs may also be studied with relative ease in the infant.

Performing orthodromic medial plantar nerve stimulation facilitates the evaluation of lower extremity sensory function in neonates and infants. This technique was suggested by a colleague, Nancy Kuntz of the Mayo Clinic, and is performed similar to that typically used in adults. Although a sural SNAP can normally be defined in older children, we often have difficulty defining this in newborns and young infants. We have not found many clinical instances in which knowledge of a sural compound SNAP instead of a medial plantar and/or a median SNAP has proved to be helpful in the differential diagnosis of infants.

In children, with the exception of some very rare childhood entrapment neuropathies, the presence of a normal SNAP provides sufficient evidence to exclude any lesion between the dorsal root ganglion and the distal sensory nerve ending. However, considerable normal variation exists in SNAP amplitudes; therefore, a "normal" value may not be representative of a healthy nerve for that individual.

Motor Nerve Conduction

Motor NCSs are performed in the newborn, but the placement of electrodes is sometimes more difficult. The inherently small hand size and the tendency of the infants to sweat more in the hand add to the technical challenge. However, lower extremity studies are not as much of a problem, particularly when recording from the intrinsic foot muscles. As in adults, the G1 pickup electrode is placed on the thenar eminence when median NCS are performed and over the hypothenar eminence for the ulnar nerve. However, the small size of the hand does not permit adequate interelectrode distance if the G2 reference electrode is placed as it is with the adult. We successfully use a new adhesive electrode placed proximally on the third digit as our G2 reference for the median CMAP or the fifth finger for the ulnar CMAP. Until we adapted this method, the G2 electrode was sometimes difficult to secure on the unrelaxed and often sweaty and fisted hand of an infant.

Equally important to a technically careful study is the ability to get the child to participate in the study. The time the electromyographer takes to encourage the child to be interested in the procedure is often well spent. At the Children's Hospital Boston, we often ask the cooperative child to observe the CMAPs as they build up and to tell us what they look like—for example, like a mountain or a pyramid. Commonly, we ask the child to see how big a "mountain" he or she can make. On other occasions, we can gain their interest by having them observe the twitching of their thumb or toes. Frequently, this gets a giggle, and, more important, good rapport is established, taking the child's attention directly away from the stimulus.

Neuromuscular Transmission

Testing for defects in neuromuscular transmission in the neonate and in the younger child (up to age

6 years) is challenged by one important difference in this age group in comparison with the older child. Infants and younger children are unable to voluntarily exercise. Electromyographers are therefore unable to use traditional techniques applied to the evaluation of possible presynaptic or postsynaptic defects. In contrast to older children and adults, in whom it is rarely necessary to use 20- to 50-Hz repetitive motor nerve stimulation, such stimulation is sometimes vitally important in an infant who has been referred with some uncommon clinical diagnoses. These diagnoses include infantile botulism (Cornblath, 1986) or other rare forms of presynaptic and postsynaptic defects seen in neonates and older children, as outlined in Chapters 93 and 94. When repetitive motor nerve stimulation is performed, it is best to immobilize the infant's arm with a pediatric arm board. Although repetitive motor nerve stimulation is sometimes well tolerated without adequate sedation, this stimulation technique may sometimes upset the child, and a technically adequate study may be impossible, necessitating a repeat evaluation later. In this setting, it is wise to go directly to general anesthesia, with the assistance of a pediatric anesthesiologist. Body surface temperature must be monitored with a thermistor while performing the study in a warm room with a blanket. With cooling, a neuromuscular transmission defect may not be identified. Therefore, it is recommended that the surface temperature be maintained above 35°C.

Because of the relatively short length of the extremities, stimuli may be delivered proximally or distally, although the latter is preferred. In general, a distance of at least 4 cm is maintained between the stimulating and recording electrodes. Some rare forms of congenital myasthenia are recognized by the characteristic evidence of a series of two or more repetitive responses to a single stimulus, as later defined in Chapter 93. The presence of these characteristic CMAPs provides another indication for proceeding with repetitive stimulation under anesthesia in the infant and younger child. In children, supramaximal stimulation is often achieved at levels that are considerably lower than those necessary in adolescents or adults. Stimulation begins with 0.5 Hz and is increased to 2 Hz. Stimulation rates of 20 to 50 Hz are used for brief trains of 1 to 5 seconds' duration in attempts to identify the presence of either postexercise facilitation or decrement.

Single-fiber EMG and the assessment of variability in amplitude of repetitively firing MUPs in adults depend on patient cooperation. These traditional techniques cannot be used adequately until children are at least age 8 to 12 years; however, stimulated single-fiber EMG has proved to be particularly useful in the evaluation of infantile botulism (Chaudhry and Crawford, 1999).

The study of facial nerve latencies in neonates demonstrated an average direct facial latency of 3.30 ± 0.44 ms (Clay and Ramseyer, 1976). The blink reflex was elicited with traditional stimulation of the supraorbital nerve. R1 and R2 components have latencies similar to adult values: R1 = 12.10 ± 0.96 ms and R2 = 35.85 ± 2.45 ms (Kimura et al., 1977). Facial nerve stimulation may be of value for the occasional child with a newborn facial palsy. We have not found much clinical use for the blink reflex in neonates and young children, particularly with the availability of magnetic resonance imaging to provide anatomic definition when there is a clinical question of a brainstem lesion. Rarely, in a instance of a patient with Guillain-Barré syndrome in whom no CMAPs are elicited, a maintained facial CMAP may be found with significant prolongation in some components of the blink reflex. Chapter 88 includes some other clinical situations in which the blink reflex may be useful.

Phrenic Nerve Stimulation

The phrenic nerve is readily stimulated at the posterior margin of the sternocleidomastoid muscle and is valuable in the study of children in the intensive care unit. Needle EMG of the diaphragm provides important additional information (Bolton, 1996). These studies are being requested more frequently. For a further discussion of the approach in the intensive care unit, see Chapter 81.

NEEDLE ELECTROMYOGRAPHY

Basic Introduction to Pediatric Needle Electromyography

Although there has been ongoing interest in the development of a noninvasive method to define the nature of the electrical signal generated by muscle cells, volume conductor effects limit the interpretation of the derived signals. A technology of this type that solves this problem will be very welcome for the electromyographic evaluation of children, especially relative to the discomfort generated by traditional electromyographic techniques. To successfully use surface techniques, a methodology needs to be developed that preserves the diagnostic specificity and sensitivity of traditional needle EMG. A study reports the use of a 16-channel surface electrode array that was able to demonstrate a statistically significant difference between the MUPs of normal control subjects and patients with motoneuron disease (Wood et al., 2001). This technique may eventually have a clinical potential, particularly for motor neuronopathies. However, just as the electromyographic differentiation is difficult between normal and infantile myopathic MUPs, the technology to accurately make this discrimination with surface EMG may be an even greater challenge before a clinically applicable means is available. Early in our pediatric careers, we anticipated that new technologies were imminent and that the use of needle

EMG in children might soon become a historical footnote. However, now, more than two decades later, we continue to use traditional concentric needle electrodes. Further, although surface techniques may become accurate in the identification of infants with spinal muscular atrophies, more accurate DNA testing is widely available to make this diagnosis. Thus, we are evaluating many fewer floppy babies who later prove to have a spinal muscular atrophy (Darras and Jones, 2000).

Maturational and Technical Factors

Voluntarily activated muscles are relatively easy to study in older children, as in adults, once one gains the child's interest and participation. In contrast, needle EMG of infants and toddlers is a much greater challenge. The pediatric electromyographer often needs to depend on eliciting reflex muscle contractions, such as stroking the plantar surface of the foot, to activate the tibialis anterior and/or the iliopsoas muscles. Considerable experience and patience are required to analyze MUPs properly in this setting. Individual MUPs are typically characterized by their amplitude, duration, number of phases, and firing rate. MUP recording characteristics are influenced by the electrical conducting properties of the intervening tissues (Daube, 1978). In children, MUPs typically have a triphasic configuration and a recruitment frequency that varies from 5 to 15 Hz (Sacco et al., 1962). MUPs are often just biphasic in normal infants, with an average duration of 1 to 4 ms and an amplitude of less than 100 μV (do Carmo, 1960). Normal MUP duration and amplitude values from birth to adulthood are established in 2- to 3-year intervals (Feinstein et al., 1955). At any age, 10% to 15% of MUPs in a normal muscle are beyond the normal range. Slight contraction of the muscle initially activates type I muscle fibers. Larger MUPs are recruited when initial MUPs fire between 5 and 10 Hz.

When individual motoneurons are lost, this is characterized by a reduced recruitment of MUPs. This occurs most commonly in an infant with spinal muscular atrophy or a child who had prior poliomyelitis. In these clinical settings, there is a very rapid recruitment of large individual MUPs at rates of 15 to 30 Hz before additional MUPs are recruited (Daube, 1978). The concomitant collateral reinnervation, widening the territorial distribution of an individual anterior horn cell, classically leads to an increase in both amplitude and duration of these neurogenic MUPs.

Myopathies, in contrast, typically lead to a partial loss of individual muscle fibers within each motor unit, so the surviving portion of the individual MUP is diminished in size. Consequently, large numbers of short-duration, low-amplitude MUPs need to be activated during minimal voluntary muscle contraction in children with a myopathy. Because normal infants typically have relatively small, low-amplitude, short-duration MUPs, it is often difficult to distinguish normal immature infantile MUPs from those of the infant with a subtle myopathy. This characteristic limits the ability of the pediatric electromyographer to differentiate more than the most profound myopathies from the "immature" MUPs of the normal infant. We teach our fellows and residents that they always need to add the caveat to their clinical correlation in the report that a normal EMG does not exclude a myopathic process. Not only is it often difficult to distinguish the small MUPs of a normal infant from a myopathic process, but also certain congenital myopathies do not necessarily lead to muscle fiber destruction, and thus their MUPs may have a relatively normal size.

When we do not use anesthesia, the child's cooperation is best gained by having the youngster feel a sense of participation in the procedure itself. Most children older than 5 years and some relatively mature children aged 3 to 5 years often participate relatively easily in the study. During the procedure, we avoid using the term *needle* and instead explain to the child that we are putting a wire into the muscle that will serve as a little microphone. Of course, we tell them that to get through the skin, the insertion will pinch like a mosquito bite. If the child accepts this, we can have fun with many of them by asking what the motor units sound like. This is often a rewarding maneuver because most children frequently become interested in the noises they produce. Responses we hear include thunder, rain on the roof, motorcycles, or even the putt-putt of a lobster boat. Commenting on the noise produced, we ask the child how she or he is able to sleep at night with all the noise their muscles can make. This often produces a laugh or at least distracts the child's attention from the electrode. In contrast, children who are younger than 3 or 4 years usually cannot be reasoned with in this fashion. It is often heartwarming to see how one is able to develop a very significant rapport with the cooperative child and to achieve a clinically successful study. A careful and accurate examination is usually feasible if the electromyographer appreciates the limits of her or his technical abilities, especially with infants and toddlers.

Sedation

Needle EMG naturally creates anxiety in children as well as in their parents and sometimes even in the less experienced pediatric electromyographer. We strive to reassure the child and his or her parents that we are making this study both practical to the clinical question and friendly to the child. Although EMG is an uncomfortable examination, we are continuously impressed with the staying power of children with whom one can communicate. In the setting in which the child's anxieties do not permit a reasonable examination, it is much better to reschedule the study under anesthesia. Because of the basically uncomfortable nature of an EMG, colleagues have varying approaches to the use of anesthesia for children. We routinely use this form of sedation in at least three instances: (1) repetitive motor nerve stimulation testing of infants and young children, (2) toddlers who require extensive testing, and (3) mentally compromised children who are unable to understand the purposes and nature of electromyographic testing. There is a varying philosophy and approach to the use of sedation, including anesthesia, for pediatric EMG in other major pediatric hospitals.

At some centers, anesthesia is routinely used for all pediatric procedures that are inherently uncomfortable. The very rare but definite chance of a serious complication is an issue that continues to concern us with reference to the routine use of anesthesia. However, the anesthesiologists at the Children's Hospital Boston continue to reassure us of the relatively benign nature of pediatric general anesthesia under the supervision of an anesthesiologist in an operating suite environment. In addition, when EMG is performed with the patient under anesthesia in a pediatric hospital rather than in a nonhospital setting, the major cause of an adverse response to sedation in children is eliminated. Other important steps to take to avoid an untoward response to pediatric sedation include (1) adequate physiological monitoring with a rapid response to any sign of unacceptable results of pulse oximetry, (2) careful presedation medical evaluation, (3) the presence of an independent observer, (4) avoidance of medication errors, and (5) adequate recovery procedures (Jones et al., 1996). Because we and our anesthesia colleagues are ever mindful of these precautions, this knowledge is leading us to increase the indications to proceed with anesthesia in the performance of pediatric EMG. The American Academy of Pediatrics has established specific guidelines for sedation during diagnostic and therapeutic procedures (Committee on Drugs, 1992).

Early in our experience at the Children's Hospital Boston, we primarily used either chloral hydrate or meperidine/promethazine/chlorpromazine compound (Demerol/Phenergan/Thorazine [DPT]) to provide sedation, especially for the younger child. However, these sedatives were not universally successful. In fact, at times we experienced paradoxical hyperactivity with chloral hydrate. It was counterproductive from the outset to personally administer these medications while establishing an initially adversarial relationship with the child. More important, as we became increasingly concerned about the very unlikely, albeit definite, possibility of an untoward medication reaction, we discontinued the use of either of these premedication agents. This occurred in the late 1980s, when we switched to anesthesia in the surgery day care center when necessary. The great skill and cooperation of our anesthesia colleagues at Children's Hospital Boston made this important transition very easy for us.

Motor Unit Characteristics in Infants and Children

MUP parameters differ in the normal infant and young child compared with those in the older child, adolescent, or adult. Neonates and young infants have normal MUP amplitudes that typically vary between 100 and 700 μV. Healthy newborns and infants up to 3 years old generally do not have MUPs with amplitudes of greater than 1,000 μV. The normal MUP histogram amplitude is shifted to the lower side of adult MUP values (Feinstein et al., 1995; do Carmo, 1960). Characteristically infantile MUPs are typically short in duration; many are biphasic or triphasic. In most infants, the recruitment pattern of MUPs is disordered and chaotic. Occasionally, these reach values more typical of those in adults. Therefore, one has to be very careful in formulating a conclusion that an infant's or a young child's MUPs are abnormally small. In particular, with the tendency for normal MUPs to be of shorter duration and lower amplitude than those in older children, one has to be very cautious in reaching a conclusion that an infant has a myopathy. Perhaps the best clue to the presence of a myopathic process is the very full recruitment of these small MUPs with seemingly very early effort. Normally, MUPs achieve "adult" configurations by age 3 to 5 years.

Insertion Activity

Abnormalities on needle insertion are sometimes difficult to define in very young children. In comparison with adults, muscle end-plate zones have a relatively disproportionately large area of muscle distribution in young children, particularly in neonates (Jones et al., 1987). End-plate potentials, characterized by an initial negativity, must not be confused with fibrillation potentials that are typified by an initial positivity. This factor may cause confusion for the inexperienced pediatric electromyographer, making it seem that some normal muscles have abnormal insertion activity when, indeed, the activity present represents a normal physiological variation secondary to the neonate's relatively greater size of end-plates in comparison with total muscle volume. Furthermore, because infantile MUPs are smaller than those of adults, fibrillation potentials have even smaller dimensions. It is also possible, because of the inability to obtain full relaxation in many infants, that some fibrillation potentials may be masked by minimal MUP activation. When the infant is upset and vigorous crying occurs, this sound also may obscure the characteristic "tick" of subtle abnormal insertion activity, such as fibrillation potentials. This is less problematic with neurogenic processes, in which it is not possible to recruit large numbers of motor units. The most severely affected floppy infants often have weak cries, making this less of a problem.

Order of Examination

One must maintain a flexible attitude in the approach to pediatric needle EMG, particularly with the nonsedated infant. In the adult, an orderly approach is often recommended, such as first examining insertion activity, followed by single motor units and, last, recruitment patterns. In contrast, we prefer to examine MUPs initially to be certain the electrode is most precisely placed. This applies to both children and adults. The pediatric electromyographer needs to be continually prepared to examine the insertion activity whenever the child is relaxed and quiet rather than trying to routinely search for insertion activity at the beginning of the examination. MUPs are most easily evaluated when the infant is spontaneously moving; the precise order of the evaluation is not pertinent. Last, we do not find that other forms of reflex stimuli, such as the Moro reflex or the various stepping postures, add any value to the needle evaluation; these maneuvers make the study more cumbersome.

Newborn Needle Electromyography

The neonate provides special challenges, as detailed in Chapter 86. Pediatric electromyographers recognize that certain muscles do not activate spontaneously, such as the vastus lateralis or triceps brachii; therefore, these provide an opportunity to evaluate insertion activity, particularly during the evaluation of a generalized process that affects the motor unit (Jones, 1990; Jones et al., 1996). Muscles such as the tibialis anterior, iliopsoas, and biceps brachii are easily activated but in general preclude any opportunity to study insertion activity. The one exception to this is the infant with severe spinal muscular atrophy, in whom there are very few MUPs and the fibrillation potentials stand out easily, even though there is concomitant motor unit activity. This approach has been particularly well suited to the generalized diseases present in many newborns and young infants who present with the floppy infant syndrome (Jones, 1990; see also Chapter 86). In contrast, the evaluation of an infant who has a mononeuropathy or plexus lesion requires the study of both insertion activity and MUPs in each of the multiple muscles in the same extremity. To accomplish this, the electromyographer must be both patient and diligent.

Limits of Needle Electromyographic Study

Occasionally, the anxious and unhappy child cannot be reasonably encouraged to cooperate with the examiner. In this circumstance, it is best to discontinue the present study, with a plan to reschedule the child under sedation at a later date. It is *always*

essential for the pediatric electromyographer to be the child's ombudsman in this circumstance, because unfortunately some parents are immature and inappropriately angered when their child refuses to cooperate. In addition, certain cultures demand absolute child obedience, and the electromyographer must be very diplomatic when deciding to move on to anesthesia at a subsequent date. Again, the pediatric electromyographer must take care to advise the parents that this next step in their child's evaluation is logical and not because the child was in any way uncooperative. Last, but very important, when an electromyographer is not accustomed to evaluating children, difficulty in performance of the study often provides a good indication to refer the patient to a children's hospital with personnel who are familiar with the performance of electromyographic examinations in the pediatric age group.

Single-Fiber Electromyography

In general, this procedure is difficult to use in younger children. Occasionally, it is useful in the evaluation of subtle questions of a neuromuscular transmission defect in the school-aged child (Chaudhry and Crawford, 1999). However, the technique of stimulated single-fiber EMG has proved to be very helpful in defining the presence of neuromuscular transmission defects in young infants. The best illustration of this comes from the Johns Hopkins University group, for whom this technique proved to be very useful in the diagnosis of infantile botulism (Chaudhry and Crawford, 1999).

Clinical Correlations in Pediatric Needle Electromyography

Because of the sporadic recruitment of MUPs in infants, the needle electromyographic impression is often based on a gestalt clinical electromyographic overview. Spinal muscular atrophy type I in particular lends itself to this type of needle electromyographic analysis. In this instance, there is a typical neurogenic dropout observed in the number of MUPs firing, with reduced recruitment and relatively large MUP size. This contrasts with myopathic processes, where the MUPs approximate the normally small MUPs in neonates or young infants. Because the diagnosis of a diffuse process that affects motoneurons in the floppy infant is usually associated with a poor prognosis, as in the adult, the electromyographer needs to demonstrate the presence of neurogenic MUPs and concomitant fibrillation potentials in at least three extremities. With the relatively common use of DNA testing for the spinal muscular atrophy abnormality at chromosome 5q11-13, electromyographers may limit this study somewhat if the electromyographic findings strongly support the clinical diagnosis and allow one to await the DNA results.

We are aware of at least nine other specific lower

motor unit disorders separate from those involving the anterior horn cell, particularly spinal muscular atrophies and rarely poliomyelitis, wherein fibrillation potentials are identified in the clinical setting of the floppy infant (Jones, 1990). Some of these entities do not have the poor long-term prognosis typical of infantile spinal muscular atrophy I. It is always important to consider this broad differential diagnosis whenever there are well-defined fibrillation potentials present on an infant's or a child's needle EMG. *The MUP size and firing pattern,* associated with the fibrillation potential, *are the important keys to the appropriate electromyographic diagnosis.* An important note of caution is suggested when an arthrogrypotic floppy infant is evaluated. In this instance, if MUPs suggestive of spinal muscular atrophies, often with some degree of fibrillation potential, are identified, one must not make the apparent clinical correlation suggesting that this baby has spinal muscular atrophy. This clinical neurophysiological setting may be representative of a different pathological entity that does not carry a prognosis similar to spinal muscular atrophy I (David et al., 1991). DNA testing is again helpful in this setting.

The amplitude and duration of MUPs in the normal infant are substantially smaller than those in the adult (Jablecki, 1986; Jones et al., 1987). The differentiation between the lower limits of normal and a subtle myopathy is a difficult one in the neonate and young infant. When we studied our experience with floppy infants, we identified neurogenic disorders much more accurately than myopathic ones (David and Jones, 1994). On other occasions, the MUP parameters that were defined were suggestive but not diagnostic of a myopathy or sometimes appeared normal. In this setting, it is important to proceed with muscle biopsy as well whenever there is any possibility of a myopathy either clinically or with EMG. Similarly, one may also need to consider a defect in neuromuscular transmission in this setting, as discussed earlier in this chapter.

Finally, we emphasize that the pediatric electromyographer is not required to always formulate a specific neuromuscular diagnosis. This is, of course, our mission, but if equivocal data are present and do not totally support the clinical question, the electromyographer must make a nonspecific clinical correlation. It is much more important to conclude that the study is nondiagnostic or equivocal than to offer an ill-conceived diagnosis. On occasion, a follow-up examination some months later clarifies the issue when DNA testing, antibody studies, and imaging studies have not led to a specific diagnosis. Despite the uncomfortable nature of an EMG, we have successfully restudied some children, with the blessing of their parents. This is particularly useful when the parents recognize our empathy and concern in identifying a diagnosis for their child's neuromuscular disorder.

References

Baer RD, Johnson EW: Motor nerve conduction velocities in normal children. Arch Phys Med Rehabil 1965;46:698–704.

Bhatia BD, Prakash U, Singh MN, et al: Electrophysiological studies in newborns with reference to gestation and anthropometry. Electromyogr Clin Neurophysiol 1991;31:55–59.

Bhatia BD, Prakash U: Electrophysiological studies in preterm and growth retarded low birth weight babies. Electromyogr Clin Neurophysiol 1993;33:507–510.

Bolton CA: Electromyography in the critical care unit. In Jones HR, Bolton CA, Harper CM (eds): Pediatric Electromyography. Philadelphia/New York, Lippincott-Raven, 1996; 445–466.

Bryant PR, Eng GD: Normal values for the soleus H-reflex in newborn infants 31–45 weeks post conceptual age. Arch Phys Med Rehabil 1991;72:28–30.

Carpenter FG, Bergland RM: Excitation and conduction in immature nerve fibers of the developing chick. Am J Physiol 1957;190:371–376.

Chaudhry V, Crawford TO: Stimulated single-fiber EMG in infantile botulism. Muscle Nerve 1999;22:1698–1703.

Clay SA, Ramseyer JC: The orbicularis oculi reflex in infancy and childhood. Neurology 1976;26:521–524.

Committee on Drugs: Guidelines for monitoring and management of pediatric patients during and after sedation for diagnostic and therapeutic procedures. Pediatrics 1992;89:1110–1115.

Cornblath DR: Disorders of neuromuscular transmission in infants and children. Muscle Nerve 1986;9:606–611.

Cottrell L: Histologic variations with age in apparently normal peripheral nerve trunks. Arch Neurol 1940;43:1138–1150.

Cruz Martinez A, Ferrer MT, Martin MJ: Motor conduction velocity and H-reflex in prematures with very short gestational age. Electromyogr Clin Neurophysiol 1983;23:13–19.

Cruz Martinez A, Ferrer MT, Perez Conde ML, Bernacer M: Motor conduction velocity and H-reflex in infancy and childhood: II. Intra and extra uterine maturation of the nerve fibers: Development of the peripheral nerve from 1 month to 11 years of age. Electromyogr Clin Neurophysiol 1978;18:11–27.

Cruz Martinez A, Perez Conde ML, Ferrer MT: Motor conduction velocity and H-reflex in infancy and childhood: I. Study in newborns, twins, and small for dates. Electromyogr Clin Neurophysiol 1977;17:493–505.

Cruz Martinez A, Perez Conde ML, Ferrer MT: Motor conduction velocity and H-reflex in prematures with very short gestational age. Electromyogr Clin Neurophysiol 1983;23:13–19.

Darras BT, Jones HR: Diagnosis of pediatric neuromuscular disorders in the era of DNA analysis. Pediatr Neurol 2000;23:289–300.

Daube JR: The description of motor unit potentials in electromyography. Neurology 1978;28:623–625.

David WS, Jones HR: Electromyography and biopsy correlation with suggested protocol for evaluation of the floppy infant. Muscle Nerve 1994;17:424–430.

David WS, Kupsky W, Jones HR: EMG evaluation of the arthrogrypotic floppy baby [abstract]. Muscle Nerve 1991;14:897.

do Carmo RJ: Motor unit action potential parameters in human newborn infants. Arch Neurol 1960;3:136–140.

Doberczak TM, Kandall SR, Rongkapan O, et al: Peripheral nerve conduction studies in passively addicted neonates. Arch Phys Med Rehabil 1986;67:4–24.

Dubowitz V, Whittaker GF, Brown BH, Robinson A: Nerve conduction velocity: An index of neurological maturity of the newborn infant. Dev Med Child Neurol 1968;10:741–749.

Feinstein B, Lindegard B, Nyman E, Wolhfart G: Morphologic studies of motor units in normal human muscles. Acta Anat (Basel) 1955;23:127–142.

Gamble HJ, Breathnach AS: An electron-microscope study of human foetal peripheral nerves. J Anat 1965;99:573–584.

Gamstorp I, Shelburne SA Jr: Peripheral sensory conduction in ulnar and median nerves of normal infants, children, and adolescents. Acta Paediatr Scand 1965;54:309–313.

Gamstorp I: Normal conduction velocity of ulnar, median and peroneal nerves in infancy, childhood and adolescence. Acta Paediatr Scand Suppl (Stockh) 1963;146(Suppl):68–76.

Gutrecht JA, Dyck PJ: Quantitative teased-fiber and histologic studies of human sural nerve during postnatal development. J Comp Neurol 1970;138:117–130.

Harmon RL, Eichman PL, Rodriguez AA: Laboratory Manual of Pediatric Electromyography. Madison, WI, Board of Regents, University of Wisconsin, 1992.

Hays RM, Hackworth SR, Speltz ML, Weinstein P: Physicians' practice patterns in pediatric electrodiagnosis. Arch Phys Med Rehabil 1993;74:494–496.

Jablecki CK: Electromyography in infants and children. J Child Neurol 1986;1:297–318.

Jones HR Jr, Miller RG, Turk MA, Wilbourn AJ: The Pediatric EMG Examination: Practical Considerations. Panel Discussion. AAEE Course A. Myopathies, Floppy Infant, and Electrodiagnostic Studies in Children: Tenth Annual Continuing Education Course. Rochester, MN, American Association of Electromyography and Electrodiagnosis, 1987; 39–46.

Jones HR: Electromyographic evaluation of the floppy infant: Differential diagnosis and technical aspects. Muscle Nerve 1990; 13:338–347.

Jones HR, Darras B: Acute care pediatric electromyography. Muscle Nerve Suppl 2000;9:S53–S62.

Jones HR, Harmon RL, Bolton CF, Harper CM: An approach to pediatric electromyography. In Jones HR, Bolton CF, Harper CM (eds): Clinical Pediatric Electromyography. Philadelphia/New York, Lippincott-Raven, 1996; 1–37.

Kimura J, Bodensteiner J, Yamada T: Electrically elicited blink reflex in normal neonates. Arch Neurol 1977;37:246–249.

Koenigsberger MR, Patten B, Lovelace RE: Studies of neuromuscular function in the newborn: 1. A comparison of myoneural function in the full term and premature infant. Neuropediatrics 1973;4:350–361.

Kunkel LM: Analysis of deletions in DNA from patients with Becker and Duchenne muscular dystrophy. Nature 1986;322: 73–77.

Kwast O, Krajewska G, Kozlowski K: Analysis of F-wave parameters in median and ulnar nerves in healthy infants and children: Age-related changes. Electromyogr Clin Neurophysiol 1984;24: 439–456.

Mayer RF, Mosser RS: Excitability of motor neurons in infants. Neurology 1969;19:932–945.

Miller RG, Kuntz NL: Nerve conduction studies in infants and children. J Child Neurol 1986;1:19–26.

Misra UK, Tiwari S, Shukla N, et al: F-response studies in neonates, infants and children. Electromyogr Clin Neurophysiol 1989;29: 251–254.

Oh SJ: Clinical Electromyography: Nerve Conduction Studies. Baltimore, University Park Press, 1984; 115–139.

Parano E, Uncini A, De Vivo DC, Lovelace RE: Electrophysiologic correlates of peripheral nervous system maturation in infancy and childhood. J Child Neurol 1993;8:336–338.

Robinson RO, Robertson WC Jr: Fetal nutrition and peripheral nerve conduction velocity. Neurology 1981;31:327–329.

Sacco G, Buchthal F, Rosenfalck P: Motor unit potentials at different ages. Arch Neurol 1962;6:366–373.

Shahani BT, Young RR: Clinical significance of late response studies in infants and children. Neurology 1981;31:66.

Thomas JE, Lambert EH: Ulnar nerve conduction velocity and H-reflex in infants and children. J Appl Physiol 1960;15:1–9.

Turk MA: Pediatric electrodiagnosis. Phys Med Rehabil 1989;3: 791–808.

Wagner AL, Buchthal F: Motor and sensory conduction in infancy and childhood: Reappraisal. Dev Med Child Neurol 1972;14:189–216.

Wood SH, Jarratt JA, Barker AT, Brown BH: Surface Electromyography using electrode arrays: A study of motor neuron disease. Muscle Nerve 2001;24:223–230.

CHAPTER 86

The Floppy Infant

Kathryn J. Swoboda and H. Royden Jones, Jr.

The floppy infant syndrome is one of the most common reasons for the referral of infants younger than 1 year to a children's hospital electromyography (EMG) laboratory. These infants provide a major challenge for the pediatric electromyographer. In this chapter, we provide a basis for performing a prudent electromyographic analysis of the floppy infant (Fig. 86–1). Approximately 80% of floppy infants have a primary central nervous system etiological mechanism (Dubowitz, 1980). Peripheral motor unit disorders compose the other major diagnostic category for this uncommon clinical syndrome (Table 86–1).

Central and peripheral nervous system abnormalities are not mutually exclusive, as some infants have a neurological disorder that produces lesions at both sites. Examples of these disorders include infantile neuronal degeneration, certain types of congenital muscular dystrophy, and various metabolic disorders, such as mitochondrial disease. Electrophysiological evaluation of these infants is of value for two primary purposes. First, it can often distinguish between central and peripheral causes, and when a lesion of the peripheral motor unit is ascertained, EMG often provides an anatomic localization of the pathological process to the anterior horn cell,

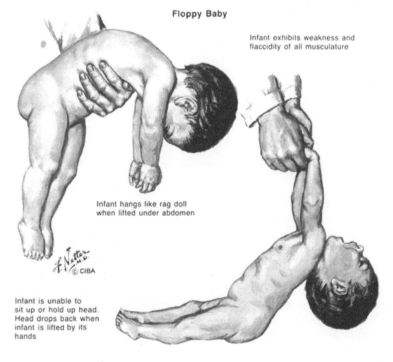

Floppy Baby

Infant exhibits weakness and flaccidity of all musculature

Infant hangs like rag doll when lifted under abdomen

Infant is unable to sit up or hold up head. Head drops back when infant is lifted by its hands

Figure 86–1. Classic means of testing for poor muscle tone in the floppy infant. (From Netter FH: The Ciba Collection of Medical Illustrations. Vol 1, Nervous System. Pt. 2, Neurologic and Neuromuscular Disorders. West Caldwell, NJ, Ciba-Geigy Medical Education, 1986.)

Table 86–1. Floppy Infant Syndrome: Disorders of the Motor Unit

Anterior horn cell
  Spinal muscular atrophy I and II
  Poliomyelitis
  Acid maltase deficiency affecting motor neurons
Polyneuropathies
  Congenital genetic
    Hypomyelinating congenital
    Axonal congenital
    Infantile neuronal degeneration
    Leukodystrophies
      Krabbe's disease
      Niemann-Pick disease
    Leigh's syndrome
    Giant axonal neuropathy
    Dysmaturation neuropathy
  Acquired
    Guillain-Barré syndrome
    Chronic inflammatory demyelinating polyneuropathy
Neuromuscular junction
  Presynaptic
    Acquired
      Infantile botulism
      Toxic
        Hypermagnesemia secondary to treatment of maternal
          eclampsia
        Aminoglycoside antibiotics
    Congenital
      Acetylcholine vesicle paucity
      Decreased quantal release
      Familial infantile myasthenia gravis
  Postsynaptic
    Acquired
      Neonatal myasthenia gravis
    Congenital
      Acetylcholinesterase deficiency
      Classic slow channel syndrome
      Acetylcholine receptor deficiency
Myopathies
  Congenital
    Nemaline rod
    Central core
    Centronuclear
    Congenital fiber type disproportion
  Dystrophies
    Myotonic dystrophy
    Congenital muscular dystrophy
  Metabolic enzymatic myopathies
    Glycogen storage disorders
    Acid maltase (type 2)
    Muscle phosphorylase (type 5)
    Phosphofructokinase (type 7)
    Lipid storage disorders (not certain to occur with floppy
      infant syndrome)
  Inflammatory
    Polymyositis (not well documented)

the peripheral nerve, the neuromuscular junction, or muscle (Jones, 1990). The results may offer therapeutic options, support the diagnosis of a specific genetic condition, or provide prognostic information. With the rapidly expanding role of DNA analysis, this more sophisticated, specific testing method will increasingly supplant the need for EMG in the evaluation of some floppy infants (Darras and Jones, 2000). This trend is evidenced in the evaluation of babies with suspected spinal muscular atrophy (SMA).

Pregnant mothers are aware of normal spontaneous fetal movements. Healthy newborns have purposeless extremity movements that are associated with well-defined muscular tone, a vigorous cry, and an excellent ability to suck and swallow. In contrast, sometimes during the pregnancy, the mother recognizes a paucity or significant diminution of fetal muscular activity. In these instances, serious motor difficulties may be evident at or soon after birth. These infants characteristically have a paucity of limb movements, poor muscle tone, and a limp appearance, leading to their designation of having the floppy infant syndrome. Lower bulbar motor dysfunction is also often present, manifested by a weak cry and suck and a compromised ability to protect the airway during feedings. Such infants are predisposed to episodes of aspiration and recurrent pneumonia. Although most floppy infants have recognizable signs of hypotonia at birth, initially such findings may be subtle. However, occasional newborns appear normal at birth but later demonstrate abnormal motor milestone development. A few months of observation by the parents, pediatrician, and pediatric neurologist may be necessary before the infant is referred for pediatric EMG. The differential diagnosis includes a broad spectrum of infantile neuromuscular disorders.

Experienced pediatric neurologists are able to select the infants who are most likely to have a peripheral motor unit disorder that may be further defined by an electromyographic evaluation. For some disorders, such as SMA type I (Werdnig-Hoffmann disease), the clinical appearance is so stereotyped that the pediatric neurologist recognizes that the clinical problem is most likely secondary to an anterior horn cell lesion. The advent of survival motor neuron gene *(SMN)* testing makes electromyographic testing unnecessary in many infants with a classic clinical presentation. However, in some of these instances, EMG is still indicated to (1) differentiate certain motor unit lesions, including disorders that may clinically mimic SMA I, such as some of the congenital neuropathies; (2) define the level of the motor unit abnormality in the rare instance of a spinal cord lesion; and (3) make an early diagnosis to determine quality-of-life issues while awaiting the DNA analysis in an infant who is quite ill in whom SMA is the apparent clinical cause (Darras and Jones, 2000). When the clinical phenotype is less well defined or when there is a combination of features that suggest both brain and peripheral motor unit involvement, the EMG also provides useful differential diagnostic information.

It is also important for the electromyographer to observe whether the floppy infant has joint contractures compatible with the clinical designation of arthrogryposis multiplex congenita (Banker, 1986). This floppy infant phenotype may result from lesions at any level of the neuraxis, including the upper and lower motor neuron, peripheral nerve, neuromuscular junction, or muscle (Smith et al., 1963; Drachman and Sokoloff, 1966; Amick et al.,

1967; Fisher et al., 1970; Bharucha et al., 1972; Holmes et al., 1980; Smit and Barth, 1980; Banker, 1985, 1986; Strehl et al., 1985; David et al., 1991). However, the concomitant presence of joint contractures is not specific to one disorder affecting any of the primary portions of the peripheral motor unit. Arthrogryposis multiplex congenita occurs in association with any long-standing process associated with limited intrauterine mobility. EMG is helpful in defining whether a peripheral motor unit problem is the etiological mechanism in these infants.

ELECTROMYOGRAPHIC PARAMETERS FOR EVALUATION OF THE FLOPPY INFANT

The basic methodology for nerve conduction study (NCS) and needle EMG in the evaluation of floppy infant syndrome is identical to that for adults. The technical evaluation and normal values for children are different from those for adults. The inexperienced pediatric electromyographer may be concerned about the floppy infant's small size. The interelectrode distances are short. Any error in measurement is amplified to the degree that erroneous conclusions, either falsely normal or pathological, may be reached; therefore, measurement of distances must be fastidious. Infants, particularly the newborn, may readily cool in the laboratory setting, so the temperature must be monitored carefully. The distal skin temperature must be maintained at 31°C to 35°C.

We can carefully evaluate most babies with the floppy infant syndrome directly in our EMG laboratory, but occasionally we evaluate infants when they are confined to an incubator in the neonatal intensive care unit. Early in our experience with infants in the neonatal intensive care unit, we had difficulties with both the confines of the incubator and electrical artifacts. The latest neonatal intensive care unit beds, with their open exposure and continuously monitored overhead heating, provide ready access to the infant. Electrical artifacts related to all the monitoring systems necessary in this setting occasionally make it difficult to perform sensory conduction studies and needle EMG. Better grounding in the newer neonatal intensive care units has significantly improved these issues. Multiple (at least two) motor and sensory nerves need to be studied in the routine NCS evaluation of an infant with floppy infant syndrome. Sensory nerve action potentials (SNAPs) are particularly valuable in consideration of the unusual neonatal polyneuropathies, which sometimes mimic more common causes of the floppy infant syndrome, such as SMA I. Obtaining SNAPs in neonates and young infants may require a longer-duration stimulus, and increased subcutaneous tissue make obtaining sural studies more challenging than they are in the older patient. Typically in the neonate and young infant, we preferentially study the median and medial plantar SNAPs

rather than try to obtain sural responses, which are more easily obtained in the somewhat older child.

Occasionally, the pediatric electromyographer must consider the possibility of a neuromuscular transmission defect when evaluating the floppy infant, particularly when the onset is acute between the ages of 1 and 6 months. Infantile botulism should be considered very seriously in any previously healthy infant in whom generalized hypotonia suddenly develops. Typically, these babies are younger than 6 months, but we evaluated a 10-month-old infant with infantile botulism. Repetitive motor nerve stimulation is required for diagnosis in this setting as well as the rare instance in which a floppy infant has a congenital neuromuscular transmission defect. In contrast, infantile autoimmune, maternally transmitted, acquired myasthenia gravis is usually a clinical diagnosis that does not require EMG. The youngest patient with autoimmune-mediated primary myasthenia gravis that we have seen at the Children's Hospital Boston was 15 months old. Hypotonia and transient respiratory depression are observed in some infants whose mothers received magnesium sulfate treatment for preeclampsia. Typically, this is short lived, on the order of several hours, but the effect can be potentiated with the use of aminoglycoside antibiotics. Although repetitive motor nerve stimulation is not routinely performed in each floppy infant, it is indicated in infants under the following clinical circumstances.

1. Ptosis, extraocular muscle weakness, or significant bulbar involvement
2. Clinical history compatible with infantile botulism (e.g., acute onset of weakness in a previously healthy infant, with constipation or other autonomic features and without routine electromyographic evidence of an acute demyelinating neuropathy or anterior horn cell disease)
3. Repetitive compound muscle action potentials (compound muscle action potentials) after single supramaximal stimuli on routine NCS, suggesting a diagnosis of either a congenital acetylcholinesterase (AChE) deficiency or slow channel syndrome (Engel, 2001)
4. Small motor unit potentials (MUPs) suggestive of a myopathy on routine needle EMG and nondiagnostic biopsy results
5. Normal routine NCS/EMG but clinical suspicion of a neuromuscular transmission defect that remains high (e.g., moderate to severe floppy infant syndrome, with normal noninvasive testing for central nervous system disorders)

Needle EMG is a challenge in the evaluation of a floppy infant. In contrast to the older child or adult, it is not possible to obtain an orderly assessment of the MUPs and insertion activity. Infantile MUPs are normally activated in an inconsistent, sporadic fashion. Often one gains a gestalt impression of the MUP amplitude, duration, phases, and firing pattern. Various technical maneuvers enhance the quality of

MUP data. Because our aim in the evaluation of a floppy infant is not to attempt to define a specific peripheral nerve or root lesion, the evaluation of both MUPs and insertion activity in the same muscles is often not essential. This approach accurately and expeditiously provides a means to evaluate the floppy infant without fastidiously defining MUPs and insertion activity in each muscle.

There are a few helpful methods to enhance the evaluation of motor units and insertion activity in babies. The tibialis anterior and iliopsoas muscles offer the most information in the leg. Gentle stimulation of the plantar surface of the foot activates both muscles as part of the withdrawal reflex. The biceps brachii muscle is frequently active in repose; on occasion, touching the volar surface of the forearm or eliciting a grasp reflex also helps to activate this muscle. Because of the spontaneous activation of MUPs in both the iliopsoas muscle and the biceps brachii, it is often difficult to evaluate insertional and abnormal forms of spontaneous activity. In contrast, the antagonists of these muscles are good muscles to evaluate for insertional activity. Sometimes in this setting, the major issue is finding a sufficient number of MUPs to analyze; this is particularly so in infants with SMA I.

Historically, opinions differ with respect to the type of insertion and spontaneous activity that may occur in normal newborns, particularly as to whether fibrillation potentials may "normally" be present at birth. We do not have any evidence to support the contention (Eng, 1976) that fibrillation potentials are normally present in the healthy newborn. The resting membrane potential in normally innervated skeletal muscle is stable. When denervation occurs, rhythmic oscillations of the muscle membrane potential occur that trigger an action potential when the oscillations exceed a threshold voltage (Purves and Sakmann, 1974). When firing in a rhythmic fashion, these are fibrillation potentials. Similar findings are present in fetal muscle as well as in noninnervated muscle cells grown in culture (Purves and Sakmann, 1974). Fibrillation potentials per se are a nonspecific finding and may be found in a number of motor unit disorders leading to the floppy infant syndrome (Table 86–2).

One frequently observes normal, spontaneous, biphasic end-plate potentials during infancy. These waveforms typically have a negative initial deflection, in contrast to the triphasic, initially positive, deflection of fibrillation potentials. End-plates account for a greater percentage of muscle bulk in the infant compared with adults (Coers and Woolf, 1959). Normal neonatal MUPs are small, and some of these units may mimic fibrillation potentials. The pediatric electromyographer must be able to distinguish normal end-plate noise from small, normal MUPs or abnormal insertional waveforms in the newborn infant. In the more vigorous infant, discomfort from the testing may cause crying, which has the potential to mask the important auditory components of the study, such as the characteristic tick-

Table 86–2. Fibrillation Potentials with the Floppy Infant Syndrome

Neuronal
　Werdnig-Hoffmann disease
　Poliomyelitis
　X-linked SMA
Spinal cord injury
Polyneuropathies
Neuromuscular transmission defects
　Infantile botulism
Myopathies
　Congenital
　　Centronuclear (myotubular) typically
　　Congenital fiber type disproportion (rarely)
　　Nemaline rod (rarely)
　Dystrophies
　　Myotonia dystrophica
　　Merosin-deficient congenital muscular dystrophy
　　Merosin-positive congenital muscular dystrophy
　Enzymatic (glycogen storage diseases)
　　Type II: Acid maltase (Pompe's disease)
　　Type IV: Myophosphorylase (McArdle's disease)
　　Type VII: Phosphofructokinase (Tarui's disease)
　Inflammatory
　　Polymyositis?

ing sound associated with typical fibrillation potentials. This can be particularly problematic in a noisy intensive care unit environment. In summary, the pediatric electromyographer must be cautious when interpreting the nature and significance of insertional potentials in newborns, especially when an infant's motor units appear to be "normal" in size with good recruitment, because the presence of such is not primarily indicative of an anterior horn cell disorder (DiMauro and Hartlage, 1978; David et al., 1991).

Normal MUP size parameters differ appreciably for infants and toddlers compared with adults. Infantile MUP amplitudes vary between 100 and 1,600 μV, with most on the lower end of the spectrum (do Carmo, 1960; Sacco et al., 1962). Normal MUPs of more than 1,000 μV are much less common than those in the older child or adult. In addition, the MUP duration in the normal newborn is shorter than that in the mature child. Such characteristics sometimes challenge the pediatric electromyographer to differentiate the MUPs of a normal infant from subtle myopathic changes or, on occasion, even fibrillation potentials when full relaxation cannot be obtained. The recruitment pattern is often sporadic, and the gestalt approach is often necessary to define such units and their firing patterns. No computerized techniques are available to provide a precise differentiation of abnormal infantile MUPs from normal, but immature, neonatal units. Because this evaluation is not precise, the pediatric electromyographer must be cautious to not overinterpret when reporting borderline or even "normal" results. Correlation studies that assess the reliability between EMG and muscle biopsy have noted that the greatest concordance occurs with the spinal muscular atrophies (David and Jones, 1994) (Table

Table 86–3. Results of Electromyographic Analyses of Floppy Infants and Correlation with Muscle and Nerve Biopsies

Study	Patients	SMA PN	NMTD	Myopathy
	ND			
Packer et al., 1982	51	21 (41%)	0 (0%)	11 (22%)
	8 (16%) 11 (64%)			
Russell et al., 1992	79	20 (40%)	0 (0%) 2 (4%)	27 (55%)
	29 (10–90%)			
Cotliar et al., 1992	122	46 (43%) 14	19 (18%)	18 (16%)
	25 (23%)			
David and Jones, 1994	41	15 (37%)	3 (7%) 2 (5%)	10 (24%)
	11 (76% [40–93%])			

ND, nondiagnostic, normal, or central hypotonia; SMA, spinal muscular atrophy; NMTDs, neuromuscular transmission defects; PN, peripheral neuropathy. From David WS, Jones HR Jr: Electromyography and biopsy correlation with suggested protocol for evaluation of the floppy infant. Muscle Nerve 1994; 17:424–431.

86–3). Concomitantly, the referring clinician must be advised that a "normal" needle EMG result does not exclude a myopathic process, especially many of the congenital myopathies. In this instance, DNA testing or a biopsy often provides the only definitive diagnostic tool.

Some motor unit disorders are unique to neonates, such as SMA I and II, some of the unusual congenital polyneuropathies, infantile botulism, and a number of the myopathies, including the infantile forms of glycogen storage disorders. In-depth electromyographic experience with infants is very helpful. Reference to standard tables of normal values for NCS and EMG in this age group provides an important foundation for neonatal EMG (Jones et al., 1996). Unless the EMG physician has experience with infants and toddlers on a fairly routine basis, it is often prudent to refer the infant to a major pediatric neuromuscular center. If the infant might have a neuromuscular transmission defect, sedation in an outpatient day surgery center makes the testing more comfortable and often provides for a technically better study. On the other hand, sedation in the EMG laboratory is ill advised, because these infants are at greater risk for respiratory depression and aspiration.

SPECTRUM OF NEUROMUSCULAR DISEASE OBSERVED WITH ELECTROMYOGRAPHIC STUDIES OF FLOPPY INFANTS

Electromyographers who evaluate the floppy infant must consider multiple disorders that affect each motor unit level from the anterior horn to the muscle cell. The accuracy and spectrum of electromyographic findings in the evaluation of floppy infants are summarized in Table 86–3 (Packer et al., 1982; Papazian et al., 1990; Russell et al., 1992; David and Jones, 1994). In two retrospective reviews, 28 and 41 hypotonic infants younger than 1 year were studied at the Children's Hospital of Philadelphia (Packer et al., 1982) or our EMG laboratory at the Children's Hospital Boston (David and Jones, 1994).

There was a 64% correlation between electromyographic and muscle biopsy results (Packer et al., 1982) and a 76% correlation between electromyographic results and muscle and nerve biopsy, a biochemical analysis, or, rarely, a microbiological definition for infantile botulism (David and Jones, 1994).

Motor Neuron Disorders

Until the advent of DNA diagnosis for SMA type I (Werdnig-Hoffmann disease), SMA I had been the most common cause for an infant to have the floppy infant syndrome. This diagnosis accounted for 21 of 51 infants (41%) seen at the Children's Hospital of Philadelphia (Packer et al., 1982) and 15 of 41 infants (37%) seen at the Children's Hospital Boston (David and Jones, 1994). Electromyography provides a very accurate means to diagnose SMA with basically no false-positive or false-negative results. This diagnosis correlated with the findings on muscle biopsy in 93% of our patients (David and Jones, 1994), similar to other studies (Papazian et al., 1990; Cotliar et al., 1992; Russell et al., 1992). To date, the 79 floppy infants studied during a 20-year period were the only ones to have a greater proportion of myopathies than SMA (Russell et al., 1992). Subsequent to the availability of DNA testing for SMA, most infants with classic clinical phenotypes are no longer referred for electromyographic evaluation. Therefore, the number of babies with SMA I who are evaluated in an EMG laboratory constitutes a smaller percentage of the total population of floppy infants. The presence of arthrogryposis in a child with the classic SMA phenotype suggests an alternative diagnosis. It is atypical for infants with classic SMA to present with joint contractures (David et al., 1991). If the EMG demonstrates abnormalities of sensory conduction, a sural nerve biopsy will often provide the means to diagnose a congenital infantile polyneuropathy (Seitz et al., 1986).

Polyneuropathies

Although motor nerve conduction studies are routinely performed in the electromyographic analysis

---

Table 86–4. Floppy Infant Syndrome and Infantile Polyneuropathies

Congenital, hereditary, and metabolic
  Hypomyelinating
  Infantile neuronal degeneration
  Infantile neuroaxonal dystrophy
  Infantile porphyria
  Dysmaturation neuromyopathy
Acquired
  Guillain-Barré syndrome
  Chronic inflammatory demyelinating polyneuropathy

---

of floppy infants, it is equally important to perform sensory conduction studies. Otherwise, some early-onset peripheral neuropathies may be confused with SMA I. For example, in electromyographic studies of floppy infants, we found three infants with a congenital peripheral neuropathy (David and Jones, 1994), whereas no neuropathies were identified in two other studies (Packer et al., 1982; Russell et al., 1992) when sensory NCS results were not reported. We routinely perform sensory NCS in every infant with floppy infant syndrome, and when these results are abnormal, a congenital neuropathy is readily differentiated from SMA. Sural nerve biopsy results were pathological in each of our floppy infants with an abnormal sensory NCS. Sensory NCSs are relatively easy to perform in infants, particularly the median SNAP and a medial plantar SNAP. The latter is more readily found with orthodromic stimulation in the infant than is a sural nerve potential, for which a lower extremity sensory study is needed (Nancy Kuntz, personal communication, 1992). A sural nerve response is often technically difficult to obtain in normal infants. In contrast to adults, in whom early signs of polyneuropathy may be limited to the lower extremities, the motor and sensory neuropathies we have seen in infants have had diffuse involvement. A broad differential diagnosis exists for the uncommon polyneuropathies that present at birth or during infancy, including Guillain-Barré syndrome (Table 86–4). In the analysis of our experience with floppy infant syndrome, only 6 infants were identified as having a polyneuropathy: 3 were found among a series of 80 infants with uncomplicated floppy infant syndrome (David and Jones, 1994), and an additional 3 were present in our group of 35 floppy infants associated with arthrogryposis multiplex congenita (David et al., 1991). It is important *not* to limit NCSs to motor studies, performed on floppy infants, entirely on the basis of the clinical phenotype. We have seen infants clinically diagnosed with Werdnig-Hoffmann disease who had the classic frog-legged, jug-handle posture; areflexia; and tongue fasciculation in whom NCS failed to demonstrate elicitable SNAPs. Sural nerve biopsy confirmed the presence of a congenital polyneuropathy (David and Jones, 1994).

When one of these infants is evaluated, the most important issue to determine is whether a poten-tially treatable condition is present (Sladky et al., 1986; Rolfs and Bolik, 1994; Jackson et al., 1996; Luijckx et al., 1997; Jones, 2000). One possibility to consider is an acquired intrauterine demyelinating neuropathy, including Guillain-Barré syndrome. In the rare instance when the electromyographic findings demonstrate dispersed compound muscle action potentials and slow motor conduction velocities, immunotherapy may be beneficial (Sladky et al., 1986). As potential therapies are developed for other forms of neonatal neuropathy, a better appreciation of their pathophysiology will be required. Possibly, those associated with arthrogryposis multiplex congenita may have long-standing developmental arrest and therefore be less prone to therapeutic intervention. However, infants without arthrogryposis multiplex congenita whose EMGs suggest a primary demyelinating process may respond to intravenous immunoglobulin (Rolfs and Bolik, 1994) or the various other therapies used for Guillain-Barré syndrome in the older child and adult.

Disorders of Neuromuscular Transmission

Rarely, a lesion at the neuromuscular junction is the cause of floppy infant syndrome (Table 86–5). In three reviews of the electromyographic experience in the evaluation of floppy infants at major children's hospitals, no instances were recorded of either a congenital neuromuscular transmission defect or autoimmune neonatal myasthenia gravis (Packer et al., 1982; Russell et al., 1992; David and Jones, 1994). Although the congenital variants are exceedingly rare, we documented a neuromuscular transmission defect, presumed to be congenital, in a 5-month-old infant with generalized hypotonia and failure to thrive. She has had a remarkable response to pyridostigmine. Infants with clinically obvious auto-

---

Table 86–5. Floppy Infants and Disorders of the Neuromuscular Junction

Presynaptic defects
  Infantile botulism
  Toxic
    Hypermagnesemia (therapy of eclampsia)
    Aminoglycoside antibiotics
  Congenital
    Familial myasthenia gravis
    Acetylcholine vesicle paucity
    Acetylcholine quantal release diminished
    Miscellaneous poorly categorized
Postsynaptic defects
  Autoimmune (antibody positive)
  Acquired myasthenia gravis
    Maternal
  Congenital (antibody negative)
  Acetylcholine receptor deficiency
  Acetylcholinesterase deficiencies
  Classic slow channel syndrome

---

immune neonatal myasthenia gravis do not require an EMG when the mother is known to have myasthenia gravis.

PRESYNAPTIC NEUROMUSCULAR TRANSMISSION DISORDERS

Presynaptic neuromuscular transmission defects are uncommon causes of the floppy infant syndrome. Infantile botulism is the most commonly acquired neuromuscular junction disorder that occurs during the first year of life (see Table 86–5). Rarely will the electromyographer see an infant with a congenital presynaptic neuromuscular transmission disorder. Even less likely is the possibility of a toxic drug mechanism, such as hypermagnesemia or aminoglycosides. It is important to realize that the incidence of botulism varies greatly from region to region. Infantile botulism is especially prevalent in certain areas of this country, particularly the mid-Atlantic states, California, and the Rocky Mountain states, where one of the authors (K.J.S.) saw 14 cases in just 5 years at Salt Lake City. *Clostridium botulinum* is clearly endemic in some geographic areas compared with other areas. Infantile botulism was present in 11 of 50 floppy infants (22%) seen at the Children's Hospital of Philadelphia (Packer et al., 1982). In contrast, no instances of infantile botulism were reported in the study of Russell and colleagues (1992) in Iowa, and we initially reported just one case among 80 infants evaluated for floppy infant syndrome in New England (David and Jones, 1994). However, we have subsequently diagnosed four additional cases, including one 10-month-old child. Therefore, it is important to always consider infantile botulism in the differential diagnosis when evaluating a previously healthy infant who has suddenly become limp (Cornblath et al., 1983).

The stereotypical set of clinical signs and symptoms of infantile botulism in a previously healthy infant primarily includes the acute onset of hypotonia, poor feeding, and constipation (Pickett et al., 1976; Clay et al., 1977; Thompson et al., 1980; Hoffman et al., 1982; Schwartz and Eng, 1982; Glauser et al., 1989; Donley et al., 1991; Gutierrez et al., 1994). However, the rapidity of progression and eventual severity of the illness vary. Some infants have a relatively benign course, and others require rapid intubation with prolonged hospitalization. Rarely, there may be a clinical relapse (Glauser et al., 1989). The differential diagnosis includes other acute disorders of the motor unit (see Table 86–4), a nonspecific encephalopathy, sepsis, or respiratory distress. Consequently, the pediatric electromyographer is sometimes asked to evaluate a broad spectrum of infants with acute hypotonia during the first 6 months of life. A diagnosis of infantile botulism may be established by appropriate repetitive nerve stimulation and needle EMG, as summarized in Table 86–6. The setting may vary from the outpatient laboratory to the intensive care unit. Compared with Lambert-Eaton myasthenic syndrome in the adult,

Table 86–6. Protocol for Suspected Presynaptic Neuromuscular Transmission Defects of Infantile Botulism

Motor/sensory nerve conduction study in one arm and leg
Repetitive motor nerve stimulation at 2 Hz to two distal muscles
Tetanizing stimulation at 50 Hz for 10 seconds followed by stimulation every 30 seconds until compound muscle action potential
Diagnostic features for infantile botulism
  Compound muscle action potential <2.0 mV in at least two muscles
  PTF >120% of baseline
  PTF prolonged >120 seconds with no PTE

Adapted from Gutierrez AR, Bodensteiner J, Gutmann L: Electrodiagnosis of infantile botulism. J Child Neurol 1994;9:362–365.

infants with infantile botulism may have a relatively modest degree of facilitation with repetitive motor nerve stimulation in contrast to the greater than 100% facilitation routinely seen with Lambert-Eaton myasthenic syndrome (Fakadej and Gutmann, 1982; Gutierrez et al., 1994). This association was illustrated by an infant seen by one of the authors (H.R.J.); this child was in respiratory distress and had a very modest 23% to 65% facilitation.

A more difficult question arises regarding when to test a floppy infant for the presence of a neuromuscular transmission defect (see Table 86–6). Although most floppy infants with either a presynaptic or a postsynaptic disorder have obvious signs of bulbar involvement, we are unaware of any study that has routinely used repetitive motor nerve stimulation to evaluate a broad spectrum of floppy infants. Because the use of 20- to 50-Hz stimulation frequencies is necessary, this is a painful procedure. Sedation under anesthesia in a surgical day care center allows the pediatric electromyographer to accomplish the best results. We suggest that the primary indications for repetitive motor nerve stimulation studies still depend on clinical judgment. The routine use of repetitive motor nerve stimulation is indicated in the floppy infant with evidence of ocular or lower bulbar dysfunction and in infants with intermittent symptoms, which occur with some of the familial neuromuscular transmission defects. However, there remains the issue of the floppy infant who has none of these indications but in whom no diagnosis is identified to explain the generalized hypotonia. These infants may also deserve this more extensive testing. As more colleagues routinely use anesthesia for EMG in these infants, this information may become available.

POSTSYNAPTIC DISORDERS OF NEUROMUSCULAR TRANSMISSION

With the exception of neonatal autoimmune maternal acquired myasthenia gravis, it is very unusual for autoimmune myasthenia gravis to present before the age of 1 year. The youngest child we have seen at the Children's Hospital Boston is a 15-month-old child. Otherwise, one is rarely confronted with the early presentation of a postsynaptic congenital neuromuscular transmission defect such as the slow channel syndrome or acetylcholinesterase deficiency. These two inborn postsynaptic disorders may be suspected on the basis of the presence of a repetitive or late component on the compound muscle action potential (Harper, 2002). (These are further defined by Harper in Chapter 76.)

Myopathies

There are a very large number of myopathies with which the patient may present in the neonatal period as a floppy infant (Table 86–7). The MUPs of normal newborn infants are shorter in duration and sometimes of lower amplitude than those observed in older children or adults and are not unlike those identified as myopathic in adults. Pediatric electromyographers usually have to form a gestalt impression of both individual MUP parameters and firing patterns that occur sporadically and unpredictably. A number of the myopathies are particularly difficult to define with EMG. Ten of the 41 floppy infants (24%) seen at the Children's Hospital Boston were found to have a myopathy (Engel, 2001). The electromyographic pathology correlation was good in four of six babies (67%) when the EMG demonstrated classic myopathic features. However, myopathies were also found in 2 of 3 floppy infants with "nonspecific" electromyographic changes and in 4 of 12 infants with normal results on EMG. Therefore, only 4 of 10 infants (40%) seen at the Children's Hospital

---

Table 86–7. Neonatal Myopathies

Congenital
   Nemaline rod
   Centronuclear
   Central core
   Fiber type disproportion
Dystrophies
   Congenital myotonia dystrophica
   Congenital muscular dystrophy
Inflammatory??
   Polymyositis
Enzymatic myopathies
   Carbohydrate cycle deficiencies
      Type II: Acid maltase, some with debrancher
      Type V: Muscle phosphorylase
      Type VII: Phosphofructokinase
   Lipid metabolism (question if cause of floppy infant syndrome)
      Infantile carnitine palmitoyltransferase deficiency
      Primary systemic carnitine deficiency
      Acetyl coenzyme dehydrogenase deficiency
   Electron transport chain disorders
      Severe infantile myopathy
         Complex II deficiency
         Complex IV deficiency
      Benign infantile myopathy
         Complex IV deficiency

Boston with histologically and clinically confirmed myopathies had EMGs compatible with that diagnosis (David and Jones, 1994). At the Children's Hospital of Philadelphia, eight children in a series of floppy infants had a myopathy (16%) (Packer et al., 1982). Four of these eight (50%) floppy infants had concordant electromyographic and biopsy results.

The disparity between the sensitivity of EMG in the definition of neurogenic processes and myopathic disorders in the newborn infant relates to several factors, including the striking diminution in the number of MUPs in patients with SMA-1 as well as the ease of identifying these isolated, somewhat enlarged, rapidly firing MUPs. These are typically found to have a widespread anatomic distribution. In contrast, in infants with myopathies, it may be more difficult to determine whether the MUPs are very predominantly abnormal. In this instance, the MUP changes are more subtle in character and more difficult to define. This is particularly so because activation requires a degree of patient cooperation that cannot be readily obtained with the neonate. In the florid neonatal myopathies, the recruitment of increased numbers of smaller MUPs is best appreciated in the iliopsoas muscle when the infant withdraws the thigh from a light stimulus to the plantar surface of the foot. However, with more subtle myopathic lesions without much fiber destruction, which occurs with the congenital myopathies, this differentiation is more difficult. One must be cautious in not overcalling a myopathic process when the findings are indeed representative of the normal immaturity of the infantile muscle fiber. Conversely, pediatric electromyographers need to emphasize to the referring clinician that "normal" results on infantile EMG do not exclude a myopathic process. If a myopathy is suspected clinically, a muscle biopsy is required to further define this possibility. In contrast, when significant neurogenic changes are present to support the diagnosis of SMA I, a muscle biopsy is not necessary because DNA testing will provide an accurate diagnosis (Darras and Jones, 2000).

Fibrillation potentials are a nonspecific finding, and their identification is not to be used to differentiate SMA from a myopathic process (see Table 86–2). Early in our experience, we were confused by the electromyographic results in some floppy infants because of the finding of a few fibrillation potentials without specific changes in the MUPs (David and Jones, 1994). We inadvertently classified these infants as having "nonspecific neurogenic changes." Later, we correlated our electromyographic results in floppy infants with muscle biopsy findings (David and Jones, 1994). Most infants with nonspecific needle electromyographic findings, such as a few fibrillation potentials, but without large motor units did not have an incipient neurogenic process such as SMA (David and Jones, 1994). In fact, these findings usually represented a myopathic process—either a congenital myopathy or dystrophy. A single case study illustrated this principle; an infant with diffuse fibrillation potentials was diagnosed as having SMA (DiMauro and Hartlage, 1978). In retrospect, this floppy infant also had increased numbers of small MUPs. Myophosphorylase deficiency was diagnosed at the age of 3 months at the time of autopsy (Di-Mauro and Hartlage, 1978).

OVERVIEW OF ELECTROMYOGRAPHIC EVALUATION OF THE FLOPPY INFANT

An electromyographic protocol for the evaluation of the floppy infant is outlined in Table 86–8. Sensory NCSs are logical initial studies because they are the least uncomfortable component of pediatric EMG. In most infants with floppy infant syndrome, including those with SMAs myopathies, and the rare infantile neuromuscular transmission defects, the SNAPs are normal. The one exception is the diffuse sensory dysfunction present with infantile polyneuropathy. In all other instances, the initial evaluation of SNAPs permits the pediatric electromyographer to test the overall function of the peripheral nervous system as well as the integrity of the testing equipment. In general, when a normal SNAP is obtained in a floppy infant, it is rare to gain more diagnostic information by testing additional sensory nerves. However, when no SNAP is defined, the presence of a primary and diffuse loss of sensory function must be confirmed by evaluating at least one other sensory nerve, usually in another extremity.

Because the compound muscle action potential amplitude may be compromised by lesions at any level of the motor unit, including the anterior horn cell, peripheral nerve, neuromuscular junction, and muscle, it is important to sample the responses of at least two peripheral motor nerves—one in an arm

---

Table 86–8. Electromyographic Protocol for Evaluation of Floppy Infant

---

Sensory NCS: At least one sensory nerve
Motor NCS: At least two motor nerves
Needle EMG: At least four to six muscles in one or two extremities, including distal and proximal sites
If spinal muscular atrophy is a consideration: At least two muscles innervated by different nerve roots, and nerves should be sampled in at least three extremities
Repetitive motor nerve stimulation (2–50 Hz) must be performed with
  Infantile botulism–type of history
  Ptosis or ophthalmoparesis
  Stimulus-linked repetitive compound muscle action potential
  Myopathy defined by EMG
  EMG/NCS normal and high suspicion of peripheral motor unit lesion

---

NCS, needle conduction study; EMG, electromyography.
Adapted from David WS, Jones HR Jr: Electromyography and biopsy correlation with suggested protocol for evaluation of the floppy infant. Muscle Nerve 1994;17:424–431.

---

and another in a leg. When no compound muscle action potential can be defined with standard sweep speeds, the time base should be extended to avoid failure to appreciate the prolonged latencies that may occur when a profound degree of dysmyelination is present. Similarly, as reported by Bolton and associates (1988), one has to carefully use maximal stimulation potential to identify the rare infant with a high motor threshold. In addition, particular attention must be paid to the configuration of the compound muscle action potential. The presence of a compound muscle action potential with a repetitive component provides a clue to the presence of an uncommon congenital defect in neuromuscular transmission at the postsynaptic level (Harper, 2002).

The most useful electromyographic parameter in the evaluation of floppy infant syndrome is the assessment of MUPs (Packer et al., 1982; David and Jones, 1994). In general, we test four to six muscles in two extremities, although on occasion we confine the needle examination to just one leg, carefully analyzing both proximal and distal muscles (Fig. 86–2). When the presence of SMA appears to be a possibility, we examine at least two muscles innervated by different nerves and nerve roots in at least three different extremities. This is especially necessary to exclude the unlikely instance of an isolated spinal injury. Nonarthrogrypotic infants with MUPs of increased duration and high amplitude that are recruited in decreased numbers and at an increased rate usually have SMA. These findings may be sufficient for a diagnosis of SMA when the clinical context is appropriate (David and Jones, 1994). Similar MUP changes have been noted in seven newborns with congenital neuropathy (unpublished data), an illness that must be strongly considered when no SNAPs are present (Engel, 2001).

Most newborns with low-amplitude, short-duration MUPs have a recognizable myopathy (Packer et al., 1982; David and Jones, 1994). However, many infantile myopathies may be associated with healthy-appearing MUPs (Packer et al., 1982; Russell et al., 1992; David and Jones, 1994). The pediatric electromyographer must always keep this in mind when dictating a clinical correlation for a floppy infant who has normal results on EMG by advising the referring physician of this particular limit of the study. Therefore, when a floppy infant shows normal results on the EMG, the pediatric neurologist should not be dissuaded from proceeding with muscle biopsy when a lesion in the peripheral motor unit is suspected on a clinical basis.

Fibrillation potentials may be associated with a disorder at any level of the motor unit, including the motor neuron, peripheral nerve, neuromuscular junction, and some myopathies (see Table 86–2). The scattered occurrence of fibrillation potentials without specific MUP abnormalities, sometimes suggesting nonspecific "neurogenic" changes, was more commonly associated with infants whose biopsies showed a myopathy, particularly congenital muscu-

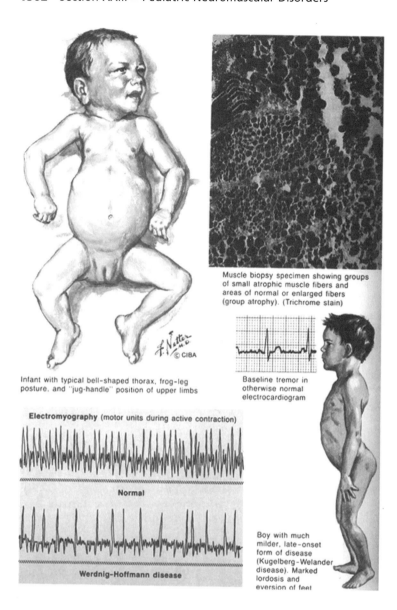

Muscle biopsy specimen showing groups of small atrophic muscle fibers and areas of normal or enlarged fibers (group atrophy). (Trichrome stain)

Baseline tremor in otherwise normal electrocardiogram

Infant with typical bell-shaped thorax, frog-leg posture, and "jug-handle" position of upper limbs

Electromyography (motor units during active contraction)

Normal

Werdnig-Hoffmann disease

Boy with much milder, late-onset form of disease (Kugelberg-Welander disease). Marked lordosis and eversion of feet

Figure 86–2. Infant with classic body posture and needle EMG and muscle biopsy findings of SMA1 (Werdnig-Hoffmann disease). (From Netter FH: The Ciba Collection of Medical Illustrations. Vol 1, Nervous System. Pt. 2, Neurologic and Neuromuscular Disorders. West Caldwell, NJ, Ciba-Geigy Medical Education, 1986.)

lar dystrophy (David and Jones, 1994). It is the characteristics of the MUP per se that are the most accurate for defining the abnormal site of disease (Jones, 1990).

To our knowledge, no study has addressed the issue of the role of routine testing for a neuromuscular junction transmission defect in the floppy infant. However, one must always keep this important portion of the peripheral motor unit in the differential diagnosis of a floppy newborn or any infant with an acutely acquired generalized hypotonia. The predominant clinical settings in which these very rare lesions must be considered and formally tested for a defect in neuromuscular transmission were outlined earlier.

An uncommon subset of floppy infants are those with the fulminant onset of diffuse hypotonia after an initially healthy first few weeks or months of life (Table 86–9). The differential diagnosis of acute infantile hypotonia includes the anterior horn cell (i.e., poliomyelitis [Moore et al., 1982; Bergeisen et

al., 1986; Robbins, 1993; Beausoleil et al., 1994] either after vaccination or due to incomplete immunization), the peripheral nerve (primarily the Guillain-Barré syndrome [Jones, 2000] or chronic inflammatory demyelinating polyneuropathy [Sladky et al., 1986]), the level of the neuromuscular junction (i.e., infantile botulism [Pickett et al., 1976; Clay et al., 1977; Cornblath et al., 1983]), familial infantile myasthenia gravis (Ohno et al., 2000; Harper, 2002), and the muscle cell per se (i.e., some glycolytic enzyme deficiencies [Hogan et al., 1969; DiMauro and Hartlage, 1978; Servidei et al., 1986; Milstein et al., 1989; Verity, 1991; Tsao et al., 1994; Swoboda et al., 1997), and possibly infantile polymyositis (Thompson, 1982; Chou and Miles, 1989; Shevell et al., 1990).

In summary, a pediatric electromyographer with knowledge of the various clinical syndromes that affect the motor unit in infancy (see Table 86–1) can provide considerable assistance to the pediatric neurologist in the evaluation of floppy infants. Occa-

Table 86–9. Acute-Onset Floppy Infant Syndrome

Anterior horn cell
  Poliomyelitis
Peripheral nerve
  Acute inflammatory demyelinating polyneuropathy
  Chronic inflammatory demyelinating polyneuropathy
  Tick paralysis
Neuromuscular junction
  Infantile botulism
  Familial infantile myasthenia gravis
  Autoimmune myasthenia gravis
Muscle
  Polymyositis
  Glycogen storage disease, muscle phosphorylase deficiency

From Jones HR, Darras B: Acute care pediatric electromyography. Muscle Nerve 2000;23:553–562.

sionally, examination of a parent may add specific diagnostic definition, especially for the diagnosis of unsuspected myotonic dystrophy. An electromyographic evaluation in the floppy infant syndrome is capable of defining specific motor unit disorders, including spinal muscular atrophy, congenital neuropathies, infantile botulism, and myotonic dystrophy. These results are helpful to the pediatric neurologist in providing a useful guide to the early management of the floppy infant. Initial results of EMG often provide encouragement to parents awaiting the muscle biopsy processing, because SMA I may be virtually excluded with a very carefully executed EMG (David and Jones, 1994). In contrast, when the EMG indicates a diffuse process affecting motor neurons, the primary pediatric neurologist can be supportive of the parents so that when results of further studies, probably including genetic testing, are available, the family may be prepared for the seriousness of their child's illness. In the future, computed analysis of MUPs may permit a more accurate definition of subtle myopathies that defy DNA classification. However, genetic definition of many of these syndromes continues to evolve rapidly. This may obviate the need for EMG in some future settings.

References

Amick LD, Johnson WW, Smith HL: Electromyographic and histo-pathologic correlation in arthrogryposis. Arch Neurol 1967; 16:512–523.

Banker BO: Arthrogryposis multiplex congenita: Spectrum of pathologic changes. Hum Pathol 1986;17:656–672.

Banker BO: Neuropathologic aspects of arthrogryposis multiplex congenita. Clin Orthop 1985;194:30–43.

Beausoleil JL, Nordgren RE, Medlin JF: Vaccine associated paralytic poliomyelitis. J Child Neurol 1994;9:334–335.

Bergeisen GH, Bauman RJ, Gilmore RL: Neonatal paralytic poliomyelitis: A case report. Arch Neurol 1986;43:192–194.

Bharucha EP, Pandya SS, Dastur DK: Arthrogryposis multiplex congenita. Part 1: Clinical and electromyographic aspects. J Neurol Neurosurg Psychiatry 1972;35:425–434.

Bolton CF, Hahn AF, Hinton GG: The syndrome of high stimulation threshold and low conduction velocity. Ann Neurol 1988;24:165.

Chou SM, Miles JM: Floppy infant syndrome with "congenital infantile polymyositis." Ann Neurol 1989;26:449.

Clay SA, Ramseyer JC, Fishman LS, Sedgwick RP: Acute infantile motor unit disorder: Infantile botulism? Arch Neurol 1977;34: 236–249.

Coers C, Woolf AL: The Innervation of Muscle: A Biopsy Study. Oxford, Blackwell Scientific, 1959; 16–17.

Cornblath DR, Sladky JT, Sumner AJ: Clinical electrophysiology of infantile botulism. Muscle Nerve 1983;6:448–452.

Cotliar R, Eng GD, Koch B, et al: Correlation of electrodiagnosis and muscle biopsy results. Muscle Nerve 1992;15:1197–1198.

Darras BT, Jones HR: Diagnosis of neuromuscular disorders in the era of DNA analysis: The role of pediatric electromyography. Pediatr Neurol 2000;23:289–306.

David WS, Jones HR Jr: Electromyography and biopsy correlation with suggested protocol for evaluation of the floppy infant. Muscle Nerve 1994;17:424–431.

David WS, Kupsky WJ, Jones HR Jr: Electromyographic and histologic evaluation of the arthrogrypotic infant [Abstract]. Muscle Nerve 1991;14:897.

DiMauro S, Hartlage PL: Fatal infantile form of muscle phosphorylase deficiency. Neurology 1978;28:1124–1129.

do Carmo RJ: Motor unit action potential parameters in human newborn infants. Arch Neurol 1960;3:136–140.

Donley DK, Knight P, Tenorio G, Oh SJ: A patient with infant botulism, improving with edrophonium. Muscle Nerve 1991; 41:201.

Drachman DB, Sokoloff L: The role of movement in embryonic joint development. Dev Biol 1966;14:401–420.

Dubowitz V: The floppy infant. In Clinics in Developmental Medicine, 2nd ed. London, Heinemann Medical, 1980; 89–94.

Eng GD: Spontaneous potentials in premature and full term infants. Arch Phys Med Rehabil 1976;57:120–121.

Engel A: Overview of the congenital myasthenic syndromes, 73rd European Neuromuscular Consortium International Workshop. Neuromusc Disord 2001;11:315–321.

Fakadej AV, Gutmann L: Prolongation of post-tetanic facilitation in infant botulism. Muscle Nerve 1982;5:727–729.

Fisher RL, Johnstone WT, Fisher WH Jr, Goldkamp OG: Arthrogryposis multiplex congenita: A clinical investigation. J Pediatr 1970;76:255–261.

Glauser TA, Maguire HC, Sladky JT: Relapse of infantile botulism [Abstract]. Ann Neurol 1989;26:449.

Gutierrez AR, Bodensteiner J, Gutmann L: Electrodiagnosis of infantile botulism. J Child Neurol 1994;9:362–365.

Harper CM: Congenital myasthenic syndromes. In Brown W, Bolton CF, Aminoff M (eds): Clinical Neurophysiology and Neuromuscular Diseases. New York/Philadelphia, WB Saunders, 2002.

Hoffman RE, Pincomb BJ, Skeels MR: Type F infant botulism. Am J Dis Child 1982;136:270–271.

Hogan GR, Gutmann L, Schmidt R, Gilbert E: Pompe's disease. Neurology 1969;19:894–900.

Holmes LB, Driscoll SG, Bradley WG: Contractures in a newborn infant of a mother with myasthenia gravis. J Pediatr 1980;96: 1067–1069.

Jackson AH, Baquis GD, Shaw BL: Congenital Guillain-Barré syndrome. J Child Neurol 1996;5:407–410.

Jones HR Jr: EMG evaluation of the floppy infant: Differential diagnosis and technical aspects. Muscle Nerve 1990;13:338–347.

Jones HR, Darras B: Acute care pediatric electromyography. Muscle Nerve 2000;23:S53–S62.

Jones HR, Harmon RL, Bolton CF, et al: Clinical Pediatric Electromyography. Philadelphia/New York, Lippincott-Raven, 1996; 1–37.

Jones HR: Guillain-Barré syndrome: Perspectives with infants and children. Semin Pediatr Neurol 2000;7:91–102.

Luijckx GJ, Vies J, de Baets M, et al: Guillain-Barré syndrome in mother and child. Lancet 1997;349:27.

Milstein JM, Herron TM, Haas JE: Fatal infantile muscle phosphorylase deficiency. J Child Neurol 1989;4:186–188.

Moore M, Katona P, Kaplan JE, et al: Poliomyelitis in the United States, 1969–1981. J Infect Dis 1982;146:558–563.

Ohno K, Engel AG, Brengman JM, et al: The spectrum of mutations causing endplate acetylcholinesterase deficiency. Ann Neurol 2000;47:162–170.

Packer RJ, Brown MJ, Berman PH: The diagnostic value of electromyography in infantile hypotonia. Am J Dis Child 1982;136:1057–1059.

Papazian O, Duenas DA, Cullen RF Jr, et al: Outcome of neonatal floppy syndrome. Ann Neurol 1990;28:430.

Pickett J, Berg B, Chaplin E, Brunstetter-Shafer M-A: Syndrome of botulism in infancy: Clinical and electrophysiologic study. N Engl J Med 1976;295:770–772.

Purves D, Sakmann B: Membrane properties underlying spontaneous activity of denervated muscle. J Physiol 1974;239:125–153.

Robbins FC: Eradication of polio in the Americas. JAMA 1993;270:1857–1859.

Rolfs A, Bolik A: Guillain-Barré syndrome in pregnancy: Reflections on immunopathogenesis. Acta Neurol Scand 1994;89:400–492.

Russell JW, Afifi AK, Ross MA: Predictive value of electromyography in diagnosis and prognosis of the hypotonic infant. J Child Neurol 1992;7:387–391.

Sacco G, Buchthal F, Rosenfalck P: Motor unit potentials at different ages. Arch Neurol 1962;6:366–373.

Schwartz RH, Eng G: Infant botulism: Exacerbation by aminoglycosides. Am J Dis Child 1982;136:952.

Seitz RJ, Wechsler W, Mosny DS, Lenard HG: Hypomyelination neuropathy in a female newborn presenting as arthrogryposis multiplex congenita. Neuropediatrics 1986;17:132–136.

Servidei S, Bonilla E, Diedrich RG, et al: Fatal infantile form of muscle phosphofructokinase deficiency. Neurology 1986;36:1465–1470.

Shevell M, Rosenblatt B, Silver K, et al: Congenital inflammatory myopathy. Neurology 1990;40:1111–1114.

Sladky JT, Brown MJ, Berman PH: Chronic inflammatory demyelinating polyneuropathy of infancy: A corticosteroid-responsive disorder. Ann Neurol 1986;20:76–81.

Smit LME, Barth PG: Arthrogryposis multiplex congenita due to congenital myasthenia. Dev Med Child Neurol 1980;22:371–374.

Smith EM, Bender LF, Stover CN: Lower motor neuron deficit in arthrogryposis: An EMG study. Arch Neurol 1963;8:97–100.

Strehl E, Vanasse M, Brochu P: EMG and needle muscle biopsy studies in arthrogryposis multiplex congenita. Neuropediatrics 1985;16:225–227.

Swoboda K, Specht L, Jones HR, et al: Infantile phosphofructokinase deficiency with arthrogryposis clinical benefit using a ketogenic diet. J Pediatr 1997;131:932–934.

Thompson CE: Infantile myositis. Dev Med Child Neurol 1982;24:307–313.

Thompson JA, Glasgow LA, Warpinski JR, Olson C: Infant botulism: Clinical spectrum and epidemiology. Pediatrics 1980;66:936–942.

Tsao CY, Boesel CP, Wright FS: A hypotonic infant with complete deficiencies of acid maltase and debrancher enzyme. J Child Neurol 1994;9:90–91.

Verity MA: Infantile Pompe's disease, lipid storage, and partial carnitine deficiency. Muscle Nerve 1991;14:435–440.

Spinal Muscular Atrophies and Other Disorders of the Motor Neuron

Thomas O. Crawford and H. Royden Jones, Jr.

SMN-ASSOCIATED SPINAL MUSCULAR ATROPHY
  Clinical Features
ELECTROMYOGRAPHY AND PATHOLOGY OF
  SPINAL MUSCULAR ATROPHY
  Clinical Course

Genetics
Diagnosis
OTHER SPINAL MUSCULAR ATROPHIES
  Differential Diagnosis
OTHER DISORDERS OF THE MOTOR NEURON

With the rapid advances in molecular medicine in the 1990s, the term *spinal muscular atrophy* has evolved into two separate connotations: one as a label for a specific monogenic disease and the other as a descriptive term for an array of presumed genetic disorders of the motor neuron. Often, the meaning of the term can be interpreted only on the basis of its context. As a precise term, *spinal muscular atrophy* (SMA) names the disorder caused by mutation of the survival motoneuron gene (*SMN*). As a generic term, *spinal muscular atrophy* applies to a range of diverse disorders, both well and poorly characterized, in which degeneration of motor neurons in the spinal cord and brainstem is a prominent feature. The bulk of this chapter considers *SMN*-associated SMA and the extraordinary advances in the science of SMA.

For the sake of completeness, the broader, very rare syndromes that also affect the motor neurons of children, which are not truly members of the SMA family of childhood neuromuscular disorders, are considered at the conclusion of the chapter. These syndromes include childhood amyotrophic lateral sclerosis, Hirayama's cervical spinal muscular atrophy, poliomyelitis, paraneoplastic disorders, some inborn errors of metabolism, syringomyelia, and arteriovenous malformations of the spinal cord as well as some traumatic entities in the newborn. Motor neuron disorders of adults and motor neuron diseases caused by infectious agents are discussed in Section XVIII.

SMN-ASSOCIATED SPINAL MUSCULAR ATROPHY

Dispute about the meaning of the term *spinal muscular atrophy* is not new, and the advances in molecular medicine of the 1990s should not be expected to have resolved all of the ambiguity. Clinicians have been engaged in vigorous nosological debate about the boundaries and coherence of several disorders that were then classed as a family of "SMAs." With linkage of the major childhood forms of SMA to chromosome 5q13 (Brzustowicz et al., 1990; Gilliam et al., 1990; Melki et al., 1990a, 1990b) and identification of *SMN* as the pathogenic gene (Lefebvre et al., 1995), the argument in favor of considering the three forms of childhood SMA (SMA type 1, also known as Werdnig-Hoffmann disease, infantile SMA, or severe SMA; SMA type 2, also known as intermediate-type SMA; and SMA type 3, also known as Kugelberg-Welander disease) as distinct disorders collapsed. Although these categorical distinctions were demoted in significance, they persist as useful descriptors of clinical severity within the spectrum of SMA.

Compared with other single-gene genetic disorders, SMA is common. Approximately 1 in 6,000 to 10,000 children have SMA, ranging across the spectrum of severity. It appears on all continents in all races in roughly equal incidence everywhere measured (Emery, 1991). As a recessive disorder, this leads to a calculated prevalence of carriers of approximately 1:40 to 1:60 individuals (McAndrew et al., 1997).

Clinical Features

With the advent of a DNA test of high sensitivity and near-perfect specificity, it is now possible to precisely define the clinical phenotype (Rudnik-Schöneborn et al., 1996). At the most severe end of the spectrum, affected infants are born profoundly weak, with arthrogryposis and immediate ventilatory insufficiency requiring assistance for survival (Bürglen et al., 1995, 1996; Bingham et al., 1997; Devriendt et al., 1997; Korinthenberg et al., 1997; MacLeod et al., 1999). At the least severe end, individuals may be asymptomatic until adult life, and indeed a few adults with an abnormal *SMN* gene have yet to develop weakness at the time of ascertainment (Brahe et al., 1995; Cobben et al., 1995; Hahnen et al., 1995; Wang et al., 1996; Bussaglia et al., 1997). Affected siblings are generally similar in phenotype severity (Feingold et al., 1977; Pearn, 1980), with a few rare exceptions (Parano et al., 1996). The clinical labels are applied with some imprecision between investigators, but in general, infants with SMA type 1 have manifested weakness before 6 months of age and never achieve the ability to maintain an independent sitting posture. Those with SMA type 2 are defined as those who at some point in their lives were able to maintain an independent sitting posture. Type 3 individuals have had the ability at some time to maintain a standing posture and walk, although the degree of bracing support and distance traveled are undefined. Some clinicians have added a "type 4" to denote those with an adult onset of weakness.

In 1990, an international consortium formulated highly specific, but not necessarily sensitive, diagnostic criteria intended to maximize the power of classic genetics to isolate the causative gene (Munsat, 1991). These criteria are now outdated but still apply to most cases and thus are useful for purposes of ascertainment; they include (1) symmetrical weakness affecting trunk and limb muscles, with proximal more than distal weakness; (2) denervation demonstrated by both electrophysiological and biopsy features; and (3) exclusion of patients with other central nervous system involvement, serious impairment of other organ systems, arthrogryposis, sensory loss, or eye or facial muscle weakness. This last criterion in particular is overly stringent, as infants with severe disease may have arthrogryposis and often more widespread neuropathology (see subsequent sections). Moreover, at any level of severity, SMA can coexist with other disorders.

One advance in the discovery of *SMN* as the causative gene is that diagnosis often no longer necessitates electromyography (EMG) and muscle biopsy. In the majority of individuals, the diagnosis is certain with the absence of detectable *SMN1* in the setting of skeletal muscle weakness. Perhaps 5% of patients with bona fide SMN-associated SMA will fail to meet this criterion (Hahnen et al., 1995; Capon et al., 1996; Somerville, 1997), however, and the complexities of identifying this small percentage of patients is discussed in the following sections.

The cardinal feature of SMA is symmetrical weakness due to muscle denervation. Across the range of severity, the legs are more affected than the arms, and the limbs are more affected than the diaphragm and cranial muscles. In the most severe cases, weakness is detectable throughout the body. In severely denervated muscles, the preservation of function in a few residual motoneurons produces several classic clinical signs that may be useful diagnostically. In infants with severe weakness, the tongue has a scalloped surface and quivers irregularly (errantly termed "fasciculations"), which reflects tonic activity in the surviving, widely spaced motor units of the tongue. The same essential physiology is expressed in the outstretched fingers of slightly stronger patients, where a fine, rapid, irregular tremor has been variously termed "contraction pseudotremor," "contraction fasciculations" (Riggs et al., 1983), and "minipolymyoclonus" (Moosa and Dubowitz, 1973; Fredericks and Russman, 1979). Wherever there is weakness, there is accompanying muscle atrophy. Sensation is normal, and muscle stretch reflexes are diminished commensurate with power. Ankle and knee reflexes may be preserved in the most mildly affected infants. Also notable is that mildly affected individuals may have pseudohypertrophy of the calf muscles (Yamada et al., 1988) and two- to fourfold elevation of serum creatine kinase activity (Bouwsma and Van Wijngaarden, 1980; Rudnik-Schöneborn et al., 1998).

ELECTROMYOGRAPHY AND PATHOLOGY OF SPINAL MUSCULAR ATROPHY

Motor nerve conduction studies demonstrate a diminished amplitude commensurate with the amount of denervation atrophy. In those with a very low compound motor action potential amplitude, especially infants with severe SMA, conduction velocity may be below normal values, but whether this reflects a technical problem in assessment, a specific loss of faster-conducting motor units (Hausmanowa-Petrusewicz and Kopec, 1973; Moosa and Dubowitz, 1976; Ryniewicz, 1977; Chien and Nonaka, 1989; Imai et al., 1990), or a specific abnormality in myelination associated with SMA (Hausmanowa-Petrusewicz et al., 1975; Ohama and Ikuta, 1977; Coers and Telerman-Toppet, 1979) is not clear. In most cases, sensory nerve studies are normal. In very severely affected newborn infants, inexcitable sensory nerves accompany an undetectable compound motor action potential (Steiman et al., 1980; Bingham et al., 1997; Korinthenberg et al., 1997; Hergersberg et al., 2000), indicating involvement of both sensory and motor neurons. Distinguishing these individuals from those with a severe congenital axonal neuropathy may be difficult with physiological and pathological studies and depends instead on the genetic analysis of *SMN*.

The electrodiagnostic hallmark of SMA is denervation on EMG. There are clear differences in the nature of denervation between severe and intermediately affected individuals. In infants with severe SMA, EMG usually detects abnormal spontaneous activity and neuropathic recruitment of voluntary motor units, reflecting their reduced numbers (Buchthal and Olsen, 1970; Hausmanowa-Petrusewicz and Karwanska, 1986). Sometimes, voluntary motor unit potentials with a moderately increased amplitude but normal duration are detected. This finding likely reflects anatomical and physiological changes in the severely denervated muscle of SMA and need not imply expansion of motor unit size by collateral sprouting. These changes may include (1) muscle fiber hypertrophy; (2) "compression" of the motor unit cross-sectional territory by atrophy of intercalated fibers from other units, bringing additional fibers of the motor unit closer to the recording electromyographic electrode; and (3) loss of smaller motor units in the recruitment array so that residual motor units that naturally innervate a larger number of muscle fibers are recruited early (Crawford et al., 1995).

In contrast to the infants severely weakened by SMA, older infants and children with milder forms of SMA have a different pattern of denervation (Buchthal and Olsen, 1970; Hausmanowa-Petrusewicz and Karwanska, 1986; Crawford et al., 1995). Abnormal spontaneous activity, either fibrillations or positive waves, is rare or absent. Voluntary motor unit potentials have increased amplitude and duration, reflecting abundant type grouping with collateral reinnervation. By the late childhood years, it is not uncommon to find motor unit potentials with prolonged duration and amplitude in excess of 10 mV. Whether these differences in collateral reinnervation have predictive prognostic value in those studied early in the first year of life is unknown.

A peculiar rhythmic spontaneous activity of motor units has been described in earlier reports (Buchthal and Olsen, 1970; Hausmanowa-Petrusewicz and Karwanska, 1986). This activity, which persists through sleep, ranges between 5 and 15 Hz and differs from fasciculations in that they are rhythmic, persist for hours, and can be activated by voluntary effort. This activity has not been the subject of much inquiry since the 1980s and generally has not had diagnostic usefulness. Its biological significance is unknown.

Obligate carriers of SMA generally have normal EMG studies, but there are some reports of group differences. This may be more apparent in mothers than in fathers (Emery et al., 1973).

Muscle biopsy is dominated by features of denervation. In more severely affected infants, the biopsy is characterized by vast numbers of small muscle fibers with a separate, sparser population of large and very large muscle fibers (Brooke and Engel, 1969). Unlike denervating conditions in adults, the small muscle fibers in childhood SMA patients are rounded, not angular, in cross section. The small fibers are marked by histochemical properties characteristic of type I, type II, and intermediate forms. The hypertrophic fibers are generally type I. The small fibers appear to remain small with development, rarely exceeding 10 to 12 μm in diameter, whereas the large fibers outpace normal developmental growth to reach sometimes massive sizes (Buchthal and Olsen, 1970). In biopsy specimens from severe infantile SMA, the large fibers often coalesce but many small fibers are intercalated, suggesting again that the capacity for collateral reinnervation is limited. Widespread muscle fiber atrophy will increase the ratio of connective to con-

tractile tissue, but this proportionate increase is not a measure of ongoing connective tissue proliferation. Muscle spindles are abundant for the same reason. The architecture within fibers is not disrupted, although occasional nemaline bodies can be seen, a feature that is common in denervated muscle (Konno et al., 1987).

In contrast with severely affected infants, the muscle biopsy of intermediate and mildly affected individuals with SMA may be less distinctive. The most common feature is type grouping, sometimes with entire fascicles displaying a single fiber type.

Most neuropathological studies in SMA have been on a limited number of specimens from poorly characterized patients and usually concentrate on a single issue (Crawford and Pardo, 1996). Nonetheless, the general findings on pathology are well accepted from widespread experience. The principal finding is the paucity of motor neurons in the spinal cord and lower brainstem. Many of the remaining motor neurons have a normal appearance, but a minority have a chromatolytic appearance, with swelling of the perikarya, dispersion of the Nissel substance, and lateral displacement and indenting of the nucleus. The cytoplasm of these "ballooned" neurons is characterized by clumps of vesicular or membranous bodies with adjacent accumulation of neurofilaments (Chou and Fakadej, 1971; Murayama et al., 1991). Immunocytochemical studies of these cells have shown concentrations of phosphorylated neurofilaments, which are usually excluded from the perikaryon and ubiquitination of the central region of the neurons (Kato and Hirano, 1990; Lippa and Smith, 1988; Murayama et al., 1991; Matsumoto et al., 1993).

Although motor neuron pathology dominates, in the most severely affected infants abnormalities are regularly found in other regions as well (Devriendt et al., 1997). In these early-onset and short-lived infants, chromatolytic neurons can be found within the sensory neurons of the dorsal root ganglion, with associated degeneration within the sensory root (Marshall and Duchen, 1975; Carpenter et al., 1978; Korinthenberg et al., 1997), the posteroventral or ventrolateral thalamus, Clarke's column, and other scattered and widespread regions (Marshall and Duchen, 1975; Towfighi et al., 1985; Peress et al., 1986; Murayama et al., 1991). The significance of these more subtle findings is not clear but suggests that the primary defect of SMA, although highly concentrated in the large motor neurons, is not exclusive to these cells.

Clinical Course

The outcome of SMA depends greatly on the severity of weakness. Mortality rates for severely affected infants are very high, with rates of 75% and 95% by the first and second birthdays, respectively (Ignatius, 1994; Thomas and Dubowitz, 1994; Zerres et al., 1997). Infants generally develop respiratory insufficiency, with either progressive atelectasis or aspiration pneumonitis due to difficulty in clearing the airway. Quite often, otherwise minor upper respiratory illnesses can be fatal. Those with milder forms of SMA survive longer. The average life span of individuals with SMA type 3 is unknown, but certainly individual survival times can be near normal. The life span of individuals with SMA type 2 was once widely reported to be limited to school years, but it is now recognized that survival and functional ability are closely linked to the vigor of palliative treatment. There are a large number of adults with SMA type 2, and their numbers and average age are likely to continue increasing.

For all but the most mildly affected individuals, the clinical course of SMA is quite different from that usually associated with a degenerative disease. Except in the mildly affected type 3 (or type 4) individuals (Carter et al., 1995), children lose muscle power and function most dramatically at the outset of the disease. With the passage of time, residual muscle power stabilizes and may even slightly improve (Souchon et al., 1999), potentially for many years or even decades (Dubowitz, 1964, 1995). This is in marked contrast to the relentlessly progressive decline that characterizes amyotrophic lateral sclerosis or more widespread neurodegenerative disorders of both children and adults. An important distinction, however, is that functional abilities decline more than does muscle power (Russman et al., 1992, 1996; Iannaccone et al., 2000). Increases in weight, size, or deformity may compromise function even while power measured in a gravity-neutral plane remains unchanged. This tendency of increasing the stability of muscle power with the passage of time is characteristic across the range of SMAs, although a caveat applies to infants with severe weakness. Because of rapid loss, the diagnosis of SMA is often made during the declining phase of disorder, and further deterioration may continue after diagnosis. Even here, different regions of the body have a more stable course than others. At the time of diagnosis, chest and bulbar innervated muscles may be near normal but thereafter weaken further, whereas the limbs that are already enfeebled at the time of diagnosis maintain about the same amount of profoundly diminished power over time.

In contrast to the relative stability of muscle power over time, many children with SMA lose functional abilities. There is no single explanation for this. There are, however, numerous complications of prolonged weakness that can have the effect of placing an additional burden on the performance of tasks. These complications, including scoliosis, secondary lung disease, obesity, malnutrition, limb deformity, and acquired pressure neuropathies, are often partially treatable or preventable and thus should be a major focus of therapy. How much of a long-term decline in function is due to these or other acquired complications and how much is due to progression of the underlying disease are unknown in individual cases. For the disorder as a whole, it is a concern of major research interest, because evaluation of the effect of any proposed specific therapy will have to accommodate these secondary effects.

Genetics

The causative gene for SMA, *SMN1*, resides in a large 500-kb inverted duplication on chromosome 5q (Lefebvre et al., 1995), which emerged in primate evolution (Rochette et al., 2001). A near-homologous copy, *SMN2*, resides in the adjacent copy of this duplication. This region of chromosome 5 is highly unstable, with multiple variation in copy number, position, and orientation of a number of markers between individuals. An intricate, and ultimately perverse, interplay at multiple levels between *SMN1* and *SMN2* is responsible for the appearance of SMA.

Absence, or intragenic mutation, of *SMN1* on both alleles is the sine qua non of SMA at the DNA level. In contrast, up to 5% of normal individuals are lacking *SMN2* (Lefebvre et al., 1995), apparently without consequence. *SMN2* is transcriptionally active, and it codes for an intact SMN protein identical to that produced by *SMN1*. The difference in the two is at the level of post-transcriptional modification. Because of a single translationally silent "wobble" base-pair change in exon 7 that alters post-transcriptional splicing (Lorson et al., 1999), most *SMN2* transcripts are missing exons 7 and 8 (Gennarelli et al., 1995). A small amount, perhaps 10%, of full-length *SMN2* mRNA, and presumably normal SMN protein, is made from *SMN2*.

SMN is constitutively expressed in all cells, and homozygous deletion of the single *SMN* gene in mice is lethal at the earliest stages of embryogenesis (Schrank et al., 1997). Similarly, although one would expect by chance that some individuals with SMA would be missing both *SMN1* and *SMN2*, no such individuals are found. Instead, there is a relationship between copy number of *SMN2* and severity of SMA (Wirth, 2000). Many affected infants have two or, sometimes in severely affected infants, only one copy of *SMN2*. Most individuals with SMA type 2 or 3 have three or more copies of *SMN2*. This relationship between copy number of human *SMN2* and severity of phenotype has been reproduced in transgenic mouse models (Monani et al., 2000). Thus, it appears that the small amount of full-length transcript that arises from the mostly aberrantly spliced *SMN2* has the effect of regulating the severity of SMA. The absence of any full-length *SMN* transcript, which occurs with the deletion of both *SMN1* and *SMN2*, is lethal in early embryonic development. Small amounts of full-length *SMN* transcript, which can be produced by a single or two copies of *SMN2*, are compatible with survival throughout gestation but manifest with severe weakness at, or just after, the time of birth. Greater amounts of full-length *SMN* transcript, from increasing copy number of *SMN2*, manifest in progressively milder forms of the disorder.

SMN2 is thus responsible for allowing the fetus with homozygous deletion of *SMN1* to survive gestation and to be born apparently normal, only to manifest a motoneuron disease later in postnatal development. In a second example of intricate perversity, *SMN2* is also apparently responsible for many of the mutations that damage *SMN1* in the first place. Two forms of mutation of *SMN1* predominate. The first is a simple deletion mutation, in which the entire *SMN1* gene is lost. The other is a conversion mutation, in which the *SMN1* gene assumes the sequence of the *SMN2* homologue during meiosis, presumably through errant sister-chromatid or intrachromosomal pairing of the duplicated regions of DNA that contain *SMN1* and *SMN2*, followed by mismatch "repair" of the sequence differences in these segments that converts the *SMN1* gene sequence to that of *SMN2*. The result is a chromosome with *SMN1* copy number reduced by one and a corresponding increase in *SMN2* copy number by one. Because copy number of *SMN2* has a role in determining disease severity, deletion mutations are associated with more severe forms of SMA, whereas conversion mutations, with the increase in *SMN2* copy number, are associated with milder forms (Burghes, 1997).

Diagnosis

In many cases, the phenotypic appearance of SMA with symmetrical, diffuse, and lower more than upper limb weakness and muscle atrophy; associated signs of reduced motor unit numbers; and absence of other neurological or systemic abnormalities is sufficiently distinctive that the diagnosis can be strongly suspected on clinical grounds alone. In such instances, confirmation of the diagnosis by testing for the presence or absence of the *SMN1* gene is highly sensitive, specific, cost efficient, and easily tolerated by children and parents alike. In circumstances where the phenotype is not distinctive or where DNA testing did not confirm the diagnosis despite strong clinical suspicion, additional electrodiagnostic and anatomic testing may be warranted.

Some affected infants and children may have features of weakness without all of the characteristic signs of motor unit depletion or with additional features not usually associated with SMA. In this instance, the demonstration of neuropathic features in a clinically weak muscle may be sufficient to raise the pretest likelihood to a sufficient level that the *SMN* gene test could be the sole additional test that is ordered. Alternatively, myopathic features on EMG would redirect the diagnostic focus away from the *SMN* gene test to muscle biopsy. The case for conducting EMG must be individualized, balancing the burden of EMG (pain and cost) against the burden of not conducting EMG (morbidity, cost and discomfort of excess tests, and prolongation of the evalua-

tion). In many cases, a limited electromyographic evaluation by an investigator who is mindful of this balance is easily justified.

The alternative situation, in which a high clinical suspicion is not confirmed by DNA testing, similarly justifies electromyographic evaluation but with a different balance of concerns. Up to 5% of patients with true *SMN*-associated SMA will not have the characteristic loss of the *SMN1* exon 7 and 8 sequence. These patients presumably have small deletions or base substitution mutations in other portions of the gene not detected by the polymerase chain reaction–based DNA test. Present technology does not allow for easy evaluation of the gene through sequencing, because it is very labor intensive to distinguish the sequence obtained from *SMN1* from that obtained from *SMN2*. However, to date, the described intragenic mutations that disable *SMN1* but are not seen on the routine test of SMA are relatively few. This suggests that identification of one of these known intragenic mutations may someday become routine when the standard polymerase chain reaction test is normal.

Until that time, however, the diagnosis of SMA in this small group of patients with a normal *SMN* DNA test reverts back to the time-tested studies of EMG and muscle biopsy. If SMA is suspected, yet the DNA test for *SMN* is normal, neurophysiological tests must be conducted meticulously. One needs to look for symmetry and diffuseness of neuropathic involvement while being certain that evidence of possible dysmyelinating or axonal congenital neuropathy is not present. Precise demonstration of a normal sensory nerve action potential (SNAP) in a nerve in which compound motor action potential amplitude is clearly reduced is an important confirmatory finding to rule out a congenital neuropathy. In these cases, sural nerve and/or muscle biopsy is appropriate. At present, the association of classic clinical, electromyographic, and muscle biopsy features is strong evidence supporting the diagnosis of SMA even in the absence of an abnormal *SMN* gene test result. Whether this triad is of sufficient certainty to permit the use of linkage data in prenatal diagnosis of siblings in such cases is controversial; such cases should probably be referred to centers specializing in the complexities of SMA genetics and clinical characterization for more detailed evaluation.

OTHER SPINAL MUSCULAR ATROPHIES

In its broadest connotation, *spinal muscular atrophy* infers a heritable disorder most prominently characterized by depletion of motor neurons. A wide array of such heritable disorders of the motor neuron exist, ranging in distinctiveness from well-characterized monogenic disorders to single cases without unique features. Not surprisingly, their classification is not easy. An ideal classification would be broadly applicable and have meaningful predictive value for each individual. To date, various classification schemes have centered on features such as age of onset, clinical course, distribution of muscle weakness, associated signs and symptoms, and mode of inheritance, and even genetic linkage to known chromosomal loci have advantages for some disorders but fail for others. Nonetheless, various combinations of these features have limited prognostic, genetic, or therapeutic predictive value for some individuals with an SMA syndrome, and even an inadequate classification is a necessary point of departure for later advances. Faulty as it is, a summary of genetic and presumed genetic disorders of the motor neuron roughly ordered by nosological integrity is given in Table 87–1.

Although heterogeneous, the diagnosis of SMA implies a disorder that is chiefly related to primary motor neuron pathology. Hence, all of the SMA syndromes manifest certain common features. Among these are weakness, muscle atrophy, and, in many cases, a fine tremor in the tongue or outstretched fingers, suggesting motor unit expansion in these regions. In most cases, the term *spinal muscular atrophy* is applied to symmetrical disorders. Weakness is the cardinal sign of motor neuron depletion and degeneration, but the early expression of weakness with chronic motor neuron depletion can be masked by residual motor unit expansion through axonal sprouting and muscle fiber hypertrophy.

Certain characteristics of a disorder weigh against the use of "SMA" as a label, because they imply a larger neurodegenerative disorder, of which motor neuronopathy is only a small part. These exclusionary features include signs, symptoms, or laboratory evidence of sensory neuropathy or neuronopathy; features of upper motor neuron degeneration; extrapyramidal or cerebellar motor impairment; and other prominent features of hemispheric dysfunction, such as seizures or dementia. It is important to emphasize that in the medical literature (and reflected in Table 87–1) authors ignore these exclusionary features and use the SMA label in a highly idiosyncratic manner.

The most important investigations to demonstrate a motor neuronopathy are EMG and nerve conduction studies. EMG must demonstrate "neuropathic" markedly reduced recruitment of voluntary motor unit potentials. These motor unit potentials are primarily of large amplitude with prolonged duration or normal sized, or even occasionally small and of short duration. These motor unit potentials may be either normal in configuration or polyphasic, depending on the ability of residual motor units to expand in the face of neighboring denervation. Spontaneous fibrillation and positive sharp wave potentials also may or may not be present, depending on the amount of denervation and on the timing of loss. Motor nerve conduction velocity must be in the normal range or only modestly reduced when compound motor action potential amplitude is substantially reduced. When there is a pattern of regional

denervation that could possibly be explained by multiple motor neuropathies, particularly when EMG shows minimal abnormal spontaneous activity, possible multiple motor nerve conduction block should be excluded specifically. Most importantly, normal sensory nerve studies are required for the diagnosis.

Differential Diagnosis

In the child with possible SMA, diagnostic considerations extend across the spectrum of neuromuscular and neuromotor disorders. The most common differential concern is for polyneuropathy, which is generally distinguished clinically from the SMAs by distal predominance and involvement of sensory as well as motor nerves. "Distal" forms of SMA cannot be clinically distinguished from heritable neuropathies without sensory nerve conduction studies. Another frequent diagnostic consideration is multilevel polyradiculopathy, which can be difficult or impossible to distinguish from motor neuronopathy by EMG and nerve conduction studies alone. In settings where the distribution and timing of weakness and electrophysiological abnormalities cannot exclude multiple radiculopathy, careful investigation with magnetic resonance imaging or metrizamide computed tomography myelography, cerebrospinal fluid examination, and somatosensory evoked responses can be helpful. In some rare cases, multilevel radiculopathy and SMA cannot be resolved on the basis of clinical studies. Various forms of myopathy may appear similar to motor neuron disorders but are usually easily distinguished by electrophysiological and pathological features. Heritable and acquired disorders of the neuromuscular junction are rarely confused with motor neuronopathy and usually can be differentiated by appropriate electrophysiological studies.

With the exception of classic *SMN*-associated SMA X-linked spinal and bulbar muscular atrophy (Kennedy's disease, of which to date no cases have been reported in infants or children), and the very rare infantile disorder spinal muscular atrophy with respiratory distress (SMARD1), there are no confirmatory tests that allow for identification of a specific diagnostic entity in a single affected individual. This is likely to change quickly, as the responsible genes for the disorders with a distinct phenotype that have an assigned chromosomal location may well be found soon. The reader is advised to consult the National Library of Medicine–supported Online Mendelian Inheritance of Man catalog OMIM (http://www3.ncbi.nlm.nih.gov/omim/) for up-to-date information on the state of these and, perhaps, other newly defined categories of SMA.

The diagnostic evaluation of a child or an infant with a motor neuron disorder starts with the history, physical examination, and electrophysiological studies to localize the source of weakness to the motor neuron. Testing for homozygous deletion of

Table 87–1. Lower Motor Neuron Syndromes

MIM No.	Inheritance	Title (Synonyms)	Linkage	Gene	Onset, Course	Distinguishing Features, Comments
Confirmed monogenic disorders						
253300, 253550, 253400	AR	SMA (SMA 1, 2, 3) (Werdnig-Hoffmann disease) (juvenile muscular atropy) (Kugelberg-Welander disease)	5q12.2-q13.3	*SMN*	SMA 1, infantile SMA 2, late infantile SMA 3, childhood through adult (also SMA 4)	Symmetrical, diffuse, subtle caudal-to-cranial gradient of weakness
313200	X	X-linked spinobulbar muscular atrophy (Kennedy's disease)	Xq11-q12		Adult, progressive	Gynecomastia, infertility, neuropathy
604320	AR	SMA with respiratory distress (SMARD1) (distal SMA type VI)	11q13-q21	*IGHMBP2*	Infantile, progressive	Prominent early respiratory muscle weakness
Presumed monogenic disorders (with distinctive semiology)						
301830, 300021	X	Distal X-linked arthrogryposis multiplex congenita (infantile X-linked SMA)	Xp11.3-q11.2		Congenital, progressive	Males, congenital joint deformity
600794	AD	Distal SMA with upper limb predominance (distal SMA type V)	7p		Late teens	Radial aspect of hand, spread to distal lower extremities
Syndromes of less certain nosology						
Diffuse or with caudal to cranial gradient						
600091, 182980, 158600	AD	Dominant proximal SMA (juvenile SMA)			Heterogeneous	Phenotype similar to *SMN*-associated SMA
271150	AR	Proximal SMA			Adult, progressive	Phenotype similar to *SMN*-associated SMA
271200	AR	SMA, Ryukyan type			Infantile, progressive	Kyphoscoliosis and pes cavus; whether separate from *SMN*-associated SMA is unknown
Distal SMA syndromes						
271120	AR	Distal SMA (distal SMA III) (distal SMA IV)			Childhood	Distally predominant denervation and weakness
182960	AD	Distal SMA type I (distal hereditary motor neuropathy)			Juvenile	Distally predominant denervation and weakness
158590	AD	Distal SMA type II (distal hereditary motor neuropathy) (SMA IV [this title is also used by some for adult-onset *SMN*-associated SMA])	Heterogeneous 12q24 (one kindred)		Adult, progressive	Distally predominant denervation and weakness; rapidly progressive in some—in these, phenotype indistinguishable from sporadic, progressive muscular atrophy form of ALS
158580	AD	Distal SMA with vocal cord paralysis (distal SMA type VII) (distal myopathy with vocal cord and pharyngeal muscular atrophy) (distal myopathy 2) (hereditary motor and sensory neuropathy type IIc)	5q31		Adult	Probably heterogeneous, distinction from MPD 1 (distal myopathy without vocal cord paralysis and a form of heritable motor and sensory neuropathy) is unclear

(Continued)

Table 87–1. (Continued)

MIM No.	Inheritance	Title (Synonyms)	Linkage	Gene	Onset, Course	Distinguishing Features, Comments
Spinal (segmental forms)						
	AR	Cervical spinal muscular atrophy			Infancy, progressive	Cranial to caudal distribution, prominent head ptosis, respiratory insufficiency[38]
	Sporadic	Congenital cervical spinal atrophy			Infancy, nonprogressive	Arthrogryposis of upper extremities, may be segmental developmental defect of cervical spinal cord[26]
158650	AR	Malignant neurogenic muscular atrophy			Adult, rapidly progressive	Indistinguishable from sporadic progressive muscular atrophy form of ALS
182970	AR	SMA, facioscapulohumeral type			Early adult, progressive	Whether distinct from FSH muscular dystrophy (MIM 158900) not clear
181405	AD	Neurogenic scapuloperoneal amyotrophy	12q24.1-q24.31 (one kindred)			Single described kindred with congenital absence of muscles, progressive scapuloperoneal atrophy, laryngeal palsy, progressive distal weakness, and atrophy
271220	AR	SMA with scapuloperoneal distribution			Childhood	
600175	AD	Congenital nonprogressive SMA of lower limbs	Heterogeneous, 12q23-q24 (one kindred)		Congenital	
Bulbar predominance with or without other cranial nerve involvement						
211500	AR (AD)	Progressive bulbar palsy of childhood (Fazio-Londe disease)			Childhood, progressive	Cranial to caudal, sparing EOMs; original case of Fazio had AD inheritance
157900	AD	Moebius syndrome (MBS1)	13q12.2-q13, sporadic		Congenital, nonprogressive	Symmetrical neurogenic defect of cranial nerves VII and VI with or without XII dysfunction, often with musculoskeletal anomalies
601471	AD	Moebius syndrome (MBS2)	3q21-q22, sporadic		Congenital, nonprogressive	Asymmetrical neurogenic defect of cranial nerve VII dysfunction
604185	AD	Moebius syndrome (MBS3)	10q21.3-q22.1, sporadic		Congenital, nonprogressive	Asymmetrical neurogenic defect of cranial nerve VII dysfunction, often with hearing loss, incomplete genetic penetrance
211530	Both AR and AD kindreds	Progressive bulbar palsy with deafness (Vialetto-van Laere syndrome) (Overlap with Madras-type motor neuron disease 48:86)			Juvenile, progressive	Early progressive deafness, bulbar weakness spreading caudally
Other forms						
605726	AR	SMA, Jerash type	9p21.1-p12		Childhood, progressive	With pyramidal signs
271110, 271109	AR	SMA with mental subnormality, with or without microcephaly	Probably heterogeneous		Infant, progressive	

Table 87–1. (Continued)

MIM No.	Inheritance	Title (Synonyms)	Linkage	Gene	Onset, Course	Distinguishing Features, Comments
	AR	SMA with pontocerebellar hypoplasia (PCH-1)	Not 5q21		Congenital, progressive	Severe cerebellar malformation; often more widespread neuropathology; phenotype may vary within kindreds 4;37;68
208100	AR	Neurogenic arthrogryposis multiplex congenita	Heterogeneous, 5q35 (one kindred)		Congenital, nonprogressive	Deformity of elbows, knees, and feet
159950	AD	Hereditary myoclonus with progressive distal muscular atrophy	Single family		Young adult, slowly progressive	Myoclonus and distal weakness at outset, dementia in 60s

Other defined disorders with prominent motor neuron degeneration

MIM No.	Inheritance	Title (Synonyms)	Linkage	Gene	Onset, Course	Distinguishing Features, Comments
272800	AR	Hexosaminidase A deficiency (Tay-Sachs disease variant)	15q23-q24	HEXA	Juvenile or adult, progressive	Dementia, spinocerebellar ataxia 49;50;72
308300	X dominant	Incontinentia pigmenti (IP2) (Block-Sulzberger syndrome)	Xq28	NEMO	Infantile	Females only (males presumed to be embryonic lethal); SMA sporadic[54]
208900	AR	Ataxia telangiectasia	11q22.3	ATM	Childhood, progressive	Motor neuronopathy reported in late stages[1]
210200, 210210	AR	3-Methylcrotonyl coenzyme A carboxylase deficiency (types 1 and 2)	3q25-127, 5q12-q13	MCCA, MCCB	Infancy, childhood; heterogeneous	Hypotonia, seizures, acidosis; widely heterogeneous
158500	AD	Muscular atrophy with ataxia, retinitis pigmentosa, and diabetes mellitus			Young adult, progressive	Similar phenotype to Refsum's except for the AD inheritance pattern

For entries with an MIM designation number, extensive reference listing can be obtained at http://www3.ncbi.nlm.nih.gov/omim.
AR, autosomal recessive; X, X-linked; AD, autosomal dominant; SMA, spinal muscular atrophy; SMN, survival motoneuron; ALS, amyotrophic lateral sclerosis; EOM, extraocular movements; FSH, facio-scapulo-humeral.

the *SMN* gene is appropriate in most cases of a symmetrical degeneration because of the wide range of expression of classic SMA and the potential that it is associated with a second disorder, confusing the presentation. Testing for the Kennedy syndrome expansion is appropriate in adults but is not necessary in infants or children. Most adult-onset cases require testing for hexosaminidase A, and all unexplained cases should have an assessment of soluble metabolism, in particular with review of the profile of excreted organic acids or the profile of acylcarnitine species. A carefully G-banded karyotype may identify novel chromosomal breaks and translocations that may be worthwhile in the targeting of new areas for potential linkage.

OTHER DISORDERS OF THE MOTOR NEURON

The eventual development of specific genetic tests is first built on the enterprise of clustering patients into distinguishable, coherent groups on the basis of their clinical features. Within the broad group of disorders that can be considered forms of SMA, these features tend to be based on the region of the body most affected, the age of onset, the pattern of progression, the association of other neurological or systemic abnormalities, and, where possible, the pattern of inheritance.

Among the SMA disorders singled out by selective regional involvement, two eponymous syndromes have defied genetic exegesis, likely because of their extreme rarity and usually sporadic occurrence. Whether they are indeed single nosological entities of a genetic nature is yet to be established. Fazio-Londe disease is a progressive disorder of children that affects first the mid to lower brainstem myotomes and in general spares the extraocular muscles. Most cases are sporadic, but a few sibling pairs are known, and one mother-daughter kindred suggests the possibility of a dominantly inherited disorder (Gomez et al., 1962; Benjamins, 1980). Onset occurs in childhood, and the course is generally progressive (Alexander et al., 1976).

The other eponymous disorder, "Moebius syndrome," is classically thought of as a congenital, symmetrical, nonprogressive motor neuronopathy of the facial and abducens nuclei, with the possible involvement of bulbar motor nuclei as well. Although dominant inheritance has been reported in some (leading to an assigned chromosomal map location for these patients, who may also have aplasia of isolated muscles), most cases are sporadic. The incidence of the disorder is too low to know whether these sporadic cases have a new dominant mutation, a possible genetic disorder with a different inheritance pattern, or a nongenetic disorder of brainstem development. The name *Moebius syndrome* has been appropriated for two additional disorders. The first (MBS2) is characterized by isolated asymmetrical facial weakness that can be distinguished from congenital facial nerve dysgenesis (congenital Bell's palsy) only by the dominant inheritance pattern in the family. The other (MBS3) is characterized by asymmetrical facial weakness and, frequently, deafness. This syndrome is also known to manifest with dominant inheritance in some kindreds but with incomplete penetrance of the mutant gene. Here also, prediction of genetic risk for first-degree relatives of an isolated case is problematic.

Another disorder defined by regional weakness that affects infants, known as spinal muscular atrophy with respiratory distress (SMARD1), has recently led to identification of the causative gene *IGHMBP2* (Grohmann et al., 2001). In direct contrast to the infantile form of *SMN*-associated SMA, the diaphragm is most significantly affected, whereas in the more common form of infantile SMA, the diaphragm is relatively spared. This form of SMA is relentlessly progressive, with death due to respiratory insufficiency in the weeks or months after diagnosis.

The various congenital cervical SMA syndromes are difficult to sort out and particularly difficult to classify appropriately compared with the well-defined variant syndromes of SMA. Three infants were evaluated in the neonatal period on the basis of hypotonia and atrophy confined to the arms and hands with otherwise normal neurological function (Darwish et al., 1981). There was no history to suggest cervical cord injury at birth. Associated findings of flexion contractures with a transverse palmar crease suggested a first trimester congenital insult (Darwish et al., 1981). Motor nerve conduction studies were normal. The EMG performed in one child during the first 2 weeks of life demonstrated fibrillation potentials present in the deltoid and triceps muscles, but none were found in the facial and lower extremity muscles. In the other two infants, EMG was performed after the age of 1 year. Although no comment was made about motor unit potentials per se with initial EMG, a repeat analysis at the age of 14 months demonstrated larger motor unit potentials with an incomplete recruitment. These abnormalities were limited to the upper extremities (Darwish et al., 1981). This combination of findings, in keeping with the normal clinical sensory examination, was compatible with a focal idiopathic motor neuronopathy at the level of the cervical spinal cord. These cases were reported in 1981, before the availability of DNA testing, so it is not possible to comment on the genetic findings, if there were any. (We studied a similar case at the Children's Hospital Boston).

Distal SMA, which probably is the most well known form of regional SMA syndrome, is heterogeneous in origin. Various distal forms of SMA may be responsible for up to 10% of cases of SMA in a population-based survey in northeastern England (Pearn and Hudgson, 1979). Without neurophysiological testing, these entities can be clinically similar to heritable axonal neuropathies and are reported under the label "spinal form of Charcot-Marie-Tooth syndrome." Harding (1993) identified seven types of distal SMA, of which four have proved sufficiently distinctive and common or have affected enough individuals of a single large kindred to achieve genetic linkage. An adult-onset, dominantly inherited, rapidly progressive distal SMA (Harding distal SMA type 2) has been linked to chromosome 12q24 in one kindred, a dominantly inherited juvenile form with initial expression in the upper extremities (Harding distal SMA type V) has been linked to chromosome 7p in multiple kindreds, a severe infantile progressive form (Harding distal SMA type VI) is now known as SMARD1 (chromosome 11q13-q21), and an adult-onset form with prominent early vocal cord paralysis (Harding distal SMA type VII) has been linked in a single large kindred to chromosome 5q31. Unfortunately, without the advantage of a positive family history, none of these disorders are sufficiently distinct on clinical grounds alone to permit a knowledgeable assessment of genetic risk. For the most part, distal forms of SMA are associated with a slowly progressive or nonprogressive course. The exception tends to be those of early onset, where progression is more common. In those with a distal SMA phenotype of congenital onset, however, distal amyotrophy may represent a nongenetic focal myelodysplasia and have a nonprogressive course.

There exists in somewhat older children an overlapping progressive disorder, commonly known as either "segmental cervical SMA" or "juvenile muscular atrophy of the distal upper extremity." This was originally described in Japan by Hirayama and associates (1963) and later by Sobue and colleagues (1978). This focal amyotrophy has been recognized in Western countries (Oryema et al., 1990; Liu and Specht, 1993). It is generally a sporadic disorder that primarily occurs in males aged 15 to 25 years (Hirayama et al., 1963; Sobue et al., 1978; Oryema et al., 1990; Liu and Specht, 1993). It may or may not be a forme fruste of SMARD1, but the unilaterality of symptoms is phenotypically distinct from the generally symmetrical involvement seen with the SMA syndromes. These patients typically present with unilateral weakness and atrophy of the fingers and hand muscles. After an initial progression of weakness in the primarily affected arm and hand and sometimes, to a lesser degree, its contralateral homologue, the clinical course usually stabilizes within 5 to 7 years. Important considerations in the differential diagnosis include juvenile amyotrophic lateral sclerosis, poliomyelitis, and syringomyelia. The prognosis for this form of segmental SMA is relatively benign, as it usually remains limited to the cervical cord, although occasionally, in India, it has been reported to predominantly affect the lumbar sacral segments (Gouri-Devi et al., 1984). The outside possibility of a multifocal motor conduction block was excluded with each of the few cases we have seen at The Children's Hospital Boston. To date, we are unaware of multifocal motor neuropathy occurring in children.

Although amyotrophic lateral sclerosis is very rare in children and adolescents, this illness also needs consideration in the evaluation of a child or an adolescent with a progressive, indeterminate motor neuronopathy. One rapidly evolving case involved a 12-year-old girl who initially developed paralysis of the arm that soon progressed to quadriparesis (Nelson and Prensky, 1972). EMG demonstrated diffuse fibrillation potentials and fasciculations. She died within 1 year. Autopsy demonstrated widespread motor neuronal cytoplasmic inclusions (Nelson and Prensky, 1972). In another instance, a 7-year-old girl initially had difficulties in keeping up with her peers (Grunnet and Donaldson, 1985). Her neurological examination at the age of 11 years demonstrated bilateral Babinski signs and pes cavus. Weakness developed by age 12, and she needed a wheelchair when she was in her 20s. Bulbar involvement led to death when she was in her 30s. At autopsy, eosinophilic cytoplasmic inclusions were present in the few remaining anterior horn cells and brainstem motor nuclei (Grunnet and Donaldson, 1985). In a review of 123 patients with amyotrophic lateral sclerosis, only one, a 17-year-old girl, had the onset of disease before the age of 20 years (Dantes and McComas, 1991). One of the authors (H.R.J.) evaluated a 19-year-old woman with 6 to 12 months of progressive arm weakness. EMG demonstrated a severe motor neurogenic process. She died within 18 months of onset; autopsy revealed typical amyotrophic lateral sclerosis.

Poliomyelitis must always be considered in the setting of a focal or asymmetrical muscle weakness with associated atrophy. Pediatric neuromuscular specialists and electromyographers occasionally evaluate a child who has an "unexplained," isolated extremity weakness. It is important to ascertain the child's poliomyelitis vaccination history as well as geographic origins. Children who immigrate from countries without modern immunization technology or who live in families who do not believe in routine immunizations may present with a poorly defined focal loss of muscle strength. EMG demonstrates low-amplitude compound motor action potentials, relatively normal motor conduction velocity, and sensory nerve action potentials. There is a marked diminution in the number of motor unit potentials. These motor unit potentials are usually enlarged, in both amplitude and duration. An acute form of postvaccinial poliomyelitis is only rarely seen during infancy.

Rarely, an acute, flaccid, asymmetrical weakness develops in children 4 to 7 days after the occurrence of an acute asthmatic attack, even though these children have had earlier poliomyelitis vaccine (Hopkins, 1974). This is usually associated with a mild cerebrospinal fluid pleocytosis. Nerve conduction studies and needle EMG demonstrated normal compound sensory nerve action potentials and severe signs of primary axonal motor neuropathy (Hopkins, 1974; Wheeler and Ochoa, 1980).

Paraneoplastic motor neuron diseases are distinctly uncommon in children as well as in adults.

Progressive bilateral weakness developed in the arms of a 14-year-old girl (Rowland and Schneck, 1963). EMG demonstrated denervation of her arms but no abnormalities of her legs. Her course was quite rapid, and she died within 14 months. At autopsy, cervical, thoracic, and upper lumbar anterior horn cells were almost totally absent, as were neurons in Clark's columns. Both central and peripheral nervous system demyelination were present. Evidence of Hodgkin's disease was found in the mediastinal lymph nodes.

Prominent progressive degeneration of motor neurons is part of a number of neurodegenerative disorders. Specific identification can generally be made on the basis of the associated characteristics. Deficiency of hexosaminidase A has been reported in association with a wide range of features, including dementia, ataxia, psychiatric abnormalities, and a retinal "cherry red spot," extending the clinical expression of Tay-Sachs disease to young adults. The associated features may be sufficiently subtle that determination of hexosaminidase A activity should be a part of the evaluation of any patient with an otherwise unexplained symmetrical progressive motor neuron degeneration.

A progressive motor neuronopathy has been associated with severe pontocerebellar hypoplasia in a number of recessive and sporadic kindreds (Barth, 1993; Gorgen-Pauly et al., 1999; Muntoni et al., 1999). The prognosis is poor, with progressive weakness and often substantial mental subnormality associated with widespread neuropathology. Pontocerebellar hypoplasia with associated SMA has been called PCH-1 by Barth (1993), but the degree of neuropathological involvement may vary within affected sibships (Gorgen-Pauly et al., 1999), raising concern about the validity of this distinction.

Rarely, various myelopathies may simulate forms of SMA. Arteriovenous malformations of the cervical region are another consideration. Transverse myelitis can produce paralysis but is usually easily distinguished by the acute course and the presence of sensory, autonomic, and long tract signs and symptoms and abnormal somatosensory evoked potentials. Electromyographic evidence of denervation may be found in paraspinal muscles at the level of the lesion.

Cervical syringomyelia can selectively affect motoneurons of the anterior horn relatively early in its progression, producing slowly progressive muscle weakness and wasting. Such patients usually have a demonstrable, suspended sensory deficit to pinprick and temperature because of the decussation of sensory fibers immediately anterior to the expanding fluid cavity that ruptures out of the central canal. Syringomyelia most often occurs at the cervicothoracic junction, producing selective hand weakness that could mimic distal SMA of the upper extremity. EMG of the lower cervical paraspinal muscles should be abnormal, however, because of the location of their respective motor neurons, immediately adjacent to the expanding cavity.

Occasionally, pediatric electromyographers evaluate floppy newborn infants who are found to be quadriparetic secondary to an unsuspected spinal injury at birth. These infants have had no return of motor function at the time of their pediatric electromyographic study. One of these infants seen at the Children's Hospital Boston appeared to lack sensation. Subsequent somatosensory evoked potential testing demonstrated no transmission below C5. Myelography and cerebral computed tomography results were normal. In this instance, nerve conduction studies were normal for median sensory nerve action potentials and for peroneal and median nerve conduction velocity and compound motor action potentials. However, needle EMG demonstrated only rare, rapidly firing motor unit potentials in muscles with C5 innervation. In contrast, there were normal motor unit potentials at C7-8, L4, and S1 myotomes. Similarly, at the Children's Hospital Boston, we evaluated another infant with denervation confined to the lower extremities. This child also had normal conduction parameters compatible with a lumbosacral cord injury. The mechanism of this spinal cord lesion was not defined.

Umbilical artery catheterization complications are another very rare consideration in the differential diagnosis of a neonate with floppy legs or even a sciatic nerve injury (Muñoz et al., 1993). Two newborn infants with acute respiratory distress required umbilical artery catheterization. The catheter in the first instance was shown radiographically to be initially at the T7 level. Five days later, the catheter had moved to the T11 level. Shortly thereafter, this baby became paraplegic, with associated loss of sensory function below T11. The other infant was catheterized through the umbilical artery at the age of 7 days. Flaccid paraplegia developed shortly thereafter from L1-2 down. Both infants had persistent paraplegia at the ages of 18 to 30 months (Muñoz et al., 1993). An electromyographic study indicated diffuse denervation of all muscles below T7 and L3, respectively (Muñoz et al., 1993). No tibial somatosensory evoked potentials were elicited. Magnetic resonance imaging 3 to 10 months later in the two infants demonstrated cord atrophy from T6-10 to L2. No other causes of acute paraplegia were found in these infants (Muñoz et al., 1993). In both infants, the paraplegia was thought to be secondary to a thromboembolic occlusion of the vascular supply of the spinal cord secondary to the umbilical artery catheterization. Possibly, the catheter was inadvertently placed near to or obstructed the artery of Adamkiewicz (or both). These two cases point to the need to be alert to this potential unusual mechanism for paraplegia when evaluating for weakness any newborn who has had an umbilical artery catheterization.

It is important to always search for the history of an acute spinal event when making a differential diagnosis of SMA and the clinical syndromes that may be confused with it. Spinal shock after an acute cervical spinal cord injury at birth may produce a flaccid tetraparesis with preservation of active facial expression. This simulates the caudal to rostral distribution of classic infantile *SMN*-associated SMA. EMG can easily distinguish these spinal injury syndromes from SMA. However, other myelopathies also directly affect the anterior horn cells and thus can be indistinguishable from SMA on EMG. Occlusion of the anterior spinal artery will injure anterior horn cells but generally will also affect adjacent spinothalamic tracts, producing associated sensory changes. Infants with severe hypoxic ischemic encephalopathy at birth manifest electrophysiological features of acute denervation and ischemic myelopathy in postmortem specimens, indicating that motoneurons may be affected along with the more diffuse and dramatic cerebral injury (Cobben et al., 1995). Hypotension can produce a border zone infarction of the T4-6 region with associated sensory and motor deficits and denervation of paraspinal muscles at the level of the lesion. Magnetic resonance imaging and somatosensory evoked potentials offer a means to distinguish these lesions.

References

Alexander MP, Emery ES, Koerner FC: Progressive bulbar paresis in childhood. Arch Neurol 1976;33:66–68.

Barth PG: Pontocerebellar hypoplasias: An overview of a group of inherited neurodegenerative disorders with fetal onset. Brain Dev 1993;15:411–422.

Benjamins D: Progressive bulbar palsy of childhood in siblings. Ann Neurol 1980;8:203.

Bingham PM, Shen N, Rennert H, et al: Arthrogryposis due to infantile neuronal degeneration associated with deletion of the SMNt gene. Neurology 1997;49:848–851.

Bouwsma G, Van Wijngaarden GK: Spinal muscular atrophy and hypertrophy of the calves. J Neurol Sci 1980;44:275–279.

Brahe C, Zappata S, Bertini E: Presymptomatic diagnosis of spinal muscular atrophy (SMA) III confirmed by deletion analysis of the survival motor neuron gene. Am J Med Genet 1995;59:101–102.

Brooke MH, Engel WK: The histographic analysis of human muscle biopsies with regard to fiber types: Children's biopsies. Neurology 1969;19:591–605.

Brzustowicz LM, Lehner T, Castilla LH, et al: Genetic mapping of chronic childhood-onset spinal muscular atrophy to chromosome 5q11.2-13. Nature 1990;344:540–541.

Buchthal F, Olsen PZ: Electromyography and muscle biopsy in infantile spinal muscular atrophy. Brain 1970;93:15–30.

Burghes AHM: When is a deletion not a deletion? When it is converted. Am J Hum Genet 1997;61:9–15.

Bürglen L, Amiel J, Viollet L, et al: Survival motor neuron gene deletion in the arthrogryposis multiplex congenita-spinal muscular atrophy association. J Clin Invest 1996;98:1130–1132.

Bürglen L, Spiegel R, Ignatius J, et al: Gene deletion in variant of infantile spinal muscular atrophy. Lancet 1995;346:316–317.

Bussaglia E, Tizzano EF, Illa I, et al: Cramps and minimal EMG abnormalities as preclinical manifestations of spinal muscular atrophy patients with homozygous deletions of the SMN gene. Neurology 1997;48:1443–1445.

Capon F, Levato C, Semprini S, et al: Deletion analysis of SMN and NAIP genes in spinal muscular atrophy Italian families. Muscle Nerve 1996:378–380.

Carpenter S, Karpati G, Rothman S, et al: Pathologic involvement of sensory neurons in Werdnig-Hoffmann disease. Acta Neuropathol 1978;42:91–97.

Carter GT, Abresch RT, Fowler WM, et al: Profiles of neuromuscular diseases: Spinal muscular atrophy. Am J Phys Med Rehabil 1995;74(Suppl):S150–S159.

Chien Y-Y, Nonaka I: Peripheral nerve involvement in Werdnig-Hoffmann disease. Brain Dev 1989;11:221–229.

Chou SM, Fakadej AV: Ultrastructure of chromatolytic motoneurons and anterior spinal roots in a case of Werdnig-Hoffmann disease. J Neuropathol Exp Neurol 1971;30:368–379.

Clancy RR, Sladky JT, Rorke LB: Hypoxic-ischemic spinal cord injury following perinatal asphyxia. Ann Neurol 1989;25:185–189.

Cobben JM, van der Steege G, Grootscholten P, et al: Deletions of the survival motor neuron gene in unaffected siblings of patients with spinal muscular atrophy. Am J Hum Genet 1995;57:805–808.

Coers C, Telerman-Toppet N: Differential diagnosis of limb-girdle muscular dystrophy and spinal muscular atrophy. Neurology 1979;29:957–972.

Crawford TO, Chaudhry V, Sladky JT: Lack of reinnervation in severe infantile spinal muscular atrophy [abstract]. Ann Neurol 1995.

Crawford TO, Pardo CA: The neurobiology of childhood spinal muscular atrophy. Neurobiol Dis 1996;3:97–110.

Dantes M, McComas A: The extent and time course of motoneuron involvement in amyotrophic lateral sclerosis. Muscle Nerve 1991;14:416–421.

Darwish H, Sarnat H, Archer C, et al: Congenital cervical spinal atrophy. Muscle Nerve 1981;4:106–110.

Devriendt K, Lammens M, Schollen E, et al: Clinical and molecular genetic features of congenital spinal muscular atrophy. Ann Neurol 1997;40:731–738.

Dubowitz V: Infantile muscular atrophy: A prospective study with particular reference to a slowly progressive variety. Brain 1964;87:707–718.

Dubowitz V: Muscle Disorders in Childhood, 2nd ed. Philadelphia: WB Saunders, 1995.

Emery AEH, Anderson AR, Noronha MJ: Electromyographic studies in parents of children with spinal muscular atrophy. J Med Genet 1973;10:8–10.

Emery AEH: Population frequencies of inherited neuromuscular diseases—a world summary. Neuromusc Disord 1991;1:19–29.

Feingold J, Arthuis M, Celers J: Genetique de l'amyotrophie spinale infantile: Existence de deux formes autosomiques recessives. Ann Genet 1977;20:19–23.

Fredericks EJ, Russman BS: Bedside evaluation of large motor units in childhood spinal muscular atrophy. Neurology 1979;29:398–400.

Gennarelli M, Lucarelli M, Capon F, et al: Survival motor neuron gene transcript analysis in muscles from spinal muscular atrophy patients. Biochem Biophys Res Commun 1995;213:342–348.

Gilliam TC, Brzustowicz LM, Castilla LH, et al: Genetic homogeneity between acute and chronic forms of spinal muscular atrophy. Nature 1990;345:823–825.

Gomez MR, Clermont V, Bernstein J: Progressive bulbar paralysis in childhood (Fazio-Londe's disease). Arch Neurol 1962;6:323.

Goodman WN, Cooper WC, Kessler GB, et al: Ataxia telangiectasia: A report of two cases in siblings presenting a picture of progressive spinal muscular atrophy. Bull Los Angeles Neurol Soc 1969;34:23–27.

Gorgen-Pauly U, Sperner J, Reiss I, et al: Familial pontocerebellar hypoplasia type I with anterior horn cell disease. Eur J Paediatr Neurol 1999;3:33–38.

Gouri-Devi M, Suresh TG, Shankar SK: Monomelic amyotrophy. Arch Neurol 1984;41:388–394.

Goutières F, Bogicevic D, Aicardi JA: Predominantly cervical form of spinal muscular atrophy. J Neurol Neurosurg Psychiatry 1991;54:223–225.

Grohmann K, Schuelke M, Diers A, et al: Mutations in the gene encoding immunoglobulin mu-binding protein 2 cause spinal muscular atrophy with respiratory distress type 1. Nat Genet 2001;29:75–77.

Grunnet ML, Donaldson JO: Juvenile multisystem degeneration with motor neuron involvement and eosinophilic intracytoplasmic inclusions. Arch Neurol 1985;42:1114–1116.

Hahnen E, Forkert R, Marke C, et al: Molecular analysis of candidate genes on chromosome 5q13 in autosomal recessive spinal muscular atrophy: Evidence of homozygous deletions of the SMN gene in unaffected individuals. Hum Mol Genet 1995;4:1927–1933.

Harding AE: Inherited neuronal atrophy and degeneration predominantly of lower motor neurons. In Dyck PJ, Thomas PK, Griffin JW, et al (eds): Peripheral Neuropathy, 3rd ed. Philadelphia, WB Saunders, 1993; 1051–1064.

Hausmanowa-Petrusewicz I, Fidzianska A, Dobosz I, et al: The foetal character of the lesion in the acute form of Werdnig-Hoffmann disease. In Bradley WG, Gardner-Medwin D, Walton JN (eds): Recent Advances in Myology. Amsterdam, Excerpta Medica, 1975; 546–556.

Hausmanowa-Petrusewicz I, Karwanska A: Electromyographic findings in different forms of infantile and juvenile proximal spinal muscular atrophy. Muscle Nerve 1986;9:37–46.

Hausmanowa-Petrusewicz I, Kopec J: Motor nerve conduction velocity in lesions of the anterior horn. In Kakulas BA (ed): Clinical Studies in Myology. Amsterdam, Excerpta Medica, 1973; 358–364.

Hergersberg M, Glatzel M, Capone A, et al: Deletions in the spinal muscular atrophy gene region in a newborn with neuropathy and extreme generalized muscular weakness. Eur J Paediatr Neurol 2000;4:35–38.

Hirayama K, Tsubaki T, Toyokura Y, Okinaka S: Juvenile muscular atrophy of unilateral upper extremity. Neurology 1963;13:373–380.

Hopkins IJ: A new syndrome: Poliomyelitis-like illness associated with acute asthma in childhood. Aust Paediatr J 1974;10:273–276.

Iannaccone ST, Russman BS, Brown RH, et al: Prospective analysis of strength in spinal muscular atrophy. J Child Neurol 2000;15:97–101.

Ignatius J: The natural history of severe spinal muscular atrophy—further evidence for clinical subtypes. Neuromusc Disord 1994;4:527–528.

Imai T, Minami R, Nagaoka M, et al: Proximal and distal motor nerve conduction velocities in Werdnig-Hoffmann disease. Pediatr Neurol 1990;6:82–86.

Jagganathan K: Juvenile motor neurone disease. In Spillane JD (ed): Tropical Neurology. London, Oxford University Press, 1973; 127–130.

Johnson WG, Wigger HJ, Glaubiger LM, Rowland LP: Juvenile spinal muscular atrophy: A new hexosaminidase deficiency phenotype. Ann Neurol 1982;11:11–16.

Karni A, Navon R, Sadeh M: Hexosaminidase A deficiency manifesting as spinal muscular atrophy of late onset. Ann Neurol 1988;24:451–453.

Kato S, Hirano A: Ubiquitin and phosphorylated neurofilament epitopes in ballooned neurons of the extraocular muscle nuclei in a case of Werdnig-Hoffmann disease. Acta Neuropathol 1990; 80:334–337.

Konno H, Iwasaki Y, Yamamoto T, Inosaka T: Nemaline bodies in spinal progressive muscular atrophy: An autopsy case. Acta Neuropathol (Berl) 1987;74:84–88.

Korinthenberg R, Sauer M, Ketelsen U-P, et al: Congenital axonal neuropathy caused by deletions in the spinal muscular atrophy region. Ann Neurol 1997;42:364–368.

Larsen R, Ashwal S, Peckham N: Incontinentia pigmenti: Association with anterior horn cell degeneration. Neurology 1987;37:446–450.

Lefebvre S, Bürglen L, Reboullet S, et al: Identification and characterization of a spinal muscular atrophy-determining gene. Cell 1995;80:155–165.

Lippa CF, Smith TW: Chromatolytic neurons in Werdnig-Hoffmann disease contain phosphorylated neurofilaments. Acta Neuropathol (Berl) 1988;77:91–94.

Liu GT, Specht LA: Progressive juvenile segmental spinal muscular atrophy. Pediatr Neurol 1993;9:54–61.

Lorson CL, Hahnen E, Androphy EJ, Wirth B: A single nucleotide in the *SMN* gene regulates splicing and is responsible for spinal muscular atrophy. Proc Natl Acad Sci USA 1999;96:6307–6311.

MacLeod MJ; Taylor JE; Lunt PW, et al: Prenatal onset spinal muscular atrophy. Eur J Paediatr Neurol 1999;3:65.

Marshall A, Duchen LW: Sensory system involvement in infantile spinal muscular atrophy. J Neurol Sci 1975;26:349–359.

Matsumoto S, Goto S, Kusaka H, et al: Ubiquitin-positive inclusion in anterior horn cells in subgroups of motor neuron diseases: A comparative study of adult-onset amyotrophic lateral sclerosis,

juvenile amyotrophic lateral sclerosis and Werdnig-Hoffmann disease. J Neurol Sci 1993;115:208–213.

McAndrew PE, Parsons DW, Simard LR, et al: Identification of proximal spinal muscular atrophy carriers and patients by analysis of SMN^t and SMN^c gene copy number. Am J Hum Genet 1997;60:1411–1422.

Melki J, Abdelhak S, Sheth P, et al: Gene for chronic proximal spinal muscular atrophies maps to chromosome 5q. Nature 1990a;344:767–768.

Melki J, Sheth P, Abdelhak S, et al: Mapping of acute (type 1) spinal muscular atrophy to chromosome 5q12-Q. Lancet 1990b; 336:271–273.

Monani UR, Sendtner M, Coovert DD, et al: The human centromeric survival motor neuron gene (SMN2) rescues embryonic lethality in SMN(−/−) mice and results in a mouse with spinal muscular atrophy. Hum Mol Genet 2000;9:333–339.

Moosa A, Dubowitz V: Motor nerve conduction velocity in spinal muscular atrophy of childhood. Arch Dis Child 1976;51:974–977.

Moosa A, Dubowitz V: Spinal muscular atrophy in childhood. Arch Dis Child 1973;48:386–388.

Muñoz ME, Roche C, Escribá R, et al: Flaccid paraplegia as a complication of umbilical artery catheterization. Pediatr Neurol 1993;9:401–403.

Munsat TL: International SMA Collaboration. Neuromusc Disord 1991;1:81.

Muntoni F, Goodwin F, Sewry C, et al: Clinical spectrum and diagnostic difficulties of infantile ponto–cerebellar hypoplasia type. Neuropediatrics 1999;30:243–248.

Murayama S, Bouldin TW, Suzuki K: Immunocytochemical and ultrastructural studies of Werdnig-Hoffmann disease. Acta Neuropathol 1991;81:408–417.

Nelson JS, Prensky AL: Sporadic juvenile amyotrophic lateral sclerosis: A clinicopathological study of a case with neuronal cytoplasmic inclusions containing RNA. Arch Neurol 1972;27:300–306.

Ohama E, Ikuta F: The morphopathogenesis of Werdnig-Hoffmann disease: Presence of axons and Schwann cells of fetal type. Shinkei Naiku (Tokyo) 1977;6:494–501.

Oryema J, Ashby P, Spiegel S: Monomelic atrophy. Can J Neurol Sci 1990;17:124–130.

Parano E, Pavone L, Falsaperla R, et al: Molecular basis of phenotypic heterogeneity in siblings with spinal muscular atrophy. Ann Neurol 1996;40:247–251.

Parnes S, Karpati G, Carpenter S, et al: Hexosaminidase—a deficiency presenting as atypical juvenile-onset spinal muscular atrophy. Arch Neurol 1985;42:1176–1180.

Pearn J: Classification of spinal muscular atrophies. Lancet 1980;1:919–922.

Pearn J, Hudgson P: Distal spinal muscular atrophy—a clinical and genetic study of 8 kindreds. J Neurol Sci 1979;43:183–191.

Peress NS, Stermann AB, Miller R, et al: "Chromatolytic" neurons in lateral geniculate body in Werdnig-Hoffmann disease. Clin Neuropathol 1986;5:69–72.

Riggs JE, Gutmann L, Schochet SS: Contraction pseudotremor of chronic denervation. Arch Neurol 1983;40:518–519.

Rochette CF, Gilchrist JM, Simard L: SMN gene duplication and the emergence of the SMN2 gene occurred in distinct hominids: SMN2 is unique to Homo sapiens. Hum Genet 2001;108:255–266.

Rowland LP, Schneck SA: Neuromuscular disorders associated with malignant neoplastic disease. J Chron Dis 1963;16:777–795.

Rudnik-Schöneborn S, Forkert R, Hahnen E, et al: Clinical spectrum and diagnostic criteria of infantile spinal muscular atrophy: Further delineation on the basis of SMN gene deletion findings. Neuropediatrics 1996;27:8–15.

Rudnik-Schöneborn S, Lutzenrath S, Borkowska J, et al: Analysis of creatine kinase activity in 504 patients with proximal spinal muscular atrophy types I–III from the point of view of progression and severity. Eur Neurol 1998;39:154–162.

Russman BS, Buncher CR, Samaha F, et al: Function changes in spinal muscular atrophy II and III. Neurology 1996;47:973–976.

Russman BS, Iannaccone ST, Buncher CR, et al: Spinal muscular atrophy: New thoughts on the pathogenesis and classification schema. J Child Neurol 1992;7:347–353.

Ryniewicz B: Motor and sensory conduction velocity in spinal muscular atrophy: Follow-up study. Electromyogr Clin Neurophysiol 1977;17:385–391.

Schrank B, Götz R, Gunnersen JM, et al: Inactivation of the survival motor neuron gene, a candidate gene for human spinal muscular atrophy, leads to massive cell death in early mouse embryos. Proc Natl Acad Sci USA 1997;94:9920–9925.

Sobue I, Saito N, Iida M, Ando K: Juvenile type of distal and segmental muscular atrophy of upper extremities. Ann Neurol 1978;3:429–432.

Somerville MJ, Hunter AG, Aubry HL, et al: Clinical application of the molecular diagnosis of spinal muscular atrophy. Am J Med Genet 1997;69:159–165.

Souchon F, Simard LR, Lebrun S, et al: Clinical and genetic study of chronic (types II and III) childhood onset spinal muscular atrophy. Neuromusc Disord 1999;6:419–424.

Steiman GS, Rorke LB, Brown MJ: Infantile neuronal degeneration masquerading as Werdnig-Hoffmann disease. Ann Neurol 1980; 8:317–324.

Summers BA, Schwartz MS, Ingram DA: Juvenile-onset bulbospinal muscular atrophy with deafness: Vialetta-Van Laere syndrome or Madras-type motor neuron disease? J Neurol 1987; 234:440–442.

Thomas NH, Dubowitz V: The natural history of type I (severe) spinal muscular atrophy. Neuromusc Disord 1994;4:497–502.

Towfighi J, Young RSK, Ward RM: Is Werdnig-Hoffmann disease a pure lower motor neuron disorder? Acta Neuropathol (Berl) 1985;65:270–280.

Wang CH, Carter TA, Ross BM, et al: Characterization of survival motor neuron (SMN^T) gene deletions in asymptomatic carriers of spinal muscular atrophy. Hum Mol Genet 1996;5:359–365.

Wheeler SD, Ochoa J: Poliomyelitis-like syndrome associated with asthma: A case report and review of the literature. Neurology 1980;37:52–53.

Wirth B: An update of the mutation spectrum of the survival motor neuron gene (SMN1) in autosomal recessive spinal muscular atrophy (SMA). Hum Mutat 2000;15:228–237.

Yamada M, Kano M, Chida K, et al: Asymptomatic benign familial spinal muscular atrophy with hypertrophy of the calves and high creatine kinase levels. J Neurol Neurosurg Psychiatry 1988; 51:452–453.

Zerres K, Wirth B, Rudnik-Schöneborn S: Spinal muscular atrophy—clinical and genetic correlations. Neuromusc Disord 1997;7:202–207.

Facial and Bulbar Weakness

Francis Renault

The electrodiagnostic study of facial, lingual, and velopharyngeal muscles is an important method for recording pathology of the brainstem and paired cranial nerves. Clinical indications for these investigations in newborns, infants, and older children include facial weakness, orofacial malformations, and dysphagia.

FACIAL WEAKNESS

Facial Nerve

The motor nucleus of cranial nerve VII is situated in the caudal portion of the pons. The taste fibers of nerve VII project to its vicinity in the upper portion of the nucleus of the tractus solitarius. Five groups of cells are described in the motor nucleus of the nerve VII corresponding to a topographical organization of motoneurons that innervate different muscles. The ventral groups of cells supply the periorbital muscles; the dorsal groups supply the perioral muscles (Courville, 1966; Chouard, 1972). The twin sensory and motor roots of the facial nerve emerge from the brainstem at the level of the bulb pontine sulcus between the sixth and eighth cranial nerves. They enter the pars petrosa ossis temporalis by the internal acoustic meatus and follow a common path in the first portion of the facial canal, at the end of which is the geniculate ganglion. The motor branch of the facial nerve alone traverses the second and third portions of the facial canal. The facial motor nerve emerges from the skull by the stylomastoid foramen and divides into two main terminal branches in the parotid gland. The inferior cervicofacial branch passes down the mandible, giving off a lower buccal branch to the risorius, the buccinator, and the orbicularis oris muscles; a mental branch to the depressor anguli oris, the depressor labii inferioris, and the mentalis muscles; and a cervical branch to the platysma muscle. The superior temporofacial branch runs horizontally forward, giving off frontal branches to the frontalis and orbicularis oculi muscles; suborbital branches to the levator labii superioris, zygomaticus, levator anguli oris, and dilator naris muscles; and buccal branches to the buccinator and orbicularis oris muscles. However, there is considerable diversity in the trajectory and divisions of the facial nerve.

Electromyographic Studies of Facial Muscles and Nerve in Children

The electromyographic activity is recorded by a fine concentric needle electrode. The skin may be previously anesthetized with lidocaine or prilocaine cream. If the infant is not fed for 4 hours, its cries allow the recording of bursts of activity with an interference pattern arising from the muscles of the orofacial region. The recording permits analysis of the recruitment pattern and the average amplitude of the trace as well as the morphology and duration of the motor unit potentials (MUPs). A brief square wave electric shock (0.2 ms) of supramaximal intensity (20 to 60 mA) is used for facial needle conduction studies (NCSs). The recruitment pattern has been analyzed in 32 normal subjects aged from 4 days to 3 years, and NCSs of the VII nerve have been performed in 344 normal subjects between birth and the age of 15 years (Raimbault, 1988; Renault and Raimbault, 1992).

FACIAL MUSCLES AND THE FACIAL NERVE

The electrode is inserted in the external portion of the orbicularis oris muscle, more than 1 cm outside the labial commissure. To perform NCSs, stimulation is applied to the cervicofacial branch at a point before the tragus and then at a point along the horizontal portion of the mandible. The orbicularis oculi muscle is approached tangentially 2 cm from the lateral angle of the eye. Stimulation to the cranial nerve VII at the pretragal point allows the measurement of motor latency. The frontalis muscle is approached tangentially above the eyebrow in a medial direction. The depressor anguli oris muscle is approached 1.5 to 2 cm below the labial commissure.

The normal mean amplitude of the interference pattern of these facial muscles is 850 µV (range, 400 to 1.2 mV). MUP duration ranges from 1 to 4.6 ms, and in more than 50% of MUPs, the duration is from 2 to 4 ms. The proportion of polyphasic potentials is above 30%. The motor response has a highly polyphasic morphology with a mean duration of 8 to 12 ms and amplitude of 0.4 to 1.2 mV (Fig. 88–1). Latencies induced by stimulation at the pretragal point do not show significant variation between birth and 15 years, ranging from 3.6 to 7.3 ms for the orbicularis oris, and from 2.3 to 4.4 ms for the orbicularis oculi (Table 88–1). Facial nerve conduction velocity increases markedly with age, particularly in the course of the first year of life, during which the average increase is 42.8%; the average increase is 11.1% in the second year, 9.1% in years 2 to 5, and 5.3% in years 5 to 10 (Table 88–2).

BLINK REFLEXES

The blink reflex results from the contraction of the orbicularis oculi muscle provoked by stimulation of a branch of the trigeminal nerve (Kugelberg, 1952). A single brief square wave electric shock (0.2 ms) of low intensity (2 to 25 mA) is applied to the supraorbital foramen to elicit blink reflexes, which can be recorded from the orbicularis oculi muscle on both sides. Stimulation of the ipsilateral nerve V provokes

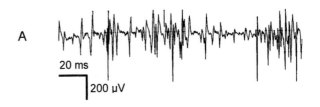

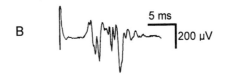

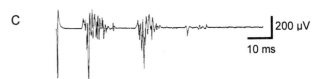

Figure 88–1. Needle electromyography of facial muscles: normal features in a full-term newborn, day 6. *A,* Orbicularis oris muscle, interference pattern on crying. *B,* Orbicularis oris muscle, response to electrical stimulation of nerve VII before the tragus. *C,* Orbicularis oculi muscle, blink reflexes provoked by electrical stimulation to the ipsilateral supraorbital nerve.

a direct response with two components: R1, which is immediate and brief, and R2, which is delayed and longer lasting (see Fig. 88–1). Stimulation of the contralateral nerve V provokes a crossed R2 response. The R1 component corresponds to an oligosynaptic reflex arc involving at least two and no more than three synapses in the pons between the main sensory nucleus of nerve V and the motor nucleus of the ipsilateral nerve VII. The R2 component follows polysynaptic medullary pathways, which are more caudal and closer to the bulbar formations: the spinal trigeminal nucleus and projections to the adjacent paramedian reticular formation and the motor nuclei of the two seventh nerves (Kimura, 1970, 1975; Boulu et al., 1981; Kiers and Carroll, 1990). Other afferent pathways are implicated in the blink reflex: sensory fibers of nerve VII

Table 88–1. Normal Values for Latencies of Orbicularis Oris, Orbicularis Oculi, and Genioglossus Muscles

Subject Age (yr)	No. of Subjects	Latency (ms ± 2 SDs)		
		Orbicularis Oris	*Orbicularis Oculi*	*Genioglossus*
0–1	120	5.3 ± 1.7	3.1 ± 0.8	3.8 ± 1.0
1–3	91	5.4 ± 1.6	3.3 ± 0.5	3.5 ± 1.1
3–9	89	5.6 ± 1.5	3.5 ± 1.0	3.3 ± 0.9
9–15	44	5.6 ± 1.7	3.5 ± 0.9	3.4 ± 0.6

Stimulation is applied to cranial nerve VII at the pretragal point and to cranial nerve XII behind the mandible.

Table 88–2. Normal Facial and Hypoglossal Nerve Conduction Velocities

Subject Age	No. of Subjects	Conduction Velocity (m/s ± 2 Sds)	
		Facial Nerve (Cervicofacial Branch)	*Hypoglossal Nerve*
0–30 d	18	19.0 ± 2.5	23.5 ± 2.2
1–2 mo	14	21.4 ± 3.4	24.1 ± 2.2
2–4 mo	12	24.5 ± 3.9	26.6 ± 2.7
4–6 mo	24	26.3 ± 2.8	28.9 ± 2.9
6–8 mo	23	29.1 ± 3.3	31.8 ± 3.4
8–10 mo	15	31.7 ± 3.7	34.3 ± 2.9
10–12 mo	14	33.3 ± 3.3	35.7 ± 3.0
12–18 mo	30	36.1 ± 3.0	37.5 ± 2.1
18 mo–2 yr	27	37.5 ± 4.7	40.6 ± 2.6
2–3 yr	34	39.5 ± 2.7	42.1 ± 3.0
3–4 yr	16	41.9 ± 4.5	43.5 ± 3.4
4–5 yr	21	43.4 ± 3.3	46.1 ± 2.5
5–6 yr	12	45.5 ± 4.8	46.5 ± 4.9
6–7 yr	12	45.8 ± 5.3	47.3 ± 2.1
7–8 yr	13	46.5 ± 4.1	48.1 ± 6.9
8–9 yr	15	48.1 ± 3.8	49.0 ± 2.6
9–11 yr	17	48.3 ± 2.8	50.2 ± 7.1
11–13 yr	12	48.7 ± 5.6	50.9 ± 6.4
13–15 yr	15	48.5 ± 2.8	50.7 ± 5.4

The distances between the two stimulation points (in mm) for facial nerve are 34.6 ± 6.6 for up to 12 mo, 48.7 ± 9.7 for 1 to 5 yr, and 56.1 ± 6 for 5 to 15 yr. The distances for hypoglossal nerve are 32.5 ± 9.3 for up to 12 mo, 36.1 ± 6.5 for 1 to 5 yr, and 38.2 ± 9.7 for 5 to 15 yr.

and the first two cervical roots (Willer and Lamour, 1979). In clinical practice, R1 and R2 studies allow differentiation between damage to the trigeminal and facial pathways; furthermore, R1 investigates the pons and R2 is abnormal in lateral medullary lesions (Cruccu and Deuschl, 2000).

Several authors (Kimura et al., 1977; Vecchierini-Blineau and Guiheneuc, 1984; Kather-Boidin and Duron, 1987; Tomita et al., 1989) have studied maturation of electrically elicited blink reflexes. The R1 response is always present regardless of the age. R1 has a polyphasic morphology with a long duration in neonates and infants; in older children, it is well synchronized and biphasic or triphasic. R1 amplitude is reduced in premature and reaches adult values at 40 to 44 weeks of gestational age. Latency of the R1 component has a very rapid maturation and achieves normal adult values before 44 weeks of gestational age. R2 responses are more difficult to elicit than are R1 responses and disappear when the rate of stimulation is above 0.5 Hz. R2 morphology is highly polyphasic. The ipsilateral R2 response can be evoked in most newborns and infants. Its latency ranges from 34 to 43 ms in full-term newborns, then increases and remains stable in early childhood, and decreases to adult values between 7 and 12 years. The contralateral R2 can be obtained in 80% of full-term newborns but may be absent up to 8 months. Its latency is longer than the ipsilateral R2 until 2 years.

ELECTRONEURONOGRAPHY

Electroneuronography uses surface electrodes placed along the nasolabial fold to record the re-

sponse of perioral muscles elicited by a brief supramaximal electrical stimulus applied to the facial nerve near the stylomastoid foramen. The amplitude of the compound muscle action potential is recorded as a percentage of the amplitude of the contralateral normal side (Esslen, 1973). Asymmetry greater than 30% is considered pathological. Electroneuronography is a technique for evaluating facial nerve motor function, which is useful in the setting of acute atraumatic unilateral facial paralysis in childhood (Eavey et al., 1989; Shapiro et al., 1996).

Congenital Facial Asymmetries and Diplegia

The incidence of congenital facial palsies ranges from 1.8‰ to 7.5‰ of births (McHugh, 1963; Levine et al., 1984; Falco and Eriksson, 1990). Congenital facial asymmetries and diplegia involve various clinical manifestations, each of which raises specific problems (Table 88–3). Comparison of clinical and neurophysiological data enables etiologies to be differentiated, pathogenesis to be evaluated, and the prognosis to be assessed. Facial paralysis due to prenatal or perinatal stress of the seventh nerve requires evaluation of severity to define the therapeutic approach. A diagnosis of agenesis of the depressor anguli oris muscle should lead to the search for an associated visceral malformation. The involvement of the seventh nerve in a hemifacial malformation syndrome is a predictive sign of a cerebral lesion. In Möbius' syndrome, neurophysiological study can shed light on the pathophysiology. Finally, electromyography (EMG) can show the absence of paralysis in congenital facial asymmetry

Table 88–3. Congenital Facial Weakness

Birth trauma
  Congenital facial palsy (with or without forceps)
  Hypoxic-ischemic encephalopathy (bulbar and/or suprabulbar)
  Posterior fossa hematoma
Developmental Defect
  First and second branchial arch syndromes (facioauriculovertebral spectrum, hemifacial microsomia, mandibulofacial dysostosis)
  Asymmetrical crying facies (hypoplasia of the depressor anguli oris muscle)
  CHARGE association (Colobomata, Heart disease, Atresia of the choanae, Retarded growth and development, Genital hypoplasia, and Ear anomalies)
  Möbius' syndrome
Neuromuscular Disease
  Congenital myotonic muscular dystrophy
  Congenital muscular dystrophy
  Facioscapulohumeral muscular dystrophy (early-onset type)
  Congenital myopathies: nemaline, centronuclear, myotubular, fiber type disproportion, cytoplasmic body
  Transient myasthenia gravis
Pseudoparalysis
  Mandibular hypoplasia
  Intrauterine postural asymmetry

resulting from intrauterine posture and in apraxic diplegia.

We carried out a retrospective study of 172 children with congenital facial palsies (Renault et al., 1993). The first clinical and electromyographic examinations were conducted from 3 to 90 days after birth in 103 patients, from 3 to 12 months in 49 patients, and from 1 to 2 years in the 20 other patients.

PERINATAL LESIONS OF THE FACIAL NERVE

In 85 cases of our series, the congenital facial asymmetry was due to unilateral facial paralysis without malformation. Review of this group shows that these congenital facial palsies were of unequal severity and that their mechanisms were not identical. In such cases, the clinical symptomatology is not always easy to interpret, especially when the paralysis is only partial. The face is often grossly symmetrical at rest, but careful observation may detect the loss of complete closure of the eyelids and overlapping of the eyelashes and the ipsilateral absence of the fine nostril dilation movements that are synchronous with breathing. Examination during crying enables the unilateral absence of puckering of the brow, the faulty closing of the eyelids, and the asymmetry of the mouth to be observed (Fig. 88–2). The asymmetrical closing of the lips on the pacifier and the asymmetry of the reaction to tactile stimulation of the perioral region may also be noted.

In 48 of 85 patients, extraction of the fetus necessitated the use of forceps. Forceps delivery, birth weight above 3500 g, and primiparity are all significant risk factors for congenital facial palsies (Falco and Eriksson, 1990). In two patients, clinical examination revealed a neonatal purulent otitis media. In the 35 other patients, no causal factor was found and, in particular, forceps had not been used; in such cases, the possible role of prenatal or perinatal compression of the extracranial portion of the seventh nerve against the myometrium and fetal shoulder or the sacral promontory should be considered, especially because there often is concordance between the side of congenital facial palsy and that of cephalic presentation (Hepner, 1951). Electromyographic results enabled the hemifacial denervation to be confirmed and the severity of congenital facial palsies to be assessed as a function of the severity and topography of the signs of axonal loss as well as alterations in NCSs and blink reflexes. Moderate forms can be distinguished in which denervation is only partial and concerns either the territories of the two branches equally or predominantly the cervicofacial. This situation was more frequent in the group delivered without forceps (71%) than in the group delivered with forceps (54%). The clinical course involves progressive recovery of hemifacial motor activity during the first few months, and EMG shows the progress of nerve regeneration, predicting a favorable outcome. The percentage values of facial function over time provided by serial electroneuronograms correlate with prognosis (Shapiro et al., 1996). In severe forms of congenital facial palsies, the lesion of the temporofacial branch is total, with inactivation and no excitability of the orbicularis oculi muscle and abolition of the blink reflexes and total or partial impairment of the cervicofacial branch. These severe forms represented 46% of cases in the forceps group and 29% in the nonforceps group. The immediate questions are whether surgical exploration is indicated and, if so, when? Surgery is useless if there is no curable local cause or if it is carried out so early that it anticipates spontaneous recovery. On the other hand, definitive nervous lesions due to a longstanding compressive process are a major worry. Even if no evidence of a lesion is found on computed tomography scanning, surgical investigation should be considered if there is no sign of clinical and electromyographic improvement. In our series, this step was taken in eight patients with no clinical improvement and after two or three successive electromyograms had shown either the persistence of a major lesion of the two branches without any sign of recovery, or partial recovery of the cervicofacial branch but persistence of total paralysis of the temporofacial branch. In two patients, surgical investigation showed that the facial nerve was compressed against a fracture line in the petrous portion of the temporal bone, associated in one patient with chronic inflammation of the mastoid antrum. In the six other patients, the seventh nerve was altered (pale, thin, flattened) without any obvious local cause. In a retrospective study of children with unilateral isolated congenital facial palsies who had not completely recovered by the age of 5 years, there was no association between this poor outcome and risk factors for birth trauma to the seventh nerve in 20 of 53 patients (Laing et al.,

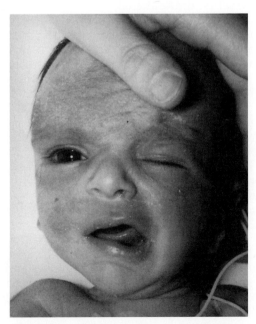

Figure 88–2. Congenital facial palsy in a full-term newborn, day 2.

1996). Clinical and electromyographic monitoring of these severe forms showed that recovery is slow. The process of nerve regeneration and muscular reinnervation proceeds very progressively. When the palsy seems to remain clinically total, EMG may indicate a more favorable prognosis by showing some MUPs and the reappearance of a low-amplitude increased-latency motor response. Electroneuronography may be repeated to show any progress in facial nerve function. Improvement in facial motor activity and electromyographic parameters may still be seen after the end of the second year.

ASYMMETRICAL CRYING FACIES

In this clinical presentation, the facial asymmetry is only evident when the child is crying and only the lower lip is involved: the labial commissure does not descend on the affected side, but the nasojugal folds are symmetrical, as is contraction of the frontalis muscle (Fig. 88–3). Among 51 children with this clinical picture, in 10 patients the EMG showed partial denervation of the depressor anguli oris, depressor labii inferioris, and mentalis muscles, leading to the diagnosis of partial facial palsy. These 10 patients were thus included in the perinatal trauma group. This very localized topography of the nervous lesions corresponds to the territory of the mental branch of the facial nerve. This branch, arising from the cervicofacial branch, has a course that in the fetus and newborn closely follows the base of the mandible and thus is easily compressed (Sammarco et al., 1966). In fact, asymmetrical crying facies was initially described as partial facial palsy (Hoefnagel and Penry, 1960). Electrodiagnostic stud-

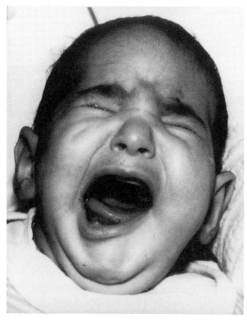

Figure 88–3. Congenital asymmetrical crying facies in a 9-month-old boy: hypoplasia of the left depressor anguli oris muscle. The lower lip is asymmetrical, but the upper face and nasojugal folds remain symmetrical.

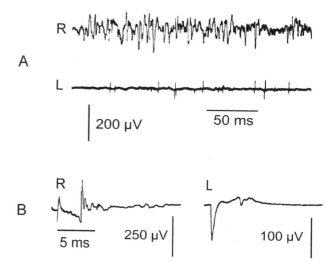

Figure 88–4. Congenital asymmetrical crying facies. Electromyography results on day 20: hypoplasia of the left depressor anguli oris muscle (DAOM). *A,* Two-channel recording of both DAOMs on crying, sparse low-amplitude, brief-duration motor unit potentials in the left hypoplasic DAOM (L) compared to normal interference pattern in the right (R). *B,* Response of DAOMs to electrical stimulation of the nerve VII before the tragus, normal-latency, low-amplitude simplified morphology response of the hypoplasic DAOM (L) compared with that of the contralateral normal muscle (R).

ies subsequently demonstrated the absence of muscle denervation with normal values for excitability and conduction of the nerve VII, but revealed signs of hypoplasia of the depressor anguli oris muscle (McHugh et al., 1969; Nelson and Eng, 1972). The lower portion of the depressor anguli oris muscle is inserted in a diffuse manner into the platysma muscle along the base of the mandible and enters as a narrow fascicle into the labial commissure, where its fibers merge with those of the orbicularis oris. Its contraction draws the labial commissure and the external portion of the lower lip down and out, producing an expression of displeasure (Duchenne de Boulogne, 1861). In all 41 patients with asymmetrical crying facies from our series, EMG showed signs of hypoplasia of the depressor anguli oris muscle: the interference pattern during crying was of low average amplitude and consisted of MUPs of brief duration and low amplitude, and the response to stimulation of the nerve VII was of low amplitude and simplified morphology (Fig. 88–4). In no case was there any question of total muscular agenesis. Hypoplasia of the depressor labii inferioris muscle was also present in six patients. Associated malformations were found in 5 of the 41 children: two septal defects, one dysmorphic syndrome, one complex cardiopathy, and one cleft palate. The association of asymmetrical crying facies with congenital cardiopathy has been reported as "Cayler cardiofacial syndrome," and the authors hypothesized that an embryopathic process was involved (Cayler et al., 1971). Prospective studies of newborns with asymmetrical crying facies confirmed a higher risk of visceral malformation, particularly of the heart, great vessels, and urinary apparatus (Perlman and Reisner, 1973; Alexiou et al., 1976). Deletion 22q11 has been reported with asymmetrical crying facies as part of the cardiofacial syndrome (Giannotti et al., 1994) and with isolated asymmetrical crying facies (Stewart and Smith, 1997). Thus, an electromyographic diagnosis of hypoplasia of the depressor anguli oris muscle should lead to the search for an associated visceral malformation.

OROFACIAL MALFORMATIONS WITH CRANIAL NERVE PALSIES

Hemifacial malformations involving tissues derived from the first and second branchial arches can indicate a lesion of cranial nerves V and VII. Facial paralysis has been reported in most cases of Goldenhar syndrome (Orobello, 1991), in 43% of cases of CHARGE (Colobomata, Heart disease, Atresia of the choanae, Retarded growth and development, Genital hypoplasia, and Ear anomalies) association (Byerly and Pauli, 1993), and in 22% cases of hemifacial microsomia (Carvalho et al., 1999). We performed bilateral facial electromyographic studies in 33 infants with asymmetrical facial motor activity associated with hemifacial hypoplasia and malformation of the ear. Clinical diagnoses were Goldenhar syndrome or facioauriculovertebral spectrum (Jones, 1997a), Treacher-Collins mandibulofacial dysostosis or Franceschetti syndrome (Jones, 1997c), and CHARGE association. Electromyographic abnormalities were either diffuse or localized to one side of the face. Electromyographic activity was either nil (10 patients), neurogenic (9 patients), or myopathic (14 patients). In these facial muscles, which are physiologically very rich in motor units and show a high level of polyphasic MUPs, we term *myopathic* those traces that have a low mean amplitude and a high level of very brief low-amplitude MUPs. In this context of facial malformation, we interpret myopathic electromyographic signs not as reflecting a definite myopathic process but as an indication of muscular hypoplasia without denervation. In all of the 14 patients with myopathic electromyographic signs, excitability thresholds, latencies, and facial NCS results were normal. In seven of nine patients with neurogenic impairment, motor latencies were increased and the facial NCSs showed slowed nerve conduction. Among the 19 infants with totally inactive or partially denervated muscles, neuroradiological investigation of the central nervous system showed a piliferous cyst of the cerebellum in 1 infant and cerebellar hypoplasia in another. In the 14 patients with myopathic electromyographic changes, no abnormalities of the central nervous system were found. Thus, for hemifacial malformations, EMG has the advantage of being able to detect whether there is involvement of the facial nerve, which is a predictive sign of an associated malformation of the central nervous system, in particular of the posterior fossa (Couly and Aicardi, 1988; Mezenes and Coker, 1990).

MÖBIUS' SYNDROME

Diagnosis of this syndrome is easy in cases of total or partial facial diplegia, whether symmetrical or asymmetrical, associated with bilateral paralysis of abduction of the eye (Sudarshan and Goldie, 1985) (Fig. 88–5). When the facial diplegia is partial, it usually involves the upper half of the face. Abducens palsy often has the appearance of esotropia (Miller and Stromland, 1999). Paralysis of the hypoglossal nerve with atrophy of the tongue is present in one third of cases. Most patients have dysphagia, drooling, malocclusion, velopharyngeal incompetence, dysarthria, and delayed speech (Meyerson and Foushee, 1978). Trigeminal nerve involvement with trismus is less frequent. Talipes equinovarus, different malformations of hands and fingers, and Poland anomaly may be associated. Most cases are sporadic, but families with autosomal dominant inheritance have been reported (Verzijl et al., 1999).

The question of pathogenesis is controversial, as different pathoanatomical data have been described (Towfighi et al., 1979): hypoplasia or atrophy of cranial nerve nuclei, hypoplasia of the facial nerve, focal brainstem necrosis, brainstem hypoplasia, and muscular dysplasia or dystrophy. Most published electromyographic data support a neurogenic origin of muscular atrophy: numerous patterns showing sparse motor units, increased latencies, slowed facial nerve conduction, and sometimes altered blink reflexes (Jaradeh et al., 1996). These data support the hypothesis of a prenatal nuclear lesion of the cranial nerves whose mechanism could be ischemic (Govaert et al., 1989). However, our electromyographic results in a series of 22 patients were hetero-

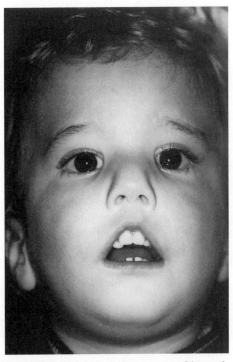

Figure 88–5. Möbius' syndrome at age 24 months.

geneous but showed the predominance of signs of axonal loss (Renault, 2000). In 17 children, generally reduced and single unit patterns were noted in several but not all facial, lingual, and/or velopharyngeal muscles; in 2 children, all patterns showed full interference and were of low amplitude, all motor responses were of low amplitude, and the latencies and conduction velocities were normal (in this 2 patients, myopathy was suspected, but deltoid muscle biopsy was normal and the course was stable); and in 3 children, all patterns in muscles of the face, tongue, and soft palate were typically neurogenic (all 3 had experienced chronic or acute fetal distress, had had severe dysphagia and respiratory complications, and might have had hypoxic-ischemic involvement of the brainstem).

Thus, in Möbius' syndrome, facial EMG is an important diagnostic tool and contributes to study of the pathogenesis, which is probably not singular. Should facial EMG be difficult to interpret due to major muscle atrophy, the study of lingual and palatal muscles can be useful in demonstrating the neurogenic process in the territories of the hypoglossal nerve and pharyngeal plexus. In the neonatal period, EMG of the limbs may be necessary to differentiate the Möbius' syndrome from congenital myotonic dystrophy or other myopathies (see the discussion on muscular dystrophies with congenital facial diplegia).

PSEUDOPARALYSIS: ASYMMETRY OF POSTURAL ORIGIN

The EMG can show the absence of paralysis in some congenital facial asymmetries noted both at rest and on crying in newborns with no apparent malformations. Such pseudoparalysis may reveal asymmetrical mandibular hypoplasia, but most often it is the result of intrauterine posture. A clinical feature that is characteristic is the lack of parallelism of the gums. Pseudoparalysis concerned 5 of 172 infants in our congenital facial asymmetry series. The EMG was strictly normal and showed the integrity of the facial muscles and nerves. The functional asymmetry resolved rapidly in all 5 infants within the first 2 months.

CONGENITAL FACIAL DIPLEGIA OF BULBAR OR SUPRABULBAR ORIGIN

Orofacial apraxia may be an early sign of cerebral palsy in newborns with prenatal or perinatal hypoxic-ischemic encephalopathy. EMG of facial muscles, facial NCSs, and blink reflexes are normal in these patients. Magnetic resonance imaging may show bilateral thalamic or opercular lesions. When prenatal or perinatal asphyxia provokes lesions of brainstem nuclei, EMG may indicate denervation in muscles of the face, tongue, and soft palate, and blink reflexes may be altered. We have reported these features in a series of 12 patients with major dysphagia at birth, complicated by early aspiration

pneumopathy and failure to thrive (Renault and Couvreur, 1992). Nasal reflux and salivary stasis were obvious in most cases. The majority (8 of 12) had facial weakness (see the discussion on dysphagia with brainstem lesions).

MUSCULAR DISEASES WITH CONGENITAL FACIAL DIPLEGIA

Facial weakness is an important diagnostic indicator of congenital myotonic muscular dystrophy, congenital muscular dystrophy, and structural or metabolic myopathies. The facial weakness is bilateral, with characteristic tent-shaped mouth, and it is associated with ptosis, dysphagia, and generalized paralytic hypotonia with amyotrophy and tendon contractures. Electrodiagnostic studies of facial muscles and nerves demonstrate the absence of electromyographic neurogenic signs and the normality of facial NCSs and blink reflexes. EMG of limb muscles is necessary for demonstrating myopathic signs.

An infantile form of facioscapulohumeral muscular dystrophy with early facial diplegia and a severe course has been described (Hanson and Rowland, 1971; Bailey et al., 1986; Yasukohchi et al., 1988). The facial diplegia is obvious in the first year of life (Korf et al., 1985): the face is expressionless; patients have a peculiar horizontal smile, and they may be unable to fully close the eyes and mouth. In some cases, mothers noticed poor sucking at birth and lack of facial expression. Sensorineural hearing loss and tortuousity of retinal arterioles have been observed. Motor milestones are not delayed, but weakness of limb and respiratory muscles regresses rapidly before adult age. Infantile forms of facioscapulohumeral muscular dystrophy seem not to be genetically distinct from late-onset type, and the histological and electromyographic findings do not differ from those of classic cases (Brouwer et al., 1994).

Acquired Facial Weakness in Infants and Children

Chapter 23 is devoted to cranial nerve palsies in the adult; thus, we discuss only briefly those pathologies common to children and adults. Certain features of pediatric practice are worth emphasizing. It may be clinically difficult to distinguish a precocious acquired facial palsy from congenital facial palsies. In such cases, EMG can date the facial palsy: recent denervation shows spontaneous activity and successive EMG will show the evolution of neuromuscular activity, excitability, and nerve conduction during the process of denervation and reinnervation; in longstanding palsy, there is no spontaneous activity, and electromyographic and NCS abnormalities are the same at repeated examinations.

UNILATERAL FACIAL WEAKNESS

Bell's idiopathic facial palsy is the most frequent cause of facial palsy in children. It may occur in the first months of life but is most frequent after the age of 8 years.

Diagnosis of idiopathic facial palsy presupposes that the clinical history and complementary examinations have excluded all other causes with known evaluations and treatments (Table 88–4). At this step, EMG of the facial muscles, facial NCSs, and blink reflex study contribute to the diagnosis of peripheral facial palsy, assess the degree of axonal loss and demyelination, and evaluate the topography and severity of the paralysis. Electroneuronography provides an estimation of the number of spared motor axons.

Complete spontaneous recovery is the rule in children. In general, the prognosis is more favorable the younger the patient. Steroid treatment, even though its efficacy in children has not yet been proved, is usually provided during the first few days. Recovery starts 2 to 3 weeks after the onset of paralysis. When paralysis is initially clinically total with abolition of the blink reflex, recovery may be late and slow but the incapacitating complications, such as crocodile tears and synkinesis, that are seen in 10% of adults are rare in children.

Table 88–4. Acquired Facial Weakness in Childhood

Idiopathic Bell's Palsy
Infection and inflammation
  Otitis media, mastoiditis
  Meningitis (viral bacterial tuberculosis, leukemia, trichinosis)
  Guillain-Barré syndrome, polyneuritis cranialis, Miller-Fisher
    syndrome
  Epstein-Barr, *Mycoplasma*, herpes zoster, Borrelia (Lyme
    disease)
  Kawasaki disease
  Vasculitis (Henoch-Schönlein purpura)
  Parotiditis
  Neurosarcoidosis
Recurrent Facial Palsies
  Melkersson-Rosenthal syndrome
  Familial alternating Bell's palsy
Trauma and Compression
  Craniofacial trauma, penetrative injury
  Iatrogenic
  Brainstem glioma and other posterior fossa tumors
  Increased intracranial pressure
  Osteopetrosis
  Histiocytosis X
  Facial tumor (e.g., vascular, osseous, parotid gland,
    myofibroma)
  Schwannoma of the seventh nerve
Malformation
  Chiari, syringobulbia
Neuromuscular Disorders
  Facioscapulohumeral dystrophy
  Progressive bulbar palsy
  Myasthenia gravis
  Botulism
Cerebral Disorders
  Traumatic, tumoral, vascular, degenerative, metabolic,
    inflammatory

As shown in the adult, the normality of motor latency (Aminoff, 1998) and preservation or return of the blink reflex in the first weeks (Kimura et al., 1976) are seen in forms where recovery is complete. When electroneuronography performed from 8 to 12 days after onset shows functional motor deficit of the facial nerve to be from 50% to 90%, recovery is normally rapid, in 7 or 8 weeks. The inexcitability of the facial nerve and the marked decrease in compound muscle action potential amplitude are correlated with a severe lesion of the seventh nerve and a poor prognosis (Aminoff, 1998). Improvement in electroneuronography at successive examinations is a useful indicator for predicting a favorable outcome when the paralysis remains clinically complete after the sixth week (Eavey et al., 1989). When the deficit in electroneuronography is from 90% to 98%, recovery is slower but is finally complete. When the deficit is from 98% to 100%, surgical decompression of the facial nerve in its pyramidal position can be indicated (Esslen, 1977), but its practice is increasingly rare.

EMG does not enable idiopathic Bell's palsy to be distinguished from other facial palsies with axonal loss.

Facial palsy is frequent in Lyme disease and may be unilateral or bilateral. Electrodiagnostic studies indicate demyelination in most cases; axonal loss has been reported to be associated with a worse prognosis in adults (Angerer et al., 1993).

Recurrent facial palsy indicates the need to rule out a neoplasm or vascular malformation. Melkersson-Rosenthal syndrome has a dominant inheritance with incomplete penetrance linked to chromosome 9p11. Patients are often of Mediterranean origin and may have fissured tongue. This entity may begin in childhood (Wadlington et al., 1984). Recurrent facial palsy is associated with red facial edema and swollen lips. Facial swelling may be the initial isolated manifestation. Residual facial weakness could increase with repeated paralyses. Recurrent alternating Bell's palsy with familial dominant inheritance has been reported (Hageman et al., 1990).

FACIAL DIPLEGIA

The main causes are, as in the adult, bilateral Bell's palsy, Guillain-Barré and Miller-Fisher syndromes, Lyme disease, multiple idiopathic cranial neuropathies, and brainstem encephalitis (Keane, 1994). Acquired facial diplegia in childhood may also reveal a tumor of the posterior fossa or meningeal leukemia. Electrodiagnostic studies contribute to the etiological diagnosis by differentiating axonal loss from demyelination.

In the course of Guillain-Barré syndrome, facial involvement is seen in 50% of cases, most often bilaterally. Facial involvement may be a revealing sign, indicating that the limb nerves should be studied to investigate the multifocal nature of the acute polyradiculoneuritis. In a clinical variant, facial diplegia may be isolated or associated with a deficit

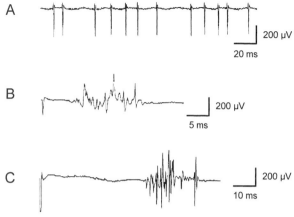

A

B

C

200 μV

20 ms

200 μV

5 ms

200 μV

10 ms

Figure 88–6. Facial electromyography in a 6-year-old girl with facial diplegia due to polyneuritis cranialis on the eighth day after onset. *A,* Reduced interference pattern in the orbicularis oris muscle. *B,* Increased latency-prolonged duration response of the orbicularis oris muscle to electrical stimulation of the nerve VII before the tragus (facial nerve conduction velocity, 18.3 m per second). *C,* Delayed and polyphasic R1 component of the blink reflex (latency, 46 ms).

of lower cranial nerves without limb pathology. In such cases of polyneuritis cranialis, electromyographic study of the facial muscles can be particularly useful to the diagnosis by showing the increase in latencies and temporal dispersion of the motor responses of the facial muscles and blink reflexes, the slowing of facial nerve conduction, and signs of denervation of the facial muscles (Polo et al., 1992) (Fig. 88–6).

Miller-Fisher syndrome is characterized by ophthalmoplegia, ataxia, and areflexia (Najim Al-Din et al., 1994). As shown by neurophysiological studies in adults, the excitability thresholds of the facial nerves and the motor latencies of the facial muscles are normal. The main anomalies are the decrease in amplitude of limb sensory nerve action potentials and the decrease in amplitude of the compound muscle action potentials of the facial muscles. The blink reflexes are either normal (Sauron et al., 1984) or altered in parallel with the decreased amplitude of the facial compound muscle action potentials (Fross and Daube, 1987) and denervation of the facial muscles. A clinical study of the general course of cranial nerve dysfunction during progression of the disease showed that overlap occurred between polyneuritis cranialis, Miller-Fisher syndrome, and classic ascending Guillain-Barré syndrome in adults as in children (Ter Bruggen et al., 1998).

BULBAR WEAKNESS AND NEUROGENIC DYSPHAGIA

Investigation of possible bulbar weakness and dysphagia is necessary for evaluation of the complications of neonatal hypotonia, orofacial malformations, and critical neurological illness. It is also an important step in the etiological assessment of res-piratory difficulties in newborns and older children with neurological conditions.

Sucking and Swallowing

Sucking and swallowing require the interaction of the face, tongue, soft palate, pharynx, larynx, and esophagus. Swallowing in human newborns and older children has been studied with manometry, cineradiography (Ardran et al., 1958; Farriaux and Milbled, 1965; Miller, 1982), ultrasonography (Smith et al., 1985; Weber et al., 1986; Bosma et al., 1990; Bu'Lock et al., 1990), and videofluoroscopy, which is the main technique in use in clinical practice (Dodds et al., 1990b; Newman et al., 1991).

The first phase is oral: the combined action of lingual muscles results in a depression in the oral cavity and the triggering of waves of contractions, which direct the bolus into the pharynx. The oral cavity is closed anteriorly by the lips and posteriorly by pressure of the tongue against the soft palate. Traversing the pharyngeal conduit constitutes the second, pharyngeal, phase. The soft palate rises, the base of the tongue projects the bolus into the laryngopharynx, and the upper esophageal sphincter relaxes. Simultaneously, the airways are protected by several means: raising the soft palate closes the nasal cavities, the larynx moves up and forward, the glottis closes, the aperture of the larynx is covered by the epiglottis and the base of the tongue, and the bolus is directed laterally and posteriorly. Respiration resumes as soon as the bolus passes into the esophagus. These first two phases, which are very interlinked, are followed by the third phase, which is purely esophageal.

In the newborn, the oral phase is inseparable from the sucking reflex: on contact with the nipple, rhythmic contractions of the tongue occur and the lips are pressed together. The pharyngeal phase occurs in a reflex manner after each suck so that the organization one suck/one swallow and its coordination with respiration occur in an entirely automatic sequence. Swallowing and respiration follow one another in an order that avoids aspiration. Deglutition apnea occurs simultaneously with the elevation of the soft palate, even before the closing of the glottis. Swallowing occurs during the natural pause between the end of inspiration and the start of expiration. Thus, the newborn can feed himself or herself without interrupting respiration, whose rate is governed by the sucking rhythm and returns to its previous value when the meal is finished (Selley et al., 1986; Weber et al., 1986).

There are no postnatal modifications of this program, which persists as long as the newborn child continues to feed at the breast or bottle. At about 4 months, swallowing begins to be influenced by the will of the infant, who can then hold the food bolus in the mouth without swallowing. This voluntary control, which results in dissociation of the oral and pharyngeal phases, inhibits the sucking-swallowing

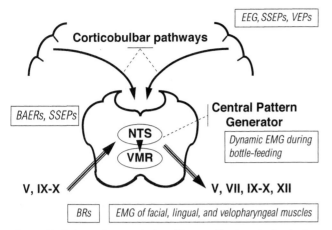

Figure 88–7. Central control of sucking-swallowing: the brainstem neuronal network involved in swallowing and the neurophysiological investigations that can be used to assess bulbar and suprabulbar involvement. NTS, nucleus of the tractus solitarius; VMR, ventromedian reticular formation.

automatism, without eliminating it entirely; it can be observed in certain pathological conditions in adults (Paulson and Gottlieb, 1968).

The regulation of sucking-swallowing involves several nervous system structures (Fig. 88–7). The central pattern generator for swallowing involves the nucleus of the tractus solitarius and adjacent ventromedian reticular formation. This center receives afferent sensory fibers from the tongue, the oral cavity, the pharynx, and the larynx via the paired V, VII, IX, and X cranial nerves. The efferent pathways are the paired V, VII, IX, and XII cranial nerves and the first two cervical roots. Suprabulbar control is exercised by the bilateral corticobulbar pathways arising from the opercular motor zones (Car, 1973; Miller, 1982; Jean, 1984).

Neurophysiological Studies

Understanding the mechanism and cause of dysphagia is essential for the management of the infant. Early research has demonstrated the role of cerebral (Worster-Drought, 1956) and bulbar (Graham, 1964) lesions. Some authors have reported the possibility that swallowing disorders may regress spontaneously after various time intervals (Franck and Gatewood, 1966). Illingworth (1969) emphasized the high incidence of dysphagia, the difficulties in authenticating swallowing disorders, and the need to know the cause to evaluate the issue of prognosis. In line with this, we developed a method of investigation (Renault and Raimbault, 1992) using several electromyographic techniques that provide convergent information on some nuclei and pathways of the brainstem involved in sucking-swallowing. Electromyographic activity of the facial muscles reflects the function of the neurons of the motor nucleus of the nerve VII. Blink reflexes investigate nerve V, the V-to-VII internuclear pathways, and the nerve VII.

Electromyographic activity of the muscles of the tongue and soft palate reflects the function of the motoneurons of the IX, X, and XII nerves. The dynamic EMG during bottle-feeding investigates the automatism generated and regulated in the central pattern generator for swallowing.

GENIOGLOSSUS MUSCLE AND THE HYPOGLOSSAL NERVE

The hypoglossal nerve is a purely motor nerve. Its nucleus consists of a column that extends for nearly the full length of the medulla oblongata. Emerging from the skull by the anterior condylar canal, the twelfth nerve crosses the pharyngomaxillary space and curves anteriorly in the carotid groove. In the sublingual region, it sends terminal branches to the ipsilateral muscles of the tongue. In addition, the twelfth nerve carries fibers from the first two cervical roots to the geniohyoid and thyrohyoid muscles.

The genioglossus is a paired paramedian muscle of the tongue; it can be recorded via the endo-oral route. After local anesthesia by touching this area with a solution of lidocaine, the needle electrode is inserted in the ventral surface of the tongue, slightly lateral to the midline. The interference pattern is recorded when the infant is crying and when the infant is sucking a nipple. The recruitment pattern was analyzed in 32 normal subjects aged from 4 days to 3 years (Renault and Raimbault, 1992). The normal mean amplitude of the interference pattern is 960 μV (range, 410 to 1.5 mV). In more than 50% of MUPs, the duration is from 1 to 2 ms. The proportion of polyphasic potentials is more than 30%.

A brief square wave electric shock (0.2 ms) of supramaximal intensity (30 to 70 mA) is used for hypoglossal NCSs. Nerve XII is stimulated proximally behind the mandible and then more distally under the chin. NCSs of nerve XII have been performed in 344 normal subjects between birth and the age of 15 years (Raimbault, 1988; Renault and Raimbault, 1992). The motor response has a polyphasic morphology, a mean duration from 6 to 10 ms, and amplitude from 0.8 to 1 mV. Latencies induced by stimulation under the angle of the mandible do not show a significant change between birth and 15 years, ranging from 2.8 to 4.6 ms (see Table 88–1). Nerve XII conduction velocity increases by 34.2% in the first year, 11.2% in the second year, 10.4% from 2 to 5 years, and 5.1% from 5 to 10 years (see Table 88–2).

MUSCLES OF THE SOFT PALATE AND THE PHARYNGEAL PLEXUS

The motor fibers of nerves IX and X that supply the muscles of the pharynx arise from the upper portion of the nucleus ambiguus. The pharyngeal branches of nerve X merge with the fibers of nerve

IX to constitute the pharyngeal plexus, which innervates muscles of the soft palate.

We record the electromyographic activity of muscles that are easily accessible via the oral route. The levator veli palatini muscle spreads into the large paramedian section of the soft palate. The electrode is inserted 1 to 1.5 cm outside the median line, about 0.5 cm under the mucous membrane. The palatoglossus muscle is recorded by placing the needle in the palatoglossal arch just under the mucous membrane. Similarly, the pharyngoglossus muscle is recorded in the palatopharyngeal arch. The normal mean amplitude of the interference pattern in these muscles of the soft palate is 1.3 mV (range, 380 to 1.8 mV). In more than 50% of MUPs, the duration is from 1 to 2 ms. The proportion of polyphasic MUPs is above 30%.

DYNAMIC STUDY OF SUCKING-SWALLOWING: ELECTROMYOGRAPHY DURING BOTTLE FEEDING

This method consists of simultaneously recording the electromyographic activity from two muscles while the infant takes formula milk or glucose solution from a bottle (Raimbault et al., 1979). For the oral phase, the genioglossus is recorded via a transcutaneous submental route, and the needle electrode traverses the mylohyoid, which is brought into play synchronously with the genioglossus (Doty and Bosma, 1956). For the pharyngeal phase, the thyrohyoid is easily accessible on the lateral face of the thyroid cartilage. Elevation of the larynx accompanies the second phase of swallowing (Dodds et al., 1990b). The recording continues during the entire feeding, permitting analysis of the activity of each of the muscles and observation of the chronology of their action and the coordination of the two phases of swallowing.

Normal results have been established in healthy term infants aged from 3 days to 18 months (Renault and Raimbault, 1992; Renault, 1998). The two muscles alternate regularly (Fig. 88–8). The electromyographic activity of the genioglossus muscle during suction is organized in bursts with a full interference pattern showing a rapid increase and then a decrease in amplitude, giving a fusiform aspect. The bursts are separated by a quiescent period. Initial frequency of sucking ranges from 0.6 to 2 Hz (mean, 1.4 Hz). Mean duration of genioglossal bursts, calculated for the first 20 sucks, ranges from 180 to 460 ms depending on the infant, without any correlation with age. The duration of the bursts and quiescent periods between sucks increases progressively (from 35% to 100%) during the course of the feeding. This probably reflects both fatigue and decreasing appetite. The electromyographic activity of the thyrohyoid muscle is also organized into bursts with the same fusiform shape, separated by a rest period, with identical frequency: each suck is followed by a swallow in the newborn and young infant before 5 months, the age at which swallowing is inseparable from the reflex of sucking. For the thyrohyoid, the mean duration of bursts calculated for the first 20 sucks is 210 to 520 ms. The start of the burst varies in relation to the end of lingual activity: the onset of thyrohyoid activity ranges from 100 ms before to 220 ms after the end of lingual activity, depending on the infant, and is unrelated to age. The timing of the two muscle contractions varies from one child to another but varies little from one swallow to another during feeding in the same child.

Abnormal results are classified in three stages of severity of sucking-swallowing disorders (Renault and Raimbault, 1992; Renault, 1998): a severe stage, in which the tongue does not perform sucking activity and the pharyngeal phase is either inactive (Fig. 88–9) or tonic; a moderate stage, in which sucking is present but the pharyngeal phase is either synchronous (Fig. 88–10) or uncertain; and a mild stage, in which the alternation between sucking and swallowing is irregular, revealing variation in the timing of the two muscles.

EMG of the facial, lingual, and velopharyngeal muscles and EMG during bottle feeding target the disturbed motor organization, assess its severity, and show whether it is isolated or associated with

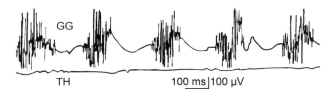

Figure 88–9. Dynamic electromyography during bottle feeding: abnormal results in a full-term newborn with isolated Pierre Robin sequence (day 11, ineffective sucking). The activity of genioglossus muscle (GG) consists of bursts of short duration, and the thyrohyoid muscle (TH) is inactive.

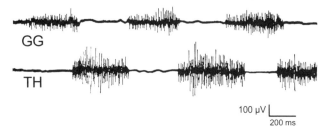

Figure 88–8. Dynamic electromyography during bottle feeding: normal alternating pattern of genioglossus (GG, upper tracing) and thyrohyoid (TH) muscles in a full-term newborn on day 10.

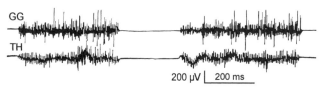

Figure 88–10. Dynamic electromyography during bottle feeding, abnormal results: synchronization of the oral and pharyngeal phases in a full-term newborn with isolated Pierre Robin sequence (day 27, poor sucking and aspiration episodes). GG, genioglossus muscle; TH, thyrohyoid muscle.

a lesion of the bulbar motor nuclei. Other neurophysiological examinations (electroencephalography, brainstem auditory evoked potentials, somatosensory and visual evoked potentials) and neuroimaging (ultrasonography, computed tomography, and magnetic resonance imaging) studies can be used to assess any anatomical or functional suprabulbar involvement (see Fig. 88–7).

Sucking-Swallowing Disorders: Congenital Dysphagia

Sucking-swallowing disorders of the newborn present as difficulty in feeding or respiratory complications, or both (Thieffry and Job, 1954; Illingworth, 1969). It is not always easy to demonstrate that pulmonary disease is due to aspiration because aspiration is often silent and chest radiographs may be normal (Le Moing et al., 1976). The diagnosis of dysphagia should immediately be considered in patients with major feeding difficulties, with salivary stasis, and at risk due to orofacial malformations or encephalopathies. Swallowing disorders should also be sought in cases of early refractory bronchopulmonary pathology and in cases with predisposing factors or anomalies with which feeding-swallowing disorders are often associated (Table 88–5).

Table 88–5. Clinical Features, Predisposing Factors, and Associated Pathologies in Sucking-Swallowing Disorders of the Newborn and Infant

Clinical features
Absence of sucking
Absence of swallowing
Salivary stasis
Slow sucking
Nasal reflux
Cyanosis and tachypnea during feeding
Apnea and/or bradycardia during feeding
Coughing
Bronchial congestion
Noisy respiration
Recurrent bronchopulmopathy
Poor weight gain

Predisposing Factors
Prematurity
Lethargy
Hypotonia
Poor cough reflex
Dyspnea
Prolonged tube feeding
Parenteral feeding
Tracheotomy
Family history of swallowing disorders, severe malaise, or unexplained sudden death

Associated Pathologies
Gastroesophageal reflux
Esophageal dysmotility
Laryngotracheomalacia
Tracheobronchial dyskinesia
Congenital heart disease
Failure to thrive

Cough is a sign that is immediately suggestive if accompanied by oropharyngeal or bronchial congestion. Coughing is often wrongly attributed to viral tracheobronchitis. It is essential to know whether the cough is precipitated by meals and whether it existed before any infection. Cough may also be completely absent.

The chest radiograph can show focal or diffuse opacities, enhancement of bronchial images, and some degree of thoracic distention. Images often vary from one radiograph to another. Findings most suggestive of aspiration pneumonia are predominance of anomalies on the right and the involvement of the right upper lobe, which may progress to atelectasis. In a series of 37 infants with congenital dysphagia aged less than 3 months, chest radiographs were normal in 20 (Baudon et al., 1997).

Videofluoroscopy is primarily used to study the pharyngeal and esophageal phases of swallowing (Newman et al., 1991). Fluoroscopic studies should be recorded on videotape to allow repeated review (Dodds et al., 1990a). In a series of 77 infants with feeding difficulties under 1 month of age, videofluoroscopic studies of swallowing demonstrated aspiration in 19 patients, including 10 with negative upper gastrointestinal series (Vazquez and Buonomo, 1999). The examination can show the entry of liquid into the trachea and reveal any mild or late aspiration at the end of the meal in the form of a narrow line; the absence of coughing indicates silent aspiration. It can also show reflux to the nasal cavity, a leakage toward the pharynx during the oral phrase, or residual food in the pharynx after the swallow. Videofluoroscopy can also reveal esophageal pathology: cricopharyngeal achalasia, esophageal dysmotility, malformation, tracheoesophageal fistula, or gastroesophageal reflux disease.

Endoscopy can demonstrate anatomical abnormalities or functional disorders of the pharynx or larynx. At the level of the trachea and bronchi, aspiration generally leads to marked edema of the mucosa, first- and second-degree inflammatory signs, and predominance of anomalies on the right, with abundant clear fluid secretions for which tests, pH, rheology, and amylase level, confirm their salivary nature. The methylene blue test verifies the absence of a tracheoesophageal fistula. Bronchoalveolar lavage can reveal alveolitis and demonstrate cell inclusions indicative of food aspiration.

Electromyographic investigations have two goals: to demonstrate the existence of swallowing disorders and to understand their mechanisms. The results of the electromyographic study enable three types of pathology to be distinguished: suprabulbar lesions, lesions of the paired cranial nerves, and isolated dysphagia (Table 88–6).

CONGENITAL DYSPHAGIA WITH SUPRABULBAR LESIONS

When the dysphagia is of suprabulbar origin, sucking-swallowing incoordination is demonstrated

---

Table 88–6. Principal Causes of Sucking-Swallowing Disorders in the Newborn and Infant

Malformations
  Atresia of the choanae
  Cleft palate
  Microretrognathia
  Pierre-Robin sequence
  Hypoglossia syndromes
  Macroglossia
  Facial microsomia
  Opitz G/BBB syndrome
  CHARGE association (*C*olobomata, *H*eart disease, *A*tresia of the choanae, *R*etarded growth and development, *G*enital hypoplasia, and *E*ar anomalies)
  Esophageal atresia or stenosis
  Cricopharyngeal achalasia
  Abnormal arterial arch

Disorders of the Nervous System
  Suprabulbar
    Prenatal encephalopathies
    Birth trauma and asphyxia
  Bulbar
    Perinatal brainstem hypoxia-ischemia
    Möbius' syndrome
    Chiari malformation
    Severe neonatal spinal muscular atrophy
    Pontocerebellar hypoplasia type I
  Congenital Isolated Dysphagia
    Isolated dysfunction or immaturity of sucking-swallowing
  Neuromuscular Disease
    Congenital muscular dystrophy
    Congenital myopathy
    Congenital myasthenic syndrome
    Dysautonomia
    Lower cranial nerve birth trauma
  Transient Dysphagia
    Transient isolated dysphagia in prematurity
    Neonate born to myasthenic mother
    Lethargy, coma
    Drug side effect
    Acute disease with general status alteration
    Stomatitis
    Dyspneic bronchopulmonary disease
    Recent tonsillectomy

---

by dynamic EMG during the bottle feeding, but there is no electromyographic sign of denervation in the facial, lingual, and velopharyngeal muscles. Electroencephalography, evoked potentials, and neuroimaging can demonstrate cerebral lesions. In such cases, the dysphagia can be considered a consequence of a cerebral disorder and is often a sign that predicts cerebral palsy (Worster-Drought, 1956; Sullivan and Rosenbloom, 1996). Sucking-swallowing disorders are one of the possible sequelae of prenatal and perinatal hypoxic-ischemic encephalopathies. These cerebral disorders lead to a suprabulbar syndrome with generalized hypotonia, lethargy, facial hypotonia with salivary incontinence, and sometimes spasm on mouth opening. Feeding difficulties and their respiratory complications are revealing signs of cerebral impairment that will subsequently manifest as poor axial tone, spastic hypertonia or dystonia of the limbs, and dysarthria. When neurophysiological and neuroradiological investigations show more or less diffuse anatomical and functional cerebral lesions, this can indicate severe spastic quadriplegia. These cerebral investigations may be normal in dystonic-athetoid forms of cerebral palsy.

In relatively moderate cases, dysphagia progressively improves over several months. In some children, difficulties may persist, in particular during ingestion of liquids, but aspiration is rare and the dysphagia has no repercussions on bronchopulmonary status or growth. In severe encephalopathies leading to multiple handicaps, swallowing disorders are a major problem with risk of malnutrition, bronchopulmonary disease, and death due to aspiration (Reilly et al., 1996). In these severe cases, aspiration of liquid foods is very frequent and usually silent; tracheobronchial dyskinesia and gastroesophageal reflux with hiatal hernia are often associated findings (Rogers et al., 1994).

Congenital dysphagia associated with facial diplegia and localized bilateral anterior opercular lesions constitute the congenital type of Foix-Chavany-Marie syndrome (Graff-Radford et al., 1986). In addition to difficulties in swallowing, then chewing, and severe dysarthria, these patients may present with psychomotor delay, cerebral palsy, epilepsy, or verbal agnosia (Christen et al. 2000).

Feeding difficulty that necessitates tube feeding is a common feature of the Prader-Willi syndrome. It tends to resolve within the first weeks of life. There is a dysmorphic facies with an open triangle-shaped mouth but no marked facial weakness. The generalized hypotonia is often profound, and the infant may appear motionless in the first few days of life (Dubowitz, 1980).

CONGENITAL DYSPHAGIA DUE TO PERINATAL BRAINSTEM INJURY

When the dysphagia is of bulbar origin, EMG shows signs of denervation in the territory of the cranial nerves and blink reflexes may be altered. Normal results of electroencephalography, evoked potentials, and neuroimaging should rule out associated cerebral lesions. In newborns with a neonatal onset of swallowing disorders and a history of prenatal pathology or acute fetal distress that subsequently have a favorable course, the hypothesis of hypoxic-ischemic lesions localized to the brainstem has been proposed. We reported these features in a series of 12 patients (Renault and Couvreur, 1992). All of these children had major dysphagia at birth, complicated by early aspiration-induced pulmonary disease and failure to thrive. Nasal reflux and salivary stasis were obvious in most cases. The majority had facial hypotonia, sometimes with asymmetry of the tongue or soft palate. They all had swallowing disorders that lasted from 9 to 26 months. Neurogenic electromyographic signs detected in the muscles of the face and in several lingual and velopharyngeal muscles indicate lesions of the VII, IX, X, and XII cranial nerves. The R2 component of blink reflexes was abolished (11 of 12) with delayed latency (3 of 12) or abolition (3 of 12) of the R1 component. Abolition or lengthening of the latency of the R1 component of blink reflexes associated with normal latency of the response of the orbicularis oculi muscle on stimulation of nerve VII suggests an ipsilateral lesion of the pons (Kimura, 1970). Abolition of the R2 component suggests a more caudal location of the lesions: the spinal trigeminal nucleus or adjacent reticular formation (Kimura, 1975; Kiers and Carroll, 1990). The perinatal histories in this series suggest that the clinical and electrodiagnostic picture of dysphagia with lesions of several cranial nerves is the consequence of perinatal anoxic ischemic injury of the brainstem. Even though the brainstem and the spinal cord are less vulnerable to anoxic ischemia than the cerebral cortex, pathological studies have shown a pattern of brainstem damage after acute asphyxia in neonatal (Leech and Alvord, 1977) or prenatal (Alvord and Shaw, 1989) anoxia ischemia. Histopathological features compatible with fetal asphyxia have been described in the thalamus and brainstem in premature newborns with respiratory failure and multiple cranial nerve palsies (Wilson et al., 1982). Hemorrhage of the brainstem and cervical spinal cord has been reported in a term newborn after meconium aspiration resulting in hypotonia, absence of sucking, lingual hemiatrophy, diaphragmatic paralysis, and electromyographic signs of denervation of the trapezius and sternomastoid muscles (Blazer et al., 1989). The diencephalon, pons, and medulla oblongata are the usual sites of neuronal loss in cases of severe neonatal asphyxia such as cardiac arrest (Govaert, 1993).

When the anoxic-ischemic lesions and/or hemorrhage involve both brainstem and hemispherical structures, the dysphagia is due to the effects of both bulbar and suprabulbar dysfunction and the condition may progress to cerebral palsy.

CONGENITAL ISOLATED DYSPHAGIA

Congenital dysphagia exists in premature and term newborns in the absence of any neuromuscular disorder, malformation syndrome, or neonatal disease (Mbonda et al., 1995; Inder and Volpe, 1998). Under suitable management, the course is usually favorable after a period ranging from several weeks to 2 years. In a series of 37 newborns with congenital dysphagia (Baudon et al., 1997), the disorder was isolated in 10 term newborns and 9 premature babies. In these 19 patients, EMG during bottle feeding showed a lack of coordination between the oral and pharyngeal phases of swallowing, but the isolated nature of the dysphagia was confirmed by the normality of all other neurophysiological and neuroradiological examinations. Swallowing disorders improved progressively: normal oral feeding could be started after the 40th week of gestational age in 7 premature infants, at 6 and 10 months in the two other premature infants, and from 2 to 15 months in term newborns. The classic hypothesis put forward to explain these cases of congenital isolated dysphagia is a transitory dysfunction of the central nervous organization of the automatism of sucking-swallowing. It is tempting to talk of the immaturity of the sucking-swallowing function, especially in prematurity. However, the possibility of a lesion that has not been detected by the investigations cannot be ruled out, and a history of acute fetal distress or the existence of minor neurological anomalies should suggest the hypothesis of an unknown perinatal cerebral event.

OROFACIAL MALFORMATIONS WITH DYSPHAGIA

In these pathologies, dysphagia and its respiratory complications can be due to both anatomical malformations and neurological disorders.

Pierre Robin sequence is characterized by glossoptosis, cleft palate, and retrognathia. The newborn with this syndrome is at risk for feeding difficulties and obstruction of the airways (Robin, 1994). In the first weeks of life, about 85% of patients with Pierre Robin sequence have feeding difficulties, which may lead to aspiration, bronchopulmonary disease, and failure to thrive (Cozzi and Pierro, 1985). Careful evaluation and management of respiratory and feeding disorders have led to an improvement in both morbidity and mortality rates (Bull et al., 1990; Caouette-Laberge et al., 1994). We have conducted blink reflex study, EMG during bottle feeding, and EMG of the face, tongue, and soft palate in 25 infants with isolated Pierre Robin sequence (Renault et al., 2000). Electromyographic recruitment pattern in facial and lingual muscles and blink reflexes were normal in all cases. The electromyographic recruitment pattern in the soft palate was normal in 14 of 25 patients, showed signs of muscular hypoplasia without denervation in 10 of 25 patients, and showed signs of denervation in 1 of 25 patients. EMG during bottle feeding showed sucking-swallowing disorders in 20 of 25 patients, including 4 patients without apparent feeding difficulties. By establishing the sucking-swallowing disorder and its severity, the EMG helped clarify whether tube feeding was indicated. In clinical practice, it is also important to bear in mind which EMG can reveal a lack of sucking-swallowing coordination even in the absence of a clinically apparent feeding disorder. From a pathophysiological point of view, our results suggest that the main neurological anomaly is a disorder of tongue and pharynx motor organization, which can by itself account for all the signs of isolated Pierre Robin sequence. At birth, the dysfunction of the lingual and pharyngeal muscles results in glossoptosis, upper airway obstruction, and dysphagia. In the prenatal period, the delay in lingual motility hampers the closure of the palate and affects mandibular growth. This sequential and interlinked pathogenesis of the dysmorphic triad is at the origin of the term *Pierre Robin sequence* (Pashayan and Lewis, 1984). Pierre Robin sequence may be associated with cardiac, skeletal, ocular, or endocrine pathologies. Associated Pierre Robin sequence occasionally reveals a specific syndrome—Stickler, DiGeorge, catch 22, fetal alcohol, or others (Cohen, 1979; Sheffield et al., 1987).

The Opitz G/BBB syndrome of dysphagia, hypertelorism, and hypospadias is an inherited disorder characterized by midline defects, which may include lip-palate-laryngotracheal clefts (Quaderi et al., 1997). Aspiration is a frequent manifestation in these infants and poses the greatest threat to life (Bershof et al., 1992). In a personal study of three infants with G syndrome, EMG was normal in facial, lingual, and velopharyngeal muscles, but EMG during bottle feeding showed a severe sucking-swallowing disorder at the ages of 3, 5, and 8 weeks, respectively.

Sucking-swallowing incoordination and multiple cranial nerve palsies are often seen in *CHARGE association* (Byerly and Pauli, 1993). The lower cranial nerves VII, VIII, IX, and X appear to be those most frequently involved. Swallowing dysfunction may be present even in the absence of obvious structural orofacial abnormalities. In a series of 44 patients, 58% had pharyngolaryngeal anomalies (dysphagia, laryngomalacia, glossoptosis, laryngeal paralysis, cleft, stenosis) leading to dyspnea with altered blood gas levels (Roger et al., 1999). Electrodiagnostic studies show denervation in the territories of the nerves involved, and EMG during bottle feeding demonstrates pharyngeal incoordination.

Dysphagia is clinically severe in *hypoglossia-hypodactyly syndrome* (Nevin et al., 1975; Jones, 1997b). We studied four infants with severe hypoglossia that was associated in one patient with upper limb malformation and isolated in the other three patients. Facial, lingual, and pharyngeal EMG showed signs of bilateral denervation of the genioglossus muscles in the four infants (Fig. 88–11) and of the muscles of

the soft palate in two patients and of the face in two patients. Facial and hypoglossal nerve conduction were normal, and the R1 component of the blink reflexes was present with normal latency in all cases. EMG during bottle feeding could be performed in only one infant and showed severe incoordination. The other three infants had a degree of dysphagia that precluded any attempt at feeding; one of them had undergone tracheostomy.

These electromyographic results in hypoglossia syndromes and CHARGE association suggest involvement of the cranial nerve nuclei and can be compared with similar abnormalities seen in the Möbius syndrome, which could have the same pathogenesis (Govaert et al., 1989).

DYSPHAGIA IN NEUROMUSCULAR DISEASES

Dysphagia may be present from birth in severe spinal muscular atrophy type I. Typical and generalized neurogenic signs are found on EMG of limb muscles (Renault et al., 1996). The same features may be shown in the genioglossus muscle as the result of associated bulbar palsy due to involvement of lower cranial nerve nuclei (Moore and Pitt, 1999). The facial muscles are not affected. Congenital dysphagia, generalized hypotonia, respiratory insufficiency, and joint contractures are main features of pontocerebellar hypoplasia type I (Barth, 1993). Electromyographic findings are diffuse neurogenic signs mimicking results observed in isolated spinal muscular atrophy, but decreased motor and sensory nerve conduction has been reported (Goutieres et al., 1977).

Some severe congenital myopathies and congenital muscular dystrophies are associated with orofacial involvement and swallowing disorders in the immediate newborn period. The problem is already present in utero, because there often is a history of hydramnios. The feeding difficulties are associated with respiratory weakness, severe diffuse paralytic hypotonia with amyotrophy, tendon contractures, and marked facial hypotonia. Ptosis and ophthalmoplegia may be found. The amyotrophy and contractures of the muscles of mastication may provoke mandibular ankylosis. The severity of feeding difficulties and their bronchopulmonary complications and persistence during growth have been reported, especially in congenital forms of myotonic muscular dystrophy (Aicardi et al., 1974) and merosin-deficient congenital muscular dystrophy (Philpot et al.,1999). Sucking and swallowing difficulties are almost constant in the severe neonatal form of nemaline myopathy, in early-onset centronuclear myopathies, and in congenital sex-linked myotubular myopathy (Fardeau and Tomé, 1994). In these pathologies, EMG of facial, lingual, and velopharyngeal muscles is often difficult to interpret. At the least, it should show the absence of neurogenic signs and the normality of facial nerve conduction and blink reflexes. EMG of the limbs may be necessary to demonstrate the myopathic origin of the muscular

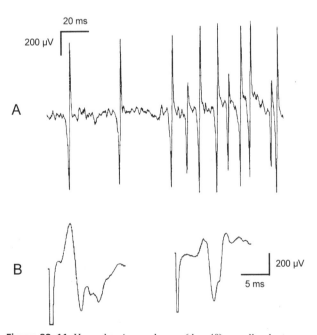

Figure 88–11. Hypoglossia syndrome (day 40): needle electromyography of the left genioglossus muscle. *A,* Neurogenic pattern on crying. *B,* Normal-latency, low-amplitude simplified morphology responses to electrical stimulation of the nerve XII on distal and proximal points with normal hypoglossal nerve conduction velocity (32.4 m per second).

weakness. Congenital myopathies should be distinguished from the Prader-Willi syndrome, which presents in the neonatal period with profound generalized hypotonia and sucking-swallowing difficulties.

Familial dysautonomia is a rare affection that results in floppy infant syndrome and dysphagia.

Feeding difficulties and aspiration may be the first signs of congenital myasthenic syndromes. Neonatal disorders of neuromuscular transmission have varying pathophysiology and expression. Typical clinical findings include feeding difficulty, respiratory dysfunction, ophthalmoparesis, ptosis, and hypotonia. Symptoms may worsen with crying and physiological activity (Engel, 1994). Electrodiagnostic studies help confirm the presence, measure the severity, and reveal the underlying mechanism of the defect of neuromuscular transmission. It also provides an objective estimate of responsiveness to therapeutic agents. The findings of NCSs, repetitive stimulation, standard needle EMG, and single-fiber EMG in major congenital myasthenic syndromes were reviewed by Harper (1996). Neurophysiological studies are not indispensable in neonates born to myasthenic mothers because dysphagia is transitory and the diagnosis is easy when the mother's disease in known. The incidence of neonatal transient myasthenia gravis is decreasing with improvement of maternal treatment. However, maternal disease may be latent, and acute choking episodes may be a presenting symptom of a floppy infant with associated bulbar weakness. There is no correlation between the severity of the disease in the mother and the infant. Decrement with low-frequency repetitive stimulation may be observed in the infant as well as in the mother. The symptoms appear within the first few hours, and the mean disease duration is 18 days. A prenatal onset results in a severe form with hydramnios, arthrogryposis, and severe hypotonia (Dinger and Prager, 1993; Barnes et al., 1995).

Congenital laryngeal paralysis results in dysphagia associated with dysphonia, which usually has a good prognosis (Aicardi, 1992). This is probably due to prenatal or perinatal compression: rotation and lateral flexion of the head results in stretching of the superior branch of the laryngeal nerve against the thyroid cartilage and that of the recurrent laryngeal nerve against the cricoid cartilage. More rarely, obstetrical paralysis of nerves IX, X, and XI (Greenberg et al., 1987) and involvement of the nerve XII associated with obstetrical paralysis of the brachial plexus (Haenggeli and Lacourt, 1989) have been reported.

Acquired Dysphagia in Infants and Children

Swallowing disorders may occur during different neuromuscular pathologies, and the findings can be diagnostic. Dysphagia associated with stomatological, otorhinolaryngological, and esophageal affections are not discussed here.

DIAGNOSIS

The diagnosis of acquired dysphagia is easy when there is a bout of coughing or choking during swallowing, indicating leakage into the larynx, or nasal regurgitation due to velopharyngeal weakness. Examination can show flaccidity of the soft palate, weakness or asymmetry of palatal reflex and voluntary contractions, and buccopharyngeal salivary congestion, sometimes with drooling. Symptoms may be more moderate, requiring attentive observation of the meal: the child may eat and drink slowly in small mouthfuls, keep food longer in the mouth, and have to swallow three or four times to empty the mouth and may avoid drinking or, on the contrary, take a sip of water after each mouthful. Flexion and extension of the neck to aid in projecting the food into the pharynx may also be seen. Auscultation should search for respiratory sounds after the ingestion of a small amount of water.

It is important to note that swallowing disorders may be subclinical and may only be revealed by the onset of bronchopulmonary complications: bronchitis, bronchopneumonia, and atelectasis. On principle, any pulmonary infection associated with a neurological condition should suggest a swallowing disorder.

Videofluoroscopy can reveal tracheal aspiration. Endoscopy can show the presence of food particles in the airways, verify the absence of anomalies of anatomical structures, and show pharyngeal muscle tone. As in the case of congenital dysphagia, facial, lingual, and velopharyngeal EMG can help clarify the pathophysiology of acquired dysphagia: paralysis of the soft palate, muscle pathology, or poor motor command (Renault and Raimbault, 1992). A dynamic electromyographic method has been developed to study the voluntary swallowing of saliva or an alimentary bolus (Ertekin et al., 1995; Ertekin et al., 1998).

ETIOLOGIES

Aspiration is most often a complication of a known neurological or muscular deficit, and when such a deficit exists, it is a good idea to search systematically for a swallowing disorder to avoid sudden aspiration accidents or repetitive silent aspiration (Wiles, 1991). The pathology involved may be acute or progressive central neurological dysfunction, coma of whatever cause, a cerebral lesion after cranial trauma (Schurr et al., 1999), a vascular accident, acute encephalitis, a degenerative disorder with bulbar or suprabulbar involvement, or cerebral palsy (Rogers et al., 1994) (see Table 88–6). The risk of aspiration is high in children who have undergone tracheostomy (Loughlin and Lefton-Greif, 1994; Kirshblum et al., 1999). Intermittent suprabulbar palsy may reveal status epilepticus of benign partial epilepsy (Fejerman and Di Blasi, 1987) or other epileptic events associated with oromotor dyspraxia (Deonna et al., 1993).

Aspiration may occur during the course of peripheral neuromuscular disorders such as myasthenia gravis and some structural or metabolic congenital myopathies and muscular dystrophies (Nowak et al., 1982; Philpot et al., 1999). Electrodiagnostic studies of the cranial nerves and limbs contribute to these etiological diagnoses. Presenting symptoms are bulbar in 16% of patients with myasthenia gravis: difficulty swallowing, nasal speech, and difficulty chewing (Grob et al., 1987). Dysphagia and ophthalmoplegia may be the presenting symptoms in children with oxidative metabolic disorders who later develop more diffuse weakness (Munnich et al., 1996). During acute polyradiculoneuritis and polydermatomyositis, the occurrence of a swallowing disorder suggests a progressive course associated with respiratory failure and necessitates very strict surveillance and withdrawal of oral food. Oculopharyngeal muscular dystrophy begins with ptosis and dysphagia. Onset is usually in middle or late adult life; a few cases with childhood-onset dysphagia and gastrointestinal involvement have been reported (Lacomis et al., 1991; Amato et al., 1995). Isolated temporary pharyngeal paralysis is characterized by acute unilateral velopharyngeal paralysis provoking rhinolalia aperta and swallowing difficulty with nasal reflux. This rare disease is considered as idiopathic or viral neuritis of the ninth and tenth cranial nerves; the complete spontaneous recovery is usually observed after a few weeks or months (Aubergé et al., 1979; Roberton and Mellor, 1982). Velopharyngeal paralysis may reveal a tumor or malformation of the posterior cranial fossa, bulbar poliomyelitis, or progressive bulbar paralysis. Impairment of the IX, X, and XII paired cranial nerves with paralysis of the soft palate and dysphagia may be seen in Chiari malformations, in particular type II (Sieben et al., 1971; Gerard et al., 1992). In a prospective study in 22 infants with congenital Chiari II malformation, 4 infants had dysphagia and aspiration resulting in respiratory complications with onset from the third to sixth month (Linder and Lindholm, 1997). In a series of 46 patients with Chiari malformations, 15 had progressive dysphagia preceding other signs of brainstem dysfunction. All 15 had normal swallowing function before the development of dysphagic symptoms. Suboccipital craniectomy and cervical laminectomy were performed; postoperative outcome with regard to swallowing function correlated with the severity of preoperative symptoms (Pollack et al., 1992). Progressive bulbar paralysis of childhood (Fazio-Londe disease) is a very rare hereditary condition, with fewer than 30 children described, including only 6 for whom an autopsy was performed (McShane et al., 1992). The age of onset ranged from 12 months to 12 years. The most frequent presenting symptoms was stridor, followed by ptosis, dysarthria, facial palsy, and dysphagia. Progressive involvement of cranial nerves and respiratory difficulties led to death in a few years. The electromyographic findings of reduced interference pattern with enlarged MUPs in bulbar muscles are an important diagnostic sign of the disease.

Diphtheria is now a rare disease in countries that apply systematic immunization programs. Local neurological complications appear 4 to 5 weeks after nasopharynx infection with *Corynebacterium diphtheriae*: soft palate, accommodation, and oculomotor paralyses. Blurred vision and swallowing difficulties mark the onset of diphtheric neuropathy. A polyneuropathic feature mimicking Guillain-Barré syndrome may appear during the following weeks (Kurdi and Abdul-Kader, 1979). Segmental demyelination predominates on the posterior roots (Solders et al., 1989). Recovery is usually complete.

In tetanus, salivary stasis and dysphagia associated with trismus and neck stiffness are the first clinical manifestations, appearing from 5 to 14 days after infection with *Clostridium tetani* introduced through the umbilical cord in a newborn baby or a wound in older infants and children. Neurophysiological studies are of little help for diagnosis: motor and sensory NCSs are normal, H wave is easily elicitable in distal muscles, F waves are of high amplitude, and EMG may show spontaneous high-frequency discharges (Khuralbet and Neubauer, 1998).

Classic botulism develops 12 to 36 hours after ingestion of the toxin-containing food. Early symptoms are blurred vision, diplopia, dizziness, dysarthria, and dysphagia followed by respiratory paralysis. Infantile botulism (Thompson et al., 1980; Schreiner et al., 1991) occurs in infants younger than 6 months and is characterized by a prodromal phase of constipation with progressive development over 4 to 5 days of complete hypotonia, areflexia, poor sucking, weak cry, ptosis, and paralysis of other cranial nerves and of the limbs. Ventilatory support may be necessary. Needle EMG may show low-amplitude and short-duration spontaneous fibrillation potentials and reduced recruitment pattern with low-amplitude and polyphasic short-duration MUPs. Sensory nerve conduction studies are normal. Motor conduction studies reveal markedly reduced amplitude of compound muscle action potentials. High-rate (25- to 30-Hz) repetitive nerve stimulation provokes incremental response from 125% to 3000%. The response to low-rate repetitive nerve stimulation (2 to 5 Hz) is more variable (Cornblath et al., 1983). Stimulation single-fiber EMG is another useful way to demonstrate the presynaptic neuromuscular junctional transmission disorder (Chaudry and Crawford, 1999).

MANAGEMENT

This consists of adaptation of feeding methods to avoid repeated aspiration. It is guided by the severity of the swallowing disorder and by the level of respiratory complications shown by clinical, radiographic, and blood gas findings. Fitting of a nasogastric tube immediately is often helpful, and the safe position and repeated pharyngeal aspiration avoid choking. Particular care must be taken in case of hematosis deficit. Antibiotics, anti-inflammatory agents, mucolytics, and physiotherapy combat infection and bronchopulmonary congestion. The decision to resume oral feeding of liquids or solids is taken as a function of the improvement in swallowing and the respiratory state. The texture of foods should be taken into account with the aid of a dietician, and it is useful for a speech therapist to watch a meal and reeducate the buccopharyngeal motor organization. If it is suspected that aspiration may recur, it is best to wait several days before attempting to reintroduce oral feeding. Generally, in children with cerebral lesions, the risk of aspiration is greater if the child is forced to eat by a caregiver who does not pay attention to correct body posture and presentation of food.

In conclusion, the earlier dysphagia is recognized, the greater the likelihood of avoiding its respiratory and nutritional complications. Clinical, radiological, and neurophysiological investigations enable the severity of swallowing disorders to be evaluated and the etiological mechanisms of dysphagia to be elucidated and thus provide a good starting point for therapeutic decisions. Electromyographic method combines several techniques: EMG of facial muscles, facial NCS, blink reflex study, EMG of the tongue, hypoglossal NCS, EMG of the soft palate, and a dynamic electromyographic study of the sucking-swallowing automatism during bottle feeding. Results observed in pathological conditions are useful in assessing the sucking-swallowing reflex, in revealing functional disturbances in the brainstem, and in evaluating orofacial malformations and congenital paralyses of cranial nerves.

References

Aicardi J: Disorders of the peripheral nerves. In Aicardi J (ed): Diseases of the Nervous System in Childhood. London, MacKeith Press, 1992; 1113–1171.

Aicardi J, Conti D, Goutières F: Les formes néonatales de la dystrophie myotonique de Steinert. J Neurol Sci 1974;22:149–164.

Alexiou D, Manolidis C, Papaevangellou G, et al: Frequency of other malformations in congenital hypoplasia of depressor anguli oris muscle syndrome. Arch Dis Child 1976;51:891–893.

Alvord EC, Shaw CM: Congenital difficulties with swallowing and breathing associated with maternal polyhydramnios: Neurocristopathy or medullary infarction? J Child Neurol 1989;4:299–306.

Amato AA, Jackson CE, Ridings LW, et al: Childhood-onset oculopharyngodistal myopathy with chronic intestinal pseudo-obstruction. Muscle Nerve 1995;18:842–847.

Aminoff MJ: Facial neuropathies. In Aminoff MJ (ed): Electromyography in Clinical Practice: Clinical and Electrodiagnostic Aspects of Neuromuscular Disease. New York, Churchill Livingstone, 1998; 513–523.

Angerer M, Pfadenhauer K, Stohr M: Prognosis of facial palsy in Borrelia burgdorferi meningopolyradiculoneuritis. J Neurol 1993;240:319–321.

Ardran GM, Kemp FH, Lind J: A cineradiography of bottle feeding. Br J Radiol 1958;31:11–22.

Aubergé C, Ponsot G, Gayraud P, et al: Les hémiparésies vélopalatines isolées et acquises chez l'enfant. Arch Fr Pédiatr 1979; 36:283–286.

Bailey RO, Marzulo DC, Harris MB: Infantile facioscapulohumeral muscular dystrophy: New observations. Acta Neurol Scand 1986;74:51–58.

Barnes PR, Kanabar DJ, Brueton L: Recurrent congenital arthrogryposis leading to a diagnosis of myasthenia gravis in an initially asymptomatic mother. Neuromuscul Disord 1995;5:59–65.

Barth PG: Pontocerebellar hypoplasia: An overview of a group of inherited neurodegenerative disorders with fetal onset. Brain Dev 1993;15:411–422.

Baudon JJ, Renault F, Tarhaoui L: Diagnostic et prise en charge des troubles de la déglutition chez le nouveau-né et le nourrisson de moins de 3 mois. In Aujard Y, Beaufils F, Chaussain JL, et al (eds): Journées Parisiennes de Pédiatrie. Paris, Flammarion Médecine-Sciences, 1997; 17–22.

Bershof JF, Guyuron B, Olsen MM: G syndrome: A review of the literature and a case report. J Craniomaxillofac Surg 1992; 20:24–27.

Blazer S, Hemli JA, Sujov PO, et al: Neonatal bilateral diaphragmatic paralysis caused by brain stem haemorrhage. Arch Dis Child 1989;64:50–52.

Bosma JF, Hepburn LG, Josell SD, et al: Ultrasound demonstration of tongue motions during suckle feeding. Dev Med Child Neurol 1990;32:223–229.

Boulu P, Willer JC, Cambier J: Analyse électrophysiologique du réflexe de clignement chez l'homme. Rev Neurol (Paris) 1981; 137:523–533.

Brouwer OF, Padberg GW, Wijmenga C, et al: Facioscapulohumeral muscular dystrophy in early childhood. Arch Neurol 1994;51: 387–394.

Bu'Lock F, Woolridge MW, Baum JD: Development of co-ordination of sucking, swallowing and breathing: Ultrasound study of term and preterm infants. Dev Med Child Neurol 1990;32:669–678.

Bull MJ, Givan DC, Sadove AM, et al: Improved outcome in Pierre Robin sequence: Effect of multidisciplinary evaluation and management. Pediatrics 1990;86:294–301.

Byerly KA, Pauli RM: Cranial nerve abnormalities in CHARGE association. Am J Med Genet 1993;45:751–757.

Caouette-Laberge L, Bayet B, Larocque Y: The Pierre Robin sequence: Review of 125 cases and evolution of treatment modalities. Plast Reconstr Surg 1994;93:934–942.

Car A: La commande corticale de la déglutition. II: Point d'impact bulbaire de la voie corticifuge déglutitrice. J Physiol 1973;66: 553–576.

Carvalho GJ, Song CS, Vargervik K, et al: Auditory and facial nerve dysfunction in patients with hemifacial microsomia. Arch Otolaryngol Head Neck Surg 1999;125:209–212.

Cayler GG, Blumenfeld CM, Anderson RL: Further studies of patients with the cardiofacial syndrome. Chest 1971;60:161–165.

Chaudry V, Crawford TO: Stimulation single-fiber EMG in infant botulism. Muscle Nerve 1999;22:1698–1703.

Chouard CH: Anatomie, Pathologie et Chirurgie du Nerf Facial. Paris, Masson et Cie, 1972.

Christen HJ, Hanefeld F, Kruse E, et al: Foix-Chavany-Marie (anterior operculum) syndrome in childhood: A reappraisal of Worster-Drought syndrome. Dev Med Child Neurol 2000;42:122–132.

Cohen MMJ: Syndromology's message for craniofacial biology. J Maxillofac Surg 1979;7:89–109.

Cornblath DR, Sladky JT, Summer AJ: Clinical electrophysiology of infantile botulism. Muscle Nerve 1983;6:448–452.

Couly G, Aicardi J: Anomalies morphologiques associées de la face et de l'encéphale chez l'enfant. Arch Fr Pediatr 1988; 45:99–104.

Courville J: The nucleus of the facial nerve: The relation between cellular groups and peripheral branches of the nerve. Brain Res 1966;1:338–354.

Cozzi F, Pierro A: Glossoptosis-apnea syndrome in infancy. Pediatrics 1985;75:836–843.

Cruccu G, Deuschl G: The clinical use of brainstem reflexes and hand-muscle reflexes. Clin Neurophysiol 2000;111:371–387.

Deonna TW, Roulet E, Fontan D, et al: Speech and oromotor deficits of epileptic origin in benign partial epilepsy of childhood with rolandic spikes. Neuropediatrics 1993;24:83–87.

Dinger J, Prager B: Arthrogryposis multiplex in a newborn of a myasthenic mother—case report and literature. Neuromuscul Disord 1993;3:335–339.

Dodds WJ, Logemann JA, Stewart ET: Radiologic assessment of abnormal oral and pharyngeal phases of swallowing. Am J Roentgenol 1990a;154:965–974.

Dodds WJ, Stewart ET, Logemann JA: Physiology and radiology of the normal oral and pharyngeal phases of swallowing. Am J Roentgenol 1990b;154:953–963.

Doty RW, Bosma JF: An electromyographic analysis of reflex deglutition. J Neurophysiol 1956;19:44–60.

Dubowitz V: The Floppy Infant, 2nd ed. London, William Heinemann Medical Books, 1980.

Duchenne de Boulogne G: De l'électrisation localisée et son application à la pathologie et à la thérapeutique, 2nd ed. Paris, JB Baillère et Fils, 1861.

Eavey RD, Herrmann BS, Joseph JM, et al: Clinical experience with electroneuronography in the pediatric patients. Arch Otolaryngol Head Neck Surg 1989;115:600–607.

Engel AG: Congenital myasthenic syndromes. Neurol Clin 1994; 12:401–437.

Ertekin C, Aydogdu I, Yüceyar N, et al: Electrodiagnostic methods for neurogenic dysphagia. Electroencephalogr Clin Neurophysiol 1998;109:331–340.

Ertekin C, Pehlivan M, Aydogdu I, et al: An electrophysiological investigation of deglutition in man. Muscle Nerve 1995;18:1177–1186.

Esslen E: Electrodiagnosis in facial palsy. In Miehlke A (ed): Surgery of the Facial Nerve. Philadelphia, WB Saunders, 1973; 45–51.

Esslen E: The Acute Facial Palsies. New York, Springer-Verlag, 1977.

Falco NA, Eriksson E: Facial nerve palsy in the newborn: Incidence and outcome. Plast Reconstr Surg 1990;85:1–4.

Fardeau M, Tomé F: Congenital myopathies. In Engel A, Franzini-Armstrong C (eds): Myology, Vol II. New York, McGraw-Hill, 1994; 1487–1532.

Farriaux JP, Milbled G: Physiologie de la déglutition. II: La succion-déglutition chez le nouveau-né. Le mécanisme nerveux de la déglutition. Presse Méd 1965;73:409–414.

Fejerman N, Di Blasi AM: Status epilepticus of benign partial epilepsies in children: Report on two cases. Epilepsia 1987; 28:351–355.

Franck MM, Gatewood OM: Transient pharyngeal incoordination in the newborn. Am J Dis Child 1966;111:178–180.

Fross RD, Daube JR: Neuropathy in the Miller Fisher syndrome: Clinical and neurophysiological findings. Neurology 1987;37: 1493–1498.

Gerard CL, Dugas M, Narcy P, et al: Chiari malformation type I in a child with velopharyngeal insufficiency. Dev Med Child Neurol 1992;34:164–181.

Giannotti A, Digilio MC, Marino B, et al: Cayler cardiofacial syndrome and del 22q11: Part of the CATCH22 phenotype. Am J Med Genet 1994;53:303–304.

Goutieres F, Aicardi J, Farkas E: Anterior horn cell disease associated with pontocerebellar hypoplasia in infants. J Neurol Neurosurg Psychiatry 1977;40:370–378.

Govaert P: Cranial Haemorrhage in the Term Newborn Infant. London, MacKeith Press, 1993.

Govaert P, Vanhaesebrouck P, De Praeter C, et al: Moebius sequence and prenatal brainstem ischemia. Pediatrics 1989;84: 570–573.

Graff-Radford NR, Bosch EP, Stears JC, et al: Developmental Foix-Chavany-Marie syndrome in identical twins. Ann Neurol 1986; 20:632–635.

Graham PJ: Congenital flaccid bulbar palsy. Br Med J 1964;2:26–30.

Greenberg SJ, Kandt RS, D'Souza BJ: Birth injury-induced glossolaryngeal paresis. Neurology 1987;37:533–535.

Grob D, Asura EL, Brunner NG: The course of myasthenia gravis and therapy affecting outcome. Ann N Y Acad Sci 1987;505:472–499.

Haenggeli CA, Lacourt G: Brachial plexus injury and hypoglossal paralysis. Pediatr Neurol 1989;5:197–198.

Hageman G, Ippel PF, Jansen ENH, et al: Familial alternating Bell's palsy with dominant inheritance. Eur Neurol 1990;30:310–313.

Hanson PA, Rowland LP: Mobius syndrome and facioscapulohumeral muscular dystrophy. Arch Neurol 1971;24:31–39.

Harper CM: Neuromuscular transmission disorders in childhood. In Jones RH, Bolton CF, Harper CM (eds): Pediatric Clinical Electromyography. Philadelphia, Lippincott-Raven, 1996; 353–385

Hepner WR: Some observations on facial paresis in the newborn infant: Etiology and incidence. Pediatrics 1951;8:494–499.

Hoefnagel D, Penry JK: Partial facial paralysis in young children. N Engl J Med 1960;262:1126–1128.

Illingworth RS: Sucking and swallowing difficulties in infancy: Diagnostic problem of dysphagia. Arch Dis Child 1969;44:655–665.

Inder TE, Volpe JJ: Recovery of congenital isolated pharyngeal dysfunction: implications for early management. Pediatr Neurol 1998;19:222–224.

Jaradeh S, D'Cruz ON, Howard JF, et al: Mobius syndrome: Electrophysiologic studies in seven cases. Muscle Nerve 1996;19:1148–1153.

Jean A: Brainstem organization of the swallowing network. Brain Behav Evol 1984;25:109–116.

Jones KL: First and second branchial arch syndrome. In Jones KL (ed): Smith's Recognizable Patterns of Human Malformation. Philadelphia, WB Saunders, 1997a; 642–645.

Jones KL: Hypoglossia-hypodactyly syndrome. In Jones KL (ed): Smith's Recognizable Patterns of Human Malformation. Philadelphia, WB Saunders, 1997b; 646–648.

Jones KL: Treacher Collins syndrome. In Jones KL (ed): Smith's Recognizable Patterns of Human Malformation. Philadelphia, WB Saunders, 1997c; 250–251.

Kather-Boidin J, Duron B: The orbicularis oculi reflexes in healthy premature and full-term newborns. Electroencephalogr Clin Neurophysiol 1987;67:479–484.

Keane JR: Bilateral seventh nerve palsy: Analysis of 43 cases and review of the literature. Neurology 1994;44:1198–1202.

Khuralbet AJ, Neubauer D: A case of neonatal tetanus with characteristic neurophysiological findings. Muscle Nerve 1998;21: 971–972.

Kiers L, Carroll WM: Blink reflexes and magnetic resonance imaging in focal unilateral trigeminal pathway demyelination. J Neurol Neurosurg Psychiatry 1990;53:526–529.

Kimura J: Alteration of the orbicularis oculi reflex by pontine lesions: Study in multiple sclerosis. Arch Neurol 1970;22:156–161.

Kimura J: Electrically elicited blink reflex in diagnosis of multiple sclerosis. Brain 1975;98:413–426.

Kimura J, Bodensteiner J, Yamada T: Electrically elicited blink reflex in normal neonates. Arch Neurol 1977;34:246–349.

Kimura J, Giron LT, Young SM: Electrophysiological study of Bell palsy: Electrically elicited blink reflex in assessment of prognosis. Arch Otolaryngol 1976;102:140–143.

Kirshblum S, Johnston MV, Brown J, et al: Predictors of dysphagia after spinal cord injury. Arch Phys Med Rehabil 1999;80:1101–1105.

Korf BR, Bresnan MJ, Shapiro F, et al: Facioscapulohumeral dystrophy presenting in infancy with facial diplegia and sensorineural deafness. Ann Neurol 1985;17:513–516.

Kugelberg E: Facial reflexes. Brain 1952;75:385–396.

Kurdi A, Abdul-Kader M: Clinical and electrophysiological studies in diphtheritic neuritis in Jordan. J Neurol Sci 1979;42:243–250.

Lacomis D, Kupsky WP, Kuban KK, et al: Childhood onset oculopharyngeal muscular dystrophy. Pediatr Neurol 1991;7:382–384.

Laing JH, Harrison DH, Jones BM, et al: Is permanent congenital facial palsy caused by birth trauma? Arch Dis Child 1996;74:56–58.

Le Moing G, Raimbault J, Laget P, et al: Pneumopathies récidivantes et inhalations alimentaires liées à un déficit des structures buccopharyngées. An Pédiatr 1976;23:471–480.

Leech RW, Alvord EC: Anoxic-ischemic encephalopathy in the human neonatal period: The significance of brain stem involvement. Arch Neurol 1977;34:109–113.

Levine MG, Holroyde J, Woods JR, et al: Birth trauma: Incidence and predisposing factors. Obstet Gynecol 1984;63:792–795.

Linder A, Lindholm CE: Laryngologic management of infants with the Chiari II syndrome. Int J Pediatr Otorhinolaryngol 1997; 39:187–197.

Loughlin GM, Lefton-Greif MA: Dysfunctional swallowing and respiratory disease in children. Adv Pediatr 1994;41:135–162.

Mbonda E, Claus D, Bonnier C, et al: Prolonged dysphagia caused by congenital pharyngeal dysfunction. J Pediatr 1995;126:923–927.

McHugh HE: Facial paralysis in birth injury and skull fractures. Arch Otolaryngol 1963;78:443–455.

McHugh HE, Sowaen KA, Levitt MN: Facial paralysis and muscle agenesis in the newborn. Arch Otolaryngol 1969;89:131–143.

McShane MA, Boyd S, Harding B, et al: Progressive bulbar paralysis of childhood: A reappraisal of Fazio-Londe disease. Brain 1992;115:1889–1900.

Meyerson MD, Foushee DR: Speech, language and hearing in Moebius syndrome. Dev Med Child Neurol 1978;20:357–365.

Mezenes M, Coker SB: CHARGE and Joubert syndromes: Are they a single disorder? Pediatr Neurol 1990;6:428–430.

Miller AJ: Deglutition. Physiol Rev 1982;62:129–184.

Miller MT, Stromland K: The Mobius sequence: A relook. J AAPOS 1999;3:199–208.

Moore CEG, Pitt MC: EMG of genioglossus in children. Clin Neurophysiol 1999;110:S93–S94.

Munnich A, Rotig A, Chretien D, et al: Clinical presentation of mitochondrial disorders in childhood. J Inherit Metab Dis 1996;19:521–527.

Najim Al-Din AS, Anderson M, Eeg-Olofsson O: Neuro-ophthalmic manifestations of the syndrome of ophthalmoplegia, ataxia and areflexia: Observations on 20 patients. Acta Neurol Scand 1994;89:87–94.

Nelson KB, Eng GD: Congenital hypoplasia of the depressor anguli oris muscle: Differentiation from congenital facial palsy. J Pediatr 1972;81:16–20.

Nevin NC, Burrow SD, Allen G, et al: Aglossia-adactylia syndrome. J Med Genet 1975;12:89–93.

Newman LA, Cleveland RH, Blickman JG, et al: Videofluoroscopic analysis of the infant swallow. Invest Radiol 1991;26:870–872.

Nowak TW, Ionasescu V, Anuras S: Gastrointestinal manifestations of the muscular dystrophy. Gastroenterology 1982;82:600–610.

Orobello P: Congenital and acquired facial nerve paralysis in children. Otolaryngol Clin North Am 1991;24:647–652.

Pashayan MM, Lewis MB: Clinical experience with the Robin sequence. Cleft Palate J 1984;21:270–276.

Paulson G, Gottlieb G: Developmental reflexes: The reappearance of foetal and neonatal reflexes in aged patients. Brain 1968;91:37–52.

Perlman M, Reisner SH: Asymmetric crying facies and congenital anomalies. Arch Dis Child 1973;48:627–629.

Philpot J, Bagnall A, King C, et al: Feeding problems in merosin deficient congenital muscular dystrophy. Arch Dis Child 1999;80:542–547.

Pollack IF, Pang D, Kocoshis S, et al: Neurogenic dysphagia resulting from Chiari malformations. Neurosurgery 1992;30:709–719.

Polo A, Manganotti P, Zanette G, et al: Polyneuritis cranialis: Clinical and electrophysiological findings. J Neurol Neurosurg Psychiatry 1992;55:398–400.

Quaderi NA, Schweiger S, Gaudenz K, et al: Opitz G/BBB syndrome, a defect of midline development, is due to mutations in a new RING finger gene on Xp22. Nat Genet 1997;17: 285–291.

Raimbault J: Les Conductions Nerveuses Chez l'enfant Normal. Paris, Expansion Scientifique Française, 1988.

Raimbault J, Le Moing G, Laget P: Enquête sur l'électromyographie des troubles de la déglutition chez l'enfant. Pédiatrie 1979;34:681–693.

Reilly S, Skuse D, Poblete X: Prevalence of feeding problems and oral motor dysfunction in children with cerebral palsy: A community survey. J Paediatr 1996;129:877–880.

Renault F: EMG during bottle feeding: A method of studying neonatal dysphagia. Muscle Nerve 1998;21:1587.

Renault F: Cranial nerve studies in 22 children with Mobius syndrome. Muscle Nerve 2000;23:1631.

Renault F, Chartier JP, Harpey JP: Apport de l'électromyogramme au diagnostic d'amyotrophie spinale infantile en prériode néonatale. Arch Pédiatr 1996;3:319–323.

Renault F, Couvreur J: Trouble congénital de la déglutition révélateur d'une atteinte du tronc cérébral. Arch Fr Pediatr 1992;49:511–517.

Renault F, Flores-Guevara R, Soupre V, et al: Neurophysiological brainstem investigations in isolated Pierre Robin sequence. Early Hum Dev 2000;58:141–152.

Renault F, Garabedian EN, Harpey JP: Diagnostic des paralysies et asymétries faciales congénitales. In Arthuis M, Beaufils F, Caille B, et al (eds): Journées Parisiennes de Pédiatrie. Paris, Flammarion Médecine-Sciences, 1993; 155–161.

Renault F, Raimbault J: Electromyographie faciale, linguale et pharyngée chez l'enfant: Une méthode d'étude des troubles de succion-déglutition et de leur physiopathologie. Neurophysiol Clin 1992;22:249–260.

Roberton DM, Mellor DH: Asymmetrical palatal paresis in childhood: A transient cranial mononeuropathy? Dev Med Child Neurol 1982;24:842–849.

Robin P: A fall of the base of the tongue considered as a new cause of nasopharyngeal respiratory impairment: Pierre Robin sequence, a translation. 1923. Plast Reconstr Surg 1994;93: 1301–1303.

Roger G, Morisseau-Durand MP, Van Den Abbeele T, et al: The CHARGE association: The role of tracheotomy. Arch Otolaryngol Head Neck Surg 1999;125:33–38.

Rogers B, Arvedson J, Buck G, et al: Characteristics of dysphagia in children with cerebral palsy. Dysphagia 1994;9:69–73.

Sammarco J, Ryan RF, Longenecker CG: Anatomy of the facial nerve in fetuses and stillborn infants. J Plast Reconst Surg 1966; 37:556–574.

Sauron B, Bouche P, Cathala HP, et al: Miller-Fisher syndrome: Clinical and electrophysiological evidence of peripheral origin in 10 cases. Neurology 1984;34:953–956.

Schreiner MS, Field E, Ruddy R: Infantile botulism: A review of 12 years' experience at the Children's Hospital of Philadelphia. Pediatrics 1991;87:159–165.

Schurr MJ, Ebner KA, Maser AL, et al: Formal swallowing evaluation and therapy after traumatic brain injury improves dysphagia outcomes. J Trauma 1999;46:817–821.

Selley WG, Ellis RE, Flack FC, et al: Ultrasonographic study of sucking and swallowing by newborn infants [letter]. Dev Med Child Neurol 1986;28:821–823.

Shapiro NL, Cunningham MJ, Parikh SR, et al: Congenital unilateral facial paralysis. Pediatrics 1996;97: 261–264.

Sheffield LJ, Reiss JA, Strohm K, et al: A genetic follow-up study of 64 patients with the Pierre Robin complex. Am J Med Genet 1987;28:64–71.

Sieben RL, Ben Hamida M, Shulman K: Multiple cranial nerve deficits associated with the Arnold-Chiari malformation. Neurology 1971;21:673–681.

Smith WL, Erenburg A, Nowak A, et al: Physiology of sucking in the normal term infant using real-time US. Radiology 1985; 156:379–381.

Solders G, Nennesmo I, Persson A: Diphtheritic neuropathy: An analysis based on muscle and nerve biopsy and repeated neurophysiological and autonomic function tests. J Neurol Neurosurg Psychiatry 1989;52:876–880.

Stewart HS, Smith JC: Two patients with asymmetric crying facies, normal cardiovascular systems and deletion of chromosome 22q11. Clin Dysmorphol 1997;6:165–169.

Sudarshan A, Goldie WD: The spectrum of congenital facial diplegia (Moebius syndrome). Pediatr Neurol 1985;1:180–184.

Sullivan PB, Rosenbloom L: The causes of feeding difficulties in disabled children. In Sullivan PB, Rosenbloom L (eds): Feeding the Disabled Child. London, MacKeith Press, 1996; 23–32.

Ter Bruggen JP, Van der Meche FGA, De Jager AEJ, et al: Ophthalmoplegic and lower cranial nerve variants merge into each other and into classical Guillain-Barré syndrome. Muscle Nerve 1998;21:239–242.

Thieffry S, Job JC: Troubles de déglutition pharyngée en pathologie infantile. Sem Hop Paris 1954;30:131–135.

Thompson JA, Glasgow LA, Warpinski JR, et al: Infantile botulism: Clinical spectrum and epidemiology. Pediatrics 1980;66:936–942.

Tomita Y, Schichida K, Takeshito S, et al: Maturation of blink reflex in children. Brain Dev 1989;11:389–393.

Towfighi J, Marks K, Palmer E, et al: Möbius syndrome: Neuropathologic observations. Acta Neuropathol 1979;48:11–17.

Vazquez JL, Buonomo C: Feeding difficulties in the firsts days of life: Findings on upper gastrointestinal series and the role of the videofluoroscopic swallowing study. Pediatr Radiol 1999; 29:894–896.

Vecchierini-Blineau MF, Guiheneuc P: Maturation of the blink reflex in infants. Eur Neurol 1984;23:449–458.

Verzijl HT, Van den Helm B, Veldman B, et al: A second gene for autosomal dominant Mobius syndrome is localized to chromosome 10q, in a Dutch family. Am J Human Genet 1999;65:752–756.

Wadlington WB, Riley HD, Lowbeer L: The Melkersson-Rosenthal syndrome. Pediatrics 1984;73:502–506.

Weber F, Woolridge MW, Baum JD: An ultrasonographic study of the organisation of sucking and swallowing by newborn infants. Dev Med Child Neurol 1986;28:19–24.

Wiles CM: Neurogenic dysphagia. J Neurol Neurosurg Psychiatry 1991;54:1037–1039.

Willer JC, Lamour Y: Electrophysiological evidence for a facio-facial reflex in the facial muscles in man. Brain Res 1979;119:459–464.

Wilson ER, Mirra SS, Schwartz JF: Congenital diencephalic and brain stem damage: Neuropathologic study of three cases. Acta Neuropathol 1982;57:70–74.

Worster-Drought C: Congenital suprabulbar paresis. J Laryngol 1956;70:453–463.

Yasukohchi S, Yagi Y, Akabane T, et al: Facioscapulohumeral dystrophy associated with sensorineural hearing loss, tortuosity of retinal arterioles, and an early onset and rapid progression of respiratory failure. Brain Dev 1988;10:319–324.

C H A P T E R 89

Disorders of Plexus and Nerve Root

Thomas A. Miller and H. Royden Jones, Jr.

BRACHIAL PLEXOPATHIES

Introduction

A factor in the common occurrence of traumatic lesions of the brachial plexus is its superficial anatomical location in close proximity to bony and vas-cular structures in the shoulder and neck. In children, similar to the case in adults, traumatic lesions to the plexus remain the most common form of brachial plexopathy. Obstetrical brachial plexus palsy complicates a very small proportion of births. However, despite this relatively low frequency and concomitant major advances in prenatal planning

1601

and assessment, obstetrical brachial plexus palsies continue to be one of the most devastating complications resulting from a difficult labor and childbirth. Sever's seminal study of 1,100 newborns with brachial plexopathies provided the first large-scale and detailed description of obstetrically related birth palsy (Sever, 1925). The reported incidence varies ranging from 0.5 to 2 per 1,000 livebirths in industrialized countries (Vassalos et al., 1968; Brown, 1984; Bager, 1997a; Kay, 1998a; Rust, 2000). There is no delineation of the frequency of other mechanisms of pediatric brachial plexopathies. Of the 65 brachial plexopathies diagnosed at the Children's Hospital Boston (CHB), electromyography (EMG) laboratory between 1979 and 2001, 48 (74%) were present at birth. The brachial plexus lesion in the other 17 children (26%) was of acute onset, between age 3 weeks and 18 years. Overall, trauma or presumed trauma is the primary pediatric mechanism. Postinfectious (osteomyelitis) and inflammatory (immune-related) mechanisms (neuralgic amyotrophy) and, rarely, neoplasms account for the remaining causes. A unique and rare presentation in children is related to a genetic predisposition of hereditary brachial plexus neuropathy (HBPN) (Dunn et al., 1978a; Chance et al., 1994a; Gouider et al., 1994a). Trauma to the peripheral nervous system is usually due to compression, traction, ischemia, or laceration and is seen secondary to motorcycle and other motor vehicle accidents, sporting activities ("burners" or "stingers"), gunshot or knife wounds, and, rarely, falls. Child abuse is an all-too-frequent cause of neurological trauma. Unfortunately, the brachial plexus is not immune to this mechanism and, so, needs consideration in any presumed idiopathic lesion.

The purpose of this chapter is to outline the unique characteristics of pediatric plexopathies in both the brachial and the lumbosacral distribution. The discussions highlight the various clinical challenges in the assessment and treatment of pediatric brachial plexus lesions. The importance of electrodiagnostic testing and its relationship to clinical assessment, imaging, rehabilitation, and surgical options are emphasized.

Brachial Plexus Anatomy

The rather complex brachial plexus anatomy always provides diagnostic and therapeutic challenges to the electromyographer. The nerve supply to the entire upper extremity and most of the shoulder girdle originates in the brachial plexus and its contiguous nerve roots C5 to T1. This consists of the following five components: (1) five roots (C5 to T1), (2) three trunks (upper, middle, and lower), (3) two divisions (consisting of six elements in all), (4) three cords (lateral, posterior, and medial), and (5) the various terminal nerves, particularly the axillary, musculocutaneous, radial, median, and ulnar (Fig. 89–1A).

Three clinically significant peripheral nerves originate supraclavicularly or very proximally in the brachial plexus: First, The *dorsal scapular nerve* arises from the C5 anterior primary ramus, near the intervertebral foramen, and innervates the rhomboid muscle. Denervation in the rhomboids is often a poor prognostic sign for a child with a brachial plexus lesion. This finding suggests a very proximal lesion, particularly one including the possibility of C5 root avulsion. Second, the *long thoracic nerve* originates from the C5, C6, and C7 anterior primary rami. It innervates primarily the serratus anterior muscle. Scapula winging is the usual manifestation of weakness of this muscle secondary to long thoracic nerve injury. This is often difficult to recognize in newborns but, again, is associated with a proximal lesion. Third, the *suprascapular nerve* innervates both the supraspinatus and the infraspinatus muscles.

The three major brachial plexus cords each provide the primary source for the various individual nerves of the arm, with the exception of the conjoint origin of the median nerve from both the lateral and the medial cords. The lateral cord (C5-6 source) of the brachial plexus is the origin for the *musculocutaneous nerve,* the *lateral head of the median nerve,* and *the lateral pectoral nerves.* The *ulnar and medial heads of the median nerves* as well as the *medial pectoral, medial brachial,* and *antebrachial cutaneous nerves* are each derived from the medial cord (C8-T1 source) of the brachial plexus. Finally, the posterior cord (C6-7 source) gives rise to the *subscapular, thoracodorsal, axillary,* and *radial nerves* (see Fig. 89–1). Thus, the predominant terminal branches of the three brachial plexus cords are the axillary, musculocutaneous, radial, median, and ulnar nerves.

At or very near its origin, the anterior primary ramus receives a contribution, the gray ramus communicans, from the corresponding sympathetic trunk ganglion. In addition, the first thoracic anterior primary ramus contributes preganglionic sympathetic fibers to the inferior cervical (stellate) ganglion via a white ramus communicans. Injury to these fibers produces Horner's syndrome (unilateral miosis, ptosis, enophthalmos, and facial anhydrosis). It is crucial to look for evidence of a Horner's syndrome in any child with a brachial plexus lesion, as, unfortunately, this is consistent with the very poor prognosis of an avulsion of the preganglionic spinal root and nerve entry zone at the T1 level.

General Principles of the Electromyography Evaluation

When one evaluates the infant or child with a possible brachial plexus lesion, the goals are similar to those in the adult population. These include the following: (1) establishing the level and extent of involvement of the individual components of the plexus, (2) accurate identification of a preganglionic lesion and/or root avulsion, and (3) defining the

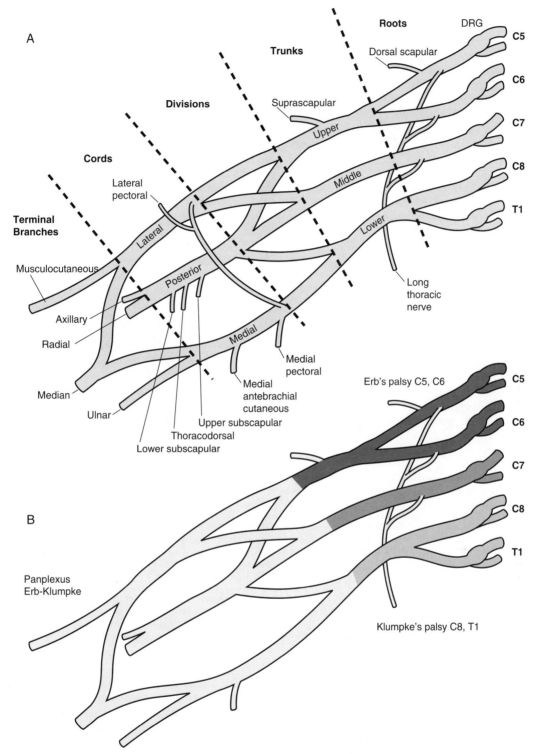

Figure 89–1. *A,* Schematic representation of the brachial plexus with its terminal branches. *B,* The most common pediatric plexus injury is that of the C5-6 palsy also known as Erb's palsy; occasionally, C7 is also affected. The second most common palsy is a panplexus injury (Erb-Klumpke). A rare isolated palsy of the C8-T1 segment is commonly referred to as a Klumpke's palsy.

nature of the lesion in terms of its underlying patho-physiological response to injury, as described by Seddon and Sunderland (i.e., neurapraxia, or an axo-notmetic and/or a neurotmetic lesion). These results provide information that allows the electromyographer to form a prognostic opinion (Fig. 89–2).

Unfortunately, one of the main criteria for differentiation between a nerve root (i.e., preganglionic) and a postganglionic plexus lesion is often technically impossible in the pediatric population, especially in newborns. Traditionally, nerve root avulsion or preganglionic lesions are suggested by the preserva-

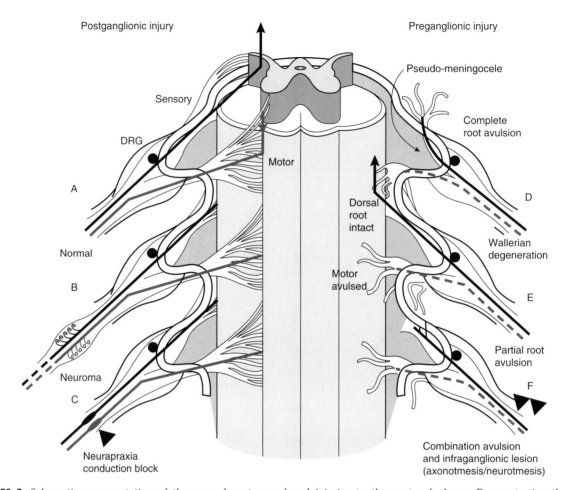

Figure 89–2. Schematic representation of the normal anatomy of and injuries to the roots of plexus. Demonstrating the typical preganglionic and postganglionic abnormalities that are possible. *A,* Normal ventral (motor) rootlets and dorsal (sensory) rootlets. *B,* Postganglionic injury (axonotmesis/neurotmesis) with neuroma formation and partial and or complete disconnection of neural elements. Continuity can be determined only by intraoperative neurophysiology across damaged segments. The compound muscle action potential (CMAP) and sensory nerve action potentials (SNAPs) from the corresponding territory will be abnormal (amplitude decreased due to axonal loss). *C,* A neurapraxic lesion resulting in abnormal sensation and weakness but normal SNAPs and CMAPs distal to the area of focal conduction block. Conduction intraoperatively across the segment may be blocked. *D,* Preganglionic injury with complete avulsion and traumatic pseudomeningocele seen on imaging. The cell body of the sensory neuron is intact (dorsal root ganglion), and therefore a normal SNAP is recorded in an asensate territory. CMAPs will be absent or nonrecordable. *E,* Partial root avulsion with dorsal root intact and ventral (motor) root avulsed. This produces weakness and normal sensation and a normal SNAP with absent or abnormal CMAPs in respective segmental distribution. *F,* Combination of a preganglionic and postganglionic lesion, which often can be determined only intraoperatively and correlated with imaging. The roots (motor and sensory) have been avulsed, but the infraganglionic component is also abnormal (axonotmesis-neurotmesis), similar to *B.* Therefore, the SNAPs and CMAPs are absent or abnormal. This can mislead the electromyographer into thinking that the lesion is infraganglionic, and he or she will potentially miss the preganglionic injury (*see text*).

tion of sensory nerve action potentials (SNAPs) in an asensate area and/or in the area of a significant clinical loss of sensory function. However, in most infants and toddlers, the determination of sensory loss on clinical examination is difficult, if not impossible. Additionally, it is more common for neonatal plexus lesions to have conjoint preganglionic and postganglionic components. Therefore, an avulsion, with its inherently poor prognosis, may be present despite the absence of SNAPs in the appropriate segment. This makes it difficult to provide an absolute opinion based on EMG findings as to whether a root avulsion is present (see Fig. 89–2*E*); Yilmaz et al., 1999). Furthermore, the use of paraspinal needle EMG is almost always technically impossible in the

pediatric and neonatal age groups because of the baby's inherent inability to relax these muscles. In most instances, it is at best challenging, if not technically infeasible, for an electromyographer to provide a definitive opinion about the presence of denervation potentials in this setting. Lastly, even in the ideal case, one cannot comment on the specific cervical level, owing to the significant segmental overlap within the paravertebral musculature. Therefore, in order to determine a precise level (i.e., C5 versus C8), complementary testing, such as magnetic resonance imaging, is required.

The technical challenges of recording infantile motor and sensory nerve action potentials are described in Chapter 85. An attempt at recording motor and sensory conduction studies from the median and ulnar nerves allows a comment on the lower trunk and medial cord. Radial motor and sensory studies allow comment on the posterior cord and stimulation at Erb's point, recording from the musculocutaneous nerve–innervated biceps muscle, can allow comment on the continuity of the upper trunk and, specifically, that of the lateral cord. Wilbourn has emphasized the value of using the thumb to record median sensory fibers of the upper trunk, knowing that this is equally as effective as the lateral antebrachial cutaneous nerve of the volar aspect of the radial forearm (Ferrante and Wilbourne, 2000). However, this is sometimes a technically difficult study in small children younger than 6 to 9 months of age. These include volume conduction and issues of impedance. In the older child (i.e., 18 to 24 months of age), it has generally been the authors' experience that the thumb provides an excellent site for evaluating the sensory function of this portion of the brachial plexus.

A good starting point is the evaluation of sensory function of the median nerve, recording from the middle finger (a digit that is large enough to permit the use of two electrodes at sufficient distance for a technically adequate response). It is important to emphasize that a comparative study between the involved and the uninvolved contralateral limb often provides the most accurate information.

Because of the wide range of normal CMAP and SNAP amplitude values (outlined in the appendix), the precise definition of an abnormality in an individual case is sometimes difficult to determine, even in comparison with the apparently normal opposite side. One of the authors (TM) has confirmed that the use of nerve action potentials (NAPs) of the median and ulnar nerves provides a technique that is more robust than digital sensory nerve recording in small infants (Smith, 1996; Pollack et al., 2000). Supramaximal stimulation is used to obtain a mixed NAP, providing a more definite means of comparing amplitudes (i.e., axonal loss) with those of the contralateral limb. This is a good complementary technique for determining axonal continuity in the neonatal period (Smith, 1996).

The precise temporal profile of the insult and its resulting effect on the brachial plexus is crucial in understanding the character of nerve damage. CMAPs usually disappear within 4 or 5 days, and definitely within a week, of complete axonal disruption (Chaudhry and Cornblath, 1992). The temporal relationship for the timing or disappearance of SNAPs is even longer—up to 10 to 11 days in adults (Chaudhry and Cornblath, 1992), although such a relationship is not defined in the newborn.

As with the adult brachial plexopathy, needle EMG is of the utmost importance for defining the degree of brachial plexus injury. With infants and children, the examiner needs to be both careful and economical in the performance of the study. Concomitantly, it is important to be thorough enough to provide the referring clinician with an adequate study. Ide-ally, EMG provides both anatomical and functional information as to the presence or absence of axonal damage. The precise timing of the onset of positive waves and fibrillation potentials in the older child is similar to that of the adult; namely, 10 to 14 days; (Luco and Eyzaguirre, 1955; Ferrante and Wilbourne, 2000). However, in the neonate and young infant, few studies have attempted to define the first appearance of EMG signs of denervation with sequential needle EMG analysis. In a single case, Mancias and colleagues documented the results of such an evaluation in a 4-day-old infant (Mancias, 1994). This baby had both an avulsion and concomitant plexus damage. Their results suggest that positive waves are seen in the newborn as early as the fourth day after injury. These findings have also been reproduced in an animal model. Gonik and colleagues (1998) demonstrated denervation at 24 hours after transection in a newborn pig. They also found a proximal-to-distal gradient and correlation with nerve length (Gonik et al., 1998). Two possible mechanisms may account for the earlier appearance of denervation potentials in the neonate. These include short distances from the site of the injury and an immature or poorly myelinated peripheral nervous system. It is important to stress that a few other authors have demonstrated signs of very early denervation and EMG patterns consistent with a "prenatally" occurring lesion (Koenigsberger, 1980; Ouzounian et al., 1997; Paradiso et al., 1997). This important and controversial subject is addressed in greater detail later in the chapter. Both animal and human data emphasize that it is inappropriate to extrapolate the anticipated timing of needle electrode examination (NEE) changes in the newborn on the basis of adult non–brachial plexus data.

Neonatal Brachial Plexus Lesions (Obstetrical, Congenital, and Perinatal BP Palsy)

HISTORICAL ASPECTS

Obstetrical brachial palsy was first described in 1768 by Smellie, who cited a case of bilateral arm paralysis at birth that rapidly resolved in a matter of days. It was Duchenne de Boulogne, in her treatise on localized electrical stimulation, who described the typical unilateral obstetrical brachial plexus palsy (1872), attributing the injury to traction on the arm that had occurred in four neonates (Robotti et al., 1995). In an 1874 paper devoted to the electrical stimulation of the brachial plexus in normal individuals, as well as in those with obstetrical-birth plexus palsies, Erb described the typical upper root palsy in an adult, anatomically localizing the lesion to the junction of the C5 and C6 roots with the upper trunk of the brachial plexus. In a postscript to this description, he acknowledged Duchenne's prior description and cited one of his own obstetrical cases that he attributed to pressure on the plexus during the Prague maneuver of version and extraction (Robotti et al., 1995). Thus, the classic upper brachial plexus palsy, described first by Duchenne, bears the name of *Erb's palsy,* although some still refer to this entity as Erb-Duchenne palsy. A few years later, in 1885, Klumpke described the paralysis of the lower roots of the brachial plexus, also highlighting the concomitant involvement of the sympathetic fibers. She described lesions of roots C8 through T1 and an associated Horner's sign to the lower trunk lesions of the BP (Robotti et al., 1995). When the entire plexus is involved (i.e., a panplexus injury), leading to the total limb being affected, it is often referred to as Erb-Klumpke paralysis (see Fig. 89–1*B*)

INCIDENCE

Obstetrical brachial plexus lesions have an incidence varying from 0.9 to 2.3 per 1,000 livebirths (Gordon et al., 1973; Hardy, 1981; Sjoberg et al., 1988; Bager, 1997). Adler and Patterson reported decreasing incidents of this condition between the years of 1938 (1.56 per 1,000 livebirths) and 1963 (0.38 per 1,000 livebirths) in New York (Adler et al., 1967). In a 1973 report from the United States, Gordon and colleagues reported 60 brachial plexus lesions among 31,700 livebirths in an "anterospective" collective perinatal study from 12 centers primarily caring for low-income families with an incidence of 1.89 per 1,000 livebirths. These pregnancies were associated with a markedly increased incidence of antepartum complications, including preeclampsia, diabetes, and hypertension and an increased number of large babies (Gordon et al., 1973). In a 1978 study, Eng and colleagues estimated that neonatal brachial plexopathies occur much less frequently (i.e., 0.4 per 1,000 births). In 1992, Jennett described 39 neonatal brachial plexopathies among 57,597 livebirths occurring from 1977 through 1990, representing an incidence of 0.67 per 1,000 livebirths (Jennett et al., 1992). Gilbert and colleagues reviewed all deliveries in the state of California between 1994 and 1995. In more than 1,000,000 deliveries, the incidence of OBP was 1.5 in 1,000 (Gilbert et al., 1999). A recent meta-analysis categorized the incidence of plexopathies related to birthweights. Deliveries were compartmentalized into three groups: (1) less than 4,000 g, (2) 4,000 g to 4,500 g, and (3) more than 4,500 g. There was an overall incidence of 0.9 in 1,000 livebirths; however, this was almost three times more common (2.6 in 1,000) for the newborns weighing more than 4,500 g. (Rouse et al., 1996).

CLASSIFICATION

The anatomical classification of brachial plexus injuries is the most common classification system used for defining perinatal brachial plexopathy (Table 89–1). Narakas eventually classified obstetrical brachial plexus lesions into four groups, outlined in Table 89–1. These are based on the neurological

Table 89–1. Classification of Obstetrical Brachial Plexus Palsy

Group I	C5-6	Paralysis of the shoulder and biceps
Group II	C5-7	Paralysis of the shoulder biceps and forearm extensors
Group III	C5-T1	Complete paralysis of the limb
Group IV	C5-T1	Complete paralysis of the limb with Horner's syndrome

examination at 2 to 3 weeks after birth (Narakas, 1987; Egloff et al., 1995).

Paralysis of the upper roots (group I) and complete paralysis (group IV) are the predominant types of obstetrical brachial plexus injury, whereas Klumpke's palsy is an exceedingly rare type (see Fig. 89–1*B*). A recent study from Toronto, Canada, examined the distribution of Klumpke's birth palsy, as cited in the English language literature over the last decade, and reported a value of 0.6% of all birth plexus injuries. The incidence of Klumpe's palsy in 3,508 cases of brachial plexus injury in the English language literature over the last 10 years was 20 in 3,508 (0.6%). They noted that in their 235 consecutive cases seen at The Hospital for Sick Children in Toronto there was an incidence of 204 Erb's palsies, 31 total brachial plexus palsies, and no Klumpke's palsy. They concluded that isolated C8-T1 lesions in birth injuries of the brachial plexus are extremely rare (0.6%) in modern obstetric practice and may be related to vaginal breech deliveries with hyperabduction of the arm. (Al Qattan et al., 1995).

ERB'S PALSY

An infant with a classic Erb palsy lies with the affected arm limp at the side with the shoulder adducted and internally rotated, the elbow extended, the forearm pronated, and the fingers and wrists flexed (Fig. 89–3). This characteristic posture is commonly referred to as *waiter* or *porter's tip.* The shoulder is adducted as the result of paralysis of both the deltoid and the supraspinatus muscles. Internal rotation of the shoulder occurs, owing to the unopposed contraction of pectoralis and latissimus dorsi as well as the unopposed pull of the subscapularis concomitant with a flaccid teres minor and infraspinatus. Elbow extension occurs owing to the effect of gravity as well as paralysis of the elbow flexors (biceps, brachialis, and brachioradialis (C5 or C6). The pronated forearm is due to paralysis of the supinator and bicep muscles (C5 or C6). The flexed wrist and fingers occur because the wrist extensors are weakened (C5 or C6).

This form is the predominant type of deficit in most major series of neonatal brachial plexopathy. In four different studies, the incidence of the classic Erb palsy (upper trunk and lateral cord) versus the other types of brachial plexus injuries ranges from 81.5% to 99.8%—167 of 169 infants (Vassalos et al., 1968); 55 of 58 infants (Gordon et al., 1973); 110 of

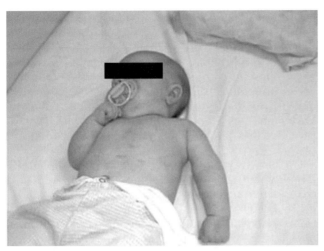

Figure 89–3. The classic posture of an infant with Erb's palsy (upper trunk C5-6). A large macrosomic baby (>4,200g) at 6 weeks of age. The extremity is held adducted, in internal rotation and pronated, and extended at the elbow. The wrist, fingers, and thumb are flexed.

135 infants (Eng et al., 1978a); and 204 of 235 (Al Qattan et al., 1995).

RISK FACTORS AND THE BRACHIAL PLEXUS ASSESSMENT

A thorough obstetrical history must be obtained from the parents. The important facts regarding prior pregnancies, deliveries, history of the pregnancy, gestational diabetes, and duration of labor are usually easily obtained. This information contrasts with the parents' perception of the method and difficulty of delivery. It is common that in the "stressful environment" of a difficult birth one or both parents cannot provide a full account of the details during delivery. Other relevant postnatal information, including respiratory difficulties, evidence of fracture (clavicular), and/or Horner's syndrome as well as the extent of the paralysis during the first few days after birth, are crucial in this assessment.

The large baby (>4,000 g), with a vertex delivery and associated shoulder dystocia, is the most common association for an obstetrical brachial plexus palsy (Laurent and Lee, 1994a). Other risk factors include multiparity, prolonged labor, high birthweight, assisted delivery (forceps, extraction), breech delivery, and previous child with obstetrical brachial plexus palsy and shoulder dystocia (Benjamin and Khan, 1993; Laurent and Lee, 1994; Ubachs et al., 1995; Ballock and Song, 1996; Rouse et al., 1996; Gilbert et al., 1999; Dodds and Wolfe, 2000).

The knowledge of risk factors is most useful when it provides a means of preventing a neonatal brachial plexopathy. Prenatal diagnosis of large birthweight and prediction of the risk of shoulder dystocia is difficult and imprecise. As summarized by Kay: "It seems unlikely that we are any nearer preventative strategies for this rare complication"

(Kay, 1998). A number of studies have demonstrated the limited usefulness of fetal weight in predicting neonatal brachial plexus injury (Rouse et al., 1996a; Ecker et al., 1997; Bryant et al., 1998). Bryant and colleagues evaluated a policy of cesarean delivery for macrosomic infants. In mothers who do not have diabetes, they argue that to prevent a single case of permanent injury 155 to 588 cesarean deliveries are required at the currently recommended cut-off weight of 4,500 g. Although McFarland and colleagues demonstrated a 52-fold increased rate of brachial plexopathy in macrosomic newborns of diabetic mothers delivered by instrumentation, 92% of these babies were delivered vaginally without complications (McFarland et al., 1996). Obstetrical palsy can occur after cesarean section, although it is rare and should provoke a careful search for other causes of limb paralysis (Al Qattan et al., 1994).

A number of large population-based studies provide important and useful data about specific factors that place babies at increased risk for a neonatal brachial plexopathy (Gilbert et al., 1999). Gestational diabetes had an associated brachial plexopathy odds ratio of 1.9 in a review of 1,611 cases of obstetrical brachial plexopathy in California (Gilbert et al., 1999). They also noted an increased risk of brachial plexopathy with an odds ratio of 2.7 for vacuum extraction, 3.4 for forceps delivery, and 76.1 for shoulder dystocia. McFarland and associates noted newborns at greatest risk for obstetrical brachial plexopathy were macrosomic (>4,500 g), born to mothers with diabetes, and delivered by instrumented vaginal delivery: 7.8% of these high-risk infants had an obstetrical brachial plexopathy (McFarland et al., 1986). This represents a 52-fold increase compared with the baseline population rate.

Very rarely, specific intrauterine anatomical factors are identified as the pathophysiological basis of neonatal brachial plexopathy. These include fetal positioning and amniotic bands. These and otherwise unidentified mechanisms are carefully discussed in the obstetrical and medical-legal literature (Iffy and Mcardle, 1996; Pollack et al., 2000). Mathematical modeling of forces associated with shoulder dystocia demonstrate that the pressures of endogenous forces (uterine and maternal expulsive efforts), in contrast with exogenous forces (clinically applied traction to the fetal head), are four to nine times greater than the values calculated for clinically applied exogenous forces (Gonik et al., 2000).

Additionally, EMG reports also support the potential of some neonatal obstetrical brachial paralyses to have an intrauterine onset. These studies make the presumption that the presence of fibrillation potentials, in the first few days of life, suggests a prenatal cause. The first such suggestion was reported in abstract form only, and the fine details are lacking (Koenigsberger, 1980). He describes two babies: the first was a newborn with Erb's palsy that demonstrated fibrillation potentials immediately. Their second infant, with an Erb-Klumpke lesion, had fibrillation potentials in the hand muscles when the first electromyogram was performed at age 4 days. This suggested that brachial plexus injury may have taken place in utero before the delivery (Koenigsberger, 1980). Ten years later, another study noted similar findings (Peterson and Peterson, 1991). Paradiso and colleagues (1997) described their findings in 78 patients suffering congenital brachial plexus palsy of the Erb type and argued that in the infant who was assessed on day 18 with findings primarily consistent with a postganglionic Erb palsy the polyphasic high-voltage motor unit potential (MUP) and the absence of denervation activity, together with the reduced amplitude of digit 1 SNAPs, indicated collateral reinnervation after postganglionic partial denervation that took place several weeks before delivery.

However, very few studies define the temporal profile for the initial appearance of EMG signs of axonal damage in the neonate. Because of the very short distances from the site of injury to the muscle, as well as the immature, poorly myelinated peripheral nervous system, the classic adult findings of 10 to 14 days for the first signs of fibrillation potentials and the 4 to 5 days for the loss of CMAPs, with 10 days for the disappearance of SNAPs, cannot be transferred to the neonate. This is exemplified by Mancias and colleagues' (1994) report demonstrating clear evidence that *"early denervation"* does indeed occur secondarily in an infant with a traumatic brachial plexopathy. Their seminal case was a macrosomic (4,030 g) infant with shoulder dystocia who after a delayed delivery was born with Erb-Klumpke palsy and associated Horner's syndrome. The nerve conduction studies in this infant were performed at age 4 days. These failed to demonstrate any CMAPs or SNAPs in the affected arm. Profuse runs of positive waves were present in the deltoid, biceps, and wrist extensors on day 4 and in the first dorsal interosseous at day 5 of life. Imaging studies at 3 weeks of age demonstrated pseudomeningoceles at C6 and C7 compatible with root avulsion. This baby had no clinical or electrophysiological improvement at this time. Therefore, the presence of positive waves at 4 days of age in this infant with an avulsion-type injury "presumably" occurring at the time of delivery for the first time suggests that acute signs of denervation may occur in neonates much earlier than in older individuals. These findings have also been confirmed in animal models. In a 2-day-old pig, denervation can occur by 24 hours after nerve disruption, in contrast with the adult pig in which 5 to 8 days are required (Gonik et al., 1998).

Johnson and colleagues (1977) reviewed 32 infantile brachial plexopathies, including 11 infants who had undergone EMG. Only one infant was examined during the first week, and this was at age 4 days. No fibrillation potentials were present in a proximal muscle. In reference to the timing of onset of fibrillation potentials in the newborn infant, another pertinent observation is outlined in a careful study by

Clay. She examined a 9-week-old infant who, 2 weeks earlier, had acute onset of a flaccid arm. The mechanism in this instance was "an unusual infiltrative" lesion of the brachial plexus secondary to osteomyelitis. This pathological process contrasts with the precipitous onset of root avulsion and plexus injury at birth in the other sequentially studied neonate. Clay's findings were more consistent with that of the adult literature, demonstrating denervation not present at day 14 but seen at day 20 (Clay, 1982).

Further information regarding the onset of fibrillation potentials in the neonate can be seen in a case of peroneal mononeuropathy defined by EMG at 18 hours of age. This baby had no peroneal CMAPs and no motor unit potentials, with profuse fibrillations isolated to a peroneal nerve–innervated muscle. These findings strongly support the possibility of an intrauterine cause of peripheral nerve damage (Jones et al., 1996). Some newborns with infantile radial nerve lesions also have an apparent intrauterine onset, as at birth they evidence an eschar over the radial nerve course within the triceps muscle (Ross et al., 1983).

Ideally, electromyographers need the opportunity to analyze serial EMG studies from birth in other infants with brachial plexopathies or focal neuropathies who prove to have axonal damage. These may provide better-defined future standards for assigning a more accurate temporal profile vis-à-vis the onset of denervation potentials in the newborn. However, until more in-depth data are available, the authors currently have evidence to support the hypothesis that some neonatal mononeuropathies, as well as brachial plexopathies, have an intrauterine onset and thus are totally unrelated to any obstetrical trauma (Koenigsberger, 1980; Ross et al., 1983; Jones et al., 1996). Although one author admonishes pediatricians not to send newborns with brachial plexopathies for EMG until age 3 months, to distinguish neurapraxic lesions from those with axonal damage, this suggestion cannot be supported in many of these instances because, unfortunately, there often are significant medical-legal issues (Molnar, 1984).

THE MEDICAL-LEGAL DEBATE

Frequently, obstetricians are cited as being responsible for a brachial plexus injury, presumably because of their having placed lateral traction on the baby's head to facilitate the delivery of the shoulder (Fig. 89–4). This is most commonly an issue when the scenario involves a macrosomic baby whose delivery is complicated by shoulder dystocia, although the lack of this potentially compromising feature does not dissuade some litigation from being initiated (see Fig. 89–4). However, the definition of alternative in utero etiologies for both a brachial plexopathy and a mononeuropathy, as well as in those babies whose Erb's palsy occurred concomitant with a cesarean section, provide support for alternative mechanisms rather than direct obstetrician-induced injury (Dunn and Engle, 1985; Jennett

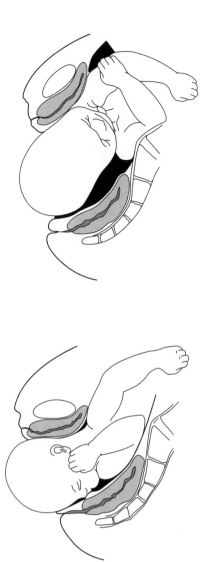

Figure 89–4. Possible mechanisms proposed in birth-related plexopathies. *A,* The mechanism includes a fractured clavicle. *B,* The resulting lateral traction on the head increases traction on the plexus.

and Tarby, 1997; Jennett et al., 1992; Ouzounian et al., 1997; Allen, 1999; Gherman et al., 1999). In the future, the authors suggest that obstetricians and pediatricians who are concerned about the possibility of litigious concerns request sequential EMG beginning within 24 hours of birth. The electromyography laboratory not only will be able to further define the timing of the onset of the signs of denervation in these neonates, but also to provide a means of accurately supplying a clinical correlation as to whether a baby's Erb's palsy is truly a birth-related process, and not a potentially intrauterine antenatal process. When enough of these data are compiled, the findings will allow us to provide a more accurate comment regarding the natural history of neonatal brachial plexopathies. It is clear that the medical-legal implications of these EMG observations, regarding the timing of fibrillation potentials and the

loss of CMAPS occurring in neonates younger than age 1 week of age with a brachial plexus injury, merit further study.

PROGNOSTIC FACTORS AND NATURAL HISTORY

Excluding the relatively rare, unfortunate infant with rupture and avulsion of each affected nerve root, significant recovery is usually seen with the most common form of obstetrical brachial paralysis. However, there is an extensive debate in the literature vis-à-vis the timing and degree of effective re-innervation. The reported incidence of complete recovery varies enormously, as different authors report different populations selected at different stages of recovery and have applied different criteria for the diagnosis of full or complete recovery.

A number of presentations, however, are considered unfavorable prognostic signs and include (1) lower plexus lesions, (2) total plexus involvement lacking some improvement within the first week or so, and (3) the absence of appreciable recovery by age 6 months. Other potential prognostic indicators are the nature of the injury (avulsion or rupture), the extent of the injury (upper, middle, or lower plexus lesion), associated Horner's syndrome, and associated fracture (e.g., ribs, clavicle, and humerus). Narakas reported that recovery in group IV patients (panplexus injury with Horner's sign) was especially poor, with more than 50% having little or no function (Narakas, 1987). Others agree that the presence of a concomitant Horner sign carries a very poor prognosis, as also is the case with an associated phrenic nerve palsy (Narakas 1987; Jeffery et al., 1998; Kay 1998; Al Qattan et al, 2000).

Although a concurrent clavicular fracture in a newborn supports a traumatic process, when this lesion is associated with an obstetrical brachial plexus palsy, it surprisingly holds no prognostic value in predicting spontaneous recovery (Al Qattan et al., 1994). These authors' retrospective review of 183 consecutive newborns, in Toronto, had specifically defined poor outcomes as "insufficient spontaneous return of motor function necessitating primary BP [brachial plexus] surgery." It is true, however, that the finding of a clavicular fracture in a neonate born with a shoulder dystocia must lead the obstetrician or pediatrician to iniate a careful and thorough neurological assessment to ensure that there has not been a brachial plexus injury (Oppenheim et al., 1990; Al Qattan et al., 1994).

NATURAL HISTORY

The prognosis is clearly the best for infants with brachial plexus lesions confined to the upper trunk and lateral cord. Overall, 70% of 131 infants with neonatal brachial plexopathy had a good to excellent result when followed over a long-term period: in 22% moderate residual damage was present, and in 8% a severe incapacity occurred (Eng et al., 1996). In summarizing the literature to date, close to 15%

of infants with obstetrical brachial plexopathy experience significant permanent disability (Michelow et al., 1994; Eng et al., 1996; Kay, 1998; Rust, 2000). In another review of 63 patients with obstetrical brachial plexopathy, Michelow and colleagues (1994) note spontaneous recovery in 92% of these infants. In contradistinction, other clinical researchers are somewhat less optimistic. Bager and colleagues, in a Swedish study, showed that complete recovery occurred in only 49% and severe impairment in 22% (Bager, 1997). Eng and her group, in an assessment of long-term prognosis, evaluated 186 patients between 1981 and 1993. They were interested in defining a general trend of improvement or deterioration. They found that 72% of children had no change over time. Of those, 28% (41 of 149) of infants showed a change from baseline over time—77% showed improvement and 4% deteriorated (Eng et al., 1996).

Assessment and Follow-Up

Affected infants should be followed at a clinic with expertise in peripheral nerve injuries. Ideally, this has to occur over a period of months, at regular intervals, in order to assess the extent of recovery, if any. A reliable and reproducible method of quantifying motor function is probably the most challenging aspect of assessing the newborn. It is unanimously agreed that the Medical Research Council muscle grading system is insufficient for the evaluation of the young patient. Subsequently, several groups have attempted to establish their own grading scales. Gilbert and Tassin follow a grading scale from M0—no contraction—to M3—complete movement against the weight of the corresponding segment of the extremity (Gilbert, 1995). Another approach to the evaluation of children with brachial plexus lesions is the assessment of the global movement of the upper limb as proposed by Mallet (Fig. 89–5). In the brachial plexopathy clinic at the Hospital for Sick Children in Toronto, the muscle grading system is an 8-grade scale that is designed to capture the subtle but significant changes in movement of the arm. Overall, one evaluates joint movements, in contrast with individual muscle testing, which can be difficult in infants. This scale is helpful in both the preoperative and postoperative settings, providing the ability to follow individuals longitudinally (Michelow et al., 1994; Clarke and Curtis, 1995).

Sensory assessment of infants is extremely difficult and, in many cases, impossible. It may be possible only to determine whether the infant will respond to painful stimuli. The most common classification system for sensory responses is that devised by the Narakas classification system: in which 0 is no reaction to painful or other stimuli, and S3 is apparently normal sensation.

Electrodiagnostic Assessment

One of the primary aims of the EMG investigation of the neuromuscular system is to allow one to make

accurate comments regarding the physiology of the peripheral nervous system—that is, diagnosing, localizing, and defining the extent of nerve injury. The needle electrode examination is helpful in assessing the subtle axonal involvement. It also adds a further definition by providing the means of assessing several of the nerves, such as the axillary and dorsal scapular, that cannot be evaluated concomitantly with nerve conduction studies. Needle electrode examination is also valuable in documenting the presence of minimal residual innervation where severe but incomplete axonal loss lesions have occurred. It will also allow one to detect early signs of clinically occult reinnervation weeks before it becomes clinically apparent. The chronicity of the lesion is also extrapolated via MUP configurations from the results of needle EMG of separate MUPs.

However, the "benefit" of EMG and nerve conduction studies remains controversial. In the surgical literature, Gilbert proposed that if there is no shoulder and/or biceps recovery by age 3 months consideration be given to surgical exploration. Furthermore, it is his group's opinion that although they routinely use EMG prior to surgery, they believe that the preoperative EMG findings produce excessive optimism. Two theories are offered in an attempt to rationalize the above discrepancy. Firstly, Vandijk noted that the muscle fiber diameter of a 3-month-old baby is 3.3 times smaller than that of an adult. This means that a cross-sectional area of the muscle contains about 11 times more muscle fiber in the infant than in the adult. This then implies that if a needle with similar pick-up territory is used a greater number of MUAPs (about 11 times) will be recorded in an infant for the same portion of functional motor units and discharge rates. Second, a novel Canadian concept is one of apraxia. Brown and colleagues set out to determine whether motor unit activation is impaired in patients with persisting disability arising from neonatal brachial plexopathy (NBPP). Using techniques of motor unit number estimation and twitch interpolation, these Canadian colleagues coined the term *apraxia* for the interesting observed phenomenon of an individual who has a significant number of motor units that are lessened in the biceps. However, the ability of these patients to recruit this full complement of MUPs is secondary to a lack of normal central nervous system maturation (Brown et al., 2000). The hypothesis of impaired motor program development is consistent with the well-known importance of normal visual input for the development of sight. The authors' hypothesis is supported by the rapidly growing evidence of activity-dependent plasticity in the sensory motor system involving the brain and spinal cord (i.e., the absence early in life of normal movements and their accompanying patterns of proprioceptive and cutaneous sensory input). The brain and spinal cord do not undergo the activity-dependent changes that lead to normal motor neuron recruitment into skilled movements (Brown et al., 2000; Rapalino and Levine, 2000). The concept of a lack of coordinated

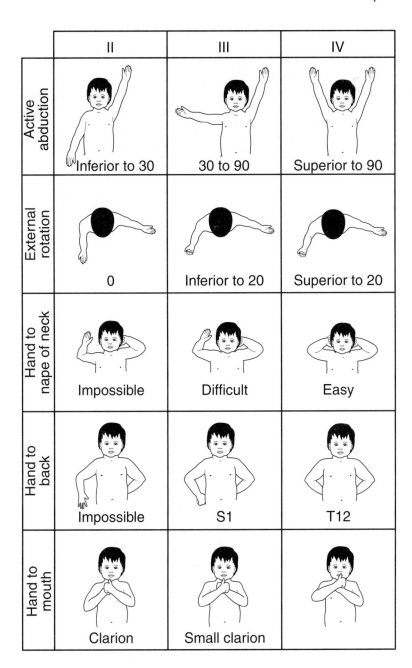

Figure 89–5. Grading system as proposed by Mallet. The Mallet system grades the amount of usable abduction and shoulder rotation, as well as bringing the hand to the mouth. Grade 0 is no movement, and Grade V is full movement. (Modified from Gilbert A: Obstetrical brachial plexus palsy. In Tubiana R [ed]: The Hand, vol IV. Philadelphia, WB Saunders, 1993; 579)

movement of the upper limb was proposed by Johnson in the Erb engram (Johnson et al., 1977). Furthermore, recent work using *Botulinum* toxin to lessen the co-contractions associated with the agonist-antagonist biceps-triceps co-contraction in birth-related brachial plexus lesions suggests that the contractions were due to a central abnormality, rather than to peripheral regeneration (Rollnik et al., 2000).

ELECTRODIAGNOSIS AND PROGNOSIS

The question of whether EMG and nerve conduction studies can help with prognosis and/or indica-

tions for surgery remains controversial. A number of centers comment on the undue optimism provided by the electromyogram. However, the vast majority of brachial plexus clinics support the use of preoperative EMG (Eng et al., 1978; Clarke and Curtis 1995; Smith et al., 1996; Terzis and Papakonstantinou, 1999). It is generally thought that the neurophysiology is complementary. In combination with the clinical assessment, EMG allows one to make accurate objective comments about the nerve pathophysiology, including a significant ability to suggest the presence of nerve root avulsion and to localize the lesion to preganglionic or postganglionic, and upper plexus versus lower. It may also provide useful information regarding the early possibility of potential recovery of function in children. For example, there is an interesting small but important subgroup of obstetrical brachial plexopathy infants who continue to have a lack of return of function at age 4 months (Smith, 1996). Without an EMG evaluation, one may assume that these babies have a poor prognosis and, otherwise nominally fulfill Gilbert's criteria for early surgical intervention. However, with stimulation at Erb's point, each baby's EMG demonstrated a neurapraxic lesion with conduction block (Smith, 1996). In fact, 16% of their infants fit into this neurapraxic category. With a conservative therapeutic approach, a full functional recovery occurred in each child by age 12 months. In general, electromyographic evidence of return of function usually precedes the clinical evidence of return of function by at least 1 month (Eng, 1971; Eng et al., 1978; Eng, 1981; Terzis and Papakonstantinou, 1999). Although the role of EMG in the prediction of prognosis retains some controversy among various clinicians, it is helpful for the determination of lesion severity (Jahnke et al., 1991; Laurent and Lee, 1994; Smith, 1996; Terzis and Papakonstantinou, 1999; Papazian et al., 2000).

NEUROIMAGING

The recent advances in microneurosurgical exploration with attempts to repair birth-related plexus palsies stresses the need for adequate surgical planning, including the differentiation between preganglionic and postganglionic lesions. Avulsion of ventral or dorsal nerve rootlets from the spinal cord results in preganglionic nerve root injury, with no potential for nerve regeneration (see Fig. 89–2D, E, and F). In these cases, surgical treatment consists of neurotization or microsurgical reinnervation of the distal portion of the plexus by nerve transfer from the spinal accessory, cervical plexus, or intercostal nerves (Laurent et al., 1993; Kay, 1998; Terzis and Papakonstantinou, 1999; Grossman 2000). The difficulty in arriving at definitive diagnosis in the pediatric population in relation to root avulsion is due to certain limitations of EMG and nerve conduction studies. These highlight the need for appropriate complementary imaging of the plexus. Magnetic resonance imaging or computed tomography myelography are the neuroradiological examinations of choice for evaluation of the obstetrical brachial plexus lesions. The diagnosis of nerve root avulsion (Fig. 89–6) has generally been based on showing deformity of the subarachnoid space or a pseudomeningocele. Although a strong association exists between nerve root avulsion and pseudomeningoceles, a significant percentage of avulsions show no evidence of pseudomeningocele, and pseudomeningoceles do occur without root avulsion (Hashimoto et al., 1991; Trojaborg, 1994; Birchansky and Altman, 2000). Ashimot and colleagues examined 47 nerve roots in a series of 9 patients with obstetrical brachial plexus palsy. The correlation between pseudomenin-

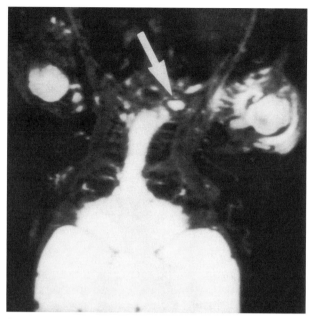

Figure 89–6. Imaging procedures. Axial T2-weighted magnetic resonance image of pseudomeningocele from nerve root avulsion as well as high signal in the right axilla. (Mancias P, Slopis JM, Yeakley JW, et al: Combined brachial plexus injury and root avulsion after complicated delivery. Muscle Nerve 1994;17:1238.)

gocele and absent intraoperative evoked responses from this series was 0.9. In a similar study, Laurent and Lee reviewed the cases of 50 operated infants and found the correlation between pseudomeningoceles and intraoperative somatosensory evoked potentials to be 0.5. Laurent and Lee (1993) also examined pseudomeningoceles with absent rootlets, and when they were compared with intraoperative somatosensory evoked potentials the correlation rose to 0.7 (Laurent and Lee, 1994). Chow and associates determined that root avulsions were better predicted by identifying the absence of rootlets in the pseudomeningocele. This absence on CT myelography may be used to suggest an extraforaminal nerve root avulsion due to its high specificity (0.98) but corresponding very low sensitivity. In other words, the sensitivity or proportion of root avulsions correctly associated with a pseudomeningocele vary between 63% and 37%, respectively—that is, the absence of rootlets versus the presence of rootlets in the pseudomeningocele. The corresponding specificity (or findings of a normal root) that were negative on the imaging procedure of 85% and 98%, respectively, demonstrates the ability to prove a negative (Chow et al., 2000). In other words, the test is not a sensitive indicator of root avulsion, but a very specific one. In children, partially avulsed roots are very common and cannot be seen; they can only be supposed during surgical exploration. Other authors concur that as a predictor of root avulsion, the presence of a pseudomeningocele on CT myelography (with thin slices less than 1.5 mm) and the absence of rootlets is far more important than is the presence of pseudomeningoceles alone (Hashimoto et al., 1991; van Ouwerkerk et al., 2000).

The advantage of magnetic resonance imaging allows observations regarding the spinal cord, including spinal cord displacement or spinal cord deformity. There have been no reports in children comparing CT myelography with magnetic resonance imaging (Bartlett et al., 1998). Although computed tomography myelography may currently provide higher spatial resolution and is considered the standard, magnetic resonance imaging is noninvasive and gives excellent delineation of pseudomeningoceles. Magnetic resonance imaging also directly aids in spinal cord evaluation as well as the peripheral soft tissue surrounding the brachial plexus. With the continued advances in instrumentation and improvement in special resolution, the authors expect that magnetic resonance imaging will soon supplant computed tomography myelography for the investigation and occasional preoperative evaluation of obstetrical brachial plexus palsy (Miller et al., 1993; Francel et al., 1995; Nakamura et al., 1997; Uetani et al., 1997; Azouz and Oudjhane, 1998; Hems et al., 1999; Yilmaz et al., 1999; Birchansky and Altman, 2000; Gomez-Anson, 2000).

A study in 13 infants compared the clinical assessment, magnetic resonance imaging, and EMG in congenital brachial plexus palsy. This report noted that the complementary nature of clinical, neurophysiology, and imaging correlated best with prediction of outcome (Yilmaz et al., 1999). This descriptive and "anterospective" Turkish study evaluated magnetic resonance imaging (performed at age 7 to 41 days and at age 3 months) with electromyography (the first study at age 27 to 50 days and the second at age 3 months) and the muscle scoring system of the Hospital for Sick Children at 3, 6, and 9 months (Table 89–2). They were then correlated with the clinical status at age 12 months. In this small study, the existence of pseudomeningocele delineated in all planes during the first days after birth is predictive of a poor prognosis. EMG evidence of root

avulsion was suggested in three individuals and correlated with the clinical examination (i.e., poor outcome) and the magnetic resonance imaging (PM) in two of the three. The authors concluded that if the EMG findings are suspicious for root avulsion (i.e., profuse fibrillations and positive waves on NEE, with nonrecordable or "scanty" motor unit potentials, no muscle response with stimulation of motor nerves, and no improvement at the second EMG but normal sensory conduction studies), EMG is reliable in predicting a poor outcome. However, EMG alone cannot be used to predict a poor outcome and or root avulsion (Yilmaz et al., 1999).

DECISION FOR EARLY OPERATIVE INTERVENTION

When one considers the possible interventional therapeutic options for neonatal brachial plexopathies, the typically good prognosis for the common upper trunk or lateral cord presentation suggests that a significant period, of usually at least 6 months, of clinical observation is certainly the baseline standard (Eng, 1971; Eng et al., 1978; Eng et al., 1996; Kay, 1998; Grossman, 2000). Surgical intervention initially fell out of favor, owing to serious complications and the lack of a benefit in the 1920s and 1930s. New microsurgical techniques that enabled primary plexus repair and perhaps promising a better rate of recovery, returned during the last two decades of the twentieth century. The challenge now lies in identifying the children who will have a very significant spontaneous recovery while concomitantly selecting the infants, if any, who require direct nerve surgery to aid their progress.

Gilbert and Razboni proposed three specific indications for proceeding with the surgical repair of a brachial plexus lesion: (1) A complete brachial plexopathy with a flail arm and Horner's syndrome; (2) a complete C5-6 brachial plexopathy without any clinical muscle contraction in the C5-6 innervated muscles by 3 months and an EMG consistent with an axonal lesion (not defined as but presumed to be profuse denervation with no recordable MUAPs); and (3) C5-6 palsy with no clinical recovery in the biceps by 3 months (the biceps alone is chosen as the clinical muscle to assess because examination of other C5-6 musculature, such as the deltoid to the exclusion of pectoralis major, is difficult at this age). For the third indication, EMG findings are not needed or used—it is strictly a clinical assessment. In C5-6 palsies at 5 years, the authors describe good to near-normal results with surgery in 80%, compared with 0% spontaneous recovery. These figures are 45% versus 0% for the C5, C6, and C7 group (Gilbert and Tassin, 1987; Gilbert et al., 1988a; Gilbert 1995). In a study of 72 brachial plexus palsies at a secondary referral center, Boome and Kay reported that of the six patients (with C5-6 lesions) whose first signs of muscle recovery were delayed until age 4 months and were not selected for surgery, only one made a full recovery. Boome and Kay concluded that if the beginning of recovery in the

---

Table 89–2. Hospital for Sick Children (HSC) Muscle Grading System

Motion	Score	Muscle Grade Score
Gravity Eliminated		
No contraction	0	0
Contraction, no motion	0.3	1
Motion ≤$\frac{1}{2}$ range	0.3	2
Motion ≥$\frac{1}{2}$ range	0.6	3
Full motion	0.6	4
Against Gravity		
Motion ≤$\frac{1}{2}$ range	0.6	5
Motion ≥$\frac{1}{2}$ range	1.3	6
Full motion	2	7

The scores for elbow flexion, together with elbow, wrist, thumb, and finger extension at 3–12 months of age are then added (maximum 10). If the score was less than 3.5, of a possible 10 at 3 months, poor recovery could be expected. (Clarke and Curtis, 1995; Michelow et al., 1994.)

muscles innervated by C5-6 was delayed beyond 3 months, root disruption was probable, agreeing with Gilbert and Razboni's criteria for surgery and that one should consider exploration (Boome and Kaye, 1988; Kay, 1998). Terzis and Papakonstantinou (1999) are often more aggressive and include the following indications for surgery: (1) global paralysis (surgery earlier than 3 months) and (2) a failure of the function of the biceps or deltoid to return to normal by 3 months (then surgery indicated) Laurent and colleagues (1993) reported their own system that used the three muscles of the upper brachial plexus (i.e., biceps, triceps, and deltoid). Surgery was indicated if there was no improvement of at least one grade in two of the three muscle groups. Improvement had to occur by age 4 to 6 months, and improvement had to continue and be maintained at a level greater than M3 for another 4 months for surgery to be avoided.

Proposals from Toronto are based on an experience scheduling children for primary brachial plexus surgery predicated on the infant's degree of recovery between ages 9 months and 1 year. These investigators analyzed the records of 39 babies over a 3-year period. Each child was examined at 3-month intervals from the time of recognition of the injury at birth. A selection of movements were scored on a simple grading and scoring system (Table 89–3). In this study, absent elbow flexion at 3 months wrongly predicted recovery quality in 13% of the cases. However, when five different functions (see Table 89–3) were scored and these scores added up to less than 3.5 at 3 months, the error was reduced to 5% and no child with a lower score went on to a good recovery (Michelow et al., 1994). They proposed that assessment of elbow flexion together with elbow, wrist, thumb, and finger extension at age 3 months provides a better prediction of expected recovery at 12 months than does elbow flexion or shoulder abduction alone. Although this group concluded that most children without biceps contraction at 3 to 4 months of age may require surgery, there is a small percentage of obstetrical brachial plexopathy infants who do not achieve this milestone until 4 to 6 months but do proceed to a spontaneous recovery (Michelow et al., 1994; Eng et al., 1996; Kay, 1998; Grossman 2000). Al-Qattan, in his obstetrical brachial plexus clinic in Saudia Arabia, used a similar end point of lack of active elbow flexion against gravity, at age 4 months, to decide on a surgical repair. Only three of the 43 infants in the analysis did not have active elbow flexion at age 4 months. He opined that 5 of 11 children, who later progressed to a satisfactory recovery, would have undergone an unnecessary operation if they had utilized the Gilbert criteria. Another very important aspect of the obstetrical brachial plexopathy natural history relates to the finding that all infants who recovered elbow flexion by age 2 months eventually had full recovery of normal limb function. Furthermore, the babies who recovered elbow flexion by 3 months of age also developed an "almost normal" function (not defined) without the need for any secondary surgery (Al Qattan, 2000).

In addition to the various prognostic studies noted, most authors accept that Narakas' group IV lesions (C5 to T1 with Horner's syndrome) represent an indication for surgery. Furthermore, some authors state that an upper brachial plexus lesion, combined with a phrenic nerve palsy, represents an indication for early exploration, as does the presence of a phrenic nerve palsy following breech delivery (Kay, 1998).

The decision to use surgical therapy versus nonsurgical management in infants with an obstetrical brachial plexus palsy continues to be controversial. The incidence of obstetrical brachial plexopathy in Sweden is 2 in 1,000 births, or about 40 per year. In 2000, Strombeck and colleagues reported a very carefully designed obstetrical brachial plexopathy study, initiated in 1986, and based on their experience with 247 of 470 children. Each infant was evaluated at the Karolinska Clinic and had at least a 5-year follow-up. Nonoperative therapy was compared with microneurosurgical sural or nerve-root graft repair. The traditional outcome measures utilized for children with obstetrical brachial plexopathy included primarily shoulder and elbow range of movement in the various series reviewed earlier in this chapter. Strombeck's group were the first to provide

Table 89–3. Summary of Obstetrical Brachial Plexopathy Prognostic Factors

Poor Prognostic Factors	Good Prognostic Factors	Unknown and Indeterminate Factors
Completely flail upper limb with Horner's syndrome (Narakas group IV)	Recovery of elbow flexion by 2 mo	Motor unit recovery MUAPs volitional in biceps at 4/12 mo, but not antigravity elbow flexion
Horner's syndrome	Antigravity strength of elbow flexion by 3/12 mo	Clavicle fracture
Phrenic nerve paralysis	No EMG evidence of axonal loss	Narakas group II (C5, C6, C7)
No recovery of biceps function (elbow flexion) by 3 to 4 mo	Scores of >3.5 at 3 mo (HSC) scale	Early recovery of elbow flexion but less than antigravity (by 4/12) mo, and then plateau
Score of <3.5 at 3 mo (HSC scale)	No root avulsion; no pseudomeningoceles with magnetic resonance imaging	
Root avulsion		
Pseudomeningocele (nerve rootlets absent)		

For further details see text.

a detailed analysis of "functional outcome." Their 247 children with obstetrical brachial plexopathy are now at least 5 years old. Interestingly, on follow-up, they demonstrated some functional impairment in grip strength and bimanual function in children who had the most common obstetrical brachial plexopathy—that is, the proximal C5-6 palsies. This is thought to be due to decreased shoulder rotation and increased shoulder instability. Of the babies with obstetrical brachial plexopathy, only eight predominant C5-6 and 24 C5-7 infants of the total of 214 infants with C5-6 or C5-7 had surgery. The surgical selection criteria for 32 of the 214 C5-6 or C5-7 infants are not well defined. In contrast, most (27 of 33) C5-T1 Erb-Klumpke infants had surgery. The authors conclude, "A significantly better shoulder movement is apparent in C5-6 palsies that have been operated on but otherwise there are no significant differences between the operated and the non-operated groups." Later, they state, "This study does not support operating on children with no biceps and deltoid activity at age 3 months." "We believe few patients with upper OBP lesions need nerve graft during their first year." It is important to note that Strombeck and colleagues' basic study design excludes all obstetrical brachial plexopathy infants with early recovery, defined as some movement in the deltoid and biceps muscle at age 3 months. These infants, in retrospect, 67 of 135 children with the most common C5-6 obstetrical brachial plexus lesion, achieved full recovery by age 6 months. This important analysis of functional outcome in obstetrical brachial plexopathy from Sweden has some interesting observations:

1. All children with complete recovery by 5 years had some recovery by 2 months.
2. All C5-6 children had normal hand and wrist movement. However only half (4 of 8) of those operated on, 11 of 15 of those not operated on, and 29 of 32 of the early recovery group performed the "pick-up" test well.
3. Children with late recovery had higher grip strength and bimanual activity than those who were operated on among the C5-7 group.
4. In the infants who were operated on for their obstetrical brachial plexopathy, early intervention, before 6 months, was no more effective than later surgery.
5. Surgery provided no advantage in the most severely affected children; that is, those with Erb-Klumpke–type lesions. This is the group for whom one needs to find the most help! It is important to note their analyses, "Do not include the performance of these 67/135 children with the most common C5-6 obstetrical brachial plexus lesion who achieved full recovery by age 6 months." Retrospectively, most of these infants had recovered by age 6 months. This flaw, in addition to small operative numbers (32 of 214 of C5-6 or C5-7 lesions), *biases* the study's opening discussion comment that

"a significantly better shoulder movement is apparent in C5-6 palsies that have been operated on."

INTRAOPERATIVE ELECTROPHYSIOLOGY

Nerve Action Potentials

The procedure of recording compound nerve action potentials (CNAPs) intraoperatively developed by Kline and colleagues can be invaluable in determining nerve axon continuity (Kline and Happel, 1993; Tiel et al., 1996; Kline and Hudson, 1997). This is valuable for both pediatric and adult plexus injuries. If a nerve axon potential (NAP) can be recorded, a substantial number of adjoining large fibers have traversed the lesion site (neuroma), which is then left intact. Conversely, if no action potentials are elicited, the abnormal segment is resected because there is a poor likelihood of a spontaneous recovery (Tiel et al., 1996). Intraoperative CNAPs, CMAPs, somatosensory evoked potentials (SSEPs), and motor evoked potentials all are useful tools for assisting in understanding the primary nerve pathophysiology. The decision to remove a neuroma or perform neurolysis is based partially on the demonstration of preserved conductivity through the neuroma per se. If the amplitude of the CMAPs obtained from stimulation proximal to the neuroma is greater than 50% of the CMAP amplitude elicited distal to the neuroma, regenerating axons are presumed to be present. Consequently, the neuroma is left alone; it is understood that the CMAP is obtained without neuromuscular paralytic agents (Tiel et al., 1996; Papazian et al., 2000). It is important to appreciate the technical factors contributing to CMAP amplitude, and many authors are reluctant to use distal CMAP amplitude alone to determine nerve continuity. Furthermore, there are no studies addressing this small but important surgical dilemma. Technical aspects aside, if the distal CMAP is less than 50%, the neuroma is excised.

Somatosensory evoked potentials are also useful in the assessment of nerve root continuity in the evaluation of brachial plexus lesions. Intraoperative stimulation of the plexus and/or exposed nerves and/or nerve roots during nerve surgery is also purported to be helpful. The early hope that SSEPs would provide information that is more accurate than that supplied by nerve conduction studies for incomplete brachial plexopathies has not been verified (Landi et al., 1980; Sugioka et al., 1982). The clinical applicability of SSEPs is limited by the fact that SSEPs assess only the dorsal root—and therefore only indirectly the presence or absence of injury to the ventral root. Additionally, SSEPs carry technical limitations with regard to their utilization in the anesthetized child. It is one of the author's (Miller) opinion that SSEPs are helpful in demonstrating nerve continuity, but, unfortunately, their technical limitations include the facts that (1) only a small portion of the dorsal root needs to be intact for a response to occur owing to magnification within the central nervous system; (2) the absence of SSEPs are often fraught with technical difficulties; and (3) they have a specificity of only 50% to 60%, which has led to their discontinuation in the intraoperative neurophysiological assessment of brachial plexus lesions.

Recent work has made use of intraoperative transcranial electrical motor evoked potentials in evaluating the functional status of anterior spinal roots and spinal nerves during brachial plexus surgery. This has been utilized primarily in adult populations. Their clinical utility awaits further analysis, particularly in children (Turkof et al., 1997; Papazian et al., 2000).

FUNCTIONAL OUTCOME

In the newborn with obstetrical brachial palsy, prognostication is difficult. The parents of these children are commonly offered reassurance that spontaneous and even complete recovery is to be expected. Such reassurance may delay referral of the patient for evaluation and, if necessary, treatment. In 1966, Gjorup reviewed 103 adults with obstetrical brachial plexopathy and found that one third had made a good or excellent recovery, but that, of these, half felt that they had some disability. In a more recent study, Bager found that nearly half the patients had significant or serious residual deficits (Gjorup, 1966; Bager 1997). In Strombeck and associates' recent study, in addition to the traditional primary attention to deltoid and biceps brachii function, the authors noted some almost paradoxical impairment in grip strength and bimanual function in children who had the most common but relatively limited C5-6 palsies at birth. This is postulated to be secondary to decreased shoulder rotation and increased shoulder instability. Of a total of 214 C5, C6, and C7 obstetrical brachial plexus lesions, just 32 babies were operated on. Unfortunately, the surgical selection criteria for the obstetrical brachial plexopathy infants are not clearly defined. Although the authors concluded there is "significantly better shoulder movement apparent in C-5/6 palsies that have been operated on, but otherwise there are no significant differences between the operated and the non-operated groups," in contradistinction, they later state, "This study does not support operating on children with no biceps, deltoid activity at age 3 months." "We believe few patients with upper OBP lesions need nerve grafting during their first year." Additionally, the basic design of this study excludes all obstetrical brachial plexopathy infants with early recovery defined as some movement in the deltoid and biceps muscle at the age of 3 months, who in retrospect achieved full recovery by age 6 months. This occurred in 67 of 135 children with the most common C5-6 obstetrical brachial plexopathy. It is also important to note that their analyses "do not include the performance of these children," most of whom, retrospectively, recovered at age 6 months. This flaw, in addition to small operative numbers

(32 of 214), biases the studies' opening discussion comment "significantly better shoulder movement is apparent in C-5/6 palsies that have been operated on." Otherwise, this functional analysis has some interesting observations. All children who had a complete recovery by 5 years had evidenced some recovery by at least age 2 months. Each C5-6 child had normal hand and wrist movement. Just half (4 of 8) of those C5-6 infants who were operated on, 11 of 15 of those who were not operated on, and 29 of 32 of the early recovery group performed their "pick-up" test well. Children with late recovery had higher grip strength and bimanual activity than those who were operated on from the C5-7 group.

Interestingly, most of Strombeck and colleagues' C5 to T1 infants (27 of 33) had surgery. However, "surgery offered no advantage in these most severely affected children, i.e., those with C-5 to T-1 lesion" (Strombeck, et al., 2000).

Gilbert and Razaborn, who operated on 178 obstetrical brachial plexopathy infants between 1977 and 1986, report good or near-normal shoulder results in 80%. Useful hand function returned in just 30% of cases with lower trunk involvement (Gilbert et al., 1988; Gilbert et al., 1991; Gilbert, 1995). Narakas' OBP classification (according to the number of roots affected) provides a means for dividing these babies into groups that are likely to benefit from surgery. Group I shows evidence of only C5 and C6 damage, whereas group IV has loss of function in all roots (C5-T1) and Horner's syndrome. All Group I and II (C5-7 lesions) patients will make some recovery, but in a few cases ultimate function will be poor. In general, their patients with group IV lesions had a very poor prognosis, if untreated. In contrast with Strombeck and colleagues, Narakas stated that there is a strong probability that surgery will reveal a lesion that benefits from repair. The question remains whether neurophysiological and/or imaging investigations improve this prognostic ability. In the authors' experience, neurophysiological and electrodiagnostic assessments have indeed indicated recovery before clinical recovery and can be very helpful in "predicting" outcome. This is corroborated by others (Smith, 1996; Terzis and Papakonstantinou, 1999; Yilmaz et al., 1999b).

The prognostic studies are, to date, the best indicators of surgery, although as previously noted it is difficult to find well-defined surgical indications based on the largest study to date (Strombeck et al., 2000). Assessments performed at 3 months are the most helpful. The approach refined in the Toronto group with the greater number of key muscles and reliance on movement, rather than power, allows a more accurate assessment (Clarke and Curtis, 1995). Waters has reported a large personal series of cases of obstetrical brachial plexopathy (Waters, 1999). He has reconfirmed that this lesion has a range of severity, and the extent of recovery is indeed related to the timing of onset and the rate of return of muscle function in key groups. He has reported that for the children with the worst lesions in whom surgery was undertaken, the outcome (in terms of shoulder function) was better than that for a more mildly injured group who did not have surgical repair (Waters, 1999). Although this report speaks to the benefits that might be expected in such a subset of obstetrical brachial plexopathy, the authors caution the reader to accept these conclusions in reference to whether there is enough convincing data to generally support primary nerve surgery for this condition. Kay eloquently discussed this issue by noting that Water's group analyzed only the babies who underwent nerve repair, universally acknowledged to have a poor prognosis. Additionally, this was a cohort in whom surgery was the least controversial (Kay, 1998). "That this very select group may obtain better shoulder function after nerve repair is not totally surprising."

Kay has proposed that the opportunity exists for a prospective trial of nerve repair for the obstetrical brachial plexopathy groups for whom recovery is predicted to be poor by the Toronto criteria and/or Gilbert criteria to be poor. "This should be done in super-regional centers suitably staffed, equipped, and experienced" (Kay, 1998). This is further echoed in the recent paper by Strombeck and co-workers (2000) and others (Bodensteiner et al., 1994). A review of early operative intervention for birth injuries to the brachial plexus summarizes the aforementioned information and concludes that in the "appropriate" patient surgery is indicated (Grossman, 2000).

ELECTRODIAGNOSTIC ASSESSMENT FOR PLANNING SURGICAL INTERVENTION

The preganglionic root avulsion is an irreparable brachial plexus injury. Functional restoration is best accomplished by the transfer of a "donor" nerve to the distal portion of the plexus or nerve soon after the injury, instead of late palliative surgery, such as tendon, muscle, or bone surgery. This procedure is referred to as neurotization, or a nerve transfer procedure. The understanding and use of these procedures is crucial in assisting the surgeon in deciding whether the donor nerve is indeed viable and normal. Neurotization procedures of the avulsed BP include the hypoglossal nerve (XII), spinal accessory nerve (XI), phrenic nerve (C3, C4, and C5), and the intercostal nerve, long thoracic nerve, and the ipsilateral C7 and contralateral C7 root (Chuang et al., 1993: Chuang, 1995; Grossman, 2000; Narakas, 1987; Terzis and Papakonstantinou, 1999). Nerve transfers to assist in shoulder abduction include multiple or double neurotization to the axillary and/ or suprascapular nerve. Nerve transfers for elbow flexion often use the intercostal nerves to the musculocutaneous nerve. More recent work has suggested that assistance with elbow flexion and extension can be accomplished by using the upper trunk transfer or contralateral C7 nerve transfer with or without functioning free muscle transplantation

(Chuang, 1995; Terzis and Papakonstantinou, 1999; Grossman, 2000).

The phrenic nerve is the motor nerve to the diaphragm, originating chiefly from the fourth cervical nerve but augmented by fibers from the third and fifth cervical nerves. It is frequently used in combination with intercostal nerve transfer for neurotization in adult brachial plexus palsy. Because the diaphragm in adults is fixed to the vertebra, sacrificing the phrenic nerve results in only mild elevation of the diaphragm, with no marked respiratory complications except mild dyspnea. However, in infants, the diaphragm is not yet fixed to the vertebral bodies, and once the phrenic nerve is sacrificed the diaphragm will elevate and occupy half the hemithorax, causing severe respiratory distress. Its use, therefore, in children younger than 2 years of age is questionable (Chuang, 1995).

Isolated C7 severance for neurotization procedures does not result in a significant loss of any specific muscle function. This has been reported primarily in the Chinese literature and has recently appeared in the North American literature (Holland and Belzberg, 1997).

In the author's opinion, this technique, although interesting from a physiological perspective, still awaits further analysis. It has now been performed on more than 130 individuals, primarily adults. Theoretically, its value in children may be greater, owing to their development and adaptation skills. It is difficult for one to imagine that the C7 root was given to us to be used for a neurotization procedure without any significant functional deficit. The literature, to date, and proponents of this technique may question this premise (Chuang et al., 1993; Chuang, 1995; Terzis and Papakonstantinou, 1999).

Assessment for concomitant injuries to the aforementioned nerves including cranial nerve XI (trapezius), to the phrenic nerve–innervated diaphragm, and to the contralateral C7-innervated musculature allows the electromyographer to provide helpful information to the surgeon. If EMG analysis of the aforementioned muscles demonstrates abnormalities consistent with axonal loss, their use in neurotization and/or as a donor is therefore put into question. Furthermore, the addition of intraoperative stimulation and recording of the appropriate donor nerve complements the aforementioned studies.

REHABILITATION ISSUES

It is important for physiotherapy to be initiated early to help prevent joint contractures. Many studies attest to a greater than 90% recovery, especially in upper plexus lesions. Appropriate management, typified by the preservation of a free and mobile glenohumeral joint, prevents the need for delayed secondary reconstructive surgery (Gilbert et al., 1988a; Grossman, 2000; Hoeksma et al., 2000; Hoffer, 1999; Kay, 1998; Laurent and Lee, 1994). The goal of physiotherapy is to focus on gently maintaining mobility of the elbow and forearm with flexion, extension, and full rotation (Gilbert and Tassin, 1987; Hoeksma et al., 2000; Ramos and Zell, 2000).

EMERGING CONCEPTS

Carlstedt and colleagues are pioneering experimental and clinical research for severe stretch and avulsion injury to the plexus. They performed intraspinal implants in seven adults and two infants with avulsed roots, usually by placing a graft into a slit in the spinal cord and connecting it more distally to the avulsed root. This work suggests that patients with severe intraspinal brachial plexus injury may, for the first time, experience some modest recovery of function. This procedure, at least in these authors' hands, can be done with minimal risk to spinal cord function. At the present time, it must be stated that this surgery is still very experimental; however, it does show the possibility of some fiber growth, from cord to replanted roots, or grafts to roots, albeit not yet very functional (Carlstedt et al., 1995; Glasby and Hems, 1995; Carlstedt et al., 2000; Kline, 2000).

Nonobstetrical Infantile and Childhood Brachial Plexopathies

Acquired brachial plexopathies are uncommon among neonates and infants beyond the immediate neonatal period, with the exception of acute trauma. However, occasionally, unusual types of brachial plexopathies are seen in the pediatric EMG laboratory. In addition to the various, hereditary, postinflammatory, and traumatic mechanisms, the differential diagnosis of brachial plexus palsy includes other peripheral nerve lesions, pseudoparesis, and amyoplasia as well as congenital lesions involving anterior horn cells and the pyramidal tract (Agboatwalla et al., 1993; Beausoleil et al., 1994; Bell 1996; Escolar and Jones, 1996; Felice and Jones, 1996; Gabriel et al., 1996; Alfonso et al., 2000).

HEREDITARY BRACHIAL PLEXUS NEUROPATHY (HBPN)

The sporadic brachial plexopathies, such as IBPN or neuralgic amyotrophy, must be differentiated from the familial form, hereditary brachial plexus neuropathy (HBPN) (Geiger et al., 1974; Bradley et al., 1975; Dunn et al., 1978; Chance et al., 1994; Gouider et al., 1994). Dunn and associates (1978) described HBPN, also known as *hereditary neuralgic amyotrophy* (HNA), in 12 members of three families. The detailed evaluation of three boys noted that their initial episodes of brachial plexus weakness occurred between age 3 and 4.3 years. Chance and colleagues noted that the onset of HBPN may also occur this early; however, most commonly, this is first seen in older teenagers. Typically, these children have repetitive episodes of shoulder and arm pain, weakness, and atrophy and eventually gradual recovery. Interestingly, when one of these children was an infant, an isolated phrenic nerve paralysis occurred at age 7 weeks (Dunn et al., 1978). The characteristic physiognomy of slender-faced youths characterized by close-set eyes (i.e., hypotelorism), long nasal bridge, and facial asymmetry are typical features of HBPN (Dunn et al., 1978; Chance et al., 1994; Pellegrino et al., 1997). Children with HBPN have painful brachial plexopathies similar to idiopathic brachial plexus neuropathy (neuralgic amyotrophy). This contrasts with the exclusively painless presentation of another hereditary neuropathic process, sometimes presenting as a recurrent plexus lesion; namely, hereditary liability to pressure palsies (HNPP). The attacks were multiple in three of seven patients, and recovery was incomplete in 8 of the 13 instances (Chance et al., 1994; Gouider et al., 1994; Stogbauer et al., 2000).

Children with HBPN have an autosomal dominant inheritance pattern. The gene for HBPN is localized on chromsome 17q (Pellegrino et al., 1997). The primary tissue involved is a non-neuronal one. Pellegrino and colleagues suggest that connective tissue is the possible pathological site in these patients (Pellegrino et al., 1997). Thus, genes coding for connective tissue could lead to brachial plexus neuropathy due to direct pressure, diminished blood supply, or an as yet to be determined immune mechanism (Stogbauer et al., 2000). The tissue inhibitor of metalloproteinase 2 (TIMP2) is another intriguing gene on chromosome 17. Matrix metalloproteinases are involved in the pathogenesis of experimental autoimmune neuritis, an animal model of immune-mediated neuropathies (Stogbauer et al., 2000).

In the differential diagnosis of nontraumatic childhood brachial plexopathies, factors favoring the familial form include the equal appearance in both boys and girls. In contrast, neuralgic amyotrophy (IBPN) occurs more commonly with boys. Mothers, who are also HBPN affected, sometimes report exacerbations subsequent to pregnancy and parturition (Gouider et al., 1994). HBPN has a tendency to have a broader distribution of plexus involvement, in contrast with the predominantly upper trunk, lateral cord damage seen with neuralgic amyotrophy (Geiger et al., 1974). Genetic testing provides better characterization of these disorders (Gouider et al., 1994; Pellegrino et al., 1997).

To date, characteristic nerve conduction studies are not well described in HBPN. There are a few reports. NCSs demonstrated predominantly median and radial sensory fiber involvement with low-amplitude SNAPs (Dunn et al., 1978). In contrast, motor conduction velocity was usually normal or only mildly slowed. Fibrillation potentials, in the affected muscles, are compatible with an axonal process in some of the HBPN children.

HEREDITARY NEUROPATHY WITH LIABILITY TO PRESSURE PALSY (HNPP)

Hereditary neuropathic pressure palsy (HNPP) is a second genetic disorder affecting the brachial plexus that occurs in childhood. It needs to be differentiated from HBPN. In contrast with HBPN, HNPP is usually painless. About 10% of patients with HNPP have brachial plexus involvement (Verhagen et al., 1993). The generic locus for HNPP is on 17P11.2 and differs from that for HBPN (17q25) (Pellegrino et al., 1997). This locus is similar to that for Charcot-Marie-Tooth (type 1A) hereditary motor sensory neuropathy. With HNPP, the genetic abnormality is a duplication at 17P11.2 in contrast with the deletion located at 17P11.2. with Charcot-Marie-Tooth disease (Chance et al., 1994; Gouider et al., 1994; Stogbauer et al., 2000). This interstitial deletion causes the complete loss of one allele of the peripheral myelin protein 22 (*PMP22* gene). Current molecular genetic tests and clinical guidelines allow improved diagnosis, prognosis, and genetic counseling for patients with HNPP (see Chapters 90 and 91). In general, these family members tend to have isolated mononeuropathies, particularly affecting nerves known to be sensitive to compression (i.e., median, radial, and peroneal nerves). However, occasionally, some children with HNPP may have, on presentation, a broad distribution of difficulty manifested by painless brachial plexopathy or even a mononeuritis-type picture confined to one arm. The inciting trauma is often minimal to coincidental. An example is seen in a 16-year-old boy in whom paresis of the posterior and lateral portions of the BP developed as a result of sleeping with his arm tucked under his head (Behse et al., 1972).

IDIOPATHIC BRACHIAL PLEXUS NEUROPATHY (NEURALGIC AMYOTROPHY)

Although this idiopathic acute brachial plexopathy has had multiple previous terminologies—Parsonage-Turner syndrome, neuralgic amyotrophy, and brachial neuritis—the nonspecific nomenclature of *idiopathic brachial plexus neuropathy* is more appropriate because no etiological or pathophysiological implications are inherent in this designation. Others have suggested that the most appropriate name is that of *neuralgic amyotrophy,* given the fact that it is often associated with pain followed by weakness in the girdle and limb (Parsonage and Turner, 1948; Turner and Parsonage, 1957; Tsairis et al., 1972; To and Traquina, 1999). This is much more commonly recognized in the adult; however, in the major Mayo Clinic review, seven of the 99 patients were younger than 20 years of age (Tsairis et al., 1972). The youngest child was age 3 months.

This plexopathy affects predominantly nerves supplying the muscles of the shoulder girdle; however, all portions of the brachial plexus and its terminal branches may be involved (England and Sumner, 1987). About one third of patients with idiopathic brachial plexus neuropathy often have bilateral but asymmetrical involvement (Tsairis et al., 1972; Wilbourn, 1993). The most important aspect is to exclude other pathophysiological mechanisms. Clearly, this is a diagnosis of exclusion, particularly

when there is no evidence of any hereditary component in this rare clinical presentation. In at least three nonfamilial instances, the onset occurred in children between the ages of 16 months and 9 years. The youngest child had a painless, diffuse brachial plexitis with flaccid weakness of the entire arm and weak grasp 4 days after a febrile illness. Limited nerve conduction studies demonstrated such a low-amplitude median nerve CMAP that these did not allow accurate calculation of nerve conduction velocity (Bale et al., 1979a). This 16-month-old infant had a poor recovery at 8 months, in contrast with the excellent recovery at 6 months in another 3 ½-year-old child whose findings were confined to the proximal arm (Bale et al., 1979). None of the 82 patients with neuralgic amyotrophy reported by Parsonage and Turner were younger than 16 years, and only 5 were 16 to 20 years of age (Parsonage and Turner, 1948).

PSEUDOPARESIS

Pseudopalsy secondary to limb pain or deformity is sometimes diagnostically difficult because of the subtlety of other clinical findings.

OSTEOMYELITIS-RELATED BRACHIAL PLEXOPATHY

There are a few case reports of an infantile brachial plexopathy secondary to occult osteomyelitis (Clay, 1982; Gainor and Olson, 1990; Gabriel et al., 1996; Jones et al., 1996; Sadleir and Connolly, 1998). Failure to consider osteomyelitis in the differential diagnosis of an acutely acquired brachial plexopathy in a previously healthy infant may lead to a serious plexus insult as well as delay the institution of appropriate antibiotic therapy. The criteria for differentiating this from idiopathic brachial plexus neuropathy includes the presence of a fever, elevated erythrocyte sedimentation rate (ESR), streptococcal infection, and a positive result on a bone scan. Normal or equivocal changes on bone scan should not dissuade one from challenging the clinical diagnosis of infantile osteomyelitis brachial plexopathy because the onset or recognition of subtle changes of early osteomyelitis can be delayed. Therefore, any febrile infant with acute brachial plexopathy requires a search for proximal humeral osteomyelitis (Clay, 1982; Jones et al., 1996; Sadleir and Connolly, 1998; Alfonso et al., 2000). One of us (HRJ) evaluated a previously healthy 19-day-old infant girl who had had fever and rhinorrhea for 5 days and decreased right arm movement for 1 day. This baby's right arm was almost flaccid, with absent muscle stretch reflexes and a possibility of tenderness noted with arm extension. Her white blood cell count (WBC) was 16,400, with a left shift. Shoulder, elbow, and chest radiographs were normal, as was a bone scan. Examination of the cerebrospinal fluid revealed glucose of 45 mg/ml, protein of 160 mg/ml, and no increase in the WBC. Repeat cerebrospinal fluid examination a few days later demonstrated a lower glucose of 28 mgm% and 7 lymphocytes. Blood and CSF cultures demonstrated group B streptococci. Electromyography 3 weeks after the onset of arm weakness demonstrated normal motor and sensory conduction studies. However there was a markedly diminished number of MUPs, with many fibrillation potentials and positive waves confined to the affected deltoid and biceps, compatible with an upper brachial plexus lesion. She was treated with penicillin G. Repeat bone scan on the fifth day after admission demonstrated a proximal right humerus osteomyelitis near the shoulder.

Clay later reported two febrile infants with a 2-week history of an acutely flaccid arm. There was "an unusual infiltrative" lesion of the brachial plexus secondary to an occult osteomyelitis. This pathological process contrasts with the precipitous onset of root avulsion and plexus injury at birth. Clay's EMG findings demonstrated active denervation at day 20, but this was not present 6 days earlier (Clay, 1982). Full recovery did not occur for 8 months. Both children had ESRs of 90 and 81 mm/hr, modest leukocytosis, and positive cultures for group B β-hemolytic streptococci—one from blood culture and the other on shoulder tap after blood culture was negative. Bone scan may be diagnostic; however, a delay in the onset of a specific change should not dissuade one from making the clinical diagnosis. The pathophysiology of this relationship awaits elucidation. Therefore, when one is confronted with the onset of an acute infantile brachial plexopathy in a febrile neonate, a search is indicated for a proximal *humeral osteomyelitis,* especially with a markedly elevated ESR and positive culture for streptococci.

An unusual case of pyogenic *cervical osteomyelitis* with paraspinal abscess and resulting Erb's palsy is reported from Oman. *Staphylococcus aureus* is the organism in the majority of cases; however, rarely, gram-negative organisms are isolated (Sharma et al., 2000).

OTHER NONGENETIC BRACHIAL PLEXUS LESIONS IN CHILDREN

Infant Seats and Backpacks

Compressive injuries to the brachial plexus are relatively uncommon. However, two potential areas where such an injury can occur are defined in children. These are primarily traumatic (Piatt et al., 1988; Piatt, 1991). With the introduction of mandatory automobile infant safety seats to prevent free-flight injuries of the unrestrained infant, the potential for a compressive injury to the brachial plexus is more frequent (Peterson and Peterson, 1991). A previously healthy 9-month-old infant was confined in a rear-facing infant-restraint device and self-retracting shoulder harnesses during a 7-day, 2500-mile journey. The infant was never confined to the seat for more than 4 hours. On the last day of the trip, the infant had loss of function in the left arm. Neurological examination documented weakness in

the distribution of the lateral and posterior cord to the brachial plexus. No other etiological mechanisms were defined. Unfortunately, no EMG was performed. The infant had a full recovery, suggesting neurapraxic injury to the brachial plexus secondary to the harness. The manufacturer had sold more than 3,000,000 of these devices in 1991 and was unaware of similar instances (Peterson and Peterson, 1991).

Despite the increasing use of backpacks by school-aged children, an increased incidence of previously described rucksack palsies has yet to be found. These were initially noted by the Cleveland Clinic group (Rothner et al., 1975) in children participating in scouting. In a study from Japan, 15 of 16 sports-related peripheral neuropathies affecting the brachial plexus were secondary to mountain climbing with packs as heavy as 40 kg. It is suggested that these lesions occurred secondary to nerve compression in the axilla. None of these injuries were further defined by EMG (Hirasawa and Sakakida, 1983). In the authors' experience, this seemingly infrequent type of adolescent brachial plexopathy may be the result of better-quality back-packing equipment, such as padding. It is also the authors' opinion that when these youngsters are evaluated, the electromyographer needs to look for other causes of neuropathy, including HNPP and HBPN in the aforementioned cases.

Postneonatal Traumatic Brachial Plexopathies

There are a number of traumatic etiological mechanisms for brachial plexopathy in the older child, particularly the teenager. These are similar to those seen in the adult population and includes trauma, particularly motorcycles, other accidents, war injuries, gunshot wounds, surgery, and, rarely, sporting events (Kline, 1972; Hirasawa and Sakakida 1983; Kline and Judice, 1983; Kline, 1989; Barisic et al., 1994; Menegaux et al., 1994; Dumitru, 1995; Kline and Hudson, 1997; Mehlman et al., 2000; Schwartz et al., 2000).

Sports injuries are a major setting known to predispose adolescents to brachial plexus injuries (Chrisman et al., 1965; Clancy et al., 1977; Robertson et al., 1979; Clancy, 1982; Rockett, 1982; Di Benedetto and Markey, 1984; Poindexter and Johnson, 1984; Watkins, 1986; Wroble and Albright, 1986; Wilbourn, 1990; Pellegrino et al., 1997). The typical clinical presentation in the sports venue includes injuries related to football, lacrosse, and rugby. In football, these injuries are often referred to as a *burner* or *stinger* (Robertson et al., 1979; Poindexter and Johnson, 1984; Wilbourn, 1993; Dumitru, 1995a). Despite the frequency with which these injuries occur, the exact pathophysiology of so-called burners and stingers is unclear. The two major proposed etiologies are compression with traction of the C5-6 cervical nerve roots and a mild stretch injury to the upper trunk of the brachial plexus. Because the clinical presentation is consistent with either or both, no definite study has defined the etiology of these lesions. If neurological weakness persists, and EMG defines these lesion sites, this type of brachial plexopathy is better referred to as a *brachial plexopathy* than simply a sports-related burner or stinger. Because neither injury has any long-term sequelae, few EMG attempts have been made to define evidence of axonal loss.

Needle electromyography is the most sensitive examination. The most common abnormal findings include abnormalities in the muscles innervated by the upper trunk of the brachial plexus. However, in most cases, the EMG is within normal limits or is only suggestive of a decreased recruitment and interference pattern (i.e., neurapraxia). Anatomically, based on the location of the "weak link" at the root level (because of the lack of supporting connective tissue structures), a number of authors suggest that the nerve root is a prime consideration for the lesion (Dumitru, 1995). The electrodiagnostic examination is of value in individuals who sustain more than a period of episodic pain and weakness or are unable to "shake it off" (Chrisman et al., 1965; Clancy et al., 1977; Robertson et al., 1979; Clancy, 1982; Rockett, 1982; Di Benedetto and Markey, 1984; Poindexter and Johnson, 1984; Watkins, 1986; Wroble and Albright, 1986; Wilbourn, 1990a; Pellegrino et al., 1997). Shoulder-girdle weakness and a normal NEE, particularly in supraspinatus and infraspinatus muscles, alerts the clinician to consider musculoskeletal causes. These include a rotator cuff tear and fracture.

Child Abuse

The possibility of the battered child syndrome always needs careful consideration with any acute pediatric brachial plexus lesion. This is especially true with the youngster in whom no definable predisposing reported trauma, infection, or febrile illness is present, as occurs with IBPN or HBPN. To illustrate this point, one of the editors (HRJ) encloses his experience with one toddler (Jones et al., 1996).

A 15-month-old infant with sickle cell disease had been otherwise healthy when she was first evaluated at CHB after her mother noted the child "fell on her arm," was unable to use it for about a day, and began preferentially to use the opposite arm. It was uncomfortable for the patient to move the affected arm. Pain had awakened her the previous night. Neurological examination demonstrated that she was unable to abduct the arm at the shoulder or flex the arm, and her biceps muscle stretch reflex was diminished. Fibrillations and positive sharp waves were present and confined to the right biceps and deltoid muscles. When an anemia with stippled red blood cells was documented, a history of plumbism (lead poisoning) was elicited. The blood lead level was mildly elevated. Both arms moved equally well 2 months later. One initial diagnostic consideration was the unlikely possibility that the plexopathy may have been secondary to the blood lead level.

Just 5 months later, the mother returned with this youngster because of recurrent weakness of the same arm. Although the mother denied a history of trauma, the social worker later confirmed recurrent parental abuse. This child's mother occasionally picked her up by the arm, twirled her overhead, and then threw her in the manner of performing the hammer throw. The authors are unaware of plumbism (i.e., pica or sickle cell disease) having also occurred in this case as a cause of recurrent brachial plexopathy. The authors were unable to detect any of the other usual causes of brachial plexus neuropathy here, including genetic mechanisms. As always, "atypical" presentations of neurological deficits, especially with poorly defined histories, should alert the astute clinician or pediatric electromyographer to the possibility of child abuse.

Thoracic Outlet Syndrome

The authors have each seen only one adolescent, one 13-year-old, and one 16-year-old, whose condition fit the strict electromyographic definition of neurological thoracic outlet syndrome (TOS) described by Gilliatt (Gilliatt et al., 1978; Roos, 1990; Wilbourn, 1990, 1993; Roos, 1999).

Most TOS patients present with hand weakness and/or atrophy. In Gilliatt's group, pain was also present in 12 of the 14 patients; however, it was usually mild and was the primary complaint in only five individuals. Each patient had either a cervical rib or an increased length of the C7 transverse process.

Classic EMG findings include (1) NCS with low-amplitude fifth-finger ulnar SNAPs, (2) normal median digit 2 SNAPs, and (3) a low-amplitude CMAP from the primarily median nerve–innervated thenar eminence compared with the (4) normal ulnar nerve–innervated CMAP of the hypothenar eminence. Conduction velocities are preserved. Wilbourn advises that clinicians utilize the medial antebrachial cutaneous nerve of the forearm in patients with "true" or neurogenic TOS (Chapter 47). An excellent discussion of the topic, including its controversial nature and clinical findings, was discussed by Wilbourn and Roos (Roos, 1999; Wilbourn, 1999).

Ouvrier and colleagues reported one 4-year-old child with thenar atrophy and weakness who, on cervical spine radiography, demonstrated a congenital Klippel-Feil anomaly associated with small cervical ribs. The amplitude of the ipsilateral median SNAP was low-normal, but still only 50% of that of the opposite unaffected side. The ipsilateral sensory evoked responses (SNAPs) from the ulnar nerve were of low amplitude compared with the normal median nerve and needle findings, consistent with chronic denervation in thenar muscles. An elongated C7 transverse process articulating with the first rib was found at surgery. There was only a little improvement over the next 5 years (Ouvrier et al., 2001).

NEOPLASMS

In contrast with adults, it is extremely rare for a neoplasm to be the cause of brachial plexopathy in the pediatric population. Important features that distinguish these children with a tumor from those with idiopathic brachial plexopathy include the following: (1) onset of weakness after the first postpartum day; (2) progressive course; (3) history of normal delivery and birth weight; (4) the appearance of a mass in the supraclavicular area without radiographic evidence of clavicle fracture; and (5) scratch marks on a weak arm (Inoue et al., 1983; Alfonso et al., 2000).

MISCELLANEOUS BRACHIAL PLEXUS MECHANISMS

There are a few other very rare causes of a pediatric brachial plexopathy. These include neonatal hemangiomatosis (Lucas et al., 1995; Sadleir and Connolly, 1998), neck compression (Turner and Parsonage, 1957), and an exostosis of the first rib (Alfonso et al., 2000). A brachial plexopathy is also described as having occurred following therapy for childhood acute lymphoblastic leukemia (Inoue et al., 1983; Harila-Saari et al., 1998; Alessandri et al., 1999).

LUMBOSACRAL PLEXOPATHIES

Lesions of the lumbosacral plexus (LSP) are the most uncommon peripheral nerve problems seen in our pediatric EMG laboratories. Most occur secondary to trauma, a mechanism similar to that in the adult population. These mechanisms include motor vehicle accident, pelvic fracture, and gunshot wounds (Jellis and Helal, 1970; Kline, 1972; Christie and Jamieson, 1974; Stoehr, 1978; Barquet, 1982; Marra, 1983; Chad and Bradley, 1987; Rai et al., 1990; Egel et al., 1995; Kline et al., 1998; Switzer et al., 2000; Chiou-Tan et al., 2001). However, on rare occasions, a postviral (immune-related) plexitis occurs (Evans et al., 1981; Chad and Bradley, 1987; Thomson, 1993). Very rarely, a tumor is found, and this lesion always needs to be considered (Pasternak and Volpe, 1980). At CHB, a distal sacral plexopathy was one child's presenting sign of lymphoma. Rarely, some iatrogenic etiologies occur (Brown et al., 1988); Villarejo and Pascual 1993; MacDonald, 1994; MacDonald and Marcuse, 1994; Marin et al., 1994). LSP have also been linked to trauma associated with an underlying predisposing factor, including hereditary liability to pressure palsy and Ehlers-Danlos syndrome (Gabreels-Festen et al., 1992; Galan and Kousseff, 1995).

Anatomy

Although it is important to recognize that the generic term *lumbosacral plexus* is used as a means of logical organization, on occasion the clinical le-

sion may predominate in either the lumbar or the sacral plexus (Fig. 89–7). This is more clearly defined in adults than in children, in whom these LSP variants sometimes appear to be almost separate anatomical structures. However, in pediatric patients, a significant overlap is seen, probably the result of the relatively small body size. This emphasizes the contiguous nature of this plexus of nerves in the infant and the young child.

The femoral nerve is the predominant nerve that arises from the lumbar portion of the lumbosacral plexus, innervating primarily the iliopsoas and the quadriceps femoris muscles. It also innervates the superficial sensory branches to the anterior and lateral thigh as well as the medial foreleg. The obturator is the other major nerve derived from the lumbar portion of this plexus. It innervates the proximal 80% of the adductor magnus. The latter muscle also receives some distal innervation from the sciatic nerve. This mixed innervation of the adductor is particularly important when one evaluates potential sciatic nerve lesions. The clinician should not be misled by signs of denervation in the distal adductor, as well as other primary sciatic nerve–innervated muscles, and then falsely conclude that a plexus lesion is present.

The sacral portion of the lumbosacral plexus innervates the remainder of the leg, including the posterior thigh and buttocks muscles as well as the entire leg below the knee. These nerves include the superior and inferior gluteal nerves, which innervate the gluteus medius, and gluteus minimus and gluteus maximus, respectively. The medial and lateral hamstrings are supplied by the sciatic nerve (peroneal and tibial sources). It then functionally divides into the peroneal and tibial nerves, and most of the remaining motor innervation is below the knee, with the exception of the short head of the biceps femoris. The short head of biceps is a useful muscle electromyographically, as it is innervated by the peroneal nerve (lateral portion of the sciatic nerve) proximal to the knee.

This nerve then proceeds to bifurcate below the knee into the superficial and the deep peroneal nerves. These two branches of the peroneal nerves supply all of the anterior compartment of the lower leg. In contrast, the tibial nerve, the other primary derivative of the sciatic nerve, supplies the posterior compartment. The primary superficial sensory nerves derived from the peroneal and tibial, respectively, are the superficial peroneal and the sural and plantar nerves.

Histologically, the lumbosacral plexus is similar to that of other peripheral nerves (Sunderland, 1965, 1970). The epineurium occupies approximately 45% to 65% of the total cross-sectional area of the nerve roots of the lumbosacral plexus and is more condensed toward the periphery (Ebraheim et al., 1997). The relatively higher connective tissue content in the L5 and S1 roots as well as the lumbosacral trunk may contribute to their inherent strength. These factors provide a cushion against any untoward de-

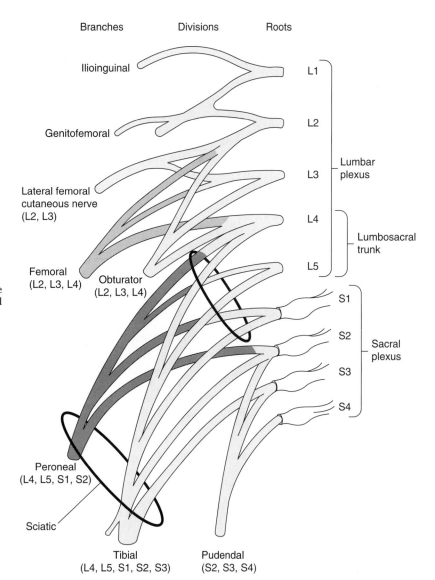

Figure 89–7. The lumbosacral plexus. The most common sites affected include femoral and the lumbosacral trunk.

forming forces. The relatively higher incidence of injury to L5, the lumbosacral trunk, and the S1 trunk probably is not due to any microscopic differences, but rather to the close proximity of these structures to the sacrum and sacroiliac joint (Ebraheim et al., 1997).

General Principles of the Electromyography Evaluation for Pediatric Lumbosacral Plexopathies

None of the nerves originating in the lumbar plexus lend themselves to direct stimulation for conventional NCS. This is especially true in children. Therefore, the clinician must depend on the results of needle EMG to assess the function of the femoral and obturator nerves. In contrast, the sacral sciatic-derived peroneal and tibial nerve components are available for routine NCS. Occasionally, a child does not tolerate stimulation in the popliteal fossa, and

the authors are content to study only the distal component. In the infant, sural stimulation is sometimes technically difficult (Bye and Fagan, 1988). As in the cervical spine, a normal SNAP amplitude in an area of abnormal sensation (peripheral nerve and/or dermatome) may suggest a preganglionic lesion and help to differentiate a root or intraspinal (i.e., preganglionic) lesion from a plexus (postganglionic) abnormality (see Fig. 89–2A to F). To further differentiate a plexus lesion, especially from the more common proximal sciatic nerve defect, examination of multiple muscles is required, including the gluteus medius and gluteus maximus. Additionally, one must exclude an intraspinal or nerve root process by examining the paraspinal muscles. These investigations are demanding in children. It is also difficult to obtain appropriate relaxation here, especially in infants and young children. Therefore, when there is a possible LSP diagnosis, one may best perform the EMG with the help of an anesthetic in the day surgery center.

Experience at the Children's Hospital of Boston

Lumbar and sacral plexus lesions are exceedingly uncommon, especially in comparison with brachial plexopathies. Nerve root lesions are equally less prevalent, and the rare cases we evaluate are in older teenagers, in whom the evaluation is similar to that of the adult patient. During the years 1979 to 1995, the authors evaluated just six children found to have damage involving primarily the lumbosacral plexus (Jones, 1996). During the same time period, the authors examined nine times as many children with brachial plexopathies (n = 54) among 1,924 EMGs in newborns to children 18 years of age. All but one of the few lumbosacral lesions occurred secondary to trauma. The sixth child was thought to have a progressive idiopathic plexopathy.

Neonatal Lumbosacral Plexopathies

Trauma to the lumbosacral plexus is rare in newborns (Dumitru, 1995b; Hope et al., 1985). Eng summarized her experience with three neonates seen during a 7-year period who sustained lumbosacral "traction" injuries after breech delivery. She emphasized the importance of differentiating these lesions from an asymmetrical myelomeningocele, infantile poliomyelitis, parenteral injection injury, or a central nervous system process. Unfortunately, no precise details of the clinical or EMG findings were described. None of these three infants experienced a complete recovery; however, the length of follow-up time is not reported (Eng, 1981). In contrast, another infant is reported who had a precise EMG performed after a precipitous double-footed breech delivery (Hope et al., 1985). At birth, this infant was unable to extend the knee or to rotate it internally. A follow-up evaluation at 4 months of age demonstrated the inability to extend the knee or internally rotate the leg, atrophy and hypotonia of the quadriceps muscle, mild flexion contracture at the knee, and an absent quadriceps muscle stretch reflex. Radiographic examination of the lumbar spine and hip were normal. No pelvic or paravertebral masses were found on ultrasonography of the pelvis and spine. An EMG study demonstrated denervation confined to the quadriceps and adductor magnus muscles. Excessive birth traction was suggested as a possible cause of the injury to the lumbar plexus; however, an isolated injury to the L2-4 nerve roots was not excluded. Slight improvement occurred 2 months later (Hope et al., 1985). Volpe described one similar infant who experienced a good recovery (Volpe, 1987).

Postneonatal Lumbosacral Traumatic Plexopathies

Infants are susceptible to stretch injuries at the lumbosacral plexus, similar to the case with the brachial plexus. Traumatic lumbosacral nerve root avulsion rarely occurs. (Volpe, 1987; Chin and Chew, 1997). It is variously associated with flexion-abduction injury to the hip, hyperextension of the thigh with pelvic fracture (Verstraete et al., 1989), posterior dislocation of the hip, and sacral fractures (Barnett and Connolly, 1975; Kolawole et al., 1988). According to pathological studies at a postmortem examination (Huittinen, 1972), the L3-S3 roots will rupture proximal to the spinal ganglion but distal to their origin at the cord. This contrasts with the more common root avulsion that occurs directly from the spinal cord in the cervical spine (Verstraete et al., 1989).

Stretch injuries to the LSP are more common than are root avulsions, but they are still relatively rare (Christie and Jamieson, 1974; Barquet, 1982; Young et al., 1993; Kline et al., 1998). The sciatic is the more predominant nerve involved. This has been reported subsequent to pelvic-sacral fractures and hip dislocations (Jones et al., 1988; Yuen et al., 1994; Kline et al., 1998). Potentially serious lumbosacral plexopathies may result from unusual, seemingly innocent activities of children, particularly babies, as illustrated by one *Raggedy-Anne–like* case seen at CHB (Jones et al., 1996). A 4-month-old infant's sister playfully but vigorously pulled him across the floor by his leg. Later that day, his leg was limp, lacked spontaneous motion, and was cool. Examination demonstrated a flaccid leg with no muscle stretch reflexes. Orthopedic evaluation, including appropriate radiographs, was normal. NCS demonstrated a low-amplitude posterior tibial CMAP but normal tibial nerve conduction velocity, and distal latencies (DLs) with normal peroneal nerve function. The EMG study demonstrated fibrillation potentials in the tibialis anterior and medial gastrocnemius, with a diminished number of MUPs in these muscles and the vastus lateralis. Seven months later, proximal strength was normal; however, there was some residual distal weakness.

Another lumbosacral plexopathy seen at the CHB EMG laboratory occurred secondary to surgical trauma during a lengthening procedure for idiopathic leg-length discrepancy. EMG documented injury primarily to the lumbar plexus. The piriformis syndrome (sciatic nerve palsy at the piriformis level), an often disputed entity, is a very rare condition. This was postulated to have occurred as a complication of posterior fossa surgery performed in the seated position in one 10-year-old boy (Brown et al., 1988). Other traumatic mechanisms include knife injuries, gunshot wounds, and motor vehicle accidents (Kline, 1972; Kline et al., 1998; Chiou-Tan et al., 2001).

Infantile Lumbosacral Injuries Related to Abdominal Trauma

Infants rarely sustain crush injuries that result in pressure lumbosacral plexopathies. One 13-month-old developed a flaccid leg, with the exception of preserved iliopsoas function. This was secondary to an acute abdominal crush injury (Egel et al., 1995). During the next few days, the loss of function ensued in the opposite leg, with the iliopsoas and quadriceps being the only muscles with preserved strength. Muscle stretch reflexes were absent bilaterally. An magnetic resonance imaging of the lumbosacral spine was normal. EMG performed 72 hours after injury demonstrated bilaterally absent peroneal F-wave and tibial H reflexes but otherwise normal peroneal motor conduction parameters. No MUPs were activated, however; and no signs of denervation were demonstrated in the leg and the lumbosacral paraspinal muscles. Within 1 month, the child had clinically recovered. Repeat EMG demonstrated normal MUPs in the previously silent muscles. The only signs of axonal damage were noted in the tibialis anterior muscles. F waves returned 3 months after injury. The clinical and EMG courses were thought to be compatible primarily with a neurapraxic injury (Egel et al., 1995).

Iliopsoas hemorrhage can also result in a femoral neuropathy, especially in the context of a bleeding diathesis. This occurred in a 15-year-old boy with hemophilia (Gertzbein and Evans, 1972).

Lumbosacral Plexus Neuropathy

Primary lumbosacral plexus neuropathy, unassociated with underlying disease, has been and remains a controversial subject. However, a lumbosacral plexus neuropathy (LSPN) has been reported in six children 2 to 16 years of age. This neuropathy presented with rapid onset of pain, weakness, and atrophy in the leg. A viral illness preceded the onset by 3 to 10 days in five of these six children. The lumbar plexus was predominantly involved in five children. The diagnosis of lumbosacral plexopathy was confirmed by EMG; however, details of these studies were not reported. Four children recovered within 3 months, and two had mild residual weakness (Chad and Bradley, 1987; Awerbuch et al., 1989a, 1989b; Thomson, 1993). In their report of 10 LSPN cases, Evans and colleagues described patients who presented with pain and weakness (age range, 15 to 81) and had no associated predisposing condition. The illness presented with inguinal pain associated with midthigh paresthesias. Leg weakness, manifested by decreased strength in the iliopsoas, quadriceps, and adductor muscles, occurred 1 day later. EMG demonstrated denervation in the femoral- and obturator-innervated muscles with a normal paraspinal evaluation. Significant recovery occurred in 3 months. The researchers likened this condition to the well-described counterpart of idiopathic brachial plexus neuropathy, *neuralgic amyotrophy* (Bale et al., 1979; Evans et al., 1981).

There are a few other rare etiologies to consider in the differential diagnosis of sudden leg weakness in children. Poliomyelitis is usually not a problem in North America. In the mid-1990s, when the live vaccine was the primary form of immunization, there were at least three cases of postimmunization infantile poliomyelitis, two of which one of the authors (HRJ) was consulted (Beausoleil et al., 1994; Goldstein, 1995; David et al., 1997). The authors also occasionally see newly arrived immigrants from developing countries in whom weakness of the leg developed just before embarkation from their native lands, who are referred to us after arrival here. Evaluation was also compatible with a primary anterior horn cell disorder (i.e., poliomyelitis) and not with LSPN.

When the onset of weakness is more insidious, the possibility of a retroperitoneal mass also needs consideration. One author (HRJ) evaluated a 14-year-old boy at CHB, who, based on needle EMG findings, had a combined sciatic as well as an inferior and superior gluteal neuropathy. A pelvic lymphoma was found when systemic symptoms developed soon after the onset of the leg difficulties. Cancer, metastatic disease, and a primary tumor affecting the lumbosacral plexus are rare conditions in children (Harila-Saari et al., 1998; Kline et al., 1998).

PEDIATRIC NERVE ROOT LESIONS

Cervical or lumbosacral radiculopathies are an unusual reason for referral to a pediatric EMG laboratory. The authors have evaluated more than 2,700 children, from newborns to 18-year-olds. Only a very few of these have unexplained neck, back, or extremity discomfort that might be secondary to a radiculopathy. One patient 18 years of age, in whom severe back spasms developed after a sudden turning movement, had isolated L5-S1 paraspinal denervation. This was the only possible nerve root lesion identified in the authors' pediatric EMG laboratory between 1979 and 1995. No specific mechanism was identified. It is possible that occult lesions may be masked because it is difficult in children to obtain relaxation in the lumbosacral paraspinal muscles. It is still important to consider the rare possibility of a nerve root process in the differential diagnosis of any child with cervical or lumbosacral pain, especially those with a radicular component.

Cervical Root Disease

Children rarely have primary cervical nerve root lesions. In a review of 561 Mayo Clinic patients with a cervical radiculopathy, only 41 individuals (7%) were 15 to 29 years of age. (Radharkrishnan et al., 1994). No more specific breakdown of the adolescents included in this report is available. The study excluded one 13-year-old girl with a cervical radiculopathy. This exclusion further supports the rarity of this lesion in children and adolescents.

ELECTROMYOGRAPHY

It is often difficult to make a differential diagnosis between the more common brachial plexus lesions and the rare case of cervical root damage while one performs a pediatric EMG. As nerve root avulsions and brachial plexus injury often occur concomitantly, particularly in children, the presence of EMG findings compatible with a primary plexus lesion does not exclude damage at the nerve root level (Mancias et al., 1994). Because it is much more difficult to obtain cervical paraspinal muscle relaxation in children, this EMG differential diagnosis is sometimes a problem in the setting of a possible traumatic mechanism. The finding of normal median and ulnar SNAPs lends support to the diagnosis of a C7-8 intraspinal lesion. When one attempts to differentiate lesions at C6 from those involving the brachial plexus, normal median SNAPs recorded from the thumb (Wilbourne, 1993) or lateral antebrachial cutaneous SNAPs provide a useful means of localizing lesions to the C6 roots, especially when paraspinal muscle EMG is unreliable (Flaggman and Kelly, 1980). The converse does not apply—that is, the absence of SNAPS, implying a postganglionic plexus lesion—does not exclude a concomitant nerve root lesion (Mancias et al., 1994).

IMAGING STUDIES AND CERVICAL RADICULOPATHIES

Magnetic resonance imaging is currently the most useful means of defining a radiculopathy. In general, in adults we find that there is little need for EMG in the evaluation of a possible nerve root lesion per se. In 1994, Trojaborg (1994) compared EMG results with myelography in patients with cervical spinal root avulsions. His study included just one adolescent, a 17-year-old boy, with a motorcycle accident–induced total loss of motor and sensory function in the left arm. Both EMG and myelography demonstrated a combined plexus and nerve root lesion. In 9 of these 17 instances, there was a discrepancy between the EMG and the myelographic findings. Myelography suggested that 4 of these 9 patients had sustained an avulsion. However, both clinical and neurophysiological follow-up studies failed to confirm total loss of root continuity. Trojaborg (1994) suggests that occasionally surgical exploration is necessary to best define these lesions. Additionally, he counseled that the anatomical appearance is sometimes still misleading, even at operation.

DIFFERENTIAL DIAGNOSIS OF PEDIATRIC CERVICAL ROOT LESIONS

Congenital Cervical Stenosis

Although the authors' experience has not included any typical cervical radiculopathies secondary to disk or uncal osteophyte-induced foraminal stenosis mechanisms (Radharkrishnan et al., 1994),

they have evaluated two children with congenital cervical spine lesions. One was a 13-year-old child with a short history of pain in the right shoulder and arm exacerbated by swimming. Electromyography demonstrated C7-T1 denervation. Cervical spine radiography demonstrated anomalous hypoplastic vertebral bodies with incompletely developed interspaces. The other was a 16-year-old boy with a 3-month history of progressive painless arm weakness, but no pain or paresthesias, or any neurological symptoms that suggested spinal cord involvement. This was apparent when he played basketball. The clinical diagnosis prior to the EMG was a possible brachial plexus lesion (Jones, 1993). Weakness affected predominantly the infraspinatus, the supraspinatus, the serratus anterior, the deltoid, and, possibly, the opposite deltoid muscles. Muscle stretch reflexes were normal, and no sensory loss was detected.

Motor and sensory NCSs were normal. Needle EMG demonstrated active denervation in the C5-8 dermatomes; contralateral changes were confined to C5. The authors were not able to obtain total relaxation of the cervical paraspinal muscles. The remaining EMG examination was normal. Cervical spine radiography demonstrated en bloc C2-3 vertebrae, with diminished diameter of the spinal canal from C4 to C7, and with spinal stenosis from C2 to C7 demonstrated on myelography. Decompressive cervical laminectomy was performed. The outcome of this patient was unknown, as he was lost to follow-up review shortly after the operation.

Hirayama's Cervical Spinal Atrophy

In addition to congenital spinal stenosis, Hirayama's cervical spinal atrophy is another very rare cause for an adolescent to present with painless arm weakness. Initially, this disorder usually affects hand function and thus can be confused with a C8 radiculopathy, medial brachial plexus lesion, or, even, an ulnar neuropathy if one does not perform a careful clinical examination as well as a detailed needle EMG. In contrast with amyotrophic lateral sclerosis (ALS), the teenaged male usually, but not always, of western Pacific Rim heritage who develops this insidiously progressive disorder has the good fortune for this process to affect predominantly just one upper extremity, and to a lesser extent its contralateral homologue (Hirayama, 2000). The cervical spinal cord is the primary site of pathology. After a 3- to 5-year progressive course, this illness often stabilizes when the patient reaches the third decade. The authors have recognized just four instances of this at CHB during more than two decades. This disorder is discussed in greater detail in Chapter 87.

Motor Neuron Disease

Fortunately in our patient population, this disorder is even less frequent than is Hirayama's disease.

One 19-year-old female basketball player presented to the Lahey Clinic with a similar 1-year history of a progressively painless and, now, flaccid left arm (Jones, 1993). Needle EMG demonstrated diffuse fibrillation potentials with almost no definable MUPs, in addition to absent median and ulnar CMAPs, but normal SNAPs. The patient refused further study, including needle EMG of the other extremities. Eighteen months later after she died, an autopsy demonstrated classic ALS. Fortunately, there was only one patient, a 17-year-old, who had symptoms commence before age 20 years in one review of 123 ALS patients (Dantes and McComas, 1989).

Grisel's Syndrome

This uncommon infectious process produces primarily subluxation of the atlantoaxial joint. It is found in both children and adults (Mathern and Batzdorf, 1991). Typically, these patients present with unrelenting neck or throat pain. This is followed often by torticollis and, sometimes, by subluxation at this joint. Fifteen percent of these patients develop a cervical radiculopathy. There is often a preceding history of a flulike illness, otitis, tonsillitis, or pharyngitis, subsequently followed by the insidious onset of a progressively severe and very localized spinal pain. Eventually, this pain becomes unremitting, sometimes radiating into the shoulder. A torticollis may occur with a relatively precipitous onset. Other neurological manifestations include greater occipital nerve paresthesias, myelopathy with transient or fixed quadriparesis (tetraparesis), and, rarely, death (Mathern and Batzdorf, 1991).

Despite the infectious nature of this illness, it is uncommon for these children to appear very septic. Spinal percussion tenderness and restriction of neck movement, including torticollis, are the primary findings with physical examination. No EMG studies are mentioned in the review by Mathern and Batzdorf (1991). However, their report points to the importance of considering this potentially serious illness in the rare instance of a child referred to the EMG laboratory with severe neck pain and symptoms of a cervical radiculopathy.

EMG CHARACTERISTICS WITH OTHER INTRASPINAL LESIONS

When one performs EMG on a teenager with a cervical radiculopathy with the symptoms of painless arm weakness, the typical findings are similar to those of the various radiculopathies, congenital spinal stenosis, or some primary intramedullary lesions, including Hirayama's disorder, and early motor neuron disease. Each entity demonstrates evidence of a primary neurogenic process at the preganglionic level. In the authors' experience, both congenital spinal stenosis and Hirayama's disorder exhibit modest chronic neurogenic changes in the clinically silent, or less affected, contralateral ex-

tremity. This differentiates these processes from the various types of brachial plexus lesions or the even more rare possibility of hereditary tendency to pressure palsies (HNPP) (Infante et al., 2001). There is a similar, also genetically linked, process of an acute, recurrent, painful brachial plexopathy that may also mimic a nerve root lesion (Stogbauer et al., 1998).

Lumbosacral Root Disease

INTRODUCTION

On the rare occasions when herniation of the nucleus pulposus occurs in children, it usually occurs in the lumbosacral area. Among surgically proven cases of lumbar radiculopathies at the Mayo Clinic, the estimated prevalence in children was between 0.8% and 3.2% (Weinert and Rizzo, 1992). There may be a much higher incidence of juvenile disk herniation in Japan. One Japanese study reported 70 patients, aged 9 to 19 years, who represented 15.4% of 456 patients who underwent lumbar disk surgical repair between 1951 and 1977 (Kurihara and Kataoka, 1980). Most of these patients (55 of 70) were boys. Twenty-one of these children were younger than 15 years of age. Another combined surgical experience at Rutgers and Dartmouth in the United States reported 43 patients 11 to 21 years of age. (Fischer and Saunders, 1981). These included 10 adolescents, 11 to 17 years of age, who had lumbar disk disease. These patients were seen over a 30-year period, or essentially one teenager with lumbosacral disk herniation every 3 years! The youngest reported case is a 27-month-old who fell from his cradle and, over 2 weeks, developed back pain, irritability, and gait difficulty. Magnetic resonance imaging demonstrated the abnormality. Surgery was successful (Revuelta et al., 2000).

At the Mayo Clinic, 1,368 patients, 16 years of age or younger, were evaluated for back, disk, or sciatic pain between 1950 and 1975 (DeOrio and Bianco, 1982). In many patients, a diagnosis of lumbar disk herniation was considered a possibility, and most of these responded well to conservative, nonoperative forms of therapy. However, 50 (3.7%) required surgical removal of one or more disks. These children who underwent lumbar disk procedures represented 0.5% of lumbar laminectomies performed at the Mayo Clinic during that time span.

CLINICAL PRESENTATION

Back pain and/or sciatica is the typical clinical presentation. It is important to note that although all children had sciatica, 12 (17%) in Japan (Kurihara and Kataoka, 1980) and 17 (34%) at the Mayo Clinic had sciatica without back pain (DeOrio and Bianco, 1982). Trauma related to athletic injuries, lifting, falls, or back injury occurring at work accounted for at least half of the cases in two series (Fisher and Saunders, 1981; Kurihara and Kataoka, 1980). In the

Mayo study, in which there was a 36% incidence of trauma, the athletic injuries occurred in a variety of sports, including football, basketball, baseball, soccer, cheerleading, tennis, and running (DeOrio and Bianco, 1982).

Clinical examination demonstrated that the neurological deficits were usually relatively subtle. Although focal weakness was detected in some, in one series no footdrop was noted in any child (Fisher and Saunders, 1981). Primary findings did include some degree of muscle weakness in 32% to 60% of patients. This involved primarily the tibialis anterior and/or toe extensors. There was recognizable, sensory loss in 10% (lateral foot 8% and medial foot 2%) to 58% of these adolescents. Severe paravertebral muscle spasm was also present, along with limited spinal motion, cough-sneeze exacerbation in many (76%), and a positive Lasègue sign in up to 86% of children (DeOrio and Bianco, 1982). Only one instance of bowel and urinary tract disturbance occurred, in a 14-year-old boy with a cauda equina syndrome, from among the 155 children reported in four studies of adolescent lumbar disk disease who eventually underwent surgical repair (Fisher and Saunders, 1981; Kurihara and Kataoka, 1980; DeOrio and Bianco, 1982; Weinert and Rizzo, 1992).

IMAGING STUDIES

Today, magnetic resonance imaging (MRI) is the diagnostic study of choice. A total of 11 of 20 patients in a 37-year retrospective study at the Children's Hospital of Boston, had MRI for disk disease. In 1996, Shillito thought that computed tomography was the best modality because it was simple, briefer, and kinder to the child. It gave a clear differentiation between bone, disk, ligaments, and ossified ligaments (Shillito, 1996). Myelography was the primary means of diagnosis in the other previously noted studies. Interestingly, standard spinal radiography demonstrated a 30% incidence of congenital bony abnormalities (DeOrio and Bianco, 1982). These included spina bifida occulta in 16% and sacralization of the last lumbar vertebra in 14%, and the presence of six lumbar vertebrae in 10%. The value of a combined diagnostic approach that included lumbosacral radiographs, spinal computed tomography, and, today, MRI, along with EMGs and NCSs is emphasized for the diagnosis of lumbar nerve root disease in teenaged children (Epstein et al., 1984). There is a value to spinal computed tomography in the diagnosis of adolescent lumbar disk disease (Ghabriel et al., 1989). They studied 25 children 12 to 19 years of age, including 14 girls who had been symptomatic for 1 to 36 months.

ELECTROMYOGRAPHY

The results of EMG were positive in five instances in which these studies were performed, including one child with normal results on myelography (Epstein et al., 1984). In this one instance with negative myelography, computed tomography suggested superior facet entrapment. This was confirmed surgically. No data are included as to whether more than five EMG s were performed and, if so, what the false-negative rate was with this procedure. Today, the authors rarely evaluate children in the CHB EMG laboratory with back and/or sciatic pain. When we do, these patients present very atypical clinical pictures, not infrequently having a significant suggestion of a complex regional pain syndrome (i.e., reflex sympathetic dystrophy).

DIFFERENTIAL DIAGNOSIS

Pediatric lumbosacral disk disease is uncommon; thus, unusual mechanisms need to be considered in children with lumbar nerve root symptoms. One 6-year review from the Orthopaedic Surgery Department of Royal Manchester Children's Hospital evaluated their clinicians' experience with low back pain in children 15 years of age or younger. This group of patients represented 2% of nontrauma referrals to this clinic (Turner et al., 1989). They defined a specific diagnosis in 32 of these 61 children. The variety of pathological mechanisms included various infections (n = 5), tumors (n = 4), spondylosis including spondylolisthesis (n = 8), Scheuermann's disease (n = 9), and miscellaneous processes (n = 2).

Routine spine radiographs were diagnostic in 18 (58%) of the 32 children with a specific final diagnosis. An elevated white cell count or ESR was found in four (13%) children. A "disk prolapse" was documented in only 4 (6%) of the total of 61 children in this group. Nerve root symptoms, including sciatic symptoms associated with limited straight leg raising, and a neurological deficit were highly suggestive of serious and treatable neurological disease. Computed tomography of the spine proved diagnostic in patients suspected of having neurological disorders, and of course, today, the same will apply to magnetic resonance imaging. This large series did not include any EMG studies.

Diskitis

Disk protrusion may sometimes be secondary to diskitis (Kurihara and Kataoka, 1980). This same diagnosis was also considered in one 3-year-old boy who was seen because of acute, severe low back pain, fever, and refusal to walk, sit, or stand (King, 1959). The neurological examination was difficult to perform because he kept his legs tightly flexed on his abdomen. Straight leg testing was markedly positive bilaterally. The right patellar muscle stretch reflex was absent. No other focal signs were detected. He was managed conservatively, but no improvement occurred. Myelography demonstrated a protruded L4-5 disk. Surgery failed to identify any unusual mechanism for the nerve root lesion. He had an excellent surgical result. The fever subsided spontaneously, and no cause for it was identified.

Today, magnetic resonance imaging and/or computed tomography helps exclude spontaneous disk space infections, as these lesions have a presentation similar to that of classic disk disease (Conforti et al., 1993; Garcia et al., 1993).

SCOLIOSIS SURGERY

Primary spinal scoliosis surgery also predisposes to the occurrence of pediatric lumbosacral radiculopathies. A 29% incidence of these postoperative lesions was reported (Dunne et al., 1991). EMG signs of myotomal weakness (not otherwise defined) were found in 4 of these 14 patients (mean age, 16 years). Direct surgical trauma affected 50% of these children. The remaining injuries were secondary to traction in the lumbosacral area. Intraoperative EMG monitoring techniques, developed at the Mayo Clinic, may be now helping to prevent these various forms of surgically induced neurological complications.

ANKYLOSING SPONDYLITIS

In older children, especially adolescents, the possibility of early ankylosing spondylitis always deserves consideration in the differential diagnosis of sciatica. This is particularly true for adolescent boys who present with classic sciatica. Routine radiographs and/or bony computed tomography of the sacroiliac joints is often the diagnostic tool of choice in these young men, especially one with a positive human leukocyte antigen (HLA) B27 study. The electromyographer needs to be alert to this possibility in any adolescent presenting to the laboratory with sciatica, as this illness is eventually crippling if not recognized early in its course. Often, these patients have a concomitant history of early-morning stiffness and "jelling" associated with diminished chest excursion on examination.

TUMORS PRESENTING WITH PEDIATRIC RADICULOPATHY

Nerve root tumors, although quite uncommon, always need consideration in the differential diagnosis of lumbosacral disk disease. One 16-year-old high school wrestler experienced 1 year of pain in the left buttock radiating into the thigh and calf. Computed tomography of the lumbosacral spine demonstrated a mass at L5-S1. At laminectomy, this was an S1 schwannoma (Lahat et al., 1984). Electromyography was not performed. A 13-year-old girl had a 6-month history of vague low back pain precipitated by gymnasium class. She had hypoesthesia in the L3 dermatome, weakness of the quadriceps, and absent knee jerk. EMG demonstrated an L3 radiculopathy. Simple palpation detected a paravertebral mass that proved to be an osteoblastoma (Rothschild et al., 1984).

Occasionally, congenital tumors, such as lipomas, often associated with a tethered cord, need to be considered in the differential diagnosis of lumbar radiculopathies presenting with footdrop or foot deformities. In the two instances we evaluated at Lahey and the CHB, there was no associated back pain. One was a 13-year-old boy with 2 years of progressive footdrop. He had 3/5 MRC weakness of the tibialis anterior, 0.5-cm calf atrophy, and pes cavus. Peroneal and tibial NCS and sural SNAPs were normal. EMG demonstrated findings of L5-S1 nerve root involvement, including abnormal insertional activity in the lumbar paraspinal muscles. The EMG served to exclude the much more common possibility of an evolving peroneal or peroneal division sciatic nerve lesion in this youngster with no back pain. This case emphasizes the need for thorough EMG, especially when the findings do not fit the usual pattern. Spinal magnetic resonance imaging demonstrated a tethered cord and congenital tumor. Magnetic resonance imaging is the diagnostic study of choice.

SACRAL BONE TUMORS

Primary sacral bone tumors may present with radicular pain, paresthesias, progressive weakness, and later paresis of the extremity (Kozlowski et al., 1990). Magnetic resonance imaging and computed tomography are the best diagnostic studies. Standard spinal radiographs often demonstrate normal results in the early stages of these lesions. In Kozlowski's review of 16 children, 13 had Ewing's sarcoma and the other 3 each had an osteoblastoma, a hemangiopericytoma, and a chordoma, respectively.

PEDIATRIC GYNECOLOGICAL LESION MIMICKING LUMBAR RADICULOPATHY

A 12-year-old girl who had not begun to menstruate presented with symptoms mimicking a lumbar radiculopathy. This was characterized by an 8-month history of intermittent low back pain, usually lasting 1 to 3 weeks. She then had 6- to 8-week symptom-free intervals, only to once again have a recurrence. Her right sacroiliac pain interfered with sleeping and sitting, but it was relieved by bending forward or lying on the side. There were typical findings of an L5 radiculopathy on examination. However, gynecological examination demonstrated no vaginal opening. Pelvic ultrasonography showed a 13 by 10 cm midpelvic mass that at surgery proved to be a congenital absence of the lower third of the vagina. A vaginoplasty released 750 mL of menstrual fluids. Her low back pain was relieved immediately. Six months later, all signs of an L5 radiculopathy disappeared (Deathe, 1993). The dilated imperforate vagina with the hematometra was thought to have compressed the lumbosacral plexus, mimicking a nerve root lesion. Noting that only about half of the referrals to an orthopedic children's hospital outpatient clinic proved to have spinal disease, and that no diagnosis was reached in the other children, Deathe (1993) suggested that pelvic ultrasonography needs to be part of the evaluation of indeterminate back pain and lumbar radiculopathy, especially in adolescent girls. This is especially pertinent, when one notes that the incidence of this type of congenital anomaly is about 1 in 5,000 phenotypic females.

THERAPY

Conservative management was successful as the primary therapy in the Mayo series, with fewer than one in 25 children having lumbar disk disease requiring surgery. (DeOrio JK, Bianco AJ Jr, 1982). In the Australian study of 87 adolescents with disk disease, 57 were successfully managed with conservative therapy (Ghabriel YAE, Tarrant MJ, 1989). Although a similar therapeutic approach was initially emphasized in each of 10 adolescents in one series, it was futile in each instance. (Fisher RG, Saunders RL, 1981). In contrast, 40% of the Japanese children initially improved with conservative therapy; however, symptoms tended to recur when these youngsters returned to school or work (Kurihara A, Kataoka O, 1980). The results of disk surgery in children and adolescents were good. However, reoperation was needed in about 10% to 25% of cases (Kurihara A, Kataoka O, 1980; DeOrio JK, Bianco AJ Jr, 1982).

References

Agboatwalla M, Kirmani SR, Sonawalla A, Akram DS: Nerve conduction studies and its importance in diagnosis of acute poliomyelitis. Indian J Pediatr 1993;60:265–268.

Al Qattan MM: The outcome of Erb's palsy when the decision to operate is made at 4 months of age. Plast Reconstr Surg 2000; 106:1461–1465.

Al Qattan MM, Clarke HM, Curtis CG: The prognostic value of concurrent clavicular fractures in newborns with obstetric brachial plexus palsy. J Hand Surg Br 1994;19:729–730.

Al Qattan MM, Clarke HM, Curtis CG: Klumpke's birth palsy: Does it really exist? J Hand Surg Br 1995;20:19–23.

Al Qattan MM, Clarke HM, Curtis CG: The prognostic value of concurrent Horner's syndrome in total obstetric brachial plexus injury. J Hand Surg Br 2000;25:166–167.

Alessandri AJ, Pritchard SL, Massing BG, et al: Misleading leads: Bone pain caused by isolated paraspinal extramedullary relapse of childhood acute lymphoblastic leukemia. Med Pediatr Oncol 1999;33:113–115.

Alfonso I, Alfonso DT, Papazian O: Focal upper extremity neuropathy in neonates. Semin Pediatr Neurol 2000;7:4–14.

Allen RH: Brachial plexus palsy: An in utero injury? Am J Obstet Gynecol 1999;181:1271–1272.

Awerbuch G, Levin GR, Dabrowski E: Lumbosacral plexus neuropathy of children. Ann Neurol 1989a;26:452.

Awerbuch GI, Nigro MA, Dabrowski E, Levin JR: Childhood lumbosacral plexus neuropathy. Pediatr Neurol 1989b;5:314–316.

Azouz EM, Oudjhane K: Disorders of the upper extremity in children. Magn Reson Imaging Clin North Am 1998;6:677–695.

Bager B: Perinatally acquired brachial plexus palsy: A persisting challenge. Acta Paediatr 1997;86:1214–1219.

Bale JF Jr, Thompson JA, Petajan JH, Ziter FA: Childhood brachial plexus neuropathy. J Pediatr 1979;95:741–742.

Ballock RT, Song KM: The prevalence of nonmuscular causes of torticollis in children. J Pediatr Orthop 1996;16:500–504.

Barisic N, Mitrovic Z, et al: Electrophysiological assessment of children with peripheral nerve injury due to war or accident. Pediatr Neurol 1994;11:180.

Barnett HG, Connolly ES: Lumbosacral nerve root avulsion: Report of a case and review of the literature. J Trauma 1975; 15:532–535.

Barquet A: Traumatic anterior dislocation of the hip in childhood. Injury 1982;13:435–440.

Bartlett RJ, Hill CR, Gardiner E: A comparison of T2 and gadolinium-enhanced MRI with CT myelography. Br J Radiol 1998; 71:11–19.

Beausoleil JL, Nordgren RE, Modlin JF: Vaccine-associated paralytic poliomyelitis. J Child Neurol 1994;9:334–335.

Behse F, Buchthal F, Carlsen F, Knappeis GG: Hereditary neuropathy with liability to pressure palsies: Electrophysiological and histopathological aspects. Brain 1972;95:777–794.

Bell WE: Acquired immobility of the right arm. Semin Pediatr Neurol 1996;3:173–176.

Benjamin B, Khan MR: Pattern of external birth trauma in southwestern Saudi Arabia. J Trauma 1993;35:737–741.

Birch R: Surgery for brachial plexus injuries. J Bone Joint Surg Br 1993;75:346–348.

Birch R: Brachial plexus injuries. J Bone Joint Surg Br 1996; 78:986–992.

Birch R, Achan P: Peripheral nerve repairs and their results in children. Hand Clin 2000;16:579–595.

Birchansky S, Altman N: Imaging the brachial plexus and peripheral nerves in infants and children. Semin Pediatr Neurol 2000; 7:15–25.

Bodensteiner JB, Rich KM, Landau WM: Early infantile surgery for birth-related brachial plexus injuries: Justification requires a prospective controlled study. J Child Neurol 1994;9:109–110.

Boome RS, Kaye JC: Obstetric traction injuries of the brachial plexus: Natural history, indications for surgical repair and results. J Bone Joint Surg Br 1988;70:571–576.

Bradley WG, Madrid R, Thrush DC, Campbell MJ: Recurrent brachial plexus neuropathy. Brain 1975;98:381–398.

Brown JA, Braun MA, Namey TC: Pyriformis syndrome in a 10-year-old boy as a complication of operation with the patient in the sitting position. Neurosurgery 1988;23:117–119.

Brown KL: Review of obstetrical palsies: Nonoperative treatment. Clin Plast Surg 1984;11:181–187.

Brown T, Cupido C, Scarfone H, et al: Developmental apraxia arising from neonatal brachial plexus palsy. Neurology 2000; 55:24–30.

Bryant DR, Leonardi MR, Landwehr JB, Bottoms SF: Limited usefulness of fetal weight in predicting neonatal brachial plexus injuries. Am J Obstet Gynecol 1998;179:686–689.

Bye A, Fagan E: Nerve conduction studies of the sural nerve in childhood. J Child Neurol 1988;3:94–99.

Carlstedt T, Anand P, Hallin R, et al: Spinal nerve root repair and reimplantation of avulsed ventral roots into the spinal cord after brachial plexus injury. J Neurosurg 2000;93:237–247.

Carlstedt T, Grane P, Hallin RG, Noren G: Return of function after spinal cord implantation of avulsed spinal nerve roots. Lancet 1995;346:1323–1325.

Chad DA, Bradley WG: Lumbosacral plexopathy. Semin Neurol 1987;7:97–107.

Chance PF, Lensch MW, Lipe H, et al: Hereditary neuralgic amyotrophy and hereditary neuropathy with liability to pressure palsies: Two distinct genetic disorders. Neurology 1994;44: 2253–2257.

Chaudhry V, Cornblath DR: Wallerian degeneration in human nerves: Serial electrophysiological studies. Muscle Nerve 1992; 15:687–693.

Chin CH, Chew KC: Lumbosacral nerve root avulsion. Injury 1997; 28:674–678.

Chiou-Tan FY, Kemp K, Elfenbaum M, et al: Lumbosacral plexopathy in gunshot wounds and motor vehicle accidents: Comparison of electrophysiologic findings. Am J Phys Med Rehabil 2001;80:280–285.

Chow BC, Blaser S, Clarke HM: Predictive value of computed tomographic myelography in obstetrical brachial plexus palsy. Plast Reconstr Surg 2000;106:971–977.

Chrisman OD, Snook GA, Stanitis JM, et al: Lateral flexion neck injuries in athletic competition. JAMA 1965;192:613–615.

Christie J, Jamieson EW: Traction lesion of the lumbosacral plexus. J R Coll Surg Edinb 1974;19:384–385.

Chuang DC: Neurotization procedures for brachial plexus injuries. Hand Clin 1995;11:633–645.

Chuang DC, Wei FC, Noordhoff MS: Cross-chest C7 nerve grafting followed by free muscle transplantations for the treatment of total avulsed brachial plexus injuries: A preliminary report. Plast Reconstr Surg 1993;92:717–725.

Clancy WG: Brachial plexus and upper extremity peripheral nerve injuries. In Torg JS (ed): Athletic Injuries to the Head, Neck, and Face. Philadelphia, Lea & Febiger, 1982; 215–220.

Clancy WG, Brand RL, Bergfield JA: Upper trunk brachial plexus injuries in contact sports. Am J Sports Med 1977;5:209–216.

Clarke HM, Curtis CG: An approach to obstetrical brachial plexus injuries. Hand Clin 1995;11:563–580.

Clay SA: Osteomyelitis as a cause of brachial plexus neuropathy. Am J Dis Child 1982;136:1054–1056.

David WS, Doyle JJ: Acute infantile weakness: A case of vaccine-associated poliomyelitis. Muscle Nerve 1997;20:747–749.

Di Benedetto M, Markey K: Electrodiagnostic localization of traumatic upper trunk brachial plexopathy. Arch Phys Med Rehabil 1984;65:15–17.

Dodds SD, Wolfe SW: Perinatal brachial plexus palsy. Curr Opin Pediatr 2000;12:40–47.

Dumitru D (ed): Brachial plexopathies and proximal mononeuropathies. In Electrodiagnostic Medicine. Philadelphia, Hanley & Belfus, 1995a; 585–642.

Dumitru D (ed): Lumbosacral plexopathies and proximal mononeuropathies. In Electrodiagnostic Medicine. Philadelphia, Hanley & Belfus, 1995b; 643–88.

Dunn DW, Engle WA: Brachial plexus palsy: Intrauterine onset. Pediatr Neurol 1985;1:367.

Dunn HG, Daube JR, Gomez MR: Heredofamilial branchial plexus neuropathy (hereditary neuralgic amyotrophy with branchial predilection) in childhood. Dev Med Child Neurol 1978;20:28–46.

Ebraheim NA, Lu J, Yang H, et al: Lumbosacral plexus: A histological study. Acta Anat (Basel) 1997;158:274–278.

Ecker JL, Greenberg JA, Norwitz ER, et al: Birth weight as a predictor of brachial plexus injury. Obstet Gynecol 1997;89:643–647.

Egel RT, Cueva JP, Adair RL: Posttraumatic childhood lumbosacral plexus neuropathy. Pediatr Neurol 1995;12:62–64.

Egloff DV, Raffoul W, Bonnard C, Stalder J: Palliative surgical procedures to restore shoulder function in obstetric brachial palsy: Critical analysis of Narakas' series. Hand Clin 1995;11:597–606.

Eng GD: Brachial plexus palsy in newborn infants. Pediatrics 1971;48:18.

Eng GD: Neuromuscular disease. In Avery GB (ed): Neonatology: Pathophysiology and Management of the Newborn. Philadelphia, WB Saunders, 1981; 989–992.

Eng GD, Binder H, Getson P, O'Donnell R: Obstetrical brachial plexus palsy (OBPP) outcome with conservative management. Muscle Nerve 1996;19:884–891.

Eng GD, Koch B, Smokvia M: Brachial plexus palsy in neonates and children. Arch Phys Med Rehabil 1978;59:458.

England JD, Sumner AJ: Neuralgic amyotrophy: An increasingly diverse entity. Muscle Nerve 1987;10:60–68.

Escolar DM, Jones HR: Pediatric radial mononeuropathies: A clinical and electromyographic study of sixteen children with review of the literature. Muscle Nerve 1996;19:876–883.

Evans BA, Stevens JC, Dyck PJ: Lumbosacral plexus neuropathy. Neurology 1981;31:1327–1330.

Felice KJ, Jones HR: Pediatric ulnar mononeuropathy: Report of 21 electromyography-documented cases and review of the literature. J Child Neurol 1996;11:116–120.

Ferrante MA, Wilbourne AJ: Plexopathies. In Levin KH, Lüders HO: Comprehensive Clinical Neurophysiology. Philadelphia, WB Saunders, 2000; 201–214.

Flaggman PD, Kelly JJ, Jr: Brachial plexus neuropathy: An electrophysiologic evaluation. Arch Neurol 1980;37:160–164.

Francel PC, Koby M, Park TS, et al: Fast spin-echo magnetic resonance imaging for radiological assessment of neonatal brachial plexus injury. J Neurosurg 1995;83:461–466.

Gabreels-Festen AA, Gabreels FJ, Joosten EM, et al: Hereditary neuropathy with liability to pressure palsies in childhood. Neuropediatrics 1992;23:138–143.

Gabriel SR, Thometz JG, Jaradeh S: Septic arthritis associated with brachial plexus neuropathy: A case report. J Bone Joint Surg Am 1996;78:103–105.

Gainor BJ, Olson S: Combined entrapment of the median and anterior interosseous nerves in a pediatric both-bone forearm fracture. J Orthop Trauma 1990;4:197–199.

Galan E, Kousseff BG: Peripheral neuropathy in Ehlers-Danlos syndrome. Pediatr Neurol 1995;12:242–245.

Geiger LR, Mancall EL, Penn AS, Tucker SH: Familial neuralgic amyotrophy: Report of three families with review of the literature. Brain 1974;97:87–102.

Gertzbein SD, Evans DC: Femoral nerve neuropathy complicating iliopsoas haemorrhage in patients. J Bone Joint Surg Br 1972;54:149–151.

Gherman RB, Ouzounian JG, Goodwin TM: Brachial plexus palsy: An in utero injury? Am J Obstet Gynecol 1999;180:1303–1307.

Gilbert A: Long-term evaluation of brachial plexus surgery in obstetrical palsy. Hand Clin 1995;11:583–594.

Gilbert A, Brockman R, Carlioz H: Surgical treatment of brachial plexus birth palsy. Clin Orthop 1991;Mar:39–47.

Gilbert A, Razaboni R, Amar-Khodja S: Indications and results of brachial plexus surgery in obstetrical palsy. Orthop Clin North Am 1998;19:91–105.

Gilbert A, Razaboni R, Amar-Khodja S: Indications and results of brachial plexus surgery in obstetrical palsy. Orthop Clin North Am 1988;19:91–105.

Gilbert A, Tassin JL: Obstetrical palsy: A clinical, pathologic, and surgical review. In Terzis JK (ed): Microreconstruction of Nerve Injuries. Philadelphia, WB Saunders, 1987; 529–553.

Gilbert WM, Nesbitt TS, Danielsen B: Associated factors in 1611 cases of brachial plexus injury. Obstet Gynecol 1999;93:536–540.

Gilliatt RW, Willison RG, Dietz V, Williams IR: Peripheral nerve conduction in patients with a cervical rib and band. Ann Neurol 1978;4:124–129.

Gjorup L: Obstetrical lesion of the brachial plexus. Acta Neurol Scand 1966;42:1–80.

Glasby MA, Hems TE: Repairing spinal roots after brachial plexus injuries. Paraplegia 1995;33:359–361.

Goldstein J: Infantile poliomyelitis in a recently immunized baby seen at Yale. *Personal communication,* 1995.

Gomez-Anson B: MR imaging of the brachial plexus. J Neurol Neurosurg Psychiatry 2000;68:801.

Gonik B, McCormick EM, Verweij BH, et al: The timing of congenital brachial plexus injury: A study of electromyography findings in the newborn piglet. Am J Obstet Gynecol 1998;178:688–695.

Gonik B, Walker A, Grimm M: Mathematic modeling of forces associated with shoulder dystocia: A comparison of endogenous and exogenous sources. Am J Obstet Gynecol 2000;182:689–691.

Gordon M, Rich H, Deutschberger J, Green M: The immediate and long-term outcome of obstetric birth trauma. I. Brachial plexus paralysis. Am J Obstet Gynecol 1973;117:51–56.

Gouider R, LeGuern E, Emile J, et al: Hereditary neuralgic amyotrophy and hereditary neuropathy with liability to pressure palsies: Two distinct clinical, electrophysiologic, and genetic entities. Neurology 1994;44:2250–2252.

Grossman JA: Early operative intervention for birth injuries to the brachial plexus. Semin Pediatr Neurol 2000;7:36–43.

Hardy AE: Birth injuries of the brachial plexus: Incidence and prognosis. J Bone Joint Surg Br 1981;63-B:98–101.

Harila-Saari AH, Vainionpaa LK, Kovala TT, et al: Nerve lesions after therapy for childhood acute lymphoblastic leukemia. Cancer 1998;82:200–207.

Hashimoto T, Mitomo M, Hirabuki N, et al: Nerve root avulsion of birth palsy: Comparison of myelography with CT. Radiology 1991;178:841–845.

Hems TEJ, Birch R, Carlstedt T: The role of magnetic resonance imaging in the management of traction injuries to the adult brachial plexus. J Hand Surg 1999;24B:550–555.

Hirasawa Y, Sakakida K: Sports and peripheral nerve injury. Am J Sports Med 1983;11:420–426.

Hoeksma AF, Wolf H, Oei SL: Obstetrical brachial plexus injuries: Incidence, natural course and shoulder contracture. Clin Rehabil 2000;14:523–526.

Hoffer MM: The shoulder in neonatal brachial palsy. Clin Orthop 1999;368:101–104.

Holland NR, Belzberg AJ: Intraoperative electrodiagnostic testing during cross-chest C7 nerve root transfer. Muscle Nerve 1997; 20:903–905.

Hope EE, Bodensteiner JB, Thong N: Neonatal lumbar plexus injury. Arch Neurol 1985;42:94–95.

Huittinen VM: Lumbosacral nerve injury in fracture of the pelvis: A postmortem radiographic and patho-anatomical study. Acta Chir Scand Suppl 1972;429:3–43.

Iffy L, Mcardle JJ: The role of medico-legal reviews in medical research. Med Law 1996;15:399–406.

Inoue M, Kawano T, Matsumura H, et al: Solitary benign schwannoma of the brachial plexus. Surg Neurol 1983;20:103–108.

Jahnke AH Jr, Bovill DF, McCarroll HR Jr, et al: Persistent brachial plexus birth palsies. J Pediatr Orthop 1991;11:533–537.

Jeffery AR, Ellis FJ, Repka MX, Buncic JR: Pediatric Horner syndrome. J AAPOS 1998;2:159–167.

Jellis JE, Helal B: Childhood sciatic palsies: Congenital and traumatic. Proc R Soc Med 1970;63:655–656.

Jennett RJ, Tarby TJ: Brachial plexus palsy: An old problem revisited again. II. Cases in point. Am J Obstet Gynecol 1997; 176:1354–1356.

Jennett RJ, Tarby TJ, Kreinick CJ: Brachial plexus palsy: An old problem revisited. Am J Obstet Gynecol 1992;166:1673–1676.

Johnson EW, Alexander MA, Koenig WC: Infantile Erb's palsy (Smellie's palsy). Arch Phys Med Rehabil 1977;58:175–178.

Jones HR, Gianturco LE, Gross PT, Buchhalter J: Sciatic neuropathies in childhood: A report of ten cases and review of the literature. J Child Neurol 1988;3:193–199.

Jones HR, Herbison GJ, Jacob SR, et al: Intrauterine onset of a mononeuropathy: Peroneal neuropathy in a newborn. Muscle Nerve 1996;19:88–91.

Jones HR: Plexus and nerve root lesions. In Jones HR, Bolton CF, Harper CK: Pediatric Clinical Electromyography. Philadelphia, Lippincott-Raven, 1996; 123–169.

Kawabata H, Shibata T, Matsui Y, Yasui N: Use of intercostal nerves for neurotization of the musculocutaneous nerve in infants with birth-related brachial plexus palsy. J Neurosurg 2001;94:386–391.

Kay SP: Obstetrical brachial palsy. Br J Plast Surg 1998;51:43–50.

Kay SP, Yaszemski MJ, Rockwood CA Jr: Acute tear of the rotator cuff masked by simultaneous palsy of the brachial plexus: A case report. J Bone Joint Surg Am 1988;70:611–612.

Kline DG: Operative management of major nerve lesions of the lower extremity. Surg Clin North Am 1972;52:1247–1265.

Kline DG: Civilian gunshot wounds to the brachial plexus. J Neurosurg 1989;70:166–174.

Kline DG: Spinal nerve root repair after brachial plexus injury. J Neurosurg 2000;93:336–338.

Kline DG, Happel LT: Penfield Lecture. A quarter century's experience with intraoperative nerve potential action recording. Can J Neurol Sci 1993;20:3–10.

Kline DG, Hudson AR: Diagnosis of root avulsions. J Neurosurg 1997;87:483–484.

Kline DG, Judice DJ: Operative management of selected brachial plexus lesions. J Neurosurg 1983;58:631–649.

Kline DG, Kim D, Midha R, et al: Management and results of sciatic nerve injuries: A 24-year experience. J Neurosurg 1998; 89:13–23.

Koenigsberger MR: Brachial plexus palsy at birth: Intrauterine or due to delivery trauma? Ann Neurol 1980;8:228.

Kolawole TM, Hawass ND, Shaheen MA, et al: Lumbosacral plexus avulsion injury: Clinical, myelographic and computerized features. J Trauma 1988;28:861–865.

Landi A, Copeland SA, Parry CB, Jones SJ: The role of somatosensory evoked potentials and nerve conduction studies in the surgical management of brachial plexus injuries. J Bone Joint Surg Br 1980;62-B:492–496.

Laurent JP, Lee R, Shenaq S, et al: Neurosurgical correction of upper brachial plexus birth injuries. J Neurosurg 1993;79:197–203.

Laurent JP, Lee RT: Birth-related upper brachial plexus injuries in infants: Operative and nonoperative approaches. J Child Neurol 1994;9:111–117.

Liggio FJ, Tham S, Price A, et al: Outcome of surgical treatment for forearm pronation deformities in children with obstetric brachial plexus injuries. J Hand Surg Br 1999;24:43–45.

Lucas JW, Holden KR, Purohit DM, Cure JK: Neonatal hemangiomatosis associated with brachial plexus palsy. J Child Neurol 1995;10:411–413.

Luco JV, Eyzaguirre C: Fibrillation and hypersensitivity to ACh in denervated muscle: Effect of length and degenerating nerve fibers. J Neurophysiol 1955;18:65–73.

MacDonald NE: Does immunization in the buttocks cause sciatic nerve injury? Pediatrics 1994;93:351.

MacDonald NE, Marcuse EK: Neurologic injury after vaccination: Buttocks as injection site. CMAJ 1994;150:326.

Mancias P, Slopis JM, Yeakley JW, Vriesendorp FJ: Combined brachial plexus injury and root avulsion after complicated delivery [letter]. Muscle Nerve 1994;17:1237–1238.

Marcuse EK, MacDonald NE: Neurologic injury after vaccination in buttocks. CMAJ 1996;155:374.

Marcuse EK, MacDonald NE: Vaccine injury—no reports. Pediatrics 1997;99:144.

Marin R, Bryant PR, Eng GD: Lumbosacral plexopathy temporally related to vaccination. Clin Pediatr (Phila) 1994;33:175–177.

Marra TA: Recurrent lumbosacral and brachial plexopathy associated with schistosomiasis. Arch Neurol 1983;40:586–587.

McFarland LV, Raskin M, Daling JR, Benedetti TJ: Erb/Duchenne's palsy: A consequence of fetal macrosomia and method of delivery. Obstet Gynecol 1986;68:784–788.

McFarland MB, Langer O, Piper JM, Berkus MD: Perinatal outcome and the type and number of maneuvers in shoulder dystocia. Int J Gynaeco! Obstet 1996;55:219–224.

Mehlman CT, Scott KA, Koch BL, Garcia VF: Orthopaedic injuries in children secondary to airbag deployment. J Bone Joint Surg Am 2000;82:895–898.

Menegaux F, Keeffe EB, Andrews BT, et al: Neurological complications of liver transplantation in adult versus pediatric patients. Transplantation 1994;58:447–450.

Michelow BJ, Clarke HM, Curtis CG, et al: The natural history of obstetrical brachial plexus palsy. Plast Reconstr Surg 1994; 93:675–680.

Miller SF, Glasier CM, Griebel ML, Boop FA: Brachial plexopathy in infants after traumatic delivery: Evaluation with MR imaging. Radiology 1993;189:481–484.

Molnar GE: Brachial plexus injury in the newborn infant. Pediatr Rev 1984;6:110–115.

Nakamura T, Yabe Y, Takayama S: Magnetic resonance myelography in brachial plexus injury. J Bone Joint Surg Br 1997;79:764–769.

Narakas AO: Obstetrical brachial plexus injuries. The Paralysed Hand. Edinburgh, Churchill Livingstone, 1987; 116–135.

Oppenheim WL, Davis A, Growdon WA, et al: Clavicle fractures in the newborn. Clin Orthop 1990;Jan:176–180.

Ouvrier RA, McLeod JG, Pollard JD: Peripheral neuropathy in childhood. 2001.

Ouzounian JG, Korst LM, Phelan JP: Permanent Erb palsy: A traction-related injury? Obstet Gynecol 1997;89:139–141.

Papazian O, Alfonso I, Yaylali I, Velez IJP: Neurophysiological evaluation of children with traumatic radiculopathy. Semin Pediatr Neurol 2000;7:26–35.

Paradiso G, Granana N, Maza E: Prenatal brachial plexus paralysis. Neurology 1997;49:261–262.

Parsonage MJ, Turner JWA: Neuralgic amyotrophy: The shoulder-girdle syndrome. Lancet 1948;1:973–978.

Pasternak JF, Volpe JJ: Lumbosacral lipoma with acute deterioration during infancy. Pediatrics 1980;66:125–128.

Pellegrino JE, George RA, Biegel J, et al: Hereditary neuralgic amyotrophy: Evidence for genetic homogeneity and mapping to chromosome 17q25. Hum Genet 1997;101:277–283.

Peterson CR, Peterson CM: Brachial-plexus injury in an infant from a car safety seat. N Engl J Med 1991;325:1587–1588.

Piatt JH: Neurosurgical management of birth injuries of the brachial plexus. Neurosurg Clin North Am 1991;2:175–185.

Piatt JH, Hudson AR, Hoffman HJ: Preliminary experiences with brachial plexus exploration in children: Birth injury and vehicular trauma. Neurosurgery 1988;22:715–723.

Poindexter DP, Johnson EW: Football shoulder and neck injury: A study of the "stinger." Arch Phys Med Rehabil 1984;65:601–602.

Pollack RN, Buchman AS, Yaffe H, Divon MY: Obstetrical brachial palsy: Pathogenesis, risk factors and prevention. Clin Obstet Gynecol 2000;43:236–246.

Rai SK, Far RF, Ghovanlou B: Neurologic deficits associated with sacral wing fractures. Orthopedics 1990;13:1363–1366.

Ramos LE, Zell JP: Rehabilitation program for children with brachial plexus and peripheral nerve injury. Semin Pediatr Neurol 2000;7:44–51.

Rapalino OA, Levine DN: Developmental apraxia arising from neonatal brachial plexus palsy. Neurology 2000;55:1761.

Robertson WC, Eichman PL, Clancy WG: Upper trunk brachial plexopathy in football players. JAMA 1979;241:1480–1482.

Robotti E, Longhi P, Verna G, Bocchiotti G: Brachial plexus surgery: An historical perspective. Hand Clin 1995;11:517–533.

Rockett FX: Observation on the "burner": Traumatic cervical radiculopathy. Clin Orthop 1982;Apr:18–19.

Rollnik JD, Hierner R, Schubert M, et al: *Botulinum* toxin treatment of co-contractions after birth-related brachial plexus lesions. Neurology 2000;55:112–114.

Roos DB: The thoracic outlet syndrome is underrated. Arch Neurol 1990;47:327–328.

Roos DB: Thoracic outlet syndrome is underdiagnosed. Muscle Nerve 1999;22:126–129.

Ross D, Jones R, Fisher J, Konkol RJ: Isolated radial nerve lesion in the newborn. Neurology 1983;33:1354–1356.

Rothner AD, Wilbourn A, Mercer RD: Rucksack palsy. Pediatrics 1975;56:822–824.

Rouse DJ, Owen J, Goldenberg RL, Cliver SP: The effectiveness and costs of elective cesarean delivery for fetal macrosomia diagnosed by ultrasound. JAMA 1996;276:1480–1486.

Rust RS: Congenital brachial plexus palsy: Where have we been and where are we now? Semin Pediatr Neurol 2000;7:58–63.

Sadleir LG, Connolly MB: Acquired brachial-plexus neuropathy in the neonate: A rare presentation of late-onset group-B streptococcal osteomyelitis. Dev Med Child Neurol 1998;40:496–499.

Schwartz DM, Drummond DS, Hahn M, et al: Prevention of positional brachial plexopathy during surgical correction of scoliosis. J Spinal Disord 2000;13:178–182.

Sever JW: Obstetric paralysis: Report of eleven hundred cases. JAMA 1925;85:1862–1865.

Sharma RR, Sethu AU, Mahapatra AK, et al: Neonatal cervical osteomyelitis with paraspinal abscess and Erb's palsy: A case report and brief review of the literature. Pediatr Neurosurg 2000;32:230–233.

Sjoberg I, Erichs K, Bjerre I: Cause and effect of obstetric (neonatal) brachial plexus palsy. Acta Paediatr Scand 1988;77:357–364.

Smith SJ: The role of neurophysiological investigation in traumatic brachial plexus lesions in adults and children. J Hand Surg Br 1996;21:145–147.

Stoehr M: Traumatic and postoperative lesions of the lumbosacral plexus. Arch Neurol 1978;35:757–760.

Stogbauer F, Young P, Kuhlenbaumer G, et al: Hereditary recurrent focal neuropathies: Clinical and molecular features. Neurology 2000;54:546–551.

Strombeck C, Krumlinde-Sundholm L, Forssberg H: Functional outcome at 5 years in children with obstetrical brachial plexus palsy with and without microsurgical reconstruction. Dev Med Child Neurol 2000;42:148–157.

Sugioka H, Tsuyama N, Hara T, et al: Investigation of brachial plexus injuries by intraoperative cortical somatosensory evoked potentials. Arch Orthop Trauma Surg 1982;99:143–151.

Sunderland S: The connective tissues of peripheral nerves. Brain 1965;88:841–854.

Sunderland S: Anatomical features of nerve trunks in relation to nerve injury and nerve repair. Clin Neurosurg 1970;17:38–62.

Switzer JA, Nork SE, Routt ML: Comminuted fractures of the iliac wing. J Orthop Trauma 2000;14:270–276.

Terzis JK, Papakonstantinou KC: Management of obstetric brachial plexus palsy. Hand Clin 1999;15:717–736.

Thomson AJ: Idiopathic lumbosacral plexus neuropathy in two children. Dev Med Child Neurol 1993;35:258–261.

Tiel RL, Happel LT Jr, Kline DG: Nerve action potential recording method and equipment. Neurosurgery 1996;39:103–108.

To WC, Traquina DN: Neuralgic amyotrophy presenting with bilateral vocal cord paralysis in a child: A case report. Int J Pediatr Otorhinolaryngol 1999;48:251–254.

Trojaborg W: Clinical, electrophysiological, and myelographic studies of 9 patients with cervical spinal root avulsions: Discrepancies between EMG and X-ray findings. Muscle Nerve 1994;17:913–922.

Tsairis P, Dyck PJ, Mulder DW: Natural history of brachial plexus neuropathy: Report on 99 patients. Arch Neurol 1972;27:109–117.

Turkof E, Millesi H, Turkof R, et al: Intraoperative electroneurodiagnostics (transcranial electrical motor evoked potentials) to evaluate the functional status of anterior spinal roots and spinal nerves during brachial plexus surgery. Plast Reconstr Surg 1997;99:1632–1641.

Turner JWA, Parsonage MJ: Neuralgic amyotrophy (paralytic brachial neuritits), with special reference to prognosis. Lancet 1957;2:209–212.

Ubachs JM, Slooff AC, Peeters LL: Obstetric antecedents of surgically treated obstetric brachial plexus injuries. Br J Obstet Gynaecol 1995;102:813–817.

Uetani M, Hayashi K, Hashmi R, et al: Traction injuries of the brachial plexus: Signal intensity changes of the posterior cervical paraspinal muscles on MRI. J Comput Assist Tomogr 1997;21:790–795.

van Ouwerkerk WJ, van der Sluijs JA, Nollet F, et al: Management of obstetric brachial plexus lesions: State of the art and future developments. Childs Nerv Syst 2000;16:638–644.

Vassalos E, Prevedourakis C, Paraschopoulou-Prevedourakis P: Brachial plexus paralysis in the newborn: An analysis of 169 cases. Am J Obstet Gynecol 1968;101:554–556.

Verhagen WI, Gabreels-Festen AA, van Wensen PJ, et al: Hereditary neuropathy with liability to pressure palsies: A clinical, electroneurophysiological and morphological study. J Neurol Sci 1993;116:176–184.

Verstraete KL, Martens F, Smeets P, et al: Traumatic lumbosacral nerve root meningoceles: The value of myelography in the assessment of nerve root. Neuroradiology 1989;31:425–429.

Villarejo FJ, Pascual AM: Injection injury of the sciatic nerve (370 cases). Childs Nerv Syst 1993;9:229–232.

Volpe JJ: Injuries of extracranial, cranial, intracranial, spinal cord, and peripheral nervous system structures. In Neurology of the Newborn. Philadelphia, JB Lippincott, 1987; 638–658.

Waters PM: Comparison of the natural history, the outcome of microsurgical repair, and the outcome of operative reconstruction in brachial plexus birth palsy. J Bone Joint Surg Am 1999; 81:649–659.

Watkins RG: Nerve injuries in football players. Clin Sports Med 1986;5:215–246.

Wilbourne AJ: Electrodiagnosis of plexopathies. Neurol Clin 1985; 3:511–529.

Wilbourne AJ: Electrodiagnostic testing of neurologic injuries in athletes. Clin Sports Med 1990a;9:229–245.

Wilbourne AJ: Brachial plexus disorders. In Dyck PJ, Thomas PK, Griff MJ, et al: Peripheral Neuropathy, 3rd ed. Philadelphia, WB Saunders, 1993; 903–950.

Wilbourn AJ: The thoracic outlet syndrome is overdiagnosed. Arch Neurol 1990b;47:328–330.

Wilbourn AJ: Thoracic outlet syndrome is overdiagnosed. Muscle Nerve 1999;22:130–136.

Wroble RR, Albright JP: Neck and low back injuries in wrestling. Clin Sports Med 1986;5:295–325.

Yilmaz K, Caliskan M, Oge E, et al: Clinical assessment, MRI, and EMG in congenital brachial plexus palsy. Pediatr Neurol 1999; 21:705–710.

Young NL, Davis RJ, Bell DF, Redmond DM: Electromyographic and nerve conduction changes after tibial lengthening by the Ilizarov method. J Pediatr Orthop 1993;13:473–477.

Yuen EC, Olney RK, So YT: Sciatic neuropathy: Clinical and prognostic features in 73 patients. Neurology 1994;44:1669–1674.

Nerve Root References

Radharkrishnan K, Litchy WJ, O'Fallo, Kurland LT: Epidemiology of cervical radiculopathy: A population based study from Rochester, Minnesota, 1976 through 1990. Brain 1994;117:325–335.

Trojaborg W: Clinical, electrophysiological, and myelographic studies of 9 patients with cervical spinal root avulsions: Discrepancies between EMG and x-ray findings. Muscle Nerve 1994;17:913–922.

Hirayama K: Juvenile muscular atrophy of the upper extremity (Hirayama disease). Intern Med 2000;39:283–290.

Jones HR Jr: Pediatric case studies. American Association of Electrodiagnostic Medicine (AAEM) Plenary Session: New Developments in Pediatric Neuromuscular Disease. Rochester, MN, AAEM, 1993;51–60.

Dantes M, McComes A: The extent and time course of motor neuron involvement in amyotrophic lateral sclerosis. Muscle Nerve 1991;14:416–421.

Mathern GW, Batzdorf U: Grisel's syndrome: Cervical spine clinical, pathologic, and neurologic manifestations. Clin Orthop 1989;244:131–146.

Weinert AM, Rizzo TD: Nonoperative management of multilevel lumbar disc herniations in an adolescent athlete. Mayo Clin Proc 1992;67:137–141.

Kurihara A, Kataoka O: Lumbar disc herniation of children and adolescents: A review of 70 operated cases and their minimum 5-year follow-up studies. Spine 1980;5:443–451.

Fisher RG, Saunders RL: Lumbar disc protrusions in children. J Neurosurg 1981;54:480–483.

DeOrio JK, Bianco AJ Jr: Lumbar disc excision in children and adolescents. J Bone Joint Surg Am 1982;64:991–996.

Epstein JA, Epstein NE, Marc J, et al: Lumbar intervertebral disk herniation in teenage children: Recognition and management of associated anomalies. Spine 1984;9:427–432.

Ghabriel YAE, Tarrant MJ: Adolescent lumbar disc prolapse. Acta Orthop Scand 1989;60:174–176.

Turner PG, Green JH, Galasko CSB: Back pain in childhood. Spine 1989;14:812–814.

King AB: Surgical removal of a ruptured intervertebral disc in early childhood. J Pediatr 1959;55:57–62.

Garcia FF, Semba CP, Sartoris DJ: Diagnostic imaging of childhood spinal infection. Orthop Rev 1993;22:321–327.

Conforti R, Scuotto A, Muras I, et al: Les hernies discales de adolescents. [Herniated disk adolescents.] J Neuroradiol 1993;20:60–69.

Dunne JW, Silbert PL, Wren M: A prospective study of acute radiculopathy after scoliosis surgery. Clin Exp Neurol 1991;28:180–190.

Lahat E, Rothman AS, Aron AM: Schwannoma presenting as lumbar disc disease in an adolescent girl. Spine 1984;9:695–701.

Rothschild EJ, Savitz MH, Chang T, et al: Primary vertebral tumor in an adolescent girl. Spine 1984;9:695–701.

Kozlowski K, Barylak A, Campbell J, et al: Primary sacral bone tumours in children (report of 16 cases with a short literature review). Aust Radiol 1990;34:142–149.

Deathe AB: Hematometra as a cause of lumbar radiculopathy: A case report. Spine 1993;18:1920–1921.

Revuelta R, Juambelz PP, Fernandez B, Flores JA: Lumbar disc herniation in a 27-month-old child. Case report. J Neurosurg 2000;92(1 Suppl):98–100.

Shillito J, Jr: Pediatric lumbar disc surgery: 20 patients under 15 years of age. Surg Neurol 1996;46:14–18.

Upper Extremity Mononeuropathies in Infants and Children

Kevin J. Felice and H. Royden Jones, Jr.

Mononeuropathies in children differ from those in adults mainly by the frequency of occurrence, individual nerve involvement, and mechanisms of nerve injury. First, mononeuropathies in infants and children are exceedingly rare. Of 1,679 pediatric patients seen by both of us at two pediatric electromyography (EMG) laboratories, mononeuropathies were present in only 113 (7%) children (Jones, 1996). In contrast, mononeuropathies account for 28% to 30% of the referrals to our adult EMG laboratories. Second, nerve involvement in children is nearly equal in distribution among the median, ulnar, radial, peroneal and sciatic nerves (Fig. 90–1). In contrast, median mononeuropathies account for the overwhelming majority of focal nerve lesions in adults. The major reason for this difference is the much lower incidence of carpal tunnel syndrome in children. Third, trauma is the most common mechanism of nerve injury in children, and it accounts for 37% to 76% of cases. Traumatic injuries from fractures and lacerations are a major cause of mononeuropathies in children, and many are related to sports injuries. Compression injuries are the second most common cause of pediatric mononeuropathies, whereas nerve entrapment injuries are relatively uncommon. In distinction, entrapment and compression injuries account for most injuries in adults.

This chapter discusses the upper extremity mononeuropathies in children, whereas Chapter 91 reviews lower extremity mononeuropathies. Tables summarizing the various causes of pediatric mononeuropathies are provided in both chapters for quick review. In addition to this information, the reader is advised to review a good general text on mononeuropathies when he or she is confronted with these problems in children (Stewart, 2000). Finally, given the relative rarity of mononeuropathies in children, the examining physician and the electromyographer always need to consider the diagnosis of hereditary neuropathy with liability to pressure palsies in a child presenting with a mononeuropathy resulting from compression or one that is unexplained, especially if localization appears to be at a common site of compression or entrapment. In the author's (KJF) series of 27 children, 4 (15%) were subsequently diagnosed with hereditary neuropathy with liability to pressure palsies after presenting with various mononeuropathies, one each including the radial, musculocutaneous, spinal accessory, and peroneal nerve (unpublished data). In each patient, the mechanism of nerve injury was poorly understood, the mononeuropathy was associated with EMG evidence of a more diffuse demyelinating peripheral neuropathy, the diagnosis was not previously known in the family, and the diagnosis was subsequently confirmed with DNA studies.

MEDIAN NERVE

Distal Median Mononeuropathies

Carpal tunnel syndrome is the most common focal mononeuropathy in adults, with an incidence of 0.99 to 3.46 cases per 1,000 person-years (Stevens et al., 1988; Nordstrom et al., 1998). In children, carpal tunnel syndrome is exceedingly rare and, when present, is usually associated with an underlying disor-

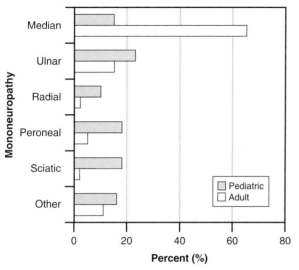

Figure 90–1. Types of mononeuropathies in 113 pediatric and 712 adult patients.

Table 90–1. Causes of Distal Median Mononeuropathies

Carpal tunnel syndrome
 Idiopathic
 Activity-related (e.g., skiing, bicycling, golfing, computer games)
 Trauma
 Inborn errors of metabolism (e.g., mucopolysaccharidosis, mucolipidosis)
 Scleroderma
 Poland's syndrome
 Cerebral palsy with dystonic hand movements
 Schwartz-Jampel syndrome
 Trigger finger
 Lipofibromatous hamartoma
 Rubella
 Hereditary neuropathy with liability to pressure palsies
 Familial carpal tunnel syndrome
Other distal median mononeuropathies
 Hematoma (e.g., radial artery puncture)
 Constriction bands
 Compression from cast

der. In a large epidemiological study of carpal tunnel syndrome in the general population over a 2-year period in Marshfield, Wisconsin, the diagnosis of probable or definite carpal tunnel syndrome was made in 309 patients (Nordstrom et al., 1998). Of these, seven (2.3%) were children, ages 0 to 17 years, thus establishing an incidence rate of 0.26 per 1,000 person-years. The specific pediatric ages in this large study were not reported. However, case reports have documented carpal tunnel syndrome in infants as young as 7 months with a positive albeit previously unrecognized family history of the disorder (Swoboda et al., 1998) and in children as young as 2 years with mucopolysaccharidosis IV (Haddad et al., 1997). In contradistinction, idiopathic carpal tunnel syndrome is usually reported in older children or teens (Jones, 1996; Ouvrier and Shield, 1999). The causes of carpal tunnel syndrome are shown in Table 90–1. As in adults, idiopathic carpal tunnel syndrome is a diagnosis of exclusion. The symptoms of carpal tunnel syndrome in older children are similar to those in adults and include bilateral hand pain and numbness, occasional radiating pain into the upper arm and shoulder, nocturnal tingling in the fingers, morning hand paresthesias, and worsening of symptoms with certain activities (e.g., skiing, computer games) (Jones, 1996). Clinical signs may be absent or may range in severity from mild sensory loss in the distribution of the median nerve (usually sparing the palm) to thenar muscle weakness and atrophy. In infants and small children with carpal tunnel syndrome, the signs may include reduced movement of the fingers and insensitivity to pain (Jones, 1996; Swoboda et al., 1998); an unusual tremor in a 9-month-old infant was presumably secondary to disconcerting paresthesias (Brown J, unpublished data, personal communication to HRJ, 2001).

The carpal tunnel syndrome is the result of median nerve entrapment and compression within the tight confines of the carpal tunnel. Predisposing factors in pediatric carpal tunnel syndrome include congenital canal stenosis (e.g., familial carpal tunnel syndrome) (Danta, 1975; McDonnell et al., 1987; Stoll and Maitrot, 1998; Swoboda et al., 1998; De Smet and Fabry, 1999), wrist trauma or injuries (Koenigsberger and Moessinger, 1977; Deymeer and Jones, 1994; Jones, 1996), thickening of the flexor retinaculum (e.g., mucopolysaccharidoses, mucolipidoses, trigger finger) (McArthur et al., 1969; Miner and Schimke, 1975; Starreveld and Ashenhurst, 1975; MacDougal et al., 1977; Haddad et al., 1997; Cruz Martinez and Arpa, 1998), repetitive hand and wrist movements (e.g., sports-related injury, work-related injury, cerebral palsy with dystonic hand movements) (Alvarez et al., 1982; Senveli et al., 1987; Deymeer and Jones, 1994; Jones, 1996; Cruz Martinez and Arpa, 1998), tenosynovitis (e.g., scleroderma, rubella) (Blennow et al., 1982; Jones, 1996), the Schwartz-Jampel syndrome (Cruz Martinez et al., 1984; Cruz Martinez and Arpa, 1998), hereditary neuropathy with liability to pressure palsies (Felice et al., 1999), and pyogenic infections (Williams and Greer, 1963). Carpal tunnel syndrome has also been associated with Poland's syndrome (Harpf et al., 1999). In addition to carpal tunnel syndrome, distal median mononeuropathies may result from congenital constriction bands (Weeks, 1982), hematoma from radial artery puncture for blood gas determination (Pape et al., 1978), compression from a cast (Deymeer and Jones, 1994), or compression from a calcified flexor digitorum tendon (Hotta et al., 1970), or may be secondary to burns at the wrist (Fissette et al., 1981).

Acquired thenar muscle atrophy occurring as the result of severe carpal tunnel syndrome is unusual in children. However, there are rare cases of thenar atrophy associated with inborn errors of metabolism, pseudoneuroma of the median nerve, congenital constriction bands, foreshortened index finger, and trigger finger (Jones, 1996). In the last two conditions, the median nerve appears to be compressed by idiopathic thickening of the flexor retinaculum. These conditions are usually associated with concomitant involvement of the median sensory fibers. In distinction, Cavanagh syndrome, a hypoplastic disorder of the thenar muscles and hand bones, is not associated with median nerve compression or sensory fiber involvement (Cavanagh et al., 1979).

Proximal Median Mononeuropathies

Trauma is the most common cause of proximal median nerve injury in children (Table 90–2). In the series of 17 patients reported by Deymeer and Jones, 10 (59%) developed median mononeuropathies as a direct result of limb trauma. Bone fractures seem to be the most common cause of nerve trauma (Deymeer and Jones, 1994). Median nerve compression, entrapment, or laceration injuries have resulted from traumatic fractures of the supracondylar humerus, midradius, and radioulnar joint. Most of these injuries involve the main trunk of the median nerve; however, the anterior interosseous nerve is sometimes also traumatized in isolation as the result of a supracondylar fracture (Fearn and Goodfellow, 1965). Traumatic median nerve injuries have also resulted from elbow dislocations, lacerations, blunt nerve trauma from athletic activities, and trauma inflicted by arterial or venous puncture (Sumner and Khuri, 1984; Floyd et al., 1987; Jones, 1996).

Proximal median nerve entrapment lesions are as uncommon in children as in adults. Rare cases of median mononeuropathy resulting from entrapment by the ligament of Struthers (Bilge et al., 1990), congenital fibromuscular bands (Marlow et al., 1981;

Table 90–2. Causes of Proximal Median Mononeuropathies

Trauma
  Fractures
  Blunt nerve trauma
  Lacerations
  Trauma following arterial or venous puncture
Entrapment
  Ligament of Struthers
  Fibromuscular bands
  Pronator syndrome
  Bicipital aponeurosis
Tumors
  Lipofibromas
  Hamartomas
  Neurofibromas
  Hemangiomas
Other causes
  Osteoid osteoma
  Juvenile cutaneous mucinosis
  Abscess
  Idiopathic
  Calcified flexor digitorum superficialis tendon

Weeks, 1982; Uchida and Sugioka, 1991), pronator teres (Danielsson, 1980; Hartz et al., 1981), and bicipital aponeurosis (Gessini et al., 1983) do occur in children. The ligament of Struthers, a fibrous band extending from a small supracondylar spur to the medial epicondyle of the humerus, forms the roof of a tunnel through which the median nerve and brachial artery pass. Despite the common occurrence of the spurs, visible on plain radiographs in about 2% of the population, the ligament of Struthers is a rare cause of median nerve entrapment (Stewart, 2000). In pronator syndrome, the median nerve is compressed by the hypertrophied heads or thickened tendinous bands of the pronator teres muscle. Given that involvement is distal to the motor branch innervating the pronator teres, this muscle is usually not involved; this is in contradistinction to more proximal median lesions (e.g., ligament of Struthers entrapment). Congenital constriction bands may cause proximal median nerve entrapment injuries, occasionally with concurrent involvement of the radial and ulnar nerves (Weeks, 1982).

Compression of the proximal and distal segments of the median nerve has resulted from lipofibromas (Louis et al., 1985; Amadio et al., 1988), hamartomas (Callison et al., 1968), neurofibromas (Barfred and Zachariae, 1975), and hemangiomas (Patel et al., 1986). Other causes of median nerve compression include osteoid osteoma (Jones, 1996), juvenile cutaneous mucinosis (Jones, 1996), calcified flexor digitorum superficialis tendon (Hotta et al., 1970), and abscess (Williams and Greer, 1963). Anterior interosseous neuropathy has been reported in several children, either of spontaneous onset possibly secondary to atypical brachial neuritis (Fearn and Goodfellow, 1965; Nakano et al., 1977) or associated with a supracondylar fracture of the humerus (Spinner and Schreiber, 1969; Nakano et al., 1977).

Evaluation

The EMG evaluation of median mononeuropathies in infants includes obtaining a sensory nerve action potential from either the index or the middle finger (preferable in newborns and infants), compound muscle action potential from the thenar muscles, median motor conduction velocity across the forearm segment, comparative ulnar sensory and nerve motor conduction studies, and needle examination of the minimal number of necessary muscles. In older children with mild symptoms, the examination also needs to include median and ulnar mixed nerve action potentials, that is, "palmar" studies.

In cases of mild carpal tunnel syndrome, one may expect to find prolonged peak latencies of the median mixed nerve action potential and the sensory nerve action potential. Prolongation of the median compound muscle action potential distal latency and attenuation of the sensory nerve action potential amplitude indicate more moderate disease. Severe carpal tunnel syndrome is associated with an absence of attenuated thenar compound muscle action potential and needle examination abnormalities demonstrating both ongoing and chronic changes of denervation and reinnervation in the abductor pollicis brevis. In cases of proximal median mononeuropathy, the distal motor latencies are normal; however, the sensory nerve action potential may be prolonged (Jones, 1966). It is important to study conduction velocities across the forearm segment because these may be reduced with demyelinating injuries. Needle examination abnormalities often extend into median nerve–innervated forearm muscles with axonal or mixed injuries. In congenital thenar hypoplasia (e.g., Cavanagh syndrome), the median sensory nerve action potential amplitude and peak latency are normal, the compound muscle action potential is of low amplitude or absent, and thenar motor unit action potentials are reduced in number without associated denervation potentials.

The clinical findings and EMG results may sometimes dictate the need for additional studies in the evaluation of median mononeuropathies. Plain roentgenograms of the hand may be indicated in suspected cases of thenar hypoplasia (Cavanagh et al., 1979), to assess for hypoplasia of the hand bones. Moreover, roentgenograms of the distal humerus are recommended in suspected cases of ligament of Struthers entrapment to identify the bony spur often seen in that disorder. Magnetic resonance imaging may offer more precise anatomical assessment of suspected soft tissue infiltrative or compressive lesions, especially in patients with symptoms of slowly progressive dysfunction or with signs of palpable focal tenderness of fullness (Jones, 1996; Stewart, 2000). Metabolic studies for the mucopolysaccharidoses and mucolipidoses are indicated in suspected cases of carpal tunnel syndrome associated with dysmorphic features, organomegaly, and other-system disease. This is particularly so in those children in whom the primary abnormalities are thenar atrophy and EMG changes characterized by motor abnormalities with relatively preserved sensory responses.

Treatment and Prognosis

Traumatic mononeuropathies require prompt attention. As with all peripheral nerves, the main questions in cases of acute median nerve trauma include whether the nerve is continuous, the type of nerve injury (i.e., demyelinating, axonal or mixed), and prognosis for meaningful recovery. Within 7 to 10 days of acute nerve injury, wallerian degeneration is complete. EMG studies are recommended in cases with severe dysfunction or when nerve function cannot be assessed clinically because of other factors related to the trauma (e.g., immobilization, casting) (Robinson, 2000). In neurapraxia (focal demyelinating injury), the distal median sensory nerve action potential and compound muscle action potential are preserved; however,

stimulation proximal to the site of injury evokes an attenuated response, or a response may be absent (partial or complete conduction block). In mild or moderate axonotmesis (axonal injury), initially the compound muscle action potential (within the first 9 days) and later the distal sensory nerve action potential (within the first 11 days) (Chaudry et al., 1992) become attenuated or absent. In addition, abnormal insertional needle examination findings develop 10 to 14 days after injury in older children and as early as a few days after injury in babies with fibrillations and positive waves in median nerve–innervated muscles that are distal to the site of injury. In severe axonotmesis or neurotmesis, the distal median sensory nerve action potential and the compound muscle action potential are usually absent. Because nerve continuity may be uncertain in these cases, early surgical exploration and, if necessary, repair are usually recommended. Often, traumatic nerve injuries show EMG evidence of both demyelinating and axonal injuries (mixed nerve injury). In patients with preserved continuity and slow return of function, periodic EMG evaluation may be helpful in understanding the degree and types of reinnervation. Treatment in mild idiopathic and activity-related carpal tunnel syndrome is often focused on conservative measures with avoidance of compromising hand positions and activities. Median nerve decompression surgery is reserved for patients with continued or progressive symptoms refractory to conservative measures or in patients with EMG evidence of an axon-loss disorder. Surgical decompression is indicated in distal median mononeuropathy associated with the inborn errors of metabolism, pseudoneuroma, trigger finger, and congenital constriction bands. Distal mononeuropathies related to trauma or activity may resolve with primary conservative therapy. Surgical decompression usually affords some relief of symptoms and return of function, with ultimate recovery related to the degree of axonal loss.

In general, children with median mononeuropathies tend to have a good prognosis. Of 17 patients with various types of pediatric median mononeuropathy described by Deymeer and Jones, 12 (70%) had documented improvement at follow-up (Deymeer and Jones, 1994). Improvement was noted with traumatic, compressive, and entrapment injuries. A poor outcome occurred in four children, two with entrapment resulting from supracondylar fractures and two with carpal tunnel syndrome. One of the 17 children, an adolescent boy, was lost to follow-up.

ULNAR NERVE

Ulnar Mononeuropathies

Trauma is the most common cause of ulnar mononeuropathy in children (Table 90–3). Of the 21 pediatric ulnar mononeuropathy cases we described in

Table 90–3. Causes of Ulnar Mononeuropathies

Trauma
  Fractures: supracondylar, medial epicondylar, forearm, distal
    radial
  Lacerations, puncture and stab wounds
  Blunt trauma
  Superficial burns
  Repetitive throwing movements
  Nerve ischemia
Entrapment
  Cubital tunnel syndrome
  Persistent epitrochleoanconeus muscle
  Congenital constriction bands
Compression
  Surgical compression
  Wheelchair arm rests
  Bicycle hand rests
  Weightlifting bar
  Hemorrhage related to hemophilia
  Infiltration of intravenous fluids
  Compartment syndrome
  Following fracture or dislocation
Tumors
  Hamartomas
  Neurofibromas
  Neurilemomas
Other causes
  Leprosy
  Focal hypertrophic neuropathy
  Recurrent dislocation
  Hereditary neuropathy with liability to pressure palsies

1996, 11 (52%) resulted directly from nerve trauma. Proximal ulnar mononeuropathies caused by trauma resulted from supracondylar fractures, medial epicondylar fracture, forearm fracture, elbow laceration, stab wound, and an elbow puncture wound (Felice and Jones, 1996). Distal radial fractures are a cause of ulnar mononeuropathies at the wrist. Fractures may cause nerve damage via blunt injury, entrapment or compression, or laceration. The ulnar nerve may also be damaged as the result of surgical procedures to repair an elbow or forearm fracture. Delayed or "tardy" ulnar nerve palsy is described in children after elbow trauma, presumably from posttraumatic bony changes and fibrosis (Ouvrier and Shield, 1999).

Entrapment at the cubital tunnel was a surgically documented cause of ulnar mononeuropathy in two children in our series (Felice and Jones, 1996). A third case of presumed cubital tunnel syndrome occurred in an 18-year-old hockey goalie during one season when he carried heavy equipment with his arm in flexion; the symptoms subsided at the end of the season. Other causes of ulnar nerve entrapment include persistent epitrochleoanconeus muscle (Gessini et al., 1981) and congenital constriction bands (Weeks, 1982). We have not seen a documented case of ulnar mononeuropathy resulting from entrapment within the Guyon canal at our centers.

Five children suffered from compressive ulnar mononeuropathy in our series (Felice and Jones, 1996). Of these, two had compressive mononeuropa-

thies at the elbow during the course of surgery, one developed a transient dorsal cutaneous branch neuropathy resulting from a sleep palsy, one had bilateral compressive mononeuropathies at the forearm or elbow resulting from wheelchair rests, and one had compression at the wrist from bicycle hand rests. Felice (unpublished data) recently evaluated an 18-year-old man who developed severe conduction block ulnar mononeuropathy involving the terminal motor branch proximal to the innervation of the hypothenar muscles after weightlifting; the mechanism of injury is presumed to be nerve compression in the proximal palm segment. Other causes of ulnar nerve compression include hemorrhage from hemophilia (Cordingley and Crawford, 1984), extravasation of intravenous fluids with subsequent compartment syndrome (Dunn and Wilensky, 1984), fractures and dislocations (Uchida and Sugioka, 1990), and compression from bicycle hand rests (Noth et al., 1980). Other causes of ulnar mononeuropathy include leprosy (Saxena et al., 1990), focal hypertrophic neuropathy (Phillips et al., 1991), burns (Marquez et al., 1993), repetitive throwing injuries in baseball pitchers (Godshall and Hansen, 1971), tumors (Cavanagh and Pincott, 1977), and hamartomas (Drut, 1988).

Evaluation

The EMG evaluation of pediatric ulnar mononeuropathy needs to include an ulnar sensory nerve action potential from the little finger, ulnar motor nerve conduction studies from the hypothenar muscles, motor conduction velocities across the forearm and elbow segments, comparative median sensory and motor nerve conduction studies, and needle examination of the first dorsal interosseous, abductor digiti minimi, and flexor carpi ulnaris muscles. Occasionally, ulnar motor nerve conduction studies recorded from the first dorsal interosseous are required as a more sensitive test for demyelinating injuries at the wrist or elbow segments (Kothari et al., 1998). Additional studies including the dorsal ulnar cutaneous and medial antebrachial cutaneous sensory nerve action potentials may be required to help further in the localization of ulnar lesions and to assess for lower brachial plexus involvement, respectively. Ulnar mononeuropathies localized at the wrist or hand may involve the terminal motor branch, proximal or distal to the innervation of the hypothenar muscles, the terminal sensory branch, or both. These lesions spare the dorsal ulnar cutaneous sensory nerve action potential and are associated with preservation of motor conduction velocities across the elbow segment. Demyelinating ulnar mononeuropathies at the elbow segment are associated with the following: focal motor conduction block or conduction slowing; axonal mononeuropathies with absent or attenuated distal sensory nerve action potential and compound muscle action potential amplitudes and evidence of variable changes of denervation and reinnervation on needle examination of ulnar hand and forearm muscles; and mixed injuries with a combination of demyelinating and axonal features.

Treatment and Prognosis

The management of pediatric ulnar mononeuropathies includes nerve decompression and repair of fractures following trauma, surgical nerve repair and grafting following nerve lacerations and severe traumatic injuries (e.g., axonotmesis or neurotmesis), resection of compressive masses and tumors, nerve decompression in cubital tunnel syndrome, and nerve transposition and decompression with progressive lesions localized to the elbow. Twelve surgical procedures were performed in our series of 21 children with ulnar mononeuropathy, five to repair acute fractures and lacerations, two to decompress the nerve in cubital tunnel syndrome, one to decompress the nerve following a medial epicondylar fracture, one transposition surgery, two resections of neuromas, and one nerve graft procedure following a laceration (Felice and Jones, 1996).

In our series of 21 patients, 15 (71%) children with pediatric ulnar mononeuropathy were seen in follow-up, with a range of 2 months to 6 years subsequent to the initial evaluation. Follow-up examinations documented that only 56% of children with traumatic versus 83% with nontraumatic ulnar mononeuropathies had a favorable outcome (Felice and Jones, 1996). Two children with cubital tunnel syndrome improved following ulnar nerve decompression and anterior transposition surgeries.

RADIAL NERVE

Radial Mononeuropathies

Of 15 children with radial mononeuropathy reported by Escolar and Jones, eight (53%) had traumatic injuries, five from fractures and three from lacerations (Escolar and Jones, 1993). The fractures included three supracondylar, one Monteggia, and one lateral epicondylar. All these were axon-loss injuries, four involving the main trunk of the radial nerve distal to the spiral groove and one caused by a supracondylar fracture involving the posterior interosseous nerve fibers only. Of the lacerations, two involved the upper arm, and the other involved the forearm. All were axon-loss injuries including isolated posterior interosseous neuropathies in two cases and distal radial neuropathy in the other. Other causes of radial nerve trauma include injection injuries and arthroscopic elbow surgery (Papilion et al., 1988) (Table 90–4).

As in adults, the radial nerve in children is most susceptible to compression injury at the spiral groove segment. In the series by Escolar and Jones, compression injuries of the radial nerve were docu-

Table 90–4. Causes of Radial Mononeuropathies

Trauma
  Fractures: Monteggia, supracondylar, lateral condylar
  Lacerations
  Injection injuries
  Arthroscopic elbow surgery
Compression
  Neonatal
  Perioperative
  Compartment syndrome
  Sleep palsy
  Crutch palsy
Tumors
  Lipomas
  Ganglia
  Fibromas
  Neuromas
  Hemangiomas
Other causes
  Multiple septal entrapment
  Hereditary neuropathy with liability to pressure palsies

mented in six children (40%), including four postnatal and two neonatal injuries (Escolar and Jones, 1993). Two of the four postnatal injuries occurred within the spiral groove segment, one a conduction block injury from nerve compression sustained during a surgical procedure and the other a mixed injury resulting from a sleep palsy. The other two postnatal compression injuries were a demyelinating posterior interosseous injury resulting from an acute compartment syndrome from infiltration of intravenously administered chemotherapy in a child with Hodgkin's disease and bilateral axon-loss proximal trunk radial mononeuropathies from improper use of crutches. Radial mononeuropathy may be the presenting feature of hereditary neuropathy with liability to pressure palsies, and up to 3% of patients with this disorder who are younger than 10 years of age have documented radial nerve involvement (Meier and Moll, 1982). Neonatal radial mononeuropathy may result from intrauterine compression by uterine contraction rings (Morgan, 1948; Feldman, 1957), prolonged labor, subcutaneous fat necrosis (Lightwood, 1951), and subcutaneous abscess or hematoma (Ross et al., 1983). At birth, the radial nerve is at risk for injury secondary to humeral fracture, hematoma, blood pressure monitoring (Tollner et al., 1980), and prolonged birth-related external compression (Jones, 1996).

The radial nerve may also be injured by benign tumors and other compressive lesions including lipomas, ganglia, fibromas, neuromas, and hemangiomas (Jones, 1996). Entrapment of the radial nerve within the triceps muscle has also been reported (Lotem et al., 1971; Manske, 1977). Radial mononeuropathy developed in a 3-year-old girl because of a surgically documented entrapment of the nerve within the interseptal fascia (Jones, 1996).

Evaluation

The EMG evaluation of the radial nerve needs to include the radial sensory nerve action potential from the affected limb, the comparative radial sensory nerve action potential from the unaffected limb (or ipsilateral median sensory nerve action potential if both limbs are affected), and needle EMG of a proximal (e.g., triceps) and a distal (e.g., brachioradialis) radial nerve–innervated muscle and a muscle innervated by the posterior interosseous nerve (e.g., extensor indicis). Radial motor nerve conduction studies are technically difficult in neonates and small children. However, we find the radial motor study, recording from the extensor indicis with stimulation at three sites (the forearm and below and above the spiral groove), to be relatively easy to perform and reliable in demonstrating conduction abnormalities across the spiral groove segment in adolescents and older children. Pure demyelinating injuries at the spiral groove segment are associated with the following: motor conduction block, slowing, or both; normal distal radial sensory nerve action potentials and compound muscle action potentials; and reduced recruitment of motor unit action potentials without abnormal spontaneous activity in affected muscles. Axonal injuries are associated with reduced or absent radial sensory nerve action potentials and compound muscle action potentials and with reduced recruitment of motor unit action potentials with fibrillations and positive waves in affected muscles. Posterior interosseous neuropathies are associated with a normal radial sensory nerve action potential, a low-amplitude or absent compound muscle action potential from the extensor indicis, and needle examination abnormalities limited to radial nerve–innervated muscles distal to the supinator.

Treatment and Prognosis

Traumatic injuries require prompt repair of fractures and soft tissue. Early EMG studies are indicated in patients with lacerations and fractures to assess for nerve continuity. Absent sensory nerve action potentials, compound muscle action potentials, and motor unit action potentials distal to the site of injury at 7 to 10 days after trauma indicate severe axonotmesis or neurotmesis, suggest the possibility of a radial nerve laceration or severe disruption, and warrant surgical exploration and, if necessary, nerve repair. Seven of the eight (88%) children with traumatic radial mononeuropathies reported by Escolar and Jones improved or completely recovered within 7 to 17 months (Escolar and Jones, 1993). A 6-year-old boy with a severe axon-loss posterior interosseous nerve injury following a supracondylar fracture showed no clinical improvement after 4 years. Acute compression injuries at the spiral groove segment, usually associated with demyelinating or mixed nerve injuries, afford a more favorable prognosis for full recovery. All six patients with neonatal and postnatal radial mononeuropathy resulting from nerve compression injuries had complete recoveries at follow-up. Slowly progressive ra-

dial or posterior interosseous nerve dysfunction may require magnetic resonance imaging studies and surgical exploration to search for possible tumors, fascial bands, or other sources of nerve compression or entrapment.

OTHER UPPER EXTREMITY NERVES

Axillary Nerve

Causes of other upper extremity mononeuropathies in children are listed in Table 90–5. In addition to the radial nerve, the axillary nerve is the other major derivation of the posterior cord of the brachial plexus and lies in close proximity to the surgical neck of the humerus. The major branches of the axillary nerve include motor branches to the deltoid and teres minor muscles and the lateral cutaneous nerve of the arm. Axillary nerve injuries cause weakness of arm abduction, deltoid muscle atrophy with severe axonal injuries, and sensory loss along the upper lateral arm. The most common causes of axillary mononeuropathies in adults are blunt trauma, dislocations, and fractures of the shoulder and humerus (Stewart, 2000). In children, axillary mononeuropathies are reported in sports-related shoulder trauma and exostosis of the humerus (Witthout et al., 1994; Jones, 1996). The EMG evaluation of axillary mononeuropathies in children is usually limited to the needle examination of the deltoid muscle. Recording a compound muscle action potential latency from the deltoid muscle with stimulation at the supraclavicular fossa may be considered in a cooperative child with a slowly progressive deficit in which a compressive demyelinating lesion is suspected.

Table 90–5. Causes of Other Upper Extremity Mononeuropathies

Axillary nerve
  Exostosis of the humerus
  Sports-related injuries
  Trauma
Long thoracic nerve
  Milwaukee brace
  Trauma
  Sports-related
  Idiopathic
Musculocutaneous nerve
  Body cast
  Hereditary neuropathy with liability to pressure palsies
  Idiopathic
Suprascapular nerve
  Entrapment within transverse ligament at suprascapular notch
  Compression by ganglion
  Trauma
Thoracodorsal nerve
  Chest wall empyema
Spinal accessory nerve
  Surgical injury
  Hereditary neuropathy with liability to pressure palsies
  Idiopathic

Long Thoracic Nerve

The long thoracic nerve originates from cervical roots 5, 6, and 7 and descends in the axilla, posterior to the brachial plexus, to innervate the serratus anterior muscle, which anchors the scapula to the chest wall. Injuries to the long thoracic nerve cause winging of the scapula, especially with the arms in anterior abduction. Reported causes of long thoracic mononeuropathies in children include sports-related injuries (e.g., tennis, weightlifting), shoulder trauma, compression from a Milwaukee brace, association with hereditary neuropathy with liability to pressure palsies, and idiopathic lesions of the nerve (Gregg et al., 1979; Foo and Swann, 1983; Jones, 1996; Felice et al., 1999). The EMG evaluation is usually limited to needle examination of the serratus anterior at its digitations over the ribs at the mid-axillary line.

Musculocutaneous Nerve

The musculocutaneous nerve is derived from the lateral cord of the brachial plexus; innervates the biceps brachii, brachialis, and coracobrachialis muscles; and terminates as the lateral cutaneous nerve of the forearm. Injuries to the musculocutaneous nerve are associated with weakness of arm flexion and sensory loss along the lateral forearm. Three cases were reported by Jones in 1986, including a child with compression of the nerve by a body cast, another child with an idiopathic lesion causing biceps muscle atrophy, and a third child with isolated involvement of lateral antebrachial cutaneous nerve (Jones, 1986). We were referred a 16-year-old boy with painless right biceps weakness and atrophy who was found to have musculocutaneous mononeuropathy superimposed on diffuse demyelinating sensorimotor polyneuropathy (Felice et al., 1999). DNA studies later confirmed the diagnosis of hereditary neuropathy with liability to pressure palsies. The cause of the musculocutaneous mononeuropathy was unknown because no known injury was identified. The EMG evaluation of the musculocutaneous nerve may include the lateral cutaneous sensory nerve action potential, a biceps brachii compound muscle action potential, and needle examination of the biceps brachii and coracobrachialis.

Suprascapular Nerve

The suprascapular nerve originates from the superior trunk of the brachial plexus and innervates the supraspinatus and infraspinatus muscles. Injuries to this nerve cause shoulder abduction and external rotation weakness. Lesions of this nerve usually result from entrapment injuries or trauma. Laulund et al. reported on a 14-year-old girl who sustained a blow to her shoulder as she stumbled in gymnastics and was later found to have entrapment of the nerve by the transverse ligament in the suprascapular notch (Laulund et al., 1984). Other reported causes of suprascapular mononeuropathy in children include sports-related injuries and compression by a ganglion cyst (Okino et al., 1991; Montagna and Colonna, 1993). The EMG evaluation includes needle examination of the supraspinatus and infraspinatus. In a cooperative child, the clinician may consider obtaining compound muscle action potentials from both muscles with needle recording electrodes.

Thoracodorsal Nerve

The thoracodorsal nerve is derived from the posterior cord of the brachial plexus and innervates the latissimus dorsi. We were referred an 8-year-old girl who developed right latissimus dorsi atrophy following insertion of a chest tube and subsequent development of chest wall empyema. Needle examination of the latissimus dorsi revealed low-amplitude fibrillations and positive waves and markedly reduced recruitment of motor unit action potentials. We have not seen other reported cases of thoracodorsal mononeuropathy in children.

Spinal Accessory Nerve

The spinal accessory nerve is derived from cranial nerve XI and innervates the sternocleidomastoid and trapezius muscles. Injury to the spinal accessory nerve occurs rarely and usually results as a complication of surgical procedures involving the posterior triangle of the neck (Jones, 1996). We have seen two children with isolated spinal accessory mononeuropathy. One was a 12-year-old girl with an idiopathic spinal accessory mononeuropathy. The other was a 13-year-old girl who had a left shoulder droop during a school scoliosis screening evaluation (Felice et al., 1999). The examination was remarkable for left trapezius weakness and atrophy, mild left scapular winging, diffusely hypoactive reflexes, and pes cavus deformities. The EMG study documented left spinal accessory mononeuropathy superimposed on diffuse sensorimotor polyneuropathy. Subsequent DNA studies confirmed the diagnosis of hereditary neuropathy with liability to pressure palsies. The EMG evaluation included recording the compound muscle action potential from the trapezius and needle examination of the trapezius and sternocleidomastoid.

References

Alvarez N, Larkin C, Roxborough J: Carpal tunnel syndrome in athetoid-dystonic cerebral palsy. Arch Neurol 1982;39:311–312.

Amadio PC, Reiman HM, Dobyns JH: Lipofibromatous hamartoma of nerve. J Hand Surg [Am] 1988;13:67–75.

Barfred T, Zachariae L: Neurofibroma in the median nerve treated with resection and free nerve transplantation: Case reports. Scand J Plast Reconstr Surg 1975;9:245–248.

Bilge T, Yalaman O, Bilge S, et al: Entrapment neuropathy of the median nerve at the level of the ligament of Struthers. Neurosurgery 1990;27:787–789.

Blennow G, Bekassy AN, Eriksson M, Rosendahl R: Transient carpal tunnel syndrome accompanying rubella infection. Acta Paediatr Scand 1982;71:1025–1028.

Callison JR, Thomas OJ, White WL: Fibrofatty proliferation of the median nerve. Plast Reconstr Surg 1968;42403–413.

Cavanagh NP, Pincott JR: Ulnar nerve tumours of the hand in childhood. J Neurol Neurosurg Psychiatry 1977;40:795–800.

Cavanagh NP, Yates DAH, Sutcliffe J: Thenar hypoplasia with associated radiologic abnormalities. Muscle Nerve 1979;2:431–436.

Chaudhry V, Cornblath DR: Wallerian degeneration in human nerves: Serial electrophysiological studies. Muscle Nerve 1992;15:687–693.

Cordingley FT, Crawford GP: Ulnar nerve palsy in a haemophiliac due to intraneural haemorrhage. BMJ 1984;289:18–19.

Cruz Martinez A, Arpa J: Carpal tunnel syndrome in childhood: Study of 6 cases. Electroencephalogr Clin Neurophysiol 1998;109:304–308.

Cruz Martinez A, Arpa J, Perez Conde MC, Ferrer MT: Bilateral carpal tunnel in childhood associated with Schwartz-Jampel syndrome. Muscle Nerve 1984;7:66–72.

Danielsson LG: Iatrogenic pronator syndrome. Scand J Plast Reconstr Surg 1980;14:201–203.

Danta G: Familial carpal tunnel syndrome with onset in childhood. J Neurol Neurosurg Psychiatry 1975;38:350–355.

Deymeer F, Jones HR: Pediatric median mononeuropathies: A clinical and electromyographic study. Muscle Nerve 1994;17:755–762.

De Smet L, Fabry G: Carpal tunnel syndrome: Familial occurrence presenting in childhood. J Pediatr Orthop 1999;8:127–128.

Drut R: Ossifying fibrolipomatous hamartoma of the ulnar nerve. Pediatr Pathol 1988;8:179–184.

Dunn D, Wilensky M: Median and ulnar nerve palsies after infiltration of intravenous fluid. South Med J 1984;77:1345.

Escolar DM, Jones HR Jr: Pediatric radial mononeuropathy: A clinical and electromyographic study. Muscle Nerve 1993;16:1100.

Fearn CB, Goodfellow JW: Anterior interosseous nerve palsy. J Bone Joint Surg Br 1965;47:91–93.

Feldman GV: Radial nerve palsies in the newborn. Arch Dis Child 1957;32:469–471.

Felice KJ, Jones HR: Pediatric ulnar mononeuropathy: Report of 21 electromyography-documented cases and review of the literature. J Child Neurol 1996;11:116–120.

Felice KJ, Leicher CR, DiMario FJ: Hereditary neuropathy with liability to pressure palsies in children. Pediatr Neurol 1999;21:818–821.

Fissette J, Onkelinx A, Fandi N: Carpal and Guyon tunnel syndrome in burns at the wrist. J Hand Surg [Am] 1981;6:13–15.

Floyd WE 3rd, Gebhardt MC, Emans JB: Intra-articular entrapment of the median nerve after elbow dislocation in children. J Hand Surg [Am] 1987;12:704–707.

Foo CL, Swann M: Isolated paralysis of the serratus anterior: A report of 20 cases. J Bone Joint Surg Br 1983;65:552–556.

Gessini L, Jandolo B, Pietrangeli A: Entrapment neuropathies of the median nerve at the elbow. Surg Neurol 1983;19:112–116.

Gessini L, Jandolo B, Pietrangeli A, Occhipinti E: Ulnar nerve entrapment at the elbow by persistent epitrochleoanconeus muscle: Case report. J Neurosurg 1981;55:830–831.

Godshall RW, Hansen CA: Traumatic ulnar neuropathy in adolescent baseball pitchers. J Bone Joint Surg Am 1971;53:359–361.

Gregg JR, Labosky D, Harty M, et al: Serratus anterior paralysis in the young athlete. J Bone Joint Surg Am 1979;61:825–832.

Haddad FS, Jones DHA, Vellodi A, et al: Carpal tunnel syndrome in the mucopolysaccharidoses. J Bone Joint Surg Br 1997;79:576–582.

Harpf C, Schwabegger A, Hussl H: Carpal median nerve entrapment in a child with Poland's syndrome. Ann Plast Surg 1999;42:458–459.

Hartz CR, Linscheid RL, Gramse RR, Daube JR: The pronator teres

syndrome: Compressive neuropathy of the median nerve. J Bone Joint Surg Am 1981;63:885–890.

Hotta T, Kanbara H, Soto S, et al: Case of carpal tunnel syndrome due to calcification of the flexor digitorum sublimis II in a child. Orthop Surg (Tokyo) 1970;21:948–950.

Jones HR: Compressive neuropathy in childhood: A report of 14 cases. Muscle Nerve 1986;9:720–723.

Jones HR: Mononeuropathies. In Jones HR, Bolton CF, Harper CM (eds): Pediatric Clinical Electromyography. Philadelphia, Lippincott-Raven, 1996; 171–250.

Koenigsberger MR, Moessinger AC: Iatrogenic carpal tunnel syndrome in the newborn infant. J Pediatr 1977;91:443–445.

Kothari MJ, Heistand M, Rutkove SB: Three ulnar nerve conduction studies in patients with ulnar neuropathy at the elbow. Arch Phys Med 1998;79:87–89.

Laulund T, Fedders O, Sogaard I, Kornum M: Suprascapular nerve compression syndrome. Surg Neurol 1984;22:308–312.

Lightwood R: Radial nerve palsy associated with localized subcutaneous fat necrosis in the newborn. Arch Dis Child 1951;26:436–437.

Lotem M, Fried A, Levy M: Radial nerve palsy following muscular effort: A nerve compression syndrome possibly related to a fibrous arch of the lateral head of the triceps. J Bone Joint Surg Br 1971;53:500–506.

Louis DS, Hankin FM, Greene TL, Dick HM: Lipofibromas of the median nerve: Long-term follow-up of four cases. J Hand Surg [Am] 1985;10:403–408.

MacDougal B, Weeks PM, Wray RC Jr: Median nerve compression and trigger finger in the mucopolysaccharidosis and related disorders. Plast Reconstr Surg 1977;59:260–263.

Manske PR: Compression of the radial nerve by the triceps muscle: A case report. J Bone Joint Surg Am 1977;59:835–836.

Marlow N, Jarratt J, Hosking G: Congenital ring constrictions with entrapment neuropathies. J Neurol Neurosurg Psychiatry 1981;44:247–249.

Marquez S, Turley JJE, Peters WJ: Neuropathy in burns patients. Brain 1993;116:471–483.

McArthur RG, Hayles AB, Gomez MR, Bianco AJ Jr: Carpal tunnel syndrome and trigger finger in childhood. Am J Dis Child 1969;117:463–469.

McDonnell JM, Makley JT, Horwitz SJ: Familial carpal-tunnel syndrome presenting in childhood: Report of two cases. J Bone Joint Surg Am 1987;69:928–930.

Meier C, Moll C: Hereditary neuropathy with liability to pressure palsies: Report of two families and review of the literature. J Neurol 1982;228:73–95.

Miner ME, Schimke RN: Carpal tunnel syndrome in pediatric mucopolysaccharidoses: Report of four cases. J Neurosurg 1975;43:102–103.

Montagna P, Colonna S: Suprascapular neuropathy restricted to the infraspinatus muscle in volleyball players. Acta Neurol Scand 1993;87:248–250.

Morgan L: Radial nerve paralysis in the newborn. Arch Dis Child 1948;23:137–139.

Nakano KK, Lundergran C, Okihiro MM: Anterior interosseous nerve syndromes: Diagnostic methods and alternative treatments. Arch Neurol 1977;34:477–480.

Nordstrom DL, DeStefano F, Vierkant RA, Layde PM: Incidence of diagnosed carpal tunnel syndrome in a general population. Epidemiology 1998;9:342–345.

Noth J, Dietz V, Mauritz KH: Cyclist's palsy: Neurological and EMG study in 4 cases with distal ulnar lesions. J Neurol Sci 1980;47:111–116.

Okino T, Minami A, Kato H, et al: Entrapment neuropathy of the suprascapular nerve by a ganglion. J Bone Joint Surg Am 1991;73:141–147.

Ouvrier RA, Shield L: Focal lesions of peripheral nerves. In Ouvrier RA, McLeod JG, Pollard JD (eds): Peripheral Neuropathy in Childhood, 2nd ed. London, MacKeith Press, 1999; 244–264.

Pape KE, Armstrong DL, Fitzhardinge PM: Peripheral median nerve damage secondary to brachial arterial blood gas sampling. J Pediatr 1978;93:852–856.

Papilion JD, Neff RS, Shall LM: Compression neuropathy of the radial nerve as a complication of elbow arthroscopy: A case report and review of the literature. Arthroscopy 1988;4:284–286.

Patel CB, Tsai T-M, Kleinert HE: Hemangioma of the median nerve: A report of two cases. J Hand Surg [Am] 1986;11:76–79.

Phillips LH 2nd, Persing JA, Vandenberg SR: Electrophysiological findings in localized hypertrophic mononeuropathy. Muscle Nerve 1991;14:335–341.

Robinson LR: Traumatic injury to peripheral nerves. Muscle Nerve 2000;23:863–873.

Ross D, Jones R Jr, Fisher J, Konkol RJ: Isolated radial nerve lesion in the newborn. Neurology 1983;33:1354–1356.

Saxena U, Ramesh V, Misra RS, Mukherjee A: Giant nerve abscesses in leprosy. Clin Exp Dermatol 1990;15:349–351.

Senveli ME, Turker A, Arda MN, Altinors MN: Bilateral carpal tunnel syndrome in a young carpet weaver. Clin Neurol Neurosurg 1987;89:281–282.

Spinner M, Schreiber SN: Anterior interosseous nerve paralysis as a complication of supracondylar fractures of the humerus in children. J Bone Joint Surg Am 1969;51:1584–1590.

Starreveld E, Ashenhurst EM: Bilateral carpal tunnel syndrome in childhood: A report of two sisters with mucolipidosis III (pseudo-Hurler polydystrophy). Neurology 1975;25:234–238.

Stevens JC, Sun S, Beard CM, et al: Carpal tunnel syndrome in Rochester, Minnesota, 1961 to 1980. Neurology 1988;38:134–138.

Stewart JD: Focal Peripheral Neuropathies. Philadelphia, Lippincott Williams & Wilkins, 2000.

Stoll C, Maitrot D: Autosomal dominant carpal tunnel syndrome. Clin Genet 1998;54:345–348.

Sumner JM, Khuri SM: Entrapment of the median nerve and flexor pollicis longus tendon in an epiphyseal fracture-dislocation of the distal radioulnar joint: A case report. J Hand Surg [Am] 1984;9:711–714.

Swoboda KJ, Engle EC, Scheindlin B, et al: Mutilating hand syndrome in an infant with familial carpal tunnel syndrome. Muscle Nerve 1998;21:104–111.

Tollner U, Bechinger D, Pohlandt F: Radial nerve palsy in a premature infant following long-term measurement of blood pressure. J Pediatr 1980;96:921–922.

Uchida Y, Sugioka Y: Ulnar nerve palsy after supracondylar humerus fracture. Acta Orthop Scand 1990;61:118–119.

Uchida Y, Sugioka Y: Peripheral nerve palsy associated with congenital constriction band syndrome. J Hand Surg [Br] 1991; 16:109–112.

Weeks PM: Radial, median, and ulnar nerve dysfunction associated with a congenital constricting band of the arm. Plast Reconstr Surg 1982;69:333–336.

Williams LF, Greer T: Acute carpal tunnel syndrome secondary to pyogenic infection of the forearm. JAMA 1963;185:409–410.

Witthout J, Steffens KJ, Koob E: Intermittent axillary nerve palsy caused by humeral exostosis. J Hand Surg [Br] 1994;19:422–423.

CHAPTER 91

Pediatric Mononeuropathies of the Lower Extremity

Diana M. Escolar and H. Royden Jones, Jr.

Mononeuropathies are relatively uncommon in childhood, but these focal neuropathies occur in all ages from the neonate to the adolescent. In contrast to adults, in whom carpal tunnel syndrome and ulnar neuropathy at the elbow are far more frequent than isolated neuropathies in the lower limb, mononeuropathies in children affect nerves in the arm and leg with equal frequency. The evaluation of upper extremity mononeuropathies is considered in Chapter 90. Some very unusual mononeuropathies occur secondary to either compression or entrapment in the pediatric population. These mechanisms particularly involve the sciatic and peroneal nerves (Jones, 2000). In contrast, trauma is the most common etiological mechanism for focal neuropathies of the arm. Another important difference between children and adults in this regard is that it is very rare in children to find that a focal neuropathy is the presenting sign of an underlying generalized peripheral neuropathy. However, during a period of 15 years at Children's Hospital in Boston, we rarely saw a case of a sciatic or peroneal neuropathy secondary to a lymphoma, hypereosinophilic syndrome, and a vasculitis. When evaluating a child with a seemingly isolated weakness or sensory loss, the presence of a more proximal lesion must also be considered, including a plexopathy, an intraspinal lesion, or an intraparenchymal muscle lesion such as a soft tissue sarcoma (David and Jones, 1994). Once a mononeuropathy is defined with electromyography (EMG), the precise nature and localization of the nerve lesion must be investigated with appropriately targeted imaging studies. This diagnostic paradigm at times has to include surgical exploration for sites of entrapment not identified by even the most modern imaging studies.

SCIATIC NEUROPATHY

Anatomy

The sciatic nerve is derived from the L5 and S1-2 nerve root portions of the lumbosacral plexus. There are two primary divisions: the laterally situated peroneal and medially placed tibial nerves. Isolated involvement of the peroneal division of the sciatic nerve occasionally has a clinical presentation similar to that of the much more common peroneal lesion at the fibula head. This occurs because the laterally placed peroneal division of the sciatic nerve is more prone to early compression. Electromyographers must always consider a possible sciatic nerve lesion in the differential diagnosis of any child with a footdrop. From the electromyographic standpoint, it is also important to recognize that the gluteus maximus and gluteus medius are not innervated by the sciatic nerve. Evaluation of these two gluteal muscles is very useful for differentiating a primary lesion of the sciatic nerve from a more proximal process that involves the lumbosacral plexus or a nerve root lesion. One must recall that the distal adductor magnus muscle also has a primary sciatic nerve innervation. Therefore, neurogenic changes may be found in this medial thigh muscle, with no need to exclude a sciatic neuropathy.

Twenty children with sciatic mononeuropathy

were evaluated between 1979 and 1994 and represented 1.2% of the 1710 electromyographic studies that were performed (Escolar and Jones, 1994). On review of the entire population of patients with pediatric mononeuropathies at Children's Hospital of Boston, we found sciatic neuropathy at a frequency of 24%, a very disproportionate percentage for children in contrast to the rare occurrence of a sciatic mononeuropathy in adults. The anatomic level was proximal in the region of the sciatic notch in 11 children, distal in the thigh in 4 children, and not identified in the remaining 5 children. The prognosis varied from complete to no recovery. The outcome was not directly related to the primary mechanism. Children with sciatic neuropathies secondary to nerve compression had either improvement or total resolution. In contrast, the prognosis was mixed with regard to the other causes. Surprisingly, in our series, sciatic neuropathies occur as commonly as peroneal neuropathies. Some years ago, neonatal and infantile sciatic neuropathies were relatively even more common. This was related to the previously higher incidence of breech vaginal deliveries with increased risk for sciatic mononeuropathy, parenteral intragluteal medications and, rarely, umbilical artery injections (Combes and Clark, 1960; Pedrocca et al., 1968; Schneegans et al., 1968; Schneegans et al., 1969; Jellis and Helal, 1970; Sharrard, 1973; Sriram, 1981; Fok et al., 1986; Merkulov, 1987; Goven'ko and Babin, 1990; Villarejo and Pascual, 1993; MacDonald and Marcuse, 1994; de Sanctis et al., 1995; Marcuse and MacDonald, 1996; Bhatia and Jindal, 1996).

Sciatic mononeuropathies occur in all pediatric age groups. These neuropathies may occur with an acute, a subacute, or a chronic clinical course and may be located proximally in the pelvis or sciatic notch or more distally in the thigh.

The sciatic nerve and its two major branches, the peroneal and tibial nerves, supply innervation to the hamstrings, the distal adductor magnus, all of the posterior compartment leg muscles, and the intrinsic foot muscles. The sciatic nerve provides sensation to the skin of the entire foot and the posterior lower leg through sensory branches of the tibial nerve (sural, medial, and lateral plantar and calcaneus) and the superficial peroneal nerve (Stewart, 1987). The clinical manifestations of sciatic neuropathies include weakness of foot dorsiflexion, inversion, eversion and plantar flexion, knee flexion, and decreased sensation over the entire foot. The muscle stretch reflex at the ankle is usually absent or decreased. Children usually present acutely with weakness and sensory changes in this distribution or with a chronic progressive footdrop or a progressive pes cavus deformity (Bassett et al., 1997). Sciatic nerve tumors are often associated with pain in the posterior aspect of the leg, sometimes extending into the foot, and often causing initial suspicion of a nerve root disorder rather than a primary sciatic nerve lesion (Thomas et al., 1983). Back pain, although most commonly associated with a spinal or

an intraspinal lesion, is also rarely associated with pure sciatic neuropathies, including nerve tumors (Thomas et al., 1983; Bodack et al., 1999). Therefore, in children with back or leg pain (or both) who have signs suggestive of an L5 or S1 root lesion (or both), a sciatic nerve lesion must always be thoroughly investigated when the results of a lumbosacral spine magnetic resonance imaging study are normal.

Sciatic neuropathies in children will often mimic peroneal nerve palsy, due to the higher susceptibility of the more superficial anatomic localization of the peroneal trunk fibers to stretch and other injuries (Sunderland, 1978). Nerve conduction studies in these situations can be deceptive. The peroneal compound muscle action potential (CMAP) is often diminished in face of a normal tibial nerve CMAP, as well as the sural sensory nerve action potential (SNAP) mimicking a primary peroneal nerve lesion at the fibula head. However, a careful needle EMG, as well as clinical examination and documentation of neurogenic changes within the short head of the biceps femoris muscle, will help to correctly localize the lesion proximal to the common peroneal nerve on the peroneal trunk.

Etiological Mechanisms

Sciatic neuropathies in children have a broad set of mechanisms. A nontraumatic mechanism was present in 16 of 20 (80%) children diagnosed during a 15-year period at our pediatric EMG laboratory (Escolar and Jones, 1994). Seven (35%) were secondary to a compressive lesion. Other causes for pediatric sciatic neuropathies include rare vasculitides, hematological or hemorrhagic lesions, tumors, and idiopathic postlithotomy perioperative lesions. This differs somewhat from the adult population, with a majority due to traumatic and stretch injuries secondary to pelvic fractures-dislocations or hip replacement surgery (Stewart, 1987; Stewart, 1993; Yuen et al., 1995).

COMPRESSION

The causes of compression included long leg and body casts, prolonged pressure on the nerve in a pavulonized newborn, and pressure by the ipsilateral heel of a child in congestive heart failure who slept sitting up with his leg tucked under his buttock (Escolar and Jones, 1994). This was similar to a 20-year-old student who developed a sciatic neuropathy while sitting for a long time in a lotus position during a yoga retreat (Vogel et al., 1991). Other reports of compressive sciatic neuropathy in children include external compression by sitting on a hard surface (Deverall and Ferguson, 1968), in the setting of severe weight loss (Lee et al., 1998), by prolonged sitting position during surgery (Brown et al., 1988; Gozal and Pomeranz, 1994; Yuen et al., 1995; Yuen and So, 1999), or by prolonged pressure in critical ill patients in intensive care unit settings (Yuen et al., 1994, 1995; Goh et al., 1996). A lithotomy position occasionally leads to sciatic neuropathies in adults (Kubiak et al., 1998; Warner et al., 2000); we had two such cases in our pediatric series (Escolar and Jones, 1994). The mechanism of injury is unclear and has been postulated to be ischemic (Romfh and Currier, 1983), stretching injury (Burkhart and Daly, 1966), or external compression.

Sciatic compressive neuropathies secondary to hematomas in hemophilic individuals was described in 6 of 36 nerve injuries secondary to intraneural bleeding (Ehrmann et al., 1981). A pelvic mass from an occult hematocolpos was related to a sciatic neuropathy in an adolescent girl with long-standing back pain and leg weakness (London and Sefton, 1996). Endometriosis compressing the sciatic nerve can cause cyclic sciatic pain and a progressive sciatic neuropathy (Dhote et al., 1996). Very rarely, a persistent sciatic artery will compress the sciatic nerve at the pelvic notch. Magnetic resonance imaging is useful in identifying the congenital anomaly (Gasecki et al., 1992).

ISCHEMIA

An acute sciatic neuropathy occurred in 2 of the 20 children in our series, probably due to ischemia of the sciatic nerve. In one child, a distal sciatic neuropathy developed secondary to hypereosinophilic vasculitis. The other instance occurred in a child with purpura fulminans due to meningococcemia (Escolar and Jones, 1994). The pathophysiological mechanism in allergic vasculitis is postulated to be either an embolic event to the vasa nervorum or a toxic effect of the eosinophilic granules on the peripheral nerve (Dorfman et al., 1983). In both patients in our series, the peroneal and tibialis CMAP had low amplitude but the sural SNAPS were preserved (Escolar and Jones, 1994). The greater compromise of the motor fibers in ischemic insults to the sciatic nerve is not novel, as it has been previously described by Sunderland (1978). It behooves the electromyographer to also consider a vascular mechanism and not always a radiculopathy with this set of electromyographic findings. In a study of 119 sciatic neuropathies involving children, 10 patients had ischemic injuries due to vasculitis, aortofemoral arterial bypass surgery, iliac artery thrombosis, and diabetes (Yuen et al., 1995).

NEOPLASMS

The most common presentation of sciatic nerve tumors is lower extremity pain that sometimes involves the foot. There may be significant nocturnal exacerbation. Paradoxically, most of these patients have minimal or no weakness (Thomas et al., 1983; Oberle et al., 1997; Gominak and Ochoa, 1998; Bickels et al., 1999). These nerve tumors are very uncommon. A review of a 60-year experience at the Mayo Clinic identified only 35 primary sciatic tumors, including neurilemomas, neurofibromas, and neurofibrosarcomas (Thomas et al., 1983). These in-

volved patients at all ages, with the youngest being a 5-year-old child. The only patient in the series by Thomas and associates (1983) without pain was this 5-year-old child who presented with progressive pes cavus deformity. This was similar to a 10-year-old boy who presented with painless progressive footdrop due to a localized perineuroma (localized hypertrophic mononeuropathy) of the peroneal trunk of the sciatic nerve (Katirji and Wilbourn, 1994). Fortunately, these previously difficult-to-diagnose tumors can be localized with magnetic resonance imaging (Emory et al., 1995).

Sciatic neurofibromas are sometimes the primary manifestation of neurofibromatosis (Gelain et al., 1988; Hruban et al., 1990). Often, these tumors can be readily diagnosed by palpation of a mass; this occurred in two thirds of the patients in different series (Barber et al., 1962; Thomas et al., 1983; Benyahya et al., 1997; Bickels et al., 1999).

Primary lymphomas may present with a sciatic neuropathy in children as well as in adults (Roncaroli et al., 1997; Misdraji et al., 2000; Quinones-Hinojosa et al., 2000). At the Children's Hospital of Boston, a 15-year-old boy had a chronic progressive sciatic neuropathy secondary to invasion of the sciatic nerve by a diffuse lymphoma (Jones et al., 1988; Escolar and Jones, 1994). Rarely, local tumors, including pelvic neuroblastomas (Escolar and Jones, 1994; Cruccetti et al., 2000), chloromas (Stillman et al., 1988), and bone tumors (sessile osteochondromas, osteosarcoma), can enlarge and compress the sciatic nerve (Lester and McAlister, 1970; Favier et al., 1993; Bickels et al., 1999).

The diagnosis of sciatic nerve tumor has been elusive. In one series, most patients were symptomatic for 3 to 5 years before the diagnosis was made, even for the patients with malignant neurofibrosarcomas (Thomas et al., 1983). This experience has raised the question as to whether a malignant transformation of some tumors may occur, making it essential to get an accurate diagnosis for each child who presents with a chronic sciatic neuropathy even if surgical exploration is needed. Fortunately, most primary or secondary nerve tumors are diagnosed with computed tomography scanning (Thomas et al., 1983) or magnetic resonance imaging (Almanza et al., 1982; Tachi et al., 1995; Uetani et al., 1998; Simmons et al., 1999; Weig et al., 2000) and with more sophisticated technology, including magnetic resonance neurography (Filler et al., 1996; Kuntz et al., 1996; Aagaard et al., 1998) and ultrasonography (Martinoli et al., 2000; Taniguchi et al., 2000).

ENTRAPMENT

Entrapment of the sciatic nerve is extremely rare. However, there are reports in the literature of progressive sciatic neuropathies caused by myofascial or fibrovascular bands or congenital iliac anomalies (Sogaard, 1983; Tada et al., 1984; Venna et al., 1991; Sayson et al., 1994; Tani, 1995). Abnormal fibrous bands are difficult to diagnose because they elude detection on magnetic resonance imaging. There is insufficient information in the literature regarding magnetic resonance neurographic diagnosis of these lesions, but this new technology can certainly help in the detection of focal constriction of the nerve (Filler et al., 1996; Kuntz et al., 1996; Aagaard et al., 1998; Weig et al., 2000). If all measures fail, surgical exploration of the nerve may be indicated. We have not identified any children with this form of sciatic neuropathy at the Children's Hospital of Boston (Escolar and Jones, 1994); however, in one instance with a negative exploration, we thought the surgeon should have been more aggressive in search of a potential entrapment site. Idiopathic pediatric sciatic neuropathies occasionally occur, defying pathological explanation even after surgical exploration at other centers (Jones et al., 1988; Engstrom et al., 1993; Sawaya, 1999).

TRAUMA

Traumatic sciatic nerve injuries are less common in children, representing only 20% of our series. This contrasts with the Children's Hospital of Boston peroneal neuropathy experience as well as the upper extremity mononeuropathies seen in our EMG laboratory (Deymeer, 1994; Escolar and Jones, 1996). In our series, two children had sciatic nerve lacerations, a third child had a crush injury, and in a fourth instance, an adolescent injured the sciatic nerve in relation to a hip dislocation (Escolar and Jones, 1994). Traumatic dislocation and fracture-dislocation of the hip can cause sciatic nerve injury, with an incidence of 5% in children (Cornwall and Radomisli, 2000). Acute sciatic nerve lacerations, stretch, or compression may occur during hip surgery in children with juvenile rheumatoid arthritis (Cornwall and Radomisli, 2000) or as a result of athletic injuries (Lorei and Hershman, 1993). The latter may lead to sciatic nerve entrapment secondary to heterotopic ossification. Stretch injury of the sciatic nerve also occurs during the repair of open fractures (Cullen et al., 1996). Victims of an earthquake who experienced crush injuries to peripheral nerves, including the sciatic, had a good recovery (Yoshida et al., 1999). In the past, infantile traumatic sciatic nerve injuries occurred more frequently due to breech deliveries, intragluteal injections (Combes and Clark, 1960; Pedrocca et al., 1968; Clark et al., 1970; Merkulov, 1987; MacDonald and Marcuse, 1994; Marcuse and MacDonald, 1996), and toxic injuries during umbilical vessel injections (Fok et al., 1986; Goven'ko and Babin, 1990; Villarejo and Pascual, 1993; de Sanctis et al., 1995). Breech delivery with prolonged labor and forceful extraction resulted in poor prognosis in the infants with complete sciatic palsy (Sriram, 1981).

Neonatal and Prenatal Sciatic Neuropathies

Neonatal sciatic palsies are very rare (Sharrard, 1973; Sriram, 1981; Rombouts et al., 1993; Ramos-

Fernandez et al., 1998). When these perinatal sciatic neuropathies do occur, the causes are usually not self-evident. Careful evaluation is in order, just as noted for the older child. One 3-day-old infant who was seen at the Children's Hospital of Boston developed a sciatic neuropathy secondary to compression after having been given Pavulon (pancuronium bromide) (Jones et al., 1988). A study of 21 neonates with a sciatic neuropathy attempted to define specific perinatal pathophysiological factors, but no mechanism was identified (Ramos-Fernandez et al., 1998). Nevertheless, most infants (16 of 21) had an excellent recovery. The infants who had an incomplete recovery were all delivered by cesarean section (Ramos-Fernandez et al., 1998).

Prenatal sciatic nerve lesions occasionally occur at birth (Sheth et al., 1994; Yilmaz et al., 2000). These have been documented with EMG just as with radial Escolar and Jones, 1994) and peroneal (Jones et al., 1996) intrauterine neuropathies. Prenatal nerve injuries are usually associated with reduced fetal activity, especially when associated with oligohydramnios, abnormal uterine contractions during prolonged labor, amniotic fluid bands, or uterine abnormalities found with Asherman's syndrome (Rombouts et al., 1993; Sheth et al., 1994). One infant had a necrotic ischemic lesion (eschar) on the site of compression as evidence of intrauterine onset (Sheth et al., 1994; Escolar and Jones, 1996). EMG is indicated during the first 1 to 2 days of life; this provides important medicolegal information with documentation of the prenatal onset of the affected nerve (Jones et al., 1996).

Diagnosis

The diagnosis of a sciatic neuropathy in a child initially requires a clinical examination, targeted to exclude pathologies at other sites. However, in an infant, this is problematic; an older child can cooperate enough to allow a meticulous clinical examination. Either EMG or imaging studies are the fundamental diagnostic procedures available to complete the evaluation.

ELECTROMYOGRAPHY

Fifteen of 20 children with sciatic mononeuropathies demonstrated diminished or absent peroneal CMAPs (Escolar and Jones, 1994). The tibial CMAPs were low in amplitude or absent in 12 of the 20 patients, including 6 with lesions in the proximal thigh or sciatic notch. In these children, the H reflex was absent when tested. Sural SNAPs were absent or low in amplitude (10 μV) in all except two children (Escolar and Jones, 1994). The experienced pediatric electromyographer usually finds sural SNAP amplitudes of at least 50 μV in young children. Thus, a 10-μV response represents a response that often is 20% of that of the contralateral normal extremity, providing important information of the postganglionic nature of the nerve injury. Control values useful in the study of pediatric mononeuropathies are often best obtained by testing the unaffected homologous nerve.

In our pediatric population, only 20% of the children had disproportionate peroneal trunk involvement (Escolar and Jones, 1994). The tibial and sural nerves were normal in 12% of the cases (Yuen et al., 1995). This correlates with other reports (Katirji and Wilbourn, 1994; Goh et al., 1996) and confirms the higher susceptibility to injury of the peroneal nerve fibers of the sciatic nerve (Sunderland, 1978). However, in children, the needle examination of paraspinal muscles, normally useful to differentiate a rare pediatric nerve root or other intraspinal lesion from a more peripheral plexus or focal nerve lesion, may be clouded by the child's poor relaxation.

Needle examination requires careful design to localize these rather complicated lesions. Rarely, infants, as well as anxious older children, may require sedation, particularly day surgery anesthesia, to accurately accomplish a sufficiently detailed examination for careful differential diagnosis. Neurogenic changes limited to the peroneal supplied distal muscles and the short head of the biceps femoris help to localize a sciatic neuropathy lesion to the peroneal trunk of the sciatic nerve (Escolar and Jones, 1994; Katirji and Wilbourn, 1994). Evaluation of the short head of the biceps femoris muscle is essential for the differentiation of a proximal sciatic nerve lesion from a peroneal neuropathy. In our experience, only 1 of 20 children with sciatic neuropathy had a pure peroneal involvement. He had an acute compressive lesion at the sciatic notch that resolved spontaneously (Escolar and Jones, 1994). The involvement of both the tibial and peroneal innervated muscles distally in the leg, not involving the short head of the biceps femoris, localizes the lesion to the distal sciatic nerve near the knee. We localized four sciatic neuropathy injuries to the distal thigh (Escolar and Jones, 1994). Involvement of the hamstring muscles, but not the glutei or the vastus lateralis, localizes the lesion to the proximal thigh, as seen in 4 of our 20 patients with sciatic mononeuropathy at the Children's Hospital of Boston (Escolar and Jones, 1994). If the gluteus muscles are involved, the lesion site is either directly at the sciatic notch or proximally; this was found in six children in our series (Escolar and Jones, 1994). The involvement of either femoral or obturator supplied muscles in addition to sciatic innervated muscles points to a lumbosacral plexus lesion, especially if accompanied by abnormal sural and peroneal SNAPs.

NERVE IMAGING STUDIES

Once the lesion has been defined and localized, magnetic resonance neurography or magnetic resonance imaging with contrast medium can be very helpful in disclosing nerve enlargements or compressions by masses or tumors (Tachi et al., 1995; Filler et al., 1996; Kuntz et al., 1996; Aagaard et al.,

1998; Ramos-Fernandez et al., 1998; Uetani et al., 1998; Yokoyama et al., 1998; Almanza et al., 1999; Marom and Helms, 1999; Weig et al., 2000). Due to its large size, the sciatic nerve is one of the best visualized by this technique. However, some lesions that cause sciatic neuropathy are not necessarily visible on magnetic resonance imaging. These sometimes require surgical exploration to define and relieve the problem. These very unusual causes for a childhood sciatic neuropathy include congenital myofascial bands and perineuromas (a focal nerve hypertrophy). With the technical improvement of magnetic resonance neurography and ultrasonography, perineuromas can more likely be diagnosed by experienced radiologists (Emory et al., 1995; Simmons et al., 1999; Martinoli et al., 2000).

Treatment and Prognosis

The prognosis for children with a sciatic neuropathy is guarded, just as it is for adults. In our experience at the Children's Hospital of Boston, the electromyographic findings did not correlate well with the prognosis (Escolar and Jones, 1994). Although normal peroneal and tibial motor CMAPs occurred in some children who had a good recovery, this was not universally the case. The presence or absence of active denervation on needle examination also did not indicate a specific prognosis. In general, the prognosis also had little relationship to the primary pathophysiological mechanism. Seven of 16 children did not improve with long-term follow-up. This also applied to those who underwent both exploratory surgery and nerve repair. At the Children's Hospital of Boston, the outcome for pediatric sciatic neuropathies is worse than that for the other mononeuropathies that occur in children, wherein the prognosis is relatively good for these other more distal, albeit disparate, focal neuropathies (Escolar and Jones, 1994).

In a much larger series of 380 adult and pediatric patients with sciatic neuropathies, surgical repair was performed only in individuals with persistent deficits in the peroneal or tibialis distribution (Kline et al., 1998). Management was guided by nerve action potential recordings that indicated whether neurolysis or resection of the lesion was required. Useful peroneal function was achieved when nerve action potentials were recorded distal to the lesion, but overall improvement for a pediatric sciatic neuropathy was only 36%. The tibialis division was associated with a much better recovery, regardless of the level or mechanism of injury (Kline et al., 1998).

PERONEAL NEUROPATHY

Clinical Manifestations

The clinical manifestations of pediatric peroneal mononeuropathies do not differ from those of adults

(Katirji and Wilbourn, 1988). Their incidence, however, is far less. In a retrospective study of 1463 electromyographic studies the Children's Hospital of Boston pediatric EMG laboratory performed during a 12-year period, only 17 peroneal focal neuropathies were identified (Jones et al., 1993). Despite this seemingly small number, peroneal neuropathies remain one of the most common focal neuropathies in children, second in frequency to sciatic neuropathies (Escolar and Jones, 1994). Children with peroneal mononeuropathies present with weakness and footdrop in the majority of the cases, representing 93% in our experience. Less commonly, pain and paresthesia may occur on the dorsum of the foot in the distribution of the superficial peroneal nerve (Jones et al., 1993).

The site of involvement of focal peroneal neuropathies is similar to that for adults (Katirji and Wilbourn, 1988), being at the fibular head in 94% and at the ankle in 6% in one series (Jones et al., 1993). The common peroneal nerve was affected in 59% of the cases, the deep peroneal nerve was affected in 12%, and the superficial peroneal nerve was affected in 6%. In the remaining 23% in this series, a precise localization was limited by technical factors (Jones et al., 1993).

Etiology

COMPRESSION

Pediatric peroneal neuropathies are in most instances secondary to compression, representing 10 of 17 cases in a pediatric series (Jones et al., 1993). The mode of onset was acute in four patients, yet indeterminate in the other six (Jones et al., 1993). Half of the compressive pediatric peroneal mononeuropathies were iatrogenic, caused by casts, Buck's traction, Velcro straps, and intravenous footboard tape in a newborn.

Three girls with anorexia nervosa had compression at the fibular head due to severe weight loss (Jones et al., 1993). This type of peroneal neuropathy, or "slimmer's palsy," has been well characterized in the adult and adolescent population (Sotaniemi, 1984; Cruz Martinez, 1987; Streib, 1993; Constanty et al., 2000; Cruz Martinez et al., 2000). Nerve conduction studies in most of these lesions show conduction block at the fibular head, and the degree of conduction block correlates with clinical weakness (Cruz Martinez, 1987; Jones et al., 1993; Cruz Martinez et al., 2000). A controversy exists regarding the metabolic versus compressive nature of these neuropathies; however, the reports in favor of the first failed to document peroneal nerve conduction values across the fibular head, so the evaluation of a focal nerve injury is not possible (Sherman and Easton, 1977; Sotaniemi, 1984). A pure demyelinating lesion was documented in a child who woke up with a footdrop and had a rapid resolution of symptoms (Jones et al., 1993), but no conduction block could be found. In this and the cases associated with severe weight loss, the clinician should always exclude an underlying peripheral neuropathy, although this association is less common in children than in adults. Sotaniemi (1984) reported a child with slimmer's palsy who also had a polyneuropathy secondary to thiamin deficiency. Peroneal palsy can also be the first manifestation of a peripheral neuropathy in diabetic children (Lawrence and Locke, 1963; Barkai et al., 1998; el Bahri-Ben et al., 2000) and neuropathy with hereditary liability to pressure palsy (Mouton et al., 1999; Cruz Martinez et al., 2000). The presence of underlying hereditary liability to pressure palsy, however, would more likely lead to recurrent mononeuropathies or plexopathy than to isolated peroneal mononeuropathies (Pareyson et al., 1998).

Multiple case reports in the literature expand the compressive pediatric peroneal mononeuropathy etiologies.

Compression of the peroneal nerve by synovial cysts, intraneural ganglion cysts, and a ganglion in the anterior compartment of the leg have all been reported (Gurdjian et al., 1965; Nucci et al., 1990; Antonini et al., 1991; Martins et al., 1997; Gayer et al., 1998; Uetani et al., 1998), often presenting with a painful footdrop (Nicholson et al., 1995). An unusual clinical presentation of an intraneural peroneal cyst was described in a 15-year-old girl who had a fluctuating footdrop worsen by sporting activities (Aulisa et al., 1998). Another possible presentation of such pathology was reported in a 3-year-old child with "in-toeing" caused by a ganglion cyst over the fibula head (Beck et al., 1998).

Chronic leg crossing (Wilburn et al., 1990) and prolonged compression during water skiing on a kneeboard (Vaccaro et al., 1998) have been documented etiologies of pediatric peroneal mononeuropathies. Spontaneous nontraumatic anterior tibial compartment syndrome caused a transient deep peroneal neuropathy in an adolescent girl (Sloane et al., 1994). In a girl aged 2½ years, a common peroneal neuropathy developed as a complication of anaphylactoid purpura with knee joint swelling (Ritter et al., 1983).

ENTRAPMENT

Less commonly, as in adults, a child presents with chronic progressive footdrop, repeated ankle sprains secondary to peroneal muscle weakness, or a cavus foot deformity due to entrapment of the common or deep peroneal nerve. The causes of entrapment reported in children include bony exostoses at the fibular head (Levin et al., 1991) and talotibial exostosis (Edlich et al., 1987) deriving from osteochondromas. Another proximal site of entrapment of the common peroneal nerve is at the splitting of the tendinous arch of origin of the peroneus longus muscle at the fibula (Sidi, 1969). These and myofascial bands that arise from the same muscle and entrap the peroneal nerve can be difficult to diagnose (Jones et al., 1993). Although computed tomography scanning and magnetic resonance imaging can assist in uncovering the pathology, on occasion these lesions can be diagnosed only through surgical exploration (Edlich et al., 1987; Jones et al., 1993; Levin et al., 1991).

The superficial peroneal nerve can be affected as a result of entrapment by scarring due to repetitive ankle sprain (Daghino et al., 1997). Magnetic resonance imaging can help make the diagnosis, and limited fasciectomy relieves the symptoms (Daghino et al., 1997; Styf and Morberg, 1997). Another site of entrapment is at the fascia where the superficial peroneal nerve leaves the lateral compartment (McAuliffe et al., 1985).

TUMORS

Occult nerve tumors can present with protracted symptoms of common, superficial, or deep peroneal neuropathy. A child with a schwannoma of the superficial peroneal nerve presented with chronic paresthesias of the calf and toes for 1 year, until diagnosis was made at surgical exploration (Jones et al., 1993). Other rare nerve tumors include hemangiomas (Bilge et al., 1989).

Localized hypertrophic neuropathy or intraneural perineuromas have been documented to cause pediatric peroneal mononeuropathies (Johnson and Kline, 1989; Emory et al., 1995). This benign condition was very difficult to diagnose in the past, frequently requiring surgical exploration (Jones et al., 1993). However, magnetic resonance neurography has improved the diagnosis of nerve tumors and made possible localization of the lesion before surgery (Emory et al., 1995; Housahian and Freund, 1999; Simmons et al., 1999; Weig et al., 2000).

TRAUMATIC PEDIATRIC PERONEAL MONONEUROPATHIES

Trauma to the peroneal nerve occurs less frequently. The series of Jones and colleagues (1993) included three traumatic pediatric peroneal mononeuropathies. Laceration of the deep peroneal nerve at the fibula head occurred in one child. Shevell and Stewart (1988) reported a similar injury in an adolescent who lacerated the nerve with a skate blade. Another child experienced a traumatic pediatric peroneal mononeuropathy during a motor vehicle accident (Jones et al., 1993), and a third child experienced a traumatic pediatric peroneal mononeuropathy during repetitive blunt trauma during martial arts (Jones et al., 1993). Similar traumatic injuries have been reported as a result of surfing (Watemberg et al., 2000).

SYSTEMIC AND IDIOPATHIC

Peroneal neuropathy in children can rarely be the presenting sign of a systemic disease, as discussed previously with diabetic neuropathy or hereditary liability to pressure palsy (Lawrence and Locke, 1963; Kruger et al., 1987; Gabreels-Festen et al., 1992; Barkai et al., 1998; Pareyson et al., 1998; Mouton et al., 1999; el Bahri-Ben et al., 2000). Leprosy involving the peroneal nerve, common in other countries, was reported in an immigrant boy from Vietnam who presented with a 1-year history of unilateral footdrop (Choe, 1994). In some children, the cause of pediatric peroneal mononeuropathies, as in pediatric sciatic mononeuropathy, remains unknown despite surgical exploration and pathological analysis of the nerve (Engstrom et al., 1993).

NEONATAL AND CONGENITAL PEDIATRIC PERONEAL MONONEUROPATHIES

Iatrogenic compression of the peroneal nerve in newborns has been reported to result from intravenous fluid infiltration (Kreusser and Volpe, 1984) and compression by tape used to secure a footboard (Fischer and Strasburger, 1982; Jones et al., 1993).

Peroneal neuropathy has also been documented in newborns with a possible antenatal onset (Crumrine et al., 1975; Jones et al., 1996; Godley, 1998; Yilmaz et al., 2000). The cause in these children is unclear, but the rapid and complete recovery in most of them points to a neurapraxic lesion. Two of the infants had abnormal intrauterine positions with a breech presentation, and a stretching mechanism was postulated (Crumrine et al., 1975; Godley, 1998; Yilmaz et al., 2000). In other infants, uterine contraction rings might have caused a compressive lesion with axonal injury, as demonstrated by the presence of fibrillation potentials 18 hours after delivery (Jones et al., 1996). The early electromyographic evaluation of this infant demonstrated the antenatal onset of the injury. The role of early electromyographic evaluation in newborns with mononeuropathies remains to be determined, but early electrophysiological testing can clearly differentiate an antenatal onset from a trauma on delivery, with its obvious legal implications.

Diagnosis

ELECTRODIAGNOSTIC STUDIES

The diagnosis of a pediatric peroneal neuropathy relies heavily on electromyographic studies. The nerve conduction evaluation is similar to that in adults and should include evaluation of the superficial and motor peroneal nerves, sural nerve, and posterior tibialis nerves. In a pediatric series, peroneal CMAP was reduced in amplitude in 60% and was normal on 40%; the latter included four of five children with conduction block at the fibular head (Jones et al., 1993). Two of 17 children had absent peroneal CMAP when recorded distally on the extensor digiti brevis (EDB) muscle, but a tibialis anterior response was evoked in both (Jones et al., 1993). Conduction block at the fibular head was present in

5 of 17 children: 3 associated with anorexia nervosa, 1 associated with a cast, and 1 associated with bony exostosis (Jones et al., 1993). Conduction block at the fibula head is not common in pediatric peroneal mononeuropathies, contrasting with the adult peroneal neuropathies, in which this is found in 45% of the patients (Katirji and Wilbourn, 1988). Like in adults, when a peroneal CMAP is not obtainable from distal muscles (EDB), attempts to record a CMAP from the tibialis anterior or peroneus longus should be done, because it might show a conduction block or conduction slowing at the fibular head (Sourkes and Stewart, 1991).

The peroneal superficialis SNAP was tested in 6 of 17 children in the series of Jones and associates (1993) and found to be absent in 2. Sensory deficits vary in common peroneal neuropathies according to the degree of involvement of the different fascicles of the nerve (Sourkes and Stewart, 1991), so peroneal superficialis could be present even in common peroneal nerve injuries. Sural responses should be normal in peroneal neuropathies, and this was the case in all pediatric peroneal mononeuropathies in this series (Jones et al., 1993).

Needle evaluation performed in the pediatric sciatic mononeuropathy series showed axonal changes in 88% of the patients, with the most severe changes in the deep peroneal innervated muscles (Jones et al., 1993), as have been shown in other studies (Sourkes and Stewart, 1991). It is essential on the needle examination of a child with a presumptive peroneal neuropathy to evaluated tibialis innervated muscles as well as the short head of the biceps femoris. This muscle was studied in 10 of 17 children with pediatric peroneal mononeuropathies and found to be normal in all (Jones et al., 1993). As discussed for pediatric sciatic mononeuropathy, lesions of the peroneal trunk of the sciatic nerve are not uncommon and can present clinically as a peroneal neuropathy. Because sciatic neuropathies are more common than peroneal neuropathies in children, even the anxious child should have evaluation of at least this proximal muscle.

NERVE IMAGING STUDIES

Imaging studies of the affected limb have revolutionized the diagnosis and management of young patients with progressive mononeuropathies of unknown cause. Magnetic resonance imaging can assist in identifying the etiology of the nerve injury and can guide the management options, including surgery. Magnetic resonance imaging of the limbs can identify ganglion cysts (Nucci et al., 1990; Uetani et al., 1998), tumors (Loredo et al., 1998; Weig et al., 2000), large neuromas, and rarer entities, such as localized hypertrophic mononeuropathy or perineuromas (Emory et al., 1995; Simmons et al., 1999). In the absence of clear pathology, more sophisticated technology, such as magnetic resonance neurography, can add in identifying abnormal signals on the nerve and might help to localize the site of nerve

injury and to reduce nerve exposure during surgery (Kuntz et al., 1996; Aagaard et al., 1998; Weig et al., 2000). This technique can also distinguish intraneural from extraneural masses and can detect discontinuity at the fascicular level in traumatic injuries, verifying the need for surgical repair (Filler et al., 1996).

With improvements in ultrasound equipment, ultrasonography adds to the imaging diagnostic techniques for evaluation of peripheral nerves, helping in pathology localization and characterization. Normal nerve morphology has been characterized with ultrasonography (Silvestri et al., 1995), as well as other pathological conditions, including nerve tumors (Martinoli et al., 2000), traumatic injuries, nerve entrapments (Martinoli et al., 2000), intraneural mucous cysts (Marchiodi et al., 1994; Aulisa et al., 1998), and nerve inflammation (Taniguchi et al., 2000).

Treatment and Prognosis

The prognosis of peroneal mononeuropathies varies. In series from the Children's Hospital of Boston, 13 of 17 patients had complete or significant improvement (Jones et al., 1993). The mechanisms for the four patients who had poor recovery included two blunt traumas, one perioperative lesion, and one entrapment lesion in which the surgical release was delayed (Jones et al., 1993).

EMG results might provide useful prognostic information, because absent or low-amplitude CMAP was related to unfavorable outcome (Jones et al., 1993). The best prognosis was in children with conduction block at the fibula head (Jones et al., 1993). Skillful primary repair of peripheral nerves in children is often followed by significant recovery (Birch and Achan, 2000). Near-nerve intraoperative recording can help to detect early nerve injury and avoid more severe damage during surgery (Wexler et al., 1998). As in the adult population (Piton et al., 1997; Fabre et al., 1998), surgery for peroneal neuropathies that fail to improve by 3 to 4 months appears to be more successful if performed early. The most significant variable in determining the results of surgery is delay in repair (Birch and Achan, 2000).

When improvement is not achieved despite surgical release or decompression of the nerve, a tendon transfer operation can reestablish functional foot dorsiflexion and enable the child to have a normal gait (Breukink et al., 2000).

FEMORAL NEUROPATHY

Clinical Manifestations

Femoral neuropathies are extremely rare in children. In a retrospective study at the Children's Hospital of Boston, only three children were diagnosed in a period of 16 years. These were the result of postoperative lesions in two, with one patient undergoing a posterior iliac osteotomy and the other a complication of a lower extremity stretch procedure (D. Escolar, unpublished data). In a teenaged girl who was reported to have intermittent thigh cramping related to exercise and muscle atrophy, EMG was used to diagnose an isolated femoral neuropathy to the vastus lateralis muscle of unidentified etiology despite surgical exploration and imaging studies (Carter et al., 1995). Children with similar idiopathic progressive mononeuropathies of the lower extremity were described by Engstrom and associates (1993).

Perineuromas or localized hypertrophic mononeuropathy affecting the femoral nerve has been identified by magnetic resonance imaging in children presenting with isolated femoral neuropathy (Emory et al., 1995; Takao et al., 1999).

Intraneural hematomas or iliopsoas muscle hematomas in hemophilic patients can cause external compression of the femoral nerve. This nerve was the one most commonly affected in a retrospective study of neurological complications in hemophiliacs, including children (Ehrmann et al., 1981). Neurofibromas of the femoral nerve have been reported in two children presenting with progressive thigh pain and weakness (Sharma, 1988).

Diagnosis: Electrodiagnostic Studies

EMG is extremely useful to localize these symptoms to the femoral nerve and differentiate from a plexopathy or an intraspinal lesion. Children with symptoms of pain and weakness in the quadriceps muscle have to undergo a complete evaluation to rule out intraspinal processes causing an upper lumbar polyradiculopathy, which would be more common than an isolated mononeuropathy. At Children's National Medical Center, in Washington, DC, four children were referred over a period of 7 years for pain, cramping, or weakness focally on the thigh. None of these children had a femoral neuropathy. One child had acute onset of lumbar radiculopathy as the first manifestation of Lyme disease, another had a transverse myelitis with asymmetrical onset of symptoms, and a third teenaged girl had idiopathic cramping. A fourth adolescent girl was referred for evaluation of progressive unilateral quadriceps weakness. On examination, this girl had clear characteristics of fascioscapulohumeral muscular dystrophy (present but undiagnosed in the family) and was not brought to medical attention until she had a rapid weakening of the right thigh muscle over a period of 3 months (D. Escolar, unpublished data). This stepwise deterioration is characteristic of facioscapulohumeral muscular dystrophy. The EMG showed clear myopathic motor unit potentials.

Nerve conduction studies of the femoral nerve, stimulating at the groin and recording from the vastus lateralis or rectus femoris, can give useful information only if compared with the unaffected side, because normal CMAP amplitude values for children are not determined for this nerve. It is also possible to record a sensory nerve action potential from the lateral femorocutaneous nerve, as it is done in adults. However, needle examination is the most useful tool to determine axonal damage and rule out obturator involvement, which would be suggestive of a lumbar plexopathy.

OTHER LOWER EXTREMITY MONONEUROPATHIES

Lateral Femorocutaneous Nerve of the Thigh

An extremely rare neuropathy in children, this has been observed as an idiopathic lesion (H. R. Jones, unpublished information), caused by compression with an orthopedic harness (Ouvrier, 1990) and by sports injuries, either by direct blunt trauma to the thigh in high-energy sports (Lorei and Hershman, 1993) or in female gymnasts due to the repetitive impact on the thigh by the uneven bars (Macgregor and Moncur, 1977). Its clinical manifestations are similar to those of adults, with numbness in the lateral thigh, or pain in the same area.

It is possible to obtain conduction studies of the femorocutaneous nerve in the thigh, but the absence of the response is only significant when unilateral in the symptomatic side. Diagnosis can also be made by local anesthetic nerve block.

Sural Neuropathy

Sural mononeuropathies in adults or children are extremely uncommon. We have not had any instances at Children's National Medical Center or the Children's Hospital of Boston.

A sural neuropathy in a girl caused by a tight ankle bracelet with complete resolution over 1 month is the only pediatric report (Reisin et al., 1994). Sural nerve entrapment in athletes presenting with chronic calf pain exacerbated by physical exertion has been reported, but there were no children or adolescents in these series (Husson et al., 1989; Fabre et al., 2000). The sural neuropathy is confirmed with nerve conduction studies, and the nerve is found entrapped on its passage through the superficial sural aponeurosis (Fabre et al., 2000).

Tibial Neuropathy

Tibial mononeuropathies are rare, but the tibial nerve can be concomitantly affected with the peroneal nerve at the popliteal fossa. One report of tarsal tunnel syndrome in girls with foot pain was not confirmed by nerve conduction studies or EMG (Albrektsson et al., 1982).

References

Aagaard BD, Maravilla KR, Kliot M: MR neurography: MR imaging of peripheral nerves. Magn Reson Imaging Clin North Am 1998; 6:179–194.

Albrektsson B, Rydholm A, Rydholm U: The tarsal tunnel syndrome in children. J Bone Joint Surg Br 1982;64:215–217.

Almanza MY, Poon-Chue A, Terk MR: Dual oblique MR method for imaging the sciatic nerve. J Comput Assist Tomogr 1999; 23:138–140.

Antonini G, Bastianello S, Nucci F, et al: Ganglion of deep peroneal nerve: Electrophysiology and CT scan in the diagnosis. Electromyogr Clin Neurophysiol 1991;31:9–13.

Aulisa L, Tamburrelli F, Padua R, et al: Intraneural cyst of the peroneal nerve. Childs Nerv Syst 1998;14:222–225.

Barber K, Bianco A, Soule E, MacCarty C: Benign extraneural soft-tissue tumors of the extremities causing compression of the nerves. J Bone Joint Surg Am 1962;44:98–104.

Barkai L, Kempler P, Vamosi I, et al: Peripheral sensory nerve dysfunction in children and adolescents with type 1 diabetes mellitus. Diabet Med 1998;15:228–233.

Bassett GS, Monforte-Munoz H, Mitchell WG, Rowland JM: Cavus deformity of the foot secondary to a neuromuscular choristoma (hamartoma) of the sciatic nerve: A case report. J Bone Joint Surg Am 1997;79:1398–1401.

Beck TD Jr, Miller KE, Kruse RW: An unusual presentation of intoeing in a child. J Am Osteopath Assoc 1998;98:48–50.

Benyahya E, Etaouil N, Janani S, et al: Sciatica as the first manifestation of a leiomyosarcoma of the buttock. Rev Rhum Engl Ed 1997;64:135–137.

Bhatia M, Jindal AK: Injection induced nerve injury: An iatrogenic tragedy. J Assoc Physicians India 1996;44:532–533.

Bickels J, Kahanovitz N, Rubert CK, et al: Extraspinal bone and soft-tissue tumors as a cause of sciatica. Clinical diagnosis and recommendations: Analysis of 32 cases. Spine 1999;24: 1611–1616.

Bilge T, Kaya A, Alatli M, et al: Hemangioma of the peroneal nerve: Case report and review of the literature. Neurosurgery 1989; 25:649–652.

Birch R, Achan P: Peripheral nerve repairs and their results in children. Hand Clin 2000;16:579–595.

Bodack MP, Cole JC, Nagler W: Sciatic neuropathy secondary to a uterine fibroid: A case report. Am J Phys Med Rehabil 1999; 78:157–159.

Breukink SO, Spronk CA, Dijkstra PU, et al: [Transposition of the tendon of M. tibialis posterior an effective treatment of drop foot; retrospective study with follow-up in 12 patients.] Ned Tijdschr Geneeskd 2000;144:604–608.

Brown JA, Braun MA, Namey TC: Pyriformis syndrome in a 10-year-old boy as a complication of operation with the patient in the sitting position. Neurosurgery 1988;23:117–119.

Burkhart F, Daly J: Sciatic and peroneal nerve injury: A complication of vaginal operations. Obstet Gynecol 1966;28:99–102.

Carter GT, McDonald CM, Chan TT, Margherita AJ: Isolated femoral mononeuropathy to the vastus lateralis: EMG and magnetic resonance imaging findings. Muscle Nerve 1995;18:341–344.

Choe W: Leprosy presenting as unilateral footdrop in an immigrant boy. Postgrad Med J 1994;70:111–112.

Clark K, Williams PE, Willis W, McGavran WL III: Injection injury of the sciatic nerve. Clin Neurosurg 1970;17:111–125.

Combes M, Clark W: Sciatic nerve injury following intragluteal injection: Pathogenesis and prevention. Am J Dis Child 1960; 100:579.

Constanty A, Vodoff MV, Gilbert B, et al: [Peroneal nerve palsy in anorexia nervosa: Three cases.] Arch Pediatr 2000;7:316–317.

Cornwall R, Radomisli TE: Nerve injury in traumatic dislocation of the hip. Clin Orthop 2000;381:84–91.

Cruccetti A, Kiely EM, Spitz L, et al: Pelvic neuroblastoma: Low mortality and high morbidity. J Pediatr Surg 2000;35:724–728.

Crumrine PK, Koenigsberger MR, Chutorian AM: Footdrop in the neonate with neurologic and electrophysiologic data. J Pediatr 1975;86:779–780.

Cruz Martinez A: Slimmer's paralysis: Electrophysiological evidence of compressive lesion. Eur Neurol 1987;26:189–192.

Cruz-Martinez A, Arpa J, Palau F: Peroneal neuropathy after weight loss. J Peripher Nerv Syst 2000;5:101–105.

Cullen MC, Roy DR, Crawford AH, et al: Open fracture of the tibia in children. J Bone Joint Surg Am 1996;78:1039–1047.

Daghino W, Pasquali M, Faletti C: Superficial peroneal nerve entrapment in a young athlete: The diagnostic contribution of magnetic resonance imaging. J Foot Ankle Surg 1997;36:170–172.

David W, Jones H: Soft tissue sarcoma presenting as atypical extremity pain. Muscle Nerve 1994;17:1071–1072.

de Sanctis N, Cardillo G, Nunziata Rega A: Gluteoperineal gangrene and sciatic nerve palsy after umbilical vessel injection. Clin Orthop 1995;321:180–184.

Deverell WF, Ferguson JH: An unusual case of sciatic nerve paralysis. JAMA 1968;205:699–700.

Deymeer F, Jones HR: Pediatric median mononeuropathies: A clinical and electromyographic study. Muscle Nerve 1994;17: 755–762.

Dhote R, Tudoret L, Bachmeyer C, et al: Cyclic sciatica: A manifestation of compression of the sciatic nerve by endometriosis. A case report. Spine 1996;21:2277–2279.

Dorfman LJ, Ransom BR, Forno LS, Kelts A: Neuropathy in the hypereosinophilic syndrome. Muscle Nerve 1983;6:291–298.

Edlich HS, Fariss BL, Phillips VA, et al: Talotibial exostoses with entrapment of the deep peroneal nerve. J Emerg Med 1987; 5:109–113.

Ehrmann L, Lechner K, Mamoli B, et al: Peripheral nerve lesions in haemophilia. J Neurol 1981;225:175–182.

el Bahri-Ben Mrad F, Gouider R, Fredj M, et al: Childhood diabetic neuropathy: A clinical and electrophysiological study. Funct Neurol 2000;15:35–40.

Emory TS, Scheithauer BW, Hirose T, et al: Intraneural perineurioma: A clonal neoplasm associated with abnormalities of chromosome Am J Clin Pathol 1995;103:696–704.

Engstrom JW, Layzer RB, Olney RK, Edwards MB: Idiopathic, progressive mononeuropathy in young people. Arch Neurol 1993;50:20–23.

Escolar DM, Jones HR: Pediatric radial mononeuropathies: A clinical and electromyographic study of sixteen children with review of the literature. Muscle Nerve 1996;19:876–883.

Escolar DM, Jones HR: Pediatric sciatic mononeuropathies: A clinical and electromyographic analysis [abstract]. Muscle Nerve 1994;17:108.

Fabre T, Montero C, Gaujard E, et al: Chronic calf pain in athletes due to sural nerve entrapment: A report of 18 cases. Am J Sports Med 2000;28:679–682.

Fabre T, Piton C, Andre D, et al: Peroneal nerve entrapment. J Bone Joint Surg Am 1998;80:47–53.

Favier T, Menei P, Rizk T, et al: Osteosarcoma of the sacrum: Apropos of a case in a 14 year old girl. Rev Rhum Ed Fr 1993; 60:365–366.

Filler AG, Kliot M, Howe FA, et al: Application of magnetic resonance neurography in the evaluation of patients with peripheral nerve pathology. J Neurosurg 1996;85:299–309.

Fischer AQ, Strasburger J: Footdrop in the neonate secondary to use of footboards. J Pediatr 1982;101:1003–1004.

Fok TF, Ha MH, Leung KW, Wong W: Sciatic nerve palsy complicating umbilical arterial catheterization. Eur J Pediatr 1986;145: 308–309.

Gabreels-Festen AA, Gabreels FJ, Joosten EM, et al: Hereditary neuropathy with liability to pressure palsies in childhood. Neuropediatrics 1992;23:138–143.

Gasecki AP, Ebers GC, Vellet AD, Buchan A: Sciatic neuropathy associated with persistent sciatic artery. Arch Neurol 1992; 49:967–968.

Gayet LE, Morand F, Goujon JM, et al: Compression of the peroneal nerve by a cyst in a seven-year-old child. Eur J Pediatr Surg 1998;8:61–63.

Gelain A, Formica C, Segantini L: von Recklinghausen's neurofibromatosis: Case report with extensive involvement of the sciatic nerve. Ital J Orthop Traumatol 1988;14:529–532.

Godley DR: Neonatal peroneal neurapraxia: A report of two cases and review of the literature. Am J Orthop 1998;27:803–804.

Goh KJ, Tan CB, Tjia HT: Sciatic neuropathies—a retrospective review of electrodiagnostic features in 29 patients. Ann Acad Med Singapore 1996;25:566–569.

Gominak SC, Ochoa JL: Sciatic schwannoma of the thigh causing foot pain mimicking plantar neuropathy. Muscle Nerve 1998; 21:528–530.

Goven'ko FS, Babin AV: [Lesions of the sciatic nerve in newborn infants after administration of various drugs into the umbilical arteries.] Akush Ginekol (Mosk) 1990;5:61–63.

Gozal Y, Pomeranz S: Sciatic nerve palsy as a complication after acoustic neurinoma resection in the sitting position. J Neurosurg Anesthesiol 1994;6:40–42.

Gurdjian ES, Larsen RD, Lindner DW: Intraneural cyst of the peroneal and ulnar nerves: Report of two cases. J Neurosurg 1965;23:76–78.

Houshian S, Freund KG: Gigantic benign schwannoma in the lateral peroneal nerve. Am J Knee Surg 1999;12:41–42.

Hruban RH, Shiu MH, Senie RT, Woodruff JM: Malignant peripheral nerve sheath tumors of the buttock and lower extremity: A study of 43 cases. Cancer 1990;66:1253–1265.

Husson JL, Mathieu M, Briand B, et al: [Syndrome of compression of the external saphenous nerve (or the sural nerve).] Acta Orthop Belg 1989;55:491–497.

Jellis JE, Helal B: Childhood sciatic palsies: Congenital and traumatic. Proc R Soc Med 1970;63:655–656.

Johnson PC, Kline DG: Localized hypertrophic neuropathy: Possible focal perineurial barrier defect. Acta Neuropathol 1989; 77:514–518.

Jones H: Mononeuropathies of infancy and childhood. Clin Neurophysiol 2000;53:396–407.

Jones HR, Felice KJ, Gross PT: Pediatric peroneal mononeuropathy: A clinical and electromyographic study. Muscle Nerve 1993;16:1167–1173.

Jones HR, Gianturco LE, Gross PT, Buchhalter J: Sciatic neuropathies in childhood: A report of ten cases and review of the literature. J Child Neurol 1988;3:193–199.

Jones HR, Herbison GJ, Jacobs SR, et al: Intrauterine onset of a mononeuropathy: Peroneal neuropathy in a newborn with electromyographic findings at age one day compatible with prenatal onset. Muscle Nerve 1996;19:88–91.

Katirji B, Wilbourn AJ: High sciatic lesion mimicking peroneal neuropathy at the fibular head. J Neurol Sci 1994;121:172–175.

Katirji MB, Wilbourn AJ: Common peroneal mononeuropathy: A clinical and electrophysiologic study of 116 lesions. Neurology 1988;38:1723–1728.

Kline DG, Kim D, Midha R, et al: Management and results of sciatic nerve injuries: A 24-year experience. J Neurosurg 1998; 89:13–23.

Kreusser KL, Volpe JJ: Peroneal palsy produced by intravenous fluid infiltration in a newborn. Dev Med Child Neurol 1984; 26:522–524.

Kruger M, Brunko E, Dorchy H, Noel P: Femoral versus peroneal neuropathy in diabetic children and adolescents—relationships to clinical status, metabolic control and retinopathy. Diabetes Metab 1987;13:110–115.

Kubiak R, Wilcox DT, Spitz L, Kiely EM: Neurovascular morbidity from the lithotomy position. J Pediatr Surg 1998;33:1808–1810.

Kuntz C, Blake L, Britz G, et al: Magnetic resonance neurography of peripheral nerve lesions in the lower extremity. Neurosurgery 1996;39:750–756; discussion 756–757.

Lawrence D, Locke S: Neuropathy in children with diabetes mellitus. Br Med J 1963;5333:784–785.

Lee R, Fann AV, Sobus K: Bilateral sciatic nerve entrapment due to weight loss. J Ark Med Soc 1998;95:153–155.

Lester P, McAlister W: Congenital iliac anomaly with sciatic palsy. Radiology 1970;96:397–399.

Levin KH, Wilbourn AJ, Jones HR: Childhood peroneal neuropathy from bone tumors. Pediatr Neurol 1991;7:308–309.

London N, Sefton G: Hematocolpos: An unusual cause of sciatica in an adolescent girl. Spine 1996;21:1381–1382.

Loredo R, Hodler J, Pedowitz R, et al: MRI of the common peroneal nerve: Normal anatomy and evaluation of masses associated with nerve entrapment. J Comput Assist Tomogr 1998; 22:925–931.

Lorei MP, Hershman EB: Peripheral nerve injuries in athletes. Treatment and prevention. Sports Med 1993;16:130–147.

MacDonald NE, Marcuse EK: Neurologic injury after vaccination: Buttocks as injection site. CMAJ 1994;150:326.

Macgregor J, Moncur JA: Meralgia paraesthetica—a sports lesion in girl gymnasts. Br J Sports Med 1977;11:16–19.

Marchiodi L, Mignani G, Stilli S: Mucous cysts of the external popliteal sciatic nerve during childhood: Presentation of two cases and a review of the literature. Chir Organi Mov 1994; 79:175–179.

Marcuse EK, MacDonald NE: Neurologic injury after vaccination in buttocks. CMAJ 1996;155:374.

Marom EM, Helms CA: Fibrolipomatous hamartoma: Pathognomonic on MR imaging. Skeletal Radiol 1999;28:260–264.

Martinoli C, Bianchi S, Derchi L: Ultrasonography of peripheral nerves. Semin Ultrasound CT MR 2000;21:205–213.

Martins RS, Martinez J, de Aguiar PH, et al: [Intraneural synovial cyst of the peroneal nerve. Case report.] Arq Neuropsiquiatr 1997;55:831–833.

McAuliffe T, Fiddian N, Browett J: Entrapment neuropathy of the superficial peroneal nerve: A bilateral case. J Bone Joint Surg Am 1985;67:62–63.

Merkulov VN: [Sciatic nerve injuries in children as a complication of intramuscular injections.] Feldsher Akush 1987;52:21–24.

Misdraji J, Ino Y, Louis DN, et al: Primary lymphoma of peripheral nerve: Report of four cases. Am J Surg Pathol 2000;24:1257–1265.

Mouton P, Tardieu S, Gouider R, et al: Spectrum of clinical and electrophysiologic features in HNPP patients with the 17p11.2 deletion. Neurology 1999;52:1440–1446.

Nicholson TR, Cohen RC, Grattan-Smith PJ: Intraneural ganglion of the common peroneal nerve in a 4-year-old boy. J Child Neurol 1995;10:213–215.

Nucci F, Artico M, Santoro A, et al: Intraneural synovial cyst of the peroneal nerve: Report of two cases and review of the literature. Neurosurgery 1990;26:339–344.

Oberle J, Kahamba J, Richter HP: Peripheral nerve schwannomas—an analysis of 16 patients. Acta Neurochir 1997; 139:949–953.

Ouvrier RA, McLeod JG, Pollard JD: Peripheral Neuropathy in Childhood. New York, Raven Press, 1990.

Pareyson D, Solari A, Taroni F, et al: Detection of hereditary neuropathy with liability to pressure palsies among patients with acute painless mononeuropathy or plexopathy. Muscle Nerve 1998;21:1686–1691.

Pedrocca A, Nicosia U, De Guidi G: [Neonatal paralysis of the sciatic nerve caused by intragluteal injections.] Minerva Pediatr 1968;20:818–825.

Piton C, Fabre T, Lasseur E, et al: [Common fibular nerve lesions. Etiology and treatment: Apropos of 146 cases with surgical treatment.] Rev Chir Orthop Reparatrice Appar Mot 1997;83: 515–521.

Quinones-Hinojosa A, Friedlander RM, Boyer PJ, et al: Solitary sciatic nerve lymphoma as an initial manifestation of diffuse neurolymphomatosis: Case report and review of the literature. J Neurosurg 2000;92:165–169.

Ramos-Fernandez JM, Oliete-Garcia FM, Roldan-Aparicio S, et al: [Neonatal sciatic palsy: etiology and outcome of 21 cases.] Rev Neurol 1998;26:752–755.

Reisin R, Pardal A, Ruggieri V, Gold L: Sural neuropathy due to external pressure: Report of three cases. Neurology 1994;44: 2408–2409.

Ritter FJ, Seay AR, Lahey ME: Peripheral mononeuropathy complicating anaphylactoid purpura. J Pediatr 1983;103:77–78.

Rombouts JJ, Debauche C, Verellen G, Lyon G: [Congenital paralysis due to compression: Apropos of 4 cases.] Ann Chir Main Memb Super 1993;12:39–44.

Romfh JH, Currier RD: Sciatic neuropathy induced by the lithotomy position. Arch Neurol 1983;40:127.

Roncaroli F, Poppi M, Riccioni L, Frank F: Primary non-Hodgkin's lymphoma of the sciatic nerve followed by localization in the central nervous system: Case report and review of the literature. Neurosurgery 1997;40:618–621; discussion, 621–622.

Sawaya RA: Idiopathic sciatic mononeuropathy. Clin Neurol Neurosurg 1999;101:256–259.

Sayson SC, Ducey JP, Maybrey JB, et al: Sciatic entrapment neuropathy associated with an anomalous piriformis muscle. Pain 1994;59:149–152.

Schneegans E, Amar G, Isch C, Schneegans D: [Sciatic nerve

paralysis in newborn and premature infants.] Therapeutique 1969;45:382–388.

Schneegans E, Amar G, Isch C, Schneegans D: [Sciatic paralysis of newborn and premature infants.] Ann Pediatr (Paris) 1968; 15:657–663.

Sharma SC, Ray RC: Femoral pain of solitary neurofibromatous origin. Indian Pediatr 1988;12:1221–1223.

Sharrard WJ: Neonatal sciatic paralysis (two cases). Proc R Soc Med 1973;66:218–219.

Sherman D, Easton J: Dieting and peroneal nerve palsy. JAMA 1977;238:230–231.

Sheth D, Gutmann L, Blumenthal DT, et al: Compressive sciatic neuropathy due to uterine abnormality. Muscle Nerve 1994;17: 1486–1488.

Shevell MI, Stewart JD: Laceration of the common peroneal nerve by a skate blade. CMAJ 1988;139:311–312.

Sidi J: Weak ankles: A study of common peroneal entrapment neuropathy. Br Med J 1969;3:623–626.

Silvestri E, Martinoli C, Derchi LE, et al: Echotexture of peripheral nerves: Correlation between US and histologic findings and criteria to differentiate tendons. Radiology 1995;197:291–296.

Simmons Z, Mahadeen ZI, Kothari MJ, et al: Localized hypertrophic neuropathy: Magnetic resonance imaging findings and long-term follow-up. Muscle Nerve 1999;22:28–36.

Sloane AE, Vajsar J, Laxer RM, et al: Spontaneous non-traumatic anterior compartment syndrome with peroneal neuropathy and favorable outcome. Neuropediatrics 1994;25:268–270.

Sogaard I: Sciatic nerve entrapment: Case report. J Neurosurg 1983;58:275–276.

Sotaniemi KA: Slimmer's paralysis—peroneal neuropathy during weight reduction. J Neurol Neurosurg Psychiatry 1984;47:564–566.

Sourkes M, Stewart JD: Common peroneal neuropathy: A study of selective motor and sensory involvement. Neurology 1991; 41:1029–1033.

Sriram K, Sakthivel A: Sciatic nerve palsy in the newborn. Ann Acad Med Singapore 1981;10:472–475.

Stewart JD: Focal Peripheral Neuropathies. New York, Elsevier Science, 1987.

Stewart JD: Compression and entrapment neuropathies. In Dyck PJ, Thomas PK (eds): Peripheral Neuropathy. Philadelphia, WB Saunders, 1993.

Stillman MJ, Christensen W, Payne R, Foley KM: Leukemic relapse presenting as sciatic nerve involvement by chloroma (granulocytic sarcoma). Cancer 1988;62:2047–2050.

Streib E: Weight loss and footdrop. Iowa Med 1993;83:224–225.

Styf J, Morberg P: The superficial peroneal tunnel syndrome. Results of treatment by decompression. J Bone Joint Surg Br 1997;79:801–803.

Sunderland S: Nerve and Nerve Injuries. London, Churchill-Livingstone, 1978.

Tachi N, Kozuka N, Ohya K, et al: Magnetic resonance imaging of peripheral nerves and pathology of sural nerves in hereditary motor and sensory neuropathy type III. Neuroradiology 1995; 37:496–499.

Tada K, Yonenobu K, Swanson AB: Congenital constriction band syndrome. J Pediatr Orthop 1984;4:726–370.

Takao M, Fukuuchi Y, Koto A, et al: Localized hypertrophic mononeuropathy involving the femoral nerve. Neurology 1999;52: 389–392.

Tani JC: Fibrous band compression of the tibial nerve branch of the sciatic nerve. Am J Orthop 1995;24:910–912.

Taniguchi N, Itoh K, Wang Y, et al: Sonographic detection of diffuse peripheral nerve hypertrophy in chronic inflammatory demyelinating polyradiculoneuropathy. J Clin Ultrasound 2000; 28:488–491.

Thomas JE, Piepgras DG, Scheithauer B, et al: Neurogenic tumors of the sciatic nerve: A clinicopathologic study of 35 cases. Mayo Clin Proc 1983;58:640–647.

Uetani M, Hashmi R, Hayashi K, et al: Peripheral nerve intraneural ganglion cyst: MR findings in three cases. J Comput Assist Tomogr 1998;22:629–632.

Vaccaro AR, Ludwig SC, Klein GR, et al: Bilateral peroneal nerve palsy secondary to a knee board: Report of two cases. Am J Orthop 1998;27:746–748.

Venna N, Bielawski M, Spatz EM: Sciatic nerve entrapment in a child: Case report. J Neurosurg 1991;75:652–654.

Villarejo FJ, Pascual AM: Injection injury of the sciatic nerve (370 cases). Childs Nerv Syst 1993;9:229–232.

Vogel CM, Albin R, Alberts JW: Lotus footdrop: Sciatic neuropathy in the thigh. Neurology 1991;41:605–606.

Warner MA, Warner DO, Harper CM, et al: Lower extremity neuropathies associated with lithotomy positions. Anesthesiology 2000;93:938–942.

Watemberg N, Amsel S, Sadeh M, Lerman-Sagie T: Common peroneal neuropathy due to surfing. J Child Neurol 2000;15:420–421.

Weig SG, Waite RJ, McAvoy K: MRI in unexplained mononeuropathy. Pediatr Neurol 2000;22:314–317.

Wexler I, Paley D, Herzenberg JE, Herbert A: Detection of nerve entrapment during limb lengthening by means of near-nerve recording. Electromyogr Clin Neurophysiol 1998;38:161–167.

Wilburn A, Levin K, Sweeney P: Peroneal neuropathies in children and adolescents [abstract]. Can J Neurol Sci 1990;17:227.

Yilmaz Y, Oge AE, Yilmaz-Degpirmenci S, Say A: Peroneal nerve palsy: The role of early electromyography. Eur J Paediatr Neurol 2000;4:239–242.

Yokoyama T, Horiuchi E, Uesaka Y, et al: [Acute compression neuropathy of the proximal sciatic nerve in a patient with facioscapulohumeral muscular dystrophy.] Rinsho Shinkeigaku 1998;38:958–960.

Yoshida T, Tada K, Uemura K, Yonenobu K: Peripheral nerve palsies in victims of the Hanshin-Awaji earthquake. Clin Orthop 1999;366:208–217.

Yuen EC, Olney RK, So YT: Sciatic neuropathy: Clinical and prognostic features in 73 patients. Neurology 1994;44:1669–1674.

Yuen EC, So YT, Olney RK: The electrophysiologic features of sciatic neuropathy in 100 patients. Muscle Nerve 1995;18:414–420.

Yuen EC, So YT: Sciatic neuropathy. Neurol Clin 1999;17:617–631, viii.

Polyneuropathies in Children

Matthew Pitt and H. Royden Jones, Jr.

INTRODUCTION

The various polyneuropathies that affect infants and children do not occur as frequently in a pediatric practice as in an adult practice. Genetically de- termined mechanisms account for a very high percentage of the childhood polyneuropathies (Hagberg, 1990). The implications of an initially in- gravescent, symmetrical, hereditary polyneuropathy vary widely. A number of these pediatric neuropa-

---

Table 92–1. Pediatric Polyneuropathy Classification Categories

Temporal profile: acute onset versus chronic
Primary pathology: demyelinating versus axonal
Symptomatic predominance: motor, sensory, mixed
Etiology: acquired versus genetic
   Immunologically mediated
   Systemic illness; metabolic/endocrine, infectious
   Toxic mechanisms

---

thies are relatively benign and minimally limiting during childhood. The various forms of Charcot-Marie-Tooth (CMT) disease are the most common of these childhood polyneuropathies and are often relatively benign. Nevertheless, these various neuropathies have profound implications, particularly in two very different clinical settings.

Initially, we discuss the acutely acquired potentially life-threatening polyneuropathies. Children with these conditions require urgent hospitalization because of a rapidly progressive weakness, such as typifies Guillain-Barré syndrome. Clinical evaluation is still key, as failure to search for a tick in a child who presents with a Guillain-Barré syndrome may prevent an immediate cure and, if unrecognized, may rarely lead to death. (The other clinical setting in which a childhood polyneuropathy has very significant prognostic implications are those hereditary neuropathies, such as seen in metachromatic leukodystrophy, where the neuropathic process represents the first manifestation of a lethal disease.) It is important to recognize that sometimes seemingly benign clinical presentations, initially thought to represent relatively modest disorders such as Charcot-Marie-Tooth disease, may also have a very serious outlook. It is here that the pediatric or adult neurologist, who frequently evaluates these children in an electromyography (EMG) laboratory, must be particularly fastidious in evaluating the child and making appropriate clinical correlations.

Various clinical nosological approaches are useful for the differential diagnosis of pediatric polyneuropathies (Table 92–1). The clinical temporal profile, either acute or chronic, provides the most useful means for initial categorization and is used in this chapter with further breakdown into those that are primarily demyelinating (Tables 92–2 and 92–3) and

---

Table 92–3. Differential Diagnosis for Childhood Guillain-Barré Syndrome

Immediate consideration
   Tick paralysis
   Spinal cord compression
   Transverse myelitis
Infectious
   Poliomyelitis
   Chinese motor neuronopathy (*Campylobacter jejuni*)
   Diphtheria
   Human immunodeficiency virus (?)
   Lyme disease (more likely a polyradiculopathy and very rare)
Other dysimmune processes
   Vasculitis, mononeuritis multiplex
   Acute viral myositis
   Graft-versus-host post–bone marrow transplantation
Toxins
   Vincristine
     Occult hereditary motor and sensory neuropathy
     Immunocompromised host (?)
   Glue sniffing
   Heavy metals: mercury, lead, arsenic, thallium
   Agriculture related: insecticides, buckthorn
   Fish toxins
Nutritional
   Thiamine deficiency with vigorous dieting
Critical illness polyneuropathy
Inborn errors of metabolism
   Leigh's disease

---

those that have a primary axonal loss (Tables 92–4 and 92–5). The evaluation of a child with a pediatric neuropathy compatible with Guillain-Barré syndrome differs significantly from that of the child presenting with the insidious onset of a chronic polyneuropathy. As one considers this classification template, Guillain-Barré syndrome fits the initial portion of each major category; that is, it is an acute, demyelinating motor neuropathy that is acquired and immunologically mediated. Guillain-Barré syndrome is the most common cause for an acute, acquired polyneuropathy in children just as it is in adults.

Children with a gradual, often insidiously developing, chronic peripheral neuropathy have a very high incidence of genetic mechanisms (Hagberg, 1990). However, a small percentage of these neuropathies do have an acquired etiological basis. Therefore, a careful family history is one of the most

---

Table 92–2. Acquired Autoimmune Demyelinating Neuropathies

Guillain-Barré syndrome
Chronic inflammatory demyelinating polyneuropathy
Toxins
   Arsenic
Metabolic
   Leigh's disease
Infectious
   Diphtheria

Table 92–4. Recurrent Childhood Neuropathies

Chronic inflammatory demyelinating polyneuropathy
Glue sniffing
Porphyria
Tangier's disease
Dejerine-Sottas disease*
Refsum's disease*
Lead intoxication*

*Classically, these polyneuropathies are thought of as having a remitting-relapsing course, but in children, actual documentation of this clinical temporal profile is difficult to find. (The author would be most pleased to hear of well-documented cases of such.)

Table 92–5. Acute Nonautoimmune Polyneuropathies

Inborn errors of metabolism
  Tyrosinemia type 1
  Porphyria
  Leigh's syndrome
Pharmacological toxins
  Oncological
    Vincristine
    Cis-platinum
  Antimicrobials
    Chloramphenicol
    Metronidazole
  Miscellaneous
    Sodium dichloracetate
    Thalidomide
Heavy metal toxins
  Lead
  Arsenic
  Mercury
  Thallium
Agriculture-related toxins
  Buckthorn (*Karwinskia humboldtiana*)
  Organophosphate pesticide
Industrial toxins
  n-Hexane (glue sniffing)
Postvaccinal
  Rubella
  Smallpox

useful initial investigations in the evaluation of a chronic childhood polyneuropathy (Hagberg, 1990). It is in this instance that the neurological examination of child and parent alike, often followed by EMG of both, provides the most important initial clues to the differential diagnosis. In our sister organization, the Institute of Child Health, Prof. Robin Winter and Dr. Michael Barisiter from The Department of Genetics produced an electronic database of neurogenetic diseases (The London Neurogenetics Database, Oxford University Press). This is used as the source for the hereditary section of this chapter.

Even when inherited mechanisms are not operative, the etiology of pediatric subacute and chronic neuropathies differs significantly from that in adults. Systemic mechanisms, such as diabetes, endocrinopathies, uremia, and vasculitis, rarely occur in children. Infectious processes such as poliomyelitis and diphtheria still need consideration when evaluating children from underdeveloped countries that lack appropriate immunization programs. Many toxins, such as alcohol, are not pertinent to the evaluation during infancy and childhood. However, one still needs to consider the rare possibility of a toxic mechanism with either an unexplained acute or chronic pediatric neuropathy.

Today DNA analysis is often the next step in the investigation of most chronic neuropathies. This is particularly important for those children whose neurophysiological studies demonstrate a primary demyelinating process. In contrast, genetic determinations have been less helpful in the approach to a hereditary axonal process. Rarely, if there remains a question as to the primary pathology, including the presence of a systemic process, such as a vasculitis, a sural nerve biopsy may be indicated (Wilmshurst and Ouvrier, 2002). Before the genetic diagnostic breakthroughs, a sural nerve biopsy might be the essential diagnostic procedure.

Anatomical maturation factors specific to infancy and early childhood need appreciation for the appropriate interpretation of both EMG and sural nerve biopsy. Nerve conduction parameters and motor unit potentials evolve in a newborn from less than 50% of adult normal values to reach the standard mature values between the ages of 3 to 5 years (Jones et al., 1996). The evolving myelination process documented by sural nerve studies of young children, wherein full adult parameters are not present until the third to the fifth year (Gutrecht and Dyck, 1970), explains the well-recognized evolution in the normal values for motor and sensory needle conduction studies (NCSs) during infancy and the preschool period.

Although many pediatric polyneuropathies have a number of similarities to their adult counterparts, the clinical presentation with infants and toddlers is sometimes quite different. When a neuropathy presents acutely in a previously healthy infant, the parents often notice a change in the infant's previously acquired motor milestones. Guillain-Barré syndrome, infantile botulism, or, rarely, infantile poliomyelitis require careful diagnostic consideration even as early as the age of 10 days. There is no documentation that the common genetically determined polyneuropathies, such as Charcot-Marie-Tooth disease, are significantly symptomatic during infancy. In other instances, the clinician may not initially suspect a polyneuropathy. For example, a floppy infant, seen during the neonatal period, occasionally has an uncommon congenital peripheral neuropathy. These babies are often initially identified by the absence of the classic DNA changes for spinal muscular atrophy or, if more acutely ill, are sent directly to the EMG laboratory in a search for other mechanisms of congenital hypotonia (David and Jones, 1994).

Some pediatric peripheral neuropathies present as a gait disorder, and a central nervous system process is initially suspected. Not until central nervous system imaging studies are negative and cerebrospinal fluid analysis is performed do the responsible physicians turn their attention to the possibility of a motor unit abnormality, particularly at the level of the peripheral nerve. An acute pseudoencephalopathic syndrome presumably secondary to a very painful neuropathy is another relatively uncommon Guillain-Barré syndrome clinical variant. In this setting, the child becomes so uncomfortable and subsequently so difficult to deal with that a primary central nervous system infection or mass lesion is initially suspected. This Guillain-Barré syndrome variant usually occurs with toddlers and preschool-aged children (Bradshaw and Jones, 2001).

A child who has a more slowly evolving peripheral

neuropathy often has a more subtle clinical presentation, sometimes characterized by an actual regression of already acquired motor skills. Toddlers may lose their confidence in their ability to mobilize and become increasingly dependent on their parents or siblings for help getting around the house. Parents may first come to the pediatrician concerned by their child's decreasing ability to walk, problems climbing stairs, or clumsiness handling various toys or eating utensils. Very rarely, insensitivity to pain is evidenced by self-mutilation with the appearance of ulcerations of the digits. In the older child, symptoms of numbness, muscle pains or cramps, weakness, or increasing difficulty performing skilled athletic activities may be the first clinical signs of a polyneuropathy.

The pediatric electromyographer may want to use various components of this classification algorithm (see Table 92–1) in the differential diagnosis of infantile and childhood peripheral neuropathies. The temporal profile of symptoms, either acute or chronic, provides the most useful means for initial categorization. The evaluation of an acute neuropathy compatible with Guillain-Barré syndrome differs significantly from that of the child presenting with the insidious onset of a chronic polyneuropathy. As the clinician considers the classification template, Guillain-Barré syndrome fits the initial portion of each major category (i.e., it is an acute, demyelinating, motor neuropathy that is acquired and is immunologically mediated). The etiology of pediatric subacute and chronic neuropathies differs significantly from that of adults.

Increasingly, DNA analysis is either the first or the second step for the initial investigation of many chronic childhood neuropathies. If EMG is performed first and demonstrates a primary demyelinating process, it is more likely that DNA analysis will demonstrate a specific genetic defect. Less frequently, sural nerve biopsy supplements EMG when there is a question as to the primary pathology, particularly the rare instance of a possible systemic process. Previously, a sural nerve biopsy was often a very useful and sometimes a definitive study. However, with the diagnostic breakthroughs provided by DNA genetic testing, disorders such as metachromatic leukodystrophy are good examples of when sural nerve biopsy and, often, EMG are no longer indicated. When there is evidence of concomitant central nervous system dysfunction in a child with an autosomal recessive demyelinating polyneuropathy, DNA analysis usually is sufficient to make the diagnosis of metachromatic leukodystrophy. Sural nerve is no longer necessary. We anticipate that DNA testing will increasingly provide a specific diagnostic role in the investigation of chronic pediatric polyneuropathies. This chapter is divided into discussions of the acquired and hereditary polyneuropathies.

ACQUIRED POLYNEUROPATHIES

This section begins with an in-depth review of Guillain-Barré syndrome, because it is the most common acute polyneuropathy seen at our respective hospitals, Great Ormond Street, London, and the Children's Hospital Boston. Because Guillain-Barré syndrome is a treatable neurological illness not only in older children but also in infants, it is very important to place significant emphasis on this neuropathy. We conclude the first major section of this chapter with an analysis of the clinical-electromyographic approach to the evaluation of the youngster who has a chronic acquired peripheral neuropathy.

Although EMG continues to have its most significant use for the diagnosis of acute weakness related to peripheral nerve disease, colleagues are beginning to evaluate the reliability and diagnostic specificity of magnetic resonance imaging for the diagnosis of Guillain-Barré syndrome. Naturally, this imaging modality does not provide evidence of the classic neurophysiological signs of an acquired neuropathy, including conduction block and conduction slowing. Enhancement of the proximal nerve roots, although a nonspecific finding, may still offer sufficient information to obviate the need for this somewhat unpleasant testing method in the already unhappy child.

Autoimmune Acquired Polyneuropathies

CLINICAL PRESENTATION

Guillain-Barré syndrome is the most common cause for an acute, acquired polyneuropathy in children (see Table 92–2). Typically, these youngsters present with a rapidly evolving symmetrical weakness associated with pain and ataxia. In the older child, varying degrees of distal paresthesias and numbness, muscle pains or cramps, or increasing difficulty in performing skilled athletic activities may be the first clinical signs of an acute polyneuropathy. This was reported in 13 of 24 children (54%) with Guillain-Barré syndrome seen at the Children's Hospital Boston (Bradshaw and Jones, 1992). Cranial nerve palsies, particularly the facial nerve, may also be a presenting sign of Guillain-Barré syndrome in some children. Bell's palsy is the most common Guillain-Barré syndrome cranial neuropathy in children. Other cranial nerve palsies also occur, particularly affecting nerve III, IV, or VI. In our experience at the Children's Hospital Boston, we found lesions in these cranial nerves in 20% of children (Bradshaw and Jones, 2001)

An acute ataxia is another means of childhood Guillain-Barré syndrome presentation (Gieron-Korthals et al., 1994); this is particularly common in toddlers. Parents or teachers often first note a subtle gait change, which then rapidly progresses. The initial clinical impression may focus at the level of the central nervous system. It is not until central nervous system imaging studies are negative that the clinician proceeds with cerebrospinal fluid analysis. When the classic albuminocytological dissociation is found, the possibility of a peripheral motor unit abnormality is first suspected. Associated weakness and hyporeflexia usually develop eventually. In a survey of 40 children who presented to an emergency department with acute ataxia, five had Guillain-Barré syndrome (12.5%), and two also had Miller Fisher syndrome (Gieron-Korthals et al., 1994).

Autonomic abnormalities may occur and often are rather labile; these include supraventricular tachycardia, bradycardia, and postural hypotension. There may be prominent swings in blood pressure. Rarely, these symptoms are the primary manifestation of childhood Guillain-Barré syndrome. These are sometimes associated with painful sensory involvement but not with weakness (Jackman and Klig, 1998). Symptoms of upper airway obstruction, manifested by dyspnea, with inability to handle secretions and dysphagia, associated with hyporeflexia, occurred in a 14-year-old boy (Larsen and Tobias, 1994). Spinal fluid analysis and EMG led to a diagnosis of Guillain-Barré syndrome.

There are a number of Guillain-Barré syndrome variants; the best known is Miller Fisher syndrome. Here, the child presents with an acute ataxia, extraocular palsies, and areflexia. In contrast to the typical Guillain-Barré syndrome profile, none of these children have significant muscle weakness. At the Children's Hospital Boston, just 1 of 24 children presented in this manner (Bradshaw and Jones, 1992). Many Miller Fisher syndrome patients have a very specific immunological profile. Miller Fisher syndrome has been associated with an IgG antibody directed at the ganglioside GQ1b. This is very specific and was demonstrated in 24 of 25 patients (Kusunoki et al., 1994). This antibody is specifically related to the Miller Fisher syndrome pathogenesis. It binds to an epitope on the surface of some *Campylobacter jejuni* strains and later cross-reacts with cranial nerve GQ1b ganglioside (Jacobs et al., 1994). Two children with typical Miller Fisher syndrome had *C. jejuni* isolated on stool culture. An anti-GQ1b antibody is found in almost every affected child (Buchwald et al., 2001).

An acute pseudoencephalopathic syndrome, presumably secondary to a very painful ganglioradiculoneuropathy, is another clinical variant of Guillain-Barré syndrome (Bradshaw and Jones, 2001). This is more frequently noted with toddlers and preschool-aged children. This variant is relatively common in our experience at the Children's Hospital Boston. In this setting, these children are so uncomfortable that they become very difficult to evaluate secondary to this very painful form of Guillain-Barré syndrome. Often, the initial physician first considers a primary central nervous system infection or mass lesion.

Occasionally, extremity pain is another presenting sign of Guillain-Barré syndrome (Nass and Chutorian, 1982). At times, the pain is severe and episodic, lasting from 5 to 20 minutes every 1 to 2 hours. One child lay in the fetal position even during sleep. At times, this youngster had nocturnal screaming

paroxysms (Wong et al., 1998). Occasionally, the pain is initially unilateral, sometimes focused at one joint. Later, the pain may become bilateral and more generalized and interferes with ability to sit, stand, or walk (Jackman and Klig, 1998).

There are axonal forms of Guillain-Barré syndrome. One variant is an acute motor axonal neuropathy seen predominantly in China. It is quite common there, affecting mainly children and young adults, and has a high incidence of respiratory insufficiency that requires care in the intensive care unit, but it usually results in early recovery (McKhann et al., 1993). This form has a much less common worldwide distribution. There are occasional instances in North and South America and in Europe. Even less common in children is acute axonal motor sensory polyneuropathy (Feasby et al., 1986). Very rarely, an acute-onset primary sensory neuropathy with loss of pain sensation occurs.

Another group of infants seen at Great Ormond Street had a rapidly progressive and ultimately fatal axonal motor sensory neuropathy (Pitt et al., 1998). All had diaphragmatic weakness at presentation. The diaphragm showed chronic denervation or reinnervation, as did the distal muscles. Absent or abnormal sensory studies and slow motor nerve conduction velocities indicated a demyelinating neuropathy. Sural nerve biopsy samples showed absence of the largest diameter fibers. Clinically, the patients resemble children with diaphragmatic paralysis and distal spinal muscular atrophy (McWilliam et al., 1985; Bertini et al., 1989; Novelli et al., 1995), but we found no evidence of anterior horn cell disease when sought. A similar patient described by Appleton and associates (1994) is still alive but is ventilated and fully dependent.

Not all cases of Guillain-Barré syndrome are easy to recognize. There are two reports of the initial misdiagnosis of brain death in an acutely paralyzed child who suddenly becomes immobilized. One author (M.P.) saw this happen in a 14-year-old child who was in a relapse during treatment for acute lymphoblastic leukemia (Heckmatt et al., 1993). A clinical picture of brain death also occurred in a 6-year-old child admitted to an intensive care unit after a respiratory arrest (Bakshi et al., 1997). Interestingly, the child had also received chemotherapy for a brain tumor but had received no medication in the past few months. The child was unable to walk for 2 days. He suddenly developed respiratory distress and became unresponsive. On examination, his pupils were fixed and dilated, and he had no corneal, oculocephalic, gag, muscle stretch, or plantar responses. His only preserved reactivity to noxious stimuli was with sternal rub. An electroencephalogram surprisingly demonstrated 4- to 6-Hz activity with normal sleep rhythms. An electromyogram 2 days later demonstrated complete absence of compound motor action potentials and sensory nerve action potentials, no motor unit potentials, and profound active denervation. This child had been previously treated for a brainstem neoplasm but had received no vincristine for more than 2 months. The association of Guillain-Barré syndrome and hematopoietic cancer is also reported (Geetha et al., 1999).

Infantile Acute Hypotonia

The typical clinical presentation of Guillain-Barré syndrome seen in infants and toddlers rarely occurs in the neonate. An acute profound muscle weakness occurring at or immediately after birth must lead the clinician to consider an intrauterine onset of Guillain-Barré syndrome. On one occasion, the mother noted a significant decrease in fetal movements in the 30th week of her pregnancy (Jackson et al., 1996). This infant was floppy at birth. Another infant had severe leg weakness and moderate proximal arm paresis, with absent muscle stretch reflexes. Electromyography demonstrated profound conduction block and temporal dispersion in many motor nerves with active denervation in many muscles. No specific treatment was provided; he had gradual but complete recovery by the age of 1 year. Very rarely, Guillain-Barré syndrome develops concomitantly in the mother and the infant (in utero) (Rolfs and Bolik, 1994; Luijckx et al., 1997). A 33-year-old mother developed severe Guillain-Barré syndrome during the 29th week of her pregnancy. She became tetraplegic and was on a respirator when her baby was born at 38 weeks' gestation. Severe hypotonia, marked respiratory distress, and feeding problems developed in the infant at 12 days postpartum. His cerebrospinal fluid protein concentration was 243 mg/dL. Electromyography was typical of Guillain-Barré syndrome. Treatment with intravenous immunoglobulin was associated with a complete resolution 2 weeks later (Rolfs and Bolik, 1994).

Guillain-Barré syndrome also occurs in infants shortly after birth (as soon as 10 days to 3 weeks), seemingly unrelated to maternal exposure (Al-Quadah et al.; Carroll et al.; Gilmartin and Ch'ien, 1977). One case of infantile Guillain-Barré syndrome went on to follow a course consistent with chronic inflammatory demyelinating neuropathy (Pasternak et al., 1982). The proportions of younger children with Guillain-Barré syndrome have varied from one third of 43 children with Guillain-Barré syndrome being younger than 3 years (Delanoe et al., 1998) to just three instances of Guillain-Barré syndrome in infants younger than 2 years (Bar-Joseph et al., 1991) and to one 14-month-old infant (Paradiso et al., 1999). The differential diagnosis of Guillain-Barré syndrome is presented in Table 92–3.

Differential Diagnosis of Guillain-Barré Syndrome

OLDER CHILDREN

Tick Paralysis

Each child who presents with the classic findings of Guillain-Barré syndrome must have her or his scalp immediately inspected for the presence of a tick. If identified, a dramatic clinical improvement often follows its removal (Grattan-Smith et al., 1997). Pupillary involvement may help to differentiate tick paralysis from Guillain-Barré syndrome, although this rarely occurs with very severe axonal Guillain-Barré syndrome (Bakshi et al., 1997) and rarely with diphtheria. We are unaware of reports of tick paralysis in infants and toddlers.

Typical electromyographic findings in tick paralysis include very low amplitude compound motor action potentials but with preserved motor nerve conduction velocities and distal latencies, normal repetitive motor nerve stimulation, and sensory nerve action potentials. Fibrillation potentials are found as soon as 24 to 48 hours (Swift and Ignacio, 1975; Donat and Donat, 1981).

Spinal Cord Tumors

Both spinal cord tumors and transverse myelitis may initially be confused with Guillain-Barré syndrome and must be immediately differentiated (Delhaas et al., 1998; Hesketh et al., 1998; Knebusch et al., 1998). Either entity may present with a rapidly progressive paralysis, hyporeflexia, and back pain. Sphincter dysfunction is common with spinal cord lesions, in contrast to its rare occurrence with Guillain-Barré syndrome. These symptoms are usually transient with Guillain-Barré syndrome. Four children with a malignant spinal cord tumor were initially not recognized to have a serious condition, let alone a myelopathy (Hesketh et al., 1998). Severe pain and asymmetrical lower extremity weakness, with a clear-cut sensory level on neurological examination, helped to differentiate these patients from the typical Guillain-Barré syndrome individual. It is important to recognize that magnetic resonance imaging studies may lead to confusion. Spinal cord swelling with increased signal intensity, but without contrast enhancement, occasionally occurs with acute Guillain-Barré syndrome (Delhaas et al., 1998).

Transverse Myelitis

This is another spinal entity that may occasionally lead to confusion in the differential diagnosis of Guillain-Barré syndrome (Knebusch et al., 1998). Four of eight children with acute transverse myelitis had equal motor and sensory symptoms: three with predominant motor loss and one with mainly sensory symptoms (Knebusch et al., 1998). Sphincter control was lost in six of eight children. The cerebrospinal fluid protein was very elevated (570 to 2,130 mg/L) in four of eight children with transverse myelitis. Only two had a pleocytosis was very modest in the two children with abnormal values.

Electromyography is generally normal in children with transverse myelitis. However, both compound motor action potentials and F waves may be abnormal if there is damage to the segmental anterior horn cells for the nerves originating from anterior horn cells in the affected segments. Therefore, the clinician must be cautious with the diagnosis if the only abnormalities on EMG are F waves that depend on just a few adjacent spinal cord segments (Bradshaw and Jones, 1992). An abnormal magnetic resonance image was obtained for 50% of these children (Knebusch et al., 1998).

Infectious Diseases

Infectious diseases occasionally must be considered in the diagnosis of an acute polyneuropathy that mimics Guillain-Barré syndrome. Diphtheria rarely presents with a recent severe sore throat, fever, and accompanying bulbar palsy before the onset of an acute peripheral neuropathy (Logina and Donaghy, 1999). Sometimes, as with our one adolescent case, the mother may recall an incomplete diphtheria, pertussis, and tetanus immunization history. Neither acquired immunodeficiency syndrome nor Lyme disease is reported to primarily present with a peripheral neuropathy that mimics childhood Guillain-Barré syndrome.

Toxins

Toxins, including glue sniffing and shellfish toxins, always warrant consideration. Children who live within agricultural communities are at risk for intoxication from heavy metals and organophosphate pesticide poisoning. Children who have been in northern Mexico or the adjacent American Southwest must be considered for buckthorn wild cherry poisoning (Dirik and Uysal, 1994; Hart et al., 1994). A few inborn metabolic errors, porphyria, or Leigh's disease, enhanced by medications, particularly barbiturates, may also precipitate symptoms that resemble childhood Guillain-Barré syndrome (Coker, 1993). Vincristine toxicity may present with an acute motor and sensory neuropathy that mimics Guillain-Barré syndrome in children who have unsuspected Charcot-Marie-Tooth type I (CMT1) hereditary neuropathy (Graf et al., 1996). Testing for the 17p11.2-12 gene duplication should be considered in any child administered vincristine who develops an acute Guillain-Barré syndrome–like motor neuropathy. An immunocompromised child may have had a similar mechanism although the family history was not reported. Children with overwhelming sepsis or status asthmaticus sometimes develop a critical illness neuromuscular syndrome mimicking Guillain-Barré syndrome (Sheth et al., 1995).

Recurrent Polyneuropathies

In the rare instance of a recurrent Guillain-Barré syndrome, in addition to chronic inflammatory demyelinating polyneuropathy (Pasternak et al., 1982), some rare toxic, metabolic, and possibly hereditary neuropathies should be considered (see Table 92–4).

Inflammatory Myopathies

These rarely mimic acute Guillain-Barré syndrome. Acute childhood myositis may involve severe calf pain that keeps the child from walking, not unlike with Guillain-Barré syndrome. This disorder is self-limited and usually confined to the calf muscles. Often, these children do not have very significant weakness. Dermatomyositis and periodic paralysis may also have subacute or even acute onsets of paralysis similar to Guillain-Barré syndrome. Electromyography can be helpful in making this differentiation.

Weakness in the Intensive Care Unit

A patient in the pediatric intensive care unit who has unexplained weakness presents some of the greatest challenges to the pediatric electromyographer. Among intensivists and others, there is a tendency to describe all such cases incorrectly as critical illness neuropathy. Some children most commonly acquire acute generalized weakness due to persistence of the neuromuscular blockade. Critical illness polyneuropathy (Bolton et al., 1984) is very rare, indeed, in the pediatric population. Petersen and co-workers (1999) reported two cases; one patient was 6 years 6 months old but the other was only 2 years 6 months old. Pitt (1996) has seen only two possible cases over about 10 years. One occurred in a child of 12 years who had cancer; the neuropathy developed in the context of multiorgan failure, but the patient was administered several neurotoxic drugs as chemotherapy. Another patient aged 9 years was in relapse of acute lymphoblastic leukemia, and pneumocystis pneumonia developed. The weakness persisted after neuromuscular blocking agents were stopped, and EMG showed changes consistent with an axonal neuropathy. Persistence of abnormalities of the repetitive stimulation was a feature. Schwarz and associates (1997) demonstrated abnormalities of jitter, suggesting that the disease focused on the terminal axon.

It is also quite possible that many neuromuscular conditions go unrecognized in pediatric intensive care units as they have in adult intensive care units. Although sepsis and multiple organ failure are less common in pediatric intensive care units, they still occur. In such cases, several neuromuscular complications should be sought: critical illness polyneuropathy, critical illness (thick filament) myopathy, necrotic myopathy, pyomyositis, and Hopkins' syndrome (monoplegia associated with asthma) (Bolton, 1996).

INFANTS AND TODDLERS

A number of relatively uncommon illnesses that, with the exception of Guillain-Barré syndrome, primarily occur only during infancy, need consideration in somewhat older infants (Jones, 2000). These illnesses include infantile botulism and, rarely, poliomyelitis or familial myasthenia gravis and possibly polymyositis. In one 7-week-old infant with acute Guillain-Barré syndrome, chronic inflammatory demyelinating polyneuropathy developed later (Pasternak et al., 1982).

Infantile Botulism

This is a very uncommon presynaptic neuromuscular transmission defect that may also mimic Guillain-Barré syndrome in infants (Pickett et al., 1976; Clay et al.; Thompson et al., 1980). Typically, this toxin affects infants primarily between the ages of 10 days and 6 months, although we had a case in a 10-month-old child at the Children's Hospital Boston. These infants are healthy at birth and subsequently develop normal motor milestones. Suddenly or over just a period of a few days, the child begins to have difficulty in feeding. Mothers may note that the infant's ability to suck has significantly diminished. "Constipation" follows. The cry becomes weak, and head control is lost in the majority of children. Some infants may have a relatively mild illness and do not require hospitalization. In other children, hypotonia rapidly becomes more prominent. The weakness is profound, and respiratory crisis suddenly ensues, often severe enough to be potentially life threatening.

A very profound clinical course occurred in one 2-week-old infant (Shukla et al., 1991). Respiratory arrest developed just 5 hours after the first symptoms were recognized. At times, a preliminary diagnosis of sepsis leads to the use of aminoglycoside antibiotics. These may inadvertently precipitate a respiratory crisis in an infant not initially suspected to have a disease at the neuromuscular junction. *Clostridium botulinum* toxin interferes with acetylcholine release at the neuromuscular junction. Although there has been an association between ingestion of honey and the infantile form of botulism, often no specific food source is defined. Infantile botulism must be considered in the differential diagnosis of both acute respiratory distress and acute hypotonia.

Electromyography is the primary method of immediately diagnosing infantile botulism (Cornblath et al., 1983). Routine motor conduction studies may be normal with the nonspecific exception of low-amplitude compound motor action potentials. Repetitive motor nerve stimulation at 20 to 50 Hz demonstrates incremental responses ranging between 23% to 313% in 23 of 25 infants with infantile botulism. The post-tetanic facilitation persists much longer than in adult Lambert-Eaton syndrome (Fakadej and Gutmann, 1982). Rarely, the classic electromyographic findings may not be evident (Sheth et al., 1999). Bacteriological confirmation usually requires a few weeks to document the presence of botulinum spores on stool analysis.

Poliomyelitis

Poliomyelitis may also mimic Guillain-Barré syndrome. If the child comes from outside the United States or from countries in which the oral live polio vaccine is still the primary form of immunization, it is important to ask about the child's recent immunization status. Rarely, infants who have just received their first type 3 polio vaccine immunization present with an acute generalized hypotonia (Beausoleil et al., 1994; David and Doyle, 1997). These infants became febrile and were irritable and at times lethargic. Subsequently, each infant soon developed symptoms that, taken in isolation, had many similarities to Guillain-Barré syndrome. Progressive generalized weakness, which was sometimes asymmetrical, and associated head lag were seen in each infant. On one occasion, there was a significant asymmetry of motor loss (J. Goldstein, personal communication). Cerebrospinal fluid protein concentrations mimicked those found in Guillain-Barré syndrome, with modest elevations of 82 to 143 mg/dL. A significant cerebrospinal fluid pleocytosis is one of the most important differential diagnostic laboratory indicators; values in these three cases ranged from 100 to 500 white blood cells.

Electromyography demonstrates a pure motor neuronopathy secondary to the primary damage to the anterior horn cells. Motor NCSs may have no or very low amplitude compound motor action potentials in the most severely affected extremities. In contrast to Guillain-Barré syndrome, the sensory nerve action potentials are normal. Active denervation with significant loss of motor unit potentials characterizes the needle examination.

Other Disorders

Tick paralysis is the only other acutely acquired presynaptic defect. Although it is well known to mimic Guillain-Barré syndrome in older children, we are unaware of an infantile case. However, any infant with an acute onset of generalized muscle weakness must undergo a search for a tick, especially in the scalp. There have been a few reports of infantile polymyositis as well as muscle-phosphorylase deficiency presenting as an acute floppy infant syndrome.

Diagnostic Studies in Guillain-Barré Syndrome

ELECTROMYOGRAPHY

Electromyography continues to be the most accurate method to precisely determine the presence of Guillain-Barré syndrome in children (Bradshaw and Jones, 1992). One of its foremost advantages is to define the nature of the primary insult—that is, whether the lesion is primarily demyelinating or axonal. The electromyographic diagnosis rests on the accurate identification of patchy demyelination. Isolated loss or prolongation of F waves and H reflexes were the most common findings that we found in our children with Guillain-Barré syndrome at the

Children's Hospital Boston. Other findings included slowing of conduction velocity to less than two thirds of normal (i.e., 15 to 30 m per second) and with distal latencies of two to three times normal. Children younger than 10 years demonstrated decidedly greater degrees of motor conduction velocity slowing than did those older than 10 years. Delanoe and colleagues (1998) use sensory as well as motor nerve abnormalities to fulfill the diagnosis of demyelinating Guillain-Barré syndrome. They suggest that this added study improves the sensitivity of this study.

It is important to be aware of the occasional instance in which the only electromyographic abnormality is the absence of F waves confined to either the legs or the arms. This finding is typical for transverse myelitis (Knebusch et al., 1998) when the primary spinal damage is localized to either L4-S1 or C6-8 cord levels, where the anterior horn cells innervating the fibers responsible for the F waves originate. Electromyography of most children with acute flaccid paralysis at Beijing Children's Hospital had very low amplitude compound muscle action potentials with normal conduction velocities and distal latencies. These findings are typical for an acute motor axonal neuropathy (McKhann et al., 1993).

The electromyographic information provided is less clearly defined regarding prognosis than in the adult population. In general, however, pediatric Guillain-Barré syndrome is a more benign condition (Korinthenberg and Monting, 1996; Delanoe et al., 1998). In adults, the prognosis is worse if the compound nerve action potential is reduced initially (Winer et al., 1985), but this is not so well documented in children (Bradshaw and Jones, 1992).

ANTIBODIES

The association between the differing forms of acute inflammatory demyelinating polyneuropathy and particular antibodies against the myelin proteins is particularly helpful in the Miller Fisher syndrome, where an association with GQ1b antiganglioside antibody is found (Jacobs et al., 1994; Kusunoki et al., 1994). Antiganglioside GM1 antibodies are present in a high proportion of patients with the axonal motor neuropathy or have nerves that are inexcitable (Hadden et al., 1998). Bulbar palsy as part of Guillain-Barré syndrome is strongly associated with anti-GT1a antibodies, and if these studies are sent early in the disease, it may be possible to have forewarning of complications (Yoshino et al., 2000). Antibodies against *Campylobacter* and other infectious agents are also commonly identified.

CEREBROSPINAL FLUID

Cerebrospinal fluid analysis usually demonstrates the classic albuminocytological dissociation with protein values between 80 and 200 mg/dL. The presence of more than 50 lymphocytes per milliliter

makes the diagnosis of Guillain-Barré syndrome suspect; poliomyelitis (David and Doyle, 1997) or even central nervous system lymphoma should be considered in the differential diagnosis (Gucuyener et al., 1994; Toren et al., 1994).

Prognosis

Children with Guillain-Barré syndrome tend to have a more dramatic response to treatment and general capacity for recovery compared with adults (Bradshaw and Jones, 1992). The axonal form of childhood Guillain-Barré syndrome is well appreciated worldwide, although it is seen primarily in China (McKhann et al., 1993). In Buenos Aires, Paradiso and associates (1999) classified 18 of their 61 cases as acute motor axonal neuropathy. Clinically, this group had all the poor prognostic indicators normally associated with this pathology, including increased needs for ventilation, slower improvement, and worse residual deficit. We have seen a few cases at the Children's Hospital Boston.

CHRONIC INFLAMMATORY DEMYELINATING POLYNEUROPATHY

Chronic inflammatory demyelinating polyneuropathy is significantly less common than Guillain-Barré syndrome in children. In only 1 of 24 cases, with careful follow-up, seen at the Children's Hospital Boston did chronic inflammatory demyelinating polyneuropathy develop in the patient (Bradshaw and Jones, 1992). It can occur in very young children (Pasternak et al., 1982). Bird and Sladky (1991) reported three children who had a corticosteroid-responsive chronic inflammatory demyelinating polyneuropathy superimposed on a dominantly inherited familial neuropathy. These children were aged 4 to 14 years. Each child had pes cavus and a family history compatible with type I or type II CMT, and possibly even Friedreich's ataxia. Proximal weakness was a prominent finding in all three children. One child, diagnosed with Charcot-Marie-Tooth disease 14 years earlier, presented with a history of 4 months of deteriorating gait. In two of the three children, NCSs demonstrated the presence of multifocal demyelination compatible with a diagnosis of chronic inflammatory demyelinating polyneuropathy. The third child had uniform motor conduction velocity (MCV) slowing. This was the only patient with even a moderate cerebrospinal fluid protein elevation (82 mg/dL). It has been suggested that some hereditary neuropathies have a genetic susceptibility to chronic inflammatory demyelinating polyneuropathy (Bird and Sladky, 1991). Although each child's condition responded to the administration of corticosteroids, with improved proximal strength, two children showed no distal improvement. Relapses followed the tapering of medication in two children (Bird and Sladky, 1991). Clinicians who care for children with Charcot-Marie-Tooth disease must be alert to the possibility that a superimposed and treatable chronic inflammatory demyelinating polyneuropathy may have sudden neurological deterioration.

In children with chronic inflammating polyneuropathy whose polyneuropathy does not respond to corticosteroids, intravenous immuno-globulin or plasmapheresis may produce dramatic improvement (Cornblath et al., 1977; Vermeulen et al., 1985; Faed et al., 1989; Vedanarayanan et al., 1991). Drugs such as azathioprine, cyclophospha-mide, and cyclosporin may be considered. One 4-year-old with a 6-month history of chronic inflam-matory demyelinating polyneuropathy was unre-sponsive to prednisone therapy. Treatment with cy-clophosphamide resulted in total remission and increased MCV (Ouvrier et al., 1999).

One of the authors (M.P.) evaluated a child at the age of 2 months who presented with a possible radial nerve palsy, but the mother reported definite reduction in fetal movements in the last few weeks before delivery. There was evidence of a patchy demyelinating polyneuropathy when other nerves were examined (Figs. 92–1 and 92–2). It is always worth looking for the gene for hereditary liability to pressure palsies. However, it was absent in this case, whose pathology was confirmed on nerve biopsy.

The differing subgroups of chronic inflammatory demyelinating polyneuropathy, such as relapsing-re-mitting, occur rarely in children. A presumed mono-

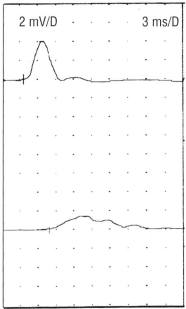

Figure 92–2. Recordings of the compound motor action potential from the abductor hallucis with stimulation of the medial popli-teal nerve at the ankle and popliteal fossa of a child with chronic inflammatory demyelinating polyneuropathy (same patient as in Fig. 92–1), showing severe dispersion on proximal stimulation. Conduction velocity is 22 m per second.

melic chronic inflammatory demyelinating polyneu-ropathy occurred in a West Indian child who was referred by an orthopedic surgeon for demonstra-tion of nerve entrapment with a view to surgical release. Electromyography showed multifocal con-duction block in all nerves in one arm with wasting and evidence of secondary axonal degeneration. All other limbs were clear. This condition may have a variety of presentations that are either purely motor or sensory or a combination of the two types (Thomas et al., 1996). Chronic inflammatory demye-linating polyneuropathy in children tends to more rapidly fluctuate and to be associated with a better prognosis (Simmons et al., 1997).

Chronic inflammatory demyelinating polyneuropa-thy is the most common recurrent childhood neu-ropathy. Various relatively rare mechanisms must be considered in the differential diagnosis.

RECURRENT CHILDHOOD NEUROPATHIES

Acute Nonautoimmune

Many of the recurrent neuropathies that are not classified as chronic inflammatory demyelinating polyneuropathy are related to an inborn error of metabolism (see Table 92–4). However, it is im-portant to always consider one toxic compound in the differential diagnosis: surreptitious glue sniffing can clinically mimic recurrent autoimmune-medi-

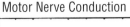

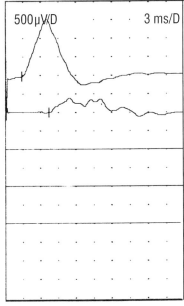

Figure 92–1. Recordings of the compound motor action potential from the abductor digiti minimi with stimulation of the ulnar nerve at wrist and elbow of a child with chronic inflammatory demyelinating polyneuropathy, showing severe dispersion at both sites. Conduction velocity is 15 m per second.

ated neuropathies as a result of intermittent abuse of this substance. This compound is covered in greater detail in the discussion of toxic neuropathies.

DEJERINE-SOTTAS DISEASE (HEREDITARY MOTOR SENSORY NEUROPATHY III)

Classically, Dejerine-Sottas disease is considered to have a remitting-relapsing course; however, a Mayo Clinic review of 11 children with Dejerine-Sottas disease failed to demonstrate any child with a remitting-relapsing course. Each child became symptomatic within 0 to 2 years of life (Benstead et al., 1990). NCSs demonstrated severe MCV slowing (less than 6 m per second in all except one child). In contrast to other hereditary neuropathies such as Charcot-Marie-Tooth disease, conduction block with greater than 50% reduction in compound motor action potential was present. Distal latencies were up to three times longer than normal. The authors emphasized that these slow conduction parameters might be mistaken for absent responses had slower-than-normal sweep speeds not been used. The hypertrophied nerves had a high threshold for stimulation. These findings illustrate the need to not assume a lack of response without first giving maximal stimuli and using prolonged sweep speeds. This was emphasized earlier when three of five children with very high stimulation thresholds were found to have Dejerine-Sottas disease, a fourth had a metachromatic leukodystrophy variant, and the fifth had chronic inflammatory demyelinating polyneuropathy (Bolton et al., 1988).

REFSUM'S DISEASE

This exceedingly uncommon autosomal recessive paroxysmal disorder is associated with a progressive hypertrophic demyelinating polyneuropathy sometimes referred to as hereditary motor sensory neuropathy type IV. These patients present with recurrent symmetrical episodic weakness. Associated clinical findings include retinal pigmentary degeneration, cerebellar ataxia, sensorineural hearing loss, cardiomyopathy, and ichthyosis. Elevated levels of serum phytanic acid, secondary to a deficit in β-oxidation degradation, distinguish Refsum's disease from chronic inflammatory demyelinating polyneuropathy or Friedreich's ataxia. The cerebrospinal fluid protein is abnormally elevated just as in chronic inflammatory demyelinating polyneuropathy. NCSs may demonstrate considerable slowing in both motor and sensory fibers (Torvik et al., 1988). We performed an NCS on one 4-year-old child with Refsum's disease but no clinically apparent peripheral neuropathy. The results were normal with no evidence of a polyneuropathy in this preschool-aged child.

PORPHYRIA

This is an exceedingly rare cause for a peripheral neuropathy in children. One girl had her first epi-

sodes of recurrent abdominal pain occur at the age of 8 years (Ford, 1966b). Two years later, she had bilateral wristdrop and footdrop, intense muscle tenderness, and cutaneous hyperesthesia. During the next 20 years, she had a few more acute neurological events, but NCSs were never performed. Bolton (personal communication, 1992) performed NCSs on a child with porphyria. He demonstrated a pure axonal motor neuropathy similar to findings reported by Albers and associates in 1978. Their study demonstrated a similar neuropathy in eight patients with acute quadriparesis that developed with an acute porphyria.

TANGIER'S DISEASE

This disorder of high-density lipoprotein is associated with low high-density lipoprotein levels as well as with apolipoprotein AI and AII in the plasma. Episodic weakness occurs in this metabolic illness associated with the important clinical hallmark of orange-colored tonsils. Two sisters with Tangier's disease, aged 12 and 14 years, had episodic extremity weakness and nonprogressive asymmetrical sensory symptoms. There was no anatomical relation of these sensory complaints to their motor abnormalities (Engel et al., 1967). The levels of plasma cholesterol were low, with nearly absent α-lipoproteins. In the one child studied, the results of NCSs were normal, and EMG showed denervation. Three of four other patients with Tangier's disease had a remitting-relapsing multifocal mononeuropathy (Pollock et al., 1983). Sural nerve biopsy demonstrated prominent demyelination and remyelination.

Nonautoimmune Acute Polyneuropathies

INBORN ERRORS OF METABOLISM

Acquired neuropathies of this type are most commonly axonal (see Table 92–5). Tyrosinemia type 1, resulting from an inborn error in the final step of tyrosine metabolism, may present with acute peripheral nerve involvement and should be considered in the differential diagnosis of Guillain-Barré syndrome. There is a predilection for phrenic nerve involvement in addition to the generalized polyneuropathy. These patients' electromyographic findings are indistinguishable from those of patients with Guillain-Barré syndrome (Gibbs et al., 1993). In a large study of 48 children, Mitchell and colleagues (1990) reported 20 who had neurological crises that began at the mean age of 1 year. Eight of these children (40%) required mechanical ventilation. However, in contrast to EMG, when pathological studies were performed, in three of the children, a primarily axonal degeneration with secondary demyelination was found.

Both porphyria (Ford, 1966b) and Leigh's syndrome (Coker, 1993), which are enhanced by medications, particularly barbiturates, may also have precipitate symptoms and findings that resemble childhood Guillain-Barré syndrome. The porphyrias are an important but rare cause of axonal, predominantly motor, neuropathy in childhood. They have an autosomal dominant inheritance. All types are caused by disturbances of the porphyrin metabolism. Acute intermittent porphyria is caused by a reduction in uroporphyrinogen synthase (porphobilinogen deaminase). Usually, the first attack occurs in adolescence or early adult life, and the attack may have been precipitated by drugs, notably the barbiturates, or alcohol. Behavioral problems, abdominal pain, and nausea and vomiting may herald the attack, which presents as acute weakness. This may be distal and proximal, and respiratory and bulbar muscles may be affected (Lip et al., 1993). Coproporphyria associated with an excess of fecal and urinary coproporphyrins is even rarer than acute intermittent but presents similarly (Barohn et al., 1994). Variegate porphyria shares the clinical presentation of the other two varieties, with its basic defect a reduction of protoporphyrinogen oxidase in skin fibroblasts. It is common in South Africa (Jenkins, 1996).

Leigh's syndrome, which is also known as subacute necrotizing encephalomyelopathy, is a hereditary process most commonly of mitochondrial origin (DiMauro et al., 1989). Commonly, these youngsters are hypotonic with symptoms that begin in the second year, usually with feeding and swallowing problems, vomiting, ataxia, and weakness. Although the associated peripheral neuropathy is often clinically unimportant, it occasionally mimics Guillain-Barré syndrome.

Toxins

The discussion that follows comments on those medicinal, industrial (including heavy metals), or naturally occurring compounds that may cause a polyneuropathy in a child. One must be ever cautious that these known pharmacological agents represent only a fraction of the compounds that may have potential to damage the peripheral nervous system. It is remarkable how infrequently children are referred for investigation of suspected peripheral neuropathy given the frequency with which they are exposed to these agents, particularly if one considers the chemotherapeutic agents. There may be a number of reasons for this. First, the neuropathy may be reversible as soon as the medication is stopped. Second, it may already be well recognized and be dose related. Finally, it may be considered unkind to subject very ill children to investigations that, unless the child is demonstrating a most severe neuropathy that is therefore likely detectable on clinical examination, are not likely to influence treatment options.

Additional information is given in Chapter 63 and on the Internet. The Pharmacological Society of Great Britain (http://www.spib.axl.co.uk) maintains one such site.

Pharmacological Preparations

Oncological Medications. The chemotherapy agents such as vincristine and cisplatin are well recognized as important causes of an ingravescent primary sensory neuropathy in children. However, vincristine toxicity also rarely presents with an acute motor polyneuropathy in children who have an unsuspected CMT1 hereditary neuropathy (Graf et al., 1996). Testing for the CMT1 gene, a 17p11.2-12 duplication, requires consideration in any child who sustains an acute motor polyneuropathy shortly after just one or two doses of vincristine.

Antimicrobials

Long-term antibiotic therapy is rarely associated with a neuromuscular syndrome mimicking Guillain-Barré syndrome or poliomyelitis. This is perhaps a peculiarity in children more than in adults, particularly for children with cystic fibrosis who take chloramphenicol for long periods. They are at risk of the development of a predominantly sensory axonal polyneuropathy, as may also occur if metronidazole is used for long periods.

Children with overwhelming sepsis (Sheth et al., 1995) or status asthmaticus (Hopkins, 1974) may develop a critical neuropathy (see Chapter 75).

Sodium dichloroacetate is used for the treatment of various inborn errors of mitochondrial function. It has the potential for peripheral nerve damage (Spruijt et al., 2001). Twenty-seven patients with chronic lacticacidemia received sodium dichloroacetate for 1 year. More than 50% of the patients had a decline in nerve conduction velocity (NCV) and compound motor action potential amplitude. In just three of these individuals, symptoms of a peripheral neuropathy developed (more in the adolescent population). This occurred in contradistinction to the patients' report of improved muscle strength. A few children who receive this medication are undergoing monitoring in our EMG laboratory at the Children's Hospital Boston. With use for just a few years, the parents report improvement in the child's basic neurological difficulties. However, we are beginning to note very significant loss of compound motor action potential amplitude with preservation of motor NCVs and distal latencies.

Thalidomide has been reintroduced for a variety of conditions, most often dermatological, that include Behçet's disease as well as lupus erythematosus, graft-versus-host disease, ulcerative colitis, and the esophageal ulcers seen in patients with acquired immunodeficiency syndrome or Crohn's disease. The reported incidence of neurotoxicity diagnosed electrophysiologically varies from 1% to 50% (Burley, 1961; Amelung and Puntmann, 1966), using the amplitude of the compound sensory nerve action potential. Thalidomide neurotoxicity is much less than that of the previous drugs discussed, such as vincristine. Its mechanism of action is the downregulation of tumor necrosis factor α. There also are well-documented cases of peripheral neuropathy (Burley, 1961; Fullerton and Kremer, 1961; Simpson, 1961; Clemensen et al., 1984); in fact, it was the early reports of peripheral neuritis that delayed its approval by the Food and Drug Administration in 1960, not the fetal abnormalities that were first reported in the next year. Pathological studies have demonstrated that the dorsal root ganglia are the primary site of the pathology. The neuropathy so produced may be slow to recover, if it does so at all.

Lack of awareness of the test-retest variability of the amplitude of sensory nerve action potential, when decreases in amplitude are more likely thought due to drug effect than to measurement error, may in part explain the varying incidence of neurotoxicity of thalidomide. The patient may then be denied a valuable medication and the incidence of neurotoxicity of the drug is falsely elevated. Without explanation of the variability observed in sensory nerve action potentials recorded routinely using surface electrodes, even a guideline such as the 40% drop of an index of three sensory nerve action potentials, indicating a neuropathy (Gardner-Medwin and Powell, 1994), may be in error.

One approach is to use alternative methods of sensory testing, other than NCSs, such as quantitative sensory testing and to include tests for autonomic function. In an editorial, Olney (1998) extols the value of quantitative sensory testing as being able to screen the broadest range of fiber types and maintains that modern equipment that use the "4-2-1" stepping algorithm (Dyck et al., 1991) have high reproducibility. They do require patient collaboration and therefore are associated with difficulties in use in some children.

Heavy Metals

Lead

This is an exceedingly rare cause of childhood motor polyneuropathy, especially in comparison to pica encephalopathy. These neuropathies are predominantly characterized by axonal degeneration. Acute exposure more likely results in an encephalopathy than in a neuropathy. However, Ford (1966a) noted that lead polyneuritis may complicate pica encephalopathy in older children. Rarely, this neuropathy occurs without any cerebral symptoms. The legs are disproportionately affected and associated with muscle tenderness (Ford, 1966a). One child died from a severe generalized neuropathy associated with profound bulbar dysfunction subsequent to ingesting lead-based paint (Ford, 1966a). The only laboratory abnormality reported was a moderately increased cerebrospinal fluid protein level. Apparently, EMG was not performed. A 3-year-old child with 2 years of pica experienced two episodes of nausea, vomiting, thigh pain, and recurrent subacute

motor neuropathy. Importantly, lead levels in both the blood and urine were normal (Windebank et al., 1995). The child was anemic. Urinary levels of coproporphyrins were positive, and δ-aminolevulinic acid levels were nine times normal. Electromyography demonstrated denervation, but NCSs were not performed. Treatment with calcium disodium edetate caused a 1000-fold increase in the excretion of lead, and the child was normal in 6 months. Lead-induced neuropathies with varying clinical pictures are reported by the same author in eight other children. In general, there was an acute motor greater than sensory neuropathy associated with the history of pica and anemia, usually with basophilic stippling of erythrocytes. The authors hypothesized that the child's blood and urine lead levels were normal because of slow absorption of the lead. The removal of lead-based paint and the more widespread use of lead-free petrol make this an exceedingly rare etiology for a polyneuropathy. We have not seen this as an identified cause of a childhood neuropathy during one of the author's 22-year experience at the Children's Hospital Boston.

Arsenic

Arsenic poisoning rarely enters into the pediatric differential diagnosis of Guillain-Barré syndrome or chronic inflammatory demyelinating polyneuropathy because, in general, arsenic intoxication is primarily seen secondary to industrial exposure. When it does occur, it is most commonly an axonal degeneration, although demyelination has been reported (Donofrio et al., 1987). One 17-year-old girl, with serious clinical depression, chose to ingest arsenious oxide powder. This resulted in a progressive motor-sensory painful neuropathy (Le Quesne and McLeod, 1977). Peroneal MCV was 36 m per second. Sural sensory nerve action potentials were absent. An examination of the urine, hair, and nails is important for the diagnosis.

Mercury

Mercury may also, very rarely, cause a peripheral neuropathy in children. Two siblings developed generalized weakness, ataxic gait, areflexia, and abdominal pain after exposure to mercury vapor (Windebank et al., 1995). NCSs demonstrated some reduction in compound motor action potentials, normal to minimally reduced motor NCV, and normal sensory nerve action potentials. Neuropathies (motor greater than sensory) also developed in two other children treated with ammoniated mercury ointments for dermatological conditions (Swaiman and Flagler, 1971). One child had an elevated level of cerebrospinal fluid protein (Ross, 1964). Electromyography was not performed for either child. A 4-year-old child had acrodynia secondary to exposure to fumes in a home that was recently painted with a latex paint containing an organic mercury preservative (Agocs et al., 1990). Inorganic mercury produced a severe sensorimotor neuropathy in an adult who ingested herbal drugs (Chu et al., 1998); we are not aware of this in the pediatric population.

Organic mercury can enter the food chain when fish becomes contaminated by toxic effluents, such as occurred in Minamata Bay. The primary effects of acute exposure are on the brain. However, a motor neuropathy with axonal degeneration occurs rarely.

Thallium

The accidental ingestion of rat poison has been identified to occur more frequently among children than adults. When this contains thallium, it may produce a polyneuropathy that affects motor-sensory fibers about 1 week after exposure. Thallium ingestion may also mimic arsenic poisoning, with concomitant symptoms of gastrointestinal distress and findings even of Mees' lines (Windebank et al., 1995). This is very rare and especially uncommon in children. An adolescent attempted suicide with ingestion of thallium (Davis et al., 1981). Attempted motor NCSs failed to demonstrate any compound motor action potentials in the legs or distal arms; however, a proximal median nerve motor NCS demonstrated a conduction velocity of 20 m per second. This is compatible with the primary demyelinating effects of the thallium. In the adolescent who ingested thallium in a suicide attempt, the changes suggested a primary demyelinating neuropathy.

Other Toxins

Biological (Buckthorn, Wild Cherry [Karwinskia humboldtiana])

This poisonous "fruit" is found on shrubs in northern Mexico, the southwestern United States, Central America, Columbia, and the Caribbean countries. If an unsuspecting child accidentally ingests this toxic fruit, an acute symmetrical motor polyneuropathy may develop within 1 to 15 days that totally mimics Guillain-Barré syndrome (Calderon-Gonzalez and Rizzi-Hernandez, 1967).

If the intoxication is severe, a bulbar paralysis with potential for a fatal outcome is a possibility. Some of the most severely affected children also had associated diarrhea and vomiting. In 1997, Martinez and associates reviewed their experience with 22 children admitted with an acute flaccid paralysis to the University Hospital in Monterrey, Mexico. Six of the 22 had buckthorn cherry paralysis. Three of these six children lived in the countryside, and each had a history of fruit ingestion.

Diagnosis was based on the findings of a semiquantitative determination of the T-514 (Tullidinol) Karwinskia humboldtiana toxin in the blood of all six children. In contrast to Guillain-Barré syndrome, the cerebrospinal fluid protein was normal in all six children. No cerebrospinal fluid analysis for this toxin per se was performed. Sural nerve biopsy demonstrated segmental demyelination with loss of myelin over the length of one or more internode segments. Other diagnoses were documented in these 22 Mexican children who presented with acute flaccid paralyses, in addition to buckthorn poisoning and Guillain-Barré syndrome. These primarily included other toxins, particularly glue and adhesive solvent exposure.

Industrial

Glue Sniffing (n-Hexane). Addiction to n-hexane occasionally occurs in adolescents in response to glue sniffing, sometimes resulting in either an acute or a subacute, occasionally recurrent, peripheral neuropathy. This unusual, almost exclusive adolescent addiction always should be considered in the differential diagnosis of chronic inflammatory demyelinating polyneuropathy. With glue, there is an exposure to n-hexane and n-butyl ketone when solvents are used. Both substances produce a mixed axonal and demyelinating neuropathy. Electromyography demonstrates slow motor NCV, also compatible with a primary demyelinating process (Korobkin et al., 1975; Ouvrier et al., 1999). In the case of Ouvrier and colleagues (1999), sural nerve biopsy demonstrated paranodal demyelination and large giant axons. Neurofilamentous axonal masses are quite specific for this toxin but are also found in neuroaxonal dystrophy, as subsequently discussed, and are found with sural nerve biopsy. Ouvrier and colleagues evaluated one adolescent who had sniffed glue.

Kuwabara and colleagues (1993) reported a teenager with a 3-week period of benzene (n-hexane) abuse who became unable to walk on discontinuation of the chemical. His symptoms evolved over a 3-month period. He became tetraplegic. Motor NCSs demonstrated moderate conduction slowing with median nerve conduction block between the wrist and the elbow. Active denervation was noted. Sural nerve biopsy revealed scattered swollen axons surrounded by thin myelin. Full recovery was gradually achieved in 14 months.

The n-hexane component of glue is also found in cements used in the shoe industry. Generalized weakness with areflexia, nausea, anorexia, and weight loss rapidly developed in four girls aged 14 to 16 years (Rizzuto et al., 1977). Each adolescent was employed in a poorly ventilated shoe factory and concomitantly had direct contact with n-hexane leather cements. Their peroneal MCVs were fine except for considerable prolongation of distal latency in one patient. After their toxic exposure was discontinued, improvement began at 2 months. A complete resolution occurred in three of the girls; one girl had residual distal weakness.

Postvaccinial Peripheral Neuropathy

On very rare occasions, a peripheral neuropathy is a complication of rubella immunization. In 36 prepubertal children, rather specific reactions developed 6 weeks after vaccination as either an arm or a leg syndrome (Schaffner et al., 1974). Some of these children with the primary "arm syndrome" abruptly awakened with dysesthesias of the hands that lasted 0.5 to 30 minutes. Their symptoms tended to recur throughout the night. In contrast, the "leg syndrome" was usually first noted on awakening. This was characterized by posterior leg pain, which led to a characteristic gait in which the children walked on their toes with the digits flexed. Slow distal sensory nerve conduction velocity was demonstrated on NCSs in 11 of the 13 children, with mild median nerve MCV slowing in 2 children (Gilmartin et al., 1972). One year later, these values were normal.

Five of 39 patients had a symmetrical polyneuritis as their neurological complication from the smallpox vaccination. An additional two had a brachial plexitis (Spillane and Wells, 1964). Only 1 of the 39 patients was a child, aged 2 years. This toddler developed a foot-slapping gait that cleared within 1 week. Electromyography was not performed.

HEREDITARY NEUROPATHIES

Leukodystrophies

The literature on peripheral neuropathy in leukodystrophy reflects a bygone age before specific DNA diagnostic tests became available. As a consequence, in our respective laboratories, it has been many years since such a case was referred for EMG. With these reservations in mind, several points are important to note.

Metachromatic leukodystrophy has a demyelinating peripheral neuropathy as a feature of all of the major clinical groups: late infantile (Aicardi, 1993), early juvenile (Yatziv and Rusell, 1981), and juvenile (Clark et al., 1979). Rarely, the demonstration of a demyelinating polyneuropathy is an important clue to the diagnosis in an infant with loss of previously achieved motor and intellectual development. At the upper end of the typical age range, there are instances where the unexpected discovery of a demyelinating neuropathy in a patient who was dementing (Percy et al., 1977; Bosch and Hart, 1978; Wulff and Trojaborg, 1985) or one with an adolescent-onset movement disorder (Scully et al., 1984) has led to the correct diagnosis. Deficiencies in the sphingolipid activator protein (SAP) or saposins give rise to atypical forms of the metachromatic leukodystrophies or Gaucher's disease. SAP B deficiency gives rise to accumulation of sulfatides in the peripheral nerve (Hensler et al., 1996) and cerebral white matter.

Krabbe's leukodystrophy caused by deficiency of the lysosomal enzyme galactocerebrosidase β-galactosidase usually presents before the age of 6 months (early infantile form). A peripheral neuropathy has been demonstrated at 7 weeks in an antenatally diagnosed case (Lieberman et al., 1980). Although NCSs and magnetic resonance images of the brain may be normal early, they usually become abnormal beyond 3 months (Zafeiriou et al., 1997). The late infantile form presents between 6 to 18 months with the floppiness secondary to a mixture of central and peripheral demyelination (Aicardi, 1993). The peripheral neuropathy is less consistently present in the late-onset or juvenile form. It was seen in only one of the four cases reported by Phelps and associates (1991), who demonstrated highly variable presentations—some patients were wheelchair bound and others were in active employment. Others may present with scoliosis; the importance of finding a demyelinating neuropathy in a 13-year-old girl was not appreciated at the time, 4 years before the diagnosis was finally made (Marks et al., 1997). One case presented acutely in the context of an influenza A infection (McGuinness et al., 1996).

Cockayne's syndrome is associated with a demyelinating peripheral neuropathy (Moosa and Dubowitz, 1970; Sasaki et al., 1992). Caused by a defective chromosome or DNA repair, there is a wide spectrum of severity, with increasing severity in the peripheral and central demyelination with age (Smits et al., 1982).

Adrenoleukomyeloneuropathy characterized by a change in the normal ratio of C26:C22 long-chain fatty acids is variably associated with a demyelinating neuropathy. The neonatal form of the condition may present with signs and neurophysiological findings that sometimes suggest an infantile spinal muscular atrophy (Paul et al., 1993). Some clinicians believe it is still important to identify the phenotype more accurately, for which EMG may help. To others, it may provide the chance to monitor treatment.

Pelizaeus-Merzbacher leukodystrophy is not presently possible to identify from blood tests. The changes on the magnetic resonance image may point to the diagnosis. It is due to a mutation in the *PLP* gene coding for the proteolipid protein. This is found only in the central nervous system, and unlike so many other leukodystrophies, the peripheral nerve is not usually involved. The absence of a peripheral neuropathy used to be an important diagnostic pointer in this context. However, a family study (Garbern et al., 1997) demonstrated that a peripheral demyelinating neuropathy is seen, albeit with a unique mutation that leads to the absence of *PLP* expression.

Other Hereditary Metabolic Conditions

ASSOCIATION WITH A DEMYELINATING POLYNEUROPATHY

β-Mannosidase deficiency is a rare condition in humans with clinical features similar to those of the mucopolysaccharidoses with coarse features and developmental delay. A demyelinating polyneuropathy is sometimes encountered (Levade et al., 1994).

Carbohydrate-deficient glycoprotein deficiency syndrome type 1 is an autosomal recessive condition that has four stages (Jaeken et al., 1987). The teenage stage, or stage 3, is the one associated with the demyelinating neuropathy accompanied by marked muscle atrophy, which suggests that there may be some axonal degeneration as well (Blenow et al., 1991). The infant cases may be associated with olivopontocerebellar hypoplasia and anterior horn cell fallout, which are features they share in common with type 1 pontocerebellar hypoplasia (Barth, 1993). Fumarase deficiency is another rare cause of lethargy, vomiting, and failure to thrive in the neonatal period. A proportion of these children have a polyneuropathy (Narayanan et al., 1996).

Sialidosis type 1, or cherry-red spot myoclonus, is an autosomal recessive condition with juvenile- or even adult-onset of mild dementia, myoclonus, and a macular cherry-red spot with a neuropathy, described by Steinman and associates (1980).

The finding of a peripheral neuropathy in a suspected case of Leigh's disease may be valuable. The hypotonia from the neuropathy (Jacobs et al., 1990) often does not develop until the third stage (van Coster et al., 1991) of the disease, between the ages of 2 and 10 years, when it is accompanied by dysphagia. Niemann-Pick disease type A, another autosomal recessive condition, is also known as the neuronopathic form with an associated neuropathy (Gumbinas et al., 1975). The presence of large Niemann-Pick cells with foamy cytoplasm in the bone marrow and low levels of sphingomyelinase make the diagnosis.

ASSOCIATION WITH AN AXONAL POLYNEUROPATHY

There are other metabolic conditions that are associated with axonal degeneration; two relate to the lipoproteins. Abetalipoproteinemia (Bassen-Kornzweig syndrome) usually presents in infancy with symptoms related to malabsorption. In the teenage years, a peripheral neuropathy, predominantly sensory (Wichman et al., 1985), cerebellar ataxia, and a pigmentary retinopathy develop. Hypobetalipoproteinemia shares many of the clinical characteristics of abetalipoproteinemia, including the presence of a neuropathy.

Glucocorticoid deficiency–achalasia–deficient tear production is an autosomal recessive condition. There is associated hyperreflexia, muscle weakness, and dysarthria. A peripheral neuropathy and autonomic involvement emerged when a cohort of patients initially reported by Allgrove and colleagues (1978) were reviewed by Grant and colleagues (1992). Santer and colleagues (1993) described the neuropathy in pseudo–neonatal adrenoleukodystrophy diagnosed by the presence of reduced activity of the peroxisomal enzyme acyl coenzyme A oxidase. Metachromatic leukodystrophy due to activator defect is also unusual in having an axonal degeneration found on nerve studies.

HEREDITARY MOTOR AND SENSORY NEUROPATHIES

These most common causes for childhood polyneuropathy have had clear genetic identification in some of the most prevalent examples of these disorders, as outlined in Table 92–6. In the relatively common form, there has been a return to the original name, Charcot-Marie-Tooth disease, for the classification of the hereditary motor sensory neuropathies (Table 92–7). A detailed discussion of these neuropathies is given in Chapter 57. Here, we comment just on those aspects that have been pertinent to us in our care of children. Lewis and colleagues (2000) reviewed the ability of NCSs to distinguish between the hereditary, such as CMT1a, and the acquired demyelinating conditions, principally chronic inflammatory demyelinating polyneuropathy. The presence or absence of conduction block or temporal dispersion is a point of some controversy. Lewis and Sumner (1982) thought this did not occur in CMT1a, but Oh and Chang (1987) found this in 60% of their 22 patients. Our personal experience

---

Table 92–6. Hereditary Demyelinating Neuropathies

Charcot-Marie-Tooth disease (see Table 92–7)
Leukodystrophies
  Adrenoleukodystrophy
  Adrenoleukodystrophy, presenting as a cerebellar ataxia or dementia
  Adrenoleukodystrophy, neonatal
  Cockayne's syndrome
  Metachromatic leukodystrophy, compound allele, heterozygous
  Metachromatic leukodystrophy, with retinitis pigmentosa
  Metachromatic leukodystrophy (spurious), pseudo–arylsulfatase deficiency
  Metachromatic leukodystrophy, late infantile type, early juvenile onset, juvenile, adult onset
  Krabbe's disease, early infantile form, late infantile type, late onset or juvenile type
Other Metabolic Conditions
  β-mannosidase deficiency
  Carbohydrate-deficient glycoprotein syndrome type I
  Sphingolipid activator protein B deficiency
  Sialidosis type 1 (cherry-red spot)
  Fumarase deficiency
  Leigh's disease, classic
  Niemann-Pick type A
Miscellaneous
  Chediak-Higashi syndrome
  Farber's disease, lipogranulomatosis
  Lemieux-Neemeh syndrome, deafness
  Lowe's syndrome, oculocerebrorenal
  Multisystem neuronal degeneration, abnormal arachidonic acid
  Muscle hypertrophy with neuropathy
  Myotonic dystrophy and a neuropathy
  Pandysautonomia
  Pressure palsy, tomaculous neuropathy
  Retinitis pigmentosa, ataxia, peripheral neuropathy
  Rosenberg-Chutorian syndrome, optic atrophy
  Rud's syndrome, ichthyosis, hypogonadism, mental retardation, retinitis pigmentosa
  Spinal muscular atrophy, pontocerebellar hypoplasia
  Werner's syndrome
  X-linked cerebellar ataxia

Table 92–7. Genetic Classification of Charcot-Marie-Tooth Disease

Type	Genetics	Inheritance
Type I (demyelinating with severely reduced conduction velocities)		
CMT1A	Duplication of chromosome 17p11.2 or point mutation of *PMP22* gene	AD
CMT1B	Point mutation in myelin protein-22 (*Po*) gene; linkage to chromosome 1q21-q23	AD
CMT1C	Unknown	AD
CMT4	Unknown	AR
Type II (neuronal with low-normal conduction velocities)		
CMT2A	Maps to chromosome 1p36	AD
CMT2B	Maps to chromosome 3q	AR
CMT2C (associated with diaphragmatic weakness and vocal cord paralysis)	No association	
Dejerine-Sottas disease (severely reduced conduction velocities)		
DSD subdivisions	Point mutations in *PMP22* or *Po* gene	AR
X-linked	Mutations of connexin 32 gene	X-linked
Hereditary neuropathy with liability to pressure palsies	1.5-mb deletion in chromosome 17p11.2-12 (likely a result of reduced expression of the *PMP22 gene*)	AD

AD, autosomal dominant; AR, autosomal recessive; CMT, Charcot-Marie-Tooth.

with metachromatic leukodystrophy also lends support to their findings in that some of our children had NCS signs of conduction block and dispersed compound motor action potentials (Cameron and Jones, 1996).

Charcot-Marie-Tooth Disease

A clinician may be called on to examine young members of families affected with CMT type I. The available evidence indicates that abnormalities are present from very early on in the clinical course. Looking primarily at the progressive atrophy in the extensor digitorum brevis in a group of children with the CMT1 duplication, Berciano and associates (2000) reported a child as young as 1 month showing nerve conduction abnormalities. Others (Emeryk-Szajewska et al., 1998) have shown that there is no worsening of the nerve conduction abnormality with age, that the degree of abnormalities of the changes tends to be uniform within families, and that there may be clear nerve conduction slowing with little clinical change. However, in personal experience, one of us (R.J.) has seen an exception to this temporal guideline.

CMT1a usually presents with a generalized peripheral neuropathy. This is typically characterized by distal weakness, absent muscle stretch reflexes, and pes cavus with cock-up toes. Usually, children with this abnormality do not come to medical attention until their inherent pes cavus or second decade–onset changes in gait lead an orthopedic surgeon or a neurologist to inquire as to whether the child has CMT1a. From experience at the Children's Hospital Boston, about 35% of children who come to the EMG laboratory with this concern are found to have a demyelinating polyneuropathy (Hsu and Jones,

1997). We have not seen CMT1a present clinically in infants or toddlers.

Hereditary Neuropathy with Liability to Pressure Palsies

Hereditary neuropathy with liability to pressure palsies may be the occasional explanation for an unexplained mononeuropathy or mononeuropathy multiplex variant (Cruz-Martinez and Arpa, 1998; Pareyson et al., 1998; Stogbauer et al., 1998). There is sensory nerve conduction velocity slowing and prolongation of distal motor latencies but only relatively infrequent minor reduction in the motor nerve conduction velocities (Andersson et al., 2000). Outside of these major groupings, there are complex forms that do not yet have chromosome abnormalities described. Those with a demyelinating neuropathy are shown in Table 92–8.

There also is a large group of very unusual inherited polyneuropathies for which no specific genetic mechanism has been identified to date (see Table 92–8). The complex forms of CMT type 2 are very uncommon. Cardiac involvement is described. This may be conduction defect (Littler, 1970) or cardiomyopathy (Lascelles et al., 1970). A severe form of CMT2 is recognized. Ouvrier and associates (1981) report one of their patients who had onset at birth and an additional six children with an onset within the first 2 years of life. Despite the early onset, the children maintained some independence from wheelchairs until the end of the second decade of life. There is thought to be a variety of CMT2 in older patients that may be associated with diaphragm and vocal cord paresis (Dyck et al., 1994). An X-linked recessive motor sensory neuropathy is also described with axonal degeneration associated with

Table 92–8. Complex Hereditary Motor and Sensory Demyelinating Neuropathies Without Identifiable Chromosome Abnormality

Description	Inheritance	Chromosome	Study
HMSN, deafness	AD	17	Pinhas Hamiel et al., 1993
HMSN, deafness, infantile onset	AR	?	Cornell et al., 1984
HMSN, cerebellar atrophy	AR		Fukuhara et al., 1995
HMSN, extrapyramidal features	AR	?	Jaradeh and Dyck, 1992
HMSN, focally folded myelin	AR	11q23	Barbieri et al., 1994
HMSN, Navajo neuropathy type I	AR	?	Appenzeller et al., 1976
HMSN type VI, optic atrophy, deafness	AR	?	Sommer and Schroder, 1989
HMSN, type V with spasticity	AR or AD	?	Harding and Thomas, 1984
HMSN, with acetabular dysplasia	AD	?	Fuller and DeLuca, 1995

AD, autosomal dominant; AR, autosomal recessive; HMSN, hereditary motor and sensory neuropathy.

deafness and mental retardation (Cowchock et al., 1985); it maps to Xq24-q26 (Priest et al., 1995).

There has been an attempt to distinguish a form of *scapuloperoneal* wasting associated with sensory nerve abnormalities only as Davidenkow's syndrome (Schwartz and Swash, 1975). In reporting three members of an affected family who showed different manifestations, Harding and Thomas (1980) thought that all three would fall within the phenotypic variation seen in hereditary motor sensory neuropathy type I.

The *X-linked form* of Charcot-Marie-Tooth disease begins early in childhood with difficulty in running, pes cavus deformity, peroneal atrophy, atrophy of hand muscles, and distal sensory loss. Males are more severely affected than are females, although females are affected twice as often as are males. Male-to-male transmission does not occur. Affected females transmit to half of their sons and half of their daughters. Affected males transmit to all of their daughters and none of their sons. Conduction velocity slowing is intermediate between CMT1 and CMT2. The long arm of the X chromosome near Xq 13 is affected, with point mutation of the connexin 32 gene. This gene is an integral part of gap junctions. This may compromise Schwann cells and Schwann cell–axon interactions, causing pathology in both myelin and axons (Nicholson and Nash, 1993; Hahn et al., 2001).

Hereditary Sensory and Autonomic Neuropathies

These rare neuropathies were originally called the *hereditary sensory neuropathies* and were first thought to be the related to syringomyelia because of their clinical presentation with predominant involvement of pain and temperature nerve fibers. All forms are very rare (Dyck, 1984). The neurophysiological testing for these conditions is understandably difficult given the well-documented deficiencies of standard sensory nerve studies in the diagnosis of small fiber abnormalities. Both Dyck (1984) and Thomas (1993) thought these deficiencies have been a major reason for the slowness of the classification

of these disorders. Dyck and colleagues (2000) called for better case ascertainment but recognize that the sensitivity and specificity of tests for early large-diameter sensory nerve fiber involvement are unproved. Tests of small-diameter sensory nerve fibers are time consuming, expensive, and invasive and therefore may not be appropriate for pediatric patients whether symptomatic or asymptomatic although at risk for the disease.

All are recessively inherited except the X-linked form and the dominantly inherited type I. This was originally known as *Denny-Brown's hereditary sensory radicular neuropathy* and has an onset at around 20 years. There is loss of pain and temperature appreciation with ulcerating painless lesions on hands and feet. Sometimes, there is significant wasting, and occasionally, there is sensorineural deafness (Horoupian, 1989). Motor conduction studies are normal, but sensory nerve responses are absent.

Type II presents at birth or infancy with ulcers and fractures in the peripheral parts of the limbs. Sweating is impaired distally. Nerve biopsy samples will show almost complete absence of myelinated fibers and a decrease in the number of unmyelinated fibers. There are absent sensory nerve studies but near-normal or low-normal responses from the motor nerves.

Type III (Riley-Day syndrome) presents in early childhood and is usually seen in Ashkenazi Jews. The dysautonomic components manifest as absence of overflow tears, poor sweating vasomotor instability, and labile temperature control. There is reduced pain and taste sensation, absent tear production, corneal ulceration, vomiting, episodic fever, smooth tongue with loss of the fungiform tongue papillae, severe gastrointestinal symptoms, and skeletal dysplasia. The gene is mapped to chromosome 9q.

Type IV is the anhidrotic congenital sensory neuropathy and has a congenital onset. There is universal insensitivity to pain with anhidrosis but normal tear production. Biopsy shows a severe paucity of unmyelinated fibers, often detectable only on electron microscopy. Neurophysiological studies are normal, particularly motor and sensory NCSs.

Type V presents with congenital insensitivity to

pain. It is detectable only by careful morphometry of the peripheral nerve. In contradistinction to type IV, there are plentiful normal unmyelinated fibers. The particular deficiency is of A delta fibers. Only one large pedigree of the X-linked form has been published to date (Jestico et al., 1985). Sensory changes were restricted to the feet. Sural nerve action potentials were reduced or absent and pathologic examination showed loss of all myelinated fibers but particularly those of the smallest diameter.

Other Hereditary Sensory Neuropathies

Sensory neuropathy with spastic paraplegia, possibly recessively inherited, can occur around the age of 3 to 4 years (Cavanagh et al., 1979). The sural nerve biopsy demonstrates loss of both myelinated and unmyelinated fibers and involvement of the dorsal root ganglia as well. Hereditary motor sensory neuropathy type V is also associated with spasticity, but the motor nerves are clearly involved, so there is no difficulty differentiating them with EMG.

Navajo Indians can have two types of recessive primary sensory neuropathies. The *type I* form involves a global loss of perception of pain leading to painless fractures and cutaneous ulcers (Appenzeller et al., 1976). Sensory nerve action potentials are abnormal and are associated with slow motor conduction velocities. Sensory nerve biopsy shows involvement of both myelinated and unmyelinated fibers. The *type II* form involves normal muscle stretch reflexes (Johnsen et al., 1993). Some patients have very little sensory loss. Nerve biopsy demonstrates marked selective loss of small myelinated and unmyelinated fibers.

Other Hereditary Neuropathies That Are Primarily Axonal

These are the conditions that are primarily diseases of the peripheral nerves but that do not fall under the Charcot-Marie-Tooth disease classification (Table 92–9).

Giant axonal neuropathy, with an onset in the first 7 years of life, is associated with tight curly hair. The neuropathy present pathologically may be not detectable neurophysiologically in the first few years (Donaghy et al., 1988; Kumar et al., 1990). Berg and colleagues (1972) described an unusual chronic polyneuropathy in a 6-year-old child with a history of clumsy gait. She had kinky hair, distal greater than proximal muscle weakness, and areflexia. Sural nerve biopsy demonstrated abnormally large argentophilic masses of tightly woven neurofilaments. A summary of 21 patients with giant axonal neuropathy noted that motor milestones were delayed, and

Table 92–9. Hereditary Axonal Neuropathy

Metabolic
  Abetalipoproteinemia (Bassen-Kornzweig syndrome)
  Glucocorticoid deficiency–achalasia-deficient tear production
  Adrenoleukodystrophy, pseudoneonatal
  Metachromatic leukodystrophy due to activator defect
  Hypobetalipoproteinemia
Structural
  Agenesis of corpus callosum
Associated with abnormalities of the skin
  Erythrokeratoderma (Beare, 1972)
  Ataxia-telangiectasia (Louis-Bar's syndrome)
  Schindler's disease or α-N-acetylgalactosaminidase deficiency
  Brachial palsy, familial congenital
  Trichomegaly-chorioretinopathy
    cerebellar ataxia
  Glutamate dehydrogenase deficiency
    Other neurological deficits with hyperuricemia
    With retained reflexes
  Vitamin E deficiency
  Spinocerebellar ataxia–Machado-Joseph, 14q linked
Hematologic
  Chorea, acanthocytosis
  Ataxia, pancytopenia
Primarily nerve disorders (other than the Charcot-Marie-Tooth type II; see Table 92–7)
  Giant axonal neuropathy
  Hereditary motor and sensory neuropathy type II
  AD, normal conduction
    With neurofilament
    With cardiac involvement
  Amyloidosis type V, cranial neuropathy, Finnish type
  Dysautonomia, distal, familial
  Infantile axonal polyneuropathy, X-linked
  X-linked motor and sensory neuropathy type II, deafness, and MR
  Hereditary spastic paraplegia with amyotrophy (AR), axon degeneration
  Porphyria, coproporphyria, variegate
  Neuropathy, dementia, retinitis pigmentosa, dysautonomia
Primarily nerve disorders with myoclonus
  Myoclonic epilepsy, with ataxia (Ramsay Hunt) and neuropathy
  Myoclonus, progressive distal muscular atrophy—AD
  Ramsay Hunt, AR (dyssynergia cerebellaris myoclonica)
Primarily nerve disorders with myopthy
  Myopathy, multicore, intermediate filaments, cardiomyopathy
  Congenital muscular dystrophy, occidental type, merosin negative
  Lipid neuromyopathy (AD)
  Mitochondrial myopathy–encephalopathy–lactic acidosis–stroke (MELAS)
Miscellaneous nerve disorders
  De Sanctis-Cacchione syndrome
  Diabetes insipidus–diabetes mellitus–optic atrophy–deafness (DIDMOAD)
  Spinal muscular atrophy–diaphragmatic paralysis
  Spinal muscular atrophy, distal, with a hoarse voice
  Infantile neuroaxonal dystrophy, or Seitelberger's disease
  Lipomatosis, symmetrical
  Möbius sequence, peripheral neuropathy, hypogonadism
  Ventricular calcification and amentia
  X-linked spastic paraplegia, neuropathy, optic atrophy, deafness

AD, autosomal donimant; AR, autosomal recessive; MR, mental retardation.

gait became clumsy consistent with either a polyneuropathy or spinocerebellar degeneration (Ouvrier, 1989). Nystagmus and dementia eventually developed. Giant axonal neuropathy may rarely be the presenting mechanism for the floppy infant syndrome (Kinney et al., 1985). NCSs in eight children with giant axonal neuropathy demonstrated absent sensory nerve action potentials in five, low-amplitude sensory nerve action potentials in two, and varied motor NCSs with axonal and/or demyelinating features (Tandan et al., 1987). Abnormal visual, auditory, and somatosensory potentials are also typical (Majnemer et al., 1986). Characteristic magnetic resonance imaging findings include cerebellar and cerebral white matter changes (Donaghy et al., 1988). Autopsy findings have included evidence of olivocerebellar, cerebellar peduncle, corticospinal, and posterior column abnormalities (Thomas et al., 1987).

Amyloidosis types I (dominant Portuguese, Swedish, and Japanese) and type V (Finnish) are associated with peripheral neuropathies. Neither are likely to present problems in the pediatric population. Type I usually has an onset in the third decade with a progressive neuropathy starting in the legs. Sobue and associates (1990) reported that on occasion there are very slow conduction velocities. The Finnish type also presents in the third decade, with the cranial nerve palsies presenting before the peripheral neuropathy. A corneal lattice dystrophy also develops in these patients.

Peripheral Neuropathy Association with Hereditary Spastic Paraplegia

Autosomal dominant hereditary spastic paraplegia has a variable onset from 1 to 68 years with a mean of around 29 years (Durr et al., 1994) and is known to be associated with peripheral nerve involvement (Tredici and Minoli, 1979). Spastic paraplegia with amyotrophy is inherited as either autosomal dominant, Silver syndrome (Silver, 1966), or recessive forms (Bruyn et al., 1993). The recessive form presents at 10 years, approximately one decade before the dominant form. The axonal neuropathy is seen in the hands rather than the feet. It resembles juvenile motor neuron disease and the hereditary motor sensory neuropathy type V (Harding and Thomas, 1984), which has slow motor conduction velocities.

Peripheral Neuropathy Association with Ataxia

Friedreich's ataxia is the most important of the recessive hereditary ataxias. There are also X-linked and autosomal dominant cerebellar ataxias—formerly classified as olivopontocerebellar atrophy. The determination of the genotype has greatly eased their classification and diagnosis. Many have trinucleotide repeat expansions, leading to a "loss of function" in Friedreich's ataxia but "gain of function" in the dominant ataxia most likely through the accumulation of intranuclear polyglutamine inclusions (Evidente et al., 2000).

Discovery of the FRDA gene on chromosome 9, which leads to reduced levels of the protein frataxin (Delatycki et al., 2000), has eliminated the need for NCSs in Friedreich's ataxia. Classically, these children present with clumsiness (i.e., ataxia) usually associated with pes cavus, slurred speech, absent muscle stretch reflexes, and definite Babinski signs. The typical electromyographic findings include reduced amplitudes or complete loss of sensory nerve action potentials with normal compound motor action potentials and other motor conduction parameters. Cerebellar ataxia with retained reflexes is similar in many respects to Friedreich's but may be allelic. There are retained reflexes not only in arms but at the knees as well, although one half have lost ankle jerks (Harding, 1981).

Autosomal dominant cerebellar ataxias are divided into three clinical types. *Type 1* is variably associated with optic atrophy, cranial nerve deficit, pyramidal and extrapyramidal signs, peripheral neuropathy, and sometimes dementia. It is subdivided by genotype into the six spinocerebellar atrophies, with spinocerebellar atrophy 3 often combined with the Machado-Joseph disease. A study by Kubis and colleagues (1999), looking at spinocerebellar atrophy 1 to spinocerebellar atrophy 3, concluded that axonal polyneuropathy was often associated with type 1 but that its frequency varies according to the locus responsible and the number of CAG repeats. These authors reported no peripheral neuropathy in *type 2*. Klockgether and associates (1999), looking at spinocerebellar atrophy 3/Machado-Joseph disease, could not satisfy themselves of the relationship to CAG repeat length or indeed the age of onset or disease duration. Soong and Lin (1998) confirmed the peripheral nervous system is affected, most probably at the level of the dorsal root ganglia and the anterior horn cells in the spinal cord. In the past when autosomal dominant cerebellar ataxia was still classified as olivopontocerebellar atrophy, peripheral nerve involvement, along with brainstem auditory evoked response abnormality (prolongation of wave 1 latency), was reported only in those patients in whom glutamate dehydrogenase deficiency was seen (Chokroverty et al., 1985).

VITAMIN E DEFICIENCY SYNDROMES

Selective Vitamin E Malabsorption

Harding and associates (1985) made the very important observation that a selective vitamin E malabsorption is sometimes associated with a spinocerebellar syndrome in an adolescent. This has subsequently been mapped to chromosome 8q (Ben Hamida et al., 1993) when investigated in families from the Mediterranean littoral. These syndromes are usually caused by malabsorption, with subsequent cerebellar disturbance, posterior column loss, and peripheral neuropathy. The 13-year-old patient studied by Harding and associates (1985) had no evidence of abetalipoproteinemia, steatorrhea, or cholestatic liver disease, in contrast to the other vitamin E–associated spinocerebellar syndromes. Absent tibial and prolonged median somatosensory evoked responses were associated with normal visual evoked responses, brainstem auditory evoked responses, and motor/sensory NCSs. Her symptoms improved with vitamin E therapy. This case emphasizes the importance of measuring vitamin E levels in all children who have a spinocerebellar ataxia, particularly those found to have normal sensory nerve action potentials.

Abetalipoproteinemia

Children with abetalipoproteinemia clinically mimic Friedreich's ataxia, with pes cavus, scoliosis, ataxia, and areflexia (Bassen and Kornzweig, 1950; Miller et al., 1980; Wichman et al., 1985). Characteristically, vitamin E deficiency is a coexistent finding. Many of these patients have malabsorption secondary to steatorrhea or chronic cholestasis. Bassen and Kornzweig (1950) noted the association between abetalipoproteinemia, prominent acanthocytes, and atypical retinitis pigmentosa. Neurological involvement varies and increases with age.

Children with abetalipoproteinemia may have either preserved or just mild diminution in sensory nerve action potential amplitudes. This contrasts with children with Friedreich's ataxia, who usually lose sensory nerve action potentials early in their illness (Miller et al., 1980). At the Children's Hospital Boston, we recall one child with abetalipoproteinemia who developed steatorrhea at age 11 and ataxia just 1 year later. Although vitamin E supplementation was initiated, retinitis pigmentosa developed. NCSs demonstrated low-amplitude sensory nerve action potentials with normal latency, absent H waves, and normal motor NCSs. Evoked potentials were studied in five children with abetalipoproteinemia. Somatosensory evoked responses were the most sensitive electrophysiological study, being abnormal in all except one child (Fagan and Taylor, 1987). Normal visual evoked responses and brainstem auditory evoked responses are usually found with abetalipoproteinemia, although one patient had consistent delay in the P-100 value. Vitamin E was less than 3 mg/L (normal, 7 to 12 mg/L).

Chronic Cholestatic Liver Disease

This is another childhood illness associated with vitamin E deficiency (Rosenblum et al., 1981). Gait ataxia, distal weakness, areflexia, diminished proprioceptive sensation, and sometimes gaze paresis develop in these children. Hyporeflexia is often the first sign; muscle stretch reflexes disappear between the ages of 2 and 10 years. Four children with chronic steatorrhea and cholestasis had a spinocer-ebellar syndrome with appendicular and gait ataxia, areflexia, extensor toe signs, and ophthalmoplegia (Elias et al., 1981). An unusual variant occurred in an adolescent, who presented with a 7-year history of ataxia as well as ophthalmoplegia and severe tongue, sternocleidomastoid, and trapezius muscle atrophy (Larsen et al., 1985).

Initiation of vitamin E therapy normalized neurological function in three children in whom this therapy was started before the age of 3 years (Sokol et al., 1985); however, these investigators had limited success when vitamin E treatment was first administered to nine other children between the ages of 5 and 17 years. In another study, vitamin E therapy prevented progression, but no clinical improvement occurred (Perlmutter et al., 1987). Motor NCVs are normal, but compound motor action potentials and sensory nerve action potentials may be of low amplitude. A superimposed median neuropathy at the wrist was noted in two children.

Protein-Losing Enteropathy

Another spinocerebellar syndrome associated with vitamin E deficiency occurred in a 9-month-old infant found to have a protein-losing enteropathy secondary to intestinal lymphangiectasia (Gutmann et al., 1986). Gait ataxia developed at the age of 13 years; areflexia with Babinski and Romberg signs subsequently followed. Electromyography demonstrated findings of a primary axonal motor sensory neuropathy. Levels of vitamin E were low; consequently, the patient was administered vitamin E therapy. Her neurological symptoms had improved at 6 months later. The effect of this treatment on motor and sensory NCSs was not studied.

MYOPATHIES ASSOCIATED WITH A PERIPHERAL NEUROPATHY

Patients with merosin-deficient congenital muscular dystrophy are deficient in the α2 subunit of the merosin heterotrimer (Shorer et al., 1995). This same α2 subunit is expressed in the *S*-merosin found in Schwann cells. Subsequently, these investigators demonstrated that 8 of the 10 merosin-deficient patients demonstrated reduced motor nerve conduction velocities (Shorer et al., 1995). All of the other 15 merosin-positive cases had normal results.

Mitochondrial myopathies are clinically heterogeneous disorders. Mizusawa and colleagues (1991) reported that peripheral neuropathy may be relatively common. A wide range of mitochondrial myopathies, including **M**yopathy, **E**ncephalopathy, **L**actic **A**cidosis, and **S**troke-like episodes (MELAS) and **M**yoclonic **E**pilepsy and **R**agged **R**ed **F**ibers (MERRF), have similar clinical and laboratory features—usually a mild sensorimotor neuropathy with the sensory fibers most affected. The motor studies demonstrate both slow conduction and neurogenic changes on EMG. Schroder (1993) found alterations in the mitochondria of peripheral nerves in most cases of mitochondrial myopathy.

Multicore myopathy with intermediate filaments and cardiomyopathy presents in late childhood or early adult life with toe-walking (Bertini et al., 1990; Fardeau et al., 1990). On biopsy, the muscle and nerve show evidence of desmin-like filaments and axonal degeneration on EMG. The associated cardiomyopathy can be life threatening and is possibly restrictive. Myotonic dystrophy in some families is rarely associated with a demyelinating peripheral neuropathy (Spaans et al., 1986).

Distal muscle hypertrophy can be seen in Charcot-Marie-Tooth disease (Sakashita et al., 1992). True muscle hypertrophy occurs in Isaacs' syndrome, otherwise known as neuromyotonia, stiff man syndrome, or continuous muscle fiber activity syndrome. It is probably not a single condition. Some autosomal forms have an underlying demyelinating neuropathy (Hahn et al., 1991). Other forms develop as a complication of an associated chronic inflammatory demyelinating neuropathy (Odabasi et al., 1996). There is a further condition with an association with neuropathy, myasthenia, and thymoma (Perini et al., 1994; Martinelli et al., 1996). Newsom-Davis and Mills (1993) characterized a sporadic or even an acquired form.

The co-occurrence of neuropathy and myopathy influences the investigative strategy of a weak child. Often, these represent a mitochondrial abnormality. Muscle biopsy and EMG may be used together, but at Great Ormond Street Hospital, there is a tendency not to perform muscle biopsies if EMG identifies a clear cause for any weakness, such as anterior horn cell disease or peripheral neuropathy. In these instances with the coexistence of two pathologies, this strategy may lead to the misdiagnosis of the underlying cause. However, with these conjoint findings, often a serum lactate test and concomitant muscle biopsy, looking for the telltale signs of a mitochondrial process, namely ragged red fibers, are important. The neuropathy seen in these cases is usually mild in the presence of significant weakness and should prompt the search for other conditions.

DERMATOLOGICAL CONDITIONS ASSOCIATED WITH NEUROPATHIES

Skin and nerve are both ectodermal in origin. Ataxia-telangiectasis is a multiple system condition in whom prominent telangiectases are present in the conjunctiva and over the ear, face, and neck. Walking is delayed, and these children develop a dysarthria, extrapyramidal signs, and cerebral deterioration. These patients typically are of short stature. Many are prone to infection due to the concomitant absence of or very low IgA levels (Woods and Taylor, 1992). A sensorimotor axonal neuropathy, sensory more than motor, develops in the second decade (Kwast and Ignatowicz, 1990). Neuropathy has also been reported in ataxia without telangiectasia (Willems et al., 1993).

De Sanctis-Cacchione syndrome, an autosomal recessive process, includes xeroderma pigmentosum with subsequent mental and physical retardation. The severity of the neuropathy is age dependent. The development of cutaneous malignancy means that most children do not survive to adulthood.

Beare's syndrome is a combination of erythrokeratodermia, deafness, and neuropathy (Beare et al., 1972). The skin lesions begin within the first months of life. Eventually, the whole body is covered by fine white scales. Pes cavus heralds the peripheral neuropathy (Baden et al., 1988). The retinal abnormalities are consistent with ocular albinism.

ASSOCIATIONS WITH MYOCLONUS

Ramsay Hunt syndrome, or dyssynergia cerebellaris myoclonia, is an autosomal condition in which an axonal neuropathy has been identified, although the incidence varies (Smith et al., 1978).

OTHER HEREDITARY CONDITIONS ASSOCIATED WITH PERIPHERAL NEUROPATHY

Axonal Degeneration

Swift and associates (1990) found a neuropathy in DIDMOAD (Diabetes Insipidus, Diabetes Mellitus, Optic Atrophy, and Deafness), also known as Wolfram's syndrome.

Infantile neuroaxonal dystrophy, or Seitelberger's disease, is an important neurodegenerative condition to pediatric neurophysiologists because it is one of a dwindling number of conditions in which the abnormalities of neurophysiological tests can point to a diagnosis and this ability has not been superseded by a blood test (characteristic fast activity that is seen on the electroencephalogram after the age of 2 years, abnormalities of the visual evoked response, and marked neurogenic change on EMG) (Ramaeckers et al., 1987). These neurogenic changes likely reflect motor nerve involvement rather than anterior horn cell disease. Skin biopsy can be performed to look for spheroids, having replaced the conjunctival biopsy.

Schindler's disease, caused by a deficiency of α-N-acetylgalactosaminidase, may present with an identical clinical picture (Desnick and Wang et al., 1990; Wolfe et al., 1995).

X-linked spastic paraplegia associated with neuropathy, optic atrophy, and deafness presents in the first decade of life (Omer et al., 1996). It is very similar clinically to Rosenberg-Chutorian syndrome, which differs in having a demyelinating neuropathy and no spasticity (Hagemoser et al., 1989).

Nine of a group of 29 patients with juvenile Parkinson's disease were shown to have changes consistent with axonal degeneration (Taly and Muthane, 1992).

Demyelination

Lemieux and Neemeh (1967) described in two Canadian families an association between nephritis and Charcot-Marie-Tooth disease with slow velocities.

Lowe's (oculocerebrorenal) syndrome is another renal condition in which there is peripheral nerve involvement (Charnas et al., 1988). X-linked recessive affected males have cataracts, hypotonia, mental retardation, generalized aminoaciduria, and renal tubular acidosis with hypophosphatemia.

Rosenberg-Chutorian syndrome describes an association between optic atrophy, peroneal muscular atrophy, and deafness that was first recognized in 1967 (Rosenberg and Chutorian, 1967). The deafness and the slow conduction velocities are seen initially, and the optic atrophy develops later at around 20 years. Inheritance is not clearly established. Pauli (1984) made the case for X-linkage, whereas autosomal dominance and even recessive inheritance have been described. The eyes are also affected in **P**olyneuropathy, **O**rganomegaly, **E**ndocrinopathy, **M**onoclonal protein (M-protein), and **S**kin changes (POEMS syndrome). This syndrome has been found to be associated with optic disc swelling in a significant number of patients (Bolling and Brazis, 1990).

Rud's syndrome, a skin condition with a demyelinating hypertrophic neuropathy (Labrisseau and Carpenter, 1982), is characterized by a combination of mental retardation, ichthyosis, hypogonadism, epilepsy, and retinitis pigmentosa.

"Disparate" Electromyographic Findings Versus Neuropathological Results

The most common reason for confusion between findings occurs when an affliction of the anterior horn cells is associated with involvement of the dorsal root ganglia. This is of particular concern in the floppy infant (David and Jones, 1994) and rarely occurs in the spinal muscular atrophy type 1 phenotype (Marshall and Duchen, 1975). We have seen a few of these instances in which the infant has the classic severe hypotonia, frog leg, and jug handle posture of the lower and upper extremities with tongue fasciculations and paradoxical breathing, as well as lack of sensory nerve action potentials with NCSs. At postmortem, there is a diffuse affectation of much of the peripheral and central nervous systems. On other occasions with a similar phenotype, we have seen NCSs compatible with an acquired demyelinating neuropathy, and in these cases, the

SMN deletion is particularly helpful (Korinthenberg et al., 1997). Similar diagnostic difficulties have been reported in Kennedy's syndrome and X-linked bulbospinal atrophy (Ferrante and Wilbourn, 1997), albeit in older patients. Albers and Bromberg (1994) reported a case masquerading as a lead neuropathy.

FUTURE EVALUATION OF PEDIATRIC POLYNEUROPATHIES: ELECTROMYOGRAPHIC CHALLENGES

Significant breakthroughs in the molecular pathogenesis of peripheral neuropathies and myopathies have resulted in an evolving genetic classification of neuromuscular disorders. This remarkable progress has introduced new genetic tests and has changed the indications for certain invasive diagnostic procedures in the evaluation of children with presumed conditions that affect the peripheral nerve as well as other portions of the motor unit. The genetic testing revolution, although highly effective, has added another level of complexity to an already challenging diagnostic field. These advances have left some pediatric neurologists uncertain about the indications for EMG and other relevant invasive procedures. This review discussed the traditional diagnostic role of pediatric EMG in reference to the evaluation of children with the many forms of pediatric polyneuropathies. The major advances in this field have sometimes negated the need for EMG in the evaluation of genetically determined disorders such as Charcot-Marie-Tooth disease and metachromatic leukodystrophy, where very specific DNA tests have become routinely available.

However, EMG is indicated (1) in children with acute polyneuropathies such as Guillain-Barré syndrome, (2) where genetic analysis has failed to confirm an initial suspected clinical diagnosis, and (3) to narrow down a neuropathy to either demyelinating or axonal to determine the type of DNA analysis and/or biochemical study required. At the Children's Hospital Boston, EMG continues to play a major role in the evaluation of many children referred to the neuromuscular service. Overall, personnel in our EMG laboratory continue to perform approximately 140 to 160 electromyograms per year (Darras and Jones, 2000). This is essentially the annual rate for the 1980s and the 1990s. Although there has been a diminution in the numbers of electromyographic evaluations performed due to the use of DNA testing, more for myopathies than for neuropathies, this change is increasingly made up by the recognition of the ever-increasing value of EMG in new circumstances, particularly in the critical care units (Jones and Darras, 2000).

Ideally, a proper investigation tool for the diagnosis and monitoring of a pediatric peripheral neuropathy has the following features: (1) it is painless or the discomfort produced is tolerable, (2) it has no

Table 92–10. Comparison of Existing Methods of Investigating Peripheral Nerve Function with the Ideal Method

	Ideal Method	Clinical Examination	Electromyography	Sensory Nerve Thresholds	Nerve Biopsy
Pain	None	Some	Moderate	Minimal	Moderate
Permanent sequelae	None	None	None	None	Scar
Specificity	High	Low/moderate	High	High	High
Sensitivity	High	Low/moderate	Moderate	Moderate/high	High
Variability	Low	High	High	High	Low
Objectivity	High	Low	High	Low	High

significant sequelae, (3) the results are highly specific and sensitive, with low variability comparing test to test, operator to operator, and subject to subject, and (4) the data derived are very objective and need no collaboration from the child's history. Table 92–10 attempts to evaluate existing techniques against these criteria.

Although the "gold standard" for the evaluation of a peripheral neuropathic process is ideally a nerve biopsy, there are only a very few circumstances where this methodology is indicated in children (Wilmshurst and Ouvrier, 2002). The one pertinent pediatric setting is the rare instance of a mononeuritis multiplex secondary to vasculitis. Other indications traditionally indicated in adults, such as amyloidosis, sarcoidosis, and lymphomatous infiltration, are not significant issues among children with polyneuropathies (Wilmshurst and Ouvrier, 2002). As a method of screening, sural nerve biopsy is totally unsuitable because of its invasive nature. Sural nerve biopsy is also exceptionally difficult technically in the very smallest infants except at major pediatric teaching hospitals, where one surgeon is selected to routinely be available to perform this procedure.

Last, it is important not to relegate the clinical evaluation to being an outmoded tool in this technological age. A careful neurological history and examination by an experienced clinician, especially with an emphasis on possible family members with similar difficulties, remains the standard keystone to successful diagnosis. Accurate quantification is still somewhat difficult to achieve in adults, let alone children. Various sensory threshold automated detection devices have attempted to correct this deficiency. These require significant patient collaboration for routine use in any but the most cooperative children and certainly can never be used for infants and toddlers. NCSs, despite their detractors, do offer the best compromise at present, provided that experienced and sympathetic practitioners perform these studies and especially if they are able to diminish the amount of discomfort perceived by the child. However, NCSs still have two major limitations: (1) routine NCSs evaluate only the function of the largest diameter nerve fibers and (2) they cannot be used to screen for small-fiber nerve dysfunction.

References

Agocs MM, Etzel RA, Parrish RG, et al: Mercury exposure from interior latex paint. N Engl J Med 1990;323:1096–1101.

Aicardi J: The inherited leukodystrophies: A clinical overview. J Inherit Metab Dis 1993;16:733–743.

Albers JW, Bromberg MB: X-linked bulbospinomuscular atrophy (Kennedy's disease) masquerading as lead neuropathy. Muscle Nerve 1994;17:419–423.

Albers JW, Donfrio PD, McGonagle TK: Sequential electrodiagnostic abnormalities in acute inflammatory demyelinating polyradiculoneuropathy. Muscle Nerve 1985;8:528–539.

Albers JW, Kelly JJ Jr: Acquired inflammatory demyelinating polyneuropathies: Clinical and electrodiagnostic features. Muscle Nerve 1989;12:435–451.

Albers JW, Robertson WC Jr, Daube JR: Electrodiagnostic findings in acute porphyric neuropathy. Muscle Nerve 1978;1:292–296.

Allgrove J, Clayden GS, Grant DB, et al: Familial glucocorticoid deficiency with achalasia of the cardia and deficient tear production. Lancet 1978;1:1284–1286.

Amelung W, Puntmann E: Clinical aspects and therapy of the so-called Contergan-polyneuropathy. Nervenarzt 1966;37:189–199.

Andersson PB, Yuen E, Parko K, So YT: Electrodiagnostic features of herditary neuropathy with liability to pressure palsies. Neurology 2000;54:40–44.

Appenzeller O, Kornfeld M, Snyder R: Acromutilating, paralyzing neuropathy with corneal ulceration in Navajo children. Arch Neurol 1976;33:733–738.

Appleton R, Riordan A, Tedman B, et al: Congenital peripheral neuropathy presenting as apnoea and respiratory insufficiency. Dev Med Child Neurol 1994;36:547–553.

Baden HP, Bronstein BR: Ichthyosiform dermatosis and deafness: Report of a case and review of the literature. Arch Dermatol 1988;124:102–106.

Bakshi N, Maselli R, Gospe SM, et al: Fulminating demyelinating neuropathy mimicking cerebral death. Muscle Nerve 1997;20:1595–1597.

Barbieri F, Santangelo R, Capparelli G, Crisci C: Autosomal recessive motor and sensory neuropathy with excessive myelin outfolding in two siblings. Can J Neurol Sci 1994;21:29–33.

Bar-Joseph G, Etzioni A, Hemli J, Gershoni-Baruch R: Guillain-Barre syndrome in siblings less than 2 years old. Arch Dis Child 1991;66:1078–1079.

Barohn RJ, Sanchez JA, Anderson KE: Acute peripheral neuropathy due to hereditary coproporphyria. Muscle Nerve 1994;17:793–799.

Barth PG: Pontocerebellar hypoplasias: An overview of a group of inherited neurodegenerative disorders with fetal onset. Brain Dev 1993;15:411–422.

Bassen FA, Kornzweig AL: Malformation of the erythrocytes in a case of atypical retinitis pigmentosa. Blood 1950;5:381–387.

Beare JM, Nevin NC, Froggal P, et al: Atypical erythrokeratoderma with deafness, physical retardation, and peripheral neuropathy. Br J Dermatol 1972;87:308–314.

Beausoleil JL, Nordgren RE, Modlin JF: Vaccine-associated paralytic poliomyelitis. J Child Neurol 1994;9:334–335.

Behse F, Buchthal F: Sensory nerve action potentials and biopsy of the sural nerve in neuropathy. Brain 1978;101:473–493.

Ben Hamida C, Doerflinger N, Belal S, et al: Localization of Friedreich ataxia phenotype with selective vitamin E deficiency to chromosome 8q by homozygosity mapping. Nat Genet 1993; 5:195–200.

Benstead TJ, Kuntz NL, Miller RG, Daube JR: The electrophysiologic profile of Dejerine-Sottas disease (hereditary motor sensory neuropathy type III). Muscle Nerve 1990;13:586–592.

Berciano J, Garcia A, Calleja J, Combarros O: Clinico-electrophysiological correlation of extensor digitorum brevis muscle atrophy in children with Charcot-Marie-Tooth disease 1A duplication. Neuromusc Disord 2000;10:419–424.

Berg BO, Rosenberg SH, Asbury AK: Giant axonal neuropathy. Pediatrics 1972;49:894–899.

Bertini E, Bosman C, Bevilacqua M, et al: Cardiomyopathy and multicore myopathy with accumulation of intermediate filaments. Eur J Pediatr 1990;149:856–858.

Bertini E, Gadisseux JL, Palmieri G, et al: Distal infantile spinal muscular atrophy associated with paralysis of the diaphragm: A variant of infantile spinal muscular atrophy. Am J Med Genet 1989;33:328–335.

Bird SJ, Sladky JT: Corticosteroid-responsive dominantly inherited neuropathy in childhood. Neurology 1991;41:437–439.

Blenow G, Jaeken J, Wiklund LM: Neurological findings in the carbohydrate-deficient glycoprotein syndrome. Acta Paediatr Scand 1991;375:14–19.

Bolling JP, Brazis PW: Optic disk swelling with peripheral neuropathy, organomegaly, endocrinopathy, monoclonal gammopathy, and skin changes (POEMS syndrome). Am J Ophthalmol 1990; 15:503–510.

Bolton CF, Gilbert JJ, Hahn AF, Sibbald WJ: Polyneuropathy in critically ill patients. J Neurol Neurosurg Psychiatry 1984;47:1223–1231.

Bolton CF, Hahn AF, Hinton GG: The syndrome of high stimulation threshold and low conduction velocity. Ann Neurol 1988;24:165.

Bolton CF: Electromyography in the critical care unit. In Jones HR, Bolton CF, Harper CM (eds): Pediatric Clinical Electromyography. Philadelphia, Lippincott-Raven, 1996.

Bosch EP, Hart MN: Late adult onset metachromatic leukodystrophy dementia and polyneuropathy in a 63-year-old man. Arch Neurol 1978;35:475–477.

Bradshaw DY, Jones HR Jr: Guillain-Barré syndrome in children: Clinical course, electrodiagnosis, and prognosis. Muscle Nerve 1992;15:500–506.

Bradshaw DY, Jones HR: Pseudoencephalopathic Guillain-Barré Syndrome. J Child Neurol 2001;16:505–508.

Bril V, Ellison R, Ngo M, et al: Electrophysiological monitoring of clinical trials. Roche Neuropathy Study Group. Muscle Nerve 1998;21:1368–1373.

Bruyn RP, Scheltens P, Lycklama-a-Nijeholt J, de-Jong JM: Autosomal recessive paraparesis with amyotrophy of the hands and feet. Acta Neurol Scand 1993;87:443–445.

Buchwald B, Bufler J, Carpo M, et al: Combined pre- and postsynaptic action of IgG antibodies in Miller Fisher syndrome. Neurology 2001;56:67–74.

Burley D: Neuropathy after thalidomide ('Distaval'). Br Med J 1961;2:1286–1287.

Calderon-Gonzalez R, Rizzi-Hernandez H: Buckthorn polyneuropathy. N Engl J Med 1967;277:69–71.

Cameron CL, Jones HR: Metachromatic leukodystrophy: Clinical and EMG characteristics in eight children. Muscle Nerve 1996; 19:1207–1208.

Cavanagh NP, Eames RA, Galvin RJ, et al: Hereditary sensory neuropathy with spastic paraplegia. Brain 1979;102: 79–94.

Charnas L, Bernar J, et al: MRI findings and peripheral neuropathy in Lowe's syndrome. Neuropediatrics 1988;19:7–9.

Chokroverty S, Duvoisin RC, Sachdeo R, et al: Neurophysiologic study with or without glutamate dehydrogenase deficiency. Neurology 1985;35:652–659.

Chu CC, Huang CC, Ryu SJ, Wu TN: Chronic inorganic mercury–induced peripheral neuropathy. Acta Neurol Scand 1998;98:461–465.

Clark JR, Miller RG, Vidgoff JM: Juvenile-onset leukodystrophy: Biochemical and electrophysiological study. Neurology 1979; 29:346–353.

Clemensen OJ, Olsen PZ, Andersen KE: Thalidomide neurotoxicity. Arch Dermatol 1984;120:338–341.

Coker SB: Leigh disease presenting as Guillain-Barré syndrome. Pediatr Neurol 1993;9:61–63.

Cornblath DR, Chaudhry V, Griffin JW: Treatment of chronic inflammatory demyelinating polyneuropathy with intravenous immunoglobulin. Ann Neurol 1977;1;30:104–106.

Cornblath DR, Sladky JT, Sumner AJ: Clinical electrophysiology of infantile botulism. Muscle Nerve 1983;6:448–452.

Cornell J, Sellars S, Beighton P: Autosomal recessive inheritance of Charcot-Marie-Tooth disease associated with sensorineural deafness. Clin Genet 1984;25:163–165.

Cowchock FS, Duckett SW, Stretz LJ: X-linked motor-sensory neuropathy type II with deafness and mental retardation: A new disorder. Am J Med Genet 1985;20:307–315.

Cruz-Martinez A, Arpa J: Pediatric bilateral carpal tunnel syndrome as first manifestation of hereditary neuropathy with liability to pressure palsies (HNPP). Eur J Neurol 1998;5:316–317.

Darras BT, Jones HR: Diagnosis of pediatric neuromuscular disorders in the era of DNA analysis. Pediatr Neurol 2000;23:289–300.

David WS, Doyle JJ: Acute infantile weakness: A case of vaccine associated poliomyelitis. Muscle Nerve 1997;20:747–749.

David WS, Jones HR: Electromyography and biopsy correlation with suggested protocol for evaluation of the floppy infant. Muscle Nerve 1994;17:424–430.

Davis LE, Standefer JC, Kornfeld M, et al: Acute thallium poisoning, toxicological and morphological studies of the nervous system. Ann Neurol 1981;10:38–44.

Delanoe C, Sebire G, Landrieu P, et al: Acute inflammatory demyelinating polyradiculopathy in children: Clinical and electrodiagnostic studies. Ann Neurol 1998;44:350–356.

Delatycki MB, Williamson R, Forrest SM: Friedreich ataxia: An overview. J Med Genet 2000;37:1–8.

Delhaas T, Kamphuis DJ, Witkamp TD: Transitory spinal cord swelling in a 6-year-old boy with Guillain-Barre syndrome. Pediatr Radiol 1998;28:544–546.

Desnick RJ, Wang AM, et al: Schindler disease: An inherited neuroaxonal dystrophy due to alpha-N-acetylgalactosaminidase deficiency. J Inherit Metab Dis 1990;13:549–559.

DiMauro S, Zeviani M, Moraes CT, et al: Mitochondrial encephalomyopathies. Prog Clin Biol Res 1989;306:117–128.

Dirik E, Uysal KM: Organophosphate-induced delayed polyneuropathy. Pediatr Neurol 1994;11:111.

Donaghy M, Brett EM, Ormerod IEC, et al: Giant axonal neuropathy: Observations on a further case. J Neurol Neurosurg Psychiatry 1988;51:991–994.

Donat JR, Donat JF: Tick paralysis with persistent weakness and electromyographic abnormalities. Arch Neurol 1981;38:59–61.

Donley DK, Knight P, Tenorio G, Oh SJ: A patient with infant botulism, improving with edrophonium. Muscle Nerve 1991; 41:201.

Donofrio PD, Wilbourn AJ, Albers JW, et al: Acute arsenic intoxication presenting as Guillain-Barré–like syndrome. Muscle Nerve 1987;10:114–120.

Durr A, Brice A, Serdaru M, et al: The phenotype of "pure" autosomal dominant spastic paraplegia. Neurology 1994;44: 1274–1277.

Dyck PJ, Dyck JB, Schaid DJ: Genetic heterogeneity in hereditary sensory and autonomic neuropathies: The need for improved ascertainment. Muscle Nerve 2000;23:1453–1455.

Dyck PJ, Litchy WJ, Minnerath S, et al: Hereditary motor and sensory neuropathy with diaphragm and vocal cord paresis. Ann Neurol 1994;35:608–615.

Dyck PJ, Kratz KM. Lehman KA, et al: The Rochester Diabetic Neuropathy Study: Design, criteria for types of neuropathy, selection bias, and reproducibility of neuropathic tests. Neurology 1991;41:799–807.

Dyck PJ: Neuronal atrophy and degeneration predominantly affecting peripheral sensory and autonomic neurons. In Dyck PJ, Thomas PK, Lambert EH, Burge R (eds): Peripheral Neuropathy, vol. II. Philadelphia, WB Saunders, 1984; 1557.

Elias E, Muller DPR, Scott J: Association of spinocerebellar disorders with cystic fibrosis or chronic childhood cholestasis and very low serum vitamin E. Lancet 1981;2:1319–1321.

Emeryk-Szajewska B, Badurska B, Kostera-Pruszczyk A: Electrophysiological findings in hereditary motor and sensory neuropathy type I and II—a conduction velocity study. Electromyogr Clin Neurophysiol 1998;38:95–101.

Engel WK, Dorman JD, Levy RI, Frederickson DS: Neuropathy in Tangier disease: Alpha lipoprotein deficiency manifesting as familial recurrent neuropathy and intestinal lipid storage. Arch Neurol 1967;17:1–9.

Evidente VG, Gwinn-Hardy KA, Caviness JN, Gilman S: Hereditary ataxias. Mayo Clin Proc 2000;75:475–490.

Faed JM, Day B, Pollock M, et al: High-dose intravenous human immunoglobulin in chronic inflammatory demyelinating poly-neuropathy. Neurology 1989;39:422–425.

Fagan ER, Taylor MJ: Longitudinal multimodal evoked potential studies in abetalipoproteinemia. Can J Neurol Sci 1987;14:617–621.

Fakadej AV, Gutmann L: Prolongation of post-tetanic facilitation in infant botulism. Muscle Nerve 1982;5:727–729.

Fardeau M, Godet-Guillain J, Tome F: Une nouvelle affection mus-culaire familiale definie par accumulation intra-sarco-plasmique d'un materiel granulo-filamentaire dense en microscopie elec-tronique. Rev Neurol 1990;131:411–425.

Feasby TE, Gilbert JJ, Brown WF, et al: An acute axonal form of Guillain-Barre syndrome. Brain 1986;100:1115–1126.

Ferrante MA, Wilbourn AJ: The characteristic electrodiagnostic features of Kennedy's disease. Muscle Nerve 1997;20:323–329.

Fisher MA: Nerve conduction biopsy correlation in over 100 con-secutive patients with suspected neuropathy. Muscle Nerve 1995;18:1078–1079.

Ford FR: Diseases of the Nervous System in Infancy, Childhood, and Adolescence, ed 5. Springfield, Ill, Charles C Thomas, 1966a; 635.

Ford FR: Diseases of the Nervous System in Infancy, Childhood, and Adolescence, ed 5. Springfield, Ill, Charles C Thomas, 1966b; 765–767.

Fukuhara N, Nakajima T, Sakajari KI, et al: Hereditary motor and sensory neuropathy associated with cerebellar atrophy (HMSNCA): A new disease. J Neurol Sci 1995;133:140–151.

Fuller JE, DeLuca PA: Acetabular dysplasia and Charcot-Marie-Tooth disease in a family. J Bone Joint Surg A 1995;77:1087–1091.

Fullerton PM, Kremer M: Neuropathy after intake of thalidomide ('Distaval'). Br Med J 1961;2:855–858.

Garbern JY, Cambi F, Tang X-E, et al: Proteolipid is necessary in peripheral as well as central myelin. Neuron 1997;19:205–218.

Gardner-Medwin JM, Powell RJ: Thalidomide—the way forward. Postgrad Med J 1994;70:860–862.

Geetha N, Hussain BM, Lali VS, et al: Guillain-Barre syndrome occurring as a complication of acute non-lymphoblastic leuke-mia. Am J Med 1999;107:100–101.

Gibbs TC, Payan J, Brett EM, et al: Peripheral neuropathy as the presenting feature of tyrosinaemia type I and effectively treated with an inhibitor of 4-hydroxyphenylpyruvate dioxygenase. J Neurol Neurosurg Psychiatry 1993;56:1129–1132.

Gieron-Korthals MA, Westberry KR, Emmanuel PJ: Acute child-hood ataxia: 10 Year experience. J Child Neurol 1994;9:381–384.

Gilmartin RC, Ch'ien LT: Guillain-Barré syndrome with hydroceph-alus in early infancy. Arch Neurol 1977;34:567–569.

Gilmartin RC Jr, Jabbour JT, Duenas DA: Rubella vaccine myelora-diculoneuritis. J Pediatr 1972;80:406–412.

Graf WD, Chance PF, Lensch W, et al: Severe vincristine neuropa-thy in Charcot-Marie-Tooth disease type 1A. Cancer 1996;77:1356–1362.

Grant DB, Dunger DB, Smith I, Hyland K: Familial glucocorticoid deficiency with achalasia of the cardia associated with mixed neuropathy, long-tract degeneration and mild dementia. Eur J Pediatr 1992;151:85–89.

Grattan-Smith PJ, Morris JG, Johnston HM, et al: Clinical and neurophysiologic features of tick paralysis. Brain 1997;121:1975–1987.

Gucuyener K, Keskil S, Baykaner MK, et al: Co-incidence of Guil-lain-Barré syndrome and spinal cord compression in non-Hodg-kins lymphoma. Neuropediatrics 1994;24:36–38.

Gumbinas M, Larsen M, Liu H: Peripheral neuropathy in classic Niemann-Pick disease: Ultrastructure of nerves and skeletal muscles. Neurology 1975;25:107–113.

Gutmann L, Shockcor W, Gutmann L, Kien CL: Vitamin E-deficient

spinocerebellar syndrome due to intestinal lymphangiectasia. Neurology 1986;36:554–556.

Gutrecht JA, Dyck PJ: Quantitative teased-fiber and histologic studies of human sural nerve during postnatal development. J Comp Neurol 1970;138:117–130.

Hadden RD, Cornblath DR, Hughes RA, et al: Electrophysiological classification of Guillain-Barre syndrome: Clinical associations and outcome. Plasma Exchange/Sandoglobulin Guillain-Barre syndrome Trial Group. Ann Neurol 1998;44:780–788.

Hagberg B: Polyneuropathies in pediatrics. Eur J Pediatr 1990;149:296–305.

Hagemoser K, Weinstein J, Bresnick G, et al: Optic atrophy, hear-ing loss, and peripheral neuropathy. Am J Med Genet 1989;33:61–65.

Hahn AF, Ainsworth PJ, Bolton CF, et al: Pathologic findings in the x-linked form of Charcot-Marie-Tooth disease: A morpho-metric and ultrastructural analysis. Acta Neuropathol 2001;101:129–139.

Hahn AF, Parkes AW, Bolton CF, Stewart SA: Neuromyotonia in hereditary motor neuropathy. J Neurol Neurosurg Psychiatry 1991;54:230–235.

Harding AE, Matthews S, Jones S, et al: Spinocerebellar degenera-tion associated with selective defect of vitamin E absorption. N Engl J Med 1985;313:32–35.

Harding AE, Thomas PK: Distal and scapuloperoneal distributions of muscle involvement occurring within a family with type I hereditary motor and sensory neuropathy. J Neurol 1980;224:17–23.

Harding AE, Thomas PK: Peroneal muscular atrophy with pyrami-dal features. J Neurol Neurosurg Psychiatry 1984;47:168–172.

Harding AE: Friedreich's ataxia: A clinical and genetic study of 90 families with an analysis of early diagnostic criteria and intrafamilial clustering of clinical features. Brain 1981;104:589–620.

Hart DE, Rojas LA, Rosario JA, et al: Childhood Guillain-Barré syndrome in Paraguay, 1990 to 1991. Ann Neurol 1994;36:859–863.

Heckmatt JZ, Pitt MC, Kirkham F: Peripheral neuropathy and neuromuscular blockade presenting as prolonged respiratory paralysis following critical illness. Neuropediatrics 1993;24:123–125.

Hensler M, Klein A, Reber M, et al: Analysis of a splice-site mutation in the sap-precursor gene of a patient with metachro-matic leukodystrophy. Am J Hum Genet 1996;58:65–74.

Hesketh E, Eden OB, Gattamaneni HR, et al: Spinal cord compression—do we miss it? Acta Paediatr 1998;87:452–454.

Hopkins IJ: A new syndrome: Poliomyelitis-like illness associated with acute asthma in childhood. Aust Paediatr J 1974;10:273–276.

Horoupian DS: Hereditary sensory neuropathy with deafness: A familial multisystem atrophy. Neurology 1989;39:244–248.

Hsu P, Jones HR: Pes Cavus as the Presenting Sign of Childhood Neuropathies: EMG Evaluation in 23 Otherwise Asymptomatic Children. San Diego, American Association of Electrodiagnostic Medicine, 1997.

Jackman NL, Klig JE: Lower extremity pain in a three year old: Manifestations of Guillain-Barre syndrome. Pediatr Emerg Care 1998;14:272–274.

Jackson AH, Baquis GD, Shaw BL: Congenital Guillain-Barre syn-drome. J Child Neurol 1996;5:407–410.

Jacobs BC, Endtz HP, van Doorn PA, van der Meché FGA: Serum anti-GQ1b IgG antibodies can specifically bind to Campylo-bacter jejuni strains from Miller Fisher patients [abstract]. Mus-cle Nerve 1994;17(Suppl 1):S235.

Jacobs JM, Harding BN, Lake BD, et al: Peripheral neuropathy in Leigh's disease. Brain 1990;113:447–462.

Jaeken J, Eggermont E, Stibler H: An apparent homozygous X-linked disorder with carbohydrate-deficient serum glycopro-teins. Lancet 1987;12:1398.

Jaradeh S, Dyck PS: Hereditary motor and sensory neuropathy with treatable extrapyramidal features. Arch Neurol 1992;49:175–178.

Jenkins RB, Toole JF: Polyneuropathy following exposure to insec-ticides: Two cases of polyneuropathy with albuminocytologic dissociation in the spinal fluid following exposure to DDD and aldrin and DDT and endrin. Arch Intern Med 1964;113:691–695.

Jenkins T: The South African malady. Nat Genet 1996;13:7–9.

Jestico JV, Orry PA, Efphimiou J: An hereditary sensory and autonomic neuropathy transmitted as an X-linked recessive trait. J Neurol Neurosurg Psychiatry 1985;48:1259–1264.

Johnsen SD, Johnson PC, Stein SR: Familial sensory autonomic neuropathy with arthropathy in Navajo children. Neurology 1993;43:1120–1125.

Jones HR: Guillain-Barre syndrome: Perspectives with infants and children. Semin Pediatr Neurol 2000;7:91–102.

Jones HR, Jr, Darras BT: Acute care pediatric electromyography. Muscle Nerve 2000;Suppl 9:S53–S62.

Jones HR, Harmon RL, Bolton CF, et al: Clinical Pediatric Electromyography. Philadelphia/New York, Lippincott-Raven, 1996; 1–37.

Kinney RB, Gottfried MR, Hodson AK, et al: Congenital giant axonal neuropathy. Arch Pathol Lab Med 1985;109:639–641.

Klockgether T, Schols L, Abele M, et al: Age related axonal neuropathy in spinocerebellar ataxia type 3/Machado-Joseph disease (SCA3/MJD). J Neurol Neurosurg Psychiatry 1999;66:222–224.

Knebusch M, Strassburg HM, Reiners K: Acute transverse myelitis in childhood: Nine cases and review of the literature. Dev Med Child Neurol 1998;40:631–639.

Korinthenberg R, Monting JS: Natural history and treatment effects in Gullain-Barre syndrome: A multicentre study. Arch Dis Child 1996;74:281–287.

Korinthenberg R, Sauer M, Ketelsen U-P, et al: Congenital axonal neuropathy caused by deletions in the spinal muscular atrophy region. Ann Neurol 1997;42:364–368.

Korobkin R, Asbury AK, Sumner AJ, Nielsen SL: Glue-sniffing neuropathy. Arch Neurol 1975;32:158–162.

Kubis N, Durr A, Gugenheim M, et al: Polyneuropathy in autosomal dominant cerebellar ataxia: Phenotype-genotype correlation. Muscle Nerve 1999;22:712–717.

Kumar K, Barre P, Nigro M, Jones MZ: Giant axonal neuropathy: Clinical, electrophyiologic, and neuropathologic features in two siblings. J Child Neurol 1990;5:229–234.

Kusunoki S, Chiba A, Kanazawa I: GQ1b antibody in Fisher syndrome and immunohistochemical studies. Muscle Nerve 1994; 17(Suppl 1):S44.

Kuwabara S, Nakajima M, Tsuboi Y, Hiryama K: Multifocal conduction block in n-hexane neuropathy. Muscle Nerve 1993;16:1416–1417.

Kuwabara S, Ogawara K, Mizobuchi K, et al: Isolated absence of F waves and proximal axonal dysfunction in Guillain-Barre syndrome with antigangliosidase antibodies. J Neurol Neurosurg Psychiatry 2000;68:191–195.

Kwast O, Ignatowicz R: Progressive peripheral neuron degeneration in ataxia-telangiectasia: An electrophysiological study in children. Dev Med Child Neurol 1990;32:800–807.

Labrisseau A, Carpenter S: Rud syndrome: Congenital ichthyosis, hypogonadism, mental retardation, retinitis pigmentosa and hypertrophic polyneuropathy. Neuropediatrics 1982;13:95–98.

Larsen A, Tobias JD: Landry-Guillain-Barré syndrome presenting with symptoms of upper airway obstruction. Pediatr Emerg Care 1994;10:347–348.

Larsen PD, Mock DM, O'Connor PS: Vitamin E deficiency associated with vision loss and bulbar weakness. Ann Neurol 1985; 18:725–727.

Lascelles RG, Baker IA, Thomas PK: Hereditary polyneuropathy of Roussy-Levy type with associated cardiomyopathy. Guy's Hosp Rep 1970;119:253–262.

Le Quesne PM, McLeod JG: Peripheral neuropathy following a single exposure to arsenic: Clinical course in four patients with electrophysiological and histological studies. J Neurol Sci 1977; 32:437–451.

Lemieux G, Neemeh JA: Charcot-Marie-Tooth disease and nephritis. Can Med Assoc J 1967;97:1193–1198.

Levade T, Graber D, Flurin V, et al: Human beta-mannosidase deficiency associated with peripheral neuropathy. Ann Neurol 1994;35:116–119.

Lewis RA, Sumner AJ, Shy ME: Electrophysiological features of inherited demyelinating neuropathies: A reappraisal in the era of molecular diagnosis. Muscle Nerve 2000;23:1472–1487.

Lewis RA, Sumner AJ: The electrodiagnostic distinctions between chronic familial and acquired demyelinative neuropathies. Neurology 1982;32:592–596.

Lieberman JS, Oshtory M, Taylar RG, et al: Peripheral neuropathy as an early manifestation of Krabbe's disease. Arch Neurol 1980;37:446–447.

Lip GY, McColl KE, Moore MR: The acute porphyrias. Br J Clin Pract 1993;47:38–43.

Littler WA: Heart block and peroneal muscular atrophy. Q J Med 1970;39:431–440.

Logigian EL, Kelly JJ Jr, Adelman LS: Nerve conduction and biopsy correlation in over 100 consecutive patients with suspected polyneuropathy. Muscle Nerve 1994;17:1010–1020.

Logina I, Donaghy M: Diphtheritic polyneuropathy: A clinical study and comparison with Guillain-Barre syndrome. J Neurol Neurosurg Psychiatry 1999;67:433–438.

Luijckx GJ, Vies J, de Baets M, et al: Guillain-Barre syndrome in mother and child. Lancet 1997;349:27.

Majnemer A, Rosenblatt B, Watters G, Andermann F: Giant axonal neuropathy: Central abnormalities demonstrated by evoked potentials. Ann Neurol 1986;19:394–396.

Marks HG, Scavina MT, Kolodny EH, et al: Krabbe's disease presenting as a peripheral neuropathy. Muscle Nerve 1997;20: 1024–1028.

Marshall A, Duchen LW: Sensory system involvement in infantile spinal muscular atrophy. J Neurol Sci 1975;26:349–359.

Martinelli P, Patuelli A, Minardi C, et al: Neuromyotonia, peripheral neuropathy and hypotonia and areflexia. J Child Neurol 1996;11:252–255.

Martinez HR, Bermudez MV, Rangel-Guerrs RA, de Leon Flores L: Clinical diagnosis in *Karwinskia humboldtiana* polyneuropathy. J Neurol Sci 1998;154:49–54.

McGuinness OE, Winrow AP, Smyth DPL: Juvenile Krabbe's leukodystrophy precipitated by influenza A infection. Dev Med Child Neurol 1996;38:460–461.

McKhann GM, Cornblath DR, Ho T, et al: Clinical and electrophysiologic aspects of acute paralytic disease of children and young adults in northern China. Lancet 1991;338:593–597.

McKhann GM, Cornblath DR, Griffin JW, et al: Acute motor axonal neuropathy: A frequent cause of flaccid paralysis in China. Ann Neurol 1993;33:333–342.

McWilliam RC, Gardner-Medwin D, Doyle D, Stephenson JB: Diaphragmatic paralysis due to spinal muscular atrophy: An unrecognised cause of respiratory failure in infancy? Arch Dis Child 1985;60:145–149.

Miller RG, Davis CJF, Illingworth DR, Bradley W: The neuropathy of abetalipoproteinemia. Neurology 1980;30:1286–1291.

Mitchell G, Larochelle J, Lambert M, et al: Neurologic crises in hereditary tyrosinemia. N Engl J Med 1990;32:432–437.

Mizusawa H, Ohkoshi N, Watanabe M, Kanazawa I: Peripheral neuropathy of mitochondrial myopathies. Rev Neurol 1991; 147:501–507.

Moosa A, Dubowitz V: Postnatal maturation of peripheral nerves in preterm and full-term infants. J Pediatr 1971;79:915–922.

Moosa A, Dubowitz V: Peripheral neuropathy in Cockayne's syndrome. Arch Dis Child 1970;45:674–677.

Narayanan V, Diven W, Ahdab-Barmada M: Congenital fumerase deficiency presenting with myasthenia gravis. Muscle Nerve 1996;19:505–510.

Nass R, Chutorian A: Dysaesthesias and dysautonomia: A self-limited syndrome of painful dysaesthesias and autonomic dysfunction in children. J Neurol Neurosurg Psychiatry 1982;45: 162–165.

Newsom-Davis J, Mills KR: Immunological associations of acquired neuromyotonia (Isaacs' syndrome): Report of five cases and literature review. Brain 1993;116:453–469.

Nicholson G, Nash J: Intermediate nerve conduction velocities define X-linked Charcot-Marie-Tooth neuropathy families. Neurology 1993;43:2558–2564.

Novelli G, Capon F, Tamisari L, et al: Neonatal spinal muscular atrophy with diaphragmatic paralysis is unlinked to 5q11.2–q13. J Med Genet 1995;32:216–219.

Odabasi Z, Joy JL, Claussen GC, et al: Isaacs syndrome associated with chronic inflammatory demyelinating neuropathy. Muscle Nerve 1996;19:210–215.

Oh SJ, Chang CW: Conduction block and dispersion in hereditary motor and sensory neuropathy. Muscle Nerve 1987;10:656.

Olney RK: Neurophysiologic evaluation and clinical trials for neuromuscular disease. Muscle Nerve 1998;21:1365–1367.

Omer S, Bohlega S, Al-Zimaiti E: X-linked spastic paraparesis, axonal neuropathy, optic atrophy and sensorineural deafness: A new entity [abstract]. J Neurol 1996;243:S114.

Op de Coul AAW, Lambregts PCLA, Koeman J, et al: Neuromuscular complications in patients given Pavulon (pancuronium bromide) during artificial ventilation. Clin Neurol Neurosurg 1985; 87:17–22.

Ouvrier RA, McLeod JG, Pollard JD: Peripheral Neuropathy in Childhood, 2nd ed. London, MacKeith Press, 1999.

Ouvrier RA: Giant axonal neuropathy. A review. Brain Dev 1989; 11:207–214.

Ouvrier RA, McLeod JG, Morgan GJ, et al: Hereditary motor and sensory neuropathy of neuronal type with onset in early childhood. J Neurol Sci 1981;51:181–197.

Paradiso G, Tripoli J, Galicchio S, Fejerman N: Epidemiological, clinical and electrodiagnostic findings in childhood Guillain-Barre syndrome: A reappraisal. Ann Neurol 1999;46: 701–707.

Pareyson D, Solari A, Taroni F, et al: Detection of hereditary neuropathy with liability to pressure palsies among patients with acute painless mononeuropathy or plexopathy. Muscle Nerve 1998;21:1686–1691.

Pasternak JF, Fulling K, Nelson J, Prensky AL: An infant with chronic relapsing polyneuropathy responsive to steroids. Dev Med Child Neurol 1982;24:505–524.

Paul DA, Goldsmith LS, Miles DK, et al: Neonatal adrenoleukodystrophy presenting as infantile progressive spinal muscular atrophy. Pediatr Neurol 1993;9:496–497.

Pauli RM: Sensorineural deafness and peripheral neuropathy. Clin Genet 1984;26:383–384.

Percy AK, Kaback MM, Herndon RM: Metachromatic leukodystrophy: Comparison of early and late-onset forms. Neurology 1977; 27:933–941.

Perini M, Ghezzi A, Basso PF, Montanini R: Association of neuromyotonia with peripheral neuropathy, myasthenia gravis and thymoma: A case report. Ital J Neurol Sci 1994;15:307–310.

Perlmutter DH, Gross P, Jones HR, et al: Intramuscular vitamin E repletion in children with chronic cholestasis. Am J Dis Child 1987;141:170–174.

Petersen B, Schneider C, Strassburg HM, Schrod L: Critical illness neuropathy in pediatric intensive care patients. Pediatr Neurol 1999;21:749–759.

Phelps M, Aicardi J, Vanier MT: Late onset Krabbe's leukodystrophy: A report of four cases. J Neurol Neurosurg Psychiatry 1991;54:293–296.

Pickett J, Berg B, Chaplin E, Brunstetter-Shafer M-A: Syndrome of botulism in infancy: Clinical and electrophysiologic study. N Engl J Med 1976;295:770–772.

Pinhas Hamiel O, Raas-Rothschild A, Upadhyaya M, et al: Hereditary motor–sensory neuropathy (Charcot-Marie-Tooth disease) with nerve deafness: A new variant. J Pediatr 1993;123:431–434.

Pitt MC, Kearney K, Oware A, et al: An unusual neuropathy presenting with severe respiratory difficulty in the neonatal period with distinctive clinical, neurophysiological and pathological findings and poor prognosis. Electroencephalogr Clin Neurophysiol 1998;106(Suppl 1001):84.

Pitt MC: A system based study of the variation of the amplitude of the compound sensory nerve action potential recorded using surface electrodes. Electroencephalogr Clin Neurophysiol 1996; 101:520–527.

Pollock M, Nukada H, Frith RW, et al: Peripheral neuropathy in Tangier disease. Brain 1983;106:911–928.

Priest JM, Fischbeck KH, Nouri N, Keats BJB: A locus for axonal motor-sensory neuropathy with deafness and mental retardation maps to Xq24-q26. Genomics 1995;29:409–412.

Raimbault J: Les Conductions Nerveuses Chez l'Enfant Normal. Paris, Expansion Scientifique Francaise, 1988.

Ramaeckers Th V, Lake BD, Harding B, et al: Diagnostic difficulties in infantile neuroaxonal dystrophy—a clinicopathological study of eight cases. Neuropediatrics 1987;18:170–175.

Reardon W, Boyd S, Pitt MC, et al: Disordered peripheral nerve conduction in DOOR(S) syndrome. Neuropediatrics 1994;25:33–35.

Rizzuto N, Terzian H, Galiazzo-Rizzuto S: Toxic polyneuropathies in Italy due to leather cement poisoning in shoe industries: A light- and electron-microscopic study. J Neurol Sci 1977;31:343–354.

Rolfs A, Bolik A: Guillain-Barré syndrome in pregnancy reflections on immunopathogenesis. Acta Neurol Scand 1994;89:400–492.

Ropper AH: Management of Guillain-Barre syndrome. In Ropper AH, Kennedy SK, Zervas NT (eds): Neurological and Neurosurgical Intensive Care. Baltimore, University Park Press, 1983; 163–174.

Rosenberg RN, Chutorian A: Familial opticoacoustic nerve degeneration and polyneuropathy. Neurology 1967;17:827–832.

Rosenblum JL, Keating JP, Prensky AL, Nelson JS: A progressive neurologic syndrome in children with chronic liver disease. N Engl J Med 1981;304:503–508.

Ross AT: Mercuric polyneuropathy with albumino-cytologic dissociation and eosinophilia. JAMA 1964;188:830b.

Sakashita Y, Sakato S, Komai K, Takamori M: Hereditary motor and sensory neuropathy with calf muscle enlargement. J Neurol Sci 1992;113:118–122.

Santer R, Claviez A, Oldigs HD, et al: Isolated defect of peroxisomal beta-oxidation in a 16 year-old patient. Eur J Pediatrics 1993;152:9–42.

Sasaki K, Tachi N, Shinoda M, et al: Demyelinating peripheral neuropathy in Cockayne syndrome: A histopathologic and morphometric study. Brain Dev 1992;14:114–117.

Schaffner W, Fleet WF, Kilroy AW, et al: Polyneuropathy following rubella immunization. Am J Dis Child 1974;127:684–688.

Schroder JM: Neuropathy associated with mitochondrial disorders. Brain Pathol 1993;3:177–190.

Schwartz MS, Swash M: Scapuloperoneal atrophy with sensory involvement: Davidenkow's syndrome. J Neurol Neurosurg Psychiatry 1975;38:1063–1067.

Schwartz RH, Eng G: Infant botulism: Exacerbation by aminoglycosides. Am J Dis Child 1982;136:952.

Schwarz J, Planck J, Briegal J, Straube A: Single-fiber electromyography, nerve conduction studies, and conventional electromyography in patients with critical-illness polyneuropathy: Evidence for a lesion of terminal motor axons. Muscle Nerve 1997; 20:696–701.

Scully RE, Mark EJ, McNeeley BU (eds): Case records of the Massachusetts General Hospital. N Engl J Med 1984;310:445–455.

Seto DSY, Freeman JM: Lead neuropathy in childhood. Am J Dis Child 1964;107:337–342.

Sheth RD, Lotz BP, Hecox KE, Waclawik AJ: Infantile botulism: Pitfalls in diagnosis. J Child Neurol 1999;14:156–158.

Sheth RD, Pryse-Phillips WEM, Riggs JE, Bodensteiner JB: Critical illness neuromuscular disease in children manifested as ventilatory dependence. J Pediatr 1995;126:259–261.

Shorer Z, Philpot J, Muntoni F, et al: Demyelinating peripheral neuropathy in merosin-deficient congenital muscular dystrophy. J Child Neurol 1995;10:472–475.

Shukla AY, Marsh W, Green JB, Hurst D: Neonatal botulism. Neurology 1991;41(Suppl 1):202.

Silver JR: Familial spastic paraplegia with amyotrophy of the hands. J Neurol Neurosurg Psychiatry 1966;29:135–144.

Simmons Z, Wald JJ, Albers JW: Chronic inflammatory demyelinating polyradiculopathy in children: II. Long-term follow-up, with comparison to adults. Muscle Nerve 1997;20:1569–1575.

Simpson JA: Neuropathy after thalidomide ('Distaval'). Br Med J 1961;2:1287.

Smith NJ, Espir MLE, Mathews WB: Familial myoclonic epilepsy with ataxia and neuropathy with additional features of Friedreich's ataxia and peroneal muscular atrophy. Brain 1978;101:461–472.

Smits MG, Gabreels FJ, Renier WO, et al: Peripheral and central myelinopathy in Cockayne's syndrome: Report of 3 siblings. Neuropediatrics 1982;13:161–167.

Sobue G, Nakao N, Murakami K, et al: Type I familial amyloid polyneuropathy: A pathological study of the peripheral nervous system. Brain 1990;113:903–919.

Sokol RJ, Guggenheim M, Iannaccone ST, et al: Improved neurologic function after long-term correction of vitamin E deficiency in children with chronic cholestasis. N Engl J Med 1985;313: 1580–1586.

Sommer C, Schroder JM: Hereditary motor and sensory neuropathy with optic atrophy: Ultrastructural and morphometric observations on nerve fibers, mitochondria and dense-cored vesicles. Arch Neurol 1989;46:973–977.

Soong BW, Lin KP: An electrophysiologic and pathologic study of peripheral nerves in individuals with Machado-Joseph disease. Chung Hua I Hsueh Tsa Chih (Taipei) 1998;61:181–187.

Spaans F, Jennekens FGI, Mirandolle J, et al: Myotonic dystrophy associated with hereditary motor and sensory neuropathy. Brain 1986;109:1149–1168.

Spillane JD, Wells CEC: The neurology of Jennerian vaccination. Brain 1964;87:1–44.

Spruijt L, Naviaux RK, McGowan KA, et al: Nerve conduction changes in patients with mitochondrial disease treated with dichloracetate. Muscle Nerve 2001;24:916–924.

Steinman L, Tharp BR, Dorfman LJ, et al: Peripheral neuropathy in the cherry-red-spot-myoclonus syndrome (sialidosis type I). Ann Neurol 1980;7:450–456.

Stogbauer F, Young P, Kerschensteiner M, et al: Recurrent brachial plexus palsies as the only clinical expression of hereditary neuropathy with liability to pressure palsies associated with a de novo deletion of the peripheral myelin protein-22 gene. Muscle Nerve 1998;21:1199–201.

Swaiman KF, Flagler DG: Mercury poisoning with central and peripheral nervous system involvement treated with penicillamine. J Pediatr 1971;48:639–642.

Swift RG, Sadler DB, Swift M: Psychiatric findings in Wolfram syndrome homozygotes. Lancet 1990;2:667–669.

Swift TR, Ignacio OJ: Tick paralysis: Electrophysiologic studies. Neurology 1975;25:1130–1133.

Taly AB, Muthane UB: Involvement of peripheral nervous system in juvenile Parkinson's disease. Acta Neurol Scand 1992;85:272–275.

Tandan R, Little BW, Emery ES, et al: Childhood giant axonal neuropathy: Case report and review of the literature. J Neurol Sci 1987;82:205–228.

Thomas C, Love S, Powell HC, et al: Giant axonal neuropathy: Correlation of clinical findings with postmortem neuropathology. Ann Neurol 1987;22:79–84.

Thomas PK, Claus D, Jaspert A, et al: Focal upper limb demyelinating neuropathy. Brain 1996;119:765–774.

Thomas PK: Hereditary sensory neuropathies. Brain Pathol 1993;3:157–163.

Thompson JA, Glasgow LA, Warpinski JR, Olson C: Infant botulism: Clinical spectrum and epidemiology. Pediatrics 1980;66:936–942.

Toren A, Mandel M, Shahar E, et al: Primary central nervous system Burkitt's lymphoma presenting as Guillain-Barré syndrome. Med Pediatr Oncol 1994;23:372–375.

Torvik A, Torp S, Kase BF, et al: Infantile Refsum's disease: A generalized peroxisomal disorder. Case report with postmortem examination. J Neurol Sci 1988;85:39–53.

Tredici G, Minoli G: Peripheral nerve involvement in familial apsatic paraplegia. Arch Neurol 1979;36:236–239.

Van Coster R, Lombres A, De Vivo DC, et al: Cytochrome c oxidase-associated Leigh syndrome: Phenotypic features and pathogenetic speculations. J Neurol Sci 1991;104:97–111.

Vedanarayanan VV, Kandt RS, Lewis DV Jr, DeLong GR: Chronic inflammatory demyelinating polyradiculoneuropathy of childhood: Treatment with high-dose intravenous immunoglobulin. Neurology 1991;41:828–830.

Vermeulen M, van der Meché FGA, Speelman JD, et al: Plasma and gamma-globulin infusion in chronic inflammatory polyneuropathy. J Neurol Sci 1985;70:317–326.

Wheeler DJ: Understanding Variation: The Key to Managing Chaos. Tennessee, SPC Press, 1993.

Wichman A, Buchthal F, Pezeshkpour GH, Gregg RE: Peripheral neuropathy in abetalipoproteinemia. Neurology 1985;35:1279–1289.

Willems PJ, Van Roy BC, Kleijer WJ, et al: Atypical clinical presentation of ataxia telangiectasia. Am J Med Genet 1993;45:777–782.

Wilmshurst JM, Ouvrier RA: Nerve biopsy. In Jones HR, DeVivo D, Darras BT (eds): Neuromuscular Disorders of Infancy, Childhood and Adolescence. Boston, Butterworth-Heinemann, 2002.

Windebank AJ, McCall JT, Dyck PJ: Metal neuropathy. In Dyck PJ, Thomas PK, Lambert EH, Bunge R (eds): Peripheral Neuropathy, Vol 2, ed 3. Philadelphia, WB Saunders, 1995.

Winer JB, Hughes RA, Greenwood RJ, et al: Prognosis in Guillain-Barre syndrome. Lancet 1985;5:1202–1203.

Wolfe DE, Schindler D, Desnick RJ: Neuroaxonal dystrophy in infantile alpha-N-acetylgalactosaminidase deficiency. J Neurol Sci 1995;132:44–56.

Wong BL, deGrauw T, Togelson MH: Pain in pediatric Guillain-Barré syndrome: Case report. J Child Neurol 1998;13:184–185.

Woods CG, Taylor AMR: Ataxia telangiectasia in the British Isles: The clinical and laboratory features of 70 affected individuals. Q J Med 1992;82:169–179.

Wulff CH, Trojaborg W: Adult metachromatic leukodystrophy: Neurophysiologic findings. Neurology 1985;35:1776–1778.

Yatziv S, Rusell A: An unusual form of metachromatic leukodystrophy in three siblings. Clin Genet 1981;19:222–227.

Yokata T, Inaba A, Yuki N, et al: The F wave disappears due to impaired excitability of motor neurons or proximal axons in inflammatory demyelinating neuropathies. J Neurol Neurosurg Psychiatry 1996;60:650–654.

Yoshino H, Harukawa H, Asano A: IgG antiganglioside antibodies in Guillain-Barre syndrome with bulbar palsy. J Neuroimmunol 2000;105:195–201.

Zafeiriou DI, Anastasiou AL, Michelakaki EM, et al: Early infantile Krabbe disease: Deceptively normal magnetic resonance imaging and serial neurophysiological studies. Brain Dev 1997;19:488–491.

Congenital Myasthenic Syndromes

C. Michel Harper

Disorders of the neuromuscular junction are an uncommon but important cause of weakness in children. Normally, the safety margin of neuromuscular transmission allows for the generation of a muscle fiber action potential in response to an action potential in the motor axon even at high firing frequencies. Failure of muscle activation with clinical weakness results when a disease process interferes with the synthesis, storage, or release of acetylcholine; disrupts the three-dimensional architecture of the synapse; or interferes with the function of either the acetylcholine receptor (AChR) or the acetylcholinesterase (AChE) molecule. The congenital myasthenic syndromes (CMSs) are a group of diseases characterized by a genetic defect in one or more molecular mechanisms of neuromuscular transmission. The site and mechanism of the defect classify the CMSs (Table 93–1).

GENERAL FEATURES AND APPROACH TO DIAGNOSIS

Genetics

All of the CMSs are autosomal recessive disorders except for slow channel CMS, which is autosomal dominant. Many patients have a family history of an affected sibling, spontaneous abortions, or sudden infant death syndrome. Slow channel syndrome is associated with affected relatives in multiple generations. Variable expression is common, but clinical and electrodiagnostic evaluation of parents of affected individuals confirms the diagnosis in some cases.

Clinical Manifestations

CMSs are present at birth, but some patients do not seek evaluation until later in childhood or adult life because the symptoms are mild or not recognized. In infants, disorders of neuromuscular transmission produce generalized hypotonia and weakness. Ptosis, strabismus, feeding difficulties, and respiratory insufficiency are common. Symptoms are often made worse by crying, feeding, or other motor activities. Motor development is often delayed. Abnormalities of pupillary constriction, reduced muscle bulk, hyporeflexia, and skeletal deformities may also occur. Later in childhood, manifestations are similar to those seen in adults with fluctuating and exertion-induced weakness of ocular, bulbar, axial, and proximal limb muscles.

The similarity of these symptoms to those of other disorders of the peripheral nervous system may make it difficult to differentiate disorders of neuromuscular transmission from other diseases of the motor unit, particularly in children. A defect of neuromuscular transmission is suspected when increased weakness with exertion (e.g., ptosis or extraocular weakness with upgaze, forward arm ele-

Table 93–1. Congenital Myasthenic Syndromes

Presynaptic defects
   Congenital myasthenic syndrome with episodic apnea*
   Congenital Lambert-Eaton myasthenia syndrome
   Paucity of synaptic vesicles
Synaptic defects
   Congenital end-plate acetylcholinesterase deficiency
Postsynaptic defects
   Primary kinetic abnormality with or without acetylcholine
     receptor deficiency
     Slow channel syndrome
     Fast channel syndrome
   Primary acetylcholine receptor deficiency without or with only
     minor kinetic abnormality
   Myasthenic syndrome with plectin deficiency

*Formerly known as familial infantile myasthenia.

vation, or repeated deep knee bends) is demonstrated. Scoliosis or lumbar lordosis that worsens with prolonged standing suggests CMS, rather than an acquired defect of neuromuscular transmission.

Some clinical manifestations suggest a specific subtype of CMS. Episodic respiratory failure triggered by infections or physical activity in early childhood with improvement during later childhood is characteristic of CMS with episodic apnea. Delayed pupillary response to light and a lack of clinical response to AChE inhibitors suggest end-plate AChE deficiency. Worsening of symptoms with AChE inhibitors and relatively selective weakness of cervical and distal upper limb extensor muscles occur in the slow channel CMS.

Laboratory Studies

Serological tests for AChR antibodies are negative in all cases of CMS. Creatine kinase and other muscle enzymes are normal. One patient has been described with CMS associated with a muscular dystrophy caused by plectin deficiency, but no specific abnormalities were noted on blood tests in this individual (Banwell et al., 1999). Some patients have subclinical respiratory compromise with carbon dioxide retention and a compensated respiratory acidosis. Pulmonary function studies frequently demonstrate a restrictive pattern, and oximetry studies may show desaturation with exercise or sleep.

Electrodiagnosis

Electrodiagnostic studies are very useful in the evaluation of patients with a suspected CMS (Harper, 1999). First, they are invaluable in detecting the presence and measuring the severity of the neuromuscular transmission defect. In the majority of cases, disorders of the motoneuron, peripheral nerve, and muscle can be excluded. Second, in conjunction with the clinical manifestations, serological studies, and the response to AChE inhibitors, electrodiagnostic studies frequently allow CMSs to be

distinguished from acquired defects of neuromuscular transmission and classified into specific subtypes (see Table 93–1). This information is often sufficient to provide useful information regarding the natural history, prognosis, genetic transmission, and symptomatic therapy. In selected cases, detailed microphysiological, ultrastructural, histochemical, and molecular genetic studies are required for accurate diagnosis and classification (Engel et al., 1999).

NERVE CONDUCTION STUDIES

Standard motor and sensory nerve conduction studies are normal in most patients with CMS. The amplitude of the compound muscle action potential (CMAP) is reduced in some cases (e.g., congenital Lambert-Eaton–like syndrome, severe cases of other subtypes). In the majority of cases of end-plate AChE deficiency or slow channel syndrome, a single supramaximal stimulus evokes two or more CMAPs at 3- to 8-ms intervals (Fig. 93–1). The first CMAP is the main M wave. The subsequent smaller "repetitive" CMAPs are caused by an abnormally prolonged end-plate potential, whose amplitude remains above threshold longer than the muscle fiber action potential refractory period. Each consecutive repetitive CMAP is smaller than the preceding one. Exercise or repetitive stimulation at rates between 0.5 and 2 Hz will abolish the repetitive CMAP (Fig. 93–2). Thus, the repetitive potentials can be easily missed when stimuli are delivered every 1 to 2 seconds in the routine process of obtaining a supramaximal response. This can be avoided by delivering a single supramaximal stimulus 5 to 10 seconds after the initial supramaximal stimulus intensity is determined. Cholinesterase inhibitors can also produce one or more repetitive CMAPs. These medications should be discontinued several hours before the study is performed. A characteristic finding in slow channel CMS is an increase in number and amplitude of repetitive CMAPs after the administration of an AChE inhibitor (Fig. 93–3). This feature can be used to distinguish slow channel CMS from congenital AChE deficiency, in which the number and size

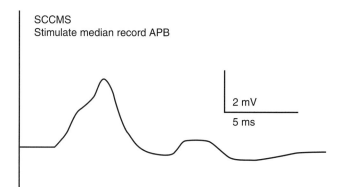

SCCMS
Stimulate median record APB

2 mV

5 ms

Figure 93–1. Repetitive compound muscle action potential (CMAP) in congenital myasthenic syndromes. A single repetitive potential is noted approximately 6 ms after the peak of the main compound muscle action potential. APB, abductor pollicis brevis; SCCMS, slow channel congenital myasthenic syndrome.

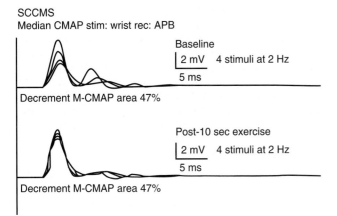

Figure 93–2. Repetitive stimulation at 2 Hz or brief exercise eliminates the repetitive compound muscle action potentials in a patient with slow channel congenital myasthenic syndrome.

of repetitive CMAPs is unchanged by AChE inhibitor administration (Fig. 93–4).

Repetitive stimulation studies performed in areas of clinical weakness in CMS produce a pattern of decrement that is similar to that observed in autoimmune myasthenia gravis. At rates of 2 to 5 Hz, the decrement is greatest in relative terms between the first and second potentials, peaks by the fourth or fifth potential, and then shows gradual repair with continued stimulation. The decrement is partially or completely repaired by exercise, AChE inhibitors (except in AChE deficiency and slow channel syndrome), and 3,4-diaminopyridine in most types of CMS. Higher rates of repetitive stimulation (10–50 Hz) may produce a rate-dependent decrement in many patients with CMS (Fig. 93–5), which, if present, helps distinguish this condition from autoim-

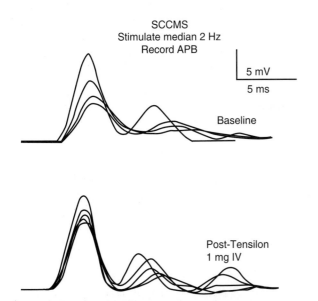

Figure 93–3. Administration of a cholinesterase inhibitor increases the number and amplitude of repetitive compound muscle action potentials in a patient with slow channel congenital myasthenic syndrome.

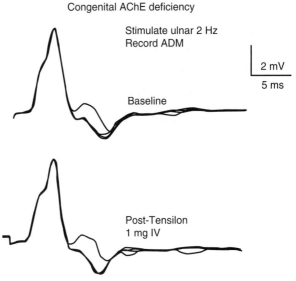

Figure 93–4. Administration of a cholinesterase inhibitor has no effect on the repetitive compound muscle action potential in a patient with congenital acetylcholinesterase (AChE) deficiency. ADM, abductor digiti minimi.

mune myasthenia gravis. Rarely, a pattern of low-amplitude baseline CMAP with facilitation after higher rates of repetitive stimulation is observed in congenital Lambert-Eaton–like syndrome. Although the abnormalities on repetitive stimulation are typically widespread, sometimes the decrement is confined to facial muscles or cannot be demonstrated in any muscle, even in the setting of objective clinical weakness. Single-fiber EMG and/or microelectrode studies are often helpful in these rare instances. If the diagnosis of CMS with episodic apnea is suspected on clinical grounds, prolonged repetitive stimulation at 10 Hz (or exercise) for 5 to 10 minutes may be required to demonstrate a decrement.

NEEDLE EXAMINATION

Standard concentric needle examination typically reveals normal insertional activity and prominent motor unit potential amplitude variation in all CMS patients. Fibrillation potentials or other abnormal spontaneous activity may be observed very rarely,

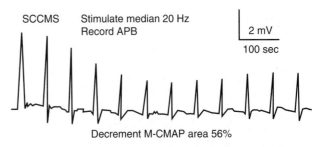

Figure 93–5. The decrement in slow channel congenital myasthenic syndrome typically increases with higher rates of repetitive stimulation. The decrement at 2-Hz repetitive stimulation of the median nerve in this patient was 18% (not shown).

usually in association with an additional disorder of muscle (e.g., CMS with plectin deficiency). Small, rapidly recruited motor unit potentials are typical. In most cases, the motor unit potentials are fairly simple in configuration, but in disorders with an associated end-plate myopathy (e.g., slow channel syndrome) or muscular dystrophy (e.g., CMS with plectin deficiency), complex polyphasic motor unit potentials may also be observed. Voluntary or stimulated single-fiber EMG shows increased jitter and blocking in all patients with CMS. Stimulated single-fiber EMG may reveal an increase in blocking with higher rates of stimulation in some types of CMS.

MUSCLE BIOPSY STUDIES

Morphological and microelectrode studies performed on intercostal or anconeus muscle biopsy specimens allow definitive determination of the mechanism of the neuromuscular transmission defect in the majority of patients with CMS (Engel et al., 1999). Morphological studies include evaluation of the end-plate regions by light and electron microscopy and estimation of the number of AChRs and amount of AChE per end-plate. Microelectrode studies include assessment of the miniature end-plate potential, quantal release, and the end-plate potential, and patch-clamp recordings of currents flowing through single AChR channels. The latter provide precise information about the conductance and kinetic properties of the AChR channel.

MOLECULAR GENETIC STUDIES

When clinical, electrodiagnostic, and/or muscle biopsy studies suggest a candidate gene or protein, molecular genetic analysis can be attempted. Because the genetic defect of many CMS subtypes has been elucidated, molecular genetic testing on peripheral blood DNA can often confirm the diagnosis in suspected cases. When a novel mutation is discovered, expression studies using the genetically engineered mutant molecule have been used to confirm pathogenicity and to analyze the properties of the mutant molecule (Fukodome et al., 1998). This has led to specific treatment strategies in at least one of the major forms of CMS (slow channel CMS) (Harper and Engel, 1998).

SPECIFIC CONGENITAL MYASTHENIC SYNDROMES

Presynaptic Congenital Myasthenic Syndromes

CONGENITAL MYASTHENIC SYNDROME WITH EPISODIC APNEA

This disorder is also known as *familial infantile myasthenia*, but this is a misnomer because all forms of CMS can be familial and present in infancy. *CMS with episodic apnea* emphasizes a key clinical feature that helps distinguish the disorder from other types of CMS. CMS with episodic apnea is an autosomal recessive disorder that has been associated with defects in the function of choline acetyltransferase, producing reduced reserves of acetylcholine in the presynaptic nerve terminal (Ohno et al., 2001). The disorder presents in infancy or early childhood with intermittent hypotonia and fatigable generalized weakness, ptosis, dysphagia, weak suck and cry, and respiratory insufficiency. Intermittent acute crises associated with severe weakness and respiratory failure precipitated by infection or excitement are characteristic of CMS with episodic apnea (Robertson et al., 1980). Sudden infant death or anoxic encephalopathy can occur. The crises lessen in frequency and severity in early to mid-childhood, leading to a clinical syndrome that is very similar to autoimmune myasthenia gravis. Deep tendon reflexes are normal. In mild cases or between crises, exercise of 5 to 10 minutes' duration may be useful in eliciting weakness. The symptoms respond to AChE inhibitors in patients of all ages.

On nerve conduction studies, the amplitude of the baseline CMAP is normal, and there are no repetitive CMAPs with single supramaximal stimuli. The results of repetitive stimulation vary. In clinically weak muscles, there usually is a decrement of the CMAP at rest that repairs with brief exercise or high-frequency stimulation, shows postactivation exhaustion for 2 to 5 minutes, and then gradually recovers over 5 to 10 minutes. In infants who are between crises or in older patients who are mildly affected, exercise or repetitive stimulation at 10 Hz may have to be continued for 5 to 10 minutes before a decrement of the CMAP is observed (Fig. 93–6). The decrement also improves after the administration of AChE inhibitors.

Microelectrode studies show a normal miniature end-plate potential amplitude and quantal content at rest but a gradual fall in both with 10-Hz stimulation for 5 to 10 minutes (Mora et al., 1987). A similar pattern of decrement is seen when hemicolinium, an inhibitor of choline uptake, is added to normal muscle. Ultrastructural and histochemical studies show normal morphology of the synapse and normal concentration of both AChE and AChRs. Based on these studies, it has been postulated that CMS with episodic apnea is caused by a defect in either the reuptake of choline into the nerve terminal or the synthesis, storage, or mobilization of acetylcholine. Mutations in the enzyme responsible for synthesis of acetylcholine in the nerve terminal, choline acetyltransferase, have been described in patients with CMS with episodic apnea (Ohno et al., 2001).

CONGENITAL LAMBERT-EATON–LIKE SYNDROME

The first reported case occurred in an infant with severe hypotonia and generalized weakness (Albers et al., 1984). Nerve conduction studies revealed a low-amplitude CMAP, a decrement at slow and fast

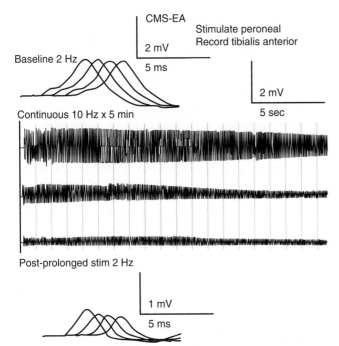

Figure 93–6. Prolonged repetitive stimulation in congenital myasthenic syndrome with episodic apnea (CMS-EA). There is little or no decrement on baseline repetitive stimulation at 2 Hz. Continuous repetitive stimulation at 10 Hz produces a gradual fall in the compound muscle action potential. Immediately after 5 minutes of continuous stimulation, a brief train of 2-Hz repetitive stimulation produces a decrement of 25%.

rates in the neonatal period, and facilitation of 50% to 740% after brief tetanic stimulation at the age of 2 months. AChE inhibitors and guanidine had no effect. Morphological and histochemical studies showed a slight decrease in the mean diameter of the synaptic vesicles as the only abnormality. Although microelectrode studies were not performed, the findings suggested a congenital presynaptic defect of neuromuscular transmission. The authors postulated that this represented a defect in the synthesis, mobilization, or storage of acetylcholine.

An infant with hypotonia, generalized weakness, and delayed motor development since birth who had electrodiagnostic abnormalities identical to those of Lambert-Eaton–like syndrome has also been reported (Bady et al., 1987). Nerve conduction studies performed at 3 years of age showed a low-amplitude CMAP at rest with a decrement of 50% with 3-Hz stimulation and facilitation of over 2000% with 50-Hz stimulation. Guanidine increased the amplitude of the CMAP and reduced the amount of facilitation by five-fold. Microelectrode studies were not performed. We studied a similar patient who presented with infantile hypotonia and respiratory insufficiency in the first few months of life. Nerve conduction studies revealed very low baseline CMAP and facilitation after repetitive stimulation at high rates (Fig. 93–7). Microelectrode studies showed a presynaptic defect with very low quantal release. The amplitude of the CMAP improved on combination therapy with 3,4-diaminopyridine and

pyridostigmine, but the clinical response was not dramatic and the patient continued to require mechanical ventilation.

PAUCITY OF SYNAPTIC VESICLES AND REDUCED QUANTAL RELEASE

A single case of this subtype has been described (Walls et al., 1993). The patient presented in the neonatal period with feeding difficulties and a weak cry. Later in childhood, she developed fatigable ptosis, ocular and bulbar weakness, and a delay in motor development. Electrodiagnostic evaluation at the age of 23 years showed normal CMAP amplitude at rest and a decrement at 2 Hz in multiple muscles. No facilitation was observed with exercise or 50-Hz stimulation. The patient responded partially to AChE inhibitors. Overall, the features suggested antibody-negative autoimmune myasthenia gravis or CMS secondary to a postsynaptic defect of neuromuscular transmission. This case illustrates that in some cases of CMS, the clinical and electrodiagnostic findings are misleading. Specifically, patients with presynaptic defects may have findings that suggest a postsynaptic defect of neuromuscular transmission on repetitive stimulation studies. This important point is illustrated by the findings on microelectrode studies in this patient. The amplitude and the frequency of the miniature end-plate potential were normal. The quantal content of the end-plate potential at 1 Hz was reduced to 20% of normal. The probability of release was normal, but the number of available quanta was reduced. This was correlated with a reduction in the density of synaptic vesicles within the nerve terminal. The authors postulated that the presynaptic defect in this disorder was caused by impaired synthesis, transport, or recycling of synaptic vesicles.

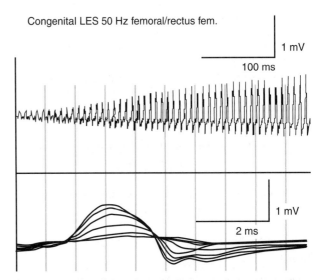

Figure 93–7. Congenital Lambert-Eaton myasthenic syndrome (LES). Low-amplitude baseline compound muscle action potential and facilitation during 50-Hz repetitive stimulation.

Synaptic Congenital Myasthenic Syndromes

Congenital End-Plate Acetylcholinesterase Deficiency

This is an autosomal recessive disease characterized by a deficiency in the asymmetrical form of AChE at the neuromuscular junction (Engel et al., 1977). The globular form of the enzyme is normal. Genetic studies have indicated that there is a defect in the collagen-like tail that anchors the AChE to the basal lamina (Ohno et al., 1998).

Clinical manifestations are usually present in the neonatal period but may be delayed into later infancy or childhood. Congenital AChE deficiency can cause severe generalized weakness and hypotonia with poor feeding, weak cry, and respiratory insufficiency requiring mechanical ventilation. Developmental delay of motor milestones is common. In older children and adults, manifestations include fatigable asymmetrical ptosis, ophthalmoparesis, dysarthria, dysphagia, and weakness of both axial and limb musculature. The extraocular muscles can be spared, and distal upper extremity muscles (wrist and finger extensors) can be involved (Hutchinson et al., 1993). There often is a diffuse reduction in muscle bulk with either normal or hypoactive reflexes. Scoliosis and lumbar lordosis that worsen after standing for 30 to 60 seconds, unresponsiveness to AChE inhibitors, and a delay in the pupillary response to light are all constant and characteristic findings in congenital AChE deficiency (Hutchinson et al., 1993).

Standard motor nerve conduction studies reveal the presence of a repetitive CMAP in response to single supramaximal stimuli (Fig. 93–8). This phenomenon has been described only with pharmacological inhibition of AChE (Besser et al., 1989), in congenital AChE deficiency (Harper, 1999) and in the slow channel CMS (Engel et al., 1982; Harper, 1999). All of these conditions are associated with prolonged duration of the end-plate potential, which in a subset of muscle fibers remains above threshold beyond the refractory period and produces one or more additional action potentials. The repetitive CMAPs are lower in amplitude than the main CMAP and follow it by 3 to 8 ms. With repetitive stimulation at rates of 0.5 to 2 Hz, the second CMAP decreases more rapidly than the main CMAP, disappearing by the second to fifth stimulus (see Fig. 93–8). The repetitive CMAP with single stimulus may be absent in young infants and in severely affected patients with congenital AChE deficiency (Hutchinson et al., 1993). This results from a severe reduction in the safety margin of neuromuscular transmission, which overshadows the effect of the prolonged end-plate potential duration. Repetitive stimulation at 2 Hz produces a 10% to 50% decrement of the main CMAP that shows minimal repair with exercise and no repair after the administration of AChE inhibitors. Stimulation at rates of 20 Hz or higher for more

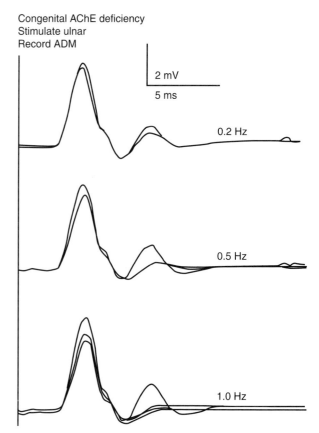

Figure 93–8. Effect of slow rates of repetitive stimulation on the repetitive compound muscle action potential (small response 6 ms after the main compound muscle action potential) in a patient with congenital acetylcholinesterase (AChE) deficiency. The repetitive potential decreases significantly even at rates as slow as 0.5 Hz. ADM, abductor digiti minimi.

than 10 to 15 seconds produces a decrement (Fig. 93–9), probably secondary to depolarization block of the AChR.

The findings on needle electromyography in AChE deficiency are nonspecific. Standard concentric needle examination reveals normal insertional activity with no fibrillation potentials or other abnormal spontaneous discharges. With voluntary muscle activation, low-amplitude, short-duration motor unit potentials that vary in amplitude and morphology

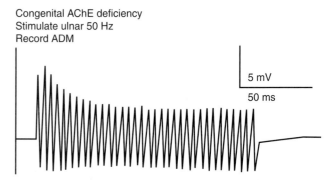

Figure 93–9. Decrement with high-frequency repetitive stimulation in acetylcholinesterase (AChE) deficiency.

are recorded in all muscles. Single-fiber EMG shows increased jitter and blocking.

An abnormal delay in contraction of the iris has been demonstrated using quantitative pupillography in patients with AChE deficiency (Hutchinson et al., 1993). Other tests of autonomic function, including quantitative sudomotor axon reflex test and cardio-vascular reflexes, were normal.

Ultrastructural, histochemical, and microphysiological studies have helped determine the pathogenesis of AChE deficiency (Engel et al., 1977; Hutchinson et al., 1993). The asymmetrical form of AChE is absent at the end-plate. Most of the nerve terminals are small in size, and the Schwann cell often extends into the synaptic space. These two factors could explain why both the quantal content and miniature end-plate potential amplitude are reduced in most patients. The three-dimensional configuration of the synaptic space is usually altered, with widening of the synaptic cleft, reduction in the number and complexity of the junction folds, and degeneration of the subcellular components of the junctional sarcoplasm. These findings probably result from the toxic effects of calcium, which enters the end-plate region of the muscle fiber in excess owing to the prolonged duration of the miniature end-plate current. In addition to the aforementioned factors, AChR desensitization and depolarization block of the end-plate may contribute to the low safety margin of neuromuscular transmission in this disease.

Postsynaptic Congenital Myasthenic Syndromes

PRIMARY KINETIC ABNORMALITY WITH OR WITHOUT ACETYLCHOLINE RECEPTOR DEFICIENCY

Slow Channel Congenital Myasthenic Syndrome

This is the only CMS described to date that has an autosomal dominant pattern of inheritance (Engel et al., 1982; Oosterhuis et al., 1987). Slow channel CMS is caused by mutations of the AChR that increase the affinity of the receptor for the acetylcholine molecule. This increases the open time of the receptor, producing prolonged end-plate currents and excess calcium leakage into the end-plate region of the muscle fiber. Mutations causing the slow channel CMS phenotype have been described in the α, β, and ε subunits of the AChR (Engel et al., 1996, 1999). Most of these are concentrated in the M2 segment that lines the channel pore. These mutations are thought to stabilize the open state of the receptor, whereas other slow channel CMS mutations in the M1 segment of the α channel are thought to enhance the affinity of acetylcholine through changes in its binding site on the α subunit.

The age at onset and clinical severity of slow channel CMS vary. Some patients are asymptomatic but have characteristic abnormalities on electrophysiological studies (Oosterhuis et al., 1987). Fluc-

tuating and fatigable ptosis, ophthalmoparesis, and trunk and extremity weakness are common. Many patients have prominent involvement of neck, wrist, and finger extensor muscles (Harper and Engel, 1998; Engel et al., 1999). The muscle weakness may be asymmetrical and does not respond to AChE inhibitors. Assays for AChR antibodies are negative. One patient has been reported who responded to the calcium channel antagonist flunarizine (Oosterhuis et al., 1987). Quinidine sulfate has shown to be clinically effective in the treatment of slow channel CMS (Harper and Engel, 1998).

On motor needle conduction studies, one or more repetitive CMAPs are observed with single supramaximal stimuli (Fig. 93–10). As with AChE deficiency, the repetitive CMAPs are lower in amplitude, occur at a latency of 3 to 8 ms, and usually decrease to a greater degree than the main CMAP at stimulus rates of 0.5 to 2 Hz. The repetitive CMAPs may be recorded in muscles that show no signs of weakness. Stimulation at 2 Hz produces a decrement of the main CMAP, which worsens on progressively higher rates of stimulation (see Fig. 93–5). The administration of AChE inhibitors has no effect on the decrement of the main CMAP but causes an increase in the amplitude and number of repetitive CMAPs (see Fig. 93–4). In contrast, the repetitive CMAP observed in congenital AChE deficiency is unchanged by AChE inhibitors. Thus, when used in conjunction with the pattern of inheritance and clinical manifestations, the effect of AChE inhibitors on the repetitive CMAP helps distinguish between the slow channel CMS and congenital AChE deficiency. Needle examination in slow channel syndrome shows normal spontaneous activity with short-duration, low-amplitude varying motor unit potentials.

Microphysiological studies show prolonged duration of the end-plate potential and the miniature end-plate current that is caused by a prolonged open time of the AChR ion channel. In addition to sodium, excess calcium passes through the AChR, leading to activation of catabolic enzymes and degeneration of the junctional folds and junctional sarcoplasm. This "end-plate myopathy" alters the configuration of the synapse and produces a secondary reduction in the number of AChRs, which in turn reduces the safety margin of neuromuscular transmission (Engel et al., 1999).

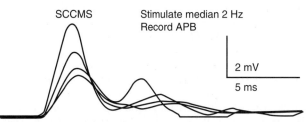

Figure 93–10. Repetitive compound muscle action potential in slow channel congenital myasthenic syndrome (SCCMS). The smaller repetitive potential occurs 7 ms after the main M wave, and there is a greater degree of decrement.

Fast Channel Syndrome (Low Affinity of Acetylcholine for Acetylcholine Receptor)

This is an autosomal recessive disorder caused by mutations that shorten the open time of the AChR. Symptoms typically begin in the neonatal or infantile period. Manifestations include hypotonia, ptosis, dysphagia, dysarthria, and generalized fatigable weakness. Most patients have a significant response to a combination of pyridostigmine and 3,4-diaminopyridine (Harper and Engel, 2000).

Repetitive stimulation studies resemble those for autoimmune myasthenia gravis with a decrement at low frequencies and partial repair after exercise. Unlike congenital end-plate AChE deficiency and slow channel CMS, high-frequency repetitive stimulation does not produce a decrement in the fast channel syndrome. Needle examination shows normal insertional activity with small varying motor unit potentials, and single-fiber EMG shows increased jitter and blocking.

Three different mutations that act via different mechanisms have been associated with the fast channel syndrome. The first is caused by a mutation in the extracellular domain of the ε subunit, εP121L, which results in a decreased rate of channel opening and a reduced affinity of the receptor for acetylcholine in the open and desensitized states (Ohno et al., 1996). The number of AChRs are normal, but there is a decrease in the size and duration of the miniature end-plate potential with an increased resistance to acetylcholine desensitization. The fast channel syndrome is also caused by a missense mutation, αV285I, which affects channel gating rather than the AChR binding affinity (Wang et al., 1998). In contrast to the low-affinity fast channel syndrome, there is a significant reduction in the number of AChRs at the motor end-plate. The miniature end-plate potentials and currents are small, with infrequent and brief channel openings. The third fast channel mutation is an inframe duplication in the long cytoplasmic loop of the ε subunit ε1254ins18 (Milone et al., 1998). This causes a reduced number of AChRs and inefficient switching of the receptor between open and closed states.

PRIMARY ACETYLCHOLINE RECEPTOR DEFICIENCY WITHOUT OR WITH ONLY MINOR KINETIC ABNORMALITY

The unifying feature of this genetically heterogeneous group is reduced expression of the AChR at the neuromuscular junction. More than 50 mutations have been described after either an autosomal recessive or a sporadic pattern (Engel et al., 1999). Most of the mutations occur in the ε subunit. This subunit has a high GC content, which predisposes to gene rearrangements. In addition, when the ε subunit is structurally deficient, the fetal γ subunit is substituted. This allows the formation of a functional AChR, whereas structural mutations of other subunits may be incompatible with survival past the fetal stage of development.

The age at onset of AChR deficiency ranges from infancy to adulthood. Clinical manifestations include hypotonia, respiratory insufficiency, weakness of ocular and bulbar muscles, and skeletal deformities. The majority of patients respond to AChE inhibitors, and some have a modest response to 3,4-diaminopyridine (Harper and Engel, 2000).

The findings on electrodiagnostic studies are indistinguishable from those for autoimmune myasthenia gravis. The amplitude of the CMAP at rest is normal. There are no repetitive CMAPs observed with single stimuli. With repetitive stimulation at low rates, there is a decrement of the CMAP in weak muscles. The decrement is partially repaired with exercise, tetanic stimulation, or AChE inhibitors (Fig. 93–11). Severe cases may look like a presynaptic defect of neuromuscular transmission (Fig. 93–12). These cases demonstrate that the findings on repetitive stimulation depend more on the severity of the neuromuscular transmission defect than on the

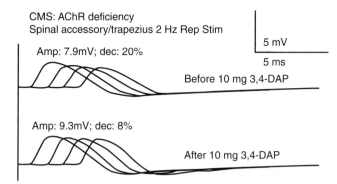

Figure 93–11. Decrement of the compound muscle action potential in congenital myasthenic syndrome (CMS) secondary to acetylcholine receptor (AChR) deficiency, without an associated kinetic abnormality. The pattern of decrement and repair with exercise, acetylcholinesterase inhibitors (not shown), or 3,4-diaminopyridine (DAP) is similar to that seen in autoimmune myasthenia gravis.

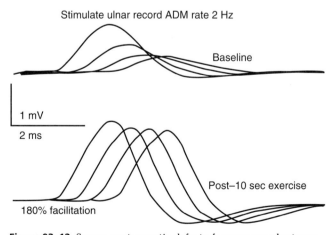

Figure 93–12. Severe postsynaptic defect of neuromuscular transmission (NMT) in a patient with congenital acetylcholine receptor deficiency. Microelectrode studies showed a normal quantal content and reduced size of the miniature end-plate potential. Despite the postsynaptic origin of the NMT defect, the amplitude of the baseline compound muscle action potential is reduced, and there is significant facilitation after exercise.

mechanism of the defect. The needle examination in AChR deficiency reveals normal spontaneous activity and rapidly recruited short, low-amplitude varying motor unit potentials.

A reduction in the number of α-bungarotoxin–binding sites on the postsynaptic membrane is the unifying feature of the congenital AChR deficiency syndrome. Poorly developed junctional folds with a paucity of secondary synaptic clefts is a common additional feature (Engel et al., 1999). The miniature end-plate potential is reduced, but the quantal release is often increased as a compensatory phenomenon. More sophisticated studies show mild kinetic abnormalities of the AChR, usually due to expression of the fetal γ subunit in most patients. One patient has been described who had the combination of congenital AChR deficiency and muscular dystrophy secondary to plectin deficiency (Banwell et al., 1999). The patient had epidermolysis bullosa since birth with progressive weakness and fatigability of ocular, facial, limb, and trunk muscles noted at the age of 9 years. Repetitive stimulation studies revealed a moderate decrement of 25% in weak muscles. Needle examination showed fibrillation potentials and small, polyphasic, rapidly recruited motor unit potentials. The serum creatine kinase level was five times the upper limit of normal, and AChR antibodies were absent. Muscle biopsy showed dystrophic changes and normal AChR density but focal degeneration of the junctional folds and expression of the fetal AChR. Microelectrode studies showed a normal quantal content but low-amplitude miniature end-plate potentials. The authors concluded that plectin probably plays an important role in the structural integrity of the neuromuscular junction in addition to other areas of the muscle and skin (Banwell, 1999). The patient responded partially to pyridostigmine and 3,4-diaminopyridine but demonstrated continued progression of weakness related to the underlying muscular dystrophy (Harper and Engel, 2000).

SUMMARY

CMSs should be considered in all patients with clinical or electrodiagnostic evidence of a defect of neuromuscular transmission when the results of tests for AChRs and calcium channel antibodies are negative. A careful history will usually reveal symptoms in infancy or early childhood and possible CMS in siblings or other family members. The combination of clinical examination, response to AChE inhibitors, and findings on electrodiagnostic studies is often sufficient to make a definitive diagnosis of CMS and in many cases to characterize the subtype. In selected cases, genetic studies or specialized morphological and electrophysiological studies performed on muscle biopsy specimens are required to completely characterize the molecular mechanisms underlying the disorder. Effective symptomatic therapy is available for most CMSs.

References

Albers JW, Faulkner JA, Dorovini-Zis K: Abnormal neuromuscular transmission in an infantile myasthenic syndrome. Ann Neurol 1984;16:28–34.
Bady B, Chauplannaz G, Carrier H: Congenital Lambert-Eaton myasthenic syndrome. J Neurol Neurosurg Psychiatry 1987;50:476–478.
Banwell BL, Russel J, Fukudome T, et al: Myopathy, myasthenic syndrome, and epidermolysis bullosa simplex due to plectin deficiency. J Neuropathol Exp Neurol 1999;58:832–846.
Besser R, Gutmann L, Dillman U, et al: End-plate dysfunction in acute organophosphate intoxication. Neurology 1989;39:561–567.
Engel AG, Lambert EH, Gomez MR: A new myasthenic syndrome with end-plate acetylcholinesterase deficiency, small nerve terminals, and reduced acetylcholine release. Ann Neurol 1977;1:315–330.
Engel AG, Lambert EH, Mulder DM: A newly recognized congenital myasthenic syndrome attributed to a prolonged open time of the acetylcholine-induced ion channel. Ann Neurol 1982;11:553–569.
Engel AG, Ohno K, Milone M, et al: New mutations in acetylcholine receptor subunit genes reveal heterogeneity in the slow-channel congenital myasthenic syndrome. Hum Mol Genet 1996;5:1217–1227.
Engel AG, Ohno K, Sine SM: Congenital myasthenic syndromes. In Engel AG (ed): Myasthenia Gravis and Myasthenic Disorders. New York, Oxford University Press, 1999; 251–297.
Fukudome T, Ohno K, Brengman JM, Engel AG: Quinidine normalizes the open duration of slow-channel mutants of the acetylcholine receptor. Neuroreport 1998;9:1907–1911.
Harper CM: Electrodiagnosis of endplate disease. In Engel AG (ed): Myasthenia Gravis and Myasthenic Disorders. New York, Oxford University Press, 1999; 65–87.
Harper CM, Engel AG: Quinidine sulfate therapy for the slow-channel congenital myasthenic syndrome. Ann Neurol 1998;43:480–484.
Harper CM, Engel AG: Treatment of 31 congenital myasthenic syndrome (CMS) patients with 3,4-diaminopyridine (DAP). Neurology 2000;54:A395.
Hutchinson DO, Engel AG, Walls TJ, et al: The spectrum of congenital end-plate acetylcholine receptor deficiency. Ann N Y Acad Sci 1993;681:469–486.
Milone M, Wang H-L, Ohno K, et al: Mode switching kinetics produced by a naturally occurring mutation in the cytoplasmic loop of the human acetylcholine receptor ε subunit. Neuron 1998;20:575–588.
Mora M, Lambert EH, Engel AG: Synaptic vesicle abnormality in familial infantile myasthenia. Neurology 1987;37:206–214.
Ohno K, Brengman J, Tsujino A, Engel AG: Human endplate acetylcholinesterase deficiency caused by mutations in the collagen-like tail subunit (ColQ) of the asymmetric enzyme. Proc Natl Acad Sci U S A 1998;4:9654–9659.
Ohno K, Tsujino A, Brengman J, et al: Choline acetyltransferase mutations cause myasthenic syndrome associated with episodic apnea in humans. Proc Natl Acad Sci U S A 2001;98:2017–2022.
Ohno K, Wang H-L, Milone M, et al: Congenital myasthenic syndrome caused by decreased agonist binding affinity due to a mutation in the acetylcholine receptor ε subunit. Neuron 1996;17:157–170.
Oosterhuis JGH, Newsom-Davis J, Wokke JHJ, et al: The slow channel syndrome: Two new cases. Brain 1987;110:1061–1079.
Robertson WC, Chun RWM, Kornguth SE: Familial infantile myasthenia. Arch Neurol 1980;37:117–119.
Wall TJ, Engel AG, Nagel AS, et al: Congenital myasthenic syndrome associated with paucity of synaptic vesicles and reduced quantal release. Ann N Y Acad Sci 1993;681:461–468.
Wang H-L, Milone M, Ohno K, et al: Acetylcholine receptor M3 domain: Stereochemical and volume contributions to channel gating. Nat Neurosci 1998;2:226–233.

Infantile Botulism and Other Acquired Neuromuscular Junction Disorders of Infancy and Childhood

H. Royden Jones, Jr.

INFANTILE BOTULISM
  Clinical Picture
  Electrodiagnosis
  Summary
NEONATAL MAGNESIUM TOXICITY RELATED TO
MATERNAL TREATMENT OF ECLAMPSIA

ACQUIRED POSTSYNAPTIC NEUROMUSCULAR
TRANSMISSION DISORDERS
  Acquired Neonatal Myasthenia Gravis
  Juvenile Autoimmune Myasthenia Gravis

A group of very interesting and relatively uncommon to very rare disorders of the neuromuscular junction occur in infants and children (Table 94–1). Juvenile onset myasthenia gravis is by far the most common of these entities. The adult version of the illness is covered elsewhere. Infantile botulism is an illness unique to infants and is the primary emphasis of this chapter. This is a potentially life-threatening illness that depends on early electromyographic evaluation to make the diagnosis. In addition, this chapter discusses neonatal autoimmune neonatal myasthenia gravis with brief commentaries made about some other nongenetic neuromuscular transmission disorders that are primarily identified during the neonatal period. These are mainly pharmacological intoxications such as hypermagnesemia and

antibiotic effects. The exceedingly rare various congenital neuromuscular transmission disorders are carefully described in Chapter 93.

INFANTILE BOTULISM

Pickett and associates (1976) originally described infantile botulism as one of the distinct causes for the very unusual occurrence of an acute onset of severe hypotonia in a previously healthy infant. Each of the infants seen by the authors was normal at birth. Motor milestone development had proceeded as anticipated, with the acquisition of normal skills, such as holding up the head, rolling over in the crib, and more purposeful use of the hands. Suddenly, over just a few days, difficulty in feeding with inability to suck strongly and constipation ensued. The cry became weak, head control was lost, and a variable degree of generalized hypotonia developed. When a previously healthy baby develops an acute floppy infant syndrome (David and Jones, 1994) or is admitted with a diagnosis of sepsis, respiratory distress, possible encephalitis, dehydration, or failure to thrive, often with associated constipation, the possibility of infantile botulism must be kept high on the differential diagnosis.

Usually, these infants are younger than 6 months, although we diagnosed this illness in a 10-month-old child at the Children's Hospital of Boston. Very rarely, the typical picture of infantile botulism occurs in an adult patient in the intensive care unit (Ly et al., 1999), where the gut flora may be changed by the use of various medications, including antibiotics. Infantile botulism is more common within certain geographical settings; in the United States,

---

Table 94–1. Neuromuscular Junction Disorders

Presynaptic defects
  Infantile botulism
  Toxic
    Hypermagnesemia (therapy for eclampsia)
    Aminoglycoside antibiotics
  Congenital*
    Familial myasthenia gravis
    Acetylcholine vesicle paucity
    Acetylcholine quantal release diminished
    Miscellaneous poorly categorized
Postsynaptic defects
  Myasthenia gravis
  Maternal autoimmune (antibody positive)
  Congenital (antibody negative)*
    Acetylcholine receptor deficiency
    Acetylcholinesterase deficiencies
    Classic slow channel syndrome

*See Chapter 93.

---

these include the Philadelphia/Baltimore area, the Rocky Mountain States, and California. Eleven of 50 floppy infants (22%) seen at the Children's Hospital of Philadelphia (Packer et al., 1982) had infantile botulism. In contrast, at the Children's Hospital of Boston, we have documented only five instances of infantile botulism during an electromyographic experience that includes more than 2800 children seen between 1979 and 2001. Two of these infants had traveled outside of New England just a few weeks before the onset of their acute illness—one to Louisiana and the other was visiting from Montana. A large series of floppy infants evaluated in Iowa included no cases of infantile botulism (Russell et al., 1992). Similarly, colleagues from the Mayo Clinic in Minnesota (C. M. Harper, personal communications) and the University of Western Ontario (C. F. Bolton, personal communications) have not seen any cases of this illness. This suggests that *Clostridium botulinum* spores do not survive or are at least significantly impeded in their growth by the very cold climates of upper North America. European colleagues have also not seen this illness (Olofsson K, Pitt M, Renault M, personal communication, 1999).

Infantile botulism results from the ingestion of *C. botulinum* spores. This is a sometimes ubiquitous, gram-positive anaerobe (Muensterer, 2000). The bacterium is found in soil, agricultural products, and sometimes even household dust. These organisms have the propensity to grow very well in the confines of the human gastrointestinal tract, particularly in children younger than 6 months. At this age, the composition of the intestinal flora may be varied compared with that of adults (Muensterer, 2000). The spores per se will multiply within the child's gut, wherein the potentially deadly botulinum toxin is then produced. This contrasts with the adult variant of botulism, in which ingestion of the toxin occurs from already spoiled and contaminated foods, particularly canned meats, fish, and vegetables that permit the development of the toxin in their anaerobic environs. The spores of *C. botulinum* grow at this young age but in general not later in life (Muensterer, 2000). Early on, the ability to culture this organism from honey suggested a potential source for some cases or outbreaks of infantile botulism (Pickett et al., 1976). The spores of *C. botulinum* are more heat resistant than its toxin and may be resistant to even a few hours of boiling (Muensterer, 2000). Therefore, processed honey may host these spores. However, further epidemiological studies demonstrated that *C. botulinum* spores were found in only 10% of 90 samples of honey (Arnon et al., 1979); it is thought that only 15% to 30% of all infantile botulism cases are related to ingested honey (Muensterer, 2000). Other sources for infantile botulism have not been well defined, in particular because no spores have been found in either human or canned milk, commercial formulas, fruit juices, or baby foods (Muensterer, 2000).

Clinical Picture

Severe quadriparesis and respiratory failure often develop rapidly in some infants, as occurred in one infant who was transferred to our hospital for intensive care after an initial diagnosis of indeterminate acute respiratory distress (Pickett et al., 1976; Clay et al., 1977). The clinical onset may be quite precipitous. One 2-week-old infant developed respiratory arrest with just 5 hours of prodromal symptoms (Hoffman et al., 1982). The prolonged subsequent course may have been potentiated by the concomitant administration of aminoglycoside antibiotics, which are known to have a deleterious effect on acetylcholine release at the neuromuscular junction (Schwartz and Eng, 1982).

Rarely, children with infantile botulism may experience a relapse, as was noted in 3 of 63 children seen at Children's Hospital of Philadelphia (Glauser et al., 1989). These three infants, as well as another infant (Ravid et al., 2000), seemingly had recovered after an average 30-day hospitalization when, at 6 to 13 days after discharge, symptoms of infantile botulism returned. The course of the relapse was severe enough to require mechanical ventilatory support in two infants (Glauser et al., 1989). No factor predisposing to relapse could be identified (Glauser et al., 1989). In other infants, infantile botulism may be a relatively mild illness that does not require hospitalization.

The neurological examination of infants with infantile botulism is rather characteristic. Typically, these children have diffuse hypotonia, with ptosis, and occasionally enlarged, sluggishly reactive pupils. In addition, they frequently are observed by their mothers to have lost their previously vigorous suck. Concomitantly, they often have a decreased gag reflex, dysphagia, and weak cry (Thompson et al., 1980). In only 1 of 12 infants were the muscle stretch reflexes not demonstrable (Thompson et al., 1980). However, later in the clinical course, they can become progressively hypoactive. Ventilatory support was necessary in six of nine hospitalized infants within 2 to 34 days of onset (Thompson et al., 1980). It is important to be aware of the potential for aminoglycoside antibiotics to produce acute respiratory distress, particularly when evaluating a child not yet suspected of having infantile botulism (Thompson et al., 1980; Schwartz and Eng, 1982). One study noted that three infants initially thought to have infantile sepsis and treated with antibiotics were later diagnosed with botulism. One of these infants sustained a respiratory arrest subsequent to being treated with antibiotics (Thompson et al., 1980).

The clinical diagnosis of infantile botulism primarily occurs in 3- to 6-month-old infants, but this disorder must be considered in infants as young as 10 days (Donley et al., 1991; Shukla et al., 1991), as well as late in their first year of life; we made this diagnosis in a 10-month-old child. Three infants with onset during the first 2 to 3 weeks had a classic and fulminating presentation with acute hypotonia (Shukla et al., 1991). In each infant, respiratory difficulties developed and led to respiratory arrest in two. The electromyographic results in each of these three infants were diagnostic, meeting the criteria of Cornblath and colleagues (1983). An edrophonium (Tensilon; ICN Pharmaceuticals Inc., Costa Mesa, Calif) test was also positive in one of these neonates (Donley et al., 1991). A positive edrophonium test result does not provide differentiation between infantile botulism and some of the congenital myasthenic syndromes (Harper, 2001); however, the clinical history is only acute with infantile botulism. A stool toxin evaluation for one of the specific botulinum toxins is the most definitive diagnostic study available. Unfortunately, these techniques do not provide a rapid means of diagnosis, so electromyography (EMG) continues to provide the most reliable clinical means to achieve an early diagnosis.

Electrodiagnosis

For any previously healthy infant in whom, during the first year of life, diffuse weakness, a feeble cry, difficulty feeding, associated constipation, and occasionally respiratory distress develop, EMG must be performed with particular attention to signs of a neuromuscular transmission defect. This test must include repetitive motor nerve stimulation. Almost all infants with infantile botulism have low-amplitude compound muscle action potentials with preserved motor conduction velocities (MCVs), distal latencies, and sensory nerve action potentials (Cornblath et al., 1983; Gutierrez et al., 1994). It is distinctly unlikely for an infant with infantile botulism, especially those who are seriously ill, to have normal compound muscle action potential amplitudes (Gutierrez et al., 1994). Normal infantile compound muscle action potentials range between 1.6 and 3.5 mV for the various motor nerves.

Repetitive motor nerve stimulation is crucial to an accurate and early diagnosis of the presynaptic neuromuscular transmission disorder typical of infantile botulism. The response to low-frequency (2- to 5-Hz) stimulation produces varying changes. A decremental response was present in 14 of 25 infants (56%) (Cornblath et al., 1983). The most important finding in this seminal infantile botulism EMG study of Cornblath and colleagues (1983) was a significant incremental response to stimulation rates of 20 to 50 Hz. This occurred in 23 of 25 infants (92%). The degree of increment ranged from 23% to 313%, with a mean of 73%. This increment was achieved with 20-Hz stimulation in 19 of 23 babies. However, 50-Hz stimulation was required to document the presence of an increment in the other four infants.

A distinct feature of both infantile and adult botulism is a prolonged period of post-tetanic facilitation with a concomitant absence of post-tetanic exhaustion (Fakadej and Gutmann, 1982; Sheth et al., 1999). For example, one 3-month-old child with infantile botulism had a 21-minute post-tetanic facilitation after 10 seconds of "exercise" (Sheth et al., 1999). In contrast to adults, in whom a "tetanic" state can be achieved with 10 seconds of brief exercise, it is suggested that 10 seconds of 50-Hz tetanic stimulation is the only suitable technique to define the classic post-tetanic facilitation of infantile botulism (Gutierrez et al., 1994). This is technically accomplished by stimulating the ulnar or median nerves (or both) at the elbow, avoiding shock artifacts. Surface electrodes can be used if the arm is carefully immobilized. Because this technique is painful, it is best to obtain anesthesiological support during this procedure. A tetanic facilitation of greater than 120% is abnormal for infants (Gutierrez et al., 1994). Pseudofacilitation will not produce a response of this size.

Stimulation single-fiber EMG is another technique reported to be helpful in making the diagnosis of infantile botulism. Four infants with classic clinical and repetitive motor nerve stimulation findings were studied with the use of a single fiber in an intrinsic hand muscle (Chaudhry and Crawford, 1999). Each study demonstrated improvement in jitter rates with sequentially higher rates of stimulation. The issue yet to be studied is whether stimulation single-fiber EMG will help to diagnose those occasional infants in whom standard repetitive motor nerve stimulation results are negative (Sheth et al., 1999).

Abnormal spontaneous activity with fibrillation potentials and positive waves compatible with a functional form of denervation secondary to impaired acetylcholine quanta release was noted with needle EMG in 13 of 24 infants (54%) (Cornblath et al., 1983). Short-duration, low-amplitude motor unit potentials were found in 22 of 24 infants (90%) (Cornblath et al., 1983). To provide a logical and practical guide to the electromyographic study of infants with acute hypotonia, Gutierrez and associates (1994) proposed a protocol for evaluation and specific diagnostic requirements for definition of the presynaptic neuromuscular transmission disorder of infantile botulism (Table 94–2).

Summary

Infantile botulism has a fairly stereotypical clinical presentation characterized by an acute onset of hypotonia, poor feeding, and constipation in a previously healthy infant. The eventual severity of this illness and the rapidity of progression vary. Some infants have a relatively benign course, whereas others require rapid intubation with prolonged hospitalization because of the need for respiratory support. The differential diagnosis includes other acute disorders of the motor unit, as well as nonspecific respiratory distress, sepsis, and even an encephalopathy, as outlined in Chapter 86.

Consequently, during the ages of 0 to 6 months, and very rarely through the age of 1 year, pediatric electromyographers are occasionally asked to evalu-

Table 94–2. Electromyographic Protocol for Suspected Presynaptic Neuromuscular Transmission Defects of Infantile Botulism

Protocol to evaluate suspected infantile botulism
1. Motor/sensory nerve conduction studies in one arm and leg
2. Repetitive motor nerve stimulation at 2 cm/s to two distal muscles
3. Tetanizing stimulation at 50 cm/s for 10 s followed by stimulation every 30 s until compound muscle action potential is baseline
4. Stimulated single-fiber electromyography*

Primary diagnostic features for infantile botulism
1. Compound muscle action potentials <2.0 mV in at least two muscles
2. Post-tetanic facilitation > 120% of baseline
3. Post-tetanic facilitation prolonged >120 s with no post-tetanic exhaustion

Adapted from Gutierrez AR, Bodensteiner J, Gutmann L: Electrodiagnosis of infantile botulism. J Child Neurol 1994; 9:362–365.

*Adapted from Chaudhry V, Crawford TO: Stimulation single-fiber EMG in infant botulism. Muscle Nerve 1999; 1698–1703.

ate an infant with acute hypotonia in whom the possibility of an infantile botulism diagnosis always must be considered. Repetitive motor nerve stimulation as well as routine needle conduction studies and needle EMG are often very useful for identifying and localizing the site of motor unit involvement (see Table 94–2). Children with infantile botulism may have a relatively modest degree of facilitation with repetitive motor nerve stimulation and not the 100% plus that is so typical for the other clinically relevant presynaptic neuromuscular transmission disorder—Lambert-Eaton myasthenic syndrome. The last four infants we evaluated with confirmed infantile botulism had only a moderate degree of facilitation, ranging between just 23% to 65%.

NEONATAL MAGNESIUM TOXICITY RELATED TO MATERNAL TREATMENT OF ECLAMPSIA

Another very rare form of a presynaptic infantile neuromuscular transmission disorder may occur in infants who are observed to be hypotonic immediately after delivery from eclamptic mothers who had been treated with magnesium sulfate (Lipsitz, 1971; Sokal et al., 1972). However, during my 22-year affiliation with the Children's Hospital of Boston, we have not been asked to perform EMG in such circumstances. A newborn with neonatal hypermagnesemia, reported in 1972, had *myoneurodepression* (a term no longer used) with potentiation greater than normal (Sokal et al., 1972). Hypermagnesemia-related infantile hypotonia is a relatively short-lived process, so EMG is not necessary to differentiate this process from other mechanisms for a floppy neonate. One study of hypermagnesemia in adults demonstrated a prolonged post-tetanic facilitation that lasted several minutes, not unlike infantile botulism (Swift, 1979).

ACQUIRED POSTSYNAPTIC NEUROMUSCULAR TRANSMISSION DISORDERS

Acquired Neonatal Myasthenia Gravis

Autoimmune myasthenia gravis occurs in two primary settings during childhood. During infancy, acquired neonatal myasthenia gravis is the only noncongenital form of a postsynaptic neuromuscular transmission disorder. The very rare postsynaptic categories of congenital structural or biochemical defects in the acetylcholine receptor end-plates are carefully discussed in Chapter 93 (Harper, 2001). Although acquired neonatal myasthenia gravis is the most common cause for a postsynaptic neuromuscular transmission disorder in a newborn, because this diagnosis is self-evident, we have not been asked to study these children in the pediatric EMG laboratory.

Autoimmune neonatal myasthenia gravis is a transitory illness secondary to the transfer of maternal acetylcholine receptor antibodies across the placenta, producing rapidly increasing weakness shortly after birth (Lefvert and Osterman, 1983; Morel et al., 1988; Papazian, 1992; Gardnerova et al., 1997). The diagnosis is obvious when the mother reports a past history of myasthenia gravis. This condition develops in 10% to 20% of infants whose mothers have myasthenia gravis (Papazian, 1992). The risk of the development of neonatal myasthenia gravis in a subsequent sibling of an infant with clinical acquired neonatal myasthenia gravis is twice that of the first-born of a mother with autoimmune myasthenia gravis (Morel et al., 1988). In most infants with acquired neonatal myasthenia gravis, the presence of acetylcholine receptor antibodies can be documented. Of the 17 infants born to 15 mothers with myasthenia gravis, only 2 had clinical acquired neonatal myasthenia gravis (Lefvert and Osterman, 1983). However, 16 of the 17 infants had acetylcholine receptor antibodies present at birth (Lefvert and Osterman, 1983). The mother of the one acetylcholine receptor antibody–negative infant was also antibody negative.

The typical symptoms of acquired neonatal myasthenia gravis develop within the first 3 days of life or never appear (Papazian, 1992). These infants have clinical features that are indistinguishable from those of the congenital neuromuscular transmission disorders of infancy (Harper, 2001). These features include generalized hypotonia, feeble cry, bilateral facial paresis, poor suck, and impaired swallowing with resultant difficulty feeding.

On rare occasions, acquired neonatal myasthenia gravis may be associated with arthrogryposis, severe hypotonia, and polyhydramnios, all indicative of a long-standing prenatal evolution (Holmes et al., 1980). Although most infants with acquired neonatal myasthenia gravis recover in 1 to 7 weeks, the course may be more prolonged, with some infants not totally improving for 1 year (Branch et al., 1978; Morel et al., 1988).

The clinical diagnosis of acquired neonatal myasthenia gravis is made on the basis of the combination of the maternal history, typical clinical findings, elevated levels of acetylcholine receptor antibodies in both mother and infant, and a positive response to anticholinesterase medications.

Two drugs are primarily used. Edrophonium chloride is administered either intramuscularly or subcutaneously at 0.04 to 0.15 mg/kg or intravenously at 0.1 mg/kg (Wise and McQuillen, 1970; Papazian, 1992). When larger doses of edrophonium chloride are administered to infants with acquired neonatal myasthenia gravis, cardiac arrhythmias and respiratory arrest have been rarely noted (Fenichel, 1978; Papazian, 1992). Edrophonium has the advantage of rapid action with improvement onset in 3 to 5 minutes and a 10- to 15-minute duration of action. The muscarinic side effects are relatively minimal. Neostigmine methylsulfate may also be administered either intramuscularly or subcutaneously. It has a 10- to 15-minute delay in action but provides a longer period of symptomatic relief than does edrophonium, usually lasting 1 to 3 hours. However, muscarinic side effects are more prevalent than with edrophonium (Papazian, 1992). In particular, neostigmine may promote a marked increase in tracheal secretions in some infants. False-negative results may occur with either edrophonium or neostigmine; therefore, negative pharmacological results do not exclude acquired neonatal myasthenia gravis (Koenigsberger et al., 1973; Papazian, 1992).

Except perhaps in the infant and mother who are antibody negative, there is little need for EMG to diagnose acquired neonatal myasthenia gravis. There is sparse literature in reference to repetitive motor nerve stimulation in infants with acquired neonatal myasthenia gravis. One infant had a 54% decrement at 50 Hz, and the clinically unaffected sibling had none (Wise and McQuillen, 1970). A control study of three infants born to mothers without myasthenia gravis demonstrated no neuromuscular transmission disorder with 3-Hz stimulation for 10 seconds and at 10 and 50 Hz for 5 seconds (Wise and McQuillen, 1970). These results in a few normal control infants contrasted with another study that used more prolonged periods of repetitive motor nerve stimulation to demonstrate a significant decrement in normal infants with 15-second stimulation (Koenigsberger et al., 1973).

There is one report that describes the successful use of EMG with 3-Hz repetitive motor nerve stimulation in a 10-day-old male infant born to a mother with antibody-negative myasthenia gravis. Her illness had commenced early in this pregnancy (Hays and Michaud, 1988). At birth, the infant was hypotonic with a bell-shaped chest and hypoactive muscle stretch reflexes. Intubation was required because of respiratory distress. When he did not respond to either intramuscular or intravenous edrophonium

on the second day of life, the physicians considered other diagnostic possibilities. When he was 10 days old, EMG documented a 20% neuromuscular transmission defect. A trial of pyridostigmine was initially unsuccessful. EMG was repeated, confirming a 23% neuromuscular transmission decrement. When edrophonium was subsequently administered intravenously at 0.15 mg/kg versus the initial 0.1 mg/kg dose, there was a complete repair of the electromyographic decrement. Subsequent to this, the dose of pyridostigmine was further increased. The electromyographic results provided the physicians with a margin of further therapeutic safety that, when the medication was further increased, permitted withdrawal of the respirator (Hays and Michaud, 1988).

In summary, this single case points to the value of EMG in the diagnosis and management of infants with acquired neonatal myasthenia gravis. The repetitive motor nerve stimulation provided diagnostic confirmation of the neuromuscular transmission disorder seen in neonatal myasthenia gravis. In addition, EMG allowed precise quantification of the need for an increased dose of anticholinesterase agents. The clinician must also appreciate that the customary clinical parameters that are so important in evaluating and monitoring the older child and adult, such as ptosis and other cranial nerve signs, are not as apparent in the neonate with myasthenia gravis. Therefore, repetitive motor nerve stimulation sometimes provides a more accurate and reproducible means to diagnose and monitor the effects of therapy in infants with neonatal myasthenia gravis (Hays and Michaud, 1988).

Mechanical ventilation support was necessary in 7 of 14 infants in one major study (Morel et al., 1988). Anticholinesterase medications are usually effective therapy (Papazian, 1992). There have been attempts to ascertain the potential value of intravenous immunoglobulin in two infants with acquired neonatal myasthenia gravis who had not responded to traditional anticholinesterase therapy and were dependent on a respirator. In the first instance, there was a suggestion that this treatment may have been effective (Bassan et al., 1998; Bassan and Spirer, 1999). In the second infant, however, intravenous immunoglobulin had no beneficial response until the infant received a double-volume exchange transfusion 5 days after the completion of 5 days of daily intravenous immunoglobulin (Tagher et al., 1999).

Juvenile Autoimmune Myasthenia Gravis

In general, when immune-mediated myasthenia gravis develops in toddlers and older children, it is very similar to the illness seen in adult patients (Seybold and Lindstrom, 1981; Rodriguez et al., 1983; Andrews, 1998; Seybold, 1998; Mullaney et al., 2000). Occasionally, an issue arises as to whether the child has congenital or autoimmune myasthenia gravis. This diagnostic challenge is accelerated some with the finding that the rate of antibody positivity is lower in children than in adults. However, the study must be sent to a well-respected laboratory. We have had the experience of receiving a negative report from the commercial laboratory only to have workers at the laboratory of Dr. Vanda Lennon at the Mayo Clinic return consistently positive results. We now routinely send all our studies to her group. When there remains a question regarding the diagnosis, we proceed with standard EMG, including repetitive motor nerve stimulation. In young children, we usually perform this in the day surgery center with the child under anesthetic sedation.

More than half of the children with juvenile myasthenia gravis have ocular symptoms (Mullaney et al., 2000). No thymomas were found in 14 consecutive patients undergoing therapeutic thymectomy (Mullaney et al., 2000). A variety of treatment options are used (Andrews, 1998; Seybold, 1998). One issue we confronted was the advisability of performing a thymectomy on a 15-month-old child with autoimmune juvenile myasthenia gravis. The overall experience suggests that this can be safely carried out with no long-term immune consequences (Seybold, 1998).

References

Andrews PI: A treatment algorithm for autoimmune myasthenia gravis. Ann N Y Acad Sci 1998;841:789–802.

Arnon SS, Midura TF, Damus K, et al: Honey and other environmental risk factors for infant botulism. J Pediatr 1979;94:331–336.

Bassan H, Muhlbaur B, Tomer A, Spirer Z: High-dose intravenous immunoglobulin in transient neonatal myasthenia gravis. Pediatr Neurol 1998;18:181–183.

Bassan H, Spirer Z: Intravenous immunoglobulin in neonatal myasthenia gravis. J Pediatr 1999;135:790.

Branch CE Jr, Swift TR, Dyken PR: Prolonged neonatal myasthenia gravis: Electrophysiological studies. Ann Neurol 1978;3:416–418.

Chaudhry V Crawford TO: Stimulation single-fiber EMG in infant botulism. Muscle Nerve 1999;22:1698–1703.

Clay SA, Ramseyer JC, Fishman LS, Sedgwick RP: Acute infantile motor unit disorder: Infantile botulism? Arch Neurol 1977;34:236–249.

Cornblath DR, Sladky JT, Sumner AJ: Clinical electrophysiology of infantile botulism. Muscle Nerve 1983;6:448–452.

David WS, Jones HR: Electromyography and biopsy correlation with suggested protocol for evaluation of the floppy infant. Muscle Nerve 1994;17:424–430.

Donley DK, Knight P, Tenorio G, Oh SJ: A patient with infant botulism, improving with edrophonium. Muscle Nerve 1991;41:201.

Fakadej AV, Gutmann L: Prolongation of post-tetanic facilitation in infant botulism. Muscle Nerve 1982;5:727–729.

Fenichel GM: Clinical syndromes of myasthenia gravis in infancy and childhood. Arch Neurol 1978;35:97–103.

Gardnerova M, Eymard B, Morel E, et al: The fetal/adult acetylcholine receptor antibody ratio in mothers with myasthenia gravis as a marker for transfer of the disease to the newborn. Neurology 1997;48:50–54.

Glauser TA, Maguire HC, Sladky JT: Relapse of infantile botulism. Ann Neurol 1989;26:449.

Gutierrez AR, Bodensteiner J, Gutmann L: Electrodiagnosis of infantile botulism. J Child Neurol 1994;9:362–365.

Harper CM: Congenital neuromuscular transmission defects. In Brown W, Bolton CF, Aminoff M (eds): Clinical Electromyography. Philadelphia, WB Saunders, 2001.

Hays RM, Michaud LJ: Neonatal myasthenia gravis: Specific advantages of repetitive stimulation over edrolphonium testing. Pediatr Neurol 1988;4:245–247.

Hoffman RE, Pincomb BJ, Skeels MR: Type F infant botulism. Am J Dis Child 1982;136:270–271.

Holmes LB, Driscoll SG, Bradley WG: Contractures in a newborn infant of a mother with myasthenia gravis. J Pediatr 1980;96:1067–1069.

Koenigsberger MR, Patten B, Lovelace RE: Studies of neuromuscular function in the newborn: 1. A comparison of myoneural function in the full term and premature infant. Neuropediatrics 1973;4:350–361.

Lefvert AK, Osterman PO: Newborn infants to myasthenic mothers: A clinical study and an investigation of acetylcholine receptor antibodies in 17 children. Neurology 1983;33:133–138.

Lipsitz PJ: The clinical and biochemical effects of excess magnesium in the newborn. Pediatrics 1971;47:501–509.

Ly L, Kelkar P, Exconde RE, et al: Adult-onset "infant" botulism: An unusual cause of weakness in the intensive care unit. Neurology 1999;53:891.

Morel E, Eymard B, Vernet-der Garabedian B, et al: Neonatal myasthenia gravis: A new clinical and immunologic appraisal of 30 cases. Neurology 1988;38:138–142.

Muensterer OJ: Infantile botulism. Pediatr Rev 2000;21:427.

Mullaney P, Vajsar J, Smith R, Buncic JR: The natural history and ophthalmic involvement in childhood myasthenia gravis at the Hospital for Sick Children. Ophthalmology 2000;107:504–510.

Packer RJ, Brown MJ, Berman PH: The diagnostic value of electromyography in infantile hypotonia. Am J Dis Child 1982;136:1057–1059.

Papazian O: Transient neonatal myasthenia gravis. J Child Neurol 1992;7:135–141.

Pickett J, Berg B, Chaplin E, Brunstetter-Shafer M-A: Syndrome of botulism in infancy: Clinical and electrophysiologic study. N Engl J Med 1976;295:770–772.

Ravid S, Maytal J, Eviatar L: Biphasic course of infantile botulism. Pediatr Neurol 2000;23:338–339.

Rodriguez M, Gomez MR, Howard FM, Taylor WF: Myasthenia gravis in children: Long-term follow-up. Ann Neurol 1983;13:504–510.

Russell JW, Afifi AK, Ross MA: Predictive value of electromyography in diagnosis and prognosis of the hypotonic infant. J Child Neurol 1992;7:387–391.

Schwartz RH, Eng G: Infant botulism: Exacerbation by aminoglycosides. Am J Dis Child 1982;136:952.

Seybold M: Thymectomy in childhood myasthenia gravis. Ann N Y Acad Sci 1998;841:733–741.

Seybold ME, Lindstrom JM: Myasthenia gravis in infancy. Neurology 1981;31:476–480.

Sheth RD, Lotz BP, Hecox KE, Waclawik AJ: Infantile botulism: Pitfalls in diagnosis. J Child Neurol 1999;14-156–158.

Shukla AY, Marsh W, Green JB, Hurst D: Neonatal botulism [abstract]. Neurology 1991;41(Suppl 1):202.

Sokal MM, Koenigsberger MR, Rose JS, et al: Neonatal hypermagnesemia and the meconium-plug syndrome. N Engl J Med 1972;286:823–825.

Swift TR: Weakness from magnesium-containing cathartics: Electrophysiologic studies. Muscle Nerve 1979;2:295–298.

Tagher RJ, Baumann R, Desai N: Failure of intravenously administered immunoglobulin in the treatment of neonatal myasthenia gravis. J Pediatr 1999;134:233–235.

Thompson JA, Glasgow LA, Warpinski JR, Olson C: Infant botulism: Clinical spectrum and epidemiology. Pediatrics 1980;66:936–942.

Wise GA, McQuillen MP: Transient neonatal myasthenia: Clinical and electromyographic studies. Arch Neurol 1970;22:556–565.

Myopathies and Arthrogryposis Multiplex Congenita

Basil T. Darras and H. Royden Jones, Jr.

INTRODUCTION

The term *myopathy* covers the entire spectrum of diseases of muscle and implies that the disorder is, in fact, a disease of muscle and does not involve the central nervous system or other portions of the peripheral motor unit, including the anterior horn cell, peripheral nerve, or neuromuscular junction. An infant with myopathy typically presents with generalized hypotonia, with or without suppression of muscle stretch reflexes, and sometimes with associated arthrogryposis multiplex congenita. Older children can present in a more varied fashion with proximal, distal, generalized, or focal weakness, fatigability, periodic paralysis, myotonia, intermittent weakness with or without muscle aches, or myoglobinuria.

The spectrum of electromyography (EMG) findings in a myopathy are outlined in Tables 95–1 and 95–2. The most important needle EMG finding in children with a myopathy is the presence of many low-amplitude, short-duration, sometimes polyphasic motor unit potentials recruited in increased numbers with relatively minimal effort. In contrast to the high level of accuracy of EMG in the evaluation of lesions at the level of the motor neuron and peripheral nerve in children, EMG is not as sensitive in defining subtle myopathies, particularly the many types of congenital myopathies. In many of these instances, there is no overt destruction of muscle fibers per se, as typically seen in inflammatory myopathy or severe muscular dystrophy.

A *motor unit potential* represents the summated electrical activity generated from all muscle fibers innervated by the terminal branches of a single α motor neuron. Individual motor units may contain from less than 10 to several thousand muscle fibers

---

Table 95–1. Nerve Conduction Study Findings in Myopathy

Normal sensory nerve conduction studies
Normal or low-amplitude CMAP
Normal CMAP duration without temporal dispersion
Normal conduction velocities and distal latencies
Normal late reflexes, including H reflex and F wave
No repetitive CMAP with single stimulus
Little or no decrement of CMAP with low rates of repetitive stimulation
No facilitation or decrement of CMAP with rapid rates of repetitive stimulation

CMAP, compound muscle action potential.

Table 95–2. Motor Unit Potential Changes in Myopathy

Finding	Mechanism
Short-duration, low-amplitude MUP	Fewer muscle fibers per MUP
Increased proportion of polyphasic MUP (>4 phases) or satellite potentials	Spatial dispersion of end-plates, changes in fiber diameter (mm), changes in length and diameter of nerve terminal, loss of individual components causing loss of fusion of MUP, increased fiber density, fiber splitting
Long duration ± high amplitude	Increased fiber density with firing MUP synchrony maintained (some chronic myopathies), associated neuropathy
MUP amplitude variation	Intermittent blocking of conduction in nerve terminal, neuromuscular junction, or muscle fiber
Early rapid recruitment	Lower capacity for force generation per motor unit
Reduced recruitment	Severe myopathy with destruction of motor units

MUP, motor unit potential.

(Feinsstein et al., 1955). Our standard method for recording motor unit potentials involves the use of an intramuscular concentric needle electrode during voluntary or reflex muscle contraction. Motor unit potentials are characterized by their amplitude, duration, number of phases or complexity, and firing rate in relation to force or recruitment of other motor units (Daube, 1979). With the recording electrode at a fixed distance from the motor unit, the size and shape of the motor unit potential depend on many factors. These include the number, size, density, conduction velocity, and synchrony of muscle fibers firing within the recording area of the electrode. Other important contributors to the final electric signal include the conductivity characteristics of the intervening tissue, the recording electrode, and the recording equipment (Daube, 1978).

Normal motor unit potentials are triphasic and have a recruitment frequency of 5 to 15 Hz. When they are recorded in a standard fashion with minimal voluntary activation, the duration and amplitude of motor unit potentials in neurologically normal persons vary with the muscle tested and with the age of the subject (Sacco et al., 1962). Normal values for motor unit potential duration and amplitude have been well established in 2- to 3-year intervals from birth to adulthood (Feinsstein et al., 1955). Infants typically have motor unit potentials that are often biphasic, having an average duration of 1 to 4 ms and an amplitude of 100 to 800 μV (do Carmo, 1960). In adults, normal motor unit potentials have two to four phases, with amplitudes ranging from 100 μV to 5 mV and durations from 3 to 15 ms. At any age, 10% to 15% of motor unit potentials in a healthy muscle are beyond the normal range for amplitude, duration, and number of phases. In most

infants, the muscles evaluated are superficial, and some are easy to activate by tactile or reflex stimulation. Slight contraction of the muscle initially activates type I muscle fibers. Larger motor unit potentials are recruited when initial motor unit potentials fire between 5 and 10 Hz. Rapid recruitment of many individual motor unit potentials occurs when the child activates large numbers of motor unit potentials during relatively minimal voluntary contraction of the affected muscle. This typically occurs in myopathies because individual portions of the muscle fibers within each motor unit are lost (Daube, 1979). Concomitant motor nerve conduction studies usually demonstrate low- to normal-amplitude compound muscle action potentials with normal conduction velocities and distal latencies. All sensory conduction parameters are also normal.

PRACTICAL CONSIDERATIONS

The performance of needle EMG examination creates increasing anxiety and consequent diminished levels of cooperation in most young children. However, careful and accurate examination can usually be accomplished, provided the electromyographer appreciates the limits of his or her technical abilities, especially with infants and toddlers.

One of the best ways to gain the cooperation of a child is to try to make the study fun by asking the child what the motor units sound like. This is often a rewarding maneuver because children frequently become interested in the noise their muscles produce. Responses frequently given include rain on the roof, thunder, motorcycles, or even the putt-putt of a lobster boat. Commenting on the noise produced, we ask how the child is able to sleep at night with all the noise the muscles are making. This often produces a laugh or at least distracts the child's attention from the electrode.

Toddlers or even most children 3 to 4 years old usually are unable to appreciate this type of approach. Therefore, one has to engage the parents so they understand the precise aim as well as the reasonable time limits of this study. We make it clear that we will stop the EMG whenever it is apparent that the child is not consolable. Additionally, we emphasize that although the pediatric electromyographer is empathetic with the child's discomfort, the study is best completed in an expeditious fashion. It is important that the initial interactions with the child and the parents allay their own anxieties as much as possible. Furthermore, parents need to recognize that the pediatric electromyographer is a compassionate and concerned physician. Finally, the pediatric electromyographer needs to have a preconceived plan regarding the precise question each EMG is designed to answer. Only then can one proceed expeditiously without unnecessary testing or delay.

With this approach in mind, the electromyographer has to tailor the number of muscles examined.

Compared with adults, this part of the EMG examination may need to be limited in children. However, whenever possible, the pediatric electromyographer needs to design an examination that addresses the clinician's concerns. Because infants do not cooperate, it is usually not possible to observe individual motor units in isolation, with the exception of a severe neurogenic process, such as spinal muscular atrophy type I, in which there are only a few remaining motor unit potentials. For this and other reasons, as detailed in Chapter 86, one has less likelihood of precisely defining the presence of a myopathic process, particularly in young children, compared with the relative ease of identification of a neurogenic process (Eng, 1992).

MOTOR UNIT MATURATIONAL FACTORS AND CHARACTERISTICS WITH A MYOPATHY

Normal motor unit potential parameters differ in the infant and young child compared with those in an adult. The histogram amplitude is shifted to the left or the lower side of adult motor unit potentials, with normal amplitudes varying between 100 and 700 μV. Motor unit potentials greater than 1,000 μV in 0- to 3-year-old infants are rare (do Carmo, 1960; Sacco et al., 1962). Infantile motor unit potentials are often shorter in duration; many are biphasic or triphasic. The recruitment pattern of infantile motor unit potentials is disordered and chaotic but on occasion similar to that of adults. Therefore, assessment of motor unit potential characteristics in young children is difficult.

When individual muscle fibers or nerve terminals within each motor unitare lost, these motor unit potentials are classically of short duration and of low amplitude, and are often polyphasic (Daube, 1979). These are usually found in the most proximal muscles. Infants with blatant infantile myopathy also often have a rapid recruitment of myopathic motor unit potentials with minimal effort; however, this classic finding is not always well appreciated in some infantile myopathies. Because of the infant's tendency to contract the iliopsoas muscle either spontaneously or on withdrawal to a subtle stimulus to the plantar surface of the foot, this muscle is one of the most useful muscles for EMG identification of myopathic motor units in our pediatric experience. This finding contrasts with the older child or adult, in whom numerous motor unit potentials from different muscles can be sampled, particularly the vastus lateralis in the leg or the triceps, biceps, or deltoid muscles in the upper extremity and sometimes the paraspinal muscles. Because of our inability to obtain relaxation successfully in the paraspinal muscles of infants, we did not previously include this set of muscles in our survey of possible signs of infantile myopathy. Noting the 10% to 50% range of positive correlation between EMG results and biopsy findings (Packer et al., 1982; Russell et al., 1992;

David and Jones, 1994), it is possible that needle examination of the paraspinal musculature in some floppy infants may enhance the diagnostic accuracy of infantile EMG.

The finding of myopathic units per se does not end the neurophysiological evaluation. One always needs to consider the possibility of a neuromuscular transmission defect in each of these infants. As an example, babies with infantile botulism often have myopathic motor unit potentials with abnormal insertional activity. Repetitive motor nerve stimulation is necessary to demonstrate the characteristic facilitatory response that leads to this rare diagnosis (Mayer and Mosser, 1969; Gutierrez et al., 1994).

GENERAL LABORATORY APPROACH

Until the mid-1980s, EMG was foremost among the three primary tools used during the initial diagnostic workup of a suspected myopathy. The laboratory investigation of a child and adult with a possible myopathy included, in sequential order: (1) serum enzymes (e.g., creatine phosphokinase, aldolase), (2) EMG and nerve conduction studies, and (3) muscle biopsy. In most instances, the EMG examination was usually performed before the patient proceeded to muscle biopsy. At that time, our knowledge of muscle pathogenesis was limited. We were aware that muscular dystrophies were genetically determined conditions and knew their modes of inheritance. Nonetheless, the precise chromosomal localization of these genetic defects and the specific genes involved were as yet unknown. These are now being identified in rapid succession. As more genes are defined with the subsequent development of a specific, clinically available DNA test, there is an ever-decreasing need for EMG in the evaluation of an infant or child suspected to have a myopathy.

In this section, we discuss the current diagnostic approach to the more common childhood myopathies. When one is unable to define a specific myopathy, the additional relevant clinical differential diagnostic considerations are reviewed, including other motor unit disorders still requiring an EMG examination for appropriate diagnosis. These include spinal muscular atrophy, chronic inflammatory demyelinating polyneuropathies, and rare disorders of the neuromuscular junction. Each one may clinically mimic a proximal myopathy. EMG still provides the best means to differentiate disorders affecting other primary regions of the motor unit. Although spinal muscular atrophy is now diagnosable by DNA testing, it may not be clinically suspected until an EMG is actually performed (Darras and Jones, 2000). Initially, we discuss the important myopathies that are seen during infancy, and thereafter we discuss those myopathies most likely occurring among toddlers and older children.

INFANTILE MYOPATHIES

Although most floppy infants have a pathophysiological mechanism at the central nervous system

Table 95–3. Neonatal Myopathies

Congenital
  Nemaline
  Centronuclear
  Central core
  Fiber-type disproportion
Dystrophies
  Congenital myotonic dystrophy
  Congenital muscular dystrophy
Inflammatory
  Polymyositis
Metabolic myopathies
  Carbohydrate metabolism defects
    Type II: acid maltase, rarely with debrancher
    Type V: muscle phosphorylase
    Type VII: phosphofructokinase
  Lipid metabolism defects
    Infantile carnitine palmitoyltransferase deficiency
    Primary systemic carnitine deficiency
    Acyl-CoA dehydrogenase deficiency
  Electron transport chain disorders
    Severe infantile myopathy
      Complex II deficiency
      Complex IV deficiency
Benign congenital hypotonia

level, another 20% of these babies have an abnormality at the peripheral motor unit level. Neonatal myopathies are one of the two most common peripheral causes of the floppy infant syndrome (Table 95–3). In our 11-year review of 80 nonarthrogrypotic floppy infants evaluated by EMG examination at the Children's Hospital of Boston (David and Jones, 1994), 41 were selected for special analysis, including 38 who underwent muscle biopsy. Myopathic processes were almost as common as the most frequent mechanism for floppy infant syndrome; 10 (24%) of these infants had a histologically and clinically confirmed myopathy versus 15 (37%) with spinal muscular atrophy (Table 95–4). Congenital myopathies, including infants with nemaline, centronuclear fiber–type disproportion, and central core disease, were the most common myopathies defined. Congenital muscular dystrophies were the next most common myopathic mechanism defined among these floppy infants (David and Jones, 1994).

The EMG study is less precise as a means of diagnosis of neonatal myopathies than it is for neurogenic lesions (David and Jones, 1994). Overall, in nonarthrogrypotic floppy infants, there was a 76% concordance between the EMG and the various other corollary studies; this concordance was almost perfect (93%) with anterior horn cell disorders. In contrast, the EMG was only compatible with the presence of myopathy in just 4 of 10 infants with histologically confirmed myopathy. This finding is comparable to that of the Philadelphia experience (Packer et al., 1982), in which four of eight infants with myopathic biopsy had EMG findings suggestive of myopathy. Another study reported that EMG predicted the clinical and biopsy diagnosis of myopathy in only 10% of floppy infants (Russell et al., 1992). We reviewed our experience with false-negative EMG studies among floppy infants whose myopathy was later diagnosed by biopsy. The EMG had initially demonstrated nonspecific changes in three infants, two of whom later were proven by biopsy to have a myopathy and one of whom had normal findings (David and Jones, 1994). Of the 11 infants with normal results on EMG who underwent biopsy, four had myopathy, and seven were normal (see Table 95–4) (David and Jones, 1994). Multiple reasons account for the finding that neonatal myopathies are not as easily diagnosed by pediatric EMG as by biopsy. First, in contrast to neurogenic processes, which produce striking and widespread changes in motor unit size and firing pattern, myopathic changes are often electrically subtle, especially in infants, in whom the normal motor unit size is considerably smaller than in an older child or an adult (do Carmo, 1960; Sacco et al., 1962). Therefore, the ability to distinguish slight motor unit potential myopathic changes from normal infantile motor units is a challenge. Additionally, another important EMG sign of a myopathic process, namely, the early recruitment of many motor unit potentials with minimal effort, is often only appreciated with the most profound infantile myopathies. Pediatric electromyographers do not have the cooperation of the infant to permit this assessment in any but the most blatant examples. Furthermore, because newborns do not consistently contract their muscles, infantile needle EMG is prone to a time sampling error.

Another possible error relates to our awareness that some infants who were initially thought on EMG to have nonspecific "neurogenic" changes characterized by occasional positive sharp waves or fibril-

Table 95–4. Results of Electromyographic Analyses of Floppy Infants and Correlation with Muscle and Nerve Biopsy

Reference	Cases (no.)	SMA	PN	NMTD	Myopathy	ND	Electromyography-Pathology Biopsy Correlation
Packer et al., 1982	51	21 (41%)	0 (0%)	11 (22%)	8 (16%)	11	64%
Russell et al., 1992	79	20 (40%)	0 (0%)	2 (4%)	27 (55%)	29	10%–90%
Cotliar et al., 1994	122	46 (43%)	19 (18%)	18 (16%)	25 (23%)	14	?
David and Jones, 1994	41	15 (37%)	3 (7%)	2 (5%)	10 (24%)	11	76% (range, 40%–93%)

ND, nondiagnostic, normal, or central hypotonia; NMTD, neuromuscular transmission defects; PN, peripheral neuropathy; SMA, spinal muscular atrophy.
Adapted from David WS, Jones HR Jr: Electromyography and biopsy correlation with suggested protocol for evaluation of the floppy infant. Muscle Nerve 1994;17:424–430.

lation potentials, when motor units could not be identified more precisely, were later identified to have a myopathic lesion by biopsy (David et al., 1991; David and Jones, 1994). Although profound fibrillation potentials are characteristically seen in spinal muscular atrophy and some congenital neuropathies, fibrillation potentials are also seen in at least nine non-neurogenic processes related to floppy infant syndrome, including eight myopathies (Table 95–5) and one neuromuscular transmission defect, that is, infantile botulism (Jones, 1990).

Evaluation of the patient's parents, especially the mother, may on occasion provide diagnostic information. This is particularly important with a floppy infant who may have some stigmata of infantile myotonic dystrophy but in whom definite myotonia is not present on the initial EMG study, as discussed later in this chapter. Therefore, when the clinical examination of a floppy infant is compatible with a peripheral motor unit defect, appropriate evaluation needs to include a muscle biopsy even when the EMG is normal or shows mild "nonspecific pseudoneurogenic" changes. The differential diagnosis of EMG myopathic findings demonstrated on evaluation of the floppy infant is broad based. Most commonly, this includes the various congenital myopathies or the dystrophies, either congenital muscular or infantile myotonic dystrophy. Rarely, we have seen an infant with an inborn error of glycogen metabolism present as a floppy baby with arthrogryposis and a myopathic EMG. Some myopathies commonly seen in the older child, such as the dystrophin deficiencies of Duchenne and Becker, and less commonly endocrine myopathies and periodic paralyses, have not been reported as a mechanism for floppy infants. We have yet to identify an instance of a floppy infant with an inflammatory myopathy; however, this uncommon entity has been implicated by other investigators in the differential diagnosis of floppy infant syndrome.

Dystrophies

CONGENITAL MUSCULAR DYSTROPHY

In our experience at the Children's Hospital of Boston (David and Jones, 1994), *congenital muscular dystrophy* is the most common myopathic cause of the floppy infant, with the exception of the diverse group of congenital myopathies. This includes those babies with or without an associated arthrogryposis. Serum creatine kinase levels are variably elevated in some infants with congenital muscular dystrophy (Lazaro et al., 1979). Motor unit potentials are of short duration and low amplitude. It is rare for abnormalities to be demonstrated on insertion, even though, in Bolton's experience (personal communication), muscle necrosis may be demonstrated pathologically. Muscle biopsy is necessary to make the precise diagnosis; immunohistochemistry with antimerosin antibodies shows no staining of the sarcolemma in a subset of patients with merosin or laminin-α_2–deficient congenital muscular dystrophy.

MYOTONIC MUSCULAR DYSTROPHY

Myotonic dystrophy is the other dystrophy that presents as floppy infant syndrome. The genetic mutation is an expanded trinucleotide repeat at chromosome 19q13.3 (Aslanidis et al., 1992; Brook et al., 1992; Harley et al., 1992). Mothers are primarily the genetic source, although an occasional report of paternal transmission has appeared (Bergoffen et al., 1994). Phenotypically, these infants are characterized by severe hypotonia, poor feeding, clubbed feet, and facial weakness associated with a characteristic "tenting" of the mouth (Harper, 1989). The family history may not have been recognized previously, and the parents, particularly the mother, may not realize that she has a subtle form of the disease. In any floppy infant, it is always important to question the mother carefully about any history of clinical myotonia or whether she may have had premature cataract surgery. The mother also may have noted diminished fetal movements, polyhydramnios, and neonatal feeding problems with respiratory distress. Neurological examination of the mother may show evidence of subtle ptosis, a typical myopathic facies, or grip or percussion myotonia sometimes requiring EMG for a precise definition. When maternal evaluation is unrewarding, paternal investigation is in order (Bergoffen et al., 1994).

Newborns with myotonic dystrophy may have two forms of this disorder (Swift et al., 1975). The most severe form has maternal transmission and is typified by severe generalized hypotonia and weakness, often requiring respiratory support early in life. Infants who survive this neonatal crisis may later be found to have an intelligence quotient that is lower

---

Table 95–5. Fibrillation Potentials with the Floppy Infant Syndrome

Neurogenic disorders
  Werdnig-Hoffmann disease
  Poliomyelitis
  Spinal cord injury
Polyneuropathies
  Hypomyelinating congenital neuropathy
  Axonal congenital neuropathy
Neuromuscular transmission defects
  Infantile botulism
Congenital myopathies
  Congenital
  Centronuclear myotubular (typically)
  Congenital fiber type disproportion (rarely)
  Nemaline rod (rarely)
Dystrophies
  Myotonic dystrophy
Enzymatic disorders
  Type II: acid maltase (Pompe's disease)
  Type IV: myophosphorylase (McArdle's disease)
  Type VII: phosphofructokinase (Tarui's disease)
Inflammatory disorders
  Polymyositis

than normal. In the other form (Swift et al., 1975), the infant presents with facial diplegia and various arthrogrypotic deformities. Transmission can be by either parent.

Clinical myotonia is defined as delayed muscle relaxation or involuntary stiffness accompanied by the finding of myotonic discharges on needle EMG. The EMG examination of newborns with myotonic dystrophy may demonstrate myotonic potentials that fire at high rates and wax and wane in frequency and amplitude (Swift et al., 1975). Although some infants have the classic dive-bomber sound, often the infantile form of myotonic potentials are somewhat higher pitched, quieter, and less sustained than those in the adult. Myotonic discharges are induced by needle insertion or, occasionally, by manual percussion over the adjacent muscle (Swift et al., 1975). At times, some positively configured myotonic discharges may be confused with endplate noise. Sometimes, myotonic discharges are not as widespread in newborns as in adults.

Profuse fibrillation potentials were the most prominent finding in six EMG studies of four infants with myotonia evaluated at the Mayo Clinic in Rochester, Minnesota (Kuntz and Daube, 1984). Myotonic discharges were found in three of the four infants, the earliest noted at 5 days. One infant had no myotonia present at age 3 weeks. In another infant, myotonic discharges increased in degree when the infant was between birth and age 17 months. Concomitantly, the numbers of fibrillation potentials diminished. In some infants, myotonic discharges may not even appear for several months or years. Because of the profuse spontaneous activity, it is often difficult to assess motor unit potentials satisfactorily (Kuntz

and Daube, 1984). EMG examinations of some mothers demonstrated myotonia that was previously unsuspected (Kuntz and Daube, 1984). On occasion, when an EMG examination of a floppy infant is normal, a brief maternal needle EMG evaluation identifies previously unsuspected myotonic dystrophy and subsequently the need for a DNA test in the mother as well as the baby (Darras and Jones, 2000).

The myotonic dystrophy phenotype is usually obvious in older children and adults with the typical temporalis and sternocleidomastoid paresis and atrophy leading to the hatchet-like appearance of the face, as well as distal weakness. In the older patient with myotonic dystrophy, temporal and frontal balding may also occur; however, balding does not occur in children of either sex. When myotonic dystrophy is clinically suspected, DNA testing is 98% to 99% accurate (Brunner et al., 1992; Suthers et al., 1992). Therefore, when there is clinical suspicion of myotonic dystrophy in a baby or older child, DNA testing is the preferred modality before performance of an EMG (Table 95–6).

Congenital Myopathies

These genetically determined myopathies include some pathoanatomically distinct entities usually having similar phenotypic expression. These children's clinical presentation includes early floppy infant syndrome, with a slowly progressive or nonprogressive course, or delayed motor milestones often associated with various skeletal abnormalities (Dubowitz, 1980). Infants who also have evidence of ptosis and extraocular muscle weakness most likely

Table 95–6. Recommended Protocol for Presumed Childhood Neuromuscular Disorders

Suspected Clinical Diagnosis	Diagnostic Test or Procedure			
	Option	First	Second	Third
Duchenne-Becker muscular dystrophy		DNA	MBx	
Limb-girdle muscular dystrophy		DNA*	MBx	EMG/NCS†
Emery-Dreifuss muscular dystrophy		DNA	MBx	EMG/NCS†
Facioscapulohumeral muscular dystrophy		DNA	EMG/NCS‡	
Myotonic dystrophy		DNA	EMG/NCS	
Periodic paralysis and myotonias		DNA	EMG/NCS	
Metabolic disorders		MBx	DNA	EMG/NCS‡
Congenital myopathies		EMG/NCS	MBx	DNA§
Dermatomyositis and polymyositis		MRI	MBx	EMG/NCS‡
Indeterminate proximal weakness		EMG/NCS	RMNS	MBx/DNA
Spinal muscular atrophy		DNA	EMG/NCS	MBx¶
Chronic inflammatory demyelinating polyneuropathy		EMG/NCS	CSF	
(Guillain-Barré syndrome) acute inflammatory demyelinating polyneuropathy		CSF	EMG/NCS	
Hereditary motor and sensory neuropathies		EMG/NCS	DNA	
Neuromuscular transmission disorders		EMG/NCS	RMNS	Antibodies

*To exclude Duchenne-Becker muscular dystrophy (if positive).
†In atypical, sporadic cases with low creatine phosphokinase values.
‡Optional.
§Not commercially available.
¶If EMG/NCS consistent with spinal muscular atrophy but DNA test is negative.
AIDP, acute inflammatory demyelinating polyneuropathy; CIDP, chronic inflammatory demyelinating polyneuropathy; CSF, cerebrospinal fluid examination; DNA, DNA or genetic testing; EMG, electromyography; GBS, Guillain-Barré syndrome; MBx, muscle biopsy; MRI, magnetic resonance imaging; NCS, nerve conduction studies; RMNS, repetitive motor nerve stimulation.

will have myotubular (centronuclear) myopathy at muscle biopsy. This is predicated on the assumption that some of the various infantile neuromuscular transmission defects or neonatal myotonic dystrophy have been excluded, because these disorders often have similarities of clinical presentation during infancy. In contrast to some other infantile myopathies, the *congenital myopathies* are not usually associated with elevated levels of serum creatine phosphokinase.

The characteristic EMG motor unit potential abnormalities identified with congenital myopathies include short-duration, low-amplitude motor unit potentials that are often rapidly recruited; however, certain of the congenital myopathies have normal motor unit amplitude, duration, and configuration. There are a few reasons for the lack of good correlation between EMG and biopsy results with these congenital myopathies. Often, it is difficult to distinguish the normally small motor unit potential found in the healthy neonate from motor unit potentials with subtle myopathic changes. Additionally, some of the anatomical changes found in the congenital myopathies do not have enough of an impact on the muscle fiber to affect motor unit potential size on EMG. This appears to have been the case in 4 of the 12 infants seen in our pediatric EMG laboratory at the Children's Hospital of Boston (David and Jones, 1994). These infants had normal results on EMG; however, subsequent muscle biopsy demonstrated a myopathic process.

In most congenital myopathies, abnormalities are not present at rest or on needle insertion. An important exception to this statement is the presence of abundant fibrillation potentials in some infants later found to have myotubular (centronuclear) myopathy (Torres et al., 1985). Rarely, this finding is associated with concomitant myotonic discharges (Munsat et al., 1969). Two other congenital myopathies may also have fibrillation potentials. These are nemaline myopathy (Norton et al., 1983) and congenital fiber–type disproportion (Kimura, 1983; see Table 95–5).

Congenital myopathies are usually present at birth and manifest with generalized infantile hypotonia, weakness with or without feeding, respiratory difficulties, and some dysmorphic features. To date, no specific DNA tests are available to diagnose congenital myopathies unequivocally; however, some testing is available in research laboratories. These children have distinctive features on muscle biopsy. When there is a clinical possibility of a congenital myopathy, especially with a floppy infant who has normal or mildly elevated creatine phosphokinase levels, we continue to order EMG studies before doing a muscle biopsy (see Table 95–6). One needs to be cautious if there is abnormal spontaneous activity present. As discussed earlier, these findings may lead to diagnostic errors, especially if they are misinterpreted as a neuropathic sign (see Table 95–5) (David and Jones, 1994). The motor unit potential per se is the key to differentiating between a neurogenic and myopathic disorder with EMG (David and Jones, 1994). Until specific DNA testing becomes available, a muscle biopsy needs to be performed to make a specific histological diagnosis.

Infantile Polymyositis

There are two reports of six infants with floppy infant syndrome who were subsequently diagnosed with *polymyositis* (Thompson, 1982; Shevell et al., 1990). Five of the six infants were floppy at birth, and each had an elevated creatine phosphokinase value. In retrospect, their mothers had noticed decreased intrauterine fetal movements. By age 6 months, all but one infant had elevated serum creatine phosphokinase levels ranging between 14 to 40 times higher than normal. Three of the five infants who had an EMG performed had myopathic motor unit potentials demonstrated. One infant had generalized increased insertional activity with prolonged high-frequency discharges (Thompson, 1982). In addition to an inflammatory myopathy, three other conditions, including congenital muscular dystrophy and two rare glycogen storage disorders (McArdle's disease and Pompe's disease), need consideration in the differential diagnosis of floppy infant syndrome with abnormal creatine phosphokinase values. Another infant with severe hypotonia and the phenotypical characteristics of Werdnig-Hoffmann disease (spinal muscular atrophy type I) had a creatine phosphokinase value three to four times normal (Chou and Miles, 1989). This baby had an inflammatory myopathy without myonecrosis on muscle biopsy at 1 month of age. The cellular infiltrates were predominantly phagocytic and monocytic and not T or B lymphocytes. These investigators suggested that these cells were essential for myofiber maturation but were not an inflammatory response. This may explain why some of the previously reported cases of infantile "polymyositis" have been refractory to steroid therapy (Chou and Miles, 1989). In contrast to the other six cases in the literature, this abstract did not contain any specific EMG findings that, if performed, could have easily differentiated a neurogenic process from a myopathic one.

Metabolic Myopathies

The *metabolic myopathies* comprise a group of muscle disorders secondary to failed energy production. Primarily, these enzymatic disorders are related to defects in glycogen, lipid, or mitochondrial metabolism. Typically, these myopathies present with either dynamic symptoms including exercise intolerance, myalgias, or myoglobinuria or static symptoms such as fixed muscle weakness.

We do not routinely perform EMG examinations in infants and older children with suspected metabolic myopathies. DNA testing is currently available for some enzymatic defects (e.g., myophosphorylase deficiency). Occasionally, a newborn with generalized infantile hypotonia and arthrogryposis whose EMG examination is characterized by myopathic motor units subsequently has a muscle biopsy that shows myophosphorylase deficiency (DiMauro and Hartlage, 1978) or phosphofructokinase deficiency (Swoboda et al., 1997). Rarely, the detection of myotonic discharges in children with an otherwise myopathic EMG may be useful in suspecting the diagnosis of infantile or juvenile cases of acid maltase deficiency, early-onset myotonic dystrophy or, later in adolescence, hyperkalemic periodic paralysis. Otherwise, in most metabolic myopathies, a muscle biopsy for light microscopy, electron microscopy, immunohistochemistry, and biochemistry remains the mainstay of the laboratory investigation.

GLYCOGEN STORAGE DISEASES

Acid Maltase Deficiency
(Pompe's Disease: Glycogenosis II)

This autosomal recessive disorder caused by the deficiency of lysosomal acid α-glucosidase affects both skeletal and cardiac muscle and subclinically motor neurons. Hypotonia may be apparent at birth or may not develop until 3 months of age. In one infant (Finegold and Bergman, 1988; Verity, 1991), creatine phosphokinase values were elevated 6 to 20 times. Although EMG was not performed in either of these infants, acid maltase deficiency may be suspected during EMG by the appearance of many complex repetitive discharges, particularly in the paraspinal muscles, concomitant with the appearance of myopathic motor unit potentials (Hogan et al., 1969).

Acid Maltase and Debrancher
Enzyme Deficiency

There is one example of this rare combined deficiency of two enzymes in the glycolytic pathway, also having an autosomal recessive pattern of inheritance (Tsao et al., 1994). This infant was normal at birth and had normal maturation during his first 2 months, but by the fourth month generalized hypotonia and profound weakness developed. In addition, he had facial diplegia, a high-pitched cry, poor suck, areflexia, macroglossia, and hepatomegaly. Cardiac failure and respiratory distress developed 1 month later associated with biventricular hypertrophy on electrocardiography.

EMG was performed at age 4 months. Needle examination demonstrated myotonic discharges, positive sharp waves, and fibrillation potentials (no comment was made about the motor unit potentials). Motor nerve conduction study results were normal. Muscle biopsy at age 5 months demonstrated vacuolar myopathy with abundant glycogen storage that, on biochemical analysis, was five times the upper limit of normal. No acid maltase or debrancher en-

zyme was present. This infant died of pneumonia at age 6 months (Tsao et al., 1994).

Myophosphorylase Deficiency
(McArdle's Disease: Glycogenosis V)

This condition is also an autosomal recessive, inherited glycogen storage disease. One infant with McArdle's disease had a gradually progressive floppy infant syndrome that began at age 4 weeks. EMG examination demonstrated many polyphasic motor unit potentials with profuse fibrillation potentials. The initial diagnosis of spinal muscular atrophy was presumably made because of the insertional abnormalities. One week later, severe respiratory distress developed. The child died at age 2 months. At autopsy, muscle histochemical evaluation demonstrated complete lack of myophosphorylase (DiMauro and Hartlage, 1978). Another infant with myophosphorylase deficiency had some increased polyphasic units but no fibrillation potentials (Milstein et al., 1989). Levels of creatine phosphokinase were twice normal in one infant (DiMauro and Hartlage, 1978) and were low normal in the other infant (Milstein et al., 1989).

Phosphofructokinase Deficiency
(Tarui's Disease: Glycogenosis VII)

A fatal form of phosphofructokinase deficiency, an autosomal recessive illness, also presented in a floppy infant who developed respiratory distress (Servidei et al., 1986). An EMG suggested a myopathic process with the presence of full motor unit potential recruitment with slight effort, combined with abundant fibrillation potentials and positive sharp waves. This infant died at age 7 months.

We studied another instance of infantile phosphofructokinase deficiency presenting in a floppy infant associated with arthrogryposis. This baby's creatine phosphokinase value was normal; the EMG had many low-amplitude, short-duration motor unit potentials, particularly in the proximal muscles. There were no fibrillation potentials or other unusual insertional activities (Swoboda et al., 1997).

LIPID STORAGE DISORDERS

Although carnitine palmitoyltransferase deficiency may occur in infancy, we are unaware of infants having this illness who presented with floppy infant syndrome.

ELECTRON TRANSPORT CHAIN DISORDERS IN COMPLEX II AND IV DEFICIENCIES

Electron transport chain defects may involve the central nervous system, peripheral nervous system, and muscles to varying clinical degrees (DiMauro et al., 1985). Characteristically, muscle biopsy demonstrates ragged red fibers.

Severe infantile myopathy was identified in two

infants with complex II deficiency (Sengers et al., 1983; Behbehani et al., 1984). These infants had associated lactic acidosis, seizures, and secondary carnitine deficiency. Cytochrome-c oxidase, that is, complex IV deficiency, may produce variably severe myopathy. One child had a fatal outcome (Minchom et al., 1983), whereas others had a more benign infantile myopathic process (Heiman-Patterson et al., 1982; DiMauro et al., 1983). In one of these infants, the EMG was normal (Heiman-Patterson et al., 1982); however, the muscle biopsy was abnormal. This EMG–muscle biopsy result disparity again emphasizes the need to pursue a muscle biopsy in any infant who clinically appears to have a myopathic process even though the EMG results are normal.

Sometimes with electron transport chain disorders, the EMG may only have nonspecific myopathic changes in concert with abnormal results on nerve conduction studies. However, these patients may not have any associated signs of clinical neuropathy (DiMauro et al., 1983). Another report studied 20 patients with mitochondrial myopathy (Yiannikas et al., 1986). Ten, including four children, had nerve conduction study evidence of peripheral neuropathy. Only five patients were symptomatic; however, all 10 patients had mild peroneal MCV slowing with low-amplitude compound sensory nerve action potentials. Nine of the ten patients with abnormal nerve conduction studies had EMG evidence of myopathy. Sural nerve biopsy in four of the five patients with clinical peripheral neuropathy demonstrated decreased density of myelinated nerve fibers with axonal degeneration (Yiannikas et al., 1986).

Benign Congenital Hypotonia

Benign congenital hypotonia is a poorly defined syndrome that may present as floppy infant syndrome (Brooke et al., 1979). Results of muscle enzyme studies, nerve conduction studies, EMG, and biopsy are normal. When a similar family history is elicited, a benign course can be predicted.

Duchenne-Becker Muscular Dystrophies

In 1986, the *Duchenne-Becker muscular dystrophy* gene was isolated by Kunkel's group at the Children's Hospital of Boston, and within another year the protein product, named dystrophin, was characterized (Hoffman et al., 1987). These major discoveries introduced the methods of Southern and Western blots and later the polymerase chain reaction to the diagnosis of the common dystrophinopathies, Duchenne's muscular dystrophy and Becker's muscular dystrophy.

Patients with classic Duchenne's or Becker's muscular dystrophy do not need an EMG for diagnostic purposes. When a "molecular" means for the diagnosis of Duchenne's and Becker's muscular dystro-

phy became available, most neurologists stopped using EMG in the evaluation of children with possible Duchenne's or Becker's muscular dystrophy. Children with probable Duchenne's or Becker's muscular dystrophy usually present with a proximal weakness, lordosis, and pseudohypertrophy of the calves with a high creatine phosphokinase level (in the thousands). Some pediatric neurologists recommend an EMG examination for "atypical phenotypes." However, atypical phenotypes are highly unusual. In the clinical setting of classic Duchenne's or Becker's muscular dystrophy, we currently proceed directly with a DNA test and sometimes, but not always, with a muscle biopsy. Many pediatric neuromuscular specialists believe that one does not need a muscle biopsy if the polymerase chain reaction DNA test is positive for a deletion, especially if the in-frame/out-of-frame status of the deletion is known (Monaco et al., 1988). Deletions are detected in about 65% to 70% of the cases. When the DNA analysis is not positive in a child with a typical phenotype for a dystrophinopathy, one then proceeds to a muscle biopsy for histology as well as immunostaining specifically for the presence or absence of dystrophin (Darras and Jones, 2000).

Limb-Girdle Muscular Dystrophies

Limb-girdle muscular dystrophies may be either autosomal recessive or autosomal dominant (Bonnemann et al., 1996). Most patients with autosomal recessive cases have earlier onset, rapid progression, and relatively high creatine phosphokinase values. Children with autosomal recessive limb-girdle muscular dystrophies may be clinically indistinguishable from those with Duchenne's or Becker's muscular dystrophy. However, in contrast to Duchenne's muscular dystrophy, cognitive function is normal in all patients with these dystrophies, particularly in the subset characterized as sarcoglycanopathies. If the creatine phosphokinase level is at least a few thousand units per liter in a child with a myopathic phenotype, thus excluding other nonmyopathic motor unit disorders, we next go directly to a dystrophin DNA test to exclude Duchenne's or Becker's muscular dystrophy. If that is negative, and because genetic or DNA testing for limb-girdle muscular dystrophies is not yet available, the next appropriate step is a muscle biopsy for immunohistochemistry with antibodies against α, β, γ, and δ sarcoglycans, dystroglycans, and merosin (Darras and Jones, 2000).

Patients with autosomal dominant limb-girdle muscular dystrophy have a later age at onset and a slower clinical progression; the creatine phosphokinase values in these patients may not be as grossly elevated. However, in limb-girdle muscular dystrophy type 1C, creatine phosphokinase values are elevated four- to 25-fold, and the clinical onset of this form of dystrophy may begin earlier in childhood (Minetti et al., 1998). Some patients with dominant cases, and even autosomal recessive cases with modest creatine phosphokinase elevation, may be clinically indistinguishable from those with spinal muscular atrophy type III, the Kugelberg-Welander form of spinal muscular atrophy. Because patients with spinal muscular atrophy type III also may have a modest creatine phosphokinase elevation, in this setting an EMG examination is used to rule out or rule in a neuropathic process.

Emery-Dreifuss Muscular Dystrophy

Emery-Dreifuss muscular dystrophy is an X-linked recessive (Xq28) or autosomal dominant condition (1q21) with onset in late childhood or adult life. Emery-Dreifuss muscular dystrophy is characterized by humeroperoneal distribution of muscle weakness typically associated with fixed contractures, particularly at the elbows and neck, cardiac arrhythmias, and a slowly progressive clinical course. This form of muscular dystrophy is caused by mutations in the emerin (Xq28) (Bione et al., 1994) and lamin *A/C* genes (1q21) (Bonne et al., 1999). In the X-linked variety of Emery-Dreifuss muscular dystrophy, DNA testing for emerin gene X chromosome mutations is now available, and, therefore, EMG is not required when this phenotype is recognized and the appropriate DNA testing is positive. In patients with autosomal dominant cases with relatively low creatine phosphokinase values, EMG to confirm the myopathic nature of the process is useful before a muscle biopsy is performed. DNA testing for the lamin *A/C* genes is now commercially available.

Facioscapulohumeral Dystrophy

Facioscapulohumeral dystrophy is an autosomal dominant dystrophy with a distinct phenotype (Munsat et al., 1972; Taylor et al., 1982). The precise genetic defect in this major form of facioscapulohumeral dystrophy is not known yet. Clinically, the diagnosis of facioscapulohumeral dystrophy can be made easily in most children and adults with this disorder. Typically, these patients have prominent facial as well as scapulohumeral muscle weakness. Parenthetically, striking asymmetry of muscle involvement occurs and is a typical feature of facioscapulohumeral dystrophy. Because of the occasional occurrence of this phenotype with asymmetrical involvement, the differential diagnosis often includes the possibility of mononeuropathy or plexopathy. Nevertheless, clinicians not familiar with this type of facioscapulohumeral dystrophy may order electrodiagnostic studies, which will fail to confirm the occurrence of a focal neuropathic process but instead will demonstrate the presence of many low-amplitude, short-duration motor unit potentials consistent with the unexpected finding of myopathy. Neuropathic findings related, in most instances, to secondary nerve injuries from stretching of the bra-

chial plexus or to focal compression neuropathies of branches of the radial, median, or ulnar nerves may be documented concomitantly by EMG. EMG is also useful in differentiating facioscapulohumeral dystrophy from the non–chromosome 5 form of spinal muscular atrophy that is characterized by a scapuloperoneal distribution of the weakness similar to that seen in facioscapulohumeral dystrophy.

A commercially available DNA test detects a deleted DNA repeat in the long arm of chromosome 4 in patients with facioscapulohumeral dystrophy. It is extremely accurate and thus can confirm the diagnosis in almost 100% of the cases (Griggs et al., 1993; Kohler et al., 1999; Ricci et al., 1999). DNA testing also provides another option for the study of patients with atypical cases of facioscapulohumeral dystrophy. However, in certain atypical patients, the exact gene defect is still not identified, and thus the sensitivity of the DNA repeat deletion test for atypical cases remains uncertain.

Myotonic Disorders and Periodic Paralyses

Myotonia is not a specific clinical or EMG finding that is diagnostic for myotonic dystrophy per se; it occurs clinically and electrophysiologically in other genetic conditions such as myotonia congenita, paramyotonia congenita, hyperkalemic periodic paralyses, and myotonia fluctuans (Moxley, 1997). Myotonic discharges have also been seen in the EMG studies of children who have centronuclear myopathy, acid maltase deficiency, and some nongenetic entities such as dermatomyositis-polymyositis, in hypothyroid myopathy in adults, and in patients receiving lipid-lowering drugs. Genetic research has identified a host of channelopathies affecting the sodium, calcium, and chloride channels. Despite the availability of DNA tests for the diagnosis of many of the myotonic disorders as well as the hyperkalemic and hypokalemic periodic paralyses, these mutations are not detected in all cases. In the absence of a family history, obvious clinical presentation, or availability of DNA testing, an EMG is often useful to confirm the presence of some myotonic disorders, particularly myotonia congenita, myotonia fluctuans, and hyperkalemic periodic paralysis. In older children suspected of possibly having periodic paralysis and in whom available genetic testing does not provide a diagnosis, the 45-minute McManis EMG test for exertional fatigue may be useful in the cooperative older child (McManis et al., 1986). The details for the performance of this EMG procedure are carefully outlined in the original article.

Inflammatory Myopathies

Most of our patients having the classic clinical and laboratory findings of *inflammatory myopathy* undergo EMG or muscle biopsy to confirm the diagnosis. However, the one exception is the child whose clinical presentation also includes the classic dermatological changes. In these instances, magnetic resonance imaging of the proximal lower extremities demonstrates areas consistent with inflammation. In this setting, experienced clinicians may sometimes initiate immunosuppressive treatment without either EMG or muscle biopsy data (Miller et al., 1996). These immunologically mediated inflammatory myopathies have no genetic predisposition. Results of EMG in the acute clinical phase commonly demonstrate the classic myopathic characteristics of inflammatory myopathy. Typically, these EMG findings are detected in the most superficial layers of the muscle. This distribution correlates with the classic histopathological findings of perifascicular atrophy so typical of dermatomyositis. These motor unit potentials are low in amplitude, of short duration, polyphasic, and easily recruited in large numbers. One sees abnormal spontaneous activity ranging from positive waves to dense fibrillation potentials, firing at slow rates, occasional myotonic discharges, or complex repetitive discharges, again with a perifascicular predominance throughout the muscle. In mild cases, the EMG abnormality may be detectable only in paraspinal muscles. In patients with chronic cases, neuropathic EMG changes are also sometimes demonstrated (Darras and Jones, 2000).

Differential Diagnosis of Indeterminate Proximal Weakness in Children

It is important to discuss the differential diagnosis of the child presenting with proximal weakness in whom no obvious myopathic mechanism is identified. In many children, a primary pathophysiological process affecting other major divisions of the motor unit is identified, including the anterior horn cell, peripheral nerve, and neuromuscular junction. EMG is valuable in this setting.

Kugelberg-Welander disease, spinal muscular atrophy type III, typically presents with proximal weakness between 2 and 14 years of age (Dubowitz, 1995), and it is often associated with mild elevations of creatine phosphokinase. These children have the same chromosomal abnormality (5q 11-13) as do those with types I and II spinal muscular atrophy (Lefebvre et al., 1995). If spinal muscular atrophy type III is considered in the differential diagnosis of childhood myopathy, this DNA test is the diagnostic tool of choice. However, often these children present to the EMG laboratory for delineation of an indeterminate proximal weakness. The findings are well defined, with a major diminution in the number of motor unit potentials recruited. These are typically of high amplitude and longer duration than normal. No other disorders in this age group have these EMG characteristics unless the child has had poliomyelitis.

Occasionally, we see a child with chronic inflammatory demyelinating neuropathy who presents with a slowly evolving proximal or distal weakness (or both) initially thought to be a dystrophy (Sladky et al., 1986). Usually, in this setting, the best clinical clue to the diagnosis of chronic inflammatory demyelinating polyneuropathy is the presence of significantly diminished muscle stretch reflexes. However, even when it is not suspected clinically, chronic inflammatory demyelinating polyneuropathy is clearly defined by EMG. Typically, these children have pronounced nerve conduction velocity slowing, with prolonged distal latencies, dispersed compound muscle action potentials, and evidence of conduction block and slowing. It is important to recognize this illness, because it is treatable.

Neuromuscular transmission defects, primarily myasthenia gravis, usually present with bulbar weakness. However, rare patients with myasthenia gravis present primarily with proximal weakness. Lambert-Eaton myasthenic syndrome is another rare neuromuscular transmission defect that may present as a myopathy in childhood. In the few examples reported, it was not until the performance of careful EMG with repetitive motor nerve stimulation that the appropriate diagnosis was appreciated (Darras and Jones, 2000).

Although one may suggest that we are now performing significantly fewer EMG examinations, with the availability of DNA analysis and muscle biopsy, the number of EMG studies performed per year at the Children's Hospital of Boston has not changed significantly. This is because the overall proportion of patients seen in a pediatric neuromuscular program with genetically determined myopathies is small. Furthermore, there is increasing interest in the use of EMG in the setting of the intensive care unit (Jones and Darras, 2000). Therefore, we are still performing a significant number of EMG examinations. Referrals to the EMG laboratory also continue to include infants and children with hypotonia with or without creatine phosphokinase elevation, as well as patients with developmental delay of unknown origin. It is estimated that approximately 20% of cases of infantile hypotonia are produced by disease of the motor unit. However, in the remaining 80%, the central origin of the hypotonia or weakness is not always obvious, and many EMG examinations are ordered to see whether the infant has a peripheral process and also to distinguish myopathies from disorders of the motor neuron, peripheral nerve, and neuromuscular junction.

EMG is an extension of the clinical neurological examination that provides an important modality for the study of the floppy infant. In most instances, it can usually, but not always (as in the case of some congenital myopathies), detect the presence of a pathological process within the peripheral motor unit. This study then provides the clinician a relatively useful means to distinguish between a central and a peripheral motor unit hypotonia (Jones, 1990). During needle EMG, a flexible gestalt approach is

Table 95–7. Electromyographic Protocol for Evaluation of a Floppy Infant

Sensory nerve conduction studies: at least one sensory nerve
Motor nerve conduction studies: at least two motor nerves
Needle electromyography: at least four to six muscles in one or
two extremities, including distal and proximal sites
If spinal muscular atrophy is a consideration: at least two
muscles innervated by different nerve roots, and nerves
should be sampled in at least three extremities
Repetitive motor nerve stimulation (2–50 Hz) should be
performed with
Infantile botulism type of history
Ptosis or ophthalmoparesis
Stimulus-linked repetitive compound muscle action potential
Myopathy defined by electromyography
Electromyography/nerve conduction studies

important. Certain muscles are not easily activated in the newborn and thus provide good sources to look for fibrillation potentials and positive sharp waves. In contrast, other muscles may be so easily activated that insertion activity is difficult to define. However, these muscles are good to use for analyzing motor unit potential parameters (Kuntz and Daube, 1984; David and Jones, 1994). Our recommended protocol for the EMG evaluation of floppy infants is shown in Table 95–7 (Jones, 1990).

Arthrogryposis Multiplex Congenita

Some infants with floppy infant syndrome also have multifocal congenital joint contractures and are classified as having *arthrogryposis multiplex congenita*. These infants have variable degrees of deformity ranging in degree from equinovarus with bilateral clubfeet to diffuse contractures at all major joints associated with varying degrees of infantile hypotonia, as defined by Banker (1986). Often, these infants have many associated congenital anomalies with prominent facial dysmorphism, including a flat nose, low-set ears, micrognathia, and a high arched palate. Concomitantly, some of these infants have systemic developmental abnormalities affecting the heart, lungs, and testes.

Multiple neurogenic or myopathic pathophysiological processes may lead to a common arthrogryposis multiplex congenita phenotype (Drachman and Banker, 1961). Experimental studies demonstrate that limited intrauterine fetal movements are the common denominator leading to the varying degrees of contractures (Drachman and Sokoloff, 1966). A congenital lesion at any level of the peripheral motor unit that predisposes to intrauterine immobility may result in the clinical picture of arthrogryposis multiplex congenita. These lesions include processes affecting motor neurons (David et al., 1991), congenital polyneuropathies (David et al., 1991), congenital myasthenia gravis (Holmes et al.,

1980; Smit and Barth, 1980), and myopathies (Banker, 1985; David et al., 1991). In a 25-year prospective study by Banker of 74 infants with arthrogryposis multiplex congenita (Banker, 1985), 69 (93%) had "neurogenic" findings on analysis of muscle tissue. Dysgenesis of the anterior horn cells was the most common pathological feature. Interestingly, just two of these infants had clinical findings and a course compatible with spinal muscular atrophy type I (Banker, 1985). In the future, DNA studies for the 5q 11-13 defect will be important to evaluate in this subgroup.

Previous EMG studies of infants with arthrogryposis multiplex congenita reported variable results. Smith et al. studied 17 randomly selected children; only 4 were infants younger than 1 year of age at the time of the EMG (Smith et al., 1963). There was a reduced number of motor unit potentials. The amplitude and duration of motor unit potentials varied; however, none were myopathic. Most of these 17 children with arthrogryposis multiplex congenita, including the 4 infants younger than 4 months of age, had fibrillation potentials. Motor or sensory conduction studies were not performed in any of these four infants (Smith et al., 1963). Other EMG studies also support the primacy of neurogenic mechanisms for arthrogryposis multiplex congenita; however, not many infants were evaluated (Amick et al., 1967; Fisher et al., 1970; Bharucha et al., 1972).

Amick et al. found giant motor unit potentials (up to 20 mV) in areas in which only a single motor unit potential was recruited, despite maximal effort (Amick et al., 1967). This finding was compatible with an anterior horn cell lesion in 9 of the 10 children, including 4 infants. In contradistinction to our experience with spinal muscular atrophy type I, fibrillation potentials were rarely detected in these nine children (Amick et al., 1967). Interestingly, the one child with myopathic motor unit potentials had well-defined fibrillation potentials in several muscles.

Strehl et al. published the largest EMG study of arthrogryposis multiplex congenita and evaluated 22 infants, 20 of whom were younger than 1 year of age (Strehl et al., 1985). Fourteen of the infants had an EMG or muscle biopsy performed. Unfortunately, this study did not contain precise EMG details (Strehl et al., 1985). Ten infants were thought to have arthrogryposis multiplex congenita secondary to a neurogenic process; however, only five were considered to be of spinal origin. These included just three infants with typical neurogenic EMGs with neurogenic abnormalities on muscle biopsy. Two other infants thought to have neurogenic arthrogryposis multiplex congenita of cerebral origin had normal results on EMG. Three infants had a combined cerebral and spinal source for their arthrogryposis multiplex congenita. Only 1 of their 10 infants assigned to the neurogenic category had a clinical picture compatible with a diagnosis of spinal muscular atrophy (Strehl et al., 1985). Nine other infants had a myopathic process. These included three with congenital muscular dystrophy, three with myotonic dystrophy, two of unknown cause, and one related to an inheritable connective tissue disorder. A myopathic EMG was defined in the six infants with either congenital muscular dystrophy or congenital myotonic dystrophy, two of whose mothers had not previously been diagnosed with myotonia (Strehl et al., 1985). Congenital muscular dystrophy is the most common myopathic mechanism associated with arthrogryposis multiplex congenita (Banker, 1985; David et al., 1991).

David et al. correlated the results of EMG and muscle and nerve biopsies in 35 infants with arthrogryposis multiplex congenita who were younger than 1 year of age when they were first examined in our pediatric EMG laboratory (David et al., 1991). Results of the EMG studies were abnormal in 28 of the 35 infants (80%). These EMG findings were similar to those associated with spinal muscular atrophy type I in nine infants, a congenital polyneuropathy in one infant, a myopathy in six infants, nonspecific changes in 11 infants, and a mixed pattern in one infant. Twenty-three infants had muscle and nerve biopsy performed. Neurogenic changes were present in four infants, myopathic abnormalities in five, indeterminate changes (probably neurogenic) in one, indeterminate changes (probably myopathic) in three other infants, dysmature end-stage muscle disease in two infants, and nonspecific changes in eight children. In contrast to a greater than 76% concordance between the results of EMG and muscle biopsy in nonarthrogrypotic floppy infants (David and Jones, 1994), our results with infants with arthrogryposis multiplex congenita were concordant in only 12 of 23 (52%) (David et al., 1991). Results of autopsy altered the diagnosis in three infants.

Only three of our nine infants with arthrogryposis multiplex congenita whose EMG initially was compatible with an anterior horn cell lesion had neurogenic results on biopsy (David et al., 1991). The other six infants with arthrogryposis multiplex congenita and "neurogenic" results on EMG included infants with indeterminate, probably myopathic or dysmature, end-stage muscle disease on biopsy. These latter infants with arthrogryposis multiplex congenita had long-term survivals that contrasted greatly with the usual nonarthrogrypotic floppy infant who has spinal muscular atrophy type I. Early on in our pediatric EMG experience with floppy infants with arthrogryposis multiplex congenita who had evidence of greatly diminished motor unit potential recruitment with rare, long-duration, sometimes high-amplitude, rapidly firing motor units associated with diffuse fibrillation potentials, we erroneously concluded that they had classic spinal muscular atrophy type I. However, some of these infants have had a more benign, static course. In fact, sometimes they have long-term, albeit handicapped, survival.

Our initial pediatric EMG experience documented just 1 of 35 infants with arthrogryposis multiplex congenita with an infantile polyneuropathy. Subsequently, we noted that most of our infants with either hypomyelinating or axonal congenital neuropathies had associated arthrogryposis multiplex congenita. One infant had a diffuse neuronal degeneration concomitantly affecting the central and peripheral nervous systems. This combination of pathological findings suggests a generalized process of neuronal maldevelopment (Steiman et al., 1980).

Our EMG, biopsy, and clinical correlation results were much better for infantile arthrogryposis multiplex congenita when the EMG demonstrated myopathic changes (David et al., 1991). This finding contrasts with the nonarthrogrypotic floppy infant in whom the EMG diagnosis of a myopathy was limited, in contrast to spinal muscular atrophy, with which we are much more accurate (David and Jones, 1994). However, some infants with arthrogryposis multiplex congenita who had myopathic results on biopsy had previously had EMG results elsewhere that were reported as either normal or nonspecific. In conclusion, neither EMG nor muscle or nerve biopsy alone is reliably diagnostic in the evaluation of the infant with arthrogryposis multiplex congenita. This includes infants whose EMG results are compatible with a disorder at the level of the anterior horn cell. The definitive diagnosis of infants with arthrogryposis multiplex congenita depends on the collation of all data, including careful ongoing follow-up examinations and occasionally a complete autopsy.

References

Amick LD, Johnson WW, Smith HL: Electromyographic and histopathologic correlations in arthrogryposis. Arch Neurol 1967;16:512–523.

Aslanidis C, Jansen G, Amemiya C, et al: Cloning of the essential myotonic dystrophy region and mapping of the putative defect. Nature 1992;355:548–551.

Banker BQ: Neuropathologic aspects of arthrogryposis multiplex congenita. Clin Orthop 1985;194:30–43.

Banker BQ: Arthrogryposis multiplex congenita: Spectrum of pathologic changes. Hum Pathol 1986;17:656–672.

Behbehani AW, Goebel H, Osse G, et al: Mitochondrial myopathy with lactic acidosis and deficient activity of muscle succinate cytochrome-c-oxidoreductase. Eur J Pediatr 1984;143:67–71.

Bergoffen J, Kant J, Sladky J, et al: Paternal transmission of congenital myotonic dystrophy. J Med Genet 1994;31:518–520.

Bharucha EP, Pandya SS, Dastur DK: Arthrogryposis multiplex congenita. I. Clinical and electromyographic aspects. J Neurol Neurosurg Psychiatry 1972;35:425–434.

Bione S, Maestrini E, Rivella S, et al: Identification of a novel X-linked gene responsible for Emery-Dreifuss muscular dystrophy. Nat Genet 1994;8:323–327.

Bonne G, Di Barletta MR, Varnous S, et al: Mutations in the gene encoding lamin A/C cause autosomal dominant Emery-Dreifuss muscular dystrophy. Nat Genet 1999;21:285–288.

Bonnemann CG, McNally EM, Kunkel LU: Beyond dystrophin: Current progress in the muscular dystrophies. Curr Opin Pediatr 1996;8:569–582.

Brook JD, McCurrach ME, Harley HG, et al: Molecular basis of myotonic dystrophy: Expansion of a trinucleotide (CTG) repeat at the 3′ end of a transcript encoding a protein kinase family member. Cell 1992;68:799–808.

Brooke MH, Carroll JE, Ringel SP: Congenital hypotonia revisited. Muscle Nerve 1979;2:84–100.

Brunner HG, Nillesen W, van Oost BA: Presymptomatic diagnosis of myotonic dystrophy. J Med Genet 1992;29:780–784.

Chou SM, Miles JM: Floppy infant syndrome with "congenital infantile polymyositis." Ann Neurol 1989;26:449.

Cotliar R, Eng GD, Koch B, et al: Correlation of electrodiagnosis and muscle biopsy results. Muscle Nerve 1992;15:1197–1198.

Darras BT, Jones HR: Diagnosis of pediatric neuromuscular disorders in the era of DNA analysis. Pediatr Neurol 2000;23:289–300.

Daube JR: The description of motor unit potentials in electromyography. Neurology 1978;28:623–625.

Daube JR: Needle examination in electromyography. Electrodiagnosis. Rochester, MN, Mayo Clinic, 1979.

David WS, Jones HR Jr: Electromyography and biopsy correlation with suggested protocol for evaluation of the floppy infant. Muscle Nerve 1994;17:424–430.

David WS, Kupsky WJ, Jones HR Jr: Electromyographic and histologic evaluation of the arthrogrypotic infant [Abstract]. Muscle Nerve 1991;14:897.

DiMauro S, Hartlage P: Fatal infantile form of muscle phosphorylase deficiency. Neurology 1978;28:1124–1129.

DiMauro S, Nicholson JF, Hays AP, et al: Benign infantile mitochondrial myopathy due to reversible cytochrome c oxidase deficiency. Ann Neurol 1983;14:226–234.

DiMauro S, Bonilla E, Zeviani M, et al: Mitochondrial myopathies. Ann Neurol 1985;17:521–538.

do Carmo RJ: Motor unit action potential parameters in human newborn infants. Arch Neurol 1960;3:136–140.

Drachman DB, Banker BO: Arthrogryposis multiplex congenita. Arch Neurol 1961;5:77–93.

Drachman DB, Sokoloff L: The role of movement in embryonic joint development. Dev Biol 1966;14:401–420.

Dubowitz V: The floppy infant. In Clinics in Developmental Medicine. London, Heinemann Medical, 1980; 89–94.

Dubowitz V: Disorders of the lower motor neurone: The spinal muscular atrophies. In Dubowitz V (ed): Muscle Disorders in Childhood. Philadelphia, WB Saunders, 1995; 325–369.

Eng GD: Electrodiagnosis. In Molnar GE (ed): Pediatric Rehabilitation. Baltimore, Williams & Wilkins, 1992; 143–165.

Feinsstein B, Lindegard B, Nyman E, Wolhfart G: Morphologic studies of motor units in normal human muscles. Acta Anat (Basel) 1955;23:127–142.

Finegold DN, Bergman I: High-protein feeding in an infant with Pompe's disease. Neurology 1988;38:824–825.

Fisher RL, Johnstone WT, Fisher WH, Goldkamp OG: Arthrogryposis multiplex congenita: A clinical investigation. J Pediatr 1970;76:255–261.

Griggs RC, Tawil R, Storvick D, et al: Genetics of facioscapulohumeral muscular dystrophy: New mutations in sporadic cases. Neurology 1993;43:2369–2372.

Gutierrez AR, Bodensteiner J, Gutmann L: Electrodiagnosis of infantile botulism. J Child Neurol 1994;9:362–365.

Harley HG, Rundle SA, Reardon W: Unstable DNA sequence in myotonic dystrophy. Lancet 1992;339:1125–1128.

Harper PS (ed): Myotonic dystrophy: The clinical picture. In Myotonic Dystrophy, 2nd ed. Philadelphia, WB Saunders, 1989; 13–36.

Heiman-Patterson TD, Bonilla E, DiMauro S, et al: Cytochrome-c–oxidase deficiency in a floppy infant. Neurology 1982;32:898–901.

Hoffman EP, Brown RH Jr, Kunkel LM: Dystrophin: The protein product of the Duchenne muscular dystrophy locus. Cell 1987;51:919–928.

Hogan GR, Gutmann L, Schmidt R, Gilbert E: Pompe's disease. Neurology 1969;19:894–900.

Holmes LB, Driscoll SG, Bradley WG: Contractures in a newborn infant of a mother with myasthenia gravis. J Pediatr 1980;96:1067–1069.

Jones HR Jr: EMG evaluation of the floppy infant: Differential diagnosis and technical aspects. Muscle Nerve 1990;13:338–347.

Jones HR, Darras BT: Acute care pediatric electromyography. Muscle Nerve Suppl 2000;(suppl 9):S53–S62.

Kimura J: Myopathies. In Electrodiagnosis in Diseases of Nerve

and Muscle: Principles and Practice. Philadelphia, FA Davis, 1983; 527–548.

Kohler J, Rohrig D, Bathke KD, Koch MC: Evaluation of the facioscapulohumeral muscular dystrophy (FSHD1) phenotype in correlation to the concurrence of 4q35 and 10q26 fragments. Clin Genet 1999;55:88–94.

Kuntz NL, Daube JR: Electrophysiology of Congenital Myotonic Dystrophy: AAEE Course. Rochester, MN, American Association of Electromyography and Electrodiagnosis, 1984.

Lazaro RP, Fenichel GM, Kilroy AW: Congenital muscular dystrophy: Case reports and reappraisal. Muscle Nerve 1979;2:349–355.

Lefebvre S, Burglen L, Reboullet S, et al: Identification and characterization of a spinal muscular atrophy-determining gene. Cell 1995;80:155–165.

Mayer RF, Mosser RS: Excitability of motoneurons in infants. Neurology 1969;19:932–945.

McManis PG, Lambert EH, Daube JR: The exercise test in periodic paralysis. Muscle Nerve 1986;9:704–710.

Miller LC, Tucker LB, Schaller JG: Dermatomyositis and polymyositis. In Burg FD, Ingelfinger JR, Wald ER, Polin RA (eds): Gellis and Kagan's Current Pediatric Therapy. Philadelphia, WB Saunders, 1996; 386–387.

Milstein J, Herron T, Haas J: Fatal infantile muscle phosphorylase deficiency. J Child Neurol 1989;4:186–188.

Minchom PE, Dormer RL, Hughes IA, et al: Fatal infantile mitochondrial myopathy due to cytochrome c oxidase deficiency. J Neurol Sci 1983;60:453–463.

Minetti C, Sotgia F, Bruno C, et al: Mutations in the caveolin-3 gene cause autosomal dominant limb-girdle muscular dystrophy. Nat Genet 1998;18:365–368.

Monaco AP, Bertelson CJ, Liechti-Gallati S, et al: An explanation for the phenotypic differences between patients bearing partial deletions of the DMD locus. Genomics 1988;2:90–95.

Moxley RT 3rd: Carrell-Krusen Symposium Invited Lecture—1997. Myotonic disorders in childhood: Diagnosis and treatment. J Child Neurol 1997;12:116–129.

Munsat TL, Piper D, Cancilla P, Mednick J: Inflammatory myopathy with facioscapulohumeral distribution. Neurology 1972;22:335–347.

Munsat TL, Thompson LR, Coleman RF: Centronuclear ("myotubular") myopathy. Arch Neurol 1969;20:120–131.

Norton A, Ellison P, Sulaiman AR, Harb J: Nemaline myopathy in the neonate. Neurology 1983;33:351.

Packer RJ, Brown MJ, Berman PH: The diagnostic value of electromyography in infantile hypotonia. Am J Dis Child 1982;136:1057–1059.

Ricci E, Galluzzi G, Deidda G, et al: Progress in the molecular diagnosis of facioscapulohumeral muscular dystrophy and correlation between the number of KpnI repeats at the 4q35 locus and clinical phenotype. Ann Neurol 1999;45:751–757.

Russell JW, Afifi AK, Ross MA: Predictive value of electromyography in diagnosis and prognosis of the hypotonic infant. J Child Neurol 1992;7:387–391.

Sacco G, Buchthal F, Rosenfalck P: Motor unit potentials at different ages. Arch Neurol 1962;6:366–373.

Sengers RC, Fischer JC, Trijbels JM, et al: A mitochondrial myopathy with a defective respiratory chain and carnitine deficiency. Eur J Pediatr 1983;140:332–337.

Servidei S, Bonilla E, Diedrich RG: Fatal infantile form of muscle phosphofructokinase deficiency. Neurology 1986;36:1465–1470.

Shevell M, Rosenblatt B, Silver K, et al: Congenital inflammatory myopathy. Neurology 1990;40:1111–1114.

Sladky JT, Brown MJ, Berman PH: Chronic inflammatory demyelinating polyneuropathy of infancy: A corticosteroid-responsive disorder. Ann Neurol 1986;20:76–81.

Smit LM, Barth PG: Arthrogryposis multiplex congenita due to congenital myasthenia. Dev Med Child Neurol 1980;22:371–374.

Smith EM, Bender LF, Stover CN: Lower motor neuron deficit in arthrogryposis: An EMG study. Arch Neurol 1963;8:97–100.

Steiman GS, Rorke IR, Brown MI: Infantile neuronal degeneration masquerading as Werdnig-Hoffmann disease. Ann Neurol 1980;8:317–324.

Strehl E, Vanasse M, Brochu P: EMG and needle muscle biopsy

studies in arthrogryposis multiplex congenita. Neuropediatrics 1985;16:225–227.

Suthers GK, Huson SM, Davies KE: Instability versus predictability: The molecular diagnosis of myotonic dystrophy. J Med Genet 1992;29:761–765.

Swift TR, Ignacio OJ, Dyken PR: Neonatal dystrophia myotonica: Electrophysiologic studies. Am J Dis Child 1975;129:734–737.

Swoboda KJ, Specht L, Jones HR, et al: Infantile phosphofructokinase deficiency with arthrogryposis: Clinical benefit of a ketogenic diet. J Pediatr 1997;131:932–934.

Taylor DA, Carroll JE, Smith ME, et al: Facioscapulohumeral dystrophy associated with hearing loss and Coats syndrome. Ann Neurol 1982;12:395–398.

Thompson CE: Infantile myositis. Dev Med Child Neurol 1982; 24:307–313.

Torres CF, Griggs RC, Goetz JP: Severe neonatal centronuclear myopathy with autosomal dominant inheritance. Arch Neurol 1985;42:1011–1014.

Tsao CY, Boesel CP, Wright FS: A hypotonic infant with complete deficiencies of acid maltase and debrancher enzyme. J Child Neurol 1994;9:90–91.

Verity MA: Infantile Pompe's disease, lipid storage, and partial carnitine deficiency. Muscle Nerve 1991;14:435–440.

Yiannikas C, McLeod JG, Pollard JD, Baverstock J: Peripheral neuropathy associated with mitochondrial myopathy. Ann Neurol 1986;20:249–257.

CHAPTER 96

Role of Electromyography for the Acutely Paralyzed Child and the Intensive Care Unit

H. Royden Jones, Jr., Basil T. Darras, and Charles F. Bolton

This chapter provides an electromyographic approach to the previously healthy infant in whom an acute floppy infant syndrome develops or the older child and adolescent who has acute generalized weakness. Pediatric electromyographers are consulted by the intensive care unit staff to provide potential diagnostic guidance in this interesting group of illnesses. Some of these disorders either are not seen in the adult or have a different *clinical phenotype* in children (Jones and Darras, 2000). In this setting, it is sometimes quite difficult to make the clinical distinction between a primary central nervous process and a lesion of the peripheral motor unit in an infant or a child. The differentiation in children between acute Guillain-Barré syndrome and transverse myelitis (Jones, 1996) or a menin-goencephalopathic process is a good example (Bradshaw, 2001). Electromyography (EMG) often provides pivotal diagnostic and, consequently, therapeutic guidance. Because the electromyographic spectrum of motor unit disorders involves a different clinical set for infants and toddlers (David and Jones, 1994; Jones and Darras, 2000) than for school-aged children and adolescents, we present this data apropos to these two respective age groups. The reader will find greater detail on each illness in Chapters 86 and 92 to 95 of this pediatric neuromuscular section.

INFANTS AND TODDLERS

Babies may present with an acute respiratory distress or a flaccid paralysis. This occasionally occurs in neonates, or it can occur acutely during infancy after the child had been healthy since birth. A variety of congenital, developmental, or acquired lesions, at any level of the peripheral motor unit, may lead to respiratory compromise or extremity weakness in the immediate neonatal period or during the first year of life. Some of the better known clinical causes include Guillain-Barré syndrome, infantile botulism, familial myasthenia gravis, and even poliomyelitis.

Electromyography in Infants

As outlined in Chapter 85, it is very important to always consider the maturational norms for needle conduction studies and needle EMG to arrive at accurate clinical correlations for infants and toddlers (Jones and Darras, 2000). Peripheral myelination advances gradually after birth, not reaching mature "adult" values until about the age of 3 years. With this knowledge, the clinician can discriminate between a demyelinating versus an axonal lesion. There are very few, if any, well-defined normative standards derived for neuromuscular junction evaluation in newborns and young infants with the use of repetitive motor nerve stimulation (Bolton, 1996). However, well-defined standards of abnormality have been established for infantile botulism, the most common neuromuscular junction disorder seen in babies, as discussed later.

Similarly, there is a definite maturation process in the definition of motor unit potential size (Jones and Darras, 2000). Needle EMG is the most helpful means for differentiating lesions at the anterior horn cell from a primary myopathic process. We are careful not to primarily rely on insertional findings that are in fact very nonspecific. The presence of fibrillation potentials is a nonspecific, albeit usually abnormal, finding. Fibrillation potentials are found in a number of infantile lesions that affect each pathoanatomical level of the motor unit (David and Jones, 1994). When confronted in the pediatric EMG laboratory or intensive care unit with an infant or a toddler presenting with an acute flaccid paralysis or respiratory distress, it is very important to always keep in mind these neurophysiological maturational changes. If not, the clinician can inappropriately conclude that an infant has a motor unit disorder when indeed the findings are normal for age. In addition, the clinician must always consider whether there is any other clinical or electromyographic evidence to suggest that some infectious or metabolic process is superimposed on one of the various milder motor unit disorders. In that instance, the underlying motor unit dysfunction may have temporarily decompensated, secondary to some acute "stress," and a more serious neuromuscular lesion may not be operative. If this premise is correct and the inciting mechanism is corrected, the infant will return to baseline level of function with routine supportive measures.

Anterior Horn Cell Disorders

Most anterior horn cell disorder cases seen during infancy represent the classic Werdnig-Hoffmann form of spinal muscular atrophy (type 1) (Jones, 1996). These children usually present as a floppy infant between the ages of 1 and 3 months. Very occasionally, this disorder has not been clinically recognized, especially with first-time parents. It is not until a respiratory infection, such as acute bronchiolitis, leads to the need for hospitalization that the underlying illness becomes apparent. At that time, the infant's limited motor reserve is recognized when there is prolonged need for respiratory support. The primary motor unit diagnosis is usually first defined by the combination of EMG and chromosomal DNA analysis (Darras and Jones, 2000). This setting is an example of when EMG still has an important diagnostic role in the early diagnosis of spinal muscular atrophy type 1. This study can rapidly provide an accurate diagnosis for the clinician trying to make important therapeutic and long-term prognostic determinations as well as provide parental guidance while awaiting the results of definitive DNA testing for the defect in the survival motoneuron (SMN1) gene at chromosome 5q11-13.

Poliomyelitis is an acute anterior horn cell infectious disease that must always be considered in the differential diagnosis of acute infantile flaccid paralysis (Beausoleil et al., 1994; David and Doyle, 1997; J. Goldstein, personal communication on infantile poliomyelitis in a recently immunized baby seen at Yale, 1995). Typically, in these babies, a febrile illness develops, with irritability, asymmetrical weakness, a weak cry, lethargy, and head lag. Brain imaging studies are usually normal. Cerebrospinal fluid analysis demonstrates a mixed pleocytosis of 100 to 580 white blood cells, with cerebrospinal protein values ranging between 82 to 143 mg/dL and essentially normal glucose values (Beausoleil et al., 1994; J. Goldstein, personal communication on infantile poliomyelitis in a recently immunized baby seen at Yale, 1995; David and Doyle, 1997). EMG can be very useful in this setting. Often, the median, ulnar, and peroneal compound muscle action potentials (CMAPs) are of low amplitude or absent (David and Doyle, 1997). In important diagnostic contrast with Guillain-Barré syndrome, all sensory nerve action potentials are well defined. The most-affected muscles have no motor unit potential activation and a mild-to-moderate degree of fibrillation potentials. Stool cultures will usually confirm this diagnosis. Recovery may be poor and can include long-term ventilator dependency.

The risk of the development of paralytic poliomyelitis from the attenuated live Sabin oral vaccine is stated to be 1 in 2.5 million immunizations, with 57% due to the type 3 oral vaccine usually occurring subsequent to their first polio vaccine and within 2 to 3 weeks of immunization (Robbins, 1993). New Centers for Disease Control and Prevention guidelines were established in the United States in January 2000. These guidelines changed the initial immunization protocol to require the Salk killed vaccine as the primary immunization method for all children. It is hoped, as with poliomyelitis in older children, that this new infantile immunization protocol will make postvaccination-related poliomyelitis of historical interest in the economically privileged nations. However, in the underdeveloped nations, oral vaccine remains the primary means of immunization. Thus, poliomyelitis still requires consideration in the differential diagnosis of an acutely floppy infant, particularly one from other health cultures.

Polyneuropathies

There are a few very provocative reports that support the concept that Guillain-Barré syndrome must be considered in the differential diagnosis of acute flaccid paralysis in neonates as well as in older infants and toddlers. These individual case reports support the concept that the intrauterine Guillain-Barré syndrome may develop in a preterm fetus.

In one instance, the mother had noted a significant decrease in fetal movements during the 30th week of her pregnancy (Jackson et al., 1996). Her baby was quadriparetic when delivered at 37 weeks, and the Apgar score was 6 at 10 minutes. A neurological examination at the age of 3 days demonstrated severe leg and moderate proximal arm weakness, with generalized absence of muscle stretch reflexes. The cerebrospinal fluid protein concentration was just 38 mg/dL. However, the needle conduction studies demonstrated profound motor nerve conduction velocity slowing (3 to 15 m per second [normal, 20 to 30 m per second]). Conduction block and temporal dispersion were present. Many muscles had active denervation on needle EMG. He received support measures with no specific therapy and had complete recovery by the age of 1 year (Jackson et al., 1996).

Another instance of neonatal Guillain-Barré syndrome occurred in the setting of a mother in whom Guillain-Barré syndrome developed during the third trimester (Rolfs and Bolik, 1994; Luijckx et al., 1997). The 33-year-old woman became quadriparetic with Guillain-Barré syndrome during the 29th week of her pregnancy. She required a respirator and remained intubated during her baby's delivery at 38 weeks' gestation (Luijckx et al., 1997). Generalized hypotonia, marked respiratory distress, and feeding problems developed in her baby at 12 days postpartum. His cerebrospinal fluid protein level was 243 mg/dL. The results of EMG were typical for Guillain-Barré syndrome. The authors suggested that Guillain-Barré syndrome developed in the infant in utero (Luijckx et al., 1997). Importantly, a trial of intravenous immunoglobulin therapy was associated with a complete resolution of all neurological deficits within just 2 weeks (Luijckx et al., 1997). At delivery, the baby of another mother with preterm Guillain-Barré syndrome had poor spontaneous ventilation that required brief intubation. No other possible signs of Guillain-Barré syndrome occurred during 5 days of observation (Rolfs and Bolik, 1994). Both the infant and the mother had high antibody titers to human peripheral nerve myelin glycolipids (Rolfs and Bolik, 1994). Symptoms of Guillain-Barré syndrome may also occur shortly after birth without any relation to known intrauterine events. Typically, these previously healthy babies have an acute rapidly progressive, often severe hypotonia, possible respiratory distress, and feeding difficulties. In one 7-week-old infant with acute Guillain-Barré syndrome, a chronic inflammatory demyelinating polyneuropathy syndrome developed later (Pasternak et al., 1982).

An EMG is particularly helpful for the differential diagnosis of Guillain-Barré syndrome from other acute floppy infant syndromes, in addition to the many other causes of a floppy infant at birth (see Chapter 86). The absence of sensory nerve action potentials with profound motor conduction slowing and dispersed CMAPs are the important electromyographic clues to the diagnosis of these rare instances of neonatal Guillain-Barré syndrome. We have seen a similar instance on EMG. This baby was phenotypically similar to spinal muscular atrophy type 1, even including tongue fasciculations (Jones and Darras, 2000). He also had severe arthrogryposis. Median and peroneal CMAPs were widely dispersed and of very low amplitude (0.02 mV) with very prolonged distal latencies (up to 8.2 ms) and very slow motor nerve conduction velocity of 6 to 8 m per second. There were no median sensory nerve

action potentials. These electromyographic findings were very similar to those of the infantile Guillain-Barré syndrome cases; however, sural nerve biopsy demonstrated hypomyelination with abortive onion bulb formation. This biopsy result with the combination of arthrogryposis suggesting a long-standing intrauterine process is more in keeping with one of the unusual congenitally determined peripheral neuropathies rather than with an acquired neuropathy such as Guillain-Barré syndrome.

Although tick paralysis is well known to mimic Guillain-Barré syndrome in older children (Grattan-Smith et al., 1997), we are unaware of an infantile case. However, any infant with an acute onset of generalized muscle weakness always warrants a search for a tick, with special care taken when searching the scalp (Grattan-Smith et al., 1997).

Neuromuscular Junction Disorders

Newborn infants may rarely have presynaptic or postsynaptic neuromuscular junction disorders. Most commonly, this occurs in babies with neonatal autoimmune myasthenia gravis born to mothers with autoimmune myasthenia gravis. Fifteen percent of babies born to mothers with autoimmune myasthenia gravis will develop transient neonatal myasthenia gravis during the first 3 days of life. These neonatal autoimmune myasthenia gravis babies typically have severe hypotonia and respiratory distress, with 50% of infants requiring respiratory support (Lefvert and Osterman, 1983; Papazian, 1992). Because *all* infants born to mothers with antibody-positive myasthenia gravis also have circulating antibodies, the presence or absence of a positive antibody test does not prove or disprove the diagnosis of neonatal autoimmune myasthenia gravis. Because the maternal history confirms the diagnosis, EMG is not usually indicated. However, an EMG may rarely be useful to monitor the response to anticholinesterase medications. Although most neonatal autoimmune myasthenia gravis infants respond well to anticholinesterase medications, sometimes there is a question as to whether the infant requires more or less medication. In this setting, an EMG with edrophonium chloride (Tensilon) testing provides an excellent means to guide the clinician when there is concern whether the anticholinesterase medication dosage is correct (Hays and Michaud, 1988).

Primary juvenile autoimmune myasthenia gravis usually does not occur until about the age of 1 year (Hays and Michaud, 1988) (see Chapter 94). These toddlers are usually well until some acute antecedent respiratory or gastrointestinal infectious process develops. Last year, we evaluated a 15-month-old girl in whom bilateral ptosis and generalized hypotonia developed. Her edrophonium chloride test was strongly positive. Here, EMG was very useful to confirm the clinical and pharmacological impression of myasthenia gravis, because the antibody studies performed at a commercial laboratory were normal. With the definitively positive edrophonium chloride test and the confirmatory EMG, a subsequent blood sample was sent to the Mayo Clinic, where the workers in the laboratory of Dr. Lennon confirmed the diagnosis of autoimmune myasthenia gravis.

Congenital myasthenia gravis with episodic apnea is the one very rare congenital neuromuscular transmission defect that has the propensity to occur acutely in babies (see Chapter 93).

Magnesium treatment for mothers with eclampsia has the potential to cause an acute infantile presynaptic neuromuscular junction disorder (Lipsitz, 1971; Sokal et al., 1972). These unusual neuromuscular junction disorders rarely come to the attention of the pediatric electromyographer, because the clinician recognizes the problems and provides appropriate supportive care.

Infantile botulism is the one presynaptic neuromuscular junction disorder of infancy for which EMG is often crucial to provide an early diagnosis. There is concern that infantile botulism may be more common than recognized; this is especially likely in consideration of the varying presentations of this illness (see Chapter 94).

Infantile botulism usually has a stereotypical clinical presentation. Typically, a previously healthy infant, between the age of 10 days and 10 months, has the acute onset of generalized hypotonia and weakness, poor feeding, and constipation. This diagnosis also requires consideration for any baby with unexplained acute respiratory distress, which may require ventilatory support (Pickett et al., 1976; Clay et al., 1977; Thompson et al., 1980; Hoffman et al., 1982; Schwartz and Eng, 1982; Donley et al., 1991; Shukla et al., 1991).

EMG is the most useful early diagnostic tool, because bacteriological confirmation usually requires a few weeks. Most babies with infantile botulism have clear-cut evidence of a neuromuscular junction disorder. Low-rate repetitive motor nerve stimulation at 2 to 5 Hz demonstrated a decremental response in 14 of 25 babies (56%) with infantile botulism (Cornblath et al., 1983). However, 11 infants (44%) had no decrement. Therefore, the inability to document a decrement on initial study does not exclude the need to perform the more uncomfortable rapid techniques. More rapid rates of repetitive motor nerve stimulation at 20 to 50 Hz is the best electrophysiological technique for diagnosing infantile botulism (Cornblath et al., 1983). Twenty-three of 25 babies had a post-tetanic facilitation that varied between 23% to 313%, with a mean of 73% (Cornblath et al., 1983). Another useful repetitive motor nerve stimulation finding, characteristic of infantile botulism, is that the post-tetanic facilitation duration is often very prolonged. It was recorded, in one instance, to last as long as 21 minutes (Fakadej and Gutmann, 1982). This contrasts with the post-tetanic facilitation of a few seconds in the most common adult presynaptic neuromuscular junction defect—Lambert-Eaton myasthenic syndrome.

EMG does not always confirm a diagnosis of infantile botulism. Two infants in two separate studies had no documented repetitive motor nerve stimulation facilitation (Cornblath et al., 1983; Gutierrez et al., 1994). In most instances, babies with infantile botulism have a typical electromyographic diagnostic triad; these include (1) low-amplitude CMAPs, (2) tetanic/post-tetanic facilitation, and (3) absence of post-tetanic exhaustion (Gutierrez et al., 1994).

Myopathies

Children with congenital myopathies rarely have acute flaccid paralysis or respiratory distress at birth. However, on occasion, we are asked to visit the neonatal intensive care unit to evaluate such a child, who later is proved to have a primary myopathy (Swift et al., 1975). Myotonic dystrophy occasionally presents in the neonate with severe generalized hypotonia. Some of these babies require immediate intubation. Sometimes the diagnosis is suspected clinically on the basis of their classic facies with tenting of the mouth that resembles an inverted V. Although most of these infants are found to have a positive family history of myotonic dystrophy, it may not have been previously diagnosed. Typically, the mother has a milder unrecognized form of the illness that first manifests as premature cataract removal or myotonia on clinical examination.

If there is clinical suspicion of congenital myotonia, DNA testing for the triplicate repeat is indicated. However, a concomitant EMG is often indicated to provide earlier diagnosis. Well-defined myotonia occurs in these newborn floppy infants as early as the age of 5 days (Swift et al., 1975; Kuntz and Daube, 1984). The myotonia seen with infants is somewhat atypical with a higher pitch, tending to be less sustained than that in adults (Kuntz and Daube, 1984). Profuse fibrillations may be the most predominant finding. In such cases, the clinician must carefully search for the myotonia. Some floppy infants have no myotonia on EMG and demonstrate only nonspecific changes. In these circumstances, we occasionally find that a maternal EMG defines previously unsuspected myotonia (Jones, 1996).

Glycogen storage disorders represent the other congenital myopathy that rarely presents as a floppy neonate (DiMauro and Hartlage, 1978; Swoboda et al., 1997). A fatal case of phosphorylase deficiency, presented at the age of 4 weeks with problems in feeding, fatigue, and respiratory distress, had a rapidly downhill course, with the patient becoming very hypotonic with generalized weakness. The child had increased numbers of motor unit potentials and fibrillations, which were interpreted as being consistent with spinal muscular atrophy (DiMauro and Hartlage, 1978). Such cases point to the importance of paying careful attention to the motor unit profile, and not the insertional finding per se. The motor unit potentials in these babies were typically myopathic, as found in our case of phosphofructokinase deficiency, particularly in the iliopsoas (Swoboda et al., 1997).

ACUTE NEUROMUSCULAR CRISES IN THE OLDER CHILD

Anterior Horn Cell

The pediatric electromyographer must keep poliomyelitis within the differential diagnosis of any child with an acute, particularly asymmetrical, flaccid paralysis. Fortunately, we have not seen any instances of acute poliomyelitis in 22 years since the inception of our EMG laboratory at the Children's Hospital of Boston. However, because some parents still decline to have their children appropriately immunized, the clinician must always keep this possibility in mind. In addition, with the increased use of air travel and the immigration or visiting of children from all parts of the world, it is important to always consider the possibility of poliomyelitis. We have seen a few instances of subacute polio in children who come from countries where standard immunization is not routinely available.

Peripheral Nerve

The Guillain-Barré syndrome is one of a number of primary peripheral nerve lesions that may lead to an acute generalized paralysis in the toddler as well as in the older child. EMG is particularly useful for defining the presence of, as well as the specific type of, neuropathy (Bradshaw and Jones, 1992). In most instances with toddlers and older children, Guillain-Barré syndrome presents in a fashion similar to that in adolescents and adults. However, some interesting variants occur in the acute care setting. Occasionally, children with clinical findings suggestive of an acute spinal cord lesion, including positive Babinski signs, do not have imaging studies compatible with the initial diagnosis. Because a definite spinal sensory level is difficult to define in some younger children, EMG is sometimes a useful additional study. Occasionally, EMG may demonstrate an atypical Guillain-Barré syndrome (Jones and Darras, 2000).

A pseudo-meningoencephalopathy is another pediatric Guillain-Barré syndrome variant (Bradshaw and Jones, 2001). Nine children proved by EMG to have Guillain-Barré syndrome were initially thought to have an acute encephalopathy during their emergency department evaluations (Swoboda et al., 1997). Each patient presented with severe pain, drowsiness, headache, irritability, and meningismus. The classic features of Guillain-Barré syndrome (weakness, hyporeflexia) were also present, but the other symptoms overshadowed these clinical findings. A central nervous system infection or inflammation was the initial diagnosis in the majority, and the atypical presentation caused diagnostic delay. Some initially had brain computed tomography scanning or magnetic resonance imaging, followed by cerebrospinal fluid examination, with an infection anticipated. When the albuminocytological dissociation was found, neurological consultation and EMG followed. The elevated cerebrospinal fluid protein with areflexia and severe pain provided the clinical clues suggesting Guillain-Barré syndrome. It is important to recognize this Guillain-Barré syndrome variant to ensure expeditious diagnosis and treatment.

There are two very rare axonal forms of Guillain-Barré syndrome, which are seen predominantly in China; although they have a much less common worldwide distribution, they also occur in North and South America, Europe, and Japan. One is an acute *motor axonal* neuropathy, and the other an even less common acute *motor sensory* axonal neuropathy (McKhann et al., 1991). Here, the initial immunological reaction is against epitopes specific to the axonal membrane rather than the more typical primary demyelination. In one instance, a child with the latter form presented acutely to an intensive care unit with respiratory distress, total body paralysis including external ophthalmoplegia, fixed dilated pupils, and absent caloric responses (Bakshi et al., 1997). He was initially thought to be brain dead. The electroencephalogram was normal. EMG failed to demonstrate any motor or sensory responses, and a severe axonal Guillain-Barré syndrome was diagnosed (Bakshi et al., 1997). Any child with acute flaccid paralysis who has fixed and dilated pupils must also have the diagnoses of diphtheria and botulism excluded (Jones, 2000). Each of these illnesses is also associated with predominant bulbar involvement. When pupillary responses are preserved in a child with rapidly developing flaccid weakness, the presence of bulbar symptoms suggests the possible diagnosis of either myasthenia gravis or poliomyelitis.

In general, electromyographic signs of significant axonal damage may not always carry the more profound prognosis in children compared with adults (Bradshaw and Jones, 1992), although the child with the "brain death" presentation had a recovery period of more than 1 year (Bakshi et al., 1997). This case exemplifies those with a more serious prognosis, including the child who requires a respirator, those in whom the clinician cannot define a CMAP, and the child who has widespread active denervation on needle EMG. Rare instances of pediatric death have occurred (Honavar et al., 1991).

Very uncommonly in children when the clinician is unable to obtain any CMAPs, it is important to note that there are pathological settings in which their peripheral nerves are remarkably resistant to electrical stimulation (Bolton et al., 1988). Five children had either no response or very low amplitude

CMAPs despite very long duration high-voltage stimuli. Motor nerve conduction velocity was very slow, ranging from just 3 to 10 m per second (Bolton et al., 1988). Although none of these children had an acute onset of symptoms, this electrical possibility must be considered. These cases serve notice that occasionally, severe hypomyelination may lead to a set of electromyographic findings that in many respects mimic acute motor axonal neuropathy. Sural nerve biopsy demonstrated severe chronic demyelination and remyelination with absent or very thin myelin sheaths (Bolton et al., 1988).

Other pediatric causes of an acute peripheral neuropathy also need consideration. When vincristine toxicity presents with a severe acute demyelinating motor and sensory neuropathy in children, the patient may have an unsuspected concomitant Charcot-Marie-Tooth type I hereditary neuropathy (Graf et al., 1996). This differential diagnosis also includes certain toxins such as glue sniffing and, rarely, buckthorn wild cherry ingestion, insecticides, and thallium (Jones, 2000). If there is concomitant gastrointestinal distress, porphyria, arsenic, lead, or mercury poisoning also enter the differential diagnosis (Jones, 2000).

Neuromuscular Junction Disorders

When the pediatric electromyographer is asked to aid in the differential diagnosis of acute childhood bulbar and generalized weakness or ataxia, it is important to consider a neuromuscular transmission disorder. Usually, this differential diagnosis is primarily between myasthenia gravis and the Miller-Fisher variant of Guillain-Barré syndrome. Although myasthenia gravis occurs in children (Mullaney et al., 2000), it is quite similar in presentation to that seen in adults, and we will not elaborate further here, because this is well known to electromyographers of adults.

Tick paralysis is a rare and dramatic, presumed atypical, neuromuscular transmission disorder that always requires consideration in the differential diagnosis of Guillain-Barré syndrome, particularly among children from the preschool age on (Cherington and Snyder, 1968; Haller and Fabara, 1972; Swift and Ignacio, 1975; Cooper and Spence, 1976; Donat and Donat, 1981; Kincaid, 1990; Grattan-Smith et al., 1997; Swift, 2000). Any child who presents with acute generalized weakness requires careful inspection of the scalp to exclude this unusual diagnosis. Tick paralysis evolves more slowly than other biological toxins, but it may actually be more deadly (Grattan-Smith et al., 1997). Prolonged respiratory paralysis occurred in two of six Australian children (Grattan-Smith et al., 1997). The responsible tick, *I. holocyclus,* is a different species than *D. andersoni* or *D. variabilis,* which are common to North America (Grattan-Smith et al., 1997). The latter is associated with a rapid improvement once the tick is removed, in contrast to a continued deterioration for up to 48

hours for the Australian variety. Early pupillary involvement is one of the most helpful clinical clues in the differentiation of tick paralysis from Guillain-Barré syndrome (Grattan-Smith et al., 1997). Total ophthalmoplegia may also occur. Such findings may suggest the Miller-Fisher Guillain-Barré syndrome variant as well as diphtheria (Jones, 2000).

Typical electromyographic findings in tick paralysis include very diminished CMAP amplitudes with preserved motor conduction velocities, motor distal latencies, and sensory nerve action potentials (Grattan-Smith et al., 1997). This clinical electromyographic set of findings is not dissimilar to acute motor axonal neuropathy or even some early demyelinating forms of Guillain-Barré syndrome. Sequential needle conduction studies immediately before the removal of a tick, a few days hence, and in 6 months demonstrated that the reduced CMAP improved dramatically after the tick was removed (Cherington and Snyder, 1968; Swift and Ignacio, 1975). No neuromuscular transmission defect is demonstrated with standard electromyographic techniques (Cherington and Snyder, 1968; Swift and Ignacio, 1975); however, experimental data suggest that tick paralysis may be related to pathology at the presynaptic neuromuscular junction with decreased acetylcholine release (Cooper and Spence, 1976). In some children, fibrillation potentials appear very early in the course of the illness—as soon as 24 to 48 hours (Cherington and Snyder, 1968; Swift and Ignacio, 1975).

Children in agricultural communities are at risk for organophosphate pesticide poisoning (Dirik and Uysal, 1994; Hart et al., 1994). In Paraguay, there was a 30% incidence of organophosphate pesticide exposure in patients with otherwise typical childhood Guillain-Barré syndrome (Hart et al., 1994). A few inborn metabolic errors, such as porphyria or Leigh's disease (Coker, 1993), enhanced by medications, particularly barbiturates, may also precipitate symptoms that resemble those of childhood Guillain-Barré syndrome. In adults, Guillain-Barré syndrome may be the presenting manifestation of acquired immunodeficiency syndrome (AIDS) (Hart et al., 1994). In a 6-year-old boy with congenital AIDS, Guillain-Barré syndrome also developed (Price et al., 1991). However, to date, on the basis of a complete National Library of Medicine computer search, Guillain-Barré syndrome has not been the presenting illness that led to a diagnosis of childhood AIDS (Price et al., 1991; Amit et al., 1994). Lyme disease may be associated with a painful neuropathy in adults. However, we are unaware of an instance of a Guillain-Barré syndrome–like illness in children who have Lyme disease.

Acute spinal cord lesions including tumors or transverse myelitis are other major immediate diagnostic considerations in the differential diagnosis of Guillain-Barré syndrome (Delhaas et al., 1998; Hesketh et al., 1998; Knebusch et al., 1998). Both of these disease entities may acutely produce a rapidly progressive paralysis, hyporeflexia, and back pain.

More commonly, spinal cord lesions and, rarely, Guillain-Barré syndrome are associated with early sphincter dysfunction. However, in contrast to spinal lesions, these symptoms are usually transient with Guillain-Barré syndrome (Bradshaw and Jones, 1992). Primary physicians did not initially recognize either a cord lesion or a possible Guillain-Barré syndrome in four children (Hesketh et al., 1998). Each child had severe pain, asymmetrical lower extremity weakness, and a clear-cut sensory level secondary to a malignant spinal cord tumor (Hesketh et al., 1998). Magnetic resonance images were abnormal in four of the eight children (Hesketh et al., 1998). Imaging studies may also cause confusion because of swelling and increased signal intensity of the spinal cord. In one 6-year-old child, progressive weakness and areflexia developed (Delhaas et al., 1998). Both the clinical and electromyographic findings were commensurate with a diagnosis of Guillain-Barré syndrome. However, magnetic resonance imaging demonstrated spinal cord swelling with increased signal intensity of the cord (Delhaas et al., 1998). If there is enlargement of the spinal cord and no contrast enhancement, a diagnosis of Guillain-Barré syndrome is not excluded (Delhaas et al., 1998).

We evaluated a 12-year-old child who had acute onset of leg weakness, areflexia, and back pain. Initially, EMG demonstrated absent F waves, suggesting a diagnosis of Guillain-Barré syndrome with predominant involvement at the nerve root level; however, the lack of evolving arm weakness, persistent sphincter involvement, and the more precise definition of a saddle sensory level led to a diagnosis of transverse myelitis. EMG is generally normal in transverse myelitis. Although absent F waves are one of the most common early signs of Guillain-Barré syndrome, similar findings occur with transverse myelitis when the segmental anterior horn cells are affected. In this instance, the related F waves, CMAPs, or both are also abnormal, leading to diagnostic confusion with early Guillain-Barré syndrome (Bradshaw and Jones, 1992).

Myopathies and Critical Care Neuromuscular Syndromes

Some of the various channelopathies, particularly hyperkalemic and hypokalemic periodic paralysis, always warrant consideration in the differential diagnosis of acute Guillain-Barré syndrome. These are autosomal dominant calcium or sodium channelopathies; there usually is a well-documented family history. Clinically, the episodes of paralysis are relatively short lived on most occasions. Routine needle conduction study findings are normal, but prolonged periods of exercise with electromyographic monitoring can evoke a diminution in CMAP amplitudes (McManis et al., 1986). Needle EMG often demonstrates significant myotonic-like discharges with the hyperkalemic variant. Because the presentation in

children is not significantly different from that in adults, we will not add further detail here (see Chapter 80 on channelopathies).

Occasionally, dermatomyositis develops in children relatively acutely with profound proximal weakness. More commonly, this illness has a more ingravescent temporal profile and does not require evaluation in the acute care setting. The essential electromyographic findings include the classic low-amplitude, short-duration, polyphasic motor unit potentials with very active abnormal insertion activity, including many fibrillation potentials and complex repetitive discharges. It is important to recall that perifascicular atrophy is the essential neuropathological change secondary to the underlying primary immunovasculitic pathophysiological mechanism. Therefore, the predominant electromyographic findings are often close to the surface and may be missed with more traditional electrode placement deeper in the muscle.

In children with overwhelming sepsis (Bolton et al., 1986) or status asthmaticus (Goulden et al., 1989) and those who have undergone organ transplantation, a *critical illness neuromuscular syndrome* sometimes develops. The severity of this disorder sometimes mimics a hospital-acquired Guillain-Barré syndrome. These children often present with a failure to wean from the respirator (Sheth et al., 1995; Goulden et al., 1989; Lacomis et al., 2000). The initial work of Bolton and associates (1986) suggested that these were secondary to a polyneuropathy (Bolton et al., 1986). However, a myopathy appears to be the more common of the two processes (Lacomis et al., 2000). Serum creatine kinase levels may be mildly elevated or even normal. In one study of 14 patients with intensive care unit myopathy, only 3 of 14 patients had an elevated creatine kinase level (Lacomis et al., 2000).

EMG demonstrates CMAPs that are sometimes mildly diminished in amplitude with normal motor nerve conduction velocities. Motor unit potentials are often very abnormal with increased percentages of low-amplitude, short-duration, and, at times, polyphasic motor unit potentials. Scattered fibrillation potentials are present on needle insertion. These findings are similar to an inflammatory myopathy, especially noting that the abnormal motor unit potentials are best defined on the surface of the muscle fiber. However, muscle biopsy demonstrates thick filament fiber loss typical of a critical care myopathy. These critical care motor syndromes were initially considered to be a primary neuromuscular transmission defect, but that is relatively uncommon. Nevertheless, we recently evaluated a 5-month-old child with failure to wean who had a very rare congenital neuromuscular transmission disorder.

CONCLUSIONS

When an acute flaccid paralysis develops in infants and children, EMG provides a very useful diagnostic modality to assess a number of primary motor unit lesions; these include some syndromes that are unusual for the electromyographer who usually conducts studies in adults, especially infantile botulism. We question whether this illness is more common than currently recognized. This is particularly relevant among babies with acute indeterminate respiratory distress. Guillain-Barré syndrome is another example of a possibly underrecognized illness in the evaluation of the floppy infant syndrome. There are some cases with an intrauterine onset (Rolfs and Bolik, 1994; Jackson et al., 1996; Luijckx et al., 1997). At times, the clinical presentations of these acute pediatric motor unit disorders mimic various central nervous system lesions; these include encephalopathies (Bradshaw and Jones, 2001) and those that mimic brain death, such as an axonal form of Guillain-Barré syndrome (Bakshi et al., 1997) or even infantile botulism. In addition, Guillain-Barré syndrome may mimic spinal cord lesions, such as transverse myelitis and spinal cord tumors (Delhaas et al., 1998; Hesketh et al., 1998; Knebusch et al., 1998). Therefore, the clinician must always keep the use of EMG in mind in the intensive care setting when dealing with an acute generalized weakness in any infant or older child.

References

Amit R, Parker M, Newman G, et al: Guillain-Barré syndrome in an immunosuppressed child. Pediatr Neurol 1994;11:107.

Bakshi N, Maselli R, Gospe SM, et al: Fulminating demyelinating neuropathy mimicking cerebral death. Muscle Nerve 1997;20:1595–1597.

Beausoleil JL, Nordgren RE, Modlin JF: Vaccine associated paralytic poliomyelitis. J Child Neurol 1994;9:334–335.

Bolton CF: Electromyography in the acute care setting. In Jones HR, Bolton CF, Harper CM (eds): Pediatric Clinical Electromyography. Philadelphia, Lippincott-Raven, 1996; 445–466.

Bolton CF, Hahn A, Hinton GG: The syndrome of high stimulation threshold and low conduction velocity. Ann Neurol 1988;24:165

Bolton CF, Laverty DA, Brown JD, et al: Critically ill polyneuropathy: Electrophysiological studies and differentiation from Guillain-Barré syndrome. J Neurol Neurosurg Psychiatry 1986;49:563–573.

Bradshaw DY, Jones HR Jr: Guillain-Barré syndrome in children: Clinical course, electrodiagnosis and prognosis. Muscle Nerve 1992;15:500–506.

Bradshaw DY, Jones HR: Pseudoencephalopathic Guillain-Barre syndrome. J Child Neurol 2001;16:505–508.

Centers for Disease Control and Prevention: Recommendations of the advisory committee on immunization practices: Revised recommendations for routine poliomyelitis vaccination. MMWR 1999;48:590.

Cherington M, Snyder RD: Tick paralysis: Neurophysiologic studies. N Engl J Med 1968;278:95–97.

Clay SA, Ramseyer JC, Fishman LS, Sedgwick RP: Acute infantile motor unit disorder: Infantile botulism? Arch Neurol 1977;34:236–249.

Coker SB: Leigh disease presenting as Guillain-Barré syndrome. Pediatr Neurol 1993;9:61–63.

Cooper BJ, Spence I: Temperature-dependent inhibition of evoked acetylcholine release in tick paralysis. Nature 1976;263:693–695.

Cornblath DR, Sladky JT, Sumner AJ: Clinical electrophysiology of infantile botulism. Muscle Nerve 1983;6:448–452.

Darras BJ, Jones HR: Diagnosis of neuromuscular disorders in the era of DNA analysis: The role of pediatric electromyography. Pediatr Neurol 2000;23:289–300.

David WS, Doyle JJ: Acute infantile weakness: A case of vaccine associated poliomyelitis. Muscle Nerve 1997;20:747–749.

David WS, Jones HR Jr: Electromyography and biopsy correlation with suggested protocol for the evaluation of the floppy infant. Muscle Nerve 1994;15:424–431.

Delhaas T, Kamphuis DJ, Witkamp TD: Transitory spinal cord swelling in a 6-year-old boy with Guillain-Barre syndrome. Pediatr Radiol 1998;28:544–546.

DiMauro S, Hartlage PL: Fatal infantile form of muscle phosphorylase deficiency. Neurology 1978;28:1124–1129.

Dirik E, Uysal KM: Organophosphate-induced delayed polyneuropathy. Pediatr Neurol 1994;11:111.

Donat JR, Donat JF: Tick paralysis with persistent weakness and electromyographic abnormalities. Arch Neurol 1981;38:59–61.

Donley DK, Knight P, Tenorio G, Oh SJ: A patient with infant botulism, improving with edrophonium. Muscle Nerve 1991;41:201.

Fakadej AV, Gutmann L: Prolongation of post-tetanic facilitation in infant botulism. Muscle Nerve 1982;5:727–729.

Felz MW, Smith CD, Swift TR: A six-year-old girl with tick paralysis. N Engl J Med 2000;342:90–94.

Goulden KJ, Dooley JM, Peters S, Ronen GM: Critical illness polyneuropathy: A reversible cause of paralysis in asthmatic children. Ann Neurol 1989;26:451.

Graf WD, Chance PF, Lensch W, et al: Severe vincristine neuropathy in Charcot-Marie-Tooth disease type 1A. Cancer 1996;77:1356–1362.

Grattan-Smith PJ, Morris JG, Johnston HM, et al: Clinical and neurophysiologic features of tick paralysis. Brain 1997;121:1975–1987.

Gutierrez AR, Bodensteiner J, Gutmann L: Electrodiagnosis of infantile botulism. J Child Neurol 1994;9:362–365.

Haller JS, Fabara JA: Tick paralysis: Case report with emphasis on neurological toxicity. Am J Dis Child 1972;124:915–917.

Hart DE, Rojas LA, Rosariio JA, et al: Childhood Guillain-Barré syndrome in Paraguay, 1990 to 1991. Ann Neurol 1994;36:859–863.

Hays RM, Michaud LJ: Neonatal myasthenia gravis: Specific advantages of repetitive stimulation over edrophonium testing. Pediatr Neurol 1988;4;245–247.

Hesketh E, Eden OB, Gattamaneni HR, et al: Spinal cord compression—do we miss it? Acta Paediatr 1998;87:452–454.

Hoffman RE, Pincomb BJ, Skeels MR: Type F infant botulism. Am J Dis Child 1982;136:270–271.

Honavar M, Tharakan KJ, Hughes RAC, et al: A clinicopathological study of the Guillain-Barré syndrome: Nine cases and literature review. Brain 1991;114:1245–1269.

Jackson AH, Baquis GD, Shaw BL: Congenital Guillain-Barre syndrome. J Child Neurol 1996;5:407–410.

Jones HR, Darras B: Acute care pediatric electromyography. Muscle Nerve 2000;23:S56–63.

Jones HR: Guillain-Barre syndrome: Perspectives with infants and children. Semin Pediatr Neurol 2000;7:91–102.

Jones HR: Childhood Guillain-Barre syndrome: A review: Clinical presentation, diagnosis and therapy. J Child Neurol 1996;11:4–12.

Jones HR: Evaluation of the floppy infant. In Jones HR, Bolton CF, Harper CM (eds): Pediatric Clinical Electromyography. Philadelphia, Lippincott-Raven, 1996; 37–104.

Kincaid JC: Tick bite paralysis. Semin Neurol 1990;10:32–34.

Knebusch M, Strassburg HM, Reiners K: Acute transverse myelitis in childhood: Nine cases and review of the literature. Dev Med Child Neurol 1998;40:631–639.

Kuntz NL, Daube JR: Electrophysiology of congenital myotonic dystrophy. AAEE Course E 1984; 23.

Lacomis D, Zochodne DW, Bird SJ: Critical illness myopathy. Muscle Nerve 2000;23:1785–1788.

Lefvert AK, Osterman PO: Newborn infants to myasthenic mothers: A clinical study and an investigation of acetylcholine receptor antibodies in 17 children. Neurology 1983;33:133–138.

Lipsitz PJ: The clinical and biochemical effects of excess magnesium in the newborn. Pediatrics 1971;47:501–509.

Luijckx J, Vies J, de Baet M, et al: Guillain-Barre syndrome in mother and child. Lancet 1997;349:27.

McKhann GM, Cornblath DR, Ho T, et al: Clinical and electrophysiologic aspects of acute paralytic disease of children and young adults in northern China. Lancet 1991;338:593–597.

McManis PG, Lambert EH, Daube J: The exercise test in periodic paralysis. Muscle Nerve 1986;9:704–710.

Mullaney P, Vajsar J, Smith R, Buncic JR: The natural history and ophthalmic involvement in childhood myasthenia gravis at the hospital for sick children. Ophthalmology 2000;107:504–510.

Papazian O: Transient neonatal myasthenia gravis. J Child Neurol 1992;7:135–141.

Pasternak JF, Fulling K, Nelson J, Prensky AL: An infant with chronic, relapsing polyneuropathy responsive to steroids. Dev Med Child Neurol 1982;24:504–524.

Pickett J, Berg B, Chaplin E, Brunstetter-Shafer M-A: Syndrome of botulism in infancy: Clinical and electrophysiologic study. N Engl J Med 1976;295:770–772.

Price L, Gominak S, Raphael SA, et al: Acute demyelinating polyneuropathy in childhood human immunodeficiency virus infection [abstract]. Ann Neurol 1990;28:459–460.

Price L, Raphael SA, Lischner HW, et al: Inflammatory, demyelinating polyneuropathy in a child with symptomatic human immunodeficiency virus infection. J Pediatr 1991;118:242–245.

Robbins FC: Eradication of polio in the Americas. JAMA 1993;270: 1857–1859.

Rolfs A, Bolik A: Guillain-Barré syndrome in pregnancy reflections on immunopathogenesis. Acta Neurol Scand 1994;89:400–492.

Schwartz RH, Eng G: Infant botulism: Exacerbation by aminoglycosides. Am J Dis Child 1982;136:952.

Sheth RD, Lotz BP, Hecox KE, Waclawik AJ: Infantile botulism: Pitfalls in diagnosis. J Child Neurol 1999;14:156–158.

Sheth RD, Pryse-Phillips WEM, Riggs JE, Bodensteiner JB: Critical illness neuromuscular disease in children manifested as ventilatory dependence. J Pediatr 1995;126:259–261.

Shukla AY, Marsh W, Green JB, Hurst D: Neonatal botulism. Neurology 1991;41(Suppl 1):202.

Sokal MM, Koenigsberger MR, Rose JS, et al: Neonatal hypermagnesemia and the meconium-plug syndrome. N Engl J Med 1972; 286:823–825.

Swift TR, Ignacio OJ, Dyken PR: Neonatal dystrophica myotonica: Electrophysiologic studies. Am J Dis Child 1975;129:734–737.

Swift TR, Ignacio OJ: Tick paralysis: Electrophysiologic studies. Neurology 1975;25:1130–1133.

Swoboda K, Specht L, Jones HR, et al: Infantile phosphofructokinase deficiency with arthrogryposis clinical benefit using a ketogenic diet. Pediatrics 1997;131:932–934.

Thompson JA, Glasgow LA, Warpinski JR, Olson C: Infant botulism: Clinical spectrum and epidemiology. Pediatrics 1980;66: 936–942.

SECTION **XXIV**

CENTRAL MOTOR DISORDERS

CHAPTER **97**

Voluntary Movement Disorders

Alfredo Berardelli and Antonio Currà

To produce a voluntary movement, the human nervous system must solve two problems: the first is to prepare the movement, and the second is to execute it. Disorders of voluntary movement commonly alter motor preparation or motor execution, or both. During the motor preparation phase, the nervous system has to plan the movement and code the motor programs; during movement execution, it transforms the motor commands into action. The modern laboratory can study voluntary movements by analyzing the ongoing electromyographic (EMG) activity and various kinematic variables, including reaction time, movement time, velocity, and acceleration of the moving limb.

Kinematic studies conducted for clinical and research purposes usually classify voluntary movements as follows: simple or complex (according to the complexity of the motor action and the trajectory), single-joint or multijoint (according to the number of joints activated), fast and slow (according to the speed and accuracy requirements), and externally triggered or self-initiated (according to the modality of execution).

MOTOR PREPARATION

Normal Subjects

Movement initiation involves motor planning (the selection of a suitable motor strategy) and motor programming (the assembly of motor commands for specifying the kinematic variables). The usual way of investigating initiation for a voluntary movement is to study the reaction time.

The *reaction time* is the time elapsing between the go stimulus and the onset of a voluntary movement. Reaction time paradigms investigate two situations: simple reaction time and choice reaction time. In the *simple reaction time* condition, before receiving the go signal, the subject receives full information on the motor task. The movement can therefore be fully planned in advance, and the motor program can be stored in memory until the appearance of the go signal (Fig. 97–1). The *choice reaction time* condition has at least two possible stimuli that require two distinct responses. Before moving, sub-

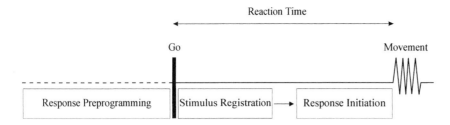

Figure 97–1. Diagram of the processing stages involved in a simple reaction time task.

jects have only partial advance information on the movement variables, and the remaining information is delivered together with the go signal. Part of the programming process therefore occurs during the reaction time (Fig. 97–2). In normal subjects, the choice reaction time is always longer than the simple reaction time. The time difference is related to the difficulty in generating the correct response or to the complexity of the required motor task. The stages of movement processing differ in simple and choice reaction time paradigms. Simple reaction time tasks require the motor set to recognize the stimulus and then immediately initiate a preprogrammed response. Choice reaction time tasks require the motor set to recognize the stimulus and immediately select, program, and initiate the response. Simple and choice reaction time tasks can be simplified by cuing the forthcoming movement. In the simple reaction time tasks, the movement is already programmed, and therefore the precue is only a warning signal with a general alerting effect that speeds up the motor response. Choice reaction time can be partially cued or fully cued, depending on the amount of advance information given before the starting signal. In cued choice reaction time tasks, when the precue provides complete advance information about the required response and the subjects are given sufficient time to process this information (fully cued choice reaction time), the preparatory processes of recognizing the stimulus and selecting and programming the response are unified, as they are in the simple reaction time.

In normal subjects, the reaction time varies from 200 to 500 ms according to the complexity of the task. Pascual-Leone and colleagues (1992a) expanded a theoretical model of response preparation (Requin, 1985; Gratton et al., 1988) to explain how the motor system prepares the response to delineate the various phases of the reaction time. These investigators divided the processes required for movement preparation into a stimulus evaluation system, a task-specific circuitry, and a response channel. The stimulus evaluation system has to detect, interpret, and extract information from the stimulus in order for the motor response to occur. It completes these processes in the *time for recognition*. The task-specific circuitry prepares the motor program for the required motor response, holds it in memory, and then transfers it to the response channel. All these processes take place during the *time of initiation*. The response channel produces the motor response in the *time of development*. The relative involvement of the various systems obviously varies according to the type of reaction time task. In simple reaction time paradigms, the task-specific circuitry is completed in advance, and the prepared motor program is stored in memory until it is transferred to the response channel for movement execution. In cued reaction time paradigms, the cuing signal to detect the go stimulus prepares the stimulus evaluation system. This preactivation is subserved by attentional processes. Although the stimulus evaluation system, the task-specific system, and the response channel are not necessarily activated serially, the various reaction time phases (i.e., recognition, initiation, and development) are completed serially.

The changes in the duration of reaction time in-

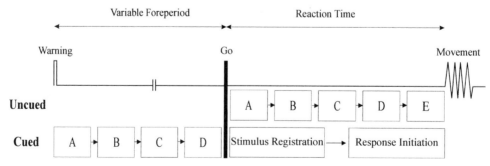

Figure 97–2. Diagrams of the various motor processing stages involved in cued and uncued choice reaction time tasks. In the diagram for the uncued choice reaction time task, *A* indicates the processing stage for identifying the go stimulus (stimulus identification), *B* indicates the mapping processing stage for the go stimulus with the possible motor responses (stimulus response mapping), *C* indicates the processing stage for selecting the response (response selection), and *D* indicates the processing stage for programming the response (response programming). In the diagram for the cued choice reaction time task, *A* indicates the processing stage of warning stimulus identification, *B* indicates the processing stage for warning stimulus and response mapping, *C* indicates the processing stage for response selection, and *D* indicates the processing stage for response preprogramming.

duced by increasing the complexity of the motor task provide useful information on motor programming. When the number of submovements in the motor sequence is increased, the subject takes longer to initiate motor execution (the sequence length effect on reaction time). Normal subjects show a sequence length effect proportionate to the complexity of the required motor sequence (Rafal et al., 1987; Stelmach et al., 1987).

Studies in humans have shown that reaction time tasks activate cortical motor areas. During the first part of the reaction time—after the go signal—the motor cortex remains unexcitable, whereas during the second part motor cortical excitability increases (Starr et al., 1988). In normal subjects, subthreshold cortical magnetic shocks delivered shortly before or after the go signal shorten the duration of reaction time to auditory, visual, and somatosensory stimuli (Pascual-Leone et al., 1992b). They do so by activating the corticocortical connections and thus transferring the motor program from the task-specific circuitry to the response channel earlier or faster.

Another way of investigating the neurophysiological mechanisms underlying reaction time in humans is to assess the various regions of the cerebral cortex by neuroimaging techniques. Using positron emission tomography to measure the regional cerebral blood flow as an index of cerebral activity, Deiber and associates investigated cortical activation during delayed motor reaction time paradigms (Deiber et al., 1996). Motor preparation invariably led to increased flow in the contralateral frontal cortex (sensorimotor, premotor, cingulate, and supplementary motor cortex), the contralateral parietal association cortex (anterior and posterior regions), the ipsilateral cerebellum, the contralateral basal ganglia, and the thalamus. The internal selection of movement preferentially activated the anterior part of the supplementary motor area. The regional cerebral blood flow increased in the anterior parietal cortex (Brodmann's area 40) according to the differing amounts of movement information processed, a finding suggesting that this area is involved in the use of visual instructions contained in the preparatory signal. The greater activation of the posterior parietal cortex (Brodmann's area 7) during conditions of restricted advance information suggests its involvement in guiding the spatial attention to the response signal and in selecting the correct movement. The nonprimary motor areas (i.e., premotor cortex, cingulate cortex, and supplementary motor area) had a similar degree of activation regardless of the level of preparation. The nonprimary motor areas may therefore participate in the anatomical substrate for motor preparation independent of the information context.

Parkinson's Disease

Although some studies have reported normal simple reaction time in patients with *Parkinson's disease*

(Zimmermann et al., 1992; Harrison et al., 1993; Revonsuo et al., 1993), most showed that simple reaction time is prolonged (Heilman et al., 1976; Evarts et al., 1981; Rafal et al., 1984; Bloxham et al., 1987; Sheridan et al., 1987; Jahanshahi et al., 1992;). Choice reaction time studies provided equally contradictory results. Some researchers reported that the choice reaction time is normal (Evarts et al., 1981; Bloxham et al., 1984; Mayeux et al., 1987; Sheridan et al., 1987; Rafal et al., 1989), whereas others found it increased (Wiesendanger et al., 1969; Lichter et al., 1988; Reid et al., 1989; Jahanshahi et al., 1992; Praamstra et al., 1996). More recently, Kutukcu and coworkers studied simple and choice reaction time tasks of differing complexity in patients with Parkinson's disease (Kutukcu et al., 1999). These investigators found longer reaction times in patients than in controls in all tasks, but particularly in the more difficult tasks, with a greater percentage change in relative magnitude in the more complex choice tasks than in simple reaction time tasks.

Exactly why patients with Parkinson's disease have prolonged reaction times is difficult to explain (Harrison et al., 1995). The observation that the delayed reaction time was improved when the go signal in reaction time tasks was preceded by a warning stimulus that had a general alerting effect (Bloxham et al., 1987; Jahanshahi et al., 1993) excluded nonspecific disturbances of arousal (Heilman et al., 1976; Jahanshahi et al., 1992). Because the motor task is known in advance in simple reaction time studies, the slowed simple reaction time may have depended on a parkinsonian-induced deficit in preprogramming (Evarts et al., 1981; Bloxham et al., 1987; Sheridan et al., 1987; Pullman et al., 1988).

A preprogramming deficit may depend at least in part on the amount of information provided by a preparatory signal and the time available to process it. When patients with Parkinson's disease had to preprogram motor responses, they made normal use of the precues (Stelmach et al., 1986; Jahanshahi et al., 1992). In a set of experiments designed to give precues at various intervals before the go signal, Jahanshahi and colleagues showed that when full advance information was given about the required response, normal subjects and patients could reduce the duration of the fully cued choice reaction time to that of the simple reaction time, but patients needed longer to process the information (Jahanshahi et al., 1992). Therefore, given sufficient time, patients with Parkinson's disease could preprogram the motor responses, but they still had slowed reaction times. The simple reaction time slowing in Parkinson's disease therefore involves the processing step of response initiation, whereas the choice reaction time slowing must also involve other processing steps (Jahanshahi et al., 1992, 1993).

Praamstra and associates used a movement precuing task to study the spatial and temporal distributions of movement-related potentials (Praamstra et al., 1996). Subjects were required to execute precued and uncued movements involving the middle and index fingers of the left or right hand. Cued and uncued reaction times were both slower in patients with Parkinson's disease than in controls. In both groups, the advance information provided by the precue reduced the reaction time similarly. Recording motor-related potentials including the lateralized motor readiness potential and the EMG activity, Praamstra and coworkers found that the lateralized motor readiness potential and the EMG onset began earlier for cued than for uncued movements (Praamstra et al., 1996). For cued movements, the lateralized motor readiness potential occurred even earlier in patients than in controls, a finding indicating that patients used advance information as effectively as the controls. For uncued movements, the lateralized motor readiness potential time delay in patients was small and was similar in duration to the EMG onset delay. The sum of the time delays accounted for the reaction time difference between groups. Overall, these findings indicated that the prolonged reaction time in Parkinson's disease may be related to a central delay, possibly because of the later initiation of motor cortex activity. This interpretation is in line with the finding of longer premovement excitability buildup in patients with Parkinson's disease (Pascual-Leone et al., 1994a).

Other possible mechanisms responsible for reaction time slowing in Parkinson's disease include difficulty in holding in memory or delivering appropriate motor programs in response to the go signal. To address this problem, Labutta and colleagues used a delayed response paradigm to study the storage of motor programs (Labutta et al., 1994). They asked parkinsonian patients to point to a target light that could be displayed either throughout the period preceding the go signal or for a brief interval followed by a delay before the go signal. These experiments showed that parkinsonian patients could hold a motor program in memory normally. Delayed responses in patients have been interpreted as indicating a disturbance in the cerebral processing of the auditory stimuli after their occurrence and before the initiation of motor activity (Kutukcu et al., 1999). One hypothesis (Berry et al., 1999) suggested that the slowed response speed may result from attentional deficits occurring only in patients who had additional frontal lobe impairment. In a study of patients with Parkinson's disease with and without frontal dysfunction and a matched control group, the investigators therefore used tests of visual attention designed to dissociate baseline response speed from central information processing speed (Berry et al., 1999). All groups had similar error rates, and a generalized slowing of response time was present only in those parkinsonian patients who had additional frontal lobe impairment, confirming previous findings (Harrison et al., 1993).

Pascual-Leone and coworkers reported that transcranial magnetic stimulation (TMS) of the motor cortex of the motor cortex improved the simple reaction time in patients with Parkinson's disease (Pascual-Leone et al., 1994a). The task consisted of a rapid elbow flexion in response to a visual go signal. Subthreshold TMS of the motor cortex was randomly delivered to the motor cortex contralateral to the moving limb at varying delays after the go signal. As in normal subjects (Pascual-Leone et al., 1992b), TMS of the motor cortex shortens the reaction time primarily by influencing the time of initiation. Pascual-Leone and colleagues suggested that in patients with Parkinson's disease, TMS of the motor cortex shortens reaction time by reducing the time needed for movement initiation and development (Pascual-Leone et al., 1994a). The same researchers also studied the effects of repetitive TMS of the motor cortex on choice reaction time, movement time, and error rate in a serial reaction time task in patients with Parkinson's disease (Pascual-Leone et al., 1994b). In normal subjects, subthreshold 5-Hz repetitive TMS of the motor cortex left choice reaction time almost unchanged and slightly shortened the movement time, but increased the error rate. In the patients, repetitive TMS of the motor cortex significantly shortened choice reaction time and movement time without affecting the error rate. In normal subjects who had no premovement excitability buildup defect, the accelerated transfer of the motor program to the response channel increased the error rate because the subjects prematurely chose the wrong motor response before they had completely discriminated the go signal. Conversely, in patients with Parkinson's disease, repetitive TMS of the motor cortex, by accelerating the abnormally slow buildup of premovement cortical excitability, reduced the choice reaction time without inducing premature selection of wrong responses.

Changes in reaction time in Parkinson's disease have also been studied during preparation for motor sequences. Rafal and associates investigated the programming of sequential finger movements in patients with Parkinson's disease (Rafal et al., 1987). They analyzed the sequence length effect on reaction time by investigating a one-step movement (pressing key with the index finger), a two-step sequence (pressing key first with the index and then with the ring finger), and a three-step sequence (pressing key with the index finger, then the ring finger, and finally the middle finger). The absence of a sequence length effect indicated that the first submovement of the sequence was executed independent of the programming requirements of the other components. In contrast, an abnormally long sequence length effect indicated slowed processing of preparatory mechanisms. Reaction times for initiating the first movement of the three tasks were longer in the patients. However, patients with Parkinson's disease showed a normal sequence length effect. During the sequential tasks studied, in patients and controls the interresponse latencies between submovements were shorter than the reaction times. Analysis of the interresponse latencies led the investigators to conclude that the programming of sequential movement was normal in Parkinson's disease. In contrast, studying a group of parkinsonian patients who were performing serial taps with the index finger with an increasing number of movements, Stelmach and coworkers had opposite results (Stelmach et al., 1987). Their patients, unlike normal subjects, showed no sequence length effect in a task of repetitive finger taps. This finding provided evidence of a programming deficit in parkinsonian disease. To clarify these inconsistent results, Harrington and Haaland examined motor programming before and during the execution of repetitive and nonrepetitive sequences requiring an increasing number of hand movements (Harrington and Haaland, 1991). For all tasks, subjects received complete information on the type of sequence they had to perform during a delay interval preceding the starting signal. Regardless of whether the sequence was nonrepetitive or repetitive, reaction time shortened similarly in both groups as the duration of the delay interval increased, a finding indicating the normal use of advance information to initiate motor sequences in Parkinson's disease. In contrast, the first interresponse time, that is, the interval from the end of the reaction time to that of the first response, was shortened as a function of the delay interval only in the patients. The observation that the first response and not the overall complexity of the sequence benefited from additional time suggested a specific deficit in programming the first response in parkinsonian patients.

The findings reviewed earlier make it clear that reaction time is a composite measure of response speed that depends on the complex intervention of attentional, perceptual, and motor operations. The preparatory activities operating during reaction time include stimulus processing, the use of working memory for the retrieval of stimulus mappings, and the generation of predictions and decision making. The ability of reaction time measures to detect changes in specific processes depends on the experimental manipulation of task variables including medication effect (Harrison et al., 1995). Whether a reaction time task is capable of detecting abnormalities in the subjects studied depends on the type of movement studied, its planning requirements, and the complexity of the response (owing to stimulus decoding, compatibility matching, and selecting the correct motor program).

Huntington's Disease

Nearly all studies investigating motor initiation in patients with *Huntington's disease* have found slowed reaction times (Girotti et al., 1988; Jahanshahi et al., 1993; Georgiou et al., 1995; Sprengelmeyer et al., 1995; Tsai et al., 1995). Slowed reaction times have also been found in complex movements such as three-dimensional sequential rapid arm movements in response to external cues (Currà et al., 2000a).

Jahanshahi and colleagues studied simple reaction time and choice reaction time for single movements and found that patients had similarly delayed motor responses in both tasks (Jahanshahi et al., 1993). By providing a warning signal before the tasks, these investigators showed that patients with Huntington's disease used advance information. The next question was whether patients with Huntington's disease relied on advance information. In a study of serial choice reaction time tasks, a pathway of illuminated lights was presented along a response board that presented two-choice points at each of 10 sequential pairs of buttons (Georgiou et al., 1995). Subjects were required to press the illuminated buttons along the board as quickly as possible while advance visual information on the forthcoming presses was systematically and increasingly reduced by extinguishing an increasing number of consecutive buttons as the current button was released. Although patients with Huntington's disease were slow in initiating and executing the sequential presses during the three conditions, they showed added difficulty only when advance information was moderately or highly reduced. Hence patients with Huntington's disease apparently rely heavily on external cues to guide initiation and performance of sequential movements.

No definitive conclusion on slowed reaction times in patients with Huntington's disease can ignore the cognitive processes involved in motor preparation and occurring during the reaction time, for example, selective attention. Girotti and associates investigated the relationship between motor and cognitive impairment in nondemented patients with Huntington's disease (Girotti et al., 1988). Nearly all of the cognitive and motor functions studied were severely impaired. Slowed reaction time and movement time correlated with cognitive impairment, whereas hyperkinesia did not. Prolonged reaction time and movement time therefore seem to be important signs in Huntington's disease and proceed at the same rate as mental decay. In a study designed to compare frontal and parietal lobe functions, Tsai and coworkers concluded that slowed reaction time in Huntington's disease depends on factors other than the inability to direct visual attention (Tsai et al., 1995).

The studies reviewed earlier point to the delayed reaction time as a definite kinematic abnormality in patients with Huntington's disease. Whether the slowed motor responses reflect a pure motor abnormality or result from the influence of concurrent factors (motor, cognitive, and attentional failure) is still unclear.

Dystonia

Only a few studies have investigated motor reaction time tasks in patients with *dystonia*. Inzelberg and colleagues studied arm-reaching movements of the upper limb to targets placed distally and proximally (Inzelberg et al., 1995). The task, holding a stylus, consisted of movements confined to the elbow joint accomplished with and without visual feedback of the moving limb. In both visual and nonvisual feedback conditions, patients showed normal reaction time during movements to both targets. Patients and normal subjects had shorter reaction times for proximal targets than for distal targets, a finding confirming that in a reaction time paradigm, the type of motor task but not the visual feedback influences movement preparation. Useful data on reaction times in patients with dystonia also come from studies primarily designed to investigate a premotor potential called *contingent negative variation* and recorded during stimulus response paradigms. Kaji and associates reported normal reaction time for head rotations and finger extensions in patients with cervical dystonia (Kaji et al., 1995), and Ikeda and coworkers reported similar reaction times for wrist extension in normal subjects and patients with writer's cramp (Ikeda et al., 1996).

To investigate whether the type of movement cuing influences the motor performance in dystonia, Currà and colleagues studied zig-zag motor sequences performed by externally cuing each submovement separately (sequential reaction times) or by externally cuing only the first submovement (single reaction time for a complex movement) (Currà et al., 2000b). The investigators compared sequential and single rapid arm movements executed in three-dimensional space in patients with generalized or focal dystonia (see also the discussion of motor execution). Patients with focal dystonia had normal reaction times in all the tasks studied. Patients with generalized dystonia had normal reaction times for single and complex movements. However, when the motor task required sequential motor responses, patients had slower reaction times for each submovement. Similar reaction times in the single and complex tasks suggested that patients coped normally with an increasing programming load. The investigators attributed the slowed serial reaction times to an impaired motor set, the function that enables subjects to perform consecutive submovements as a sequence.

Cerebellar Disease

Early reaction time findings in patients with *cerebellar damage* come from studies designed to investigate the EMG and the kinematic variables of voluntary movements. In patients with cerebellar damage who perform elbow flexion tasks, the simple reaction time is prolonged, and the onset of the first agonist burst is delayed (Hallett et al., 1975a). Similar abnormalities have also been reported during tracking movements (Beppu et al., 1984, 1987) and arm-pointing movements (Bonnefoi-Kyriacou et al., 1995; Day et al., 1998). A prolongation of choice reaction time was also found (Jahanshahi et al., 1993; Bonnefoi-Kyriacou et al., 1995), but patients

with cerebellar disease had a normal increase in the reaction time duration from simple reaction time to choice reaction time tasks (Bonnefoi-Kyriacou et al., 1995). This latter finding suggests that the mechanisms underlying the selection of motor programs are preserved in patients with cerebellar disease. Jahanshahi and colleagues investigated precued reaction time paradigms in patients with cerebellar disease (Jahanshahi et al., 1993). Patients performed unwarned simple reaction time tasks faster than uncued and unwarned choice reaction time tasks. They also did simple reaction time and choice reaction time tasks faster when they received a warning signal before the stimulus. In addition, patients performed fully cued tasks faster than uncued choice reaction time tasks, a finding showing that they made use of the advance information.

Studying the sequence length effect on reaction time, Inhoff and colleagues analyzed the programming of motor sequences consisting of single, double, or triple key press components (Inhoff et al., 1989). Patients with mild cerebellar dysfunction increased reaction time normally with the sequence length. In contrast, patients with moderate cerebellar dysfunction showed a negligible or absent sequence length effect. These findings suggest that the integrity of cerebellar structures is necessary to schedule the programmed sequence of responses before transforming them into action.

To understand the role played by attention on motor abnormalities, Yamaguchi and coworkers recorded event-related evoked potentials and reaction time in patients with cerebellar degenerative disorders affecting mainly the lateral cerebellum (Yamaguchi et al., 1998). These investigators studied the response to valid, invalid, peripheral, and central cues. The reaction time data for central and peripheral cues showed that all subjects responded faster to valid cues than to invalid ones. Consistent with the reaction time data, the event-related evoked potential data for the central and the peripheral cue experiments showed a comparable generation of attention shift–related negativity during the cue-target interval. The early component of the event-related evoked potential, which reflects the neural activities that allocate spatial attention, changed similarly in both groups as a function of cue validity. The late negative deflection preceding the imperative target stimulus and the late sustained positivity following target presentation—components reflecting the neural activities that prepare and select the motor response—were reduced in the cerebellar group. The lateral cerebellum therefore contributes poorly to visuospatial attention shifts, but it mainly participates in the processes of response preparation and selection.

MOTOR PERFORMANCE
Normal Subjects

In 1926, Wacholder and Altenburger reported that slow movements of the upper arm were characterized by continuous EMG activity in both agonist and antagonist muscles, whereas rapid movements were characterized by alternating EMG bursts (Wacholder and Altenburger, 1926). Numerous subsequent reports confirmed that surface EMG recordings obtained during the performance of rapid, simple movements show two bursts of phasic muscle activity in the agonist muscle (first and second agonist bursts) separated by an almost complete electrical silence. During this pause, a burst of phasic activity occurs in the antagonist muscle. This pattern of EMG activity results in a smooth movement, with a bell-shaped velocity profile showing roughly equal acceleration and deceleration times (Hallett et al., 1975a; Berardelli et al., 1996) (Fig. 97–3). The EMG triphasic pattern is recorded not only during the execution of proximal or distal limb movements but also during automatic postural adjustments of the trunk. This generality means that even minor disturbances of the triphasic pattern may profoundly influence motor behavior.

The first agonist burst provides the impulse force to start the movement. In a certain range of movement amplitudes, the duration of the first agonist burst remains constant, whereas the size increases. During movements executed with increasing distances or with increasing loads, however, the duration and the size of the first agonist burst increase. To describe changes in the duration and amplitude of the first agonist burst induced by changes in movement variables, two main models have been proposed (Corcos et al., 1989; Gottlieb et al., 1989; Berardelli et al., 1996). The pulse-height control model assumes the constant duration of the input to the agonist motor neuron pool, with the amount of excitation graded only by changes in the height of the pulse. The pulse-width control model assumes a constant excitatory pulse delivered to the motor

neurons for different lengths of time. The pulse-width and the pulse-height strategies are modulated according to the kinematic requirements of the task and the physiological constraints imposed by muscle mechanisms; the result is a graduated system for performing diverse movements.

During the electrical silence between the first and second agonist bursts, the activation of the antagonist muscle produces the antagonist burst. The function of the antagonist burst is to decelerate movement. Its size is therefore adjusted for the level of force needed to halt the limb at the intended end position. This force is determined by the speed of movement, the inertia of the load, and the passive mechanical braking forces acting at the joint. The latency and duration of the antagonist burst are related to movement constraint variables (Brown and Cooke, 1981; Berardelli et al., 1996).

The second agonist burst follows the antagonist burst and is more variable than the other EMG bursts of the triphasic pattern. The latency of the second agonist burst shortens with faster movements, whereas its amplitude increases with longer movement distances. The function of the second agonist burst is to dampen oscillations stabilizing the limb at the end of the movement (Brown and Cooke, 1981, 1990; Berardelli et al., 1996).

Numerous observations support the notion that the triphasic EMG pattern originates centrally (Garland et al., 1972; Hallett et al., 1975a; Waters and Strick, 1981), although it can be modulated by afferent inputs (Rothwell et al., 1982; Sanes et al., 1985; Berardelli et al., 1996). Abnormalities of the EMG triphasic pattern result in slowness of movements, trajectory irregularities, and loss of accuracy.

Normal human motor behavior during everyday life, however, rarely consists of simple, single movements alone. It usually requires more complex, goal-

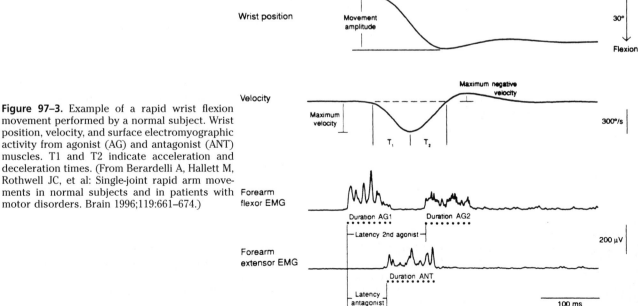

Figure 97–3. Example of a rapid wrist flexion movement performed by a normal subject. Wrist position, velocity, and surface electromyographic activity from agonist (AG) and antagonist (ANT) muscles. T1 and T2 indicate acceleration and deceleration times. (From Berardelli A, Hallett M, Rothwell JC, et al: Single-joint rapid arm movements in normal subjects and in patients with motor disorders. Brain 1996;119:661–674.)

directed arm motor acts. The activities of daily life necessitate various movements that have to be accomplished simultaneously or sequentially or both. Many movements involve numerous joints in more than one limb. In programming and performing a complex voluntary movement, the human nervous system must complete a variety of processes. First it must identify, order, and group all the responses, then program the physical variables for each response, solve the problem of how the movement ends (i.e., end-point control), and finally control switching between sequential motor acts.

A physiological insight into the performance of complex movements has also come from experiments using functional imaging techniques to describe brain activation in humans. At least four areas of the human frontomesial cortex are involved in motor control: the anterior supplementary motor area, the posterior supplementary motor area, the rostral cingulate zone, and the caudal cingulate zone. Neuroimaging data suggest that the frontomesial motor areas mediate specific functions according to the movement type (simple or sequential), the movement rate (slow or fast, rhythmic or nonrhythmic) and the mode of movement initiation (self-initiated or externally triggered) (Roland and Zilles, 1996; Deiber et al., 1999).

We now briefly report the findings in normal subjects of those kinematic variables analyzed in studies investigating complex movements in pathological conditions. The numerous neurophysiological investigations have done much to clarify the temporal and spatial processes underlying the normal execution of simultaneous and sequential movements. Studies investigating the timing of these motor tasks have shown that normal subjects perform submovements in sequential tasks and the same submovement as a simple task at similar speeds. Because the various durations of the submovements composing either the sequence or the simultaneous motor task do not correlate, the performance of the sequential or simultaneous motor task comes under the control of different motor programs that are superimposed or sequentially assembled (Benecke et al., 1986a). When normal subjects have to draw simple planar geometric figures such as lines, triangles, or squares that differ in size but belong to the same class, the movement time remains relatively constant (the isochrony principle). In addition, also during motor sequences, the duration of the single submovements remains unchanged with task completion (Berardelli et al., 1986a; Agostino et al., 1992). Finally, normal subjects always optimize the performance of rapid, complex movements. Accordingly, their movement speed is not increased by the provision of external visual or auditory cues (Georgiou et al., 1994, 1995).

Studies investigating the spatial features of voluntary movements show that when normal subjects have to move the hand toward a target on a frontal plane, they preferentially use straight trajectories independent of the movement speed or the load, and their movements characteristically yield bell-shaped velocity profiles. When required to accomplish three-dimensional, unconstrained movements, normal subjects try to restrict movement to a single plane. When they change from one movement plane to another, their movement trajectories become segmented.

Parkinson's Disease: Simple Movements

Kinematic analysis shows that unlike normal subjects, patients with Parkinson's disease are unusually slow in executing arm movements, and their difficulty increases for movements of large amplitude. Flowers reported that parkinsonian patients perform movements of different amplitude with similar velocity, whereas normal subjects increase their velocity when they execute movements of increasing amplitude (Flowers, 1975, 1976). Patients with Parkinson's disease are also slow in performing movements that require high levels of accuracy (Sheridan and Flowers, 1990), as well as when they track moving targets. Although parkinsonian patients activate agonist and antagonist muscles in the correct order, in contrast to normal subjects—who perform simple movements with a single triphasic pattern, they accomplish these movements with multiple cycles of EMG bursts (Hallett and Koshbin 1980; Berardelli et al., 1984). This finding led Hallett and Khoshbin to suggest that in Parkinson's disease the multiple cycles of EMG bursts serve to compensate for the lack of initial first agonist burst activation (Hallett and Khoshbin, 1980). By studying changes in the first agonist burst during movements of varying amplitude and load, we showed that the mechanisms that generate the first agonist bursts do not saturate in patients with Parkinson's disease, and we concluded that patients with Parkinson's disease are unable to scale first agonist burst activation according to the movement requirements (Berardelli et al., 1986b) (Fig. 97–4).

Various hypotheses have been put forward to explain the mechanisms underlying movement slowness in patients with Parkinson's disease. One is that slow movements could result from a reduced production of force (Stelmach et al., 1989). An early study designed to investigate force in patients with Parkinson's disease found that patients who were off medication had reduced strength, particularly in the extensor muscles (Corcos et al., 1996). Reduced muscle strength could therefore be one component of bradykinesia. A further hypothesis is that patients with Parkinson's disease move slowly to maintain the required level of accuracy (Sheridan and Flowers, 1990). Yet this abnormal speed-accuracy trade-off fits in poorly with the observation that parkinsonian patients move slowly even when the spatial accuracy constraints of the tasks are removed (Teasdale et al., 1990).

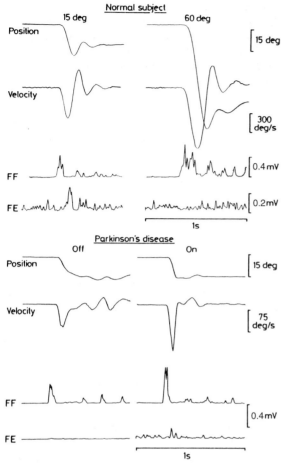

Figure 97–4. Rapid wrist movements of different amplitude in a normal subject and in a patient with Parkinson's disease (on and off therapy). The size and duration of the first agonist burst increase during movements of larger amplitude. Electromyographic signals are recorded from forearm flexor and extensor muscles. (From Berardelli A, Dick JPR, Rothwell JC, et al: Scaling of the size of the first agonist EMG burst during rapid wrist movements in patients with Parkinson's disease. J Neurol Neurosurg Psychiatry 1986;49:1273–1279.)

Parkinson's Disease: Complex Movements

Abnormalities of the triphasic EMG pattern recorded during single-joint movements correlate poorly with the clinical estimates of mobility in patients with Parkinson's disease. In addition, clinical observation shows that parkinsonian patients have greater difficulty in performing complex movements. For this reason, in clinical practice, bradykinesia is commonly assessed by testing simultaneous and sequential movements. In the Unified Parkinson's Disease Rating Scale, sequential arm movements are generally assessed by means of three repetitive tasks: finger tapping, hand opening and closing, and forearm pronation and supination. One study focused on these three sequential tasks in parkinsonian patients who were off therapy (Agostino et al., 1998). Finger, hand, and forearm tasks all test motor sequences, but they differ in the agonist and antago-

nist muscles used, the force exerted and the limb positions required for executing the movements, and the presence of relatively independent finger movements. Clinical scores showed that nearly all patients had impaired motor performance of all three tasks, but finger tapping was significantly more severely impaired than the other two tasks. Greater impairment in executing individual finger movements than gross hand movements suggests that the finger task demands finer cortical motor control or a greater cortical facilitation, both processes that in patients are defective owing to abnormal basal ganglia output.

Early studies attempting a quantitative analysis of complex movements in Parkinson's disease addressed simultaneous movements. Schwab and colleagues first observed that patients had difficulty when they were required to press a sphygmomanometer bulb repeatedly with one hand while drawing a triangle with the other (Schwab et al., 1954). Although patients accomplished the drawing task relatively well, they often interrupted the pressing task so it resulted in gaps during which patients did not press for a few seconds. Talland and Schwab asked subjects to press a tally counter with one hand while using tweezers to pick up beads with the other (Talland and Schwab, 1964). The simultaneous performance of the two tasks decreased the rate of counter pressing significantly more than the rate of bead picking. Schwab and associates coined the term *asynkinesia* to describe patients' inability to execute simultaneous motor tasks; although this term has not been adopted, various subsequent studies consistently reported that patients with Parkinson's disease had difficulty in accomplishing bimanual movements (Schwab et al., 1954). Although these early studies indicated severe temporal and spatial disruption in the organization of simultaneous movement, they may have been biased by the occurrence of learning processes or by differences in the timing or complexity of the two tasks. The experimental design of later studies took these factors into account. Benecke and co-workers required patients to perform three different types of rapid movements: an isotonic flexion of the elbow (flex), an isometric opposition of the thumb and the index finger against a strain gauge (squeeze), and an isotonic finger flexion (cut) (Benecke et al., 1986b). Movements were executed separately and were combined simultaneously in the "flex and squeeze" and the "flex and cut" tasks. The simultaneous motor tasks could be accomplished with the same arm or the two limbs. Neither in normal subjects nor in parkinsonian patients did the movement times of the two acts composing the task correlate. This finding suggests that the two motor tasks were implemented by assembling two distinct motor programs. Patients did the flex, the squeeze, and the cut tasks more slowly than controls. However, in contrast to normal subjects, when the movements executed separately were compared with those executed during the simultaneous task, in parkinsonian patients the movement speed decreased. This reduction was small when the simultaneous task involved the combination of two isotonic movements (flex and cut) and when the task was executed with the two limbs. The reduction was much larger when the task involved movements differing in the type of muscle activation (isometric versus isotonic flex and squeeze) and when the task was executed with the same limb. In patients with Parkinson's disease, the impairment in executing the simultaneous motor task is greater for more complex movements involving activation of the motor system on the same side of the brain. This deficit was related to the functional abnormality in the connection between the basal ganglia and the cortical motor areas.

By comparing the simultaneous execution of Purdue pegboard and finger button presses with the performance of each task separately, Jahanshahi and colleagues found that pegboard performance in patients with Parkinson's disease remained unchanged, whereas their finger tapping deteriorated (Jahanshahi et al., 1993). This distinction implied that patients were able to maintain performance of a task requiring visual control, whereas a repetitive non–visually guided task suffered. Oliveira and colleagues investigated whether the size of movement changed when parkinsonian patients were distracted by a secondary task other than a motor task (Oliveira et al., 1998). Patients had to make a lexical decision during paced and unpaced repeated oppositions of the thumb and forefinger. When they did both tasks together, patients with Parkinson's disease executed hypometric movements, and the movement amplitude further decreased. In addition, movements were more undershot during the unpaced motor task. At first glance, this finding suggested that because the unpaced task was less automatic for patients with Parkinson's disease than for normal subjects, it was more prone to interference from a secondary task. Johnson and associates investigated the bimanual coordination of patients with Parkinson's disease (Johnson et al., 1998). These investigators required subjects to perform a bimanual cranking task at different speeds (1 and 2 Hz) and phase relationships (in-phase, antiphase). Both patients and normal subjects were able to perform the bimanual in-phase movement on a pair of cranks at fast and slow speeds. When coping with the antiphase movements, in which rotation of the cranks differed by 180 degrees, patients with Parkinson's disease were unable to perform the asymmetrical antiphase movement at either speed and reverted to the in-phase symmetrical movement. In addition, whereas an external timing cue given before in-phase movements helped them to perform the movement more accurately, a cue given before antiphase movements facilitated patients' tendency to revert to the more symmetrical, in-phase movements.

The conclusion from studies on simultaneous movements is that patients with Parkinson's disease

have extra difficulty when they have to run two motor programs simultaneously, particularly when the motor tasks involve the same arm. This abnormality indicates an inability to superimpose motor programs for separate joint movements that is out of proportion to the difficulty in performing the single movements separately.

An experimental motor task similar to that described for simultaneous movements has been used for investigating sequential arm movements. Benecke and coworkers instructed patients to squeeze with the right hand and then flex with the right elbow, to squeeze the left hand and then flex with the right elbow, to cut with the right hand and then flex with the right elbow, and flex the right elbow and then squeeze the right hand (Benecke et al., 1987a). Subjects had to move as rapidly as possible and to start the second movement immediately after terminating the first. Finally, they also did each submovement separately. The kinematic variables measured were the duration of movement, the time interval between the onset of the first and the onset of the second movement (interonset latency), and the time elapsing between movements, that is, the pause. In patients and controls, the durations of movements and pauses in each pair of motor tasks were not correlated, and this finding indicated that the sequential movements were guided not by a common motor plan, but by two separate motor programs. The interonset latency proved critical in determining the faster performance of the second movement in normal subjects, because normal subjects produced slower movements for interonset latency that were shorter than 200 ms. This finding indicated that normal subjects automatically switch between subsequent motor tasks with an optimal minimal delay. In parkinsonian patients, this switching process was slowed, so interonset latency and pauses increased (Fig. 97–5). Benecke and colleagues concluded that there is a disturbance in running two motor programs sequentially in patients with Parkinson's disease (Benecke et al., 1987a), an abnormality that can be improved by dopaminergic treatment (Benecke et al., 1987b). When we investigated rapid two-joint arm movements during the continuous tracing of triangles and squares of different sizes, we found that patients were slower in tracing the geometrical patterns and paused longer at the vertices. When normal subjects traced each side of the figure, the EMG recording showed a single burst of activity in the agonist and antagonist muscles; however, when patients did the same tasks, the EMG showed a larger number of bursts, which did not correlate with the number of sides in the geometric figures. Because of the different pattern of combination of shoulder and arm muscles in tracing sides at various positions of figures, we concluded that subjects had to assemble more than one motor program during tracing. The prolonged pauses at the vertices reflected parkinsonian patients' difficulty in switching from one program to another (Berardelli et al., 1986a).

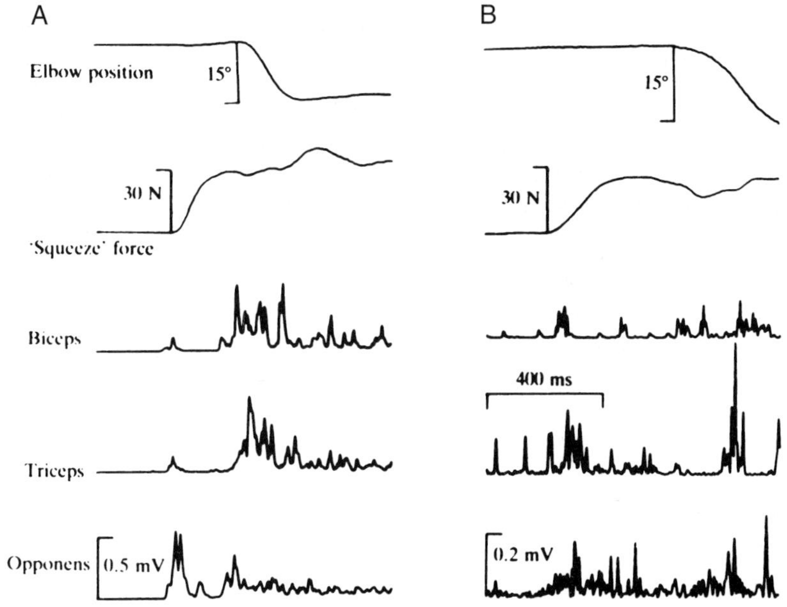

A   B

Figure 97–5. Unilateral "squeeze then flex" task in a normal subject *(A)* and in a patient with Parkinson's disease *(B)*. From *top to bottom,* force tracings and rectified electromyographic activity. Movement time and interonset latency are prolonged in the patient. (From Benecke R, Rothwell JC, Dick JPR, et al: Disturbance of sequential movements in patients with Parkinson's disease. Brain 1987;110:361–379.)

Simple clinical examination of common sequential limb movements reveals that in patients with Parkinson's disease sequential motor acts are slow and undershot, and these abnormalities become more and more evident as the motor sequence progresses. In a quantitative experiment, Agostino and associates recorded arm movements by means of a two-joint articulated structure, with one end fixed on a table (Agostino et al., 1992). Subjects had to grasp the handle at the free end of the structure and trace geometrical figures marked on the table. These figures had an increasing number (from two to five) of segments of identical length. Patients were slow in completing each sequence, and the movement time progressively lengthened as the sequence progressed (the sequence effect on movement time). These findings specified that the progressive fading of patients' performance depended on the sequential feature of the task and not on the different position of the segments in the workspace or the different direction of each single movement in the sequences. Although parkinsonian patients paused longer than normal subjects at the vertex of the figures, the duration of the pauses did not lengthen as the sequence progressed. This finding confirmed that parkinsonian patients were slow in switching from one movement to the next. It also showed that their slowness remained regardless of the number of submovements in the motor sequence. The progressive worsening of bradykinesia during the drawing of a pentagon may be equated to the fatigue phenomenon described clinically for repetitive tasks. However, the performance of repetitive motor sequences implies repeating the same movement in opposite directions, thus activating a similar pattern of muscle groups in an alternating fashion. In contrast, nonrepetitive sequential tasks, such as that of drawing a pentagon, imply a continual change in the direction of the movement and the pattern of muscle

activation. A subsequent study (Agostino et al., 1994) investigated whether the sequence effect seen during the nonrepetitive task also occurred during a repetitive task consisting of similar arm movements. The performance of the sequential drawing of a pentagon was compared with a repetitive task requiring the subject to draw the same side of the pentagon five times. Because movement time at the end of the sequence lengthened similarly in both tasks, the sequence effect appears not to depend on whether the sequential task involves nonrepetitive or repetitive movements. In parkinsonian patients, the switching difficulties occur not only between two movements in a sequence but also between two successive sequences of finger movements (Jones et al., 1992). This problem was more evident when the switching process meant transferring the motor activity to the fingers on the opposite side of the body than when it meant transferring activity to the fingers on the same side of the body.

Abnormalities in motor sequence execution have also been shown in parkinsonian patients engaged in natural everyday motor tasks such as the act of drinking (Bennett et al., 1995). Subjects were required to reach and grasp a half-filled glass and to take a sip of water. Although patients with Parkinson's disease often began to open the hand later than controls and paused between the first and the second parts of the drinking action, both groups showed similar proportional organization of the action. Parkinsonian patients therefore seemed to develop a compensatory mechanism. More information on compensatory mechanisms came from a study investigating the movement kinematics of a bilateral, nonhomologous reach-to-grasp action (Castiello and Bennett, 1997). The task was to reach and grasp a cylinder with one hand (gross grasp) while reaching to grasp the cylinder handle with the contralateral hand (precision grasp). Patients with

Parkinson's disease showed more pronounced left-right hand control differences than controls, but they also showed independent and appropriate kinematic parameterization of each limb. Therefore, compensatory mechanisms operate so natural, non-homologous reach-to-grasp actions can be performed in a functional, coordinated, and appropriate manner.

During the performance of repetitive sequential acts, a prominent role in the generation and maintenance of the rhythm may be played by temporal discrimination between two successive sensory stimuli and time perception. In parkinsonian patients, somesthetic temporal discrimination (Artieda et al., 1992) and time perception (Pastor et al., 1992) are abnormal, and these abnormalities could account for impaired sequence execution. Patients with Parkinson's disease can apparently compensate for their motor impairment when they receive external cues that direct their attention to the task. Early studies showed that the lack of visual guidance during movement causes the patients' performance to deteriorate (Flowers, 1978b; Stern et al., 1983, 1984). A later study investigated the importance of visual guidance in patients performing a task of sequential button pressing with the index finger, with the buttons illuminated or not illuminated (Georgiou et al., 1993). In the first experimental condition, the performance was visually guided, and it relied on an external cue; in the second, it relied on an internal control. Normal subjects did the two tasks equally well. When the buttons were illuminated, patients took longer than normal subjects to execute each step of the sequence and to switch between consecutive submovements. When the lights were off, their performance worsened. The novel finding was that when the patients performed the sequence with the light off, the motor execution of each submovement and the switching process were improved by providing auditory cues. The improvement was greatest when the patients executed the task while keeping time with a metronome. This effect also applies to other motor tasks, including daily life activities and gait. Patients with Parkinson's disease are less micrographic if they are presented with visual targets or are constantly reminded to write using large letters (Oliveira et al., 1997). Patients can improve their walking if they are shown the desired stride length, and if they are constantly required to remind themselves of the amplitude of the movement to perform (Morris et al., 1998). Therefore, during the performance of a motor sequence, the reliance on external cues is related not only to visual cues but also to other sensory information. This finding confirms the suggestion that cues have a role in the internal or external control of attention during motor performance (Brown and Marsden, 1988).

All of these data strongly support the idea that the basal ganglia have a pivotal role in implementing the internal motor representation normally needed to guide movement. In addition, the observation that the manipulation of external cues leads to changes in motor execution in patients with Parkinson's disease (but not in normal subjects) indicates that, as already suggested by Flowers (1976), Parkinson's disease primarily accentuates the difficulty in executing internally generated movements. Seeking more information on the effect of external cues on the kinematics of arm movements, we studied the execution of a sequential task in free space under two experimental conditions (Currà et al., 1997). First, the subjects did a motor sequence without knowing the movement steps beforehand. They then did the same sequence, but during this session they knew the pathway before starting to move. Interestingly, patients had more difficulty in executing the known sequences than the unknown. The two experimental conditions differed in more than one respect, however, because they imposed a different mode of movement selection. In the known sequences, movements were self-initiated, whereas in the unknown condition, they were externally triggered. Parkinsonian patients' performance deficits may thus depend more on the mode of movement selection than on an advance knowledge of the sequence path. This hypothesis has been tested by investigating the execution of a ball grasp during two task conditions and measuring whether parkinsonian patients could move faster when their movement speed was externally rather than internally driven (Majsak et al., 1998). During the first condition, patients and controls had to reach a stationary ball as fast as possible. They therefore used their own internal drive to generate a self-determined, maximal speed. In the second condition, the subjects had to grasp a rapidly rolling ball. When patients had to reach the moving ball, they were able to exceed their self-determined maximal speed while maintaining movement accuracy. This finding suggests that in Parkinson's disease the slowness of movement is not the result of a basic defect in force production capacity, but rather reflects patients' inability to maximize their movement speed when they are required to drive their motor output internally. The occasional failure of patients to grasp the rolling ball successfully was attributed to errors of coincident anticipation and difficulty in grasping but not to limitations in the speed or accuracy of the reaching movements.

The mode of movement selection is often interconnected with the predictability of the movement end point. Studies on the manual trackings of unpredictable and predictable targets with a similar number of external cues showed that parkinsonian patients took less advantage of the predictability of the target path than normal subjects (Flowers, 1978a; Day et al., 1984). In contrast, in another study, patients and controls took equal advantage of predictability (Bloxham et al., 1984). This discrepancy raised the question of a specific programming deficit for sequential movements in Parkinson's disease, a topic already covered in the discussion of reaction time. The processes of planning (Frith et al., 1986) and executing an action have also been addressed in a kinematic study in patients with Parkinson's disease (Gentilucci and Negrotti, 1999). Patients had to accomplish two successive motor acts: reaching-grasping an object (first target) and placing it on a second target of the same shape and size with and without visual control of the targets and the arm. The findings indicate that patients with Parkinson's disease are able to compute the general program of an action by taking into account the extrinsic properties of the final target. However, to improve their motor performance, they reprogram the reaching component by taking into account the extrinsic properties of the first target alone. The decay in the program during its time course is strong evidence of the conclusion that the basal ganglia are involved in storing the plan of an action and in controlling its correct execution.

Some studies investigated whether abnormalities of sensorimotor integration are responsible for slowness of movement in Parkinson's disease. Among the tasks studied were the lifting and holding of an object in a precision grip between thumb and the forefinger and holding of the object in this grip at a fixed height above a table (Fellows et al., 1998). The first motor task was complicated by unwarned changes in object loading between lifts, and the second motor task was complicated by unexpected step load changes applied to the object with a torque motor. All perturbations could be delivered with or without visual control of the hand and the object. Parkinsonian patients generated abnormally high grip forces and required periods of time longer than those needed by normal subjects to complete a lift, particularly with lighter loads. In addition, patients took longer than normal to develop peak grip force and showed a pronounced slowing in the rate at which grip force was generated. The internal parameter set for lifting an object in a precision grip and the automatic processes that adapt the precision grip to actual conditions therefore seem to be intact in Parkinson's disease. The deterioration in performance nevertheless reflects impairments in sensorimotor processing and in the rate of force development in Parkinson's disease. In two-point discrimination and the proprioceptive position sense, patients with Parkinson's disease have decreased precision (Schneider et al., 1986). In a study of arm movements testing the effects of both visual and kinesthetic information, patients showed impaired peripheral afferent feedback (Klockgether and Dichgans, 1994). When parkinsonian patients used kinesthetic information to match a visual target, they perceived the distances as shorter than they were (Demirci et al., 1997). All of these observations imply that impairment of sensorimotor integration participates in the generation of hypometria or bradykinesia and that kinesthesia may have a role in the pathophysiology of Parkinson's disease. Two questions remaining unclear are its importance and whether the movement deficit originates from altered cutaneous peripheral receptors or from abnormal central processing resulting from a physiological disturbance in the basal ganglia.

In summary, patients with Parkinson's disease are slow in performing simple movements. They accomplish simple movements not with a single triphasic pattern, as normal subjects do, but with multiple cycles of EMG bursts. The amount of EMG activation is inadequate not because the generating mechanism is saturated, but because patients are unable to scale it to the movement variables. Studies of complex movements have provided evidence that patients with Parkinson's disease have difficulty in switching from one movement to the next, and as the execution of a motor sequence progresses, they become slower in completing each step. Patients can compensate for abnormal motor execution by using external cues to guide movement, a finding indicating a predominant impairment of internally guided movements. Yet despite intensive research, no consensus has been reached on the abnormality of motor programming in patients with Parkinson's disease. Among the factors contributing to the discrepant results, we include the type of patients and motor task studied, the effects of learning during practice trials before movement recordings, and the methods used for statistical analysis. Current knowledge argues in favor of a deficit in the sequential and simultaneous running of motor programs. Finally, rigidity, tremor, and weakness, though not fully responsible, unquestionably contribute to the pathophysiology of movement slowness in Parkinson's disease (Stelmach et al., 1989; Johnson et al., 1991; Corcos et al., 1996).

Huntington's Disease

The main feature of surface EMG recordings of choreic movements is the high variability. Muscle activation shows variable and random patterns, the EMG bursts have variable duration, and the agonist and antagonist muscle pairs are activated in variable combinations and patterns including cocontraction (Thompson et al., 1988). This variability in the generation of muscle activity interferes with the correct performance of voluntary movement. In a study on simple and complex movements, Hefter and coworkers reported a significant slowing of the movement time in patients with Huntington's disease who were executing self-paced, single isometric forefinger movements (Hefter et al., 1987). In a more extensive investigation, Thompson and associates studied fast, simple wrist flexion movements to 15 or 60 degrees (Thompson et al., 1988). In those patients with Huntington's disease who were able to execute the tasks, these investigators found that individual movements were slower and showed greater variability than those seen in normal subjects. Kinematic variables such as movement velocity, amplitude, and the final position varied more in patients than in controls. Electromyographic recordings during movement showed a disorganized pattern of activity with EMG bursts of variable duration—often prolonged—and a disrupted sequence of agonist and antagonist contraction. In particular, the first agonist burst is poorly defined, and the antagonist burst starts either before or after the first agonist burst; these bursts often coactivate (Fig. 97–6). These features were more pronounced in akinetic and rigid patients, but they were also seen in patients with chorea alone. In addition, kinematic and EMG abnormalities were independent of the drug treatment that the patients were receiving and therefore were not the result of drug-induced parkinsonism. Prolonged EMG bursts during movement were also described previously in patients with Sydenham's chorea (Hallett and Kaufman, 1981).

The experimental techniques used for investigating motor disturbance in patients with Parkinson's disease have also been used for studying the pathophysiology of voluntary movements in patients with Huntington's disease. Thompson and coworkers studied sequential hand squeezing and elbow flexing (Thompson et al., 1988). Some patients were unable to combine two movements in a simultaneous or sequential movement task. However, those who could perform these complex movements exhibited reduced velocity of movement and increased pauses

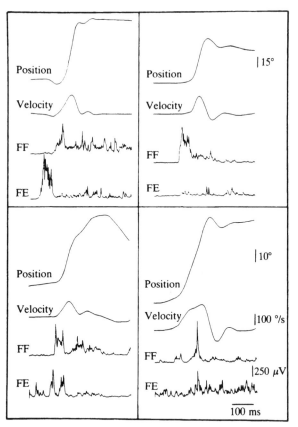

Figure 97–6. Rapid wrist flexion movements in patients with Huntington's disease. Electromyographic signals are recorded from forearm flexor (FF) and extensor (FE) muscles. Movement trajectory and agonist and antagonist muscle activation are variable. (From Berardelli A, Hallett M, Rothwell JC, et al: Single-joint rapid arm movements in normal subjects and in patients with motor disorders. Brain 1996;119:661–674.)

between movements. These abnormalities probably result from impaired motor programming of complex movements, over and above the defect in executing simple movements. Agostino and colleagues required patients to trace geometrical figures with an increasing number of segments of identical length in counterclockwise and clockwise directions (Agostino et al., 1992). Patients with Huntington's disease were slow in executing submovements and in switching from one to the next, but their motor performance remained unchanged throughout the task. In contrast, performing a kinematic analysis of handwriting, huntingtonian patients showed progressive changes in the sequential writing of the letter *l* in a linked cursive script (Phillips et al., 1995). A similar finding was also reported from the same group of investigators during a serial button-pressing task designed to investigate the reliance on external advance information in movement sequencing in patients with Huntington's disease (Georgiou et al., 1995). A pathway of illuminated lights was presented along a response board that displayed two-choice points at each of 10 sequential pairs of buttons. Subjects were required to press the illuminated buttons along the board as quickly as possible. The advance visual information on the forthcoming presses in the sequence was systematically and increasingly reduced by extinguishing an increasing number of consecutive buttons as the current button was released. Although the patients with Huntington's disease were slower than controls in initiating and executing the sequential presses during the three conditions, they showed no added difficulty when they received normal or moderately reduced advance information, whereas they demonstrated significantly progressive slowing when they received moderately or highly reduced advance information. Studying the performance of sequential button presses under varying conditions of visual advance information, Bradshaw and associates had already shown that Huntington's disease causes difficulties in incorporating and using advance information during sequential movements (Bradshaw et al., 1992). However, the novel finding of Georgiou and coworkers was that patients with Huntington's disease require external visual cues to sequence motor programs effectively, as a result of the abnormalities in a central mechanism that controls the switching between submovements within a motor plan (Georgiou et al., 1995). In a further study, Phillips and colleagues investigated whether bradykinesia in patients with Huntington's disease was the result of impaired force production or an increased requirement for terminal visual guidance (Phillips et al., 1996). These investigators studied drawing movements with varying precision requirements executed on a graphics tablet. In patients with Huntington's disease, movements were slower, and their kinematic profiles showed multiple cycles of acceleration and deceleration. Patients were not disproportionately affected by variations in target size or separation, however. The investigators concluded that slowness of movement in Huntington's disease does not depend on impaired force production or increased reliance on terminal visual guidance, because neither accelerative nor decelerative phases were specifically affected.

Bimanual tasks have also been investigated in Huntington's disease. In a study requiring subjects to place pegs in a vertical row of holes and to tap a button repetitively with the index finger (Brown et al., 1993), each task had to be performed as quickly as possible with each hand separately, bimanually, and then concurrently with the other task. Patients with Huntington's disease generally performed worse than did controls, but they had low impairment in the combined bimanual task. Interestingly, an identical pattern of performance was shown by a group of patients with both cerebellar disease and Parkinson's disease. The hypothesis concerning whether a concurrent task (the digit span) would affect the kinematics of goal-directed movements in patients with Huntington's disease has been tested (Georgiou et al., 1997). Using a graphics tablet, subjects performed vertical zig-zag movements, with both the left and the right hands, to large or small circular targets at long or short distances. The motor sequence was executed with and without the concurrent task. In both groups, the concurrent task yielded shorter movement times and reduced right-hand superiority. Normal subjects performed movements with symmetrical velocity profiles and tuned kinematic variables according to target distance and dimension. Patients with Huntington's disease were slow, especially when they executed long strokes. During movements directed to large and small targets, they exhibited similar peak velocities. In addition, these patients had longer decelerative phases, particularly when they moved to small targets. With the concurrent task, however, the behavior of the left hand differed in the two groups. In patients, it became more force efficient with short strokes and less efficient with long strokes, whereas in controls, it became more efficient with long strokes. In our opinion, controls may be able to divert attention away from the left hand and to increase its automaticity, whereas patients with Huntington's disease may be forced to engage even further on-line visual control under the demands of a concurrent task and therefore to rely increasingly on terminal visual guidance.

The studies reviewed earlier provide evidence that in patients with Huntington's disease, bradykinesia during complex motor tasks may be related to a breakdown in the ability to link one component of a movement to the next (as in Parkinson's disease). Similar abnormalities have been observed at both low and high levels of provision of advance information. Providing high levels of advance information means that external cues are available to drive subjects' motor performance, whereas the absence of advance information requires subjects to peform movements from memory. This overreliance on advance information has been related to the lack of

the internally generated cues to guide movement that would normally be provided by intact basal ganglia. We investigated whether the mode of submovement cuing during the execution of motor sequences influences the speed of movement in patients with Huntington's disease (Currà et al., 2000a). In a kinematic analysis of externally triggered and self-initiated sequential, rapid free arm movements, we found that patients with Huntington's disease performed both externally triggered and self-initiated tasks more slowly than normal subjects. Both groups executed externally triggered sequences more slowly than self-initiated sequences, but movement times for the two tasks differed less in patients than in controls. Patients paused normally between submovements during the self-initiated task, but they had slower reaction times for all of the submovements of the externally triggered task. We concluded that the smaller movement time difference in patients than in controls in the performance of self-initiated and externally triggered movements suggests that Huntington's disease impairs internal more than external timing mechanisms.

In conclusion, EMG recordings in chorea show variable and random patterns of muscle activation. Patients with Huntington's disease perform simple voluntary movements more slowly than normal subjects and with an abnormal triphasic EMG pattern. In addition, the final position and the peak velocity vary more in patients than in normal subjects. When performing simultaneous and sequential movements, patients with Huntington's disease are slow and also exhibit difficulty in switching from one movement to the next. These abnormalities tend to be more evident during internally determined than externally triggered motor tasks. In the presence of external cues, patients with Huntington's disease can improve their motor performance.

Dystonia

Clinical examination of patients with dystonia shows motor disturbances characterized by involuntary movements (dystonic, myoclonic movements, and tremor) and abnormal execution of voluntary movements. Early EMG studies showed that dystonic postures result from periods of continuous activity lasting several seconds, sometimes accompanied by repeated shorter bursts (Herz, 1944). The duration and regularity of these superimposed bursts are responsible for the associated motor signs in dystonia, such as postural and action tremors, slow myorhythmia, and myoclonus (myoclonic dystonia) (Berardelli et al., 1998).

Among the abnormalities that interfere with voluntary movement in patients with dystonia is the lack of selectivity in attempts to perform discrete independent movements (Cohen and Hallett, 1988) (Fig. 97–7). This deficit results in the overflow of activity to remote muscle groups that are not normally activated in the movement (van der Kamp et

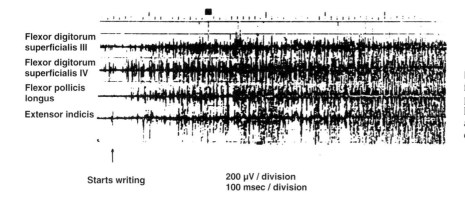

Flexor digitorum
superficialis III
Flexor digitorum
superficialis IV
Flexor pollicis
longus
Extensor indicis

Starts writing

200 μV / division
100 msec / division

Figure 97–7. Electromyographic activity from finger muscles during writing in a patient with hand cramp. (From Cohen G, Hallett M: Hand cramp: Clinical features and electromyographic patterns in a focal dystonia. Neurology 1988;38:1005–1012.)

al., 1989). Studies of rapid elbow flexion movements in patients with dystonia affecting the upper arm showed that the first agonist burst lasted longer in these patients than in normal subjects. Finally, movement amplitude varied more (as measured by the coefficient of variation) in patients than in normal subjects even when the latter moved at a slow velocity. Despite these abnormalities, acceleration and deceleration times were approximately equal, and the velocity profile was symmetrical, a finding suggesting that this aspect of motor programming is intact in dystonic patients (van der Kamp et al., 1989). During elbow flexion movements, the EMG abnormalities similar to those observed in patients with dystonia have also been found in patients with athetosis (Hallett and Alvarez, 1983).

Inzelberg and associates studied the kinematic properties of time-constrained arm-reaching movement in patients with dystonia (Inzelberg et al., 1995). As with single-joint tasks, these free arm movements were slower and more variable than normal, and they had a prolonged deceleration phase. Deceleration worsened when subjects had no visual feedback of the moving limb, a finding suggesting defective integration of sensory feedback corrections in dystonia. In a study of sequential planar movements, dystonic patients were slower than controls in completing individual movements and took longer than controls to switch from one submovement to the next. However, dystonic patients did not show progressive slowing with sequence completion. In addition, when performing a single movement as a submovement of a motor sequence, patients with dystonia became even slower *(extra slowness)* (Agostino et al., 1992). More recently, we investigated whether the type of movement cuing influences motor performance in patients with dystonia (Currà et al., 2000b). Patients with generalized or focal dystonia had to perform sequential, rapid zig-zag arm movements under various conditions of cuing. The externally triggered task required subjects to initiate each submovement in response to consecutive visual cues. The self-initiated task allowed subjects to start the motor sequence at will. A condition of mixed cuing required subjects to initiate the entire sequence in response to a single cue given before the first submovement. Controls

performed the SI task significantly faster than the externally triggered task. Their single externally triggered movements and first externally triggered sequential submovements had similar speeds. Patients with focal dystonia had normal reaction times, but they performed single and sequential tasks slowly, made long pauses during self-initiated tasks, and also executed the first externally triggered submovement more slowly than the single externally triggered movement. Patients with generalized dystonia had longer reaction times during the externally triggered sequences and made long pauses between self-initiated sequential submovements. They were slow in performing single and sequential tasks, and they performed the first externally triggered submovement more slowly than the single externally triggered movement. Patients with generalized dystonia had disproportionate slowness during the self-initiated sequence. Patients with dystonia therefore have a general impairment of sequential movements, but the more marked slowness in executing self-initiated than externally triggered movements observed in patients with generalized dystonia shows that dystonia impairs internal cuing more than external cuing mechanisms. These findings provide evidence confirming abnormal activation of primary and nonprimary motor areas during movement in dystonia.

In summary, voluntary movement, like dystonic movement, is characterized by excessive and overlapping activity in agonist and antagonist muscles together with an overflow of activity to muscles not normally involved in the task. As a result, voluntary movement is slow and variable in amplitude. The movement time becomes even longer during sequential movements, and patients also take longer to switch between submovements. Finally, in dystonia, the performance of complex movements worsens when patients are required to self-initiate the subcomponents of the motor task.

Cerebellar Disease

Earlier EMG studies in patients with cerebellar ataxia showed that movement execution was characterized by cocontraction activity, prolonged duration of first agonist and antagonist bursts, and reduced or absent antagonist inhibition before the onset of the first agonist burst (Altenburger, 1930; Hallett et al., 1975b). Abnormalities of movement amplitude and the velocity profile are present during rapid movements performed at different joints (finger, wrist, and elbow) and at different distances (5, 30, and 60 degrees) (Hore et al., 1991). Patients with cerebellar disease were hypermetric during all tasks, in particular for the shortest movements. In addition, patients were slower, more hypermetric, and more variable than controls, and their motor performance varied most during the shortest movements. Hallett and coworkers first proposed that abnormalities of first agonist and antagonist bursts may underlie the clinical sign of dysmetria (Hallett et al., 1975b), whereas abnormalities of antagonist inhibition may be responsible for the sign of dysdiadochokinesia and the rebound phenomenon. During movements about the elbow executed at different velocities and amplitudes as fast or as fast and as accurately as possible, patients with cerebellar disease could scale the peak velocity with movement amplitude normally (Brown et al., 1990). In addition, when they were required to perform fast movements of short distances without regard for accuracy, they had normal kinematic profiles. In contrast, for larger and accurate movements, their velocity profiles had shorter acceleration and longer deceleration phases. The temporal structure of voluntary movements in cerebellar patients was therefore altered. However, whether long deceleration was the result of an abnormality of the phasic voluntary EMG burst (not recorded) or caused by changes in movement strategy remained unsolved. To study this question further, rapid elbow movements of increasing amplitude were investigated (Hallett et al., 1991). In patients with cerebellar disease, the duration of the first agonist burst was longer than that of normal subjects executing movements of similar amplitude and velocity (Fig. 97–8). In contrast to the findings of Brown and colleagues (1990), patients had longer acceleration phases than controls, and the lengthening correlated with the longer duration of the first agonist burst. These abnormalities correlated with the clinical severity of ataxia in cerebellar patients. Patients with cerebellar disease may therefore move slowly in the attempt to be more accurate. Independent of speed, however, their movements have asymmetrical velocity profiles and altered duration of agonist and antagonist EMG bursts. Possible mechanisms proposed to explain prolonged acceleration time include an inability to turn off agonist activation and a difficulty in implementing muscle force phasically. In conclusion, EMG and kinematic analysis of simple movements suggests that the cerebellum contributes to the shaping of the agonist command and to the braking process of the moving limb.

In patients with cerebellar disease, however, the inability to perform movements accurately does not always result in hypermetria but sometimes also in hypometria. This is probably the result of overcompensation for the altered production of appropriate acceleration during rapid movements. Investigation of wrist flexion movements and the associated EMG activities in cerebellar patients showed that the mechanisms for generating hypometria differed according to the anatomical site of the lesion (Manto et al., 1998). In patients with lesions involving the efferent dentatothalamocortical pathway, hypometria was associated with an imbalance between the rate of the rise of the agonist and antagonist EMG activity. In patients with lesions located at the level

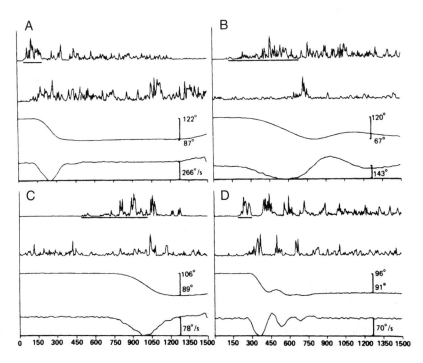

Figure 97–8. Individual rapid flexion movements at the elbow in a patient with moderate ataxia *(A and D)* and in two patients with severe ataxia *(B and C).* From *top to bottom,* each panel shows rectified biceps and triceps electromyographic activity, angular position, and velocity. The first agonist burst is *underlined* (mildly prolonged in *A,* markedly prolonged in *B* and *C,* and tremulous movement in *D).* (From Berardelli A, Hallett M, Rothwell JC, et al: Single-joint rapid arm movements in normal subjects and in patients with motor disorders. Brain 1996;119:661–674.)

of the middle cerebellar peduncle (disrupting the crossed pontocerebellar projections), hypometria was accompanied by reduced agonist EMG activity and increased duration of the antagonist EMG activity. In patients having either diffuse cerebellar atrophy or a stroke involving a large parenchymatous area, hypometria was found, together with prolonged duration of the antagonist EMG burst. The efferent dentatothalamocortical pathway therefore determines the rate of rise of muscle EMG activity, whereas the pontocerebellar projections are more concerned with the relative duration of such activity in the antagonist muscle groups. Overall, hypometria and hypermetria—the two types of errors reflecting dysmetria—result from motor control deficits in force-rate production and movement amplitude scaling.

Patients with cerebellar disease also perform abnormally multijoint, simple movements because of their deficit in the coordination of joint rotations (dyssynergy). During the execution of multijoint movements, subjects have to compensate rapidly for the effects deriving from multiple interaction torques between the body segments. Patients with cerebellar disease decompose multijoint movements into multistep single-joint submovements to simplify programming by minimizing interaction torque between joints (Thach et al., 1993; Massaquoi and Hallett, 1996). This process causes multijoint trajectory errors as a result of the abnormal compensation of interaction torque (Bastian et al., 1996; Topka et al., 1998).

Complex movements have also been studied. Patients with cerebellar disease perform arm-pointing movements slowly, and the duration of movement does not correlate with the extent of the pointing surface (Bonnefoi-Kyriacou et al., 1995), as in normal subjects. In addition, patients with cerebellar disease are hypermetric. A retrospective analysis of movement studies on patients with cerebellar disease performing arm movements suggests that hypermetria can be caused by the absence of an early antagonist EMG component, a delayed late component, or both (Wild and Corcos, 1997).

Tracking movements toward a target displayed on a screen have also been studied (Beppu et al., 1984, 1987). The process of tracking comprises an initial catchup phase, a middle pursuit phase, and a terminal phase. Patients with cerebellar disease had difficulty in all the three phases of tracking. During the initial catch-up phase, these patients failed in selecting the appropriate amplitude of initial peak velocity in proportion to the target velocity. During the middle pursuit phase, they transformed the smooth, continuous movement into a segmented and jerky movement (a motor abnormality called the saccadic pattern). During the terminal phase, ataxic patients initiated the deceleration phase late and performed numerous further corrective adjustments in approaching the movement end point. Bonnefoi-Kyriacou and associates studied patients with cerebellar limb ataxia who performed three-dimensional complex arm-pointing movements in a double-step paradigm (Bonnefoi-Kyriacou et al., 1998). Subjects moved to visual stimuli during four paradigms. Two of these consisted of one single-step and one double-step movement toward the same target. The remaining tasks involved two double-step movements toward a second target, the first using a straight trajectory and the second moving in an initial direction toward the previous position. Patients with cerebellar disease were able to modify their motor programs almost as well as the controls. However, they did it with impaired timing and movement accuracy and marked anomalies in the direction and amplitude of the changed movement trajectories. In a study of ball-throwing movements, Becker and coworkers observed that patients had high variability in reproducing consistent limb trajectories across trials, so hand directions and throws were inaccurate (Becker et al., 1990). The main abnormal finding was in the timing of antagonist muscle contraction. The investigators concluded that impairment in ball throws was the result of a defect of visual-motor coordination. Timmann and colleagues analyzed the execution of ball throws, with a special focus on the timing of finger opening during the throw (Timmann et al., 1999). Subjects were seated and instructed to throw tennis balls at three different speeds. Patients with cerebellar disease threw more slowly, were markedly less accurate, had more variable hand trajectories, and showed increased variability in the timing, amplitude, and velocity of finger opening compared with controls. Patients took four to five times as long as controls to open the fingers and release the ball. Because of this abnormal timing, they released the tennis ball during flattened-arc hand trajectories, so throwing became inaccurate. The cerebellum therefore plays an important role in timing the central command that initiates finger opening in this fast, skilled multijoint arm movement.

Clinical examination shows that ataxic patients try to improve their motor performance by visually guiding the movement. In patients with cerebellar disease, the importance of vision for the control of voluntary movement has been studied during tracking (Beppu et al., 1987) and reaching (Day et al., 1998) movements of the upper limb. As previously reported, patients with cerebellar ataxia perform slow elbow tracking movements with irregular undulations of pursuit velocity (Beppu et al., 1984). In a subsequent study, the same group of investigators tested the tracking ability when either the tracking cursor or the target cursor was suddenly erased from the screen during pursuit, thus depriving subjects of visual information (Beppu et al., 1987). In control subjects, the erase procedure left performance practically unchanged. In patients, however, it significantly reduced the velocity undulation so that they produced smoother continuous pursuits independent of erasing the target or the tracking cursor. An effect on velocity pursuit similar to that induced by vision deprivation can be obtained by adding a viscous load to the wrist, by feedback of the wrist velocity to a torque motor coupled to the moving limb (Morrice et al., 1990). Day and associates asked patients with cerebellar ataxia to reach out and touch a visually presented target either in the dark or with the target and their moving finger visible (Day et al., 1998). Patients moved more slowly than controls during all tasks, and their fingertips described unusually long and circuitous spatial paths. This kinematic feature was uninfluenced by visual conditions. Ataxic movements showed early and late kinematic spatial abnormalities that were differentially influenced by vision. Early in the movement trajectory, patients showed greater spatial path variability that visual feedback did not correct. Later abnormalities were the large, constant errors at the end of movement, which were present only when subjects moved in darkness. The finding that patients made spatial errors indicated that the cerebellum influences the preparatory processes of reaching motor acts. However, visual guidance allowed patients to make midflight adjustments to their movements to improve accuracy. This finding indicated that the cerebellum computed the pattern of muscle activity required to launch the limb accurately toward a target on the basis of proprioceptive information from the limb and the retina. However, the visual correction mechanism was abnormal, and the end phase of movement was often prolonged and characterized by excessive deviations or directional changes in the path. These deviations probably arise when the motor system has misjudged the initial pattern of muscle activity and has tried to produce corrections. However, the corrections themselves contain errors requiring further correction.

The inability of patients with cerebellar disease to correct abnormal motor performance without further errors suggests that these patients have difficulty in adapting their motor output to the constraints of the task. In fact, patients with cerebellar disease show poor adaptation when they are required to rearrange their movement execution according to the lateral displacement of vision induced by prism glasses (Weiner et al., 1983; Martin et al., 1996) or to the changed visual-motor gain during a matching movement task (Deuschl et al., 1996). Adaptation is one of the main aspects of the process of motor learning. Therefore, the finding of impaired motor learning in patients with cerebellar disease indicates that, together with other brain structures, the cerebellum plays a pivotal role in the process of acquiring new strategies of motor behavior and of improving the motor performance with practice.

In summary, EMG studies in patients with cerebellar disease show that the abnormal timing and recruitment of agonist and antagonist muscle contraction produce movements that are slow in starting, progress irregularly and jerkily, and are slow in stopping. The velocity profile is asymmetrical, owing to changes in the duration and magnitude of the decelerative phases, and movements are either hypermetric or hypometric, depending on the level of compensation operated by patients. These motor abnormalities result from deficits in force-rate production and movement amplitude scaling. Kinematic abnormalities are also present during tracking movements and are influenced by kinesthetic and visual information. Most difficulties arise from abnormal compensation of interaction torque between joints resulting in the inability to coordinate multiple joint activation. In patients with cerebellar disease, complex movements are characterized by the abnormal timing of antagonist muscle contraction, marked movement inaccuracy, and variable trajectories.

Essential Tremor

Britton and coworkers studied the single movement in patients with essential tremor who exhibited postural and action tremor (Britton et al., 1994). Kinematic analysis showed normal or faster peak velocities in patients, a finding explaining why they often overshot the target. The velocity profile was asymmetrical, owing to higher peak deceleration. The EMG recordings showed that the triphasic pattern was preserved, but the onset of the second agonist burst was repeatedly delayed. This delay correlated with the frequency of the tremor. The delayed second agonist burst left the antagonist contraction unopposed, thereby leading to inappropriate and excessive deceleration and causing movement inaccuracy. In an attempt to correct this inaccuracy, the subsequent agonist bursts produced tremor. The similarities in movement execution abnormalities between patients with essential tremor and those with cerebellar disease suggest that the second agonist burst or other subsequent bursts may be generated or timed by central mechanisms involving the cerebellum.

Upper Motor Neuron Syndrome

In early EMG studies conducted in a patient with traumatic cerebral palsy who executed rapid shoulder abductions, Angel found prolonged first agonist burst durations (Angel, 1975). A similar abnormality was found in patients with spasticity deriving from various causes, who were required to perform rapid alternating movements (Sahrmann and Norton, 1977). In a study of rapid elbow flexions in patients with amyotrophic lateral sclerosis, Hallett interpreted the prolonged duration of the first agonist and first antagonist bursts as a compensatory mechanism that patients with pyramidal tract damage used to reduce the motoneuronal recruitment (Hallett, 1979). By studying the elbow movements of increasing amplitude in patients with stroke-induced upper motor neuron syndrome, Fagioli and colleagues confirmed prolonged EMG bursts in patients, but they also showed that first agonist burst size and duration increased normally with movement amplitude (Fagioli et al., 1988). These findings suggest that because the duration of the first agonist burst is determined by a certain level of motor neuron recruitment, these two variables vary in parallel.

References

Agostino R, Berardelli A, Currà A, et al: Clinical impairment of sequential finger movements in Parkinson's disease. Mov Disord 1998;13:418–421.

Agostino R, Berardelli A, Formica A, et al: Sequential arm movements in patients with Parkinson's disease, Huntington's disease and dystonia. Brain 1992;115:1481–1495.

Agostino R, Berardelli A, Formica A, et al: Analysis of repetitive and nonrepetitive sequential arm movements in patients with Parkinson's disease. Mov Disord 1994;57:368–370.

Altenburger H: Untersuchungen zur Physiologie und Pathologie der Koordination. 2. Mitteilung. Die willkurlichen Einzebewegungen bei Kleinhirnlasionen. Zeitschrift fur die gesamate Neurologie und Psychiatrie 1930;124:679–713.

Angel RW: Electromyographic patterns during ballistic movement of normal and spastic limbs. Brain Res 1975;99:387–392.

Artieda J, Pastor MA, Lacruz F, et al: Temporal discrimination is abnormal in Parkinson's disease. Brain 1992;115:199–210.

Bastian AJ, Martin TA, Keating JG, Thach WT: Cerebellar ataxia: Abnormal control of interaction torques across multiple joints. J Neurophysiol 1996;76:492–509.

Becker WJ, Kunesch E, Freund HJ: Coordination of a multi-joint movement in normal humans and in patients with cerebellar dysfunction. Can J Neurol Sci 1990;17:264–274.

Benecke R, Rothwell JC, Day BL, et al: Motor strategies involved in the performance of sequential movements. Exp Brain Res 1986a;63:585–595.

Benecke R, Rothwell JC, Dick JPR, et al: Disturbance of sequential movements in patients with Parkinson's disease. Brain 1987a;110:361–379.

Benecke R, Rothwell JC, Dick JPR, et al: Performance of simultaneous movements in patients with Parkinson's disease. Brain 1986b;109:739–757.

Benecke R, Rothwell JC, Dick JPR, et al: Simple and complex movements off and on treatment in patients with Parkinson's disease. J Neurol Neurosurg Psychiatry 1987b;50:296–303.

Bennett KM, Marchetti M, Iovine R, et al: The drinking action of Parkinson's disease subjects. Brain 1995;118:959–970.

Beppu H, Nagaoka M, Tanaka R: Analysis of cerebellar motor disorders by visually guided elbow tracking movement: II. Contribution of the visual cues on slow ramp pursuit. Brain 1987;110:1–18.

Beppu H, Suda M, Tanaka R: Analysis of cerebellar motor disorders by visually guided elbow tracking movement. Brain 1984;107:787–809.

Berardelli A, Accornero N, Argenta M, et al: Fast complex arm movements in Parkinson's disease. J Neurol Neurosurg Psychiatry 1986a;49:1146–1149.

Berardelli A, Dick JPR, Rothwell JC, et al: Scaling of the size of the first agonist EMG burst during rapid wrist movements in patients with Parkinson's disease. J Neurol Neurosurg Psychiatry 1986b;49:1273–1279.

Berardelli A, Hallett M, Rothwell JC, et al: Single-joint rapid arm movements in normal subjects and in patients with motor disorders. Brain 1996;119:661–674.

Berardelli A, Rothwell JC, Day BL, et al: Movements not involved in posture are abnormal in Parkinson's disease. Neurosci Lett 1984;47:47–50.

Berardelli A, Rothwell JC, Hallett M, et al: The pathophysiology of primary dystonia. Brain 1998;121:1195–1212.

Berry EL, Nicolson RI, Foster JK, et al: Slowing of reaction time in Parkinson's disease: The involvement of the frontal lobes. Neuropsychologia 1999;37:787–795.

Bloxham CA, Dick DJ, Moore M: Reaction times and attention in Parkinson's disease. J Neurol Neurosurg Psychiatry 1987;50:1178–1183.

Bloxham CA, Mindel TA, Firth CD: Initiation and execution of

predictable and unpredictable movements in Parkinson's disease. Brain 1984;107:371–384.

Bonnefoi-Kyriacou B, Legallet E, Lee RG, et al: Spatio-temporal and kinematic analysis of pointing movements performed by cerebellar patients with limb ataxia. Exp Brain Res 1998;119:460–466.

Bonnefoi-Kyriacou B, Trouche E, Legallet E, et al: Planning and execution of pointing movements in cerebellar patients. Mov Disord 1995;10:171–178.

Bradshaw JL, Phillips JG, Dennis C, et al: Initiation and execution of movement sequences in those suffering from and at-risk of developing Huntington's disease. J Clin Exp Neuropsychol 1992;14:179–192.

Britton TC, Thompson PD, Day BL, et al: Rapid wrist movements in patients with essential tremor: The critical role of the second agonist burst. Brain 1994;117:39–47.

Brown RG, Jahanshahi M, Marsden CD: The execution of bimanual movements in patients with Parkinson's, Huntington's and cerebellar disease. J Neurol Neurosurg Psychiatry 1993;56:295–297.

Brown RG, Marsden CD: Internal versus external cues and the control of attention in Parkinson's disease. Brain 1988;111:323–345.

Brown SH, Cooke JD: Amplitude- and instruction-dependent modulation of movement-related EMG activity in humans. J Physiol 1981;316:97–107.

Brown SH, Cooke JD: Movement-related phasic muscle activation: I. Relations with temporal profile of movement. J Neurophysiol 1990;63:455–464.

Brown SH, Hefter H, Mertens M, et al: Disturbances in human arm movement trajectory due to mild cerebellar dysfunction. J Neurol Neurosurg Psychiatry 1990;53:306–313.

Castiello U, Bennett KM: The bilateral reach-to-grasp movement of Parkinson's disease subjects. Brain 1997;120:593–604.

Cohen G, Hallett M: Hand cramp: Clinical features and electromyographic patterns in a focal dystonia. Neurology 1988;38:1005–1012.

Cooke JD, Brown S, Forget R, et al: Initial agonist burst duration changes with movement amplitude in a deafferented patient. Exp Brain Res 1985;60:184–187.

Corcos DM, Chen CM, Quinn NP, et al: Strength in Parkinson's disease: Relationship to rate of force generation and clinical status. Ann Neurol 1996;39:79–88.

Corcos DM, Gottlieb GL, Agarwal GC: Organizing principle for single-joint movements: II. A speed-sensitive strategy. J Neurophysiol 1989;62:358–368.

Currà A, Agostino R, Galizia P, et al: Sub-movement cuing and motor sequence execution in patients with Huntington's disease. Clin Neurophysiol 2000a;111:1184–1190.

Currà A, Berardelli A, Agostino R, et al: Movement cuing and motor execution in patients with dystonia: A kinematic study. Mov Disord 2000b;15:103–112.

Currà A, Berardelli A, Agostino R, et al: Performance of sequential arm movement with and without advance knowledge of motor pathways in Parkinson's disease. Mov Disord 1997;12:646–654.

Day BL, Dick JPR, Marsden CD: Patients with Parkinson's disease can employ a predictive motor strategy. J Neurol Neurosurg Psychiatry 1984;47:1299–1306.

Day BL, Thompson PD, Harding AE, et al: Influence of vision on upper limb reaching movements in patients with cerebellar ataxia. Brain 1998;121:357–372.

Deiber MP, Honda M, Ibanez V, et al: Mesial motor areas in self-initiated versus externally triggered movements examined with fMRI: Effect of movement type and rate. J Neurophysiol 1999;81:3065–3077.

Deiber MP, Ibanez V, Sadato N, et al: Cerebral structures participating in motor preparation in humans: A positron emission tomography study. J Neurophysiol 1996;75:233–247.

Demirci M, Grill S, McShane L, et al: A mismatch between kinesthetic and visual perception in Parkinson's disease. Ann Neurol 1997;41:781–788.

Deuschl G, Toro C, Zeffiro T, et al: Adaptation motor learning of arm movements in patients with cerebellar disease. J Neurol Neurosurg Psychiatry 1996;60:515–519.

Evarts EV, Teravainen H, Calne DB: Reaction time in Parkinson's disease. Brain 1981;104:167–186.

Fagioli S, Berardelli A, Hallett M, et al: The first agonist and antagonist burst in patients with an upper motor neuron syndrome. Mov Disord 1988;3:126–132.

Fellows SJ, Noth J, Schwarz M: Precision grip and Parkinson's disease. Brain 1998;12:1771–1784.

Flowers K: Ballistic and corrective movements on an aiming task. Neurology 1975;25:413–421.

Flowers K: Visual "closed-loop" and "open-loop" characteristics of voluntary movements in patients with parkinsonism and intention tremor. Brain 1976;99:269–310.

Flowers K: Lack of prediction in the motor behaviour of parkinsonism. Brain 1978a;101:35–52.

Flowers K: Some frequency response characteristics of parkinsonism on pursuit tracking. Brain 1978b;101:19–34.

Frith CD, Bloxham CA, Carpenter KN: Impairment of motor planning in patients with Parkinson's disease. J Neurol Neurosurg Psychiatry 1986;49:661–668.

Garland H, Angel RW, Moore WE: Activity of triceps brachii during voluntary elbow extension: Effect of lidocaine blockade of elbow flexors. Exp Neurol 1972;37:831–835.

Gentilucci M, Negrotti A: Planning and executing action in Parkinson's disease. Mov Disord 1999;14:69–79.

Georgiou N, Bradshaw JL, Iansek R, et al: Reduction in external cues and movement sequencing in Parkinson's disease. J Neurol Neurosurg Psychiatry 1994;57:368–370.

Georgiou N, Bradshaw JL, Phillips JG, et al: Reliance on advance information and movement sequencing in Huntington's disease. Mov Disord 1995;10:472–481.

Georgiou N, Iansek R, Bradshaw JL, et al: An evaluation of the role of internal cues in the pathogenesis of parkinsonian hypokinesia. Brain 1993;116:1575–1587.

Georgiou N, Phillips JG, Bradshaw JL, et al: Impairments of movement kinematics in patients with Huntington's disease: A comparison with and without a concurrent task. Mov Disord 1997; 12:386–396.

Girotti F, Marano R, Soliveri P, et al: Relationship between motor and cognitive disorders in Huntington's disease. J Neurol 1988; 235:454–457.

Gottlieb GL, Corcos DM, Agarwal GC: Organizing principles for single-joint movements: I. A speed-insensitive strategy. J Neurophysiol 1989;62:342–357.

Gratton G, Coles MGH, Sirevaag EJ, et al: Pre- and post-stimulus activation of the response channel: A psychophysiological analysis. J Exp Psychol 1988;14:331–344.

Hallett M: Ballistic elbow flexion movements in patients with amyotrophic lateral sclerosis. J Neurol Neurosurg Psychiatry 1979;42:232–237.

Hallett M, Alvarez N: Attempted rapid elbow movements in patients with athetosis. J Neurol Neurosurg Psychiatry 1983;46: 1273–1279.

Hallett M, Berardelli A, Matheson J, et al: Physiological analysis of simple rapid movements in patients with cerebellar deficits. J Neurol Neurosurg Psychiatry 1991;54:124–133.

Hallett M, Kaufman C: Physiological observations in Sydenham's chorea. J Neurol Neurosurg Psychiatry 1981;44:829–832.

Hallett M, Khoshbin S: A physiological mechanism of bradykinesia. Brain 1980;103:301–314.

Hallett M, Shahani BT, Young RR: EMG analysis of stereotyped voluntary movements in man. J Neurol Neurosurg Psychiatry 1975a;38:1154–1162.

Hallett M, Shahani BT, Young RR: EMG analysis of patients with cerebellar deficits. J Neurol Neurosurg Psychiatry 1975b; 12:1163–1169.

Harrington DL, Haaland KY: Sequencing in Parkinson's disease: Abnormalities in programming and controlling movements. Brain 1991;114:99–115.

Harrison J, Goodrich S, Kennard C, et al: The consequence of "frontal" impairment for reaction times in Parkinson's disease. J Neurol Neurosurg Psychiatry 1993;56:726–727.

Harrison J, Henderson L, Kennard C: Abnormal refractoriness in patients with Parkinson's disease after brief withdrawal of levodopa treatment. J Neurol Neurosurg Psychiatry 1995; 59:499–506.

Hefter H, Homberg V, Lange HW, et al: Impairment of rapid movement in Huntington's disease. Brain 1987;110:585–612.

Heilman KM, Bowers D, Watson RT, et al: Reaction times in Parkinson's disease. Arch Neurol 1976;33:139–140.

Herz E: Dystonia: I. Historical review: Analysis of dystonic symptoms and physiologic mechanisms involved. Arch Neurol Psychiatry 1944;51:305–318.

Hore J, Wild B, Diener HC: Cerebellar dysmetria at the elbow, wrist and fingers. J Neurophysiol 1991;65:563–571.

Ikeda A, Shibasaki H, Kaji R, et al: Abnormal sensorimotor integration in writer's cramp: Study of contingent negative variation. Mov Disord 1996;11:683–690.

Inhoff AW, Diener HC, Rafal RD, et al: The role of cerebellar structures in the execution of serial movements. Brain 1989; 112:565–581.

Inzelberg R, Flash T, Schechtman E, et al: Kinematic properties of upper limb trajectories in idiopathic torsion dystonia. J Neurol Neurosurg Psychiatry 1995;58:312–319.

Jahanshahi M, Brown RG, Marsden CD: Simple and choice reaction time and the use of advance information for motor preparation in Parkinson's disease. Brain 1992;115:539–564.

Jahanshahi M, Brown RG, Marsden CD: A comparative study of simple and choice reaction time in Parkinson's, Huntington's and cerebellar disease. J Neurol Neurosurg Psychiatry 1993;56: 1169–1177.

Johnson KA, Cunnington R, Bradshaw JL, et al: Bimanual coordination in Parkinson's disease. Brain 1998;121:743–753.

Johnson MT, Kipnis AN, Lee MC, et al: Modulation of the stretch reflex during volitional sinusoidal tracking in Parkinson's disease. Brain 1991;114:443–460.

Jones DL, Phillips JG, Bradshaw JL, et al: Impairment in bilateral alternating movements in Parkinson's disease? J Neurol Neurosurg Psychiatry 1992;55:503–506.

Kaji R, Ikeda A, Ikeda T, et al: Physiological study of cervical dystonia: Task-specific abnormality in contingent negative variation. Brain 1995;118:511–522.

Klockgether T, Dichgans J: Visual control of arm movement in Parkinson's disease. Mov Disord 1994;9:48–56.

Kutukcu Y, Marks WJ Jr, Goodin DS, et al: Simple and choice reaction time in Parkinson's disease. Brain Res 1999;815:367–372.

Labutta JR, Miles RB, Sanes JN, et al: Motor program memory storage in Parkinson's disease patient tested with a delayed response task. Mov Disord 1994;9:218–222.

Lichter DG, Corbett AJ, Fitzgibbon GM, et al: Cognitive and motor dysfunction in Parkinson's disease: Clinical, performance, and computed tomographic correlations. Arch Neurol 1988;45:854–860.

Majsak MJ, Kaminski T, Gentile AM, et al: The reaching movements of patients with Parkinson's disease under self-determined maximal speed and visually cued conditions. Brain 1998; 121:755–766.

Manto MU, Setta F, Jacquy J, et al: Different types of cerebellar hypometria associated with a distinct topography of the lesion in cerebellum. J Neurol Sci 1998;158:88–95.

Martin TA, Keating JG, Goodkin HP, et al: Throwing while looking through prisms: I. Focal olivocerebellar lesions impair adaptation. Brain 1996;119:1183–1198.

Massaquoi S, Hallett M: Kinematics of initiating a two-joint arm movement in patients with cerebellar ataxia. Can J Neurol Sci 1996;23:3–14.

Mayeux R, Stern Y, Sano M, et al: Clinical and biochemical correlates of bradyphrenia in Parkinson's disease. Neurology 1987; 37:1130–1134.

Morrice BL, Becker WJ, Hoffer JA, et al: Manual tracking performance in patients with cerebellar incoordination: Effects of mechanical loading. Can J Neurol Sci 1990;17:275–285.

Morris M, Iansek R, Matyas T, et al: Abnormalities in the stride length-cadence relation in parkinsonian gait. Mov Disord 1998; 13:61–69.

Oliveira RM, Gurd JM, Nixon P, et al: Micrographia in Parkinson's disease: The effect of providing external cues. J Neurol Neurosurg Psychiatry 1997;63:429–433.

Oliveira RM, Gurd JM, Nizon P, et al: Hypometria in Parkinson's disease: Automatic versus controlled processing. Mov Disord 1998;13:422–427.

Pascual-Leone A, Brasil-Neto JP, Valls-Solé J, et al: Simple reaction time to focal transcranial magnetic stimulation: Comparison with reaction time to acoustic, visual and somatosensory stimuli. Brain 1992a;115:109–122.

Pascual-Leone A, Valls-Solé J, Brasil-Neto JP, et al: Akinesia in Parkinson's disease: I. Shortening of simple reaction time with focal single pulse transcranial magnetic stimulation. Neurology 1994a;44:884–891.

Pascual-Leone A, Valls-Solé J, Brasil-Neto JP, et al: Akinesia in Parkinson's disease: II. Effects of subthreshold repetitive transcranial motor cortex stimulation. Neurology 1994b;44:892–898.

Pascual-Leone A, Valls-Solé J, Wassermann EM, et al: Effects of focal transcranial magnetic stimulation on simple reaction time to acoustic, visual and somatosensory stimuli. Brain 1992b;115:1045–1059.

Pastor MA, Artieda J, Jahanshahi M, et al: Time estimation and reproduction is abnormal in Parkinson's disease. Brain 1992;115:211–225.

Phillips JG, Bradshaw JL, Chiu E, et al: Bradykinesia and movement precision in Huntington's disease. Neuropsychologia 1996;34:1241–1245.

Phillips JG, Chiu E, Bradshaw JL, et al: Impaired movement sequencing in patients with Huntington's disease: A kinematic analysis. Neuropsychologia 1995;33:365–369.

Praamstra P, Meyer AS, Cools AR, et al: Movement preparation in Parkinson's disease: Time course and distribution of movement related potentials in movement precuing task. Brain 1996;119:1689–1704.

Pullman SL, Watts RL, Juncos JL, et al: Dopaminergic effects on simple and choice reaction time performance in Parkinson's disease. Neurology 1988;38:249–254.

Rafal RD, Friedman JH, Lannon MC: Preparation of manual movements in hemiparkinsonism. J Neurol Neurosurg Psychiatry 1989;52:399–402.

Rafal RD, Inhoff AW, Friedman JH, et al: Programming and execution of sequential movements in Parkinson's disease. J Neurol Neurosurg Psychiatry 1987;50:1267–1273.

Rafal RD, Posner MI, Walker JA, et al: Cognition and the basal ganglia: Separating mental and motor components of performance in Parkinson's disease. Brain 1984;107:1083–1094.

Reid WGJ, Broe GA, Hely MA, et al: The neuropsychology of de novo patients with idiopathic Parkinson's disease: The effect of age of onset. Int J Neurosci 1989;48:205–217.

Requin J: Looking forward to moving soon: Ante factum selective processes in motor control. In Posner MI, Marin OSM (eds): Attention and Performance, No. 11. Hillsdale, NJ, Lawrence Erlbaum, 1985; 147–167.

Revonsuo A, Portin R, Koivikko L, et al: Slowing of information processing in Parkinson's disease. Brain Cogn 1993;21:87–110.

Roland PE, Zilles K: Functions and structures of the motor cortices in humans. Curr Opin Neurobiol 1996;6:773–781.

Rothwell JC, Traub MM, Day BL, et al: Manual motor performance in a deafferented man. Brain 1982;105:515–542.

Sahrmann SA, Norton BJ: The relationship of voluntary movement to spasticity in the upper motor neurone syndrome. Ann Neurol 1977;2:460–465.

Sanes JN, Mauritz KH, Dalakas MC, et al: Motor control in humans with large-fiber sensory neuropathy. Hum Neurobiol 1985;4:101–114.

Schneider JS, Diamond SG, Markham CH: Deficits in orofacial sensorimotor function in Parkinson's disease. Ann Neurol 1986;19:275–282.

Schwab RS, Chafetz ME, Walker S: Control of two simultaneous voluntary motor acts in normals and in parkinsonism. Arch Neurol 1954;72:591–598.

Sheridan MR, Flowers KA: Movement variability and bradykinesia in Parkinson's disease. Brain 1990;113:1149–1161.

Sheridan MR, Flowers KA, Hurrel J: Programming and execution of movement in Parkinson's disease. Brain 1987;110:1247–1271.

Sprengelmeyer R, Canavan AG, Lange HW, et al: Associative learning in degenerative neostriatal disorders: Contrasts in explicit and implicit remembering between Parkinson's and Huntington's diseases. Mov Disord 1995;10:51–65.

Starr A, Caramia M, Zarola F, et al: Enhancement of motor cortical excitability in humans by non-invasive electrical stimulation appears prior to voluntary movement. Electroencephalogr Clin Neurophysiol 1988;70:26–32.

Stelmach GE, Worringham CJ, Strand EA: Movement preparation in Parkinson's disease: The use of advance information. Brain 1986;109:1179–1194.

Stelmach GE, Worringham CJ, Strand EA: The programming and execution of movement sequences in Parkinson's disease. Int J Neurosci 1987;35:51–58.

Stelmach GE, Teasdale N, Phillips J, et al: Force production characteristics in Parkinson's disease. Brain Res 1989;76:165–172.

Stern Y, Mayeux R, Rosen J, et al: Perceptual motor dysfunction in Parkinson's disease: A deficit in sequential and predictive voluntary movement. J Neurol Neurosurg Psychiatry 1983;46:145–151.

Stern Y, Mayeux R, Rosen J: Contribution of perceptual motor dysfunction to construction and tracing disturbances in Parkinson's disease. J Neurol Neurosurg Psychiatry 1984;47:983–989.

Thach WT, Perry JG, Kane SA, Goodkin HP: Cerebellar nuclei: Rapid alternating movement, motor somatotopy, and a mechanism for the control of muscle synergy. Rev Neurol (Paris) 1993;149:607–628.

Talland GA, Schwab RS: Performance with multiple sets in Parkinson's disease. Neuropsychologia 1964;2:45–53.

Teasdale N, Phillips J, Stelmach GE: Temporal movement control in patients with Parkinson's disease. J Neurol Neurosurg Psychiatry 1990;53:862–868.

Thompson PD, Berardelli A, Rothwell JC, et al: The coexistence of bradykinesia and chorea in Huntington's disease, and its implications for theories of basal ganglia control of movement. Brain 1988;111:223–244.

Timmann D, Watts S, Hore J: Failure of cerebellar patients to time finger opening precisely causes ball high-low inaccuracy in overarm throws. J Neurophysiol 1999;82:103–114.

Topka H, Konczak J, Schneider K, et al: Multijoint arm movements in cerebellar ataxia: Abnormal control of movement dynamics. Exp Brain Res 1998;119:493–503.

Tsai TT, Lasker A, Zee DS: Visual attention in Huntington's disease: The effect of cuing on saccade latencies and manual reaction times. Neuropsychologia 1995;33:1617–1626.

van der Kamp W, Berardelli A, Rothwell JC, et al: Rapid elbow movements in patients with torsion dystonia. J Neurol Neurosurg Psychiatry 1989;52:1043–1049.

Wacholder K, Altenburger H: Beitrage zur Physiologie der willkurlichen Bewegung 10: Einzelbewegungen. Pflugers Arch Gesamte Physiol Menschen Tiere 1926;213:642–661.

Waters P, Strick PL: Influence of "strategy" on muscle activity during ballistic movements. Brain Res 1981;207:189–194.

Weiner MJ, Hallett M, Funkenstein HH: Adaptation to lateral displacement of vision in patients with lesions of the central nervous system. Neurology 1983;33:766–772.

Wiesendanger M, Schneider P, Villoz JP: Electromyographic analysis of a rapid volitional movement. Am J Phys Med 1969;48:17–24.

Wild B, Corcos DM: Cerebellar hypermetria: Reduction in the early component of the antagonist electromyogram. Mov Disord 1997;12:604–607.

Yamaguchi S, Tsuchiya H, Kobayashi S: Visuospatial attention shift and motor responses in cerebellar disorders. J Cogn Neurosci 1998;10:95–107.

Zimmermann P, Sprengelmeyer R, Fimm B, et al: Cognitive slowing in decision tasks in early and advanced Parkinson's disease. Brain Cogn 1992;18:60–69.

Myoclonus and Other Involuntary Movements

Mark Hallett

When the clinician in approaches a patient with an involuntary movement, the first steps are the usual neurological history and physical examination. If the movement is rhythmical (other than a few exceptions), it would usually be considered to be tremor, the topic of Chapter 99. The involuntary movements considered here are generally irregular. Some voluntariness suggests tic, and unusual features and psychopathology suggest a psychogenic movement disorder. If the movement is completely involuntary, a neurophysiological assessment may be helpful. One reason is that small differences in timing, easily measured with simple techniques, can be impossible to tell by eye. For example, there are important differences in the millisecond range for the burst duration of electromyogram (EMG) underlying an involuntary movement and the latency of a muscle jerk after a stimulus. The EMG pattern evaluation is the first and often the most important step. Subsequent electroencephalography (EEG) and reflex testing may have additional value.

METHODS

Involuntary movements can be characterized by the body part affected, the frequency of the movements, the triggers for the movements, and the duration of each movement. The last feature is best studied with EMG methods. Because mechanical events take so long compared with the electrical events that control them, sorting out observations of the mechanical events by themselves can be difficult. Additionally, EMG can determine the relationship between the activity in antagonist muscle pairs, another difficult observation to make only clinically.

EMG data can be measured with surface, needle, or wire electrodes (Hallett et al., 1994; Hallett, 1999). The advantages of surface electrodes are that they are not painful and they record from a relatively large volume of muscle. The advantage of needle electrodes is that they are more selective, sometimes a necessity when one records from small or deep muscles. Traditional needle electrodes are stiff, and it is best to use them for recording from muscles during movements that are close to isometric. Pairs of fine wire electrodes have the advantage of selectivity similar to that of needle electrodes and are flexible, thus permitting free movement with only minimal pain. In any case, it is important to avoid movement artifact, which can contaminate the EMG signal. Wire movement should be limited. Low-frequency content of the EMG signal can be restricted with filtering. The EMG has the highest power in the range of direct current to 150 Hz. Movement artifact has most of its power at less than 10 Hz. If the low-frequency filter is set at 10 to 20 Hz, most movement artifact will be eliminated.

When one uses surface electrodes, it is extremely important to reduce skin impedance. Values should be less than 10 kohm and certainly less than 20 kohm. This makes a major difference, and it may even make restricting the filter settings unnecessary.

For the purposes of timing, the EMG can be used as recorded without further processing. The amplitude of the EMG signal is roughly proportional to force, and to extract this information further processing is needed. Generally, the EMG signal needs to be integrated. This can be accomplished by rectifying the EMG and measuring the area under the curve. The EMG is typically smoothed after rectifying to make a cleaner envelope.

ELECTROMYOGRAPHIC PATTERNS

Three EMG patterns may underlie involuntary movements (Hallett et al., 1987, 1994; Hallett, 1997,

---

1999). One pattern, which can be called *tonic,* resembles slow voluntary movements and is characterized by continuous or almost continuous EMG activity lasting for the duration of the movement, from 200 to 1,000 ms or longer. Activity can be solely in the agonist muscle, or there can be some cocontraction of the antagonist muscle with the agonist. Another pattern, which can be called *ballistic,* resembles voluntary ballistic movements with a triphasic pattern; there is a burst of activity in the agonist muscle lasting 50 to 100 ms, a burst of activity in the antagonist muscle lasting 50 to 100 ms, and then return of activity in the agonist, often in the form of another burst. The third pattern, which can be called *reflex,* resembles the burst occurring in many reflexes, including H reflexes and stretch reflexes (Fig. 98–1). The EMG burst duration is 10 to 40 ms, and EMG activity in the antagonist muscle is virtually always synchronous.

MYOCLONUS

Myoclonus is characterized by quick muscle jerks, either irregular or rhythmical (Hallett et al., 1987; Hallett, 1997, 1999). There are many types of myoclonus, and no common etiological, physiological, or therapeutic features bind them together. Myoclonus can be focal, involving only a few adjacent muscles; generalized, involving many or most of the muscles in the body; or multifocal, involving many muscles but in different jerks. Myoclonus can be spontaneous, activated or accentuated by voluntary movement *(action myoclonus),* and activated or accentuated by sensory stimulation *(reflex myoclonus).* *Rhythmical (segmental) myoclonus* has the appearance of a rest tremor but is typically unaffected by

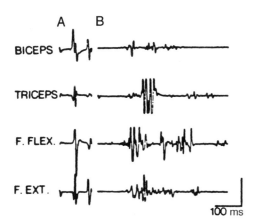

Figure 98–1. Comparison of "reflex" *(A)* and "ballistic" *(B)* electromyographic appearance underlying different types of myoclonus. *A* is from a patient with reticular reflex myoclonus, and *B* is from a patient with ballistic movement overflow myoclonus. Vertical calibration is 1 mV for *A* and 0.5 mV for *B.* (From Chadwick D, Hallett M, Harris R, et al: Clinical, biochemical, and physiological features distinguishing myoclonus responsive to 5-hydroxytryptophan, tryptophan with a monoamine oxidase inhibitor, and clonazepam. Brain 1977;100:455–487.)

action, stimulation, or even sleep. In this disorder, a segment of the spinal cord *(spinal myoclonus)* or brainstem *(palatal myoclonus)* produces persistent rhythmical repetitive discharges usually unaffected by sleep. Contiguous muscles produce synchronous contractions at a rate of 1 to 3 Hz. Because of the slow speed of the movements, palatal myoclonus is now preferentially called *palatal tremor.*

By defining *epileptic myoclonus* as myoclonus that is a fragment of epilepsy, it is possible to divide irregular myoclonus into epileptic and nonepileptic myoclonus (Hallett et al., 1987; Hallett, 1997, 1999). The physiological characteristics of epileptic myoclonus are (1) EMG burst length of 10 to 50 ms, (2) synchronous antagonist activity, and (3) an EEG correlate (the technique of EMG-EEG correlation is described later). The EMG shows a reflex pattern. Nonepileptic myoclonus shows (1) EMG burst lengths of 50 to 300 ms, (2) synchronous or asynchronous antagonist activity, and (3) no EEG correlate. The EMG patterns are either ballistic or tonic.

Examples of epileptic myoclonus are cortical reflex myoclonus, reticular reflex myoclonus, and primary generalized epileptic myoclonus; these are discussed later. Examples of nonepileptic myoclonus include dystonic myoclonus, essential myoclonus such as ballistic movement overflow myoclonus, exaggerated startle, physiological phenomena such as hypnic jerks, and periodic movements of sleep. Frequent myoclonus may have the appearance of tremor. In the case of action myoclonus, this may be confusing clinically, but EMG analysis is definitive.

For sorting out the different types of myoclonus, it can be useful to look for EEG events at the time of a movement (Hallett, 1999). Events in the ongoing EEG can be correlated with EMG events, but it is more informative to average the EEG with respect to the EMG (Hallett et al., 1994). Just as sensory evoked cerebral potentials are time-locked to the stimulus, these movement-related EEG potentials must be time-locked to a phase of the EMG, such as its onset. Much attention is devoted to that part of the potential preceding movement onset because it may relate to generation of the movement; the part of the potential after movement onset includes feedback from the movement itself. The movement potential can be analyzed for the presence of consistent positive and negative waves, and the topography and time relationship of these to the movement can be determined.

Stimulation may produce involuntary movements, such as reflex myoclonus, and evoke responses in the EEG. The waves in the evoked response that precede the provoked movement can be analyzed for their relationship with the movement. If the timing and topography of an event in the movement potential before a spontaneous involuntary movement are similar to the timing and topography of an event in the evoked response before the provoked movement, a similarity of the physiological mechanism can be suggested.

With reflex myoclonus, a late response may ap-

male, 10 y.o.

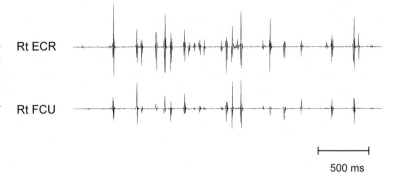

Figure 98–2. Electromyographic recording from a 10-year-old boy with Gaucher's disease with cortical myoclonus. The *top trace* is from the right extensor carpi radialis, and the *bottom trace* is from the right flexor carpi ulnaris. Note the short electromyographic bursts that are often synchronous in antagonist muscles. (Courtesy of K. Toma.)

Rt ECR

Rt FCU

|——————|
500 ms

pear in a relaxed muscle after stretch, mixed nerve stimulation, or cutaneous nerve stimulation. This response, which would not normally be present, may also be seen in muscles outside the region of the nerve stimulated or even throughout the body. This additional response, sometimes called a *C reflex,* is a myoclonic movement produced by the stimulation (Hallett, 1997; Toro and Hallett, 1997). Such responses are manifestations of hyperexcitability of the nervous system and typically reflect exaggerations of a normal reflex.

Epileptic Myoclonus

The use of these techniques can distinguish the three types of *epileptic myoclonus* described earlier (Hallett, 1997, 1999; Toro and Hallett, 1997). *Cortical reflex myoclonus* is a fragment of focal or partial

epilepsy. Each myoclonic jerk involves only a few adjacent muscles, but larger jerks with involvement of more muscles can be seen (Fig. 98–2). The disorder is commonly multifocal and is accentuated by action and sensory stimulation. The genesis of cortical reflex myoclonus is thought to be hyperexcitability of sensorimotor cortex, with each jerk representing the discharge of a small region activated by a paroxysmal depolarization shift. The EEG recognizes the discharge as a focal negative event preceding spontaneous and reflex-induced myoclonic jerks (Figs. 98–3 and 98–4). The event with reflex jerks is a giant P1-N2 component of the somatosensory evoked potential. Detailed studies with magnetoencephalography show that the exaggerated component of the EEG, with both spontaneous and reflex jerks, comes from the motor cortex (Mima et al., 1998a, 1998b).

Cortical control of muscular activity can be dem-

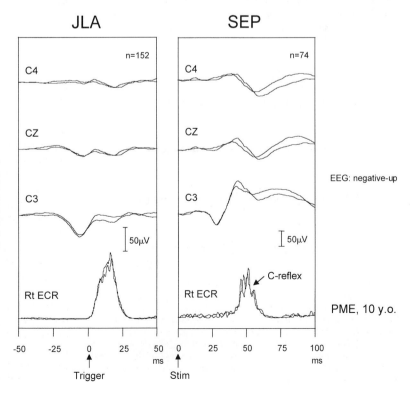

Figure 98–3. Jerk-locked average (JLA) and somatosensory evoked potentials (SEP) tracing from the same patient as in Figure 98–1. In each part of the figure, there are three electroencephalographic channels recorded referenced to linked ears and electromyography from the right extensor carpi radialis. The SEP tracing was produced by mechanical stimulation of the palm. (Courtesy of K. Toma.)

JLA

SEP

C4   n=152

CZ

C3

50µV

Rt ECR

C4   n=74

CZ

C3

50µV

Rt ECR   C-reflex

EEG: negative-up

PME, 10 y.o.

-50   -25   0   25   50
ms
Trigger

0   25   50   75   100
ms
Stim

onstrated by showing coherence between the EEG over the motor cortex region and the EMG (Mima and Hallett, 1999). This coherence is seen in discrete frequency bands, with the highest coherence generally in the β range. Several observations show that in some patients with cortical myoclonus, there is also coherence at high frequencies, not typical of neurologically normal persons (Brown et al., 1999; Marsden et al., 2000). This finding may indicate abnormal functioning of the motor cortex in this condition.

Cortical myoclonus can be rhythmical and may be confused with essential tremor. This condition has been called *cortical tremor* (Ikeda et al., 1990; Toro et al., 1993; Terada et al., 1997). The EEG correlate can be helpful to make the diagnosis if there is ambiguity.

Reticular reflex myoclonus is a fragment of a type of generalized epilepsy. These jerks are usually generalized with proximal more than distal and flexor more than extensor predominance. Voluntary action and sensory stimulation increase the jerking. The genesis of the myoclonus is thought to be hyperexcitability of a portion of the caudal brainstem reticular formation. A spike can be seen in the EEG often associated with the myoclonic jerk, but because it follows the first EMG manifestation and is not time-locked to the jerk, it does not seem responsible for the jerk. The first activated muscles are those innervated by cranial nerve XI; this finding strongly suggests the brainstem origin. The somatosensory evoked potential is not enlarged, but there can be a C reflex.

In both human investigations and animal studies, reticular reflex myoclonus and cortical reflex myoclonus can coexist (Hallett, 1997). In one case of posthypoxic myoclonus, the action myoclonus was cortical, and the sensory-induced myoclonus was reticular (Brown et al., 1991c).

In two patients with posthypoxic myoclonus who were thought on clinical and electrophysiological grounds to have reticular reflex myoclonus, thyrotropin-releasing hormone enhanced the onset of myoclonus, shortened the latency of the C reflex, and increased its amplitude, but it produced no change in the somatosensory evoked potential (Takeuchi et al., 1992). These results are consistent with the concept that thyrotropin-releasing hormone stimulates medullary reticular neurons and thereby enhances reticular reflex myoclonus. No such changes are seen in cortical reflex myoclonus. Hence, the thyrotropin-releasing hormone test may be helpful as a diagnostic aid.

Primary generalized epileptic myoclonus is a fragment of primary generalized epilepsy. The most common clinical manifestation is a small, focal jerk that often involves only the fingers and has sometimes been called *minipolymyoclonus.* Generalized body jerks can also be seen. This type of myoclonus is thought to arise from the firing of a hyperexcitable cortex driven synchronously by ascending subcortical impulses. The EEG correlate is a slow, bilateral, frontocentrally predominant negativity similar to the wave of a primary generalized paroxysm. In this circumstance, there is neither an enlarged somatosensory evoked response nor a C reflex.

Asterixis

Asterixis is a brief lapse in tonic innervation (Shibasaki, 1995; Tassinari et al., 1998 Hallett, 1999). It appears as an involuntary jerk superimposed on a postural or intentional movement. Careful observation often reveals that the jerk is in the direction of gravity, but this determination can be difficult because the lapse is frequently followed by a quick compensatory antigravity movement to restore limb position. The involuntary movement is usually irregular, but when asterixis comes rapidly, there may be the appearance of tremor. EMG analysis shows characteristic synchronous pauses in antagonist muscles (Fig. 98–5). Asterixis is also called *negative myoclonus* (Shibasaki, 1995). When there is an EEG correlate, then the physiology is likely similar to epileptic myoclonus, as described previously.

Essential Myoclonus

This term can be used for those patients whose sole neurological abnormality is myoclonus and who specifically do not have seizures, dementia, or ataxia. The EEG and other laboratory investigations

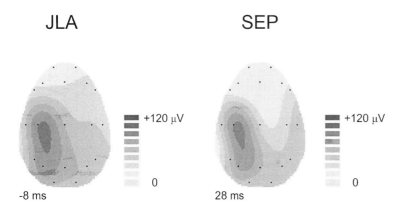

JLA   SEP

+120 µV

+120 µV

0

0

-8 ms   28 ms

Figure 98–4. Topographic map of the jerk-locked average (JLA) and somatosensory evoked potential (SEP) signals from which selected traces are shown in Figure 98–2. Note the similarity of the topography of the positive event that occurs just before the electromyographic discharge of the myoclonic jerk. (Courtesy of K. Toma.)

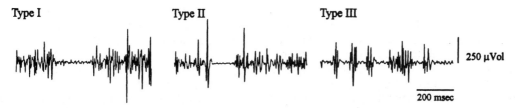

Figure 98–5. The electromyographic silent periods in negative myoclonus. Type I silent periods are characterized by abrupt cessation of electromyographic activity without a preceding positive event. In type II silent periods, a brief, variable-amplitude burst of electromyographic activity precedes the silence. Type III silent periods are briefer and follow typical positive myoclonus. (From Toro C, Hallett M, Rothwell JC, et al: Physiology of negative myoclonus. Adv Neurol 1995;67:211–217.)

should be normal. Familial cases as well as sporadic cases are seen. The most common features of the familial cases are autosomal dominant inheritance with variable severity, equal involvement of males and females, onset in the first or second decade of life, and benign course compatible with normal life span. *Essential myoclonus* can be generalized or multifocal. The myoclonus is variable in amplitude, and in some cases the jerks are so small that the disability can be minimal. Jerks can be present at rest and may be improved or worsened by action. Reflex myoclonus has not been described in this group.

In some families with essential myoclonus, some involved patients also have essential tremor, and some family members have essential tremor without myoclonus. Some of these patients also may exhibit elements of dystonia. The essential tremor, myoclonus, and dystonia may all be sensitive to alcohol in these patients (Quinn, 1996).

Startle

The *startle reflex* is a rapid, generalized motor response to a sudden, surprise stimulus (Brown et al., 1991a; Matsumoto et al., 1992; Matsumoto and Hallett, 1994; Hallett, 1999). The most extensively studied human startle response is that which occurs to loud noises. It is an oligosynaptic reflex mediated in the brainstem. The startle response is distinctive on EMG testing with surface electrodes. The pattern is bilaterally symmetrical with an invariable blink; other craniocervical muscles almost always are activated, but recruitment in the limbs is variable. The onset latency of EMG activity is 30 to 40 ms in orbicularis oculi, 55 to 85 ms in masseter and sterno-cleidomastoid, 85 to 100 ms in biceps brachii, 100 to 125 ms in hamstrings and quadriceps, and 130 to 140 ms in tibialis anterior. Careful observation shows that the latencies of the responses in the hand and foot muscles are much longer than would be expected from the latencies of more proximal muscles, and this may be a hallmark of startle. Detailed analysis shows that there is often a quick response in the orbicularis oculi separable from a second response. Assuming that the second is the "startle component," it appears that the reflex spreads up the brainstem similar to reticular reflex

myoclonus (Fig. 98–6). This is likely, in fact, because the startle reflex appears to be mediated in the nucleus reticularis pontis caudalis, a neighbor of the nucleus reticularis gigantocellularis that mediates reticular reflex myoclonus. There is synchronous activation of antagonist muscles with an EMG burst duration of 50 to 400 ms. Habituation generally occurs after four or five stimuli. Increased startle responses are recognized by being excessive or being evoked by stimuli that would not be effective in most people. This is most easily identified by loss of habituation. Increased startle reflexes are characteristic of a variety of disorders including hereditary hyperekplexia.

Spinal Myoclonus

In *spinal myoclonus,* a segment of the spinal cord produces spontaneous, persistent rhythmical repetitive discharges usually unaffected by sleep. Some contiguous muscles produce synchronous contractions at a rate of 0.5 to 3 Hz, and this seems to result from heightened spinal excitability (Di Lazzaro et al., 1996). Involved regions can be one limb, one limb and the adjacent trunk, or both legs. Lesions of the spinal cord giving rise to focal movements include infection, degenerative disease, tumor, cervical myelopathy, and demyelinating disease, and the disorder may follow spinal anesthesia or the introduction of contrast media into the cerebrospinal fluid.

Propriospinal myoclonus is a special type of spinal myoclonus (Brown et al., 1991b; Chokroverty et al., 1992). It is clinically characterized by axial jerks that are nonrhythmical and that lead to symmetrical flexion of neck, trunk, hips, and knees. Jerks can be spontaneous or induced by a stimulus. The myoclonus can be induced by drowsiness and relaxation (Montagna et al., 1997). The myoclonus is identified with electrodiagnostic studies that show the myoclonus starting in midthoracic region and propagating slowly, at about 5 m per second, both rostrally and caudally.

Nocturnal Myoclonus

Various types of myoclonus occur during drowsiness or sleep and are described in detail in subse-

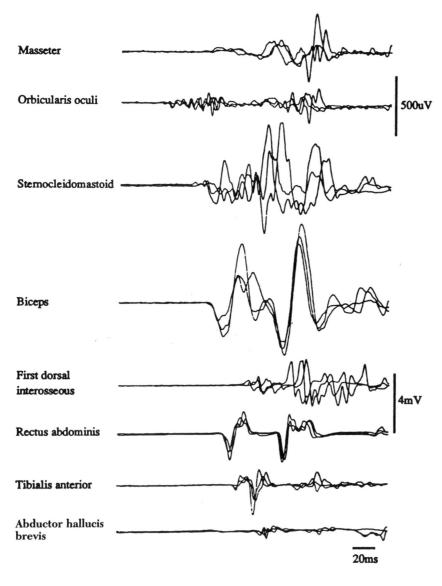

Masseter

Orbicularis oculi

500uV

Sternocleidomastoid

Biceps

First dorsal
interosseous

4mV

Rectus abdominis

Tibialis anterior

Abductor hallucis
brevis

20ms

Figure 98–6. Electromyographic activity in an abnormal startle response elicited by auditory stimulation in a patient with symptomatic hyperexplexia. The unrectified electromyographic activity in three single trials is superimposed. Discounting the initial auditory blink response, electromyographic activity was recorded first in sternocleidomastoid and then in masseter and trunk and limb muscles. The latencies to the intrinsic muscles of the hand and foot were disproportionately long. (From Brown P, Rothwell JC, Thompson PD, et al: The hyperekplexias and their relationship to the normal startle reflex. Brain 1991a;114:1903–1928.)

quent chapters. There are two physiological forms, the *hypnic jerk* (Dagnino et al., 1969) and *physiological fragmentary myoclonus,* which is characterized by small, multifocal jerks maximal in hands and face, but present diffusely (Broughton et al., 1985; Montagna et al., 1988). Pathological types of myoclonus include isolated periodic movements in sleep, restless legs syndrome with periodic movements in sleep, and excessive fragmentary myoclonus in nonrapid eye movement sleep (Broughton et al., 1985). Myoclonus associated with epilepsy, intention myoclonus associated with semivolitional movements, and segmental myoclonus also occur in sleep, but they are not primarily nocturnal.

Periodic movements of sleep, or periodic limb movement disorder, occurs in virtually all groups of patients referred to a sleep disorder laboratory, and the clinical correlation is not always clear. Although often classified as myoclonus, the movement is typically too long in duration to fit this category. Patients with the restless legs syndrome often have

periodic movements of sleep (Walters, 1995; Trenkwalder et al., 1996). Certainly, periodic movements of sleep can be asymptomatic for the patient, although, as with all types of nocturnal myoclonus, the disorder may cause distress to the patient's sleeping partner. On some occasions, however, periodic movements of sleep can induce sleep fragmentation and excessive daytime sleepiness. The origin of periodic movements of sleep seems to be increased excitability of the flexor reflex mechanism of the spinal cord (Bara-Jimenez et al., 2000).

TIC

Tics are quick, involuntary, repetitive movements that occur at irregular intervals (Hallett, 1999). The unique feature of a tic is that it is not completely involuntary. Most patients describe a psychic tension that builds up inside them and can be relieved by the tic movement. Hence the tics can be volunta-

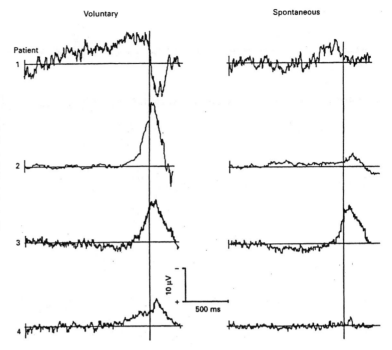

Figure 98–7. Movement-related cortical potentials accompanying voluntarily imitated and spontaneous tics. All tracings are from Cz referenced to linked ears. The *horizontal line* represents the baseline, and the *vertical line* indicates the time of electromyographic onset. Only in patients 1 and 3 is there a brief negativity preceding the tic movement. (From Karp BI, Porter S, Toro C, Hallett M: Simple motor tics may be preceded by a premotor potential. J Neurol Neurosurg Psychiatry 1996;61:103–106.)

rily suppressed for some time at the expense of increasing psychic tension; patients "let the tic happen" (or perhaps even "make the tic") to relieve the tension. Tic movements, which can be simple or complex, look like quick, voluntary movements both clinically and by EMG. EMG bursts vary from 50 to 200 ms in duration and may have a ballistic or tonic pattern. The EMG has more complex patterns and longer bursts of activity associated with dystonic or complex tics. The EMG pattern of a dystonic tic is not clearly separable from a dystonic movement. These findings differ from certain types of myoclonus, for example, in which the EMG bursts are shorter than can be produced voluntarily. They also differ from chorea, which is characterized by EMG bursts that appear with random length in random muscles and is associated with paroxysmal lapses in EMG activity when there is an attempted tonic contraction.

Obeso et al. reported that there was no normal premotor activity before simple tics (Obeso et al., 1981), but the premotor activity was normal for similar movements produced voluntarily by the same patients. Five of six patients had no activity at all before the tics, and in the sixth patient only a small potential was recognized. These findings were interpreted to mean that tics differed from voluntary movements because of their lack of cortical preparatory activity. Karp et al. repeated this study and found similar results (Karp et al., 1994). Three of five patients showed no premotor activity, and the other two showed a small negativity before tics (Fig. 98–7). The negativity, when present, was brief, and it is possible to interpret their findings that there was only the late component of the premotor activity. This pattern of activity may be helpful in differential diagnosis because, for example, normal pre-

motor activity occurs in most patients with psychogenic movement disorders (Terada et al., 1995a).

CHOREA, DYSKINESIA, AND BALLISM

The most appropriate adjective to describe *chorea* is "random" (Hallett, 1999). Random muscles throughout the body are affected at random times and make movements of random duration. Movements can be brief, such as myoclonus, or long, such as dystonia. Usually, they are totally beyond voluntary control, but in some mild cases, the movements can be temporarily suppressed. EMG patterns are reflex, ballistic, and tonic. *Dyskinesia* describes choreic movements seen in selected circumstances, such as a late consequence of neuroleptic drugs or with levodopa toxicity. *Ballism* describes wild, large-amplitude choreic movements; these usually involve one side of the body and are then called *hemiballismus*.

Sometimes there are rhythmical movements in dyskinesias. Stereotyped repetitive alternating movements of the legs have been described in dyskinesia resulting from levodopa. The EMG pattern of the repetitive alternating movements is an asynchronous, alternating, rhythmical pattern at about 1 Hz (Luquin et al., 1992). In vascular chorea (Hashimoto and Yanagisawa, 1994), caused by infarcts in the basal ganglia, and in tardive dyskinesia (Bathien et al., 1984), there can be some rhythmical bursting as well as the random bursts, and perhaps this bears some relation to the repetitive alternating movements.

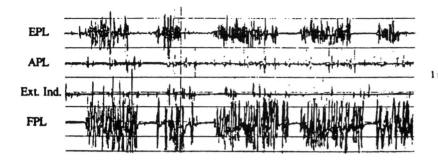

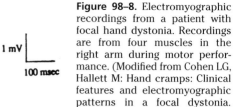

Figure 98–8. Electromyographic recordings from a patient with focal hand dystonia. Recordings are from four muscles in the right arm during motor performance. (Modified from Cohen LG, Hallett M: Hand cramps: Clinical features and electromyographic patterns in a focal dystonia. Neurology 1988;38:1005–1012.)

DYSTONIA AND ATHETOSIS

The involuntary movements of dystonia and athetosis are similar, and the use of one term rather than the other seems more a matter of situation and semantics than physiology (Hallett, 1999). The movements are typically slow but can be quick and may be "sustained for a second or longer at the height of the involuntary contraction." *Dystonia* is often used to describe proximal "twisting" movements; *athetosis* is often used to describe distal "flowing" movements. Dystonic and athetotic movements are frequently characterized by cocontraction of antagonist muscles (Hallett, 1998b). Although normal voluntary movement is often characterized by reciprocal inhibition, there may be some cocontraction. The cocontraction of dystonia and athetosis is excessive, with the appearance of increased tension at the joint. Some dystonic and athetotic movements are fully involuntary and arise at rest independent of will. Other movements arise as excessive, unwanted concomitants to voluntary movements. This phenomenon is called *overflow,* with the implication that the motor control command is sent to too many muscles with too much intensity. EMG studies can document these phenomena (Fig. 98–8). The shortest EMG bursts seen even with dystonic myoclonus are in the range of 100 to 300 ms.

The physiology of dystonia has been studied in detail and generally can be characterized by loss of inhibition at all levels of the neuraxis (Berardelli et al., 1998; Hallett, 1998a, 1998b). Some clinical neurophysiological tests are frequently abnormal in patients with dystonia, but none have specificity. Hence, such studies can be employed to see whether a consistent abnormality is present. Three tests are worthy of mention in this regard.

Reciprocal inhibition can be assessed at the spinal cord level. It is evaluated in the upper extremity by studying the effect of stimulating the radial nerve at various times before producing an H reflex with median nerve stimulation. The radial nerve afferents come from muscles that are antagonist to median nerve muscles. Via various pathways, the radial afferent traffic can inhibit motoneuron pools of median nerve muscles. Reciprocal inhibition is reduced in patients with dystonia, including those with generalized dystonia, writer's cramp, spasmodic torticollis, and blepharospasm (Fig. 98–9) (Nakashima et

al., 1989; Panizza et al., 1989, 1990; Deuschl et al., 1992; Chen et al., 1995).

The *blink reflex* can be used to assess inhibition at the level of the brainstem. Abnormalities of blink reflex recovery were first identified for blepharospasm (Berardelli et al., 1985), and they have also been demonstrated in generalized dystonia, spasmodic torticollis, and spasmodic dysphonia (Cohen et al., 1989). In the last two conditions, abnormalities can be found even without clinical involvement of the eyelids.

Inhibition can also be shown to be deficient at the level of the motor cortex. Ridding et al. studied *intracortical inhibition* with the "double pulse paradigm" (Ridding et al., 1995). Motor evoked potentials were inhibited when they were conditioned by a prior subthreshold transcranial magnetic stimulation stimulus to the same position at intervals of 1 to 5 ms. Inhibition was less in both hemispheres of patients with focal hand dystonia, a finding showing that the test is sufficiently sensitive to detect subclinical abnormality.

PSYCHOGENIC MOVEMENT DISORDERS

Psychogenic movements can mimic virtually any involuntary movement disorder. In their report of

Controls/affected side of patients

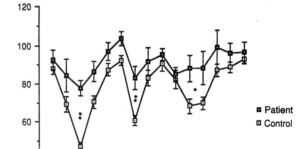

Figure 98–9. Reciprocal inhibition study of the affected hands of patients with focal hand dystonia compared with a group of normal control subjects. (From Panizza ME, Hallett M, Nilsson J: Reciprocal inhibition in patients with hand cramps. Neurology 1989;39:85–89.)

patients with psychogenic myoclonus, Monday and Jankovic pointed to the following clinical findings that help to make this diagnosis: features incongruous with "organic" myoclonus, evidence of underlying psychopathology, an improvement with distraction or placebo, and the presence of incongruous sensory loss or false weakness (Monday and Jankovic, 1993). Thompson et al. proposed five neurophysiological criteria suggesting psychogenic movements: (1) variable latencies to the onset of stimulus-induced jerks, (2) latencies greater than those seen in reflex myoclonus of cortical or brainstem origin and (3) longer than the fastest voluntary reaction times of normal subjects, (4) variable patterns of muscle recruitment within each jerk, and (5) significant habituation with repeated stimulation (Thompson et al., 1992).

As noted earlier, psychogenic involuntary movements are generally preceded by normal-looking premotor activity on the EEG (Terada et al., 1995b). Conversely, some physiological findings rule out a psychogenic movement disorder: (1) short EMG burst with a reflex pattern and (2) reflex myoclonus (C reflex) latency shorter than voluntary reaction time.

Acknowledgment

This chapter has drawn heavily on earlier chapters on the clinical neurophysiology of motor control (Hallett, 1999, 2000).

References

Bara-Jimenez W, Aksu M, Graham B, et al: Periodic limb movements in sleep: State-dependent excitability of the spinal flexor reflex. Neurology 2000;54:1609–1616.
Bathien N, Koutlidis RM, Rondot P: EMG patterns in abnormal involuntary movements induced by neuroleptics. J Neurol Neurosurg Psychiatry 1984;47:1002–1008.
Berardelli A, Rothwell JC, Day BL, Marsden CD: Pathophysiology of blepharospasm and oromandibular dystonia. Brain 1985;108:593–608.
Berardelli A, Rothwell JC, Hallett M, et al: The pathophysiology of primary dystonia. Brain 1998;121;1195–1212.
Broughton R, Tolentino MA, Krelina M: Excessive fragmentary myoclonus in NREM sleep: A report of 38 cases. Electroencephalogr Clin Neurophysiol 1985;61;123–133.
Brown P, Farmer SF, Halliday DM, et al: Coherent cortical and muscle discharge in cortical myoclonus. Brain 1999;122;461–472.
Brown P, Rothwell JC, Thompson PD, et al: The hyperekplexias and their relationship to the normal startle reflex. Brain 1991a;114:1903–1928.
Brown P, Thompson PD, Rothwell JC, et al: Axial myoclonus of propriospinal origin. Brain 1991b;114;197–214.
Brown P, Thompson PD, Rothwell JC, et al: A case of postanoxic encephalopathy with cortical action and brainstem reticular reflex myoclonus. Mov Disord 1991c;6;139–144.
Chadwick D, Hallett M, Harris R, et al: Clinical, biochemical, and physiological features distinguishing myoclonus responsive to 5-hydroxytryptophan, tryptophan with a monoamine oxidase inhibitor, and clonazepam. Brain 1977;100:455–487.
Chen RS, Tsai CH, Lu CS: Reciprocal inhibition in writer's cramp. Mov Disord 1995;10;556–561.
Chokroverty, S, Walters A, Zimmerman T, Picone M: Propriospinal

myoclonus: A neurophysiologic analysis. Neurology 1992;42;1591–1595.
Cohen LG, Hallett M: Hand cramps: Clinical features and electromyographic patterns in a focal dystonia. Neurology 1988;38:1005–1012.
Cohen LG, Ludlow CL, Warden M, et al: Blink reflex excitability recovery curves in patients with spasmodic dysphonia. Neurology 1989;39;572–577.
Dagnino N, Loeb C, Massazza G, Sacco G: Hypnic physiological myoclonias in man: An EEG-EMG study in normals and neurological patients. Eur Neurol 1969;2;47–58.
Deuschl G, Seifert G, Heinen F, et al: Reciprocal inhibition of forearm flexor muscles in spasmodic torticollis. J Neurol Sci 1992;113;85–90.
Di Lazzaro V, Restuccia D, Nardone R, et al: Changes in spinal cord excitability in a patient with rhythmic segmental myoclonus. J Neurol Neurosurg Psychiatry 1996;61;641–644.
Hallett M: Myoclonus and myoclonic syndromes. In Engel JJ, Pedley TA (eds): Epilepsy: A Comprehensive Textbook, vol 3. Philadelphia, Lippincott–Raven, 1997; 2717–2723.
Hallett M: The neurophysiology of dystonia. Arch Neurol 1998a;55;601–603.
Hallett M: Physiology of dystonia. Adv Neurol 1998b;78:11–18.
Hallett M: Electrophysiologic evaluation of movement disorders. In Aminoff MJ (ed): Electrodiagnosis in Clinical Neurology. New York, Churchill Livingstone, 1999; 365–380.
Hallett M: Electrodiagnosis in movement disorders. In Levin KH, Lüders HO (eds): Comprehensive Clinical Neurophysiology. Philadelphia, WB Saunders, 2000; 281–294.
Hallett M, Berardelli A, Delwaide P, et al: Central EMG and tests of motor control: Report of an IFCN Committee. Electroencephalogr. Clin Neurophysiol 1994;90;404–432.
Hallett M, Marsden CD, Fahn S: Myoclonus. In Vinken PJ, Bruyn GW, Klawans HL (eds): Handbook of Clinical Neurology, vol 5. Amsterdam, Elsevier Science, 1987; 609-625.
Hashimoto T, Yanagisawa N: A comparison of the regularity of involuntary muscle contractions in vascular chorea with that in Huntington's chorea, hemiballism and parkinsonian tremor. J Neurol Sci 1994;125;87–94.
Ikeda A, Kakigi R, Funai N, et al: Cortical tremor: A variant of cortical reflex myoclonus. Neurology 1990;40;1561–1565.
Karp BI, Porter S, Toro C, Hallett M: Simple motor tics may be preceded by a premotor potential. J Neurol Neurosurg Psychiatry 1996;61:103–106.
Karp BI, Toro C, Hallett M: Simple motor tics in Tourette's syndrome may be preceded by a premotor potential [Abstract]. Mov Disord 1994;9(suppl 1):34.
Luquin MR, Scipioni O, Vaamonde J, et al: Levodopa-induced dyskinesias in Parkinson's disease: Clinical and pharmacological classification. Mov Disord 1992;7;117–124.
Marsden JF, Ashby P, Rothwell JC, Brown P: Phase relationships between cortical and muscle oscillations in cortical myoclonus: Electrocorticographic assessment in a single case. Clin Neurophysiol 2000;111;2170–2174.
Matsumoto J, Fuhr P, Nigro M, Hallett M: Physiological abnormalities in hereditary hyperekplexia. Ann Neurol 1992;32;41–50.
Matsumoto J, Hallett M: Startle syndromes. In Marsden CD, Fahn S (eds): Movement Disorders 3. Oxford, Butterworth-Heinemann, 1994; 418–433.
Mima T, Hallett M: Corticomuscular coherence: A review. J Clin Neurophysiol 1999;16;501–511.
Mima T, Nagamine T, Ikeda A, et al: Pathogenesis of cortical myoclonus studied by magnetoencephalography. Ann Neurol 1998a;43;598–607.
Mima T, Nagamine T, Nishitani N, et al: Cortical myoclonus: Sensorimotor hyperexcitability. Neurology 1998b;50;933–942.
Monday K, Jankovic J: Psychogenic myoclonus. Neurology 1993;43;349–352.
Montagna P, Liguori R, Zucconi M, et al: Physiological hypnic myoclonus. Electroencephalogr Clin Neurophysiol 1988;70;172–176.
Montagna P, Provini F, Plazzi G, et al: Propriospinal myoclonus upon relaxation and drowsiness: A cause of severe insomnia. Mov Disord 1997;12;66–72.
Nakashima K, Rothwell JC, Day BL, et al: Reciprocal inhibition in

writer's and other occupational cramps and hemiparesis due to stroke. Brain 1989;112;681–697.

Obeso JA, Rothwell JC, Marsden CD: Simple tics in Gilles de la Tourette's syndrome are not prefaced by a normal premovement potential. J Neurol Neurosurg Psychiatry 1981;44;735–738.

Panizza M, Lelli S, Nilsson J, Hallett M: H-reflex recovery curve and reciprocal inhibition of H-reflex in different kinds of dystonia. Neurology 1990;40;824–828.

Panizza ME, Hallett M, Nilsson J: Reciprocal inhibition in patients with hand cramps. Neurology 1989;39;85–89.

Quinn NP: Essential myoclonus and myoclonic dystonia. Mov Disord 1996;11;119–124.

Ridding MC, Sheean G, Rothwell JC, et al: Changes in the balance between motor cortical excitation and inhibition in focal, task specific dystonia. J Neurol Neurosurg Psychiatry 1995;59;493–498.

Shibasaki H: Pathophysiology of negative myoclonus and asterixis. In Fahn S, Hallett M, Lüders HO, Marsden CD (eds): Negative Motor Phenomena. Philadelphia, Lippincott-Raven, 1995; 199–209.

Takeuchi H, Touge T, Miki H, et al: Electrophysiological and pharmacological studies of somatosensory reflex myoclonus. Electromyogr Clin Neurophysiol 1992;32;143–154.

Tassinari CA, Rubboli G, Shibasaki H: Neurophysiology of positive and negative myoclonus. Electroencephalogr Clin Neurophysiol 1998;107;181–195.

Terada K, Ikeda A, Mima T, et al: Familial cortical myoclonic tremor as a unique form of cortical reflex myoclonus. Mov Disord 1997;12;370–377.

Terada K, Ikeda A, Nagamine T, Shibasaki H: Movement-related cortical potentials associated with voluntary muscle relaxation. Electromyogr Clin Neurophysiol 1995a;95;335–345.

Terada K, Ikeda A, Van Ness PC, et al: Presence of Bereitschafts-potential preceding psychogenic myoclonus: Clinical application of jerk-locked back averaging. J Neurol Neurosurg Psychiatry 1995b;58;745–747.

Thompson PD, Colebatch JG, Brown P, et al: Voluntary stimulus-sensitive jerks and jumps mimicking myoclonus or pathological startle syndromes. Mov Disord 1992;7;257–262.

Toro C, Hallett M: Pathophysiology of myoclonic disorders. In Watts RL, Koller WC (eds): Movement Disorders: Neurologic Principles and Practice. New York, McGraw-Hill, 1997; 551–560.

Toro C, Hallett M, Rothwell JC, et al: Physiology of negative myoclonus. Adv Neurol 1995;67:211–217.

Toro C, Pascual-Leone A, Deuschl G, et al: Cortical tremor: A common manifestation of cortical myoclonus. Neurology 1993; 43;2346–2353.

Trenkwalder C, Walters AS, Hening W: Periodic limb movements and restless legs syndrome. Neurol Clin 1996;14;629–650.

Walters AS: Toward a better definition of the restless legs syndrome: The International Restless Legs Syndrome Study Group. Mov Disord 1995;10;634–642.

Tremor

Rodger J. Elble and Günther Deuschl

Neurophysiological techniques have been applied to the study of *tremor* for more than a century. Available techniques provide insight into the mechanisms of tremor, but, with few exceptions, they do not provide the investigator with a specific diagnosis. Nevertheless, the neurophysiological techniques described in this chapter are employed with increasing regularity in the quantification and diagnosis of tremor disorders and in the elucidation of their pathophysiology. Here the most widely used techniques are described in some detail, with emphasis on their pitfalls and limitations. Methods of less certain utility are briefly summarized and referenced.

QUANTIFICATION OF TREMOR

Accelerometry

Many types of transducers are used to record the force, displacement, velocity, and acceleration of tremor. Each transducer has advantages and disadvantages, which are reviewed elsewhere (Elble and Koller, 1990; Stiles and Hahs, 1991).

Miniature *accelerometers* are the most popular devices for recording tremor because they are lightweight (less than 15 g) and extremely sensitive (greater than 6 mV per acceleration of gravity). Accelerometers have been used extensively in clinical and basic research since the mid-1960s, and accelerometry has become a standard for measuring tremor amplitude and frequency. A uniaxial accelerometer costs less than $1,000 and is easily interfaced with a personal computer that is equipped with an analog-to-digital converter.

The most popular accelerometers are the piezoresistive devices. Piezoresistive accelerometers are sensitive to gravity, and this gravitational artifact can impede the recording of low-amplitude tremor. Consequently, the accelerometer signal is often filtered to remove frequencies lower than 1.0 Hz (van Someren et al., 1996).

At least six uniaxial accelerometers are required to measure three-dimensional translation and rotation of a body segment (Padgaonkar et al., 1975), and accelerometers must be mounted on each body segment to provide a complete recording of tremor that emerges from multiple joints. Thus, a hand-mounted uniaxial or triaxial accelerometer provides only a crude measure of tremor in an upper extremity that is free to move at the shoulder, elbow, and wrist. Changes in tremor amplitude can be obscured by changes in tremor direction, and it is impossible to identify the joint from which a tremor is emerging unless the limb is splinted or supported to restrict motion to a single joint.

Another limitation of accelerometry stems from the mathematical relationship between acceleration and displacement. For a sinusoidal displacement of amplitude A, the velocity and acceleration are the first and second derivatives of displacement, as given in the equations

$$displacement = A \sin(\omega t),$$
$$velocity = A\omega \cos(\omega t),$$

and

$$acceleration = -A\omega^2 \sin(\omega t),$$

where ω is the frequency of oscillation in radians per second (1 cycle per second equals 1 Hz equals 2π radians per second) and t is time. Thus, for two tremors of identical displacement amplitude but different frequencies, the tremor with the higher frequency will have a larger acceleration, as measured with an accelerometer. The displacement amplitude of tremor is generally symptomatic, not the velocity or acceleration. Consequently, it is reasonable to convert tremor acceleration to displacement amplitude at a particular frequency by dividing tremor acceleration by the squared tremor frequency in radians per second. This may improve the correlation between accelerometry and ordinal clinical ratings of tremor, which are often quite poor (Bain et al., 1993). Additional improvement in the correlation between accelerometry and clinical ratings is obtained by log-transformation of these measures to accommodate their nonlinear relationship (Bain et al., 1993; Elble et al., 1996; Matsumoto et al., 1999).

Digitizing Tablet

Writing and drawing are particularly useful tasks for assessing action tremor in the upper extremities (Bain et al., 1993). *Computerized digitizing (graphics) tablets* can be used to quantify the amplitude and frequency of tremor and to obviate the need for subjective, imprecise rating scales (Elble et al., 1990b, 1996). The horizontal and vertical displacement of a pen is recorded by the tablet and is fed to a digital computer for subsequent analyses. Estimates of velocity and acceleration can be obtained through numerical differentiation of displacement, using methods such as those described by Savitzky and Golay (1964). Available digitizing tablets with accuracies better than 0.25 mm and sampling frequencies greater than 70 per second are

suitable for measuring pathological (i.e., visible) tremor in handwriting and drawings but are not suitable for measuring physiological tremor.

Force Transducers

Force transducers are advantageous when the principal aim is to measure changes in isometric force resulting from motor unit entrainment while minimizing the influence of mechanical resonant properties of a limb. Force transducers use a strain gauge mounted on a cantilever beam that is anchored to a fixed platform, so they are suitable only for measuring tremor during isometric contractions.

Measurement of Limb Position and Rotation

Measurements of joint rotation and limb position have been accomplished with precision potentiometers (goniometers) and a variety of optical devices. Most of these devices have a sensitivity that is suitable only for measuring pathological tremor. However, Beuter and colleagues used a modern laser system to measure finger tremor, and they obtained recordings comparable to those achieved with an accelerometer (Beuter et al., 1994). Such laser systems are portable and are easily interfaced with a personal computer. The finger or other recording site must remain in the recording volume of the laser. Therefore, voluntary limb motion during a recording must be limited.

Photogrammetrical methods have been used for decades in the analysis of gait and now have a precision and accuracy suitable for studies of pathological tremor (Bastian and Thach, 1995; Cappello et al., 1997; Quintern et al., 1999). The resolution and accuracy depend on the reference volume (distance of the cameras from the patient), and the size of the reference volume determines the extent of the body and its movement that can be recorded. Spatial accuracies better than 1 mm are possible. This spatial accuracy is satisfactory for moderate to severe pathological tremors but is not sufficient for the study of extremely mild pathological tremors and physiological tremor. Sampling frequencies of 50 per second or more are common and are adequate for the quantification of all pathological tremors.

Photogrammetry is the best available method for studying the motion of multiple joints in three-dimensional space. Modern photogrammetrical systems use either active or passive topographic markers and a set of two or more computer-controlled cameras. The active markers are infrared light–emitting diodes that emit pulses of light at specified intervals. A computer controls the timing of light emission. Computer-controlled cameras record the light emissions over time, and three-dimensional translation and rotation of body segments are computed from these data. The passive markers are hemispheres of plastic that reflect stroboscopic infrared light emitted from computer-controlled cameras.

Acoustic Myogram

The sounds produced by single motor units in superficial muscles can be detected with a *sound transducer* (microphone or electronic stethoscope) applied over a muscle (Gordon and Holbourn, 1948; Oster and Jaffe, 1980; Rhatigan et al., 1986). This technique has been used to detect rhythmical motor activity, which tends to occur at 10, 20, and 40 Hz (Oster and Jaffe, 1980; Rhatigan et al., 1986; Brown, 1997; McAuley et al., 1997). It is unclear whether this approach has any advantage over conventional electromyography (EMG), which provides a more direct measure of rhythmical motor unit entrainment. Indeed, Ouamer and coworkers found that most of the acoustic myogram bears no relationship with motor unit firing or tremor but is mainly a resonant bending vibration of contracting muscle (Ouamer et al., 1999). Cross-talk and low signal-to-noise ratio are problems in acoustic myography, just as they are in EMG (Orizio, 1993).

ELECTROMYOGRAPHIC ANALYSIS OF TREMOR

Single Motor Unit Recordings

Single motor unit spike trains can be recorded continuously with needle or fine wire electrodes. Bipolar and unipolar electrodes of both types have been used successfully in the study of tremor and motor unit synchronization (Elble and Randall, 1976; Logigian et al., 1988; De Luca et al., 1993; Wessberg and Kakuda, 1999). Holding one or two motor units is difficult during voluntary movement and during steady posture when tremor is severe. Low-frequency motion artifact is common and must be removed with a high-pass filter.

Surface Electromyography

Recording EMG with skin electrodes is a noninvasive, painless method of sampling a large population of motor units. Surface EMG is preferable to needle and wire EMG when information is desired about the global behavior of motor units in a particular muscle. This approach is particularly useful when the details of individual motor unit behavior are not required and when the muscle is located immediately beneath the skin. Deeper muscles are recorded with needle or wire electrodes (Perry et al., 1981).

Cross-talk is the volume-conducted spread of electrical activity from one muscle to the electrodes overlying a neighboring muscle (Perry et al., 1981; Journée et al., 1983; De Luca and Merletti, 1988). This problem should always be suspected when extremely high amplifier gains are used and when multiple neighboring muscles are active. Cross-talk can occur between neighboring extensors or flexors and between extensors and flexors on opposite sides of a limb segment (e.g., the forearm). Reducing the size of and spacing between surface electrodes will reduce cross-talk but will also reduce the amplitude of the EMG. Flexible wire electrodes can be used when cross-talk is a problem. With wire electrodes, much lower amplifier gains are required because the attenuation of EMG by the skin impedance is not a problem. The surface area on the wires that is stripped of insulation governs the number of motor units recorded.

Spectral analysis of surface EMG reveals activity from 0 to 200 Hz or more, depending on the low-pass filtering properties of the electrodes, skin, and other soft tissues between the muscle and the electrodes (Kwatny et al., 1970; Hogan and Mann, 1980). Activity greater than 40 Hz largely reflects the shapes and durations of the motor unit action potentials, which are not relevant to the study of tremor (Basmajian and De Luca, 1985). Often, there is an ill-defined peak at 10 to 30 Hz that is caused by the prevailing motor unit firing frequencies (Hogan and Mann, 1980; Basmajian and De Luca, 1985). To investigate tremor, the EMG is full-wave rectified (equivalent to taking the absolute value of the EMG) and low-pass filtered, producing a so-called *demodulated EMG* (Journée et al., 1983). The cutoff frequency of the low-pass filter is usually less that 60 Hz, depending on the frequency range of interest. Demodulation can be performed with analog devices or with a digital computer after the EMG is digitized. A slightly different approach to demodulation is to square the digitized signal, low-pass filter the squared signal, and then take the square root of the result (Bacher et al., 1989; Spieker et al., 1997). It is unclear whether this approach and other alternative approaches (Kreifeldt and Yao, 1974) have any practical advantages over the traditional approach of full-wave rectification (Hogan and Mann, 1980). Before rectification, the EMG is high-pass filtered to remove baseline artifact caused by motion of the limb and recording electrodes. This is usually accomplished by setting the lower frequency limit of the amplifier to 10 to 25 Hz.

The demodulated EMG is proportional to the force generated by the muscle, but this relationship is nonlinear and varies among subjects (Hogan and Mann, 1980; Solomonow et al., 1991). Consequently, rectified-filtered EMG provides only a crude measure of tremor amplitude that cannot be compared across different subjects. Spectral analysis of the rectified-filtered EMG is most useful in revealing entrainment of motor unit activity at the frequency of tremor. The fraction of the total spectral power from 1 Hz to the upper frequency of interest (12 to 60 Hz) that is contained in the tremor spectral peak provides a measure of the intensity of motor unit entrainment.

LONG-TERM AMBULATORY RECORDINGS OF TREMOR

In most clinical and basic experimental studies, tremor has been recorded for a minute or so during one or more trials in an experimental session. This approach does not capture the hourly or daily fluctuations that occur in physiological and pathological tremors (Tyrer and Bond, 1974; Koller and Royse, 1985; Cleeves et al., 1986; Cleeves and Findley, 1987). For example, parkinsonian rest tremor is notoriously intermittent in some patients and may be influenced by drug-induced fluctuations. Essential tremor may also be intermittent, particularly in milder cases. A random recording for a minute or so may not reflect a patient's peak or average disability and may not capture the abnormal tremor (Elble et al., 1992a; Boose et al., 1995). Consequently, long-term ambulatory recording devices using accelerometry (van Someren et al., 1998) and EMG (Bacher et al., 1989; Boose et al., 1995; Spieker et al., 1997) are becoming increasingly popular methods of quantifying tremor.

Long-term recording of tremor in a freely moving patient is hampered by mechanical and electromagnetic artifact. Accelerometric systems are prone to mechanical artifact caused by bumping and extraneous vibrations. Filtering the artifact may distort the recording because tremor and mechanical artifact often have similar frequencies. Mechanical artifacts are less of a problem in recording EMG because their frequency content is much lower than the high-frequency activity of the interference pattern. Mechanical artifact in EMG consists of deviations in the EMG baseline caused by inadvertent jarring of the electrodes or by the tremor itself, and this artifact is usually easily identified and removed with high-pass filters having cutoff frequencies of 10 to 25 Hz. The filtered EMG is demodulated before spectral analysis, and spectra of successive time segments are computed to determine the intensity (ratio of spectral peak to background noise) and occurrence (percentage of recording time) of EMG modulation by tremor. The phase between EMG modulations of antagonistic muscles is also computed (Boose et al., 1995). Spieker and coworkers found that tremor occurrence, but not intensity, correlated well with clinical ratings of parkinsonian tremor and essential tremor (Spieker et al., 1997).

Redmond and Hegge developed a self-contained activity monitor *(actigraph)* that was worn on the wrist and used a miniature accelerometer (Redmond and Hegge, 1985). This device had no receiver to restrict the patient's activity. The frequency response, sensitivity, and vulnerability to mechanical artifact have been refined to the point that these devices are useful in recording tremor outside a laboratory (van Someren et al., 1998). The frequency content of voluntary movement overlaps with that of physiological and pathological tremors (van Someren et al., 1996), so the actigraphs often contain a software algorithm for identifying tremor on the basis of rhythmicity (van Someren et al., 1998). Tremor duration, frequency, and amplitude are estimated with this algorithm. It is also possible to use an actigraph to record a continuous sample of tremor during a particular activity, and the digitized time series could then be downloaded to a personal computer for analysis. The duration of the time series is limited by the memory capacity of the actigraph.

SIGNAL ANALYSIS

Spectral Analysis

Spectral analysis is a mathematical process that decomposes a digitized signal into its frequency components. The most popular method of spectral analysis is the *fast Fourier transform,* which produces series of sine and cosine waves that in sum provide an approximation of the recorded signal. The frequencies of the sine and cosine waves reflect the frequency content of tremor, and the amplitudes of the sine and cosine waves reflect the amplitude of tremor at each frequency. The sum of the squared sine and cosine amplitudes at each frequency plotted versus frequency is called the *autospectrum* (also known as the power spectrum).

Tremor consists of one or more oscillations that are superimposed on a background of broad-frequency activity, which is often regarded as noise. Consequently, tremor is ideally suited for spectral analysis. The principles and mathematical methods of spectral analysis have been reviewed in the context of tremor (Elble and Koller, 1990; Timmer et al., 1996) and in other contexts (Kay and Marple, 1981; Miller and Sigvardt, 1998; Muthuswamy and Thakor, 1998), and a detailed description of these methods is beyond the scope of this chapter. Spectral methods have been applied extensively to the analysis of tremor and associated spike trains recorded from muscle (Elble and Randall, 1976; Halliday et al., 1999), peripheral nerve, and the central nervous system (Elble et al., 1984; Hua et al., 1998; Zirh et al., 1998; Lemstra et al., 1999). Alternative methods of spectral smoothing have been developed for the study of tremor (Timmer et al., 1996; Lauk et al., 1999). The *autoregressive method* of spectral analysis has been applied to short data segments (Cappello et al., 1997; Muthuswamy and Thakor, 1998; Spyers-Ashby et al., 1998).

It is frequently desirable to determine the timing or phase relationship between two signals and to determine the degree to which one signal is linearly correlated (coherent) with the other. Mere visual inspection of data is notoriously unreliable. Therefore, cross-spectral, phase, and coherence analyses have been applied extensively to pairs of signals such as EMG and accelerometry, EMG and electroencephalography (EEG), EMG and a neuronal spike train, and two neuronal spike trains. The coherence spectrum is the squared linear correlation between two signals (time series) versus frequency (Benignus, 1969). The coherence spectrum is bounded by values ranging from zero (no linear relationship) to one (perfect linear relationship). Amjad and co-workers described a method for computing the coherence of data from two or more experimental trials (Amjad et al., 1997).

The fast Fourier transform and autoregressive methods are used with the assumption that the signal is statistically stationary or slowly varying (Muthuswamy and Thakor, 1998). A stationary signal has first-, second-, and higher-order statistical properties (e.g., mean, variance) that do not change with time. Intermittent (nonstationary) tremor can be explored using short-time Fourier analysis or the relatively new methods of wavelet analysis (Thakor et al., 1993; Thakor and Sherman, 1995; Muthuswamy and Thakor, 1998).

Spectral analysis and related methods of signal analysis are performed easily with commercially available software such as Matlab (MathWorks, Inc., Natick, MA). Quantitative signal analysis is both an art and a science. Each approach has important assumptions and methods of statistical analysis that may affect the results and their interpretation. Consultation with a person experienced in these methods is advisable.

Time Domain Analysis

Cross-correlation of motor unit spike trains has been useful in the quantification of short-term synchronization (i.e., motor units firing within a few milliseconds of each other). The techniques and application of cross-correlation were reviewed by Farmer and colleagues (1997). The cross-spectrum is the Fourier transform of the cross-correlation function. Coherence, the normalized cross-spectrum, is better suited for quantifying synchronous rhythmical modulation of two spike trains, whereas short-term synchronization is best revealed in the cross-correlogram (Farmer et al., 1997). Furthermore, the shape and duration of the cross-correlogram are believed to reflect the time course of excitatory postsynaptic potentials (Datta and Stephens, 1990; Farmer et al., 1997).

Other Methods of Time Series Analysis

Randall found that normal wrist tremor could be modeled by a second-order autoregressive equation with a residual variance consisting of white noise (Randall, 1973). This result is consistent with the hypothesis that the principal rhythmical component of physiological tremor emerges from the agitation of a linear second-order mechanical system (inertia, damping, and stiffness) by random motor unit irreg-

ularities and cardioballistics (white noise). This and other methods of linear and nonlinear time series analysis have been applied to physiological tremor, essential tremor, and parkinsonian tremor, with the aim of identifying distinguishing characteristics for each form of tremor (Gantert et al., 1992; Timmer et al., 1993, 2000; Deuschl et al., 1995; Elble, 1995). This approach to tremor analysis is still experimental.

MECHANISTIC CLASSIFICATION OF TREMOR

Overview of Tremor Pathophysiology

Normal postural tremor in the upper extremity consists primarily of two rhythmical oscillations, *mechanical reflex* and *8- to 12-Hz* (Elble and Randall, 1978; Timmer et al., 1998). The 8- to 12-Hz oscillation is produced by rhythmical motor unit entrainment at 8 to 12 Hz. Its frequency is not affected significantly by changes in limb mechanics (inertia and stiffness) or reflex arc length (latency), and it is therefore believed to emerge from a central source of oscillation. The mechanical reflex component is so named because its frequency is a function of the inertia and stiffness of the limb and its reflex arc, and when the stretch reflex is enhanced, the frequency of tremor is also a function of reflex arc length. Irregularities in motor unit firing and cardioballistics provide a broad-frequency forcing to the limb that results in mechanical reflex oscillation. The mechanical reflex oscillation is associated with motor unit entrainment when its amplitude becomes great enough to induce reflex modulation of motor unit discharge or when the sensitivity of the reflex arc is increased by such factors as drugs, fatigue, and anxiety.

Several reviews of tremor pathophysiology have been published in the literature (Elble and Koller, 1990; Elble, 1996, 1998, 2000; Wilms et al., 1999), and a detailed review is beyond the scope of this chapter. Here, we provide a brief summary of what is known, while acknowledging that no pathological tremor has been elucidated completely.

Parkinsonian tremor emerges from the death of dopaminergic nigrostriatal neurons that causes abnormal oscillation in cortical–basal ganglia–thalamocortical pathways; however, the principal origin of oscillation is unknown. Essential tremor is hypothesized to emerge from abnormal olivocerebellar oscillation, but thalamocortical oscillation is equally likely (Bucher et al., 1997; Wilms et al., 1999). Little is known about the anatomy of primary orthostatic tremor, task-specific tremors (e.g., primary writing tremor), and position-specific tremors, except that cerebellar activation is seen in positron emission tomography scans. Dystonic tremor is believed to emerge from dysfunction of cortical–basal ganglia–thalamocortical pathways, but the principal locus of oscillation is unknown. Symptomatic palatal tremor (palatal myoclonus) is most probably a result of pathological oscillation in the hypertrophied inferior olives, produced by lesions in the dentatorubro-olivary pathway (Deuschl et al., 1990, 1994). Myorhythmia is possibly a related phenomenon. Lesions in the deep cerebellar nuclei or brachium conjunctivum produce cerebellar intention tremor. Such lesions produce a loss of feed-forward control of antagonistic muscles during the execution of target-directed movements, and this leads to excessive reliance on sensorimotor feedback control, which is incapable of preventing abnormal mechanical reflex oscillation as the target is approached. Central oscillation from a reverberating thalamocortical loop or cerebellar-brainstem loop may also contribute. Rubral tremor (Holmes tremor, midbrain tremor) is usually caused by combined damage to the brachium conjunctivum and nigrostriatal pathway in the vicinity of the red nucleus, which causes an unusual mixture of rest tremor and intention tremor. Thus, Holmes tremor appears to combine the pathophysiological mechanisms of parkinsonian tremor and cerebellar tremor (Holmes, 1904; Friedman, 1992; Remy et al., 1995; Deuschl et al., 1999). It is unclear why most forms of tremor respond to ventrolateral thalamotomy and produce cerebellar hyperactivity in positron emission tomography scans (Boecker and Brooks, 1998). Parkinsonian tremor is suppressed by pallidotomy, but one case report illustrates that pallidotomy may also be effective in the treatment of cerebellar intention tremor (Miyagi et al., 1999).

Electrophysiological studies of physiological and pathological tremors have led to two broad mechanistic classifications, *mechanical reflex oscillation* and *central oscillation*. Essential tremor, parkinsonian tremor, primary orthostatic tremor, position- and task-specific tremors, dystonic tremor, palatal tremor, and myorhythmia are believed to be central oscillator tremors because each tremor has a frequency that changes less than 1 Hz with changes in limb inertia, limb stiffness, or reflex loop time (Elble, 1986, 1996, 1998; Hömberg et al., 1987; Boroojerdi et al., 1999; Wilms et al., 1999). Studies of laboratory primates have shown that cerebellar intention tremor has a frequency that is predictably altered by inertia and stiffness (Vilis and Hore, 1977; Elble et al., 1984), but a systematic study of cerebellar tremor in humans has not been done. Such a study of cerebellar tremor must distinguish classic intention tremor resulting from a brachium conjunctivum lesion from tremors caused by more extensive cerebellar and brainstem disease. Rubral tremor is probably a combination of central and mechanical reflex oscillation, but definitive mechanistic studies have not been done. Peripheral neuropathies cause mechanical reflex tremors but may also cause central oscillator tremor, presumably through secondary tremorogenic changes in central pathways. The limitations of this classification scheme are now discussed.

Distinguishing Central Oscillation from Mechanical Reflex Oscillation

MECHANICAL LOADING

Mechanical reflex tremors, by definition, emerge from the oscillatory properties of limb mechanics and sensorimotor loops. Most body parts have mechanical properties that produce damped oscillations in response to pulsatile perturbations. The frequency ω (radians per second) of these oscillations depends on limb inertia I and stiffness K, according to the equation $\omega = \sqrt{K/I}$ (Lakie et al., 1986). Consequently, adding inertia or stiffness readily changes the frequency of mechanical reflex tremor when there is little involvement of segmental or long-loop reflexes. The principal rhythmical component of physiological and enhanced physiological postural tremor has these properties (Fig. 99–1). The addition of mass to the hand, for example, causes the frequency of physiological hand (wrist) tremor to decrease, whereas the addition of stiffness (e.g., a spring attached to the hand) produces an increase in frequency.

The use of mechanical loading in distinguishing central oscillation from mechanical reflex oscillation has limitations. In most situations, the stretch-reflex stiffness and damping are small relative to the stiffness and damping of passive limb mechanics and active muscle contraction. Under these circumstances, the frequency of mechanical reflex tremor is increased with the addition of mechanical stiffness and is decreased with the addition of an inertial load. With greater reflex stiffness and damping, the influence of limb mechanics on tremor frequency diminishes. For example, the greater involvement of segmental and long-loop (e.g., transcortical) stretch-reflex pathways in enhanced mechanical reflex tremor results in tremor frequencies that are less dependent on limb mechanics and more dependent on reflex loop properties (Stiles, 1980; Elble et al., 1984). This is nicely illustrated in mathematical models of mechanical reflex tremor (Stein and Oguztöreli, 1976; Bock and Wenderoth, 1999). In these models, the frequency of mechanical reflex tremor is nearly independent of limb stiffness and inertia when the limb damping and stiffness are small relative to the damping and stiffness provided by the stretch reflex. Therefore, in situations of large reflex stiffness (gain) and damping, a mechanical reflex oscillation may be difficult to distinguish from a central oscillation on the basis of the frequency response to mechanical loading. However, such an enhanced mechanical reflex tremor should have a frequency that is a function of reflex arc length (latency) (Bock and Wenderoth, 1999). *A tremor whose frequency varies predictably with mechanical load or reflex arc length is produced, at least in part, by mechanical reflex mechanisms. A tremor whose frequency is independent of both mechanical load and reflex arc length most probably emerges from a central source of oscillation.*

Physiological tremor | Enhanced physiological tremor

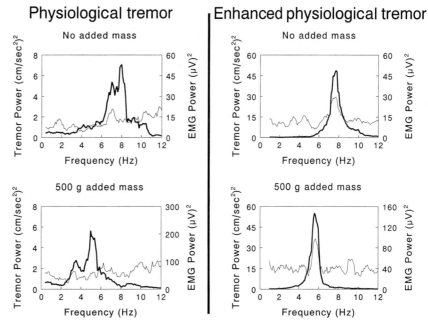

Figure 99–1. Autospectra of hand tremor *(thick lines)* and rectified-filtered extensor carpi radialis brevis electromyogram *(thin lines)*, recorded with an accelerometer and surface electrodes during horizontal extension of the hand, with the forearm supported. The frequency of physiological tremor decreased with 500-g loading, and there was no associated peak in the electromyographic spectrum (i.e., no evidence of motor unit entrainment). The frequency of enhanced physiological tremor in a patient with thyrotoxicosis also decreased with mass loading, but this tremor was associated with a significant peak in the electromyographic spectrum.

In the case of a central oscillator tremor, the presence of strong sensory feedback could entrain the central oscillator at the frequency of mechanical reflex oscillation, if the natural frequencies of the central oscillator and mechanical reflex oscillation were not too dissimilar and if the strength of central oscillation was relatively weak compared with the strength of mechanical reflex oscillation (Wenderoth and Bock, 1999). Therefore, a weak central oscillator could conceivably exhibit small changes in frequency with mechanical loading or with changes in reflex latency.

Physiological and pathological tremors exhibit spontaneous frequency fluctuations of less than 1 Hz (O'Suilleabhain and Matsumoto, 1998), and changes in limb posture or movement can affect tremor frequency (Elble et al., 1996). These factors must be considered in deciding how much change in frequency with mechanical loading can be accepted as insignificant. A change in frequency of at least 1 Hz should be regarded as significant, but it is best to apply three or more magnitudes of inertia I or stiffness K and to demonstrate changes in frequency ω according to the equation $\omega = \sqrt{K/I}$. For hand (wrist) tremor, loads of 100 to 1000 g have been used, with the change in moment of inertia depending on the distance of the mass load from the axis of rotation (i.e., the wrist) (Stiles and Randall, 1967; Deuschl, 1999a). Larger loads are needed for joints such as the elbow with greater natural moment of inertia (Fox and Randall, 1970), and much smaller loads are required for low-inertia joints, as in the measurement of finger tremor (Stiles and Randall, 1967; Halliday et al., 1999).

All tremors vary in amplitude among joints, and tremor frequency may also vary, particularly when the tremor has a mechanical reflex mechanism. The manner in which tremor frequency varies among joints can provide an important clue to the mechanism of tremor because joints vary in their mechanical properties (inertia and stiffness) and reflex arc length. If tremor frequency does not vary with the mechanical and reflex properties of different joints, then the tremor probably emerges from a central oscillator mechanism (e.g., parkinsonian tremor and essential tremor) (Hunker and Abbs, 1990; Elble, 1994). The frequency of mechanical reflex tremor tends to be lower in joints with greater inertia, and the frequency of enhanced mechanical reflex tremor tends to be lower in more distal joints with greater reflex arc length.

PERTURBATION (PHASE RESETTING) AND FREQUENCY ENTRAINMENT STUDIES

A nonlinear oscillator will exhibit phase resetting if it receives a pulsatile stimulus (perturbation) of sufficient strength. Similarly, the frequency of a nonlinear oscillator can be entrained at the frequency of a sinusoidal forcing if the amplitude of forcing is adequate and if the frequency of forcing is near the natural frequency of the oscillator. The principles of phase resetting and frequency entrainment were discussed in the context of tremor by Elble and Koller (1990), and they were discussed in a more theoretical context by Winfree (1980). It was originally hoped that tests of phase resetting and frequency entrainment with stretch reflex forcings would be useful in distinguishing tremors caused by central oscillators from those caused by mechanical reflex oscillation (Oguztöreli and Stein, 1979). The assumption was that a central oscillator should be relatively refractory to phase resetting and to frequency entrainment by stretch-reflex perturbations or sinusoidal forcings, whereas oscillations emerging from the stretch reflex should be easily reset or entrained.

This approach failed for three reasons. First, this approach was based on a model of tremor in which the central source of oscillation was autonomous or not significantly influenced by sensory feedback pathways. However, virtually all candidate sources of central oscillation in tremorogenesis (e.g., thalamus, inferior olive, sensorimotor cortex, spinal cord) are strongly influenced by sensory feedback and therefore could be reset with a reflex perturbation of adequate strength. Second, a nonlinear mechanical reflex oscillation could be so strong that stretch-reflex perturbations and sinusoidal forcings would not be sufficient to achieve phase resetting or frequency entrainment. In other words, there is no guarantee that stretch-reflex perturbations will reset a tremor that emerges from mechanical reflex oscillation. The third reason for failure of this approach stems from the difficulty of determining the steady-state phase of a tremor oscillation that has random variability in amplitude and frequency. The new phase or phase shift cannot be computed until the transient response to a perturbation is fully dissipated. However, by this time, there is usually too much uncertainty in the computation of phase to determine whether steady-state phase resetting has occurred. Consequently, the temptation is to compute phase from one of the first three cycles of oscillation after a perturbation, and these cycles are usually part of the transient response to perturbation, not the steady-state oscillation. These limitations of phase resetting and frequency entrainment are amply illustrated in experimental studies (Lee and Stein, 1981; Rack and Ross, 1986; Elble and Koller, 1990; Britton et al., 1992a, 1993a; Elble et al., 1992b) and in mathematical models of mechanical reflex tremor (Bock and Wenderoth, 1999).

Thus, the demonstration of phase resetting or frequency entrainment of a tremor with stretch reflex perturbations is proof of an influential pathway from the periphery to the tremor oscillator, but phase resetting does not distinguish tremors of peripheral origin from those of central origin. Parkinsonian tremor and essential tremor are reset by peripheral mechanical and electrical stimuli (Lee and Stein, 1981; Elble and Koller, 1990; Britton et al., 1992a, 1993a; Elble et al., 1992b), but orthostatic tremor is uniquely refractory to phase resetting by these methods of stretch reflex perturbation (Thompson et al., 1986; Britton et al., 1992b). Consequently, the central oscillator of orthostatic tremor is either too strong to be reset by sensory feedback or, less likely, does not receive sensory feedback. The strength of the oscillator of orthostatic tremor is reflected in the unique coherence between upper and lower body segments and between the right and left sides of the body (Köster et al., 1999; Raethjen et al., 2000b). Phase resetting with stretch-reflex perturbation has not been examined in patients with cerebellar outflow tract lesions, but such perturbations readily induce abnormal joint oscillation (Richard et al., 1997).

Transcranial magnetic stimulation of motor cortex is capable of resetting the phase of essential tremor, parkinsonian postural tremor, and orthostatic tremor (Britton et al., 1993b; Pascual-Leone et al., 1994; Tsai et al., 1998; Pfeiffer et al., 1999). This approach suffers from the same limitations as for phase resetting with stretch-reflex stimuli. However, Britton and coworkers observed two subtle differences in the transient responses of parkinsonian postural tremor and essential tremor to magnetic stimulation of motor cortex (Britton et al., 1993b). First, the time to reappearance of the tremor rhythm, following stimuli at 10% higher than threshold, correlated significantly with the tremor period in Parkinson's disease but not in essential tremor. Second, the stimuli had a tendency to shorten the tremor period by 17 ms in Parkinson's disease but not in essential tremor. More studies are needed to establish the sensitivity and specificity of these observations, which could prove useful in distinguishing parkinsonian and essential postural tremors.

Mechanical and Neural Resonance

It is doubtful that any source of tremor is completely isolated from the effects of sensory feedback and segmental sensorimotor loops, and body mechanics constitute the final common pathway for all forms of tremor. Consequently, a centrally generated tremor could resonate with the mechanical reflex system, if their natural frequencies were similar (Elble et al., 1992b). For example, parkinsonian and essential hand tremors have frequencies that are similar to the mechanical reflex frequency of the wrist, so there is less mechanical attenuation of the tremor than would occur if these tremors had much higher frequencies. The 13- to 18-Hz frequency of orthostatic tremor, by contrast, is much higher than the natural mechanical reflex frequency of the lower limbs, so this tremor is not visible to the examiner until the tremor frequency undergoes subharmonic reduction to 7 to 9 Hz (Thompson et al., 1986; Kelly and Sharbrough, 1987; Britton et al., 1992b). Similar dynamic interactions undoubtedly occur between the central oscillators of pathological tremors and central neural pathways to which the oscillators are connected. Resonance between a tremor oscillator and other parts of the central nervous system could be as important as the strength of the tremor oscillator in determining the amplitude of pathological tremors. Stereotactic surgery and pharmacological treatment of tremor could control the tremor oscillator directly or could impede the entrainment of other neural pathways, thereby limiting the clinical expression of the tremor oscillator. The latter mechanism could explain the nonspecific benefits of thalamotomy and pallidotomy.

MOTOR UNIT ENTRAINMENT AND SYNCHRONIZATION

Physiological Tremor

For the most part, normal steady muscle contractions are produced by asynchronous motor unit firing. Two or more motor units may discharge nearly synchronously (within a few milliseconds) during steady voluntary contractions by neurologically normal people, but this short-term synchronization affects only 8% of motor unit discharges (Dietz et al., 1976; Dengler et al., 1984; Datta et al., 1991; De Luca et al., 1993; Semmler and Nordstrom, 1998). The mechanism of short-term synchronization is uncertain. Some authors have postulated that this synchronization results from the joint occurrence of excitatory postsynaptic potentials evoked in multiple motor neurons by branches of a corticospinal fiber (Sears and Stagg, 1976; Datta and Stephens, 1990; Datta et al., 1991; Farmer et al., 1997), whereas others favor a role for central oscillatory drive to the motor neuron pool (De Luca et al., 1993). Sensory feedback is not necessary for short-term synchronization (Farmer et al., 1993a, 1997).

Short-term synchronization of motor units does not contribute significantly to the *8- to 12-Hz component of physiological tremor* (Farmer et al., 1993a). This tremor in the upper limb is produced by bursts of motor unit discharge at 8 to 12 Hz, and the individual motor unit frequencies typically range from 8 to 22 spikes per second. Motor unit firing is synchronously modulated at the frequency of tremor (Elble and Randall, 1976; Wessberg and Kakuda, 1999). This modulation of motor unit activity is such that double (paired) discharges, with interspike intervals of 10 to 40 ms, tend to occur during a cycle of tremor. Most people exhibit 8- to 12-Hz bursts of EMG activity during slow voluntary movements, particularly in the wrist and finger extensors during slow wrist or finger flexion (Wessberg and Vallbo, 1996). However, this tendency for 8- to 12-Hz motor unit entrainment is too weak in most healthy adults to produce an EMG spectral peak during steady horizontal extension of the hand or finger (Elble, 1986).

Elble and coworkers quantified hand tremor and forearm EMG activity in 100 healthy volunteers, ages 20 to 40 years, and 100 older adults, ages 70 to 90 years (Elble et al., unpublished data). During horizontal extension of the hand with the forearm pronated and supported, 62% of neurologically normal adults exhibited no evidence of motor unit entrainment in their wrist extensors or flexors. This ultranormal tremor behaves as a linear second-order mechanical system forced by white noise (unsynchronized motor unit activity) and cardioballistics (Elble and Randall, 1978; Timmer et al., 1998). Approximately 27% exhibited motor unit entrainment in association with the mechanical resonant peak. The EMG signal was entrained by somatosensory feedback, and the frequency of tremor was governed primarily by limb inertia and stiffness. The re-

maining 11% of neurologically normal adults had rhythmical entrainment of motor unit activity at a frequency that was not altered significantly by mechanical loading, nor was it a function of reflex arc length. This frequency-invariant motor unit entrainment has a frequency of 8 to 12 Hz in most adults (Fig. 99–2). However, the frequency may be as low as 5 to 8 Hz in people older than 70 years, and these people have action tremor that is indistinguishable from mild essential tremor.

The relationship of the 8- to 12-Hz component of physiological tremor to pathological postural tremors seen in essential tremor and Parkinson's disease is unclear. Young adults and adolescents with extremely mild essential tremor (Elble, 1986) and many patients with Parkinson's disease exhibit prominent 8- to 12-Hz entrainment of motor unit activity (Lance et al., 1963; Brown et al., 1997, 1998). The frequency of this tremor is independent of reflex arc length, and it is not reduced by increasing limb inertia (Fox and Randall, 1970; Stephens and Taylor, 1974; Elble and Randall, 1976, 1978). Furthermore, the stretch-reflex response to joint perturbation is too weak and too delayed to account for this tremor (Wessberg and Vallbo, 1996). Thus, this tremor appears to emerge from a central oscillator, but the source of this oscillation is unknown. The inferior

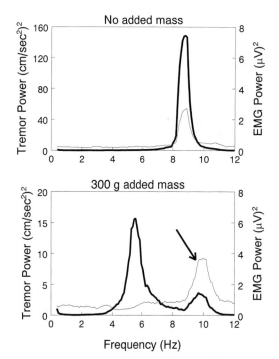

Figure 99–2. Autospectra of hand tremor *(thick lines)* and rectified-filtered extensor carpi radialis brevis electromyogram *(thin lines)*, recorded with an accelerometer and surface electrodes from a normal 32-year-old woman with an asymptomatic 8- to 12-Hz tremor. Tremor was recorded from the horizontally extended hand, with the forearm supported. In the absence of mass loading, the 8- to 12-Hz activity was so irregular and intermittent that it simply perturbed the wrist and produced a single oscillation at the mechanical resonance frequency (8 to 10 Hz). Mass loading separated the mechanical resonance oscillation and the 8- to 12-Hz oscillation *(arrow)*.

olive is the most frequently hypothesized source, but this hypothesis is largely conjectural, based on the similarities between this tremor and the 8- to 12-Hz harmaline tremor in laboratory primates (Elble, 1998). The olivary hypothesis is consistent with the observation of weak coherence between 10-Hz oscillations in the human eye and finger during slow tracking tasks (McAuley et al., 1999). However, other sources of rhythmicity (e.g., thalamus and cortex) are also possible.

Halliday and coworkers demonstrated the presence of *15- to 30-Hz motor unit entrainment* that was estimated to explain approximately 20% of finger tremor in this frequency band (Halliday et al., 1999). The contribution of 15- to 30-Hz motor unit entrainment to tremor in body parts with greater inertia (e.g., hand, forearm) will be much smaller. Consequently, its presence may be evident in the rectified-filtered EMG spectrum but not in the acceleration spectrum. This component of physiological tremor is believed to emerge from cortical rhythmicity (Conway et al., 1995; Baker et al., 1997, 1999; Salenius et al., 1997; Halliday et al., 1998).

Enhanced Physiological Tremor

Enhanced mechanical reflex tremor occurs when the stretch reflex is enhanced by fatigue, anxiety, voluntary movement, or β-adrenergic drugs (Stiles, 1976; Logigian et al., 1988; Stiles and Hahs, 1991). The amplitude of tremor is increased by a factor of 5 to 20, and there is rhythmical entrainment of motor unit activity at the tremor frequency (Hagbarth and Young, 1979; Stiles, 1980). This modulation of motor unit activity is such that double (paired) discharges, with interspike intervals of 10 to 40 ms, tend to occur during a cycle of tremor (Logigian et al., 1988). Short-term synchronization of motor units does not contribute significantly.

The frequency of enhanced mechanical reflex oscillation decreases as the amplitude increases. The reasons for this frequency-amplitude relationship are unclear. A reduction in the mechanical stiffness of the joint with increasing amplitude of oscillation is one explanation (Gottlieb and Agarwal, 1977; Agarwal and Gottlieb, 1984; Lakie et al., 1984; Zahalak and Pramod, 1985; Milner and Cloutier, 1998). Regardless, the reduction in tremor frequency with increased amplitude should be advantageous because it produces a greater phase advance of sensory feedback on tremor, which results in greater reflex damping (Stiles and Hahs, 1991). By contrast, stretch-reflex responses can destabilize the wrist and similar joints at frequencies of 7 Hz or greater (Milner and Cloutier, 1998). People with deafferented limbs exhibit irregular broad-band errors in limb position that exceed the amplitude of physiological and enhanced physiological tremor, but they do not exhibit the increased tremor with rhythmical motor unit entrainment seen in patients with enhanced mechanical reflex tremor (Sanes, 1985). Thus, the

presence of somatosensory feedback is not deleterious in terms of the overall amplitude of positional error; rather, somatosensory feedback seems to entrain or concentrate error at a particular frequency and results in rhythmical oscillation. The stretch reflex probably contributes to most, if not all, pathological tremors in this manner, even when a tremor emerges from a central source of oscillation.

If motor unit entrainment by a central oscillator is intermittent, it may do little more than perturb the ever-present mechanical reflex system and may thus produce damped mechanical oscillations that induce a reflex modulation of motor unit activity at a frequency that is sensitive to mechanical loading. An extreme example of this phenomenon occurs in patients with symptomatic palatal tremor (Elble, 1991; Deuschl et al., 1994). Brief 50- to 80-ms silent periods in the forearm EMG occur intermittently at the frequency of palatal tremor (~2 Hz), and these periods of motor unit inhibition perturb the wrist enough to cause an enhanced mechanical reflex tremor (Fig. 99–3). The same phenomenon occurs in patients with mild irregular essential tremor. The essential tremor rhythm can be so intermittent that it creates little or no frequency-invariant spectral peak, but the irregular bursts of motor unit activity perturb the mechanical reflex system and cause a spectral peak that varies predictably with spring and inertial loads.

Pathological Tremors

All forms of *pathological tremor* are associated with bursts of motor unit activity at the frequency

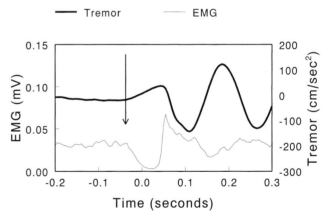

Figure 99–3. Computed average transient of rectified-filtered electromyogram (extensor carpi radialis brevis) and hand tremor (acceleration), recorded from a 74-year-old woman with the syndrome of progressive ataxia and palatal myoclonus. The electromyogram and tremor were averaged, time-locked to silent periods in the forearm electromyogram that occurred synchronously with the 2-Hz palatal myoclonus. These silent periods *(arrow)* perturbed the hand and produced damped mechanical oscillation that was asymptomatic. Any burst of muscle activity, electromyographic silent period, or cardioballistic impulse could have this effect, thereby enhancing mechanical reflex oscillation. Tremor was recorded with an accelerometer on the horizontally extended hand, with the forearm supported.

of oscillation. Early investigators hypothesized that synchronized motor units firing at the frequency of tremor produced most tremors, but this hypothesis proved to be untrue in most instances. Short-term synchronization of motor units occurs in patients with pathological tremors (Davey et al., 1986; Datta et al., 1991), but the contribution of short-term synchronization to pathological tremors is much less than the contribution of rhythmical modulation and entrainment of motor neuron firing. The frequency modulation of motor unit activity is such that double or triple discharges (paired or grouped discharges), with interspike intervals of 10 to 40 ms, tend to occur during a cycle of tremor. This pattern of motor unit firing occurs in parkinsonian tremor (Das Gupta, 1963; Dietz et al., 1974; Shahani and Young, 1977; Davey et al., 1986; Dengler et al., 1986; Elek et al., 1991) and essential tremor (Shahani and Young, 1977; Dengler et al., 1989; Elek et al., 1991) and is similar to that which occurs in the 8- to 12-Hz component of physiological tremor (Elble and Randall, 1976) and enhanced physiological mechanical reflex tremor (Logigian et al., 1988). Paired motor unit discharges with short interspike intervals produce stronger muscle contraction than is observed with single spikes and therefore contribute more substantially to tremor amplitude (Renou et al., 1970; Elek et al., 1991). Thus, although some motor units fire at the frequency of tremor, many other motor units with greater firing frequencies contribute more substantially to tremor by virtue of a modulation in their firing frequency at the frequency of tremor.

OTHER MECHANISTIC AND DIAGNOSTIC METHODS

Normal Versus Abnormal Tremor Amplitude and Frequency

Mild parkinsonian and essential tremors intermittently fall within the amplitude range of physiological tremor (Deuschl, 1999b). Similar overlap exists for tremor frequency. Consequently, neither amplitude nor frequency is a completely reliable measure of disease. The frequency range of most pathological tremors is 4 to 10 Hz. Orthostatic tremor has a uniquely high frequency (13 to 18 Hz) (Thompson et al., 1986; McManis and Sharbrough, 1993). Myorhythmia and Holmes (rubral) tremor typically have uniquely low frequencies of less than 4 Hz, and cerebellar tremor can also fall into this frequency range (Deuschl, 1999b).

Parkinsonian action tremor and essential tremor have virtually identical frequency ranges (Deuschl, 1999b; Jankovic et al., 1999). The rest tremor of Parkinson's disease typically decreases or stops during voluntary muscle contraction in a posture or movement, but this cessation in tremor is commonly transient, such that the tremor re-emerges 1 to 50 seconds later, despite continued voluntary muscle

contraction (Jankovic et al., 1999). The tremor frequencies of the rest tremor and re-emergent tremor are the same in a given patient (Jankovic et al., 1999). A delay in the onset of postural tremor was found in 12 of 18 patients with Parkinson's disease who were studied by Jankovic and coworkers (Jankovic et al., 1999). By contrast, 1 of 20 patients with essential tremor had a delay in onset, which was only 1.29 seconds.

Antagonistic Muscle Interaction

The rhythmical bursts of motor unit activity tend to occur synchronously in the antagonistic forearm muscles of patients with essential tremor and tend to occur reciprocally (180 degrees out of phase) in parkinsonian tremor (Shahani and Young, 1976; Raethjen et al., 2000b). However, these patterns of activity are not consistent among patients with the same disease, nor are they consistent in the same patient performing a variety of motor tasks (Elble, 1986; Boose et al., 1996; Deuschl et al., 1996). Reciprocal, synchronous, and random antagonistic muscle interactions occur in both groups of patients, as revealed by cross-spectral analysis of rectified-filtered EMG signals. Therefore, the pattern of antagonistic muscle interaction is of no diagnostic value in distinguishing these two forms of tremor.

Coherence of Tremor in Muscles of Different Body Segments (Polyelectromyography)

The simultaneous recording of EMG activity from multiple muscles *(poly-EMG)* is useful in the differential diagnosis of tremor. Köster and coworkers found significant side-to-side coherence in drug-induced enhanced physiological tremor of patients with persistent mirror movements (Köster et al., 1998b). However, orthostatic tremor is the only condition that produces consistent coherence between muscles on both sides of the body and among muscles of different limbs on the same side (Fig. 99–4) (Köster et al., 1999; Lauk et al., 1999; Raethjen et al., 2000b). Thus, the strength and left-right connectivity of the oscillator in orthostatic tremor are uniquely capable of producing widespread entrainment of motor pathways.

Poly-EMG is also useful in the differential diagnosis of asterixis. The 7- to 14-Hz action tremor in asterixis is mixed with irregular EMG silent periods of 50 to 500 ms that are responsible for the well-known wrist flap. These silent periods occur synchronously in the muscles of the arm and are followed by damped mechanical oscillations of the wrist. Rhythmical myoclonias can be misinterpreted as tremors, and EMG is diagnostically helpful if the burst activity is time-locked in muscles of different extremities.

Poly-EMG is extremely useful in the diagnosis of psychogenic tremor. Psychogenic tremor is often produced by a voluntary coactivation of muscles *(coactivation sign),* which can be documented by EMG (Deuschl et al., 1998b). The frequencies of organic tremors typically fluctuate less than 1 Hz in a given posture or movement, but the frequency of psychogenic tremor fluctuates more widely (more than 1 Hz) and erratically (O'Suilleabhain and Matsumoto, 1998). In most cases, distraction with mental or motor tasks suppresses psychogenic tremor or changes its frequency (Deuschl et al., 1998b; Kim et al., 1999), and the erratic fluctuations in frequency and amplitude occur simultaneously in different limbs. In addition, patients with psychogenic tremor cannot voluntarily oscillate the same or opposite extremity at a frequency different from the frequency of their psychogenic tremor. Attempts to do so either suppress the psychogenic tremor (Fig. 99–5) or cause the psychogenic tremor to shift to the frequency of voluntary repetitive movement. Patients with pathological tremor can easily perform repetitive movements with the same or opposite limb without changing the frequency of their invol-

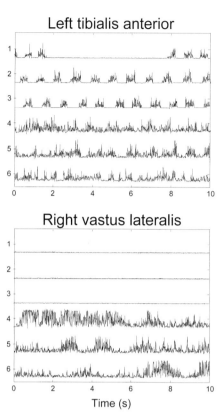

Figure 99–5. Rectified surface electromyographic recordings from a 49-year-old woman with a long history of depression and multiple somatic complaints. She abruptly developed an irregular intermittent tremor in her right lower limb that interfered with her ability to work. Her psychogenic tremor consisted of intermittent tremulous extension of the right knee and ankle. While she was seated in a chair, she was asked to tap her left foot on the floor at approximately 1 Hz. The six consecutive 10-second sweeps of electromyographic activity illustrate the cessation of right vastus lateralis "tremor" whenever she voluntarily tapped her left foot. Spectral analysis (not shown) revealed a widely fluctuating 3- to 8-Hz tremor frequency.

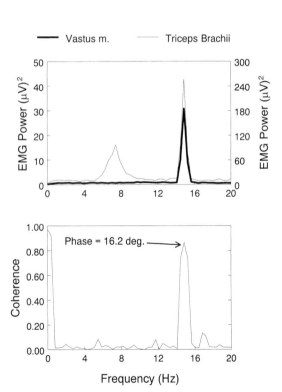

Figure 99–4. Orthostatic tremor recorded from an 83-year-old woman who complained of nervousness and fear of falling whenever she stood. Rectified-filtered electromyograms were recorded while she stood erect and leaned on a table with her upper limbs. Power spectra of the right vastus medialis *(left axis)* and the triceps brachii *(right axis)* are shown *(upper graph)* with their coherence spectrum *(lower graph).* Note the well-tuned 14.8-Hz spectral peaks, which were strongly coherent with a phase difference of 16.2 degrees. The 7.4-Hz peak in the triceps spectrum was produced by intermittent subharmonic reduction in the tremor frequency. She had only normal physiological tremor (i.e., no motor unit entrainment) in the upper and lower limbs when she was seated.

untary tremor more than 1 Hz. This electrophysiological approach to the diagnosis of psychogenic tremor is clearly illustrated in a report by McAuley and coworkers (1998).

Finally, poly-EMG has been used in the differential diagnosis of dystonic and essential head tremors. Nearly all patients with dystonic head tremor exhibit reduced tremor activity in the prime movers of the head during so-called *antagonistic gestures* (e.g., touching the chin with a hand). This manifestation of *geste antagonistique* is not seen in essential head tremor (Deuschl et al., 1992). Although the effect of *geste antagonistique* is often demonstrable clinically without EMG, multichannel EMG recordings are helpful when this phenomenon is subtle.

Evoked Potentials and Long-Latency Reflex Studies

Cortical tremor is an irregular 7- to 14-Hz action tremor that resembles essential tremor and that occurs in patients with cortical reflex myoclonus. Major motor seizures, myoclonus, and a family history of these disorders and tremor are characteristic of cortical tremor (Ikeda et al., 1990; Toro et al., 1993; Oguni et al., 1995). An enhanced C reflex (long-latency transcortical muscle reflex) and giant sensory evoked potentials are demonstrable in more than half of these patients, a finding consistent with the presence of enhanced cortical irritability and transcortical reflexes. Despite the enhanced C reflex, cortical tremor probably emerges from enhanced cortical rhythmicity, rather than from oscillation in a transcortical sensorimotor loop (Toro et al., 1993; Brown and Marsden, 1996).

Giant sensory evoked potentials and an enhanced C reflex also may be found in patients with asterixis (Ugawa et al., 1989; Artieda et al., 1992). The characteristic negative myoclonus (wrist flap) is produced by EMG silent periods of 50 to 500 ms. Patients also exhibit an irregular 7- to 14-Hz action tremor that is probably a form of cortical tremor, although enhanced mechanical reflex oscillation may also contribute.

Long-latency reflexes of hand muscles are abnormal in various movement disorders (Deuschl and Lücking, 1990). Approximately 10% of normal adults have a small long-latency reflex in the thenar muscles at 40 ms (long-latency reflex I) in response to median nerve stimulation, but an increased long-latency reflex I was found in 53% of patients with Parkinson's disease and about one third of patients with essential tremor (Deuschl and Lücking, 1990). An increased long-latency reflex I was associated with rest and postural tremor in the patients with Parkinson's disease and with a beneficial response to primidone in the patients with essential tremor. An increased long-latency reflex I was also found in some patients with cortical myoclonus. Thus, an increased long-latency reflex I lacks specificity in the diagnosis of tremor disorders but may be useful in subgrouping patients with particular clinical characteristics.

Reciprocal Inhibition of the H Reflex

Mercuri and coworkers measured reciprocal inhibition of the H reflex in the forearm muscles of 11 patients with essential tremor and found normal disynaptic inhibition, but presynaptic inhibition at 10 to 30 ms between the test and conditioning stimuli was reduced (Mercuri et al., 1998). H-reflex amplitude and the H_{max}/M_{max} ratios were normal. Botulinum injection into the wrist extensors and flexors produced normal reciprocal inhibition of the H reflex and reduced tremor (Modugno et al., 1998). Similar results have been found in patients with occupational dystonias of the upper limb (Nakashima et al., 1989; Priori et al., 1995). Bain and coworkers found that patients with primary writing tremor had normal reciprocal inhibition of the median nerve H reflex (Bain et al., 1995). A test for distinguishing primary writing tremor from tremulous writer's cramp would be useful because these conditions can be clinically similar (Elble et al., 1990a; Bain et al., 1995). However, the specificity and sensitivity of reciprocal inhibition of the H reflex are unknown in these and other tremor disorders.

Triphasic Electromyographic Pattern in Ballistic Joint Rotations

Rapid (ballistic) movement of a single joint is produced by an initial burst of agonist muscle activity. This is followed by a burst of antagonist muscle activity that decelerates the limb as it approaches its intended target. A second burst of agonist activity attenuates mechanical reflex oscillation at the end of movement. These muscle activities produce the so-called triphasic EMG pattern (first agonist–first antagonist–second agonist) of ballistic movement (Berardelli et al., 1996). These bursts of EMG activity are programmed centrally but are modified by sensory feedback. Parkinsonian tremor and essential tremor entrain voluntary movements of the hand (Logigian et al., 1991; Wierzbicka et al., 1993; Elble et al., 1994; Staude et al., 1995), and in both conditions, the tremor entrains the first agonist activity, which impedes rapid movement and alters its timing. When patients with essential tremor perform ballistic wrist flexion from complete rest, the second agonist activity is delayed in proportion to the tremor period, and this delay is conducive to oscillation about the target (Britton et al., 1994). Köster and coworkers studied ballistic elbow flexion in patients with essential tremor and found that the first antagonist activity and the second agonist activity were delayed. These delays were greatest in those patients with intention tremor during visually guided movements to a target, as in finger-nose-finger testing (Köster et al., 1998a). These delays could be caused by entrainment of the triphasic pattern by the tremor rhythm (Elble et al., 1994), a disturbance of cerebellar feed-forward control (Britton et al., 1994; Köster et al., 1998a), or possibly other mechanisms.

Measuring Cortical Rhythms with Electroencephalography and Magnetoencephalography

The search for tremor-related activity in EEG and magnetoencephalography (MEG), using quantitative methods of signal analysis, is still highly investigational and is currently of no diagnostic utility. Nevertheless, scientifically important observations have been made in studies of physiological and pathological tremors.

In a study of five neurologically normal people, Halliday and coworkers looked for correlation between EEG and forearm EMG during wrist flexion and extension (Halliday et al., 1998). EEG recordings from sensorimotor cortex and rectified EMG recordings were coherent only in the 15- to 30-Hz frequency band. Conway and coworkers (1995) studied six healthy adults and found spectral peaks in their MEG recordings at 10, 20, and 40 to 50 Hz during steady isometric contraction. Statistically significant coherence between MEG and contralateral EMG recordings (first dorsal interosseous muscle) was found in all subjects at 14 to 35 Hz. The observed MEG-EMG coherence mapped to the hand area of primary sensorimotor cortex. Other investigators confirmed these observations in the first dorsal interosseous and in other muscles of the upper and lower limbs (Salenius et al., 1997). In addition, Hari and Salenius found coherence at 30 to 60 Hz during strong voluntary contractions (Hari and Salenius, 1999). Thus, it appears that corticospinal input to motor neurons contributes to the broadband peaks at 14 to 35 Hz and at 35 to 60 Hz in the rectified-filtered EMG spectra of neurologically normal adults. The MEG-EMG coherence at these frequencies reflects corticospinal rhythmicity that modulates motor neuron firing frequencies and possibly contributes to short-term synchronization of motor units (Farmer et al., 1993a, 1993b; Hari and Salenius, 1999). The purpose of this cortical rhythmicity is unclear, but it could enhance the activation of other cortical neurons (Murthy and Fetz, 1992) and spinal motor neurons (Hari and Salenius, 1999) required for a particular activity.

Corticomuscular coherence in the frequency range of most tremors (less than 14 Hz) has not been found consistently in neurologically normal people. Conway and coworkers (1995) found significant MEG-EMG coherence at 1 to 14 Hz (7 Hz) in only one of six healthy adults, and Mima and coworkers (2000) found no significant coherence between cortical EEG and contralateral forearm 8- to 12-Hz tremor in seven healthy adults. The cortical 10-Hz μ rhythm originates from the rolandic cortex. It is initially suppressed by voluntary muscle activation of an upper limb but reappears with sustained contraction (Hari and Salenius, 1999). Coherence studies have found no relationship between this rhythm and the 8- to 12-Hz modulation of EMG activity (Hari and Salenius, 1999). These negative results must be interpreted cautiously because it is possible that the amplitude of tremor and the intensity and breadth of cortical neuronal and motor neuronal entrainment are less than the sensitivity of scalp recordings and existing analysis techniques. In support of this hypothesis, Raethjen and coworkers recorded EEG activity with an epidural electrode grid and found significant coherence between motor cortical activity and the 8- to 12-Hz component of physiological tremor (Raethjen et al., 2000a).

Coherent EEG-EMG rhythmicity has not been found consistently in patients with cortical tremor (Brown et al., 1999), but EEG transients preceding the EMG bursts of cortical tremor have been demonstrated with EEG back-averaging (Toro et al., 1993; Terada et al., 1997; Elia et al., 1998; Okuma et al., 1998). Patients with cortical myoclonus exhibit increased EEG-EMG coherence at 15 to 30 Hz and at 30 to 60 Hz (Brown et al., 1999).

Evidence of corticomuscular coherence has been found in patients with parkinsonian tremor. Alberts et al. recorded rhythmical activity from the surface of sensorimotor cortex that correlated with contralateral parkinsonian rest tremor (Alberts et al., 1969), but Mäkelä and coworkers found no cortical MEG correlate of parkinsonian rest tremor, except that the μ rhythm was suppressed during periods of shaking (Mäkelä et al., 1993). However, Volkmann and coworkers found tremor-related MEG activity in the regions of the contralateral thalamus and lateral premotor, somatomotor, and somatosensory cortices (Volkmann et al., 1996). These results are consistent with the widely recognized participation of the thalamocortical loop in parkinsonian tremorogenesis.

Studies of essential tremor have produced conflicting results. Halliday and coworkers failed to find coherent MEG-EMG rhythmicity at less than 12 Hz in patients with essential tremor, but these investigators recorded only from the first dorsal interosseous muscle (Halliday et al., 2000). By contrast, highly coherent EEG-EMG rhythmicity was found by Hellwig and coworkers (2000), who recorded from the wrist extensors and flexors in the forearm. Thus, corticomuscular coherence cannot be used to distinguish parkinsonian tremor from essential tremor. Nevertheless, the pathophysiological role of sensorimotor cortex may be different in these two forms of tremor, and future studies, perhaps with phase analysis, may reveal distinguishing features.

Hellwig and coworkers found no coherence in patients with low-amplitude essential tremor and in mildly symptomatic patients with prominent 8- to 12-Hz tremor (Hellwig et al., 2000). These negative results were attributable to low signal-to-noise ratios in the rectified EMG power spectrum, and these negative results illustrate the caution that is needed in interpreting negative results in this type of study. As in studies of physiological tremor, the amplitude of tremor and the intensity and breadth of cortical neuronal and motor neuronal entrainment may fall below the sensitivity of present recording and analysis techniques (Elble, 2000). More direct cortical recording, as performed by Raethjen and coworkers (2000a), would probably reveal significant corticomuscular coherence in patients with mild essential tremor.

EEG-EMG and MEG-EMG coherence values often fall in the extremely low range of 0.03 to 0.1 (Volkmann et al., 1996; Halliday et al., 2000). Although statistically significant, these coherence values indicate that, at best, only 3% to 10% of the cortical activity is linearly related to tremor. Spuriously significant coherencies at these low values are always a concern.

Visual and Proprioceptive Feedback

If parkinsonian tremor, essential tremor, and the 8- to 12-Hz component of physiological tremor emerge from central sources of oscillation that are influenced by sensory feedback (Elble, 1996), the loss of sensory feedback may reduce tremor amplitude and rhythmicity, with little or no change in tremor frequency. Lippold reported that limb cooling reduced both amplitude and frequency of the 8- to 12-Hz component of physiological tremor (Lippold, 1970). However, subsequent investigators found that limb cooling and limb ischemia reduced the amplitude of physiological tremor and essential tremor but did not change tremor frequency (Elble and Randall, 1976; Lakie et al., 1994). Limb cooling reduced essential tremor by more than 50% and therefore has potential therapeutic utility. Focal and task-specific tremors have not been studied in this manner. Parkinsonian tremor is reduced but not abolished by deafferentation (Walshe, 1924), but the effects of limb cooling and ischemia have not been studied.

If cerebellar intention tremor is produced by a loss of cerebellar feed-forward motor control and an excessive reliance on sensorimotor feedback control (Elble, 1998), then reducing sensory feedback may reduce tremor amplitude. Indeed, limb cooling, limb ischemia, and the elimination of visual feedback have been found to reduce tremor amplitude (Chase et al., 1965; Dash, 1995; Mitoma, 1996; Liu et al., 1997; Quintern et al., 1999). No change in tremor frequency was reported, but tremor frequency was not studied adequately in some of these investigations (Chase et al., 1965; Dash, 1995; Mitoma, 1996). The elimination of visual feedback increased the amplitude of physiological tremor (Quintern et al., 1999).

The prevailing impression is that cerebellar intention tremor is uniquely reliant on visual feedback (Sanes et al., 1988; Mitoma, 1996; Liu et al., 1997; Quintern et al., 1999), and clinical observation has revealed little or no dependence of other pathological tremors on visual feedback. Consequently, the current definition of intention tremor includes the requirement that tremor increases during visually guided movement toward a target (Diener and Dichgans, 1992; Deuschl et al., 1998a). Therefore, quantifying the effect of visual feedback could prove useful in the differential diagnosis of tremor disorders. Liu and coworkers found that visual feedback had no effect on the amplitude or frequency of parkinsonian action tremor (Liu et al., 1999). Additional quantitative studies comparing cerebellar intention tremor with other forms of action tremor are needed.

The cooling and ischemia experiments are difficult to interpret because the effects of these maneuvers on muscle function, reflex loop times, and sensory receptors must be considered and are poorly understood. The effect of temperature on tremor amplitude could result from changes in the strength and speed of muscle contraction, as suggested by Lakie and coworkers (1994). However, altered sensory feedback to a central source of oscillation could have profound effects on tremor amplitude, and such a mechanism must also be considered. Cooling and ischemia suppress the stretch reflex and reduce primary spindle afferent input (Eldred et al., 1960; Mense, 1978). Furthermore, cooling and ischemia could lead to an alteration of central pathway gains such that oscillation and neuronal entrainment are reduced. More information on the underlying mechanisms of these procedures and their effects on other forms of tremor (e.g., parkinsonian tremor) is needed before these procedures can be used diagnostically.

SUMMARY

Here we summarize the electrophysiological methods that are useful in specific differential diagnoses encountered in clinical neurology.

Distinguishing a central source of oscillation from one that emerges from a neuromuscular reflex loop: If tremor frequency is independent of mechanical load (inertia and stiffness) and reflex loop latency (long-loop or segmental), then the tremor most probably emerges from a central source of oscillation. The involvement of mechanical reflex mechanisms is assumed when tremor frequency is predictably altered by changes in limb inertia or stiffness or when tremor frequency is a function of reflex loop time.

Distinguishing enhanced physiological mechanical reflex tremor from mild essential tremor or another form of mild action tremor: Moderate and severe essential tremors exceed normal tremor in amplitude and invariably exhibit strong entrainment of EMG activity at a frequency that is not influenced by mechanical loading or reflex loop time. However, mechanical loading and all other neurophysiological tests are incapable of reliably distinguishing enhanced physiological tremor from mild essential tremor. In general, there are four possible outcomes of inertial loading:

1. No entrainment of the EMG activity (flat rectified-filtered EMG spectrum) occurs despite rhythmical oscillation of the limb, recorded with accelerometry. The frequency of oscillation decreases when an inertial load is applied to the limb. These results are characteristic of normal mechanical reflex tremor. The EMG spectrum is flat because there is no significant contribution from the stretch reflex or central oscillation at the time of tremor recording. However, this outcome is possible when essential tremor or some other pathological action tremor is mild and intermittent.

2. Motor unit entrainment is found in the EMG recording (statistically significant spectral peak in the rectified-filtered EMG spectrum), and the frequency of the hand oscillation (accelerometry) and EMG entrainment both decrease and are equal. Hence, the oscillating musculoskele-

tal system dictates the frequency of motor unit entrainment through somatosensory feedback. This is the outcome in most patients with enhanced physiological tremor, but it may also occur in when essential tremor or other pathological action tremor is so irregular and intermittent that the bursts of EMG activity simply perturb the mechanical reflex system and result in enhanced mechanical reflex oscillation.

3. Inertial loading discloses the presence of two oscillations. In the unloaded condition, limb oscillation and EMG entrainment may have the same frequencies, but inertial loading causes the frequency of mechanical reflex oscillation to decrease away from an oscillation with associated EMG entrainment (Fig. 99–6). The latter oscillation is interpreted as a central oscillation because its frequency does not decrease with inertial loading and bears no obvious relationship with reflex arc length (loop conduction time). This is the most common outcome in patients with mild essential tremor, but identical results are obtained from neurologically normal people with prominent 8- to 12-Hz tremor.

4. The mechanical oscillation and EMG entrainment have the same frequency in the loaded and unloaded conditions (see Fig. 99–6). This result is interpreted as a sign of pathological central oscillation and is most common in advanced tremor or when the mechanical resonance frequency of the joint and the tremor oscillator frequency are nearly the same.

All patients with moderate or severe essential tremor exhibit outcome 4, although several recordings may be needed to demonstrate this outcome. Outcomes 1, 2, and 3 commonly occur in patients with mild essential tremor and other forms of mild action tremor (e.g., Parkinson's disease). The frequencies of essential tremor and parkinsonian postural tremor may vary with posture and movement (Elble et al., 1992a); therefore, they are not as constant as the literature may seem to suggest.

Distinguishing parkinsonian postural tremor from essential tremor: The frequency of parkinsonian postural tremor overlaps significantly with that of essential tremor, and the frequencies of both tremors do not vary with reflex loop time or mechanical loading. No electrophysiological method can reliably distinguish these two forms of postural tremor. In many patients with Parkinson's disease, the postural tremor appears to be the rest tremor that may cease with voluntary muscle contraction, only to reemerge 1 to 50 seconds later (Jankovic et al., 1999).

Distinguishing orthostatic tremor from essential tremor, parkinsonian tremor, and other tremors that may affect the lower limbs while the patient is standing: The frequency of orthostatic tremor is uniquely high (14 to 18 Hz), and there is consistently high coherence between muscles of different limbs on the same and opposite sides of the body (see Fig. 99–4).

Distinguishing cortical tremor from other action tremors: An enhanced C reflex and giant sensory evoked potentials are found in patients with cortical tremor associated with cortical reflex myoclonus. Asterixis can be separated from enhanced physiological tremor by poly-EMG identification of synchronous EMG silent periods in forearm muscles associated with characteristic wrist flap.

Distinguishing advanced essential tremor from intention tremor caused by cerebellar outflow tract lesions: Studies in laboratory primates and limited studies in humans have shown that cerebellar intention tremor has a frequency that is predictably altered by adding inertia or stiffness to the affected limb. However, a systematic study of cerebellar tremor in humans has

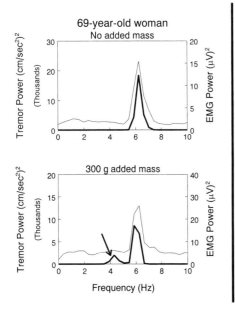
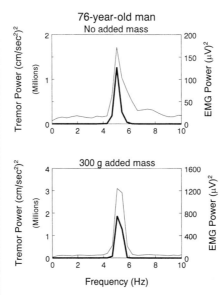

Figure 99–6. Examples of essential tremor in which the mechanical reflex oscillation was disclosed by mass loading (in a 69-year-old woman) and obscured by advanced essential tremor (in a 76-year-old man). With no mass loading, both patients exhibited only one peak in the tremor acceleration spectrum *(thick lines)* and rectified-filtered electromyographic spectrum *(thin lines)* because the mechanical reflex oscillation and essential tremor resonated at the same frequency. Mass loading reduced the natural frequency of the wrist mechanics, but a mechanical reflex peak *(arrow)* was evident only in the tremor spectrum of the woman, who had milder tremor. The rectified-filtered electromyogram was obtained from the extensor carpi radialis brevis, and tremor was recorded with an accelerometer during horizontal extension of the hand, with the forearm supported.

not been done. Cerebellar intention tremor, resulting from lesions in the brachium conjunctivum, is associated with other signs of ataxia, except in rare instances when the lesion is in or near the ventrolateral thalamus. The frequency of essential tremor changes less than 1 Hz when additional inertia or stiffness is applied to the limb, and nearly all patients with essential tremor have no other signs of ataxia or eye movement abnormalities.

Distinguishing essential and dystonic head tremor: Poly-EMG of neck muscles during antagonistic gestures can be useful in this differential diagnosis because complete or incomplete suppression of rhythmical EMG activity is seen in dystonic head tremor but not in essential tremor. The effect of antagonistic gestures on dystonic tremors of the extremities and trunk is too inconsistent to be useful diagnostically.

Distinguishing focal and task-specific tremors from focal and task-specific dystonic tremor: This differentiation can be difficult when the dystonia is mild. Reciprocal inhibition of the median nerve H reflex may be useful, but the sensitivity and specificity of this test are unknown.

Distinguishing organic tremor from psychogenic tremor: Poly-EMG is useful in demonstrating the identical frequencies of oscillation in the two upper or lower limbs of patients with psychogenic tremor and in demonstrating the large and erratic fluctuations in tremor amplitude and frequency. The performance of voluntary rapid repetitive movements either suppresses psychogenic tremor or causes its frequency to shift to that of the voluntary movement. By contrast, the frequencies of physiological and pathological tremors change less than 1 Hz when rapid repetitive movements are performed with the same or contralateral limb. Voluntary coactivation of antagonistic muscles is often present.

Acknowledgments

This work was supported by the Spastic Research Foundation of Kiwanis International (R.J.E.), National Institute of Neurological Disorders and Stroke grant 20973 (R.J.E.), and the Deutsche Forschungsgemeinschaft and the Bundesministerium für Forschung und Bildung (G.D.).

References

Agarwal GC, Gottlieb GL: Mathematical modeling and simulation of the postural control loop. Part III. Crit Rev Biomed Eng 1984;12:49–93.

Alberts WW, Wright EW, Feinstein B: Cortical potentials and parkinsonian tremor. Nature 1969;221:670–672.

Amjad AM, Halliday DM, Rosenberg JR, Conway BA: An extended difference of coherence test for comparing and combining several independent coherence estimates: Theory and application to the study of motor units and physiologic tremor. J Neurosci Methods 1997;73:69–79.

Artieda J, Muruzabal J, Larumbe R, et al: Cortical mechanisms mediating asterixis. Mov Disord 1992;7:209–216.

Bacher M, Scholz E, Diener HC: 24 hour continuous tremor quantification based on EMG recording. Electroencephalogr Clin Neurophysiol 1989;72:176–183.

Bain PG, Findley LG, Atchison P, et al: Assessing tremor severity. J Neurol Neurosurg Psychiatry 1993;56:868–873.

Bain PG, Findley LJ, Britton TC, et al: Primary writing tremor. Brain 1995;118:1461–1472.

Baker SN, Kilner JM, Pinches EM, Lemon RN: The role of synchrony and oscillations in the motor output. Exp Brain Res 1999;128:109–117.

Baker SN, Olivier E, Lemon RN: Coherent oscillations in monkey motor cortex and hand muscle EMG show task-dependent modulation. J Physiol (Lond) 1997;501:225–241.

Basmajian JV, De Luca CJ: Muscles Alive: Their Functions Revealed by Electromyography. Baltimore: Williams & Wilkins, 1985.

Bastian AJ, Thach WT: Cerebellar outflow lesions: A comparison of movement deficits resulting from lesions at the levels of the cerebellum and thalamus. Ann Neurol 1995;38:881–892.

Benignus VA: Estimation of the coherence spectrum and its confidence intervals using the fast Fourier transform. IEEE Trans Audio Electroacoustics 1969;17:145–150.

Berardelli A, Hallett M, Rothwell JC, et al: Single-joint rapid arm movements in normal subjects and in patients with motor disorders. Brain 1996;119:661–674.

Beuter A, de Geoffroy A, Cordo P: The measurement of tremor using simple laser systems. J Neurosci Methods 1994;53:47–54.

Bock O, Wenderoth N: Dependence of peripheral tremor on mechanical perturbations: Modeling study. Biol Cybern 1999;80:103–108.

Boecker H, Brooks DJ: Functional imaging of tremor. Mov Disord 1998;13:64–72.

Boose A, Jentgens C, Spieker S, Dichgans J: Variations on tremor parameters. Chaos 1995;5:52–56.

Boose A, Spieker S, Jentgens C, Dichgans J: Wrist tremor: Investigation of agonist-antagonist interaction by means of long-term EMG recording and cross-spectral analysis. Electroencephalogr Clin Neurophysiol 1996;101:355–363.

Boroojerdi B, Ferbert A, Foltys H, et al: Evidence for a non-orthostatic origin of orthostatic tremor. J Neurol Neurosurg Psychiatry 1999;66:284–288.

Britton TC, Thompson PD, Day BL, et al: "Resetting" of postural tremors at the wrist with mechanical stretches in Parkinson's disease, essential tremor, and normal subjects mimicking tremor. Ann Neurol 1992a;31:507–514.

Britton TC, Thompson PD, Day BL, et al: Modulation of postural tremors at the wrist by supramaximal electrical median nerve shocks in essential tremor, Parkinson's disease and normal subjects mimicking tremor. J Neurol Neurosurg Psychiatry 1993a;56:1085–1089.

Britton TC, Thompson PD, Day BL, et al: Modulation of postural wrist tremors by magnetic stimulation of the motor cortex in patients with PD and essential tremor and in normal subjects mimicking tremor. Ann Neurol 1993b;33:473–479.

Britton TC, Thompson PD, Day BL, et al: Rapid wrist movements in patients with essential tremor: The critical role of the second agonist burst. Brain 1994;117:39–47.

Britton TC, Thompson PD, van der Kamp W, et al: Primary orthostatic tremor: Further observations in six cases. J Neurol 1992b;239:209–217.

Brown P: Muscle sounds in Parkinson's disease. Lancet 1997;349:533–535.

Brown P, Corcos DM, Rothwell JC: Does parkinsonian action tremor contribute to muscle weakness in Parkinson's disease? Brain 1997;120:401–408.

Brown P, Corcos DM, Rothwell JC: Action tremor and weakness in Parkinson's disease: A study of the elbow extensors. Mov Disord 1998;13:56–60.

Brown P, Farmer SF, Halliday DM, et al: Coherent cortical and muscle discharge in cortical myoclonus. Brain 1999;122:461–472.

Brown P, Marsden CD: Rhythmic cortical and muscle discharge in cortical myoclonus. Brain 1996;119:1307–1316.

Bucher SF, Seelos KC, Dodel RC, et al: Activation mapping in essential tremor with functional magnetic resonance imaging. Ann Neurol 1997;41:32–40.

Cappello A, Leardini A, Benedetti MG, et al: Application of stereophotogrammetry to total body three-dimensional analysis of human tremor. IEEE Trans Rehabil Eng 1997;5:388–393.

Chase RA, Cullen JK, Sullivan SA: Modification of intention tremor in man. Nature 1965;206:485–487.

Cleeves L, Findley LJ: Variability in amplitude of untreated essential tremor. J Neurol Neurosurg Psychiatry 1987;50:704–708.

Cleeves L, Findley LJ, Gresty M: Assessment of rest tremor in Parkinson's disease. Adv Neurol 1986;45:349–352.

Conway BA, Halliday DM, Farmer SF, et al: Synchronization between motor cortex and spinal motoneuronal pool during the performance of a maintained motor task in man. J Physiol (Lond) 1995;489:917–924.

Das Gupta A: Paired response of motor units during voluntary contraction in parkinsonism. J Neurol Neurosurg Psychiatry 1963;26:265–268.

Dash BMS: Role of peripheral inputs in cerebellar tremor. Mov Disord 1995;10:622–629.

Datta AK, Farmer SF, Stephens JA: Central nervous pathways underlying synchronization of human motor unit firing studied during voluntary contractions. J Physiol (Lond) 1991;432:401–425.

Datta AK, Stephens JA: Synchronization of motor unit activity during voluntary contraction in man. J Physiol (Lond) 1990;422:397–419.

Davey NJ, Ellaway PH, Friedland CL: Synchrony of motor unit discharge in humans with Parkinson's disease. J Physiol (Lond) 1986;377:30P.

De Luca CJ, Merletti R: Surface myoelectric signal cross-talk among muscles of the leg. Electroencephalogr Clin Neurophysiol 1988;69:568–575.

De Luca CJ, Roy AM, Erim Z: Synchronization of motor-unit firings in several human muscles. J Neurophysiol 1993;70:2010–2023.

Dengler R, Gillespie J, Argenta M, et al: The impact of paired motor unit discharges on tremor. Electromyogr Clin Neurophysiol 1989;29:113–117.

Dengler R, Wolf W, Birk P, Struppler A: Synchronous discharges in pairs of steadily firing motor units tend to form clusters. Neurosci Lett 1984;47:167–172.

Dengler R, Wolf W, Schubert M, Struppler A: Discharge pattern of single motor units in basal ganglia disorders. Neurology 1986;36:1061–1066.

Deuschl G: Differential diagnosis of tremor. J Neural Transm Suppl 1999a;56:211–220.

Deuschl G: Neurophysiological tests for the assessment of tremors. Adv Neurol 1999b;80:57–65.

Deuschl G, Bain P, Brin M: Consensus statement of the Movement Disorder Society on tremor: Ad hoc scientific committee. Mov Disord 1998a;13:2–23.

Deuschl G, Heinen F, Kleedorfer B, et al: Clinical and polymyographic investigation of spasmodic torticollis. J Neurol 1992;239:9–15.

Deuschl G, Köster B, Lücking CH, Scheidt C: Diagnostic and pathophysiological aspects of psychogenic tremors. Mov Disord 1998b;13:294–302.

Deuschl G, Krack P, Lauk M, Timmer J: Clinical neurophysiology of tremor. J Clin Neurophysiol 1996;13:110–121.

Deuschl G, Lauk M, Timmer J: Tremor classification and tremor time series analysis. Chaos 1995;5:48–51.

Deuschl G, Lücking CH: Physiology and clinical applications of hand muscle reflexes. Electroencephalogr Clin Neurophysiol 1990;Supplement 41:84–101.

Deuschl G, Mischke G, Schenck E,et al: Symptomatic and essential rhythmic palatal myoclonus. Brain 1990;113:1645–1672.

Deuschl G, Toro C, Valls-Sole J, et al: Symptomatic and essential palatal tremor. I. Clinical, physiological and MRI analysis. Brain 1994;117:775–788.

Deuschl G, Wilms H, Krack P, et al: Function of the cerebellum in parkinsonian rest tremor and Holme's tremor. Ann Neurol 1999;46:126–128.

Diener H-C, Dichgans J: Pathophysiology of cerebellar ataxia. Mov Disord 1992;7:95–109.

Dietz V, Bischofberger E, Wita C, Freund H-J: Correlation between the discharges of two simultaneously recorded motor units and physiological tremor. Electroencephalogr Clin Neurophysiol 1976;40:97–105.

Dietz V, Hillesheimer W, Freund H-J: Correlation between tremor, voluntary contraction, and firing pattern of motor units in Parkinson's disease. J Neurol Neurosurg Psychiatry 1974;37:927–937.

Elble RJ: Physiologic and essential tremor. Neurology 1986;36:225–231.

Elble RJ: Inhibition of forearm EMG by palatal myoclonus. Mov Disord 1991;6:324–329.

Elble RJ: Mechanisms of physiologic tremor and relationship to essential tremor. In Findley LJ and Koller WC (eds): Handbook of Tremor Disorders. New York, Marcel Dekker, 1994; 51–62.

Elble RJ: The role of aging in the clinical expression of essential tremor. Exp Gerontol 1995;30:337–347.

Elble RJ: Central mechanisms of tremor. J Clin Neurophysiol 1996;13:133–144.

Elble RJ: Animal models of action tremor. Mov Disord 1998;13:35–39.

Elble RJ: Origins of tremor. Lancet 2000;355:1113–4.

Elble RJ, Brilliant M, Leffler K, Higgins C: Quantification of essential tremor in writing and drawing. Mov Disord 1996;11:70–78.

Elble RJ, Higgins C, Hughes L: Longitudinal study of essential tremor. Neurology 1992a;42:441–443.

Elble RJ, Higgins C, Hughes L: Phase resetting and frequency entrainment of essential tremor. Exp Neurol 1992b;116:355–361.

Elble RJ, Higgins C, Hughes L: Essential tremor entrains rapid voluntary movements. Exp Neurol 1994;126:138–143.

Elble RJ, Koller WC: Tremor. Baltimore: Johns Hopkins University Press, 1990.

Elble RJ, Moody C, Higgins C: Primary writing tremor: A form of focal dystonia? Mov Disord 1990a;5:118–26.

Elble RJ, Randall JE: Motor-unit activity responsible for 8- to 12-Hz component of human physiological finger tremor. J Neurophysiol 1976;39:370–83.

Elble RJ, Randall JE: Mechanistic components of normal hand tremor. Electroencephalogr Clin Neurophysiol 1978;44:72–82.

Elble RJ, Schieber MH, Thach WT Jr: Activity of muscle spindles, motor cortex and cerebellar nuclei during action tremor. Brain Res 1984;323:330–4.

Elble RJ, Sinha R, Higgins C: Quantification of tremor with a digitizing tablet. J Neurosci Methods 1990b;32:193–198.

Eldred E, Lindsley DF, Buchwald JS: The effect of cooling on mammalian muscle spindles. Exp Neurol 1960;2:144–157.

Elek JM, Dengler R, Konstanzer A, et al: Mechanical implications of paired motor unit discharges in pathological and voluntary tremor. Electroencephalogr Clin Neurophysiol 1991;81:279–283.

Elia M, Musumeci SA, Ferri R, et al: Familial cortical tremor, epilepsy, and metal retardation: A distinct clinical entity? Arch Neurol 1998;55:1569–1573.

Farmer SF, Bremner FD, Halliday DM, et al: The frequency content of common synaptic inputs to motoneurons studied during voluntary isometric contraction in man. J Physiol (Lond) 1993a;470:127–155.

Farmer SF, Halliday DM, Conway BA, et al: A review of recent applications of cross-correlation methodologies to human motor unit recording. J Neurosci Methods 1997;74:175–187.

Farmer SF, Swash M, Ingram DA, Stephens JA: Changes in motor unit synchronization following central nervous lesions in man. J Physiol (Lond) 1993b;463:83–105.

Fox JR, Randall JE: Relationship between forearm tremor and the biceps electromyogram. J Appl Physiol 1970;29:103–108.

Friedman JH: "Rubral" tremor induced by a neuroleptic drug. Mov Disord 1992;7:281–282.

Gantert C, Honerkamp J, Timmer J: Analyzing the dynamics of hand tremor time series. Biol Cybern 1992;66:479–484.

Gordon G, Holbourn AHS: The sounds from single motor units in a contracting muscle. J Physiol (Lond) 1948;107:456–464.

Gottlieb GL, Agarwal GC: Physiological clonus in man. Exp Neurol 1977;54:616–621.

Hagbarth K-E, Young RR: Participation of the stretch reflex in human physiological tremor. Brain 1979;102:509–526.

Halliday DM, Conway BA, Farmer SF, Rosenberg JR: Using electroencephalography to study functional coupling between cortical activity and electromyograms during voluntary contractions in humans. Neurosci Lett 1998;241:5–8.

Halliday DM, Conway BA, Farmer SF, Rosenberg JR: Load-independent contributions from motor-unit synchronization to human physiological tremor. J Neurophysiol 1999;82:664–675.

Halliday DM, Conway BA, Farmer SF, et al: Coherence between low-frquency activation of the motor cortex and tremor in patients with essential tremor. Lancet 2000;355:1149–1153.

Hari R, Salenius S: Rhythmical corticomotor communication. Neuroreport 1999;10:1–10.

Hellwig B, Häussler S, Guschlbauer B, et al: Tremor-correlated EEG activity in essential tremor detected by coherence analysis. Mov Disord 2000;15[Suppl 3]:97.

Hogan N, Mann RW: Myoelectric signal processing: optimal estimation applied to electromyography. Part II. Experimental demonstration of optimal myoprocessor performance. IEEE Trans Biomed Eng 1980;27:396–410.

Holmes G: On certain tremors in organic cerebral lesions. Brain 1904;27:327–375.

Hömberg V, Hefter H, Reiners K, Freund H-J: Differential effects of changes in mechanical limb properties on physiological and pathological tremor. J Neurol Neurosurg Psychiatry 1987;50:568–579.

Hua SE, Lenz FA, Zirh TA, et al: Thalamic neuronal activity correlated with essential tremor. J Neurol Neurosurg Psychiatry 1998;64:273–276.

Hunker CJ, Abbs JH: Uniform frequency of parkinsonian resting tremor in the lips, jaw, tongue and index finger. Mov Disord 1990;5:71–77.

Ikeda A, Kakigi R, Funai N,et al: Cortical tremor: A variant of cortical reflex myoclonus. Neurology 1990;40:1561–1565.

Jankovic J, Schwartz KS, Ondo W: Re-emergent tremor of Parkinson's disease. J Neurol Neurosurg Psychiatry 1999;67:646–650.

Journée HL, van Manen J, van der Meer JJ: Demodulation of EMGs of pathological tremours: Development and testing of a demodulator for clinical use. Med Biol Eng Comput 1983;21:172–175.

Kay SM, Marple SL: Spectrum analysis: A modern perspective. Proc IEEE 1981;69:1380–1419.

Kelly JJ, Sharbrough FW: EMG in orthostatic tremor. Neurology 1987;37:1434.

Kim YJ, Pakiam AS-I, Lang AE: Historical and clinical features of psychogenic tremor: A review of 70 cases. Can J Neurol Sci 1999;26:190–195.

Koller WC, Royse VL: Time course of a single oral dose of propranolol in essential tremor. Neurology 1985;35:1494–1498.

Köster B, Lauk M, Timmer J, et al: Evidence for a cerebellar dysfunction in essential tremor. Mov Disord 1998a;13:269.

Köster B, Lauk M, Timmer J, et al: Involvement of cranial muscles and high intermuscular coherence in orthostatic tremor. Ann Neurol 1999;45:384–388.

Köster B, Lauk M, Timmer J, et al: Central mechanisms in human enhanced physiological tremor. Neurosci Lett 1998b;241:135–138.

Kreifeldt JG, Yao S: A signal-to-noise investigation of nonlinear electromyographic processors. IEEE Trans Biom Eng 1974;21:298–308.

Kwatny E, Thomas DH, Kwatny HG: An application of signal processing techniques to the study of myoelectric signals. IEEE Trans Biomed Eng 1970;17:303–313.

Lakie M, Walsh EG, Arblaster LA, et al: Limb temperature and human tremors. J Neurol Neurosurg Psychiatry 1994;57:35–42.

Lakie M, Walsh EG, Wright GW: Resonance at the wrist demonstrated by the use of a torque motor: An instrumental analysis of muscle tone in man. J Physiol (Lond) 1984;353:265–285.

Lakie M, Walsh EG, Wright GW: Passive mechanical properties of the wrist and physiological tremor. J Neurol Neurosurg Psychiatry 1986;49:669–676.

Lance JW, Schwab RS, Peterson EA: Action tremor and the cogwheel phenomenon in Parkinson's disease. Brain 1963;86:95–110.

Lauk M, Köster B, Timmer J, et al: Side-to-side correlation of muscle activity in physiological and pathological human tremor. Clin Neurophysiol 1999;110:1774–1783.

Lee RG, Stein RB: Resetting of tremor by mechanical perturbations: A comparison of essential tremor and parkinsonian tremor. Ann Neurol 1981;10:523–531.

Lemstra AW, Verhagen Metman L, Lee JI, et al: Tremor-frequency (3–6 Hz) activity in the sensorimotor arm representation of the internal segment of the globus pallidus in patients with Parkinson's disease. Neurosci Lett 1999;267:129–132.

Lippold OCJ: Oscillation in the stretch reflex arc, and the origin of the rhythmical 8–12 c/s component of physiological tremor. J Physiol (Lond) 1970;206:359–382.

Liu X, Miall C, Aziz TZ, et al: Analysis of action tremor and impaired control of movement velocity in multiple sclerosis during visually guided wrist-tracking tasks. Mov Disord 1997;12:992–999.

Liu X, Tubbesing SA, Aziz TZ, et al: Effects of visual feedback on manual tracking and action tremor in Parkinson's disease. Exp Brain Res 1999;129:477–481.

Logigian E, Hefter H, Reiners K, Freund H-J: Does tremor pace repetitive voluntary motor behavior in Parkinson's disease? Ann Neurol 1991;30:172–179.

Logigian EL, Wierzbicka MM, Bruyninckx F, et al: Motor unit synchronization in physiologic, enhanced physiologic and voluntary tremor in man. Ann Neurol 1988;23:242–250.

Mäkelä JP, Hari R, Karhu J, et al: Supression of magnetic mu rhythm during parkinsonian tremor. Brain Res 1993;617:189–193.

Matsumoto JY, Dodick DW, Stevens LN, et al: Three-dimensional measurement of essential tremor. Mov Disord 1999;14:288–294.

McAuley JH, Farmer SF, Rothwell JC, Marsden CD: Common 3 and 10 Hz oscillations modulate human eye and finger movements while they simultaneously track a visual target. J Physiol (Lond) 1999;515:905–917.

McAuley JH, Rothwell JC, Marsden CD: Frequency peaks of tremor, muscle vibration and electromyographic activity at 10 Hz, 20 Hz and 40 Hz during finger muscle contraction may reflect rhythmicities of central neural firing. Exp Brain Res 1997;114:525–541.

McAuley JH, Rothwell JC, Marsden CD, Findley LJ: Electrophysiological aids in distinguishing organic tremor from psychogenic tremor. Neurology 1998;50:1882–1884.

McManis PG, Sharbrough FW: Orthostatic tremor: Clinical and electrophysiologic characteristics. Muscle Nerve 1993;16:1254–1260.

Mense S: Effects of temperature on the discharges of muscle spindles and tendon organs. Pflugers Arch 1978;374:159–166.

Mercuri B, Berardelli A, Modugno N, et al: Reciprocal inhibition in forearm muscles in patients with essential tremor. Muscle Nerve 1998;21:796–799.

Miller WL, Sigvardt KA: Spectral analysis of oscillatory neural circuits. J Neurosci Methods 1998;80:113–128.

Milner TE, Cloutier C: Damping of the wrist joint during voluntary movement. Exp Brain Res 1998;122:309–317.

Mima T, Goldstein S, Toma K, et al: The lack of cortico-muscular coupling of 8–12 Hz central component of human physiologic tremor. Mov Disord 2000;15[Suppl 3]:79.

Mitoma H: Intention tremor exaggerated by visually guided movement. Eur Neurol 1996;36:177–178.

Miyagi Y, Shima F, Ishido K, et al: Posteroventral pallidotomy for midbrain tremor after a pontine hemorrhage. J Neurosurg 1999;91:885–888.

Modugno N, Priori A, Berardelli A, et al: Botulinum toxin restores presynaptic inhibition of group Ia afferents in patients with essential tremor. Muscle Nerve 1998;21:1701–1705.

Murthy VN, Fetz EE: Coherent 25- to 35-Hz oscillations in the sensorimotor cortex of awake behaving monkeys. Proc Natl Acad Sci USA 1992;89:5670–5674.

Muthuswamy J, Thakor NV: Spectral analysis methods for neurological signals. J Neurosci Methods 1998;83:1–14.

Nakashima K, Rothwell JC, Day BL, et al: Reciprocal inhibition between forearm muscles in patients with writer's cramp and other occupational cramps, symptomatic hemidystonia and hemiparesis due to stroke. Brain 1989;112:681–697.

Oguni E, Hayashi A, Ishii A, et al: A case of cortical tremor as a variant of cortical reflex myoclonus. Eur Neurol 1995;35:63–64.

Oguztöreli MN, Stein RB: Interactions between centrally and peripherally generated neuromuscular oscillations. J Math Biol 1979;7:1–30.

Okuma Y, Shimo Y, Shimura H, et al: Familial cortical tremor with epilepsy: An under-recognized familial tremor. Clin Neurol Neurosurg 1998;100:75–78.

Orizio C: Muscle sound: Bases for the introduction of a mechanomyographic signal in muscle studies. Crit Rev Biomed Eng 1993;21:201–243.

Oster G, Jaffe JS: Low frequency sounds from sustained contraction of human skeletal muscle. Biophys J 1980;30:119–127.

O'Suilleabhain PE, Matsumoto JY: Time-frequency analysis of tremors. Brain 1998;121:2127–2134.

Ouamer M, Boiteux M, Petitjean M, et al: Acoustic myography during voluntary isometric contraction reveals non-propagative lateral vibration. J Biomech 1999;32:1279–1285.

Padgaonkar AJ, Krieger KW, King AI: Measurement of angular acceleration of a rigid body using linear accelerometers. J Appl Mech 1975;42:552–556.

Pascual-Leone A, Valls-Solé J, Toro C, et al: Resetting of essential tremor and postural tremor in Parkinson's disease with transcranial magnetic stimulation. Muscle Nerve 1994;17:800–807.

Perry J, Easterday CS, Antonelli DJ: Surface versus intramuscular electrodes for electromyography of superficial and deep muscles. Phys Ther 1981;61:7–15.

Pfeiffer G, Hinse P, Humbert T, Riemer G: Neurophysiology of orthostatic tremor: Influence of transcranial magnetic stimulation. Electromyogr Clin Neurophysiol 1999;39:49–53.

Priori A, Berardelli A, Mercuri B, Manfredi M: Physiological effects produced by botulinum toxin treatment of upper limb dystonia: Changes in reciprocal inhibition between forearm muscles. Brain 1995;118:801–807.

Quintern J, Immisch I, Albrecht H, et al: Influence of visual and proprioceptive afferences on upper limb ataxia in patients with multiple sclerosis. J Neurol Sci 1999;163:61–69.

Rack PMH, Ross HF: The role of reflexes in the resting tremor of Parkinson's disease. Brain 1986;109:115–141.

Raethjen J, Lindemann M, Dümpelmann M, et al: Cortical correlates of physiologic tremor. Mov Disord 2000a;15[Suppl 3]:90–91.

Raethjen J, Lindemann M, Schmaljohann H, et al: Multiple oscillators are causing parkinsonian and essential tremor. Mov Disord 2000b;15:84–94.

Randall JE: A stochastic time series model for hand tremor. J Appl Physiol 1973;34:390–395.

Redmond DP, Hegge FW: Observations on the design and specification of a wrist-worn human activity monitoring system. Behav Res Methods Instr Comput 1985;17:659–669.

Remy P, de Recondo A, Defer G, et al: Peduncular "rubral" tremor and dopaminergic denervation: A PET study. Neurology 1995;45:472–477.

Renou G, Rondot P, Metral S: Analyse de décharges itératives d'une même unité motrice dans les bouffées de tremblement. Rev Neurol (Paris) 1970;122:420–423.

Rhatigan BA, Mylrea KC, Lonsdale E, Stern LZ: Investigation of sounds produced by healthy and diseased human muscular contraction. IEEE Trans Biomed Eng 1986;33:967–971.

Richard I, Guglielmi M, Boisliveau R, et al: Load compensation tasks evoke tremor in cerebellar patients: The possible role of long latency stretch reflexes. Neurosci Lett 1997;234:99–102.

Salenius S, Portin K, Kajola M, et al: Cortical control of human motoneuron firing during isometric contraction. J Neurophysiol 1997;77:3401–3405.

Sanes JN: Absence of enhanced physiological tremor in patients without muscle or cutaneous afferents. J Neurol Neurosurg Psychiatry 1985;48:645–649.

Sanes JN, LeWitt PA, Mauritz K-H: Visual and mechanical control of postural and kinetic tremor in cerebellar system disorders. J Neurol Neurosurg Psychiatry 1988;51:934–943.

Savitzky A, Golay MJE: Smoothing and differentiation of data by simplified least squares procedures. Anal Chem 1964;36:1627–1639.

Sears TA, Stagg D: Short-term synchronization of intercostal motoneurone activity. J Physiol (Lond) 1976;263:357–381.

Semmler JG, Nordstrom MA: Motor unit discharge and force tremor in skill- and strength-trained individuals. Exp Brain Res 1998;119:27–38.

Shahani BT, Young RR: Physiological and pharmacological aids in the differential diagnosis of tremor. J Neurol Neurosurg Psychiatry 1976;38:772–783.

Shahani BT, Young RR: Specific abnormalities of single motor unit discharge patterns in tremor. Neurology 1977;27:354.

Solomonow M, Baratta RV, D'Ambrosia R: EMG-force relations of a single skeletal muscle acting across a joint: Dependence on joint angle. J Electromyogr Kinesiol 1991;1:58–67.

Spieker S, Ströle V, Sailer A, et al: Validity of long-term electromyography in the quantification of tremor. Mov Disord 1997;12:985–991.

Spyers-Ashby JM, Bain PG, Roberts SJ: A comparison of fast fourier transform (FFT) and autoregressive (AR) spectral estimation techniques for the analysis of tremor data. J Neurosci Methods 1998;83:35–43.

Staude G, Wolf W, Ott M, et al: Tremor as a factor in prolonged reaction times of parkinsonian patients. Mov Disord 1995;10:153–162.

Stein RB, Oguztöreli MN: Tremor and other oscillations in neuromuscular systems. Biol Cybern 1976;22:147–157.

Stephens JA, Taylor A: The effect of visual feedback on physiological muscle tremor. Electroencephalogr Clin Neurophysiol 1974;36:457–464.

Stiles RN: Frequency and displacement amplitude relations for normal hand tremor. J Appl Physiol 1976;40:44–54.

Stiles RN: Mechanical and neural feedback factors in postural hand tremor of normal subjects. J Neurophysiol 1980;44:40–59.

Stiles RN, Hahs DW: Muscle-load oscillations: Detection, analysis and models. In Wise DL (ed): Bioinstrumentation and Biosensors. New York, Marcel Dekker, 1991; 75–119.

Stiles RN, Randall JE: Mechanical factors in human tremor frequency. J Appl Physiol 1967;23:324–330.

Terada K, Ikeda A, Mima T, et al: Familial cortical myoclonic tremor as a unique form of cortical reflex myoclonus. Mov Disord 1997;12:370–377.

Thakor NV, Sherman D: Wavelet (time-scale) analysis in biomedical signal processing. In Bronzino JD (ed): The Biomedical Engineering Handbook. Boca Raton, FL, CRC, 1995; 886–906.

Thakor NV, Xin-Rong G, Yi-Chun S, Hanley DF: Multiresolution wavelet analysis of evoked potentials. IEEE Trans Biomed Eng 1993;40:1085–1094.

Thompson PD, Rothwell JC, Day BL, et al: The physiology of orthostatic tremor. Arch Neurol 1986;43:584–587.

Timmer J, Gantert C, Deuschl G, Honerkamp J: Characteristics of hand tremor time series. Biol Cybern 1993;70:75–80.

Timmer J, Häussler S, Lauk M, Lücking CH: Pathological tremors: Deterministic chaos or nonlinear stochastic oscillators? Chaos 2000;10:278–288.

Timmer J, Lauk M, Deuschl G: Quantitative analysis of tremor time series. Electroencephalogr Clin Neurophysiol 1996;101:461–468.

Timmer J, Lauk M, Pfleger W, Deuschl G: Cross-spectral analysis of physiologic tremor and muscle activity. I. Theory and application to unsynchronized electromyogram. Biol Cybern 1998;78:349–357.

Toro C, Pascual-Leone A, Deuschl G, et al: Cortical tremor: A common manifestation of cortical myoclonus. Neurology 1993;43:2346–2353.

Tsai CH, Semmler JG, Kimber TE, et al: Modulation of primary orthostatic tremor by magnetic stimulation over the motor cortex. J Neurol Neurosurg Psychiatry 1998;64:33–36.

Tyrer PJ, Bond AJ: Diurnal variation in physiological tremor. Electroencephalogr Clin Neurophysiol 1974;37:35–40.

Ugawa Y, Shimpo T, Mannen T: Physiological analysis of asterixis: Silent period locked averaging. J Neurol Neurosurg Psychiatry 1989;52:89–93.

van Someren EJW, Lazeron RHC, Vonk BFM, et al: Gravitational artefact in frequency spectra of movement acceleration: Implications for actigraphy in young and elderly subjects. J Neurosci Methods 1996;65:55–62.

van Someren EJW, Vonk BFM, Thijssen WA, et al: A new actigraph for long-term registration of the duration and intensity of tremor and movement. IEEE Trans Biomed Eng 1998;45:386–395.

Vilis T, Hore J: Effects of changes in mechanical state of limb on cerebellar intention tremor. J Neurophysiol 1977;40:1214–1224.

Volkmann J, Joliot M, Mogilner A, et al: Central motor loop oscillations in parkinsonian resting tremor revealed by magnetoencephalography. Neurology 1996;46:1359–1370.

Walshe FMR: Observations on the nature of the muscular rigidity of paralysis agitans, and on its relationship to tremor. Brain 1924;47:159–177.

Wenderoth N, Bock O: Load dependence of simulated central tremor. Biol Cybern 1999;80:285–290.

Wessberg J, Kakuda N: Single motor unit activity in relation to pulsatile motor output in human finger movements. J Physiol (Lond) 1999;517:273–285.

Wessberg J, Vallbo ÅB: Pulsatile motor output in human finger movements is not dependent on the stretch reflex. J Physiol (Lond) 1996;493:895–908.

Wierzbicka MM, Staude G, Wolf W, Dengler R: Relationship between tremor and the onset of rapid voluntary contraction in Parkinson's disease. J Neurol Neurosurg Psychiatry 1993; 56:782–787.

Wilms H, Sievers J, Deuschl G: Animal models of tremor. Mov Disord 1999;14:557–571.

Winfree AT: The Geometry of Biological Time. New York, Springer-Verlag, 1980.

Zahalak GI, Pramod R: Myoelectric response of human triceps brachii to displacement-controlled oscillations of the forearm. Exp Brain Res 1985;58:305–317.

Zirh TA, Lenz FA, Reich SG, Dougherty PM. Patterns of bursting occurring in thalamic cells during parkinsonian tremor. Neuroscience 1998;83:107–121.

Tone and Its Disorders

Reiner Benecke, Joseph Classen, and Dirk Dressler

The term *muscle tone* was introduced about 150 years ago to describe the continuous contractile tension that was first clearly detected in a variety of experimental animal preparations. It was suggested by Sherrington (1894, 1898, 1909) that muscle tone might play an important role in the maintenance of posture. For the clinician, the presence of normal and abnormal muscle tone is difficult to assess simply by observation of the patient under resting conditions. In practice, clinicians test muscle tone by stretching the muscles, thus measuring passive resistance to the stretch by their own skin and muscle receptors. Furthermore, abnormal muscle tone can be recognized by eye, especially in dystonia, when the abnormal exaggerated tone leads to twisting and repetitive movements or abnormal postures (Fahn et al., 1987b; Fahn, 1988). A more stable abnormal positioning of the limbs can also be observed in rigid and spastic patients. Rigid parkinsonian patients often show generalized flexion of the neck, trunk, hips, and knees at rest that is increased during walking. Spastic patients may develop abnormal flexion of the elbow joints or abnormal adduction of the hip joints, especially when performing voluntary movements.

This chapter reviews the neural mechanism important to an understanding of increased muscle tone, outlines new and promising developments in clinical neurophysiology, and, finally, presents reliable methods for assessing muscle tone in patients. The chapter is divided into three parts that deal with the most important forms of abnormally increased muscle tone—dystonia, spasticity, and rigidity.

While the methods of clinical neurophysiology have helped a great deal in elucidating the patho-physiological principles of motor disturbances in disorders of muscle tone, a major consequence has been the opinion that it is much too simple to view such motor disorders only in terms of abnormal spinal reflexes. Therefore, classical methods of clinical neurophysiology have their limits in promoting the understanding of, the ability to differentiate among, and the monitoring of these motor abnormalities. Dystonia, spasticity, and rigidity are induced by complex disturbances of sensorimotor integration on the supraspinal level that can be only partially envisioned by neuroscientists, even when modern neurophysiological methods are used. Furthermore, the general problem exists that the detectable neurophysiological signals in these diseases may be epiphenomena, rather than valid clues to the pathophysiology underlying them.

DYSTONIA

Today, the term *dystonia* is applied in the description of a number of clinical symptoms that run together, that is, a syndrome, and it is also used to delineate specific diseases (e.g., idiopathic torsion dystonia, tardive dystonia, dopa-responsive dystonia). Oppenheim was responsible for introducing the word *dystonia* (Oppenheim, 1911). While Gowers (1888) and Thompson (1896) presented their patients as suffering from an organic disorder, in 1908 Schwalbe (1908) suggested that a family with a "chronic cramp syndrome" had hysterical features. Despite further clinical descriptions of dystonia (Oppenheim, 1911; Herz, 1944), it took more than half a century before neuroscientists accepted that this bizarre syndrome was due to an organic brain disease (Marsden et al., 1976). Since Marsden and colleagues published the series of papers that demonstrated, beyond all reasonable doubt, that most patients with dystonia are suffering from an organic disorder, research into dystonia has been vigorous and highly productive. In both Jewish (Bressman et al., 1989) and non-Jewish groups (Zeman and Dyken, 1967), dystonia can be inherited as an autosomal dominant disorder, and advances in the molecular genetics of dystonia have led to the recent identification of a 3-basepair deletion in the *DYT1* gene, causing early-onset generalized torsion dystonia, and to the detection of mutations in the GTP cyclohydrolase I and the tyrosine hydroxylase genes, causing dopa-responsive dystonia (Ichinose et al., 1994; Ozelius et al., 1997). Animal models of dystonia are beginning to contribute to our limited understanding of the pathophysiology and neurochemistry of dystonia. Postmortem studies and new techniques for imaging the brain indicate that the putamen may be a common site of the causal pathology, especially in symptomatic forms of dystonia (Burton et al., 1984; Marsden et al., 1985).

Yet despite the substantial achievements that have taken place in the study of dystonia, there remains a long list of unanswered questions, many of which are of fundamental importance. The following section is an attempt to summarize recent knowledge on the pathophysiology of dystonia, to describe the clinical spectrum of the syndrome, and to introduce the neurophysiological methods available for detecting and quantifying the various aspects of dystonia.

Classifications

Dystonia is defined as a movement disorder characterized clinically by involuntary twisting and repetitive movements and abnormal postures (Marsden, 1976; Fahn et al., 1987b; Fahn, 1988). According to this definition, *dystonia*, as the term would imply, is not only a form of abnormal muscle tone but also a hyperkinetic motor disturbance presenting with phasic muscle activities, such as tremor and myoclonus. The original simple classification of dystonia categorizes the disorder as either primary, in which there is no identifiable underlying cause, or secondary to other neurological conditions, which includes structural lesions of the basal ganglia, exposure to drugs and toxins, and cerebral palsy. It was from the study mainly of secondary dystonia that it became clear that disruption of basal ganglia motor circuits produces dystonia. Primary dystonia is distinguished by the lack of other neurological involvement and the absence of distinct neuropathology. In some forms of dystonia, disturbed central dopaminergic pathways have been implicated in the production of dystonic movements. This seems to be of importance, especially in tardive dystonia and dopa-responsive dystonia. Dystonia was further simply categorized according to some clinical findings, such as age at onset, distribution of symptoms, or drug responsiveness (Fahn et al., 1998).

In recent years, advances in molecular genetic techniques have led to exciting discoveries that have expanded our knowledge of the pathogenesis of dystonia and resulted in revision of its classification. This classification incorporates the genetics and etiology of dystonia, and also the increasing number of distinguishable clinical phenotypes. Fahn and coworkers (1998) have proposed a new classification that contains the following subgroups: primary (dystonia only), dystonia-plus (e.g., dystonia with parkinsonism, and dystonia with myoclonic jerks), secondary (due to an environmental insult), and heredodegenerativity (with hereditary dystonia as the prominent clinical feature, secondary to neural degeneration). Within the primary dystonia and the dystonia-plus diseases, the more traditional classification of the dystonias is increasingly being replaced by the genetic one because various gene loci have been found to be associated with autosomal dominant, X-linked recessive, and autosomal recessive forms of dystonia. Currently, at least 12 different types of dystonia can be distinguished genetically, which are designated dystonias 1 through 12 (DYT1–DYT12) (Müller et al., 1998). The new classification of dystonic syndromes is summarized in Table 100–1.

Most types of hereditary dystonic syndromes tend to be associated with a relatively well-defined phenotype, although there is a substantial phenotypic overlap in individual cases. The traditional clinical classification by distribution of symptoms remains useful and is somewhat related to the genetic scheme (Table 100–2). In general, dystonia with onset in childhood or adolescence starts in the lower limbs, tends to generalize, and is often hereditary (DYT1 dystonia); various adult-onset forms of dystonia rarely involve the lower limbs, and they stay focal and frequently appear sporadic.

Table 100–1. Modern Classification of Dystonic Syndromes

Primary Dystonia
  Phenotype of dystonia alone; tremor may be present in individual cases; mostly hereditary; penetrance varies; autosomal dominant: DYT1, DYT4, DYT6, DYT7; autosomal recessive: DYT2

Dystonia-Plus Syndromes
  Phenotype of dystonia plus additional neurological features
  Paroxysmal dystonia: Autosomal dominant, DYT8, DYT9, DYT10
  Myoclonus-dystonia: Autosomal dominant, DYT11
  Dystonia-parkinsonism: Autosomal dominant, DYT5a, DYT12; autosomal recessive, DYT5b; X-linked recessive, DYT3

Secondary Dystonia Induced by Environmental Factors (e.g., drugs, toxins, stroke, perinatal asphyxia, encephalitis, tumor)
  Heredodegenerative diseases with dystonia: Present as dystonia-plus syndromes often associated with known enzyme defect or chemical marker (e.g., Wilson's disease, Hallervorden-Spatz disease, Parkinson's disease)

Table 100–2. Traditional Clinical Classification of Dystonia

By Age at Onset
Early Onset: Usually starts in a leg or an arm and frequently progresses to involve other limbs and the trunk.
Late Onset: Usually starts in the neck, cranial muscles, or arm and tends to remain localized, with restrictive spread to adjacent muscles.

By Distribution
Focal: Only one part of the body is affected (e.g., writer's cramp, blepharospasm, spasmodic dysphonia, cervical dystonia).
Segmental: Contiguous body regions are affected (e.g., the face and jaw in Meige's syndrome, cervical dystonia plus writer's cramp).
Multifocal: Noncontiguous body regions are affected (e.g., one arm and one leg, blepharospasm and writer's cramp).
Generalized: All parts of the body can be affected, especially the trunk and both legs.

Genetic and Clinical Aspects of Primary Dystonias

Most of the neurophysiological studies in dystonia have been performed in patients suffering from primary torsion dystonia, and so the main clinical aspects of these syndromes are summarized in the following. Primary dystonias, also known as idiopathic torsion dystonias, are the most common form of dystonia. The estimated prevalence of cases is 329 per million, of which focal dystonia accounted for 294 per million (Nutt et al., 1988). The range of severity is wide, and the number of affected muscle groups is large, including severe generalized dystonia, also called dystonia musculorum deformans; segmental and multifocal dystonia; and focal dystonia (cervical dystonia, blepharospasm, and writer's cramp). Dystonia in primary torsion dystonia can develop at almost any age, and this often determines the severity. Onset in childhood, particularly in a limb, is strongly predictive of subsequent generalization, and this form of dystonia is reported to be more prevalent in the Ashkenazi Jewish population. By contrast, dystonia arising in muscles of the cranium or upper limbs or in axial muscles tends to develop in adult life and remains focal or segmental in distribution.

The *DYT1* gene has been cloned and analyzed for mutations (Ozelius et al., 1997). A 3-basepair deletion in the coding sequence was found in all affected and obligate carriers with chromosome 9–linked primary dystonia. The mutation specifically causes early-onset generalized dystonia. The deletion results in the loss of a pair of glutamic acid residues near the carboxy terminus of a novel protein named torsin A. Torsin A contains an ATP-binding domain and a putative N-terminal leader sequence. For focal and segmental primary dystonia, the role of *DYT1* and the other genes is less clear. Like early-onset primary dystonia, late-onset, focal, or cervical-cranial primary dystonia also appears to be inherited in an autosomal dominant fashion (Waddy et al.,

1991; Defazio et al., 1993; Leube et al., 1996; Bressman et al., 1998). Most studies of late-onset focal dystonia showed that penetrance is even more greatly reduced compared with early-onset dystonia (12% versus 30%).

The dystonic movements in primary dystonias are sustained contractions that typically are twisting in nature and usually increase with action. Often phasic movements can be rapid, as in myoclonic disorders, and a repetitive recurring pattern may be rhythmical, thus giving rise to dystonic tremor. Dystonic activities and consecutive abnormal postures differ in different parts of the body.

In early-onset dystonia in children, abnormal posture and movements usually begin in the legs and arms. In the legs, action dystonia results in a peculiar twisting of the leg when the child walks forward; sometimes, walking backward, running, or dancing may still be normal. As the disorder progresses, dystonia not only may appear during action but also may be noted when the leg is at rest. The foot is plantar-flexed and turns inward, and the knee and hip often assume a flexed posture. In the arms, action dystonia tends to interfere with writing very early in the disease. The fingers curl, the wrist flexes and pronates, and the elbow elevates. The dystonic tremor of the arm includes features of both a postural and an action tremor. During walking, the arm often moves backward behind the body. Later, arm dystonia may be present even when the arm is at rest. As a single part of the body becomes more severely affected, the dystonia spreads beyond the initially involved limb to other limbs and axial muscles of the trunk and results in scoliosis, lordosis, tortipelvis, torticollis, retrocollis, antecollis, and laterocollis. Dystonia progresses from focal to segmental to generalized manifestation. In advanced disease, the contractions become constant, so that instead of moving, the affected part of the body remains in a fixed dystonic posture.

Adult-onset dystonia typically begins in the arms as writer's cramp, in the neck mostly as torticollis, in the face as blepharospasm, in the jaw muscles as oromandibular dystonia, in the tongue as lingual dystonia, or in laryngeal muscles as spasmodic dysphonia. With adult onset, the disease tends to remain limited as focal or segmental dystonia, it does not usually become generalized.

Blepharospasm is caused by tonic and/or myoclonic contractions of the orbicularis oculi muscles. It usually begins with increased blinking, followed by involuntary closure of the eyelids and then more firm and prolonged closure of the lids. Untreated blepharospasm in a severe form usually causes functional blindness. Blinking and lid closure can be intermittent, and often the dystonic activities are temporarily suppressed by talking, humming, or singing. It normally worsens during walking and with exposure to bright sunlight. The common sensory trick that relieves contractions is the placement of a finger just lateral to the orbit. Blepharospasm usually is accompanied by dystonic activities in lower facial muscles, such as the platysma and the mentalis muscle. When dystonia clearly spreads to a number of cranial and cervical muscles, the picture is called Meige's syndrome.

Writer's cramp of adult onset usually remains limited to one limb, usually the dominant side. However, in about 15% of cases, it spreads to the other arm. The abnormal posturing of the arm and the fingers during writing shows an individual reproducible pattern, and the interindividual variation of patterns is extreme. The abnormal posturing during writing can involve all joints of the arm but also can be limited to only one finger. Dystonia can be more pronounced in flexor muscles or extensor muscles, and the flexor-extensor pattern can vary between the joints and even individual finger positioning. Two forms of writer's cramp have been described: simple and dystonic. Simple writer's cramp is defined as the occurrence of dystonic features only during writing, while in dystonic writer's cramp dystonia appears with other tasks as well, for example, shaving, applying make up, using eating utensils, buttoning buttons, or playing a musical instrument. In about one third of cases of simple writer's cramp, over a period of months or years, a change of the manifestations into the picture of dystonic writer's cramp can be observed. Further extensions of the clinical picture to segmental or even generalized dystonia is also possible. Many patients find that they can write normally on a vertically amounted wall board despite the complete inability to write on a table. Such patients are able to activate the proximal shoulder muscles to write without any major problems. If they can relax the wrist and hand sufficiently, they may be able to train themselves to write using proximal shoulder movements. This style of writing with proximal muscles appears to employ a motor program different from the one employed for the usual writing with distal wrist and finger movements. Simple writer's cramp is a typical example of task-specific limb dystonia. This kind of dystonia, a subset of action dystonia, occurs exclusively or primarily when the patient is performing a specific task. The majority of task-specific dystonias involve the upper limb. It is noteworthy that these tasks, almost without exception, require either highly repetitive movements or extreme motor precision. Focal task-specific dystonia appears to be particularly frequent in professional musicians—the prevalence may be as high as 15% (Lockwood, 1989). It may well be that musicians execute extremely precise and complicated motor skills. Such condition has been reported in almost every kind of instrumentalist, but pianists and other keyboardists appear to be inordinately represented.

Cervical dystonia may develop in patients of all ages, but the peak age at onset falls within the 40- to 49-year range. The onset is usually insidious, although in some patients the onset has been described as sudden. The most prominent feature is sustained abnormal posture of the head and neck. The head may exhibit lateral rotation (torticollis spasmodicus), tilting (laterocollis), flexion (antecollis), or extension (retrocollis). The most frequent type of cervical dystonia is torticollis spasmodicus (48%), 19% show a combination of torticollis and laterocollis; antecollis or retrocollis can be observed in about 8% of patients (Kessler et al., 1999). The abnormal postures may fluctuate throughout the day, and they may be aggravated, usually by stress and anxiety. The symptoms may vary with posture, with some patients noting that the cervical dystonia is worse when they stand up and walk, while others find it most bothersome to sit and lie down. As in other focal dystonias, the symptoms of cervical dystonia disappear during sleep. In patients with a long-standing cervical dystonia, continuous contractions may develop and fixed deformities may be present. Sustained abnormal head-posturing may by associated with intermittent fast or slow movements. These movements may be jerky and irregular, or they may be regular and lead to head tremor. About 70% of patients show some improvement in their dystonia when they use a sensory trick. Typically, the patient has great difficulty in maintaining the head straight; however, if certain parts of the head, especially the chin, are touched, the head can be kept straight with much less effort. In some patients, the improvement with the use of a sensory trick can already be observed when they perform the reaching movement of the arm to the chin.

Spasmodic dystonia of the vocal cords occurs in two forms. In the more common type, the vocalis muscles contract, thereby bringing the vocal cords together and causing the voice to sound restricted, strangled, and coarse, with pauses often breaking up speech. The abductor type of spasmodic dystonia is caused by contractions of the posterior cricoarytenoids, so that the patient cannot talk in a loud voice and tends to run out of air while trying to speak. Spasmodic dysphonia, especially of the adductor type, is often associated with tremor of the vocal cords.

General Pathophysiology of Primary Dystonias

From the observations in patients suffering from symptomatic dystonia it can be concluded that dystonia is a disorder mainly of basal ganglia circuits. Most of the lesions responsible for symptomatic dystonia involve some of the basal ganglia or thalamus (Marsden et al., 1985; Pettigrew and Jankovic, 1985). In a meta-analysis of 240 patients with lesions affecting basal ganglia and causing movement disorders, 36% exhibited dystonia (Bhatia and Marsden, 1994). The putamen and globus pallidus were the most frequent sites affected in these patients. Dystonia was also observed in 30% of patients with movement disorders associated with lesions of the thalamus and subthalamic region (Lee and Marsden, 1994). Thalamic lesions producing dystonia involve the posterior and midline thalamic nuclei. Since no consistent anatomical pathology has been found in primary dystonia, it is reasonable to assume that functional abnormalities of the basal ganglia and thalamus without cell degeneration are responsible for the genesis of primary dystonia. Functional imaging studies lend support to the concept of abnormal neural activity in basal ganglia loops, as does the evidence provided by studies of levodopa-induced dystonia in human and subhuman primates with parkinsonism. Perlmutter and colleagues (1997) suggest that dystonia may occur following striatal dopamine deficiency. Baboons treated with intracarotid MPTP developed transient hemidystonia. This dystonia corresponded temporarily with a decreased striatal dopamine content and a transient decrease in D_2-like receptor number. Additional lines of evidence suggest that patients with primary dystonia have either decreased D_2-like receptor function or decreased D_2-like receptor binding. It is well known that acute blockade of D_2-like receptors with neuroleptics may produce acute dystonic reactions. Furthermore, it was found that patients with idiopathic focal dystonias, including dystonic hand cramp in clinical dystonia, have a mean 29% decrease in putaminal binding of [^{18}F]spiperone, a radioligand that binds predominantly to dopaminergic D_2-like and serotoninergic S_2 receptors (Perlmutter et al., 1997). A relative decrease in D_2-like inhibitory function would increase the activity of the inhibitory neurons projecting from putamen to external pallidum. On the basis of the well-known basal ganglia circuitry, this abnormality will eventually decrease the activity of excitatory neurons projecting from the thalamus to the cortex. If this projection under normal conditions predominantly activates intracortical interneurons, it can be hypothesized that a decreased surround inhibition results in the inability to depress unwanted overflow movements in other parts of the body. Clinically, this is typical of dystonia in which involuntary postures and muscle spasms frequently occur, especially during specific motor activity and not at rest. This phenomenon is commonly seen in writer's cramp, as the muscle spasms tend to spread from hand to wrist to arm as writing persists. This specific function of basal ganglia was first discussed by Mink and Thach (1993). It is, however, not clear why the proposed malfunction of the indirect pathway of the basal ganglia, important for the inhibition of excessive movements and which has been proposed to be due to a functional decrement in postsynaptic D_2-like receptor activity, can be normalized in dopa-responsive dystonia by levodopa, but not in the other forms of primary dystonia. Berardelli and associates (1998) proposed another abnormality of the basal ganglia circuitry in dystonia. They assumed an overactivity of the direct putaminopallidal pathway that leads to an increased thalamic input to cortex that could project mainly to motor output cells of the primary motor cortex. The authors, however, gave no clear explanation of why the direct pathway should be overactive in dystonia. The concept of disturbed

intracortical surround inhibition first discussed by Mink and Thach (1993) was recently supported by findings obtained by Ridding and colleagues (1995). One method of examining intracortical inhibition is by giving paired magnetic shocks delivered at varying interstimulus intervals in a conditioning-test design (Kujirai et al., 1993). Ridding and associates (1995) found that there was less initial inhibition (conditioning-test interval shorter than 6 ms) in patients with focal, task-specific primary dystonia when tested at rest. It was proposed that under normal circumstances one role of the inhibition was to focus the motor command within the motor cortex so that the correct muscles can be activated. Experiments in monkeys have shown that application of the GABA antagonist bicuculline to the motor cortex increased the contraction of antagonist muscles in a simple wrist-movement task (Matsumura et al., 1991). Although a hyperactivity of the direct putaminopallidal pathway was first favored as the mechanism (Berardelli et al., 1998), a later study confirmed the role of an abnormal intracortical inhibitory mechanism and showed that this inhibitory action can be renormalized by intramuscular botulinum toxin injections in patients with generalized dystonia, segmental dystonia, and focal dystonia (Gilio et al., 2000). Renormalization of intracortical inhibitory action was paralleled by clinical improvement in these patients.

When it is accepted that abnormal neuronal activity within the basal ganglia circuitry is the cause of the generation of abnormal dystonic muscle tone and dystonic movements, the question arises as to how this abnormal signaling is induced. In dystonia-plus syndromes with nerve cell and fiber degeneration and in secondary dystonias, it can be suggested that an imbalance of excitatory and inhibitory activities occurs. What, however, is the mechanism behind the rise of abnormal activity in primary dystonia? One possible explanation is that the various genetic abnormalities with consecutive abnormal protein formation change the excitability of neurons in the sense of subcortical epileptoid disturbances. Another hypothesis is that by a change in synaptic connectivity within the basal ganglia an abnormal central processing of proprioceptive information from muscle spindles and also of other peripheral afferent systems results. Indeed, there have been reports of abnormal somatosensory responses to vibratory stimuli in focal dystonia (Tempel and Perlmutter, 1990); vibratory stimuli preferentially stimulate muscle spindle afferents. Vibratory stimuli also induce dystonic symptoms in subjects with writer's cramp (Kaji et al., 1995), whereas intramuscular injection of lidocaine, which blocks γ-motoneurons and also afferent activity, may temporarily relieve symptoms. Furthermore, it was demonstrated by Grünewald and colleagues (1997) that there is abnormal perception of motion, but not of position, in dystonic subjects. Dystonic subjects showed bilateral abnormalities of perception of the tonic vibration reflex. It is also of interest that injection of botulinum toxin often achieves extremely good responses, especially in patients with writer's cramp, although the muscles injected show only slight paresis. It could be argued that it is the paresis of the intrafusal muscles of the muscle spindles that is followed by a decrease in type Ia afferent activity—and not the paresis of the extrafusal muscle fibers—that induces clinical improvement. All this information supports the view that dystonia is a sensory or sensorimotor disorder, rather than a pure motor disorder. The role of abnormal processing of sensory information, however, may not be dominant for all types of primary dystonias. Facial muscles do not have any muscle spindles; nevertheless, in blepharospasm and in Meige's disease, dystonia occurs in these muscles.

From a pathophysiological point of view also, task-specific dystonia is of major interest. In these patients (e.g., those with writer's cramp), who belong to a family with genetically determined dystonia, it can be suggested that overactivity or overtraining may be just an additional trigger mechanism that makes a subclinical abnormality within the basal ganglia circuitry symptomatic. In single separate cases, however, either there may be a low prevalence of the disease, or overuse of a certain muscle group in a specific task alone is able to induce abnormal synaptic connectivity in the basal ganglia and/or the sensorimotor cortex. Experiments performed by Merzenich and colleagues (Byl et al., 1996, 1997) favor the latter explanation. Monkeys were trained to perform hundreds of hand movements per day and developed motor coordination disorders in the hand with posturing reminiscent of dystonia.

In summary, dystonia seems to be induced either by an inherited abnormal synaptic connectivity or synaptic excitability due to abnormalities of specific proteins, which have a certain role in interacting with neurons in the basal ganglia, or by an acquired abnormality induced by overuse of a specific motor act (Fig. 100–1). Thus, various pathophysiological mechanisms can be combined in patients with a task-specific dystonia who belong to a genetically affected family. The pathophysiological mechanisms in neurodegenerative diseases with dystonia-plus syndromes and in symptomatic dystonia may be more simple and may arise from an imbalance of excitatory and inhibitory neural activities within the basal ganglia circuitry. Abnormal processing of sensory information from muscle spindles and other receptor systems obviously is not a prerequisite

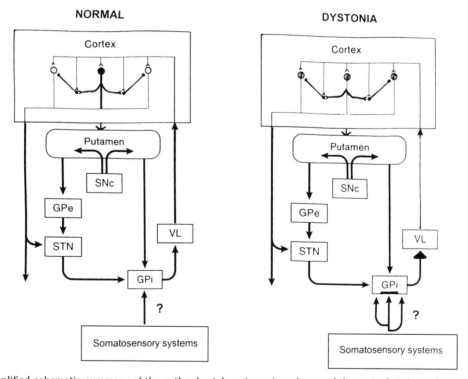

Figure 100–1. Simplified schematic summary of the pathophysiology in various forms of dystonia. It is hypothesized that a decreased activity of the thalamocortical pathway projecting to motor cortex output cells and cortical inhibitory interneurons is the final outcome of various dysfunctions within the basal ganglia circuitry in dystonia. A decrease in cortical output cells would lead to bradykinesia, and a decrease in local inhibitory activity leads to deficient surround inhibition, with an inability to depress unwanted overflow movements. Underactivity of thalamocortical projections may be caused by hyperactive inhibitory GPi, induced by an imbalance of excitatory and inhibitory activities within the circuitry (secondary dystonias), by exaggerated activation of GPi induced by somatosensory influences (plastic changes induced by overuse; task-specific dystonia), or by an enhanced excitability of GPi neurons due to a hereditary metabolic disturbance. So far, it is not clear via which pathways the somatosensory systems influence the basal ganglia loop in detail. GPi, medial globus pallidus; GPe, lateral globus pallidus; STN, subthalamic nucleus; VL, ventrolateral thalamic nucleus; SNc, substantia nigra pars compacta.

for the development of dystonia but may induce dystonia in some task-specific focal forms.

The primary abnormality within the basal ganglia circuitry induces changes in secondary neuronal activity within motor cortices, brainstem reflex pathways, and spinal cord reflex activities. It is not clear whether these changes play an important role in the development of dystonia or whether they represent epiphenomena that are not directly linked to dystonia itself. Researchers found a decrease in the amplitude of the movement-related cortical potential with a deficiency in the NS′ component (Deuschl et al., 1995) and an overactive striatum and premotor and rostral supplementary motor area, but depressed activity in the caudal supplementary motor area and bilateral sensorimotor cortex on positron emission tomography activation studies (Ceballos-Baumann et al., 1997). Eidelberg and associates (1995) described relative bilateral increases in activity in lateral, frontal, and paracentral cortices, associated with relative covariate hypermetabolism of the contralateral lentiform nucleus, pons, and midbrain. In dystonia, in contrast with Parkinson's disease, lentiform metabolism and thalamic metabolism were dissociated, suggesting excess activity of the direct putaminopallidal pathway. In another study by Eidelberg and coworkers (1998), it was demonstrated that DYT1 dystonia is mediated by the expression of two independent regional metabolic covariance patterns. With [18F]fluorodeoxyglucose positron emission tomography, it could be shown that an abnormal pattern—even when the patients were at rest—could be characterized by increased metabolic activity in the lentiform nuclei, cerebellum, and supplementary motor areas. This abnormal metabolic pattern was present in DYT1 carriers with and without clinical manifestations. The findings indicated that the penetrance of the *DYT1* gene is considerably greater than was previously assumed.

Studies with brain stimulation (Mavroudakis et al., 1995; Ridding et al., 1995; Ikoma et al., 1996; Byrnes et al., 1998; Currà et al., 2000) suggest that although the resting level of corticospinal excitability is normal, there is an increase in the gain of the input-output relationship of the motor cortex and accompanying change in the excitability of local cortical inhibitory systems.

In addition to the changes in cortical activities, many reflex abnormalities have also been described in dystonia. Reflex abnormalities can be observed in affected and nonaffected muscles, although they are greatest in the affected muscles. Common tendon jerks, as tested in routine clinical examination, are normal in primary dystonia. Recovery of the H reflex at intervals of 200 ms is increased in patients with spasmodic torticollis or generalized dystonia (Panizza et al., 1990). A long-latency reflex (LLR2 reflex) in the thenar muscles is reduced in amplitude in patients with writer's cramp (Naumann and Reiners, 1997). In the light of abnormal co-contraction of agonists and antagonists in dystonia, it was suggested that there is an abnormal reciprocal spinal inhibition. Indeed, Panizza and associates (1989) and Chen and colleagues (1995) observed abnormalities of reciprocal inhibition more pronounced in patients with dystonic than in those with simple writer's cramp. Although abnormal reciprocal inhibition could foster understanding of the abnormal co-contractions seen in dystonia, the findings that similar changes can also been seen in the unaffected normal arms of patients with writer's cramp and in the unaffected arms of patients with spasmodic torticollis put in question a primary pathophysiological role of abnormal reciprocal inhibition (Deuschl et al., 1992; Chen et al., 1995).

Practical Neurophysiology in the Assessment of Dystonia

Careful clinical examination is certainly sufficient for the recognition of dystonia in a patient. Measurements of cortical activity by means of transcranial magnetic stimulation or by obtaining sensory evoked potentials or the various event-related potentials are not helpful in detecting dystonia. The field of cortical neurophysiology requires that practitioners have a better understanding of the pathophysiology of this area. The same holds true for measurements of brainstem reflexes, testing of spinal reflexes, and measurements of inhibitory phenomena in the motor cortex, the brainstem, and the spinal cord. However, after the introduction of botulinum toxin as a first-line treatment, especially in cases of focal dystonia, polyelectromyographic recordings are of extreme value. By means of concentric needle recordings, it is possible to better identify and localize the dystonic muscles that have to be injected, and in cervical dystonia the sternocleidomastoid muscle can easily be identified. When neck muscles are evaluated, exact positioning of the injection is markedly improved with the use of electromyographic recordings. Also, in patients with the opening-type of oromandibular dystonia especially, injections into the pterygoid muscles should be performed under electromyographic guidance. Beyond the problem of the correct positioning of the injecting needle, in some forms of focal dystonia the muscles involved cannot be sufficiently identified just by inspection of the patient with abnormal posturing of the head, the jaw, or the arm muscles in writer's cramp. In these clinical situations, polyelectromyographic recordings have to differentiate the muscles with dystonia from those that are not affected and those that are tonically active for compensation of abnormal posturing (Fig. 100–2) (Dressler, 2000a). Dystonic muscle activities are characterized by fluctuating tonic activity that is superimposed by phasic jerky or tremulous activities, by abnormal crescendo-like activities in writer's cramp, and also by cessation of the geste antagonistique in cervical dystonia.

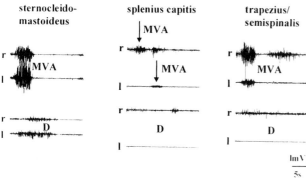

Figure 100–2. Abnormal electromyographic patterns in cervical dystonia. The patient has torticollis spasmodicus to the right. The upper rows of each panel show surface electromyograms at maximal voluntary isometric activation (MVA) of the right sternocleidomastoid muscle (*left panel*) of, first, the right and, then, the left splenius capitis muscles (*middle panel*) and the right trapezius-semispinalis complex (*right panel*). Note abnormal involuntary cocontraction of the left sternocleidomastoideus and the left trapezius-semispinalis complex. The lower rows of each panel show spontaneous dystonic (D) muscle activities. (From Dressler D, Rothwell JC: Electromyographic quantification of the paralysing effect of botulinum toxin in the sternocleidomastoid muscle. Eur Neurol 2000;43:13–16.)

SPASTICITY

With lesions of the corticofugal system (Thilmann et al., 1993) at various levels, a multitude of motor phenomena and deficits are induced. One phenomenon that is easily clinically recognized is increased velocity-dependent resistance on passive limb movements, or spastic muscle tone. In contrast with dystonia, and still markedly different from rigidity, spastic muscle tone virtually always occurs with other abnormalities. Among these are "negative signs," including weakness, increased fatigability, loss of dexterity and coordination, and loss of cutaneous (abdominal) reflexes, and "positive signs," such as increased tendon jerks, clonus, and release of cutaneomotor reflexes, such as the plantar response (Babinski's sign), spasms, and the clasp-knife phenomenon, which designates an initial increase of resistance to passive movement followed by a sudden loss of resistance. Other phenomena, such as dystonia, postural abnormalities, and pain, may be associated with, or may represent secondary consequences of, the aforementioned clinical signs and symptoms (Table 100–3). Much of the confusion surrounding the term *spasticity* arises from the fact that it sometimes refers to spastic muscle tone alone, and sometimes to various motor syndromes that, in turn, are not unequivocally defined themselves.

A popular definition by Lance (1980) defines *spasticity* as "a motor disorder characterized by a velocity-dependent increase in tonic stretch reflexes resulting from hyperexcitability of the stretch reflex as one component of the upper motoneurone syndrome." Although this definition is popular, one can argue that it adds to the confusion because it does not delineate the borders between the (syndromic)

Table 100–3. Symptoms and Signs Associated with Spasticity

Increased resistance of a limb to passive movements (spastic muscle tone)
Weakness, increased fatigability, loss of dexterity and coordination, slowness
Increased tendon jerks, spread of tendon reflex to neighboring muscles, clonus
Release of cutaneomotor reflexes (extending big toe [Babinski's sign]; ankle, knee, and hip flexion; contraction of abdominals)
Flexor and extensor spasms
Loss of cutaneous (abdominal) reflexes
Clasp-knife phenomenon
Dystonia, postural abnormalities
Autonomic hyperreflexia

spastic motor disorder, the details of which are not included in the definition, and a larger motor syndrome. A second problem results from the fact that this definition combines clinical phenomenology and pathophysiological concepts ("hyperexcitability of the stretch reflex," "upper motoneurone syndrome"), rendering it dependent on the truth of the latter. Indeed, as will be seen later, there is considerable evidence that hyperexcitability of the tonic stretch reflex may not be the single factor leading to enhanced muscle tone, and that the many symptoms and signs of spasticity do not reflect a lesion primarily of the corticospinal motoneurons.

To avoid confusion, we shall use the term *spastic muscle tone* to refer to the clinical phenomenon of a velocity-dependent increase in resistance on passive stretching. Thus, we specifically eliminate all pathophysiological connotations with this observation. *Spasticity* is widely used in neurology—thus, we do not propose to abandon this term; rather, we suggest its use in a statistical sense. Spasticity may then designate the motor syndrome frequently associated with the clinical phenomenon of spastic muscle tone. Restricting the basis of the definition to a statistical association would avoid making inferences about a possible causal relationship between a symptom and any underlying physiological mechanism. In particular, this usage of the term *spasticity* does not imply causality of a symptom and hyperexcitability of the tonic stretch reflex. The threshold of a statistical association should be low enough to include spasms and dystonia in the meaning of *spasticity*.

Characteristics and Differential Diagnosis of Spastic Muscle Tone

As shown in Table 100–4, virtually any pathology of the central nervous system can be associated with spastic muscle tone. Therefore, spastic muscle tone is a sign frequently encountered in neurological patients.

In most patients, detection of spastic muscle tone is relatively easy clinically. However, spastic muscle

---

Table 100–4. Neurological Disorders Leading to Spasticity

Cerebral birth trauma, including asphyxia
Traumatic brain injury
Stroke
Spinal cord injury
Neurodegenerative diseases (e.g., amyotrophic lateral
  sclerosis, primary lateral sclerosis, spastic paraparesis)
Demyelinating disorders (e.g., multiple sclerosis)

Table 100–6. Some Factors Influencing the Results of Pathophysiological Studies of Spasticity

Location of lesion (cortical, subcortical, bulbar, spinal)
Age of lesion (acute, subacute, chronic)
Extremity (upper, lower)
Principal direction of action (antigravity, collinear with gravity)
Motor task (e.g., rest; isometric, isotonic contraction; postural
  activity, precision movements, complex movements)

---

tone may be so severe that it may be difficult to perform passive movements on the patient. In these cases, it may be difficult to distinguish between spastic muscle tone and fixed contractures or severe dystonia (Table 100–5). In rare cases, it may be difficult to differentiate spastic muscle tone from the stiffness found in the stiff-person syndrome.

Additional difficulty arises because spastic muscle tone and dystonia may be present simultaneously in the same limb. Spastic muscle tone can be found more readily in certain muscle groups (adductors and flexors in the upper limb; adductors and extensors in the lower limb). Several scores are available for clinically grading spastic muscle tone. Of these, the Ashworth scale (Ashworth, 1964) is the most widely used despite several shortcomings.

General Pathophysiology of Spasticity

Although numerous studies have been devoted over the past century to the elucidation of the pathophysiology of spasticity, very few principles have emerged that could safely be regarded as generalizable. This is probably partially due to the considerable heterogeneity (both within a study and between studies) of the patient populations, whose pathology involves a large variety of lesions at different levels of the neuraxis and at different stages in the course of disease (Table 100–6). In addition, the scarcity of generalizable principles probably reflects the complexity of human motor control, which has yet to be matched by an adequate complexity of physiological and pathophysiological models.

In a completely relaxed subject, a joint will resist movement as the result of three physical processes: (1) inertia of the limb, producing reaction forces proportional to acceleration; (2) viscoelastic proper-

---

Table 100–5. Clinical Differential Diagnosis of Spastic Muscle Tone

Spastic muscle tone
Rigidity
Dystonia
Contractures
Stiff-person syndrome and related
  disorders

---

ties of the muscle and joint that oppose movement in a complex way, as a function of both muscle length and rate of change; and (3) reflex activity, if any is evoked. The combination of these components produces the total stiffness that is perceived as muscle tone externally (Pisano et al., 1996).

Most clinical neurophysiologists would agree that the velocity-dependent increase of resistance toward passive movement is, at least to a substantial extent, the result of a pathologically enhanced stretch reflex. This concept is supported by early findings demonstrating that spastic muscle tone in the gastrocnemius muscle is abolished by pharmacological blockade of the tibial nerve (Herman et al., 1974). It is important to realize that the term *stretch reflex* refers to any kind of mechanical muscle stretch and involves complex physiological phenomena. Responses to passive muscle stretch may be differentiated kinematically in phasic, dynamic, and tonic responses (Nichols and Houk, 1976). These phases roughly correspond to early (phasic) and late (dynamic and tonic) electromyographic activity recordable from the stretched muscle. Healthy subjects have hardly any appreciable muscle tone, reflecting the fact that under normal circumstances the angular velocity of passive movements is below the velocity-threshold of the stretch reflex. Spastic muscle tone, as judged clinically, corresponds to an increase of the late (i.e., dynamic and tonic) phase of the stretch reflex. There is reason to believe that the tonic stretch reflex is elicited more readily in patients with spastic muscle tone because the gain of the stretch reflex is increased. However, some authors have found that the threshold of the stretch reflex is decreased, with the gain remaining unchanged (Powers et al., 1988).

It is important to briefly consider the complex nature of neuronal circuits subserving the responses to muscle stretch (Fig. 100–3). Primary afferent type Ia fibers surrounding intrafusal fibers of the muscle spindle are excited when a muscle is stretched. The type Ia fiber makes a monosynaptic excitatory connection with α-motoneurons of its muscle of origin, and it similarly connects with α-motoneurons of synergistic muscles. This monosynaptic circuit is believed to be the dominant basis of the Hoffmann (H) reflex. The type Ia fiber also monosynaptically connects with an inhibitory interneuron ("Ia inhibitory interneuron") that projects directly to the α-motoneurons of antagonist muscles ("reciprocal inhibition"). The α-motoneuron sends recurrent col-

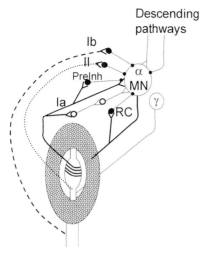

Descending
pathways

Figure 100–3. Schematic diagram summarizing the spinal pathways that control the excitability of the stretch reflex arc. Excitatory and inhibitory synapses are represented by Y-shaped bars and small black circles, respectively. Excitatory and inhibitory interneurons are represented by open and large black circles, respectively. Projections of descending tracts onto interneurons are not represented. α-MN, α-motoneuron; γ, γ-motoneuron; RC, Renshaw cell; PreInh, presynaptic inhibition; Ia, Ib, group II muscle afferents. (From Pierrot-Deseilligny E: Electrophysiological assessment of the spinal mechanisms underlying spasticity. In Rossini PN, Maugiere F [eds]: New Trends and Advanced Techniques in Clinical Neurophysiology [EEG Suppl 41]. Amsterdam, Elsevier Science Publishers, 1990.)

laterals back, targeting an inhibitory interneuron that inhibits the α-motoneuron—the "Renshaw inhibitory interneuron." Importantly, in addition to inhibiting the α-motoneuron that sends out the recurrent collateral, the Renshaw cell also inhibits the type Ia inhibitory interneuron targeting antagonistic muscles. Therefore, increased activity of the Renshaw cell may decrease reciprocal inhibition. In addition to the type Ia reflex pathway, signals from receptors located in tendon organs are transmitted to the spinal cord via type Ib afferents, where they disynaptically or oligosynaptically produce inhibition of the α-motoneuron. Furthermore, group II afferents from muscle spindle secondary endings also target interneurons inhibiting the α-motoneuron. Finally, afferents from cutaneous receptors and deep connective tissue are thought to constitute an important, if not exclusive, part of the afferent reflex arc involved in the late electromyographic responses following the mechanical perturbation necessary for stretching a muscle (Corden et al., 2000).

All spinal interneurons involved in these pathways are heavily controlled by descending pathways. In addition, at least the type Ia afferent volley is gated by powerful presynaptic inhibition of type Ia terminals. Given this spinal organization, in theory, hyperexcitability of the stretch reflex can result from hyperexcitability of the α-motoneurons (primary or secondary), hyperactivity of type Ia afferents, or insufficient inhibition at any of the aforementioned inhibitory interneurons. Most of the spinal pathways previously outlined have been studied in patients

with spastic muscle tone with the use of a variety of neurophysiological stimulation techniques. Indirect neurophysiological evidence of α-motoneuron hyperactivity came from findings demonstrating an increase in F-wave amplitudes and a greater persistence of F waves in patients with spastic muscle tone. An increased ratio of the maximal H-reflex amplitude to the maximal M-response amplitude (Hmax/Mmax) may indicate that the number of motoneurons that can be activated monosynaptically by electrical stimulation of type Ia afferents is increased. However, because this technique cannot distinguish between membrane properties and modification of synaptic input, definite evidence of α-motoneuron hyperexcitability is still lacking. No evidence has been found for increased type Ia afferent activity in patients with spastic muscle tone. Abnormalities of presynaptic inhibition of type Ia fibers, of reciprocal type Ia inhibition, of type Ib inhibition, and (under some circumstances, in some patients) of recurrent inhibition all have been demonstrated in patients with spastic muscle tone. Various combinations of abnormalities were found in individual patients with a variety of lesions. Correlation between the degrees of abnormality measured by different interneuron tests was found to be generally poor, to the extent that one test result could be normal while another was grossly abnormal in the same patient. Thus, no specific patterns of abnormalities have emerged that could be used to distinguish classes of pathophysiological mechanisms. Furthermore, as a rule, none of the abnormalities correlated well with the severity of spastic muscle tone as assessed clinically. One possible explanation of this lack of correlation is that virtually all studies investigating the aforementioned abnormalities of interneuronal function involved in stretch reflex control employ the H reflex, which engages type Ia afferent fibers almost exclusively. Since muscle stretch activate other fibers in addition to type Ia afferents, studies relying on modulation of the H reflex can provide only an incomplete measure of the hyperexcitability of the tonic stretch reflex.

Considering the fact that the neuronal circuits underlying the stretch reflex are heavily controlled by descending commands and that the stretch reflex, at least in the active muscle, may have late components that take a transcortical route, it seems surprising that very few studies have examined the relationship between neurophysiological variables of the primary motor cortex, as assessable by transcranial magnetic stimulation (TMS), and spastic muscle tone. As a rule, these studies have not revealed significant correlations of spastic muscle tone and the degree of corticospinal tract involvement, indicating that spastic muscle tone requires lesions outside the portion of the corticospinal tract that originates in the primary motor cortex. Benecke (1993) did not find a relationship between the TMS-evoked silent period and intracortical inhibition and spasticity.

An important conceptual advance with respect

to both pathophysiological and clinical issues of spasticity came through a series of papers originating to a large extent from the laboratory of Dietz. This group showed that enhancement of muscle tone in spastic patients may be caused by peripheral factors (i.e., muscular) in addition to neuronal factors. According to the results of Dietz and Berger (1983), these rheological changes in spastic muscles occur in a continuum ranging from slightly increased viscoelasticity to contractures and fibrosis. Consistent with these findings, marked morphological transformation of spastic muscle fibers have been found.

Whereas the contribution of mechanical factors to spastic muscle tone is generally accepted, there is disagreement about the relative proportions of non-neuronal and neuronal factors. One explanation for highly divergent results seems to be that the relative contribution of spastic muscle tone may vary according to the body region, with relatively more mechanical contributions in the lower limbs. Furthermore, it is recognized that the weight of the two factors contributing to spastic muscle tone changes dynamically during the first months following a lesion of the central nervous system. Whereas hyperexcitability of the tonic stretch reflex due to a variety of mechanisms may prevail during the first weeks, the changes in the mechanical properties of the muscle fibers may dominate during later stages.

Tapping on a tendon with sufficient strength is one way of stretching a muscle. If there is increased excitability of the stretch reflex, tendon reflexes will be exaggerated. However, contrary to common belief, both clinical and experimental neurophysiological studies suggest that spastic muscle tone and enhanced tendon reflexes, albeit related, are distinct from each other. For example, the two phenomena reach their respective maxima at different time periods following an ischemic brain lesion (Fellows et al., 1993b). Evidence that exaggerated tendon jerks are physiologically distinct from muscle tone also comes from observations in monkeys, in which lesions of the ventral funiculus lead to hyperreflexia in the setting of normal tone. Furthermore, in human newborns, hyperreflexia is present, while muscle tone is flaccid. At least two explanations may account for the divergent behavior of tendon reflexes and muscle tone: First, a variety of mechanoreceptive afferent fibers are involved in the stretch reflex and may be activated to a different degree by different ways of mechanical stretch. The tendon reflex engages mainly type Ia afferent fibers, whereas passive movements also activate type Ib and cutaneous afferents in addition to type Ia afferents. In addition, passive movements may engage type Ia afferents less synchronously. Second, if spastic muscle tone is significantly influenced by non-neuronal factors, as suggested by the work of Dietz and Berger (1983), muscle tone may be abnormal while tendon reflexes are normal.

Spasms may occur in spasticity as a response to cutaneous (non-noxious or noxious) stimuli or may even occur spontaneously. Physiologically, they probably correspond to released cutaneomotor reflexes (also known as flexor and extensor reflexes). In animals, short-latency excitatory pathways from cutaneous afferent fibers to hindlimb flexor motor neurons have been shown to be under inhibitory suprasegmental control by the central locomotor pattern generator and by fibers from the red nucleus and pyramidal tract. Pathological release of cutaneomotor reflexes in spasticity has been attributed to an abnormal facilitation of homologous polysynaptic pathways from type Ia afferents, as well as group II, III, and IV afferents to motoneurons. Hyperactive nociceptive reflexes have also been attributed to excessive activation of propriospinal neurons.

The clasp-knife phenomenon—a sudden decrease of resistance during sustained stretch—has been linked to the activity of high-threshold stretch-sensitive mechanoreceptor afferents that probably belong to group III and group II afferent fibers (Cleland et al., 1990).

Pathoanatomy of Spasticity

Traditionally, spasticity is ascribed to lesions in the pyramidal tract. In a strict anatomical sense, the pyramidal tract is defined as the fibers passing through the pyramids at the medulla. However, when referring to pyramidal tract lesions, most clinicians implicate lesions of the part of the corticospinal pathway arising from the primary motor cortex located in the precentral gyrus (Brodmann's area 4) that synapse directly onto α-motoneurons in the spinal cord. Both animal studies and observations in patients who had suffered lesions of the medullary pyramid, either related to disease or through surgery, suggest that isolated lesions of the corticospinal tract at the level of the pyramids, or of the part of the corticospinal tract arising from the primary motor cortex, do not produce spastic muscle tone. Rather, these lesions lead to weakness and the loss of superficial reflexes, such as the abdominal reflexes, with muscle tone being decreased. Spastic muscle tone, then, must be due to the involvement of motor tracts originating from regions other than the primary motor cortex or at least must be different from the part of the corticospinal tract that arises from the primary motor cortex. Although still somewhat debated, there is now considerable evidence to suggest that these tracts target neurons in the bulbar reticular formation (Brown, 1994). This corticobulbar system, in turn, has been shown to be heavily modulated by the premotor cortex, paramedian cerebellar cortex, and fastigial nucleus. Inhibitory influences from the bulbar reticular formation are conducted in the spinal cord by the dorsal reticulospinal tract in the dorsal half of the lateral funiculus, in close relationship with the lateral corticospinal tract. The dorsal reticulospinal tract transmits inhibitory signals to spinal stretch reflexes as well as flexor reflex afferents. Thus, in addition to enhanced stretch reflexes, flexor reflexes are released with damage to this system.

The role of other descending fiber tracts is less clear and is probably of lesser importance. The vestibulospinal tract has a weak and relatively unimportant role in maintaining spasticity. In contrast, the medial reticulospinal tract (which runs in the sulcomarginal territory, along with the median longitudinal bundles) has a pronounced role in *maintaining* spasticity. Thus, surgical creation of lesions of the medial reticulospinal tract may alleviate some symptoms of spasticity.

If lesions affect all major components of the descending pathways that modulate the spinal reflex circuitries, a disturbance of the delicate balance between inhibitory and excitatory influences ensues. As previously described in more detail, the net effect of this disturbance can be viewed as a shift of spinal motor neuron excitability toward a lowered firing threshold—in response either to the remaining descending facilitatory influences or to excitation as part of spinal reflex activity.

Pathophysiology of Motor Disability in Spasticity

An obvious "candidate" mechanism underlying weakness, as one of the principal "negative" signs of spasticity, is deficient motoneuronal activation, resulting from diminished corticomotoneuronal drive, occurring as a consequence of interruption of the corticomotoneuronal fiber tracts. In theory, any pathology that results in a resisting force subtracting from the force exerted by the movement agonist, and thus opposing movements in the desired direction, could also contribute to weakness, slowness, and loss of dexterity.

When increased muscle tone is so severe as to be present at rest in the absence of passive movements, its functional consequences can readily be recognized. It may, however, be impossible to decide whether continuous muscle activity in a bed-ridden or wheelchair-bound patient represents the upper extreme of the spectrum of spastic muscle tone or, alternatively, continuous spontaneous spasms. Severely enhanced muscle tone, typically present in certain muscle groups, may lead to pain, secondary contractures, and difficulties in maintaining hygiene.

Important questions that continue to elude many clinical neurologists is whether moderately enhanced muscle tone is related to impairment of motor function in patients, and, if so, to what extent. Increased muscle tone, if also present during active movements, may well represent a resisting force that subtracts from the agonist force. Spastic muscle tone, by definition, is assessed at rest; thus, it must first be established that pathophysiological mechanisms shown to be present at rest are also operative with active movements.

As outlined previously, spastic muscle tone has two components: enhanced stretch reflex activity and altered viscoelastic properties. The question of whether enhanced stretch reflex activity, as seen in the absence of voluntary activation, is present during movement is far from being evident a priori. Indeed, one observation suggests that the level of at least the *phasic* stretch reflex activity at rest is not necessarily related to motor performance: In healthy control subjects, motor performance is not influenced by the level of tendon reflex activity, used as a marker of the phasic stretch reflex. However, this finding may be different in patients with lesions of the central nervous system, and premature and exaggerated activation of the movement antagonist by an exaggerated phasic or tonic stretch reflex theoretically may well contribute to motor disability.

Spinal reflex circuitries have been tested by applying a torque during voluntary activation. Ibrahim and co-workers found no evidence of enhanced reflexive electromyographic activity during voluntary activation of upper limb muscles that exhibited spastic muscle tone (Ibrahim et al., 1993). Patients were asked to maintain a steady elbow position while challenged by a sinusoidal torque about the elbow joint. When arm flexors were externally stretched during this procedure, reflexive electromyographic activity was found to be *decreased* compared with normal subjects. Similarly, the same investigators found decreased, instead of increased, reflexive electromyographic activity in the triceps surae when patients with spastic paraparesis were tested in a treadmill-walking task (Dietz and Berger, 1983). Thus, in some patients, there seems to be little evidence of enhanced stretch reflex activity contributing to the motor deficit in spasticity.

How about the second component of spastic muscle tone, increased viscoelasticity? The fact that the passive viscoelastic properties of muscle fibers may vary with the state of contraction makes this question, too, relevant. The mechanical resistance to a sudden torque was found to be *decreased* in voluntarily activated spastic muscles (Ibrahim et al., 1993). This decrease in mechanical resistance in the active state was entirely due to a massive reduction in reflexive electromyographic activity, since the ratio of electromyographic activity to torque was found to be increased even in active muscles of patients with spasticity (Ibrahim et al., 1993). This finding probably indicates that increased viscoelasticity may not be particularly relevant to the motor deficit, at least in circumstances in which reflexive electromyographic activity is elicited.

There are conflicting reports about the observations noted regarding whether reflexive electromyographic activity occurs *spontaneously* in voluntary movements of patients in whom spastic muscle tone is present (see the review by Fellows et al., 1993a). Some studies have provided evidence of an abnormal spontaneous reflex activity in the movement antagonist during upper limb movements; however, this finding has not been corroborated in the majority of studies that have looked at angular velocities within the range of normal movements.

Although there is still no definite answer to the question of how much spastic muscle tone contributes to the motor disability in spasticity, expert opinion holds that the contribution of exaggerated stretch reflex activity to disability with active movements is probably minor. However, it is important to realize that even minimal torques, such as those induced by minimal reflexive muscle activity, may have a significant impact on the successful completion of movements (Popescu and Rymer, 2000).

Muscle activation in spasticity may be disturbed independently from exaggerated reflex activity. Conceivably, motor disability in spasticity may be the result of inappropriately timed activation of agonists and antagonists. Is there evidence of a disturbed "pattern" of muscle activation? The "pattern" of muscle activation has been studied in natural complex motor tasks, such as bicycling at different speeds and loads, and walking at different speeds. In bicycling, the rectus femoris muscle is normally recruited in an alternating fashion on both sides at distinct pedal positions (Benecke, 1987). In patients with spasticity of the lower limbs, the rectus femoris muscles were found to be recruited prematurely, while relaxation developed later (Benecke, 1987). Thus, the total time of muscle activation was prolonged, but the magnitude of peak activation during the "window" of normal muscle activation was reduced. More recently, Beer and co-workers have provided evidence of a disturbed internal model of limb dynamics as an important factor contributing to poor motor performance in spastic hemiparesis (Beer et al., 2000).

Practical Clinical Neurophysiology

Spastic muscle tone and other "positive" signs of spasticity are amenable to pharmacological, physiotherapeutic, and surgical treatment. As outlined previously, there is little evidence that "positive" signs of spasticity contribute substantially to motor disability. Clinical evidence exists that spastic muscle tone may occasionally even be useful to the patient. Therefore, despite the seductive appeal provided by relatively powerful treatment options, it must be ascertained that spastic muscle tone does in fact interfere with function before specific treatment can be initiated. Although a variety of clinical neurophysiological methods are available that may potentially be useful in addressing relevant questions related to spasticity (Table 100–7), the majority of tests available focus merely on quantifying, objectively, the clinical diagnosis of spastic muscle tone. Another problem (not uncommon in clinical neurophysiology) is that hardly any single test, or battery of tests, has been formally evaluated in different laboratories by employing accepted test criteria.

Numerous attempts have been made to use mechanical techniques to objectify the examiner's evaluation. These mechanical methods measure torque-

---

Table 100–7. Questions Posed at Clinical Neurophysiology Built into an Algorithm Related to the Assessment of Spasticity

1. Is muscle tone increased? Is the muscle tone spastic? Can spastic muscle tone be differentiated from other types of tone disorders? Can spastic muscle tone be quantified?
2. What is the cause of spastic muscle tone? Can neuronal and non-neuronal origins of spastic muscle tone be distinguished? Is there a relevant contribution to spastic muscle tone from exaggerated tonic stretch reflex?
   a. *(mainly scientific interest)* Which is the underlying cause of an exaggerated tonic stretch reflex?
   b. Which interneuronal function involved in the tonic stretch reflex circuitry is disturbed?
3. Does an exaggerated tonic stretch reflex persist into movement? If yes, does it have a relevant functional impact? Does (e.g., pharmacologic) reduction of an exaggerated tonic stretch reflex partially improve motor function?
4. Are there signs of spinal hyperreflexia other than enhanced stretch reflexes, such as flexor reflexes?
5. Do they persist into movement? Do they have a functional impact? Does (pharmacologic) reduction of flexor reflex activity lead to functional improvement?

---

angle relationships at spastic joints during passive flexion and extension. Controlled stretches can be delivered by devices containing torque motors. The perturbation can be a single step or more complex, such as a sinusoid. The mechanical response of the limb is measured. Objective techniques are an improvement over bedside testing and theoretically may have a role in differentiating spastic muscle tone from other tone disorders, although this distinction usually is made clinically. Additionally, these techniques might provide a means of monitoring muscle tone in longitudinal studies or studies aimed at studying the effects of a therapeutic intervention. However, it is important to bear in mind that their clinical usefulness depends on the value of the parameters assessed by them.

Diagnostic nerve or motor point blocks may help to differentiate between the contributions of neural and intrinsic mechanical factors to spastic muscle tone. Quantitative differentiation of the intrinsic and neural components of spastic muscle tone can also be performed noninvasively. A simple and semiquantitative assessment is provided by multichannel surface electromyography (Pullman et al., 2000), but the most accurate assessment is provided by a combination of electromyographic and biomechanical techniques. Few approaches have been assessed with respect to validity and re-test reliability (Pisano et al., 2000). Certain indices of stiffness are derived from torque–position relationships at various angular velocities. An intrinsic stiffness index corresponds to an angular velocity in situations in which no reflexive electromyographic activity is noted. Conversely, the total stiffness index obtained at higher angular velocities would reflect both intrinsic and neuronal contributions to stiffness. The intrinsic stiffness index differs between female and male subjects, most probably owing to the sex-dependent difference in arm muscle mass. The total stiffness index is significantly higher (indicating greater stiffness) in subjects who exhibit a stretch reflex than in those who do not have a stretch reflex even at high angular velocities. The total stiffness index has been validated in stroke patients by demonstrating that it correlates well with conventional clinical scales of spasticity. Conversely, correlations with conventional neurophysiological measures, such as H-reflex latency, Hmax/Mmax ratio, stretch reflex latency, and area were poor (Pisano et al., 2000). However, the usefulness of the technique in differentiating between the intrinsic and the neuronal factors that contribute to spasticity was limited, because the lowest angular velocity (10 degrees per second) tested already evoked a stretch reflex in the flexor electromyogram (EMG) in almost two thirds of stroke patients, in marked contrast with healthy control subjects. Thus, the intrinsic stiffness was impossible to assess. In such cases, a diagnostic nerve block may be used to isolate the intrinsic muscle stiffness component of the spastic muscle tone from the stretch reflex–related component. Similar set-ups, such as those employed by Pisano and co-workers, may be used for the study of the lower limbs (Dietz and Berger, 1983) (Fig. 100–4).

As outlined previously, reflex studies employing electrical nerve stimulation are generally not needed for the proper clinical management of a patient with spasticity. They may, however, be used in a scientific context. Once it has been established that spastic muscle tone has a significant neuronal component, there are a variety of well-elaborated techniques available for determining which of the (inter)neurons involved in the stretch-reflex circuitry function abnormally. α-Motoneuronal excitability can be assessed with the use of F waves or the H reflex. An inventory of techniques available for testing human spinal reflexes is provided by Hallett and colleagues (1994), Kimura and associates (1994), Capaday (1997), Pierrot-Deseilligny (1997), and Burke and co-workers (1999). These tests characterize reciprocal inhibition, presynaptic inhibition, synergistic type Ia facilitation, and type Ib inhibition. The main principle underlying the methods is that the H reflex is used as a test reflex, and the effect of conditioning stimulation to various nerves is evaluated. (The caveats against the use of the H reflex as a measure of α-motoneuronal excitability have been addressed in preceding sections.) The conditioning effect is determined as a difference in the sizes of the conditioned and unconditioned reflexes. The conditioning effect is expressed as a percentage of the Mmax or of the unconditioned test reflex (Kimura et al., 1994). While these tests are generally performed in the resting patient, the basic principles of deficient human motor control are best determined by studying freely moving subjects during motor tasks that are as natural as possible, for reasons previously outlined.

Weakness is the leading factor that determines disability in the vast majority of patients with spastic muscle tone. In a given patient, it may be useful to quantitate and visualize the functional conse-

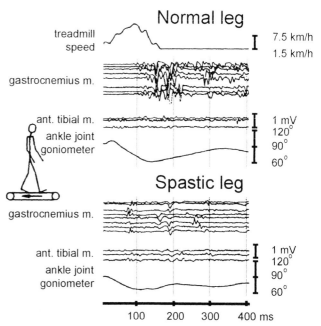

Figure 100–4. Investigation of reflexive muscle activity in the lower limbs during walking on a treadmill. Induction of compensatory leg-muscle activity in a patient with spastic hemiparesis by a sudden increase in treadmill velocity. Raw recordings from gastrocnemius and tibialis anterior muscle with ankle-joint movements after a sudden transient increase in treadmill velocity induced at the beginning of the stance phase in an unaffected or spastic leg of a patient with spastic hemiparesis. Displacement of the spastic leg was followed by a strong compensatory response in the gastrocnemius muscle at a latency of about 80 ms after the onset of stretching of the triceps surae. Displacement of the spastic leg was followed by electromyographic activity at a short latency (about 45 ms), while a polysynaptic EMG response was almost absent. Overall EMG activity in the gastrocnemius in the spastic leg was reduced compared with the unaffected one. (From Berger W, Quintern J, Dietz V: Tension development and muscle activation in the leg during gait in spastic hemiparesis: The independence of muscle hypertonia and exaggerated stretch reflex. J Neurol Neurosurg Psychiatry 1983;47:1029–1033.)

quences of a lesion of descending fiber tracts. Transcranial magnetic stimulation may be used to assess the integrity of the corticospinal tract. Needle recordings may be used both to visualize insufficient recruitment of motor units and in the assessment of a reduction in the maximal upper frequency to which motor units can be driven when the patient performs a maximal isometric contraction.

Disturbances of the muscle activation pattern may be visualized by recording surface electromyographic activity during the execution of common and natural motor tasks. If these recordings are used in a controlled setting, such as reaching for a target, or bicycling (Fig. 100–5), they may reveal abnormal co-activation of agonist and antagonist muscles, and temporally extended muscular activity (Benecke, 1987). These measures may then be used to control for the effect of therapeutic interventions, such as physiotherapy. Deficits in the control of limb dynamics may also be visualized and quantitated by using optoelectronic systems (Fig. 100–6) (Beer et al., 2000) or computer-operated robot arms.

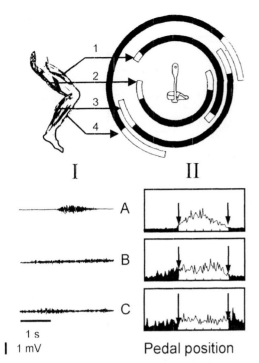

Figure 100–5. Electromyography in man bicycling on an ergometer for evaluation of spasticity of the lower limbs. *Upper Part,* Mean angle range (*black*) of four routinely examined muscles and standard deviation (*white*) presented as concentric arcs. *Lower Part I,* Representative EMG recordings of the right rectus femoris muscle in a normal subject (*A*) and in two patients with spastic paraparesis (*B* and *C*). *Lower Part II,* Corresponding average (eight rotations) of EMG in the normal subject and in the two patients with severe paraparesis. Horizontal axis shows the position of the pedal, with the origin corresponding to the lowest position of the right pedal. Note the flattening of activity and the enhanced duration of muscle recruitment in *B* and *C*. (From Benecke R: Spasticity/spasms: Clinical aspects and treatment. In Benecke R, Conrad B, Marsden CD [eds]: Motor Disturbances I. London, Academic Press, 1987.)

RIGIDITY

Rigidity is defined as a form of hypertonia characterized by a constant uniform increase in resistance to passive movement throughout the range of joint displacement while the patient attempts to relax (Lakke, 1981). This resistance consists of elastic (i.e., length-dependent), viscous (i.e., velocity-dependent), and inertial (i.e., acceleration-dependent) components. It reflects mechanical properties of the displaced limb, following the principles of Newtonian physics, as well as activity of its neuronal control. Moving a rigid limb, an examiner may identify a "leadpipe" phenomenon, when rigidity occurs continuously, or a "cogwheel" phenomenon, when there is superimposed tremor with a frequency usually in the range of action tremor (Denny-Brown, 1962). Rigidity can be facilitated by mental arithmetic or physical activity in the contralateral corresponding limb as in Froment's sign, when contralateral fist clenching is facilitating elbow rigidity. Rigidity is usually most prominent in the flexor muscles of the neck, trunk, and limbs, thus possibly contributing

to, but by no means explaining, the stooped posture of Parkinson's syndrome. Rigidity is frequently associated with akinesia, constituting the akinetic-rigid syndrome, or with akinesia and tremor, forming the clinical picture of parkinsonism. Despite its frequent association with akinesia and its contribution to akinesia, it is clearly distinct from akinesia, as demonstrated in parkinsonian patients who lose rigidity after thalamotomy or levodopa therapy and still continue to suffer from akinesia.

Differential Diagnosis

Rigidity has to be differentiated from other conditions causing muscle stiffness. All of those conditions feature continuous muscle activity at rest that does not occur in rigidity. In stiff-person syndrome, continuous muscle activity at rest is superimposed by spasms provoked by excitement, anxiety, voluntary movement, sudden noise, or peripheral stimuli (Moersch and Woltman, 1956; Thompson, 1993; Meinck et al., 1995). It is localized predominantly in the axial muscles. It is often associated with antibodies against glutamic acid decarboxylase interfering with spinal GABAergic interneuronal inhibition (Solimena et al., 1988). In progressive encephalomyelitis with rigidity or spinal interneuronitis, continuous muscle activity at rest is not associated with spasms (Campbell and Garland, 1956; Howell et al., 1979). It may occur spontaneously or paraneoplastically (Roobol et al., 1987). In spinal alpha rigidity, continuous muscle activity at rest occurs as the result of isolation of motor neurons from inhibitory interneuronal control. This is usually caused by trauma, vascular disease, tumors, inflammation, and syringomyelia in the cervical spinal cord (Gelfan and Tarlov, 1959). In tetanus, continuous muscle activity is superimposed by severe painful spasms (Ernst et al., 1997). It is caused by tetanus toxin–induced spinal inhibitory interneuron dysfunction. In neuromyotonia or Isaacs' syndrome, continuous muscle activity at rest is most probably caused by dysfunction of voltage-gated potassium channels in the peripheral nerve (Isaacs, 1961; Hayat et al., 2000). In myotonia (Thornton, 1999), Morvan's fibrillary chorea (Barber et al., 2000), rippling muscle disease (Stephan et al., 1994), and Schwartz-Jampel syndrome (Schwartz and Jampel, 1962), continuous muscle activity at rest is thought to be caused by muscular dysfunction. Other conditions that produce discontinuous muscle activity, such as dystonia, chorea, athetosis, tremor, and others, are easily distinguishable from rigidity. Decorticate rigidity with flexion and inward rotation of the arms and extension of the legs caused by hemispheric or upper brainstem lesions, and decerebrate rigidity with arm and leg extension due to lower brainstem lesions (Davis and Davis, 1982), represent exaggerated nociceptive reflexes, rather than rigidity, according to the definition introduced previously.

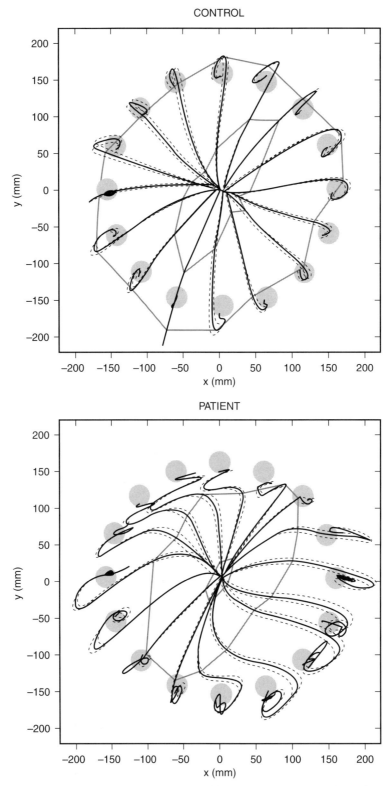

Figure 100–6. Evaluation of disturbances of higher-order motor control by optoelectronic recordings of reaching movements. Subjects performed rapid movements from a central starting point to 16 targets equidistantly around the circumference of a circle. Mean ± 1 SEM (standard error of the mean) hand paths for all target directions are shown for the dominant (right) limb of a control subject (*upper panel*) and the paretic (right, dominant) limb of a patient with spastic hemiparesis. Targets are indicated (to scale) by the shaded circles. Also shown are contour lines that indicate the mean hand position at 100 and 200 ms after movement onset. Note systematic misdirection of movements of the patient with spastic hemiparesis. (From Beer RF, Dewald JP, Rymer WZ: Deficits in the coordination of multijoint arm movements in patients with hemiparesis: Evidence for disturbed control of limb dynamics. Exp Brain Res 2000;131:305–319.)

Diseases with Rigidity

Rigidity occurs in a large number of pathological conditions that produce nigrostriatal impairment by affecting the striatum, its inputs, its outputs, and its wider hemispheric connections. All of these conditions produce akinetic-rigid syndromes or parkinsonism. The occurrence of isolated rigidity is extremely rare. By far, the most common cause of rigidity is presynaptic nigrostriatal impairment caused by Parkinson's disease with degeneration of dopaminergic cells in the pars compacta of the substantia nigra, thus affecting the striatal input. Owing to frequent association with tremor, rigidity in Parkinson's disease tends to be more of the cogwheel type. Conditions that produce predominantly postsynaptic nigrostriatal impairment with rigidity more often of the leadpipe type include progressive supranuclear palsy, with the striatal output being predominantly affected; multiple system atrophy, with the striatal output being predominantly affected; and corticobasal degeneration and parkinson-dementia complex, with the hemispheres being widely affected. Other causes include heredodegenerative parkinsonism, such as Huntington's disease and Wilson's disease, with extensive striatal damage; spinocerebellar degenerations; neuroacanthocytosis and mitochondrial encephalopathies, with the hemispheres being widely affected; and secondary parkinsonism caused by drugs, especially D_2-blocking agents, with striatal damage, and by anoxia, encephalitis, traumatic injury, intoxication, vascular disorders, especially in Binswanger's disease, and neoplasia or paraneoplasia, all producing more or less widespread hemispheric lesions. With the exception of progressive supranuclear palsy, in which rigidity tends to be milder and more axial, and parkinsonism-dementia complex, in which rigidity tends to be less common, all other forms of parkinsonism do not have exceptional or distinguishing features of rigidity.

Pathophysiology

Initially, it was believed that rigidity was caused by γ-motoneuron hyperactivity (Rushworth, 1960; Lance et al., 1963; Selby, 1968; Ward, 1968), since local anesthetic blockade of muscle spindle receptors (Walshe, 1924) and dorsal root dissection (Pollock and Davies, 1930) were able to abolish it. Gamma fiber microneurography, however, failed to demonstrate γ-motoneuron dysfunction (Burke et al., 1977; Mano et al., 1979). On the other hand, enhanced facilitation of late components of H-reflex recovery curves (Olson and Diamantopoulos, 1967; Yap, 1967; McLeod and Walsh, 1972) suggests α-motoneuron hyperactivity in parkinsonian rigidity. Together with normal tendon reflexes, but increased late components of muscle stretch reflexes (Tatton and Lee, 1975; Rothwell et al., 1983), parkinsonian rigidity was then believed to reflect increased long-loop reflex activity (Berardelli et al., 1983). With long-loop reflexes involving spinothalamocorticospinal and spinocerebellothalamocorticospinal pathways (Conrad et al., 1984), the immediate abolition of parkinsonian rigidity by ventrolateral thalamotomy might be explained by disruption of hyperactive long-loop reflexes. However, with long-loop reflexes best elucidated by rapid muscle stretch and with motor cortex excitability now believed to be decreased in parkinsonism (Alexander and Crutcher, 1990), the role of overactive long-loop reflexes in producing rigidity was challenged (Marsden, 1992). Therefore, overactive long-loop reflexes are known to be present in Parkinson's disease, but a specific role in the generation of rigidity is not apparently clear. Reduction of parkinsonian rigidity by administration of levodopa together with elucidation of parkinsonian rigidity by highly selective lesioning of the substantia nigra induced by MPTP (1-methyl-4-phenyl-1,2,3,6-tetrahydropyridine) (Burns et al., 1983) points to nigrostriatal impairment as a causal factor in rigidity. Despite some increased insight into the pathophysiology of parkinsonism (Alexander and Crutcher, 1990), it remains unclear how nigrostriatal impairment could transform into rigidity.

Treatment

Rigidity can be treated with dopaminergic drugs, including levodopa, synaptic levodopa agonists, and postsynaptic levodopa agonists, and with anticholinergic drugs. Although akinesia sometimes does not respond sufficiently, the decrease in rigidity in response to these drugs reflects the overall improvement of the condition. Depending on the pathology, rigidity due to presynaptic nigrostriatal impairment responds markedly better than rigidity due to postsynaptic nigrostriatal impairment. Thalamotomy (Moriyama et al., 1999) and thalamic stimulation (Limousin-Dowsey et al., 1999) have marked effects on tremor and rigidity and usually only mild effects on akinesia, whereas pallidotomy (Fine et al., 2000), pallidal stimulation (Barcia-Salorio et al., 1999), and subthalamic nucleus stimulation (Krack et al., 1998) exert the best effects on levodopa-associated dyskinesias and slightly milder effects on parkinsonism or akinetic-rigid conditions. Adrenal or fetal tissue transplants are still in an experimental stage, and nerve growth factor applications are still hypothetical.

Neurophysiological Assessment

Rigidity can be assessed clinically by examination of limb resistance to passive movement. This clinical assessment is biased by the variability of the mechanical properties of the examined limb, of the clinical maneuver used for limb displacement, and of the individual perception of limb resistance. The clinical impression can be reported semiquantita-

Patient 1   Patient 2

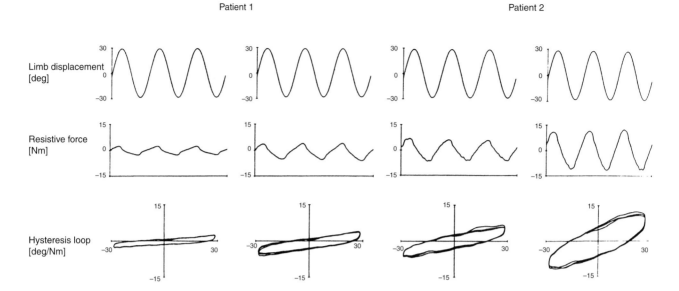

Figure 100–7. Averaged limb displacement, corresponding resistive force, and derived hysteresis loop in two patients with rigidity at rest (rest) and under standardized contralateral voluntary wrist movements (activation). The "work score," defined as the area of the hysteresis loop, represents an objective measurement of the combined elastic, viscous, and inertial components of wrist rigidity. (From Fung VS, Burne JA, Morris JG: Objective quantification of resting and activated parkinsonian rigidity: A comparison of angular impulse and work scores. Mov Disord 2000;15:48–55.)

tively by using scales and scores usually developed to measure parkinsonian syndromes, such as the Unified Parkinson's Disease Rating Scale (UPDRS) Part III (Fahn et al., 1987a), the Webster Score (Webster, 1968), the Columbia Rating Scale (Martilla and Rinne, 1977), and others.

More elaborate methodologies using torque motor pulses and measurements of the resistive limb force have been introduced over the years (Watts et al., 1986; Wieger and Watts, 1986; Teravainen et al., 1989; Ghika et al., 1993). The most advanced device records the torque motor voltage necessary for producing set cyclic wrist displacements (Fung et al., 2000). The torque motor voltage is directly correlated to the resistive force, as measured in newton-meters (Nm). As shown in Figure 100–7, wrist position and corresponding resistive force in a displacement cycle can be plotted as a hysteresis loop. The "work score," defined as the area of the hysteresis loop, represents an objective measurement of the combined elastic, viscous, and inertial components of wrist rigidity. Unfortunately, tremor interferes with these measurements, thus limiting their clinical usefulness. If one assumes a relationship between the severity of rigidity and long-loop reflex activity (Berardelli et al., 1983), measurements of long-loop reflex activity can be used for indirect quantification of rigidity. However, this relationship has been questioned (Bergui et al., 1992).

References

Alexander GE, Crutcher MD: Functional architecture of basal ganglia circuits: Neural substrates of parallel processing. Trends Neurosci 1990;13:266–221.

Ashworth B: Preliminary trials of carisoprodol in multiple sclerosis. Practitioner 1964;192:540–542.

Barber PA, Anderson NE, Vincent A: Morvan's syndrome associated with voltage-gated K+ channel antibodies. Neurology 2000; 54:771–772.

Barcia-Salorio JL, Roldan P, Talamantes F, et al: Electrical inhibition of basal ganglia nuclei in Parkinson's disease: Long-term results. Stereotact Funct Neurosurg 1999;72:202–207.

Beer RF, Dewald JP, Rymer WZ: Deficits in the coordination of multijoint arm movements in patients with hemiparesis: Evidence for disturbed control of limb dynamics. Exp Brain Res 2000;131:305–319.

Benecke R: Spasticity/spasms: Clinical aspects and treatment. In Benecke R, Conrad B, Marsden CD (eds): Motor Disturbances I. London, Academic Press, 1987.

Benecke R: The role of the corticospinal tract in spasticity studied by magnetic brain stimulation. In Thilmann AF, Burke DJ, Rymer WZ, et al (eds): Spasticity: Mechanisms and Management. Berlin, Springer-Verlag, 1993.

Benecke R: Pathophysiologische Mechanismen der Dystonien. Klin Neurophysiol 1999;30:95–103.

Berardelli A, Sabra AF, Hallett M: Physiological mechanisms of rigidity in Parkinson's disease. J Neurol Neurosurg Psychiatry 1983;46:45–53.

Berardelli A, Rothwell JC, Hallett M, et al: The pathophysiology of primary dystonia. Brain 1998;121:1195–1212.

Berger W, Quintern J, Dietz V: Tension development and muscle activation in the leg during gait in spastic hemiparesis: The independence of muscle hypertonia and exaggerated stretch reflex. J Neurol Neurosurg Psychiatry 1983;47:1029–1033.

Bergui M, Lopiano L, Paglia G, et al: Stretch reflex of quadriceps femoris and its relation to rigidity in Parkinson's disease. Acta Neurol Scand 1992;86:226–229.

Bhatia KP, Marsden DC: The behavioural and motor consequences of focal lesions of the basal ganglia in man. Brain 1994; 117:859–876.

Bressman SB, de Leon D, Brin MF, et al: Idiopathic torsion dystonia among Ashkenazi Jews: Evidence for autosomal dominant inheritance. Ann Neurol 1989;26:612–620.

Bressman SB, de Leon C, Raymond D, et al: Clinical-genetic spectrum of primary dystonia. Adv Neurol 1998;78:79–92.

Brown P: Pathophysiology of spasticity. J Neurol Neurosurg Psychiatry 1994;57:773–777.

Burke D, Hagbarth KE, Wallin BG: Reflex mechanisms in parkinsonian rigidity. Scand J Rehab Med 1977;9:15–23.

Burke D, Hallett M, Fuhr P, et al: H reflexes from the tibial and median nerves. The International Federation of Clinical Neurophysiology. Electroencephalogr Clin Neurophysiol 1999;52:259–262.

Burns RS, Chiueh CC, Markey SP, et al: A primate model of parkinsonism: Selective destruction of dopaminergic neurons in the pars compacta of the substantia nigra by N-methyl-4-phenyl-1,2,3,6-tetrahydropyridine. Proc Natl Acad Sci U S A 1983;80:4546–4550.

Burton K, Farrell K, Li D, et al: Lesions of the putamen and dystonia: CT and magnetic resonance imaging. Neurology 1984; 34:962–965.

Byl NN, Merzenich MM, Jenkins WM: A primate genesis model of focal dystonia and repetitive strain injury: I. Learning-induced differentiation of the representation of the hand in the primary somatosensory cortex in adult monkeys. Neurology 1996;47: 508–520.

Byl NN, Merzenich MM, Cheung S, et al: A primate model for studying focal dystonia and repetitive strain injury: Effects on the primary somatic sensory cortex. Phys Ther 1997;77:269–284.

Byrnes ML, Thickbroom GW, Wilson SA, et al: The cortico-motor representation of upper limb muscles in writer's cramp and changes following botulinum toxin injection. Brain 1998;121: 977–988.

Campbell AMG, Garland H: Subacute myoclonic spinal interneuronitis. J Neurol Neurosurg Psychiatry 1956;19:268–274.

Capaday C: Neurophysiological methods for studies of the motor system in freely moving human subjects. J Neurosci Methods 1997;74:201–218.

Ceballos-Baumann AO, Sheean G, Passingham RE, et al: Botulinum toxin does not reverse the cortical dysfunction associated with writer's cramp: A PET study. Brain 1997;120:571–582.

Chen RS, Tsai CH, Lu CS: Reciprocal inhibition in writer's cramp. Mov Disord 1995;10:556–561.

Cleland CL, Hayward L, Rymer WZ: Neural mechanisms underlying the clasp-knife reflex in the cat. II. Stretch-sensitive muscular-free nerve endings. J Neurophysiol 1990;64:1319–1330.

Conrad B, Dressler D, Benecke R: Changes of somatosensory evoked potentials in man as correlates of transcortical reflex mediation? Neurosci Lett 1984;46:97–102.

Corden DM, Lippold OC, Buchanan K, et al: Long-latency component of the stretch reflex in human muscle is not mediated by intramuscular stretch receptors. J Neurophysiol 2000;84:184–188.

Currà A, Romaniello A, Berardelli A, et al: Shortened cortical silent period in facial muscles of patients with cranial dystonia. Neurology 2000;54:130–135.

Davis RA, Davis L: Decerebrate rigidity in humans. Neurosurgery 1982;10:635–642.

Defazio G, Livrea P, Guanti G, et al: Genetic contribution to idiopathic adult-onset blepharospasm and cranial-cervical dystonia. Eur Neurol 1993;33:345–350.

Denny-Brown D: The Basal Ganglia and Their Relation to Disorders of Movement. London, Oxford Press, 1962; 75.

Deuschl G, Seifert G, Heinen F, et al: Reciprocal inhibition of forearm flexor muscles in spasmodic torticollis. J Neurol Sci 1992;113:85–90.

Deuschl G, Toro C, Matsumoto J, et al: Movement-related cortical potentials in writer's cramp. Ann Neurol 1995;38:862–868. Comment in: Ann Neurol 1995;38:837–838.

Dietz V, Berger W: Normal and impaired regulation of muscle stiffness in gait: A new hypothesis about muscle hypertonia. Exp Neurol 1983;79:680–687.

Dressler D, Rothwell JC: Electromyographic quantification of the paralysing effect of botulinum toxin in the sternocleidomastoid muscle. Eur Neurol 2000a;43:13–16.

Dressler D, Bigalke H, Rothwell JC: The sternocleidomastoid test: An in vivo assay to investigate botulinum toxin antibody formation in humans. J Neurol 2000b;247:630–632.

Eidelberg D, Moeller JR, Ishikawa T, et al: The metabolic topography of idiopathic torsion dystonia. Brain 1995;118:1473–1484.

Eidelberg D, Moeller JR, Antonini A, et al: Functional brain networks in DYT1 dystonia. Ann Neurol 1998;44:303–312.

Ernst ME, Klepser ME, Fouts M, et al: Tetanus: Pathophysiology and management. Ann Pharmacother 1997;31:1507–1513.

Fahn S: Concept and classification of dystonia. Adv Neurol 1988; 50:1–8.

Fahn S, Elton RL, and Members of the UPDRS Development Committee: Unified Parkinson's disease rating scale. In Fahn S, Marsden CD, Goldstein M, et al (eds): Recent Developments in Parkinson's Disease II. New York, Macmillan, 1987a; 153–163.

Fahn S, Marsden CD, Calne DB: Classification and investigation of dystonia. In Marsden CD, Fahn S (eds): Movement Disorders 2. London, Butterworths, 1987b; 332–358.

Fahn S, Bressman SB, Marsden CD: Classification of dystonia. Adv Neurol 1998;78:1–10.

Fellows SJ, Kraus C, Ross HF, et al: Disturbances of voluntary arm movement in human spasticity: The relative importance of paresis and muscle hypertonia. In Thilmann AF, Burke DJ, Rymer WZ, et al (eds): Spasticity: Mechanisms and Management. Berlin, Springer-Verlag, 1993a.

Fellows SJ, Ross HF, Thilmann AF: The limitations of the tendon jerk as a marker of pathological stretch reflex activity in human spasticity. J Neurol Neurosurg Psychiatry 1993b;56:531–537.

Fine J, Duff J, Chen R, et al: Long-term follow-up of unilateral pallidotomy in advanced Parkinson's disease. N Engl J Med 2000;342:1708–1714.

Fung VS, Burne JA, Morris JG: Objective quantification of resting and activated parkinsonian rigidity: A comparison of angular impulse and work scores. Mov Disord 2000;15:48–55.

Gelfan S, Tarlov IM: Interneurons and rigidity of spinal origin. J Physiol (Lond) 1959;146:594–617.

Ghika J, Wiegner AW, Fang JJ, et al: Portable system for quantifying motor abnormalities in Parkinson's disease. IEEE Trans Biomed Eng 1993;40:276–283.

Gilio F, Currà A, Lorenzano C, et al: Effects of botulinum toxin type A on intracortical inhibition in patients with dystonia. Ann Neurol 2000;48:20–26.

Gowers WR: A Manual of Diseases of the Nervous System. Philadelphia, P. Blakiston, 1888; 1357.

Grünewald RA, Yoneda Y, Shipman JM, et al: Idiopathic focal dystonia: A disorder of muscle spindle afferent processing? Brain 1997;120:2179–2185.

Hallett M, Berardelli A, Delwaide P, et al: Central EMG and tests of motor control. (Report of an IFCN committee.) Electroencephalogr Clin Neurophysiol 1994;90:404–432.

Hayat GR, Kulkantrakorn K, Campbell WW, et al: Neuromyotonia: Autoimmune pathogenesis and response to immune-modulating therapy. J Neurol Sci 2000;181:38–43.

Herman R, Freedman W, Mayer N: Neurophysiologic mechanisms of hemiplegic and paraplegic spasticity: Implications for therapy. Arch Phys Med Rehabil 1974;55:338–343.

Herz E: Dystonia 2: Clinical classification. Arch Neurol Psychiatry 1944;51:319–355.

Howell DA, Lees AJ, Toghill PJ: Spinal internuncial neurones in progressive encephalomyelitis with rigidity. J Neurol Neurosurg Psychiatry 1979;42:773–785.

Ibrahim IK, Berger W, Trippel M, et al: Stretch-induced electromyographic activity and torque in spastic elbow muscles: Differential modulation of reflex activity in passive and active motor tasks. Brain 1993;116:971–989.

Ichinose H, Ohye T, Takahashi E, et al: Hereditary progressive dystonia with marked diurnal fluctuation caused by mutations in the GTP cyclohydrolase 1 gene. Nat Genet 1994;8:236–242.

Ikoma K, Samii A, Mercuri B, et al: Abnormal cortical motor excitability in dystonia. Neurology 1996;46:1371–1376.

Isaacs H: A syndrome of continuous muscle-fibre activity. J Neurol Neurosurg Psychiatry 1961;24:319–325.

Kaji R, Rothwell JC, Katayama M, et al: Tonic vibration reflex and muscle afferent block in writer's cramp. Ann Neurol 1995; 38:155–162.

Kessler KR, Skutta M, Benecke R (for the German Dystonia Study Group): Long-term treatment of cervical dystonia with botulinum toxin A: Efficacy, safety, and antibody frequency. J Neurol 1999;246:265–274.

Kimura J, Daube J, Burke D, et al: Human reflexes and late responses. (Report of an IFCN committee.) Electroencephalogr Clin Neurophysiol 1994;90:393–403.

Krack P, Benazzouz A, Pollak P, et al: Treatment of tremor in Parkinson's disease by subthalamic nucleus stimulation. Mov Disord 1998;13:907–914.

Kujirai T, Caramia MD, Rothwell JC, et al: Corticocortical inhibition in the human motor cortex. J Physiol (Lond) 1993;471:501–519.

Lakke PWF: Classification of extrapyramidal disorders. J Neurol Sci 1981;51:311–327.

Lance JW: Symposium synopsis. In Feldmann RG, Young RR, Koella WP (eds): Spasticity: Disordered Motor Control. Chicago, Year Book Medical Publishers, 1980; 1303–1313.

Lance JW, Schwab RS, Peterson ER: Action tremor and the cogwheel phenomenon in Parkinson's disease. Brain 1963;86:95–110.

Lee MS, Marsden CD: Movement disorders following lesions of the thalamus or subthalamic region. Mov Disord 1994;9:493–507.

Leube B, Rudnicki D, Ratzlaff T, et al: Idiopathic torsion dystonia: Assignment of a gene to chromosome 18p in a German family with adult onset, autosomal dominant inheritance and purely focal distribution. Hum Mol Genet 1996;10:1673–1677.

Leube B, Hendgen T, Kessler KR, et al: Sporadic focal dystonia in Northwest Germany: Molecular basis on chromosome 18p. Ann Neurol 1997;42:111–114.

Limousin-Dowsey P, Pollak P, Van Blercom N, et al: Thalamic, subthalamic nucleus and internal pallidum stimulation in Parkinson's disease. J Neurol 1999;246(suppl 2):1142–1145.

Lockwood AH: Medical problems in musicians. N Engl J Med 1989; 320:221–227.

Mano T, Yamazaki Y, Takagi S: Muscle spindle activity in parkinsonian rigidity. Acta Neurol Scand 1979;73(suppl):176.

Marsden CD: Motor dysfunction and movement disorders. In Ashbury AK, McKhann GM, McDonald WI (eds): Diseases of the Nervous System, vol 1. Clinical Neurobiology. Philadelphia, WB Saunders, 1992; 309–318.

Marsden CD, Harrison MJ, Bundey S: The natural history of idiopathic torsion dystonia. In Eldridge R, Fahn S (eds): Dystonia: Advances in Neurology. New York, Raven Press, 1976; 177–187.

Marsden CD, Obeso JA, Zarranz JJ, et al: The anatomical basis of symptomatic hemidystonia. Brain 1985;108:463–483.

Martilla RJ, Rinne UK: Disability and progression in Parkinson's disease. Acta Neurol Scand 1977;56:159–169.

Matsumura M, Sawaguchi T, Oishi T, et al: Behavioral deficits induced by local injection of bicuculline and muscimol into the primate motor and premotor cortex. J Neurophysiol 1991;65:1542–1553.

Mavroudakis N, Caroyer JM, Brunko E, et al: Abnormal motor evoked responses to transcranial magnetic stimulation in focal dystonia. Neurology 1995;45:1671–1677.

McLeod JG, Walsh JC: H-reflex in patients with Parkinson's disease. J Neurol Neurosurg Psychiatry 1972;35:77–80.

Meinck HM, Rickler K, Hülser PJ, et al: Stiff man syndrome: Neurophysiological findings in eight patients. J Neurol 1995;242:134–142.

Mink JW, Thach WT: Basal ganglia intrinsic circuits and their role in behavior. Curr Opin Neurobiol 1993;3:950–957.

Moersch FP, Woltman HW: Progressive fluctuating muscular rigidity and spasm ('stiff-man' syndrome): Report of a case and some observations in 13 other cases. Mayo Clin Proc 1956; 31:421–427.

Moriyama E, Beck H, Miyamoto T: Long-term results of ventrolateral thalamotomy for patients with Parkinson's disease. Neurol Med Chir (Tokyo) 1999;39:350–357.

Mueller U, Steinberger D, Memeth A: Clinical and molecular genetics of primary dystonias. Neurogenetics 1998;1:165–177.

Naumann M, Reiners K: Long-latency reflexes of hand muscles in idiopathic focal dystonia and their modification by botulinum toxin. Brain 1997;120:409–416.

Nichols TR, Houk JC: Improvement in linearity and regularity of stiffness that results from actions of stretch reflex. J Neurophysiol 1976;39:119–142.

Nutt JG, Muenter MD, Aronson A, et al: Epidemiology of focal and generalized dystonia in Rochester, Minnesota. Mov Disord 1988; 3:188–194.

Olson PZ, Diamantopoulos E: Excitability of spinal motor neurones in normal subjects and in patients with spasticity, Parkinsonian rigidity, and cerebellar hypotonia. J Neurol Neurosurg Psychiatry 1967;30:325–331.

Oppenheim J: Über eine eigenartige Krampfkrankheit des kindlichen und jugendlichen Alters (Dysbasia lordotica progressiva, Dystonia musculorum deformans). Neurol Centralbl 1911;30:1090–1107.

Ozelius LJ, Hewett J, Page CE, et al: The early-onset torsion dystonia gene (DYT1) encodes an ATP-binding protein. Nat Genet 1997;17:40–48.

Panizza ME, Hallett M, Nilsson J: Reciprocal inhibition in pateints with hand cramps. Neurology 1989;39:85–89.

Panizza M, Lelli S, Nilsson J, et al: H-reflex recovery curve and reciprocal inhibition of H-reflex in different kinds of dystonia. Neurology 1990;40:824–828.

Perlmutter JS, Stambuk MK, Markham J, et al: Decreased [^{18}F]-spiperone binding in putamen in idiopathic focal dystonia. J Neurosci 1997;17:843–850.

Pettigrew LC, Jankovic J: Hemidystonia: A report of 22 patients and a review of the literature. J Neurol Neurosurg Psychiatry 1985;48:650–657.

Pierrot-Deseilligny E: Electrophysiological assessment of the spinal mechanisms underlying spasticity. In Rossini PN, Maugiere F (eds): New Trends and Advanced Techniques in Clinical Neurophysiology (EEG Suppl 41). Amsterdam, Elsevier Science Publishers, 1990.

Pierrot-Deseilligny E: Assessing changes in presynaptic inhibition of Ia afferents during movement in humans. J Neurosci Methods 1997;74:189–199.

Pisano F, Miscio G, Colombo R, et al: Quantitative evaluation of normal muscle tone. J Neurol Sci 1996;135:168–172.

Pisano F, Miscio G, Del Conte C, et al: Quantitative measures of spasticity in post-stroke patients. Clin Neurophysiol 2000;111:1015–1022.

Pollock LJ, Davies L: Muscle tone in Parkinsonian states. Arch Neurol Psychiatry 1930;23:303–317.

Popescu FC, Rymer WZ: End points of planar reaching movements are disrupted by small force pulses: An evaluation of the hypothesis of equifinality. J Neurophysiol 2000;84:2670–2679.

Powers RK, Marder-Meyer J, Rymer WZ: Quantitative relations between hypertonia and stretch reflex threshold in spastic hemiparesis. Ann Neurol 1988;23:115–124.

Pullman SL, Goodin DS, Marquinez AI, et al: Clinical utility of surface EMG: Report of the therapeutics and technology assessment subcommittee of the American Academy of Neurology. Neurology 2000; 55:171–177.

Ridding MC, Sheean G, Rothwell JC, et al: Changes in the balance between motor cortical excitation and inhibition in focal, task specific dystonia. J Neurol Neurosurg Psychiatry 1995;59:493–498.

Roobol TH, Kazzaz BA, Vecht CJ: Segmental rigidity and spinal myoclonus as a paraneoplastic syndrome. J Neurol Neurosurg Psychiatry 1987;50:628–631.

Rothwell JC, Obeseo JA, Traub MM, et al: The behaviour of the long-latency reflex in patients with Parkinson's disease. J Neurol Neurosurg Psychiatry 1983;46:35–44.

Rushworth G: Spasticity and rigidity: An experimental study and review. J Neurol Neurosurg Psychiatry 1960;23:99–118.

Schwalbe W: Eine eigentümliche tonische Krampfform mit hysterischen Symptomen. Inaugural Dissertation. Berlin, G. Schade, 1908.

Schwartz O, Jampel RS: Congenital blepharophimosis associated with a unique generalized myopathy. Arch Ophthalmol 1962; 68:712–715.

Selby G: Parkinson's disease. In Vincken PJ, Bruyn GW (eds): Handbook of Clinical Neurology, vol 6: Diseases of the Basal Ganglia. Amsterdam, North Holland, 1968; 173–211.

Sherrington CS: On the anatomical constitution of nerves of skeletal muscles; with remarks on recurrent fibres in the ventral spinal nerve-root. J Physiol 1894;17:211–258.

Sherrington CS: Decerebrate rigidity and reflex co-ordination of movement. J Physiol 1898;22:319–332.

Sherrington CS: On plastic tonus and proprioceptive reflexes. Q J Exp Physiol 1909;2:109–156.

Solimena M, Folli F, Denis-Donini S, et al: Autoantibodies to glutamic acid decarboxylase in a patient with stiff-man syndrome, epilepsy, and type I diabetes mellitus. N Engl J Med 1988;318:1012–1020.

Stephan DA, Buist NR, Chittenden AB, et al: A rippling muscle disease gene is localized to 1q41: Evidence for multiple genes. Neurology 1994;44:1915–1920.

Tatton WG, Lee RG: Evidence for abnormal long-loop reflexes in rigid Parkinsonian patients. Brain Res 1975;100:671–676.

Tempel LW, Perlmutter JS: Abnormal vibraton-induced cerebral blood flow responses in idiopathic dystonia. Brain 1990;113:691–707.

Teravainen H, Tsui JK, Mak E, et al: Optimal indices for testing parkinsonian rigidity. Can J Neurol Sci 1989;16:180–183.

Thilmann AF, Burke DJ, Rymer WZ: Spasticity: Mechanisms and Management. Berlin, Springer-Verlag, 1993.

Thompson JH: A wry-necked family. Lancet 1896;2:24.

Thompson PD: Stiff muscles. J Neurol Neurosurg Psychiat 1993;56:121–124.

Thornton C: The myotonic dystrophies. Semin Neurol 1999;19:25–33.

Waddy HM, Fletcher NA, Harding AE, et al: A genetic study of idiopathic focal dystonia. Ann Neurol 1991;29:320–324.

Walshe FMR: Observations on the nature of the muscluar rigidity of paralysis agitans, and on its relationship to tremor. Brain 1924;47:159–177.

Ward AA: The function of the basal ganglia. In Vinken PJ, Bruyn GW (eds): Handbook of Clinical Neurology, vol 6: Diseases of the Basal Ganglia. Amsterdam, North Holland, 1968; 90–115.

Watts RL, Wiegner AW, Young RR: Elastic properties of muscles measured at the elbow in man: II. Patients with Parkinsonian rigidity. J Neurol Neurosurg Psychiatry 1986;49:1177–1181.

Webster DD: Critical analysis of the disability in Parkinson's disease. Mod Treat 1968;5:257–282.

Wieger AW, Watts RL: Elastic properties of muscles measured at the elbow in man: I. Normal controls. J Neurol Neurosurg Psychiatry 1986;49:1171–1176.

Yap CB: Spinal segmental and long-loop reflexes on spinal motoneuron excitability in spasticity and rigidity. Brain 1967;90:887–896.

Zeman W, Dyken P: Dystonia musculorum deformans: Clinical, genetic and pathoanatomical studies. Psychiatr Neurol Neurochir 1967;70:77–121.

Recommended Reading

Mayer NH: Clinicophysiologic concepts of spasticity and motor dysfunction in adults with an upper motoneuron lesion. Muscle Nerve 1997;(suppl 6):S1–S13.

Thilmann AF, Burke DJ, Rymer WZ: Spasticity: Mechanisms and Management. Berlin, Springer-Verlag, 1993.

Botulinum Toxin Treatment

Richard M. Dubinsky

BOTULINUM TOXINS

Historical Perspective

In 1897, Van Ermengen reported the discovery of an anaerobic bacterium that was responsible for an outbreak of food-borne paralytic illness in Ellezelles, Belgium (Van Ermengen, 1897; Cherington, 1972). Twenty-three musicians became ill after performing at the funeral of another musician. They had all consumed sausage and ham that was served after the funeral. Three died from a paralytic illness, and the remaining 20 recovered. Van Ermengen was able to isolate the bacterium using the newly discovered anaerobic culture techniques and was able to reproduce the paralytic illness by injecting the toxin into laboratory animals. He named the bacterium *Bacillus botulinus* after *botulus,* the Latin term for "sausage."

Through education and public health interventions, there have been fewer cases of food-borne paralytic illness due to *Clostridium botulinum,* but rare cases of botulism still occur owing to improper home canning techniques. Years ago, *C. botulinum*

was investigated as a chemical and biological warfare agent. Through the efforts of Edward Schantz, Ph.D., and others at Camp Dietrick (later renamed Fort Dietrick), Maryland, the toxin was isolated and characterized. In the late 1960s, discussions between Dr. Schantz and Alan B. Scott, M.D., at the Smith-Kettlewell Eye Institute led to the first animal trials of botulinum toxin for the treatment of strabismus. In 1972, Fort Dietrick was closed and Dr. Schantz moved to the University of Wisconsin. In 1978, the Food and Drug Administration approved Dr. Scott's Investigational New Drug Application, and the first batch of botulinum toxin, strain A, was made in November 1979 in Dr. Schantz's laboratory. This initial lot of 150 g (79-11) was used for human trials and was the original lot approved by the Food and Drug Administration for the treatment of strabismus and facial movement disorders in December 1989 (Schantz, 1994).

Serotypes

There are eight clostridial neurotoxins: tetanus toxin, from *Clostridium tetanii,* and the seven serotypes of botulinum toxin (A, B, C, D, E, F, and G). Types A, B, E, and F have been used for clinical trials in humans. Collectively, the botulinum neurotoxins have been labeled with many different abbreviations. In this chapter, the convention BoNT is used for botulinum neurotoxins.

Botulinum progenitor toxins occur in three forms: M toxin (300 kDa), L toxin (500 kDa), and LL toxin (900 kDa) (Minton, 1995). The M toxin consists of the BoNT (150 kDa) in association with a nontoxic protein (150 kDa). The L and LL forms consists of the M form with additional proteins that have hemagglutin-like activity. All three forms are produced by type A *C. botulinum* cultures, whereas only the M and L forms are produced by types B, C, and D *C. botulinum* cultures. Types E and F produce only the M form. The progenitor toxin appears to protect the BoNT from high heat and from pH extremes.

Mechanism of Action

Proteolytic cleavage of the M form results in a light chain (50 kDa) and a heavy chain (900 kDa) joined by a disulfide bond (Halpern and Neale, 1995). The light chain is associated with an atom of zinc (DasGupta and Tepp, 1993; Schiavo et al., 1994). Three steps are involved in the paralytic action of BoNT: binding and internalization, release of the light chain, and blockade of the release of acetylcholine. The heavy chain promotes binding of the toxin to the presynaptic nerve terminal. Internalization occurs via endocytosis (DasGupta and Tepp, 1994) and is promoted by nerve stimulation (Hughes and Whaller, 1962) or activity (Eleopra et al., 1997; Chen et al., 1999). After internalization, the heavy chain promotes the opening of the endosomal vesicle and the release of the light chain. The light chain interferes with the release of acetylcholine, although the mechanism differs among the different types of BoNT. This process can take from several hours to several days before clinical effect is noticed.

Acetylcholine is manufactured in the presynaptic nerve terminal and stored in vesicles. The vesicles are linked to vesicle-associated membrane protein (VAMP), also known as synaptobrevin. This protein is used for the targeting of acetylcholine vesicles for eventual release (Benfenati and Valtorta, 1995). The 25-kDa synaptosomal-associated protein SNAP-25 and syntaxin are involved in the binding of the vesicle to the presynaptic membrane. Synaptotagmin is involved in the final step of release of acetylcholine through fusion of the vesicle to the presynaptic membrane, which is triggered by calcium influx, after membrane depolarization (Fig. 101–1).

VAMP/synaptobrevin is blocked by BoNT types B, D, F, and G. SNAP-25 is blocked by types A, D, and E, although at different sites. Type C blocks syntaxin (Schiavo et al., 1992; Huttner, 1993; Poulain et al., 1995) (Table 101–1).

The site of action of the toxin may have significant effect on the duration of induced weakness. Eleopra

and colleagues (1998) injected the extensor digitorum brevis muscles of volunteers with either BoNT A or E or a mixture of A and E. The compound muscle action potential was serially measured as a marker for recovery. Recovery was longest with injections with BoNT A; the recovery times from injection with either BoNT E or injection with a mixture of BoNT A and E were similar. Both BoNT A and E cleave SNAP-25 but at different sites, with E removing a larger portion of the protein. How the differential cleavage of SNAP-25 promotes faster recovery after type E BoNT is still unknown.

The effect of BoNT is temporary, lasting between 2 and 9 months. Nerve sprouting occurs within 2 days in mice, leading to reinnervation of isolated motor units (Pamphlett, 1989). In humans, the sprouting occurs at the nodes of Ranvier and at the nerve terminals (Holds et al., 1990; Alderson et al., 1991). In the clinical use of BoNT, the toxin induces weakness best when injected into the end-plate region of the muscle (Shaari and Sanders, 1993). The toxin does spread after injection, both within the target muscle and into adjacent muscles. In an animal model, Borodic and associates (1994) demonstrated spread of the toxin by up to 4.5 cm from the injection site.

The potency of the BoNT is measured in units (U), where 1 U is the LD_{50} equivalent for intraperitoneal injection into 18- to 20-g Swiss-Webster mice. However, the dose for human use varies greatly between the two commercially available preparations of type A—Botox and Dysport—and type B. The usual effective dose of BoNT A Botox for cervical dystonia is between 200 and 300 U, whereas that for BoNT A Dysport is 800 to 1000 U and that for BoNT B is 5,000 to 10,000 U (Brashear et al., 1999). The conversion ratio between Botox and Dysport is 1:3 (Odergren et al., 1998) or 1:4 (Sampaio et al., 1997).

The BoNT A LD_{50} for humans is calculated to be 3,000 U, on the basis of extrapolation of data from subhuman primate studies (Scott and Suzuki, 1988). The maximum recommended dose of BoNT A Botox is 300 U for injection during one session, with only one injection session in a 3-month period. Higher doses and more frequent dosing are associated with the development of resistance to the effects of BoNT. The maximum dose reported for the use of BoNT B (under development by Elan Pharmaceuticals) is 10,000 U.

Most persons develop weakness of the targeted muscles after an injection of BoNT. Those who do not are termed *primary nonresponders*. A *secondary nonresponder* is a person who has experienced benefit from two rounds of the same strain and preparation of BoNT and then fails to demonstrate clinical improvement or weakness after injection on two additional occasions. This is thought to be due to the development of antibodies to BoNT. However, of the different methods of measuring BoNT antibodies (mouse assay and enzyme-linked immunosorbent assay), none have very good clinical correlation with the response of BoNT. Subjects with cervical

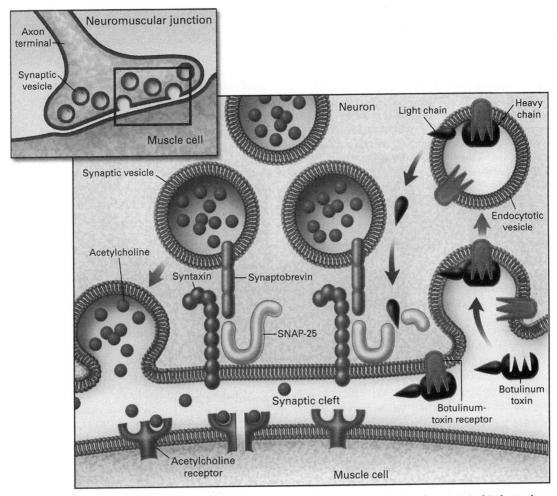

Figure 101–1. Mechanism of action of botulinum toxin. After intramuscular injection, the botulinum toxin binds to the presynaptic terminal and enters the cell via endocytosis. The disulfide bond linking the two botulinum toxin chains is broken, and the light chain is translocated out of the endocytotic vesicle into the cytoplasm. The process of exocytosis of acetylcholine is complicated, requiring the participation of many proteins, and each serotype of botulinum toxin works via enzymatic cleavage of one or more of these proteins. Botulinum toxins A, C, and E cleave the 25-kDa synaptosomal-associated protein SNAP-25; types B, D, F, and G cleave a synaptobrevin vesicle-associated membrane protein (VAMP); and type C cleaves syntaxin. Hence, acetylcholine cannot be released, and the muscle is paralyzed. The action of type A is shown here. (From Hallett M: One man's poison: Clinical application of botulinum toxin. N Engl J Med 1999;341:118–120. © Copyright 2000 Massachusetts Medical Society. All rights reserved.)

dystonia who are secondary nonresponders are reported to benefit from BoNT B injections, although the duration of benefit is shorter than that of patients treated de novo with BoNT B (Brashear et al., 1999; Brin et al., 1999).

Table 101–1. Site of Action of Botulinum Toxins

Serotype	Site of Action
A	SNAP-25
B	VAMP/synaptobrevin
C	Syntaxin
D	VAMP/synaptobrevin, SNAP-25
E	SNAP-25
F	VAMP/synaptobrevin
G	VAMP/synaptobrevin

SNAP, sensory nerve action potential; VAMP, vesicle-associated membrane protein.

Generalized weakness is rarely reported with clinical injections of BoNT. There are distant, subclinical effects of BoNT on the neuromuscular junction. Abnormal jitter, as determined by single-fiber EMG, has been found in forearm muscles after injection of BoNT into the orbicularis oculi muscle as part of the treatment of blepharospasm (Lange et al., 1991; Sanders et al., 1986).

Principles of Treatment Using Botulinum Neurotoxins

The use of BoNT as a treatment for disorders characterized by excessive contraction of skeletal or smooth muscle is relatively simple. Once the clinician is satisfied that the patient with the disorder will not respond to other treatments, careful observation is required to determine which muscles are involved. Often, the suspect muscles can be observed easily, such as the orbicularis oculi, buccinator, and mentalis muscles in hemifacial spasm, or the tibialis posterior in dystonic foot inversion. In other disorders, such as cervical dystonia or writer's cramp, detailed observation combined with a thorough knowledge of the muscular anatomy is required. For selected patients, kinesigenic electromyograms (Basmajian, 1973) with fine wire intramuscular electrodes are helpful in determining which muscles are involved in the abnormal movement (Cohen and Hallett, 1988).

There is a lack of agreement among clinicians whether electromyographic guidance is needed for the treatment of spasmodic dysphonia with BoNT and for limb dystonias, and it is controversial whether electromyographic guidance is needed for the use of BoNT for neck muscles. Some contend that electromyographic guidance is not necessary. In the one study that compared the two techniques, patients were randomized to receive injections with electromyographic guidance or based on clinical examination (Comella et al., 1992). The physicians who administered the injections were all well versed in the use of BoNT, and the evaluators were blinded. An increased magnitude of benefit was noted for patients who received electromyographically guided injections. In one short report by an experienced injector of BoNT in the treatment of cervical dystonia, initial needle placement was not always within the target muscles (Speelman and Brans, 1995). The authors found that the needle must be repositioned to reach the target muscle in 17% to 53% of the muscles in a series of 540 target muscles. The sternocleidomastoid muscle was most easily found (83%), followed by the trapezius (83%), scalenus medius (74%), splenius capitis (70%), semispinalis capitis (57%), and levator scapulae (47%) muscles. In another study, electromyography was found to be more accurate than physical examination in determining which muscles were active in patients with cervical dystonia (Brans et al., 1998). The spread of BoNT after injection (Borodic et al., 1994) may very well explain why the magnitude of the advantage of electromyographic guidance is not greater. Regardless of which view is correct, a thorough knowledge of the anatomy is required. Another concern is that muscle involvement may change after treatment with BoNT. When the movements have returned, other muscles may be involved (Buchman et al., 1993).

Adverse Events

Adverse events linked to the injection of BoNT are predominantly due to induced weakness of the targeted and adjacent muscles. Dysphagia, predominantly of sticky foods, occurs after the injection of BoNT for treatment of cervical dystonia in up to 29% of injected patients (Denislic et al., 1994). The rate of dysphagia is related to both the total dose

and the location of injections, although the frequency of dysphagia is less than originally reported. Dysphagia of thin liquids is reported after the use of BoNT in the treatment of spasmodic dysphonia. There have been only rare, anecdotal reports of generalized weakness after the injection of BoNT (Bhatia et al., 1999). In this study, three patients were described with generalized weakness after the injection of BoNT for treatment of torticollis (two patients) or hemidystonia (one patient). All had received prior injections of BoNT.

Inadvertent injection of BoNT into the brachial plexus has been reported (Glanzman et al., 1990). Dysesthesias and weakness of proximal arm muscles began 1½ days after the injection and were present for at least 5 months. BoNT type A was to be injected into the ipsilateral sternocleidomastoid and trapezius muscles, but it may have been injected into the brachial plexus. BoNT may have entered into the axons at the site of injection, or the cause of the weakness may have been mechanical disruption of the nerve trunks by the injection. It is imperative that when injecting BoNT, the clinician be certain of the placement of the tip of the needle. If a patient notices arm discomfort during injection of the lateral portion of the neck, either the needle is in the brachial plexus or the volume of toxin injectate in the scalenus medius or scalenus anterior muscle is compressing the brachial plexus.

Response and Loss of Benefit

Most patients have weakness after the injection of BoNT. The term *primary nonresponder* is used to refer to a patient in whom no weakness or denervation is induced by the injection of BoNT. The cause of the lack of response may be the dose, muscle selection, improper storage or preparation of BoNT, or prior immunization against BoNT. Some food workers and military personnel are immunized against BoNT using a toxoid of several different types of BoNT. The term *secondary nonresponder* refers to a patient in whom no weakness is induced by the injection of BoNT on two occasions, after having demonstrated weakness of injected muscles induced by BoNT on two prior occasions. This lack of response can be investigated through an antibody assay, mouse assay, or functional test. There is a lack of significant correlation between clinical response to BoNT and the presence of antibodies. The frequency of secondary nonresponders in several longitudinal cohort studies varies between 2% and 5% in cohorts of patients with cervical dystonia (Greene and Fahn, 1994; Mezaki et al., 1994; Kessler et al., 1999). Antibody formation was found in less than half of the clinical nonresponders (Zuber et al., 1993; Greene and Fahn, 1994; Kessler et al., 1999).

A commonly used functional test of BoNT response is to inject either the frontalis or the extensor digitorum brevis muscle on one side, reserving the other side as a control. Clinical inspection of the injected muscle is used to determine response or lack of response. The compound muscle action potential of the extensor digitorum brevis muscle can also be used to measure the effectiveness of the denervation from BoNT and the time course of recovery (Hamjian and Walker, 1994; Kessler et al., 1997). In a study in which this technique was used in normal volunteers, BoNT type A produced a longer lasting decrease in the M wave from the extensor digitorum brevis muscle than that obtained with BoNT type B (Sloop et al., 1997).

Loss of benefit from injections of BoNT type A is associated with the injection of more than 300 U at one time and with repeat injection at intervals of less than 3 months (Greene and Fahn, 1994; Borodic et al., 1996). However, one subject with writer's cramp developed a lack of response after receiving a total lifetime dose of BoNT type A of 140 U over a 7-month period (Cole et al., 1995).

APPLICATIONS

Strabismus

Nonsurgical treatment of strabismus was the goal of Alan Scott when he began to look at neurotoxins to alter the balance of the extraocular muscles. Traditional therapies for strabismus included muscle recession surgery to weaken the muscle, muscle resection surgery to strengthen the muscle, and the use of prisms to correct the double vision. Injection of BoNT into the extraocular muscles is performed with a hollow Teflon-coated electromyogram needle. Local or general anesthesia must be used. This technique should be performed only by trained ophthalmologists who have immediate access to the proper treatment if the globe should be punctured.

In a comparison of injection with BoNT versus repeat operation in 47 children with prior strabismus surgery, 24 were randomized to reoperation and 23 were randomized to injection with BoNT (Tejedor et al., 1998). At 1 year after treatment and at the end of follow-up (mean, 2.7 years), both groups had equal benefit in reduction of strabismus to less than 8 prism diopters. In acute sixth nerve palsies, injection of the antagonist muscle with BoNT resulted in eventual full recovery in 22 of 31 patients versus 16 of 52 control subjects (Metz and Mazow, 1988). Patients with bilateral acquired sixth nerve palsy had a poorer outcome than that in patients with unilateral sixth nerve palsy.

Dystonias

The primary clinical application of BoNT in the treatment of nervous system disorders is for dystonia. Dystonia is characterized by excessive co-contraction of antagonist muscle pairs, resulting in abnormal tone or posture (Fahn, 1988). This disorder is predominantly one of action. When the affected

Table 101–2. Types of Dystonia

Type	Description
Blepharospasm	Contraction of orbicularis oculi and other upper facial muscles
Meige's syndrome	Contraction of lower facial muscles; may result in jaw clenching, jaw opening, lip pursing, and other lower facial movements
Spasmodic dysphonia	Laryngeal muscles
Torticollis	Co-contraction of neck muscles, resulting in abnormal head and neck posture
Brachial dystonia	Involvement of the proximal arm and neck muscles
Focal limb dystonia	Involvement of arm muscles (writer's and musician's cramp) or of lower leg muscles (dystonic foot inversion)
Hemidystonia	Involvement of arm and leg
Generalized dystonia	Involvement of facial, truncal, and limb muscles
Multifocal dystonia	Two noncontiguous body parts involved

body part is at rest, the movement lessens or dissipates. Dystonia is usually characterized by the portion of the body that is involved (Table 101–2). Some dystonias are task dependent, as in organic writer's cramp, musician's cramp, and typist's cramp (Cohen and Hallett, 1988) (see Chapter 100).

BLEPHAROSPASM

Historically blepharospasm was the first form of dystonia to be treated with BoNT A (Frueh et al., 1984). Blepharospasm is characterized by an increased blink rate and sustained forceful closure of the eyelids. This is distinctly different than the myotonic contraction of myotonic muscular dystrophy or the apraxia of eyelid opening described in parkinsonian syndromes. Blepharospasm is due to contraction of the orbicularis oculi, corrugator supercilii, and procerus muscles. The typical age at onset is in the fifth decade but can be from the second decade on. The blinking can be in reaction to bright or flickering lights. Blepharospasm can be so severe that the person becomes functionally blind. As with most focal dystonias, sensory or proprioceptive tricks can be used to lessen the severity of the blepharospasm. The tricks include talking, singing, humming, and placing a finger at the outer canthus. From a physiological aspect, there is increased excitability of the blink reflex that does not change after the injection of BoNT (Valls-Sole et al., 1991).

The orbicularis oculi muscle is a circular muscle that, when activated, closes the eyelids. The facial portion is used for forceful closure. Thin strips of the muscle in the eyelid, in front of the tarsal plate and just above the eyelash margin, work to close the eyelid for blinking and for sleep. In blepharospasm, the corrugator supercilii and procerus muscles are also involved, resulting in a frowning appearance and a deep dermal crease just over the glabella. Induction of weakness in the orbicularis oculi, corrugator supercilii, and procerus muscles lessens the involuntary blinking of blepharospasm (Jankovic and Orman, 1987; Jankovic, 1988). Earlier studies with the injection of BoNT into the upper portion of the eyelid resulted in ptosis; this can be avoided by injecting 2 to 4 mm above the eyelashes in the inner and outer canthus of the eyelid. Although the inferior portion of the orbicularis oculi is involved in blepharospasm, excessive weakness of this muscle can lead to exposure keratitis of the inferior cornea. Typical doses for the treatment of blepharospasm with BoNT are 40 U of Botox and 120 to 160 U Dysport. The dose is usually distributed in several locations throughout the orbicularis oculi muscle. Careful observation is required in determining which muscles to inject and the dose to be injected. If the amount of BoNT injected into the pretarsal portion of the orbicularis oculi is excessive or if it is injected close to the center, where the levator palpebrae attaches to the tarsal plate, ptosis will occur. Diplopia can occur if the toxin spreads from the procerus and corrugator supercilii muscles to the superior oblique muscle at the trochlea.

BoNT F has been shown to be of benefit for patients who are refractory to BoNT A, although the duration of benefit was shorter (Mezaki et al., 1995). In this double-blind parallel study, the combination of BoNT A and BoNT F proved to be no different than the injection of either agent into the control eyelid muscles.

MEIGE'S SYNDROME

Meige's syndrome, or oromandibular dystonia, is in many ways an extension of blepharospasm. The syndrome consists of lower facial dystonic movements, either alone, or in combination with blepharospasm, spasmodic dysphonia, or both. The lower facial movements can be excessive jaw opening, jaw clenching or bruxism, lip pursing, grimacing, and lingual involvement (Jankovic, 1988). The lower facial movements are in many ways similar to those of tardive dyskinesia and cause significant embarrassment to the patient. The lingual movements can be severe enough to interfere with speech and swallowing. There is a variable response of Meige's syndrome to oral medications.

Jaw clenching can be alleviated by injections of BoNT into the masseter and temporalis muscles (Jankovic and Orman, 1987). From 25 to 50 U of BoNT, type A (Botox), will cause sufficient weakness of the masseter muscles to lessen jaw clenching. Excessive jaw opening responds to the injection of BoNT into the anterior belly of the digastric and the lateral pterygoid muscles. BoNT can spread from the lateral pterygoid muscle, around the pterygoid plate to the muscles of the pharynx, resulting in significant dysphagia. Lingual dyskinesias also have a variable response to denervation with BoNT, with

a substantial risk of dysphagia (Jankovic and Orman, 1987).

SPASMODIC DYSPHONIA

Spasmodic dysphonia is a disturbance of the control of the vocal apparatus. The two major types are adductor and abductor spasmodic dysphonia (Ludlow, 1990; Van Pelt et al., 1994). In the adductor type, there is inappropriate adduction of the vocal cord during phonation. This results in a strangled voice with frequent phonatory breaks after consonants and at the end of words. In the abductor type, there is inappropriate abduction of the vocal cords. This results in a whispery voice with cessation of phonation midway through vocalization. There also is a mixed type, with features of both adductor and abductor spasmodic dysphonia. Videofluoroscopy is frequently used to characterize the type of spasmodic dysphonia and to exclude other causes of abnormal vocalization. Spasmodic dysphonia can occur as a feature of generalized dystonia, as an isolated dystonia, or in conjunction with Meige's syndrome (Marsden and Sheehy, 1982).

In a larger series of patients with spasmodic dysphonia, 90% had the adductor type and 10% had abductor spasmodic dysphonia (Blitzer et al., 1998). Injections of BoNT into the thyroarytenoid for adductor spasmodic dysphonia result in a return to a near-normal voice, whereas injections into the posterior cricoarytenoid for abductor spasmodic dysphonia are beneficial but not to such an extent as in adductor dysphonia (Blitzer et al., 1998). Unlike in writer's cramp, vocalization for 30 minutes after injection of BoNT is associated with a lessened benefit compared with vocal rest for 30 minutes (Wong, 1995).

After injection with BoNT for adductor spasmodic dysphonia, many patients have a breathy voice that persists for 1 to 3 weeks. This is followed by a return to near-normal speech patterns for 12 to 16 weeks and eventual return to the original vocal pattern (Ludlow, 1990). The most common serious adverse event after injection of BoNT for spasmodic dysphonia is dysphagia for thin liquids (Holzer and Ludlow, 1996).

CERVICAL DYSTONIA

Cervical dystonia, or torticollis, usually has onset from the third decade on. It is characterized by involuntary neck turning or tilting, or both. Besides rotation of the head and neck, there may be sagittal displacement either anteriorly (anterocollis) or posteriorly (retrocollis). The neck can be shifted toward the side or toward the front, resulting in a swan neck appearance, Like all dystonias, cervical dystonia is almost exclusively manifested when the neck muscles are active in holding up the head. If the head is supported by a chair or by the subject's hand, the abnormal movements are easily overcome. This sensory trick, or geste antagoniste, lessens the excessive muscle activity (Leis et al., 1992; Buchman et al., 1998). Most cases of cervical dystonia are idiopathic. Secondary causes include tardive dystonias (Calne and Lang, 1988) and trauma, either to the central nervous system (Isaac and Cohen, 1989; Jankovic, 1994) or to the neck (Truong et al., 1991).

The magnitude of abnormal neck posture varies greatly among patients but is usually consistent for the same patient. Patients rarely have just one direction or movement. Most have combinations of rotation and tilt. As in the use of BoNT for any treatment, it is imperative that the clinician have a thorough knowledge of the muscular anatomy of the neck and the actions of the neck muscles (Clemente, 1985; Dubinsky, 1994). Most of the neck muscles have more than one action. For example, the sternocleidomastoid rotates the head to the opposite side while tilting the head to the same side. Together, both sternocleidomastoid muscles flex the head and the neck. Multiple muscles innervated by both the spinal accessory and the cervical nerve roots are involved in cervical dystonia. Multichannel surface electromyographic recordings published more than 40 years ago demonstrated the co-contraction of the ipsilateral (to the direction of rotation) splenius capitus and the contralateral sternocleidomastoid and trapezius muscles (Hertz and Hoeffer, 1949; Tournay and Paillard, 1955; Podivinsky, 1968). These studies were limited to superficial muscles. With the use of fine wire intramuscular recordings (Basmajian, 1973), a wider range of muscle involvement has been demonstrated (Vasin et al., 1988; Thompson et al., 1990; Dubinsky, 1994). Over time, the muscles involved and the direction of the cervical dystonia can change (Buchman et al., 1993; Brans et al., 1998). After a beneficial response to BoNT, many patients are found to have involvement of previously uninvolved muscles, whereas those previously injected were not active, although there was clinical evidence of the wearing off of the chemodenervation.

Muscles involved in neck rotation include the contralateral sternocleidomastoid, trapezius, ipsilateral splenius capitis, oblique capitis inferior, rectus capitis posterior major, and multifidus muscles. Bilateral sternocleidomastoid, longus capitis, scalenus medii, and scalenus anterior muscles are involved in anteroflexion of the neck. The longus capitis muscle cannot be injected easily, and attempts to inject this muscle are often complicated by severe dysphagia. Tilting of the neck involves the scalenus medius, semispinalis capitis, longissimis capitis, and levator scapulae. Retroflexion of the neck involves the bilateral splenius capitis, semispinalis capitis, longissimus capitis, and rectus capitis posterior major muscles. Although the trapezii can be involved in voluntary retroflexion, they are seldom, if ever, involved in retrocollis (personal observation). Shoulder elevation is frequently present in cervical dystonia and can be caused by contraction of the ipsilateral trapezius, scalenus medius, and levator scapulae muscles.

Several different scales have been developed for the assessment of cervical dystonia; these include the Marsden and Fahn scale (Marsden, 1988), a scale developed by Tsui (1986), and the Toronto Western Spasmodic Torticollis Scale (Comella, 1997). Of these, the Toronto Western Spasmodic Torticollis Scale is most commonly used. It consists of an observational portion for movement and a self-reported disability scale that examines how the torticollis affects the subject's life.

BoNT types A, B, and F have been used in the treatment of torticollis. Typical total doses used for the treatment of cervical dystonia are between 120 and 300 U (Tsui, 1988; Dubinsky et al., 1991; Jankovic and Brin, 1991) for type A, between 5,000 and 10,000 U (Brashear et al., 1999; Brin et al., 1999) for type B, and 250 U (Greene and Fahn, 1993; Sheean and Lees, 1995) for type F. The duration of benefit is around 20 weeks for type A (Tsui, 1988; Dubinsky et al., 1991; Jankovic and Brin, 1991), 12 to 16 weeks for type B (Brin et al., 1999), and 4 weeks for type F (Greene and Fahn, 1993; Sheean and Lees, 1995). Initially, BoNT was distributed throughout the muscle in small amounts in multiple sites (Jankovic and Orman, 1987; Tsui, 1988; Koller et al., 1990). Based on concern about the development of resistance to BoNT (Greene and Fahn, 1994) and the evidence that BoNT spreads several centimeters from a single injection site (Borodic et al., 1994), current practice is to limit the injections to one or two sites per muscle.

Common side effects of the treatment of cervical dystonia with BoNT are neck extensor weakness, muscle pain, and dysphagia. Neck extensor weakness is an extension of the desired benefit of BoNT, because the neck extensors are involved in neck rotation. Although the rare patient has an increase in neck discomfort after the injection of BoNT, the amount of pain relief was significantly better than the decrease in the severity of neck movement reported in the early studies of BoNT (Tsui, 1986; Comella et al., 1992). Some patients develop muscle aching after the development of neck extensor weakness; this is from the added workload to the other neck extensor muscles after the weakness is induced by BoNT in the targeted and adjacent muscles. Dysphagia occurred in 4% to 22% of cervical dystonia patients after the injection of BoNT (Tsui, 1986; Comella et al., 1992; Kessler et al., 1999).

WRITER'S CRAMP

Writer's cramp involves one of a group of focal limb dystonias and is action specific. Other types include musician's and typist's cramps (Calne, 1988; Lederman, 1994). At initial presentation, the involuntary movement is limited to the involved task, but not for others. A musician may have dystonic movements while playing the flute but not while playing a piano. In most cases, the focal dystonia is associated with overuse of the limb (Chen and Hallett, 1998). The involved muscles can be determined through close observation and by the use of fine wire intramuscular recordings (Cohen and Hallett, 1988). The benefit of BoNT in the treatment of writer's cramp has been proved in a double-blind placebo-controlled study (Cole et al., 1995). In the case of simple wrist flexion, the flexor carpi radialis and flexor carpi ulnaris are involved. In more complex cases with extension of some fingers, flexion of others, and movement of the wrist, intramuscular recording may be the only way to determine which muscles are involved. In either case, the patient must first be instructed to avoid using any sensory tricks or voluntary co-contraction to lessen the cramp. Alleviation of the dystonia in the first muscle to be involved in the cramp may prevent the cramp from occurring entirely (Chen and Hallett, 1998). In this form of dystonia, more so than in the others, functional weakness is needed to achieve improvement of the dystonic movement. In a person who has involuntary fisting while writing, weakness of grip strength may be needed to achieve facility while writing. Use of the limb after injection will potentiate the weakness induced by BoNT. This may eventually allow the reduction in the dose of BoNT (Chen et al., 1999).

LIMB DYSTONIA

Involuntary foot inversion is the first manifestation of juvenile-onset generalized dystonia (Fahn, 1988). This movement can also be the result of a stroke or traumatic brain injury. Denervation with BoNT of the posterior tibialis muscle decreases the tendency for the foot to invert (Reiter et al., 1998). Spread of BoNT to the tibialis anterior muscle will cause foot drop. In patients with poststroke hemidystonia, there may be underlying weakness of the tibialis anterior that is masked by the dystonic foot inversion. This form of focal limb dystonia must also be distinguished from the fixed foot position, due to contracture, that is seen in complex regional pain syndrome (Bhatia et al., 1993).

TRUNCAL DYSTONIA

Truncal extensor dystonia is difficult to treat using oral medications. In a study of five patients, benefit was found from the injection of 25 to 50 U of BoNT type A (Botox) into the lumbar and thoracic paraspinal muscles (Comella et al., 1998).

Hemifacial Spasm

Hemifacial spasm is characterized by irregular, involuntary contraction of muscles innervated by the facial nerve. Typically, the orbicularis oculi, buccinator, and mentalis muscles are involved. Onset is from the fourth decade on. Hemifacial spasm is usually associated with compression of the facial nerve by an ectatic basilar artery or branch of the basilar artery. Rarely, hemifacial spasm is caused by compression by a posterior fossa mass. Microvascular

decompression of the facial nerve can result in complete resolution of hemifacial spasm, but there is a small risk of deafness and facial weakness (McLaughlin et al., 1999). Ephaptic conduction can be demonstrated between the branches of the facial nerve (Geller et al., 1989). Like blepharospasm, the involuntary blinking can be triggered by external stimuli such as a bright flickering light, but hemifacial spasm does not improve with the use of sensory tricks. Hemifacial spasm persists in sleep, whereas blepharospasm, like most dystonias, does not. This disorder is almost exclusively unilateral, although rare bilateral cases due to extremely tortuous vertebrobasilar arteries have been reported (Tan and Jankovic, 1999).

Injection of the orbicularis oculi for the treatment of hemifacial spasm is similar to that for blepharospasm. The procerus and corrugator supercilii muscles are rarely involved in hemifacial spasm. The buccinator muscle is located at the corner of the mandible and inserts into the corner of the mouth. This band-like muscle can be easily palpated in the cheek. Although the levator labialis and zygomaticus muscles are often involved in hemifacial spasm (Geller et al., 1989), inducing weakness in these muscles with BoNT can cause drooping of the lip or the cheek. This would cause an appearance similar to that due to facial weakness after a cerebrovascular accident. Improvement in hemifacial spasm is reported in up to 97% of patients in large, longitudinal studies (Jitpimolmard et al., 1998).

Spasticity

Spasticity is operationally defined as the velocity-dependent increase in tone in response to muscle stretch. From a physiological standpoint, there is diminished supraspinal inhibition of the alpha and gamma motoneurons (please see Chapter 109).

In an electrophysiological comparison of the effects of denervation with phenol versus BoNT, it was found that phenol predominantly affects the alpha motoneuron, whereas BoNT primarily affects the fusimotor system and the muscle spindles (On et al., 1999). In the patients who underwent tibial nerve blockade with phenol, the M response had the greater decrease, whereas those who received BoNT A had a greater decrease in the response to tendon tap and in the ratio of tendon tap to H reflex. The authors concluded that BoNT acted on the fusimotor system, whereas phenol blocked the alpha motoneuron. Both induce weakness and decrease the tone in spasticity, but they act through different mechanisms. In a study of reciprocal inhibition in patients with upper limb spasticity after a stroke, there was no difference in the two phases of reciprocal inhibition after the use of BoNT, showing that the effect was peripheral and not central (Girlanda et al., 1997).

UPPER LIMB

In open-label studies (Dunne et al., 1995) and in double-blind studies (Simpson et al., 1996), injection of BoNT A has been found to reduce the tone in spastic upper limbs. Typical muscles injected are the biceps, brachioradialis, and wrist flexors. Several dosage paradigms have been tried. Improved benefit is reported when 300 U of BoNT A (Botox) is used compared with lower doses (Simpson et al., 1996).

LOWER LIMB

Early studies of BoNT for lower limb spasticity focused on hip adduction. Denervation of the hip adductor group resulted in increased ease of hygiene in patients with severe lower limb spasticity in both open-label (Borg-Stein et al., 1993; Calne, 1993) and double-blind studies (Snow et al., 1990). Studies have concentrated on the treatment of increased tone in the gastrocnemius and soleus muscles in both adults and children (Heinen et al., 1997; Viriyavejakul et al., 1998; Wissel et al., 1999; Wong, 1998). In adults, treatment instituted soon after the onset of spasticity yields a greater degree of improvement compared with that obtained with treatment started for long-standing spasticity (Burbaud et al., 1996). It is not clear whether this is a direct effect of BoNT combined with physical therapy, coincident with a rapid improvement in clinical status, or is due to muscle shortening and fibrosis.

DETRUSOR-SPHINCTER DYSSYNERGIA

Detrusor-sphincter dyssynergia is the involuntary contraction of the internal urethral sphincter during contraction of the detrusor muscle; this usually occurs as a result of high spinal cord lesions. If the condition is left untreated, hydronephrosis can develop, but chronic indwelling catheters carry a significant risk of urinary tract infection. Open studies of BoNT have shown that when toxin is injected into the urethral sphincter by a transperineal approach, voiding problems are decreased (Gallien, 1998). In a double-blind, placebo-controlled study, BoNT A was found to significantly reduce urethral pressure, pressure during voiding, and postvoid residual in men with high spinal cord lesions (Dykstra and Sidi, 1990).

Other Hypertonic Disorders

Benefit has been reported in one patient for the alleviation of dystonic neck stiffness in progressive supranuclear palsy and in the paraspinal muscles of a subject with stiff person syndrome (Davis and Jabbari, 1993; Polo et al., 1994).

Tremor

Clinically evident tremor disorders are caused by rhythmical contraction of the limb muscles in one of three patterns: co-contraction of agonist/antagonist pairs, alternating contraction of agonist/antagonist pairs, or contraction of the agonist muscles (Deuschl et al., 1987). With any of these mechanisms as the underlying physiology, it appears that treatment with BoNT would readily be of benefit for tremor disorders. However, the magnitude of benefit is not as great as that in the dystonias. Subjective improvement, but not objective improvement, was reported when BoNT A was used for head nodding tremor (Pahwa et al., 1995; Wissel et al., 1997). A single-center, double-blind placebo-controlled study reported improvement in hand tremor when BoNT was injected into the wrist flexors and extensors (Jankovic et al., 1996). A multicenter study, using the same treatment paradigm for a double-blind, placebo-controlled study, reported only slight subjective benefit and no objective benefit (Koller, 1999).

Myokymia, Muscle Hypertrophy, and Muscle Cramps

Myokymia is a rare cause of painless muscle twitching that can result in muscle hypertrophy. Two cases of unilateral tibialis anterior hypertrophy secondary to focal myokymia have been reported (Nix et al., 1992). Both patients improved after the injection of BoNT.

Two small studies reported decreased masseter hypertrophy in patients after the injection of BoNT (Moore and Wood, 1994; Smyth, 1994). The benefit lasted at least 6 months and was not associated with difficulties with mastication. Bertolasi and associates (1997) reported improvement in subjects with the benign cramp fasciculation syndrome. Not only did the painful cramps of their subjects abate, but the ability to induce cramp by rapid electrical stimulation was decreased as well.

Myoclonus

Myoclonus is an extremely rapid contraction of skeletal muscle, faster than can be achieved with volitional muscle activation, yet the difference cannot be appreciated by eye (Hallett, 1983). The origin can be from the cortex, brain stem, or spinal cord. Often, myoclonus is refractive to therapy with oral medications. An initial study reported benefit for myoclonus due to a spinal cord infarct (Polo et al., 1994). In an open-label study of BoNT A in patients with myoclonus refractory to oral medications, benefit was reported in eight of the nine patients, with reduction in painful myoclonus and improvement in functional skills (Awaad et al., 1999). The dose of Dysport ranged from 8 to 20 U/kg in seven patients and from 32 to 45 U in two patients. The injections were repeated every 4 to 8 months, with preserved benefit in eight subjects.

Tourette's Syndrome

The motor and vocal tics of Tourette's syndrome constantly change, typically being present for 4 to 6 weeks. This would seem to prevent benefit from the use of BoNT. However, several studies have shown lessening of the severity of the motor tics after the injection of BoNT A, either alone or in combination with the use of oral baclofen (Jankovic, 1994; Poungvarin et al., 1995; Awaad et al., 1999). Vocal tics and coprolalia also diminish after the injection of BoNT A. Severe coprolalia improved after injections of the vocal cord (Scott et al., 1996), and vocal tics and coprolalia improved after injections of the thyroarytenoid (Salloway et al., 1996; Trimble et al., 1998). In a report by Trimble and colleagues, the decrease in vocal volume allowed the affected patient to blend the utterance into other words. He did not report a lessening of the sensory premonition, stating that the feeling was in his brain. The reports of Scott (1996) and Salloway (1996) and their associates noted a decrease in the premonitory sensation as well as a decrease in the vocal tics.

Palatal Tremor

Formerly known as *palatal myoclonus,* palatal tremor is a rhythmical contraction of the muscles of the soft palate, Usually, this occurs at a frequency between 40 and 200 times per minute. The tremor can spread to other structures innervated by the brain stem and upper spinal cord (Dubinsky, 1988). Palatal tremor can be divided into two types: symptomatic palatal tremor, associated with brain stem or cerebellar pathology, and essential palatal tremor (Deuschl et al., 1994a, 1994b). The palatal tremor in and of itself is not bothersome to the patient. Many patients with essential palatal tremor have an associated ear click. The click is heard by the patient and can be heard by an examiner listening closely to the patient's auditory meatus. The click is synchronous with the palatal tremor and is due to contraction of the tensor veli palatini muscle, which rapidly opens the eustachian tube, causing the click (Deuschl, 1991). Therapy of palatal tremor has been successful with the injection of BoNT into the tensor veli palatini muscle either using a transpalatal approach or under fiberoptic guidance with an intranasal approach (Deuschl et al., 1994). The doses of BoNT A used have been between 17 U of Dysport and 25 U of Botox (Deuschl et al., 1991).

Gastrointestinal Disorders

ACHALASIA

Achalasia is delayed emptying of the esophagus due to contraction of the lower esophageal sphincter. The contraction may be mechanical or may be due to excessive contraction of the sphincter. In a randomized, controlled trial of BoNT, pneumatic dilatation (the usual treatment), and placebo, the greatest improvement was noted in the pneumatic dilatation group, whereas the BoNT-treated group had significant improvement as measured by intrasphincteric pressure, and esophageal emptying compared with placebo injection (Annese et al., 1996). In a comparison of injection of BoNT versus pneumatic dilatation, the usual treatment of achalasia, pneumatic dilatation was found to be associated with a greater rate of improvement after 1 year of therapy (Vaezi et al., 1999). However, endoscopic injection of BoNT into the esophageal sphincter may be the preferred treatment in older patients (Wehrmann et al., 1999).

SPHINCTER OF ODDI SPASM

Spasm of the sphincter of Oddi causes severe abdominal pain owing to biliary obstruction, without evidence of mechanical obstruction. Endoscopic manometry demonstrates increased intersphincteric pressure. In an open-label study of 22 patients, injection of 100 U of BoNT into the papilla of Vater provided relief that lasted an average of 6 months (Wehrmann et al., 1998). The only complication occurred in a patient who developed pancreatitis after the injection.

ANISMUS

Anismus is an unusual condition characterized by contraction, instead of relaxation, of the external anal sphincter and the puborectalis portion of the levator ani during defecation. Patients with this condition rely on laxatives and other exogenous methods to assist in defecation. BoNT has been tried in open-label pilot studies. From 10 to 15 U of BoNT A was injected into either the external anal sphincter or the puborectalis muscle. Benefit lasted from 3 months to 1 year in patients who were resistant to biofeedback, the usual mode of therapy (Joo et al., 1996).

ANAL FISSURE

Chronic anal fissure is associated with increased contraction of the anal sphincters, with resultant increased anal pressure at rest. Traditional therapy has been to decrease the anal pressure by severing a portion of the fibers of the internal or external anal sphincter. Fecal incontinence can be avoided by preserving the pubococcygeus and puborectalis portions of the levator ani muscle and a portion of one of the sphincters. BoNT, instead of surgery, has been used to weaken the anal sphincter. Total doses have varied from 10 to 20 U of BoNT A (Botox). In a double-blind, placebo-controlled study, 20 U of BoNT A injected into the internal anal sphincter resulted in healing of the anal fissure in 8 of 10 BoNT-treated subjects and a decrease in the anal pressure by 25% in the treated group (Maria et al., 1998). In a follow-up study, the same group reported an increased improvement rate for a dose of 25 U versus a dose of 20 U (Maria et al., 1998). Repeat injections in patients who failed to have complete healing of the fissure are also of benefit (Jost and Schrank, 1999).

Cosmetic Concerns

Excessive contraction of facial muscles, either from involuntary movement disorders such as blepharospasm or from habit, can result in dermal creases. The furrowing of the brow associated with contraction of the procerus and corrugator supercilii muscles yields a facial expression interpretable as anger, whereas the sharp horizontal forehead lines due to excessive frontalis contraction can give the appearance of anger. The excessive contraction is termed *hyperfunctional animation* when dystonia is not present as an underlying disorder (Ellis and Tan, 1997; Ellis et al., 1997). In many open-label studies, the injection of BoNT has decreased or eliminated dermal creases associated with hyperfunctional animation of the frontalis, lateral orbicularis oculi, procerus, and corrugator supercilii muscles (Lowe et al., 1996). In a double-blind, placebo-controlled study of 11 patients, 9 had a significant decrease in the facial wrinkling on the injected side, compared with baseline and with the placebo-injected side (Keen et al., 1994).

Headache Disorders

During the initial use of BoNT for the cosmetic treatment of hypertrophic frown lines, several patients anecdotally reported improvement in their migraine headaches. Based on these reports, trials were undertaken to test the hypothesis that weakness induced by BoNT would reduce the severity of headache disorders.

CHRONIC DAILY HEADACHE

Injection of BoNT into the temporalis and frontalis muscles has been reported to lessen the duration and severity of muscle tension headaches in patients who were refractory to other treatment modalities (Wheeler, 1998).

MIGRAINE

In an open-label study of BoNT for migraine headaches, injection of BoNT into the glabella, temporalis, corrugator, and occipital muscles resulted in partial or complete improvement in 77% of 96 subjects (Binder et al., 1998). In a double-blind placebo (vehicle)-controlled study, a dose of 25 U of BoNT A significantly reduced the severity and frequency of migraine headaches compared with a dose of 75 U and with placebo (Silberstein et al., 2000).

Myofascial Pain Syndrome

The pathophysiology of myofascial pain syndrome is poorly understood. Clinically, there is muscle tenderness, with the presence of trigger points, which are focal spots of increased tenderness. Often, this disorder occurs after peripheral trauma or with overuse of the muscle. From an electromyographic standpoint, the painful muscles are electrically silent at rest. The hypothesis that forced resting of a painful muscle using BoNT can reduce the pain of myofascial pain syndrome has been tested in several studies. In an initial double-blind, placebo-controlled, randomized, crossover study of six patients, four experienced at least a 30% decrease in their pain (Cheshire et al., 1994).

In a double-blind, placebo-controlled, pilot study of BoNT in cervicothoracic myofascial pain, comparison was made between doses of 50 and 100 U of BoNT A and placebo. Thirty-three patients were studied who had myofascial pain resistant to medical therapy. All three groups had significant improvement over the course of the study, compared with baseline, but none of the treatments had a significant benefit over the others (Wheeler, 1998).

Temporomandibular Joint Disorder

Temporomandibular joint disorder is a painful dental condition consisting of crepitus with movement of the jaw, pain at the temporomandibular joint, and limitation of jaw opening. In an open-label study of 15 patients, injection of BoNT was found to be of benefit in reducing the pain, tenderness of the temporomandibular joint, frequency of jaw opening, but not bite force (Freund et al., 1999). In this study, 50 U was injected into each masseter muscle and 25 U was injected into each temporalis muscle. No adverse effects were reported.

Hyperhidrosis

Sweat glands consist of a secretory coil connected to the skin by a duct. The apocrine and eccrine glands are the two types of sweat glands. The eccrine glands are distributed throughout the skin and are used for thermoregulation. They provide moisture to the fingertips, which is required for fine dexterity. The eccrine glands are innervated by postganglionic cholinergic sympathetic neurons. The apocrine glands are located in the axillae and in the perianal regions, are active after puberty, and are under adrenergic control. The eccrine glands are involved in hyperhidrosis. The average density of eccrine glands is 60/cm^2, but in the palms and soles the density is increased to 600/cm^2 (Sato, 1997).

Hyperhidrosis usually occurs in the second and third decades of life. Approximately half of the cases are familial. The amount of sweat production can vary greatly among patients. The excessive sweat leads to social embarrassment and isolation. Hyperhidrosis has been defined clinically as the production of 50 mg per minute, or more, of sweat from one palm or axilla (Naumann et al., 1999).

The first human trial of BoNT to diminish sweating in humans was performed in 1994. Sweating was abolished in the axillae and on the dorsum of the hand for up to 11 months after injection in normal volunteers (Bushara and Park, 1994). Several open-label (Naver and Aquilonius, 1997; Naumann, 1998; Shelley et al., 1998) and a double-blind controlled study (Schnider, 1997) have demonstrated the efficacy of injections of small amounts in BoNT A in the treatment of palmar and axillary hyperhidrosis. In these studies, total doses of 40 to 78 U of BoNT A (Botox) were injected subcutaneously on a grid over the affected region. Decreased sweating lasted between 4 and 12 months. The discomfort of palmar injections can be lessened with ulnar and median nerve blocks. Several subjects had transient hand weakness that resolved well before the return of hyperhidrosis.

Gustatory sweating is an unusual form of autonomic nervous system disorder that can occur after parotid gland surgery. The area of hyperhidrosis is usually on the face. Injection of BoNT at 1 to 2 U/ 2.25 cm^2 was reported to be of benefit in 45 patients, with half having complete resolution and the other half reporting a substantial decrease in gustatory sweating (Naumann et al., 1997).

CONCLUSION

BoNT is a potent inhibitor of the release of acetylcholine at the neuromuscular junction and at the postganglionic cholinergic sympathetic nerve endings. It is useful in the treatment of wide range of neurological disorders characterized by excessive muscle contraction, either involuntary or voluntary. Future uses of BoNT may include the use of hybrids toxins, combining the heavy chain, which is specific for binding to the presynaptic nerve terminal, and other toxins, which then can be delivered to the nerve terminal or even delivered to the axon through retrograde transport.

References

Alderson K, Holds JB, Anderson RL: Botulinum-induced alteration of nerve-muscle interactions in the human orbicularis oculi following treatment for blepharospasm. Neurology 1991;41: 1800–1805.

Annese V, Basciani M, Perri F, et al: Controlled trial of botulinum toxin injection versus placebo and pneumatic dilation in achalasia. Gastroenterology 1996;111:1418–1424.

Awaad Y: Tics in Tourette syndrome: New treatment options. J Child Neurol 1999;14:316–319.

Awaad Y, Tayem H, Elgamal A, Coyne MF: Treatment of childhood myoclonus with botulinum toxin type A. J Child Neurol 1999; 14:781–786.

Basmajian JV: Electrodes and electrode connectors. In Desmedt JE (ed): New Developments in EMG and Clinical Neurophysiology. Basel, Karger, 1973; 502–510.

Benfenati F, Valtorta F: Neuroexocytosis. Curr Top Microbiol Immunol 1995;195:195–219.

Bertolasi L, Priori A, Tomelleri G, et al: Botulinum toxin treatment of muscle cramps: A clinical and neurophysiological study. Ann Neurol 1997;41:181–186.

Bhatia KP, Bhatt MH, Marsden CD: The causalgia-dystonia syndrome. Brain 1993;116:843–851.

Bhatia KP, Munchau A, Thompson PD, et al: Generalized muscular weakness after botulinum toxin injections for dystonia: A report of three cases. J Neurol Neurosurg Psychiatry 1999;67:90–93.

Binder W, Brin MF, Blitzer A, et al: Botulinum toxin type A (BTX-A) for migraine: An open label assessment. Mov Disord 1998; 13(suppl 2):241.

Blitzer A, Brin MF, Stewart CF: Botulinum toxin management of spasmodic dysphonia (laryngeal dystonia): A 12-year experience in more than 900 patients. Laryngoscope 1998;108:1435–1441.

Borg-Stein J, Pine ZM, Miller JR, Brin MF: Botulinum toxin for the treatment of spasticity in multiple sclerosis: New observations. Am J Phys Med Rehabil 1993;72:364–368.

Borodic G, Johnson E, Goodnough M, Schantz E: Botulinum toxin therapy, immunologic resistance, and problems with available materials. Neurology 1996;46:26–29.

Borodic GE, Ferrante R, Pearce LB, Smith K: Histologic assessment of dose-related diffusion and muscle fiber response after therapeutic botulinum A toxin injections. Mov Disord 1994; 9:31–39.

Brans JW, Aramideh M, Koelman JH, et al: Electromyography in cervical dystonia: Changes after botulinum and trihexyphenidyl. Neurology 1998;51:815–819.

Brashear A, Lew MF, Dykstra DD, et al: Safety and efficacy of NeuroBloc (botulinum toxin type B) in type A–responsive cervical dystonia. Neurology 1999;53:1439–1446.

Brin MF, Lew MF, Adler CH, et al: Safety and efficacy of NeuroBloc (botulinum toxin type B) in type A–resistant cervical dystonia. Neurology 1999;53:1431–1438.

Buchman AS, Comella CL, Leurgans S, et al: The effect of changes in head posture on the patterns of muscle activity in cervical dystonia (CD). Mov Disord 1998;13:490–496.

Buchman AS, Comella CL, Stebbins GT, et al: Quantitative electromyographic analysis of changes in muscle activity following botulinum toxin therapy for cervical dystonia. Clin Neuropharmacol 1993;16:205–210.

Burbaud P, Wiart L, Dubos JL, et al: A randomised, double blind, placebo controlled trial of botulinum toxin in the treatment of spastic foot in hemiparetic patients. J Neurol Neurosurg Psychiatry 1996;61:265–269.

Bushara KO, Park DM: Botulinum toxin and sweating. J Neurol Neurosurg Psychiatry 1994;57:1437–1438.

Calne DB, Lang AE: Secondary dystonia. Adv Neurol 1988;50:9–33.

Calne S: Local treatment of dystonia and spasticity with injections of botulinum-A toxin. Axone 1993;14:85–88.

Chen R, Hallett M: Focal dystonia and repetitive motion disorders. Clin Orthop 1998:102–106.

Chen R, Karp BI, Goldstein SR, et al: Effect of muscle activity immediately after botulinum toxin injection for writer's cramp. Mov Disord 1999;14:307–312.

Cherington M: Botulism, clinical and therapeutic observations. Rocky Mtn Med J 1972;69:55–58.

Cheshire WP, Abashian SW, Mann JD: Botulinum toxin in the treatment of myofascial pain syndrome. Pain 1994;59:65–69.

Clemente CD: Gray's Anatomy, 30th American Edition. Philadelphia, Lea & Febiger, 1985.

Cohen LG, Hallett M: Hand cramps: Clinical features and electromyographic patterns in a focal dystonia. Neurology 1988;38: 1005–1012.

Cole R, Hallett M, Cohen LG: Double-blind trial of botulinum toxin for treatment of focal hand dystonia. Mov Disord 1995; 10:466–471.

Comella CL, Buchman AS, Tanner CM, et al: Botulinum toxin injection for spasmodic torticollis: Increased magnitude of benefit with electromyographic assistance. Neurology 1992;42:878–882.

Comella CL, Shannon KM, Jaglin J: Extensor truncal dystonia:

Successful treatment with botulinum toxin injections. Mov Disord 1998;13:552–555.

Comella CL, Stebbins GT, Goetz CG, et al: Teaching tape for the motor section of the Toronto Western Spasmodic Torticollis Scale. Mov Disord 1997;12:570–575.

Comella CL, Tanner CM, DeFoor-Hill L, Smith C: Dysphagia after botulinum toxin injections for spasmodic torticollis: Clinical and radiologic findings. Neurology 1992;42:1307–1310.

DasGupta BR: Structures of botulinum neurotoxin, its functional domains, and perspectives on the crystalline type A toxin. In Jankovic J, Hallett M. (eds): Therapy with Botulinum Toxin. New York, Marcel Dekker, 1994;15–39.

DasGupta BR, Tepp W: Protease activity of botulinum neurotoxin type E and its light chain: Cleavage of actin. Biochem Biophys Res Commun 1993;190:470–474.

Davis D, Jabbari B: Significant improvement of stiff-person syndrome after paraspinal injection of botulinum toxin A. Mov Disord 1993;8:371–373.

Denislic M, Pirtosek Z, Vodusek DB, et al: Botulinum toxin in the treatment of neurological disorders. Ann N Y Acad Sci 1994;710:76–87.

Deuschl G, Lohle E, Heinen F, Lucking C: Ear click in palatal tremor: Its origin and treatment with botulinum toxin. Neurology 1991;41:1677–1679.

Deuschl G, Lohle E, Toro C, et al: Botulinum toxin treatment of palatal tremor (myoclonus). In Jankovic J, Hallett M (eds): Therapy with Botulinum Toxin. New York, Marcel Dekker, 1994a;567–576.

Deuschl G, Lücking CH, Schenk E: Essential tremor: Electrophysiological and pharmacological evidence for a subdivision. J Neurol Neurosurg Psychiatry 1987;50:1435–1441.

Deuschl G, Toro C, Hallett M: Symptomatic and essential palatal tremor. 2. Differences of palatal movements. Mov Disord 1994b;9:676–678.

Deuschl G, Toro C, Valls-Sole J, et al: Symptomatic and essential palatal tremor. 1. Clinical, physiological and MRI analysis. Brain 1994;117:775–788.

Dubinsky RM: Anatomy and neurophysiology of neck muscles. In Jankovic J, Hallett M (eds): Therapy with Botulinum Toxin. New York, Marcel Dekker, 1994; 239–256.

Dubinsky RM, Gray CS, Vetere-Overfield B, Koller WC: Electromyographic guidance of botulinum toxin treatment in cervical dystonia. Clin Neuropharmacol 1991;14:262–267.

Dubinsky RM, Hallett M: Palatal myoclonus and facial involvement in other types of myoclonus. Adv Neurol 1988;49:263–278.

Dunne JW, Heye N, Dunne SL: Treatment of chronic limb spasticity with botulinum toxin A. J Neurol Neurosurg Psychiatry 1995;58:232–235.

Dykstra DD, Sidi AA: Treatment of detrusor-sphincter dyssynergia with botulinum A toxin: A double-blind study. Arch Phys Med Rehabil 1990;71:24–26.

Eleopra R, Tugnoli V, De Grandis D: The variability in the clinical effect induced by botulinum toxin type A: The role of muscle activity in humans. Mov Disord 1997;12:89–94.

Eleopra R, Tugnoli V, Rossetto O, et al: Different time courses of recovery after poisoning with botulinum neurotoxin serotypes A and E in humans. Neurosci Lett 1998;256:135–138.

Ellis DA, Chi PL, Tan AK: Facial rejuvenation with botulinum. Dermatol Nurs 1997;9:329–333, 365.

Ellis DA, Tan AK: Cosmetic upper-facial rejuvenation with botulinum. J Otolaryngol 1997;26:92–96.

Fahn S: Concept and classification of dystonia. In Fahn S, Marsden CD, Calne DB (eds): Dystonia 2. New York, Raven Press, 1988; 1–8.

Freund B, Schwartz M, Symington JM: The use of botulinum toxin for the treatment of temporomandibular disorders: Preliminary findings. J Oral Maxillofac Surg 1999;57:916–920; discussion 920–921.

Frueh BR, Felt DP, Wojno TH, Musch DC: Treatment of blepharospasm with botulinum toxin: A preliminary report. Arch Ophthalmol 1984;102:1464–1468.

Gallien P, Robineau S, Verin M, et al: Treatment of detrusor sphincter dyssynergia by transperineal injection of botulinum toxin. Arch Phys Med Rehabil 1998;79:715–717.

Geller BD, Hallett M, Ravits J: Botulinum toxin therapy in hemifacial spasm: Clinical and electrophysiologic studies. Muscle Nerve 1989;12:716–222.

Girlanda P, Quartarone A, Sinicropi S, et al: Botulinum toxin in upper limb spasticity: Study of reciprocal inhibition between forearm muscles. Neuroreport 1997;8:3039–3044.

Glanzman RL, Gelb DJ, Drury I, et al: Brachial plexopathy after botulinum toxin injections. Neurology 1990;40:1143.

Greene P, Fahn S, Diamond B: Development of resistance to botulinum toxin type A in patients with torticollis. Mov Disord 1994;9:213–217.

Greene PE, Fahn S: Use of botulinum toxin type F injections to treat torticollis in patients with immunity to botulinum toxin type A. Mov Disord 1993;8:479–483.

Hallett M: Analysis of abnormal voluntary and involuntary movements with surface electromyography. Adv Neurol 1983;39:907–914.

Hallett M: One man's poison—clinical applications of botulinum toxin. N Engl J Med 1999;341:118–120.

Halpern JL, Neale EA: Neurospecific binding, internalization, and retrograde axonal transport. Curr Top Microbiol Immunol 1995;195:221–241.

Hamjian JA, Walker FO: Serial neurophysiological studies of intramuscular botulinum-A toxin in humans. Muscle Nerve 1994;17:1385–1392.

Heinen F, Wissel J, Philipsen A, et al: Interventional neuropediatrics: Treatment of dystonic and spastic muscular hyperactivity with botulinum toxin A. Neuropediatrics 1997;28:307–313.

Hertz E, Hoeffer PFA: Spasmodic torticollis. I. Physiologic analysis of involuntary motor activity. Arch Neurol Psychiatry 1949;61:129–136.

Holds JB, Alderson K, Fogg SG, Anderson RL: Motor nerve sprouting in human orbicularis muscle after botulinum A injection. Invest Ophthalmol Vis Sci 1990;31:964–967.

Holzer SE, Ludlow CL: The swallowing side effects of botulinum toxin type A injection in spasmodic dysphonia. Laryngoscope 1996;106:86–92.

Hughes R, Whaller BC: Influence of nerve ending activity and of drugs on the rate of paralysis of rat diaphragm preparations by *Clostridium botulinum* type A toxin. J Physiol 1962;160:221–223.

Huttner WB: Cell biology: Snappy exocytoxins. Nature 1993;365:104–105.

Isaac K, Cohen JA: Post-traumatic torticollis. Neurology 1989;39:1642–1643.

Jankovic J: Blepharospasm and oromandibular-laryngeal-cervical dystonia: A controlled trial of botulinum A toxin therapy. Adv Neurol 1988;50:583–591.

Jankovic J: Cranial-cervical dyskinesias: An overview. Adv Neurol 1988;49:1–13.

Jankovic J: Botulinum toxin in the treatment of dystonic tics. Mov Disord 1994;9:347–349.

Jankovic J: Post-traumatic movement disorders: Central and peripheral mechanisms. Neurology 1994;44:2006–2014.

Jankovic J, Brin MF: Therapeutic uses of botulinum toxin. N Engl J Med 1991;324:1186–1194.

Jankovic J, Orman J: Botulinum A toxin for cranial-cervical dystonia: A double-blind, placebo-controlled study. Neurology 1987;37:616–623.

Jankovic J, Schwartz K, Clemence W, et al: A randomized, double-blind, placebo-controlled study to evaluate botulinum toxin type A in essential hand tremor. Mov Disord 1996;11:250–256.

Jitpimolmard S, Tiamkao S, Laopaiboon M: Long term results of botulinum toxin type A (Dysport) in the treatment of hemifacial spasm: A report of 175 cases. J Neurol Neurosurg Psychiatry 1998;64:751–757.

Joo JS, Agachan F, Wolff B, et al: Initial North American experience with botulinum toxin type A for treatment of anismus. Dis Colon Rectum 1996;39:1107–1111.

Jost WH, Schrank B: Repeat botulinum toxin injections in anal fissure: In patients with relapse and after insufficient effect of first treatment. Dig Dis Sci 1999;44:1588–1589.

Keen M, Blitzer A, Aviv J, et al: Botulinum toxin A for hyperkinetic facial lines: Results of a double-blind, placebo-controlled study. Plast Reconstr Surg 1994;94:94–99.

Kessler KR, Benecke R: The EDB test: A clinical test for the detection of antibodies to botulinum toxin type A. Mov Disord 1997;12:95–99.

Kessler KR, Skutta M, Benecke R: Long-term treatment of cervical dystonia with botulinum toxin A: Efficacy, safety, and antibody frequency. German Dystonia Study Group. J Neurol 1999;246: 265–274.

Koller W, Brin M, Lyons K, et al: Double blind assessment of botulinum toxin (Botox®) for essential hand tremor. Neurology 1999;52(Suppl 2):A456.

Koller W, Vetere-Overfield B, Gray C, Dubinsky R: Failure of fixed-dose, fixed muscle injection of botulinum toxin in torticollis. Clin Neuropharmacol 1990;13:355–358.

Lange DJ, Rubin M, Greene PE, et al: Distant effects of locally injected botulinum toxin: A double-blind study of single fiber EMG changes. Muscle Nerve 1991;14:672–675.

Lederman RJ: AAEM Minimonograph #43: Neuromuscular problems in the performing arts. Muscle Nerve 1994;17:569–577.

Leis AA, Dimitrijevic MR, Delapasse JS, Sharkey PC: Modification of cervical dystonia by selective sensory stimulation. J Neurol Sci 1992;110:79–89.

Lowe NJ, Maxwell A, Harper H: Botulinum A exotoxin for glabellar folds: A double-blind, placebo-controlled study with an electromyographic injection technique. J Am Acad Dermatol 1996; 35:569–572.

Ludlow CL: Treatment of speech and voice disorders with botulinum toxin. JAMA 1990;264:2671–2675.

Maria G, Brisinda G, Bentivoglio AR, et al: Botulinum toxin injections in the internal anal sphincter for the treatment of chronic anal fissure: Long-term results after two different dosage regimens. Ann Surg 1998;228:664–669.

Maria G, Cassetta E, Gui D, et al: A comparison of botulinum toxin and saline for the treatment of chronic anal fissure. N Engl J Med 1998;338:217–220.

Marsden CD: Investigation of dystonia. Adv Neurol 1988;50:35–44.

Marsden CD, Sheehy MP: Spastic dysphonia, Meige disease, and torsion dystonia. Neurology 1982;32:1202–1203.

McLaughlin MR, Jannetta PJ, Clyde BL, et al: Microvascular decompression of cranial nerves: Lessons learned after 4400 operations. J Neurosurg 1999;90:1–8.

Metz HS, Mazow M: Botulinum toxin treatment of acute sixth and third nerve palsy. Graefes Arch Clin Exp Ophthalmol 1988; 226:141–144.

Mezaki T, Kaji R, Hamano T, et al: Optimisation of botulinum treatment for cervical and axial dystonias: Experience with a Japanese type A toxin. J Neurol Neurosurg Psychiatry 1994;57: 1535–1537.

Mezaki T, Kaji R, Kohara N, et al: Comparison of therapeutic efficacies of type A and F botulinum toxins for blepharospasm: A double-blind, controlled study. Neurology 1995;45:506–508.

Minton NP: Molecular genetics of clostridial neurotoxins. Curr Top Microbiol Immunol 1995;195:161–194.

Moore AP, Wood GD: The medical management of masseteric hypertrophy with botulinum toxin type A. Br J Oral Maxillofac Surg 1994;32:26–28.

Naumann M, Hamm H, Kinkelin I, Reiners K: Botulinum toxin type A in the treatment of focal, axillary and palmar hyperhydrosis and other hyperhydrotic conditions. Eur J Neurol 1999;6:S111–S115.

Naumann M, Hofmann U, Bergmann I, et al: Focal hyperhidrosis: Effective treatment with intracutaneous botulinum toxin. Arch Dermatol 1998;134:301–304.

Naumann M, Zellner M, Toyka KV, Reiners K: Treatment of gustatory sweating with botulinum toxin. Ann Neurol 1997;42:973–975.

Naver H, Aquilonius S-M: The treatment of focal hyperhidrosis with botulinum toxin. Eur J Neurol 1997;4:S75–S79.

Nix WA, Butler IJ, Roontga S, et al: Persistent unilateral tibialis anterior muscle hypertrophy with complex repetitive discharges and myalgia: Report of two unique cases and response to botulinum toxin. Neurology 1992;42:602–606.

Odergren T, Hjaltason H, Kaakkola S, et al: A double blind, randomised, parallel group study to investigate the dose equivalence of Dysport and Botox in the treatment of cervical dystonia. J Neurol Neurosurg Psychiatry 1998;64:6–12.

On AY, Kirazli Y, Kismali B, Aksit R: Mechanisms of action of phenol block and botulinum toxin Type A in relieving spasticity: Electrophysiologic investigation and follow-up. Am J Phys Med Rehabil 1999;78:344–349.

Pahwa R, Busenbark K, Swanson-Hyland EF, et al: Botulinum toxin treatment of essential head tremor. Neurology 1995;45:822–824.

Pamphlett R: Early terminal and nodal sprouting of motor axons after botulinum toxin. J Neurol Sci 1989;92:181–192.

Podivinsky F: Torticollis. In Vinken PJ, Bruyn GW (eds): Handbook of Clinical Neurology. Amsterdam, North Holland, 1968; 567–603.

Polo KB, Jabbari B: Botulinum toxin-A improves the rigidity of progressive supranuclear palsy. Ann Neurol 1994;35:237–239.

Polo KB, Jabbari B: Effectiveness of botulinum toxin type A against painful limb myoclonus of spinal cord origin. Mov Disord 1994;9:233–235.

Poulain B, Molgo J, Thesleff S: Quantal neurotransmitter release and the clostridial neurotoxins' targets. Curr Top Microbiol Immunol 1995;195:243–255.

Poungvarin N, Devahastin V, Viriavejakul A: Treatment of various movement disorders with botulinum A toxin injections: An experience with 900 patients. J Med Assoc Thai 1995;78:281–288.

Reiter F, Danni M, Lagalla G, et al: Low-dose botulinum toxin with ankle taping for the treatment of spastic equinovarus foot after stroke. Arch Phys Med Rehabil 1998;79:532–535.

Salloway S, Stewart CF, Israeli L, et al: Botulinum toxin for refractory vocal tics. Mov Disord 1996;11:746–748.

Sampaio C, Ferreira JJ, Simoes F, et al: DYSBOT: A single-blind, randomized parallel study to determine whether any differences can be detected in the efficacy and tolerability of two formulations of botulinum toxin type A—Dysport and Botox—assuming a ratio of 4:1. Mov Disord 1997;12:1013–1018.

Sanders DB, Massey EW, Buckley EG: Botulinum toxin for blepharospasm: Single fiber EMG studies. Neurology 1986;36:545–547.

Sato K: The physiology, pharmacology and biochemistry of the eccrine sweat gland. Rev Physiol Biochem Pharmacol 1997; 79:51–131.

Schantz EJ: Preparation and characterization of botulinum toxin type A for human treatment. In Jankovic J, Hallett M (eds): Therapy with Botulinum Toxin. New York, Marcel Dekker, 1994; 41–50.

Schiavo G, Benfenati F, Poulain B: Tetanus and botulinum toxin-B neurotoxins block neuromuscular transmitter release by proteolytic cleavage of synaptobrevin. Nature 1992;359:832–835.

Schiavo G, Rossetto O, Benfenati F, et al: Tetanus and botulinum neurotoxins are zinc proteases specific for components of the neuroexocytosis apparatus. Ann N Y Acad Sci 1994;710:65–75.

Schnider P, Binder M, Auff E, et al: Double-blind trial of botulinum A toxin for the treatment of focal hyperhidrosis of the palms. Br J Dermatol 1997;136:548–552.

Scott AB, Suzuki D: Systemic toxicity of botulinum toxin by intramuscular injection in the monkey. Mov Disord 1988;3:333–335.

Scott BL, Jankovic J, Donovan DT: Botulinum toxin injection into vocal cord in the treatment of malignant coprolalia associated with Tourette's syndrome. Mov Disord 1996;11:431–433.

Shaari CM, Sanders I: Quantifying how location and dose of botulinum toxin injections affect muscle paralysis. Muscle Nerve 1993;16:964–969.

Sheean GL, Lees AJ: Botulinum toxin F in the treatment of torticollis clinically resistant to botulinum toxin A. J Neurol Neurosurg Psychiatry 1995;59:601–607.

Shelley WB, Talanin NY, Shelley ED: Botulinum toxin therapy for palmar hyperhidrosis. J Am Acad Dermatol 1998;38:227–229.

Silberstein S, Mathew N, Saper J, Jenkins S: Botulinum toxin type A as a migraine preventative treatment. Headache 2000; 40:445–450.

Simpson DM, Alexander DN, O'Brien CF, et al: Botulinum toxin type A in the treatment of upper extremity spasticity: A randomized, double-blind, placebo controlled study. Neurology 1996;46:1306–1310.

Sloop RR, Cole BA, Escutin RO: Human response to botulinum toxin injection: Type B compared with type A. Neurology 1997; 49:189–194.

Smyth AG: Botulinum toxin treatment of bilateral masseteric hypertrophy. Br J Oral Maxillofac Surg 1994;32:29–33.

Snow BJ, Tsui JK, Bhatt MH, et al: Treatment of spasticity with botulinum toxin: A double-blind study. Ann Neurol 1990;28:512–515.

Speelman JD, Brans AWM: Cervical dystonia and botulinum treatment: Is electromyographic guidance necessary? Mov Disord 1995;10:802.

Tan EK, Jankovic J: Bilateral hemifacial spasm: A report of five cases and a literature review. Mov Disord 1999;14:345–349.

Tejedor J, Rodriguez, JM: Retreatment of children after surgery for acquired esotropia: Reoperation versus botulinum injection. Br J Ophthalmol 1998;82:110–114.

Thompson PD, Stell R, Maccabe JJ, et al: Electromyography of neck muscles and treatment in spasmodic torticollis. In Berardelli A, Benecke R, Manfredi M, Marsden CD (eds): Motor Disturbances II. London, Harcourt Brace Jovanovich, 1990; 289–304.

Tournay A, Paillard J: Torticollis spasmodique et électromyographie. Rev Neurol 1955;93:347–355.

Trimble MR, Whurr R, Brookes G, Robertson MM: Vocal tics in Gilles de la Tourette syndrome treated with botulinum toxin injections. Mov Disord 1998;13:617–619.

Truong DD, Dubinsky R, Hermanowicz N, et al: Posttraumatic torticollis. Arch Neurol 1991;48:221–223.

Tsui JK, Eisen A, Stoessl AJ, et al: Double-blind study of botulinum toxin in spasmodic torticollis. Lancet 1986;2:245–247.

Tsui JKC, Eisen A, Calne DB: Botulinum toxin in spasmodic torticollis. In Fahn S, Marsden CD, Calne DB (eds): Dystonia 2. New York, Raven Press, 1988; 593–597.

Vaezi MF, Richter JE, Wilcox CM, et al: Botulinum toxin versus pneumatic dilatation in the treatment of achalasia: A randomised trial. Gut 1999;44:231–239.

Valls-Sole J, Tolosa ES, Ribera G: Neurophysiological observations on the effects of botulinum toxin treatment in patients with dystonic blepharospasm. J Neurol Neurosurg Psychiatry 1991; 54:310–313.

Van Ermengen E: Uber einen anaeroben Bacillus und seine Beziehungen zum Botulismus. Z Hygiene Infektions 1897;26:1–56.

Van Pelt F, Ludlow CL, Smith PJ: Comparison of muscle activation patterns in adductor and abductor spasmodic dysphonia. Ann Otol Rhinol Laryngol 1994;103:192–200.

Vasin NI, Safronov VA, Medzhidov MR, Shabalov VA: Voluntary activity of the neck muscles in patients with spastic torticollis. Nevropatol Psikhiatr 1988;88:7–10.

Viriyavejakul A, Vachalathiti R, Poungvarin N: Botulinum treatment for post-stroke spasticity: low dose regime. J Med Assoc Thai 1998;81:413–422.

Wehrmann T, Kokabpick H, Jacobi V, et al: Long-term results of endoscopic injection of botulinum toxin in elderly achalasic patients with tortuous megaesophagus or epiphrenic diverticulum. Endoscopy 1999;31:352–358.

Wehrmann T, Seifert H, Seipp M, et al: Endoscopic injection of botulinum toxin for biliary sphincter of Oddi dysfunction. Endoscopy 1998;30:702–707.

Wheeler AH: Botulinum toxin A, adjunctive therapy for refractory headaches associated with pericranial muscle tension. Headache 1998;38:468–471.

Wheeler AH, Goolkasian P, Gretz SS: A randomized, double-blind, prospective pilot study of botulinum toxin injection for refractory, unilateral, cervicothoracic, paraspinal, myofascial pain syndrome. Spine 1998;23:1662–1666; discussion 1667.

Wissel J, Heinen F, Schenkel A, et al: Botulinum toxin A in the management of spastic gait disorders in children and young adults with cerebral palsy: A randomized, double-blind study of "high-dose" versus "low-dose" treatment. Neuropediatrics 1999;30:120–124.

Wissel J, Masuhr F, Schelosky L, et al: Quantitative assessment of botulinum toxin treatment in 43 patients with head tremor. Mov Disord 1997;12:722–726.

Wong DL, Adams SG, Irish JC, et al: Effect of neuromuscular activity on the response to botulinum toxin injections in spasmodic dysphonia. J Otolaryngol 1995;24:209–216.

Wong V: Use of botulinum toxin injection in 17 children with spastic cerebral palsy. Pediatr Neurol 1998;18:124–131.

Zuber M, Sebald M, Bathien N, et al: Botulinum antibodies in dystonic patients treated with type A botulinum toxin: frequency and significance. Neurology 1993;43:1715–1718.

ELECTROPHYSIOLOGICAL STUDIES IN THE OPERATING ROOM

C H A P T E R 102

Cranial Nerve Monitoring

Jeffrey A. Strommen and Jasper R. Daube

The integrity of cranial nerves and surrounding structures, such as the brainstem and spinal cord, can be monitored effectively with multimodal techniques during intra-axial and extra-axial procedures. Various techniques are used to preserve function and to prevent injury to vital neural structures when clinical examination is not possible. These techniques identify and locate nerves, warn of potential nerve injury, quantify the degree of nerve injury,

help investigate the mechanism of injury, potentially shorten the procedure, and improve future surgical techniques.

The usefulness of electrodiagnostic testing is well established in routine clinical practice. The use of similar procedures, with minor modifications, to protect the integrity of neurological function intra-operatively is also not a new concept. For many years, surgeons have used the presence or absence of a visible muscle twitch after electrical stimulation of a nerve as an indicator of nerve integrity (Daube and Harper, 1989). In the last 20 years, more useful techniques have been developed for patients undergoing procedures involving the cerebral cortex, brainstem, spinal cord, and cranial or peripheral nerves. There have been many modifications of the basic techniques, with significant variation in their use among institutions and individuals. Ongoing development of intraoperative techniques continues, with advances in technology and surgical technique and improvement in the identification of disease at an earlier stage.

GENERAL CONSIDERATIONS

The ideal monitoring system includes a mechanism for providing the surgeon with rapid feedback of reliable, easily interpreted data while not interfering with the surgical procedure. The surgeon or anesthesiologist then can take appropriate action to prevent or to reverse a potential neurological injury. Even recognition of irreversible changes can be useful when it teaches the surgeon about the mechanism of injury and helps predict the nature and severity of the postoperative deficit (Daube and Harper, 1989). Additionally, the use of monitoring not only assists the surgical team with immediate preservation but also substantially speeds the learning of future procedures (Ebersold et al., 1992).

Many methods have been developed to measure neural function electrically in patients during anesthesia. Most of these have been derived from routine clinical neurophysiology and, with minor modification, have been helpful in the intraoperative setting. Cortical function can be monitored with electroencephalography (EEG) and surface recording of somatosensory evoked potentials (SSEPs). Thalamic nuclei can be located by direct recording during stereotactic procedures. Functions of the eighth cranial nerve and the brainstem can be monitored with brainstem auditory evoked potentials (BAEPs). Peripheral and central sensory pathways are monitored with recording SSEPs. Peripheral and cranial motor nerve function can be monitored with electromyography (EMG) and by studying compound muscle action potentials (CMAPs). Nerve action potentials (NAPs) can be recorded directly from peripheral nerves, the trigeminal nerve, and the eighth cranial nerve. The use of visual evoked potentials (VEPs) for monitoring has been limited because of problems in identifying an adequate stimulus and appropriate applications. Motor evoked potentials (MEPs) from the spinal cord can be used to evaluate central motor pathways.

Selection of the appropriate modalities is customized to the patient's clinical status and the structures thought to be at potential risk. This is especially true for procedures involving the posterior fossa, where several structures, including the cranial nerves, the brainstem, and, occasionally, the spinal cord, are at risk for inadvertent injury. In this setting, one must be able to perform multimodal recordings, including EMG, CMAP recordings, BAEPs,

and potentially SSEPs. By monitoring several structures as well as monitoring the same structure with multiple techniques, the neurophysiologist can provide rapid and accurate feedback to the surgeon.

During the procedure, changes may occur rapidly and irreversibly. Therefore, it is desirable to have a way of learning whether the patient is at risk for such damage before the damage occurs, even if the technique used to identify the risk does not give information about whether the damage will result in a clinical deficit. Alternatively, some lesions, such as those from compression, may be reflected in a gradual change in potentials. Given this, the system must also be able to provide reliable information in the relatively hostile electrical environment so that relatively subtle changes can be detected and conveyed accurately to the surgeon.

Any monitoring system has inherent limitations. False-positive results are not infrequent and probably reflect either a subclinical lesion or, more likely, technical factors that have artificially affected the potentials. Identifying changes requires that a well-defined set of baseline values be obtained during the initial, low-risk portions of the operation. The variation due to extraneous factors must be identified so that the surgeon can be assured that if he or she is told of a change, it is related to the surgical procedure—and not to changes in blood pressure, artifacts, anesthesia, or other factors. Much less frequent are false-negative results, in which the patient experiences a neurological deficit without an identifiable change in the recording. In most cases, a false-negative result is probably related to involvement of critical structures that were not monitored directly during the procedure. An example of this would be paralysis after a spinal operation when the SSEPs remained stable and MEPs were not monitored. This also can occur when monitoring is discontinued prematurely. Abnormalities may be seen immediately after an injury; others, particularly those indicative of mild nerve compression, may not become manifest for up to an hour after the step in the procedure that caused the injury. Therefore, monitoring must continue throughout the surgical procedure, even after a so-called critical period in the operation has passed.

Intraoperative monitoring differs from routine electrodiagnostic studies in many technical ways and with regard to interpretation. The most prominent factor is related to a hostile electrical environment in which cautery, 60-Hz artifact, respirators, or warmers may attenuate or completely obliterate the response. Additionally, a normal control value is relatively useless in the intraoperative setting. Extrinsic factors, such as the concentration of anesthetic agents and the patient's temperature and blood pressure, prolong many evoked responses (Cheek, 1993; Harper and Daube, 1998; Sloan, 1998). The underlying disease process itself is likely to have affected the baseline responses to the degree that the findings are outside the normal range. Owing to these factors, the practitioner generally views the

Table 102–1. Cranial Nerve Monitoring

Nerve	Evoked Potentials	EMG	CMAP	NAP
Optic	+			+
Oculomotor		+	+	
Trigeminal (motor)		+	+	+
Facial		+	+	+
Acoustic	+			+
Vagus		+	+	
Spinal accessory		+	+	+
Hypoglossal		+	+	

CMAP, compound muscle action potential; EMG, electromyography; NAP, nerve action potential.

patient as his or her own control, with a change in values during the procedure indicating potential neurological injury rather than using an absolute value. Therefore, reliable baseline recordings must be established before critical portions of the procedure are performed, and all potential confounding factors must be monitored so that the surgeon can be informed of a true potential change due to surgical manipulation.

CRANIAL NERVE MONITORING

Techniques

Techniques have been developed to monitor cranial nerves and surrounding structures: EMG, CMAPs, BAEPs, NAPs, electrocochleography (EChG), VEPs, and SSEPs (Table 102–1). Generally, the intraoperative monitoring scheme involves several mo-

dalities that need to be monitored simultaneously and continuously. This requires the capability of multiple channels (four to eight) that can be viewed at different sweep speeds, amplifications, and filter settings (Fig. 102–1). Additionally, effective monitoring requires the capability to average responses, to provide a triggered stimulus, and to record free-running potentials. There must be adequate auditory output to provide the surgeon with immediate feedback and the ability to store, retrieve, and report the information in an efficient manner. Finally, there must be appropriate shielding and attention to technical detail to minimize artifact.

ELECTROMYOGRAPHY

Electromyography records electrical potentials in muscle fibers. In the diagnostic laboratory, it is used to record evidence of denervation in the form of fibrillation potentials and to assess voluntary motor unit potentials by means of morphological changes and recruitment patterns. Intraoperatively, the primary potentials of interest are neurotonic discharges and motor unit potentials. Neurotonic potentials occur in response to mechanical, thermal, or metabolic irritation of the nerve that innervates a muscle. Motor unit potentials reflect reflex activity of anterior horn cells.

Neurotonic discharges are distinctive discharges of a motor unit that appear as rapid, irregular bursts lasting several milliseconds or prolonged trains lasting up to 1 minute. Each discharge may contain 1 to 10 individual motor unit potentials, which discharge at frequencies of 50 to 200 Hz (Daube and Harper, 1989; Harper and Daube, 1998). They are distin-

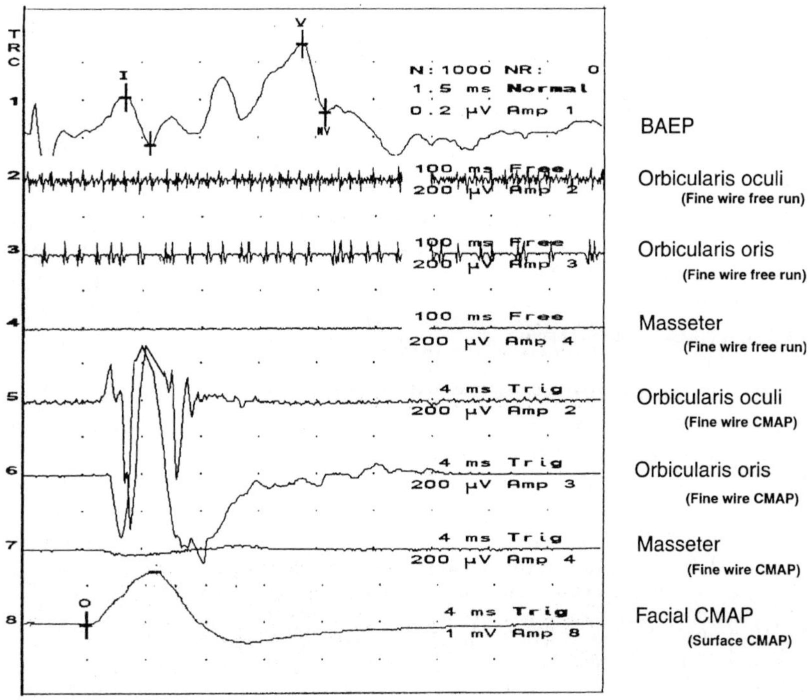

Figure 102–1. Acoustic neuroma resection. Multimodal recording with brainstem auditory evoked potentials (BAEP), free-run electromyography, triggered electromyography, and facial compound muscle action potentials (CMAP).

guished from motor unit potentials by this burst pattern and their relationship to mechanical, thermal, or metabolic irritation of the nerve membrane. By contrast, a motor unit potential has a semirhythmical pattern, which can occur in response to irritation of the motor axon or to voluntary activity from incomplete muscle relaxation.

Neurotonic discharge may be noted, with stretching, contusing, compressing, rubbing, or manipulating of the nerve, thus providing a sensitive means of informing the surgeon of impending damage. Neurotonic discharges occur more often with cranial nerve manipulation than with peripheral nerve manipulation (Harner et al., 1987). Although a discharge alone is not predictive of neurological deficit, the number of discharges and particularly the long neurotonic discharges do appear to correlate with postoperative functional deficit (Harner et al., 1987). Conversely, the absence of neurotonic discharge does not exclude injury, because a sudden, sharp laceration may be associated with minimal or no neurotonic discharges. Long neurotonic discharges are also common during benign events such as irrigation, when the nerve is irritated by a combination of temperature and mechanical stimulation. The neurophysiologist must be aware of the surgical manipulation, by either frequent communication with others involved with the procedure or video feedback from the surgical field.

Neurotonic discharges and motor unit potentials must be distinguished from other physiological and artifactual waveforms. Generally, 60-Hz interference can be controlled with adequate grounding and proper shielding of the equipment. Movement artifact can be recognized as triangular waves that occur irregularly and have a characteristic popping sound. Interference from respirators, cautery, Cavitron dissectors, warmers, and gas humidifiers can be recognized easily (Fig. 102–2). Interference from cautery is best suppressed with a switch attached directly to the cautery control switch. Electromyographic activity cannot be monitored during cautery.

Muscle activity that must be distinguished from neurotonic discharges includes motor unit potentials that may occur in patients not deeply anesthetized so that their reflexes remain active, fibrillation potentials in muscles that have been partially denervated, myokymic discharges, muscle end-plate noise and spikes, and complex repetitive discharges. Each of these types of activity is seen intraoperatively, but they can be distinguished readily from neurotonic discharges by the firing patterns and action potential characteristics typical of each. Neurotonic discharges may take various forms, but all are rapid bursts that occur irregularly (Fig. 102–3).

Technique

Electromyographic activity can be recorded with various electrodes. Surface electrodes usually are

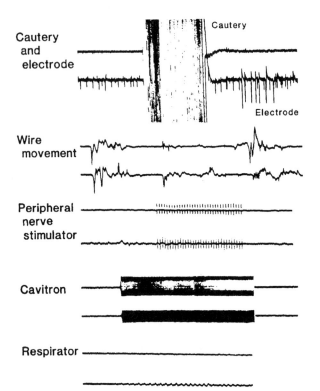

Figure 102–2. Artifacts recorded with electromyography fine-wire electrodes during surgical monitoring. (From Daube JR, Harper CM: Surgical monitoring of cranial and peripheral nerves. In Desmedt JE [ed]: Neuromonitoring in Surgery. Amsterdam, The Netherlands, Elsevier Science, 1989; 115–138. By permission of JE Desmedt.)

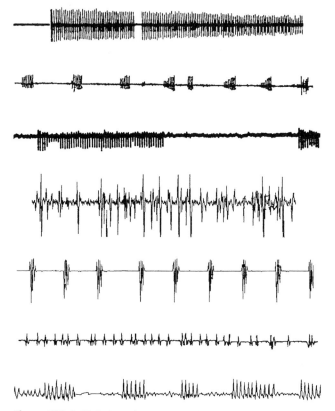

Figure 102–3. Variation of neurotonic discharges.

Figure 102–4. Fine-wire recording electrode.

inadequate because they cannot record deep activity or clearly identify the specific muscle responsible. Electroencephalograph needles placed subcutaneously are commonly used, but they do not appear as sensitive for the detection of neurotonic discharges. Standard monopolar or concentric needle electrodes can record EMG activity reliably but are bulky and difficult to keep in place and out of the way of the surgeon and anesthesiologist.

Teflon-coated Nichrome wires (0.01 mm) placed percutaneously with a 26-gauge, hollow needle do not have these limitations and work well. A 2- to 3-mm, hooked tip allows the wire to remain securely in the muscle when the needle is removed (Fig. 102–4). Generally, two wires are placed approximately 5 mm apart in each muscle. In small muscles, such as extraocular muscles, two wires can be placed simultaneously through a single 30-gauge needle if the tips are bared in different areas to avoid shorting of the signal. Two wires can be placed in separate muscles, which broadens the field of recording but has the disadvantage of being unable to identify specific muscle involvement as well as imparting more distant artifact. The wires in loops are taped securely to the skin to prevent dislodging the wires during surgical manipulations. They are connected to the amplifier through a spring-loaded connector or a modified integrated circuit connector held in its socket by circuit pins (Fig. 102–5). The leads from the probes to the preamplifier must be kept as short as possible to reduce interference from external sources. Perfect placement and stabilization are required initially to ensure the high quality of the recording throughout the surgical procedure. After the patient has been scrubbed and draped, there is no opportunity to replace or reconnect wires that are dislodged. This often requires electrode placement before the surgical procedure, with the patient awake to ensure proper placement. Although some consider such presurgical placement a major disadvantage, it adds only 10 to 15 minutes to the preparation and ensures excellent recordings.

The EMG recordings are made with standard gains of 100 to 500 μV: with a low-frequency filter at 20 to 30 Hz, a high-frequency filter at 20 kHz, and a sweep speed of 10 to 200 ms/division. Electromyographic recordings from several muscles can be presented simultaneously over a loudspeaker and on a digital or analog display. The EMG activity of interest can be printed or stored for later review.

Neuromuscular blockade significantly attenuates this activity and should be avoided as much as possible. Alternative inhalational agents or narcotic anesthesia is preferred, although neurotonic discharges can be recorded if short-acting, nondepolar-

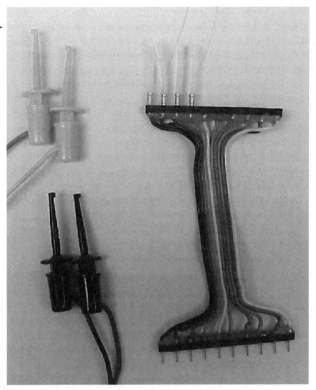

Figure 102–5. Probit and circuit jacks.

izing neuromuscular blocking agents are titrated to produce a 50% reduction of the baseline motor action potentials. Although such a level of muscle relaxation increases the possibility of unwanted movement during the operation, movements of the patient can be prevented with adequate levels of narcotic or inhalational anesthesia. At times, additional agents, such as fentanyl or midazolam, must be administered to reduce background muscle contractions and associated MUPs. If partial neuromuscular blockade is used, monitor the degree of blockage continuously.

Application

The EMG recording has diverse applications for peripheral, spinal, and cranial procedures. Recordings can be made from any somatic muscle, including extraocular, facial, laryngeal, intercostal, abdominal, anal sphincter, and limb muscles. Any procedure that requires manipulation or dissection of a nerve can be performed more safely and effectively with intraoperative EMG monitoring. This simple technique provides a means of rapid feedback to the surgeon to warn of potential nerve trauma. The presence of these discharges warns the surgeon that a nerve is being affected by surgical activity, and the absence of these discharges can usually reassure the surgeon that the nerve remains unaffected. Additionally, this technique can be used for nerve localization when the tissue is not clearly identified as the result of altered anatomy from a tumor that displaces or encases the nerve. Facial nerve monitoring is the most common application of cranial nerve monitoring. Others include the oculomotor, trochlear, and abducens nerves during operations in the region of the orbit, cavernous sinus, or petrous portion of the temporal bone; the trigeminal nerve during posterior fossa tumor resection or microvascular decompression surgery; the vagus nerve, with intraoperative recording of the vocalis or cricothyroid during brainstem or laryngeal procedures; and the spinal accessory and hypoglossal nerves during vascular or tumor cases involving the lower brainstem or region of the foramen magnum.

COMPOUND MUSCLE ACTION POTENTIALS

Compound muscle action potentials represent the summated activity of all axons or muscle fibers recorded over a muscle when the nerve is stimulated. The integrity of motor axons can be tested directly by stimulating the nerve in the surgical field and recording CMAPs in one or more of the muscles innervated by the nerve.

Technique

The CMAPs can be recorded over the muscle with surface, subcutaneous, or intramuscular electrodes. When recorded with fine-wire intramuscular electrodes, the responses are multispike waveforms that vary in size and configuration. These electrodes record from only a small area of muscle and, thus, cannot be used as a quantitative measure, but they suffice to help localize nerve fibers during dissection and to ensure gross integrity of the nerve. Intramuscular electrodes are also useful in monitoring deep muscles that would not otherwise be recorded by surface electrodes or muscles that are close to one another. In contrast, surface or subcutaneous electrodes provide a quantitative means of assessment. The potentials are recorded as stable biphasic potentials that can be measured and compared directly with recordings later in the procedure or from a different site along the nerve. If surface or subcutaneous electrodes are used, they are placed on the muscle, with the active electrode over the central end-plate region of the muscle and the reference electrode generally 3 to 5 cm distally over the tendon or at an electrically inactive site. Intramuscular electrode placement is similar but avoids the end-plate region.

The variables in CMAP recording are similar to those used in routine neurophysiological studies. Sweep speeds of 1 to 10 ms/cm are usually satisfactory. The amplification of the response varies, but it is usually between 500 μV and 5 mV/cm; filter settings are 2 Hz to 20 kHz.

Stimulating techniques differ markedly from routine studies in that various stimulators are necessary, depending on the structures and confines of the surgical field. Most stimulators are hand held by the surgeon to ensure the proper placement of the stimulus and to ease the movement of the stimulator during the operation. Stimulators may be either bipolar or monopolar, each with distinct advantages and disadvantages. Bipolar stimulation has the active electrode (cathode) distal and the anode proximal along the length of the nerve. This may take the form of two adjacent 1-mm wires (insulated except for their tips), a central wire in an insulated cannula, insulated forceps tips that allow the surgeon to dissect tissue with the stimulator, or a hand-held hook electrode that can retract the nerve slightly from the wet surgical field. In contrast, for a monopolar stimulator, the cathode is placed directly on the nerve and the anode is some distance away from the nerve; usually a small needle electrode is inserted in surrounding muscle or subcutaneous tissue (Fig. 102–6). The advantage of the bipolar stimulator is that it can provide a focal stimulus, thus minimizing current spread to surrounding nerves. The disadvantage is that if the nerve is distant from the stimulator or there is fluid in the operative field, there may be inadequate activation of the nerve and thus a falsely decreased amplitude of response. A monopolar stimulator reduces this likelihood but increases the possibility of current spread, with resultant excess shock artifact and stimulation of surrounding nerves. The size of the stimulating electrodes varies, depending on the nerve that is stimulated. Small cranial nerves require stimulator tips that are as small as 1 mm.

Stimulation intensity is much lower than that used in routine studies, because of the direct proximity to the nerve. A healthy nerve can be maximally activated, with a stimulus duration of 0.05 ms and an intensity of 0.5 to 5 mA (2.5 to 25 V). The failure to record a response can result from the use of a muscle relaxant, shorting of the stimulus current because of fluid in the stimulating field, stimulating electrodes either not connected or not on the nerve, amplifiers not on, disconnected recording electrodes, or recording electrodes not working properly. Higher stimulus intensities may be necessary for a diseased nerve or nerve segment or because of overlying tissue, such as tumor. Threshold measures may provide important localizing information for the surgeon. An intensity greater than 5 mA (>25 V) should be avoided because it can lead to current spread and inaccurate interpretation.

Application

Compound muscle action potential recordings are used to monitor the integrity of peripheral and cranial nerves and to localize lesions that may not be identified easily on routine studies. In peripheral nerve surgery, this technique provides valuable information to help the surgeon perform neurolysis,

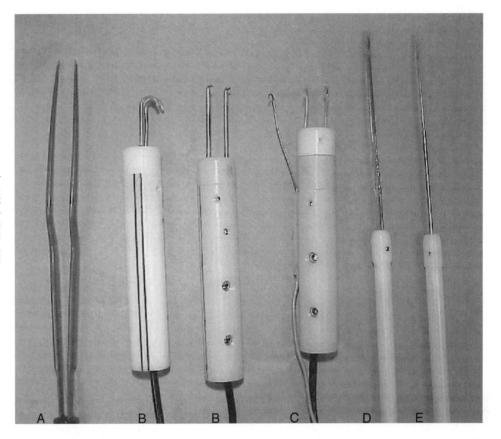

Figure 102–6. Hand-held stimulating and recording electrodes. *A*, Stimulating forceps. *B*, Hook electrodes. *C*, Recording electrode with active, reference, and ground. *D*, Bipolar 1-mm wires insulated except at the tips. *E*, Monopolar 1-mm wire insulated except at the tip.

decompression, or grafting to the appropriate nerve segment. In extracranial or intracranial surgery, this same technique aids in the identification of neural tissue and the assessment of its functional integrity.

The most frequent application of CMAPs is related to identifying the facial nerve during resection of an acoustic neuroma. For this purpose, intramuscular electrodes placed in appropriate muscles innervated by the facial nerve suffice to identify neural tissue. This technique can also be used for cranial nerve surgery, such as parotid tumor resection or identification of the recurrent laryngeal nerve during neck dissection.

Prognostic information is provided with quantitative measurements of the CMAPs from different segments of the nerve or during different stages of the procedure. Specifically, a gradual reduction of the response during an operation suggests axonal injury if the level of neuromuscular blockade has been stable and other technical or physiological factors are controlled. More importantly, in cranial nerve operations, stimulation proximal to the site of surgical manipulation and comparison of this response with the distal response determine nerve integrity. If the proximal response is lost or significantly decreased but the distal response is preserved, either physiological or anatomical disruption of the nerve has occurred. Routine studies after 5 days help determine the degree of axonal injury. A reduction in both the proximal and the distal responses immediately after the operation is probably the result of a technical problem.

NERVE ACTION POTENTIALS

Nerve action potentials are similar to CMAPs in that they represent the summated activity of all axons but differ in that they are recorded over a nerve. Currently, there is little application for this technique in routine studies, but it can provide valuable information during operative procedures on peripheral or cranial nerves.

Technique

For larger peripheral nerves, the response is recorded by hook electrodes that allow the surgeon to retract the nerve from the field (see Fig. 102–6). For smaller nerves, a small pledget of cotton can be secured to a coated silver wire that is placed directly on the nerve and referenced to a distant electrode. The stimulation may be either electrical or, in the case of the acoustic nerve, a click stimulation to the tympanic membrane. Either monopolar or bipolar hand-held stimulators can be used in the surgical field in an attempt to keep the stimulator as dry as possible to avoid shorting or current spread. For acoustic NAPs, a cotton-tipped electrode is placed directly on the acoustic nerve after exposure, and broadband click stimulation is provided through earplug or headset devices. The NAP is smaller in amplitude than the corresponding CMAP and, thus, generally requires the averaging of many responses.

Application

The technique of recording NAPs has applications similar to those for CMAPs. Nerve action potentials can be used in cranial nerve procedures to help localize nerve lesions and to provide important information about potential nerve trauma and prognosis. In the realm of cranial nerve monitoring, this technique has gained wide acceptance for auditory monitoring since being described by Moller and Jannetta (1983). This technique has the advantage of providing well-formed potentials with minimal averaging, but it also requires involvement of the surgeon to place and to maintain the position of the electrode, which may be difficult with large tumors. Facial NAPs have also been described as an alternative method of preserving facial function (Colletti and Fiorino, 1998).

EVOKED POTENTIAL MONITORING

Brainstem Auditory Evoked Potentials

Short-latency BAEPs are far-field potentials that are recorded within 10 seconds after auditory stimulation. BAEPs have gained acceptance in routine neurophysiology for diagnosing insults to the peripheral and brainstem auditory pathways. More recently, they have been used extensively in the intraoperative setting to monitor closely the acoustic nerve and brainstem function. Five to seven waveforms are generally recorded that are positive at the vertex when referenced to the ipsilateral ear. The first two waves are thought to arise from the acoustic nerve, with wave I generated from the most lateral portion and wave II probably generated from the intracranial proximal acoustic nerve near the cochlear nucleus (Moller et al., 1988; Moller et al., 1994). Waves III through V reflect central, intracranial far-field potentials. Wave III is probably generated from the superior olivary nucleus, whereas waves IV and V arise from the region of the lateral lemniscus and inferior colliculus, respectively (Markand, 1994).

TECHNIQUE

Routinely, BAEPs are recorded from the vertex referenced to an ipsilateral surface or subcutaneous electrode on the earlobe. Broadband click stimulation is provided through a headset with condensation, rarefaction, or alternating polarity at a frequency of 10 to 30 Hz. The tested ear is stimulated at 60 to 70 dB above threshold, while white masking noise is provided to the contralateral ear at 60 dB. With this technique, five well-formed waveforms generally can be recorded and the peak latencies, interpeak latencies, and amplitudes determined.

Intraoperatively, many challenges make recording reliable responses more difficult. Apart from the inherent difficulty presented by electrical interference, anesthetic effects, and temperature effects, the waveforms generally are poorly defined because of the underlying pathogenic process.

Also, routine recording and stimulating equipment cannot be used because of space confines and altered recording characteristics. Various stimulating and recording electrodes can be used. A convenient electrode is a gold foil–covered sponge with a central tube for transmitting the click stimuli (Nicolet Biomedical, Madison, WI). This electrode is inserted into the external ear canal, and the canal is sealed with bone wax. This is referenced to the vertex with a tin disk electrode. The ear is covered with tape to maintain a dry environment. Molded ear inserts or commercial earphones, such as those used for portable radios, also can be used to provide the stimulus (Moller, 1996).

Intraoperatively, surface or subcutaneous needle electrodes are referenced to the vertex. Broadband click stimulation with alternating polarity is provided at a frequency of 10 to 30 Hz. Factors of 60 are avoided to minimize 60-Hz artifact. A short polyvinyl tube between the transducer and the ear insert reduces stimulus artifact by producing a delay between the stimulus and its arrival at the tympanic membrane. Adequate filtering reduces background artifact. White noise is provided to the contralateral ear at a 60-dB level. The response is generally an average of 500 to 1,000 sweeps. If more rapid acquisition is desired, the frequency can be increased, but this generally leads to attenuation of the waveforms. Some investigators provide stimulation up to a rate of 30 to 40 Hz, but they have noted that stimulation rates greater than 50 Hz can significantly alter the amplitude. The earlier peaks are generally more affected by high rates of stimulation. Thus, if only wave V is being followed, rates as high as 80 Hz could be used (Moller, 1996). BAEPs are elicited every 5 to 10 minutes during opening of the dura mater to establish a stable baseline, and then the responses are monitored continuously. In most patients, waves I and V are readily identifiable, though significantly more delayed than awake patients. The patient serves as his or her own control. Stable baseline studies are obtained, and the responses are followed either periodically or continuously, with comparison to baseline or studies of the contralateral side.

APPLICATION

BAEPs are the mainstay of acoustic nerve monitoring because the method is a relatively simple and noninvasive technique that can monitor the entire pathway throughout the procedure without surgical interruption. They provide a means of reducing the risk of hearing loss when the intracranial portions of the acoustic nerve or brainstem pathways are at risk from surgical manipulation. This is particularly important during tumor resection from the cerebellopontine angle, but BAEPs also have applications in microvascular decompression, nerve section, and therapy for other brainstem tumors, such as meningiomas, epidermoid tumors, or metastatic tumors. Stable baseline recordings are made, and the surgeon is informed of any change during a critical stage when the acoustic nerve is at risk or when there is a 50% reduction or 1-ms latency prolongation of the waveform (Radtke et al., 1989; Slavit et al., 1991; Harper et al., 1992; Harner et al., 1996).

Somatosensory Evoked Potentials

SSEPs are widely used in routine clinical practice and have extensive application in intraoperative monitoring. They provide a simple means of monitoring spinal cord and brainstem structures during various procedures. Removal of tumors of the clivus, tumors anterior to the brainstem, brainstem gliomas, and intraventricular tumors can alter SSEPs, warning the surgeon of potential brainstem compromise or injury.

In the authors' experience, median nerve SSEPs are the most reliable and most readily recorded SSEPs for brainstem monitoring. Independent monitoring with stimulation of the median nerve on each side is more important to use if sufficient channels are available to record both sides. Although it is possible for lesions to selectively damage the axons in the brainstem that come from the legs, such damage is so unlikely to occur during an operation that tibial SSEPs are often not monitored during brainstem procedures. However, tibial SSEPs are critical for operations that involve the spine.

TECHNIQUE

As in routine studies, an electrical stimulus is applied to a nerve and responses are recorded at several sites over the peripheral nerve, spinal cord, and cerebral cortex. With minor modification, standard SSEPs can be recorded relatively easily in the operating room. Stimulation is provided to the median nerve at the wrist with either a subcutaneous needle or a block electrode held in place with a rubber strap. Surface electrodes suffice for scalp recordings, being placed with a standard C3' or C4'-Fz montage and firmly attached with collodion and filled with conductive gel. The cervical response can be recorded with either standard surface electrodes or, more commonly, with monopolar needles that are placed on the lamina of the spine. Esophageal or nasal electrodes may be required if the surgical field extends into the region of the cervical spine. Peripheral recording sites ensure stimulus input. Maximizing the signal-to-noise ratio is an ongoing challenge in the electrically hostile environment of the operating room, but with proper electrode placement, impedance matching, and filtering, reproducible recordings generally can be obtained with 250 stimuli. As with other evoked potentials, stable baseline studies must be done before critical stages and then followed continuously when these structures are at risk.

APPLICATION

The variability of intraoperative evoked potentials makes interpretation difficult. In addition to the inherent variability due to muscle and electrical artifact, most anesthetic agents have a significant attenuating effect on cortical responses (Sloan, 1998). In most circumstances, a decrease in the amplitude of the scalp potential by more than 50% or an increase in latency by 1 ms for median nerve responses or 2 ms for tibial responses is probably significant if the concentration of anesthetic and other physiological factors have remained stable (Cheek, 1993). Subcortical potentials are less likely to be affected by anesthetic and, thus, provide a means of interpreting the significance of cortical changes (Sloan, 1998). Although in most spinal operations a decrease in the amplitude of the scalp potential with preservation of the cervical spine potential suggests anesthetic effects, this is not necessarily true in upper cord or brainstem procedures, in which the cervical response will be maintained despite a clinically important insult. Because of this, the neurophysiologist must be aware of the anesthetic levels and physiological variables and also must be in communication with the surgeon at all times, because mild changes during critical portions of the procedure may reflect substantial neural compromise.

Although the most frequent application is related to spinal surgery, especially surgery for deformity, evoked potentials may be a useful adjunct for monitoring brainstem structures during intracranial procedures or procedures at the base of the skull (Gentili et al., 1985; Schramm et al., 1989). Median nerve SSEPs may be used in conjunction with BAEPs to monitor brainstem structures, especially in patients who have large tumors involving the posterior fossa or foramen magnum. Because the BAEPs monitor primarily the region between the lower pons and the caudal midbrain, SSEPs provide information about medullary structures when these more caudal structures are at risk. SSEPs may be useful in patients who have large tumors of the posterior fossa, where BAEPs are absent or there is a potential for vascular injury in regions not served by auditory pathways (Piatt et al., 1985), and for peripheral nerve operations, especially to identify the continuity of nerve roots with suspected avulsion as well as to assist with cortical localization during resection of a tumor or seizure site.

CRANIAL NERVE MONITORING

The most frequent application of intraoperative monitoring of cranial nerves is related to posterior fossa operations, most commonly acoustic neuromas, but similar monitoring techniques are used for other extrinsic and intrinsic tumors, hemifacial spasm, trigeminal neuralgia, and vascular brainstem lesions. Procedures in the region of the orbit, cavernous sinus, or petrous region of the temporal bone pose a risk to upper cranial nerves, whereas tumors of the foramen magnum, jugular foramen, or clivus impart significant risk to lower cranial nerve function. Finally, the cranial nerve can be readily monitored in the peripheral, extracranial portion, such as the facial nerve in parotid tumors.

Cranial nerves III through XII and surrounding structures are monitored with the techniques described in the previous section (see Table 102–1). Multimodal monitoring generally is required because of the number of structures potentially at risk. The same structure may be monitored with more than one technique to maximize sensitivity and to reduce the potential of false-positive results that may have been due to anesthesia or other technical artifact. Given the complexity, each case is unique and an individual intraoperative plan must be developed, depending on the clinical findings and structures most at risk. The following section describes the techniques most helpful during operations at the Mayo Medical Center over many years; e.g., in more than 400 procedures since 1984 with the use of intraoperative monitoring during acoustic neuroma resection via the retrosigmoid approach (Ebersold et al., 1992). Although the application and efficacy of intraoperative monitoring have been well documented over the last 20 years, new monitoring techniques, surgical techniques, and anesthesia regimens continue to be developed.

POSTERIOR FOSSA ACOUSTIC NEUROMA

Cranial nerve involvement in tumors affecting the cerebellopontine angle is common, and these same structures are at high risk during surgical resection. The most common tumor in this region is an acoustic neuroma that arises from the vestibular portion of cranial nerve VIII. Cranial nerve involvement occurs frequently with acoustic neuromas, especially when the tumor is more than 2 cm in diameter (Harner and Laws, 1983; Harner et al., 1984). Although acoustic nerve involvement with hearing loss is the most frequent presenting symptom, trigeminal involvement occurs often, with facial sensory symptoms in 29% and sensory loss in 26% (Harner and Laws, 1983). Facial weakness occurs in only 13% overall, but of patients with tumors larger than 4 cm, 56% have loss of facial sensation and 31% have facial weakness (Harner and Laws, 1981). Electrophysiological signs of facial nerve damage are present in an even higher proportion of patients, often without clinical symptoms or signs. Normand and Daube (1994) reported that 73% of patients had abnormal electrophysiological studies despite only 16% with clinical facial weakness. Large tumors can even impinge on the accessory and hypoglossal nerves, but clinical symptoms or signs have not been reported.

Monitoring Techniques

FACIAL NERVE MONITORING

Although the primary surgical goal is total resection of the tumor, increasing emphasis has been placed on preservation of facial nerve function and, more recently, attempted preservation of hearing. In the past, many of these tumors were discovered only when they became large enough to cause significant clinical symptoms. By the time of diagnosis and subsequent removal, there was already significant cranial nerve involvement, which probably led to a more severe postoperative deficit. With new high-resolution imaging, these tumors frequently are identified at an early stage, when preservation of facial function and hearing becomes a realistic goal. With regard to facial function, the outcome depends mainly on tumor size, location, adherence to underlying structures, and, to a lesser extent, specific surgical techniques (Harner et al., 1987; Harner et al., 1988; Hardy et al., 1989).

Initial studies by Harner and colleagues (1987) reported that with large tumors (larger than 4 cm), nearly 100% of patients had complete facial paralysis postoperatively, even though in 12% the nerve was intact after the operation. The nerve was intact after the operation in 85% of patients who had medium-sized tumors and in all patients who had small (less than 2 cm) tumors. Nonetheless, 95% of patients who had medium-sized tumors had some postoperative weakness, and 50% had complete paralysis. Of patients with small tumors, 21% had complete paralysis and 68% had some weakness after the operation (Harner et al., 1986). If the nerve is left anatomically intact, recovery of function eventually occurs in as many as two thirds of patients (Harner and Laws, 1981).

The same authors expanded their experience to 255 patients and reported anatomical preservation of the facial nerve in 92.6% of patients. There was again a clear association with tumor size. Specifically, at 1 year after surgical resection, facial function was nearly normal in those with tumors smaller than 2 cm, and 50% of those with medium-sized tumors had clear facial deficit; the deficit was more severe when the tumor was larger than 4 cm in diameter. Only 9 of 178 patients who had follow-up at 1 year had complete absence of facial function, and this was evenly distributed among those with medium and large tumors (Ebersold et al., 1992). The trigeminal nerve suffers less damage at operation, with only a small percentage of patients having increased deficit (Harner et al., 1987). Lower cranial nerve damage occurs even less frequently (Harner et al., 1987; Ebersold et al., 1992). Clearly, preservation of motor nerve function can be improved in these difficult surgical procedures.

The benefit of intraoperative monitoring of facial nerve integrity during posterior fossa operations has been shown in many studies. In 1979, Sugita and colleagues reported an improvement in the preservation of facial nerve function when electrophysiological monitoring was used intraoperatively for acoustic neuroma. In their series of 22 cases in which 20 tumors were larger than 4 cm in diameter, they applied direct electrical stimulation to the nerve via insulated bipolar coagulating forceps. With these techniques, the authors preserved anatomical and physiological function in 86% of their patients. Compared with historical controls, Harner and co-workers (1987, 1988) reported improved facial nerve preservation with the use of intraoperative monitoring techniques. In patients with small tumors, the facial nerve was preserved in all patients, but anatomical preservation was 91% in those with medium-sized tumors and 67% in those with tumors larger than 4 cm. In comparison, the facial nerve was preserved in only 33% of unmonitored patients with large tumors. Although facial function was not markedly different immediately postoperatively, the degree of improvement in the monitored group exceeded that in the nonmonitored group, especially those with medium-sized and large tumors.

Three electrophysiological monitoring approaches can be used to complement each other in providing different types of information for monitoring the facial nerve. These techniques monitor facial function with the primary goal of preservation but also with the goals of predicting long-term outcome and advancing the surgical technique. First, preoperative EMG, blink reflexes, and facial nerve conduction studies define the amount of preoperative nerve damage and identify any spontaneous discharges. Second, inadvertent mechanical stimulation of the facial nerve is monitored by visual and auditory feedback of EMG activity in muscles innervated by the facial nerve. Third, the location and function of the nerve in the operating field are monitored by record the CMAPs over cranial muscles in response to direct electrical stimulation of the nerve by the surgeon (Harner et al., 1986).

Baseline studies are performed preoperatively. These include routine facial nerve conduction studies recording over the nasalis with a surface electrode, blink reflexes recorded in a standard fashion with supraorbital stimulation, and standard needle EMG of facial muscles, most commonly the orbicularis oris, orbicularis oculi, and masseter. Harner and co-workers (1986) showed that 6% of patients with acoustic neuromas have abnormal facial nerve conduction studies, 44% have abnormal blink reflexes, and 78% have abnormal EMG findings. This was confirmed by Normand and Daube (1994), who were able to identify facial neuropathies by electrophysiological testing five times more frequently than by clinical examination. These studies can identify abnormalities of nerve function preoperatively (Harner et al., 1986; Pavesi et al., 1992) and reliably predict the likelihood of further loss of function

during operation (Harner et al., 1986; Harner et al., 1987; Catalano et al., 1996). Harner clearly showed that preoperative abnormalities are the most accurate predictor of postoperative facial nerve function. More specifically, those with no evidence of facial neuropathy on preoperative studies had excellent facial function, whereas 75% of those with moderate to severe preoperative facial neuropathies had poor results at 3 months (Harner et al., 1987).

The second method of facial nerve monitoring is EMG activity recorded directly from the muscles in response to mechanical, metabolic, or thermal irritation. Nichrome wires (0.01 mm) are placed in the appropriate muscle 5 mm apart through 26-gauge hollow needles. Two wire electrodes can be inserted together through a single needle if the tips are exposed at different locations to avoid short-circuiting the wires. Placement of two wires separately in a muscle monitors a broader area of muscle but may show more artifact. It is possible to place wires in two different muscles, which would then be monitored simultaneously. The disadvantage of this method is that the specific muscle giving rise to neurotonic discharges cannot be identified. However, if the muscles have the same innervation, this may be satisfactory and allow monitoring of more muscles with fewer recording channels. Surface recordings or subcutaneous EEG needles generally do not provide the specificity necessary, nor do they monitor deeper areas of the muscles. Although several facial muscles can be monitored, the orbicularis oris and orbicularis oculi are of greatest clinical significance and are the most commonly monitored. Activity in the mentalis and frontalis muscles is often recorded for extracranial procedures, such as parotid tumor resection. These channels are run continuously, with immediate feedback provided to the surgeon whenever a neurotonic discharge is noted.

The third method used to monitor facial nerve function is to record the CMAPs evoked by direct stimulation of the nerve by the surgeon. CMAPs are recorded by surface electrodes, because the amplitude of the response can be monitored more reliably with this method than with intramuscular recording electrodes. A baseline preoperative response is recorded with routine nerve conduction techniques for the facial nerve for comparison with responses recorded during the operation. Subcutaneous needle electrodes are placed anterior to the lower tip of the mastoid to stimulate the facial nerve and to provide a peripheral monitor of the recording system as well as to monitor the amplitude of the distal CMAP. This method provides the advantage of being able to stimulate the facial nerve distal to the operative field and the ability to stimulate the nerve at any time without distracting the surgeon.

The mentalis muscle gives the most reliable, easily measurable responses in most patients, but the nasalis muscle is used occasionally. If possible, the surgeon stimulates a distal segment of the nerve early in the procedure to determine the threshold

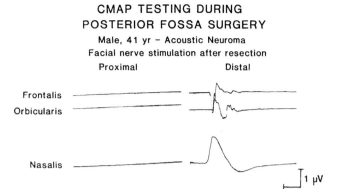

**CMAP TESTING DURING
POSTERIOR FOSSA SURGERY**

Male, 41 yr – Acoustic Neuroma

Facial nerve stimulation after resection

Figure 102–7. Facial nerve stimulation after tumor removal. Note the complete absence of the proximal response and preservation of the distal response, suggesting significant axon injury. CMAP, compound muscle action potential. (From Daube JR, Harper CM: Surgical monitoring of cranial and peripheral nerves. In Desmedt JE [ed]: Neuromonitoring in Surgery. Amsterdam, The Netherlands, Elsevier Science, 1989; 115–138. By permission of JE Desmedt.)

for activation and the voltage needed for a supramaximal response and to compare with the baseline. Normal nerve can be activated with less than 20 mV at 0.05 ms (<4 mA). Stimulation greater than 25 mV (>5 mA) may cause current spread, especially with a monopolar stimulator, and activate other nerves in the surgical field. Stimulation of the nerve can be performed at intervals as the surgeon requests, either to localize the nerve or to evaluate the integrity of the nerve. In large tumors involving several nerves, the individual nerves can be identified by electrical stimulation with either CMAPs or fine-wire EMG recordings. At the end of the operation, the nerve is stimulated proximally in the surgical field and the amplitude is compared with that of the distal stimulation site. By this means, one can quantitate the degree of axon disruption. If the nerve has been damaged or completely transected during dissection, it can still be activated distally, but no response will be obtained from proximal portions (Fig. 102–7).

The correlation between the preservation of an evoked response intraoperatively and the preservation of facial function postoperatively has been excellent. In one study, no patient who retained an evoked response had total facial paresis, and all those who lost the response had complete paralysis (Harner et al., 1986). Also, facial nerve function generally improves in 60% to 70% of patients when a proximal response is evoked at the end of the operation (Fig. 102–8) (Harner et al., 1988). Furthermore, Ebersold and colleagues (1992) reported that if the proximal amplitude is 90% of the distal response at the completion of the operation, the patient is expected to have a good early recovery, whereas those with proximal amplitudes of less than 50% of the distal response are expected to have various degrees of permanent weakness.

TRIGEMINAL NERVE MONITORING

Involvement of the trigeminal nerve is not uncommon; approximately 30% of patients present with facial sensory symptoms or clinical facial sensory loss (Harner and Laws, 1983; Normand and Daube, 1994). This nerve can be damaged further during dissection, especially in cases of larger tumors, leading to potential postoperative pain syndromes. Although the sensory division cannot be monitored reliably, the motor division can be monitored easily with fine-wire EMG recordings from the masseter or temporalis muscle. As in the facial nerve, these wires can be used to record neurotonic discharges during dissection or to record CMAPs with intraoperative stimulation by the surgeon. Stimulation of the trigeminal nerve with small needle electrodes adjacent to the nerve in the supraorbital or infraorbital foramina can elicit NAPs with a minimum of artifact if the stimulus voltage (current) is kept low. Antidromic NAPs also can be recorded with stimulation of the nerve in the surgical field while one is recording from the peripheral nerve. The latter technique is more often marred by excess shock artifact, precluding reliable measurement of the NAPs.

Distal Stimulation

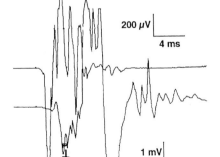

Proximal Stimulation

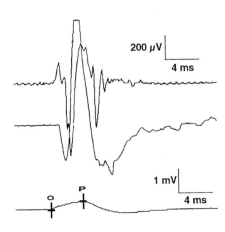

Figure 102–8. Facial nerve stimulation after tumor removal. Note approximately 60% conduction block of facial compound muscle action potential with proximal stimulation.

ACOUSTIC NERVE MONITORING

The acoustic nerve is involved most frequently in tumors of the cerebellopontine angle. Harner et al. (1984) reported preoperative hearing loss in 95% of patients with acoustic neuromas. Preservation of hearing is a reasonable goal but is often difficult, especially if there are preoperative hearing deficits or tumors greater than 2 cm in diameter (Ojemann et al., 1984; Silverstein et al., 1986; Nadol et al., 1987; Kanzaki et al., 1989; Slavit et al., 1991; Ebersold et al., 1992; Harper et al., 1992). Other factors, such as the lateral extent of the tumor in the internal auditory canal, the relationship of the tumor to the blood supply to the cochlea and cochlear nerve, and the differences in biologic characteristics such as "adhesiveness" to nerves in the internal auditory canal, also have a role in determining hearing preservation (Slavit et al., 1991).

Early controlled studies comparing monitored patients with unmonitored ones showed a clear benefit of preservation of hearing in patients who had small tumors when these monitoring techniques were used. Specifically, Harper and co-workers (1992) showed that in tumors less than 1.1 cm in diameter, 79% of the monitored group had preserved hearing postoperatively, compared with only 42% in the unmonitored group. When tumor size reached 2 cm or greater, intraoperative BAEP monitoring did not provide significant benefit, and if there was poor hearing preoperatively or poor BAEP findings the patient generally did not have hearing postoperatively (Harner et al., 1996). Others have clearly shown the benefit of acoustic nerve monitoring during posterior fossa surgery (Ojemann et al., 1984; Radtke et al., 1989). Despite this relatively poor prognosis for hearing preservation, it is of value to attempt to monitor auditory function if baseline recordings are present. Reliable potentials may not be present during preoperative baseline studies, but when they are, they can provide a guide to the preservation of nerve function during the operation. If there is no hearing preoperatively, BAEP monitoring has little to add.

The three techniques frequently used include (1) BAEPs, (2) EChG, and (3) direct recording of the NAPs. The monitoring of these evoked potentials makes it possible to recognize damage early before permanent neurological deficit, to predict postoperative hearing function, and to improve surgical technique in the future by recognizing that a particular surgical maneuver leads to an irreversible deficit.

BAEPs are the mainstay of acoustic nerve monitoring performed to preserve hearing. The recording technique differs from that with routine studies. Intraoperatively, a gold foil–covered sponge electrode (Nicolet Biomedical, Madison, WI) is inserted into the external ear canal and the canal is sealed with bone wax. This electrode is referenced to a tin disk electrode at the vertex. The ear is then covered with tape to maintain a dry environment. Broadband click stimulation with alternating polarity is provided through the central core of the sponge electrode at a frequency of 9.9 Hz. White noise is provided to the contralateral ear at a 60-dB sound level. The response generally is averaged with 500 to 1,000 sweeps, which take approximately 2 minutes to record. If more rapid acquisition is desired, the frequency can be increased, but this generally leads to attenuation of the waveforms. BAEPs are performed every 5 to 10 minutes during opening of the dura mater to establish a stable baseline. After the dura mater has been opened, the responses are monitored continuously.

In most patients, waves I and V are readily identifiable, although considerably more delayed than in the recording from an awake patient. The latency of wave V generally shows mild prolongation after dural opening, probably owing to cooling. At this point, a new stable baseline is established, and the anesthetic is maintained at as stable a level as possible. In nearly all cases, there is some gradual or sudden change in the BAEPs (Harper et al., 1992; Harner et al., 1996). In general, a latency prolongation of 1 ms or an amplitude loss of 50% is considered significant and warrants informing the surgeon. If wave V begins to decrease in amplitude or to show a prolongation early in the course of dissection, there is probably excess traction on the nerve, which can be corrected by release of the cerebellar retractor (Fig. 102–9). The loss or reduction of wave I or waves I

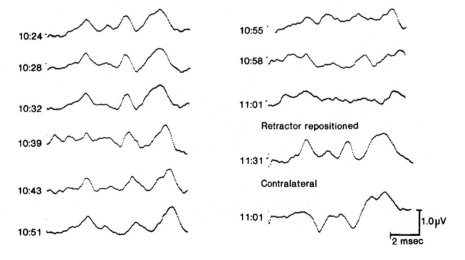

Figure 102–9. Brainstem auditory evoked response was lost during cerebellar retraction and then returned after the retractor was released during acoustic neuroma surgery.

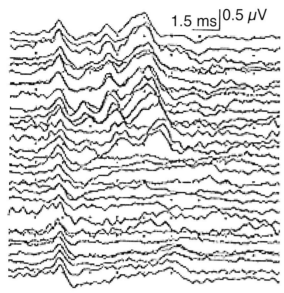

1.5 ms | 0.5 μV

Figure 102–10. Brainstem auditory evoked potentials. Waves II to V were lost during dissection. Gradual return of wave V with preservation of hearing.

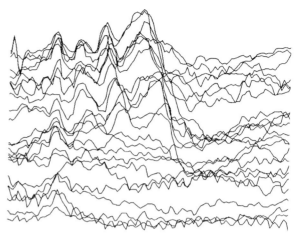

Figure 102–12. Waves II to V were lost during dissection; no return and no preservation of hearing in the patient.

and V in combination is more probably due to dissection (Watanabe et al., 1989) (Figs. 102–10 and 102–11). Extracanalicular dissection generally involves wave V to a greater degree (Fig. 102–12), whereas intracanalicular dissection generally involves both waves I and V (Ojemann et al., 1984; Luders, 1988).

Once the surgeon is aware of a significant change, the possible course of action is (1) to discontinue dissection for several minutes to see if the waveform returns, (2) to release the cerebellar retractor, (3) to move to another area, or (4) to apply a vasodilating substance, such as papaverine, to the vessels on the nerve (Harner et al., 1996). The sudden loss of

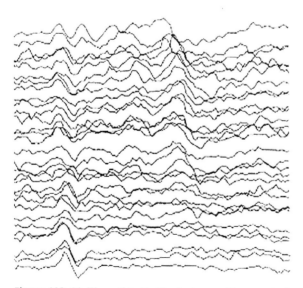

Figure 102–11. Waves II to V of brainstem auditory evoked potentials were lost during dissection; no return and no preservation of hearing in the patient.

BAEPs generally is associated with the loss of the internal auditory artery during dissection or cautery around the tumor (Nadol et al., 1987; Harper et al., 1992). By learning from intraoperative monitoring, surgeons can modify their surgical technique to separate and to preserve even the tiny vessels associated with the tumor, because they may provide arterial supply to the cochlear apparatus (Ebersold et al., 1992).

The predictive value of loss of BAEPs is not absolute but strongly suggests postoperative hearing loss. The loss of wave V generally is associated with hearing loss, as is the loss of wave I. In a study by Watanabe and colleagues (1989), 10 of 13 patients who lost wave V had hearing loss. However, preservation of wave V did not guarantee that hearing would be preserved; 2 of 68 patients with wave V present at the completion of the procedure had hearing loss. Similarly, the loss of wave I resulted in hearing loss in most patients, but 4 of 12 were deaf postoperatively despite preservation of the wave. Finally, the loss of wave V could be reversible, mostly by releasing tension on the retractor, with preservation of hearing, whereas loss of wave I was generally permanent. These findings were confirmed by Harper and co-workers (1992), who found that if waves I and V were preserved, hearing was preserved in 67% of patients. When wave I alone was preserved, useful hearing was present in 29%. However, loss of both waves I and V was always associated with hearing loss.

Thus, monitoring BAEPs is beneficial when any reproducible waveforms can be recorded during preoperative baseline studies, especially when the tumor is less than 2 cm in diameter.

NAPs have gained popularity as an alternative or a supplemental means of monitoring acoustic nerve integrity during posterior fossa operations. Moller and Jannetta initially described this procedure, and we refer the reader to their rigorous evaluation of this technique (Moller and Jannetta, 1983; Moller et al., 1994; Moller, 1996). The procedure involves

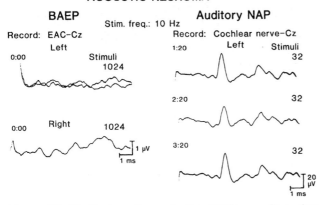

**COCHLEAR NERVE MONITORING
ACOUSTIC NEUROMA**

Figure 102–13. Nerve action potential (NAP) recording when brainstem auditory evoked potentials (BAEPs) cannot be recorded during baseline studies.

placement of a wick electrode directly on the exposed intracranial portion of the acoustic nerve after exposure. Broadband click stimulation is provided through either insert earphones or the previously described sponge electrodes. A near-field potential is generally recorded with minimal averaging and is much larger than the corresponding BAEPs (Moller, 1996) (Fig. 102–13).

This technique provides nearly real-time monitoring of the acoustic nerve from the cochlea to the brainstem. Stretching the acoustic nerve typically causes a prolongation of the latency, whereas mechanical injury causes a decrease in the amplitude of the negative peak (Moller, 1996). As with BAEPs, a sudden loss of the potential is probably due to an irreversible loss of the blood supply to the cochlea. Hearing preservation with the use of direct NAP recordings produced results similar to those of BAEP recording. Silverstein and colleagues (1986) reported 37% hearing preservation with the use of NAPs, and reported this as a valuable means of providing rapid feedback to reverse potential damage to the acoustic nerve.

Moller and Jannetta (1983) successfully applied this technique to other posterior fossa procedures, such as microvascular decompression. Latency changes of 0.5 and 1 ms should be reported to the surgeon, and an amplitude reduction of 50% is significant (Cheek, 1993). Maintaining strict criteria for abnormalities is again fraught with difficulty and error, because a small change may lead to significant nerve damage. A smaller change during a critical portion of the procedure should be reported to the surgeon, especially if baseline studies have been stable to that point.

Electrocochleography is the least-used method of monitoring acoustic nerve integrity during posterior fossa operations. These are also click-evoked potentials that are generated from the acoustic nerve, but they differ in that they are recorded near the cochlear apparatus. The electrocochleogram consists of a short latency response that corresponds to the

cochlear microphonics and a major negative waveform that correlates roughly with wave I of the BAEP (Luders, 1988). The electrode generally is placed through the tympanic membrane to lie on the bony promontory of the middle ear. Tympanic and extra-tympanic approaches have been described for acoustic neuroma and vestibular nerve section operations (Winzenburg et al., 1993). Although this technique appears to predict damage to the distal nerve or the cochlear apparatus (Ojemann et al., 1984; Nadol et al., 1987; Winzenburg et al., 1993; Mullatti et al., 1999), it monitors only the lateral portion of the nerve. The medial intracranial portion can be damaged substantially without effect on the potential (Moller, 1996).

The decision of which technique or, often, combination of acoustic nerve monitoring techniques to use must be made on an individual basis, depending on the clinical deficit, tumor size, surgical approach, and personal preference. BAEPs are the most useful technique for monitoring the acoustic nerve during posterior fossa procedures with the retrosigmoid approach. BAEPs have the advantage of being a simple, noninvasive technique that monitors the entire auditory pathway, including the acoustic nerve and brainstem pathways, throughout the procedure. The disadvantages of BAEP monitoring include the frequency of poor baseline studies and longer acquisition time. Although these studies are sensitive, their predictive value is not absolute.

NAPs recorded directly from the acoustic nerve have the advantage of rapid acquisition but require that the electrode be placed and maintained directly within the field, which may be difficult with larger tumors. An alternative technique, recording the potentials near the floor of the fourth ventricle, has been described and may be useful with these large tumors (Moller, 1996). Also, these potentials monitor the intracranial portion of the acoustic nerve but do not provide information about the brainstem pathways. A combination of these techniques may provide the most ideal monitoring system. BAEPs can be monitored initially, followed by combined monitoring of BAEPs and NAPs after the tumor has been exposed. Alternatively, NAP monitoring certainly has a role when BAEPs either are not obtainable or are poorly reproducible (Roberson et al., 1999). Reliable EChG requires considerable experience with electrode placement and has not been shown to add information to what can be obtained with the alternative techniques. The general setup of the various recordings obtained during resection of an acoustic neuroma via the suboccipital approach is shown in Figure 102–14.

MICROVASCULAR DECOMPRESSION

Microvascular decompression for facial pain, pharyngeal pain, disabling positional vertigo, or hemifacial spasm is not an infrequent procedure and poses significant risk to the cranial nerves being decom-

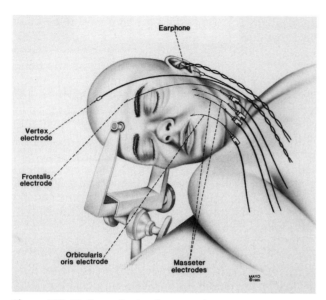

Figure 102–14. General setup for acoustic neuroma resection via the suboccipital approach. Note the fine-wire recordings in facial and trigeminal muscles. In this illustration, a single fine-wire electrode was placed in facial muscles. Pairs of electrodes generally allow better recordings if the channels are available. (From Daube JR, Harper CM: Surgical monitoring of cranial and peripheral nerves. In Desmedt JE [ed]: Neuromonitoring in Surgery. Amsterdam, The Netherlands, Elsevier Science, 1989; 115–138. By permission of Mayo Foundation.)

pressed and to surrounding structures. Treatment of hemifacial spasm is the most frequent microvascular decompression procedure that requires the assistance of the neurophysiologist to warn of impending nerve trauma and also to ensure adequate decompression. The latter is assessed by means of the lateral spread response, which was described initially by Nielsen (1984b) and Moller and Jannetta (1985).

In patients with hemifacial spasm, a unique response occurs in muscles innervated by a facial nerve branch when another facial nerve branch is stimulated. Specifically, Nielsen (1984b) described a technique in which the zygomatic or temporal branch was stimulated and a response was recorded from the mentalis muscle. The response, not seen in normal subjects, is a brief 1- to 5-ms burst of spikes, 100 to 200 µV in amplitude, that follows the stimulus by 7 to 12 ms. This response has been called the "lateral spread response," because it may arise by ephaptic activation of facial nerve axons at a site of vascular compression either outside the brainstem or in the facial nucleus (Nielsen, 1984a; Moller and Jannetta, 1985). The lateral spread response varies somewhat in appearance from one stimulus to the next. The usefulness of this response for intraoperative monitoring is that when the offending vessel has been removed from the nerve, the lateral spread response disappears completely, almost immediately. If the vessel is allowed to touch the nerve again, the lateral spread response returns quickly (Moller and Jannetta, 1985, 1987; Harper, 1991). Furthermore, if the lateral spread response is present

at the completion of the procedure, the likelihood that the spasm will remain is high; conversely, if the response is absent, the likelihood of cure is high (Nielsen and Jannetta, 1984). Specifically, hemifacial spasm was eliminated in 95% of patients when the lateral spread response disappeared intraoperatively. Conversely, 4 of 7 patients in whom the response remained had persistent spasm that required reoperation (Moller and Jannetta, 1987).

Technique

Recordings from both the orbicularis oculi and the orbicularis oris muscles give greater flexibility. Two fine wires are inserted approximately 5 mm apart into each of these muscles while the patient is awake to ensure proper placement. At the same time, subcutaneous EEG electrodes are inserted over the zygomatic and mandibular branches of the facial nerve to provide the stimulation. A standard 50- to 150-V (5- to 15-mA) stimulus is applied for 0.05 to 0.1 ms. With stimulation of the mandibular branch, a lateral spread response is recorded over the orbicularis oculi muscle. Similarly, stimulation over the zygomatic branch may produce a response recorded in the orbicularis oris muscle (Fig. 102–15). The sites of stimulation and recording, with the appropriate values, are determined best by preoperative EMG and a nerve conduction study. During exploration and decompression, these responses are recorded frequently, with communication to the surgeon about their presence or disappearance (Fig. 102–16). This technique is especially important when several vessels are in contact with the nerve, and only the disappearance of the lateral spread response helps identify the vessel that is causing the spasm. Continuous EMG recordings with fine wires are also performed to warn of potential damage of the facial nerve by identifying neurotonic discharges.

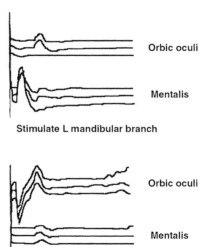

Figure 102–15. Lateral spread response. Orbic, orbicularis.

Stimulate Zygomatic   **Record Orb. oris**

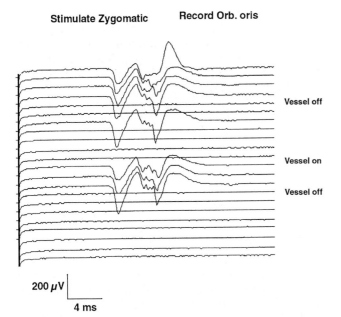

200 µV

4 ms

Figure 102–16. Lateral spread response recorded over the orbicularis (Orb.) oris muscle while the zygomatic branch of the facial nerve was being stimulated. Note the disappearance during decompression, with return of the response when the aberrant vessel is placed back on the nerve.

SELECTIVE STIMULATION OF CRANIAL NERVE

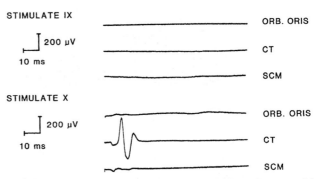

Figure 102–17. Intraoperative fine-wire recordings from cranial nerve–innervated muscles to identify the appropriate nerve during glossopharyngeal nerve sectioning. Stimulation of the glossopharyngeal nerve (IX) failed to elicit a response, but direct stimulation of vagus nerve (X) rootlets produced a well-defined compound muscle action potential from the cricothyroid (CT). ORB., orbicularis; SCM, sternocleidomastoid. (Modified from Lagerlund TD, Harper CM Jr, Sharbrough FW, et al: An electroencephalographic study of glossopharyngeal neuralgia with syncope. Arch Neurol 1988;45:472–475. By permission of the American Medical Association.)

Acoustic nerve monitoring is also important in these cases, because as many as 15% of the patients operated on for hemifacial spasm have hearing loss postoperatively (Auger et al., 1986). The value of monitoring BAEPs in microvascular decompression for hemifacial spasm was demonstrated by Radtke and colleagues (1989), when they showed a clear decrease in the frequency and severity of hearing loss in patients who were monitored compared with a historical age-matched control group. Subsequent studies also have reported success with auditory monitoring during hemifacial spasm surgery (Moller and Moller, 1989; Sindou et al., 1992; Acevedo et al., 1997).

Sectioning of individual cranial nerves has been necessary for some intractable pain syndromes when medical therapy, injection procedures, and microvascular decompression are inadequate in controlling symptoms. Incapacitating vertigo may also require sectioning of the vestibular nerve. In each operation, monitoring of electromyographic activity or CMAPs can help identify the critical segments of the nerve for sectioning and warn of irritation of other surrounding nerves.

Monitoring for sectioning of the sensory branches of the trigeminal nerve can include recordings from the motor and the sensory divisions. Motor branch monitoring is similar to that described for acoustic neuroma. Fine-wire or monopolar needle electrodes are placed in the masseter and temporalis muscles. The surgeon stimulates the branches of the trigeminal nerve, sectioning only those that do not produce a motor response. The facial nerve is monitored during these procedures as well as the acoustic

nerve. In patients undergoing sectioning of the glossopharyngeal nerve for glossopharyngeal neuralgia, spontaneous and stimulus-evoked EMG responses can be recorded from the cricothyroid muscle to avoid sectioning of any nerve rootlets contributing to the vagus nerve (Lagerlund et al., 1988) (Fig. 102–17).

SPINAL ACCESSORY NERVE

The spinal accessory nerve is monitored most often during removal of large meningiomas and glomus jugulare tumors, although resection of some carcinomas of the neck may be an indication for monitoring this nerve. The spinal accessory nerve is monitored in the same way as the facial nerve, with wire electrodes placed in the trapezius or sternocleidomastoid muscle or both. The electrodes usually are placed after the patient is asleep to ensure that they are not dislodged during positioning and intubation. CMAPs can be recorded from the wire electrodes to assist with nerve identification and tumor dissection. Less often, the spinal accessory nerve is directly involved in tumors requiring direct dissection and, thus, is less often the source of neurotonic discharges. When this nerve does produce such discharges, they are similar to those of other nerves.

HYPOGLOSSAL NERVE

Neurotonic discharges arising in the hypoglossal nerve can be recorded readily from the tongue muscles with fine-wire electrodes inserted by a submandibular approach near the midline to a depth of 3 to 5 cm. Wires can be placed selectively in the right or left side of the tongue from this location. Recording

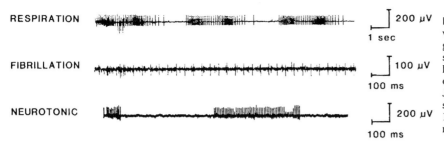

Figure 102–18. Activity recorded from the vocalis muscle with fine-wire electromyographic electrodes (EMG) during neck dissection for metastatic thyroid cancer. (From Daube JR, Harper CM: Surgical monitoring of cranial and peripheral nerves. In Desmedt JE [ed]: Neuromonitoring in Surgery. Amsterdam, The Netherlands, Elsevier Science, 1989; 115–138. By permission of JE Desmedt.)

is usually performed only during resection of large posterior fossa meningiomas, clivus tumors, or foramen magnum tumors. Tumors in this region generally involve more diffuse brainstem structures that may require the use of BAEPs as well as SSEPs.

Glossopharyngeal and Vagus Nerves

Few surgical procedures involve the glossopharyngeal and vagus nerves. The most frequent application of intraoperative monitoring is related to their peripheral course, as in neck dissection. They may also be involved in large brainstem tumors or vascular structures in the lower brainstem. Recordings could be made from posterior pharyngeal muscles to monitor the glossopharyngeal nerve, but electrode placement is difficult in an intubated patient. The vagus nerve is monitored most readily by evaluating EMG responses from the cricothyroid or vocalis muscle. The cricothyroid electrodes can be placed easily by a routine percutaneous technique while the patient is awake to ensure proper placement. Although the vocalis muscle can be approached by a standard percutaneous technique, the assistance of an otolaryngologist can ensure proper placement through direct laryngoscopy.

The use of this technique to monitor the recurrent laryngeal nerve during an operation to resect an invasive thyroid carcinoma in the neck is shown in Figure 102–18. Fine wires were placed in the vocalis muscle after intubation. Spontaneous EMG activity was observed and included fibrillation potentials and rhythmical bursts of motor unit activity related to respirations. These types of spontaneous activity and artifacts due to wire movement and cautery could readily be distinguished from neurotonic discharges, which occurred intermittently during dissection in and around the recurrent laryngeal nerve.

Oculomotor, Abducens, and Trochlear Nerves

Surgical procedures in the region of the cavernous sinus, supraorbital ridge, or intraventricular tumors pose a risk for the oculomotor, trochlear, and abducens nerves. In large tumors such as meningiomas, pituitary tumors, or lymphomas, the anatomy may be substantially disrupted, which makes identification of these nerves difficult (Sekhar and Moller, 1986). Fine Nichrome wire electrodes can be placed in the medial rectus (oculomotor nerve), lateral rec-

tus (abducens nerve), and superior oblique (trochlear nerve) muscles to monitor EMG activity and CMAPs. When the patient is asleep, the electrodes can be inserted percutaneously by the neurophysiologist or with the assistance of an ophthalmologist. After the electrodes have been inserted, free-run responses are recorded to identify neurotonic discharges, and triggered CMAP responses are obtained with selective stimulation by the surgeon for nerve identification.

For most surgical procedures in the posterior fossa or the neck, monitoring of several channels of electrical activity is necessary, as defined by the nerves at risk in the operation. It is usual to monitor several different cranial motor nerves on different channels. These recordings are often combined with a median nerve SSEP to monitor the central pathways or an auditory evoked response to monitor the acoustic nerve. The monitoring is selected for each patient for assessment of the structures at risk intraoperatively for that patient. No single protocol can be used to define the monitoring that will be optimal for all patients.

References

Acevedo JC, Sindou M, Fischer C, Vial C: Microvascular decompression for the treatment of hemifacial spasm: Retrospective study of a consecutive series of 75 operated patients—electrophysiologic and anatomical surgical analysis. Stereotact Funct Neurosurg 1997;68:260–265.

Auger RG, Piepgras DG, Laws ER Jr: Hemifacial spasm: Results of microvascular decompression of the facial nerve in 54 patients. Mayo Clin Proc 1986;61:640–644.

Catalano PJ, Post KD, Sen C, Simpson D: Preoperative facial nerve studies predict paresis following cerebellopontine angle surgery. Am J Otol 1996;17:446–451.

Cheek JC: Posterior fossa intraoperative monitoring. J Clin Neurophysiol 1993;10:412–424.

Colletti V, Fiorino FG: Advances in monitoring of seventh and eighth cranial nerve function during posterior fossa surgery. Am J Otol 1998;19:503–512.

Daube JR, Harper CM: Surgical monitoring of cranial and peripheral nerves. In Desmedt JE [ed]: Neuromonitoring in Surgery. Amsterdam, The Netherlands, Elsevier Science, 1989; 115–138.

Ebersold MJ, Harner SG, Beatty CW, et al: Current results of the retrosigmoid approach to acoustic neuroma. J Neurosurg 1992;76:901–909.

Gentili F, Lougheed WM, Yamashiro K, Corrado C: Monitoring of sensory evoked potentials during surgery of skull base tumours. Can J Neurol Sci 1985;12:336–340.

Hardy DG, Macfarlane R, Baguley D, Moffat DA: Surgery for acoustic neuroma: An analysis of 100 translabyrinthine operations. J Neurosurg 1989;71:799–804.

Harner SG, Laws ER Jr: Posterior fossa approach for removal of acoustic neurinomas. Arch Otolaryngol 1981;107:590–593.

Harner SG, Laws ER Jr: Clinical findings in patients with acoustic neurinoma. Mayo Clin Proc 1983;58:721–728.

Harner SG, Laws ER Jr, Onofrio BM: Hearing preservation after removal of acoustic neurinoma. Laryngoscope 1984;94:1431–1434.

Harner SG, Daube JR, Ebersold MJ: Electrophysiologic monitoring of facial nerve during temporal bone surgery. Laryngoscope 1986;96:65–69.

Harner SG, Daube JR, Beatty CW, Ebersold MJ: Intraoperative monitoring of the facial nerve. Laryngoscope 1988;98:209–212.

Harner SG, Daube JR, Ebersold MJ, Beatty CW: Improved preservation of facial nerve function with use of electrical monitoring during removal of acoustic neuromas. Mayo Clin Proc 1987; 62:92–102.

Harner SG, Harper CM, Beatty CW, et al: Far-field auditory brainstem response in neurotologic surgery. Am J Otol 1996;17:150–153.

Harper CM Jr: AAEM case report #21: Hemifacial spasm: Preoperative diagnosis and intraoperative management. Muscle Nerve 1991;14:213–218.

Harper CM, Daube JR: Facial nerve electromyography and other cranial nerve monitoring. J Clin Neurophysiol 1998;15:206–216.

Harper CM, Harner SG, Slavit DH, et al: Effect of BAEP monitoring on hearing preservation during acoustic neuroma resection. Neurology 1992;42:1551–1553.

Kanzaki J, Ogawa K, Shiobara R, Toya S: Hearing preservation in acoustic neuroma surgery and postoperative audiological findings. Acta Otolaryngol 1989;107:474–478.

Lagerlund TD, Harper CM Jr, Sharbrough FW, et al: An electroencephalographic study of glossopharyngeal neuralgia with syncope. Arch Neurol 1988;45:472–475.

Luders H: Surgical monitoring with auditory evoked potentials. J Clin Neurophysiol 1988;5:261–285.

Markand ON: Brainstem auditory evoked potentials. J Clin Neurophysiol 1994;11:319–342.

Moller AR: Monitoring auditory function during operations to remove acoustic tumors. Am J Otol 1996;17:452–460.

Moller AR, Jannetta PJ: Monitoring auditory functions during cranial nerve microvascular decompression operations by direct recording from the eighth nerve. J Neurosurg 1983;59:493–499.

Moller AR, Jannetta PJ: Hemifacial spasm: Results of electrophysiologic recording during microvascular decompression operations. Neurology 1985;35:969–974.

Moller AR, Jannetta PJ: Monitoring facial EMG responses during microvascular decompression operations for hemifacial spasm. J Neurosurg 1987;66:681–685.

Moller AR, Moller MB: Does intraoperative monitoring of auditory evoked potentials reduce incidence of hearing loss as a complication of microvascular decompression of cranial nerves? Neurosurgery 1989;24:257–263.

Moller AR, Jannetta PJ, Jho HD: Click-evoked responses from the cochlear nucleus: A study in human. Electroencephalogr Clin Neurophysiol 1994;92:215–224.

Moller AR, Jannetta PJ, Sekhar LN: Contributions from the auditory nerve to the brain-stem auditory evoked potentials (BAEPs): Results of intracranial recording in man. Electroencephalogr Clin Neurophysiol 1988;71:198–211.

Mullatti N, Coakham HB, Maw AR, et al: Intraoperative monitoring during surgery for acoustic neuroma: Benefits of an extratympanic intrameatal electrode. J Neurol Neurosurg Psychiatry 1999;66:591–599.

Nadol JB Jr, Levine R, Ojemann RG, et al: Preservation of hearing in surgical removal of acoustic neuromas of the internal auditory canal and cerebellar pontine angle. Laryngoscope 1987; 97:1287–1294.

Nielsen VK: Pathophysiology of hemifacial spasm: I. Ephaptic transmission and ectopic excitation. Neurology 1984a;34:418–426.

Nielsen VK: Pathophysiology of hemifacial spasm: II. Lateral spread of the supraorbital nerve reflex. Neurology 1984b;34:427–431.

Nielsen VK, Jannetta PJ: Pathophysiology of hemifacial spasm: III. Effects of facial nerve decompression. Neurology 1984;34:891–897.

Normand MM, Daube JR: Cranial nerve conduction and needle electromyography in patients with acoustic neuromas: A model of compression neuropathy. Muscle Nerve 1994;17:1401–1406.

Orbemann RG, Levine RA, Montgomery WM, McGaffigan P: Use of intraoperative auditory evoked potentials to preserve hearing in unilateral acoustic neuroma removal. J Neurosurg 1984; 61:938–948.

Pavesi G, Macaluso GM, Tinchelli S, et al: Presurgical electrophysiological findings in acoustic nerve tumours. Electromyogr Clin Neurophysiol 1992;32:119–123.

Piatt JH Jr, Radtke RA, Erwin CW: Limitations of brain stem auditory evoked potentials for intraoperative monitoring during a posterior fossa operation: Case report and technical note. Neurosurgery 1985;16:818–821.

Radtke RA, Erwin CW, Wilkins RH: Intraoperative brainstem auditory evoked potentials: Significant decrease in postoperative morbidity. Neurology 1989;39:187–191.

Roberson JB Jr, Jackson LE, McAuley JR: Acoustic neuroma surgery: Absent auditory brainstem response does not contraindicate attempted hearing preservation. Laryngoscope 1999; 109:904–910.

Schramm J, Watanabe E, Strauss C, Fahlbusch R: Neurophysiologic monitoring in posterior fossa surgery. I. Technical principles, applicability and limitations. Acta Neurochir 1989;98:9–18.

Sekhar LN, Moller AR: Operative management of tumors involving the cavernous sinus. J Neurosurg 1986;64:879–889.

Silverstein H, McDaniel A, Norrell H, Haberkamp T: Hearing preservation after acoustic neuroma surgery with intraoperative direct eighth cranial nerve monitoring: Part II. A classification of results. Otolaryngol Head Neck Surg 1986;95:285–291.

Sindou M, Fobe JL, Ciriano D, Fischer C: Hearing prognosis and intraoperative guidance of brainstem auditory evoked potential in microvascular decompression. Laryngoscope 1992;102:678–682.

Slavit DH, Harner SG, Harper CM Jr, Beatty CW: Auditory monitoring during acoustic neuroma removal. Arch Otolaryngol Head Neck Surg 1991;117:1153–1157.

Sloan TB: Anesthetic effects on electrophysiologic recordings. J Clin Neurophysiol 1998;15:217–226.

Sugita K, Kobayashi S, Mutsuga N, et al: Microsurgery for acoustic neurinoma—lateral position and preservation of facial and cochlear nerves. Neurol Med Chir (Tokyo) 1979;19:637–641.

Watanabe E, Schramm J, Strauss C, Fahlbusch R: Neurophysiologic monitoring in posterior fossa surgery. II. BAEP-waves I and V and preservation of hearing. Acta Neurochir (Wien) 1989;98:118–128.

Winzenburg SM, Margolis RH, Levine SC, et al: Tympanic and transtympanic electrocochleography in acoustic neuroma and vestibular nerve section surgery. Am J Otol 1993;14:63–69.

CHAPTER 103

Monitoring Spinal Function During Surgery*

Jasper R. Daube

STRUCTURES TO MONITOR DURING SPINE AND
  AORTA SURGERY
MONITORING METHODS
  Somatosensory Evoked Potentials
    Stimulating and Recording Electrodes
    Technical Factors
  Motor Evoked Potentials
    Stimulating Electrodes
    Recording Electrodes
    Technical Factors
  Electromyographic and Nerve Conduction
  Studies

TYPES OF SURGERY
  Primary Spine Disease
    Cervical Spine Disease
    Thoracic Spine Disease
    Lumbosacral Spine Disease
  Primary Neural Disease
    Dorsal Rhizotomy
    Cauda Equina and Tethered Cord
  Primary Vascular Disease
SUMMARY

Monitoring neural function during surgery has been a long-standing tradition in anesthesia for defining the level of neuromuscular junction block with "train-of-four" stimulation. Surgical monitoring has expanded enormously over the last few years to include all levels of the central and peripheral nervous systems, and many different neural systems (Herdmann et al., 1996; Guerit, 1998). Monitoring is of benefit in many surgical procedures on the spine and spinal contents. Although a persistent neurological deficit develops immediately postoperatively in only a small proportion of patients—usually fewer than 0.5%—who have corrective operations for scoliosis or other surgical procedures on the spine, these complications can be devastating. In half of the patients, the complications produce complete paraplegia, and in the other half they produce incomplete paraplegia, with a third of the patients having no recovery of function (MacEwen et al., 1975). Careful surgical techniques and stabilization of the spine during surgery have helped to keep this complication rate small. To further decrease this possible complication of scoliosis surgery, the "wake-up test" was devised (Hall et al., 1978). To ensure continuity of the spinal cord pathways after correction of a spinal deformity, the patient is awakened during the surgical procedure and asked to voluntarily move the feet. Although this test is help-

ful, it is difficult to perform. Also, there are problems with changing the level of anesthesia. Furthermore, the test is not applicable to patients who are undergoing a surgical procedure for a disorder for which there is no well-defined time of major hazard.

Surgical monitoring allows some patients to be viewed as surgical candidates who otherwise might not have been considered because of the risks of an adverse outcome. The purposes of monitoring include the following:

Demonstrating function
Monitoring function
Warning of irritation
Identifying damage
Localizing damage
Identifying tissue

The primary goal of intraoperative monitoring is to prevent new neurological deficits by identifying impairment early enough so the cause can be corrected promptly (Dunne and Field, 1991). Such identification is best accomplished by demonstrating normal function early in a procedure and testing repeatedly in search of changes that signal impending damage. Electrophysiological testing early in a procedure distinguishes between functions that remain intact with the patient under anesthesia and those that do not, owing to normal variation, patient age, underlying disease, or other factors. Thus, monitoring can reassure the surgeon that neural function is intact during the operation, allowing greater intervention than would have been contemplated in the absence of monitoring. Continuous monitoring of neural function demonstrates physiological changes

---

*This chapter is adapted from "Spinal Cord Monitoring," by Jasper Daube, from *Clinical Neurophysiology*, 2nd ed., edited by Jasper R. Daube, copyright by the Mayo Foundation for Medical Education and Research. Used by permission of Oxford University Press, Inc.

due to alterations in temperature, anesthetic, or hypotension. These changes may be the earliest signs of such alterations, changing even before the vital signs do. Such changes typically are reversible, with these parameters returning to baseline after the alteration has been corrected.

Similar reversible alterations in recordings occur when a manipulation results in a nondestructive change in neural function that can be recognized by monitoring function continuously. Irritation of neural tissue, or mild local compression, produces changes that are reversed after the offending activity has been relieved. Early recognition of the alteration allows surgeons to modify the procedure to decrease the likelihood of a persistent deficit. Destructive manipulation—for example, severing tissue—is also readily recognizable but is not reversible. Thus, monitoring provides immediate evidence not only of damage but also of the severity of the damage. Selective recordings can localize the damage within the neural structures at risk, by demonstrating which nerves or tracts are still functional and which are not.

Intraoperative testing can assist the surgeon in identifying tissue. The identification of neural structures in the region of a tumor is aided by assessing the responses to mechanical or electrical stimulation, reassuring surgeons as they dissect and remove tissue. Intraoperative monitoring of the nervous system also provides a degree of reassurance to patients and their families. In some countries, there are medicolegal implications if adverse events occur in patients who were not being monitored intraoperatively.

Intraoperative monitoring requires the following:

Teamwork
Precautions for ensuring safety and quality
A team whose members have adequate training and experience
Flexibility of the team
A team capable of using multiple modalities of monitoring

Monitoring requires a team approach—one that strives to provide the surgeon with information that will aid in bringing about the most successful conclusion possible to the operation. Generally, the surgeon does not have the time or training to conduct the monitoring and to ensure its reliability. A physician-neurophysiologist or a medically qualified (nonphysician) neurophysiologist is best qualified to take responsibility for the monitoring. Most certified clinical neurophysiologists work with nonphysician technologists who remain in the operating room throughout the surgery to collect data (Nuwer and Nuwer, 1997). The neurophysiology team must work closely with the surgeon to define the information needed and to decide how best to present it. The anesthesiologist or anesthetist, an equally important member of the team, is not trained to perform the monitoring and does not have time to do so while maintaining the anesthesia. The effect of anesthe-

tics, blood pressure, temperature, and other variables controlled by the anesthesiologist require communication between the neurophysiologist and the anesthesiologist before and throughout the monitoring. Anesthetic agents can profoundly alter the electrical activity of the nervous system. Changes due to anesthesia must be distinguished from those due to neurological dysfunction. Therefore, it is critical that the neurophysiologist be familiar with the effects of anesthetic agents and be able to discuss these with the anesthesiologist.

Two publications of the International Federation of Clinical Neurophysiology provide specific recommendations for ensuring quality and safety during surgical monitoring (Nuwer et al., 1993; Burke et al., 1999). The equipment used for surgical monitoring usually is the same as that used in outpatient testing, with some modifications, provided that it conforms to the safety specifications of the operating room. The common-mode rejection ratio should be at least 85 dB for the elimination of 50- or 60-Hz line interference, which is a common problem in the operating room. Evoked potential equipment should include capabilities for adding, subtracting, storing, and smoothing data; automatic artifact rejection; and simultaneous display of multiple traces from several channels. Electromyographic equipment should allow both auditory and visual presentations and have automatic artifact rejection for minimizing operative interference, particularly that due to cautery.

Electrical safety is critically important. Monitoring equipment must not be able to cause currents greater than 100 μA to pass through the patient if equipment grounding fails. This is measured as the chassis leakage current across a functioning ground plug. For electrically sensitive patients—for example, with catheters leading to the heart or great vessels—the limit should be 10 μA. These current limits are substantially larger than what would occur under normal operating circumstances with properly functioning equipment. The most common danger is from improper and malfunctioning grounding. A patient should be grounded electrically at only one site, usually a large ground plate. That ground is used for the diathermy and similar routine operating room equipment. If all operating room machinery is grounded properly, a second patient ground is unnecessary.

Current neurophysiology equipment should have optical isolation for each patient contact, preventing inadvertent conduction of electrical currents between the patient and the equipment. An optically isolated isoground is used with many such pieces of equipment. Generally, this can be used safely in an operating room, even with a patient who has a true ground plate already in place. In such a patient, any ground current will travel out the true ground plate, without substantial leakage current traveling through the isoground circuit. The neurophysiologist needs to be responsible for ensuring that the leakage current of the equipment has been tested and is safe. At most hospitals, biomedical engineers are available to check equipment for proper grounding on the main power cord and for leakage current along any connection to the patient.

The ultimate surgical outcome depends primarily on the skills and experience of the surgeon, but those of the anesthesiologist and neurophysiologist are also important. The skills needed by the neurophysiologist and the neurophysiology technologist are best acquired through a combination of specific training with oversight and on-the-job experience. Such qualifications should be reviewed and substantiated. To ensure the ongoing quality of the monitoring, the recordings of each case should be documented and available for independent review. Quality assurance should be conducted periodically by having knowledgeable experts independent of the principal monitoring team review the intraoperative records.

The monitoring team must be flexible because of the variety of surgical procedures on the spine, the many diseases that require spine surgery (bony spine diseases, spinal cord diseases, or spinal nerve and root disorders), the many levels of deficit that the patient may show, and the varying anesthetic needs. It is not possible to have a single, standard protocol for monitoring. The unique problems encountered with each patient require that the monitoring be designed individually after review of the clinical problem, after discussion with the surgeon of the structures at risk, and after discussion with the anesthesiologist of the anesthetic options.

For each case, the methods of surgical monitoring are selected on the basis of the structures at risk, the optimal methods for monitoring their function, and the anticipated anesthetic regimen. The spinal cord, nerve roots, spinal nerves, and cauda equina all may need to be monitored; thus, somatosensory evoked potentials (SSEPs), motor evoked potentials (MEPs), nerve conduction studies, electromyograms (EMGs), and reflex testing may need to be used. Some surgical procedures put more than one anatomical structure at risk of damage, and all the structures warrant monitoring. This requires the simultaneous use of multiple methods of monitoring. The skills of the neurophysiologist and the capability of the equipment must provide the options for multimodality monitoring.

STRUCTURES TO MONITOR DURING SPINE AND AORTA SURGERY

Any neural structure in the region of the spine may be damaged during an operation on the spinal cord, the surrounding bony spine, or the blood supply to the neural structures. The potential risk to each of the following needs to be considered in selecting the optimal monitoring protocol. The risks to structures include the following:

Spinal cord ischemia, slow compression, stretching, and direct trauma

Nerve roots and spinal nerve stretching, blunt trauma, pinching, and ischemia
Cauda equina stretching, blunt trauma, pinching, and ischemia

Damage may occur at one or more levels of the spine. Optimal monitoring requires monitoring each level that is at risk for damage. The modalities and variables of monitoring change with each of these structures and the level. Thoracic-level monitoring is the most common, followed by lumbar and lower cervical monitoring. The levels of the spine examined with different methods of monitoring include the following:

Upper cervical—C1 to C4
Lower cervical—C5 to T1
Thoracic—T2 to L1 (two thirds of all monitoring)
Lumbar—L2 to S1
Sacral—S2 to S4

MONITORING METHODS

Several different modalities are available for monitoring each of the structures and levels mentioned in the preceding section. Each modality may be modified to meet the needs of the operation. The procedures are reviewed briefly below and are discussed more fully in textbooks and reviews of surgical monitoring (Nuwer, 1986; Ducker and Brown, 1988; Møller, 1988; Schramm and Møller, 1991; Kalkman et al., 1993; Loftus and Traynelis, 1994; Russell and Rodichok, 1995; Andrews, 1996; Stålberg et al., 1998).

1. Somatosensory Evoked Potentials (SSEPs)
   Stimulation: peripheral nerve, dermatome, cauda equina, or spinal cord
   Recording: peripheral nerve, plexus, cauda equina, directly from spinal cord (lumbar, thoracic, or cervical) or cerebral cortex
2. Motor Evoked Potentials (MEPs)
   Stimulation: cerebral cortex or spinal cord (magnetic, electric)
   Recording: spinal cord, peripheral nerve, or muscle
3. Nerve Conduction Studies
   Stimulation: root
   Recording: peripheral nerve or muscle
4. Electromyogram (EMG)
   Stimulation: mechanical or electrical
   Recording: muscle
5. Reflex Testing
   Stimulation: peripheral nerve, root, or pudendal nerve
   Recording: root, peripheral nerve, or muscle
6. Electrophysiological Modifications
   Rates and patterns of stimulation
   Recording electrode type or placement
   Facilitation of MEPs or SSEPs

Somatosensory Evoked Potentials (SSEPs)

Despite ongoing debate on the value of intraoperative electrophysiological monitoring (Daube, 1999; Gelber, 1999), animal models have clearly shown that spinal cord ischemia or compression prolongs, reduces, and finally obliterates SSEPs in proportion to the amount of cord damage (Bennett, 1983). SSEPs are an accepted method of monitoring the spinal cord during a wide range of surgical procedures on the spine or spinal cord (Forbes et al., 1991). A large multicenter study of scoliosis surgery showed that the incidence of postoperative neurological deficit was 0.46% with SSEP monitoring and 1.04% without monitoring (Nuwer et al., 1995). The numerous stimulation and recording electrode placements and stimulation and recording variables have been reviewed by Nuwer (1998, 1999).

STIMULATING AND RECORDING ELECTRODES

The most commonly used monitoring modality is SSEPs, because of the ease of application, limited susceptibility to anesthesia, and reasonable sensitivity in detecting damage. Although SSEPs may be used to monitor the spinal cord, spinal nerves, or nerve roots, they are less effective in monitoring the latter two.

Electrical stimulation evokes the centrally directed sensory action potential that can be tracked along its course from the limb to the cerebral cortex. Most commonly, stimulation is distal surface stimulation and is often performed simultaneously for the right and left sides of the body by using synchronous or asynchronous parallel averaging techniques. In the latter, averages are made from a single location on one trace with a 100-ms interval between the stimuli on the two sides. The nerves most reliable for monitoring are the median or ulnar nerve at the wrist and the posterior tibial nerve at the ankle. The ulnar nerves are particularly valuable if the low cervical spinal cord is at risk, as in cervical spondylosis surgery, because the median SSEPs can bypass the low cervical area and be normal despite local damage. The stimulation and recording techniques are similar to those used in the outpatient setting and are reviewed elsewhere in this text.

Ideally, recording electrodes should be placed proximal and distal to the site of possible damage to determine whether a loss of response is a peripheral technical problem or is related to the operation. The electrodes may be applied in various ways:

Surface electrodes on the limb, lumbar spine, cervical spine, and scalp. Larger, more reliable tibial SSEPs may be seen with C3-4 recordings than with the standard CZ-FZ recordings and should always be tested to be sure that the optimal potential is selected.
Needle electrodes adjacent to the peripheral nerve or lamina; percutaneous needle electrodes of 30

to 75 mm placed directly on the lamina outside the surgical field can record well-defined, reliable potentials, or in the intraspinous ligament at any spinal level in the surgical field.
Epidural recordings can be made at any level in the operating field with multilead electrodes, cable electrodes, strip electrodes, fine wires, or needles in the intraspinous ligament at any spinal level.
Esophageal or nasopharyngeal electrodes at the cervical levels; either of these can provide a good, stable recording anterior to the spinal cord.

Figure 103–1 illustrates a readily performed, technically reliable approach to SSEP monitoring of spinal cord function during spine surgery using tibial SSEPs recorded from the sciatic nerve, cervical cord, and scalp. Several methods of recording in the operating field have been developed so that recordings can be made closer to the neural tissue. Also, after the patient is in the operating room, electrodes can be placed at several locations near the spinal cord. Needle electrodes—the same types as those used for scalp electroencephalograms (EEGs)—can be placed into the intervertebral ligaments or spinal lamina. Epidural or interspinous ligament electrodes are usually placed after the back has been opened surgically. Several types of com-

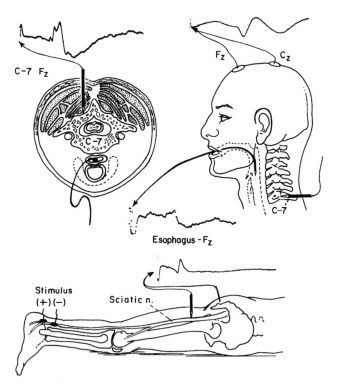

Figure 103–1. Standard placement SSEP electrodes for monitoring during thoracolumbar spine surgery. Sciatic response is recorded with a needle electrode near the nerve. Cervical responses are recorded from an electrode on the lamina of spine C7 and from an esophageal electrode. Scalp responses are recorded from standard vertex electrodes. (From Daube JR, Harper CM, Litchy WJ, Sharbrough FW: Intraoperative monitoring. In Daly DD, Pedley TA [eds]: Current Practice of Clinical Electroencephalography, 2nd ed. New York, Raven Press, 1990; 739–779. By permission of the publisher.)

mercially available, insulated wires are available for placement in the epidural space. They can be placed after the spinal column has been exposed surgically, or they can be placed preoperatively under fluoroscopic guidance. Epidural electrodes can record particularly high-amplitude, well-defined responses from lumbar and thoracic spinal levels. Thus, epidural recordings can be made either above or below the level of stimulation. The combination of epidural stimulation and epidural recordings often produces superior SSEP amplitudes with well-defined peaks (Fig. 103–2). Strips of multiple electrodes in the epidural space can be used to localize specific spinal levels for postherpetic neuralgia ablation or other localized operations (Fig. 103–3).

Direct stimulation in the operative field directly activates ascending and descending SSEPs. Often, it is not easy to tell whether the potentials are motor or sensory, because stimulation of the spinal cord may activate either or both. Thin wires implanted into the epidural space serve as stimulating electrodes. Methods for direct stimulation of the spinal cord typically use subarachnoid, epidural, spinous process, and intraspinous ligament recordings. Large, easily recorded potentials are obtained with epidural electrodes inserted between the spine and the dural sac. Similar recordings have been made of descending activity by stimulating and recording from the spinal cord directly.

Although recordings made in the surgical field provide larger responses, they are associated with the technical problems of the surgical procedure. Thus, they are subject to mechanical artifact and are limited to surgical procedures in which the spine is opened to expose the dura mater. Also, such recordings generally require more technical expertise to obtain satisfactory results and require that the surgeon be familiar with and cooperate with the recording procedure.

TECHNICAL FACTORS

Spinal cord evoked potentials differ from scalp recordings in their sensitivity to anesthetic agents. For example, scalp-recorded potentials are sensitive to inhalational anesthetic agents, such as isoflurane, and nitrous oxide decreases their amplitude by about 50%. Scalp monitoring can be performed only when the anesthesia does not abolish the cortical responses; alfentanil-propofol may be a better alternative than inhalational agents (Kalkman et al., 1991). In comparison, spinal cord evoked potentials are relatively unaffected by most anesthetic agents and drugs, but the electrodes are usually placed only after surgical exposure and must be removed when the incision is being closed. Accordingly, with electrodes in the surgical field, monitoring stops at the time it may be important to continue monitoring. The time period just before the incision is closed is a time of maximal risk for injury to the spinal cord, especially during correction of scoliosis. In contrast, percutaneous electrodes on the lamina can be left in place until the patient awakens. The combination of spinal and scalp recordings has the advantages of both types of monitoring. The percutaneous electrodes allow continuous recording of spinal potentials when reproducible scalp potentials cannot be obtained. Occasionally, because of a patient's preoperative neurological deficit, scalp potentials cannot be recorded. SSEPs may be recorded at the neck in many of these patients. The addition of a cervical spine and a peripheral recording location to the usual scalp recording allows reliable monitoring in more patients.

Both the level of anesthesia and blood pressure change the latency and amplitude of SSEPs, especially when the mean blood pressure is less than 70 mm Hg. Rarely, the scalp response is enhanced after the induction of anesthesia; generally, it is decreased. In a small proportion of cases, the response is lost immediately after the induction of anesthesia. This occurs more frequently in children and adolescents than in adults. Similarly, there is a gradual decrease in amplitude and increase in latency with long-duration anesthesia. SSEP changes due to anesthesia are much less prominent at the neck than on the scalp. The response varies, depending on the anesthetic agent. Of the common induction agents, propofol has the least effect. Nitrous oxide has some effect, but enflurane and isoflurane decrease SSEPs in more than half of the patients monitored.

Several technical factors must be considered with intraoperative recordings. The rate of stimulation cannot be as fast as when one tests an awake patient. Anesthetics make the sensory system more

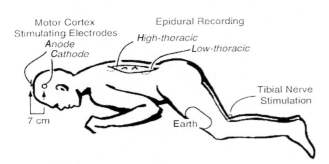

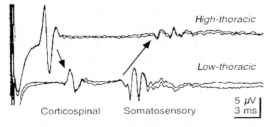

Figure 103–2. Simultaneous stimulation is applied to the scalp and peripheral nerve to evoke simultaneous MEPs and SSEPs that are recorded with epidural electrodes at two levels of the spinal cord. (From Burke D, Hicks R: Corticospinal volleys evoked by transcranial electrical and magnetic stimulation. In Stålberg E, Sharma HS, Olsson Y [eds]: Spinal Cord Monitoring. Vienna, Springer-Verlag, 1998; 446–461. By permission of the publisher.)

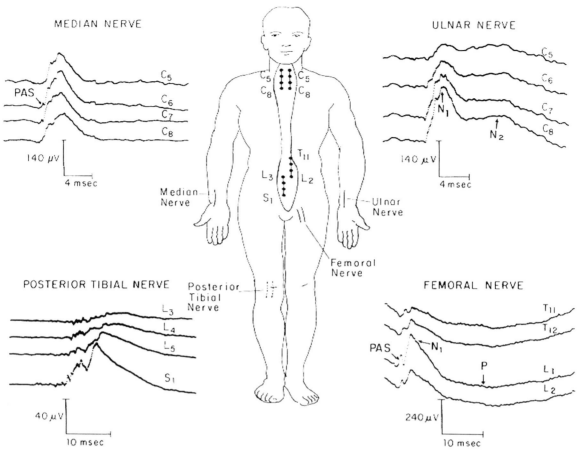

Figure 103–3. Spinal cord dorsum potentials recorded with an array of four electrodes in response to supramaximal, peripheral nerve stimulation for localizing the dorsal horn segmental response. PAS, primary afferent spike from large-diameter fibers in the dorsal column; N_1, first postsynaptic negative wave from dorsal horn neurons; N_2, second postsynaptic negative wave; P, postsynaptic positive wave. (From Nashold BS Jr, Ovelmen-Levitt J, Sharpe R, Higgins AC: Intraoperative evoked potentials recorded in man directly from dorsal roots and spinal cord. J Neurosurg 1985;62:680–693. By permission of the American Association of Neurological Surgeons.)

susceptible to fatigue. Although SSEPs can be recorded with stimulation rates of 5 Hz or even 10 Hz in most awake patients, scalp SSEPs fatigue at rates greater than 3 Hz with anesthesia. It may be necessary to stimulate at rates as low as 0.5 or 1.0 Hz, especially at deeper levels of anesthesia.

The number of stimuli that are averaged varies with the magnitude of the response and the level of background noise. Muscle activity is minimal because many of the patients are paralyzed. Under ideal conditions, responses can be obtained clearly with only 64 or 128 stimuli. However, in most cases, there are sources of artifact other than muscle, and 500 stimuli are often needed to obtain reproducible traces. Because of this variability, it is always best to record two superimposed examples of SSEPs to help determine which components are reproducible.

Technical artifacts are common in the operating room. For example, 60-Hz artifact occurs with gas warmer-humidifiers, blood warmers, and some electric drills. Movement of the recording wires must be eliminated. Wires can be disconnected, cut, dislodged, or damaged during the course of surgical procedures (especially those performed near the head or neck) and with movement of the torso.

Because stimulating electrodes can also be displaced, some type of peripheral monitor is required to ensure that they are functioning.

In children and selected adults, the core body temperature may decrease spontaneously or may be decreased for protective effects, such as spinal cord cooling. In either case, the SSEP latency increases significantly and the potential may be lost.

A frequent problem with surgical monitoring is SSEP variability in sequential recordings. SSEPs may change for many reasons other than surgical damage to the sensory pathway. During cervical surgery with the patient in the sitting position, SSEPs can decrease markedly because of the accumulation of subdural air. This change can easily be recognized by comparing the standard vertex electrode recording with that of electrodes just above the ear, where there is less subdural air. Many other nonsurgical factors, such as electrical artifact, blood pressure changes, and anesthetic level, can alter SSEPs. Differentiating these changes from those of pathway damage requires that the alteration in the amplitude or latency be consistent at both the neck and the scalp recording sites and that the peripheral response be intact. It must be shown that this change is not due to technical factors. Also, the change must be greater than the baseline variation that occurred during the initial period of the operation. In a few patients, recordings can be obtained at only one of the two cephalad sites, usually the neck. In these cases, changes need to be demonstrated with stimulation of more than one nerve before they can be considered significant. Although a 50% decrease in amplitude from baseline and a 5% change in latency generally indicate probable damage (Nuwer, 1999), no absolute change in amplitude can be considered evidence of spinal cord damage. In some patients without damage, the scalp response appears transiently lost while other responses are intact. In other patients with damage, a smaller but consistent alteration at two sites of stimulation can indicate compression before the 50% amplitude or 5% latency changes occur.

Random variability of the signals can cause unnecessary alarm during somatosensory monitoring, but generally they are infrequent (Nuwer, 1999). Such false alarms, or false-positive results, can be reduced substantially by careful attention to technique—for example, the use of a restricted filter bandpass, with the low filter increased to 30 Hz and the high filter to 2,000 Hz. With attention to technical problems and baseline variation, a decrease in amplitude of 35% or more can be used as a threshold for indicating damage, and the false-positive rate will be less than 10% (More et al., 1988). In a study of a large group of spinal cord operations, a 5% change in latency and a 60% change in amplitude were defined as outside the range of normal variation (Jones et al., 1988). Recording variables should be chosen for the individual patient to maximize the stability of the recording, and they need to be kept constant throughout the operation. The variability of the recorded potential should be assessed early in an operation so that adverse events can be distinguished from background variability. Ideally, the ordinary background variability of the potentials is no more than 30% in amplitude and 1.0 ms in latency.

Infrequent, unusual, and nonsurgical causes of rapid changes in SSEPs (e.g., the physiological changes in temperature and blood pressure noted earlier) must always be considered before one concludes that the operation is responsible. Air entering the subdural space and rising to the convexity in a patient in the seated position for cervical spine surgery may produce a rapid change in SSEPs, suggesting abnormality. Placement of an alternative electrode in the midtemporal region usually shows that the response is still intact, because the air rises to the upper areas of the cortical representation (Fig. 103–4).

The accuracy of monitoring can be improved with the appropriate use of peripheral control recordings. These include monitoring arm SSEPs over Erb's point with median or ulnar nerve stimulation and leg SSEPs from the sciatic nerve at the gluteal fold or the N22 lumbar potential from T12-L1. Monitoring median nerve responses during thoracic spinal procedures can also be helpful in differentiating changes due to anesthesia from those due to surgical problems.

Preoperative testing with SSEPs, EMGs, and nerve conduction studies or some combination of them often helps to determine the optimal combination of recordings for each patient. When SSEPs have a very low amplitude or are absent, stimulation of tibial nerves bilaterally, stimulation of the sciatic nerves, or stimulation of the cauda equina may be needed to elicit SSEPs. Recordings may have to be made from the epidural space, rather than from an extraspinal location. If the EMG or nerve conduction study demonstrates abnormalities in the distribution of particular nerve roots, these roots are more susceptible to further damage and warrant intramuscular recordings for monitoring neurotonic discharges.

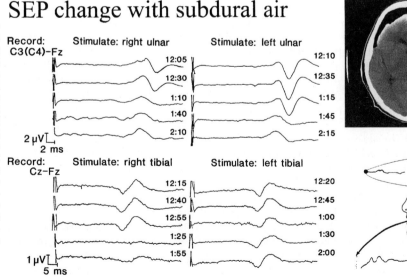

SEP change with subdural air

Figure 103–4. Left and right ulnar (C3 and C4-FZ) and tibial (CZ-FZ) SSEP recordings during monitoring in cervical spinal cord surgery with the patient in the sitting position. Ulnar and tibial responses decrease abruptly, especially on the right at 1:25 PM, because of subdural air that separated the cerebral cortex from the skull, as shown on the postoperative magnetic resonance imaging. Change in the ulnar SSEP recording electrode position to a superior temporal electrode provided a recordable potential that was monitored for the rest of the operation. No postoperative deficit occurred.

The variety of approaches available reflects differences in experience, surgical philosophy, and technical issues. None of the approaches have been compared directly for effectiveness. Each neurophysiologist in the field generally has become comfortable with a particular approach and relies on it. The differences among these approaches in preventing neural damage to the somatosensory pathways do not appear to be major. Thus, direct spinal cord stimulation and recording produce better defined potentials, but more technical expertise is required. In contrast, percutaneous recording at levels of the spinal cord and scalp are less reliable but are more readily performed.

SSEP monitoring during spine surgery has proved valuable in warning surgeons of potential damage to the spinal cord. Because such damage is uncommon, few large studies have defined the change in SSEPs in relation to spinal cord damage. In surgical monitoring of spinal cord sensory pathways, approximately 20% of patients have significant changes in SSEPs intraoperatively. As many as half of these changes may be reversed surgically (e.g., removal of hematoma, rods, spine wires). Patients with no change in SSEPs may have postoperative deficits consistent with anterior spinal artery syndrome, but this is rare. SSEP changes are similar in most patients. Ten to thirty minutes after localized spinal cord damage occurs, the amplitude begins to decrease at the neck and scalp, with an increase in latency of up to 3 ms. SSEPs can recover to baseline values within 5 to 10 minutes after correction. The abrupt loss of SSEPs is less likely to be reversible. SSEP amplitude shows improvement intraoperatively in a few patients.

In summary, several patterns of change in SSEPs have been correlated with postoperative neurological function (Dawson et al., 1991) after operative manipulation, which gradually resolve without neurological sequelae. The change may be late or gradual, emphasizing the importance of continuing the monitoring until the patient is awake. Gradual changes in SSEPs may be caused also by ischemia of the spinal cord or peripheral nerves; for example, during operations on the thoracic or abdominal aorta (Okamoto et al., 1992). Less frequently, the SSEPs change abruptly, usually in relation to contusion of the spinal cord or compression by an epidural or a subdural hematoma. When the loss of SSEPs is abrupt, the site of injury should be localized by recording with epidural or direct spinal electrodes, followed by careful inspection of the involved level for hematoma or other potentially reversible causes of spinal cord injury. If the loss of SSEPs is abrupt and nonreversible, paraplegia is probable. Improvement in the amplitude of SSEPs intraoperatively usually is associated with improved neurological status postoperatively. Postoperative motor deficits without associated changes in SSEPs intraoperatively are infrequent but well documented (Lesser et al., 1986). The motor deficits may occur as part of the anterior spinal artery syndrome or by direct injury to the ventral spinal cord, ventral horn cells, or nerve roots.

Motor Evoked Potentials

STIMULATING ELECTRODES

The integrity of corticospinal motor pathways can be monitored with MEPs evoked with stimulation of the motor cortex or spinal cord. Both electrical stimulation and magnetic stimulation have been reported for each site. In an anesthetized patient, magnetic stimulation has no advantage over electrical stimulation and has major disadvantages: the coil is cumbersome and hard to immobilize relative to the skull, the apparatus is expensive (particularly if trains of stimuli are to be given), and magnetic MEPs are more sensitive to anesthetic agents (Schramm and Kurthen, 1992; Burke and Hicks, 1998). MEPs are obtained easily and reliably with direct stimulation of the spinal cord or cerebral hemispheres with the patient receiving a combination of nitrous oxide and narcotic anesthesia. Halogenated anesthetics markedly decrease the amplitude of MEPs through effects on both cortical neurons and anterior horn cells.

Two methods are available for directly stimulating the cerebral cortex through the intact skull. Some medical centers have begun to use these methods for surgical monitoring, but in the United States they are considered experimental methods. Transcranial stimuli are best delivered at a low rate, less than 1 per 3 seconds, using a device such as the specially constructed transcranial electrical stimulator from Digitimer (D180 or D180A). The optimal stimulus is a capacitively coupled stimulus of modest intensity, 250 V to 450 V, with a time constant of 100 μs. Although the amplitude of the D wave is usually greater than 10 μV, 8 to 10 sweeps usually are averaged to improve reproducibility.

The spinal cord can be stimulated with an epidural electrode, a needle in or between spinous processes, or a combination of nasopharyngeal active and laminar reference electrodes. Interspinous or epidural electrodes in the surgical field use a distant anode in the subcutaneous tissue and are technically more difficult than the combination of laminar and esophageal electrodes. Typically, MEPs are recorded with partial neuromuscular block to reduce body movement. Spinal cord-evoked MEPs have been used successfully in thoracic and lumbar but not cervical spine surgery (Taylor et al., 1993). Cervical spine surgery requires cranial stimulation to evoke MEPs.

RECORDING ELECTRODES

MEPs can be recorded directly from the spinal cord as a cord-evoked potential, from a peripheral nerve as a nerve action potential, or from muscle as a compound muscle action potential (CMAP). Cranial-evoked MEPs can be recorded directly from the spinal cord with electrodes, similar to those used for stimulation, in either the epidural or the subarachnoid space (Gokaslan et al., 1997). The response may be mixed motor and sensory if excessive stimulation activates sensory tracts in the upper cervical cord. Spinal cord stimulation activates both motor and sensory fibers, even at threshold. Therefore, the MEPs recorded from the spinal cord in response to direct spinal cord stimulation ("cord-to-cord") are a mixture of potentials in ascending and descending pathways; cord-to-cord MEPs may be less sensitive to spinal insults than selective monitoring. Recordings performed in the surgical field are most useful for operations on the spinal cord (e.g., tumors or arteriovenous malformations); the directly recorded potentials can localize the area of damage or record responses that are too small to be obtained with other methods.

TECHNICAL FACTORS

Filter settings from 500-Hz high-pass to 2- to 5-kHz low-pass are often necessary to allow reliable recording intraoperatively, despite general interference and stimulus artifact. Epidural bipolar cardiac pacing electrodes with an interelectrode separation of 2 to 3 cm are suitable for recording descending MEPs (the same electrode can be used to record SSEPs directly from the spinal cord or to stimulate the spinal cord). The bipolar montage may not allow all I waves (i.e., indirectly generated waves of activity in corticospinal axons) to be recorded, but this is not important, because in practice only the D wave (i.e., the directly activated component of the corticospinal volley) is measured. The major advantages and disadvantages of transcranial MEP monitoring from the spinal cord are the following:

Advantages

The D wave of the corticospinal volley is large and highly reproducible; an amplitude deterioration of more than 20% would be outside the 2.5 SD of normal mean variation
The MEP is relatively immune to the effects of anesthetic agents
Full muscle relaxation is possible, indeed desirable
SSEPs can be recorded reliably in the same sweeps if the cerebral cortex and peripheral nerve are stimulated simultaneously
Often, MEPs can be recorded in patients with preexisting neural deficits
MEP change provides prompt identification of abnormality

Disadvantages

It is feasible only when epidural leads can be inserted, which normally requires a posterior approach to the cord

It does not identify the side responsible for any deterioration in the recorded volleys
MEPs are not as reliably recorded from the lumbar cord

When a preexisting lesion or the surgeon's preference prevents the recording of MEPs and SSEPs with epidural electrodes, monitoring can still be performed with other potentials.

In *peripheral nerve recordings,* neurogenic potentials can be recorded in the region of the sciatic or tibial nerve in response to stimulation of the cerebral cortex or spinal cord, but they are less well defined with cortical stimulation (Pereon et al., 1998). One hundred or more responses need to be averaged. With the patient under inhalation anesthesia, neurogenic MEPs evoked with spinal cord stimulation may be recorded primarily from posterior column axons, because spinal motor neuron activity is reduced. With the neuromuscular block typically used, neurogenic potentials may contain end-plate potentials from surrounding muscle as well as potentials from the motor and sensory fibers in the peripheral nerve.

Muscle recordings (CMAPs) are made with surface electrodes in response to either cortical or spinal cord stimulation but differ for the two modes of stimulation. Limited anesthesia is necessary for CMAPs to be elicited and even then the CMAP produced by single stimuli to the motor cortex is too variable for reliable monitoring of motor function. The variability results from the low excitability of the motor neuron when inhalation anesthesia is administered. This limitation can be overcome partly with trains of stimuli and narcotic anesthesia (Jones et al., 1996; Woodforth et al., 1996). Pairs or trains of stimuli, especially delivered to the spinal cord, produce enough temporal summation of excitatory inputs to the motor neurons to activate most of them. Large, stable CMAPs can be recorded, but this often requires partial neuromuscular block to control movement. The level of neuromuscular block is monitored best with simultaneous recording of CMAPs in response to peripheral nerve stimulation.

An optimal CMAP with spinal cord stimulation is obtained with paired stimuli at intervals of 3 to 5 milliseconds. Cortical stimulus trains of five or six stimuli are needed at intervals of 2 to 5 milliseconds, using a stimulus intensity that with cortical stimulation produces a D wave of maximal amplitude (perhaps 450 V, using the Digitimer D180 transcranial stimulator). The paired stimuli or stimulus train is repeated at low rates as needed. CMAPs are recorded best from multiple muscles in both legs. With cortical stimulation, CMAP recording improves with paired stimulation, relatively light anesthesia, and incomplete muscle relaxation (Kalkman et al., 1995; Pechstein et al., 1996), whereas with spinal cord stimulation, CMAPs can be obtained with full narcotic anesthesia (Ubags et al., 1997). A major advantage of the technique is the opportunity to adapt the monitoring by choosing muscles to suit the specific clinical need, for example, muscles innervated by specific nerve roots when the operation is low spinal or segmental or the risk is to a known nerve root. The CMAPs may need to be filtered more than they are in outpatient recordings with a high-pass filter increased to 100 Hz or 200 Hz. This distorts the CMAP and attenuates its amplitude, but it can give better baseline stability when necessary. The signal-to-noise ratio for the CMAP is sufficient for single trials to be recorded without averaging. The reproducibility of the evoked CMAP, although good, may not be as high as that of the MEP in epidural recordings. Irrigation of the operative wound with cold water can produce transient change in the responses.

It is critical for the neurophysiology team to be in constant contact with the anesthesia team to prevent loss of the evoked response due to anesthesia. The most common reason for deterioration of cortically evoked CMAPs is the administration of an anesthetic agent, such as a supplemental narcotic agent. The most common reason for the spinal CMAPs to change is an alteration in the level of neuromuscular block. The latter can be recognized readily with simultaneous peripheral monitoring of the neuromuscular block.

The major advantages and disadvantages of MEP monitoring with CMAPs are the following:

Advantages

Unilateral dysfunction can be identified
Evoked potentials with spinal cord stimulation are resistant to anesthesia
CMAPs evoked with spinal stimulation can be recorded simultaneously with SSEPs
Cortically evoked CMAPs can be adapted for virtually all spinal and cerebral operations
CMAP recording is equally useful for low spinal cord, cauda equina, and nerve root surgery
MEP monitoring with CMAPs does not intrude into the operative field

Disadvantages

CMAPs evoked with spinal stimulation cannot be used with cervical spine surgery
Cortically evoked CMAPs are intrinsically more variable and more sensitive to anesthesia
CMAPs evoked with spinal stimulation vary with level of neuromuscular block

Many neurophysiologists have found that direct spinal cord stimulation gives highly reliable motor and sensory responses when recorded directly from the spinal cord (see Fig. 103–2).

Electromyographic and Nerve Conduction Studies

Damage to cervical or lumbosacral nerve roots or motor neurons during surgical procedures on the spine can be minimized with a combination of EMG recordings and nerve conduction studies (Holland, 1998). Anterior horn cells can be damaged during dissection of intraspinal tumors or by ischemia from compression or traction. Radiculopathies are occasionally a complication of scoliosis surgery, likely because of local root compression or traction (Harper et al., 1988). Neurotonic discharges in limb muscles innervated by affected motor neurons or axons can provide a warning of potential damage due to manipulation, traction, or ischemia of nerve roots (Fig. 103–5B).

Neurotonic discharges are irregular bursts of motor unit potentials recorded in muscles in response to axonal irritation (Obi et al., 1999). (For more detailed discussion, see Chapter 102 by Strommen and Daube.) Neurotonic discharges can be recorded with surface, subcutaneous, or intramuscular electrodes. Fine wire electrodes inserted in each of the muscles at risk are the most convenient and specific. Such recordings can be made from any somatic muscle. For example, monitoring of L3-S3 muscles, including the anal sphincter, is helpful in operations for myelomeningocele. Irritation of the sensory axons in the dorsal root can also be detected with intramuscular recordings of motor unit potential firing that occurs as a reflex response (see Fig. 103–5C).

The direct stimulation of nerves in the surgical field can provide information about the location and integrity of the nerves (Kothbauer et al., 1994). In situations in which the normal anatomy is distorted, muscle recording of the response to stimulation can help to distinguish among nerve roots and differentiate them from non-neural structures. The studies record CMAPs in response to local stimulation of individual nerves (see Fig. 103–5A). Stimulation may be applied with monopolar, bipolar, or forceps electrodes. Recordings can be made with surface, subcutaneous, or intramuscular electrodes.

TYPES OF SURGERY

In many surgical procedures in infants, children, and adults, electrophysiological monitoring can help reduce the extent and duration of damage. The responsible surgeon, who can judge the risk of neural damage and the structures at risk, is best suited for selecting the patients for intraoperative monitoring. The anesthesiologist selects the optimal anesthesia. The clinical neurophysiologist selects the optimal monitoring methods after discussion with the surgeon and anesthesiologist. The largest group of patients in whom intraoperative monitoring is performed is teenagers undergoing corrective surgery for scoliosis. Another large group is elderly persons operated on for cervical or lumbar spondylosis, often with associated spinal stenosis or foraminal stenosis. Monitoring may also be performed in patients with bony spine tumors, thoracic aneurysms, trau-

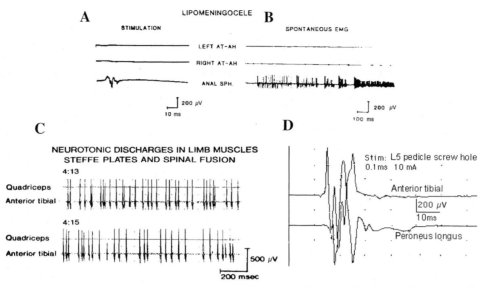

Figure 103–5. Three examples of monitoring with EMG and nerve conduction studies during lumbosacral surgery. *A,* During lipomeningocele resection, the CMAP evoked in the anal sphincter (SPH.) by direct stimulation of tissue in the surgical field identified it as axons in the L2-4 nerve roots. *B,* Neurotonic discharges in the anal sphincter during lipomeningocele dissection warned the surgeon of irritation of L2-4 axons. *C,* Motor unit potential firing during lumbar fusion warned the surgeon of irritation of dorsal root axons. *D,* CMAP evoked in L5-innervated muscles with a stimulating electrode in a pedicle screw hole with less than 20 mA current indicated to the surgeon that the pedicle screw would be close enough to the dorsal root to irritate or damage it. (From Daube JR [ed]: Clinical Neurophysiology, 2nd ed. New York, Oxford University Press [in press]. By permission of Mayo Foundation.)

matic spinal damage, or spondylitis. The commonly monitored spine surgery procedures are scoliosis, kyphoscoliosis, cervical spondylosis and stenosis, lumbar spondylosis and stenosis, spine trauma, rheumatoid arthritis, spine tumor, and herniated disk.

Primary Spine Disease

The optimal methods of monitoring differ from patient to patient depending on the patient's age, preoperative deficit, type of operation, level of spine, anesthetic agents used, and other factors regardless of the spinal level of the operation. The patient's age, surgical risk, and the spinal level of the operation are especially important in selecting the method of monitoring.

Three major factors must be considered in monitoring patients younger than 21 years, and each of these factors presents unique challenges to the clinical neurophysiologist. First, infants and small children usually require different stimulating and recording electrodes, which must be placed with great care. Second, SSEP averaging is more difficult in children, especially younger ones, than in adults because of higher amplitude slow wave activity under anesthesia. This often requires slower rates of stimulation, a larger number of averaged stimuli, or a lower level of anesthesia (or a combination of these) to obtain scalp recordings. For all children, recordings from the cervical cord are ideal for demonstrating that the spinal cord is intact, even if the scalp response is not clearly recognizable. Third, in some children and adolescents, the scalp response

is lost early during anesthesia, presumably because of an idiosyncratic reaction to the anesthetic agent. In these cases, a cervical cord recording from a nasopharyngeal, esophageal, or laminar needle electrode is necessary to monitor spinal cord function.

Surgical risk varies with every type of operation, depending on the amount of spinal cord deformity, severity of preoperative deficit, size and type of lesion to be excised, bony stability, previous operations, and other medical disorders. In some patients, the surgical risk is low enough that monitoring neural function intraoperatively is not necessary. For other patients, monitoring provides no benefit, either because the deficit is complete and cannot be made worse, or the structure has to be sacrificed to complete the operation.

For each level of operation, it is best to assess the risk to individual neural structures separately. For example, if the risk of damage is primarily to nerve roots rather than the spinal cord, the patient can be monitored with EMG and may not need spinal cord monitoring. O'Brien and colleagues (1994) assessed the risk to upper extremity nerves and plexus during thoracic and lumbar spine surgery. They found a 9% incidence of new deficits, most of which had been identified by monitoring peripheral and central pathways with SSEPs; 10% had SSEP changes that were reversed during the operation, suggesting that ulnar and median SSEPs would be useful in all spine operations. The differences in these risks are considered further with each level of surgery.

The risk to nerve roots during spine surgery increases with hardware fixation in spondylolisthesis, stenosis, scoliosis, instability, and other spinal disorders at any level. Fixation for spine fusion can be

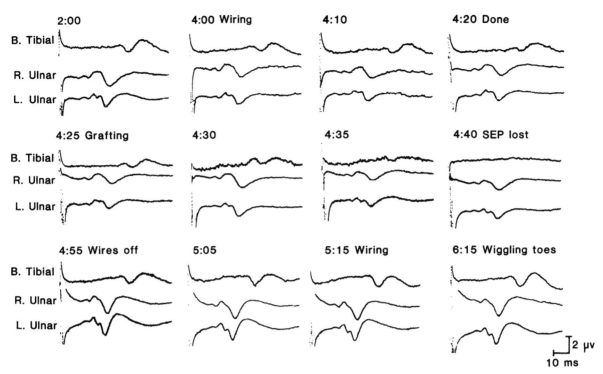

Figure 103–6. Gradual loss of SSEP during stabilization procedure for cervical spine fracture in a 60-year-old man. Responses were lost within a few minutes after wiring C5 to C7 and returned quickly after the wires were removed. Patient awoke with no deficit. (From Daube JR, Harper CM, Litchy WJ, Sharbrough FW: Intraoperative monitoring. In Daly DD, Pedley TA [eds]: Current Practice of Clinical Electroencephalography, 2nd ed. New York, Raven Press, 1990; 739–779. By permission of the publisher.)

accomplished with several different surgical approaches. At the cervical level, it is common to wire adjacent vertebrae together to obtain the stabilization needed for bone healing and fusion. The risk to neural structures can develop at any time during the procedure but particularly during fixation (Fig. 103–6). Shortly after the C6 and C7 pedicles had been wired together in the case in Figure 103–6, the scalp response was gradually lost while the nasopharyngeal response remained unchanged. The responses returned after the wires were removed. They were replaced in a different position without difficulty. The patient awoke with no deficit.

Also, the hardware is often fixed to the pedicle with a metal screw. The proximity of the pedicle to the nerve root results in the risk of root damage with pain or radiculopathy if the screw leaves the pedicle and impinges on the root. SSEPs are not sufficiently sensitive to identify such damage. Thresholds to stimulation can determine the likelihood of damage (Welch et al., 1997, Moed et al., 1998). The threshold for activation of the nerve root by stimulation within the hole drilled in the pedicle is determined by the amount of bone surrounding the hole. Thresholds less than 20 V indicate that the nerve root is close enough to the pedicle screw to be damaged by it (see Fig. 103–5D). Motor unit potential firing may occur if a screw is placed too close to the dorsal root or the root is otherwise irritated.

Although the major purpose of SSEP monitoring is to help recognize subclinical changes that could

herald a new postoperative neural deficit, occasionally SSEPs improve when the procedure reduces spinal cord compression or ischemia, as in cervical stabilization of cervical rheumatoid arthritis (Fig. 103–7).

CERVICAL SPINE DISEASE

Monitoring cervical spine surgery requires initially determining which neural structures are at risk and the level of risk. Myelopathy is the major concern with operations at the C1-4 level. Preoperative neurological deficits, multilevel operations, upper cervical surgery, and instrumentation all increase the risk, but the specificity of monitoring for recognizing the risk of damage is as high as 99% (May et al., 1996). Monitoring of tibial and median SSEPs is sufficient unless the spinal cord is already compromised. In that case, MEPs may also be needed. If the cervical spine is unstable, monitoring should begin before anesthesia, because positioning the head with the patient under anesthesia may compromise the spinal cord. The partial loss of an SSEP should not be considered a "false positive" because the loss can often be reversed by appropriate surgical action (May et al., 1996) (see Figure 103–6). Neurogenic MEPs have been reported of value in warning of possible damage in anterior cervical spine surgery (Darden et al., 1996).

Monitoring nerve roots with EMG should be considered in patients undergoing spine surgery at the C5-T1 level if there is significant preoperative radicu-

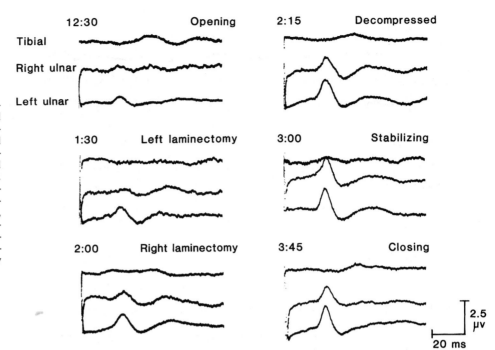

Figure 103–7. Gradual improvement of SSEP amplitude and latency during spinal cord decompression for rheumatoid arthritis. The patient's neurological deficit also showed improvement postoperatively. (From Daube JR, Harper CM, Litchy WJ, Sharbrough FW: Intraoperative monitoring. In Daly DD, Pedley TA [eds]: Current Practice of Clinical Electroencephalography, 2nd ed. New York, Raven Press, 1990; 739–779. By permission of the publisher.)

lopathy or if the roots or spinal nerves may be compromised during the operation. The value of monitoring during cervical spine surgery has been studied less well but nonetheless has been shown in a prospective study to be of benefit when specific criteria are used (Dennis et al., 1996).

THORACIC SPINE DISEASE

SSEP monitoring is sufficient for most patients undergoing thoracic spine surgery (Nuwer, 1998). However, because motor function may be lost despite intact SSEPs (Pelosi et al., 1999), a combination of MEPs and SSEPs has been suggested as the "standard of care" for scoliosis surgery (Padberg et al., 1998). In some academic centers, MEPs can be readily applied and are used routinely (Burke et al., 1992). However, anesthetic and technical considerations make MEPs more difficult to apply in many settings. In these cases, MEP monitoring should be considered if there is marked deformity, preoperative deficit, or other evidence of greater risk to the spinal cord. The possible loss of sensory function alone makes it appropriate to monitor SSEPs, even if MEPs are monitored (Lorenzini and Schneider, 1996).

LUMBOSACRAL SPINE DISEASE

With operations at the lumbosacral level, spinal nerves are often at greater risk than the spinal cord itself. Because SSEPs are less effective than EMG in identifying nerve root damage, EMG monitoring is often important in operations at this level (Calancie et al., 1992; Holland and Kostuik, 1997).

Primary Neural Disease

Tumors of the spinal cord, particularly intramedullary tumors, are high-risk procedures in which the surgeon often has little opportunity to modify the procedure—other than to stop it—in response to electrophysiological changes. Therefore, in such operations on these tumors, monitoring often is not necessary. If monitoring is performed, simultaneously monitoring MEPs and SSEPs optimizes the recognition of significant change (Nagle et al., 1996). Some groups have found that monitoring performed during intramedullary cord surgery decreases the frequency of major complications (Jones et al., 1996; Kothbauer et al., 1997; Tamaki, 1998) (Fig. 103–8). Multimodality monitoring can also include EMG recordings (Fig. 103–9).

DORSAL RHIZOTOMY

According to anecdotal reports, improvement in spasticity and function, especially in children with cerebral palsy, has been achieved by cutting a proportion of the fibers in the L2-S1 dorsal roots (McQuillan and Newberg, 1995; Gul et al., 1999). Although this procedure has been known for many years, Peacock and co-workers (Staudt et al., 1995) recently reported electrophysiological monitoring in these patients. Two to five fascicles are dissected apart in each dorsal root and stimulated with single stimuli and trains of stimuli to elicit a reflex. The character of the responses bilaterally in L2-S2–innervated limb muscles is assessed to determine which fascicle contributes to the spasticity. Repetitive firing in response to single stimuli, an increasing response to repetitive stimuli, spread of the re-

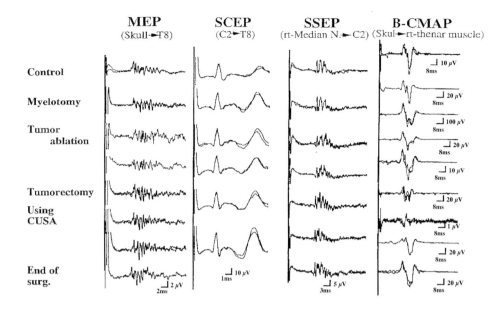

| MEP (Skull→T8) | SCEP (C2→T8) | SSEP (rt-Median N.→C2) | B-CMAP (Skull→rt-thenar muscle) |

Control
Myelotomy
Tumor ablation
Tumorectomy
Using CUSA
End of surg.

Figure 103–8. Four monitoring methods recorded simultaneously during removal of an intramedullary spinal cord tumor (astrocytoma). MEP, response to transcranial electric stimulation recorded at T8; SCEP (spinal cord evoked potential), response to C2 electrical stimulation recorded at T8; SSEP (somatosensory evoked potential), response to right median nerve stimulation recorded at C2; B (brain)-CMAP, response to transcranial electrical stimulation recorded from thenar muscle. CUSA, an ultrasonic tissue-removing instrument, produced a change in B-CMAP. No change in postoperative deficit except for slight sensory loss in the left leg. (From Tamaki, 1998. By permission of Springer-Verlag.)

sponse to other spinal cord segments, and continuation of responses after stimulation has ceased are all considered evidence of abnormal fibers, and the fascicles containing these fibers are severed (usually 30% to 60% of a dorsal root), leaving some fascicles intact to preserve sensation. Patients who primarily have spasticity have had better results than those with dystonic or ataxic forms of cerebral palsy. The extent and type of response decreases with the depth of anesthesia. If the depth of anesthesia is too shallow, many fascicles appear abnormal; if it is too deep, few fascicles appear abnormal. Also, it is critical that the motor root be identified to prevent

its being sectioned and, thus, increasing weakness. The motor and sensory roots are distinguished readily by measuring the threshold to single stimuli: motor roots are activated with less than 2.0 mA current, but sensory roots require more than 2.0 mA.

Although many have reported on the benefits of dorsal rhizotomy, no controlled studies have demonstrated that electrophysiological testing provides a better outcome than blind sectioning of 30% to 50% of the dorsal roots innervating spastic muscles. In normal children, dorsal roots show responses considered abnormal in spastic children. No correlation

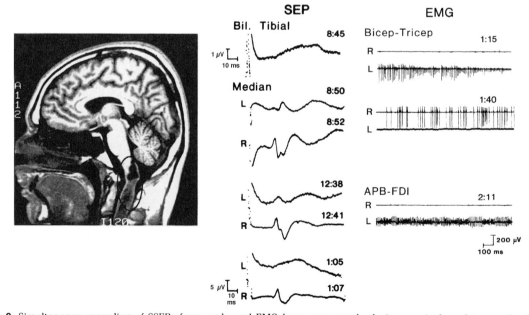

Figure 103–9. Simultaneous recording of SSEPs from scalp and EMG from arm muscle during cervical cord tumor (oval on the MRI scan) and syrinx surgery. Neurotonic discharges warned the surgeon of local root or anterior horn cell irritation. Tibial SSEPs were absent from onset. Left median SSEP was lost at 1:00. The only postoperative deficit was loss of proprioceptive sensation in the left arm. (From Daube JR [ed]: Clinical Neurophysiology, 2nd ed. New York, Oxford University Press [in press]. By permission of Mayo Foundation.)

has been found between the degree of spasticity in a muscle and the response of the dorsal roots innervating that muscle (Hays et al., 1998). One randomized, blinded study was unable to demonstrate consistent responses from single fascicles (Warf and Nelson, 1996).

Cauda Equina and Tethered Cord

Surgical procedures below spinal level L1 pose a risk to the cauda equina rather than to the spinal cord. The overlap of multiple roots innervating individual dermatomes makes SSEP monitoring insensitive to nerve root damage in the cauda equina (Tsai et al., 1997). Therefore, monitoring cauda equina function relies on a combination of EMG and nerve conduction studies. The presence and distribution of evoked responses in limb and anal sphincter muscles with direct stimulation of tissue in the area of the cauda equina allow neural tissue and the specific root to be identified. With continuous EMG monitoring of the same muscles, the occurrence of neurotonic discharges warns the surgeon that a ventral root is mechanically irritated and motor unit potential firing warns that a dorsal root is irritated (Kothbauer et al., 1994).

The most difficult operations to perform below level L1 are ones for congenital abnormalities. Several congenital abnormalities of the lumbosacral cord and cauda equina can result in progressive neurological deficit referred to as "tethered cord" (McQuillan and Newberg, 1995). The progression has been attributed to mechanical distortion of the cord, impaired cord metabolism, and cord ischemia. Surgical release of the "tether" can stop progression of the deficit. The primary purpose of electrophysiological monitoring is to preserve neural tissue by identifying and distinguishing it from other tissue that will be dissected or sectioned.

Monitoring is accomplished in two ways. Continuous EMG monitoring from multiple limb and sphincter muscles is the most effective because it identifies mechanical irritation of neural tissue during dissection and immediately warns the surgeon of possible damage. Direct stimulation of unidentified tissue elements will quickly identify whether it is neural tissue by evoking a CMAP in a limb or sphincter muscle. Although controlled studies of the value of such monitoring have not been conducted, surgeons who have used it agree that it provides valuable feedback and reduces the amount of neural damage or allows the operation to proceed more expeditiously.

Primary Vascular Disease

Electrophysiological monitoring during vascular surgery is a well-known, valuable technique during operations on cerebral aneurysms and the carotid artery and other cerebral vascular procedures. It has been applied during two spinal cord procedures: thoracoabdominal aortic aneurysm and vascular

malformation. Direct surgical ablation of arteriovenous malformations can be monitored with SSEPs or MEPs if the surgeon deems the risk sufficient. Monitoring SSEPs or MEPs during temporary occlusion of major feeder vessels to an arteriovenous malformation can provide guidance to the risk of ablating the vessel by embolization. The difficulty of performing MEPs has precluded their use during embolization of arteriovenous malformations. Because patients often are awake during embolization of an arteriovenous malformation of the spinal cord, SSEPs add limited information to the clinical assessment. Some workers have found that the continuous input of SSEPs from each leg is a more efficient manner of testing limb function than clinical testing.

Monitoring is important in thoracoabdominal aortic aneurysm operations, in which the risk of paraplegia is as high as 15%. Many modifications of the surgical procedure have been made to decrease this rate, including spinal cord cooling, cerebrospinal fluid drainage, premedication, cross-clamping at short distances to minimize the segment of spinal cord exposed to ischemia, femoral bypass, and the measurement of blood flow in the spinal cord. For each of these, the functional measures of SSEPs and MEPs are invaluable in identifying significant ischemia (North et al., 1991). Analysis of the changes in both SSEPs and MEPs requires understanding and distinguishing the effects of the ischemia that can occur at the cortical (blood pressure or carotid occlusion), peripheral nerve (femoral artery clamping), entire spinal cord (aorta clamping), and segmental spinal cord (segmental spinal artery occlusion) levels (Guerit, 1999). In all patients, pulse

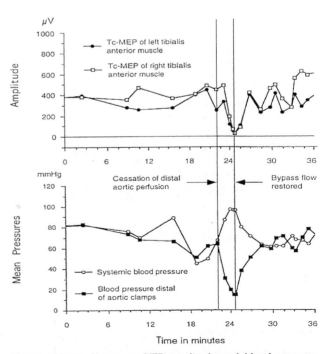

Figure 103–10. Change in MEP amplitude and blood pressure during thoracoabdominal aortic aneurysm surgery. (From Jacobs et al., 2000. By permission of Thieme Medical Publishers.)

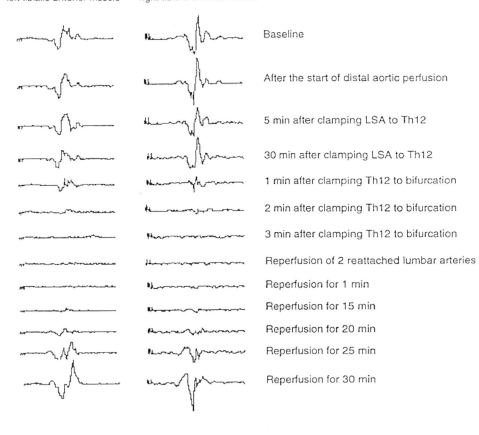

Tc-MEP recorded from the left tibialis anterior muscle / Tc-MEP recorded from the right tibialis anterior muscle

Baseline

After the start of distal aortic perfusion

5 min after clamping LSA to Th12

30 min after clamping LSA to Th12

1 min after clamping Th12 to bifurcation

2 min after clamping Th12 to bifurcation

3 min after clamping Th12 to bifurcation

Reperfusion of 2 reattached lumbar arteries

Reperfusion for 1 min

Reperfusion for 15 min

Reperfusion for 20 min

Reperfusion for 25 min

Reperfusion for 30 min

Figure 103–11. Loss of anterior tibial MEP with electric stimulation at the cerebral cortex immediately after clamping of the aorta during thoracoabdominal aortic aneurysm surgery. Responses recovered after reperfusion through reattached lumbar arteries. (From Jacobs MJ, de Haan P, Meylaerts SA, et al: Benefits of monitoring motor evoked potentials during thoracoabdominal aortic aneurysm repair. Perspectives in Vascular Surgery 2000;12:1–23. By permission of Thieme Medical Publishers.)

train MEP stimulation produces responses with a 20% coefficient of variation (Ishikawa et al., 1997; van Dongen et al., 1999). Initial studies of the benefit of revascularization using SSEPs as a guide (Griepp et al., 1996; Galla et al., 1999) were less successful than more recent studies with MEPs (Jacobs et al., 2000). The rapid alterations that can occur with occlusion and revascularization are shown in Figures 103–10 and 103–11. MEPs recorded from peripheral muscles are better indicators of dangerous ischemia, because the motor neurons in the anterior horn are more sensitive to ischemia than the motor pathways in the spinal cord (Daube and Harper, 2000). Jacobs and colleagues (2000) achieved a remarkably low spinal cord deficit rate of 3% after thoracoabdominal aneurysm operations, with careful attention to MEP changes after clamping.

SUMMARY

Continuous monitoring of the spinal cord or spinal nerve (or both) intraoperatively can minimize the potential damage that can occur during spine surgery. The easiest method to use for monitoring function is SSEPs, which have the widest application. Unless damage is caused by a vascular insult with a purely motor deficit, SSEPs are able to identify most spinal cord damage early enough to alert the surgeon. MEPs are useful as well, but technical problems limit their application in some settings. Neurotonic discharges recorded from a peripheral muscle are sensitive to nerve root irritation and, thus, can help surgeons recognize when and where damage may be occurring.

References

Andrews RJ: Intraoperative Neuroprotection. Baltimore, Williams & Wilkins, 1996.

Bennett MH: Effects of compression and ischemia on spinal cord evoked potentials. Exp Neurol 1983;80:508–519.

Burke D, Hicks R, Stephen J, et al: Assessment of corticospinal and somatosensory conduction simultaneously during scoliosis surgery. Electroencephalogr Clin Neurophysiol 1992;85:388–396.

Burke D, Hicks RG: Surgical monitoring of motor pathways. J Clin Neurophysiol 1998;15:194–205.

Burke D, Nuwer MR, Daube J, et al: Intraoperative monitoring. The International Federation of Clinical Neurophysiology. Electroencephalogr Clin Neurophysiol Suppl 1999;52:133–148.

Calancie B, Ayyar DR, Eismont FJ: Myokymic discharges: Prompt cessation following nerve root decompression during spine surgery. Electromyogr Clin Neurophysiol 1992;32:443–447.

Darden BV II, Hatley MK, Owen JH: Neurogenic motor evoked potential monitoring in anterior cervical surgery. J Spinal Disord 1996;9:485–493.

Daube JR: The role of intraoperative electrophysiologic monitoring. Muscle Nerve 1999;22:1151–1153.

Daube JR, Harper CM: Expert commentary. Perspectives in Vascular Surgery 2000;12:19–20.

Dawson EG, Sherman JE, Kanim LE, Nuwer MR: Spinal cord monitoring: Results of the Scoliosis Research Society and the European Spinal Deformity Society survey. Spine 1991;16(suppl): S361–S364.

Dennis GC, Dehkordi O, Millis RM, et al: Monitoring of median nerve somatosensory evoked potentials during cervical spinal cord decompression. J Clin Neurophysiol 1996;13:51–59.

Ducker TB, Brown RH (eds): Neurophysiology and Standards of Spinal Cord Monitoring. New York, Springer-Verlag, 1988.

Dunne JW, Field CM: The value of non-invasive spinal cord monitoring during spinal surgery and interventional angiography. Clin Exp Neurol 1991;28:199–209.

Forbes HJ, Allen PW, Waller CS, et al: Spinal cord monitoring in scoliosis surgery: Experience with 1168 cases. J Bone Joint Surg Br 1991;73:487–491.

Galla JD, Ergin MA, Lansman SL, et al: Use of somatosensory evoked potentials for thoracic and thoracoabdominal aortic resections. Ann Thorac Surg 1999;67:1947–1952.

Gelber DA: Intraoperative monitoring is of limited use in routine practice. Muscle Nerve 1999;22:1154–1156.

Gokaslan ZL, Samudrala S, Deletis V, et al: Intraoperative monitoring of spinal cord function using motor evoked potentials via transcutaneous epidural electrode during anterior cervical spinal surgery. J Spinal Disord 1997;10:299–303.

Griepp RB, Ergin MA, Galla JD, et al: Looking for the artery of Adamkiewicz: A quest to minimize paraplegia after operations for aneurysms of the descending thoracic and thoracoabdominal aorta. J Thorac Cardiovasc Surg 1996;112:1202–1213.

Guerit JM: Neuromonitoring in the operating room: Why, when, and how to monitor? Electroencephalogr Clin Neurophysiol 1998;106:1–21.

Guerit JM, Witdoeckt C, Verhelst R, et al: Sensitivity, specificity, and surgical impact of somatosensory evoked potentials in descending aorta surgery. Ann Thorac Surg 1999;67:1943–1946.

Gul SM, Steinbok P, McLeod K: Long-term outcome after selective posterior rhizotomy in children with spastic cerebral palsy. Pediatr Neurosurg 1999;31:84–95.

Hall JE, Levine CR, Sudhir KG: Intraoperative awakening to monitor spinal cord function during Harrington instrumentation and spine fusion: Description of procedure and report of three cases. J Bone Joint Surg Am 1978;60:533–536.

Harper CM Jr, Daube JR, Litchy WJ, Klassen RA: Lumbar radiculopathy after spinal fusion for scoliosis. Muscle Nerve 1988;11:386–391.

Hays RM, McLaughlin JF, Bjornson KF, et al: Electrophysiological monitoring during selective dorsal rhizotomy, and spasticity and GMFM performance. Dev Med Child Neurol 1998;40:233–238.

Herdmann J, Deletis V, Edmonds HL Jr, Morota N: Spinal cord and nerve root monitoring in spine surgery and related procedures. Spine 1996;21:879–885.

Holland NR: Intraoperative electromyography during thoracolumbar spinal surgery. Spine 1998;23:1915–1922.

Holland NR, Kostuik JP: Continuous electromyographic monitoring to detect nerve root injury during thoracolumbar scoliosis surgery. Spine 1997;22:2547–2550.

Ishikawa M, Yamaguchi N, Bertalanffy H, et al: Effects of spinal cord ischemia on the refractory period of descending spinal cord evoked potential. Electroencephalogr Clin Neurophysiol 1997;102:54–63.

Jacobs MJHM, de Haan P, Meylaerts SA, et al: Benefits of monitoring motor-evoked potentials during thoracoabdominal aortic aneurysm repair. Perspectives in Vascular Surgery 2000;12:1–23.

Jones SJ, Howard L, Shawkat F: Criteria for detection and pathological significance of response decrement during spinal cord monitoring. In Ducker TB, Brown RH (eds): Neurophysiology and Standards of Spinal Cord Monitoring. New York, Springer-Verlag, 1988; 201–206.

Jones SJ, Harrison R, Koh KF, et al: Motor evoked potential monitoring during spinal surgery: Responses of distal limb muscles to transcranial cortical stimulation with pulse trains. Electroencephalogr Clin Neurophysiol 1996;100:375–383.

Kalkman CJ, Been HD, Ongerboer de Visser BW: Intraoperative monitoring of spinal cord function: A review. Acta Orthop Scand 1993;64:114–123.

Kalkman CJ, Traast H, Zuurmond WW, Bovill JG: Differential effects of propofol and nitrous oxide on posterior tibial nerve somatosensory cortical evoked potentials during alfentanil anaesthesia. Br J Anaesth 1991;66:483–489.

Kalkman CJ, Ubags LH, Been HD, et al: Improved amplitude of myogenic motor evoked responses after paired transcranial electrical stimulation during sufentanil/nitrous oxide anesthesia. Anesthesiology 1995;83:270–276.

Kothbauer K, Deletis V, Epstein FJ: Intraoperative spinal cord monitoring for intramedullary surgery: An essential adjunct. Pediatr Neurosurg 1997;26:247–254.

Kothbauer K, Schmid UD, Seiler RW, Eisner W: Intraoperative motor and sensory monitoring of the cauda equina. Neurosurgery 1994;34:702–707.

Lesser RP, Raudzens P, Luders H, et al: Postoperative neurological deficits may occur despite unchanged intraoperative somatosensory evoked potentials. Ann Neurol 1986;19:22–25.

Loftus CM, Traynelis VC: Intraoperative Monitoring Techniques in Neurosurgery. New York, McGraw-Hill, 1994.

Lorenzini NA, Schneider JH: Temporary loss of intraoperative motor-evoked potential and permanent loss of somatosensory-evoked potentials associated with a postoperative sensory deficit. J Neurosurg Anesthesiol 1996;8:142–147.

MacEwen GD, Bunnell WP, Sriram K: Acute neurological complications in the treatment of scoliosis: A report of the Scoliosis Research Society. J Bone Joint Surg Am 1975;57:404–408.

May DM, Jones SJ, Crockard HA: Somatosensory evoked potential monitoring in cervical surgery: Identification of pre- and intraoperative risk factors associated with neurological deterioration. J Neurosurg 1996;85:566–573.

McQuillan PM, Newberg N: Intraoperative electromyography. In Russell GB, Rodichok LD: Primer of Intraoperative Neurophysiologic Monitoring. Boston, Butterworth-Heinemann, 1995; 171–187.

Moed BR, Ahmad BK, Craig JG, et al: Intraoperative monitoring with stimulus-evoked electromyography during placement of iliosacral screws: An initial clinical study. J Bone Joint Surg Am 1998;80:537–546.

Møller AR: Evoked Potentials in Intraoperative Monitoring. Baltimore, Williams & Wilkins, 1988.

More RC, Nuwer MR, Dawson EG: True and false positive amplitude attenuations during cortical evoked potential spinal cord monitoring. In Ducker TB, Brown RH (eds): Neurophysiology and Standards of Spinal Cord Monitoring. New York, Springer-Verlag, 1988; 222–225.

Nagle KJ, Emerson RG, Adams DC, et al: Intraoperative monitoring of motor evoked potentials: A review of 116 cases. Neurology 1996;47:999–1004.

North RB, Drenger B, Beattie C, et al: Monitoring of spinal cord stimulation evoked potentials during thoracoabdominal aneurysm surgery. Neurosurgery 1991;28:325–330.

Nuwer JM, Nuwer MR: Neurophysiologic surgical monitoring staffing patterns in the USA. Electroencephalogr Clin Neurophysiol 1997;103:616–620.

Nuwer MR: Evoked Potential Monitoring in the Operating Room. New York, Raven Press, 1986.

Nuwer MR: Spinal cord monitoring with somatosensory techniques. J Clin Neurophysiol 1998;15:183–193.

Nuwer MR: Spinal cord monitoring. Muscle Nerve 1999;22:1620–1630.

Nuwer MR, Daube J, Fischer C, et al: Neuromonitoring during surgery: Report of an IFCN Committee. Electroencephalogr Clin Neurophysiol 1993;87:263–276.

Nuwer MR, Dawson EG, Carlson LG, et al: Somatosensory evoked potential spinal cord monitoring reduces neurologic deficits after scoliosis surgery: Results of a large multicenter survey. Electroencephalogr Clin Neurophysiol 1995;96:6–11.

Obi T, Mochizuki M, Isobe K, et al: Mechanically elicited nerve root discharge: Mechanical irritation and waveform. Acta Neurol Scand 1999;100:185–188.

O'Brien MF, Lenke LG, Bridwell KH, et al: Evoked potential monitoring of the upper extremities during thoracic and lumbar spinal deformity surgery: A prospective study. J Spinal Disord 1994;7:277–284.

Okamoto Y, Murakami M, Nakagawa T, et al: Intraoperative spinal cord monitoring during surgery for aortic aneurysm: Application of spinal cord evoked potential. Electroencephalogr Clin Neurophysiol 1992;84:315–320.

Padberg AM, Wilson-Holden TJ, Lenke LG, Bridwell KH: Somatosensory- and motor-evoked potential monitoring without a wake-up test during idiopathic scoliosis surgery: An accepted standard of care. Spine 1998;23:1392–1400.

Pechstein U, Cedzich C, Nadstawek J, Schramm J: Transcranial high-frequency repetitive electrical stimulation for recording myogenic motor evoked potentials with the patient under general anesthesia. Neurosurgery 1996;39:335–343.

Pelosi L, Jardine A, Webb JK: Neurological complications of anterior spinal surgery for kyphosis with normal somatosensory evoked potentials (SEPs). J Neurol Neurosurg Psychiatry 1999; 66:662–664.

Pereon Y, Bernard JM, Fayet G, et al: Usefulness of neurogenic motor evoked potentials for spinal cord monitoring: Findings in 112 consecutive patients undergoing surgery for spinal deformity. Electroencephalogr Clin Neurophysiol 1998;108:17–23.

Russell GB, Rodichok LD: Primer of Intraoperative Neurophysiologic Monitoring. Boston, Butterworth-Heinemann, 1995.

Schramm J, Kurthen M: Recent developments in neurosurgical spinal cord monitoring. Paraplegia 1992;30:609–616.

Schramm J, Møller AR: Intraoperative Neurophysiologic Monitoring in Neurosurgery. Berlin, Springer-Verlag, 1991.

Stålberg E, Sharma HS, Olsson Y: Spinal Cord Monitoring: Basic Principles, Regeneration, Pathophysiology, and Clinical Aspects. Vienna, Springer-Verlag, 1998.

Staudt LA, Nuwer MR, Peacock WJ: Intraoperative monitoring during selective posterior rhizotomy: Technique and patient outcome. Electroencephalogr Clin Neurophysiol 1995;97:296–309.

Tamaki T: Intraoperative spinal cord monitoring—clinical overview. In Stålberg E, Sharma HS, Olsson Y (eds): Spinal Cord Monitoring: Basic Principles, Regeneration, Pathophysiology, and Clinical Aspects. Vienna, Springer-Verlag, 1998; 509–520.

Taylor BA, Fennelly ME, Taylor A, Farrell J: Temporal summation—the key to motor evoked potential spinal cord monitoring in humans. J Neurol Neurosurg Psychiatry 1993;56:104–106.

Tsai RY, Yang RS, Nuwer MR, et al: Intraoperative dermatomal evoked potential monitoring fails to predict outcome from lumbar decompression surgery. Spine 1997;22:1970–1975.

Ubags LH, Kalkman CJ, Been HD, et al: The use of ketamine or etomidate to supplement sufentanil/N_2O anesthesia does not disrupt monitoring of myogenic transcranial motor evoked responses. J Neurosurg Anesthesiol 1997;9:228–233.

van Dongen EP, ter Beek HT, Schepens MA, et al: Within patient variability of lower extremity muscle responses to transcranial electrical stimulation with pulse trains in aortic surgery. Clin Neurophysiol 1999;110:1144–1148.

Warf BC, Nelson KR: The electromyographic responses to dorsal rootlet stimulation during partial dorsal rhizotomy are inconsistent. Pediatr Neurosurg 1996;25:13–19.

Welch WC, Rose RD, Balzer JR, Jacobs GB: Evaluation with evoked and spontaneous electromyography during lumbar instrumentation: A prospective study. J Neurosurg 1997;87:397–402.

Woodforth IJ, Hicks RG, Crawford MR, et al: Variability of motor-evoked potentials recorded during nitrous oxide anesthesia from the tibialis anterior muscle after transcranial electrical stimulation. Anesth Analg 1996;82:744–749.

Monitoring Peripheral Nerves During Surgery

Jasper R. Daube and C. Michel Harper

Electrophysiological monitoring during surgery can be applied at each level of the nervous system. Chapters 101 and 102 discuss the applications of these techniques to the spinal cord, spinal nerves, brainstem, and cranial nerves. Monitoring also can be helpful during surgical procedures in the region of peripheral nerves and plexuses. Increasingly, surgeons are asking clinical neurophysiologists to assist them in peripheral nerve surgery. Thus, it behooves a clinical neurophysiologist to become familiar with the methods, their applications, and their value.

PURPOSE

In some patients being considered for peripheral nerve surgery, preoperative neurophysiological studies can provide the surgeon with information about the location, type, and severity of pre-existing nerve damage. Such information can aid in surgical planning. Peripheral nerve monitoring during surgery can provide several additional distinct benefits, including the following:

- Assist with the identification of nerve tissue
- Define precisely the location and severity of pre-existing nerve damage
- Warn of imminent new nerve damage
- Define the location, type, and severity of new nerve damage
- Confirm intact neural pathways that are at risk of damage
- Assist in determining the optimal surgical procedures to minimize nerve damage

The many uncommon perioperative nerve lesions that occur with a multitude of different surgical pro-

cedures have been well described by Dawson et al. (Dawson et al., 1999). A patient undergoing an operation on or near any peripheral nerve or plexus may benefit from monitoring nerve function intraoperatively. The need for monitoring is defined best by assessing both the risk of preventable nerve damage during the operation and the additional information that could be provided to the surgeon. The risk to the nerve and whether it is preventable are judgments best made by the surgeon. For example, nerves embedded in a large tumor often need to be sacrificed to remove the tumor; these generally do not need to be monitored. In contrast, the preservation of nerves less involved by tumor can be aided by monitoring. Peripheral nerve or plexus damage has been reported often enough to suggest that intraoperative monitoring may be helpful in total hip arthroplasty, cardiac surgery, ulnar nerve surgery, brachial plexus surgery, nerve tumor resection, and many other selected procedures in which nerves are known to be at particular risk.

Common applications of monitoring peripheral nerves and plexuses during surgery include nerve trauma, entrapment neuropathies, primary or metastatic neoplasm, and operations on structures adjacent to nerves. In these situations, monitoring can provide information about the number, location, type, and severity of nerve lesions (Brown and Veitch, 1994). This information can be used to answer questions that were not resolved by preoperative electrodiagnostic studies and to help surgeons to make therapeutic decisions about decompression, neurolysis, grafting, or neurotization of nerves. Standard electrodiagnostic techniques, with minor modifications of nerve conduction studies, electromyography (EMG), and somatosensory evoked potentials, singly or in combination, are used to monitor peripheral nerves and plexuses intraoperatively. Monitoring protocols are best designed individually for patients after review of the preoperative neurological examination findings, preoperative nerve conduction and EMG studies, anesthetic options, and surgical goals.

METHODS

If the surgeon has decided that monitoring may be helpful and if the anesthesiologist is able to use an anesthesia program compatible with monitoring, the monitoring procedures will need to be defined. The International Federation of Clinical Neurophysiology Recommendations for the Practice of Clinical Neurophysiology reviewed the general principles of monitoring neural function intraoperatively (Burke et al., 1999). A monitoring protocol must be designed individually for each patient based on the surgical procedure, the structures at risk, the anesthesia requirements, and the clinical neurophysiology capabilities. For example, a need for neuromuscular block makes monitoring of motor axons more difficult. Although neurotonic discharges may still be recorded, the amplitude of the compound muscle action potential is much less reliable. The selection of peripheral monitoring procedures should consider nerve conduction studies, EMG, and somatosensory evoked potentials.

Nerve Conduction

Mixed motor and sensory nerves or sensory cutaneous nerves are tested by stimulation of nerve and recording from nerve (nerve action potential), muscle (compound muscle action potentials), or brain (somatosensory evoked potentials) (Fig. 104–1) (see Chapter 101 for a more detailed description of these methods during surgery). Although standard commercial electrodes may be used, specially designed electrodes for intraoperative monitoring are optimal and give more reliable results. In general, stimulation is applied anywhere along the exposed length of the nerve with a hand-held electrical stimulator placed directly on the nerve in the surgical field. Stimulation with the cathode and anode applied to the nerve *(bipolar stimulation)* is used when a well-localized stimulus is needed to minimize current spread. Stimulation with the cathode on the nerve and the anode at some distance away *(monopolar stimulation)* is used when locating neural tissue and when the two stimulating electrodes cannot be oriented properly. Generally, bipolar stimulation is preferred for peripheral nerve stimulation in surgical monitoring. The stimulator size and type are matched to the size and location of the nerve. Larger stimulators, similar to those used in diagnostic nerve conduction studies, are used to stimulate large nerves; these nerves should be isolated from other nerves to prevent current spread. Hooked stimulating electrodes can be used to elevate nerves from surrounding tissue when better stimulus isolation is required. Small electrodes are used when individual or small groups of fascicles

are stimulated (Terzis et al., 1976; Williams and Terzis, 1976). Electrode orientation and direction of current flow are important when recording over short distances and for ensuring accurate measurements. Large shock artifacts can obliterate a small response and need to be minimized with proper electrode positioning. The cathode and anode should be aligned along the long axis of the nerve, with the cathode closer to the recording electrode than the anode.

Intraoperative stimulation requires careful consideration of the location and strength of stimulus to prevent overstimulation, current spread, and other technical problems. Normal nerve is activated with as little as 1 mA of current and 0.05 ms of pulse duration. Overstimulation can produce stimulation of surrounding nerves or stimulus spread along the course of the nerve. The latter leads to inaccurate measurements of latency and conduction velocity. Diseased nerve typically has a higher threshold for stimulation. Thus, stimulus threshold should be monitored closely during intraoperative nerve conduction studies.

Compound muscle action potentials are recorded with surface or subcutaneous needle electrodes placed over muscles distal to the stimulus. Although intramuscular needle electrodes can also record compound muscle action potentials, they sample a smaller proportion of the muscle and are difficult to measure because of irregular shapes, and muscle movement makes them considerably less stable, especially during a long operation. Compound muscle action potential recordings are large with minimal artifact, and they monitor exclusively the function of motor axons. Compound muscle action potentials can quantitate loss of motor function intraoperatively in comparison with both baseline values at the beginning of the operation and the responses at different points along the nerve. Compound muscle action potentials are reduced and more variable during neuromuscular block. Useful data can be obtained during neuromuscular block, but an anesthetic regimen that minimizes it is optimal when recording compound muscle action potentials.

Nerve action potentials are recorded from large mixed nerves with hand-held bipolar recording electrodes placed directly on the nerve or from small cutaneous nerves with needle electrodes placed next to the nerve. Compared with compound muscle action potential recordings, nerve action potential recordings are technically more difficult to perform but more sensitive in localizing abnormalities along nerves. Moreover, nerve action potentials are able to detect the amount and extent of early axonal regeneration through an area of nerve injury well before regeneration is reflected in compound muscle action potential recordings. The presence of a compound muscle action potential or nerve action potential distal to the site of stimulation indicates that some axons are in continuity. The amplitude and area of the compound muscle action potential or nerve action potential are proportional to the num-

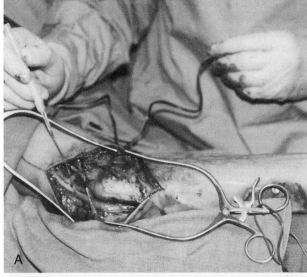

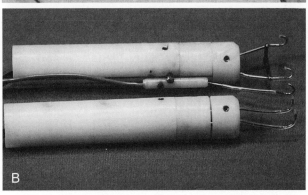

Figure 104–1. *A,* Monitoring ulnar nerve with direct nerve stimulation while recording compound muscle action potentials with subcutaneous needle electrodes. *B,* Flexible stimulating and recording hook electrodes for recording directly from nerve in the surgical field. The active and reference recording electrodes are held at a fixed distance by the *black bar.* A third hook on the recording electrode is a ground that is placed on the nerve between stimulating and recording electrodes. *C,* Intraoperative recordings from ulnar nerve and ulnar–innervated muscles in response to direct stimulation of the ulnar nerve in the surgical field. Compound muscle action potentials are recorded with subcutaneous electrodes over the muscle. Superimposed nerve action potentials are recorded directly from the ulnar nerve with hook electrodes. ADQ, abductor digiti quinti; FDI, first dorsal interosseous. (*C* from Daube JR, Harper CM: Surgical monitoring of cranial and peripheral nerves. In Desmedt JE [ed]: Neuromonitoring in Surgery. Amsterdam, Elsevier Science Publishers, 1989; 115–138. By permission of JE Desmedt.)

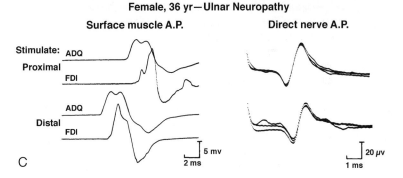

Electromyography

Intraoperatively, EMG is recorded best with small intramuscular wire electrodes. The wires are introduced percutaneously with a hollow needle, which is then withdrawn, to leave the wire in place. When intramuscular electrodes are used, nerve stimulation produces a polyphasic compound muscle ac-

ber of functioning axons. Focal slowing of conduction velocity, conduction block, or increased threshold of stimulation localizes a lesion along the nerve with 1 to 2 cm of accuracy.

tion potential that, although difficult to quantify, is less likely than surface electrodes to record nonspecific activity from adjacent muscles. Mechanical irritation of the nerve produces a high-frequency discharge of motor unit potentials *(neurotonic discharge)* that can be distinguished easily from artifact and other motor unit potential activity in EMG recordings (Daube and Harper, 1989). Neurotonic discharges can help to locate nerves within the surgical field and to warn that potential nerve injury may occur if the irritation continues (Nelson and Phillips, 1990). Rarely, clean, rapid sectioning of a nerve may not be associated with neurotonic discharges (Nelson and Vasconez, 1995).

Central Evoked Potentials

For intraoperative monitoring, somatosensory evoked potentials are recorded from surface electrodes over the cervical spine and contralateral parietal scalp following direct electrical stimulation of a peripheral nerve in the surgical field. The presence of a response indicates continuity of sensory axons between the spinal cord and the site of peripheral nerve stimulation. This technique has several advantages over standard somatosensory evoked potential recordings made in the laboratory, including increased selectivity of stimulation and enhanced sensitivity resulting from amplification of the response by the central nervous system. Somatosensory evoked potentials have been reported more frequently in peripheral nerve monitoring, likely because of the greater ease of application and technical simplicity. Generally, however, they are not as sensitive as direct nerve monitoring. A single report of motor evoked potential recording from peripheral nerve in response to cerebral stimulation suggests that this may be a useful tool, too (Turkof et al., 1997).

Applications

Nerve conduction studies, EMG, and somatosensory evoked potential studies are used alone or in combination during operations for entrapment neuropathies, repair of traumatic injuries, resection of tumors that affect peripheral nerves or a plexus, and other procedures in the region of a peripheral nerve or plexus (Kline and Happel, 1993). The most proximal segments of the peripheral nervous system (roots and spinal nerves) are monitored during spinal surgery. Distal elements (i.e., brachial and lumbar plexuses and individual nerves of the extremities) are studied to better localize peripheral nerve lesions, to determine the status of axonal regeneration, and to protect nerve fascicles from iatrogenic injury. Preoperative nerve conduction studies and needle EMG can be used to localize and to characterize most lesions affecting the peripheral nervous system (Campbell et al., 1988a). When chronic lesions produce segmental demyelination, mechanical distortion of paranodal myelin, or impaired function of ion channels at the node of Ranvier, then conduction block and focal slowing of conduction velocity are observed on routine nerve conduction studies. Two important criteria are required to demonstrate conduction block or focal slowing of conduction velocity. First, stimulation must be performed proximally and distally to the lesion (preferably in short 1- to 2-cm segments through the area of the lesion). Second, the fascicles that contain the lesion should be stimulated or recorded in isolation from fascicles belonging to other nerves in proximity. These criteria cannot always be fulfilled when a lesion affects proximal or deep nerves. In this setting, compound muscle action potential or nerve action potential recordings (or both) over short segments of exposed nerve at surgery are helpful.

Localization with preoperative nerve conduction and EMG studies is much less precise when partial or complete axon loss is the major pathological substrate. In that setting, intraoperative nerve conduction studies can often localize the main site of peripheral nerve abnormality and can identify functioning nerve fascicles that are preserved or regenerating across the site of the lesion. Precise localization of the site of median nerve damage in carpal tunnel syndrome and its relation to local increase in pressure in the tunnel were demonstrated with combined intraoperative nerve action potential and pressure recordings (Luchetti et al., 1990).

In the absence of conduction block, the compound muscle action potential amplitude does not change between proximal and distal stimulation sites. In contrast, a segmental change in nerve action potential amplitude frequently can be demonstrated even in purely axonal lesions (see Fig. 104–1). To show this, a bipolar hooked nerve electrode is placed proximal to the lesion for nerve action potential recording. Placement proximal to the lesion eliminates movement artifact and volume-conducted compound muscle action potentials caused by contraction of adjacent muscles. The stimulator is moved from distal to proximal in successive 1- to 2-cm segments. The lesion is identified by a change in amplitude and slowed conduction of the nerve action potentials over the short nerve segment. Nerve action potentials may show nerve regeneration before the nerve action potential has had a chance to reach the muscle, a time when compound muscle action potentials are absent.

Entrapment Neuropathies

Localization by clinical signs and by preoperative nerve conduction and EMG studies is adequate in most cases of entrapment neuropathy (Brown and Veitch, 1994). Carpal tunnel release and most cases of ulnar transposition do not require monitoring. However, patients with complicated cases of ulnar or median neuropathy and radial, femoral, sciatic, tibial, and peroneal neuropathy are often monitored because of inherent difficulties in defining with preoperative studies the number and location of lesions.

Ulnar neuropathy at the elbow is one of the most common mononeuropathies. The ulnar nerve can be injured by repeated trauma to the nerve in the region of the medial epicondyle, compression by bony or soft tissue deformities around the elbow joint, recurrent subluxation over the medial epicondyle, or entrapment between the heads of the flexor carpi ulnaris *(cubital tunnel syndrome)* (Dawson et al., 1983). Moreover, the ulnar nerve may be compressed in the midforearm or at the wrist. Ulnar transposition has been the most popular surgical procedure for ulnar neuropathy at the elbow. However, because transposition is not always successful and may increase morbidity, more conservative procedures such as simple cubital tunnel release have been advocated (Campbell et al., 1988b).

Often, the site of entrapment can be determined with preoperative electrodiagnostic studies. Useful findings include a localized area of motor conduction block or slowing on short segmental stimulation. The distribution of abnormalities on needle EMG also may help to localize the lesion, especially if the flexor carpi ulnaris or flexor digitorum profundus muscles are affected. Sometimes, preoperative studies provide inadequate or inaccurate information. Variability in the location of the cubital tunnel in relation to the medial epicondyle, selective damage to fascicles within the ulnar nerve, technical difficulties (e.g., overstimulation causing current spread), and lesions in unusual locations contribute to limited accuracy of preoperative testing (Campbell et al., 1988a). Many of these difficulties can be avoided with intraoperative nerve conduction studies. Conduction block and focal slowing are easier to detect and to localize accurately when the nerve is exposed. In addition, overstimulation is easier to detect and to correct intraoperatively, and areas of increased threshold can help to identify damaged nerve segments.

The sensitivity and accuracy of intraoperative nerve conduction studies may help the surgeon to choose the most appropriate treatment. A well-localized lesion in the region of the two heads of the flexor carpi ulnaris may be treated with a simple cubital tunnel release, whereas a transposition may be performed when the lesion is more diffuse or is localized at or proximal to the medial epicondyle. Lesions at unusual sites, such as the distal aspect of the cubital tunnel, can be localized and explored, thereby avoiding unnecessary decompression or transposition at more proximal sites. The results of nerve conduction studies performed during ulnar nerve exploration are shown in Figure 104–2. Preoperative nerve conduction recordings showed localized slowing with increased compound muscle action potential dispersion approximately 3 cm distal to the medial epicondyle. Compound muscle action potentials were recorded intraoperatively over the abductor digiti minimi and flexor carpi ulnaris muscles, and nerve action potentials were recorded from the proximal ulnar nerve. There were changes in amplitude and latency of both compound muscle action potentials and nerve action potentials over a 3-cm segment at the origin of the cubital tunnel. Because there was no area of slowing proximal or distal to this point, a cubital tunnel release was performed.

Localized hypertrophic mononeuropathy is a less common lesion for which intraoperative nerve action potential recording may be helpful (Gruen et

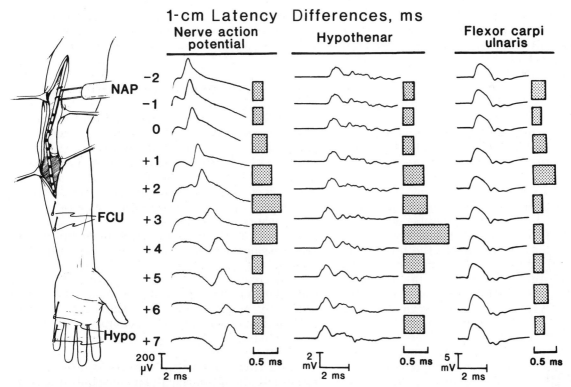

Figure 104–2. Intraoperative recording of compound muscle action potentials and nerve action potentials (NAP) during ulnar nerve exploration and stimulation at 1-cm intervals. The "0" point indicates the location of the medial epicondyle. The greatest changes in latency and amplitude occur over a 3-cm segment spanning the origin of the cubital tunnel. FCU, flexor carpi ulnaris; Hypo, hypothenar. (From Daube JR, Harper CM: Surgical monitoring of cranial and peripheral nerves. In Desmedt JE [ed]: Neuromonitoring in Surgery. Amsterdam, Elsevier Science Publishers, 1989; 115–138. By permission of JE Desmedt.)

al., 1998). The presence or absence of intact action potentials across the lesion provided guidance in determining whether to resect and graft the nerve segment in 15 patients. Of nine patients who had a graft, seven were clinically unchanged or were improved.

Repair of Traumatic Peripheral Nerve Injury

Intraoperative monitoring is particularly useful when multiple deep proximal nerves are injured and when many mechanisms of injury are involved (e.g., traction, contusion, and ischemia). The primary purpose of monitoring in this setting is to localize the injured segment and to assess the status of axonal continuity across the injured area (Kline, 1990; Tiel et al., 1996).

The usefulness of these techniques is best illustrated by examining their role in the surgical repair of traumatic injuries to the brachial plexus. The complexity of brachial plexus anatomy, the multiplicity and severity of injury to its elements, and the frequent occurrence of nerve root avulsion make lesions of this structure particularly difficult to evaluate and to treat (Davis et al., 1978; Kline et al., 1986). The presence or absence of nerve root avulsion is one of the most important factors in determining prognosis and the need for surgical intervention in brachial plexus injuries. If root avulsion is present, then repair of postganglionic elements innervated by the avulsed root will be of no benefit. The clinical examination, nerve conduction study, needle EMG, and myelogram are used preoperatively to assess the integrity of the cervical nerve roots (Davis et al., 1978; Landi et al., 1980). The combination of Horner's syndrome, denervation of paraspinal and other proximal muscles, preserved sensory nerve action potentials, and the presence of a meningocele on myelography in the setting of a paralyzed anesthetic limb are diagnostic of multiple root avulsions. However, any one of these findings in isolation is less predictive. Examples of false-positive and false-negative myelograms have been reported (Kline et al., 1986). Because the posterior primary ramus of a nerve root innervates paraspinal muscles at several levels, the distribution of fibrillation potentials may overestimate the number of roots involved (Levin et al., 1998). In addition, the presence of a postganglionic lesion with diminished sensory nerve action potentials may mask an associated lesion involving preganglionic segments. The predictive value of preoperative somatosensory evoked potentials in detecting root continuity as well as the presence of mixed preganglionic and postganglionic lesions has been disappointing (Yiannikas et al., 1983).

Sometimes, these uncertainties can be resolved with intraoperative somatosensory evoked potential recordings (Sugioka et al., 1982; Mahla et al., 1984). In this setting, the exposed spinal nerve is stimu-

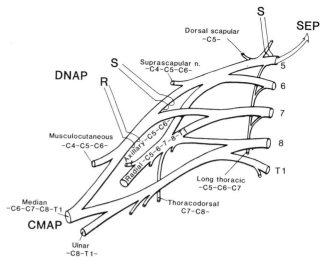

Figure 104–3. Electrophysiological techniques for monitoring brachial plexopathy. Somatosensory evoked potentials (SEP) recorded over the scalp during root stimulation. Nerve action potentials recorded directly (DNAP) from short segments of the plexus. *Bottom,* Compound muscle action potentials (CMAP) recorded from distal muscles during selective stimulation of plexus elements. R, recording electrodes; S, stimulating electrodes. (From Daube JR, Harper CM: Surgical monitoring of cranial and peripheral nerves. In Desmedt JE [ed]: Neuromonitoring in Surgery. Amsterdam, Elsevier Science Publishers, 1989; 115–138. By permission of JE Desmedt.)

lated directly by the surgeon while somatosensory evoked potential recordings are made from the cervical spine or scalp (or both) (Fig. 104–3). If sensory fibers within the root are intact, a well-defined somatosensory evoked potential will be recorded. The absence of a response confirms dorsal root avulsion at that level (Fig. 104–4). One assessment of the method compared somatosensory evoked potential responses with direct, intraoperative visualization of the spinal nerve and nerve root in 13 patients with inconclusive or erroneous radiographic findings (Oberle et al., 1998). Somatosensory evoked potentials correctly identified both intact and disrupted roots. Because this technique tests sensory function, it is theoretically possible that the ventral motor root could be avulsed with sparing of the dorsal root. If this occurred, the presence of a somatosensory evoked potential would be misleading. One report on the value of motor evoked potentials in assessing ventral root function may provide a solution (Turkof et al., 1997). However, motor evoked potential studies in this setting are technically difficult, and the results have not been confirmed by other authors. Therefore, when a well-defined somatosensory evoked potential is present, it is probably best to proceed with surgical repair of the postganglionic elements.

When root continuity is present, attention is turned to the assessment and possible repair of postganglionic elements. Injured elements of the plexus are stimulated proximally, with attempts to record a compound muscle action potential from a distal muscle or a nerve action potential from the

STIMULATE RIGHT: record C3-Fz

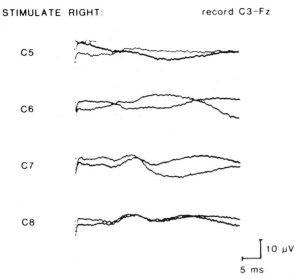

Figure 104–4. Root avulsion intraoperative recording of somatosensory evoked potentials over the scalp, with stimulation of cervical nerve roots directly in the surgical field. Well-defined responses were seen with stimulation of C7 and C8 roots. No response was obtained with stimulation of C5 or C6 roots, indicating avulsion of the root at these levels. (From Daube JR, Harper CM: Surgical monitoring of cranial and peripheral nerves. In Desmedt JE [ed]: Neuromonitoring in Surgery. Amsterdam, Elsevier Science Publishers, 1989; 115–138. By permission of JE Desmedt.)

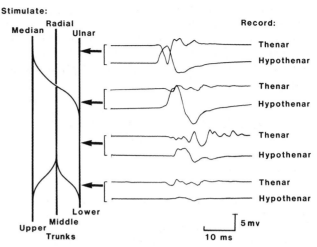

Figure 104–5. Intraoperative nerve conduction studies showing localization of conduction block along the medial cord of the brachial plexus. (From Daube JR, Harper CM: Surgical monitoring of cranial and peripheral nerves. In Desmedt JE [ed]: Neuromonitoring in Surgery. Amsterdam, Elsevier Science Publishers, 1989; 115–138. By permission of JE Desmedt.)

nerve distal to the site of injury (see Fig. 104–3). Direct electrical stimulation with a hand-held stimulator can be used to identify viable nerves or fascicles. When a compound muscle action potential is present, the surgeon can be confident that some motor axons are intact. In this setting, the lesion is left alone or, at most, a simple neurolysis is performed. Detecting conduction block or focal slowing of conduction velocity over short segments in either compound muscle action potential or nerve action potential recordings sometimes localizes lesions (Fig. 104–5). When no compound muscle action potential is recorded, the disruption of axons may be complete at the site of injury, or regeneration across the lesion may be insufficient for the regenerating axons to reach a distal muscle. Thus, recording a nerve action potential across the injured segment suggests that regeneration is occurring, whereas the absence of a nerve action potential suggests severe and complete axon loss. The latter finding suggests the need for lesion resection and subsequent grafting or a neurotization procedure (Kline and DeJonge, 1968; Kline et al., 1992). Recording nerve action potentials from individual nerve fascicles has been reported to help guide partial fascicular repair in incomplete lesions (Kline et al., 1992). Technical difficulties related to the size of the electrodes, the occurrence of shock artifact, and current spread to adjacent fascicles have limited the widespread use of fascicular recordings. Kline et al. reported the outcomes of this approach in sciatic nerve injuries (Kline et al., 1998). Nerve action potential recordings guided the decision of neurolysis versus resection

and graft of injured sciatic nerves. Although the return of tibial nerve function was good or excellent in all patients, substantial peroneal nerve recovery occurred in only 36%. In contrast, successful nerve action potential recordings across the site of severe peroneal nerve damage at the knee correctly predicted useful recovery of function in 89% of 80 patients (Kim and Kline, 1996). Similar encouraging results were obtained with nerve action potential recordings in femoral nerve injuries (Kim and Kline, 1995).

Prevention of Peripheral Nerve Injury Intraoperatively

The peripheral nerves that innervate the trunk and extremity muscles are susceptible to mechanical or ischemic injury during many surgical procedures. Both EMG monitoring and evoked potential recordings can help to prevent such injury, but the decision to use them must take into account the likelihood of injury. For example, motor neuropathy in the leg occurs in only 1 in 3,608 patients undergoing surgery in the lithotomy position, but it is more likely to occur with a prolonged operation and with thin body habitus (Warner et al., 1994).

EMG monitoring for neurotonic discharges caused by nerve irritation can localize and warn of potential injury to the nerve, as described earlier. An experimental model defined the changes in evoked potentials resulting from peripheral nerve damage in these injuries (Fowler and Gilliatt, 1981). Damage was manifested primarily by the loss of amplitude of responses caused by either axon disruption or conduction block. Thus, loss of a response conducted across susceptible nerve segments (nerve action potentials, compound muscle action potentials, somatosensory evoked potentials) can serve as an excellent monitor to prevent injury.

Definition of the mechanism of injury by monitoring during surgery has led to improvements in some cardiac and shoulder procedures. Postoperative ulnar neuropathies are uncommon (Warner et al., 1999), but somatosensory evoked potential recordings from median, radial, and ulnar nerves during brachial artery occlusion showed a greater ulnar nerve susceptibility that resulted in a higher proportion of damage to the ulnar nerve (Swenson et al., 1998).

Plexus injuries are uncommon after surgical procedures; the greatest risk is to the brachial plexus during cardiac surgery (Lederman et al., 1982). Of patients undergoing cardiac surgery, 2% to 13% may have peripheral nerve damage (Sila, 1998). Median and ulnar somatosensory evoked potentials changed during chest retraction in 21 (70%) of 30 patients undergoing coronary artery bypass surgery, but they returned to baseline during the procedure in 16 of these patients. The other five patients in whom somatosensory evoked potentials remained abnormal had postoperative deficits (Hickey et al., 1993). Subsequent studies confirmed somatosensory evoked potential changes during retraction in similar patients, but to different degrees with different methods of retraction (Seal et al., 1997; Jellish et al., 1999). Thus, somatosensory evoked potential monitoring was able to bring about improvements in surgical procedures. The application of somatosensory evoked potential monitoring has not been widespread because most patients have a reasonably good recovery from these injuries (Ben-David and Stahl, 1997).

Postoperative nerve injuries after orthopedic procedures that involve disarticulation or extensive manipulation may be reduced by monitoring (van der Linde and Tonino, 1997). EMG monitoring can help to detect and prevent injury to the axillary and musculocutaneous nerves during shoulder surgery, to the lumbosacral plexus during acetabular fracture repair, and to the femoral, obturator, and sciatic nerves during high-risk hip surgery (Helfet et al., 1997).

Somatosensory evoked potential monitoring provided benefit for 20 patients undergoing surgery for acetabular fractures, compared with a group of 21 without monitoring (Baumgaertner et al., 1994). Somatosensory evoked potential monitoring also has been reported to help prevent nerve damage in hip surgery (Rasmussen et al., 1994), and it was particularly helpful during hip revisions (Stone et al., 1985; Nercessian et al., 1989). During shoulder arthroscopy, somatosensory evoked potential monitoring appears to reduce the occurrence of postoperative deficits, especially of the musculocutaneous nerve (Pitman et al., 1988). No studies have compared somatosensory evoked potential and EMG monitoring for relative effectiveness in identifying possible nerve damage.

EMG monitoring may also be useful during resec-

tion of primary or metastatic peripheral nerve neoplasms. In this setting, the goal is to resect the tumor with as little damage to normal nerve fascicles as possible. During dissection, individual fascicles or groups of fascicles are stimulated mechanically or electrically while EMG activity is monitored in distal muscles. An attempt is made to preserve fascicles that produce a distal EMG response, whereas those that do not are sacrificed. Neurotonic discharges also warn of axonal irritation during an operation.

References

Baumgaertner MR, Wegner D, Booke J: SSEP monitoring during pelvic and acetabular fracture surgery. J Orthop Trauma 1994; 8:127–133.

Ben-David B, Stahl S: Prognosis of intraoperative brachial plexus injury: A review of 22 cases. Br J Anaesth 1997;79:440–445.

Brown WF, Veitch J: AAEM minimonograph #42: Intraoperative monitoring of peripheral and cranial nerves. Muscle Nerve 1994;17:371–377.

Burke D, Nuwer MR, Daube J, et al: Intraoperative monitoring: The International Federation of Clinical Neurophysiology. Electroencephalogr Clin Neurophysiol Suppl 1999;52:133–148.

Campbell WW, Pridgeon RM, Sahni SK: Entrapment neuropathy of the ulnar nerve at its point of exit from the flexor carpi ulnaris muscle. Muscle Nerve 1988a;11:467.

Campbell WW, Sahni SK, Pridgeon RM, et al: Intraoperative electroneurography: Management of ulnar neuropathy at the elbow. Muscle Nerve 1988b;11:75–81.

Daube JR, Harper CM: Surgical monitoring of cranial and peripheral nerves. In Desmedt JE (ed): Neuromonitoring in Surgery. Amsterdam, Elsevier Science Publishers, 1989; 115–138.

Davis DH, Onofrio BM, MacCarty CS: Brachial plexus injuries. Mayo Clin Proc 1978;53:799–807.

Dawson DM, Hallett M, Millender LH: Entrapment Neuropathies. Boston, Little, Brown, 1983; 87–122.

Dawson DM, Hallett M, Wilbourn AJ: Entrapment Neuropathies, 3rd ed. Philadelphia, Lippincott–Raven, 1999.

Fowler CJ, Gilliatt RW: Conduction velocity and conduction block after experimental ischaemic nerve injury. J Neurol Sci 1981; 52:221–238.

Gruen JP, Mitchell W, Kline DG: Resection and graft repair for localized hypertrophic neuropathy. Neurosurgery 1998;43:78–83.

Helfet DL, Anand N, Malkani AL, et al: Intraoperative monitoring of motor pathways during operative fixation of acute acetabular fractures. J Orthop Trauma 1997;11:2–6.

Hickey C, Gugino LD, Aglio LS, et al: Intraoperative somatosensory evoked potential monitoring predicts peripheral nerve injury during cardiac surgery. Anesthesiology 1993;78:29–35.

Jellish WS, Blakeman B, Warf P, Slogoff S: Somatosensory evoked potential monitoring used to compare the effect of three asymmetric sternal retractors on brachial plexus function. Anesth Analg 1999;88:292–297.

Kim DH, Kline DG: Surgical outcome for intra- and extrapelvic femoral nerve lesions. J Neurosurg 1995;83:783–790.

Kim DH, Kline DG: Management and results of peroneal nerve lesions. Neurosurgery 1996;39:312–319.

Kline DG: Surgical repair of peripheral nerve injury. Muscle Nerve 1990;13:843–852.

Kline DG, DeJonge BR: Evoked potentials to evaluate peripheral nerve injuries. Surg Gynecol Obstet 1968;127:1239–1248.

Kline DG, Hackett ER, Happel LH: Surgery for lesions of the brachial plexus. Arch Neurol 1986;43:170–181.

Kline DG, Happel LT: Penfield lecture: A quarter century's experience with intraoperative nerve action potential recording. Can J Neurol Sci 1993;20:3–10.

Kline DG, Hudson AR, Zagar E: Selection and preoperative workup for peripheral nerve surgery. Clin Neurosurg 1992;39:8–35.

Kline DG, Kim D, Midha R, et al: Management and results of sciatic nerve injuries: A 24-year experience. J Neurosurg 1998; 89:13–23.

Landi A, Copeland SA, Parry CB, Jones SJ: The role of somatosensory evoked potentials and nerve conduction studies in the surgical management of brachial plexus injuries. J Bone Joint Surg Br 1980;62:492–496.

Lederman RJ, Breuer AC, Hanson MR, et al: Peripheral nervous system complications of coronary artery bypass graft surgery. Ann Neurol 1982;12:297–301.

Levin KH, Wilbourn AJ, Maggiano HJ: Cervical rib and median sternotomy-related brachial plexopathies: A reassessment. Neurology 1998;50:1407–1413.

Luchetti R, Schoenhuber R, Alfarano M, et al: Carpal tunnel syndrome: Correlations between pressure measurement and intraoperative electrophysiological nerve study. Muscle Nerve 1990; 13:1164–1168.

Mahla ME, Long DM, McKennett J, et al: Detection of brachial plexus dysfunction by somatosensory evoked potential monitoring: A report of two cases. Anesthesiology 1984;60:248–252.

Nelson KR, Phillips LH: Neurophysiologic monitoring during surgery of peripheral and cranial nerves, and in selective dorsal rhizotomy. Semin Neurol 1990;10:141–149.

Nelson KR, Vasconez HC: Nerve transection without neurotonic discharges during intraoperative electromyographic monitoring. Muscle Nerve 1995;18:236–238.

Nercessian OA, Gonzalez EG, Stinchfield FE: The use of somatosensory evoked potential during revision or reoperation for total hip arthroplasty. Clin Orthop 1989;243:138–142.

Oberle J, Antoniadis G, Rath SA, et al: Radiological investigations and intra-operative evoked potentials for the diagnosis of nerve root avulsion: Evaluation of both modalities by intradural root inspection. Acta Neurochir (Wien) 1998;140:527–531.

Pitman MI, Nainzadeh N, Ergas E, Springer S: The use of somatosensory evoked potentials for detection of neuropraxia during shoulder arthroscopy. Arthroscopy 1988;4:250–255.

Rasmussen TJ, Black DL, Bruce RP, Reckling FW: Efficacy of corticosomatosensory evoked potential monitoring in predicting and/or preventing sciatic nerve palsy during total hip arthroplasty. J Arthroplasty 1994;9:53–61.

Seal D, Balaton J, Coupland SG, et al: Somatosensory evoked potential monitoring during cardiac surgery: An examination of brachial plexus dysfunction. J Cardiothorac Vasc Anesth 1997;11:187–191.

Sila CA: Neurologic complications of vascular surgery. Neurol Clin 1998;16:9–20.

Stone RG, Weeks LE, Hajdu M, Stinchfield FE: Evaluation of sciatic nerve compromise during total hip arthroplasty. Clin Orthop 1985;201:26–31.

Sugioka H, Tsuyama N, Hara T, et al: Investigation of brachial plexus injuries by intraoperative cortical somatosensory evoked potentials. Arch Orthop Trauma Surg 1982;99:143–151.

Swenson JD, Hutchinson DT, Bromberg M, Pace NL: Rapid onset of ulnar nerve dysfunction during transient occlusion of the brachial artery. Anesth Analg 1998;87:677–680.

Terzis JK, Dykes RW, Hakstian RW: Electrophysiological recordings in peripheral nerve surgery: A review. J Hand Surg [Am] 1976;1:52–66.

Tiel RL, Happel LT Jr, Kline DG: Nerve action potential recording method and equipment. Neurosurgery 1996;39:103–108.

Turkof E, Millesi H, Turkof R, et al: Intraoperative electroneurodiagnostics (transcranial electrical motor evoked potentials) to evaluate the functional status of anterior spinal roots and spinal nerves during brachial plexus surgery. Plast Reconstr Surg 1997;99:1632–1641.

van der Linde MJ, Tonino AJ: Nerve injury after hip arthroplasty: 5/600 cases after uncemented hip replacement, anterolateral approach versus direct lateral approach. Acta Orthop Scand 1997;68:521–523.

Warner MA, Martin JT, Schroeder DR, et al: Lower-extremity motor neuropathy associated with surgery performed on patients in a lithotomy position. Anesthesiology 1994;81:6–12.

Warner MA, Warner DO, Matsumoto JY, et al: Ulnar neuropathy in surgical patients. Anesthesiology 1999;90:54–59.

Williams HB, Terzis JK: Single fascicular recordings: An intraoperative diagnostic tool for the management of peripheral nerve lesions. Plast Reconstr Surg 1976;57:562–569.

Yiannikas C, Shahani BT, Young RR: The investigation of traumatic lesions of the brachial plexus by electromyography and short latency somatosensory potentials evoked by stimulation of multiple peripheral nerves. J Neurol Neurosurg Psychiatry 1983;46:1014–1022.

CLINICAL TRIALS AND CLINICAL ELECTROPHYSIOLOGICAL STUDIES

C H A P T E R **105**

Quantitative Motor Function Testing in Clinical Trials

Mark B. Bromberg

Clinical neurophysiology can be viewed as having three goals: (1) to help make a diagnosis, (2) to follow disease progression, and (3) to provide information on pathophysiological processes. Historically, clinical neurophysiology has focused on disease diagnosis. Measuring disease progression in clinical trials is challenging because of the need to identify clinical neurophysiology tests that are appropriate and sensitive to small and clinically meaningful change. The rewards of this challenge can be substantial because the process of assessing tests for following disease progression provides insight into pathophysiological processes.

In clinical trials, treatable neuromuscular diseases such as inflammatory neuropathies and myopathies and defects in neuromuscular junction transmission have been followed primarily by clinical observation, and objective and quantitative neurophysiological testing is less important as an informative end-point measure. Clinical neurophysiology end-point measures become important in disorders in which clinical improvement is less obvious or when progression is inexorable. Diabetic peripheral neuropathy is an example in which quantitative neurophysiological tests can be useful end-point measures to assess changes in peripheral nerve when the underlying pathophysiology is incompletely understood. Amyotrophic lateral sclerosis is an example of a progressive denervating disorder in which clinical neurophysiological end-point measures can provide quantitative information on changes that traditionally have been viewed by clinical observation. This chapter addresses the role of clinical neurophysiology as end-point measures of motor function in a variety of neuromuscular disorders.

The first part of the chapter outlines pertinent portions of anatomy, physiology, and pathophysiology of the motor system that relate to the neurophysiological measurement of motor function. The second part discusses available neurophysiological tests and focuses on advantages and limitations of specific tests. Test reproducibility is important in clinical trials, and it is discussed. The third part reviews experience with neurophysiological tests as end-point measures in clinical trials for a variety of neuromuscular disorders. The chapter concludes with a discussion on selecting informative end-point measures for clinical trials.

MOTOR UNIT

Clinical neurophysiology traditionally focuses on measurement of the lower motor neuron (Stålberg, 1991). Measurement of the upper motor neuron has proved more difficult to perform and is not considered in this chapter. The lower motor neuron or motor unit is the α-motor neuron, its axon, neuromuscular junctions, and the muscle fibers innervated by terminal branches of the axon. The α motor neurons arise from somatic motor nuclei of the brainstem and the anterior horn of the spinal cord.

Motor unit size is related to soma diameter, axon diameter, conduction velocity, and the number of innervated muscle fibers. Motor axons undergo terminal branching within muscle and innervate a variable number of muscle fibers. The innervation ratio differs between muscles and within a muscle. Muscles that require fine gradations of force, such as extraocular eye muscles, have small motor units with an innervation ratio of approximately 18 muscle fibers per axon. Muscles that are not as finely graded, such as proximal limb muscles, have high ratios of 1,000 to 2,000 muscle fibers per axon (Feinstein et al., 1955). Within a muscle, there is a gradation in the size of the motor units, and the gradation is related to the recruitment size principle (discussed later).

Although the motor unit is a readily definable entity, it is difficult to identify or view a motor unit in vivo. A muscle is innervated by several hundred motor neurons, but it is not possible to identify individual motor units on histological cross sections of muscle. Although fibers from the same motor unit will be of the same histochemical type, fibers from different motor units of the same type are intermingled. With denervation and reinnervation, histological sections will show fiber type grouping, but it is not possible to determine how many motor units are contributing to a fiber group because of intermingling. It is possible to identify a motor unit with special techniques in animal preparations (Edström and Kugelberg, 1968). If a single ventral root is identified and isolated and is repetitively stimulated electrically, muscle fibers of one motor unit will become metabolically exhausted. If the muscle is removed and sectioned, muscle fibers of the motor unit can be identified by an absence of glycogen staining. It has been found from such experiments that fibers of a motor unit occupy a circular or elliptical area 5 to 10 mm in diameter, and 20 or so motor units overlap at any given site in a muscle. Muscle fibers of the same motor unit are rarely contiguous. With denervation and reinnervation, the density of muscle fibers in the motor unit increases, but the cross-sectional area does not (Kugelberg et al., 1970).

The motor unit is the domain of clinical neurophysiology, and its elusive nature is the challenge. Individual clinical neurophysiological tests have been developed to approach the motor unit from different directions and to address different aspects. These tests are unique in their ability to accurately and meaningfully quantify changes in the motor unit with disease progression and to follow treatment.

COLLATERAL REINNERVATION

Denervation of muscle occurs in diseases causing death of the cell body, axonal destruction, or dying back of distal nerve segments. Axonal loss leaves muscle fibers of the motor unit electrically inexcitable and mechanically unable to generate force. Denervation stimulates the initiation of collateral reinnervation, the compensatory process in which nerve terminals from nearby surviving motor neurons sprout branches to make new synaptic connections with orphaned muscle fibers (Wohlfart, 1958). Each motor neuron has a limit in its ability to perform collateral reinnervation, and the distribution of new terminals is restricted by fascicular boundaries within muscle (Kugelberg et al., 1970). Accordingly, reinnervation increases the number of fibers of a motor unit but not the area of innervation. Reinnervated muscle fibers are electrically excitable and can generate force, and collateral reinnervation tends to restore function. The advantage of clinical neurophysiological testing is that it can detect and measure the process of reinnervation, even in conditions that have not changed force or function measurably.

The ability of collateral reinnervation to compensate for lower motor loss can be impressive, but the effectiveness of reinnervation depends on the rate and extent of neuron loss. Slowly progressive loss provides sufficient time for maximal reinnervation. Old poliomyelitis represents one extreme, with sufficient time for full reinnervation, and muscle strength may be preserved when only a small number of lower motor neurons survived. Rapidly progressive loss provides insufficient time for full reinnervation before reinnervating motor neurons die. Amyotrophic lateral sclerosis is an example of progressive lower motor neuron loss in which strength is often preserved until approximately 50% of lower motor neurons are lost.

The relationship between the rate of lower motor loss and the effect of collateral reinnervation on muscle strength is complex, but it has been explored with computer modeling (Kuether and Lipinski, 1988). When the rate of neuron loss is linear, the compensatory effects of collateral reinnervation results in a slow loss of strength until 50% of neurons die, at which time decompensation ensues and strength falls rapidly (Fig. 105–1). When a sigmoidal rate of loss or an exponential rate with an initial rapid loss of lower motor neurons is modeled, the loss of strength is relatively linear until 80% of neurons die, at which time strength falls rapidly.

These modeling studies have implications for choosing clinical neurophysiological end-point measures. The relationship between compensation and decompensation is not linear. The various neurophysiological tests provide the ability to assess the compensatory and decompensatory processes. Appropriate selection of end-point measures requires an understanding of the pathophysiology and time course of the particular disease.

MEASUREMENT TECHNIQUES

Accurate and meaningful quantitative electrophysiological assessment of motor function partially depends on the properties of specific tests and measurement technique. Neuromuscular diseases largely affect the motor unit, which can be assessed electrically or mechanically. The electrical view is the primary domain of clinical neurophysiological testing, and it differs from the mechanical view. Neurophysiological tests and techniques are discussed in other chapters, but a brief review is presented here, focusing on specific tests and techniques as they relate to quantitative measurement of motor function.

Electrical Recordings

Electrical activity of a motor unit represents action potentials from all muscle fibers innervated by the motor axon. Surface electrodes applied over specific muscles or muscle groups record the gross activity of many or all motor units in the muscle. Intramuscular electrodes are more selective (Fig. 105–2). Macroelectromyography (macro-EMG) electrodes record activity from a whole motor unit, concentric or monopolar electrodes record from a limited number of fibers of the motor unit, and single-fiber electrodes record activity from single muscle fibers (Bromberg, 1993a).

Mechanical Recordings

In contrast with the electrophysiological view, the mechanical view of a motor unit represents activity

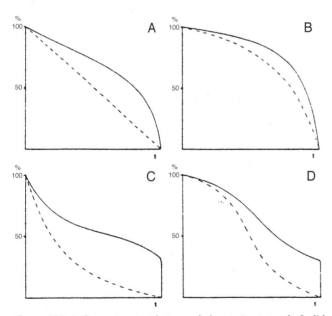

Figure 105–1. Computer simulations of change in strength *(solid lines)* with various rates of lower motor neuron loss *(dashed lines); x-axis,* time; *y-axis,* percentage of change in strength and lower motor neuron number. *A,* Linear rate of lower motor neuron loss results in rapid loss of strength when 50% of motor neurons are lost. *B,* Exponential rate (initial slow and later rapid) of lower motor neuron loss results in late rapid loss of strength. *C,* Exponential rate (initial fast and later slow) of lower motor neuron loss results in relatively linear loss of strength. *D,* Sigmoidal rate of lower motor neuron loss also results in relatively linear loss of strength. (From Kuether G, Lipinski H-G: Computer Simulation of Neuron Degeneration in Motor Neuron Disease. Amsterdam, Elsevier, 1988.)

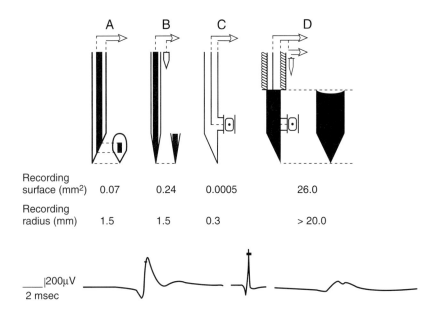

Figure 105–2. Configuration of electromyographic recording electrodes illustrating the recording surface and representative waveforms, with the recording surface area and recording radius listed in between. *A,* Concentric electrode. *B,* Monopolar electrode. *C,* Single-fiber electrode. *D,* Macroelectromyographic electrode. (From Bromberg M: Electromyographic [EMG] findings in denervation. Crit Rev Phys Rehabil Med 1993;5:83–127.)

of all innervated muscle fibers with no ability to focus on different aspects. Motor unit mechanical activity is usually recorded as maximal isometric voluntary contraction of a muscle or set of agonist muscles or of a single motor unit. Strength can be measured qualitatively using ordinal data scales such as the Medical Research Council 0 to 5 rating scale. However, quantitative interval measurement by dynamometry is preferable (Andres et al., 1986). Values may be obtained from an individual muscle or from numerous different muscles. Managing values from many muscles can be unwieldy, and values can be summed as composite or "megascores" to simplify statistical comparisons (Andres et al., 1988). Quantitative strength values are frequently converted to z-scores so each megascore value contributes equally (Andres et al., 1988).

Muscle strength is the most frequently used primary end-point measure in clinical trials. However, collateral reinnervation obscures the relationship between strength and the number of motor units innervating a muscle (see Fig. 105–1). There are advantages in direct comparison of strength data with clinical neurophysiological data, but this rarely occurs. One impediment is that most quantitative isometric strength measurements are performed on proximal limb muscles, whereas most clinical neurophysiological measurements are performed on distal limb muscles. This is largely the result of the relative ease of measuring strength from proximal muscle groups and the greater difficulty in measuring from distal muscles (Bromberg and Larson, 1996). In contrast, motor nerves and their corresponding muscles are more accessible to electrical stimulation and recording electrode placement in distal limb segments in the hands and feet. Furthermore, strength data usually represent summed values from many muscles (megascores), whereas neurophysiological data are from a limited number of muscles.

A goal of clinical neurophysiological testing is to provide more information on the state of the motor unit than can be obtained from muscle strength testing. Each neurophysiological test has limitations and advantages, and these factors need to be considered for proper selection.

Motor Nerve Conduction Studies

Motor nerve conduction studies are used to assess the number of intact nerve fibers innervating a muscle and their speed of conduction. Primary measurements are compound muscle action potential amplitude and conduction velocity. Several issues affect the accuracy and sensitivity of these measures.

COMPOUND MUSCLE ACTION POTENTIAL

The maximum *compound muscle action potential* (CMAP) represents the summed activity of all muscle fiber action potentials in a muscle or group of muscles innervated by the same nerve (Dumitru, 1995). The CMAP is elicited by supramaximal electrical stimulation of the motor nerve and is recorded by an active electrode over the muscle motor point and a reference electrode over the tendon. CMAP amplitude reflects the number of motor axons in the nerve. However, CMAP amplitude falls short as a quantitative measure of axon number because there is no proportionality constant to relate amplitude numerically to axon number. In normal nerve, CMAP amplitude varies among subjects, and abnormal values are recognized when they are less than a statistically determined lower limit of normal. In an abnormal nerve with fewer fibers innervating the muscle as a result of denervation, collateral reinnervation will obscure the relationship between CMAP amplitude because remaining motor units will be en-

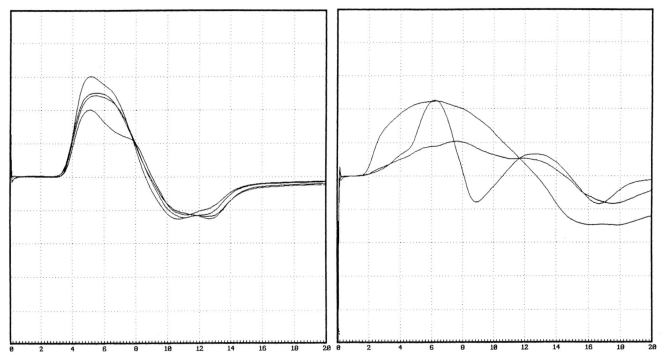

Figure 105–3. Compound muscle action potential (CMAP) recordings showing technical issues. *Left Tracings,* Thenar CMAP waveforms obtained with the recording electrode moved 0.5 mm around the motor point (largest amplitude, 15 mV; lowest amplitude, 10 mV). *Right Tracings,* Biceps brachii CMAP waveforms obtained with different stimulating electrode positions in the axilla. Different waveform shapes reflect volume conduction from neighboring muscles.

larged. CMAP amplitude may be higher than the normal limit with only a few motor units remaining.

The position of the recording electrode is a technical factor affecting accurate measurement of CMAP amplitude. Amplitude values can vary up to 40% with small changes in active electrode position over the muscle belly (Fig. 105–3), and this variability affects test-retest reliability (Bromberg and Spiegelberg, 1997; van Dijk et al., 1999). It may be appropriate during a clinical trial to verify that the CMAP amplitude is the maximal value by moving the recording electrode until the amplitude is maximized. CMAP amplitude is most commonly obtained from distal muscles, and for proximal muscles it is more difficult to ensure that the amplitude reflects a single proximal muscle because of volume conduction from other muscles innervated by the same nerve or neighboring nerves (see Fig. 105–3).

CONDUCTION VELOCITY

Motor nerve conduction velocity is determined by nerve fiber diameter and Schwann cell internode length, with larger axons having longer internode lengths (Kimura, 1989). Motor nerves contain a spectrum of fiber diameters, but conduction velocity values reflect only the speed of the fastest fibers, and, consequently, conduction velocity measurement provides limited information. In axonal neuropathies, conduction velocity is only mildly reduced and may remain higher than the lower limit of normal because sufficient numbers of large diameter

nerve fibers usually remain. In demyelinating neuropathies, remyelination is associated with Schwann cell proliferation and shorter internode lengths, and conduction velocity may not improve despite a clinical response (Kimura, 1989).

Interexaminer and intraexaminer reliability of motor nerve conduction studies has been assessed. Intraexaminer reliability is high. In a study with seven experienced electromyographers testing two normal subjects twice, no statistically significant differences were found for any nerve conduction measure (Chaudhry et al., 1991). Interexaminer reliability is lower, and significant differences are found for median CMAP amplitude, peroneal distal latency, and F-wave latency (Chaudhry et al., 1991). A probable cause of interexaminer CMAP amplitude differences is electrode placement (Bromberg and Spiegelberg, 1997; van Dijk et al., 1999). Anatomically defining recording sites can reduce variability of all measures (Tjon-A-Tsien et al., 1996). Another approach to reduce CMAP amplitude variability is use of larger recording electrodes. A comparison of traditional 10 mm in diameter disk electrodes (0.78 cm^2 area) and larger disposable rectangular electrodes (2.90 × 2.65 cm with 7.65 cm^2 area) shows reduced variability with the larger electrodes (Tjon-A-Tsien et al., 1996). Nerve temperature is a factor affecting conduction velocity, with a linear relationship of approximate 2 m per second per degree Celsius in the range of 29 to 38°C (Denys, 1991). It is preferable to warm a patient rather than to apply correction factors.

Use of a central monitoring facility to review all neurophysiological data, including waveforms, can improve interexaminer reliability in multicenter trials (Bril et al., 1998). In a multinational, 60-center trial, test-retest variability in 253 normal subjects was 10% for median and 13% for peroneal CMAP amplitude and 3% for conduction velocity in both nerves. The importance of attending to detail is highlighted by the central monitoring facility's request for changes in more than one third of tracings.

Needle Electromyography

ROUTINE ELECTROMYOGRAPHY

Needle EMG assesses the electrical activity of the motor unit, but the EMG definition of a motor unit is more restricted than the physiological definition because the uptake or recording radius of the needle electrode varies among different types of electrodes (see Fig. 105–2). Concentric and monopolar electrodes differ in shape but have similar recording radii and measure activity from approximately 7 to 15 muscle fibers of a motor unit (Thiele and Böhle, 1978).

The routine EMG study is usually divided into two portions, assessing spontaneous discharges of muscle fibers and determining properties of the motor unit. Abnormal spontaneous activity in the form of positive sharp waves and fibrillation potentials is a measure of muscle fiber denervation. These potentials can be seen in neuropathic and myopathic disorders (Buchthal and Rosenfalck, 1966), but the patient's history and clinical findings help to distinguish between the two. Abnormal spontaneous activity is usually judged qualitatively by a four-point scale, and statistically meaningful comparisons between examiners are not reliable.

The second portion of the routine EMG assesses motor unit recruitment and several aspects of the motor unit waveform, including amplitude, duration, and complexity (number of phases and turns). Motor unit recruitment is governed by the size of the motor unit, with smaller and more slowly conducting units activated before more rapidly conducting and larger units (Dengler et al., 1988). During recruitment, a given motor unit will increase its discharge rate from an initial 5 to 7 Hz to 12 to 15 Hz, at which time another motor unit will be recruited with an initial discharge rage of 5 to 7 Hz (Petajan, 1991). The process continues until new motor units cannot be distinguished in the growing interference pattern. In neuropathic disorders, recruitment is reduced because the rank order will have gaps resulting from missing motor units. Additionally, motor unit discharge rates will be 20 Hz and greater before the next motor unit is recruited, because the rank-order appropriate one is missing. Motor unit amplitude and duration will also increase because of collateral reinnervation. Motor unit recruitment is perhaps the most sensitive indicator of motor neuron loss, but

assessment is subjective. In myopathic disorders, the recruitment pattern is normal, but muscle force is reduced, and the recruitment pattern will appear greater than expected for the degree of force generated. Recruitment abnormalities are usually expressed by a four-point scale that does not lend itself to quantitation or statistical comparisons.

Several aspects of the motor unit waveform can be assessed quantitatively. The traditional or manual method is based on triggering on individual motor units, making hard copies of the waveform, and manually measuring peak-to-peak amplitude, duration, and number of phases and turns (Buchthal et al., 1954a, 1954b). Motor units within a muscle vary, and it is necessary for statistical robustness to collect a sample of 20 and report average values for each type of measurement (Engstrom and Olney, 1992). The measurement process has become automated with the development of computers within EMG machines that perform algorithms to place markers on the waveforms and to make calculations. In addition to traditional motor unit measurements of amplitude, duration, and phases and turns, derived measurements such as motor unit area and area-to-amplitude ratio can be obtained. Algorithms are proprietary and differ among EMG machine manufacturers, and measurements have been found to vary substantially among algorithms for the same data (Bromberg et al., 1999).

Computer programs have also been developed that can detect simultaneously several individual motor units in an EMG signal. Various computational techniques or algorithms are available, including waveform template matching and decomposition processes (Bischoff et al., 1994; Stålberg et al., 1996). Although computerized methods may differ, the principle is that several motor units can be analyzed at one electrode site. The advantage of such multimotor unit EMG analysis is that data from a large number of motor units can be obtained rapidly. Because the computer programs can recognize motor units within a complex interference pattern, motor units recruited at higher levels of force can also be measured. There are concerns about the accuracy of marking and measuring waveforms, and individual waveform data must be reviewed before summary data can be trusted (Bischoff et al., 1994).

Reliability of the multimotor unit analysis technique has been analyzed, and comparisons between it and individual motor unit analysis have been made (Bischoff et al., 1994). Intraexaminer differences for five subjects evaluated five times, and interexaminer differences for four investigators studying one muscle, showed no statistically significant differences for any type of measurement. A review of multimotor unit data from 72 normal subjects reveals shorter duration and higher amplitude compared with traditional manual assessment of individual motor units.

Quantitative EMG represents a statistically robust technique to assess the state of the motor unit in both neuropathic and myopathic disorders. It can provide more specific information about the pathophysiology than muscle strength measurements.

INTERFERENCE PATTERN ANALYSIS

Most motor unit data are gathered at low levels of recruitment. However, there is information in more full *interference patterns* in the form of amplitude and pattern complexity (Fuglsang-Frederiksen, 2000). Amplitude reflects the size of motor units, and complexity reflects the number of phases and turns in individual motor units (Nandedkar et al., 1986b). Quantitative assessment of the interference pattern is accomplished by computer algorithms that extract and analyze properties of the interference signal. The interference pattern increases in complexity as muscle force increases because motor units fire at faster rates and more motor units are recruited. Analysis is in terms of the number of turns the signal makes (reflecting the number of motor units firing and their complexity) and the amplitude of each turn (reflecting the amplitude of the motor units) (Nandedkar et al., 1986b). The basic analysis plots the number of turns against amplitude (Stålberg et al., 1983), but various numerical parameters have been derived to help distinguish among normal, neuropathic, and myopathic patterns (Nandedkar et al., 1986a, 1986c). Many analysis algorithms are proprietary and are limited to specific EMG equipment. Test-retest reliability of automatic interference analysis has been assessed in patients with amyotrophic lateral sclerosis and has been found to be high (Bromberg et al., 1993).

Special Electromyography Techniques

Concentric and monopolar needle electrodes used in routine EMG recording assess the activity of 7 to 14 muscle fibers of a motor unit. Although the use of these electrodes represents a compromise between selectivity of individual muscle fibers and inclusion of all muscle fibers, this approach provides a reasonable and clinically useful view of the motor unit. More detailed information is available from single-fiber EMG electrodes that have a smaller recording radius, about 300 μg or about five muscle fiber diameters, and include action potentials from one or two muscle fiber action potentials from a motor unit. Single-fiber EMG can be used to measure the relative density of muscle fibers in the motor unit and the variability of neuromuscular junction transmission. Special single-fiber EMG electrodes can be used to record activity from the whole motor unit (macro-EMG) (Bromberg, 1993a).

FIBER DENSITY

In a normal motor unit, muscle fibers are distributed relatively uniformly within the motor unit territory, with peaks and troughs of higher and lower *fiber density,* but it is rare for fibers of the same unit to be contiguous (Edström and Kugelberg, 1968). Thus, when a single-fiber EMG electrode is close to and records from one muscle fiber, it is unusual for a second fiber's action potential to be included, and it is rare for a third (Stålberg and Thiele, 1975). An average fiber density value in a muscle can be determined as a measure of motor unit remodeling. The average value is determined by recording fiber density from many motor units, usually at 20 sites in the muscle. Normal fiber density values are determined empirically and are approximately 1.3 to 1.8 (Stålberg and Thiele, 1975). Values vary among muscles and increase with age, and tables of normal values are available (Bromberg et al., 1994). In neurogenic disorders, denervation and reinnervation result in higher fiber densities. In myopathic disorders, fiber density also increases, but not to the same degree because muscle fibers both atrophy and move closer together (Hilton-Brown et al., 1985). The increase in fiber density with age occurs after 65 years and reflects age-related neuronal loss and subsequent reinnervation (Stålberg and Thiele, 1975).

Fiber density is considered to be the most sensitive and earliest measure of denervation and reinnervation in any neuropathic disorder (Thiele and Stålberg, 1975; Stålberg, 1982). Fiber density values reflect the state of the motor unit and can be used to follow disease progression. During the compensatory phase of collateral reinnervation, fiber density increases. During the decompensation phase when remaining motor units degenerate and die, density values fall (Stålberg, 1982). Fiber density values are highest in slowly progressive disorders (Stålberg et al., 1975).

Fiber density determinations have a subjective component, and guidelines are available (Stålberg and Trontelj, 1994). Experience with collection of normal single-fiber EMG data by multiple centers indicates that fiber density values are more variable than jitter values (Gilchrist and Ad Hoc Committee of the AAEM Special Interest Group on Single Fiber EMG, 1992). However, a study of fiber density values recorded five times over 30 days by five electromyographers in five normal subjects showed no statistically significant difference among examiners or over time (Straube et al., 1994). Fiber density test-retest reliability with the same observer has been assessed in patients with amyotrophic lateral sclerosis and has been found to be high (Bromberg et al., 1993).

MACROELECTROMYOGRAPHY

Macro-EMG electrodes are able to record activity from all fibers of the motor unit (Stålberg, 1980). The macro-EMG electrode is a special single-fiber EMG electrode with a large recording surface based on 15 mm of the cannula (see Fig. 105–2). There is a trade-off, however, and although the macro-EMG electrode includes all fibers of the motor unit, it records little detail. Accordingly, the primary macro-EMG measurement is amplitude, with no useful information from duration and number of phases and turns (Stålberg, 1983). Macro-EMG amplitude increases in denervating diseases and can reflect early disease progression. However, with late progression, macro-EMG amplitude values will fall as remaining motor units degenerate and die (Stålberg, 1982).

Reproducibility of macro-EMG has not been thoroughly addressed, but interexaminer retest values are 30% of test values (Bromberg et al., 1993). Bilateral macro-EMG amplitude comparisons have been made in normal subjects, and if a measure of variability can be inferred based on expected symmetry in normal subjects, the smaller macro-EMG values are within 10% to 30% of the larger values (Stålberg et al., 1989).

Neuromuscular Junction Transmission

NEUROMUSCULAR JITTER

Neuromuscular junction transmission is a complex process linking each nerve terminal action potential to a muscle fiber action potential. When this process is viewed on a fine time scale (microseconds), there is impulse-to-impulse variability of transmission across the junction in normal muscle even when transmission itself is 100%. This variability is called *jitter* and can be measured with a single-fiber EMG electrode. The single-fiber EMG electrode is positioned to record from a pair of muscle fibers from the same motor unit (fiber density value of 2). One action potential is used as the trigger signal, and the variability of the second potential is measured over 100 consecutive discharges. The variability reflects the combined variability of transmission between the two neuromuscular junctions (Sanders and Stålberg, 1996). Jitter values are calculated as a mean consecutive difference (MCD) to avoid trends of gradually increasing jitter during the 100 discharges (Ekstedt et al., 1974). An average jitter value for a muscle is calculated from 20 fiber pairs (20 different motor units). Normal jitter values are determined empirically and are approximately 35 μs (Stålberg and Trontelj, 1994). They vary among muscles and increase with age, and tables of normal values are available (Bromberg et al., 1994). Increased jitter values are sensitive for detection of abnormalities in neuromuscular junction transmission, but they are not specific for underlying disease. Abnormal jitter occurs in both presynaptic and postsynaptic neuromuscular junction disorders and during reinnervation.

Jitter measurement values are similar among normal subjects when collected by multiple examiners (Gilchrist and Ad Hoc Committee of the AAEM Special Interest Group on Single Fiber EMG, 1992). A study of jitter values recorded five times over 30 days by five electromyographers in five normal subjects showed no statistically significant difference among examiners or over time (Straube et al., 1994).

REPETITIVE NERVE STIMULATION

Pathological conditions affecting neuromuscular junction transmission may be mild or severe. When they are mild, transmission may be secure, and abnormalities may be reflected only as an increase in the variability of timing across the junction in the form of abnormal jitter values. When they are severe, there will be frank failure of transmission that can be detected by abnormalities to repetitive nerve stimulation. In *repetitive nerve stimulation,* four to five supramaximal shocks at a frequency of 2 to 3 Hz are applied to a motor nerve. The amplitude of successive CMAP responses is compared with the first response and is expressed as a percentage (Oh, 1988). A decrementing response is a reduction in CMAP amplitude with successive discharges that follows a U-shaped pattern, with the rate of decline showing a reversal by the fourth response (Bromberg, 1999). A facilitating response is an increase in successive CMAP amplitudes that may not be evident at 2 to 3 Hz or with five shocks. Facilitation is customarily assessed by delivering 50 to 100 shocks at a frequency of 50 Hz. The increment may exceed several hundred percent of the initial CMAP value, a result reflecting an initial low amplitude that increases to normal CMAP values.

The sensitivity of repetitive nerve stimulation to detect change is based on technical factors and on the degree of pathological involvement. The technical factors include patient relaxation and stable supramaximal nerve stimulation (Oh, 1988). Various muscles can be tested, with fewer technical factors associated with stimulating and recording from distal muscles compared to proximal muscles. In normal subjects, an apparent decrement can be recorded, and clinical experience suggests that a decrement of 5% to 10% may be allowable (Oh, 1988; Tim and Sanders, 1994). The pathological issue is that the percentage of decrement will be proportional to the number of neuromuscular junctions in the muscle that become blocked with repeated shocks (Bromberg, 1999). Mildly affected muscles may have abnormal jitter and may not show a decrement to repetitive stimulation, and selection of a weak muscle is important (Gilchrist et al., 1994). In a facilitating response, the maximal amplitude will equal the amplitude of a normal CMAP, and the percentage of facilitation will be inversely proportional to initial CMAP amplitude (O'Neill et al., 1988). There is little information on test-retest reproducibility of repetitive stimulation, but practical experience indicates that it is high.

Selection of end-point measures in diseases of neuromuscular transmission depends on the disease and the information desired. Decremental responses to repetitive stimulation occur in both presynaptic and postsynaptic disorders, whereas facilitation is characteristic of presynaptic disorders. Single-fiber measurement of jitter is more sensitive that repetitive nerve stimulation for defects in transmission, but it is not specific for presynaptic or postsynaptic disorders.

Motor Unit Number Estimation

Compound muscle action potential amplitude does not accurately (numerically) reflect the number of axons innervating a muscle. *Motor unit number estimation* (MUNE) is a special neurophysiological method to estimate this number (McComas et al., 1971). The principle of MUNE is based on the simple ratio:

$$\frac{\text{maximum CMAP (amplitude or area)}}{\text{average single motor unit (amplitude or area)}}$$

where CMAP is the compound motor action potential.

The maximum CMAP amplitude represents the summed activity of all motor units. Knowing the size of the contributing motor units permits calculation of the total number of motor units in the CMAP. Individual single motor units vary in size, and to achieve a representative average value, approximately 10 to 15 single motor units must be sampled (Bromberg, 1993b; Doherty and Brown, 1993). Accordingly, calculated motor unit number values represent estimates of the number of axons innervating a muscle.

There are assumptions in MUNE methodology (McComas et al., 1971; Milner-Brown and Brown, 1976; Slawnych et al., 1990; McComas, 1991, 1995). Several different MUNE techniques have been developed to address limitations and specific applications (Table 105–1). Selection among techniques is based on certain issues and requirements (Bromberg, 1998). Most techniques are readily applied to distal muscles, whereas some can be more easily applied to proximal muscles. Some include an intramuscular electrode that allows gathering data on fiber density, macro-EMG amplitude, or quantitative motor unit information (Brown et al., 1988). Many techniques rely on proprietary computer algorithms and are limited to specific EMG machines.

There is no objective method for actually counting motor units innervating a muscle. Despite the lack of a current standard, MUNE values for commonly studied muscles are similar (McComas, 1991). MUNE reliability has been assessed, and with current refinements in techniques, test-retest variability approaches 10% or less (Shefner et al., 1999; Lomen-Hoerth and Olney, 2000). In denervating diseases, variability is reduced when MUNE values are low (Bromberg, 1993b).

TESTING IN CLINICAL TRIALS

The success of quantitative motor function testing in trials using clinical neurophysiological tools depends on several principles. One is choosing an appropriate end-point measure to demonstrate a change (Stålberg, 1991). End points vary with disease, and ideally the end point should be a surrogate marker for the underlying pathophysiological process. The end point must be sensitive to meaningful change. A neurophysiological measure may lag behind clinical improvement, or it may remain permanently abnormal despite a good clinical outcome. Many clinical trials include multiple testing centers, and intraexaminer and interexaminer reliability must be good. Natural history studies of disease progression permit exploration of a variety of clinical neurophysiological measures and their comparisons with other end-point measures.

Practical experience with sensitive and informative neurophysiological end-point measures in clinical trials is limited. For diseases that clearly improve with effective treatment, strength and function are informative end points. Clinical neurophysiological testing can be informative for diseases in which an effective treatment may improve a physiological state or slow progression. However, there have been few therapeutically successful clinical trials in these diseases to assess the sensitivity and practical issues of neurophysiological end-point measures.

Peripheral Neuropathy

Inflammatory Neuropathies

Serial nerve conduction studies in *acute inflammatory demyelinating polyradiculoneuropathy* (AIDP)

Table 105–1. Motor Unit Number Estimation Techniques

Technique	Method of Motor Unit Activation	Method of Data Acquisition	Appropriate Muscle Groups	Reference
Incremental stimulation (manual)	Stimulation	Manual	Distal	McComas et al., 1971
Incremental stimulation (automated)	Stimulation	Automated, proprietary	Distal	Galea et al., 1991
Multiple point stimulation	Stimulation	Manual	Distal	Doherty and Brown, 1993
Adapted multiple point stimulation	Stimulation	Manual	Distal	Wang and Delwaide, 1995
F-wave	Stimulation	Automated, proprietary	Distal	Doherty et al., 1994
Spike triggered averaging	Voluntary	Manual	Distal/proximal	Brown et al., 1988
Decomposition-assisted spike triggered averaging	Voluntary	Automated, proprietary	Distal/proximal	Stashuk, 1999
Statistical	Stimulation	Automated, proprietary	Distal	Daube, 1995

show an evolution of abnormalities over the 3- to 4-week time course of the disease (Albers et al., 1985). However, abnormalities persist at 1 year when improvement has stabilized, and this limits the ability to document further improvement in nerve function. This situation results from Schwann cell proliferation and the formation of shorter internode lengths during remyelination that permanently affects the rate of saltatory conduction.

Chronic inflammatory demyelinating polyradiculoneuropathy (CIDP) is a chronic neuropathy characterized by natural and treatment-related relapses and remissions. The relationship between nerve conduction values and the clinical state is not predictable in uncontrolled trials (Barohn et al., 1989). However, changes in motor nerve conduction results have been useful as secondary end points in randomized, controlled trials of CIDP (Dyck et al., 1982; Dyck et al., 1986; Dyck et al., 1994; Hahn et al., 1996a; Hahn et al., 1996b). In the first of these trials, patients randomized to receive a tapering schedule of prednisone for 3 months had significant improvement in median motor nerve conduction velocity, and a trend favoring improvement in peroneal motor nerve conduction velocity and thenar CMAP amplitude, compared with those randomized to no treatment (Dyck et al., 1982). In the next trial, patients randomized to plasma exchange had improvement in motor nerve conduction studies over 3 weeks compared with those receiving sham exchange (Dyck et al., 1986). Subsequently, a similar improvement in summed CMAP amplitudes was used to support equal benefit of plasma exchange and immune globulin infusion (Dyck et al., 1994). Other investigators have also demonstrated improvement in motor nerve conduction studies as secondary end points to support benefit of plasma exchange and intravenous immunoglobulins in patients with CMAP (Hahn et al., 1996a; Hahn et al., 1996b).

These controlled trials were conducted over brief periods, which may be of insufficient duration for maximal changes from remyelination to become apparent in nerve conduction tests. The variables underlying clinical improvement in treated patients are complex and poorly understood. Routine nerve conduction testing focuses on limited aspects of nerve conduction. Accordingly, nerve conduction tests will probably remain secondary end-point measures in CMAP.

MULTIFOCAL MOTOR NEUROPATHY

Multifocal motor neuropathy is characterized by sites of focal conduction block along motor nerves. An estimate of the global degree of focal conduction block can be made by summing distal and proximal CMAP amplitudes and comparing the differences before and after treatment. Correlations between reduction in conduction block and functional clinical response are good, but not all subjects respond to treatment (Chaudhry, 1993; Federico, 2000). Furthermore, not all patients have demonstrable conduc-

tion block (Pakiam and Parry, 1998), and clinical neurophysiological testing is less inclusive than functional testing.

DIABETIC NEUROPATHIES

Nerve conduction studies have been used as endpoint measures in *diabetic neuropathy* trials. In an effort to determine a meaningful change in nerve conduction values, a consensus statement concerning controlled clinical trials for diabetic polyneuropathy proposes that a meaningful change must reflect a change in the polyneuropathy itself (Peripheral Nerve Society, 1995). Linear regression analysis has been used to equate nerve conduction values to a change in neuropathy disability score (Dyck and O'Brien, 1989). The analysis indicates that a one-point change in neuropathic signs (two-point change in disability score because each side is scored separately) corresponds to an average CMAP amplitude increase of 1.2 mV and a conduction velocity increase of 2.3 m per second.

Reproducibility of nerve conduction studies has been assessed in patients with diabetic neuropathy. When six patients with diabetes were studied twice by six experienced electromyographers, intraexaminer reliability was high, with only peroneal distal latency varying significantly among examiners. Intraexaminer assessment showed significant differences among examiners for median and peroneal CMAP amplitude and median distal latency (Chaudhry et al., 1994). Another study found reduced variability using larger recording electrodes (Tjon-A-Tsien et al., 1996). Assessment of variability in nerve conduction measurements in a multicenter setting showed no significant differences among 1,144 subjects tested at the beginning and 12 months later (Bril et al., 1998). Nerve conduction data in this study were analyzed by a central monitoring facility, and the facility probably contributed to reduced test variability.

There are few successful clinical trials in diabetic neuropathy to assess the sensitivity of motor nerve conduction studies as end-point measures. A long-term study comparing conventional insulin therapy (one or two injections per day) with intensive glucose control (three or more injections or an insulin pump) showed positive changes in motor nerve function with intensive treatment (Diabetes Control and Complications Trial Research Group, 1995). Follow-up was 3 to 9 years (median, 6.5 years). Nerve conduction data were reviewed by a study coordinating center. Median and peroneal CMAP amplitude did not change among subjects in either treatment group, but conduction velocity stabilized or increased to a statistically significant degree. Another study of the effects of pancreatic transplantation in patients with insulin-dependent diabetes showed improvement in nerve conduction studies performed at varying time intervals after transplantation compared with pretransplantation values

(Kennedy et al., 1990). Statistically significant improvement in CMAP amplitude was recorded in 61 subjects at 12 months for upper extremity nerves and in conduction velocity for upper and lower extremity motor nerves. Median, but not sural, sensory nerve amplitude and conduction velocity improved significantly. Further improvement occurred in motor and sensory nerve amplitude and conduction velocity, but changes were not significant, probably because of the small numbers of study subjects assessed at 24 (27 subjects) and 48 months (11 subjects). Both clinical studies show that motor nerve conduction study can document changes in diabetic neuropathy.

Exploratory studies indicate that fiber density and macro-EMG amplitude in anterior tibialis muscle of patients with diabetes are more sensitive for axonal loss than CMAP amplitude and conduction velocity (Bril et al., 1996; Andersen et al., 1998). Although fiber density measurement is sensitive, intraexaminer and interexaminer variability of fiber density measurements may exceed that of well-controlled nerve conduction studies in normal subjects (Gilchrist and Ad Hoc Committee of the AAEM Special Interest Group on Single Fiber EMG, 1992; Bromberg et al., 1993), they have not been assessed in patients with diabetes.

Disorders of Neuromuscular Junction Transmission

The pathophysiology of presynaptic and postsynaptic neuromuscular transmission disorders results in both clinical weakness and neurophysiological abnormalities that are readily reversible with effective treatment. Although clinical improvements in strength and function are obvious end-point measures, clinical neurophysiological tests represent good surrogate markers of disease state. Tests include repetitive nerve stimulation to assess decrement and facilitation and single-fiber EMG to measure jitter.

LAMBERT-EATON MYASTHENIC SYNDROME

The *Lambert-Eaton myasthenic syndrome* (LEMS) is a presynaptic disorder caused by antibodies directed against voltage-gated calcium channels in the presynaptic nerve terminal membrane resulting in reduced amounts of acetylcholine released with each nerve impulse (Lang et al., 1981; Lennon et al., 1995). Neurophysiological changes in Lambert-Eaton myasthenic syndrome are low CMAP amplitudes and a facilitatory response to high-frequency nerve stimulation or after a brief voluntary maximal activation of the muscle. Clinical improvement in Lambert-Eaton myasthenic syndrome is associated with an increase in CMAP amplitude and a decrease in percentage of facilitation.

Compound muscle action potential amplitude is an accurate indicator of clinical improvement in

studies comparing plasma exchange and immunosuppressive drug therapy in the Lambert-Eaton myasthenic syndrome (Dau and Denys, 1982; Newsom-Davis and Murray, 1984). Frequent CMAP testing can estimate the time course of response to plasma exchange. A subsequent fall in CMAP amplitude can herald the diagnosis of underlying cancer in Lambert-Eaton myasthenic syndrome. Two randomized controlled trials of 3,4-diaminopyridine (a drug that prolongs presynaptic depolarization and allows for a greater calcium influx) in Lambert-Eaton myasthenic syndrome confirmed clinical efficacy by showing nearly doubled CMAP amplitude with treatment (McEvoy et al., 1989; Sanders et al., 2000). In one study in which isometric strength was compared with nerve conduction studies, doubling of CMAP amplitude was equated with a 10% increase in upper extremity strength and a 20% increase in lower extremity strength (McEvoy et al., 1989).

MYASTHENIA GRAVIS

Myasthenia gravis is a postsynaptic disorder resulting from an antibody-mediated attack on acetylcholine receptors that reduces the muscle fiber's response to released acetylcholine (Lindstrom, 2000). Decrement has been used as an end-point measure in a trial of azathioprine and prednisone in myasthenia gravis, with good correlations between patient response and summed decrement from the muscles tested (Bromberg et al., 1997). Longitudinal studies of jitter show good correlations between change in clinical state and change in jitter values. Sixty-seven percent of patients with clinical worsening had increased jitter, and 85% with clinical improvement showed a fall in jitter values (Sanders and Howard, 1986).

Amyotrophic Lateral Sclerosis

Clinical neurophysiological testing has been used in *amyotrophic lateral sclerosis* (ALS), primarily in the diagnostic process, but it has also provided information on pathophysiological changes during disease progression (Stålberg, 1982). Use of neurophysiological tests as end-point measures in clinical trials has not been fully exploited. Pathophysiological processes in ALS include primary progressive loss of lower motor neurons and secondary compensation by collateral reinnervation. The relationship between these two processes is dynamic, and it is challenging to assess them separately. Most clinical neurophysiological tests and isometric muscle strength measurements assess the combined effects of these processes, whereas MUNE is unique in its ability to assess motor neuron loss separately (Table 105–2).

NERVE CONDUCTION STUDIES

Compound muscle action potential amplitude can be used as a measure of lower motor neuron loss,

Table 105–2. Relation Between Pathophysiological Processes and Clinical Neurophysiological Tests in Conditions with Lower Motor Neuron Loss

Primary Pathological Process: Lower Motor Neuron Loss	Secondary Pathological Process: Reinnervation	Combined Primary and Secondary Pathological Processes: Global
Motor unit number estimation	Quantitative electromyography Fiber density Macroelectromyography	Isometric strength Compound muscle action potential amplitude Interference analysis

although it is affected by collateral reinnervation. When measured serially in a group of subjects, averaged CMAP amplitude values fall over time, but values from individual subjects may show both decreases and increases (Kelly et al., 1990). Some of the variability of individual values probably reflects suboptimal recording electrode placement.

FIBER DENSITY

Fiber density measurements are sensitive to early denervation. Serial fiber density measurements in patients with ALS reveal increases early in the course of the disease, but late in the disease, as remaining motor neurons degenerate and die, fiber density values fall (Fig. 105–4) (Stålberg, 1982). Accordingly, fiber density values do not represent continuous variables and are not suitable as primary end-point measures in clinical trials. However, fiber density measurements can provide information about the capacity for collateral reinnervation (Yuen and Olney, 1997). Fiber density can be a complementary or co–end-point measure (Bromberg, 1998).

MACROELECTROMYOGRAPHY

Macro-EMG amplitude reflects changes in the whole motor unit from denervation and reinnervation, and serial studies indicate increasing ampli-

tudes during the early portion of the disease. The size of reinnervated motor units may reach a limit, and late in the disease macro-EMG amplitudes decline, with further degeneration of remaining motor units (see Fig. 105–4) (Stålberg, 1982). As with fiber density, macro-EMG data are not continuously variable during the course of the disease, but they can be used as a co–end-point measure.

INTERFERENCE ANALYSIS

Turns and amplitude analysis has been used to a limited degree in following ALS progression. A study of 76 patients with ALS tested 6 months apart revealed no significant changes in turns and amplitude values (Bromberg et al., 2001). Subject fatigue was prominent during forceful contractions, and it may have limited sampling across an optimal range of motor unit recruitment levels.

MOTOR UNIT NUMBER ESTIMATION

Motor unit number estimation has a unique role in measuring progression in ALS. Collateral reinnervation obscures the ability of most clinical neurophysiological tests to detect changes, and MUNE is the only measure of lower motor neuron loss unaffected by collateral reinnervation. In serial studies, MUNE values fall before CMAP amplitude (Felice,

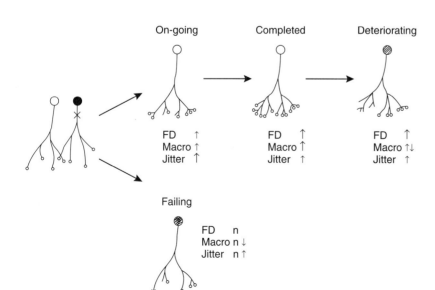

Figure 105–4. Schematic interpretation of clinical neurophysiological changes during collateral reinnervation showing initial compensation followed by decompensation in amyotrophic lateral sclerosis and other progressive denervating diseases. (From Stålberg E: Electrophysiological Studies of Reinnervation in ALS. New York, Raven, 1982.)

1997). The natural history of ALS has been studied with quantitative muscle strength testing, and mega-scores have been found to decline in a linear manner (Munsat et al., 1988; Pradas et al., 1993; Ringel et al., 1993). However, computer modeling of the effects of collateral reinnervation on the initial preservation of strength (discussed earlier; see also Fig. 105–1) indicate that lower motor neuron number and level of strength do not fall at the same rate. Rather, an exponential or sigmoidal time course of motor neuron loss is required to explain the relative linear fall in strength over the middle portion of the disease. Data from serial MUNE studies verify the computer model by showing an exponential loss of motor neurons (Fig. 105–5) (Brown and Jaatoul, 1974; Dantes and McComas, 1991).

Motor unit number estimation and other clinical neurophysiological tests were assessed as secondary end-point measures in a two-center drug trial (Bromberg et al., 2001). The drug trial was therapeutically unsuccessful, and data from all treatment arms were combined for further analysis. Neurophysiological measurements were carried out in the biceps brachii and MUNE, CMAP amplitude, average single motor unit amplitude, fiber density, macro-EMG, and elbow flexion maximal isometric voluntary contraction. All measures changed in the expected direction over the 6-month study period, but no changes were statistically significant, including maximal isometric voluntary contraction. The 6-month study duration may have been too short, but the feasibility of a battery of clinical neurophysiological tests was demonstrated.

Motor unit number estimation is sensitive to early motor neuron loss, and it can provide prognostic information. A rapid fall in MUNE values over a 3-month period in a single muscle is associated with overall rapid disease progression and short survival time (Yuen and Olney, 1997). It may be feasible to stratify subjects in a drug study by predicted rate of progression from the fall in MUNE values over a 3-month prerandomization evaluation period.

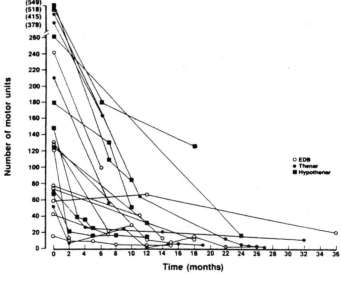

Figure 105–5. Serial motor unit number estimation studies in subjects with amyotrophic lateral sclerosis; *x-axis,* time of serial studies; *y-axis,* motor unit number estimation values. *Upper Graph,* Individual motor unit number estimation values recorded from distal muscles. *Lower Graph,* Averaged data from the *upper graph.* (From Dantes M, McComas A: The extent and time course of motoneuron involvement in amyotrophic lateral sclerosis. Muscle Nerve 1991; 14:416–421.)

SINGLE MOTOR UNIT TRACKING

One MUNE technique, the multiple point stimulation technique, activates single motor units by electrical stimulation of single axons. In some patients, individual axons are optimally positioned in the nerve and can be reliably activated at each recording session (Doherty and Brown, 1994). This technique permits longitudinal study of single motor units. Some motor units can also be voluntarily activated, thus permitting assessment of both central and peripheral changes (Gooch and Harati, 1997; Chan et al., 1998). Initial tracking studies show that motor units may undergo changes in waveform over time, a finding indicating a deterioration of the motor unit. Other motor units may remain unchanged to electrical stimulation, indicating stability, but they become difficult to activate voluntarily, a finding indicating loss of upper motor neuron drive.

Spinal Muscular Atrophy

Spinal muscular atrophy (SMA) is a disease of lower motor neurons occurring primarily in infants and young children. The natural history of motor neuron loss in spinal muscular atrophy is unknown. There is usually an initial rapid loss heralding disease onset, followed by long periods of relative stability (Crawford and Pardo, 1996). Clinical neurophysiological methods have infrequently been applied to measure progression, but MUNE is well suited to measure neuron loss. Initial MUNE studies in distal muscles indicate low motor unit counts in two thirds of patients. Spinal muscular atrophy is considered to primarily affect proximal muscles, and this may account for normal counts in one third of patients. Follow-up studies over 4 to 10 years suggest that values remain stable in some patients, fall in some, and surprisingly may increase in others (Eisen and McComas, 1993).

Spinal muscular atrophy is divided into types based on degree of weakness. Efforts to equate the degree of motor neuron loss at time of diagnosis with spinal muscular atrophy type uses refinements to the multiple point stimulation MUNE technique applied to the hypothenar muscle group in infants (Bromberg and Swoboda, 2002). Preliminary data show low MUNE values in spinal muscular atrophy type I (between five and eight motor units) and good test-retest reliability.

Old Poliomyelitis

Paralytic poliomyelitis is an infectious monophasic disease resulting in varying degrees of lower motor neuron death. The postpolio syndrome may include progressive muscle weakness beginning decades after the initial infection. Serial maximal isometric voluntary contraction testing suggests a slow loss of muscle strength associated with chronic and late

denervation and reinnervation (Dalakas et al., 1986; Cashman et al., 1987). Questions about the degree of motor neuron loss and whether there is loss greater than expected for age have been addressed with MUNE. Studies show that motor neuron loss is extensive even in clinically strong muscles (Windebank et al., 1996; McComas et al., 1997). The issue of whether there is progressive motor unit loss is less clear; although most serial MUNE studies suggest little change over 5 years, others show disease progression (Daube et al., 1995; Windebank et al., 1996; McComas et al., 1997).

Muscle Diseases

Clinical trials in *inflammatory muscle diseases* (polymyositis, dermatomyositis, inclusion body myositis) rely on clinical function or strength testing. Although clinical neurophysiological testing can provide additional information about disease status, quantitative measures have been used infrequently. A longitudinal study of the response of patients with polymyositis and dermatomyositis to steroid and immunosuppressive therapy showed improvement in a quantitative measure of the interference pattern in parallel with improvement in strength (Sandstedt et al., 1982). A comparison of patients with polymyositis at different stages showed good correlation between the degree of weakness and two aspects of the motor unit (area-to-amplitude ratio and duration) (Barkhaus et al., 1990).

CHOICE OF END-POINT MEASURES

Clinical neurophysiology has the unique ability to assess the state of the motor unit. Clinical neurophysiological testing has long been used in the diagnostic process and to understand changes in the motor unit with disease progression better. Full advantage has not been taken of neurophysiological end-point measures in clinical trials. Clinical neurophysiological tests can serve as surrogate markers of the disease. As more is known about disease mechanisms and sites of therapeutic action, endpoint measures that serve as surrogate markers will become increasingly important.

Selection of specific tests will depend on what aspect of the disease is under treatment. For some diseases, a single test is sufficient, whereas for others it may be desirable to select several neurophysiological tests to provide maximal information (Stålberg, 1991; Bromberg, 1998). Quantitative end-point measures of motor function may be divided into categories. Global measures assess the combined effects of lower motor neuron loss and collateral reinnervation and include maximal isometric voluntary contraction and CMAP amplitude. Measures focusing on collateral reinnervation include quantitative EMG, fiber density, and macro-EMG. MUNE assesses the degree of lower motor neuron loss

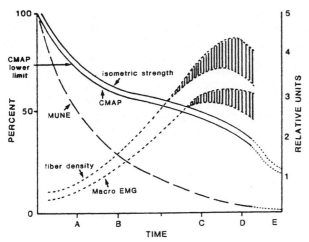

Figure 105–6. Model of temporal relationships between primary and secondary pathological processes. (From Bromberg M: Electrodiagnostic studies in clinical trials for motor neuron disease. J Clin Neurophysiol 1998;15:117–128.)

(Fig. 105–6). Measures of neuromuscular junction transmission include repetitive stimulation and jitter measures. Table 105–3 lists suggested combinations of tests for different categories of neuromuscular diseases. In general, a test of global function combined with a test of collateral reinnervation or motor unit loss is desirable.

There are questions of time, effort, and patient comfort in any clinical trial. Quantitative testing, whether clinical or neurophysiological, requires time. Maximal isometric voluntary contraction testing of certain muscles and clinical neurophysiological testing take about the same time to perform. Both must be carried out carefully and with demonstrated test-retest reliability. Patient comfort and acceptance must be considered. Clinical trials require patient commitment and goodwill. Although clinical neurophysiological testing is considered uncomfortable by some patients, maximal isometric voluntary contraction testing may leave patients sore for sev-

eral days. On balance, all tests of motor function discussed here are equal in terms of time, effort, and comfort. Selection of specific tests for inclusion in trial design is appropriately made by considering the pathophysiological process that the therapeutic agent is expected to alter.

References

Albers J, Donofrio P, McGonagle T: Sequential electrodiagnostic abnormalities in acute inflammatory demyelinating polyradiculoneuropathy. Muscle Nerve 1985;8:528–539.

Andersen H, Stålberg E, Gjerstad M, Jakobsen J: Association of muscle strength and electrophysiological measures of reinnervation in diabetic neuropathy. Muscle Nerve 1998;21:1647–1654.

Andres P, Finison L, Conlon T, et al: Use of composite scores (megascores) to measure deficit in amyotrophic lateral sclerosis. Neurology 1988;38:405–408.

Andres P, Hedlund W, Finison L, et al: Quantitative motor assessment in amyotrophic lateral sclerosis. Neurology 1986;36:937–941.

Barkhaus P, Nandedkar S, Sanders D: Quantitative EMG in inflammatory myopathy. Muscle Nerve 1990;13:247–253.

Barohn R, Kissel J, Warmolts J, Mendell J: Chronic inflammatory demyelinating polyradiculoneuropathy. Arch Neurol 1989;46:878–884.

Bischoff C, Stålberg E, Falck B, Eeg-Olofsson K: Reference values of motor unit action potentials obtained with multi-MUAP analysis. Muscle Nerve 1994;17:842–851.

Bril V, Ellison R, Ngo M, et al: Electrophysiological monitoring in clinical trials. Muscle Nerve 1998;21:1368–1373.

Bril V, Werb M, Greene D, Sima A: Single-fiber electromyography in diabetic peripheral polyneuropathy. Muscle Nerve 1996;19:2–9.

Bromberg M: Electromyographic (EMG) findings in denervation. Crit Rev Phys Rehabil Med 1993a;5:83–127.

Bromberg M: Motor unit estimation: Reproducibility of the spike-triggered averaging technique in normal and ALS subjects. Muscle Nerve 1993b;16:466–471.

Bromberg M: Electrodiagnostic studies in clinical trials for motor neuron disease. J Clin Neurophysiol 1998;15:117–128.

Bromberg M: Myasthenia gravis and myasthenic syndromes. In Younger D (ed): Motor Disorders. Philadelphia, Lippincott Williams & Wilkins; 1999.

Bromberg M, Larson W: Relationships between motor-unit number estimates and isometric strength in distal muscles in ALS/MND. J Neurol Sci 1996;139:38–42.

Table 105–3. Categories of Informative End-Point Measures for Various Neuromuscular Diseases: Choice of End-Point Measures Dependent on Disease and Clinical Trial Design (One End-Point Measure May Be Chosen from Each Category)

	Global		Speed	Reinnervation			NMJ Transmission		LMN Loss
	MVIC	CMAP	MCV	QEMG	FD	Macro	Rep Stim	Jitter	MUNE
Neuropathy	×	×	×		×				×
MND									
ALS	×	×		×	×	×			×
SMA	×	×		×	×	×			×
NMJ									
MG							×	×	
LEMS							×	×	
Myopathy	×	×		×		×			

Global, combined primary and secondary processes; Speed, motor nerve conduction velocity; NMJ, neuromuscular junction; LMN, lower motor neuron; MVIC, maximum voluntary isometric contraction; CMAP, compound muscle action potential; QEMG, quantitative EMG; FD, fiber density; Macro, macro-EMG; Rep Stim, repetitive stimulation; MUNE, motor unit number estimation; MND, motor neuron disease; ALS, amyotrophic lateral sclerosis; SMA, spinal muscular atrophy. MG, myasthenia gravis; LEMS, Lambert-Eaton myasthenic syndrome.

Modified from Stålberg E: Invited review: Electrodiagnostic assessment and monitoring of motor unit changes in disease. Muscle Nerve 1991;14:293–303.

Bromberg M, Spiegelberg T: The influence of active electrode placement on CMAP amplitude. Electroencephalogr Clin Neurophysiol 1997;105:385–389.

Bromberg M, Swoboda K: Motor unit number estimation in infants and children with spinal muscular atrophy. Muscle Nerve, in press.

Bromberg M, Scott D, Ad Hoc Committee of the AAEM Single Fiber Special Interest Group: Single fiber EMG reference values: Reformatted in tabular form. Muscle Nerve 1994;17:820–821.

Bromberg M, Smith A, Bauerle J: A comparison of two commercial quantitative electromyographic algorithms with manual analysis. Muscle Nerve 1999;22:1244–1248.

Bromberg MB, Fries TJ, Forshew DA, Tandan R: Electrophysiologic endpoint measures in a multi-center ALS drug trial. J Neurol Sci 2001;184:51–55.

Bromberg M, Forshew D, Nau K, et al: Motor unit number estimation, isometric strength, and electromyographic measures in amyotrophic lateral sclerosis. Muscle Nerve 1993;16:1213–1219.

Bromberg M, Wald J, Forshew D, et al: Randomized trial of azathioprine or prednisone for initial immunosuppressive treatment of myasthenia gravis. J Neurol Sci 1997;150:59–62.

Brown W, Jaatoul N: Amyotrophic lateral sclerosis: Electrophysiologic study (number of motor units and rate of decay of motor units). Arch Neurol 1974;30:242–248.

Brown WF, Strong MJ, Snow R: Methods for estimating numbers of motor units in biceps-brachialis muscles and losses of motor units with aging. Muscle Nerve 1988;11:423–432.

Buchthal F, Guld C, Rosenfalck P: Action potential parameters in normal human muscle and their dependence on physical variables. Acta Physiol Scand 1954a;32:200–218.

Buchthal F, Pinelli P, Rosenfalck P: Action potential parameters in normal human muscle and their physiological determinants. Acta Physiol Scand 1954b;32:219–229.

Buchthal F, Rosenfalck P: Spontaneous electrical activity of human muscle. Electroencephalogr Clin Neurophysiol 1966;20:321–336.

Cashman N, Maselli R, Wollmann R, et al: Late denervation in patients with antecedent paralytic poliomyelitis. N Engl J Med 1987;317:7–12.

Chan K, Stashuk D, Brown W: A longitudinal study of the pathophysiological changes in single human thenar motor units in amyotrophic lateral sclerosis. Muscle Nerve 1998;21:1714–1723.

Chaudhry V, Cornblath D, Mellits E, et al: Inter- and intraexaminer reliability of nerve conduction measurements in normal subjects. Ann Neurol 1991;30:841–843.

Chaudhry V, Corse A, Cornblath D, et al: Multifocal motor neuropathy: Response to human immune globulin. Ann Neurol 1993;33:237–242.

Chaudhry V, Corse A, Freimer M, et al: Inter- and intraexaminer reliability of nerve conduction measurements in patients with diabetic neuropathy. Neurology 1994;44:1459–1462.

Crawford T, Pardo C: The neurobiology of childhood spinal muscular atrophy. Neurobiol Dis 1996;3:97–110.

Dalakas M, Elder G, Hallett M, et al: A long-term follow-up study of patients with post-poliomyelitis neuromuscular symptoms. N Engl J Med 1986;314:959–963.

Dantes M, McComas A: The extent and time course of motoneuron involvement in amyotrophic lateral sclerosis. Muscle Nerve 1991;14:416–421.

Dau P, Denys E: Plasmapheresis and immunosuppressive drug therapy in the Eaton-Lambert syndrome. Ann Neurol 1982;11:570–575.

Daube J: Estimating the number of motor units in a muscle. J Clin Neurophysiol 1995;12:585–594.

Daube J, Windebank AJ, Litchy WJ: Electrophysiologic changes in neuromuscular function over five years in polio survivors. Ann NY Acad Sci 1995;753:120–128.

Dengler R, Stein R, Thomas C: Axonal conduction velocity and force of single human motor units. Muscle Nerve 1988;11:136–145.

Denys E: AAEM Minimonograph no. 14: The influence of temperature in clinical neurophysiology. Muscle Nerve 1991;14:795–811.

Diabetes Control and Complications Trial Research Group: The effect of intensive diabetes therapy on the development and progression of neuropathy. Ann Intern Med 1995;122:561–568.

Doherty TJ, Brown W: The estimated numbers and relative sizes of thenar units as selected by multiple point stimulation in young and older adults. Muscle Nerve 1993;16:355–366.

Doherty TJ, Brown W: A method for the longitudinal study of human thenar motor units. Muscle Nerve 1994;17:1029–1036.

Doherty TJ, Komori T, Stashuk DW, et al: Physiological properties of single thenar motor units in the F-response of younger and older adults. Muscle Nerve 1994;17:860–872.

Dumitru D: Electrodiagnostic Medicine. Phildelphia, Hanley & Belfus, 1995.

Dyck PJ, Daube J, O'Brien P, et al: Plasma exchange in chronic inflammatory demyelinating polyradiculoneuropathy. N Engl J Med 1986;314:461–465.

Dyck PJ, Litchy WJ, Kratz KM, et al: A plasma exchange versus immune globulin infusion trial in chronic inflammatory demyelinating polyradiculoneuropathy. Ann Neurol 1994;36:838–845.

Dyck PJ, O'Brien P: Meaningful degrees of prevention or improvement of nerve conduction in controlled clinical trials of diabetic neuropathy. Diabetes Care 1989;12:649–652.

Dyck PJ, O'Brien PC, Oviatt KF, et al: Prednisone improves chronic inflammatory demyelinating polyradiculoneuropathy more than no treatment. Ann Neurol 1982;11:136–141.

Edström L, Kugelberg E: Histochemical composition, distribution of fibers and fatiguability of single motor units. J Neurol Neurosurg Psychiatry 1968;31:424–433.

Eisen A, McComas A: Motor neuron disorders. In Brown W, Boulton C (eds): Clinical Electromyography. Boston, Butterworth-Heinemann, 1993.

Ekstedt J, Nilsson G, Stålberg E: Calculation of the electromyographic jitter. J Neurol Neurosurg Psychiatry 1974;37:526–539.

Engstrom J, Olney R: Quantitative motor unit analysis: The effect of sample size. Muscle Nerve 1992;15:277–281.

Federico P, Zochodne D, Hahn A, et al: Multifocal motor neuropathy improved by IVIg: Randomized, double-blind, placebo-controlled study. Neurology 2000;55:1256–1262.

Feinstein B, Lindegård B, Nyman E, Wohlfart G: Morphologic studies of motor units in normal human muscle. Acta Anat (Basel) 1955;23:127–143.

Felice K: A longitudinal study comparing thenar motor unit number estimates to other quantitative tests in patients with amyotrophic lateral sclerosis. Muscle Nerve 1997;20:179–185.

Fuglsang-Frederiksen A: The utility of interference pattern analysis. Muscle Nerve 2000;23:18–36.

Galea V, DeBruin H, Cavasin R, McComas A: The numbers and relative sizes of motor units estimated by computer. Muscle Nerve 1991;14:1123–1130.

Gilchrist J, Massey J, Sanders D: Single fiber EMG and repetitive stimulation of the same muscle in myasthenia gravis. Muscle Nerve 1994;17:171–175.

Gilchrist JC, Ad Hoc Committee of the AAEM Special Interest Group on Single Fiber EMG: Single fiber EMG reference values: A collaborative effort. Muscle Nerve 1992;15:151–161.

Gooch CL, Harati Y: Longitudinal tracking of the same single motor unit in amyotrophic lateral sclerosis. Muscle Nerve 1997;20:511–513.

Hahn AF, Bolton CF, Pillay N, et al: Plasma-exchange therapy in chronic inflammatory demyelinating polyneuropathy: A double-blind, sham-controlled, cross-over study. Brain 1996a;119:1055–1066.

Hahn AF, Bolton CF, Zochodne D, Feasby TE: Intravenous immunoglobulin treatment in chronic inflammatory demyelinating polyneuropathy: A double-blind, placebo-controlled, cross-over study. Brain 1996b;119:1067–1077.

Hilton-Brown P, Stålberg E, Trontelj J, Mihelin M: Causes of the increased fiber density in muscular dystrophies studied with single fiber EMG during electrical stimulation. Muscle Nerve 1985;8:383–388.

Kelly J, Thibodeau L, Andres P, Finison L: Use of electrophysiologic tests to measure disease progression in ALS therapeutic trials. Muscle Nerve 1990;13:471–479.

Kennedy W, Navarro X, Goetz F, et al: Effects of pancreatic transplantation on diabetic neuropathy. N Engl J Med 1990;322:1031–1037.

Kimura J: Electrodiagnosis in Diseases of Nerve and Muscle: Principles and Practice. Philadelphia, FA Davis, 1989.

Kuether G, Lipinski H-G: Computer Simulation of Neuron Degeneration in Motor Neuron Disease. Amsterdam, Elsevier, 1988.

Kugelberg E, Edström L, Abbruzzese M: Mapping of motor units in experimentally reinnervated rat muscle. J Neurol Neurosurg Psychiatry 1970;33:319–329.

Lang B, Newsom-Davis J, Wray D, et al: Autoimmune aetiology for myasthenic (Eaton-Lambert) syndrome. Lancet 1981;2:224–226.

Lennon V, Kryzer T, Griesmann G, et al: Calcium-channel antibodies in the Lambert-Eaton syndrome and other paraneoplastic syndromes. N Engl J Med 1995;332:1467–1474.

Lindstrom J: Acetylcholine receptors and myasthenia. Muscle Nerve 2000;23:453–477.

Lomen-Hoerth C, Olney R: Comparison of multiple-point and statistical motor unit number estimation. Muscle Nerve 2000;23: 1525–1533.

McComas A: Invited review. Motor unit estimation: Methods, results, and present status. Muscle Nerve 1991;14:585–597.

McComas A: Motor unit estimation: Anxieties and achievements. Muscle Nerve 1995;18:369–379.

McComas A, Fawcett P, Campbell M, Sica R: Electrophysiological estimation of the number of motor units within a human muscle. J Neurol Neurosurg Psychiatry 1971;34:121–131.

McComas A, Quartly C, Griggs R: Early and late losses of motor units after poliomyelitis. Brain 1997;120:1415–1421.

McEvoy K, Windebank A, Daube J, Low P: 3,4-Diaminopyridine in the treatment of Lambert-Eaton myasthenic syndrome. N Engl J Med 1989;321:1567–1571.

Milner-Brown H, Brown W: New methods of estimating the number of motor units in a muscle. J Neurol Neurosurg Psychiatry 1976;39:258–265.

Munsat T, Andres P, Finison L, et al: The natural history of motoneuron loss in amyotrophic lateral sclerosis. Neurology 1988; 38:409–413.

Nandedkar SD, Sanders DB, Stålberg EV: Automatic analysis of the electromyographic interference pattern. Part I: Development of quantitative features. Muscle Nerve 1986a;9:431–439.

Nandedkar SD, Sanders DB, Stålberg EV: Simulation and analysis of the electromyographic interference pattern in normal muscle. Part I: Turns and amplitude measurement. Muscle Nerve 1986b;9:423–430.

Nandedkar SD, Sanders DB, Stålberg EV: Automatic analysis of the electromyographic interference pattern. Part II: Findings in control subjects and in some neuromuscular diseases. Muscle Nerve 1986c;9:491–500.

Newsom-Davis J, Murray N: Plasma exchange and immunosuppressive drug treatment in the Lambert-Eaton myasthenic syndrome. Neurology 1984;34:480–485.

O'Neill J, Murray N, Newsom-Davis J: The Lambert-Eaton myasthenic syndrome: A review of 50 cases. Brain 1988;111:577–596.

Oh S: Electromyography: Neuromuscular Transmission Studies. Baltimore, Williams & Wilkins, 1988.

Pakiam A, Parry G: Multifocal motor neuropathy without overt conduction block. Muscle Nerve 1998;21:243–245.

Peripheral Nerve Society: Diabetic polyneuropathy in controlled clinical trials: Consensus report of the Peripheral Nerve Society. Ann Neurol 1995;38:478–482.

Petajan J: AAEM minimonograph no. 3: Motor unit recruitment. Muscle Nerve 1991;14:489–502.

Pradas J, Finison L, Andres P, et al: The natural history of amyotrophic lateral sclerosis and the use of natural history controls in therapeutic trials. Neurology 1993;43:751–755.

Ringel S, Murphy J, Alderson M, et al: The natural history of amyotrophic lateral sclerosis. Neurology 1993;43:1316–1322.

Sanders D, Howard J: AAEE Minimonograph no. 25: Single-fiber electromyography in myasthenia gravis. Muscle Nerve 1986; 9:809–819.

Sanders D, Stålberg E: AAEM Minimonograph no. 25: Single-fiber electromyography. Muscle Nerve 1996;19:1069–1083.

Sanders D, Massey J, Sanders L, Edwards L: A randomized trial of 3,4-diaminopyridine in Lambert-Eaton myasthenic syndrome. Neurology 2000;54:603–607.

Sandstedt P, Henriksson K, Larsson L-E: Quantitative electromyography in polymyositis and dermatomyositis. Acta Neurol Scand 1982;65:110–121.

Shefner J, Jillapalli D, Bradshaw D: Reducing intersubject variability in motor unit number estimation. Muscle Nerve 1999;22: 1457–1460.

Slawnych M, Laszlo C, Hershler C: A review of techniques employed to estimate the number of motor units in a muscle. Muscle Nerve 1990;13:1050–1064.

Stålberg E: Macro EMG, a new recording technique. J Neurol Neurosurg Psychiatry 1980;43:475–482.

Stålberg E: Electrophysiological Studies of Reinnervation in ALS. New York, Raven, 1982.

Stålberg E: Macro EMG. Muscle Nerve 1983;6:619–630.

Stålberg E: Invited review: Electrodiagnostic assessment and monitoring of motor unit changes in disease. Muscle Nerve 1991; 14:293–303.

Stålberg E, Borges O, Ericsson M, et al: The quadriceps femoris muscle in 20–70 year old subjects: Relationships between knee extension torque, electrophysiological parameters, and muscle fiber characteristics. Muscle Nerve 1989;12:382–389.

Stålberg E, Chu J, Bril V, et al: Automatic analysis of the EMG interference pattern. Electroencephalogr Clin Neurophysiol 1983;56:672–681.

Stålberg E, Nandedkar S, Sanders D, Falck B: Quantitative motor unit potential analysis. J Clin Neurophysiol 1996;13:401–422.

Stålberg E, Schwartz M, Trontelj J: Single fibre electromyography in various processes affecting the anterior horn cell. J Neurol Sci 1975;24:403–415.

Stålberg E, Thiele B: Motor unit fibre density in the extensor digitorum communis muscle. J Neurol Neurosurg Psychiatry 1975;38:874–880.

Stålberg E, Trontelj J: Single Fiber Electromyography: Studies in Healthy and Diseased Muscle. New York, Raven, 1994.

Stashuk D: Decomposition and quantitative analysis of clinical electromyographic signals. Med Eng Phys 1999;21:389–404.

Straube A, Garner C, Witt T: Repeated single fiber recordings do not affect the jitter and the fiber density. Electromyogr Clin Neurophysiol 1994;34:387–390.

Thiele B, Böhle A: Anzahl der Spike-Komponenten im Motor-Unit Potential. Z EEG-EMG 1978;9:125–130.

Thiele B, Stålberg E: Single fiber EMG findings in polyneuropathies of different aetiology. J Neurol Neurosurg Psychiatry 1975; 38:881–887.

Tim R, Sanders D: Repetitive nerve stimulation studies in the Lambert-Eaton myasthenic syndrome. Muscle Nerve 1994;17: 995–1001.

Tjon-A-Tsien A, Lemkes H, Van Der Kamp-Huyts A, Van Dijk J: Large electrodes improve nerve conduction repeatability in controls as well as in patients with diabetic neuropathy. Muscle Nerve 1996;19:689–695.

van Dijk J, van Benten I, Kramer C, Stegeman D: CMAP amplitude cartography of muscles innervated by the median, ulnar, peroneal, and tibial nerves. Muscle Nerve 1999;22:378–389.

Wang FC, Delwaide PJ: Number and relative size of thenar motor units estimated by an adapted multiple point stimulation method. Muscle Nerve 1995;18:969–979.

Windebank A, Litchy W, Daube J, Iverson R: Lack of progression of neurologic deficit in survivors of paralytic polio: A 5-year prospective population-based study. Neurology 1996;46:80–84.

Wohlfart G: Collateral regeneration in partially denervated muscles. Neurology 1958;8:175–180.

Yuen E, Olney R: Longitudinal study of fiber density and motor unit number estimate in patients with amyotrophic lateral sclerosis. Neurology 1997;49:573–578.

Quantitative Measurement of Sensory Function in Clinical Trials

Richard K. Olney

INTRODUCTION

Participation in the design and conduct of clinical trials is assuming an increasingly prominent role for clinical neurophysiologists. In designing a clinical trial, an important goal is the selection of appropriate measurements that will be able to establish objective differences between two or more groups, usually in response to a promising new therapy. In the context of clinical trials, the quantitative techniques that are discussed in this chapter may be referred to as end points or surrogate measures, depending on the specific technique and the context. A *surrogate measure* assesses a function that cannot be observed clinically. A surrogate measure is usually thought to be a highly sensitive, quantitative measurement that correlates with a clinically relevant function. An *end point* is a quantitative measure that is specified prospectively in a trial protocol as being important. The single most important measure is designated as the primary end point. The overall experimental error of a clinical trial is set so that a positive result has less than a 1 in 20 chance (a probability less than 0.05) of being produced by chance. If there is only one primary end point, then the difference between groups for this one measure needs to be less than 0.05 for the trial to be successful. If there is more than one primary measure, then the difference between groups for any one measure must be greater than this (that is, the probability [P] must be lower), so there is usually only one. Secondary end points are other prospectively designated measures that are thought to be relevant to the desired outcome but are relegated to a supportive role. Among quantitative measures of sensory function, aspects of sensory nerve conduction studies, somatosensory evoked potentials, nerve biop-

sies, and skin biopsies are types of surrogate measures that may be designated as primary or secondary end points. Quantitative measurements of sensory detection thresholds are not surrogate measures because they quantify a function that is assessed clinically. They may be designated as primary or secondary end points.

The first part of this chapter briefly reviews the anatomy, the physiology, and the pathophysiology of the sensory system that is pertinent to relate diseased conditions to the quantitative measures. The second part discusses the range of techniques that are available for quantitative measurement of sensory function, with discussion of the sensitivity, specificity, and reproducibility of each. This discussion is not limited to the electrophysiological techniques of nerve conduction studies and somatosensory evoked potentials, which are traditionally performed by clinical neurophysiologists, or the psychophysical quantitative sensory tests, which are increasingly interpreted by clinical neurophysiologists, but also includes nerve and cutaneous biopsies, which are used occasionally in clinical trials of peripheral neuropathy. The third part reviews the experience from previous clinical trials with different types of peripheral neuropathy and briefly with multiple sclerosis. The chapter concludes with a discussion of the considerations that may be relevant in the design of future clinical trials.

NORMAL SENSORY FUNCTION AND PATHOPHYSIOLOGY OF DISEASE

Normal Sensory Function

The clinically relevant aspects of quantitative sensory measurement may be appreciated by considering the normal anatomy and physiology of sensation as two parallel systems, one serving vibration and proprioception and the other pain and temperature.

Vibration primarily activates the rapidly adapting pacinian corpuscles, which are located subcutaneously. Vibration is transmitted through cutaneous nerves by relatively large-diameter myelinated axons *(large fibers)* to the spinal cord. These axons generally have diameters from 6 to 12 μm and conduction velocities from 35 to 75 m per second. These axons are classified as Aβ in cutaneous nerves or group II in muscle afferents. These are the largest-diameter axons in cutaneous nerves and are the anatomical substrate for the sensory nerve action potentials that are recorded with routine sensory nerve conduction studies. Muscle spindle afferents also contain group I (Aα) afferents, which are 10 to 18 μm in diameter and have conduction velocities of 60 to 100 m per second. These larger myelinated axons are the afferent limb of the H reflex. Muscle spindle afferents, joint receptors, and cutaneous afferents contribute to *proprioception,* the perception of joint position and joint movement. These first-order sensory neurons have their cell bodies in the dorsal root ganglia. Although collaterals synapse on neurons in laminae III and IV in the dorsal horn of the spinal cord at their entry level, the centrally projecting axons of the first-order sensory neurons ascend ipsilaterally in the posterior or dorsal column. The first-order neurons synapse in the medulla on the second-order neurons, which decussate into the contralateral medial lemniscus and transmit their signals to the thalamus, from which they are relayed to the parietal cortex.

Pain and temperature receptors are free nerve endings that extend superficially into the epidermis. Those that are polymodal nociceptors are activated by mechanical, chemical, and painful thermal stimuli (e.g., heat higher than 45°C). These signals are conveyed by unmyelinated C fibers, which have a conduction velocity of 0.5 to 2 m per second. Thermal receptors for nonpainful stimuli, especially cool, are conveyed by small myelinated Aδ fibers, which have diameters from 2 to 6 μm and conduction velocities of 5 to 30 m per second. Activity from C and Aδ fibers does not contribute to surface-recorded sensory nerve action potentials. These primary sensory neurons have their cell bodies in the dorsal root ganglia and synapse with second-order neurons located predominantly in lamina I of the dorsal horn of the spinal cord. Axons of the second-order neurons decussate and ascend in spinothalamic tracts to the brainstem reticular formation and the thalamus.

Pathophysiology of Sensory Symptoms

The symptoms of neurological disease may be divided into negative and positive ones. Positive sensory symptoms are paresthesias and various types of pain. Paresthesias may result from alter-ations in large or small fiber function, but pain usually relates more to diseases that affect the small C and Aδ fibers. The pathophysiology of paresthesias, and often pain, involves the spontaneous discharge of one or more of these sensory axons. Neurophysiological techniques have limited utility in quantifying the frequency of these positive symptoms. Although microneuronography can quantify the frequency of spontaneous discharges in peripheral axons, clinical pain scales are usually used to quantify neuropathic pain in clinical trials, and nonpainful paresthesias have limited clinical significance as a target for treatment.

Negative sensory symptoms include loss of sensation at the most basic level, with additional symptoms including lack of awareness of physical injury, imbalance, difficulty in manipulating small objects with fingers, and other functional impairments that result from loss of sensory function. The pathophysiology of loss of sensation involves decreased or absent transmission of data from receptors through the peripheral sensory axons to the central nervous systems in patients with peripheral neuropathy, or impaired conduction through the spinothalamic or posterior column pathways in patients with central nervous system disorders, such as multiple sclerosis. Peripheral neuropathy may be produced by a dying back of the most distal portion of sensory axons, by transection of axons, by demyelination that blocks conduction along the axons, or by death of the cell body in the dorsal root ganglia. Peripheral neuropathy often affects small and large fiber functions, but some types of neuropathy affect only one preferentially or exclusively. Central nervous system disorders, such as multiple sclerosis, may demyelinate and block conduction or may transect the axons in the spinothalamic or posterior column pathways.

TECHNIQUES FOR QUANTITATIVE MEASUREMENT OF SENSORY FUNCTION

Combinations of sensitivity, specificity, and reproducibility are important considerations in choosing techniques for use in clinical trials. The *sensitivity* of a test is the proportion of cases with an abnormal test result among all tested cases with the condition. For example, high diagnostic sensitivity of a test for peripheral neuropathy means that the test is abnormal with high frequency whenever peripheral neuropathy is present. The *specificity* of a test is the proportion of cases with an abnormal test result among all tested cases with a different condition present. For example, high diagnostic specificity of a test for peripheral neuropathy means that the test is rarely abnormal whenever other disorders that cause numbness, such as multiple sclerosis, are present. The concepts of sensitivity and specificity have a slightly different meaning in the context of clinical trials, because the purpose is to measure change over time, rather than to detect abnormality at one point in time. A test with high sensitivity in a clinical trial is a test whose results will change in the appropriate direction in most cases that have worsening or improvement. A test with high specificity is one for which a change in any other condition will not produce a change in the test. A major factor that determines whether the test will have this type of sensitivity and specificity is its reliability or *reproducibility*. Studies on reproducibility are important to define the limits of technical or random variation in a test, in contrast to other factors that affect sensitivity and specificity over time. Thus, the discussion of individual techniques includes review of studies that assess their sensitivity, specificity, and especially reproducibility in clinical trials.

Nerve Conduction Studies

Sensory *nerve conduction studies* quantitatively assess the function of large myelinated peripheral sensory axons. Nerve conduction studies are usually included in clinical trials for peripheral neuropathy, in which treatment is intended to improve, or to reduce the rate of progressive loss of, sensory function (American Diabetes Association, 1992a; Peripheral Nerve Society, 1995). A decrease in the amplitude of sensory nerve action potentials over time is highly specific for a decrease in the number of large myelinated sensory axons in peripheral nerve. Furthermore, a decrease in conduction velocity of sensory and motor nerves is relatively specific for a decrease in the number of large myelinated peripheral axons or for a decrease in myelination of these fibers over time, although a modest decrease in sensory and motor velocity may also be produced by metabolic factors. Inclusion of sensory and motor nerve conduction studies increases the specificity of change over time, because a decrease in amplitude of compound muscle action potentials without a change in the amplitude of sensory nerve action potentials suggests that loss of motor axons is from nerve root or anterior horn cell disease. For purposes of sensitivity and specificity, a combination of sensory and motor nerve conduction studies is generally recommended (American Diabetes Association, 1992c; Peripheral Nerve Society, 1995).

The techniques for nerve conduction studies are discussed in previous chapters of this book, so they are not reviewed in detail in this chapter. Surface recording techniques are used in preference to near-nerve needle recording in clinical trials because of their greater reproducibility and comfort. Both sensory and motor nerve conduction studies are usually a part of most protocols for assessment of peripheral neuropathy. The choice of nerves to be studied depends on various factors, not least of which is the severity of the peripheral neuropathy. For example, nerve conduction studies may be restricted to lower limb nerves, if patients are selected to have asymptomatic or mild polyneuropathy. However, upper limb nerves are included so that measur-

able responses can be recorded if the trial includes patients with moderate or severe peripheral neuropathy. Whereas the preceding is the consensus of opinion by experts in the field, the data supporting these recommendations are reviewed in this chapter.

The reproducibility of nerve conduction studies in neurologically normal subjects has been examined by several groups (Alexander and Olney, 1987; Alexander et al., 1989; Bleasel and Tuck, 1991; Chaudhry et al., 1991; Claus et al., 1993). The early work by Buchthal and Rosenfalck demonstrated that amplitude is less reproducible than conduction velocity (Buchthal and Rosenfalck, 1966). Subsequent investigators have examined this quantitatively, and some have proposed techniques for improving reproducibility. In a study that tested 20 normal subjects twice, Alexander and colleagues demonstrated that amplitude of a sensory or motor response in one individual varied by as much as 100%, but the average amplitude change of four nerves did not exceed 50% for sensory (bilateral sural and superficial peroneal nerves) and 30% for motor (bilateral tibial and peroneal nerves) for any one normal subject (Alexander and Olney, 1987; Alexander et al., 1989). The maximum change in velocity for an individual study subject approached 30% for a single nerve but was less than 15% for a four-nerve average. Thus, they demonstrated that the average change of four nerves is much more reproducible than for a single nerve, supporting the notion that technical factors contribute significantly to variability. Bleasel and Tuck performed 10 serial sensory and motor nerve conduction studies on three nerves of a single subject (Bleasel and Tuck, 1991). The coefficient of variation varied from 26.9% to 32.1% for amplitude of sensory nerve action potentials, 8.5% to 14.2% for amplitude of compound muscle action potentials, and 2.2% to 6.7% for sensory and motor velocity. Chaudhry and colleagues assessed interexaminer and intraexaminer reliability by having seven examiners each randomly assigned to study four of the other six examiners as subjects on two occasions (Chaudhry et al., 1991). These investigators found significant interexaminer variability for sural amplitude, extensor digitorum brevis compound muscle action potential amplitude, and peroneal motor velocity, but not for median sensory amplitude, thenar compound muscle action potential amplitude, or the other three velocities with analysis of variance. Furthermore, they found that intraexaminer reproducibility (retesting was performed by the same examiner) was greater than interexaminer reproducibility (retesting was performed by a different examiner). Claus and colleagues found similar test-retest correlation coefficients of 0.60 to 0.76 for sensory and motor velocities, 0.64 to 0.70 for sensory (radial and sural) amplitudes, and 0.66 to 0.78 for motor (median and peroneal) amplitude, with reproducibility studies performed on 30 normal subjects twice (Claus et al., 1993). However, they were not impressed that the reproducibility was as good for amplitude as for velocity measurements, because the 90th percentile for test-retest difference was 4.0 to 7.5 m per second for velocities, but it was 3.2 to 3.5 μV for sensory amplitude, 2.9 mV for extensor digitorum brevis compound muscle action potential amplitude, and 5.2 mV for thenar compound muscle action potential amplitude (Claus et al., 1993). Thus, these reports on neurologically normal persons demonstrate that amplitude is less reproducible than velocity for nerve conduction studies, even over short time intervals, and that reproducibility is improved by the performance of repeated measures by the same examiner, even within a single institution.

Nerve conduction studies have been used in clinical trials for peripheral neuropathy since the 1970s. Because nerve conduction study results are used as surrogate markers to indicate a therapeutic effect even when one is not apparent clinically, studies have been performed to estimate the degree of change in these studies that is likely to predict clinical improvement. Determining how much clinical improvement is necessary for this to be meaningful is a difficult question in itself. Dyck and O'Brien started with the assumption that a two-point mean change on a clinical scale of neurological disability represents a clinically meaningful change for a clinical trial (Dyck and O'Brien, 1989). Using data from a cross-sectional study of 180 patients with diabetes with and without polyneuropathy, they then calculated that a 2.2 m per second change in peroneal motor velocity or a 2.9 m per second change in the average of median, ulnar, and peroneal motor velocities would correspond to a two-point change in the neurological disability scale (Dyck and O'Brien, 1989). In a similar manner, these investigators calculated that a 0.7-mV change in peroneal compound muscle action potential amplitude, a 1.2-mV change in the average amplitude of median, ulnar, and peroneal compound muscle action potentials, or a 2.4-μV change in sural amplitude corresponds to a two-point clinical change. This group later associated changes in sural myelinated fiber density with nerve conduction results and clinical changes (Russell et al., 1996). In this cross-sectional study of 18 patients with diabetes and five control subjects, a decrease in myelinated fiber density of 150 fibers/mm² corresponds to a 1-μV reduction in the sural amplitude, and a decrease of 200 fibers/mm² corresponds to a two-point change in the neurological disability scale.

Several groups studied the reproducibility of nerve conduction studies in peripheral neuropathy in the 1990s (Dyck et al., 1991; Olney and Schleimer, 1992; Sundkvist et al., 1992; Santiago et al., 1993; Valensi et al., 1993; Chaudhry et al., 1994a; Dyck et al., 1997). Dyck and colleagues performed nerve conduction studies twice over 1 week in 20 patients with diabetes with or without polyneuropathy (Dyck et al., 1991). The correlation coefficient was more than 0.9 for sensory amplitudes of ulnar, median, and sural nerves, for summed sensory amplitudes, for compound muscle action potential amplitudes of ulnar, peroneal, and tibial nerves (but the median was less than 0.7), for summed motor amplitudes, and for all individual and summed motor velocities; however, sensory velocities, especially for the sural nerve, were less reproducible than motor velocities. In a subsequent longitudinal study, most results of nerve conduction studies assessment in patients with diabetes with and without polyneuropathy over 2 and 4 years demonstrated worsening over time, even after correction for the effects of aging (Dyck et al., 1997). The rate of worsening was greater in magnitude for the patients with diabetes with polyneuropathy over 2 and 4 years of observation than for the total group of patients with diabetes who had been observed for 2 years or longer. Many aspects of nerve conduction studies were among the measures that had the highest correlation with detecting change over time. In particular, peroneal motor velocity had a rank-order correlation with worsening over time with a value of 0.389 ($P < .0001$) in all patients with diabetes and a value of 0.235 ($P < .06$) in the smaller subgroup of patients with diabetes with polyneuropathy. Although sural amplitude had a rank-order correlation with worsening over time with a value of 0.303 ($P < .0001$) in all patients with diabetes, the correlation with worsening over time was not significant among patients with diabetes with polyneuropathy, possibly because the sural response was unrecordable in many of these patients. Ulnar sensory amplitude had a rank-order correlation with worsening over time with a value of 0.492 ($P < .0001$) in all patients with diabetes and a value of 0.373 ($P < .002$) in the smaller subgroup of patients with diabetes with polyneuropathy.

Olney and Schleimer assessed the interexaminer and intraexaminer reproducibility of nerve conduction studies in a study of 10 patients with diabetes with mild polyneuropathy who were examined three times within 1 month (Olney and Schleimer, 1992). Although amplitudes tended to be more reproducible with intraexaminer than with interexaminer comparisons, no significant differences were found for reproducibility of sural or median sensory amplitudes, median or peroneal compound muscle action potential amplitudes, sensory or motor velocities, or median or peroneal minimum F-wave latencies. Chaudhry and colleagues assessed intraexaminer and interexaminer reproducibility by having each of six examiners test and retest each of six patients with diabetes with polyneuropathy at least 1 week apart (Chaudhry et al., 1994a). These investigators found greater reproducibility for intraexaminer than interexaminer comparisons for nerve conduction studies results, especially for amplitude.

Valensi and colleagues assessed the reproducibility of nerve conduction studies in 132 patients with diabetes with moderate polyneuropathy who underwent test-retest at a 4-week interval (Valensi et al., 1993). Their studies included median and sural sensory nerve conduction, median and peroneal motor nerve conduction, and median and peroneal mean

F-wave latencies. The reproducibility was higher for velocity (except sural) and mean F-wave latency than for amplitudes. The mean variability was 26.5% for the sural velocity, but it was 3.7% to 7.7% for median sensory velocity, median and peroneal motor velocity, and median and peroneal mean F-wave latency. In contrast to the results of Dyck and colleagues, Valensi and colleagues found that the mean variation for amplitude was lowest for median compound muscle action potential at 12.3%, intermediate for median sensory at 20.9% and peroneal motor at 22.1%, and highest for sural sensory at 40.1%.

In the multicenter ponalrestat study, 340 patients with diabetic polyneuropathy were studied twice at a 1-month interval (Sundkvist et al., 1992). The coefficients of variation among the 22 centers ranged from 0.9% to 20.9% for sural velocity and 1.6% to 12.7% for median sensory velocity, whereas the coefficients of variation ranged from 8.9% to 42.8% for sural and median amplitudes. The coefficients of variation were even higher for motor than for sensory amplitude, whereas motor velocities were slightly less variable than sensory velocities. In the multicenter tolrestat withdrawal study, 372 patients with diabetic polyneuropathy were studied (Santiago et al., 1993; Bril, 1994). Among the 25 centers, the coefficients of variation in the median, ulnar, and sural nerves ranged from 5.4% to 9.1% for sensory velocities and from 28.3% to 35.6% for median sensory amplitudes.

Bril and colleagues performed a multicenter study on 253 neurologically normal persons and 1,345 patients with mild diabetic polyneuropathy, by using a carefully designed protocol and training (Bril et al., 1998). Across 60 centers internationally, these investigators were able to achieve the following coefficients of variation: 7% for controls and 10% for patients for thenar compound muscle action potential amplitude; 9% and 13%, respectively, for peroneal compound muscle action potential amplitude; 8% and 11%, respectively, for median sensory amplitude; 10% and 16%, respectively, for sural amplitude; 3% for median and peroneal motor velocities; and 3% to 5% for sensory velocities. Thus, this multicenter study demonstrated greater reproducibility for nerve conduction results than was obtainable in previous multicenter trials.

In summary, nerve conduction studies are sensitive, specific, and reproducible techniques that are strongly recommended for inclusion in the design of clinical trials for peripheral neuropathy in which treatment is intended to improve, or to reduce the rate of progressive loss of, sensory function.

Somatosensory Evoked Potentials

Somatosensory evoked potentials quantitatively assess sensory function peripherally and centrally. Because more time is required for performing somatosensory evoked potentials than for sensory nerve conduction studies, these tests are generally not included in clinical trials for peripheral neuropathy, but they may have utility in clinical trials for multiple sclerosis or other central nervous system disorders that alter sensory function. Visual and brainstem auditory evoked potentials may also be used to assess the special afferents.

Evoked potential studies have reproducible latencies over time in neurologically normal persons (Emerson, 1998). Some investigators have found that the latency does not vary by more than 2 ms in neurologically normal persons retested within 1 month, whereas other investigators have found that the mean plus 2.5 standard deviations for the upper limit of test-retest peak latency change for full-field pattern reversal visual evoked potentials in an individual normal subject is 6 ms (Hammond et al., 1987; Emerson, 1998). Group means are more reproducible than individual results, with the upper limit of test-retest peak latency change for full-field pattern reversal visual evoked potentials less than 1 ms in normal subjects (Meienberg et al., 1979). Both brainstem auditory and somatosensory short latency evoked potentials have higher reproducibility than that of visual evoked potentials in normal subjects (Lauter and Loomis, 1986; Shaw and Synek, 1987; Romani et al., 1993). Thus, the technical reproducibility of evoked potential latency is sufficient to support the potential utility of these tests in clinical trials.

The latencies of evoked potentials are more variable among patients with multiple sclerosis (Emerson, 1998). Matthews and Small found that visual evoked potential and somatosensory evoked potential abnormalities usually persisted after clinical improvement and therefore concluded that evoked potentials were not useful to monitor the course of multiple sclerosis in individual patients (Matthews and Small, 1979). Other investigators found similarly discouraging results for the utility of evoked potentials in multiple sclerosis. For example, Aminoff and colleagues recorded visual, brainstem auditory, and somatosensory evoked potentials on five occasions over 1 year in 12 patients with clinically definite multiple sclerosis (Aminoff et al., 1984). Two patients who were stable clinically over the year had at least transient worsening in their somatosensory evoked potential results, but no change in the results of their visual or brainstem auditory evoked potentials. Two who had steady clinical progression of the disease without acute relapses had at least transient improvement in their somatosensory evoked potentials, but no change in their visual or brainstem auditory evoked potentials. Another patient who had steady clinical disease progression with acute relapses had variable evoked potential results. The other seven patients had 14 acute relapses that correlated poorly with changes in the evoked potential findings. Davis and coworkers recorded median somatosensory evoked potentials seven times over $1\frac{1}{2}$ years in 12 patients with clinically definite multiple sclerosis (Davis et al., 1985). These investigators found a poor correlation between clinical changes in arm function and changes in latency of median somatosensory evoked potentials.

Thus, the variability of latency for visual, brainstem auditory, and somatosensory evoked potentials in patients with multiple sclerosis limits the utility of these tests in clinical trials for multiple sclerosis; however, an evoked potential change from normal to abnormal may be helpful in indicating a new lesion (Aminoff, 1985). In other central nervous system disorders that may have a more predictable course, the latency of evoked potentials has sufficient reproducibility that these studies may be useful in clinical trials.

Quantitative Sensory Testing

Quantitative sensory testing refers to any of several psychophysical methods for determination of the sensory threshold for reliable detection of a particular stimulus modality or a change in it. These tests are analogous to testing visual acuity and performing audiometry, which are quantitative tests of the special sensory afferents. These are not surrogate markers but an end point in clinical trials, because they are quantifying clinically assessable functions. Quantitative sensory tests are more objective and quantitative than is the sensory portion of the neurological examination. Thus, although they may be more sensitive than the clinical examination, quantitative sensory tests are less specific than nerve conduction studies for peripheral neuropathy, because changes in central sensory pathways may also affect these results.

Quantitative sensory testing has become part of the objective assessment of polyneuropathy in most clinical trials, consistent with the consensus recommendations of expert panels (American Diabetes Association, 1992b; Peripheral Nerve Society, 1995). These noninvasive tests are well tolerated and are relatively simple to perform. Different stimulus modalities, such as vibration, cool and warm temperature, pain, and touch-pressure, may be included to test different fiber-size populations. The usually recommended types of quantitative sensory tests administer stimuli that directly activate sensory receptors (American Diabetes Association, 1992b; Peripheral Nerve Society, 1995; Dyck and O'Brien, 1999). For one test at one anatomical location, one particular stimulus modality is delivered many times at various intensities. Stimulus intensity is varied in a predetermined manner by a specific algorithm. Algorithms are executed manually by a technician or automatically by a computer. Three of the most commonly used automated algorithms are the method of limits, forced choice, and 4-2-1 stepping. With the *method of limits,* the sensory stimulus is increased at a defined constant rate until the subject indicates perception. This stimulus intensity is noted as the detection threshold. Then, the stimulus intensity is decreased at a defined constant rate

until the subject no longer perceives the stimulus. This stimulus intensity is noted as the disappearance threshold. Usually, three or more trials with increasing and decreasing stimulus intensity are performed, and the results are averaged.

With the *forced choice algorithm,* there are two stimulus intervals, with the actual stimulus delivered only during one interval. The subject is cued to the intervals and is forced to choose which interval was the one during which the stimulus was delivered. The stimulus intensity is changed, depending on whether the choice is correct. If the subject correctly chooses the interval with the stimulus, then the stimulus intensity is reduced in the next presentation; if the choice is incorrect, then stimulus intensity is increased. Whether the actual stimulus is presented during the first or second interval is predetermined in a "random" manner. Thus, computer control is advantageous over manual control to prevent inadvertent cueing by the supervising technician. After multiple presentations of stimuli at systematically varied intensity, the threshold stimulus intensity is identified as the one at which the subject has a 50% probability of guessing correctly or incorrectly.

Different groups have used different methods for deciding how many stimuli to present and how much to vary the stimulus intensity. One group of investigators developed a method to reduce the number of stimulus intensity levels that were necessary for presentation (Dyck et al., 1993). They determined the magnitude of change in stimulus intensity that was necessary for a subject to notice a difference in two successive stimuli. These intensities were divided into discrete steps that they labeled *"just noticeable difference" (JND) units.* JND units are closer together at lower intensity and are farther apart at higher intensity. These investigators found that 25 steps of JND units encompassed a broad range of stimulus intensity. Even with this time-saving approach, administration of a single forced choice quantitative sensory test (one modality at one anatomical site) requires 10 to 15 minutes to complete. Because testing of two or three modalities at two or three sites is desirable in most clinical trials, 1 to 2 hours would be required on each occasion that forced choice quantitative sensory testing was to be performed. A more time-efficient method was developed, which these investigators called the *4-2-1 stepping algorithm.* With this approach, the subject reports "yes" or "no" if the stimulus is perceived during only one stimulus interval, so each stimulus presentation requires half the time of the forced choice algorithm. For the 4-2-1 algorithm, the initial stimulus is at 13 JND units (the middle of the range of intensity). If this stimulus is perceived, stimulus intensity is decreased by 4 JND units in each successive trial until it is not perceived. Then, the stimulus intensity is increased by 2 JND units in each successive trial until it is perceived again. Finally, the stimulus intensity is varied by 1 JND unit up or down until a cumulative total of four stimuli have been delivered that were not perceived. Null stimuli are delivered occasionally during the systematic variation of stimulus intensity to ensure objectivity; the results of that particular test are invalidated if a patient reports perception of a significant number of null stimuli. The 4-2-1 algorithm is considerably faster than the forced choice algorithm at 2 to 5 minutes per modality per site.

The reproducibility of quantitative sensory testing has been studied in neurologically normal persons (Claus et al., 1993). Claus and colleagues found correlation coefficients for vibratory detection threshold to be 0.92 for the method of limits and 0.96 for the forced choice method (Claus et al., 1993). Correlation coefficients reflect at least a trend in favor of greater reproducibility for vibratory detection threshold than for sensory amplitudes on nerve conduction studies, which had correlation coefficients of 0.64 to 0.70, in assessing large myelinated sensory function. The correlation coefficients were also excellent for quantitative sensory testing of warming and cooling detection thresholds at 0.77 and 0.66.

Vinik and collaborators performed a variety of quantitative sensory tests with a forced choice method on 32 neurologically normal persons and 81 patients with diabetes, who were assessed twice over 2 to 60 days (Vinik et al., 1995). Vibration, cold, and warm perception thresholds as well as current perception thresholds at three frequencies were reproducible, with coefficients of variation of repeated measures with analysis of variance ranging from 0.75 to 0.87. Although equally reproducible, vibration and cold and warm perception thresholds each had higher sensitivity and specificity than were noted for current perception threshold at any of the three frequencies in separating normal persons and patients with diabetes.

High reproducibility of quantitative sensory tests has been observed also among patients with peripheral neuropathy. Dyck and colleagues performed quantitative sensory testing twice over a week in 20 patients with diabetes with or without polyneuropathy (Dyck et al., 1991). The correlation coefficient was higher than 0.9 for vibratory detection threshold, similar to sensory amplitude on nerve conduction studies. The correlation coefficients were excellent for detection threshold of cooling and warming at 0.9 and 0.8, respectively. In their longitudinal assessment that was performed on patients with diabetes, these investigators found that the vibratory detection threshold demonstrated worsening over 2 to 4 years, even after correction for the effects of aging. The rank-order correlation for worsening had a coefficient of 0.453 ($P < .0001$) in all patients with diabetes and a coefficient of 0.453 ($P < .0001$) in the smaller subgroup of patients with diabetes with polyneuropathy.

Valensi and colleagues assessed the reproducibility of quantitative sensory testing in 132 patients with diabetes with moderate polyneuropathy who underwent test-retest at a 4-week interval with a forced choice method (Valensi et al., 1993). The mean variation values were 7.4% and 8.6% for vibratory detection thresholds at the ankle and on the great toe, respectively, 18.3% for cooling detection threshold, and 21.2% for warming detection threshold. Their multicenter study found results similar to those for the short-term study by Dyck and colleagues in that vibratory detection thresholds were more reproducible than warming and cooling detection thresholds, with slightly better results for cooling than for warming. However, unlike in the other group, vibration detection thresholds were more reproducible than sensory nerve action potential amplitudes.

Bril and collaborators compared the reproducibility of two methods for vibration detection threshold and sensory nerve conduction studies in 42 patients with diabetic polyneuropathy who were studied three times (Bril et al., 1997). The forced choice method was used to determine vibration detection threshold with the Vibratron II (Physitemp Instruments, Clifton, NJ). The method of limits was used to determine vibration detection threshold with the Horwell Neurothesiometer (Scientific Laboratory Supplies, Nottingham, UK). One examiner, using the antidromic surface recording technique, recorded the sural nerve action potential. The coefficients of variation were 31% and 34% for the vibration detection threshold with the Vibratron II on the left and right great toes, respectively, 6% and 8% for the vibration detection threshold with the Neurothesiometer on the left and right great toes, respectively, 8% for sural amplitude, and 2% for sural velocity.

In the multicenter ponalrestat trial, the 340 patients with diabetic polyneuropathy had sensory detection thresholds measured in a manner similar to the method of limits twice at a 1-month interval (Sundkvist et al., 1992). The coefficients of variation among the 22 centers ranged from 8.7% to 29.7% for vibration perception threshold at the great toe, 8.8% to 129.5% for cooling detection threshold, and 3.2% to 108.1% for warming detection threshold. Thus, the vibration detection threshold had a trend favoring slightly greater reproducibility than sensory nerve action potential amplitudes, but thermal thresholds had much poorer reproducibility, at least at some of the centers. In the multicenter tolrestat withdrawal study, the coefficients of variation for vibration threshold also had a trend favoring slightly greater reproducibility than that for sensory nerve action potential amplitudes (Santiago et al., 1993; Bril, 1994).

In summary, quantitative sensory tests, especially for vibration, are highly reproducible techniques that are strongly recommended for inclusion in the design of clinical trials for peripheral neuropathy in which treatment is intended to improve, or to reduce the rate of progressive loss of, sensory function.

Nerve Biopsy

One possible method for quantitative assessment of sensory fibers is to perform *nerve biopsies* before and at the end of a clinical trial. One potential advantage of this approach over sensory nerve conduction studies is that all sizes of sensory fibers may be assessed. Whereas surface recorded sensory nerve action potentials assess only large myelinated sensory fibers, the density of large myelinated, small myelinated, and unmyelinated sensory fibers can be measured by nerve biopsy. The large and small myelinated fibers can be counted with light microscopy. The greater expense of electron microscopy is usually required for reliable assessment of unmyelinated fibers in nerve biopsy.

Quantitative assessment of cutaneous nerve biopsies has been used as an end point in clinical trials for diabetic polyneuropathy (Sima et al., 1988; Greene et al., 1999). Sima and colleagues performed a randomized, double-blind, placebo-controlled trial with sorbinil in 16 patients with diabetes who underwent fascicular sural nerve biopsy on one side before and more proximally on the same side after 1 year of treatment (Sima et al., 1988). Compared with placebo, the fascicular biopsy specimens of the 10 sorbinil-treated patients with diabetes had a 42% decrease in nerve sorbinil and a 3.8-fold increase in the percentage of regenerating myelinated fibers, with a 33% higher number of myelinated fibers per unit of cross-sectional area. Improvement was also seen in paranodal demyelination, segmental demyelination, and myelin wrinkling.

This group subsequently assessed the reproducibility of these quantitative findings by removing four sural nerve fascicles (two from each side) at autopsy of 13 patients with diabetes and 13 persons who did not have diabetes (Sima et al., 1992). The coefficient of variation for fiber density in the patients with diabetes was 3% for ipsilateral fascicles and 0% for left versus right fascicles, whereas it was 0% for both in the persons who did not have diabetes. Fiber size and percentage of terminal myelin loops devoid of axoglial junctions were also highly reproducible. The percentage of fibers with segmental demyelination and the percentage of regenerating or remyelinating fibers were poorly reproducible measures, with coefficients of variation of 181% and 89% for side-to-side comparisons among the patients with diabetes.

Greene and coinvestigators performed a randomized, dose-ranging, placebo-controlled trial with zenarestat in which 208 patients with diabetes were randomized to one of four groups (Greene et al., 1999). These investigators used change in total myelinated fiber density of contralateral sural nerves removed after 6 weeks and 52 months of treatment as one of two coprimary end points. The total myelinated fiber density tended to decrease over the year in patients treated with placebo or 300 mg of zenarestat per day and tended to increase in patients treated with 600 or 1,200 mg per day, but differences were not statistically significant. However, statistically significant improvement was seen at the two higher doses in small (less than 5 μm) myelinated fiber density in a post hoc analysis. Although the coprimary end point of total myelinated fiber density did not demonstrate a statistically significant treatment effect, the other coprimary end point was a composite nerve conduction score, the average rank-order score of sural, median, and peroneal nerve conduction velocity. The electrophysiological end point did demonstrate statistically significant benefit from zenarestat.

Biopsy of a cutaneous nerve is an invasive procedure that may cause neuropathic pain, especially during the initial weeks after biopsy, and produces a sensory deficit. Although this is a well-known diagnostic procedure that is indicated for evaluation of neuropathies with suspected pathological alteration of vascular or interstitial tissues, the long-term morbidity was systematically assessed only recently in 30 patients with diabetes and 12 nondiabetic patients who had undergone sural nerve biopsy (Theriault et al., 1998). Postbiopsy wound infections developed in four (13%) patients with diabetes and in one (8%) patient who did not have diabetes. Wound dehiscence occurred in five patients with diabetes (17%) and in one patient without diabetes (8%). The area of complete sensory loss to pinprick gradually diminished to 10% of the initial area at 18 months in patients with diabetes and to 3% in nondiabetic patients. After 12 months, irritating but not painful sensations continued to occur in the region of the biopsy in response to mechanical stimulation in 78% of patients with diabetes and in 67% of patients who did not have diabetes. The severity of these symptoms was 3 to 4 on a 10-point scale at 12 months and better at 18 months. Allodynia persisted at 12 months in 19% of the patients with diabetes but in none of the patients who did not have diabetes.

Although assessment of unmyelinated fibers is possible in nerve biopsies, these previous studies have not performed electron microscopy for this, and experience in clinical trials has involved measurement of large and small myelinated fibers. Consensus statements that were developed in 1992 and 1994 urged caution in the use of nerve biopsy as an end point in clinical trials for diabetic polyneuropathy, because of the invasiveness, cost, and uncertain relation to clinically meaningful improvement (American Diabetes Association, 1992c; Peripheral Nerve Society, 1995). Although a subsequent study defined the quantitative change in myelinated fiber density that is required to support meaningful clinical improvement (Russell et al., 1996), the invasiveness and long-term morbidity of nerve biopsy support that continued caution is warranted in its use for quantitative assessment of sensory function.

Skin Biopsy

Punch biopsies of the skin may be used for assessment of small fiber sensory function. Nociceptors and thermal receptors are free nerve endings that extend superficially into the epidermis. These intraepidermal fibers stain with the panaxonal marker antiprotein gene product 9.5 (PGP9.5), and they can then be seen with light microscopy (McCarthy et al., 1995). These fibers were first described by Langerhans more than a century ago, but they were difficult to visualize before the immunocytochemical use of PGP9.5, except by electron microscopy. McCarthy and colleagues performed 3- or 4-mm punch biopsies on eight patients with probable idiopathic sensory polyneuropathy, five human immunodeficiency virus (HIV)–positive patients with nucleoside-induced sensory polyneuropathy, five HIV-positive patients without polyneuropathy, and seven healthy control subjects (McCarthy et al., 1995). Intraepidermal nerve fiber density was measured by counting the number of single fibers that were seen on at least three sections and by dividing this number by the length in mm of the epidermis in all counted sections. The two groups of patients with polyneuropathy had significantly lower intraepidermal nerve fiber density (linear density of 1 and 3 per mm in the distal leg) than the healthy or HIV-positive control subjects (linear density of 18 and 13 per mm in the distal leg).

The sensitivity and reproducibility of intraepidermal nerve fiber density were examined in 20 patients with painful distal symmetrical sensory polyneuropathy associated with HIV infection compared with 98 healthy control subjects (McArthur et al., 1998). Intraepidermal nerve fiber density was measured by the linear density technique as well as by an unbiased stereological method, which uses an optical fractionator (Stocks et al., 1996). These two methods had correlation coefficients of 0.79 ($P = .001$) with comparison of 16 specimens from eight healthy controls (McArthur et al., 1998). Intraobserver and interobserver correlation coefficients ranged from 0.74 to 0.94 for repeated linear density measurements, a finding supporting excellent reproducibility. Setting the lower limit of normal for linear density at the fifth percentile, distal punch biopsies had a 45% sensitivity and a 97% specificity.

The sensitivity of intraepidermal nerve fiber density was compared with that for the quantitative sudomotor afferent reflex test and quantitative sensory tests for cold and vibratory detection in 32 patients with burning feet but normal sural nerve conduction results (Periquet et al., 1999). Although punch biopsies were taken and were analyzed from only one site 10 cm proximal to the lateral malleolus and each of the other two types of testing consisted of four measurements, intraepidermal nerve fiber density was abnormal in 28 (87.5%), whereas quantitative sensory testing was abnormal in 23 (72%), and quantitative sudomotor afferent reflex testing was abnormal in 19 (59%). Intraepidermal nerve fiber density had the highest sensitivity. This study did not determine specificity, and abnormality on any one type of test did not reliably predict abnormality on either of the other two.

The reproducibility of intraepidermal nerve fiber density was also examined in a subset of patients who participated in the phase II trial of nerve growth factor in HIV-associated distal symmetrical sensory polyneuropathy (McArthur et al., 2000). Punch biopsies were performed twice at baseline and week 18 on 60 patients. No significant treatment effect on intraepidermal nerve fiber density was detected. The overall estimate of correlation was 77% in the upper thigh and 81% in the lower leg ($P < .001$).

This technique is minimally invasive with minimal morbidity, particularly in comparison with nerve biopsy. Thus, determination of intraepidermal nerve fiber density from punch biopsies of the skin is a sensitive and specific test with good reproducibility and is expected to become an important component of clinical trials that are designed to affect small fiber sensory function.

EXPERIENCE FROM PREVIOUS CLINICAL TRIALS

Peripheral Neuropathy

Few clinical trials for treatment of peripheral neuropathies that have sensory onset or sensory more than motor deficits have demonstrated unequivocal benefit, so previous experience has not yet proved the optimal design. Because diabetic polyneuropathy is the most common polyneuropathy in Western societies and because most patients with diabetes mellitus are compliant and are accustomed to regularly scheduled visits with physicians, experience in clinical trial design has accumulated more for diabetic polyneuropathy than for any other peripheral neuropathy that has sensory onset or sensory more than motor deficits.

The greatest numbers of treatment trials for diabetic polyneuropathy have been designed to demonstrate the potential benefit of aldose reductase inhibitors. In an early clinical trial, 39 patients with diabetes participated in a randomized, double-blind, crossover trial during which each patient received sorbinil 250 mg per day for one 9-week treatment period and a placebo during the alternate 9-week period (Judzewitsch et al., 1983). The primary end point was improvement in conduction velocity in peroneal motor, median motor, and median sensory nerves. All three nerves demonstrated an improvement of approximately 1 m per second during the sorbinil compared with the placebo-treatment periods. All three changes were statistically significant, with probabilities for these results occurring from chance alone being .035 for median sensory, .005 for median motor, and .008 for peroneal motor. Although the results of this study were thus unequivocally positive in demonstrating a consistent benefit on the surrogate marker of nerve conduction velocity, which incidentally many subsequent aldose reductase trials have also done, the question of clinically significant benefit from aldose reductase inhibitors has persisted from 1983 to the present. Thus, one important lesson that has been taught since the 1980s is that the trial design must ensure that a statistically significant change in the desired direction for the primary end point will be interpreted as a clinically significant benefit.

In a subsequent, small 52-month trial with 16 patients with diabetes who were treated with sorbinil or placebo, many types of measurements were explored, including clinical scales, electrophysiological measures, and quantitative changes in repeated sural fascicular nerve biopsy (Sima et al., 1988). Although treatment-related decreased levels of sorbitol and improved morphometric results were demonstrated in the nerve biopsies and treatment-related improvements in the nonbiopsied sural nerve amplitude and velocity were demonstrated electrophysiologically, the clinical significance of these results was debated. Among the 10 clinical scales, a 50% or greater improvement was demonstrated in a mean of 4.6 scales with sorbinil treatment compared with a mean of 2.4 scales with placebo treatment. Furthermore, quantitative sensory tests did not reflect benefit. At least two issues in trial design are illustrated by these results. First, the degree of improvement in nerve morphometry that supports clinically significant benefit was ambiguous. Second, although this was a small exploratory trial and not a phase III efficacy trial, the ambiguous implication of multiple clinical scales that do not uniformly demonstrate the same benefit suggests the need to have a single composite measure, for which a statistically significant change in the desired direction will be interpreted as an unambiguous clinically significant benefit.

Subsequent studies clarified these issues. Dyck and O'Brien estimated that an improvement in motor conduction velocity of 2.9 m per second for the average of ulnar and peroneal nerves or 2.2 m per second for the peroneal nerves corresponds to clinically significant benefit (Dyck and O'Brien, 1989). Sima and colleagues established that myelinated fiber density and several other morphometric measurements are reproducible (Sima et al., 1992). Russel et al. estimated that a 200 fiber/mm^2 change in myelinated fiber density corresponds to clinically significant change (Russell et al., 1996). Development of the optimal composite measure to support clinically significant benefit remains under evaluation.

One of the few clinical trials that has demonstrated unequivocal clinical benefit for treatment of diabetic polyneuropathy is the Diabetes Control and Complications Trial (DCCT) (DCCT, 1993, 1995a, 1995b). In this trial, 1,441 patients with insulin-dependent diabetes mellitus were stratified into two groups based on the absence (the primary prevention group) or presence (the secondary intervention group) of retinopathy. Within each group, patients were randomly assigned to intensive therapy (insulin pump or three or more daily insulin injections) or conventional therapy (one or two daily insulin injections) for a mean of 6.5 years. The primary end point was the prevention of retinopathy (the primary prevention group) or the slowing of progression of retinopathy (the secondary intervention group). The prevention of the development of polyneuropathy was a secondary end point in both groups. The presence of polyneuropathy was defined as abnormal neurological examination findings that were consistent with polyneuropathy and either abnormal nerve conduction results or unequivocally abnormal autonomic function testing. In the primary prevention group, diabetic polyneuropathy developed over 5 years in 28 of 291 (9.6%) patients with diabetes who received conventional therapy and in 7 of 248 (2.8%) patients with intensive therapy (69% reduced risk; $P = .006$). In the secondary intervention group, diabetic polyneuropathy developed over 5 years in 52 of 307 (16.9%) patients with diabetes with conventional therapy and in 21 of 315 (6.7%) patients with intensive therapy (57% reduced risk; $P < .001$). Nerve conduction study results also supported the benefit of intensive therapy. Thus, the only trial design strategy that has provided unequivocal benefit for diabetic polyneuropathy is a primary prevention trial design.

Although primary prevention is a definitive strategy to prove clinically significant benefit, this strategy usually requires a large sample size and long-term follow-up of a well-defined population that is at risk. Furthermore, this strategy does not work for assessing a treatment that is intended to reduce the rate of progression or to stimulate actual improvement in patients with established polyneuropathy, which is the more commonly needed trial design. A consensus developed during the 1990s concerning the general methodology for assessment of diabetic polyneuropathy in clinical trials (American Diabetes Association, 1992c; Peripheral Nerve Society, 1995). Quantitative sensory testing for detection thresholds is more sensitive and reproducible than measurement of sensory function by clinical scales (Dyck et al., 1991). Although quantitative sensory tests have the advantage of assessing function of both large and small sensory fibers, a disadvantage is that the results are affected by central as well as peripheral nervous dysfunction (American Diabetes Association, 1992b). Sensory nerve conduction studies provide a noninvasive quantitative assessment of peripheral sensory fibers that is not affected by central nervous system disease (Dyck et al., 1991; American Diabetes Association, 1992a). Although sensory amplitude measurements are less reproducible than conduction velocity measurements, nerve conduction abnormalities are specific for large-fiber peripheral nerve dysfunction (Dyck et al., 1991). Caution has been expressed regarding the use of nerve biopsies in clinical trials (American Diabetes Association, 1992c; Peripheral Nerve Society, 1995). The assessment of intraepidermal nerve fibers by punch biopsy of the skin had not yet been introduced at the time these consensus recommendations were made.

A major focus for improving the design for clinical trials on peripheral neuropathy has been the development of composite measures that combine clinical and surrogate measures, so that a single sensitive and reproducible end point can be used to support clinically significant benefit. One such measure is the Total Neuropathy Score, which was developed and validated by Cornblath and colleagues (1999). This score consists of 10 subtests, each of which is scored from 0 to 4, with 0 being normal and 4 being severely abnormal. Among the 10 subtests, three focus on symptoms, four on neurological examination findings, one on results of quantitative sensory testing, and two on attributes of nerve conduction results. In their validation study, five neurologically normal persons had total scores of 0 or 1 with assessment by two raters. Thirty patients with diabetic polyneuropathy of varying severity had scores ranging from 6 to 34. The Total Neuropathy Score had high intrarater and interrater reliability. The Total Neuropathy Score was used as the primary end point in two successful trials that were designed to detect and quantify the development of chemotherapy-induced polyneuropathy (Chaudhry et al., 1994b; Chaudhry et al., 1996). The Total Neuropathy Score has not yet been used in long-term clinical trials to assess treatments that may improve peripheral neuropathy.

Dyck and colleagues have been developing and refining composite scales to measure clinically significant changes in peripheral neuropathy since 1980 (Dyck et al., 1980). They have developed a composite score, the NIS(LL) + 7 tests, which includes the neurological examination findings in the lower limbs (LL) as scored by the Neuropathy Impairment Score (NIS) with substitution of quantitative sensory testing for vibration perception threshold in the place of clinical vibration testing and with the addition of one autonomic and five nerve conduction measures (Dyck et al., 1997). In their Rochester Diabetic Neuropathy Study cohort, the average patient with diabetes worsened by 0.34 point per year and the average patient with diabetes and polyneuropathy worsened by 0.85 point per year with the NIS(LL) + 7 tests. Based on this rate of worsening of diabetic polyneuropathy, a clinical trial that is expected to prevent progression rather than to stimulate improvement in diabetic polyneuropathy is projected to require a 3-year trial design to achieve a clinically meaningful change.

Multiple Sclerosis and Other Central Nervous System Disorders

Limited experience has been acquired with the quantitative assessment of sensory function in clinical trials for multiple sclerosis and other central nervous system disorders. In a 3-year, double-blind, placebo-controlled trial of azathioprine with or without steroids, Nuwer and colleagues found that the progressive worsening of serial peak latencies of visual evoked potentials and somatosensory evoked potentials was significantly less with treatment

(Nuwer et al., 1987). This group found that analysis of actual latency values, rather than scales that scored the results as normal or abnormal or as unchanged, worsened or improved, increased the sensitivity of serial evoked potentials to detect change over time. The utility of visual, brainstem auditory, and somatosensory evoked potentials in multiple sclerosis has also been supported by a subsequent trial (La et al., 1994). The potential use of motor evoked potentials in clinical trials for multiple sclerosis has been less thoroughly studied, but at least one group has suggested utility (Kandler et al., 1991).

Thus, evoked potentials may have utility as a surrogate measure in clinical trials for treatment of multiple sclerosis, but this has not been established. In particular, the issue of the degree of change in evoked potential latency that is necessary to support a clinically meaningful change has not been addressed.

CONSIDERATIONS IN DESIGN OF FUTURE CLINICAL TRIALS FOR NEUROLOGICAL DISORDERS THAT AFFECT SENSORY FUNCTION

Useful approaches for quantitative measurement of sensory function in clinical trials of treatment for peripheral and central nervous system disorders are summarized in Table 106–1. An effective primary end point is needed to establish clinically meaningful benefit to the treatment that is under investigation. Because the results of sensory nerve conduction studies and quantitative sensory tests are sensitive, specific, and reproducible, the role of clinical neurophysiology in the quantitative assessment of sensory function is well established in clinical trials for peripheral neuropathy. To establish clinical benefit, these measures are likely to be combined with clinical measures in a composite score. The use of punch biopsy of the skin to assess small intraepidermal nerve fibers is a highly promising approach to quantify small fiber sensory function. Among currently described composite measures, the Total Neuropathy Score and the Neuropathy Impairment Score for the Lower Limbs + 7 tests [the NIS(LL) + 7 tests] are highly promising. These com-

Table 106–1. Useful Approaches for Quantitative Measurement of Sensory Function in Clinical Trials for Peripheral and Central Nervous System Disorders

Quantitative Measure	Peripheral Neuropathy	Central Sensory Disorder
Nerve conduction studies	Yes	No
Somatosensory evoked potentials	No	Yes
Quantitative sensory tests	Yes	Yes
Intraepidermal nerve fiber density	Yes	No

posite scores or others like them that combine neurological examination findings, nerve conduction study results, quantitative sensory testing, and possibly intraepidermal nerve fiber analysis are recommended for inclusion in the design of clinical trials that quantitatively assess sensory function. The role of clinical neurophysiology in the quantitative assessment of sensory function is uncertain but promising in clinical trials of treatment for central nervous system disease.

References

Alexander LO, Olney RK: Normal variability of sensory nerve action potential amplitude. Muscle Nerve 1987;10:645.

Alexander LO, Stigler J, Olney RK: Normal variability of lower extremity compound muscle action potential measurements. Muscle Nerve 1989;12:755.

American Diabetes Association: Proceedings of a consensus development conference on standardized measures in diabetic neuropathy: Electrodiagnostic measures. Muscle Nerve 1992a; 15:1150–1154.

American Diabetes Association: Proceedings of a consensus development conference on standardized measures in diabetic neuropathy: Quantitative sensory testing. Muscle Nerve 1992b; 15:1155–1157.

American Diabetes Association: Proceedings of a consensus development conference on standardized measures in diabetic neuropathy: Summary and recommendations. Muscle Nerve 1992c;15:1167–1170.

Aminoff MJ: Electrophysiologic evaluation of patients with multiple sclerosis. Neurol Clin 1985;3:663–674.

Aminoff MJ, Davis SL, Panitch HS: Serial evoked potential studies in patients with definite multiple sclerosis: Clinical relevance. Arch Neurol 1984;41:1197–1202.

Bleasel AF, Tuck RR: Variability of repeated nerve conduction studies. Electroencephalogr Clin Neurophysiol 1991;81:417–420.

Bril V: Role of electrophysiological studies in diabetic neuropathy. Can J Neurol Sci 1994;21:S8–S12.

Bril V, Ellison R, Ngo M, et al: Electrophysiological monitoring in clinical trials. Muscle Nerve 1998;21:1368–1373.

Bril V, Kojic J, Ngo M, Clark K: Comparison of a neurothesiometer and vibration in measuring vibration perception thresholds and relationship to nerve conduction studies. Diabetes Care 1997;20:1360–1362.

Buchthal F, Rosenfalck A: Evoked action potentials and conduction velocity in human sensory nerves. Brain Res 1966;3:1–122.

Chaudhry V, Cornblath DR, Mellits ED, et al: Inter- and intraexaminer reliability of nerve conduction measurements in normal subjects. Ann Neurol 1991;30:841–843.

Chaudhry V, Corse AM, Freimer ML, et al: Inter- and intraexaminer reliability of nerve conduction measurements in patients with diabetic neuropathy. Neurology 1994a;44:1459–1462.

Chaudhry V, Eisenberger MA, Sinibaldi VJ, et al: A prospective study of suramin-induced peripheral neuropathy. Brain 1996; 119:2039–2052.

Chaudhry V, Rowinsky EK, Sartorius SE, et al: Peripheral neuropathy from Taxol and cisplatin combination chemotherapy: Clinical and electrophysiological studies. Ann Neurol 1994b;35:304–311.

Claus D, Mustafa C, Vogel W, et al: Assessment of diabetic neuropathy: Definition of norm and discrimination of abnormal nerve function. Muscle Nerve 1993;16:757–768.

Cornblath DR, Chaudhry V, Carter K, et al: Total neuropathy score: Validation and reliability study. Neurology 1999;53:1660–1664.

Davis SL, Aminoff MJ, Panitch HS: Clinical correlations of serial somatosensory evoked potentials in multiple sclerosis. Neurology 1985;35:359–365.

Diabetes Control and Complications Trial Research Group: The effect of intensive treatment of diabetes on the development

and progression of long-term complications in insulin-dependent diabetes mellitus. N Engl J Med 1993;329:977–986.

Diabetes Control and Complications Trial Research Group: The effect of intensive diabetes therapy on the development and progression of neuropathy. Ann Intern Med 1995a;122:561–568.

Diabetes Control and Complications Trial Research Group: Effect of intensive diabetes treatment on nerve conduction in the Diabetes Control and Complications Trial. Ann Neurol 1995b; 38:869–880.

Dyck PJ, Davies JL, Litchy WJ, O'Brien PC: Longitudinal assessment of diabetic polyneuropathy using a composite score in the Rochester Diabetic Neuropathy Study cohort. Neurology 1997;49:229–239.

Dyck PJ, Kratz KM, Lehman KA, et al: The Rochester Diabetic Neuropathy Study: Design, criteria for types of neuropathy, selelction bias, and reproducibility of neuropathic tests. Neurology 1991;41:799–807.

Dyck PJ, O'Brien PC: Meaningful degrees of prevention or improvement of nerve conduction in controlled clinical trials of diabetic neuropathy. Diabetes Care 1989;12:649–652.

Dyck PJ, O'Brien PC: Quantitative sensation testing in epidemiological and therapeutic studies of peripheral neuropathy. Muscle Nerve 1999;22:659–662.

Dyck PJ, O'Brien PC, Kosanke JL, et al: A 4, 2, and 1 stepping algorithm for quick and accurate estimation of cutaneous sensation threshold. Neurology 1993;43:1508–1512.

Dyck PJ, Sherman WR, Hallcher LM, et al: Human diabetic endoneurial sorbitol, fructose, and myo-inositol related to sural nerve morphometry. Ann Neurol 1980;8:590–596.

Emerson RG: Evoked potentials in clinical trials for multiple sclerosis. J Clin Neurophysiol 1998;15:109–116.

Greene DA, Arezzo JC, Brown MB: Effect of aldose reductase inhibition on nerve conduction and morphometry in diabetic neuropathy: Zenarestat Study Group. Neurology 1999;53:580–591.

Hammond SR, MacCallum S, Yiannikas C, et al: Variability on serial testing of pattern reversal visual evoked potential latencies from full-field, half-field and foveal stimulation in control subjects. Electroencephalogr Clin Neurophysiol 1987;66:401–408.

Judzewitsch RG, Jaspan JB, Polonsky KS, et al: Aldose reductase inhibition improves nerve conduction velocity in diabetic patients. N Engl J Med 1983;308:119–125.

Kandler RH, Jarratt JA, Davies-Jones GA, et al: The role of magnetic stimulation as a quantifier of motor disability in patients with multiple sclerosis. J Neurol Sci 1991;106:31–34.

La ML, Riti F, Milanese C, et al: Serial evoked potentials in multiple sclerosis bouts: Relation to steroid treatment. Ital J Neurol Sci 1994;15:333–340.

Lauter JL, Loomis RL: Individual differences in auditory electric responses: Comparisons of between-subject and within-subject variability. I. Absolute latencies of brainstem vertex-positive peaks. Scand Audiol 1986;15:167–172.

Matthews WB, Small DG: Serial recording of visual and somatosensory evoked potentials in multiple sclerosis. J Neurol Sci 1979;40:11–21.

McArthur JC, Stocks EA, Hauer P, et al: Epidermal nerve fiber density: Normative reference range and diagnostic efficiency. Arch Neurol 1998;55:1513–1520.

McArthur JC, Yiannoutsos C, Simpson DM, et al: A phase II trial of nerve growth factor for sensory neuropathy associated with HIV infection: AIDS Clinical Trials Group Team 291. Neurology 2000;54:1080–1088.

McCarthy BG, Hsieh ST, Stocks A, et al: Cutaneous innervation in sensory neuropathies: Evaluation by skin biopsy. Neurology 1995;45:1848–1855.

Meienberg O, Kutak L, Smolenski C, Ludin HP: Pattern reversal evoked cortical responses in normals: A study of different methods of stimulation and potential reproducibility. J Neurol 1979;222:81–93.

Nuwer MR, Packwood JW, Myers LW, Ellison GW: Evoked potentials predict the clinical changes in a multiple sclerosis drug study. Neurology 1987;37:1754–1761.

Olney RK, Schleimer JA: Intraexaminer and interexaminer reproducibility of nerve conduction measurements in diabetics with mild polyneuropathy. Muscle Nerve 1992;15:1195.

Peripheral Nerve Society: Diabetic polyneuropathy in controlled clinical trials: Consensus report of the Peripheral Nerve Society. Ann Neurol 1995;38:478–482.

Periquet MI, Novak V, Collins MP, et al: Painful sensory neuropathy: Prospective evaluation using skin biopsy. Neurology 1999; 53:1641–1647.

Romani A, Bergamaschi R, Versino M, et al: One-week test-retest reliability of spinal and cortical somatosensory evoked potentials by tibial nerve stimulation. Boll Soc Ital Biol Sper 1993; 69:601–607.

Russell JW, Karnes JL, Dyck PJ: Sural nerve myelinated fiber density differences associated with meaningful changes in clinical and electrophysiologic measurements. J Neurol Sci 1996; 135:114–117.

Santiago JV, Snksen PH, Boulton AJ, et al: Withdrawal of the aldose reductase inhibitor tolrestat in patients with diabetic neuropathy: Effect on nerve function. The Tolrestat Study Group. J Diabetes Complications 1993;7:170–178.

Shaw NA, Synek VM: Intersession stability of somatosensory evoked potentials. Electroencephalogr Clin Neurophysiol 1987; 66:281–285.

Sima AA, Bril V, Nathaniel V, et al: Regeneration and repair of myelinated fibers in sural-nerve biopsy specimens from patients with diabetic neuropathy treated with sorbinil. N Engl J Med 1988;319:548–555.

Sima AA, Brown MB, Prashar A, et al: The reproducibility and sensitivity of sural nerve morphometry in the assessment of diabetic peripheral polyneuropathy. Diabetologia 1992;35:560–569.

Stocks EA, McArthur JC, Griffen JW, Mouton PR: An unbiased method for estimation of total epidermal nerve fibre length. J Neurocytol 1996;25:637–644.

Sundkvist G, Armstrong FM, Bradbury JE, et al: Peripheral and autonomic nerve function in 259 diabetic patients with peripheral neuropathy treated with ponalrestat (an aldose reductase inhibitor) or placebo for 18 months: United Kingdom/Scandinavian Ponalrestat Trial. J Diabetes Complications 1992;6:123–130.

Theriault M, Dort J, Sutherland G, Zochodne DW: A prospective quantitative study of sensory deficits after whole sural nerve biopsies in diabetic and nondiabetic patients: Surgical approach and the role of collateral sprouting. Neurology 1998; 50:480–484.

Valensi P, Attali JR, Gagant S: Reproducibility of parameters for assessment of diabetic neuropathy: The French Group for Research and Study of Diabetic Neuropathy. Diabet Med 1993; 10:933–939.

Vinik AI, Suwanwalaikorn S, Stansberry KB, et al: Quantitative measurement of cutaneous perception in diabetic neuropathy. Muscle Nerve 1995;18:574–584.

Quantitative Autonomic Functional Testing in Clinical Trials

Max J. Hilz

As with any medical examination, patient history and the physical examination provide the most important guidance as to which autonomic function tests should be performed to identify and quantify the specific autonomic dysfunction (Oribe, 1999).

There is a wide variety of autonomic testing procedures and challenge maneuvers that can be used to activate the sympathetic and parasympathetic nervous systems. Many tests are not easily standardized, and it is beyond the scope of this chapter to provide a complete overview of the manifold tests that have been used to study autonomic control.

In clinical trials, quantitative assessment of autonomic function should be limited to well-standardized procedures. Intraindividual and interindividual variabilities in the results of autonomic challenge maneuvers might be high. Therefore, reproducibility of test results should be ensured, and patient data must be compared with those of age- and sex-matched healthy control subjects (Low and Pfeifer, 1997).

Study participants should be advised to avoid factors that interfere with autonomic nervous system function, such as altered patterns of sleep (particularly sleep deprivation), drinking, eating, medication, and exercise (Genovely and Pfeifer, 1988). Testing should be performed at a standardized time, preferably in the morning, in a quiet and relaxed atmosphere after a sufficient period of adjustment, such as after the patient has been in the supine position for 30 to 40 minutes. Body position influences test results (Low, 1997; Singer et al., 1999), so all participants should be examined in a standard position. We prefer to conduct all tests with the subject in the supine position on a tilt table. This approach does not require repositioning of the study participant or the testing equipment during different procedures. Room temperature and humidity should be constant and comfortable.

Specific tests are suited to assess sympathetic function, whereas others evaluate parasympathetic modulation. Finally, there are procedures that can be used to study both sympathetic and parasympathetic activities (Low and Pfeifer, 1997).

Among the methods primarily used to analyze parasympathetic function is time domain analysis of heart rate modulation at rest or during metronomic breathing, after standing up, and in response to coughing, squatting, or the Valsalva maneuver (Table 107–1). The frequency domain analysis of heart rate or blood pressure by means of fast Fourier transformation or autoregressive techniques provides measures of sympathetic and parasympathetic influences. Although the pupil cycle time is considered an index of parasympathetic activity, infrared light reflex pupillography yields parameters of both sympathetic and parasympathetic pupillary modulation. Measurement of pancreatic polypeptide levels, urologic procedures such as a cystometrogram with intravenous betanechol, and recordings of nocturnal

penile tumescence provide indicators of parasympathetic outflow, but these tests are not discussed in this chapter (Low and Pfeifer, 1997).

Sympathetic function can be determined with various sweat tests, such as the thermoregulatory sweat test, the quantitative sudomotor axon reflex test, the recording of sympathetic skin responses, or sweat imprint techniques. Other parameters of sympathetic activity are blood pressure responses to standing, handgrip, squatting, and the Valsalva maneuver; plasma norepinephrine levels, particularly after sympathetic activation; venoarteriolar reflexes; and vasomotor reflexes assessed by means of laser Doppler flowmetry of superficial skin vessels (Henriksen et al., 1983; Low et al., 1983; Baba et al., 1988; Belcaro and Nicolaides, 1989; Belcaro et al., 1989; Fealey et al., 1989; Moy et al., 1989; Baser et al., 1991; Belcaro and Nicolaides, 1991; Yokota et al., 1991; Fealey, 1997; Low, 1997).

Biosignals such as heart rate, blood pressure, cerebral blood flow velocity, and superficial skin blood flow are under the constant influence of sympathetic and parasympathetic modulation (Task Force of the European Society of Cardiology and the North American Society of Pacing and Electrophysiology, 1996); therefore, these signals are not fixed but fluctuate around a mean value. For most clinical studies, the analysis of a 5- to 10-minute time series of a signal provides a sufficient measure of autonomic modulation (Task Force of the European Society of Cardiology and the North American Society of Pacing and Electrophysiology, 1996). Signals can be analyzed in the time domain or the frequency domain (Task Force of the European Society of Cardiology and the North American Society of Pacing and Electrophysiology, 1996). Long-term recordings of up to 24 hours can be used to determine time domain parameters such as the number of successive differences in R-R intervals in the electrocardiogram that exceed 50 ms (pNN50), an index of parasympathetic activity (Task Force of the European Society of Cardiology and the North American Society of Pacing and Electrophysiology, 1996). These recordings also allow the evaluation of the spectral power of the very low frequency band (VLF) (0.003 to 0.04 Hz) and the ultralow-frequency band (ULF) (<0.003 Hz), parameters whose physiological correlates are not well known (see later) (Task Force of the European Society of Cardiology and the North American Society of Pacing and Electrophysiology, 1996). Spectral analysis should, however, be performed on recordings of stationary signals (Task Force of the European Society of Cardiology and the North American Society of Pacing and Electrophysiology, 1996). This requirement of being stationary is compromised with long-term recordings; therefore, we prefer to use short-term recordings for the spectral analysis of slow frequencies underlying a biosignal and reflecting sympathetic and parasympathetic signal modulation (Task Force of the European Society of Cardiology and the North American Society of Pacing and Electrophysiology, 1996).

Table 107–1. Useful Approaches for Quantitative Measurement of Autonomic Function in Clinical Trials for Peripheral and Central Nervous System Disorders

Quantitative Measure	Peripheral Neuropathy	Central Disorders
Heart rate variability (time domain analysis)	X	X
Analysis of heart rate and blood pressure variability in the frequency domain		
With metronomic breathing	X	X
With sustained handgrip	X	(X)
With Valsalva maneuver	X	X
Assessment of orthostatic tolerance		
By active standing	X	X
By passive head-up tilt	X	X
Venoarteriolar reflex testing	X	
Impedance plethysmography during head-up tilt	X	(X)
Baroreflex testing	X	X
Testing of peripheral hypoxic and hypercapnic chemoreceptor sensitivity using the "single-breath" method	X	
Testing of progressive hypercapnia using the rebreathing method		X
Cerebral autoregulation		X
Analysis of coherence and phase relation between blood pressure and cerebral blood flow		X
Sudomotor function testing		
Thermoregulatory sweat test	X	X
Quantitative sudomotor axon reflex test	X	
Laser Doppler flowmetry	X	(X)
Pupillography	(X)	X

TIME DOMAIN ANALYSIS OF HEART RATE VARIABILITY

Heart rate variability can be determined under resting conditions and during various challenge maneuvers by calculating *time domain parameters* from the time series of the heart rate or the R-R intervals in the electrocardiogram (Ewing, 1992; Task Force of the European Society of Cardiology and the North American Society of Pacing and Electrophysiology, 1996). We prefer to analyze R-R intervals instead of heart rate values, because the millisecond values of the R-R intervals provide more information than the beats-per-minute values of heart rate. When heart rate slows, for example, during parasympathetic stimulation, a deceleration of 20 beats per minute has a different meaning if the baseline heart rate is 60 or 150 beats per minute. In contrast to the heart rate differences, R-R differences more clearly reflect such diverse conditions.

Many parameters have been suggested to determine heart rate variability (Genovely and Pfeifer, 1988; Ewing, 1992; Stein et al., 1994; Task Force of the European Society of Cardiology and the North American Society of Pacing and Electrophysiology, 1996). Straightforward indices of the variation of the R-R intervals are the standard deviation of the R-R intervals and the coefficient of variation, both considered to reflect sympathetic and parasympathetic heart rate modulation (Stein et al., 1994; Task Force of the European Society of Cardiology and the North American Society of Pacing and Electrophysiology, 1996). The standard deviation is easy to determine, but the parameter is linked to the intrinsic heart rate of the tested person, and standard deviation values can be significantly affected by artifacts such as ectopic heartbeats or a gradual change in heart rate (Genovely and Pfeifer, 1988). Moreover, standard deviation values depend on the length of the recording and usually increase with recording time (Task Force of the European Society of Cardiology and the North American Society of Pacing and Electrophysiology, 1996). Commonly, a 5-minute recording of resting heart rate is used for the analysis of short-term heart rate variability (Ewing, 1992).

A comparison of the length of adjacent cardiac cycles is independent of long-term trends of heart rate. A simple method is to count the number of adjacent cycles with an interval difference of greater than 50 ms and to indicate the percentage of these intervals in comparison with the total number of intervals evaluated. The value, the pNN50, predominantly reflects vagal activity (Stein et al., 1994; Task Force of the European Society of Cardiology and the North American Society of Pacing and Electrophysiology, 1996).

The root-mean-square successive differences value is the square root of the averaged sum of squared differences in adjacent R-R intervals (Stein et al., 1994; Task Force of the European Society of Cardiology and the North American Society of Pac-

ing and Electrophysiology, 1996). Similar to the pNN50, the root-mean-square successive differences value is not significantly influenced by heart rate trends and reflects parasympathetic tone (Stein et al., 1994; Task Force of the European Society of Cardiology and the North American Society of Pacing and Electrophysiology, 1996). The statistical properties of this value are, however, considered to be better than those of the pNN50 (Task Force of the European Society of Cardiology and the North American Society of Pacing and Electrophysiology, 1996). The root-mean-square successive differences value can be biased by premature ventricular contractions followed by a long compensatory pause (Harry and Freeman, 1993).

When used for the assessment of long-term heart rate variability, time domain and frequency domain parameters strongly correlate with each other (Stein et al., 1994). The root-mean-square successive differences value correlates with the high-frequency (HF) power, whereas the standard deviation correlates with the total power (Task Force of the European Society of Cardiology and the North American Society of Pacing and Electrophysiology, 1996). Therefore, assessment of 24-hour heart rate variability can be based on the more readily performed time domain analysis (Stein et al., 1994).

ANALYSIS OF HEART RATE AND BLOOD PRESSURE VARIABILITY IN THE FREQUENCY DOMAIN

Frequency domain analysis of the time series of cardiovascular signals decomposes the total variance of this biosignal into the modulation arising from underlying groups of frequencies that contribute to the overall signal modulation (Stein et al., 1994). The analysis provides a measure, such as the heart rate or blood pressure variability, arising from periodic oscillations at predefined frequencies (Stein et al., 1994). Various mathematical algorithms have been used for frequency analysis and can be divided into parametric and nonparametric methods; the two methods provide a similar estimate of the signal modulation due to underlying autonomic, mechanical, and other influences (Task Force of the European Society of Cardiology and the North American Society of Pacing and Electrophysiology, 1996). Spectral analysis is mostly used for short-term recordings of 2 to 5 minutes' duration (Task Force of the European Society of Cardiology and the North American Society of Pacing and Electrophysiology, 1996). As mentioned, long-term recordings, such as those over a period of 24 hours, usually do not fulfill the requirement of being stationary which is needed to adequately interpret a frequency contribution to the signal modulation (Task Force of the European Society of Cardiology and the North American Society of Pacing and Electrophysiology, 1996). The significance of a frequency component for the signal modulation is not well defined if the mechanisms accounting for signal modulation in that particular frequency range do not remain stable during the recording time (Task Force of the European Society of Cardiology and the North American Society of Pacing and Electrophysiology, 1996).

Frequency domain analysis provides a measure of the degree of sympathetic or parasympathetic signal modulation but not necessarily of the level of sympathetic or parasympathetic tone (Task Force of the European Society of Cardiology and the North American Society of Pacing and Electrophysiology, 1996). For example, the fluctuation in a frequency range reflecting sympathetic influence on the overall modulation of heart rate might be low, even if there is an excessively high, but continuous and invariant, sympathetic tone, such as that seen during physical exercise (Bernardi et al., 1990).

The contribution of specific frequencies to the total signal variability is referred to as the *power* of these frequencies (Stein et al., 1994). For heart rate variability, the power is measured in milliseconds squared; for blood pressure variability, the power is expressed in millimeters of mercury squared (Berger et al., 1989). To assess the power, the integral under the power spectral density (ms^2/Hz or bpm^2/Hz) curve is computed for a defined frequency band and expressed as the power of that frequency range (Berger et al., 1989). Some calculate the spectral "amplitude" that is the square root of power, measured in milliseconds or millimeters of mercury (Stein et al., 1994).

The spectrum analyzed from a 2- to 5-minute recording contains three main components: the very low frequency (≤ 0.04 Hz), low-frequency (0.04 to 0.15 Hz), and high-frequency (0.15 to 0.4 Hz) ranges (Task Force of the European Society of Cardiology and the North American Society of Pacing and Electrophysiology, 1996). In short-term recordings, interpretation of the very low frequency component should be avoided, because its physiological origin is not clearly explained (Task Force of the European Society of Cardiology and the North American Society of Pacing and Electrophysiology, 1996). Similarly, the origin of fluctuations at ultralow frequencies (≤ 0.003 Hz) that occur in 24-hour recordings is not clearly defined (Hojgaard et al., 1998). The activity of the renin-angiotensin system (Akselrod et al., 1981), thermoregulation (Kitney and Rompelman, 1977), peripheral vasomotor activity (Fallen et al., 1988), and physical activity (Bernardi et al., 1996) may contribute to heart rate variability in the very low and ultralow-frequency bands. The fluctuations of heart rate in the high-frequency band are in large part due to parasympathetic efferent activity and represent respiratory variation (Saul et al., 1991; Stein et al., 1994; Bernardi et al., 1995; Sleight et al., 1995). Controlled respiration or coldface stimulation increases high-frequency modulation of heart rate (Malliani et al., 1991; Task Force of the European Society of Cardiology and the North American Society of Pacing and Electrophysiology, 1996).

Heart rate fluctuations in the low-frequency band are influenced by oscillations of the baroreceptor system (Kamath et al., 1987; Stein, et al., 1994) and are thought to reflect both sympathetic and parasympathetic modulation, particularly at rest (Akselrod et al., 1981; Pomeranz et al., 1985; Appel et al., 1989; Saul, 1990; Malliani et al., 1991; Goldstein et al., 1994; Stein et al., 1994; Task Force of the European Society of Cardiology and the North American Society of Pacing and Electrophysiology, 1996). Some consider the low-frequency component to be an index of sympathetic modulation only (Rimoldi et al., 1990; Malliani et al., 1991; Kamath and Fallen, 1993; Montano et al., 1994), especially when the low-frequency activity is presented in normalized units (Wolf et al., 1978; Appel et al., 1989). Particularly when expressed in normalized units, low frequency increases during head-up tilt, active standing, mental stress, or moderate exercise (Task Force of the European Society of Cardiology and the North American Society of Pacing and Electrophysiology, 1996).

According to the Task Force of the European Society of Cardiology and the North American Society of Pacing and Electrophysiology (1996), the calculation of normalized units (i.e., the relative value of the low- or high-frequency power component in proportion to the total power in the range from 0.04 to 0.4 Hz) has the advantage of minimizing the influences of total power changes on the value of low- or high-frequency components but should not be quoted without the absolute low- and high-frequency values.

Some consider the ratio of low- to high-frequency activity to be a suitable index of sympathovagal balance (Malliani et al., 1994; Task Force of the European Society of Cardiology and the North American Society of Pacing and Electrophysiology, 1996). Malliani and associates (1991) summarize that functional states accompanied by enhanced sympathetic activity result in a shift of the low frequency–high frequency balance toward the low-frequency component, whereas situations that enhance vagal activity have the opposite effect.

Low-frequency oscillations of systolic blood pressure are considered to be an index of sympathetic modulation of vasomotor activity, whereas blood pressure oscillations in the high-frequency band are thought to be due to the mechanical effects of changes in stroke volume, resulting from changes in venous return induced by respiration (Pagani et al., 1986; Radaelli et al., 1994; Sleight et al., 1995).

AUTONOMIC CHALLENGE MANEUVERS

A standard battery of autonomic challenge maneuvers was suggested by Ewing and Clarke (1982) to evaluate diabetic autonomic neuropathy. In a 1988 consensus statement, the American Diabetes Association and the American Academy of Neurology Consensus Committee recommended this battery for the routine screening for autonomic dysfunction and to monitor the progress of autonomic neuropathy.

Among these standard procedures are tests primarily of parasympathetic heart rate control in response to the Valsalva maneuver, metronomic breathing, and active standing, as well as tests of mainly sympathetic blood pressure control during active standing (or passive tilting) and during sustained handgrip (Consensus Commitee of the American Autonomic Society and the American Academy of Neurology, 1996). In addition, the consensus statement recommended tests of sudomotor control by means of chemically or temperature-induced sweating.

There are many easy-to-perform maneuvers, such as the cold pressor test, the cold face test, squatting, or coughing, that assess cardiovascular responsiveness to sympathetic or parasympathetic activation (Low, 1997). Other tests are more complex and provide more detailed insight into the pathophysiology of cardiovascular reflexes loops, such as baroreflexes, the chemoreflexes, and cerebral autoregulation. Techniques to evaluate the autonomic modulation of these feedback circuits are described after a discussion of straightforward tests that more directly assess autonomic outflow toward end-organs. The Valsalva and Ewing maneuvers are described in the context of methods used to assess baroreflex function, orthostatic tolerance, and cerebral autoregulation.

Metronomic Breathing

Analysis of heart rate variability during metronomic breathing is the most widely used procedure to test cardiovascular autonomic function (Freeman, 1997; Hilsted and Low, 1997). Respiratory sinus arrhythmia with inspiratory acceleration and expiratory slowing of heart rate depends on the rate of breathing and is maximal at a rate of 5 or 6 breaths per minute (Angelone and Coulter, 1964; Wheeler and Watkins, 1973; Pfeifer et al., 1982). Sinus arrhythmia decreases with age (O'Brien et al., 1986; Low et al., 1990).

Various mechanisms are thought to contribute to sinus arrhythmia: The inspiratory network might inhibit cardiovagal neurons directly (Levy et al., 1966; Richter and Spyer, 1990). Respiration and changes in carbon dioxide concentration induce central modulation of baroreflex and chemoreflex sensitivity. The baroreflex sensitivity is greatest during inspiration and early expiration and is least during late expiration and early inspiration (Eckberg et al., 1980). Respiration-related changes in central venous volume affect heart rate via the Bainbridge reflex, whereas mechanical blood pressure modulation induces baroreflex-mediated heart rate changes (Saul and Cohen, 1994). Pulmonary and chest wall stretch receptors stimulate brainstem nuclei via the vagus nerve and the nucleus of the solitary tract and induce modulation of sympathetic and parasympathetic output to the heart (Saul and Cohen, 1994).

Changes in heart rate with deep respiration can be considered a parameter of parasympathetic cardiac control. Atropinization or vagus nerve cooling in large part reduces respiratory heart rate variability (Katona and Jih, 1975; Fouad et al., 1984).

Heart rate variability can be assessed with the patient breathing metronomically at a rate of 6 cycles per minute for 180 seconds. The frequency of 6 cycles per minute is used, because it results in maximal heart rate variability in healthy individuals (Wheeler and Watkins, 1973; Pfeifer and Peterson, 1987). Inspiration causes an increase in heart rate; expiration leads to a decreased heart rate (Wheeler and Watkins, 1973; Pfeifer and Peterson, 1987). Low and colleagues (1990) recommend an analysis of the average of the five largest consecutive responses of eight respiratory cycles. Bennett and associates (1978) prefer to analyze only the first cycle, because sinus arrhythmia attenuates with hypocarbia, which is induced by continued hyperventilation (Borgdorff, 1975; Hirayama et al., 1995). The breathing cycle with the greatest difference between maximal and minimal heart rate can be chosen for analysis of respiratory arrhythmia, although the analysis of a single respiratory cycle may yield indices less reproducible than those obtained by the analysis of averaged responses (Espi et al., 1982; Wieling, 1983). Usually, the minimum and maximum heart rates during a breathing cycle are determined, and the difference between maximum and minimum heart rates (expiratory-inspiratory difference) or the expiratory/inspiratory ratio is calculated (Genovely and Pfeifer, 1988). In addition, the mean circular resultant—a parameter resistant to biases of heart rate variability such as intrinsic heart rate, a gradual change in heart rate, or ectopic heartbeats—can be calculated with the use of vector analysis (Weinberg and Pfeifer, 1984; Genovely and Pfeifer, 1988). For this determination, R-R intervals are considered to be time events and are wrapped around a circle with the periodicity of one breath. The procedure is repeated with subsequent breaths. If the points of the time intervals are clustered on the circle, the vector is large and the heart rate variability is normal. An even distribution of events around the circle results in a small vector and indicates reduced heart rate variability (Weinberg and Pfeifer, 1984).

Heart rate variability during deep breathing is influenced by the position of the study participant, the rate and depth of breathing, hypocapnia, sympathetic activity, the use of salicylates and other drugs, and body weight (Pfeifer et al., 1982; Low, 1997). The heart rate variability decreases with age and with higher resting heart rates (Smith and Smith, 1981; Ewing et al., 1985). Therefore, single reference values are often misleading, and age-matched control data are required (Freeman, 1997). An expiratory-inspiratory difference exceeding 15 beats per minute is considered normal (Mackay et al., 1980). Expiratory-inspiratory differences of less than 10 beats per minute are considered abnormal in subjects younger than 40 years (Persson and Solders, 1983). Differences of less than 5 beats per minute are abnormal in persons older than 50 years (Wheeler and Watkins, 1973). The expiratory-inspiratory ratio should be greater than 1.23 for subjects younger than 20 years or greater than 1.06 for subjects aged 76 to 80 years (Smith, 1982).

Sustained Handgrip Test

The sustained handgrip test can be used as a clinical test of sympathetic autonomic dysfunction. Handgrip is maintained for a period of 3 to 5 minutes at 30% of the maximum voluntary contraction with the use of a handgrip dynamometer. During muscle contraction, there is increased muscle sympathetic activity and vasoconstriction. Blood pressure rises due to increased peripheral resistance and cardiac output. Early heart rate acceleration results from vagal withdrawal, whereas sympathetic activation accounts for the late acceleration (Borst et al., 1972; Low, 1997). The difference between diastolic blood pressure just before release of the handgrip and that before the onset of the effort is taken as the measure of response (Ewing and Clarke, 1982, 1987; Ewing et al., 1985). Normally, the isometric muscle contraction raises diastolic blood pressure by at least 16 mm Hg; a rise of 10 mm Hg or less is considered an abnormal response. In patients with central or efferent lesions, the maneuver does not adequately elevate diastolic blood pressure (Mathias and Bannister, 1993). Subjects must avoid a Valsalva maneuver during the handgrip (Oribe, 1999). Blood pressure can be measured discontinuously (i.e., every minute), but the test is of limited reproducibility, sensitivity, and specificity (Low, 1997).

ASSESSMENT OF ORTHOSTATIC TOLERANCE BY ACTIVE STANDING AND PASSIVE HEAD-UP TILT

Orthostatic tolerance can be tested during active standing up (Ewing maneuver) or passive head-up tilt. The change from the supine to the upright position induces a rapid redistribution of 300 to 900 mL of blood from the central vessels to those of the dependent limbs (Sjostrandt, 1952; Borst et al., 1982; Blomqvist and Stone, 1984; Rowell, 1993). Commonly, the cardiovascular adjustments after the assumption of the upright position are divided into (1) an initial response, mainly occurring during the first 30 seconds; (2) an early phase of circulatory stabilization after 1 to 2 minutes of orthostatic challenge; and (3) the response to prolonged orthostasis exceeding 5 minutes (Wieling, 1993; Wieling and Lieshout, 1997).

In contrast to the initial cardiovascular responses, adjustments in the early phase of stabilization and during prolonged orthostasis are similar for active standing and the passive tilt test (Wieling and Karemaker, 1999). Therefore, passive tilt testing is preferred over active standing for the evaluation of neural control during long-duration orthostatic stress (e.g., to assess neurocardiogenic syncope) and for the examination of patients with disabilities such as lower limb weakness, because the patients are under better control and can be readily returned to the supine position if necessary (Wieling and Karemaker, 1999).

Active Standing

Active standing is better suited than passive tilt for the assessment of neural responses during the initial phase of orthostasis (Wieling and Karemaker, 1999).

In contrast to passive tilt, active standing induces a contraction of abdominal and leg muscles with a subsequent compression of resistance and capacitance vessels and an increase in intra-abdominal pressure (Blomqvist and Stone, 1984; Tanaka, 1996; Wieling and Lieshout, 1997; Wieling and Karemaker, 1999). This results in increased venous return and cardiac output, which, however, do not fully compensate for a drop in total peripheral resistance on standing but not during passive tilt. This decrease in peripheral resistance seems to be related to the muscle activation and the subsequent flow increase in the muscles (Wieling and Lieshout, 1997) and accounts for a transient fall in blood pressure on active standing (Wieling, 1993; Wieling and Lieshout, 1997). Muscle contraction induces an exercise reflex–mediated rapid withdrawal of cardiovagal activity and results in heart rate acceleration within the first 3 seconds after a change in posture. The decrease in peripheral resistance induces a brief fall in blood pressure. The subsequent reduction in baroreceptor activation results in a continued inhibition of cardiovagal tone and an increase in sympathetic tone, both generating a secondary, more gradual rise in heart rate (Wieling, 1993; Wieling and Lieshout, 1997). After approximately 7 seconds, the decreased stimulation of baroreceptors and cardiopulmonary receptors results in blood pressure recovery. In healthy adults, there even is a blood pressure overshoot.

The initial trough and the subsequent overshoot of systolic and diastolic blood pressures during the early phase after standing up can be continuously recorded by means of noninvasive radial artery tonometry (Colin Pilot; Colin Medical Instruments Corp., San Antonio, TX) or finger plethysmography (PortapressM2; TNO-TPD Biomedical Instrumentation, Amsterdam, The Netherlands). Some consider an initial fall of more than 40 mm Hg in systolic blood pressure, more than 25 mm Hg in diastolic blood pressure, or both as an abnormal response (Lindqvist et al., 1997; Wieling and Karemaker, 1999). Lindqvist and associates (1997) suggest that the absence of an overshoot after the trough is a sign of sympathetic vasomotor dysfunction. Within 30 seconds after standing up, both blood pressure and heart rate are normalized (Wieling, 1993; Wieling and Lieshout, 1997).

To evaluate the initial cardiac responses to active standing up, Ewing and colleagues introduced the 30:15 heart rate ratio (Ewing and Clarke, 1982; Ewing et al., 1985). The index calculates the ratio between the shortest R-R interval at or around the 15th heartbeat and the longest R-R interval at or around the 30th heartbeat after standing up (Ziegler et al., 1992). Atropine abolishes the bradycardiac response, indicating that the 30:15 ratio is a parameter of cardiovagal function (Ewing et al., 1980; Mitchell et al., 1983; Bellavere et al., 1987). Normal values are age dependent, but for clinical purposes, values above 1.04 can be considered normal (Ewing and Clarke, 1987; Ewing, 1990; Ziegler et al., 1992). In patients without the secondary relative bradycardia, responses can be quantified by calculating the difference between the baseline heart rate and the highest heart rate occurring within 15 seconds after standing up (Wieling and Karemaker, 1999). Again, this heart rate increase is age dependent. According to the reference data established by Wieling and Karemaker (1999), the initial heart rate increase on standing—after a 5- to 10-minute resting period—should not be less than 20 beats per minute in 10- to 14-year-old persons and not less than 11 beats per minute in 75- to 80-year-old persons.

The initial response to active standing is followed by an *early phase of stabilization during 1 to 2 minutes* of standing. The adjustments are similar for active and passive orthostatic stress and show a diastolic blood pressure increase of approximately 10 mm Hg and a sympathetically mediated heart rate acceleration of about 10 beats per minute but no major change in systolic blood pressure (Wieling, 1993).

During *prolonged, 5 to 10 minutes of standing or head-up tilt*, there is a steady-state sympathetic outflow, and the heart rate and blood pressure of healthy persons show only minor changes (Wieling and Lieshout, 1997). Although the initial cardiovascular responses to orthostatic challenge and the responses that occur during the early stabilization phase are under neural circulatory control (Wieling, 1993), humoral mechanisms play an additional role in maintaining blood pressure during a prolonged standing phase exceeding 5 minutes. The sympathetic system and the renin-angiotensin-aldosterone system are activated, and within minutes there is a rise in plasma catecholamine levels (Wieling, 1993; Wieling and Lieshout, 1997). In patients with volume depletion and increased orthostatic stress, vasopressin is also released to enhance renal fluid reabsorption and to further vasoconstriction (Wieling and Lieshout, 1997).

Ewing (1992) considers a fall in systolic blood pressure of more than 30 mm Hg to be abnormal. According to Wieling and Karemaker (1999), a persistent decrease in systolic blood pressure of more than 20 mm Hg after 1 to 2 minutes of standing, a fall in diastolic blood pressure of more than 5 to 10 mm Hg, or both are abnormal. According to the

Consensus Committee of the American Autonomic Society and the American Academy of Neurology (1996), a fall in systolic blood pressure of at least 20 mm Hg or in diastolic blood pressure of at least 10 mm Hg within 3 minutes of standing or head-up tilt is considered to define orthostatic hypotension.

Passive Head-Up Tilt

Passive head-up tilt is particularly suited to assess cardiovascular adjustments to prolonged orthostatic challenge (Wieling and Karemaker, 1999). During passive tilt, cardiovascular changes are more gradual than during active standing up (Wieling and Lieshout, 1997). Heart rate and blood pressure do not show a biphasic response, but there is a gradual increase in diastolic blood pressure and heart rate and no or little change in systolic blood pressure, resulting in an increase in mean pressure of 5 to 10 mm Hg (Wieling and Lieshout, 1997; Wieling and Karemaker, 1999).

The difference seems to be due to the effects of abdominal and lower extremity muscle contractions during active standing (Wieling and Karemaker, 1999). To avoid muscle activation, patients should not be tilted to the fully upright position. The orthostatic challenge depends on the gravitational stress (Wieling and Lieshout, 1997). The gravitational or hydrostatic effect corresponds to the sine of the tilt angle (Wieling and Karemaker, 1999). With a 70-degree tilt angle (sine 70 degrees = 0.94), the orthostatic challenge is almost equivalent to the upright position (Wieling and Karemaker, 1999). We prefer a 60-degree inclination (sine 60 degrees = 0.87), because further tilting beyond this angle does not significantly change the hemodynamic effects (Matalon and Farhi, 1979; Khurana and Nicholas, 1996), but higher tilt angles might activate muscle contraction and thereby mimic the effects of active standing. In contrast to active standing, 60- or 70-degree head-up tilting is not suited for the assessment of mild cardiovagal dysregulation during the initial phase of orthostatic adjustment but can be used to evaluate neural cardiovascular control during the phase of stabilization (after 1 to 2 minutes) and during prolonged orthostasis (5 to 10 minutes) (Wieling and Karemaker, 1999).

With the change from the supine to the upright position, Walker and Longland (1950) found an increase in venous pressure in the feet from 5 to 10 mm Hg to approximately 90 mm Hg. The increased hydrostatic pressure induces a progressive transudation of blood volume into the surrounding tissues. Although pooling of blood in the lower extremities is—at least in part—counteracted by the increase in skeletal muscle tone during active standing, passive tilt is more suited to assess shifts of blood volume to the lower body parts during prolonged orthostasis (Smith and Ebert, 1990; Wieling et al., 1993).

The volume shift during gravitational stress rapidly decreases venous return and diastolic filling of the heart (Mosqueda-Garcia, 1995; Wieling and Lieshout, 1997). Cardiac output starts to decrease after approximately six beats (Wieling and Lieshout, 1997). During prolonged orthostatic stress, stroke volume may be reduced by up to 30% or 40% (Wieling and Lieshout, 1997). However, baroreflex activation induces heart rate acceleration by approximately 20%. The higher frequency contributes to counteraction of the reduction in cardiac output; therefore, output decreases by only approximately 20% (Wieling and Lieshout, 1997).

Reduction in blood pressure and cardiac filling on tilting activates baroreceptors and cardiopulmonary receptors. Vagal withdrawal and sympathetic activation result in heart rate acceleration and vasoconstriction (Borst et al., 1982; Wieling and Lieshout, 1997). In addition, the increasing hydrostatic pressure in the veins of the lower extremities activates the venoarteriolar axon reflex. According to Henriksen and colleagues (Henriksen and Sejrsen, 1977; Henriksen and Skagen, 1988), this reflex might account for the increase in vascular resistance by up to 40% that occurs during standing (Wieling and Lieshout, 1997). The reflex reduces the effects of decreased cardiac output and slows fluid loss into the tissue (Henriksen et al., 1973). One of the most important responses to orthostatic challenge is the constriction of the splanchnic resistance vessels (Wieling and Lieshout, 1997). The expulsion of the blood reservoir from the splanchnic bed contributes to a sufficient venous return and to cardiac filling and therefore is essential for orthostatic tolerance (Low, 1978; Shepherd, 1986; Hainsworth, 1990; Rowell, 1993; Wieling and Lieshout, 1997).

During head-up tilt, not only do we monitor the standard parameters of blood pressure and heart rate, but also we assess cerebral blood flow velocity by means of transcranial Doppler sonography to determine cerebral autoregulation (see later), and we measure volume shifts to the lower extremities by means of impedance plethysmography (see later). If catecholamines are to be measured during prolonged orthostatic stress, adequate determination requires that an intravenous line be placed while the patient is in the supine position and that baseline levels be determined after a resting period of 30 to 60 minutes (Mosqueda-Garcia, 1995). Otherwise, the invasive procedure of the intravenous insertion might bias catecholamine levels and cardiovascular responses (Stevens, 1966; Hainsworth and el-Bedawi, 1994).

VENOARTERIOLAR REFLEX TESTING

The venoarteriolar reflex contributes to the increase in peripheral vascular resistance during orthostatic stress (Henriksen et al., 1983). The venoarteriolar reflex is a local, sympathetic, postganglionic C-fiber axon reflex with its receptors in small veins and its effector limb in the arterioles of dependent tissues (Henriksen et al., 1983; Belcaro and Nicolaides, 1989, 1991; Belcaro et al., 1989; Moy et

al., 1989). In addition to postural reflexes that involve the central nervous system, the veno-arteriolar reflex constricts arterial inflow to the musculocutaneous vascular bed after distention of the dependent veins above a transmural pressure of 25 mm Hg (Henriksen and Sejrsen, 1977). An increase in venous pressure induces antidromic stimulation of the postganglionic axon. The impulse travels up to axon branching points and then orthodromically to the arterioles (Henriksen et al., 1983; Moy et al., 1989; Belcaro and Nicolaides, 1991). According to Henriksen and associates (1983), the reflex partially compensates (by up to 45%) for the decrease in cardiac output after assumption of an upright posture. However, this response alone might not be sufficient to maintain blood pressure during orthostasis (Benarroch, 1997). The venoarteriolar reflex can be assessed by means of laser Doppler flowmetry (Belcaro and Nicolaides, 1989, 1991; Belcaro et al., 1989; Moy et al., 1989). The laser probe is positioned at the distal dorsum of the foot. Measurements should be taken in a quiet room with an ambient temperature of approximately 20° to 22°C after a period of at least 30 minutes for acclimatization (Belcaro and Nicolaides, 1989). Resting skin blood flow is assessed in arbitrary perfusion units while the patient is supine. The venoarteriolar reflex is elicited by lowering the leg more than 40 cm below the level of the heart or by sitting or standing up (Belcaro and Nicolaides, 1991). The combination of these stimuli allows differentiation of peripheral venoarteriolar reflex responses and responses that involve centrally mediated reflexes (Belcaro and Nicolaides, 1991). The lowest flow obtained within 5 minutes after a change in leg position (SF) is compared to the resting flow (RF), and the venoarteriolar reflex is calculated as $[(SF - RF)/RF] \times 100$ (Belcaro and Nicolaides, 1991). In addition, the time needed to reach the lowest flow after a change of leg position can be evaluated and used as an index of venoarteriolar reflex function (Belcaro and Nicolaides, 1991). Several authors have shown the venoarteriolar reflex to be impaired in diabetic neuropathy (Hilsted, 1979; Belcaro and Nicolaides, 1989, 1991; Belcaro et al., 1989; Moy et al., 1989). Belcaro and Nicolaides consider that increased skin blood flow and an impaired venoarteriolar reflex may contribute to distal edema and microangiopathy in diabetic patients (Belcaro and Nicolaides, 1989, 1991; Belcaro et al., 1989). Venoarteriolar reflex testing might be useful for the evaluation of drug effects on the microcirculation (Belcaro and Nicolaides, 1989; Belcaro et al., 1989). However, there is controversy regarding the sensitivity and specificity of venoarteriolar reflex testing and its usefulness as a clinical test (Low et al., 1983; Moy et al., 1989).

IMPEDANCE PLETHYSMOGRAPHY DURING HEAD-UP TILT

Increased transudation of plasma volume into the tissue of the lower extremities can be a major factor of impaired orthostatic tolerance (Brown and Hainsworth, 1999). Hickler and colleagues (1960) showed that this fluid loss might account for a reduction of the circulating blood volume by up to 15% after 30 minutes of quiet standing. Assessment of plasma volume changes during orthostasis helps to identify the pathophysiology of orthostatic dysregulation.

A noninvasive, easy-to-perform approach to determine volume shifts between body segments is the use of impedance plethysmography. Impedance plethysmography allows the derivation of volume changes in various body segments from the changes in electrical impedance when a small alternating current (1 mA, 50 Hz) is passed through stimulating electrodes above and below the segments of interest (Brown and Hainsworth, 1999). The length of these body segments does not change during orthostasis, so a change in impedance can be considered to result from a change in volume of the segment, because changes in impedance are inversely related to changes in volume (Nyboer, 1950; Self et al., 1996). Segments are defined by the position of the recording electrodes. Volume changes in the calf, thigh, and abdominal segment can be derived from impedance changes between electrodes placed at the lateral malleolus, lateral aspect of the knee at the midpatellar level, the trochanteric prominence of the hip, and the lateral aspect to the 12th rib with the stimulating electrodes at the wrist and ankle (Montgomery et al., 1988; Brown and Hainsworth, 1999). Volume changes can be derived from the impedance change and the initial volume of the segment (Self et al., 1996; Brown and Hainsworth, 1999). This volume is calculated by assuming that each segment has a conical geometry and by measuring the segment length and the circumferences at 3-cm intervals (Brown and Hainsworth, 1999).

There is a close correlation between volume changes determined by impedance plethysmography and those determined by water displacement plethysmography ($r = 0.93$) (Fleming et al., 1986), strain-gauge plethysmography (Schribman et al., 1975), and the invasive measurement of changes in plasma protein concentration (Brown and Hainsworth, 1999). Although impedance plethysmography tends to underestimate volume changes (Schribman et al., 1975; Fleming et al., 1986; Brown and Hainsworth, 1999), the technique provides a useful and noninvasive method of determining fluid shifts during orthostasis (Brown and Hainsworth, 1999).

ASSESSMENT OF LIMB BLOOD FLOW, VENOUS COMPLIANCE, AND POSTISCHEMIC HYPEREMIA BY VENOUS OCCLUSION PLETHYSMOGRAPHY

Venous occlusion plethysmography can be used to study blood flow in the forearm or lower leg (Hokanson et al., 1975; Hainsworth, 1983; Convertino et al., 1988; Benjamin et al., 1995). The technique reflects the bulk of influences on total limb blood flow arising from neuronal, local, or circulating mediators (Benjamin et al., 1995).

Arterial inflow into the limb can be measured during venous occlusion. Venous return from the tested extremity is obstructed by means of an inflatable cuff placed around the upper arm above the elbow or around the thigh, just above the knee. Intermittent inflation of the cuff for 10 to 15 seconds above venous pressure but significantly below arterial blood pressure—for example, at 40 mm Hg—ensures that arterial inflow into the forearm remains unimpeded while the return of venous blood is interrupted (Convertino et al., 1988; Benjamin et al., 1995; Blitzer et al., 1996). The inflow of blood during venous occlusion induces an increase in forearm volume, resulting in forearm swelling that is equal to arterial inflow (Convertino et al., 1988; Benjamin et al., 1995). The volume change could be measured, for example, as the rate of water displacement from a water-filled jacket (Benjamin et al., 1995). Nowadays, inflow is more conveniently determined as the increase of forearm circumference measured by means of a strain gauge (Hainsworth, 1983; Convertino et al., 1988; Benjamin et al., 1995). A mercury-in-Silastic strain gauge is placed around the forearm, at approximately one third of the distance from the elbow to the wrist, or around the calf at the level of maximal circumference (Convertino et al., 1988; Benjamin et al., 1995). The pharmacology and physiology of hand blood flow differ from those of forearm blood flow (Whitney, 1953; Scroop et al., 1965; Whelan, 1967; Benjamin et al., 1995). Therefore, several recommend excluding the hands from the circulation by means of a second cuff at the wrist that is permanently inflated above systolic blood pressure values (Benjamin et al., 1995; Blitzer et al., 1996).

Volume changes are calculated from the average of circumference changes during several venous occlusions repeated at 10- to 20-second intervals (Blitzer et al., 1996). The increase in circumference can be determined in millimeters per minute from the slope of the tangent to the line of the pulse waves after onset of venous occlusion. Convertino and associates (1988) recommend assessment of this slope from the first three pulse waves after the beginning of occlusion. The flow is expressed as blood flow (mL/min) per 100 mL volume of forearm (or lower leg) (Convertino et al., 1988; Benjamin et al., 1995) or as percent volume change per minute (Hokanson et al., 1975; Convertino et al., 1988; Benjamin et al., 1995).

Changes in arterial inflow are considered to reflect changes in the smooth muscle tone of small arteries and arterioles, provided that the perfusion pressure (i.e., arterial blood pressure) remains constant (Benjamin et al., 1995). To ensure stability of blood pressure and heart rate during a series of plethysmographic tests, measurements should be taken after an adequate period of adjustment in a quiet and warm room (21° to 24°C) with a comfortable and relaxed atmosphere (Benjamin et al., 1995). For follow-up examination, we consider it relevant to carefully reproduce the position of the tested subject.

Venous occlusion plethysmography allows an assessment of the compliance of an extremity. High compliance of the legs indicates that larger amounts of blood are pooled during orthostatic challenge or exposure to lower body negative pressure and predisposes to orthostatic intolerance (Klein et al., 1977; Tipton, 1983; Convertino et al., 1988).

The compliance of the forearm or leg can be determined by assessing arterial inflow at two different levels of venous occlusion pressure (Convertino et al., 1988). Arterial inflow induces forearm or leg swelling only until the veins are not fully distended. Then, a further pressure increase expels blood under the compression cuff (Benjamin et al., 1995). Leg or forearm compliance is determined by assessing the volume change (mL·100 mL^{-1}) at the plateau where venous pressure is equivalent to cuff pressure. Occlusion plethysmography is repeated at two different cuff pressures, such as 30 and 50 mm Hg. The difference in volume changes at the plateaus of each measurement is calculated and then related to the difference in cuff pressures (in this example, 20 mm Hg). The limb compliance is expressed as $\Delta vol\%/\Delta mm$ Hg (Convertino et al., 1988).

Another application of venous occlusion plethysmography is the assessment of postischemic hyperemia (Sax et al., 1987). Reduced hyperemia after forearm ischemia may indicate dysfunction of vasodilator reserve and of the regulation of vascular tone (Sax et al., 1987; Schobel and Schmieder, 1998).

After the conventional assessment of arterial inflow, circulation in the forearm is occluded by inflating the pressure cuff significantly above systolic blood pressure values—for example, at 190 mm Hg (Sax et al., 1987). Sax and associates (1987) evaluated the effects of 1, 3, 5, and 10 minutes of ischemia and found that postischemic hyperperfusion increases with the duration of the blood flow occlusion. Takeshita and Mark (1980) demonstrated that 10 minutes of ischemia induces maximal hyperemic flow responses. However, we share the experience of Sax and associates (1987) that many patients find an ischemic period of 10 minutes uncomfortable and might abort the test.

Postischemic hyperperfusion is determined after the cuff is rapidly deflated at the end of ischemia and then reinflated to a value above venous occlusion pressure, such as to 40 mm Hg. Peak flow responses during subsequent conventional venous occlusion plethysmography are assessed shortly after ischemia—for example, 5 or 15 seconds after release of the suprasystolic pressure (Sax et al., 1987). Normally, ischemia induces a rapid blood flow increase that is most pronounced during the first measurement and decreases with the following measurements. In patients with small vessel disease and reduced capability to increase capillary and small

vessel blood flow, ischemia induces less hyperemia (Sax et al., 1987; Schobel and Schmieder, 1998).

PLASMA CATECHOLAMINES

Analysis of plasma catecholamine and metabolite levels can be used to determine autonomic dysfunction (Polinsky, 1992). Plasma or urine norepinephrine levels are parameters of sympathetic activity (Wallin et al., 1981).

Norepinephrine is released from nerve terminals into the synaptic cleft and removed via different uptake mechanisms (Bevan et al., 1980). A small portion reaches the bloodstream. This spillover mainly reflects norepinephrine release from the nerve endings of blood vessels, whereas the adrenal medulla contributes only slightly to the plasma levels at rest (Brown et al., 1981).

Plasma catecholamines should be assessed under standardized conditions. An appropriate resting period of at least 30 minutes after placement of the intravenous catheter is needed to establish baseline values. Blood must be stored at $-70°C$ or processed as soon as possible after collection in a chilled tube (Robertson et al., 1979; Ziegler, 1989). Venous plasma levels of norepinephrine in the forearm and muscle sympathetic nerve activity show a close correlation (Eckberg et al., 1988), but steady-state levels of plasma norepinephrine cannot be obtained in intervals of less than 5 to 10 minutes, whereas muscle sympathetic activity can be monitored at short intervals by means of microneurography (Hjemdahl, 1993).

Fluctuations in plasma levels due to stress, daytime, caffeine, nicotine, drugs, or the menstrual cycle contribute to a high retest variability if standardization is poor (Hjemdahl, 1993; Benarroch, 1997).

Normally, supine levels of plasma norepinephrine (150 to 300 pg/mL) double in the standing or head-up tilt position (Polinsky, 1990). This increase is reduced in patients with autonomic failure and parallels the orthostatic intolerance of the patients (Bannister et al., 1977). Low resting levels (<100 pg/mL) can occur in postganglionic adrenergic failure, such as pure autonomic failure (Polinsky, 1988). In contrast, norepinephrine levels are normal or even elevated in preganglionic or central autonomic failure, such as multiple system atrophy (Polinsky et al., 1981; Polinsky, 1990). In both central and peripheral autonomic failure, levels fail to increase on standing (Polinsky et al., 1981; Cohen et al., 1987).

In postganglionic sympathetic failure, the impaired reuptake of norepinephrine and the depletion of norepinephrine stores account for a lack of norepinephrine increase with sympathomimetic stimulation by means of drugs such as the indirect sympathomimetic tyramine (Polinsky, 1990). Exaggerated pressor responses to low doses of direct adrenoreceptor agonists such as norepinephrine are due to denervation supersensitivity of adrenoreceptors and indicate postganglionic lesions (Polinsky, 1992).

In central autonomic failure such as multisystem atrophy, there might also be a hyperresponsiveness to vasoconstrictor substances. The phenomenon is due to a "decentralization" with altered baroreflex sensitivity (Polinsky, 1992).

MICRONEUROGRAPHY

Microneurography allows the direct recording of bursts of efferent muscle sympathetic nerve activity (Delius et al., 1972). Muscle sympathetic nerve activity transmits vasoconstrictor impulses to intramuscular vessels and therefore is closely related to the intramuscular vasoconstriction and vascular resistance (Wallin and Elam, 1997). There is a close correlation between muscle sympathetic nerve activity and plasma norepinephrine levels, although plasma concentration lags behind changes in muscle sympathetic nerve activity (Rea et al., 1990). Recordings can be obtained from peripheral nerves such as the median or the tibial nerve and—most commonly—the peroneal nerve at the level of the fibular head, with a tungsten recording electrode inserted through the perineural sheath into a single nerve fascicle and the reference electrode placed subcutaneously (Vallbo et al., 1979; Mosqueda-Garcia, 1995; Wallin and Elam, 1997). After preamplification and filtering with filters set at 700 Hz and 2 kHz, the signal is rectified and amplified, and the mean voltage or voltage area determined. Sympathetic nerve activity is determined as the number of bursts per minute multiplied by the mean burst amplitude or mean voltage area (Mosqueda-Garcia, 1995). For comparisons between different recording sites or between individuals, only the number of bursts is used (Wallin and Elam, 1997). Muscle sympathetic nerve activity bursts are related to the cardiac rhythm and show an individually stable latency from the R wave of the electrocardiogram, which results from the inhibitory influence of arterial baroreceptors (Sanders et al., 1988; Wallin and Elam, 1997). Baroreceptor denervation increases muscle sympathetic nerve activity but abolishes its relation to the cardiac rhythm (Delius et al., 1972), whereas baroreflex activation inhibits muscle sympathetic nerve activity (Delius et al., 1972). Unloading of arterial baroreceptors and cardiopulmonary volume receptors during head-up tilt, during lower body negative pressure challenge, or during the hypotensive phase II of the Valsalva maneuver increases muscle sympathetic nerve activity (Mosqueda-Garcia, 1995; Wallin and Elam, 1997), as do the hypoxic or hypercapnic activation of chemoreceptors and sympathoexcitatory maneuvers such as the cold pressor test or the cold face test (Wallin and Elam, 1997). In contrast to physical effort, mental stress and arousal stimuli have little or no effect on muscle sympathetic nerve activity (Wallin and Elam, 1997).

In contrast to muscle sympathetic nerve activity, sympathetic activity in nerve fascicles of the skin is difficult to quantify, because the skin sympathetic nerve activity occurs as irregular impulses with no clear relation to blood pressure changes or cardiac rhythm (Hagbarth et al., 1972; Wallin and Elam, 1997). Moreover, skin sympathetic nerve activity consists of a mixture of vasoconstrictor and sudomotor activities and possibly vasodilator and piloerector impulses to the skin (Hagbarth et al., 1972; Wallin and Elam, 1997).

MYOCARDIAL SINGLE-PHOTON EMISSION COMPUTED TOMOGRAPHY IMAGING OF CARDIAC SYMPATHETIC INNERVATION

The presynaptic postganglionic sympathetic innervation of the heart can be evaluated by means of single-photon emission computed tomography (SPECT) using iodine-123-metaiodobenzylguanidine (MIBG) as a radioactive marker (Sisson et al., 1987, 1988; Mantisaari et al., 1992, 1996; Schnell et al., 1996). MIBG is accumulated in the norepinephrine storage granules of postganglionic sympathetic neurons (Mantisaari et al., 1996; Druschky et al., 1999, 2000), and the uptake is qualitatively similar to the uptake of norepinephrine (Wieland et al., 1981; Sisson et al., 1987; Dae et al., 1989). The extraneuronal MIBG uptake is low and accounts for only 5% to 15% of the total myocardial uptake (Dae et al., 1989; Glowniak et al., 1989; Fagret et al., 1993; Rabinovitch et al., 1993). Animal studies have demonstrated that sympathetically denervated areas do not accumulate the guanidine analogue MIBG (Dae et al., 1989). In humans, transplanted hearts showed no specific neuronal MIBG uptake (Dae et al., 1989). MIBG uptake is reduced not only in areas of sympathetic denervation but also in regions of malperfusion or in other cardiac diseases (Petch and Nayler, 1979; Henderson et al., 1988; Schofer et al., 1988; Dae et al., 1989; Druschky et al., 1999, 2000). Therefore, influences of perfusion deficits of cardiac ischemia have to be ruled out, such as by means of technetium flow studies using technetium-99m sestamibi-SPECT (MIBI-SPECT) before a reduction in myocardial MIBG uptake can be interpreted as an index of presynaptic sympathetic cardiac dysfunction (Petch and Nayler, 1979; Henderson et al., 1988; Schofer et al., 1988; Dae et al. 1989; Druschky et al., 1999, 2000).

In our studies, preganglionic cardiac sympathetic innervation was assessed by means of double-nuclide SPECT (Druschky et al., 1999, 2000). After thyroid gland blocking with sodium perchlorate, 185 to 230 MBq ^{123}I-MIBG was injected intravenously. After 4 hours, 250 MBq ^{99m}Tc sestamibi was administered to identify eventual cardiac malperfusion. One hour later (i.e., 5 hours after MIBG injection), the double-nuclide SPECT study evaluated both the MIBI uptake pattern as an index of cardiac perfusion and MIBG uptake in preganglionic sympathetic terminals. The uptake was quantified in regions of interest, and myocardial uptake was related to the uptake in the mediastinum, the lung, and the liver (Druschky et al., 1999). Various studies showed impaired MIBG uptake or increased clearance in patients with severe autonomic failure, due mainly to diabetes mellitus, but also due to pure autonomic failure, multisystem atrophy, amyloid neuropathy, and myotonic dystrophy (Mantisaari et al., 1992; Claus et al., 1994; Hakusui et al., 1994; Machida et al., 1994; Hirayama et al., 1995; Langer et al., 1995; Nakata et al., 1995; Schnell et al., 1995). Mantisaari and associates (1996) showed a more significant reduction in the late, 6-hour myocardial MIBG accumulation in diabetic patients with clinically evident autonomic neuropathy than in those without autonomic neuropathy. We found reduced MIBG uptake in patients in the early stages of amyotrophic lateral sclerosis (Druschky et al., 1999), multisystem atrophy, and Parkinson's disease (Druschky et al., 2000). In agreement with Braune and colleagues, our results suggest that MIBG-SPECT facilitates the differentiation of multisystem atrophy and Parkinson's disease, because there is a more significant reduction in MIBG uptake in the latter than in the former (Braune et al., 1999; Druschky et al., 2000).

BAROREFLEX TESTING

The arterial baroreflex is the primary mechanism involved in the short-term regulation of arterial blood pressure. The baroreceptors are located in the deep layers of adventitia, mainly in the carotid sinus and aortic arch walls, and are the principal sensory regions in the reflex control of blood pressure (Smit et al., 1996). Afferent nerve fibers mediate baroreceptor impulses via the glossopharyngeus and vagus nerve to the ipsilateral nucleus tractus solitarius (Eckberg, 1977, 1980; Smit et al., 1996; Benarroch, 1997; Hilz et al., 2000). Reflex responses are modulated by various structures of the central autonomic nervous system, such as the caudal ventrolateral medulla, the dorsal nucleus of the vagus nerve, the parabrachial nuclei, the periaqueductal gray, magnocellular neurons of the supraoptic and paraventricular nuclei, the preoptic-anterior hypothalamic region, or the central nucleus of the amygdala (Benarroch, 1997). Efferent sympathetic impulses arise from the rostral ventrolateral medulla and are transferred to the heart and blood vessels; parasympathetic activity from the area of the nucleus ambiguus reaches only the heart (Smit et al., 1996; Benarroch, 1997; Hilz et al., 2000). An increase in blood pressure stretches the vessel walls and activates the baroreceptors, which in turn raise the discharge frequency in the afferent nerves. The central inhibition of sympathetic outflow and the increase in vagal activity induce heart rate deceleration and peripheral vasodilatation and ensure a rapid cardiovascular counterregulation on a beat-to-beat basis (Eckberg, 1977, 1980). The baroreceptor-induced modulation of vascular resistance through

changes in sympathetic activity (Bjurstedt et al., 1975; Linblad, 1977; Mancia et al., 1977) occurs more slowly (Eckberg, 1980). Blood pressure changes only at least 2 seconds after the stimulus onset (Eckberg, 1980). The heart rate responses to changes in carotid distending pressure follow a sigmoid relation (Eckberg, 1980). The resting level of arterial pressure is on the central, steep, and linear parts of this curve (Mancia et al., 1977); therefore, blood pressure changes induce a rapid reflex response. However, prolonged pressure elevation (or decrease) results in resetting the operational point of the baroreflex to the higher (or lower) blood pressure values within minutes (Eckberg and Sleight, 1992). Because the baroreflex is of such major importance in autonomic regulation, its assessment is highly important in the evaluation of patients at risk for autonomic disturbances. Several methods are available for the clinical evaluation of baroreflex sensitivity. Although the standard technique is still considered to be the pressor method introduced by Smyth and colleagues in 1969, several noninvasive, easy-to-apply techniques have been developed.

Baroreflex Sensitivity Testing During Challenge Maneuvers

Several techniques are used to evaluate baroreceptor function in response to changes in blood pressure. The most widely used techniques of inducing blood pressure changes are active standing and passive head-up tilt (see previous section), pharmacological blood pressure modification (Oxford method), mechanical carotid receptor stimulation by neck suction, and the Valsalva maneuver.

Pharmacological Approach

Smyth and colleagues (1969) introduced the pharmacological approach, or so-called Oxford method. Rapid changes in blood pressure are induced via pharmacological means, usually through the infusion of a bolus of phenylephrine. The resulting baroreflex activation generates bradycardia. *Baroreflex sensitivity* is defined as the slope of the linear regression between the beat-to-beat systolic blood pressure and R-R interval values. Normally, an average value is calculated from the best three of five repeated measurements (Smyth et al., 1969).

Smyth and associates showed that the baroreflex response to phenylephrine differs between wakefulness and sleep. The authors found a baroreflex sensitivity between 2 and 15.5 ms/mm Hg in awake subjects and between 4.5 and 28.9 ms/mm Hg in sleeping subjects.

Modifications of the Oxford technique are used to calculate the baroreflex sensitivity after sequential injections of depressor and pressor drugs (Ebert and Cowley, 1992; Rudas et al., 1999). This approach characterizes baroreflex responses over a wider range of arterial pressures than does the conventional method (Ebert and Cowley, 1992; Rudas et al., 1999).

The pharmacological techniques do not require patient cooperation and have the advantage that the applied stimuli are physiological—that is, ramps of increasing or decreasing arterial pulses (Eckberg and Fritsch, 1993). A limitation of the method might be its invasiveness. Moreover, drugs that elevate blood pressure should be avoided in patients with arterial hypertension, the method defines only baroreflex-mediated heart rate changes and cannot evaluate blood pressure responses to reflex activation.

Neck Suction

The noninvasive neck chamber method was first described by Ernsting and Parry (1957) and further modified by Eckberg and colleagues (Ernsting and Parry, 1957; Eckberg and Fritsch, 1993) and by Bernardi and colleagues (1994, 1995, 1997). During neck suction, the carotid sinus and the baroreceptors are mechanically deformed through the application of subatmospheric pressure. A molded lead collar is placed over the anterior part of the neck (Fig. 107–1). A reservoir, in which subatmospheric pressure is maintained by means of a modified vacuum cleaner, is connected to the neck collar and provides the vacuum for stimulation. Eckberg and colleagues recommended that the tested subject hold his or her breath at the end of normal expiration to eliminate the influences of respiratory sinus arrhythmia (Ernsting and Parry, 1957; Eckberg and Fritsch,

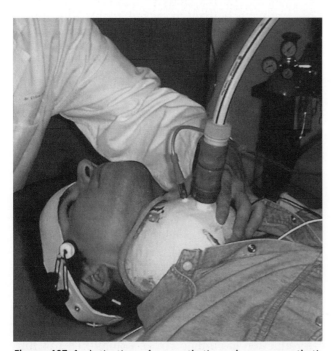

Figure 107–1. Activation of sympathetic and parasympathetic responses to 0.1-Hz baroreceptor stimulation and of sympathetic responses to 0.2-Hz baroreceptor stimulation by means of sinusoidal neck suction (0 to 30 mm Hg) using a molded lead collar.

1993). After recording a baseline for several heartbeats, neck suction is applied for a few additional beats. The changes in R-R intervals of the electrocardiogram are compared with the distending pressure. The R-R interval prolongation is calculated as the difference between the longest R-R interval during the stimulus and the mean interval during the baseline (Eckberg et al., 1975). A stimulus-response curve can be drawn after the application of several different negative pressures. Usually, pressures between −10 and −60 mm Hg are applied, and the cardiac responses to these stimuli are on the linear portion of the baroreflex curve (Eckberg et al., 1975). The slope of this curve is a measure of baroreflex sensitivity, expressed as milliseconds per millimeter of mercury.

Eckberg and Fritsch (1993) described an alternative testing algorithm. First, positive neck pressure of approximately 40 mm Hg is applied for five heartbeats. Then, neck suction is performed with stepwise (15 mm Hg) R-wave–triggered reductions in pressure to −65 mm Hg. The *control*, or *reference*, R-R interval is defined as the average of the last two R-R intervals before the onset of the pressure change. The authors determined several parameters, including the maximum, minimum, and range (maximum R-R interval minus minimum R-R interval) of R-R interval values; the maximum slope (determined from linear regression analyses applied to every set of three consecutive data pairs on the stimulus-response relationship); and the operational point of the baroreceptors (estimated as the R-R interval at resting systolic blood pressure divided by the R-R interval range, ×100%). This technique allows the study of baroreflex responses over a wider range of the baroreflex curve than does the standard approach (Eckberg and Fritsch, 1993).

The neck chamber method evaluates not only heart rate responses but also blood pressure responses to baroreflex activation. The technique does not require any medication and allows the study of the responses to blood pressure increases as well as decreases (Eckberg and Sleight, 1992; Eckberg and Fritsch, 1993). However, some patients find the chamber uncomfortable to wear. Another disadvantage arises from the superimposition of the pressure changes onto the naturally occurring arterial pulses. Finally, the extent to which the pressure changes are transmitted through the neck tissue onto the arterial wall is uncertain (Eckberg and Sleight, 1992; Eckberg and Fritsch, 1993). In addition, the responses from the carotid receptors may be buffered by opposing responses from aortic baroreceptors (Eckberg and Sleight, 1992; Eckberg and Fritsch, 1993).

Sinusoidal Neck Suction

Bernardi and colleagues (1994, 1995, 1997) developed another modification of the neck chamber method that aims at quantifying the sympathetic

Heart Rate   Blood Pressure

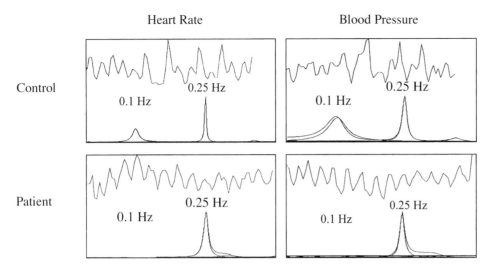

Figure 107–2. Time series and spectral powers of heart rate and blood pressure responses during baroreflex activation by 0.1-Hz sinusoidal "neck suction" (0 to −30 mm Hg) in a control and a patient with autonomic failure. The 0.25-Hz peak is due to paced breathing at this frequency. The neck suction–induced sympathetic blood pressure modulation and the sympathetic and parasympathetic heart rate modulation at 0.1 Hz are absent in the patient, whereas there is an intact response at 0.1 Hz in the control.

and parasympathetic responses to the activation of the reflex arc. Baroreceptors are activated by sinusoidal pressure changes at the neck, ranging from 0 to −30 mm Hg. The sinusoidal pressure change activates and deactivates the carotid baroreceptors; in a normal subject, the same sinusoidal change is evident in the R-R interval, in the blood pressure, and in the midcerebral artery blood flow velocity and can be identified by means of spectral analysis of these biosignals (Bernardi et al., 1994, 1995, 1997). A slow stimulus rate at a frequency of 0.1 Hz, or six cycles per minute, induces cardiovascular responses that are transmitted to both the R-R interval and the blood pressure (Fig. 107–2); a faster stimulation at 0.20 Hz, or 12 cycles per minute (i.e., at frequencies close to the respiratory rate), are transferred to only the R-R interval (Bernardi et al., 1994, 1995, 1997). Bernardi and colleagues (1997) consider the response to fast neck suction at the level of the R-R interval to be an index of vagal baroreceptor activation and the response to the slow neck suction at the blood pressure level to be an index of sympathetic baroreceptor activation, whereas the response to slow neck suction at the R-R interval level might indicate sympathetic or vagal effects, or both, of baroreceptor stimulation on the heart. The authors base this conclusion on the following facts. First, the R-R interval is modulated by both vagal and sympathetic activity, whereas blood pressure is modulated by sympathetic outflow. Second, the vagus is able to modulate both fast and slow changes in the R-R interval, whereas rapid stimuli are not transferred onto the vasculature but only to the R-R interval, because the sympathetic system is able to modulate only slow cardiovascular fluctuations (Saul et al., 1991; Bernardi et al., 1995; Sleight et al., 1995). The standardization of the stimulus at 30 mm Hg sinusoidal swings allows quantification of the number of responses to the 0.1- and 0.2-Hz baroreflex activation. The sinusoidal suction increases oscillation of heart rate (R-R interval) or blood pressure at the stimulating frequencies. The amount of

oscillation can by determined by means of spectral analysis (see Fig. 107–2). To avoid interference between signal modulation due to sinusoidal neck suction and respiratory influences, respiration is paced at 0.25 Hz (15 cycles per minute)—that is, a frequency above the rate of stimulation (Bernardi et al., 1994, 1995, 1997).

Valsalva Maneuver

The Valsalva maneuver is used to assess the afferent, central, and efferent branches of the baroreflex arc and to evaluate the sympathetic as well as the parasympathetic reactions to baroreflex activation. The study participant is asked to breathe into a mouthpiece connected to a manometer and to maintain a pressure of 40 mm Hg for 15 seconds (Benarroch, 1997).

Responses to the Valsalva maneuver occur in four phases (Benarroch, 1997).

- Phase I consists of the first 2 to 3 seconds of expiration. Due to the expiratory pressure, the aorta is compressed, which induces a short increase in blood pressure and decrease in heart rate. These changes are mainly the result of mechanical influences.
- The ongoing expiratory pressure constitutes phase II of the maneuver. In the early stage of phase II, there is a blood pressure decrease followed by an increase in late phase II. The initial blood pressure decrease triggers an increase in sympathetic activity that subsequently increases peripheral resistance and thereby induces the blood pressure increase seen in the late stage of phase II. Due to the continuing expiratory pressure, the venous return is reduced and results in a reduction in cardiac stroke volume. This in turn induces a baroreflex-mediated compensatory tachycardia and peripheral vasoconstriction.
- Phase III consists of the first 1 to 2 seconds after

release of the strain and is a mirror image of phase I. Blood pressure falls passively and heart rate increases with the release of the expiratory pressure.

- In the ensuing phase IV, the persistent increase in peripheral resistance and the normalized venous return and stroke volume result in an increase in blood pressure. The blood pressure overshoot during phase IV normally results in an increase in mean pressure by at least 10 mm Hg, but the response is blunted in patients with sympathetic failure (Mosqueda-Garcia, 1995). The increased blood pressure activates the baroreflex and results in a reflex bradycardia.

The reflex bradycardia seen in phase IV is an indicator of baroreceptor function and the vagal innervation of the heart. The blood pressure changes in phases II and IV allow for evaluation of the sympathetic vasoconstrictor activity. The baroreflex-mediated heart rate changes can be quantified using the Valsalva ratio, which is the ratio of the highest heart rate during the expiration and the lowest heart rate during the first 20 seconds after the release of strain.

Results depend on the position, age, and gender of the tested subject as well as the duration and intensity of the expiratory pressure (Low, 1997). Low recommends that the maneuver be repeated up to four times. To ensure reliability of the maneuver, two similar responses should be obtained. Low reported age- and gender-specific normative data for the Valsalva ratio. A ratio between the maximum and minimum heart rate responses below values of 1.10 is clearly pathological, whereas some even consider values below 1.2 to be abnormal (Mosqueda-Garcia, 1995).

Baroreflex Sensitivity Testing at Rest

THE "SEQUENCE" METHOD

Beat-to-beat analysis of the continuous relationship between spontaneous fluctuations in heart rate and blood pressure reveals sequences of continuous beats in which systolic arterial pressure increases and heart rate decreases, or vice versa (Bertinieri et al., 1985; Parati et al., 1988; Legramante et al., 1999). Baroreflex sensitivity can be evaluated by calculating the slope of the regression between spontaneously occurring ramps of blood pressure increase or decrease and subsequent R-R interval increase or decrease (Fritsch et al., 1986; Parati et al., 1988). With this method, Parati and associates (1988) calculated a baroreflex sensitivity of 7.6 ± 2.0 ms/mm Hg for positive sequences (i.e., when increases in blood pressure and R-R intervals were analyzed) and a sensitivity of 6.4 ± 1.5 ms/mm Hg for negative sequences.

Significant correlations have been demonstrated between baroreflex slopes assessed using the sequence method and the "gold standard" phenyleph-rine method (Pitzalis et al., 1998). In hypertensive patients, Parati showed that the slope obtained after plotting systolic blood pressure against pulse intervals was less steep and the sequences of spontaneously occurring ramps of blood pressure and heart rate changes were less frequent than those in normotensive subjects (Fritsch et al., 1986; Parati et al., 1988). The main advantage of this method is that it is simple to apply and does not require any active cooperation from the patient. However, only a small portion of the baroreflex curve is evaluated, because there is no challenge to the blood pressure and, consequently, the baroreflex arc.

SPECTRAL ANALYSIS

Spectral analysis provides another method with which to quantify "spontaneous" baroreceptor sensitivity. The gain of the transfer function between systolic blood pressure and heart rate in the low-frequency band (0.04 to 0.15 Hz) is considered to be a measure of baroreflex sensitivity (Robbe et al., 1987; Saul, 1990; Weise et al., 1993). Robbe and associates (1987) demonstrated that this index of baroreflex sensitivity correlates significantly with the results of the phenylephrine method, especially if respiration is controlled (Pitzalis et al., 1998). The authors found similar values for the baroreflex sensitivity calculated as the gain of the transfer function between the low-frequency modulation of systolic blood pressure and R-R intervals (18.1 ± 8.9 ms/mm Hg) and for the sensitivity derived from the heart rate deceleration after a phenylephrine-induced blood pressure increase (16.2 ± 7.3 ms/mm Hg) (Robbe et al., 1987). Saul and colleagues (1991) analyzed the transfer function gain between blood pressure and heart rate modulation and calculated values of 1 to 2 bpm/mm Hg.

Both the sequence method and the spectral analysis method allow testing of baroreflexes without drug administration or neck pressure changes (i.e., without perturbation of the measured reflex) (Eckberg and Sleight, 1992). However, in contrast to the application of 0.1 and 0.2 Hz neck suction (Bernardi et al., 1994, 1995, 1997), neither technique can be used to evaluate baroreflex-mediated blood pressure modulation. The analysis of the transfer function between systolic blood pressure and heart rate is merely a mathematical approach to reflect complex relations between both biosignals. These relations might not depend only on the baroreflex function but rather on many variables, such as mechanical, respiratory, movement-induced alterations of blood pressure, or heart rate. Therefore, Saul and colleagues emphasize that transfer functions may also reflect the combined effect of baroreflex-mediated heart rate changes after changes in blood pressure and of blood pressure changes resulting from heart rate changes through mechanical coupling between the left ventricle and the vasculature (Saul et al., 1991; Eckberg and Sleight, 1992).

CHEMOREFLEX TESTING

There are close interactions between baroreflex and chemoreflex functions. Input from chemoreceptors influences baroreflex function, and vice versa (Somers and Abboud, 1994; Benarroch, 1997; Henry et al., 1998). Evaluation of chemoreflex function may provide more complete information about autonomic regulation than that produced by the exclusive assessment of baroreflex sensitivity.

Chemoreflexes are stimulated by hypoxia, hypercapnia, and acidosis. Peripheral chemoreceptors that are sensitive to hypoxia and hypercapnia are located in the carotid and aortic bodies. In addition, central structures, primarily sensitive to hypercapnia, are located in the ventrolateral medulla oblongata (Berger and Hornbein, 1989). A decrease in blood oxygen saturation activates peripheral chemoreceptors, and an increase in carbon dioxide partial pressure stimulates both peripheral and central chemoreceptors (Berger and Hornbein, 1989). A transient increase in carbon dioxide concentration in the blood activates peripheral chemoreceptors, whereas the central chemoreceptors primarily respond to a prolonged increase in the blood–carbon dioxide concentration or to changes in pH of the cerebrospinal fluid (Kronenberg et al., 1972; Chua et al., 1996; Benarroch, 1997). Chemoreceptor activation induces increases in ventilation, selective sympathetically mediated vasoconstriction, and vagally mediated bradycardia (Somers and Abboud, 1994; Benarroch, 1997). The sympathetic vasoconstriction affects nonessential muscle and splanchnic and renal vascular beds, whereas the perfusion of "vital" organs such as the heart and brain is maintained (Somers and Abboud, 1994; Benarroch, 1997).

Normally, chemoreceptor-induced bradycardia is evident only in the absence of the ventilatory response, such as during apnea (Somers and Abboud, 1994). Otherwise, the increased ventilatory response inhibits the cardiovagal outflow and results in heart rate acceleration (Somers and Abboud, 1994; Benarroch, 1997).

This cardiovagal activation is not only dampened by increased ventilation but also opposed by baroreflex activation (Somers et al., 1992; Somers and Abboud, 1994). Baroreceptor activation inhibits sympathetic as well as parasympathetic responses to hypoxic chemoreflex activation. In patients with impaired baroreflex activity, the chemoreflex responses may be disinhibited, potentially leading to fatal bradyarrhythmias during apneic episodes (Somers et al., 1992; Somers and Abboud, 1994).

In patients with sleep apnea and hypertension, it has been shown that impaired baroreflex inhibition may result in exaggerated bradyarrhythmias (Somers et al., 1992; Somers and Abboud, 1994; Benarroch, 1997). In preterm and newborn infants, an imbalance between intact chemoreflex function and underdeveloped baroreflex responses can result in severe bradyarrhythmias and may contribute to sudden infant death syndrome (Somers et al., 1992;

Somers and Abboud, 1994; Benarroch, 1997). In patients with chronic heart failure, there also is an impaired baroreceptor response that might disinhibit chemoreflex-induced cardiovagal outflow, particularly during sleep apnea and hypoxia resulting in bradyarrhythmia or asystole (Somers and Abboud, 1994; Ponikowski et al., 1997).

The sensitivity of peripheral chemoreceptors can be tested using transient hypoxic or hypercapnic stimulation (Edelman et al., 1970; Chua et al., 1996). Central and peripheral chemoreceptors can be examined through progressive stimulation (Weil et al., 1972) or through prolonged stimulation, reaching a steady-state response (Chua et al., 1996).

Testing of Peripheral Hypoxic and Hypercapnic Chemoreceptor Sensitivities Using the "Single-Breath" Method

TRANSIENT HYPOXIC STIMULATION

The subjects breathe through a two-way valve that separates the expired from the inspired air (Fig. 107–3). A nose clip prevents the person from breathing additional room air. The inspiratory port receives air from a second T-valve. Depending on the position of this valve, the subject breathes either room air or air from a 4-L bag containing 100% nitrogen (Chua et al., 1996). For baseline values, the valve position ensures inspiration of room air. Minute ventilation is recorded by means of a heated pneumotachograph, and arterial oxygen saturation

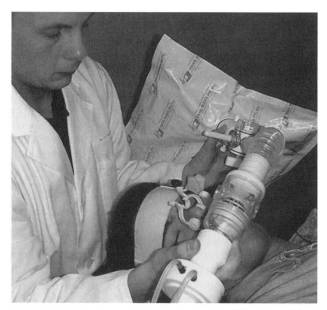

Figure 107–3. Testing of chemoreflex sensitivity using a single breathing method. The patient breathes room air through a mouthpiece until a valve (at the left hand of the examiner) connects the inspiratory port to the bag containing either 13% carbon dioxide or 100% nitrogen. Hypercapnia or hypoxia is induced by one or two breaths from the bag.

is assessed at the earlobe using pulse oximetry with a fast 2- to 3-second response time. End-tidal carbon dioxide is measured from the expiratory port at the mouth. After several minutes, the valve is turned so that the subject breathes pure nitrogen for two to eight breaths. According to Chua and associates (1996), the procedure should be repeated at least 10 times to obtain a range of oxygen saturation from 100% to 70%. Between hypoxic stimulations, there should be intervals of approximately 2 minutes of room air inhalation to ensure the return of arterial oxygen saturation and end-tidal carbon dioxide to baseline levels. Edelman and colleagues (1970) and Chua and associates (1996) recommend that the maximal ventilatory response to each stimulation be assessed as the average of the two largest consecutive breaths after each hypoxic exposure. This response is plotted against the lowest arterial oxygen saturation measured during the corresponding stimulation. The slope of the best-fit line, obtained by linear regression analysis, is a measure of transient hypoxic chemosensitivity (Chua et al., 1996). Chua and colleagues published a reference value, obtained in control subjects, of 0.293 ± 0.217 L/min per percent arterial oxygen saturation and considered a response of greater than 0.727 L/min per percent arterial oxygen saturation to be an abnormally augmented peripheral chemosensitivity (mean + 2 SDs of control value) (Chua et al., 1996; Ponikowski et al., 1997).

TRANSIENT HYPERCAPNIC STIMULATION

According to Chua and associates (1996), peripheral hypercapnic chemosensitivity can be tested using the same apparatus as described previously. After breathing room air for baseline assessment, the subject takes one (Chua et al., 1996) or two breaths from a bag containing a gas mixture of 13% carbon dioxide in air. The procedure is repeated 10 times at 2-minute intervals to ensure return to baseline of cardiorespiratory parameters. Again, minute ventilation and end-tidal carbon dioxide in the expiratory port are monitored. Baseline or control ventilation is calculated as the average of the ventilation (L/min) during the five breaths preceding carbon dioxide stimulation. The baseline or control end-tidal fraction of carbon dioxide is averaged from these same breaths. The ventilatory response to carbon dioxide stimuli is taken as the mean of the two largest consecutive breaths after the stimulus. Only breaths recorded within the first 20 seconds after hypercapnic stimulation are included in the analysis, because peripheral chemoreceptors respond to step changes in arterial carbon dioxide levels much more rapidly (within approximately 3 seconds) than do central chemoreceptors (Sorensen and Cruz, 1969). This approach avoids the inclusion of responses that might be due to central chemoreceptor activation (Chua et al., 1996). The end-tidal carbon dioxide level during the hypercapnic breaths and the ventilatory response are compared with baseline values, and the peripheral hypercapnic chemosensitivity is calculated according to the following formula (Chua et al., 1996):

$$\text{Single-breath } CO_2 \text{ response} = \frac{[V(S)] - [V(C)]}{[F_{ETCO_2}(S)] - [F_{ETCO_2}(C)] \times (Pa - 47)}$$

where CO_2 is carbon dioxide, $V(S)$ is the ventilatory response to CO_2 stimuli, $V(C)$ is control ventilation, $F_{ETCO_2}(S)$ is end-tidal CO_2 level during the hypercapnic breaths, $F_{ETCO_2}(C)$ is the control end-tidal fraction of CO_2, Pa is the atmospheric pressure (mm Hg), and 47 (mm Hg) is the saturated vapor pressure of the expiratory air (McClean et al., 1988; Chua et al., 1996).

Chua and associates (1996) consider the mean of 10 such responses to hypercapnic stimulation to be the single-breath carbon dioxide response at rest and express the hypercapnic chemosensitivity as liters per minute per millimeter of mercury.

Progressive Stimulation of Chemoreceptors

Chemoreflex responses can also be evaluated by progressive hypercapnic or hypoxic stimulation with the use of a rebreathing technique.

Study participants breathe through a closed circuit system into and from a 10-L air bag reservoir. End-tidal carbon dioxide levels are monitored in the expiratory air. A three-way valve allows redirection of the expiratory air either through a standard anesthesiology carbon dioxide calcium hydroxide filter or directly into the reservoir (Fig. 107–4). This enables adjustments of inspiratory carbon dioxide levels.

PROGRESSIVE HYPERCAPNIC STIMULATION

For progressive hypercapnic stimulation, the absorber filter can be bypassed, thereby obtaining an accumulation of expiratory carbon dioxide in the reservoir bag. The carbon dioxide concentration should be increased by 15 mm Hg. A decrease in oxygen levels should be avoided to prevent hypoxic stimulation (Chua et al., 1996). Oxygen saturation is maintained at baseline (95% to 100%) by means of an oxygen-supplying port in the inspiratory branch of the system. If the inspiratory oxygen concentration is kept at high hyperoxic levels, responses to hypercapnic stimulation are considered to result mainly from central stimulation because the sensitivity of peripheral chemoreceptors to hypercapnia is small (Chua et al., 1996).

The chemosensitivity toward progressive hypercapnia can be assessed using the slope that relates changes in minute ventilation to end-tidal carbon dioxide changes during rebreathing (L/min/mm Hg) (Bernardi et al., 1999). Results for patients and con-

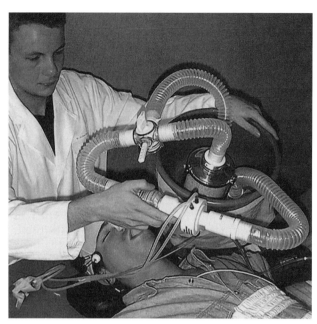

Figure 107–4. Testing of chemoreflex sensitivity for oxygen and carbon dioxide by rebreathing in a closed circuit. The filter allows the removal of carbon dioxide from the expiratory port for testing responses to increasing hypoxia. To evaluate responses to increasing hypercapnia, oxygen is maintained constant by an external oxygen supply fed into the inspiratory port.

trol subjects might require normalization by expressing values per unit body surface area or body mass index (Kronenberg et al., 1972; Bernardi et al., 1999).

PROGRESSIVE HYPOXIC STIMULATION

The rebreathing technique can also be used for progressive hypoxic stimulation. The closed circuit system with the 10-L air bag reservoir is used to steadily lower oxygen saturation. Subjects rebreathe their own expired air from the reservoir. In contrast to hypercapnic stimulation, oxygen is no longer added but steadily decreases with continued ventilation. Carbon dioxide is kept at baseline values by redirecting the expiratory air through the carbon dioxide absorber. Oxygen saturation should be lowered to 70% provided study participants can tolerate such desaturation and are not too breathless (Chua et al., 1996; Bernardi, et al., 1999). Again, the chemosensitivity toward progressive hypoxia can be determined as the slope between baseline and hypoxia-induced minute ventilation and oxygen saturation (L/min/mm Hg) (Bernardi et al., 1999).

A potential disadvantage of progressive hypoxic stimulation is that some report a hyperbolic relation of ventilation to blood deoxygenation at constant carbon dioxide levels (Lloyd et al., 1958; Weil et al., 1972), and there might be a depressant effect of prolonged hypoxia on central respiratory drive (Wade et al., 1970).

In addition to the ventilatory responses to hypercapnic or hypoxic stimulation, the various cardio-

vascular and cerebrovascular responses can be analyzed using time domain or frequency domain techniques. However, frequency domain analysis requires stationary data segments, which are not easily obtained with continuously changing blood gas levels.

CEREBRAL AUTOREGULATION

Cerebral autoregulation refers to the ability of cerebral resistance vessels to maintain a constant cerebral blood flow in the face of changing cerebral perfusion pressure, provided mean systemic blood pressure remains between 50 and 170 mm Hg (Aaslid et al., 1989; Paulson and Waldemar, 1991; Ursino, 1991; Wahl and Schilling, 1993; Low et al., 1999). Myogenic, neurogenic, metabolic, and local chemical factors contribute to cerebral autoregulation (Low et al., 1999; Hilz et al., 2000) and assure adjustment of cerebral perfusion to BP changes within only a few heartbeats (Low et al., 1999, Hilz et al., 2000). Changes in cerebral blood flow velocity (CBFV) in response to blood pressure changes can be monitored by means of transcranial Doppler sonography (Aaslid et al., 1989; Low et al., 1999). CBFV is preferably monitored from the proximal M1 segment of the middle cerebral artery. The artery is insonated at a depth of 35 to 55 mm through the temporal window above the zygomatic arch using a pulse-range gated probe emitting a 2-MHz signal (Low et al., 1999; Hilz et al., 2000). During the entire recording time, the Doppler probe must be held in a stable position by means of adjustable headbands to ensure optimal monitoring of CBFV (Low et al., 1999; Hilz et al., 2000). The integrity of cerebral autoregulation can be evaluated by various static or dynamic procedures that alter blood pressure and thus challenge the constancy of cerebral blood flow. Arterial flow equals the mean blood flow velocity in the vessel multiplied by its cross-sectional area. Various studies support the assumption that CBFV changes measured at the level of the insonated M1 segment are proportional to changes in cerebral blood flow (Lindegaard et al., 1987; Aaslid et al., 1989, 1991; Giller et al., 1993; Levine et al., 1994; Bondar et al., 1997). There is ample evidence that the caliber of the insonated segment remains invariant during challenge maneuvers (Lindegaard et al., 1987; Aaslid et al., 1989, 1991; Giller et al., 1993; Levine et al., 1994; Bondar et al., 1997).

Static and Dynamic Autoregulation Tests

Static methods assess the regression between BP as the independent variable and CBFV as the dependent variable in response to BP changes induced by infusion of pressor agents such as angiotensin or phenylephrine or by vasodilating drugs such as sodium nitroprusside (Werner et al., 1993) or by head-up tilt or lower body negative pressure (Low et al., 1999). With intact autoregulation, there is only little or no relation between blood pressure and CBFV, and flow does not regress with pressure (Low and Tuck, 1984; Takeuchi and Low, 1987; McManis et al., 1997). With deterioration of cerebral autoregulation, the relation between blood pressure and CBFV becomes curvilinear and finally linear (Low and Tuck, 1984; Takeuchi and Low, 1987; McManis et al., 1997). The slope of the regression can be used as an index of autoregulatory failure (Low et al., 1999).

Dynamic methods are based on measurement of the CBFV response to a sudden and transient BP change. The abrupt reduction of blood flow to the head challenges cerebral autoregulation. The acceleration of CBFV after the perturbation is an index of autoregulatory function (Low et al., 1999).

"Leg-Cuff" Method

Aaslid and colleagues (1989) described the *leg-cuff method*. Special blood pressure cuffs are attached to both thighs, and blood flow to the legs is interrupted for 2 to 3 minutes by inflating the cuffs to 20 mm Hg above systolic blood pressure values. Rapid cuff deflation then results in a transient hyperperfusion of the legs due to the local hypoxia and hypercapnia. This lowers systemic blood pressure by approximately 20 mm Hg (Aaslid et al., 1989). CBFV in the middle cerebral artery also decreases briefly but starts to recover immediately. After 0.5 second, there is a first significant increase in CBFV, and after 4 seconds there is a second increase in CBFV, with a consequent hyperperfusion due to the now-beginning recovery of blood pressure, which is significant only after 5 to 7 seconds (Aaslid et al., 1989). According to Aaslid and colleagues (1989), the early CBFV response used for autoregulation analysis is not influenced by hypoxic and hypercapnic blood from the legs, because the blood transport time to the cerebrovascular bed is approximately 15 seconds.

Valsalva Maneuver

Another method by which to assess cerebral autoregulation is the Valsalva maneuver. Changes in cerebral blood flow during the Valsalva maneuver closely resemble these in blood pressure described earlier. In phase I of the maneuver, cerebral blood flow increases due to the mechanically induced increase in blood pressure. However, as intrathoracic pressure increases, so does intracranial pressure. Although intracranial pressure is increased in phase II, systemic blood pressure decreases, resulting in a decrease in cerebral blood flow. In response to the decreased perfusion pressure, cerebral resistance vessels dilate due to autoregulatory mechanisms. This accounts for the increased CBFV during late phase II (Tiecks et al., 1995, 1996; Hilz et al., 2000).

Cerebral vasodilatation in late phase II coincides with an increase in systemic blood pressure re-

sulting from sympathetic peripheral vasoconstriction. Therefore, the increase in CBFV exceeds the increase in blood pressure during late phase II (Tiecks et al., 1995, 1996). The release of strain in phase III does not induce any major changes in cerebral blood flow. In phase IV, there is an overshoot of both cerebral blood flow and systemic blood pressure. Again, the cerebral blood flow overshoot results from autoregulation. After release of the strain, intracranial pressure rapidly normalizes. In contrast, blood pressure increases significantly as a result of continued constriction of peripheral resistance vessels and of increasing left-ventricular cardiac output. This increase in blood pressure induces not only baroreflex-mediated bradycardia but also an overshoot of CBFV. Cerebral resistance vessels are still dilated as a consequence of the increased intracranial pressure, whereas this pressure has already normalized. The concurrent increase in blood pressure as the driving force of cerebral perfusion therefore results in an overshoot of blood flow that exceeds the increase in blood pressure (Tiecks et al., 1995, 1996).

Tiecks and colleagues (1995, 1996) introduced indices that allow evaluation of cerebral autoregulation. They compare the CBFV increase in late phases II and IV with the respective blood pressure increases. The increase in cerebral blood flow in phase II is assessed as the difference between the early and late phase II CBFV values in relation to CBFV in early phase II. The same relation is calculated for blood pressure values. Both ratios are then compared with each other. Autoregulation is considered intact if the ratio of blood pressure to CBFV exceeds a value of 1, because the CBFV increase should be more pronounced than the blood pressure increase at the end of phase II (Tiecks et al., 1995, 1996). A similar ratio is calculated for blood pressure and CBFV increases during phase IV of the maneuver. Phase IV increases are now compared with values during phase I of the maneuver. Again, the ratio should exceed 1 if autoregulation is intact (Tiecks et al., 1996) (Fig. 107–5).

Low and associates (1999) prefer a different approach; they suggest that the parameters used by Tiecks and colleagues are biased by changes in intracranial pressure. Because intracranial pressure cannot be readily measured, it is an unknown variable.

Low and associates (1999) suggest analysis of the recovery of phase IV of the maneuver, because it is no longer biased by changes in intracranial pressure. The authors consider the restoration of CBFV from the peak of phase IV to baseline values to reflect autoregulatory function. They therefore recommend determination of the duration of this recovery interval to assess the integral from this CBFV phase IV peak to baseline and to calculate the slope of the CBFV-versus-time relationship. The authors demonstrated that the recovery of CBFV after the peak of phase IV is delayed in patients with postural

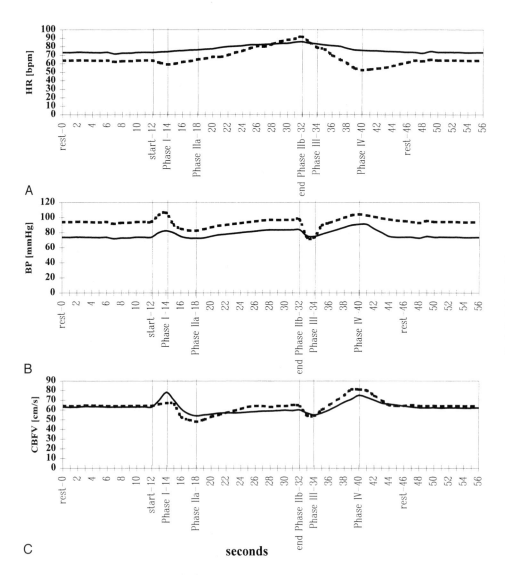

Figure 107–5. Averaged responses of heart rate (HR) *(A)*, blood pressure (BP) *(B)*, and cerebral blood flow velocity (CBFV) *(C)* during Valsalva maneuver in a group of controls *(broken line)* and attenuated responses in a group of patients with autonomic dysfunction *(continuous line)*.

orthostatic tachycardia syndrome in comparison with control subjects.

We suggest a comparison of the CBFV parameters recommended by Low and associates (1999) with corresponding parameters of the blood pressure recovery curve after the peak of phase IV of the maneuver. If the CBFV recovery from the blood pressure perturbation is a more reliable index of autoregulation than are the responses during phases II and IV (Low et al., 1999), the CBFV should normalize more rapidly than blood pressure.

Analysis of Coherence and Phase Relations Between Blood Pressure and Cerebral Blood Flow

The dynamics of autoregulation can be compared with a high-pass filter (Diehl et al., 1995). Rapid blood pressure perturbations are transferred to CBFV, whereas slow blood pressure changes are dampened (Diehl et al., 1995). Because cerebral au-

toregulation is a frequency-dependent phenomenon (Zhang et al., 1998a), its function can be evaluated by comparing blood pressure and CBFV oscillations in the frequency domain (Diehl et al., 1995; Zhang et al., 1998a). Transfer function analysis with blood pressure as the input signal and cerebral blood flow as the output signal (Nichols et al., 1996; Zhang et al., 1998) can be used to compare the gain between both variables (Zhang et al., 1998). If autoregulation is functioning effectively, spontaneously occurring changes in blood pressure should only minimally influence cerebral blood flow; that is, there should be little coherence between both variables, or the transfer function between the parameters should have only a small gain. Conversely, a high gain indicates deficient cerebral autoregulation (Nichols et al., 1996; Zhang et al., 1998b).

Diehl and associates (1995) proposed a simple clinical test for the assessment of cerebral autoregulation. Patients are instructed to breathe metronomically at a rate of six breaths per minute. This respiratory pattern induces 0.1-Hz oscillations of blood pressure. Changes in blood pressure generate similar CBVF fluctuations that are dampened and shifted to the left due to the high-pass filter characteristics of autoregulatory mechanisms (Diehl et al., 1995). Increasing blood pressure activates autoregulation, which ensures counterregulation of the vascular resistance bed with vasoconstriction. The counterregulation causes CBFV to be maximal before blood pressure oscillation has reached its maximum. While blood pressure approaches its maximum, the autoregulatory responses already start to slow CBFV. When blood pressure finally declines, CBFV declines even faster because of the continued response to the preceding blood pressure increase. As blood pressure further declines, autoregulation opposes the slowing of CBFV by dilating the resistance bed. Again, CBFV reaches its minimum before blood pressure is at its lowest value, and CBFV recovers before the next rise in blood pressure. Therefore, the relation between blood pressure and CBFV oscillations can be described by calculating the phase shift between the leading CBFV and the lagging blood pressure signal (Diehl et al., 1995). With intact autoregulation, Diehl and associates (1995) found a phase angle of approximately 70 degrees between the maxima (or minima) of blood pressure and CBFV undulations. The authors consider a phase angle of 30 degrees to be the lower normal limit. The phase angle is reduced with impaired autoregulation, such as in high-grade stenosis of the middle cerebral arteries, where CBFV is passively driven by blood pressure changes (Diehl et al., 1995). This phase angle could be determined in the time domain by calculating the interval between

the maxima or minima of the 0.1-Hz fluctuations in the CBFV and blood pressure signals (Diehl et al., 1995; Diehl and Berlit, 1996). Because an interval of 10 seconds corresponds to one full cycle of paced breathing (360 degrees), a 2-second interval between a CBFV and the blood pressure maximum would be equivalent to a 72-degree phase shift between both signals (Diehl et al., 1995; Diehl and Berlit, 1996). The calculation is more conveniently performed by means of spectral analysis provided there is sufficient coherence between the paced signals (Diehl et al., 1995; Diehl and Berlit, 1996) (Fig. 107–6).

ASSESSMENT OF AUTONOMIC FUNCTION IN OTHER ORGANS

The aforementioned procedures evaluate cardiovascular and cerebrovascular responses to autonomic challenge. Assessment of autonomic dysfunction of other organs requires additional tests, not all of which can be addressed in this chapter. Among the more important procedures are methods that evaluate sudomotor reagibility and skin blood flow changes during autonomic activation. According to the criteria of the American Diabetes Association (1988), diabetic autonomic neuropathy is characterized by both cardiovascular autonomic dysfunction and impaired sudomotor function. The evaluation of autonomic influences on skin perfusion or sweat output is an important diagnostic element for the assessment of many autonomic disorders.

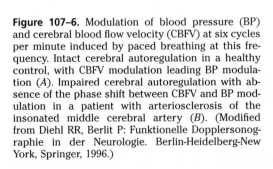

Figure 107–6. Modulation of blood pressure (BP) and cerebral blood flow velocity (CBFV) at six cycles per minute induced by paced breathing at this frequency. Intact cerebral autoregulation in a healthy control, with CBFV modulation leading BP modulation (*A*). Impaired cerebral autoregulation with absence of the phase shift between CBFV and BP modulation in a patient with arteriosclerosis of the insonated middle cerebral artery (*B*). (Modified from Diehl RR, Berlit P: Funktionelle Dopplersonographie in der Neurologie. Berlin-Heidelberg-New York, Springer, 1996.)

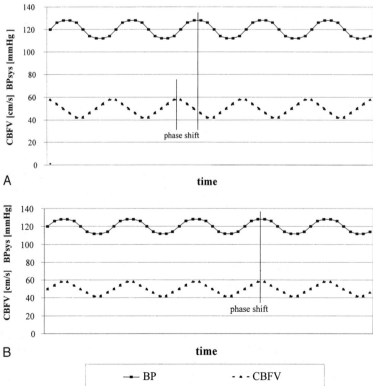

THERMOREGULATORY SWEAT TEST

The thermoregulatory sweat test evaluates the central and peripheral structures involved in sympathetic sudomotor function (Fealey et al., 1989; Fealey, 1997).

The patient's skin surface is dusted with an indicator powder that changes color when it becomes wet (Fealey et al., 1989; Fealey, 1997). In a sweat cabinet, the patient's body core temperature is elevated using overhead infrared heaters (Fealey et al., 1989; Fealey, 1997). The cabinet should have an air temperature of 45° to 50°C and humidity of 35% to 40% (Fealey et al., 1989; Fealey, 1997). After an approximate heating time of 45 to 65 minutes (Fealey, 1997), oral temperature must increase to at least 38.0°C, or by 1.0°C (Bannister et al., 1967; Cohen et al., 1987; Fealey, 1997) but should not be raised above 38.5°C (Fealey, 1997).

Areas of abnormal sweating are documented photographically or on an anatomical drawing and are estimated as anterior body surface percentage (Cohen et al., 1987; Fealey, 1997). The thermoregulatory sweat test allows assessment and monitoring of autonomic dysfunction in various disorders, such as primary autonomic failure and central and peripheral secondary autonomic dysfunction due to neuropathies, myelopathy, surgical sympathectomy, and skin or sweat gland dysfunction (Fealey et al., 1989; Fealey, 1997). In primary autonomic failure, there is widespread, global anhidrosis (Bannister et al., 1967; Cohen et al., 1987).

In central anhidrosis, the test results are abnormal, but preserved postganglionic sweating usually accounts for normal quantitative sudomotor axon reflex test results (Stewart et al., 1992). For example, global anhidrosis can be seen with hypothalamic dysfunction due to pinealism or hypothalamic tumors (Fealey, 1997). In diabetic neuropathy, sweat loss correlates with the severity of the autonomic neuropathy (Fealey et al., 1989).

QUANTITATIVE SUDOMOTOR AXON REFLEX TEST

During the quantitative sudomotor axon reflex test, acetylcholine is iontophoresed through the skin. Acetylcholine binds to muscarinic receptors on eccrine sweat glands and induces a direct sweat response. Simultaneously, acetylcholine binds to nicotinic receptors of postganglionic sympathetic sudomotor axons and activates a C-fiber impulse that travels antidromically. At branching points, the impulse travels orthodromically to C-fiber nerve terminals, where it releases acetylcholine. This acetylcholine binds to muscarinic M3 receptors of eccrine sweat glands and finally evokes an indirect (i.e., axon reflex–mediated) sweat response (Low et al., 1983, 1990, 1992; Low and Fealey, 1992; Low, 1997). Cleavage of acetylcholine by subcutaneous acetyl-cholinesterase into acetate and choline ends the sweat response (Low, 1997).

Sweat production is quantified by means of a hygrometer and a multicompartmental sweat cell. The cell contains the inner stimulus compartment, which is filled with 10% acetylcholine as well as an outer compartment that takes up the axon-induced sweat output. The sweat output in this compartment is evaporated by a nitrogen gas flow of 50 to 150 mL/min and is carried to a thermocontrolled hygrometer. There, the change in relative humidity is continuously monitored. The skin temperature in the recording area is kept constant and should be around 34.5°C for an optimal sweat response (Low et al., 1983). A constant 2-mA anodal current iontophoreses acetylcholine from the stimulus compartment into the skin. The 4 × 6-cm cathode is attached to a nearby site. The sweat response is recorded during 5 minutes of stimulation and the subsequent 5 minutes, during which the response returns to baseline. With a 1- to 2-minute latency period after stimulus onset, sweating increases rapidly. After stimulus completion, humidity returns to baseline within 5 to 10 minutes. The area under the recorded sweating curve can be calculated as a parameter of normal or abnormal response.

The quantitative sudomotor axon reflex test is highly reproducible and sensitive toward impaired postganglionic sudomotor function (Low, 1997). Standard recording sites are the proximal dorsal foot, the lateral proximal calf, the distal medial leg, and the medial forearm. Healthy men have higher sweat responses than those of healthy women (Low, 1997).

Several test responses were described by Low and Fealey (1992) and Low (1997). According to Low, the persistent response can be seen in painful (e.g., diabetic) neuropathies or in reflex sympathetic dystrophy and might arise from enhanced somatosympathetic reflexes (Low, 1997). This test evaluates the distal, postganglionic sudomotor axon in various peripheral neuropathies and usually shows normal responses in preganglionic, central disorders such as multisystem atrophy, spinal cord injuries, and others.

The combination of the thermoregulatory sweat test and the quantitative sudomotor axon reflex test allows determination of whether impaired sweating is due to a preganglionic or postganglionic lesion.

Quantitative sudomotor axon reflex testing had depended on appropriate assembly of the technical components of the test equipment. A newly developed portable multichannel system (Q-Sweat; WR Medical Electronics, Stillwater, MN) facilitates testing and allows simultaneous assessment of responses at four body sites and automatic analysis of sweat output.

SYMPATHETIC SKIN RESPONSE

Normally, any arousal stimulus induces sympathetic sweat gland activation and thereby a change in skin resistance (Baba et al., 1988; Baser et al., 1991). The central sympathetic skin response pathway includes a complex polysynaptic, not completely known circuitry (Yokota et al., 1991).

The sympathetic skin response should be recorded from the palms and soles, with the indifferent leads on the dorsum of the hands and feet. Recording filter settings should be low, such as 0.1 to 30 Hz (Levy et al., 1992). The sympathetic skin response can be elicited by electrical, acoustic, and inspiratory gasp stimulation. The stimuli should be delivered at randomized intervals and with increasing intensities, because the sympathetic skin response tends to habituate (Hoeldtke et al., 1992; Schondorf, 1997).

The sympathetic skin response is quite variable, and there are no clear criteria as to what constitutes an abnormal response (Schondorf, 1997). According to Yokota and colleagues (1991), the sympathetic skin response is abnormal if it is absent in one of four limbs or if there is a 50% left-right amplitude difference. The advantage of this testing is its easy application as a simple screening tool (Hoeldtke et al., 1992; Gutrecht, 1994; Schondorf, 1997). However, it is not particularly sensitive in the early detection of small fiber neuropathy and most likely not in the detection of peripheral or central autonomic failure (Schondorf, 1997).

LASER DOPPLER FLOWMETRY

Laser Doppler flowmetry can be used to study skin blood flow during vasomotor reflexes, the veno-arteriolar reflex, or neurogenic flare responses.

In laser Doppler flowmetry, a narrow-band laser light beam (e.g., 632 or 780 nm) is penetrated into the skin via a flexible fiberoptic light guide. In the skin, the light is scattered by static structures and by moving blood cells. Light is backscattered from static tissue without any frequency change and from moving blood cells with a shift in the frequency that is proportional to the velocity of the cells (Doppler shift). Receiving optic fibers guide the backscattered light from different tissue structures and blood cells from the tissue under study back to a photodetector. The signal can then be processed and analyzed.

The intensity of the portion of the backscattered light that underwent a Doppler shift can be interpreted as a parameter of the number of moving blood cells hit by the laser beams. The frequency distribution is a parameter reflecting the velocity of moving cells in the measured volume. The concentration of moving blood cells in the measured volume is derived from the Doppler-shifted part of the backscattered light. The mean velocity of these moving cells is derived from the frequency distribution of the shifted light. The product of the concentration and the mean velocity is expressed in arbitrary perfusion units, which are linearly related to absolute blood flow. However, a laser Doppler instrument cannot present absolute blood perfusion in mL/min/100

g (Stern et al., 1977; Nilsson et al., 1980, 1984; Low et al., 1983).

Standardized temperatures of 34° to 35°C have been recommended (Low et al., 1983). Preferably, skin vasomotor reflexes should be studied at the finger and toe pads, because these sites contain only vasoconstrictor fibers (Roddie et al., 1957). Vasoconstriction can be induced by maneuvers such as an inspiratory gasp, standing, Valsalva maneuver, or contralateral cold pressor test. Skin blood flow changes with these maneuvers can be considered to be an approximate index of sympathetic activity (Low et al., 1983). The response to such maneuvers is diminished in neuropathies that involve peripheral sympathetic function (Low et al., 1983; Low, 1997).

The hyperemia of the C-fiber–mediated neurogenic axon flare response to intradermally injected histamine or to painful stimuli can be quantified by means of laser Doppler flowmetry (Low, 1997). The technique can be used to assess afferent C-fiber dysfunction in neuropathies (Low, 1997).

PUPILLOGRAPHY

In addition to cardiovascular and sudomotor function tests, the assessment of pupillary modulation provides further insight into an autonomic reflex system that might be affected independently from other organs (Hreidarsson and Gunderson, 1985).

Pupillary function is under sympathetic and parasympathetic control (Lowenstein and Loewenfeld, 1950; Pfeifer et al., 1982). The interplay of both systems determines the spontaneous and light-induced changes in pupillary diameter. Evaluation of the hippus, that is, the spontaneous fluctuation of pupillary diameter, and of diameter changes in response to light stimuli are noninvasive methods with which to assess cranial autonomic function.

Pupillary constriction is mediated by parasympathetic outflow and results from a contraction of the circular sphincter pupillae muscle after light stimuli or near vision. The cell bodies of the preganglionic parasympathetic neurons are located in the Edinger-Westphal nuclei in the anterior midbrain (Smith, 1993). The preganglionic neurons travel in the oculomotor nerve to the ciliary ganglion, located in the orbita 10 mm anterior to the superior orbital fissure. Here, the fibers synapse with the postganglionic parasympathetic fibers that innervate the ciliary and sphincter iris muscles (Blumen, 1995).

Light stimulation of retinal ganglion cells activates axons that travel along the optic nerve, partially cross the optic chiasma, bypass the lateral corpus geniculum, and reach the pretectal nuclear complex of both sides (Hultborn et al., 1978). The pretectal neurons activate the Edinger-Westphal nuclei of both sides and induce the parasympathetic pupillary constrictor response. The response is modulated by other structures of the central nervous system, such as the cerebellum (Hultborn et al., 1973; Tsukanara et al., 1973).

Pupillary dilatation occurs during arousal and in darkness and depends on a central inhibition of the Edinger-Westphal nuclei as well as on activation of the peripheral sympathetic pathway (Lowenstein and Loewenfeld, 1950). Dilatation is also influenced by cortical areas, such as the frontal lobe (Rasmussen and Penfield, 1948; Jampel, 1960). The sympathetic pathway is unilateral and is composed of three neurons. It originates from the ipsilateral hypothalamus and descends through the subthalamus, midbrain, and brainstem to the cervical spinal cord, where it synapses in the ciliospinal center of Budge in the intermediolateral cell column at the level C8-T2 (Morris et al., 1984; Drummond and Lance, 1987; Carasso et al., 1991).

The preganglionic pupillodilating fibers leave the spinal cord with the T1 root and, to some extent, with the C8 and T2 roots (Morris et al., 1984; Drummond and Lance, 1987; Carasso et al., 1991). They reach the paravertebral sympathetic chain via the white rami communicans and then ascend through the inferior and middle cervical ganglia to the superior cervical ganglion. Here, they synapse on the postganglionic fibers. The postganglionic fibers follow the internal carotid artery to the skull and then the ophthalmic branch of the trigeminal nerve and the nasociliaris nerve, and finally they reach the dilator pupillae muscle (Smith, 1993; Blumen, 1995). The ipsilateral course of the sympathetic, dilatating pathways accounts for an uncrossed miosis in patients with lesions of the lateral diencephalon. Ipsilateral mydriasis might result from activation of the ventrolateral hypothalamus (Hess, 1957; Carmel, 1968).

Dynamic pupillary function can be assessed by means of rather costly television systems. Photography can be used to monitor static pupil size. Infrared systems have been introduced for the precise recording of pupillary diameter (Smith, 1993; Blumen, 1995). For all types of pupillometry, the subjects should fix on a distant target to avoid accommodation, and the testing room should be quiet with reproducible background lighting.

INFRARED LIGHT REFLEX PUPILLOGRAPHY

With this technique, infrared light is used to continuously illuminate the iris and pupil. Due to different degrees of absorption, the iris and pupil reflect different quantities of the infrared light. We use a pupillograph that allows us to record spontaneous fluctuations of the pupillary diameter over several minutes as well as to automatically analyze the pupillary responses to standardized light stimuli (CIP9.08; AMTech, Weinheim, Germany). A sensor of the pupillograph, a horizontal charge coupled device line, scans the reflection of the emitted infrared light and allows identification of the instantaneously

changing margin between the iris and the pupil as a breaking point in the intensity of reflected light (Katz et al., 1987; Jones et al., 1992). The momentary diameter of the pupil is automatically marked on a video screen by horizontal bars (Katz et al., 1987; Jones et al., 1992). The changes of pupillary diameter are recorded with a sampling rate of up to 250 Hz and stored on a personal computer after transmission via an analog output of the pupillograph (Katz et al., 1987; Jones et al., 1992).

We evaluate modulation of the pupillary diameter after a period of 30 minutes of dark adaptation to a background illumination of 1.25 foot-candles (13.46 lux). Subjects are instructed to look at a target point mounted at a distance of at least 3 m to prevent the pupillary near response or accommodation adjustments (Smith, 1993; Blumen, 1995).

Pupillary light reflexes can be elicited by a standardized stimulus, such as from a light-emitting diode, with a brightness of 10^4 cd and a flash duration of 200 ms (Ellis, 1981; Katz et al., 1987). Consecutive changes in pupillary diameter are recorded for 2 seconds (Katz et al., 1987). Light reflex is assessed for each eye by averaging four artifact-free responses to light stimulation.

To evaluate light reflex responses, we assess the following static and dynamic parameters: pupil size, light reflex amplitude and relative amplitude (i.e., the percentage change related to the initial diameter), the constriction velocity, and the early and late redilatation velocities (Figs. 107–7 and 107–8). The latency and velocity of constriction and dilatation depend on the constriction amplitude, which, again, is influenced by the resting diameter of the pupil. Therefore, latencies increase and velocities of constriction or dilatation decrease with decreasing amplitudes (Smith, 1993). The constriction velocity and redilatation velocities are less reproducible than the resting pupillary diameter and the constriction amplitude (Smith, 1993). The latency and constriction velocity reflect parasympathetic activity (Smith, 1993). Redilatation shows an early, rapid recovery and a secondary, more gradual return to the resting diameter (Lowenstein and Loewenfeld, 1950; Smith, 1993). The late redilatation velocity is considered to primarily reflect sympathetic activity (Smith, 1993). The time to three-quarter dilatation reflects sympathetic activity (Smith and Smith, 1990). A delay in this redilatation is a sensitive index of peripheral sympathetic dysfunction (Smith, 1993). In darkness, the resting pupillary diameter is highly reproducible, with coefficients of variation that average 3% (Plouffe and Stelmach, 1979; Smith and Smith, 1983; Miller, 1985; Hasegawa and Ishikawa, 1989; Pozzessere et al., 1996). The pupil size depends on the degree of inhibition of parasympathetic outflow and on the amount of peripheral sympathetic tone. A decrease in sympathetic tone and changes in supranuclear inhibition seem to contribute to the decrease in pupil size seen in adults with increasing age (Smith and Dewhirst, 1986; Smith, 1993). In diabetic patients, small, dark-adapted pupils suggest a

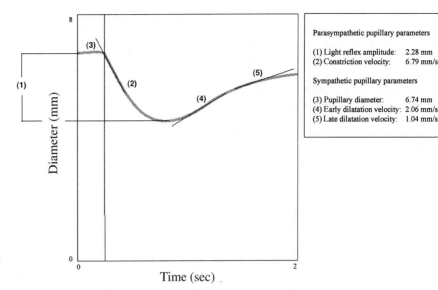

Figure 107–7. Pupillary light reflex of the dark-adapted right eye in a 45-year-old control subject.

sympathetic deficit of autonomic activity (Smith and Smith, 1983; Hreidarsson and Gunderson, 1985; Lanting et al., 1990; Smith, 1993). The absolute and relative constriction amplitudes and the constriction velocity are considered to predominantly depend on parasympathetic activity (Heller et al., 1990; Smith, 1993; Piha and Halonen, 1994). The reflex amplitude is reduced in subjects with a small resting diameter due to age or sympathetic neuropathy (Smith and Dewhirst, 1986; Smith, 1993).

An increase in the light reflex latency can be due to dysfunction of the afferent as well as the efferent limb of the light reflex arc (Blumen, 1995). The simultaneous recording of the pupillographic light reflex responses and the visual evoked responses might be useful in differentiating among afferent lesions, such as optic nerve atrophy, ischemia or inflammation, and efferent parasympathetic lesions. Afferent pregeniculate dysfunction will yield abnormal re-

sults with both tests, whereas efferent parasympathetic dysfunction will not compromise the visual evoked responses. Retrogeniculate lesions of the visual pathway will yield normal pupillography but altered visual evoked responses (Muller-Jensen and Zschocke, 1979; Lanting et al., 1990; Smith, 1993; Blumen, 1995).

In healthy persons, the pupillary diameter is not fixed, but there is an unrest, particularly when the eyes are exposed to continuous bright light (Smith, 1993). Pupils initially constrict and then redilate. During redilatation, the pupillary diameter slowly oscillates, with a predominant frequency below 0.2 Hz (Smith, 1993). This phenomenon, the *hippus* (Lowenstein and Loewenfeld, 1969), is synchronous in both eyes and seems to be centrally mediated (Smith, 1993). Hippus is reduced in patients with diabetic neuropathy, suggesting an impairment of central pupillary control (Smith, 1993).

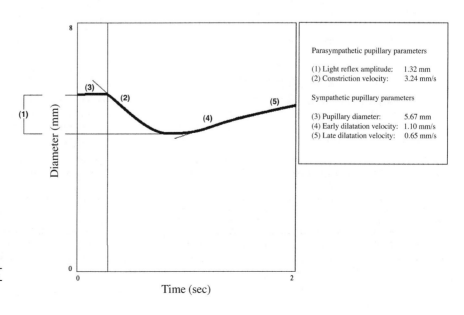

Figure 107–8. Reduced pupillary light reflex of the dark-adapted right eye in a 47-year-old diabetic patient.

Hippus can be monitored with an infrared light camera used for light reflex measurements but must be distinguished from the larger and slower pupillary fluctuations induced by fatigue and sleepiness (Yoss et al., 1969).

Pupillographic results must be interpreted with care. Abnormal parameters suggest autonomic dysfunction only if there is no concomitant pathology of the optic nerve and the pregeniculate visual pathway or of the refractory media, such as corneal scarring in the main ocular axis or cataracts. Therefore, we consider a thorough ophthalmologic assessment to be a prerequisite for a meaningful pupillographic examination. Moreover, patients should not be under any medication; for example, most blood pressure medications affect sympathetic or parasympathetic pupillary control.

SUMMARY

There are abundant additional tests with which to evaluate dysfunction of the autonomic nervous system (Low, 1997; Mathias and Bannister, 1999). In particular, disorders that affect the autonomic innervation of the gastrointestinal tract or the urogenital system require specific expertise with special techniques that are beyond the scope of this chapter.

In clinical trials, the quantitative testing of autonomic function should rely on easy-to-perform procedures with high reproducibility and low interinvestigator variability. Most of the procedures described in this chapter can be well standardized and therefore are suited for multicenter studies and studies that involve follow-up examinations of disease progression.

Acknowledgments

The author thanks Drs. C. Brown, M. Deutsch, H. Marthol, and B. Stemper for their generous assistance in the preparation of the manuscript.

References

Aaslid R, Lindegaard KF, Sorteberg W, Nornes H: Cerebral autoregulation dynamics in humans. Stroke 1989;20:45–52.

Aaslid R, Newell DW, Stooss R, et al: Assessment of cerebral autoregulation dynamics from simultaneous arterial and venous transcranial Doppler recordings in humans. Stroke 1991; 22:1148–1154.

American Diabetes Association: Report and recommendations of the San Antonio Conference on Diabetic Neuropathy. Diabetes Care 1988;11:592–597.

Akselrod S, Gordon D, Ubel FA, et al: Power spectrum analysis of heart rate fluctuation: A quantitative probe of beat-to-beat cardiovascular control. Science 1981; 213:220–222.

Angelone A, Coulter N: Respiratory sinus arrhythmia: A frequency dependent phenomenon. J Appl Physiol 1964;19:479–482.

Appel ML, Berger RD, Saul JP, et al: Beat to beat variability in cardio vascular variables: Noise or music? J Am Coll Cardiol 1989; 14:1139–1148.

Baba M, Watahiki Y, Matsunaga M, Takebe K: Sympathetic skin response in healthy man. Electromyogr Clin Neurophysiol 1988; 28:277–283.

Bannister R, Ardill L, Fentem P: Defective autonomic control of blood vessel in idiopathic hypotension. Brain 1967; 90:725–746.

Bannister R, Sever P, Gross M: Cardiovascular reflexes and biochemical responses in progressive autonomic failure. Brain 1977; 100:327–344.

Baser S, Meer J, Polinsky R, Hallett M: Sudomotor function in autonomic failure. Neurology 1991; 41:1564–1566.

Belcaro G, Nicolaides AN: Microvascular evaluation of the effects of nifedipine in vascular patients by laser-Doppler flowmetry. Angiology 1989; 40:689–694.

Belcaro G, Nicolaides AN: The venoarteriolar response in diabetics. Angiology 1991; 42:827–835.

Belcaro G, Vasdekis S, Rulo A, Nicolaides AN: Evaluation of skin blood flow and venoarteriolar response in patients with diabetes and peripheral vascular disease by laser Doppler flowmetry. Angiology 1989; 40:953–957.

Bellavere F, Cardone C, Ferri M, et al: Standing to lying heart rate variation: A new simple test in the diagnosis of diabetic autonomic neuropathy. Diabet Med 1987; 4:41–43.

Benarroch EE: Central Autonomic Network: Functional Organization and Clinical Correlations. Armonk, NY, Futura, 1997.

Benjamin N, Calver A, Collier J, et al: Measuring forearm blood flow and interpreting the responses to drugs and mediators. Hypertension 1995; 25:918–923.

Bennett T, Farquhar I, Hosking D, Hampton J: Assessment of methods for estimating autonomic nervous control of the heart in patients with diabetes mellitus. Diabetes 1978; 27:1167–1174.

Berger A, Hornbein T: Control of respiration. In Patton H, Fuchs A, Hille B (eds): Textbook of Physiology. Philadelphia, WB Saunders, 1989; 1026–1045.

Berger RD, Saul JP, Cohen RJ: Transfer function analysis of autonomic regulation. I. Canine atrial rate response. Am J Physiol 1989; 256:H142–H152.

Bernardi L, Bianchini B, Spadacini G, et al: Demonstrable cardiac reinnervation after human heart transplantation by carotid baroreflex modulation of RR interval. Circulation 1995; 92:2895–2903.

Bernardi L, Hilz M, Stemper B, et al: Resetting of chemoreflex sensitivity to carbon dioxide can explain respiratory arrest in familial dysautonomia. Clin Auton Res 1999;9:214.

Bernardi L, Leuzzi S, Radaelli A, et al: Low-frequency spontaneous fluctuations of R-R interval and blood pressure in conscious humans: A baroreceptor or central phenomenon? Clin Sci (Colch) 1994; 87:649–654.

Bernardi L, Passino C, Robergs R, Appenzeller O: Acute and persistent effects of a 46-kilometre wilderness trail run at altitude: Cardiovascular autonomic modulation and baroreflexes. Cardiovasc Res 1997; 34:273–280.

Bernardi L, Salvucci F, Suardi R, et al: Evidence for an intrinsic mechanism regulating heart rate variability in the transplanted and the intact heart during submaximal dynamic exercise? Cardiovasc Res 1990; 24:969–981.

Bernardi L, Valle F, Coco M, et al: Physical activity influences heart rate variability and very-low frequency components in Holter electrocardiograms. Cardiovasc Res 1996; 32:234–237.

Bertinieri G, di Rienzo M, Cavallazzi A, et al: A new approach to analysis of the arterial baroreflex. J Hypertens 1985; 3(suppl 3):S79–S81.

Bevan J, Bevan R, Duckles S: Adrenergic regulation of vascular smooth muscle. In Bohr D, Smylo A, Sparks H (eds): Handbook of Physiology. Section 2: The Cardiovascular System. Bethesda, MD, American Physiological Society, 1980; 515–566.

Bjurstedt H, Rosenhamer G, Tyden G: Cardiovascular responses to changes in carotid sinus transmural pressure in man. Acta Physiol Scand 1975; 94:497–505.

Blitzer ML, Lee SD, Creager MA: Endothelium-derived nitric oxide mediates hypoxic vasodilation of resistance vessels in humans. Am J Physiol 1996; 271:H1182–H1185.

Blomqvist C, Stone H: Cardiovascular adjustments to gravitational stress. In Shepherd J, Abboud F (eds): Handbook of Physiology, Section 2: The Cardiovascular System. Washington, DC, American Physiological Society, 1984; 1025–1063.

Blumen S: Light and ciliospinal reflexes: Pupil pharmacology, pupil cycle time, and pupillography. In Korczyn A (ed): Handbook of Autonomic Nervous System Dysfunction. New York, Marcel Dekker, 1995; 539–555.

Bondar RL, Dunphy PT, Moradshahi P, et al: Cerebrovascular and cardiovascular responses to graded tilt in patients with autonomic failure. Stroke 1997; 28:1677–1685.

Borgdorff P: Respiratory fluctuations in pupil size. Am J Physiol 1975; 228:1094–1102.

Borst C, Hollander AP, Bouman LM: Cardiac acceleration elicited by voluntary muscle contractions of minimal duration. J Appl Physiol 1972; 32:70–77.

Borst C, Wieling W, Brederode J, et al: Mechanisms of initial heart rate response to postural change. Am J Physiol 1982; 243:H676–H681.

Braune S, Reinhardt M, Schnitzer R, et al: Cardiac uptake of [123I] MIBG separates Parkinson's disease from multiple system atrophy. Neurology 1999; 53:1020–1025.

Brown CM, Hainsworth R: Assessment of capillary fluid shifts during orthostatic stress in normal subjects and subjects with orthostatic intolerance. Clin Auton Res 1999; 9:69–73.

Brown M, Jenner D, Allison D, Collery C: Variations in individual organ release of noradrenaline measured by improved radio-enzymatic technique: Limitations of peripheral venous measurements in the assessment of sympathetic nervous activity. Clin Sci 1981; 61:585–590.

Carasso R, Nisipeanu P, Blumen S, Korczyn A: Unilateral facial anhidrosis without Horner's syndrome. Neurology 1991; 41(suppl):310.

Carmel PW. Sympathetic deficits following thalamotomy. Arch Neurol 1968; 18:378–387.

Chua T, Clark A, Amadi A, Coats A: Relation between chemosensitivity and the ventilatory response to exercise in chronic heart failure. J Am Coll Cardiol 1996; 27:650–657.

Claus D, Feistel H, Brunholzl C, et al: Investigation of parasympathetic and sympathetic cardiac innervation in diabetic neuropathy: Heart rate variation versus meta-iodo-benzylguanidine measured by single photon emission computed tomography. Clin Auton Res 1994; 4:117–123.

Cohen J, Low P, Fealey R, et al: Somatic and autonomic function in progressive autonomic failure and multiple system atrophy. Ann Neurol 1987; 22:692–699.

Consensus Committee of the American Autonomic Society and the American Academy of Neurology: Consensus statement on the definition of orthostatic hypotension, pure autonomic failure, and multiple system atrophy. Neurology 1996;46:1470.

Convertino VA, Doerr DF, Flores JF, et al: Leg size and muscle functions associated with leg compliance. J Appl Physiol 1988; 64:1017–1021.

Dae M, O'Connell J, Botvinick E: Scintigraphic assessment of regional cardiac adrenergic innervation. Circulation 1989; 79:634–644.

Delius W, Hagbarth K, Hongell A, Wallin B: General characteristics of sympathetic activity in human muscle nerves. Acta Physiol Scand 1972; 84:65–81.

Diehl RR, Berlit P: Funktionelle Dopplersonographie in der Neurologie. Berlin (Heidelberg) New York, Springer, 1996.

Diehl RR, Linden D, Lucke D, Berlit P: Phase relationship between cerebral blood flow velocity and blood pressure: A clinical test of autoregulation. Stroke 1995; 26:1801–1804.

Drummond P, Lance J: Facial flushing and sweating mediated by the sympathetic nervous system. Brain 1987; 110:793–803.

Druschky A, Hilz M, Platsch G, et al: Differentiation of Parkinson's disease and multiple system atrophy in early disease stages by means of I-123-MIBG-SPECT. J Neurol Sci 2000; 175:3–12.

Druschky A, Spitzer A, Platsch G, et al: Cardiac sympathetic denervation in early stages of amyotrophic lateral sclerosis demonstrated by 123I-MIBG-SPECT. Acta Neurol Scand 1999; 99:308–314.

Ebert TJ, Cowley AW Jr: Baroreflex modulation of sympathetic outflow during physiological increases of vasopressin in humans. Am J Physiol 1992; 262:H1372–H1378.

Eckberg D, Rea R, Andersson O, et al: Baroreflex modulation of sympathetic activity and sympathetic neurotransmitters in humans. Acta Physiol Scand 1988; 133:221–231.

Eckberg DL: Baroreflex inhibition of the human sinus node: Impor-

tance of stimulus intensity, duration, and rate of pressure change. J Physiol (Lond) 1977; 269:561–577.

Eckberg DL: Nonlinearities of the human carotid baroreceptor-cardiac reflex. Circ Res 1980; 47:208–216.

Eckberg DL, Cavanaugh MS, Mark AL, Abboud FM: A simplified neck suction device for activation of carotid baroreceptors. J Lab Clin Med 1975; 85:167–173.

Eckberg DL, Fritsch JM: How should human baroreflexes be tested? News Physiol Sci 1993; 8:7–12.

Eckberg DL, Kifle YT, Roberts VL: Phase relationship between normal human respiration and baroreflex responsiveness. J Physiol (Lond) 1980; 304:489–502.

Eckberg DL, Sleight P: Human Baroreflexes in Health and Disease. New York, Oxford University Press, 1992.

Edelman NH, Cherniack NS, Lahiri S, et al: The effects of abnormal sympathetic nervous function upon the ventilatory response to hypoxia. J Clin Invest 1970; 49:1153–1165.

Ellis CJ: The pupillary light reflex in normal subjects. Br J Ophthalmol 1981; 65:754–759.

Ernsting J, Parry DJ: Some observations on the effects of stimulating the stretch receptors in the carotid artery of man. J Physiol 1957; 136:45–46.

Espi F, Ewing DJ, Clarke BF: Testing for heart rate variation in diabetes: Single or repeated deep breaths? Acta Diabetol Lat 1982; 19:177–181.

Ewing D: Analysis of heart rate variability and other non-invasive tests with special reference to diabetes mellitus. In Bannister R, Mathias C (eds): Autonomic Failure: A Textbook of the Autonomic Nervous System. Oxford, Oxford University Press, 1992; 312–333.

Ewing DJ: Which battery of cardiovascular autonomic function tests? Diabetologia 1990; 33:180–181.

Ewing DJ: Noninvasive evaluation of heart rate: The time domain. In Low P (ed): Clinical Autonomic Disorders. Rochester, MN, Mayo Foundation, 1992; 297–314.

Ewing DJ, Clarke BF: Diagnosis and management of diabetic autonomic neuropathy. Br Med J 1982; 285:916–918.

Ewing DJ, Clarke BF: Diabetic autonomic neuropathy: A clinical viewpoint. In Dyck PJ, Thomas PK, Asbury AK (eds): Diabetic Neuropathy. Philadelphia, WB Saunders, 1987; 66–88.

Ewing DJ, Hume L, Campbell IW, et al: Autonomic mechanisms in the initial heart rate response to standing. J Appl Physiol 1980; 49:809–814.

Ewing DJ, Martyn CN, Young RJ, Clarke BF: The value of cardiovascular autonomic function tests: 10 Years experience in diabetes. Diabetes Care 1985; 8:491–498.

Fagret D, Wolf JE, Vanzetto G, Borrel E: Myocardial uptake of metaiodobenzylguanidine in patients with left ventricular hypertrophy secondary to valvular aortic stenosis. J Nucl Med 1993; 34:57–60.

Fallen EL, Kamath MV, Ghista DN: Power spectrum of heart rate variability: A non-invasive test of integrated neurocardiac function. Clin Invest Med 1988; 11:331–340.

Fealey RD: Thermoregulatory sweat test. In Low PA (ed): Clinical Autonomic Disorders. Philadelphia, Lippincott-Raven, 1997; 245–257.

Fealey RD, Low PA, Thomas JE: Thermoregulatory sweating abnormalities in diabetes mellitus. Mayo Clin Proc 1989; 64:617–628.

Fleming JS, Hames TK, Smallwood J: Comparison of volume changes in the forearm assessed by impedance and water-displacement plethysmography. Med Biol Eng Comput 1986; 24:375–378.

Fouad F, Tarazi R, Ferrario C, et al: Assessment of parasympathetic control of heart rate by a noninvasive method. Am J Physiol 1984; 246:H838–H842.

Freeman R: Noninvasive evaluation of heart rate variability. In Low PA (ed): Clinical Autonomic Disorders. Philadelphia, Lippincott-Raven, 1997; 297–307.

Fritsch JM, Eckberg DL, Graves LD, Wallin BG: Arterial pressure ramps provoke linear increases of heart period in humans. Am J Physiol 1986; 251:R1086–R1090.

Genovely H, Pfeifer MA: RR-variation: The autonomic test of choice in diabetes. Diab Metab Rev 1988; 4:255–271.

Giller CA, Bowman G, Dyer H, et al: Cerebral arterial diameters during changes in blood pressure and carbon dioxide during craniotomy. Neurosurgery 1993; 32:737–741; discussion 741–742.

Glowniak JV, Turner FE, Gray LL, et al: Iodine-123 metaiodobenzylguanidine imaging of the heart in idiopathic congestive cardiomyopathy and cardiac transplants. J Nucl Med 1989; 30:1182–1191.

Goldstein B, Woolf PD, DeKing D, et al: Heart rate power spectrum and plasma catecholamine levels after postural change and cold pressor test. Pediatr Res 1994; 36:358–363.

Gutrecht JA: Sympathetic skin response. J Clin Neurophysiol 1994; 11:519–524.

Hagbarth K, Hallin R, Hongell A, et al: General characteristics of sympathetic activity in human skin nerves. Acta Physiol Scand 1972; 84:164–176.

Hainsworth R: The measurement of blood flow. In Linden RJ (ed): Techniques in Cardiovascular Physiology, Part 1. Ireland, Elsevier, 1983; 1–24.

Hainsworth R: The importance of vascular capacitance in cardiovascular control. News Physiol Sci 1990; 5:250–254.

Hainsworth R, el-Bedawi KM: Orthostatic tolerance in patients with unexplained syncope. Clin Auton Res 1994; 4:239–244.

Hakusui S, Yasuda T, Yanagi T, et al: A radiological analysis of heart sympathetic functions with meta-[123I]iodobenzylguanidine in neurological patients with autonomic failure. J Auton Nerv Syst 1994; 49:81–84.

Harry J, Freeman R: Assessing heart rate variability: A computer simulated comparison of methodologies. Muscle Nerve 1993; 16:267–277.

Hasegawa S, Ishikawa S: Age changes in pupillary light reflex: A demonstration by means of pupillometer. Nippon Ganka Gakkai Zasshi 1989; 93:955–961.

Heller P, Perry F, Jewett D, Levine J: Autonomic components of the human pupillary light reflex. Invest Ophthalmol Vis Sci 1990; 31:156–162.

Henderson EB, Kahn JK, Corbett JR, et al: Abnormal I-123 metaiodobenzylguanidine myocardial washout and distribution may reflect myocardial adrenergic derangement in patients with congestive cardiomyopathy. Circulation 1988; 78:1192–1199.

Henriksen O, Nielsen SL, Paaske WP, Sejrsen P: Autoregulation of blood flow in human cutaneous tissue. Acta Physiol Scand 1973; 89:538–543.

Henriksen O, Sejrsen P: Local reflex in microcirculation in human skeletal muscle. Acta Physiol Scand 1977; 99:19–26.

Henriksen O, Skagen K: Local and central sympathetic vasoconstrictor reflexes in human limbs during orthostatic stress. In Christensen N, Henriksen O, Lassen N (eds): The Sympathoadrenal System: Physiology and Pathophysiology. Copenhagen, Minksgaard, 1988; 83–94.

Henriksen O, Skagen K, Haxholdt O, Dyrberg V: Contribution of local blood flow regulation mechanisms to the maintenance of arterial pressure in upright position during epidural blockade. Acta Physiol Scand 1983; 118:271–280.

Henry R, Lu I, Beightol L, Eckberg D: Interactions between CO_2 chemoreflexes and arterial baroreflexes. Am J Physiol 1998; 274:H2177–H2187.

Hess W: The Functional Organization of the Diencephalon. New York, Grune & Stratton, 1957.

Hickler RB, Hoskins RG, Hamlin JT: The clinical evaluation of faulty orthostatic mechanisms. Med Clin North Am 1960; 44.

Hilsted J: Decreased sympathetic vasomotor tone in diabetic orthostatic hypotension. Diabetes 1979; 28:970–973.

Hilsted J, Low PA: Diabetic autonomic neuropathy. In Low PA (ed): Clinical Autonomic Disorders. Philadelphia, Lippincott-Raven, 1997; 487–507.

Hilz M, Stemper B, Heckmann JG, et al: Mechanisms of cerebral autoregulation, assessment and interpretation by means of transcranial Doppler sonography. Fortschr Neurol Psychiatr 2000; 68:398–412.

Hilz MJ, Stemper B, Neundorfer B: Baroreflex physiology and examination techniques. Fortschr Neurol Psychiatr 2000; 68:37–47.

Hirayama M, Hakusui S, Koike Y, et al: A scintigraphical qualitative analysis of peripheral vascular sympathetic function with meta-[123I]iodobenzylguanidine in neurological patients with autonomic failure. J Auton Nerv Syst 1995; 53:230–234.

Hjemdahl P: Plasma catecholamines: Analytical challenges and physiological limitations. Baillieres Clin Endocrinol Metab 1993; 7:307–353.

Hoeldtke R, Davis KM, Hshieh PB, et al: Autonomic surface potential analysis: Assessment of reproducibility and sensitivity. Muscle Nerve 1992; 15:926–931.

Hojgaard MV, Holstein-Rathlou NH, Agner E, Kanters JK: Dynamics of spectral components of heart rate variability during changes in autonomic balance. Am J Physiol 1998; 275:H213–H219.

Hokanson DE, Sumner DS, Strandness DE Jr: An electrically calibrated plethysmograph for direct measurement of limb blood flow. IEEE Trans Biomed Eng 1975; 22:25–29.

Hreidarsson A, Gunderson H: The pupillary response to light in type I (insulin-dependent) diabetes. Diabetologia 1985; 28:815–821.

Hultborn H, Mori K, Tsukahara N: The neuronal pathway subserving the pupillary light reflex and its facilitation from cerebellar nuclei. Brain Res 1973; 63:357–361.

Hultborn H, Mori K, Tsukahara N: The neuronal pathway subserving the pupillary light reflex. Brain Res 1978; 159:255–267.

Jampel S: Convergence, divergence, pupillary reactions and accommodation of the eye from faradic stimulation of the macaque brain. J Comp Neurol 1960; 115:371–399.

Jones D, Harris S, Scicinski S: Pupillometer for clinical applications using dual 256-element linear CCD arrays. Med Biol Eng Comp 1992; 30:487–490.

Kamath MV, Fallen EL: Power spectral analysis of heart rate variability: A noninvasive signature of cardiac autonomic function. Crit Rev Biomed Eng 1993; 21:245–311.

Kamath MV, Ghista DN, Fallen EL, et al: Heart rate variability power spectrogram as a potential noninvasive signature of cardiac regulatory system response, mechanisms, and disorders. Heart Vessels 1987; 3:33–41.

Katona P, Jih F: Respiratory sinus arrhythmia: Noninvasive measure of parasympathetic cardiac control. J Appl Physiol 1975; 39:801–805.

Katz B, Mueller K, Helmle H: Binocular eye movement recording with CCD arrays. Neuro-ophthalmology 1987; 7:81–91.

Khurana RK, Nicholas EM: Head-up tilt table test: How far and how long? Clin Auton Res 1996; 6:335–341.

Kitney RI, Rompelman O: Analysis of the interaction of the human blood pressure and thermal system. In Perkins WJ (ed): Biomedical Computing. London, Pitman Medical, 1977; 49–54.

Klein KE, Wegmann HM, Kuklinski P: Athletic endurance training: Advantage for space flight? The significance of physical fitness for selection and training of spacelab crews. Aviat Space Environ Med 1977; 48:215–222.

Kronenberg R, Hamilton F, Gabel R, et al: Comparison of three methods for quantitating respiratory response to hypoxia in man. Respir Physiol 1972; 16:109–125.

Langer A, Freeman M, Josse R, Armstrong P: Metaiodobenzylguanidine imaging in diabetes mellitus: Assessment of cardiac sympathetic denervation and its relation to autonomic dysfunction and silent myocardial ischemia. J Am Coll Cardiol 1995; 25:610–618.

Lanting P, Bos J, Aartsen J, et al: Assessment of pupillary light reflex latency and darkness adapted pupil size in control subjects and in diabetic patients with and without cardiovascular autonomic neuropathy. J Neurol Neurosurg Psychiatry 1990; 53:912–914.

Legramante JM, Raimondi G, Massaro M, et al: Investigating feed-forward neural regulation of circulation from analysis of spontaneous arterial pressure and heart rate fluctuations. Circulation 1999; 99:1760–1766.

Levine BD, Giller CA, Lane LD, et al: Cerebral versus systemic hemodynamics during graded orthostatic stress in humans. Circulation 1994; 90:298–306.

Levy DM, Reid G, Rowley DA: Quantitative measures of sympathetic skin response in diabetes: Relation to sudomotor and neurological function. J Neurol Neurosurg Psychiatry 1992; 10:902–908.

Levy MN, Degeest H, Zieske H: Effects of respiratory center activity on the heart. Circ Res 1966; 18:67–78.

Linblad B: Influence of age on sensitivity and effector mechanisms of carotid baroreflex. Acta Physiol Scand 1977; 101:43–49.

Lindegaard KF, Lundar T, Wiberg J, et al: Variations in middle cerebral artery blood flow investigated with noninvasive transcranial blood velocity measurements. Stroke 1987; 18:1025–1030.

Lindqvist A, Torffvit O, Rittner R, et al: Artery blood pressure oscillation after active standing up: An indicator of sympathetic function in diabetic patients. Clin Physiol 1997; 17:159–169.

Lloyd BB, Jukes MGM, Cunningham DJC: The relation between alveolar oxygen pressure and the respiratory response to carbon dioxide in man. Q J Exp Physiol 1958; 43:214–227.

Low P: The splanchnic autonomic outflow in Shy-Drager syndrome and idiopathic orthostatic hypotension. Ann Neurol 1978; 4:511–514.

Low PA: The effect of aging on the autonomic nervous system. In Low PA (ed): Clinical Autonomic Disorders. Philadelphia, Lippincott-Raven, 1997; 161–175.

Low PA: Laboratory evaluation of autonomic function. In Low PA (ed): Clinical Autonomic Disorders. Philadelphia, Lippincott-Raven, 1997; 179–208.

Low PA, Caskey PE, Tuck RR, et al: Quantitative sudomotor axon reflex test in normal and neuropathic subjects. Ann Neurol 1983; 14:573–580.

Low PA, Fealey RD: Testing of sweating. In Bannister R, Mathias CJ (eds): Autonomic Failure. New York, Oxford University Press, 1992; 413–420.

Low PA, Neumann C, Dyck PJ, et al: Evaluation of skin vasomotor reflexes by using laser Doppler velocimetry. Mayo Clin Proc 1983; 58:583–592.

Low PA, Novak V, Spies JM, et al: Cerebrovascular regulation in the postural orthostatic tachycardia syndrome (POTS). Am J Med Sci 1999; 317:124–133.

Low PA, Opfer-Gehrking TL, Kihara M: In vivo studies on receptor pharmacology of the human eccrine sweat gland. Clin Auton Res 1992; 2:29–34.

Low PA, Opfer-Gehrking TL, Proper CJ, Zimmerman I: The effect of aging on cardiac autonomic and postganglionic sudomotor function. Muscle Nerve 1990; 13:152–157.

Low PA, Pfeifer MA: Standardization of autonomic function. In Low PA (ed): Clinical Autonomic Disorders. Philadelphia, Lippincott-Raven, 1997; 287–307.

Low PA, Tuck RR: Effects of changes of blood pressure, respiratory acidosis and hypoxia on blood flow in the sciatic nerve of the rat. J Physiol (Lond) 1984; 347:513–524.

Lowenstein O, Loewenfeld I: Mutual role of sympathetic and parasympathetic [systems] in shaping of the pupillary reflex to light. Arch Neurol Psychiatr 1950; 64:341–377.

Lowenstein O, Loewenfeld I: The pupil. In Davson H (ed): The Eye. New York, Academic Press, 1969; 255–337.

Machida K, Honda N, Mamiya T, et al: Abnormal sympathetic innervation of the heart in a patient with myotonic dystrophy detected with I-123 MIBG cardiac SPECT. Clin Nucl Med 1994; 19:968–972.

Mackay JD, Page MM, Cambridge J, Watkins PJ: Diabetic autonomic neuropathy: The diagnostic value of heart rate monitoring. Diabetologia 1980; 18:471–478.

Malik M, Camm AJ: Components of heart rate variability–what they really mean and what we really measure (editorial). Am J Cardiol 1993; 72:821–822.

Malliani A, Lombardi F, Pagani M, Cerutti S: Power spectral analysis of cardiovascular variability in patients at risk for sudden cardiac death. J Cardiovasc Electrophysiol 1994; 5:274–286.

Malliani A, Pagani M, Lombardi F, Cerutti S: Cardiovascular neural regulation explored in the frequency domain. Circulation 1991; 84:482–492.

Mancia G, Ferrari A, Gregorini L, et al: Circulatory reflexes from carotid and extracarotid baroreceptor areas in man. Circ Res 1977; 41:309–315.

Mantisaari M, Kuikka J, Mustonen J, et al: Measurement of myocardial accumulation of ^{123}I-metaiodobenzylguanidine for studying cardiac autonomic neuropathy in diabetes mellitus. Clin Auton Res 1996; 6:163–169.

Mantisaari M, Kuikka J, Mustonen J, et al: Noninvasive detection of cardiac sympathetic dysfunction in diabetic patients using [^{123}I] metaiodobenzylguanidine. Diabetes 1992; 41:1069–1076.

Matalon SV, Farhi LE: Cardiopulmonary readjustments in passive tilt. J Appl Physiol 1979; 47:503–507.

Mathias C, Bannister R: Investigations of autonomic disorders. In Bannister R (ed): Autonomic Failure. Oxford, Oxford Medical Publications, 1993; 255–290.

Mathias CJ, Bannister R: Autonomic Failure: A Textbook of Clinical Disorders of the Autonomic Nervous System. Oxford, Oxford University Press, 1999.

McClean PA, Phillipson EA, Martinez D, Zamel N: Single breath of CO_2 as a clinical test of the peripheral chemoreflex. J Appl Physiol 1988; 64:84–89.

McManis PG, Schmelzer JD, Zollman PJ, Low PA: Blood flow and autoregulation in somatic and autonomic ganglia: Comparison with sciatic nerve. Brain 1997; 120:445–449.

Miller N: The autonomic nervous system: Pupillary function, accommodation and lacrimation. In Miller N (ed): Walsh and Hoyt's Clinical Neuro-ophthalmology, 4th ed. Baltimore, Williams & Wilkins, 1985; 385–556.

Mitchell EA, Wealthall SR, Elliott RB: Diabetic autonomic neuropathy in children: Immediate heart-rate response to standing. Aust Paediatr J 1983; 19:175–177.

Montano N, Ruscone TG, Porta A, et al: Power spectrum analysis of heart rate variability to assess the changes in sympathovagal balance during graded orthostatic tilt. Circulation 1994; 90:1826–1831.

Montgomery LD, Hanish HM, Burns JW: A system to measure lower body volume changes during rapid onset high-G acceleration. Aviat Space Environ Med 1988; 59:1098–1102.

Morris J, Lee J, Lim C: Facial sweating in Horner's syndrome. Brain 1984; 107:751–758.

Mosqueda-Garcia R: Evaluation of autonomic failure. In Robertson D, Biaggioni I (eds): Disorders of the Autonomic Nervous System. Luxembourg, Harwood Academic Publishers, 1995; 25–60.

Moy S, Opfer-Gehrking TL, Proper CJ, Low PA: The venoarteriolar reflex in diabetic and other neuropathies. Neurology 1989; 39:1490–1492.

Muller-Jensen A, Zschocke S: Possibilities of simultaneous analysis of phasic pupillary light reflex and visual evoked potentials. Electroencephalogr Clin Neurophysiol 1979; 47:239–242.

Nakata T, Shimamoto K, Yonekura S, et al: Cardiac sympathetic denervation in transthyretin-related familial amyloidotic polyneuropathy: Detection with iodine-123-MIBG. J Nucl Med 1995; 36:1040–1042.

Nichols JS, Beel JA, Munro LG: Detection of impaired cerebral autoregulation using spectral analysis of intracranial pressure waves. J Neurotrauma 1996; 13:439–456.

Nilsson G, Ahn H, Johannson K, Lundgren O: Signal processor for laser Doppler flowmeters. Med Biol Eng Comput 1984; 22:343–348.

Nilsson G, Tenland T, Öberg P: Evaluation of a laser Doppler flowmeter for measurement of tissue blood flow. IEEE Trans Biomed Eng 1980; BME-27:597–604.

Nyboer J: Electrical impedance plethysmography: A physical and physiologic approach to peripheral vascular study. Circulation 1950; 2:811–820.

O'Brien I, O'Hare P, Corrall R: Heart rate variability in healthy subjects: Effect of age and the derivation of normal ranges for tests of autonomic function. Br Heart J 1986; 55:348–354.

Oribe E: Testing autonomic function. In Vinken PJ, Bruyn GW, Appenzeller O (eds): Handbook of Clinical Neurology: Autonomic Nervous System. Part I, Normal Functions. Amsterdam, Elsevier, 1999; 595–647.

Pagani M, Lombardi F, Guzzetti S, et al: Power spectral analysis of heart rate and arterial pressure variabilities as a marker of sympatho-vagal interaction in man and conscious dog. Circ Res 1986; 59:178–193.

Parati G, Di Rienzo M, Bertinieri G, et al: Evaluation of the baroreceptor-heart rate reflex by 24-hour intra-arterial blood pressure monitoring in humans. Hypertension 1988; 12:214–222.

Paulson OB, Waldemar G: Role of the local renin-angiotensin system in the autoregulation of the cerebral circulation. Blood Vessels 1991; 28:231–235.

Persson A, Solders G: R-R variations: A test of autonomic dysfunction. Acta Neurol Scand 1983; 67:285–293.

Petch MC, Nayler WG: Concentration of catecholamines in human cardiac muscle. Br Heart J 1979; 41:340–344.

Pfeifer M, Cook D, Brodsky J, et al: Quantitative evaluation of sympathetic and parasympathetic control of iris function. Diabetes Care 1982; 5:518–528.

Pfeifer M, Cook D, Brodsky J, et al: Quantitative evaluation of cardiac parasympathetic activity in normal and diabetic man. Diabetes 1982; 31:339–345.

Pfeifer MA, Peterson H: Cardiovascular autonomic neuropathy. In Dyck PJ, Thomas PK, Asbury AK (eds): Diabetic Neuropathy. Philadelphia, WB Saunders, 1987; 122–133.

Piha S, Halonen J: Infrared pupillometry in the assessment of autonomic function. Diab Res Clin Pract 1994; 26:61–66.

Pitzalis MV, Mastropasqua F, Passantino A, et al: Comparison between noninvasive indices of baroreceptor sensitivity and the phenylephrine method in post-myocardial infarction patients. Circulation 1998; 97:1362–1367.

Plouffe L, Stelmach R: Neuroticism and the effect of stress on the pupillary light reflex. Percept Mot Skills 1979; 49:635–642.

Polinsky R: Neurotransmitter and neuropeptide function in autonomic failure. In Bannister R (ed): Autonomic Failure. New York, Oxford University Press, 1988; 321–347.

Polinsky R: Clinical autonomic neuropharmacology. Neurol Clin 1990; 8:77–92.

Polinsky R: Neuropharmacological investigation of autonomic failure. In Bannister R, Mathias C (eds): Autonomic Failure: A Textbook of Clinical Disorders of the Autonomic Nervous System. Oxford, Oxford University Press, 1992; 334–358.

Polinsky R, Kopin I, Ebert M, Weise V: Pharmacologic distinction of different orthostatic hypotension syndromes. Neurology 1981; 31:1–7.

Pomeranz B, Macaulay RJB, Caudill MA, et al: Assessment of autonomic function in humans by heart rate spectral analysis. Am J Physiol 1985; 248:H151–H153.

Ponikowski P, Chua TP, Piepoli M, et al: Augmented peripheral chemosensitivity as a potential input to baroreflex impairment and autonomic imbalance in chronic heart failure. Circulation 1997; 96:2586–2594.

Pozzessere G, Valle E, Rossi P, et al: Pupillometric evaluation and analysis of light reflex in healthy subjects as a tool to study autonomic nervous system changes with aging. Aging Clin Exp Res 1996; 8:55–60.

Rabinovitch MA, Rose CP, Schwab AJ, et al: A method of dynamic analysis of iodine-123-metaiodobenzylguanidine scintigrams in cardiac mechanical overload hypertrophy and failure. J Nucl Med 1993; 34:589–600.

Radaelli A, Bernardi L, Valle F, et al: Cardiovascular autonomic modulation in essential hypertension: Effect of tilting. Hypertension 1994; 24:556–563.

Rasmussen T, Penfield W: Movements of the head and eye from stimulation of human frontal cortex. Res Publ Assoc Res Nerv Ment Dis 1948; 36:346–361.

Rea R, Eckberg D, Fritsch J, Goldstein D: Relation of plasma norepinephrine and sympathetic traffic during hypotension in humans. Am J Physiol 1990; 58:R982–R986.

Richter D, Spyer K: Cardiorespiratory control. In Loewy A, Spyer K (eds): Central Regulation of Autonomic Functions. New York, Oxford University Press, 1990; 189–207.

Rimoldi O, Pierini S, Ferrari A, et al: Analysis of short-term oscillations of R-R and arterial pressure in conscious dogs. Am J Physiol 1990; 258:H967–H976.

Robbe HW, Mulder LJ, Ruddel H, et al: Assessment of baroreceptor reflex sensitivity by means of spectral analysis. Hypertension 1987; 10:538–543.

Robertson D, Johnson G, Robertson R, et al: Comparative assessment of stimuli that release neuronal and adrenomedullary catecholamines in man. Circulation 1979; 59:637–643.

Roddie I, Shepherd J, Whelan R: A comparison of the heat elimination from the normal and nerve-blocked finger during body heating. J Physiol 1957; 138:445–448.

Rowell L: Human Cardiovascular Control. Oxford, Oxford University Press, 1993.

Rowell L: Passive effects of gravity. In Rowell L (ed): Human Cardiovascular Control. New York, Oxford University Press, 1993; 1–36.

Rudas L, Crossman AA, Morillo CA, et al: Human sympathetic and vagal baroreflex responses to sequential nitroprusside and phenylephrine. Am J Physiol 1999; 276:H1691–H1698.

Sanders J, Ferguson D, Mark A: Arterial baroreflex control of sympathetic nerve activity during elevation of blood pressure in normal man: Dominance of aortic baroreceptors. Circulation 1988; 77:279–288.

Saul J, Cohen R: Respiratory sinus arrhythmia. In Levy M, Schwartz P (eds): Vagal Control of the Heart: Experimental Basis and Clinical Implications. Armonk, NY, Futura, 1994; 511–536.

Saul JP: Beat-to-beat variations of heart rate reflect modulation of cardiac autonomic outflow. News Physiol Sci 1990; 5:32–37.

Saul JP, Berger RD, Albrecht P, et al: Transfer function analysis of the circulation: Unique insights into cardiovascular regulation. Am J Physiol 1991; 261:H1231–H1245.

Sax FL, Cannon RO 3d, Hanson C, Epstein SE: Impaired forearm vasodilator reserve in patients with microvascular angina: Evidence of a generalized disorder of vascular function? N Engl J Med 1987; 317:1366–1370 (erratum in N Engl J Med 1987; 317:1674).

Schnell O, Kirsch CM, Stemplinger J, et al: Scintigraphic evidence for cardiac sympathetic dysinnervation in long-term IDDM patients with and without ECG-based autonomic neuropathy. Diabetologia 1995; 38:1345–1352.

Schnell O, Muhr D, Weiss M, et al: Reduced myocardial ^{123}I-metaiodobenzylguanidine uptake in newly diagnosed IDDM patients. Diabetes 1996; 45:801–805.

Schobel HP, Schmieder RE: Vasodilatory capacity of forearm resistance vessels is augmented in hypercholesterolemic patients after treatment with fluvastatin. Angiology 1998; 49:743–748.

Schofer J, Spielmann R, Schuchert A, et al: Iodine-123 meta-iodobenzylguanidine scintigraphy: A noninvasive method to demonstrate myocardial adrenergic nervous system disintegrity in patients with idiopathic dilated cardiomyopathy. J Am Coll Cardiol 1988; 12:1252–1258.

Schondorf R: Skin potentials: Normal and abnormal. In Low PA (ed): Clinical Autonomic Disorders. Philadelphia, Lippincott-Raven, 1997; 221–231.

Schribman IG, Mott D, Naylor GP, Charlesworth D: Comparison of impedance and strain guage plethysmography in the measurement of blood flow in the lower limb. Br J Surg 1975; 62:909–912.

Scroop GC, Walsh TA, Whelan RF: A comparison of the effects of intra-arterial and intravenous infusions of angiotensin and noradrenaline on the circulation in man. Clin Sci 1965; 29:315–326.

Self DA, White CD, Shaffstall RM, et al: Differences between syncope resulting from rapid onset acceleration and orthostatic stress. Aviat Space Environ Med 1996; 67:547–554.

Shepherd J: Role of vasoconstriction for circulatory adjustment to orthostatic stress. In Christensen N, Hendriksen O, Lassen N (eds): The Sympathoadrenal System: Physiology and Pathophysiology. Copenhagen, Minksgaard, 1986; 103–115.

Singer W, McPhee BR, Opfer-Gehrking TL, et al: Is there an effect of body position on the Valsalva-maneuver? Clin Auton Res 1999; 9:244–245.

Sisson J, Lynch J, Johnson J, et al: Scintigraphic detection of regional disruption of adrenergic neurons in the heart. Am Heart J 1988; 116:67–76.

Sisson J, Shapiro B, Meyers L, et al: Metaiodobenzylguanidine to map scintigraphically the adrenergic nervous system in man. J Nucl Med 1987; 28:1625–1636.

Sisson JC, Wieland DM, Sherman P, et al: Metaiodobenzylguanidine as an index of the adrenergic nervous system integrity and function. J Nucl Med 1987; 28:1620–1624.

Sjostrandt T: The regulation of the blood distribution in man. Acta Physiol Scand 1952; 26:312–327.

Sleight P, La Rovere MT, Mortara A, et al: Physiology and pathophysiology of heart rate and blood pressure variability in humans: Is power spectral analysis largely an index of baroreflex gain? Clin Sci (Colch) 1995; 88:103–109 (erratum in Clin Sci [Colch] 1995; 88:733).

Smit AAJ, Wieling W, Karemaker JM: Clinical approach to cardiovascular reflex testing. Clin Sci 1996; 91:108–112.

Smith J, Ebert J: General response to orthostatic stress. In Smith J (ed): Circulatory Response to the Upright Posture. Boca Raton, FL, CRC Press, 1990; 1–46.

Smith S: Reduced sinus arrhythmia in diabetic autonomic neuropathy: Diagnostic value of an age-related normal range. Br Med J 1982; 285:1599–1601.

Smith S: Pupil function: Test and disorders. In Bannister R, Mathias CJ (eds): Autonomic Failure: A Textbook of Clinical Disorders of the Autonomic Nervous System, 3rd ed. Oxford, Oxford Medical Publications, 1993; 421–441.

Smith S, Dewhirst R: A simple diagnostic test for pupillary abnormality in diabetic autonomic neuropathy. Diabet Med 1986; 3:38–41.

Smith S, Smith S: Reduced pupillary light reflexes in diabetic autonomic neuropathy. Diabetologia 1983; 24:330–332.

Smith S, Smith S: The quantitative estimation of pupillary dilatation in Horner's syndrome. In Huber A (ed): Sympathicus und Auge. Stuttgart, Enke, 1990; 152–165.

Smith SE, Smith SA: Heart rate variability in healthy subjects measured with a bedside computer-based technique. Clin Sci 1981; 61:379–383.

Smyth HS, Sleight P, Pickering GW: Reflex regulation of arterial pressure during sleep in man: A quantitative method of assessing baroreflex sensitivity. Circ Res 1969; 24:109–121.

Somers VK, Abboud FM: Chemoreflex control of cardiac vagal activity. In Levy MN, Schwartz PJ (eds): Vagal Control of the Heart: Experimental Basis and Clinical Implications. Armonk, NY, Futura, 1994; 403–416.

Somers VK, Dyken ME, Mark AL, Abboud FM: Parasympathetic hyperresponsiveness and bradyarrhythmias during apnoea in hypertension. Clin Auton Res 1992; 2:171–176.

Sorensen SC, Cruz JC: Ventilatory response to a single breath of CO_2 in O_2 in normal man at sea level and high altitude. J Appl Physiol 1969; 27:186–190.

Stein PK, Bosner MS, Kleiger RE, Conger BM: Heart rate variability: A measure of cardiac autonomic tone. Am Heart J 1994; 127:1376–1381.

Stern MD, Lappe DL, Bowen PD, et al: Continuous measurement of tissue blood flow by laser-Doppler spectroscopy. Am J Physiol 1977; 232:H441–H448.

Stevens PM: Cardiovascular dynamics during orthostasis and the influence of intravascular instrumentation. Am J Cardiol 1966; 17:211–218.

Stewart JD, Low PA, Fealey RD: Distal small fiber neuropathy: Results of tests of sweating and autonomic cardiovascular reflexes. Muscle Nerve 1992; 15:661–665.

Takeshita A, Mark AL: Decreased vasodilator capacity of forearm resistance vessels in borderline hypertension. Hypertension 1980; 2:610–616.

Takeuchi M, Low PA: Dynamic peripheral nerve metabolic and vascular responses to exsanguination. Am J Physiol 1987; 253: E349–E353.

Tanaka H: Cardiac output and blood pressure during active and passive standing. Clin Physiol 1996; 16:157–170.

Task Force of the European Society of Cardiology and the North American Society of Pacing and Electrophysiology: Heart rate variability: Standards of measurement, physiological interpretation, and clinical use. Circulation 1996; 93:1043–1065.

Tiecks FP, Douville C, Byrd S, et al: Evaluation of impaired cerebral autoregulation by the Valsalva maneuver. Stroke 1996; 27: 1177–1182.

Tiecks FP, Lam AM, Matta BF, et al: Effects of the Valsalva maneuver on cerebral circulation in healthy adults. Stroke 1995; 26: 1386–1392.

Tipton CM: Considerations for exercise prescriptions in future space flights. Med Sci Sports Exerc 1983; 15:441–444.

Tsukanara N, Kiyoara T, Iijichi Y: The mode of cerebellar control of pupillary light reflex. Brain Res 1973; 60:244–248.

Ursino M: Mechanisms of cerebral blood flow regulation. Crit Rev Biomed Eng 1991; 18:255–288.

Vallbo A, Hagbarth K, Torebjork H, Wallin B: Somatosensory, proprioceptive, and sympathetic activity in human peripheral nerves. Physiol Rev 1979; 59:919–957.

Wade JG, Larson CP Jr, Hickey RF, et al: Effect of carotid endarterectomy on carotid chemoreceptor and baroreceptor function in man. N Engl J Med 1970; 282:823–829.

Wahl M, Schilling L: Regulation of cerebral blood flow—A brief review. Acta Neurochir Suppl 1993; 59:3–10.

Walker AJ, Longland CJ: Venous pressure measurement in foot in exercise as aid to investigation of venous disease in leg. Clin Sci 1950; 9:101.

Wallin B, Elam M: Microneurography and autonomic dysfunction. In Low P (ed): Clinical Autonomic Disorders. Philadelphia, Lippincott-Raven, 1997; 233–244.

Wallin B, Sundlof G, Eriksson B, et al: Plasma noradrenaline correlates to sympathetic muscle nerve activity in normotensive man. Acta Physiol Scand 1981; 111:69–73.

Weil J, Byrne-Quinn E, Sodal J, et al: Augmentation of chemosensitivity during mild exercise in normal man. J Appl Physiol 1972; 33:813–819.

Weinberg CR, Pfeifer MA: An improved method for measuring heart rate variability: Assessment of cardiac parasympathetic function. Biometrics 1984; 40:855–861.

Weise F, Laude D, Girard A, et al: Effects of the cold pressor test on short-term fluctuations of finger arterial blood pressure and heart rate in normal subjects. Clin Auton Res 1993; 3:303–310.

Werner C, Kochs E, Hoffman WE, et al: Cerebral blood flow and cerebral blood flow velocity during angiotensin-induced arterial hypertension in dogs. Can J Anaesth 1993; 40:755–760.

Wheeler T, Watkins PJ: Cardiac denervation in diabetes. Br Med J 1973; 4:584–586.

Whelan RF: Control of the Peripheral Circulation in Man. Springfield, Ill, Charles C Thomas, 1967.

Whitney RJ: The measurement of volume changes in human limbs. J Physiol (Lond) 1953; 121:1–27.

Wieland D, Brown L, Rogers W, et al: Myocardial imaging with a radioiodinated norepinephrine storage analog. J Nucl Med 1981; 22:22–31.

Wieling W: Reduced sinus arrhythmia in diabetic autonomic neuropathy (letter). Br Med J (Clin Res Ed) 1983; 286:1285.

Wieling W: Non-invasive continuous recording of heart rate and blood pressure in the evaluation of neurocardiovascular control. In Bannister R, Mathias C (eds): Autonomic Failure. Oxford, Oxford Medical Publications, 1993; 291–311.

Wieling W, Karemaker JM: Measurement of heart rate and blood pressure to evaluate disturbances in neurocardiovascular control. In Mathias CJ, Bannister R (eds): Autonomic Failure—A Textbook of Clinical Disorders of the Autonomic Nervous System. Oxford, Oxford University Press, 1999; 196–210.

Wieling W, Lieshout JJ: Maintenance of postural normotension in humans. In Low PA (ed): Clinical Autonomic Disorders. Philadelphia, Lippincott-Raven, 1997; 73–82.

Wieling W, Lieshout JJ, Leeuwen AM: Physical manoeuvres that reduce postural hypotension in autonomic failure. Clin Auton Res 1993; 3:57–65.

Wolf MM, Varigos GA, Hunt D, Sloman JG: Sinus arrhythmia in acute myocardial infarction. Med J Aust 1978; 2:52–53.

Yokota T, Matsunaga T, Okiyama R, et al: Sympathetic skin response in patients with multiple sclerosis compared with patients with spinal cord transection and normal controls. Brain 1991; 114:1381–1394.

Yoss R, Moyer N, Ogle K: The pupillogram and narcolepsy. Neurology 1969; 19:921–928.

Zhang R, Zuckerman JH, Giller CA, Levine BD: Transfer function analysis of dynamic cerebral autoregulation in humans. Am J Physiol 1998a; 274:H233–H241.

Zhang R, Zuckerman JH, Levine BD: Deterioration of cerebral autoregulation during orthostatic stress: Insights from the frequency domain. J Appl Physiol 1998b; 85:1113–1122.

Ziegler D, Dannehl K, Muhlen H, et al: Prevalence of cardiovascular autonomic dysfunction assessed by spectral analysis, vector analysis, and standard tests of heart rate variation and blood pressure responses at various stages of diabetic neuropathy. Diabet Med 1992; 9:806–814.

Ziegler M: Catecholamine measurement in behavioral research. In Schneiderman N, Weiss S, Kaufmann P (eds): Handbook of Research Methods in Cardiovascular Behavioral Medicine. New York, Plenum Press, 1989; 167–184.

APPENDIX

Normal Values

Charles F. Bolton

A. INTRODUCTION AND OVERVIEW

A key initiative of any laboratory is to establish accurate normal values. Initially, it was advised that each laboratory should establish its own normal values, but over the years, with electrophysiological techniques becoming more standardized and equipment more accurate, many laboratories now depend on normal values reported by recognized laboratories. For the purposes of this chapter, I have chosen a number of sources that I felt were likely to be most comprehensive and accurate. The techniques are those which have involved surface electrodes for both stimulating and recording. Latencies have been measured to the onset of the first negative peak, and amplitudes from the baseline to the negative peak. The source is referenced for each set of values should the reader desire further information.

A number of variables of a physiological nature influence normal values. The wide variety of technical factors are not discussed—only the physiological values that are especially noteworthy. These physiological variables should always be kept in mind when one interprets individual results. They should probably always be incorporated into the analysis of research results (Dyck et al., 1995; Salerno et al., 1998). In time, they may be automatically calculated as correction factors in the software of EMG systems to give a more accurate result in regular clinical investigations.

Gender

Gender affects chiefly the amplitudes of certain antidromic sensory nerve action potentials (SNAPs), but not compound muscle action potentials (CMAPs). It seems to have little effect on sural or radial SNAPs or orthodromic median and ulnar SNAPs.

The following are the values (mean ± SD) for median and ulnar SNAP amplitudes (μV) in adults, stimulating at the wrist and recording at digit II (antidromic).

	Male	Female
Median-antidromic	37 ± 12	50 ± 21
Ulnar-antidromic	28 ± 10	52 ± 14

(Bolton and Carter, 1980)

Age

Age has effects on all electrophysiological measurements. Changes in childhood are especially marked during infancy. Changes in adulthood begin at about the age of 40 years. The reader is referred to the various tables in this section for changes during childhood.

In adults, conduction velocity for motor and sensory fibers declines at approximately 1 to 2 m per second per decade after the age of 40. For thenar, hypothenar, and abductor hallucis brevis CMAPs in those between the ages of 40 and 80 years, amplitude declines at 1 mV per decade. For the extensor digitorum brevis CMAP, amplitude declines 0.5 mV per decade.

Sural nerve SNAPs decline 4 μV per decade after the age of 40. However, there are more marked changes in antidromic SNAP measurements at digit II: for females 8 μV per decade, and for males 4 μV per decade. Note that the differences in median SNAP amplitudes for males and females are related to digit circumference, as discussed later.

Motor unit estimates for human thenar muscle measured by the multiple-point stimulation technique change with age: 20 to 40 years, 288 ± 95; 40 to 80 years, 139 ± 68 (Doherty and Brown, 1993).

Limb Circumference

As noted previously, the amplitudes of antidromic median and ulnar SNAPs from digit II are higher in females than in males. This can be entirely accounted for by the greater digit circumference in males than females, causing surface recording electrodes to be farther away from the underlying nerve. Thus, digit circumference affects median SNAP amplitude approximately -2 μV/mm. For median orthodromic and radial antidromic SNAP amplitudes recorded at the wrist, there is no significant relationship to wrist circumference (Bolton and Carter, 1980).

Height

There is an inverse relationship between height and conduction velocity. In heights ranging from 150 to 195 cm, peroneal conduction velocity varies by 40 to 55 m per second (Campbell et al., 1981).

Temperature

Changes in limb temperature as measured by a skin surface thermistor affect all electrophysiological measurements. Conduction velocities for motor and sensory fibers rise approximately 2 m/s/°C and latency decreases approximately 0.2 ms/°C. There are also effects on amplitude. The median SNAP amplitude of digit II for antidromic conduction changes -2 μV/°C, but there is much less change for orthodromic conduction recorded at the wrist, -0.04 μV/°C. The thenar CMAP amplitude changes -0.2 mV/°C and the duration -0.2 ms/°C (Bolton et al., 1981).

It may not be appropriate to apply correction factors for temperature, partly because in peripheral nerve pathology the changes may be different; for example, the SNAP amplitude at digit II changes only approximately -1 μV/°C (Bolton and Carter, 1982). In actual practice, most laboratories warm the limbs to above 32°C recorded in the hands and 30°C in the feet. Surface skin temperatures should be routinely recorded just before electrophysiological measurements are taken.

The Factor of Distance

The distance between stimulating and recording electrodes may play a major role. It has only a minor effect on motor conduction, since motor neurons have similar diameters and, hence, conduction velocities. Thus, temporal dispersion due to a fall in amplitude (with increased duration but no change in area) is only about 10%. However, the range of diameters of myelinated sensory fibers is much greater, with a commensurately greater range of conduction velocities and more temporal dispersion. But the main effect on amplitude is partial cancellation of the negative and positive phases of the SNAP as a result of this dispersion, the decrease in amplitude being more marked the greater the distance between stimulating and recording electrodes. Thus, in antidromic conduction studies recording SNAPs from digit II with stimulation of the median nerve, the amplitude may drop 50% when elbow stimulation is compared with wrist stimulation.

References

Bolton CF, Carter K: Human sensory nerve compound action potential amplitude: Variation with sex and finger circumference. J Neurol Neurosurg Psychiatry 1980;43:925–928.

Bolton CF, Carter K, Koval JJ: Temperature effects in conduction studies of normal and abnormal nerve. Muscle Nerve 1982;5:5145–5147.

Bolton CF, Sawa GM, Carter K: The effects of temperature on human compound action potentials. J Neurol Neurosurg Psychiatry 1981;44:407–413.

Campbell WW, Ward LC, Swift TR: Nerve conduction velocity varies inversely with height. Muscle Nerve 1981;4:520–523.

Doherty TJ, Brown WF: The estimated numbers and relative sizes of thenar motor units as selected by multiple-point stimulation in young and older adults. Muscle Nerve 1993;16:355–366.

Dyck PJ, Litchy WJ, Lehman KA, et al: Variables influencing neuropathic endpoints: The Rochester Diabetic Neuropathy Study of Healthy Subjects. Neurology 1995;45:1115–1121.

Dyck PJ, O'Brien PC, Litchy WJ, et al: Use of percentiles and normal deviates to express nerve conduction and other test abnormalities. Muscle Nerve 2001;24:307–310.

Kimura F: Electrodiagnosis in Diseases of Nerve and Muscle: Principles and Practice, 2nd ed. Philadelphia, FA Davis Company, 1989.

Krogness K: Serial conduction studies of the spinal accessory nerve used as a prognostic tool in a lesion caused by lymph node biopsy. Arch Chir Scand 1974;140:7.

Miller DW, Nelson JA, Bender LF: Measurement of latency of facial nerve in normal and uremic persons. Arch Phys Med Rehabil 1970;51:413.

Redford JWB: Conduction Time in Motor Fibers of Nerves Which Innervate Proximal Muscles of the Extremities in Normal Persons and in Patients with Neuromuscular Disease. Thesis, University of Minnesota, 1958.

Salerno DE, Fanzblau A, Werner RA, et al: Median and ulnar nerve conduction studies among workers: Normative values. Muscle Nerve 1998;21:999–1005.

B. PEDIATRIC NORMAL VALUES

Table B–1. Postmenstrual Age (mean ± SD), Ulnar and Posterior Tibial MNCV (mean ± SD), and Number of Patients at Four Points in Time

Time of Measurement	PMA (wk)	Ulnar MNCV (m/s)	Tibial MNCV (m/s)
0–3 days after birth	28.3 ± 1.3	13.3 ± 2.6 (n = 46)	11.4 ± 1.7 (n = 44)
14–17 days after birth	30.4 ± 1.3	14.4 ± 2.4 (n = 51)	13.0 ± 1.9 (n = 50)
Term age	40.6 ± 1.0	27.7 ± 3.9 (n = 52)	23.0 ± 2.5 (n = 56)
6 months corrected age	66.3 ± 1.0	44.4 ± 5.0 (n = 48)	37.5 ± 2.3 (n = 50)

MNCV, motor nerve conduction velocity; PMA, postmenstrual age.
From Smit BJ, Kok JH, De Vries LS, et al: Motor nerve conduction velocity in very preterm infants. Muscle Nerve 1999;22:372–377. Reprinted with permission from John Wiley & Sons, Inc.

Table B–2. Cortical N_1 Peak Latency in Median Nerve SEP at Postmenstrual Age (PMA)

Time of Measurement	PMA (wk)	N_1 Latency Normal US (ms)	N_1 Latency Abnormal US (ms)	N_1 Latency All Patients (ms)
2 weeks after birth	31.1 ± 0.8	69.3 ± 6.9 (n = 17)	59.0 ± 7.3 (n = 7)	66.3 ± 8.4 (n = 24)
Term age	40.7 ± 1.3	38.1 ± 10.7 (n = 30)	39.6 ± 8.7 (n = 28)	38.8 ± 9.7 (n = 58)
6 months (corrected) age	66.1 ± 1.2	19.8 ± 1.2 (n = 23)	20.3 ± 1.1 (n = 27)	20.1 ± 1.1 (n = 50)

SEP, somatosensory evoked potential; PMA, postmenstrual age; US, cranial ultrasound.
From Smit BJ, Ongerboer de Visser BW, de Vries LS, et al: Somatosensory evoked potentials in very preterm infants. Clin Neurophysiol 2000;111:901–908; with permission from Elsevier Science Ireland, Ltd.

Table B–3. Phrenic Nerve Conduction

	Latency (ms), Mean ± SD (Range)		DAP Amplitude (µV), Mean ± SD (Range)	
	Age <1 y (n = 12)	*Age >1 y (n = 8)*	*Age <1 y (n = 12)*	*Age >1 y (n = 8)*
Right	6.12 ± 0.99 (5.2–8.6)	5.80 ± 0.54 (5.2–6.5)	460.7 ± 329.8 (110–1,167)	483.0 ± 322.2 (120–920)
Left	6.17 ± 0.95 (5.0–7.8)	5.65 ± 0.56 (5.0–6.4)	414.0 ± 318.1 (120–974)	446.9 ± 328.1 (86–882)
R – L difference	0.50 ± 0.43 (0.1–1.3)	0.30 ± 0.14 (0.2–0.5)	137.0 ± 149.3 (7–370)	67.4 ± 62.5 (5–172)
% Difference*	1.9 ± 1.4 (0.4–4.1)	1.3 ± 0.6 (0.8–1.9)	8.6 ± 8.8 (0.7–26.3)	6.8 ± 8.0 (0.2–23.6)

*Percent difference calculated as % of absolute value (R – L)/(R + L)/2.
DAP, diaphragm action potential.
From Imai T, Shizukawa H, Imaizumi H, et al: Phrenic nerve conduction in infancy and early childhood. Muscle Nerve 2000;23:915–918; with permission from John Wiley & Sons, Inc.

Table B–4. Median Motor Nerve Conduction

Age	Number	Amplitude (mV)	Distal Latency	MNCV (m/s)
7 days–1 mo	20	3.00 ± 0.31	2.23 ± 0.29	25.43 ± 3.84
1–6 mo	23	7.37 ± 3.24	2.21 ± 0.34	34.35 ± 6.61
6–12 mo	25	7.67 ± 4.45	2.13 ± 0.19	43.57 ± 4.78
1–2 yr	24	8.90 ± 3.61	2.04 ± 0.18	48.23 ± 4.58
2–4 yr	22	9.55 ± 4.34	2.18 ± 0.43	53.59 ± 5.29
4–6 yr	20	10.37 ± 3.66	2.27 ± 0.45	56.26 ± 4.61
6–14 yr	21	12.37 ± 4.79	2.73 ± 0.44	57.32 ± 3.35

From Parano E, Uncini A, De Vivo DC, Lovelace RE: Electrophysiologic correlates of peripheral nervous system maturation in infancy and childhood. J Child Neurol 1993;8:336–338.

Table B–5. Median F-Wave Latencies

Age	Number	Latency (ms)
7 days–1 mo	20	16.12 ± 1.5
1–6 mo	23	16.89 ± 1.65
6–12 mo	25	17.31 ± 1.77
1–2 yr	24	17.44 ± 1.29
2–4 yr	22	17.91 ± 1.11
4–6 yr	20	19.44 ± 1.51
6–14 yr	21	23.23 ± 2.57

From Parano E, Uncini A, De Vivo DC, Lovelace RE: Electrophysiologic correlates of peripheral nervous system maturation in infancy and childhood. J Child Neurol 1993;8:336–338.

Table B–6. Median H-Reflex Latencies

Age	Latency (ms)
Premature (mean age 35.8 wk gestation)	19.5 ± 1.46
Newborn (38–42 wk gestation)	18.1 ± 1.10
0–1 mo	17.7 ± 1.01
1–3 mo	17.0 ± 1.0
3–6 mo	15.9 ± 1.14
6–12 mo	15.9 ± 1.09

From Martinez AC, Ferrer MT, Perez Conde ML, Bernacer M: Motor conduction velocity and H-reflex in infancy and childhood. II. Intra- and extrauterine maturation of the nerve fibres: Development of the peripheral nerve from 1 month to 11 years of age. Electromyogr Clin Neurophysiol 1978:18:11–27; and Martinez AC, Perez Conde ML, Ferrer MT: Motor conduction velocity and H-reflex in infancy and childhood. I. Study in newborns, twins, and small-for-dates. Electromyogr Clin Neurophysiol 1977;17:493–505.

Table B–7. Ulnar Motor Nerve Conduction

Age	Number	Amplitude (mV)	MNCV (m/s)	Distal Latency (ms)	Distance (cm)
Neonate	56	1.6 – 7.0	20.0 – 36.1	1.3 – 2.9	1.0 – 3.4
1–6 mo	22	2.5 – 7.4	33.3 – 50.0	1.1 – 3.2	1.7 – 4.4
7–12 mo	28	3.2 – 10.0	35.0 – 58.2	0.8 – 2.2	1.9 – 4.6
13–24 mo	53	2.6 – 9.7	41.3 – 63.5	1.1 – 2.2	2.4 – 4.8

From Miller RG, Kuntz NL: Nerve conduction studies in infants and children. J Child Neurol 1986;1:19–26.

Table B–8. Ulnar F-Wave Latencies

Age	Number	Latency (ms)	Distance (cm)
1–6 mo	1	17	21
7–12 mo	6	13–16	21–30
13–24 mo	10	14–17	25–39

From Shahani BT, Young RR: Clinical significance of late response studies in infants and children. Neurology 1981;31:66.

Table B–9. Ulnar H-Reflex Latencies

Age	Number	Latency (ms)
1–3 days	6	17.3 (16.0–19.0)
6–12 mo	5	15.8 (14.0–17.0)

From Mayer RF, Mosser RS: Excitability of motoneurons in infants. Neurology 1969;19:932–945.

Table B–10. Peroneal Motor Nerve Conductions

Age	Number	Amplitude (mV)	MNCV (m/s)	Distal Latency (ms)
7 days–1 mo	20	3.06 ± 1.26	22.43 ± 1.22	2.43 ± 0.48
1–6 mo	23	5.23 ± 2.37	35.18 ± 3.96	2.25 ± 0.48
6–12 mo	25	5.41 ± 2.01	43.55 ± 3.77	2.31 ± 0.62
1–2 yr	24	5.80 ± 2.48	51.42 ± 3.02	2.29 ± 0.43
2–4 yr	22	6.10 ± 2.99	55.73 ± 4.45	2.62 ± 0.75
4–6 yr	20	7.10 ± 4.76	56.14 ± 4.96	3.01 ± 0.43
6–14 yr	21	8.15 ± 4.19	57.05 ± 4.54	3.25 ± 0.51

From Parano E, Uncini A, De Vivo DC, Lovelace RE: Electrophysiologic correlates of peripheral nervous system maturation in infancy and childhood. J Child Neurol 1993;8:336–338.

Table B–11. Peroneal F-Wave Latencies

Age	No.	Latency (ms)
7 days–1 mo	20	22.07 ± 1.46
1–6 mo	23	23.11 ± 1.89
6–12 mo	25	25.86 ± 1.35
1–2 yr	24	25.98 ± 1.95
2–4 yr	22	29.52 ± 2.15
4–6 yr	20	29.98 ± 2.68
6–14 yr	21	34.27 ± 4.29

Data are presented as means ± SD or as normative ranges.
From Parano E, Uncini A, De Vivo DC, Lovelace RE: Electrophysiologic correlates of peripheral nervous system maturation in infancy and childhood. J Child Neurol 1993;8:336–338.

Table B–12. Tibial Motor Nerve Conduction

Age	Mean (range) Amplitude (mV)	MNCV (m/s)	Distal Latency (ms)
Premature (mean gestation 35.8 wk)		19.0 ± 2.73	3.6 ± 0.53
Newborn (38–42 wk gestation)		24.5 ± 2.35	3.35 ± 0.41
0–1 mo	(5–8)	25.3 ± 1.96	3.20 ± 0.61
1–3 mo		27.8 ± 3.89	2.86 ± 0.45
3–6 mo		36.3 ± 4.98	2.20 ± 0.24
6–12 mo		39.9 ± 3.89	2.46 ± 0.34
1–2 yr		42.6 ± 3.80	2.40 ± 0.27
2–4 yr		49.8 ± 5.79	2.81 ± 0.47
4–6 yr		50.0 ± 4.26	3.20 ± 0.56
6–11 yr	12 (5–20)	52.4 ± 4.19	3.60 ± 0.67

From Martinez AC, Ferrer MT, Perez Conde ML, Bernacer M: Motor conduction velocity and H-reflex in infancy and childhood. II. Intra- and extrauterine maturation of the nerve fibres: Development of the peripheral nerve from 1 month to 11 years of age. Electromyogr Clin Neurophysiol 1978;18:11–27; and Martinez AC, Perez Conde ML, Ferrer MT: Motor conduction velocity and H-reflex in infancy and childhood. I. Study in newborns, twins, and small-for-dates. Electromyogr Clin Neurophysiol 1977;17:493–505.

Table B–13. Tibial F-Wave Latencies

Age	No.	Latency (ms)	Distance (cm)
7–12 mo	2	19–24	43–48
13–24 mo	9	22–26	42–52

Data are presented as normative ranges.
From Miller RG, Kuntz NL: Nerve conduction studies in infants and children. J Child Neurol 1986;1:19–26.

Table B–14. Tibial H-Reflex Latencies

Age	No.	Latency (ms)
1–3 days	25	13–17 (mean 15.7)
4–30 days	9	13–17 (mean 14.8)
1–5 mo	13	14–15 (mean 14.3)
6–12 mo	17	13.5–16.5 (mean 14.9)
1–3 yr	10	14.0–18.5 (mean 15.8)
3–7 yr	5	16.0–19.5 (mean 17.7)
1–3 days	7	22.0–25.0 (mean 23.7)
6–12 mo	5	17.0–21.0 (mean 18.4)

From Mayer RF, Mosser RS: Excitability of motoneurons in infants. Neurology 1969;19:932–945.

Table B–15. Median Sensory and Mixed Nerve Conduction Reference Values

Age	No.	Amplitude (μV)	SNCV (m/s)	Distal Latency (ms)	Distance (cm)
(a) Miller and Kuntz					
Neonate	10	7–15 8–17	25.1–31.9	2.1–3.0	3.8–5.4
1–6 mo	11	13–52 9–26	36.3–41.9	1.5–2.3	4.3–6.3
7–12 mo	15	14–64 11–36	39.1–60.0	1.6–2.4	5.5–6.8
13–24 mo	29	14–82 7–36	46.5–57.9	1.7–3.0	5.7–9.1

Age	No.	SNCV (m/s)	Amplitude (μV)
(b) Parano et al.			
7 days–1 mo	20	22.31 ± 2.16	6.22±1.30
1–6 mo	23	35.52 ± 6.59	15.86±5.18
6–12 mo	25	40.31 ± 5.23	16.00±5.18
1–2 yr	24	46.93 ± 5.03	24.00±7.36
2–4 yr	22	49.51 ± 3.34	24.28±5.49
4–6 yr	20	51.71 ± 5.16	25.12±5.22
6–14 yr	21	53.84 ± 3.26	26.72±9.43

Table B–16. Median Sensory Conduction

	Digit I		Digit II		Digit III (Orthodromic)	
Age	NCV (m/s)	Amplitude (μV)	NCV (m/s)	Amplitude (μV)	NCV (m/s)	Amplitude (μV)
Newborn	19.4 ± 2.03	10.3 ± 4.38	19.7 ± 3.3	7.0 ± 2.64	20.8 ± 2.17	7.2 ± 2.1
1–3 mo	21.2 ± 2.3	16.2 ± 3.56	26.7 ± 5.21	12.4 ± 4.77	29.0 ± 5.24	12.2 ± 4.71
3–6 mo	29.2 ± 4.92	23.8 ± 4.19	34.9 ± 4.6	17.8 ± 5.11	37.1 ± 4.68	17.7 ± 3.75
6–12 mo	31.8 ± 4.4	27.3 ± 7.8	36.5 ± 3.79	16.7 ± 6.0	38.7 ± 4.47	18.0 ± 7.19
1–2 yr	35.5 ± 5.8	35.2 ± 10.27	43.3 ± 7.36	22.6 ± 3.81	44.0 ± 6.27	22.1 ± 4.22
2–4 yr	38.8 ± 5.27	38.3 ± 8.64	46.4 ± 4.6	22.8 ± 4.22	47.5 ± 4.33	22.0 ± 3.08
4–6 yr	38.9 ± 3.52	36.6 ± 6.41	46.1 ± 4.36	19.2 ± 5.37	46.5 ± 4.79	19.2 ± 6.59
6–14 yr	42.9 ± 3.78	36.1 ± 8.82	49.3 ± 4.65	16.8 ± 4.6	48.9 ± 4.21	19.0 ± 4.65

Wrist-Elbow Segment (Orthodromic)

		Amplitude (μV)	
Age	NCV (m/s)	Component 1	Component 2
Newborn	30.6 ± 2.93	2.9 ± 1.02	
1–3 mo	31.4 ± 0.98	2.22 ± 1.29	
3–6 mo	44.9 ± 4.92	3.5 ± 1.5	5.2 ± 1.83
6–12 mo	51.4 ± 6.85	2.78 ± 1.5	6.7 ± 1.77
1–2 yr	57.1 ± 5.72	3.37 ± 1.4	8.1 ± 1.73
2–4 yr	61.7 ± 4.95	2.6 ± 0.69	5.9 ± 1.8
4–6 yr	63.1 ± 6.26	2.7 ± 0.94	4.75 ± 1.51
6–14 yr	64.9 ± 5.39	1.7 ± 0.77	3.1 ± 1.35

Modified from Martinez AC, Perez Conde MC, del Campo F, et al: Sensory and mixed conduction velocity in infancy and childood. I. Normal parameters in median, ulnar and sural nerves. Electromyogr Clin Neurophysiol 1978;18:487–504.

Table B–17. Ulnar Sensory Conduction—Orthodromic

| Age | Digit V–Wrist Segment | | Wrist–Elbow Segment | | |
| | NCV (m/s) | Amplitude (μV) | NCV (m/s) | Amplitude (μV) | |
				Component 1	Component 2
Newborn	18.4 ± 3.97	5.5 ± 3.1	25.2 ± 3.64	2.2 ± 0.88	
1–3 mo	27.7 ± 6.37	9.4 ± 3.2	28.9 ± 1.45	2.62 ± 0.94	
3–6 mo	37.1 ± 5.25	13.2 ± 3.23	41.9 ± 3.03	3.1 ± 1.5	4.5 ± 1.0
6–12 mo	40.0 ± 5.13	13.0 ± 5.6	51.6 ± 6.6	2.8 ± 1.12	6.0 ± 1.65
1–2 yr	44.2 ± 7.79	16.3 ± 2.44	55.0 ± 6.15	3.5 ± 1.41	6.8 ± 1.19
2–4 yr	48.8 ± 3.01	16.0 ± 3.6	60.3 ± 5.25	3.0 ± 1.3	6.2 ± 1.15
4–6 yr	47.7 ± 6.75	14.2 ± 2.72	58.4 ± 2.59	2.9 ± 0.98	4.1 ± 1.17
6–14 yr	46.6 ± 5.6	13.4 ± 4.2	60.5 ± 5.38	2.4 ± 1.15	4.7 ± 1.53

Modified from Martinez AC, Perez Conde MC, del Campo F, et al: Sensory and mixed conduction velocity in infancy and childood: I. Normal parameters in median, ulnar and sural nerves. Electromyogr Clin Neurophysiol 1978;18:487–504.

Table B–18. Antidromic—Wrist to Elbow (Mixed NAP)

Age	NCV (m/s)	Amplitude (μV)
Newborn	30.5 ± 2.29	7.4 ± 2.22
1–3 mo	37.1 ± 3.72	11.3 ± 4.96
3–6 mo	45.3 ± 6.36	23.4 ± 7.73
6–12 mo	56.2 ± 4.13	31.0 ± 13.7
1–2 yr	60.0 ± 7.67	48.6 ± 13.7
2–4 yr	62.5 ± 3.51	41.8 ± 15.4
4–6 yr	62.3 ± 2.56	40.3 ± 19.5
6–14 yr	62.7 ± 4.61	45.8 ± 16.7

Modified from Martinez AC, Perez Conde MC, del Campo F, et al: Sensory and mixed conduction velocity in infancy and childhood. I. Normal parameters in median, ulnar, and sural nerves. Electromyogr Clin Neurophysiol 1978;18:487–504.

Table B–19. Sural Sensory Nerve Conduction—Antidromic

Age	No.	SNCV (m/s)	Amplitude (μV)
7 days–1 mo	20	20.26 ± 1.55	9.12 ± 3.02
1–6 mo	23	34.63 ± 5.43	11.66 ± 3.57
6–12 mo	25	38.18 ± 5.00	15.10 ± 8.22
1–2 yr	24	49.73 ± 5.53	15.41 ± 9.98
2–4 yr	22	52.63 ± 2.96	23.27 ± 6.84
4–6 yr	20	53.83 ± 4.34	22.66 ± 5.42
6–14 yr	21	53.85 ± 4.19	26.75 ± 6.59

Modified from Parano E, Uncini A, De Vivo DC, Lovelace RE: Electrophysiologic correlates of peripheral nervous system maturation in infancy and childhood. J Child Neurol 1993;8:336–338.

Table B–20. Medial Planter Sensory Nerve Conduction—Antidromic

Age	No.	Amplitude (μV)	NCV (m/s)	Distal Latency (ms)	Distance (cm)
Neonate	3	10–40		2.1–3.3	4.5–5.8
1–6 mo	2	17–26	35.4–35.7	1.5–1.9	4.5–5.5
7–12 mo	6	15–38	39.4–40.3	1.9–2.7	6.5–7.9
13–24 mo	12	15–60	42.6–57.3	1.8–2.5	6.1–9.3

Modified from Miller RG, Kuntz NL: Nerve conduction studies in infants and children. J Child Neurol 1986;1:19–26.

Table B–21. Facial Nerve Conduction and Blink Reflex Latencies in 30 Neonates

Type of Response	Latency (ms)	Latency Side-to-Side Difference in Same Subject (ms)	Amplitude (mV)	Amplitude Right-Left Ratio in Same Subject (mV)
Direct facial	3.30 ± 0.44	0.32 ± 0.33	0.48 ± 0.30	0.95 ± 0.56
R1 component	12.10 ± 0.96	0.38 ± 0.22	0.51 ± 0.18	1.00 ± 0.33
R2 component (ipsilateral to stimulus)	35.85 ± 2.45	1.79 ± 1.36	0.39 ± 0.19	1.15 ± 0.64

Modified from Kimura J, Bodensteiner J, Yamada T: Electrically elicited blink reflex in normal neonates. Arch Neurol 1977;37:246–249.

Table B–22. Motor Unit Potential Measurement

	Amplitude (μV)[a]				Duration (ms)[a]			
	Mean	*SEM*	*SD*	*Range*	*Mean*	*SEM*	*SD*	*Range*
Quadriceps femoris, newborn	507	29	290	100–1,600	6.27	0.15	1.51	2–10
Tibialis anterior, newborn	498	28	283	100–1,500	5.67	0.16	1.65	2.5–10.5
Biceps brachii								
3 mo	96	7			7.7	0.3		
16–23 yr	175	20			10.3	0.2		
Abductor digiti quinti								
3 mo	78	12			5.8	0.1		
16–23 yr	360	20			9.4	0.25		

Amplitude (μV)[b]	Duration (ms)[b]
Initially 300–500	Initially 2–3
Range, 200–2000	Range, 1–5
Range, 150–3000	Range, 2–5

[a] For muscles of pediatric patients at different ages using concentric needle electrodes with 0.04 mm2 [44] or 0.03 mm2 [43] core surface area.
[b] For infants, using monopolar needle electrodes.
SEM, standard error of the mean.
From Sacco et al., do Cormo, Eng, and Turk.

Table B–23. Single-Fiber Measurement[a]

Muscle	Age (yr)	Fiber Density	Mean MCD	Jitter (>2 of 20 potentials)
Frontalis	5	1.67	33.6	49.7
	10	1.67	33.6	49.7
	15	1.67	33.7	49.9
	20	1.67	33.9	50.1
Orbicularis oculi	5		39.8	54.6
	10		39.8	54.6
	15		39.8	54.6
	20		39.8	54.7
Orbicularis oris	5		34.6	52.5
	10		34.7	52.5
	15		34.7	52.6
	20		34.7	52.7
Deltoid	5	1.56	32.9	44.4
	10	1.56	32.9	44.4
	15	1.56	32.9	44.5
	20	1.56	32.9	44.5
Biceps	5	1.52	29.5	45.1
	10	1.52	29.5	45.2
	15	1.52	29.5	45.2
	20	1.52	29.6	45.2
Extensor digitorum communis	5	1.77	34.9	50.0
	10	1.77	34.9	50.0
	15	1.77	34.9	50.1
	20	1.78	34.9	50.1
Quadriceps	5	1.93	35.8	47.9
	10	1.93	35.9	47.9
	15	1.93	35.9	48.0
	20	1.94	36.0	48.0
Tibialis anterior	5	1.94	49.4	80.0
	10	1.94	49.4	80.0
	15	1.94	49.4	79.9
	20	1.94	49.3	79.8
Soleus	5	1.56		
	10	1.56		
	15	1.56		
	20	1.56		

MCD, mean consecutive difference.
[a] At 95% upper normal limits.
From the ad hoc committee of the AAEM special interest group on single fiber EMG, Gilchrist JM: Single fiber EMG reference values: A collaborative effort. Muscle Nerve 1992;15:151–161.

C. CRANIAL NERVE CONDUCTION STUDIES

Table C–1. Accessory Nerve

	Latency (ms)	Amplitude (mV)
To sternocleidomastoid	2.3 ± 0.4 (9.6 ± 1.4)	8.7 ± 4.6
To trapezius	3.5 ± 0.5 (12.5 ± 1.4)	10.7 ± 5.6

n = 21.
From Krogness K: Serial conduction studies of the spinal accessory nerve used as a prognostic tool in a lesion caused by lymph node biopsy. Arch Chir Scand 1974;140:7.

Table C–2. Facial Nerve Motor Conduction

Stimulation Below Ear, Recording Nasalis Muscles

Latency	3.45 ± 0.38 ms (8.8–13.1 cm)

n = 55, years 19–59.
From Miller DW, Nelson JA, Bender LF: Measurement of latency of facial nerve in normal and uremic persons. Arch Phys Med Rehabil 1970;51:413.

Table C–3. Blink Reflex Latencies (ms ± SD)

Direct response	2.9 ± 0.4
R_1	10.5 ± 0.8
R_2 (ipsilateral)	30.5 ± 3.4
R_2 (contralateral)	30.5 ± 4.4
R1D ratio	3.6 ± 0.5

n = 83.
From Kimura F: Electrodiagnosis in Diseases of Nerve and Muscle: Principles and Practice, 2nd ed. Philadelphia, FA Davis, 1989; 315.

Table C–4. Masseter Reflex

	Latency (ms)	Latency Difference (Large Value Minus Small Value)	Amplitude (mV)	Amplitude Ratio (Large Value Over Small Value)
Mean right	7.10		0.23	
Mean left	7.06		0.21	
Total	7.08	0.27	0.22	1.44
SD	0.62	0.15	0.24	0.42
Mean±3 SD	9.0	0.8	Variable	2.7

n = 20.
From Kimura F: Electrodiagnosis in Diseases of Nerve and Muscle: Principles and Practice, 2nd ed. Philadelphia, FA Davis, 1989; 362.

D. UPPER LIMB CONDUCTION STUDIES

Table D–1. Median Nerve Motor and Sensory Conduction*

Site of Stimulation	Amplitude† (mV) (μV)	Latency‡ (ms)	Difference Between Right and Left (ms)	Conduction Velocity (m/s)
Motor fibers				
Palm	6.9 ± 3.2 (3.5)§	1.86 ± 0.28 (2.4)¶	0.19 ± 0.17 (0.5)¶	48.8 ± 5.3 (38)**
Wrist	7.0 ± 3.0 (3.5)	3.49 ± 0.34 (4.2)	0.24 ± 0.22 (0.7)	57.7 ± 4.9 (48)
Elbow	7.0 ± 2.7 (3.5)	7.39 ± 0.69 (8.8)	0.31 ± 0.24 (0.8)	63.5 ± 6.2 (51)
Axilla	7.2 ± 2.9 (3.5)	9.81 ± 0.89 (11.6)	0.42 ± 0.33 (1.1)	
Sensory fibers				
Digit				
Palm	39.0 ± 16.8 (20)	1.37 ± 0.24 (1.9)	0.15 ± 0.11 (0.4)	58.8 ± 5.8 (47)
Wrist	38.5 ± 15.6 (19)	2.84 ± 0.34 (3.5)	0.18 ± 0.14 (0.5)	56.2 ± 5.8 (44)
Elbow	32.0 ± 15.5 (16)	6.46 ± 0.71 (7.9)	0.29 ± 0.21 (0.7)	61.9 ± 4.2 (53)

n = 61, yrs 11–74.
* Mean ± standard deviation (SD) in 122 nerves from 61 patients, 11 to 74 years of age (average, 40), with no apparent disease of the peripheral nerves.
† Amplitude of the evoked response, measured from the baseline to the negative peak.
‡ Latency, measured to the onset of the evoked response, with the cathode at the origin of the thenar nerve in the palm.
§ Lower limits of normal, based on the distribution of the normative data.
¶ Upper limits of normal, calculated as the mean + 2 SD.
** Lower limits of normal, calculated as the mean − 2 SD.
From Kimura F: Electrodiagnosis in Diseases of Nerve and Muscle: Principles and Practice, 2nd ed. Philadelphia, FA Davis, 1989.

Table D–2. Ulnar Nerve Motor and Sensory Conduction

Site of Stimulation	Amplitude† (mV) (μV)	Latency‡ to Recording Site (ms)	Difference Between Right and Left (ms)	Conduction Velocity (m/s)
Motor fibers				
Wrist	5.7 ± 2.0 (2.8)§	2.59 ± 0.39 (3.4)	0.28 ± 0.27 (0.8)¶	58.7 ± 5.1 (49)**
Below elbow	5.5 ± 2.0 (2.7)	6.10 ± 0.69 (7.5)	0.29 ± 0.27 (0.8)	61.0 ± 5.5 (50)
Above elbow	5.5 ± 1.9 (2.7)	8.04 ± 0.76 (9.6)	0.34 ± 0.28 (0.9)	66.5 ± 6.3 (54)
Axilla	5.6 ± 2.1 (2.7)	9.90 ± 0.91 (11.7)	0.45 ± 0.39 (1.2)	
Sensory fibers				
Digit				
Wrist	35.0 ± 14.7 (18)	25.4 ± 0.29 (3.1)	0.18 ± 0.13 (0.4)	58.8 ± 5.3 (44)
Below elbow	28.8 ± 12.2 (15)	5.67 ± 0.59 (6.90)	0.26 ± 0.21 (0.5)	64.7 ± 5.4 (53)
Above elbow	28.3 ± 11.8 (14)	7.46 ± 0.64 (8.7)	0.28 ± 0.27 (0.8)	66.7 ± 6.4 (54)

n = 65, yrs 13–74.
* Mean ± standard deviation (SD) in 130 nerves from 65 patients, 13 to 74 years of age (average, 39), with no apparent disease of the peripheral nerves.
† Amplitude of the evoked response measured from the baseline to the negative peak.
‡ Latency, measured to the onset of the evoked response with the cathode 3 cm above the distal crease in the wrist.
§ Lower limits of normal, based on the distribution of the normative data.
¶ Upper limits of normal, calculated as the mean + 2 SD.
** Lower limits of normal, calculated as the mean − 2 SD.
From Kimura F: Electrodiagnosis in Diseases of Nerve and Muscle: Principles and Practice, 2nd ed. Philadelphia, FA Davis, 1989.

Table D–3. Radial Motor and Sensory Conduction

Conduction	n	Conduction Velocity (m/s) or Conduction Time (ms)	Amplitude (mV; μV)	Distance (cm)
Motor				
Axilla–elbow	8	69 ± 5.6	11 ± 7.0	15.7 ± 3.3
Elbow–forearm	10	62 ± 5.1	13 ± 8.2	18.1 ± 1.5
Forearm–muscle	10	2.4 ± 0.5	14 ± 8.8	6.2 ± 0.9
Sensory				
Axilla–elbow	16	71 ± 5.2	4 ± 1.4	18.0 ± 0.7
Elbow–wrist	20	69 ± 5.7	5 ± 2.6	20.0 ± 0.5
Wrist–thumb	23	58 ± 6.0	13 ± 7.5	13.8 ± 0.4

Adapted from Trojaborg W, Sindrup EH: Motor and sensory conduction in different segments of the radial nerve in normal subjects. Neurol Neurosurg Psychiatry 1969;32:354–359.

Table D–4. Musculocutaneous Motor and Sensory Conduction

Age	n	Motor Nerve Conduction Between Erb's Point and Axilla — Range of Conduction Velocity (m/s)	Range of Amplitude (μV) Axilla	Range of Amplitude (μV) Erb's Point	n	Orthodromic Sensory Nerve Conduction Between Erb's Point and Axilla — Range of Conduction Velocity (m/s)	Range of Amplitude (μV)	n	Orthodromic Sensory Nerve Conduction Between Axilla and Elbow — Range of Conduction Velocity (m/s)	Range of Amplitude (μV)
15–24	14	63–78	9–32	7–27	14	59–76	3.5–30	15	61–75	17–75
25–34	6	60–75	8–30	6–26	6	57–74	3–25	8	59–73	16–72
35–44	8	58–73	8–28	6–24	7	54–71	2.5–21	8	57–71	16–69
45–54	10	55–71	7–26	6–22	10	52–69	2–18	13	55–69	15–65
55–64	9	53–68	7–24	5–21	9	49–66	2–15	10	53–67	14–62
65–74	4	50–66	6–22	5–19	4	47–64	1.5–12	6	51–65	13–59

From Trojaborg W: Motor and sensory conduction in the musculocutaneous nerve. J Neurol Neurosurg Psychiatry 1976;39:890–899.

Table D–5. Lateral and Medial Cutaneous Nerve (Mean ± SD)

Nerve	Number of Patients Seen	Age (mean)	Distance (cm)	Latency Onset (ms)	Latency Peak (ms)	Conduction Velocity (m/s)	Amplitude (μV)
Lateral cutaneous nerve	154	17–80 (45)	14		2.8 ± 0.2	62 ± 4	18.9 ± 9.9
Medial cutaneous nerve	155	17–80 (45)	14		2.7 ± 0.2	63 ± 5	11.4 ± 5.2

From Izzo KL, Aravabhumi S, Jafri A, et al: Medial and lateral antebrachial cutaneous nerves: Standardization of technique, reliability and age effect on healthy subjects. Arch Phys Med Rehabil 1985;66:592–597.

Table D–6. Brachial Plexus Latency with Nerve Root Stimulation

Plexus	Site of Stimulation	Recording Site	Latency Across Plexus (ms) Range	Mean	SD
Brachial (upper trunk and lateral cord)	C5 and C6	Biceps brachii	4.8–6.2	5.3	0.4
Brachial (posterior cord)	C6, C7, C8	Triceps brachil	4.4–6.1	5.4	0.4
Brachial (lower trunk and medial cord)	C8 and T1 Ulnar nerve	Abductor digiti quinti	3.7–5.5	4.7	0.5

From MacLean IC: Nerve root stimulation to evaluate conduction across the brachial and lumbosacral plexuses. Third Annual Continuing Education Course, American Association of Electromyography and Electrodiagnosis, September 25, 1980, Philadelphia.

E. LOWER LIMB CONDUCTION STUDIES

Table E–1. Tibial Nerve

Site of Stimulation	Amplitude† (mV)	Latency (ms)	Difference Between Two Sides (ms)	Conduction Velocity (m/s)
Ankle	5.8 ± 1.9 (2.9)§	3.96 ± 1.00 (6.0)¶	0.66 ± 0.57 (1.8)¶	48.5 ± 3.6 (41)**
Knee	5.1 ± 2.2 (2.5)	12.05 ± 1.53 (15.1)	0.79 ± 0.61 (2.0)	

* Mean ± standard deviation (SD) in 118 nerves from 59 patients, 11 to 78 years of age (average, 39), with no apparent disease of the peripheral nerves.
† Amplitude of the evoked response, measured from the baseline to the negative peak.
‡ Latency, measured to the onset of the evoked response, with a standard distance of 10 cm between the cathode and the recording electrode.
§ Lower limits of normal, based on the distribution of the normative data.
¶ Upper limits of normal, calculated as the mean + 2 SD.
** Lower limits of normal, calculated as the mean − 2 SD.
From Kimura F: Electrodiagnosis in Diseases of Nerve and Muscle: Principles and Practice, 2nd ed. Philadelphia, FA Davis, 1989.

Table E–2. Common Peroneal Nerve*

Site of Stimulation	Amplitude† (mV)	Latency (ms)	Difference Between Right and Left (ms)	Conduction Velocity (m/s)
Ankle	5.1 ± 2.3 (2.5)§	3.77 ± 0.86 (5.5)¶	0.62 ± 0.61 (1.8)¶	
Below knee	5.1 ± 2.0 (2.5)	10.79 ± 1.06 (12.9)	0.65 ± 0.65 (2.0)	48.3 ± 3.9 (40)**
Above Knee	5.1 ± 1.9 (2.5)	12.51 ± 1.17 (14.9)	0.65 ± 0.60 (1.9)	52.0 ± 6.2 (40)

n = 60, age 16–86.
* Mean ± standard deviation (SD) in 120 nerves from 60 patients, 16 to 86 years of age (average, 41), with no apparent disease of the peripheral nerves.
† Amplitude of the evoked response, measured from the baseline to the negative peak.
‡ Latency, measured to the onset of the evoked response, with a standard distance of 7 cm between the cathode and the recording electrode.
§ Lower limits of normal, based on the distribution of the normative data.
¶ Upper limits of normal, calculated as the mean + 2 SD.
** Lower limits of normal, calculated as the mean − 2 SD.
From Kimura F: Electrodiagnosis in Diseases of Nerve and Muscle: Principles and Practice, 2nd ed. Philadelphia, FA Davis, 1989.

Table E–3. Sural Nerve

Stimulation Point	Recording Site	n	Age	Amplitude (μV)	Latency (ms)	Conduction Velocity (m/s)
14 cm above lateral malleolus	Lateral malleolus	52	10–40	20.9 ± 8.0	2.7 ± 0.3	52.5 ± 5.6
			41–84	17.2 ± 6.7	2.8 ± 0.3 (onset)	51.1 ± 5.9

From Kimura F: Electrodiagnosis in Diseases of Nerve and Muscle: Principles and Practice, 2nd ed. Philadelphia, FA Davis, 1989.

Table E–4. Superficial Peroneal Nerve

Stimulation Point	Recording Site	n	Age	Amplitude (μV)	Latency (ms)	Conduction Velocity (m/s)	
5 cm above, 2 cm medial to lateral malleolus	Dorsum of foot	50	1–15	13.0 ± 4.6	1.22 ± 0.40	53.1 ± 5.3	(Distal segment)
		50	Over 15	13.9 ± 4.0	(Peak) 2.24 ± 0.49	47.3 ± 3.4	(Distal segment)
Anterior edge of fibula, 12 cm above the active electrode	Medial border of lateral malleolus	50	3–60	20.5 ± 6.1	(Peak) 2.9 ± 0.3	65.7 ± 3.7	(Proximal segment)
Anterolateral aspect of leg, 14 cm above the active electrode	Medial border of lateral malleolus	80		18.3	(Peak) 2.8 ± 0.3	51.2 ± 5.7	(Proximal segment)
					(Onset)		

Data from Di Benedetto, Jabre, and Izzo et al.
From Kimura F: Electrodiagnosis in Diseases of Nerve and Muscle: Principles and Practice, 2nd ed. Philadelphia, FA Davis, 1989.

Table E–5. Lumbosacral Plexus

Plexus	Site of Stimulation	Recording Site	Latency Across Plexus (ms)		
			Range	*Mean*	*SD*
Lumbar	L2, L3, L4 Femoral nerve	Vastus medialis	2.0–4.4	3.4	0.6
Sacral	L5 and S1 Sciatic nerve	Abductor hallucis	2.5–4.9	3.9	0.7

From MacLean IC: Nerve root stimulation to evaluate conduction across the brachial and lumbosacral plexuses. Third Annual Continuing Education Course, American Association of Electromyography and Electrodiagnosis, September 25, 1980, Philadelphia.

Table E–6. Femoral Nerve

Sitmulation Point	Recording Site	No.	Age	Onset Latency (ms)	Conduction Velocity (m/s)
Just below inguinal ligament	14 cm from stimulus point	42	8–79	3.7 ± 0.45	70 ± 5.5 between the two recording sites
	30 cm from stimulus point	42	8–79	6.0 ± 0.60	

Modified from Gasel MM: A study of femoral nerve conduction time. Arch Neurol 1963;9:57–64.

Table E–7. Saphenous Nerve

Authors	Method	Age	Inguinal Ligament—Knee			Knee—Medial Malleolus		
			Number	*Amplitude (μV)*	*Conduction Velocity (m/s)*	*Number*	*Amplitude (μV)*	*Conduction Velocity (m/s)*
Wainapel et al. (1978)[102]	Antidromic	20–79			Peak latency of 3.6 ± 1.4 for 14 cm	80	9.0 ± 3.4	41.7 ± 3.4

Adapted from Wainapel SF, Kim DJ, Ebel A: Conduction studies of the saphenous nerve in healthy subjects. Arch Phys Med Rehabil 1978;59:316–319.

Table E–8. Lateral Femoral Cutaneous Nerve

(Stimulation at inguinal ligament with needle electrodes, recorded 12 cm distal with surface electrodes)
Latency = 2.6 ± 0.2 ms
Amplitude = 10 − 25 μV

From Butler ET, Johnson EW, Kaye ZA: Normal conduction velocity in the lateral femoral cutaneous nerve. Arch Phys Med Rehabil 1974;55:31–32.

F. F WAVES AND H REFLEXES

Table F–1. Various F-Wave Measurements

Number of Nerves Tested	Site of Stimulation	F-Wave Latency to Recording Site (ms)	Difference Between Right and Left (ms)	Central Latency† to and from the Spinal Cord (ms)	Difference Between Right and Left (ms)	Conduction Velocity‡ to and from the Spinal Cord (m/s)	F Ratio§ Between Proximal and Distal Segments
122 median nerves from 61 subjects	Wrist	26.6 ± 2.2 (31)**	0.95 ± 0.67 (2.3)**	23.0 ± 2.1 (27)**	0.93 ± 0.62 (2.2)**	65.3 ± 4.7 (56)††	0.98 ± 0.08 (0.82–1.14)**,††
	Elbow	22.8 ± 1.9 (27)	0.76 ± 0.56 (1.9)	15.4 ± 1.4 (18)	0.71 ± 0.52 (1.8)	67.8 ± 5.8 (56)	
	Axilla¶	20.4 ± 1.9 (24)	0.85 ± 0.61 (2.1)	10.6 ± 1.5 (14)	0.85 ± 0.58 (2.0)		
130 ulnar nerves from 65 subjects	Wrist	27.6 ± 2.2 (32)	1.0 ± 0.83 (2.7)	25.0 ± 2.1 (29)	0.84 ± 0.59 (2.0)	65.3 ± 4.8 (55)	1.05 ± 0.09 (0.87–1.23)
	Above elbow	23.1 ± 1.7 (27)	0.68 ± 0.48 (1.6)	16.0 ± 1.2 (18)	0.73 ± 0.52 (1.8)	65.7 ± 5.3 (55)	
	Axilla¶	20.3 ± 1.6 (24)	0.73 ± 0.54 (1.8)	10.4 ± 1.1 (13)	0.76 ± 0.52 (1.8)		
120 peroneal nerves from 60 subjects	Ankle	48.4 ± 4.0 (56)	1.42 ± 1.03 (3.5)	44.7 ± 3.8 (52)	1.28 ± 0.90 (3.1)	49.8 ± 3.6 (43)	1.05 ± 0.09 (0.87–1.23)
	Above knee	39.9 ± 3.2 (46)	1.28 ± 0.91 (3.1)	27.3 ± 2.4 (32)	1.18 ± 0.89 (3.0)	55.1 ± 4.6 (46)	
118 tibial nerves from 59 subjects	Ankle	47.7 ± 5.0 (58)	1.40 ± 1.04 (3.5)	43.8 ± 4.5 (53)	1.52 ± 1.02 (3.6)	52.6 ± 4.3 (44)	1.11 ± 0.11 (0.89–1.33)
	Knee	39.6 ± 4.4 (48)	1.25 ± 0.92 (3.1)	27.6 ± 3.2 (34)	1.23 ± 0.88 (3.0)	53.7 ± 4.8 (44)	

* Mean ± standard deviation (SD) in the same patients shown in Tables 6–1, 6–3, 6–10, and 6–12.
† Central latency = F − M, where F and M are latencies of the F wave and M response, respectively.
‡ Conduction velocity = 2D/(F−M−1), where D is the distance from the stimulus point to C-7 or T-12 spinous process.
§ F ratio = (F−M−1)/2M with stimulation with the cathode on the volar crease at the elbow (median), 3 cm above the medial epicondyle (ulnar), just above
the head of the fibula (peroneal) and in the popliteal fossa (tibial).
¶ F(A) = F(E) ± M(E) − M(A), where F(A) and F(E) are latencies of the F wave with stimulation at the axilla and elbow, respectively, and M(A) and M(E) are latencies of the corresponding M response.
** Upper limits of normal calculated as mean + 2 SD.
†† Lower limits of normal calculated as mean − 2 SD.
From Kimura F: Electrodiagnosis in Diseases of Nerve and Muscle: Principles and Practice, 2nd ed. Philadelphia, FA Davis, 1989.

Table F–2. H Reflex, Stimulating Tibial Nerve at Popliteal Fossa, Recording Soleus Muscle

Amplitude[†] (mV)	Difference Between Right and Left (mV)	Latency[‡] to Recording Site (ms)	Difference Between Right and Left (ms)
2.4 ± 1.4	1.2 ± 1.2	29.5 ± 2.4	0.6 ± 0.4 (1.4)[§]

$n = 59$.
* Mean ± standard deviation (SD)
† Amplitude of the evoked response measured from the baseline to the negative peak.
‡ Latency measured to the onset of the evoked response.
§ Upper limits of normal calculated as mean + 2 SD.
From Kimura F: Electrodiagnosis in Diseases of Nerve and Muscle: Principles and Practice, 2nd ed. Philadelphia, FA Davis, 1989.

G. SINGLE-FIBER AND MACRO ELECTROMYOGRAPHY

Table G–1. Jitter in Normal Subjects*

Muscles	Number of Potential Pairs	MCD—Pooled Data		SD of MCD Values from Individual Subjects		Upper Normal Limit Close to Mean + 3 SD
		Mean	*SD*	*Mean*	*SD*	
Frontalis (range of individual means)	258	20.4 (15.7–29.2)	8.8	6.2 (5.5–8.7)	2.3	45
Biceps	125	15.6	5.9			35
Extensor digitorum communis (range of individual means)	759	24.6 (16.5–32.0)	10.6	8.3 (2.3–12.4)	3.2	55 (65)†
Rectus femoris	73	31.0	12.6			60 (75)†
Tibialis anterior	153	32.1	15.0			60
Extensor digitorum brevis	29	85.3	68.6			None

*Jitter (MCD, mean consecutive difference) measured with voluntary activation in normal subjects aged 10 to 70 years.
†Because of some extremely high values, the data deviate from a gaussian distribution. Thus, a more appropriate upper normal limit is 60 μs. In no one normal subject was there more than one value exceeding this limit.
From Stålberg E, Trontelj J: Single Fibre Electromyography. The Miraville Press Limited, Old Working, Surrey, UK, 1979.

Table G–2. Macro EMG in Normal Subjects

	Suggested Amplitude Limits (μV)											
	Biceps				*Vastus Lateralis*				*Tibialis Anterior*			
	Median		*Individual Macro-MUP*		*Median*		*Individual Macro-MUP*		*Median*		*Individual Macro-MUP*	
Age	*Min*	*Max*	*Min*	*Max*	*Min*	*Max*	*Min*	*Max*	*Min*	*Max*	*Min*	*Max*
10–19	65	100	30	350	70	150	20	350	65	200	30	350
20–29	65	140	30	350	70	240	20	525	65	250	30	450
30–39	65	180	30	400	70	240	20	550	65	260	30	450
40–49	65	180	30	500	70	250	20	575	65	330	30	575
50–59	65	180	30	500	70	260	20	575	65	375	40	700
60–69	65	250	30	650	80	370	20	1250	120	375	45	700
70–79	65	250	30	650	90	600	20	1250	120	620	65	800

From Stålberg E: AAEE Minimonograph #20, Macro EMG. Muscle Nerve 1983;6:619–630.

H. SOMATOSENSORY EVOKED POTENTIALS

Table H–1. Latency of Erb's Potential and Short-Latency Median SEP in 34 Normal Subjects

Components	Latency (Left and Right Combined)			Latency Difference (Between Left and Right)		
	Number Identified	*Mean ± SD (ms)*	*Mean + 3 SD*	*Number Identified*	*Mean ± SD (ms)*	*Mean + 3 SD*
Erb's potential	68	9.8 ± 0.8	12.2	34	0.4 ± 0.2	1.0
P_9*	68	9.1 ± 0.6	10.9	34	0.4 ± 0.2	1.0
N_{11}	43	11.2 ± 0.6	13.0	19	0.4 ± 0.3	1.3
N_{13}*	68	13.2 ± 0.9	15.9	34	0.5 ± 0.4	1.7
P_{14}	55	14.1 ± 0.9	16.8	25	0.5 ± 0.4	1.7
N_{18}	68	18.3 ± 1.5	22.8	34	0.5 ± 0.5	2.0
Interwave peaks						
P_9-P_{11}	43	2.2 ± 0.3	3.1	19	0.2 ± 0.2	0.8
N_{11}-N_{13}	43	1.9 ± 0.4	3.1	19	0.2 ± 0.2	0.8
N_{13}-P_{14}	55	1.0 ± 0.4	2.2	25	0.3 ± 0.2	0.9
P_{14}-N_{18}	55	4.2 ± 0.9	6.9	25	0.7 ± 0.5	2.2
P_9-N_{13}*	68	4.0 ± 0.4	5.2	34	0.3 ± 0.3	1.2
N_{13}-N_{18}*	68	5.1 ± 0.9	7.8	34	0.6 ± 0.5	2.1

* Consistently measurable components and interwave peaks.
From Yamada T, Shivapour E, Wilkinson JT, Kimura J: Short- and long-latency somatosensory evoked potentials in multiple sclerosis. Arch Neurol 1982;38:88–94.

Table H–2. Latency of Medium- and Long-Latency Median SEP in 34 Normal Subjects

Components	Latency (Left and Right Combined)			Latency Difference (Between C3 and C4)		
	Number Identified	*Mean ± SD (ms)*	*Mean + 3 SD*	*Number Identified*	*Mean ± SD (ms)*	*Mean + 3 SD*
N_{18} (NI)	68	18.1 ± 1.6	22.9	34	0.4 ± 0.4	1.6
P_{22} (PI)	68	22.8 ± 2.3	29.7	34	0.6 ± 0.4	1.8
N_{30} (NII)	68	31.6 ± 2.6	39.4	34	0.5 ± 0.4	1.7
P_{40} (PII)	68	43.6 ± 3.6	54.4	34	0.6 ± 0.5	2.1
P_{60} (NIII)	64	62.8 ± 9.3	90.7	32	1.5 ± 1.1	4.8

From Yamada T, Shivapour E, Wilkinson JT, Kimura J: Short and long-latency somatosensory evoked potentials in multiple sclerosis. Arch Neurol 1982; 38:88–94.

Table H–3. Latency of Short-Latency Tibial SEP (A) and Negative Peaks Along the Somatosensory Pathway (B) in 21 Healthy Subjects

Recording Site	Scalp					
(A) Components	P_{11}	P_{17}	P_{21}	P_{24}	P_{27}	P_{31}
Mean ± SD (ms)	11.4 ± 2.7	17.3 ± 1.9	20.8 ± 1.9	23.8 ± 2.0	27.4 ± 2.1	31.2 ± 2.1
Number recorded	22	40	21	39	30	40
Number tested	40	40	40	40	40	40
Recording Site		Gluteus	L-4	T-12	C-7	C-2
(B) Components		N_{16}	N_{21}	N_{23}	N_{28}	N_{30}
Mean ± SD (ms)		16.4 ± 3.2	20.9 ± 2.2	23.2 ± 2.1	27.6 ± 1.8	30.2 ± 1.9
Number recorded		20	40	40	18	25
Number tested		22	40	40	22	26

From Yamada T, Machida M, Kimura J: Far-field somatosensory evoked potentials after stimulation of the tibial nerve in man. Neurology 1982;32:1151–1158.

Table H–4. PI Latency and NI/PI Amplitude of Trigeminal SEP in 82 Healthy Subjects

Latency (ms) (Mean ± SD)	Upper Limit (ms) (Mean + 2 SD)	Side-to-Side Latency Difference (ms) (Mean ± SD)	Upper Limit (ms) (Mean + 2 SD)	Amplitude (µV) (Mean)	Side-to-Side Amplitude Difference (µV) (Mean)
18.5 ± 1.51	22.3	0.55 ± 0.55	1.93	2.6	0.51

Modified from Stohr M, Petruch F: Somatosensory evoked potentials following stimulation of the trigeminal nerve in man. Neurology 1979;220:95–98.

Table H–5. Latency Comparison Between Tibial and Pudendal Evoked Potential in Healthy Subjects (Mean ± SD)

	Onset (ms)	P$_1$ (ms)	N$_1$ (ms)	P$_2$ (ms)	N$_2$ (ms)	P$_3$ (ms)	N$_3$ (ms)
Men (13)							
Tibial	34.0 ± 2.8	41.2 ± 2.9	50.5 ± 3.0	62.7 ± 3.3	78.5 ± 4.4	99.5 ± 6.0	117.9 ± 9.0
Pudendal	35.2 ± 3.0	42.3 ± 1.9	52.6 ± 2.6	64.9 ± 3.4	79.3 ± 4.0	96.6 ± 4.7	116.0 ± 7.2
Women (7)							
Tibial	32.7 ± 1.7	39.3 ± 1.4	49.4 ± 2.1	60.0 ± 2.0	76.1 ± 4.2	96.1 ± 5.8	119.2 ± 7.9
Pudendal	32.9 ± 2.9	39.8 ± 1.3	49.1 ± 2.3	59.4 ± 2.8	73.4 ± 4.6	90.1 ± 5.8	110.0 ± 10.2

From Haldeman S, Bradley WE, Bhatia NN, Johnson BK: Pudendal evoked responses. Arch Neurol 1982;39:280–283.

I. RESPIRATORY STUDIES

Table I–1. Normal Values of Respiratory Electrophysiological Studies

Motor Central Respiratory Pathway	Mean ± SD (n = 35)	Normal Values
Transcortical Magnetic Stimulation		
Latency (ms)	13.5 ± 1.4	<16.3
Amplitude (µV)	263 ± 144	>100
Threshold (%)	49.1 ± 7.5	<65
Cervical Magnetic Stimulation		
Latency (ms)	8.3 ± 1.2	<10.7
Amplitude (µV)	281 ± 128	>100
Threshold (%)	31.4 ± 9.0	<50
Central motor conduction time (ms)	5.3 ± 1.1	<7.5

Sensory Central Respiratory Pathway	Mean ± SD (n = 3)	
Phrenic Nerve Somatosensory Evoked Potentials		
P$_1$ latency (ms)	12 ± 0.8	
N$_1$ latency (ms)	17 ± 1.3	
Amplitude (µV)	0.3 ± 0.6	

Motor Peripheral Respiratory Pathway	Mean ± SD (n = 25)	Normal Values
Phrenic Nerve Conduction		
Latency (ms)	6.5 ± 0.8	<8.1
Amplitude (µV)	669 ± 159	>300
Area (µVms)	7.3 ± 2.1	>4.0
Duration (ms)	19.4 ± 2.7	<25

	Mean ± SD (n = 6)	Normal Values
3-Hz Repetitive Phrenic Nerve Conduction		
Amplitude (%)	12.1 ± 8.3	
Area (%)	−2.2 ± 4.3	<10.8
Duration (%)	−8.7 ± 9.6	

From Zifko U, Chen R: The respiratory system. Baillieres Clin Neurol 1996a;5:477–495.

J. MOTOR UNIT ESTIMATES

Table J–1. Motor Unit Number Estimates in Younger and Older Control Subjects

Muscle	Investigator	Controls	Controls >60 years
Extensor digitorum brevis	McComas et al. (1971)	199 ± 60[a]	
	Campbell et al. (1973)	198 ± 58[a]	<210
	Ballentyne et al. (1974)	197 ± 49[a]	
	Milner-Brown and Brown (1976)	163 ± 84[b]	
	McComas (1977)	210 ± 65[a]	
	Galea et al. (1991)	131 ± 45[d]	
	Daube (1995)	158 (58, lower limit of normal)[c]	
Thenar group	Brown (1972)	253 ± 34[a]	<120
	Sica et al. (1974)	340 ± 87[a]	83 ± 46
	Lee et al. (1975)	167 ± 16[e]	
	Milner-Brown and Brown (1976)	261 ± 116[b]	
	Stein and Yang (1990)	170 ± 62[a]	
		135 ± 27[e]	
		122 ± 38[f]	
	Galea et al. (1991)	228 ± 93[d]	
	Doherty and Brown (1993)	288 ± 95[g]	139 ± 68
	Stashuk et al. (1994)	245 ± 105[h]	
	Daube (1995)	234 (95, lower limit of normal)[c]	
Hypothenar group	Sica et al. (1974)	380 ± 79[a]	139 ± 68
	Milner-Brown and Brown (1976)	300 ± 125	
	Daube (1995)	265 ± 115[c]	
Biceps brachii	Galea et al. (1991)	113 ± 40[d]	
Biceps brachii/brachialis	Doherty et al. (1993)	357 ± 97[e]	189 ± 77
Vastus medialis	Galea (1991)	229 ± 108[d]	

[a]Manual incremental stimulation.
[b]Alteration-corrected manual incremental stimulation.
[c]Statistical method.
[d]Automated incremental stimulation.
[e]Spike-triggered averaging.
[f]Intramuscular microstimulation.
[g]Multiple-point stimulation.
[h]F-response method.

Index

Note: Page numbers followed by f refer to figures; page numbers followed by t refer to tables.

A

A wave, 467f, 469
Abdomen
  crush injury of, lumbosacral plexopathy with, 1624–1625
  disorders of, in phrenic neuropathy, 1526
Abdominal cutaneous nerves, entrapment of, in thoracic radiculopathy, 807
Abdominal rectus muscle, electromyography of, in respiratory dysfunction, 584
Abducens nerve, intraoperative monitoring of, 1836
Abductor digiti minimi muscle
  central motor conduction time for, 194t
  H reflex of, 460
Abductor hallucis brevis muscle, central motor conduction time for, 194t, 196t
Abductor pollicis brevis muscle
  atrophy of, in carpal tunnel syndrome, 882
  central motor conduction time for, 194t, 196t
  fiber types of, 257, 257t
  H reflex of, 460
Abetalipoproteinemia, 240, 1672, 1677
  vitamin E deficiency in, 1118, 1120
Abscess
  epidural, thoracic radiculopathy with, 806
  iliacus, femoral neuropathy with, 997
Absolute refractory period, 10
Accelerometry, in tremor quantification, 1759–1760
Accessory nerve
  conduction study of, 1939t
  in myasthenia gravis, 766
  transcranial magnetic stimulation of, 445–446
Accessory neuropathy, 789–790
  vs. long thoracic neuropathy, 945
Accommodation, action potential and, 10
Accuracy, of electrophysiological equipment, 706–707
Acebutolol, autonomic nervous system effects of, 508t
Acetabulum, fracture of
  sciatic neuropathy with, 956
  somatosensory evoked potentials in, 1864
Acetazolamide
  in hypokalemic periodic paralysis, 653
  in sodium channelopathy, 1476
Acetylcholine, 507–508, 507t
  fibrillation potentials and, 355
Acetylcholine receptor, 404–405
  age-related changes in, 611
  antibodies to, 1346, 1350, 1700. See also Myasthenia gravis.
  density of, 405
  primary deficiency of, 1694–1695, 1694f
  structure of, 404, 1346
  turnover of, 405
Acetylcholinesterase deficiency, congenital, 1348, 1692–1693, 1692f
N-Acetylgalactosaminidase deficiency, 1678

Achalasia, 541–542
  botulinum toxin treatment in, 1812
  immune system in, 542
  pathogenesis of, 542
Achondroplasia, somatosensory evoked potentials in, 166
Acid maltase deficiency, 1432–1435
  adult, 1432–1433
  childhood, 1432, 1710
  diagnosis of, 1433, 1435
  electromyography in, 1432t, 1433
  genetics of, 1433
  infantile, 1432
  muscle histology in, 1433, 1434f
  respiratory disorders in, 1516, 1532
  serum enzymes in, 1433
Aconitase deficiency, 1449t, 1450
Acoustic myography, in tremor quantification, 1761
Acoustic nerve, intraoperative monitoring of, 1831–1833
  brainstem auditory evoked potentials for, 1831–1832, 1831f, 1832f, 1833
  electrocochleography for, 1833
  nerve action potential for, 1832–1833, 1833f
Acoustic neuroma, posterior fossa, resection of, 1821f, 1828–1833, 1834f
  acoustic nerve monitoring during, 1831–1833, 1831f–1834f
  cranial nerve monitoring during, 1821f
  facial nerve monitoring during, 1828–1830, 1830f
  trigeminal nerve monitoring during, 1830
Acoustic startle reflex. See Startle reflex.
Acquired immunodeficiency syndrome (AIDS)
  antiretroviral therapy in
    distal symmetrical polyneuropathy with, 1335
    myelopathy with, 1331
  ataxic neuropathy in, 1335t, 1339
  autonomic neuropathy in, 1335t, 1337–1338
  cranial neuropathy in, 1337
  cytomegalovirus-related myelopathy in, 1332
  diffuse infiltrative lymphocytosis syndrome in, 1335t, 1338–1339
  distal symmetrical polyneuropathy in, 1334–1335, 1335t
  enteric nervous system disorders with, 546
  herpes simplex virus type 2–related myelopathy in, 1332
  HTLV-1–related myelopathy in, 1332
  inflammatory demyelinating polyradiculoneuropathy in, 1335–1336, 1335t
  mononeuropathy multiplex in, 1335t, 1337
  motor neuron disease in, 1285, 1340–1341
  myelopathy in, 1327–1331
    assessment of, 238
    clinical manifestations of, 1328t, 1329
    diagnosis of, 1329–1331, 1330f
    highly active antiretroviral therapy effects on, 1331

Acquired immunodeficiency syndrome (AIDS) (Continued)
    motor evoked potentials in, 1331
    pathogenesis of, 1328–1329
    pathology of, 1328, 1328f, 1328t
    somatosensory evoked potentials in, 162, 1329–1331, 1330f
    treatment of, 1331
  myopathy in, 1335t, 1339–1340, 1413–1415, 1532
  neuropathy with, 1334–1339, 1335t
    quantitative sensory testing in, 139
  pediatric, Guillain-Barré syndrome in, 1723
  progressive polyradiculopathy in, 1335t, 1336–1337
  respiratory muscle weakness in, 1532
  syphilitic myelopathy in, 1332
  transverse myelitis in, 1331–1332
  wasting syndrome in, 1340
  zidovudine-associated myopathy in, 1335t, 1340, 1413–1415
Acromegaly
  carpal tunnel syndrome in, 879, 889, 1084
  myopathy in, 1405–1406
  neuropathy in, 1084–1085
Acrylamide neuropathy, 77, 78, 1161
ACTA1 gene, 652
  in nemaline myopathy, 1360
Actigraph, in tremor quantification, 1762
Actin, 644, 644f
  in muscle contraction, 389, 389f, 390f
Action potential, 2, 9–12. See also specific action potentials, e.g., Compound muscle action potential (CMAP).
  absolute refractory period of, 10
  accommodation and, 10
  conduction of, 11–16
    continuous, 11–12
    discontinuous (saltatory), 12–15, 13f–15f, 15t
    impedance mismatches and, 59
    in myelinated nerve fibers, 12–16, 13f–15f, 15t, 16t
    safety factor for, 57, 59
    speed of, 14–15, 15t. See also Nerve conduction velocity.
    temperature and, 15–16, 16f, 16t
  extracellular recording of, 17–20, 18f, 96–98, 97f, 97t, 98t, 99, 99f, 100t
    solid angle analysis of, 98–100, 98f, 99f
  generation of, 9–10, 9f, 10f
  in muscle fibers, 17, 291–297. See also Muscle fiber action potential (MFAP).
  in volume conduction, 96–100, 97t, 98f, 99f, 100t
  intracellular recording of, 96–98, 97f, 97t, 98t
  ionic basis of, 5–6, 6f
  phase I of, 9, 9f
  phase II of, 9–10, 9f, 10f
  phase III of, 9f, 10
  phase IV of, 9f, 10
  relative refractory period of, 10
  spatial distribution of, 14, 15f
  subnormal period of, 10, 11f

E

P/N 9997627822

90038

9 789997 627827